Fourth Edition

MEDICAL-SURGICAL
NURSING CARE

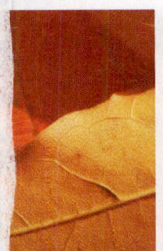
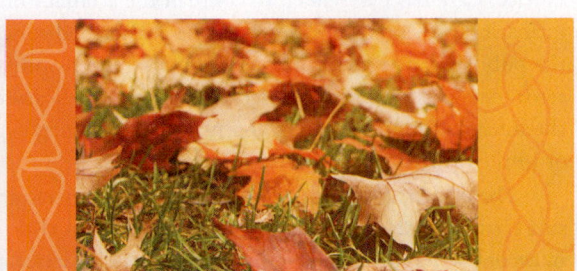
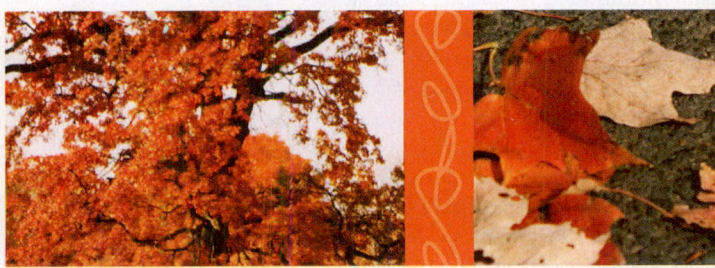

Karen M. Burke, RN, MS
Nursing Education Consultant
Astoria, Oregon

Elaine L. Mohn-Brown, RN, EdD, CMSRN
Instructor of Nursing
Chemeketa Community College
Salem, Oregon

Linda Eby, RN, MN
Instructor of Nursing
Portland Community College
Portland, Oregon

PEARSON

Boston Columbus Indianapolis New York San Francisco Hoboken
Amsterdam Cape Town Dubai London Madrid Milan Munich Paris Montreal Toronto
Delhi Mexico City Sao Paulo Sydney Hong Kong Seoul Singapore Taipei Tokyo

Library of Congress Cataloging-in-Publication Data

Burke, Karen M.
  Medical-surgical nursing care / Karen M. Burke, RN, MS, Nursing Education Consultant, Astoria, Oregon, Elaine L. Mohn-Brown, RN, EdD, Instructor of Nursing Chemeketa Community College, Salem, Oregon, Linda Eby, RN, MN, Instructor of Nursing Portland Community College, Portland, Oregon.—Fourth edition.
    pages cm
  Includes bibliographical references and index.
  ISBN 978-0-13-338978-4
  ISBN 0-13-338978-2
  1. Surgical nursing. 2. Nursing. I. Mohn-Brown, Elaine. II. Eby, Linda. III. Title.
  RT41.B89 2016
  617'.0231—dc23
                                                            2014035173

Publisher: Julie Levin Alexander
Publisher's Assistant: Regina Bruno
Senior Acquisitions Editor: Kelly Trakalo
Development Editor: Rachel Bedard
Editorial Assistant: Erin Sullivan
Project Manager: Michael Giacobbe
Program Manager: Erin Rafferty
Director of Field Marketing: David Gesell
Senior Product Marketing Manager: Phoenix Harvey
Field Marketing Manager: Debi Doyle
Marketing Coordinator: Michael Sirinides
Marketing Assistant: Amy Pfund
Production Editor: Saraswathi Muralidhar, Lumina Datamatics, Inc.
Senior Art Coordinator: Maria Guglielmo-Walsh
Digital Media Product Manager: Travis Moses-Westphal
Composition: Lumina Datamatics, Inc.
Printing and Binding: RR Donnelley/Willard
Cover Printer: Phoenix Color/Hagerstown

Notice: Care has been taken to confirm the accuracy of information presented in this book. The authors, editors, and the publisher, however, cannot accept any responsibility for errors or omissions or for consequences from application of the information in this book and make no warranty, express or implied, with respect to its contents.

The authors and publisher have exerted every effort to ensure that drug selections and dosages set forth in this text are in accord with current recommendations and practice at time of publication. However, in view of ongoing research, changes in government regulations, and the constant flow of information relating to drug therapy and drug reactions, the reader is urged to check the package inserts of all drugs for any change in indications of dosage and for added warnings and precautions. This is particularly important when the recommended agent is a new and/or infrequently employed drug.

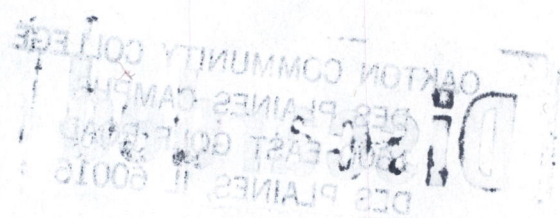

10 9 8 7 6 5 4 3 2 1

PEARSON

www.pearsonhighered.com

ISBN 10:   0-13-338978-2
ISBN 13: 978-0-13-338978-4

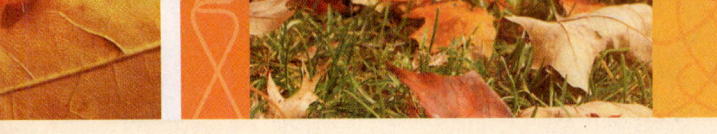

Preface

The need for nurses is greater than ever before. There are no short-term solutions to this problem. As currently practicing nurses age and retire, so does the population as a whole, further increasing the need for health care services. Today, more than ever, we need you, the nursing student, to succeed in your studies and enter the nursing profession. Today, more than ever, we need you, the nursing student, to see nursing as a career, not just a job.

This book is dedicated to your success as a student and as a practicing nurse. We believe a strong foundation in understanding the common diseases and disorders that affect adults is necessary to provide effective nursing care. We believe that nurses are an integral part of the interprofessional health care team. We believe that understanding the basis for nursing care activities is vital to providing individualized care for patients. We believe that individualized patient teaching is a crucial nursing role at all levels and in all settings. *Medical–Surgical Nursing Care* provides a strong foundation for caring through its emphasis on pathophysiology, nursing care, and patient teaching.

New to This Edition

Understanding comes not through memorization, but through practice and integration of new material into your thinking. *Medical–Surgical Nursing Care* promotes understanding in several ways. The writing style is clear, with a focus on readability. Its content is streamlined but thorough, focusing on what you need to know and be able to do. Its organization provides material in easily accessible format.

This edition of *Medical–Surgical Nursing Care* includes new content and features that will help students grow and develop as practical/vocational nurses.

- Unit 1 has been substantially revised to focus on the roles and responsibilities of the LPN/LVN including legal/ethical guidelines and settings of care in which the LPN/LVN commonly works.

- Chapter 1 introduces and elaborates on quality and safety in nursing, provision of evidence-based nursing care, and essential competencies for nurses.

- Applied Learning Outcomes at the beginning of each chapter refocus the student's attention on essential quality and safety competencies for nurses: patient-centered care, teamwork and collaboration, evidence-based practice, quality improvement, safety, and informatics.

- Key Concepts embedded within each chapter help students identify and focus on important concepts and develop an understanding of patient needs.

- Throughout the book, features such as Focus on Diversity boxes and Cultural Care Strategies build on the foundation for culturally sensitive nursing care.

- Throughout the book, drugs that are among the most frequently prescribed in the United States are italicized to help students identify and focus on those that are most likely to be encountered in nursing practice.

- The importance of the entire nursing care team—RN, LPN/LVN, and unlicensed assistive nursing personnel—is emphasized throughout the book. A new feature, Managing Nursing Care, focuses on the LPN/LVN's responsibility for assigning and supervising patient care.

- Chapter 10, Caring for Patients Having Surgery, has been extensively revised with a new focus on patient safety, National Patient Safety Goals, and effective communication during hand-offs.

- The unit on Mental Health Disorders has been updated per *DSM-5* (*Diagnostic and Statistical Manual of Mental Disorders*, 5th edition).

- End-of-unit features, **Thinking Strategically About...**, have been extensively revised to promote clinical reasoning and to provide practice in prioritizing and managing nursing care.

- **Memory Alerts** appear throughout the book. These alerts provide cues, ideas, or alternate ways of thinking about a concept to help the student learn and remember important information.

- **Safety Alerts**, which also appear throughout the book, help the student recognize threats to patients' safety.

- Clinical Reasoning Care Maps at the end of each disorders chapter have added a question about identifying patient safety risks and prioritizing nursing interventions to address the risk. To emphasize the importance of teamwork and collaboration, students also are asked to identify members of the interprofessional team likely to be involved in the patient's care.

- Nursing care sections throughout the book stress the nurse's responsibilities for promoting health, establishing priorities, and recognizing critical complications. Expected Outcomes are included for each nursing diagnosis to help the student focus on the intent of planned nursing interventions. Continuity of Care focuses on the nurse's responsibilities for teaching and communicating pertinent information to the patient, family, and caregivers as the patient moves from one setting of care to another.

Organization

Medical–Surgical Nursing Care is organized to promote learning. Unit I, Introduction to Medical–Surgical Nursing, focuses on core concepts, issues, foundational knowledge, and nursing care competencies for caring for adults in many different situations and settings. Unit I includes new information that lays the foundation for providing holistic, culturally sensitive nursing care as a practical/vocational nurse. Unit II focuses on conditions that affect many people with a variety of underlying disorders. It includes a section on disaster preparedness and response. Units III through XII focus on common diseases and disorders affecting adults. These disorders are organized by body systems (e.g., common skin problems, gastrointestinal disorders, cardiac disorders). Unit XIII, Mental Health Disorders, covers frequently encountered mental health and cognitive disorders.

Each body system unit begins with a chapter that reviews the system's structure and function, focused nursing assessment, and commonly ordered diagnostic tests, along with their nursing implications. Examples of nursing assessment documentation are included. These introductory chapters provide a foundation for learning about disorders presented in the subsequent chapters of the unit.

Diseases and disorders are presented in a consistent format: The disease or disorder is defined; its pathophysiology, signs and symptoms, and complications are explained; and **Collaborative Care** (including diagnostic tests, medications, surgery, and other treatments) for the disorder is outlined. **Nursing Care** for patients experiencing the disorder is presented in a nursing process format. When a disorder is commonly encountered (e.g., pneumonia, heart disease, certain cancers), health promotion activities to prevent the disorder are identified and major steps of the **Nursing Process** are provided. **Identifying Potential Complications**, new to this edition, alerts students to assessment data that may indicate an unexpected or critical complication of the disorder. The text provides an abbreviated, more focused discussion of less common disorders, similar to the focused assessment nurses perform. Because nursing care prioritization is a critical skill, a brief **Prioritizing Nursing Care** section is included. Recognizing the importance of the entire nursing team in caring for patients, **Managing Nursing Care** sections suggest essential activities that may be appropriately assigned to assistive personnel. Teaching and continuing care are vital nursing considerations, so discussion of each disorder concludes with **Continuity of Care** and teaching for the patient and family.

Nursing Care Plans following many major disorders bring the disorders to life. The care plans in this text emphasize the holistic aspects of nursing care.

Design and Features

Chapter Openers help focus students on what is important.

Brief Outlines preview what the chapter will cover for quick access and review.

Applied Learning Outcomes identify what you can expect to learn from each chapter and apply that learning when caring for patients.

Key Terms are listed alphabetically, with page numbers, at the beginning of the chapter. They are also boldfaced and defined where they first appear in the text.

Special Features highlight nursing care plans, clinical reasoning care maps, and other features that assist with learning chapter content.

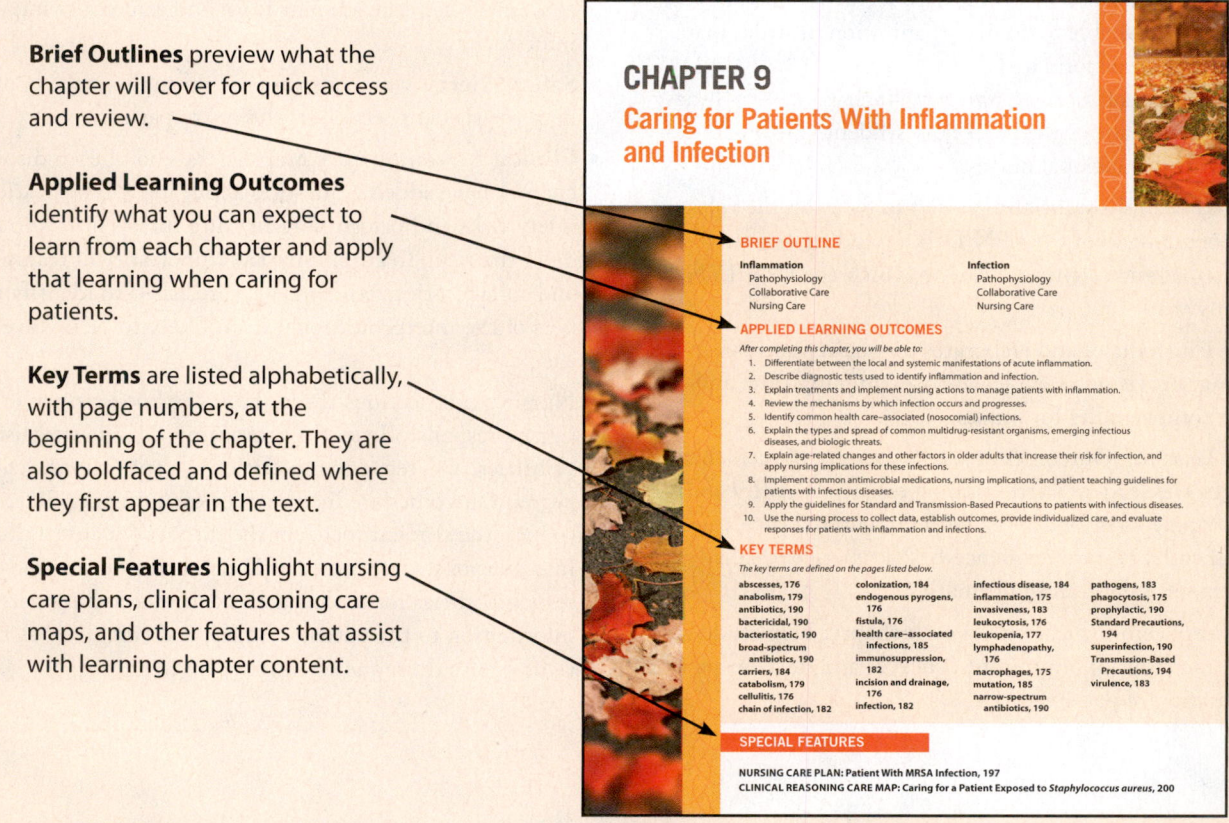

Key Concepts provide about four or five major concepts for understanding in each chapter. Concepts are repeated in the Chapter Review section to reinforce learning.

Key Concept Inflammation is the body's protective response when injured by factors such as abrasions, chemicals, pathogenic organisms, overuse, or extreme temperatures. While the acute inflammatory response is usually short term; chronic inflammation is often long term.

Patient Teaching and **Population Focus** boxes provide information on age-specific and other special needs of patient groups and help you prepare for patient instruction.

BOX 4-2 — PATIENT TEACHING

Health Promotion for the Older Adult
- Choose foods from all food groups, and eat a variety of foods. Balance food and calorie intake with physical activity to maintain an appropriate weight.
- Choose a diet that includes at least seven servings of fruits and vegetables and six servings of whole grains daily.
- Choose a diet low in fat (30% or less of total calories), saturated fat (less than 10% of calories), and cholesterol (less than 300 mg daily).
- Use sugar in moderation, and limit sodium intake to less than 1,500 mg daily. Limit intake of refined grains and prepared and processed foods.
- If possible, obtain at least 30 minutes of exposure to sunlight daily. Use sunscreen and avoid sunburn.
- Increase calcium intake to 1,200 mg and consume 600 mg of vitamin D daily.
- Limit alcohol consumption, if any, to no more than one drink per day.
- If weight loss is needed, aim for a slow, steady loss by decreasing caloric intake while maintaining a balanced nutrient intake and increasing physical activity.
- Make exercise a part of life, carrying out regular exercise that is moderately strenuous, is consistent, and avoids overexertion. Include stretching, aerobic exercise, and weight training or resistance exercises for 30 minutes or longer five or more days per week.
- Sleep 7 to 8 hours each day.
- Eliminate smoking and use of other tobacco products.
- Maintain recommended immunizations.

Focus on Diversity boxes highlight transcultural nursing issues and prepare you to deliver culturally sensitive care.

BOX 9-4 — FOCUS ON DIVERSITY

Incidence of Communicable Diseases
People who live in overcrowded urban areas and the homeless have a greater incidence of communicable disease spread among their population. Immigrants may unknowingly have diseases such as TB, dengue fever, or diarrheal disorders caused by bacteria or parasites. People living in rural areas or on Native American reservations are at risk for developing *Hantavirus*, a pulmonary infection from infected rats or mice.

TABLE 39-1 — Giving Medications Safely: Parkinson Disease

CLASS/DRUGS	PURPOSE	NURSING IMPLICATIONS	PATIENT TEACHING
Dopaminergics			
■ Levodopa (Larodopa) ■ *Carbidopa–levodopa (Sinemet)* ■ *Amantadine (Symmetrel)*	Levodopa is converted to dopamine in the brain, and carbidopa prevents levodopa from being destroyed. Levodopa is the most effective drug for PD. Amantadine, an antiviral drug, raises dopamine levels.	Check for drug interactions before giving. Do not give to patients with angle-closure glaucoma. Monitor for nausea, hypotension, confusion, and dyskinesia. Assess for "on–off" effect—symptoms may appear or improve suddenly. Hold levodopa for 8 hours before giving Sinemet to avoid toxicity.	Take the medication as directed. Do not alter dosages. Inform the physician of other drugs you are taking. Change position slowly to avoid hypotension. Increase fluid intake and exercise regularly. Report the "on–off" effect, decreased motor movements, insomnia, and rapid heartbeat to your physician.
Dopamine agonists			
■ Apomorphine (Apokyn) ■ *Bromocriptine (Parlodel)* ■ *Pramipexole (Mirapex)* ■ *Ropinirole (Requip)*	They are given to decrease tremor, rigidity, and bradykinesia.	Monitor for adverse reactions: nausea, orthostatic hypotension, and psychosis. See nursing implications under the dopaminergics.	Patient teaching information is similar to that found under the dopaminergics.
Anticholinergics			
■ Trihexyphenidyl (Artane) ■ *Benztropine (Cogentin)*	They decrease the activity of acetylcholine and are given	Do not give to patients with glaucoma, cardiac disease, and	Take the medication as prescribed. Do not suddenly

Giving Medications Safely tables highlight nursing implications and patient teaching for drugs commonly used to treat particular disorders. Drugs in the top 200 most prescribed list are *italicized* in tables to help you recognize and learn about drugs most likely to be encountered in practice.

Nursing Care Checklist boxes provide handy summaries of important nursing interventions related to specific procedures.

BOX 22-3 — NURSING CARE CHECKLIST

Controlling Influenza in Long-Term Care Settings
- ☑ Provide annual influenza vaccine to all residents and personnel unless contraindicated by allergy or health status.
- ☑ Limit potential exposure to influenza:
  - ☑ Post visual alerts asking people with symptoms of a respiratory infection to notify health care personnel.
  - ☑ Discourage people who are ill from visiting residents.
  - ☑ Exclude or reassign health care personnel with influenza symptoms or confirmed cases to nondirect care activities for 7 days after the onset of symptoms.
  - ☑ Encourage people with upper respiratory symptoms to sit at least 3 feet away from others.
  - ☑ Provide masks to residents with upper respiratory symptoms.
- ☑ Provide hand-hygiene supplies by sinks and in readily accessible locations.
- ☑ Ensure that health care personnel know and follow Standard Precautions.
- ☑ Implement droplet precautions for patients with suspected or confirmed influenza.
- ☑ Move residents with influenza symptoms to a private room.
  - ☑ If private rooms are not available, place residents with similar symptoms in one area (particularly for meals and activities).
- ☑ Provide and instruct all health care personnel to use a facemask when caring for the patient, removing and discarding the mask when leaving the patient's room.

Source: Centers for Disease Control and Prevention, 2013b.

Assessment boxes summarize data collected and manifestations you may observe.

Prioritizing Nursing Care helps you learn to identify priority nursing care needs for the patient experiencing the disease or disorder.

PRIORITIZING NURSING CARE

The nursing care needs of the patient with an inflammatory process are related to the manifestations of inflammation and altered tissue integrity. Priority nursing diagnoses include Pain, Impaired Tissue Integrity, and Risk for Infection.

Nursing Care is presented in the nursing process format and emphasizes the scope of practice for LPNs/LVNs. Rationales after each nursing intervention provide an evidence base for the intervention and explain why it is important.

Managing Nursing Care suggests actions and tasks that may be appropriate to delegate to assistive personnel.

Risk for Deficient Fluid Volume

Expected outcome: Weight, urinary output, and vital signs will remain stable and within established range.

- Maintain accurate intake and output records, including emesis and diarrheal stools. *The patient with IBD can experience significant fluid losses during an acute exacerbation of the disease. Accurate records help determine fluid replacement needs.*
- Document vital signs every 4 hours. *Elevated pulse and respiratory rates may indicate fluid volume deficit.*

MANAGING NURSING CARE

As appropriate and allowed by the designated duties and responsibilities of assistive personnel, the nurse may assign nursing care activities such as taking vital signs, recording intake and output and assisting with providing diet and fluids for the patient with inflammation. The nurse retains responsibility for providing wound care.

CONTINUITY OF CARE

Instruct the patient and family about wound care, activity level after discharge, return to work, and any other recommended restrictions or procedures. If a temporary colostomy has been created, teach the patient and family about its care. For the patient with recurrent obstructions, discuss cause, early identification of symptoms, and preventive measures.

Continuity of Care focuses on preparing patients, their families, and caregivers for discharge.

Clinical Alerts call attention to specific instances and responsibilities for heightened awareness, monitoring, and/or reporting.

clinicalALERT

Use heat or cold application cautiously in older adults who have fragile skin and are at risk for tissue injury.

Memory Alerts provide cues, ideas, or alternate ways of thinking about a concept to help you learn and remember important information.

Safety Alerts help you be aware of threats to patient safety so you can prevent problems from occurring.

Nursing Care Plans illustrate nursing care in a "real-life" scenario.

Critical Thinking Questions allow you to apply new knowledge to a specific patient. Discussion of the questions appears on the companion website.

Cultural Care Strategies include nursing implications and self-reflection questions that prepare you to deliver sensitive adult nursing care.

---

undergoes extensive surgery will require preoperative and postoperative care as discussed in Chapter 10.

Encourage patients with melanoma to schedule regular medical checkups every 3 months for the first 2 years, every 6 months for the next 5 years, and yearly thereafter. Emphasize that proper self-care combined with regular medical care can help the patient lead a fairly normal life. If assistance for home care is necessary, provide referrals to a community health or home care agency. Refer the patient to a local cancer support group if the patient believes this will be helpful.

NURSING CARE PLAN
Patient With Malignant Melanoma

Pat Malone, age 45, is an insurance broker in Washington. She frequently travels to warm, sunny vacation resorts, where she plays golf and likes to sunbathe. She has a variety of warts and moles but seldom pays attention to them. However, after taking a shower one day, she notices that a mole on her right shoulder looked bigger and darker. She sees her primary care physician, who makes a tentative diagnosis of malignant melanoma and refers her to a dermatologist.

Assessment
Ms. Malone has a family history of skin cancer; her father had several squamous cell cancers removed from his face. She states that the mole has been present for years but that she just noticed yesterday that it is larger and darker. The mole does not bleed or hurt, but sometimes it itches. A complete skin assessment reveals various freckles, warts, and moles. The mole in question is raised, is 3 cm in diameter with irregular borders, and is various shades of brown. Ms. Malone is scheduled for a biopsy of the mole under a local anesthetic the following morning. After the biopsy, histologic examination reveals lentigo maligna melanoma. Staging of the tumor shows a melanoma *in situ*, without metastasis to regional lymph nodes. Ms. Malone undergoes a wide excision of the mole the following afternoon.

Nursing Diagnosis
The following nursing diagnoses are identified for Ms. Malone:
- *Impaired Skin Integrity* related to excision of melanoma from the right shoulder
- *Risk for Infection* related to the surgical wound on the right shoulder
- *Acute Pain* related to wide excision of melanoma on the right shoulder
- *Anxiety* related to diagnosis of skin cancer

Expected Outcomes
The expected outcomes are that Ms. Malone will:
- Demonstrate complete healing of the incision without manifestations of infection.
- Verbalize relief of pain by the time the incision is healed.
- Verbalize fears and concerns about her diagnosis.

Planning and Implementation
The following nursing interventions are implemented following the wide excision of the mole:
- On discharge, provide adequate dressings and tape for the first home dressing change. Include necessary information about where to buy supplies and how many dressing supplies will be needed.
- Reinforce instructions for prescribe antibiotic and pain medication.
- Reinforce teaching about dressing change, manifestations of infection, and phone number of the physician's office. Stress the importance of calling if any abnormal symptoms occur.
- Teach ways to protect the incision from bumps and to protect the site from irritants.
- Stress the importance of lifelong regular health care evaluations to identify any recurrence or metastasis.

Evaluation
Ms. Malone returns to the physician's office 1 week after her surgical incision. Her incision is well approximated without any signs of infection. She is taking her antibiotic four times a day as prescribed and reports that her need for pain medication is decreasing. She says that she is still "scared to death" about having cancer but has joined a local cancer support group. She has gotten a list of skin care guidelines from the American Cancer Society. She plans to quit sunbathing and will use sunscreen and cover up when she plays golf. Ms. Malone makes a follow-up care appointment in 3 months.

Critical Thinking in the Nursing Process

1. Consider reasons why people who notice a change in a skin lesion put off seeking health care. How could this action affect their overall health? What can nurses do to effect change?
2. What would you suggest to Ms. Malone if she called the physician's office and said that the antibiotics are making her sick?
3. Consider nursing interventions that could be implemented for Ms. Malone for a diagnosis of *Powerlessness*.

Note: Discussion of Critical Thinking questions appears on the companion website.

CULTURAL CARE STRATEGIES
CONSIDERING CULTURAL VARIATIONS RELATED TO SPACE

A 25-year-old male Cuban American patient says to the nurse, "Everybody in this culture is so cold. When I talk up to them they are always backing away. I think the nurses think I'm going to attack them sexually or something. They keep backing away from me. It's especially noticeable if I'm in line waiting for something. I may be standing close to the person in front of me, and they turn around and glare."

All verbal communication occurs in the context of space (Giger & Davidhizar, 2012). *Personal space* is the area needed by an individual to maintain intimacy and safety in relationships. Because health care providers frequently invade a person's space when providing direct care, understanding the cultural perceptions of space is important. For example, among Americans and most Europeans, personal space is highly valued, and an unannounced invasion will often result in the patient becoming suspicious and tense (Bechtel & Davidhizar, 1988).

Proximity to Others

Hall (1966) established three different dimensions of personal space: *intimate zone* (0 to 18 in.), *personal zone* (18 in. to 3 ft), and the *social zone* (3 to 6 ft). The intimate zone is used for close, personal encounters like comforting, counseling, and direct care activities. Invading this area without the patient's acknowledgment may lead to suspicion and hostile feelings.

For most interactions not involving direct care or intimate conversation, the personal zone is considered most appropriate. In presenting patient education and information, a distance of 18 in. to 3 ft is close enough for privacy yet far enough away to avoid intimate touch. Health care providers who have the respect of their patients and families are often able to interact well in this zone.

Individuals are frequently not conscious of their personal space requirements, although they react to invasion of their territory. The nurse should always be aware of patients' and families' body language during interactions. Signs that suggest the patient's personal space is being invaded include stepping back, looking uncomfortable and tense, and not facing the nurse during communication.

Objects in the Environment

Objects in the environment can have great meaning for patients of different cultures, and the patient may feel uncomfortable when the nurse discards or moves these objects. Objects can also affect patient care and teaching. For example, when the nurse sits behind a desk, a position of authority is assumed. This may be appropriate in some cases, but usually communication is improved by sitting across from or at a 90-degree angle to the patient.

Removal of a patient's personal items can create distrust. For example, it may be necessary to remove a wedding ring before treatment, but the patient may feel this takes away a strong sense of support. Likewise, placing a Roman Catholic person's rosary on a table out of reach can cause anxiety.

Items that may seem worthless to the caregiver can be of great significance to the patient. For example, some patients collect plastic medicine cups to symbolize the adversities overcome in the treatment plan. If the nurse discards the medicine cups, the patient may lose track of how much success has taken place and may not be as motivated to comply with the treatment.

Nursing Implications

- *Provide information about the need to invade a patient's space.* When it is necessary to invade a patient's space, the nurse should provide information about what will be done and how long it will take. This information will enhance compliance and increase the patient's comfort.
- *Assess the patient for degree of comfort when invading personal space.* Personal space boundaries vary from individual to individual. Although most individuals are comfortable in a conversational space of 3 to 6 ft, some individuals need more space. It is important to be alert for reactions of patients during close physical contact.
- *Provide privacy for patients during close physical care.* Use privacy curtains, keep the patient covered whenever possible, expose only the necessary body part, and ask other persons to leave the room during close physical care. These actions increase feelings of security.

Self-Reflection Questions

1. How much space do you need to feel comfortable during interactions with strangers?
2. How much space do you prefer when you are with friends?
3. What do you do when your personal space is invaded?
4. How can you assist patients to accept your care when you must invade their personal space?

Comprehensive review at the end of each chapter!

Key Points at the end of each chapter provide a reminder of need-to-know information and concepts. The main concepts of the chapter are included in this list.

Pearson Nursing Student Resources lead you to additional materials at nursing.pearsonhighered.com including NCLEX-PN® style review questions, case studies, and more!

A **Clinical Reasoning Care Map** helps you prioritize data and nursing interventions. Each map provides a case study, nursing diagnosis, and a list of data and interventions. You select which data and nursing interventions would relate to that patient with that particular nursing diagnosis. You identify any safety issues that might arise and the priority actions to be taken in this situation. You also consider what other professionals may be involved in the patient's care. Each map sharpens reporting and charting skills by asking what you should document and by providing examples of appropriate documentation. You can compare your answers to those provided on the companion website.

Chapter Review

KEY POINTS

- **Concept:** Shock is characterized by oxygen supply that is less than demand, leading to inadequate tissue perfusion. Without immediate recognition and treatment, shock progresses through the compensatory, progressive, and irreversible stages and can result in death.
- Early signs of shock include a change in the level of consciousness and restlessness, indicating decreased blood flow to the brain.
- Hypovolemic shock, the most common type of shock, is caused by a decrease of 15% or more in circulating blood volume.
- An allergic reaction to an antigen can progress from a mild to a severe hypersensitivity response, resulting in anaphylactic shock. Anaphylactic shock is caused by blood pooling in the periphery from vasodilation of the blood vessels.
- Cardiogenic shock is caused by decreased pumping ability of the heart so that the heart cannot maintain adequate cardiac output and tissue perfusion. A serious myocardial infarction can lead to cardiogenic shock.
- Septic shock is most often caused by gram-negative infections that trigger systemic vasodilation and increased capillary permeability, resulting in relative hypovolemia.
- Fluid resuscitation and oxygen therapy are the cornerstones for managing patients with shock. Other additional measures include patient support, medications such as epinephrine, antihistamines, diuretics, antibiotics or vasopressors, and blood or blood products. Early recognition and treatment are essential to prevent shock complications such as ARDS, DIC, and renal failure.
- **Concept:** Trauma is any life-threatening occurrence, either accidental or intentional that causes injuries (American

Trauma Society, 2012). Leading causes of trauma are falls, motor vehicle accidents, and assaults. Trauma kills or disables people often during their most productive years of life.
- Traumatic injuries can be classified as minor or major, depending on the extent of the damage. Trauma is the leading cause of death in young people. It can be prevented by following common safety guidelines, such as wearing a seat belt when riding in or driving a car or a helmet when riding a bicycle.
- Airway assessment and management is the highest priority in the trauma patient, followed by assessment of breathing, circulation, disability, and exposure. It is essential to identify all life-threatening injuries and to institute immediate, priority interventions.
- Nurses in the critical care unit focus not only on the critically ill patient's life-threatening problems but also on basic needs such as comfort, communication, and emotional support. The nurse also plays an important role in providing support, assurance, and information to families of the critically ill patient.
- **Concept:** Disasters require extraordinary efforts beyond what is needed to respond to everyday emergencies. Nurses play an essential role in knowing how to respond when a disaster occurs and in providing care for disaster victims.
- Manmade disasters may result from chemical, biologic, radiologic, and nuclear terrorism; food or water contamination; transportation accidents; or building collapses. When disasters occur, a triage system focuses on providing care to those with life-threatening conditions first.
- Nurses should have their own family disaster plan in place to be able to assist others during a disaster.

PEARSON NURSING STUDENT RESOURCES

Find additional materials at **nursing.pearsonhighered.com**.

Clinical Reasoning Care Map

Caring for a Patient at an Accident Scene
NCLEX-PN® Focus Area: Physiologic Integrity

Case Study: You are driving down a rural road and see a car swerve back and forth across the road. It hits a patch of ice and strikes a utility pole. There is no one else in sight and you stop. You find a young man alone in the car who says his name is Paul Thompson. He is not wearing a seat belt.

Nursing Diagnosis: Risk for Ineffective Tissue Perfusion		
COLLECT DATA		
Subjective	Objective	

Data Collected
(use only those that apply)
- Scalp is bleeding
- Allergic to penicillin
- Skin slightly pale and dry
- Is awake
- Complains of being thirsty
- Left leg is twisted at an odd angle
- Slow, shallow respirations
- Does not drink alcohol
- Rapid radial pulse rate
- Says his dad will be really mad that he wrecked the car
- Denies any difficulty breathing
- Complains of left leg pain
- Wears glasses

Does this present a threat to the patient's safety?
If yes, the priority intervention to address this threat would be:

Nursing Care

Nursing Interventions
(use only those that apply; list in priority order)
- Splint Paul's left leg.
- Ask how the accident happened.
- Give him a few sips of water.
- Cover scalp wound with a clean cloth.
- Cover the patient with a blanket.
- Keep head and neck in neutral position.
- Assist him out of the car.
- Call for help.
- Lay him on the ground and elevate his feet and legs.
- Look for hazards in the area.

Interprofessional team members to include when planning care:

How would you document this?

Compare your answers and documentation to those provided on the companion website.

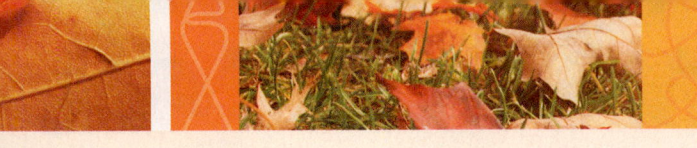
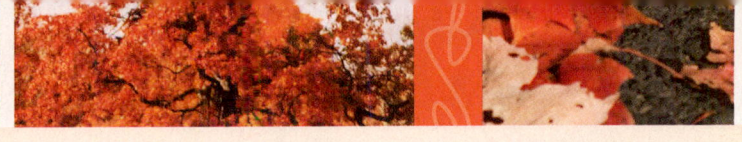

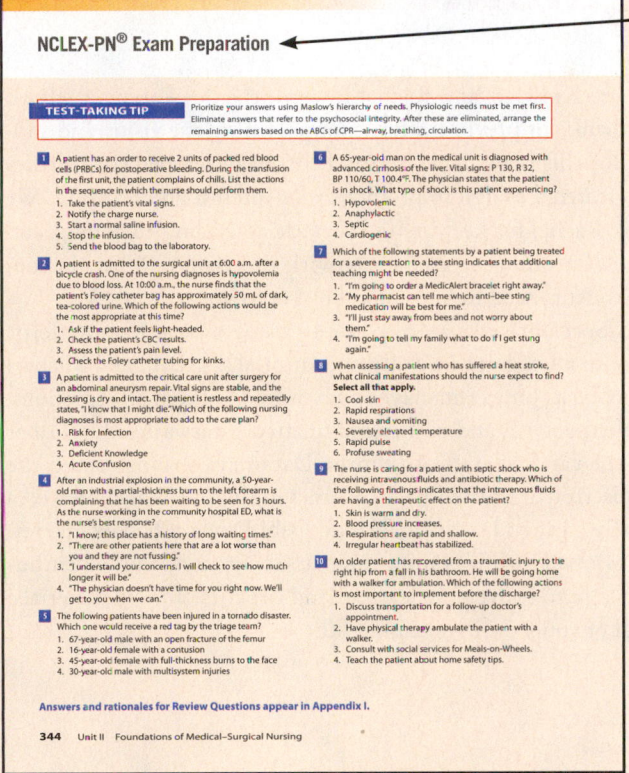

NCLEX-PN® Exam Preparation includes:

- Test-Taking Tip with a focused study hint
- NCLEX-PN® style questions for review and test practice, with both traditional and alternative formats. Answers are found in Appendix I.

NCLEX-PN® Exam Preparation

TEST-TAKING TIP   Prioritize your answers using Maslow's hierarchy of needs. Physiologic needs must be met first. Eliminate answers that refer to the psychosocial integrity. After these are eliminated, arrange the remaining answers based on the ABCs of CPR—airway, breathing, circulation.

1 A patient has an order to receive 2 units of packed red blood cells (PRBCs) for postoperative bleeding. During the transfusion of the first unit, the patient complains of chills. List the actions in the sequence in which the nurse should perform them.
1. Take the patient's vital signs.
2. Notify the charge nurse.
3. Start a normal saline infusion.
4. Stop the infusion.
5. Send the blood bag to the laboratory.

2 A patient is admitted to the surgical unit at 6:00 a.m. after a bicycle crash. One of the nursing diagnoses is hypovolemia due to blood loss. At 10:00 a.m., the nurse finds that the patient's Foley catheter bag has approximately 50 mL of dark, tea-colored urine. Which of the following actions would be the most appropriate at this time?
1. Ask if the patient feels light-headed.
2. Check the patient's CBC results.
3. Assess the patient's pain level.
4. Check the Foley catheter tubing for kinks.

3 A patient is admitted to the critical care unit after surgery for an abdominal aneurysm repair. Vital signs are stable, and the dressing is dry and intact. The patient is restless and repeatedly states, "I know that I might die." Which of the following nursing diagnoses is most appropriate to add to the care plan?
1. Risk for Infection
2. Anxiety
3. Deficient Knowledge
4. Acute Confusion

4 After an industrial explosion in the community, a 50-year-old man with a partial-thickness burn to the left forearm is complaining that he has been waiting to be seen for 3 hours. As the nurse working in the community hospital ED, what is the nurse's best response?
1. "I know; this place has a history of long waiting times."
2. "There are other patients here that are a lot worse than you and they are not fussing."
3. "I understand your concerns. I will check to see how much longer it will be."
4. "The physician doesn't have time for you right now. We'll get to you when we can."

5 The following patients have been injured in a tornado disaster. Which one would receive a red tag by the triage team?
1. 67-year-old male with an open fracture of the femur
2. 16-year-old female with a contusion
3. 45-year-old female with full-thickness burns to the face
4. 30-year-old male with multisystem injuries

6 A 65-year-old man on the medical unit is diagnosed with advanced cirrhosis of the liver. Vital signs: P 130, R 32, BP 110/60, T 100.4°F. The physician states that the patient is in shock. What type of shock is this patient experiencing?
1. Hypovolemic
2. Anaphylactic
3. Septic
4. Cardiogenic

7 Which of the following statements by a patient being treated for a severe reaction to a bee sting indicates that additional teaching might be needed?
1. "I'm going to order a MedicAlert bracelet right away."
2. "My pharmacist can tell me which anti–bee sting medication will be best for me."
3. "I'll just stay away from bees and not worry about them."
4. "I'm going to tell my family what to do if I get stung again."

8 When assessing a patient who has suffered a heat stroke, what clinical manifestations should the nurse expect to find? **Select all that apply.**
1. Cool skin
2. Rapid respirations
3. Nausea and vomiting
4. Severely elevated temperature
5. Rapid pulse
6. Profuse sweating

9 The nurse is caring for a patient with septic shock who is receiving intravenous fluids and antibiotic therapy. Which of the following findings indicates that the intravenous fluids are having a therapeutic effect on the patient?
1. Skin is warm and dry.
2. Blood pressure increases.
3. Respirations are rapid and shallow.
4. Irregular heartbeat has stabilized.

10 An older patient has recovered from a traumatic injury to the right hip from a fall in his bathroom. He will be going home with a walker for ambulation. Which of the following actions is most important to implement before the discharge?
1. Discuss transportation for a follow-up doctor's appointment.
2. Have physical therapy ambulate the patient with a walker.
3. Consult with social services for Meals-on-Wheels.
4. Teach the patient about home safety tips.

Answers and rationales for Review Questions appear in Appendix I.

After each unit in this book, use the **Thinking Strategically About …** feature as an opportunity to reflect on the topics read in the context of important themes across the LPN/LVN curriculum. Short scenarios and project ideas call for critical thinking about the unit's content from a variety of perspectives. Answers to questions appear on the companion website.

Critical Thinking questions highlight specific challenges you will face as a new nurse striving to provide the best possible care.

Management of Care questions highlight specific nursing interventions to take in different situations and the implications of care.

Delegating encourages you to think in terms of the work you must oversee as well as the hands-on work you will do.

Patient Teaching focuses on communication and educational strategies to take with the patient and family.

Priorities in Nursing Care helps you prioritize assessment and care.

UNIT II WRAP-UP

Thinking Strategically About . . .

You are an LPN working the evening shift in a rural 15-bed hospital. The usual staffing pattern is an RN, one or two LPNs depending on the census, and a CNA for each 8-hour shift. Most patients are stable and require routine care. Patients with complex or critical conditions are generally taken to the regional medical center 30 miles away. This evening there is one RN, one LPN, and one CNA to care for the three patients. You will be responsible for the following patients who have been admitted today from the ED. You receive reports on their status.

- Jane Souza, a 25-year-old married woman with two children, was involved in a car crash. Both cars were traveling approximately 35 mph. Ms. Souza was not wearing a seat belt and was thrown forward against the steering wheel. Her lower legs hit the underside of the dashboard. She is conscious, is receiving high-flow oxygen by mask, and has one intravenous line in place. Vital signs are BP 142/76, P 120, R 26. She has multiple bruises and abrasions. She has limited extremity movement because of a broken right arm and an open fracture of the left ankle. There is no active external bleeding. Surgery is planned within the hour to repair the fractured ankle and set her broken arm.

- Howard Still, a 76-year-old widower, has been receiving chemotherapy for recurrent lung cancer. He has been experiencing nausea and vomiting for the past week. His vital signs are BP 102/68, T 102, P 98, R 26. He complains of extreme fatigue and muscle cramps in his legs. His potassium level is 3.0. He has an IV of D5 ½ NS with 20 mEq of KCl at 100 mL/hr. Howard stated, "I am ready to stop this cancer treatment and join my wife in Heaven."

- Juan Martinez, a 28-year-old, came to the emergency room with his third migraine headache in the last 6 weeks. Juan milks cows on a large dairy. He admits to drinking three beers every evening. He smokes one pack of cigarettes a day. His vital signs are stable. He was medicated with 25 mg of Demerol (meperidine) intravenously 30 minutes ago. If his migraine subsides and he does not require further meperidine doses, he will be discharged the next day with instructions to see the doctor in the clinic within 2 days.

CRITICAL THINKING

- What specific observations of Jane must you make to determine whether her condition remains stable and she is not developing further complications?
- What questions should you ask Howard to add clarity to your understanding of his desire to stop cancer treatment and his wish to join his wife in Heaven?
- What questions should you ask Juan to add precision to your assessment of his headache?

PRIORITIES IN NURSING CARE

- In what order will you assess your patients?
- What is your rationale for your prioritization of care?

MANAGEMENT OF CARE

- How frequently should you monitor Jane?
- At 1530 there is 400 mL of fluid in Howard's IV bottle. When will the next bottle need to be hung?
- What nonpharmacologic interventions could you implement for Juan?

DELEGATING

- If a CNA is available to assist with your assignment, what care would you delegate?
- What information must you provide to the RN regarding the care of these patients that was delegated to you?

PATIENT TEACHING

- What preoperative teaching is a priority for Jane?
- What teaching should you provide to Howard about his treatment plan?
- What teaching will Juan require before discharge?

TEAMWORK AND COLLABORATION

- What interprofessional team members should be involved in Howard's discharge planning to address his wishes about his treatment and to "be with his wife in Heaven"?

DOCUMENTING AND REPORTING

- What SBAR report would you give to the operating room nurse regarding Jane's injuries and condition?
- What report would you expect to receive from the nurse caring for Howard during the day shift?
- Write a medical record entry, using the Focus Charting method, regarding Juan's discharge.

Note: Discussion of Unit questions appears on the companion website.

Documenting and Reporting helps you practice what and how to document and report your findings.

Cultural Care Strategies build your confidence by providing information and scenarios to familiarize you with cultural patterns and differences.

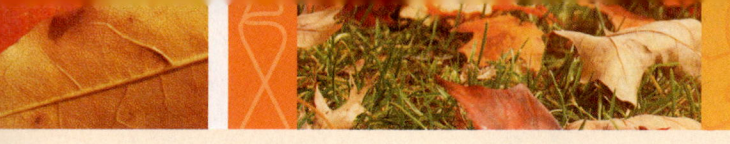
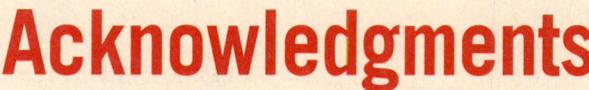

Acknowledgments

A project such as *Medical–Surgical Nursing Care* would not come into being without the contributions of many people.

First of all, we thank you, our students, past, present, and future, from whom we learn so much. Your quest for learning and your enthusiasm for the profession you have chosen stimulate us, invigorate us, and always keep us honest and humble. You are the future of our profession.

Many nursing professionals provided invaluable expertise and input into this book. Our contributors provided their knowledge, skills, and time to this project, writing selected chapters and features of this book. Reviewers provide quality assurance for the book. They validate content, attend to details, and challenge our ways of thinking and expressing ourselves. Contributors and reviewers for *Medical–Surgical Nursing Care* are listed with their current affiliations after this Preface.

A project such as this one requires the support, skills, and expertise of many people. We especially want to thank Julie Alexander, our publisher, for having the vision to create this book specifically for you, the practical/vocational nursing student.

Throughout its development, champions of this project were Kelly Trakalo, the acquisitions editor; her predecessor, Barbara Krawiec; and Rachel Bedard, the development editor. We thank our previous editors for providing the vision and support for this book. They researched and developed the features and created a design to promote your interest and learning. We thank Rachel for keeping us on track, attending to details, and forever encouraging us to stay with the vision: What do you, the student, need to know and be able to do?

Special thanks are also due to many others. Erin Rafferty, program manager; Erin Sullivan, editorial assistant; and Michael Giacobbe as project manager who moved parts in all directions, problem-solved, and monitored quality. Saraswathi Muralidhar and the capable staff of Lumina Datamatics transformed the manuscript to printed page. Maria Guglielmo Walsh created a visually clear and inviting format. Debi Doyle, Phoenix Harvey, and Michael Sirinides from the marketing team worked enthusiastically to convey the features and benefits of these materials. To all of you we are most grateful!

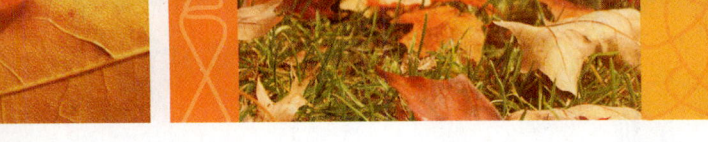

About the Authors

Karen M. Burke, RN, MS

Karen M. Burke is a nursing education consultant with experience as a nurse educator, program director, and nursing education program manager for the Oregon State Board of Nursing. She obtained her initial nursing education at Emanuel Hospital School of Nursing in Portland, Oregon, later completing baccalaureate studies at Oregon Health & Sciences University and a master's degree at University of Portland. Ms. Burke has extensive clinical nursing experience in acute care and community-based settings, as well as more than 25 years of experience in nursing education.

As a nurse educator, Ms. Burke is known as a leader and an innovator. She has been actively involved in nursing education in Oregon, participating in the development of the Oregon Consortium for Nursing Education (OCNE), an educational consortium of a public university and local community colleges to develop and deliver a competency-based nursing curriculum that prepares graduates for practice in a rapidly changing health care environment. She also has been active in helping to develop innovative clinical models. Ms.

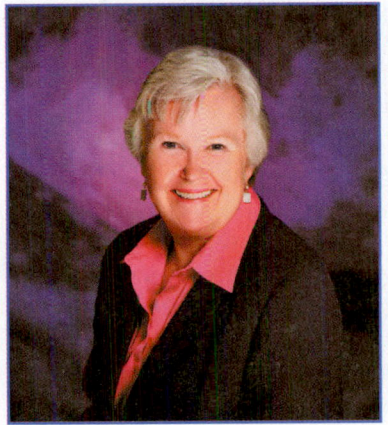

Burke values the nursing profession and believes in the importance of a strong education in the art and science of nursing for all students entering the profession. Her commitment to access to quality education and health care has led to service on the boards of directors for Clatsop Community College and Clatsop Care Center Health District, as well as Supporters of the Oregon Consortium for Nursing Education (SOCNE).

Ms. Burke and her husband Steve love to garden, travel, and spend time with their extended family. Ms. Burke also enjoys a passion for quilting and accumulating and gradually completing multiple UFOs (unfinished objects).

Elaine L. Mohn-Brown, RN, EdD, CMSRN

Elaine L. Mohn-Brown received her diploma in nursing from Akron General Medical Center School of Nursing in Akron, Ohio. She has baccalaureate and master's degrees in nursing and health education from Metropolitan State College, United States University, and University of Northern Colorado, and a doctor of education degree in higher education administration from Brigham Young University. She has worked in critical care units in Ohio and Colorado. She holds current national certification in medical–surgical nursing.

Her first teaching position was as a practical nursing instructor at Larimer County Vocational-Technical Center in Colorado. For the past 35 years, she has been on the faculty of the ADN Program at Chemeketa Community College in Salem, Oregon. Through thought-provoking classroom presentations and hands-on acute care medical–surgical experiences, she encourages students to question, use critical thinking skills, and understand the rationale for their nursing care. She has implemented an extensive orientation program for novice nursing faculty at Chemeketa Community College. In 2005 she developed *Clinical Teaching in Oregon*, a DVD to

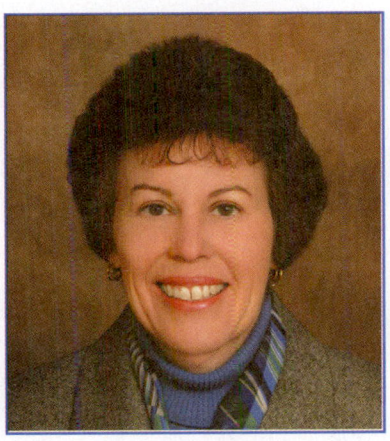

educate new clinical nursing faculty, and in 2009 she coauthored an online nursing faculty orientation program for several Oregon ADN programs.

Dr. Mohn-Brown serves as a member of the Editorial Advisory Board for *Nurse Educator* and has been a program evaluator for the Northwest Commission on Colleges and Universities. She has published nationally and conducts workshops at the national and international level. Her love of nursing and teaching has taken her to numerous international and national conferences.

When not working, she and her husband, Gene, spend time traveling. She enjoys photography, flower gardening, and needle arts.

Linda Eby, RN, MN

Linda Eby received her baccalaureate and master's degrees in nursing from Oregon Health and Sciences University. She has 39 years of experience in nursing. Her nursing practice has been in critical care, home health/hospice, and psychiatric mental health nursing. As a clinical nurse specialist in clinical genetics, she coordinated the Prenatal Genetics Clinic at OHSU. As a member of the Portland Community College Federation of Faculty and Academic Professionals, she serves as an advocate for the rights of education employees and students.

Ms. Eby has been teaching nursing at the community college level for 29 years. Her current teaching areas are nursing fundamentals, diabetes care, transcultural nursing, cardiovascular nursing, and psychiatric mental health nursing. Her special teaching interest is students who are non-native speakers of English. She is the coordinator of a

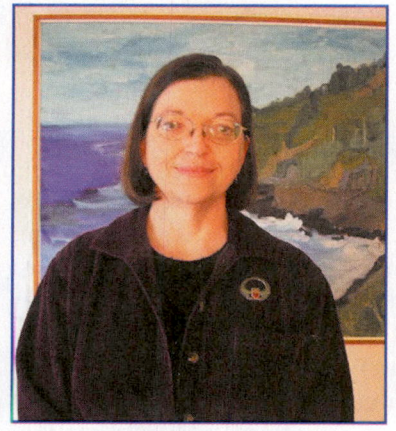

Nursing Student Success Program, which serves these as well as immigrant students, and other nontraditional students. She has consulted and conducted workshops on teaching diverse students of nursing. In 2012 she traveled to Africa to study the evolution of culture and nursing care in the third world. Fortunately, she has two wonderful daughters, Kate and Monica, a partner named John, a good dog named Benito, and a garden to provide balance in her life.

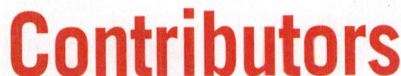

Contributors

Paul S. Smith, MN, RN, CCRN, CNE
Assistant Professor of Nursing
Linfield College
Portland, Oregon
Chapter 5 Guidelines for Patient Assessment
Chapter 13 Loss, Grief, and End-of-Life Care

Mary Ann Towle, RN, MSN
Boise State University
Boise, Idaho
Unit Wrap-Ups

Reviewers

Lisa M. Bass, MS, RN
Professor
Northern Essex Community College
Lawrence, Massachusetts

Eileen Bauer, MSN, RN
Nursing Instructor
College of Southern Nevada
Las Vegas, Nevada

Mary Cagle, RN, BSN
Assistant Professor
Dalton State College
Dalton, Georgia

Sherri Comfort, RN
Instructor
Holmes Community College
Goodman, Mississippi

Cheryl Gates, RN, MSN, PHN
Director of Vocational Nursing and Health Careers
Cerro Coso Community College
Ridgecrest, California

Evelyn Grigsby, MSN, RN
Associate Professor, Program Coordinator
Bluegrass Community & Technical College
Lexington, Kentucky

Helena Gunnell, MEd, BSN, RN
Instructor
Jones County Junior College
Ellisville, Mississippi

Jenny Holloway, BSN, RN
Instructor
Vance-Granville Community College
Henderson, North Carolina

Ruby Johnson, LPN, ADN, BSN, MSN/Ed
Professor
Ozarka College
Melbourne, Arkansas

Sharon Nowak, RN, MSN, Ed. D. (c)
Professor
Jackson College
Jackson, Michigan

Mary Russo, MSN, RN
Professor
Lincoln Land Community College
Jacksonville, Illinois

Patricia L. Schrull, MSN, MBA, MEd, RN, CNE
Associate Professor
Lorain County Community College
Elyria, Ohio

Contents

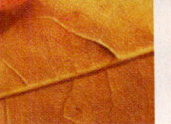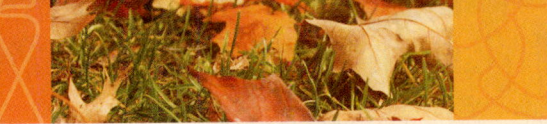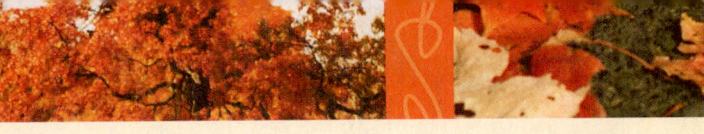

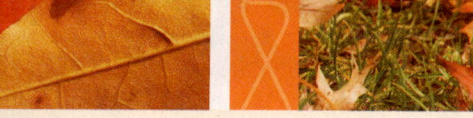
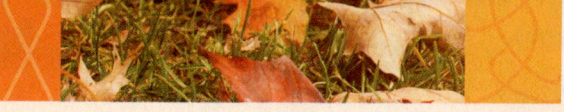
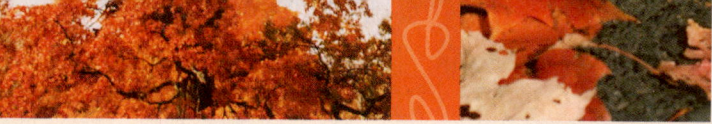

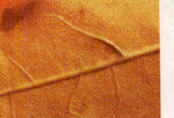
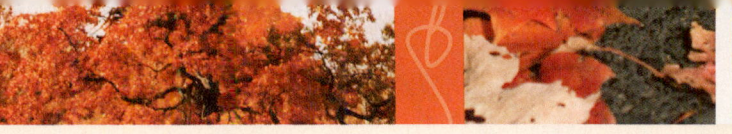

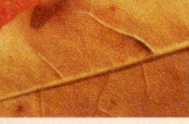
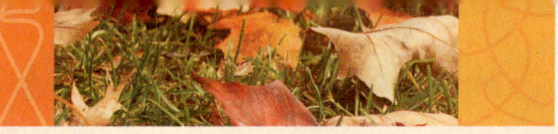
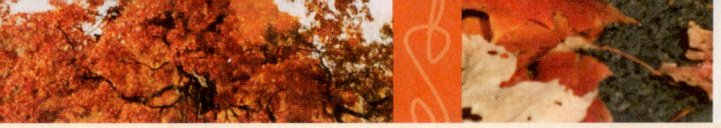

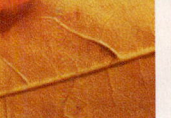
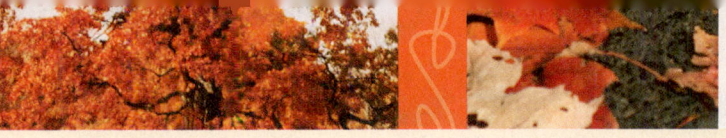

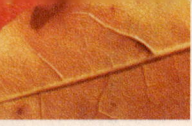
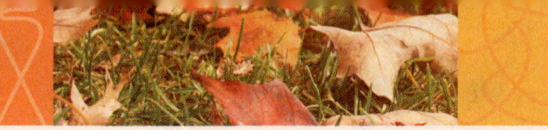
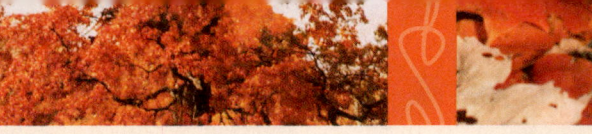

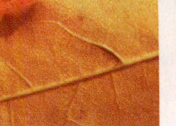
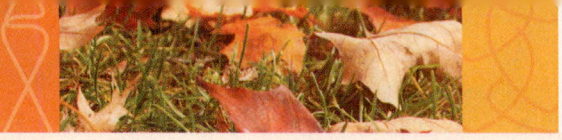
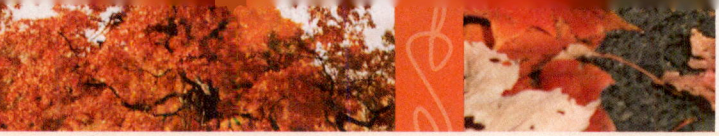

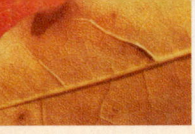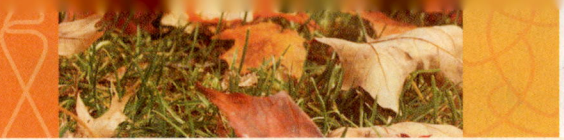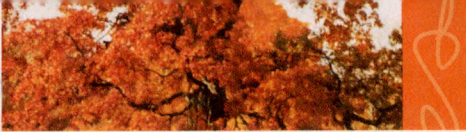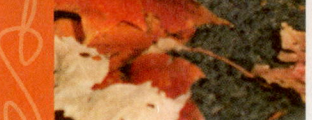

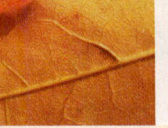
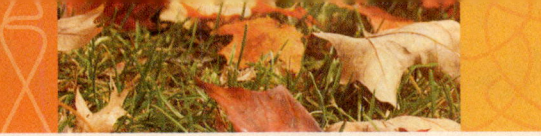
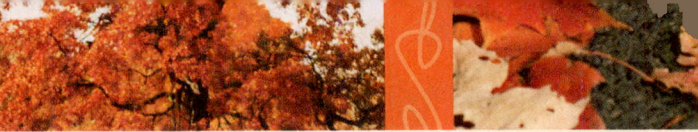
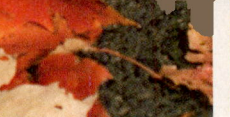

Contents   **xxiii**

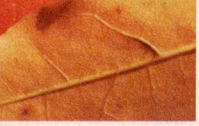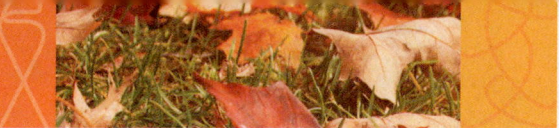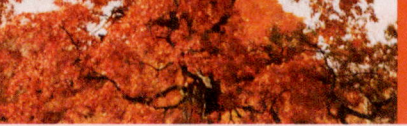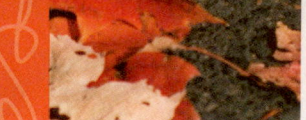

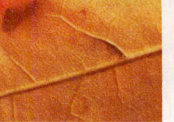
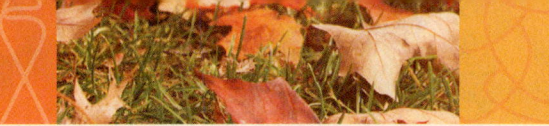
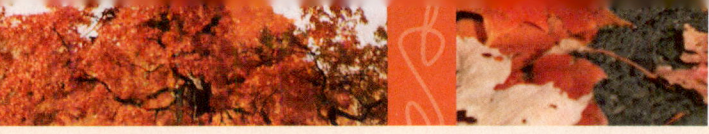

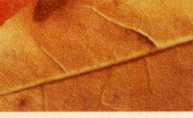
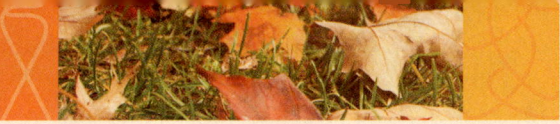
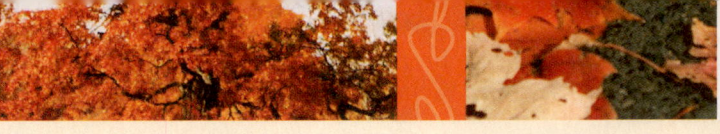

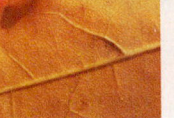
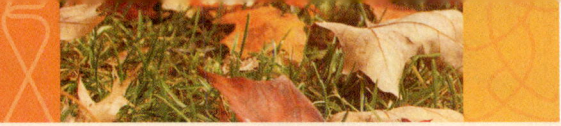
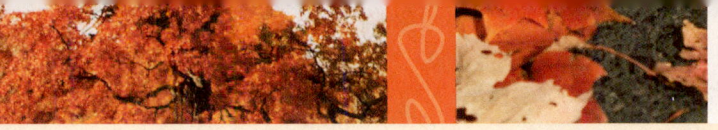

Contents   **xxvii**

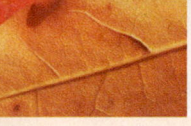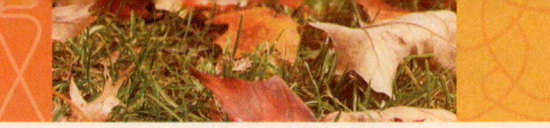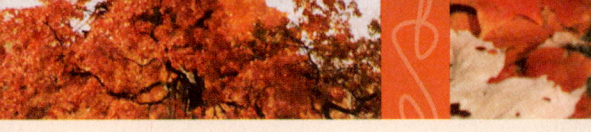

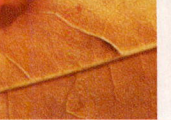
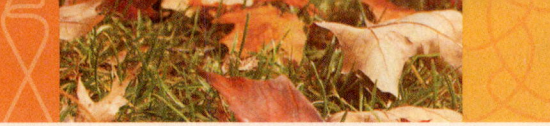
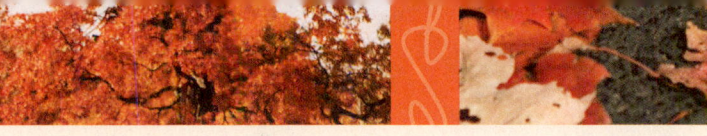

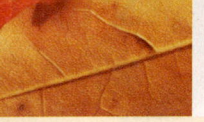
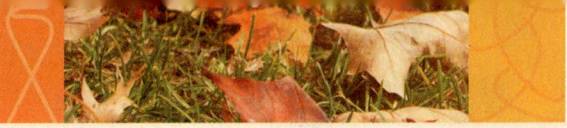
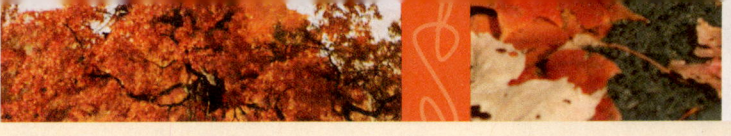

UNIT I
Introduction to Medical–Surgical Nursing

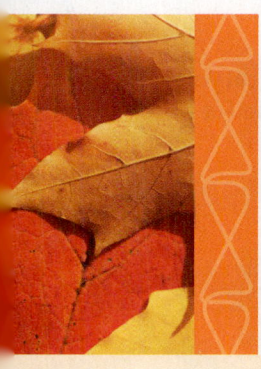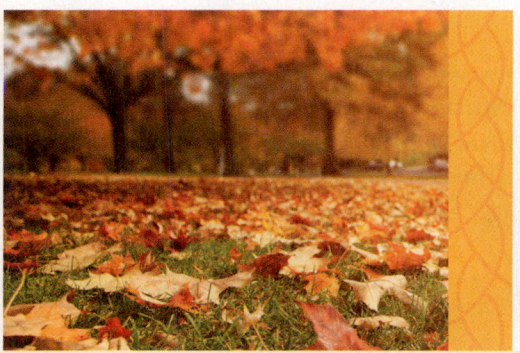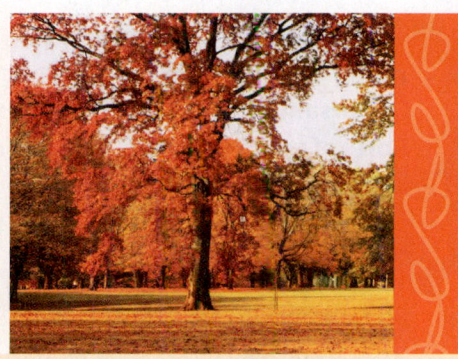

Cultural Care Strategies:

Unit I Wrap-Up

CHAPTER 1
Nursing in the 21st Century

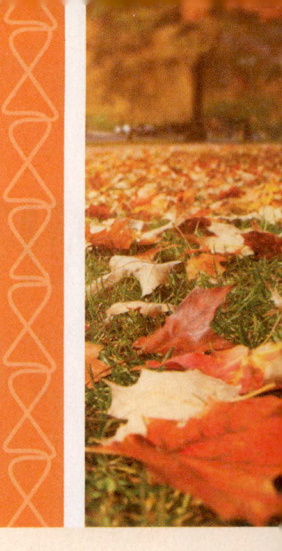

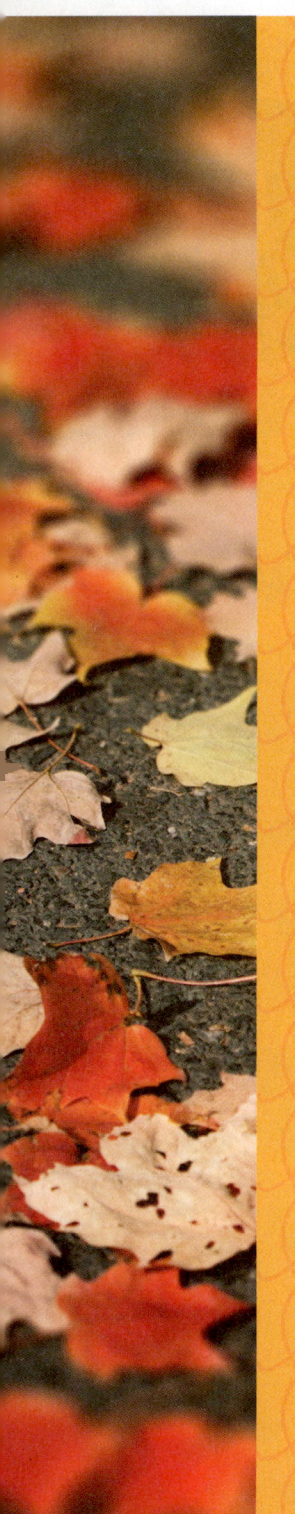

BRIEF OUTLINE

Quality and Safety in
   Nursing

Roles of the LPN/LVN in
   Medical–Surgical Nursing
   Care

Framework for Practice: The
   Nursing Process

Critical Thinking and
   Clinical Judgment

Legal and Ethical Aspects of
   Nursing Practice

APPLIED LEARNING OUTCOMES

After completing this chapter, you will be able to:

1. Discuss current trends and issues in health care and nursing.
2. Describe the essential elements of quality and safety in nursing and their impact on the nurse's role and responsibilities.
3. Describe the role of the LPN/LVN as a member of the health care team.
4. Use the nursing process to assess, plan, implement, and evaluate individualized, patient-centered care.
5. Explain how clinical reasoning, current evidence, and available standards are used to determine priorities of nursing care and to promote, maintain, or restore health.
6. Describe the nature of laws regulating nursing practice in the United States.
7. Practice within the LPN/LVN scope of practice.
8. Use ethical standards and codes as a guide in providing medical–surgical nursing care.

KEY TERMS

The key terms are defined on the pages listed below.

advocate, 6

assessment, 6

caregivers, 5

clinical judgment, 9

collaborator, 5

critical thinking, 9

dilemma, 15

ethics, 14

evaluation, 8

evidence-based
   practice, 3

health care informatics, 4

HIPAA, 14

holistic, 6

implementation, 8

interventions, 5

malpractice, 13

medical–surgical
   nursing, 3

nursing diagnosis, 7

nursing process, 6

outcomes, 7

patient-centered care, 3

planning, 7

professional boundaries,
   15

quality improvement, 4

safety, 4

standard, 12

statutory law, 11

tort law, 13

Key Concept   Medical–surgical nurses promote health and provide care to adult patients during illness or injury.

Medical–surgical nursing is the care of adults to protect, promote, and maintain health; to prevent illness and injury; and to alleviate suffering (ANA, 2013). It is based on knowledge from the arts and sciences and is shaped by the science of nursing. The focus of medical–surgical nursing is the adult patient's response to actual or potential disruptions in health. The adult requiring health care services is the *patient*. In some instances, nursing care is directed toward the family (e.g., supporting the family of a dying person) or even the community (e.g., immunizing people to prevent an outbreak of whooping cough). In these instances, the *patient* is the family or the community.

Medical–surgical nurses focus on the adult patient's responses to disease and illness. For example, when surgery is required to treat a disease, the nursing focus is on promoting the patient's comfort and healing and preventing complications that could result from surgery. This requires knowledge about the structure, function, and interrelatedness of body systems, as well as effects on the patient's social, cultural, economic, and personal life. Medical–surgical nurses provide care for people across the major part of the life span, ranging from their late teens to early 100s. The variety of individual health care needs and the wide range of patients' ages make medical–surgical nursing an ever-changing and challenging field.

This chapter serves as a broad overview of medical–surgical nursing practice. Topics include quality and safety in nursing and health care, roles of the licensed practical/vocational nurse (LPN/LVN), the nursing process, clinical reasoning, guidelines for practice, and legal and ethical issues that may arise when providing care.

Quality and Safety in Nursing

Key Concept   Nurses, as well as all health care providers, are responsible for ensuring the safety of patients and quality of the health care they receive.

Health care today is a vast and complex system. It reflects changes in society, changes in the populations that require nursing care, and an emphasis on health promotion as well as illness care. The increasing complexity of the health care system has led to a growing recognition of the need to refocus on the quality and safety of health care. In response, the National Academy of Sciences (2004) identified core competencies for all health care providers and the Quality and Safety Education for Nurses (QSEN) project developed competencies for nurses. These quality and safety competencies are the following:

- Patient-centered care
- Teamwork and collaboration
- Evidence-based practice
- Quality improvement
- Safety
- Informatics (Sherwood & Barnsteiner, 2012)

These competencies, which are further explained here, will be incorporated throughout this book.

PATIENT-CENTERED CARE

Patient-centered care is care in which the nurse attends to the uniqueness of the individual, planning and adapting care to the needs of that person. When providing patient-centered care, the nurse listens to and respects the patient's wishes and desired outcomes of the care. Care is planned with respect for the patient's culture and values (see Chapter 3 for more information about culture). Attention is paid to relieving pain and suffering. A nurse providing patient-centered care adapts the nursing care and coordinates activities to the needs of the individual (and, as appropriate, the family), not to the desires of the health care team. In patient-centered care, the nurse advocates for wellness, healthy lifestyles, and disease prevention. When the patient has a chronic disease or condition, the nurse advocates for lifestyle changes and disease management, with the patient assuming the primary role. For the dying patient, the nurse providing patient-centered care advocates for comfort care and pain relief and supports the family.

TEAMWORK AND COLLABORATION

Nurses and other health care providers work as a team to meet the health care needs of patients. The members of the team may vary, but the need to communicate effectively, cooperate, and collaborate with one another does not change. Clear and effective communication is vital for the continuity of safe, patient-centered care. Effective communication, in turn, requires that the nurse know and understand the roles and responsibilities of team members and have skills in problem solving, conflict resolution, and negotiation (Sherwood & Barnsteiner, 2012).

EVIDENCE-BASED PRACTICE

In **evidence-based practice**, the nurse uses the best current evidence together with clinical knowledge and patient values and preferences to provide optimal care (Cronenwett et al., 2007). The *science of nursing* is based on research that supports the effectiveness of specific nursing interventions to improve patient's health or reduce the risk of adverse outcomes. This science is rapidly evolving. As the body of evidence grows, it becomes increasingly clear that nursing care based on science and on current best practices can have a profound effect on the quality of nursing and the health of the patient.

Nurses have always identified problems in patient care and developed interventions to meet specific needs. Patient care should be based on current evidence and identified best practices, not on tradition or intuition. The nurse's role as a caregiver is increasingly based on evidence-based practice.

QUALITY IMPROVEMENT

Nurses should strive continuously to improve care for individuals as well as for all patients. **Quality improvement** is the use of data to evaluate the outcomes of care and to design and test changes to improve the quality and safety of health care systems (Cronenwett et al., 2007). In practice, quality improvement compares actual care with an ideal care standard and identifies strategies to bring these into alignment (Sherwood & Barnsteiner, 2012). To apply quality improvement strategies, nurses must understand and implement basic safety principles and must critically evaluate the outcomes of care. They can then identify errors and hazards in the implementation and environments of care.

Quality improvement methods also are used to evaluate the care of individual patients against established standards of care. In this process, documentation is reviewed, patient surveys are conducted, nurses are interviewed, and nurse or patient performance is directly observed. This information is then used to identify differences between actual practice and established standards and to develop a plan of action to resolve the differences. Later, the actions are assessed to determine whether they were effective in improving practice. Box 1-1■ lists selected 2014 Clinical Quality Measures identified by the Centers for Medicare & Medicaid Services (CMS).

SAFETY

Safety in health care is the effort to minimize the risk of harm to patients and to providers by examining both individual performance and system effectiveness (Cronenwett et al., 2007). Safe practice requires looking forward to identify potential risks and errors and identifying ways to prevent errors or harm from occurring. A focus on safety means that errors are addressed from an approach of not blaming the individual but examining the system in which the error occurred. In this approach, environmental conditions that may have contributed to the error are examined, and approaches to prevent errors or reduce their effects are designed (Sherwood & Barnsteiner, 2012). The Joint Commission, which accredits hospitals and health care organizations, publishes National Patient Safety Goals (Box 1-2■).

INFORMATICS

Although communications technology has become a vital part of health care, the use of information technology to support clinical decision making is relatively new. **Health care informatics** is the management and use of data, information, and knowledge through computer information systems. Health care informatics is used to manage care through documentation in electronic medical records (EMRs), support diagnosis and treatment decisions, and share information among the interprofessional care team.

BOX 1-1   SELECTED 2014 CMS CLINICAL QUALITY MEASURES

- Heart failure patients discharged home with written instructions addressing activity, diet, discharge medications, follow-up, weight monitoring, and what to do if symptoms worsen.
- Surgery patients with appropriate surgical site hair removal (no hair removal or use of clippers or depilatory for hair removal are considered appropriate).
- Surgical patients with urinary catheter removed on postoperative day 1 or day 2.
- Stroke patients who received educational materials during hospital stay addressing activation of the emergency medical system, follow-up after discharge, risk factors for stroke, and warning signs and symptoms of stroke.
- Patients screened for seasonal influenza vaccination status and were vaccinated before discharge if indicated.

Source: Centers for Medicare and Medicaid Services (CMS). (2013). Proposed Clinical Quality Measures for 2014. Retrieved from CMS website.

BOX 1-2   SELECTED 2014 NATIONAL PATIENT SAFETY GOALS

1. Improve the accuracy of patient identification.
   a. Use at least two patient identifiers when providing care, treatment, and services.
2. Improve the effectiveness of communication among caregivers.
   a. Report critical results of tests and diagnostic procedures on a timely basis.
3. Improve the safety of using medications.
   a. Maintain and communicate accurate patient medication information.
4. Reduce the risk of health care–associated infections.
   a. Comply with either the current CDC hand hygiene guidelines or the current WHO hand hygiene guidelines.
   b. Implement evidence-based practices for preventing surgical site infections.
   c. Implement evidence-based practices to prevent indwelling catheter-associated urinary tract infections (CAUTI).

Source: Data from the Joint Commission. (2013). National Patient Safety Goals Effective January 1, 2014. Hospital Accreditation Program. Retrieved from The Joint Commission website.

Roles of the LPN/LVN in Medical–Surgical Nursing Care

Key Concept   The medical–surgical nurse has multiple roles, including caregiver, manager of care, collaborator, patient advocate, and teacher.

Medical–surgical nurses are not only caregivers but also managers of care, advocates, and teachers. The nurse assumes these roles to promote and maintain health, to prevent illness, and to help patients cope with disability or death in any setting.

THE NURSE AS CAREGIVER

Nurses have always been **caregivers** (people who provide personal, individual assistance), but the activities carried out within the caregiver role have changed tremendously. From 1900 to the 1960s, the nurse was almost always female; the primary definition of her caregiver role was to provide personal care for the patient and to carry out physicians' orders. The caregiver role for the nurse today is both independent and collaborative. Registered nurses (RNs) may independently make assessments, plan, and implement patient care based on nursing knowledge and skills. LPNs/LVNs, in conjunction with RNs, carry out the same activities (Figure 1-1 ■). All licensed nurses also *collaborate* (work cooperatively) with other members of the interprofessional health care team to implement and evaluate care.

As a caregiver, the nurse practices both the science and the art of nursing. Using the nursing process as the framework for care, the nurse plans and provides **interventions** (purposeful actions) to meet the physical, psychosocial, spiritual, environmental, and cultural needs of patients and families. The science of nursing is translated into the art of nursing through caring. *Caring* is the means by which the nurse is connected with and concerned for the patient. The nurse as caregiver is knowledgeable, skilled, understanding, and caring.

THE NURSE AS MANAGER OF CARE

All nurses must learn to coordinate care and to be leaders. Their jobs may require them to manage time, resources, the environment in which they provide care, and other people, such as nursing assistants (NAs). Nurses develop the skills to direct, delegate, and coordinate activities and to evaluate the quality of care provided. In the role of leader and manager, the nurse takes responsibility for the quality of patient care by assigning or delegating nursing care activities only to persons who are qualified and competent to provide that care safely and effectively. The nurse evaluates patients' needs and plans of care, determining which require a licensed nurse and which can safely be assigned to unlicensed assistive personnel (UAP). When assigning care, the nurse supervises caregivers and the care they provide. In all cases, the licensed nurse retains responsibility for the care assigned to others.

Prioritizing is an essential skill for nurses. The needs of patients are prioritized from the most urgent to those that can be met at a later time. When managing a group or team of patients, the nurse decides the order in which care is provided by prioritizing patient needs and planned interventions.

THE NURSE AS COLLABORATOR

Patient-centered care within the complexity of the health care system requires collaboration between the patient and all members of the health care team. As a **collaborator**, the nurse works together with the patient and the interprofessional team to provide optimal patient care. Effective collaboration requires mutual respect and shared decision making (Blais & Hayes, 2011).

In the role of collaborator with the patient, the nurse supports and encourages active involvement in health care decisions, working with patients to identify health care goals that are mutually agreed upon. With the interprofessional health care team, the nurse participates in sharing information, decision making, and responsibility for implementing patient care activities. Working with nursing peers, the nurse seeks and respects the expertise of others and shares his or her personal expertise. In all instances, the nurse develops trust and mutual respect for the contributions of patients, peers, and interprofessional team members (Blais & Hayes, 2011).

THE NURSE AS ADVOCATE

The American Nurses Association (2010) includes advocacy for individuals, families, communities, and populations in its definition of nursing. The patient who enters the health care system is often unprepared to make independent

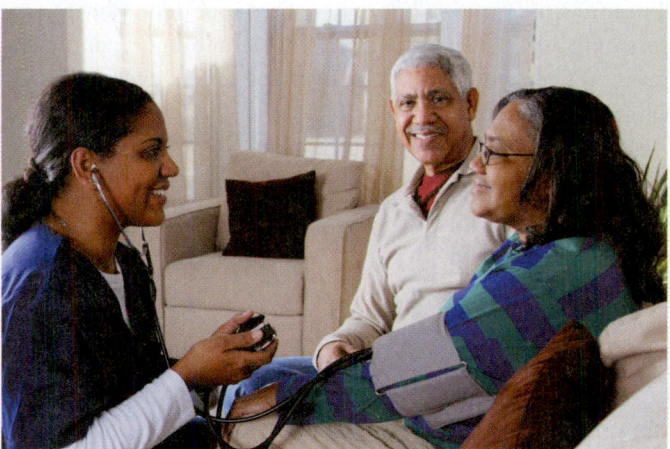

Figure 1-1. ■ In the role of caregiver, the nurse provides comprehensive, individualized care to the adult patient. (© Rob Marmion/ Shutterstock)

decisions. The nurse as **advocate** (one who speaks for another) actively promotes the patient's rights to make decisions and choices. The nurse speaks for the patient when necessary, mediates between the patient and other persons, and protects the patient's right to self-determination (even when the nurse disagrees with the patient's decision). As a patient advocate, the nurse:

- Communicates with other health care team members.
- Provides or reinforces patient and family teaching.
- Assists and supports patient decision making.
- Suggests referrals as appropriate.
- Identifies community and personal resources.

Nurses' advocacy extends beyond the individual patient to include families, communities, and population groups. The nurse who speaks for a family's expressed desires for a loved one's care in a team meeting, who works with a community health department to quell an outbreak of pertussis (whooping cough), or who promotes measures to reduce obesity is functioning in the role of advocate.

THE NURSE AS TEACHER

The teaching role of the nurse is important for many reasons. First, there is an increasing emphasis on health promotion and illness prevention. Second, hospital stays are becoming shorter, so the patient and family must provide continuing care at home. Third, as the overall population ages, more people are affected by chronic illnesses. In chronic illness, the patient and family have significant responsibility for managing the disease or condition, so they must have information. All of these make the nurse's role as a teacher increasingly important.

The framework for the role of teacher is the teaching–learning process. Within this framework, the LPN/LVN, in conjunction with the RN, assesses learning needs, plans and implements teaching to meet those needs, and evaluates the effectiveness of the teaching. The nurse must have good interpersonal skills and be familiar with adult learning principles (Figure 1-2■).

Teaching is a major part of helping patients and their families know how to provide care at home. Because patient and family education is such an important aspect of medical–surgical nursing care, we include information about what to teach for continuing care throughout this textbook.

Framework for Practice: The Nursing Process

> **Key Concept**   The nursing process is used to plan and organize care for patients. It includes five interdependent phases: assessment, diagnosis, planning, implementation, and evaluation.

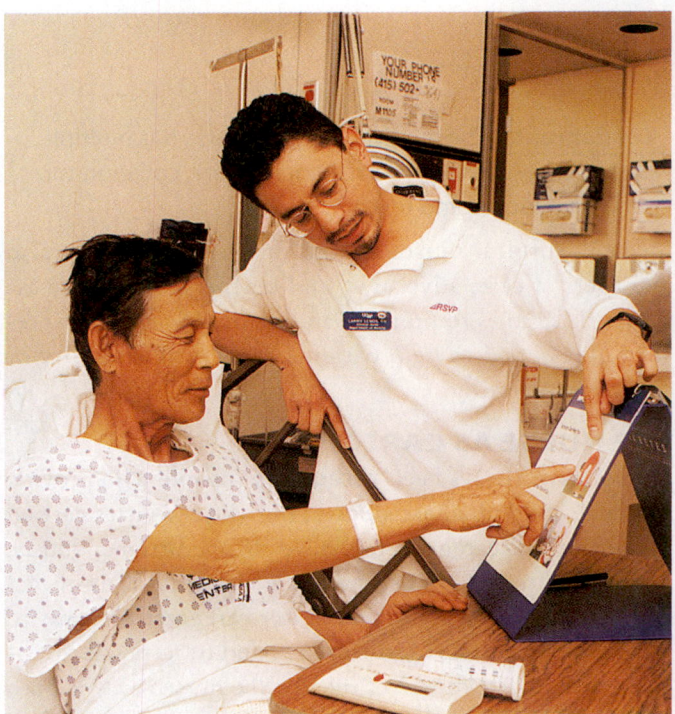

Figure 1-2. ■ The nurse's role as teacher is an essential component of care. As part of the discharge planning process, this nurse is teaching for self-care at home. (Photographer: Alain McLaughlin, Pearson Education.)

The **nursing process** is an approach to planning and organizing that nurses use as they care for patients. The nursing process is a model of care that differentiates nursing from other helping professions. It can be used in any setting in which the nurse provides care, from promoting wellness to coping with disability or death. Regardless of the situation, the nursing process includes activities that are specific, individualized, and **holistic** (concerned with the whole person—physical, emotional, and spiritual).

PHASES OF THE NURSING PROCESS

The nursing process has five interdependent phases: assessment, diagnosis, planning, implementation, and evaluation. They are most often illustrated in a cyclic manner (Figure 1-3■).

LPNs and LVNs use all phases of the nursing process. The LPN/LVN contributes to diagnosis and nursing care planning in these phases of the nursing process. The RN has ultimate responsibility for establishing nursing diagnoses and developing plans of care. LPNs and LVNs, however, provide information that supports nursing diagnoses and are often involved in identifying specific health problems of individual patients. Care plans that illustrate the nursing process are included throughout this textbook.

Assessment

Assessment, the first phase of the nursing process, begins when the patient first encounters the health care system

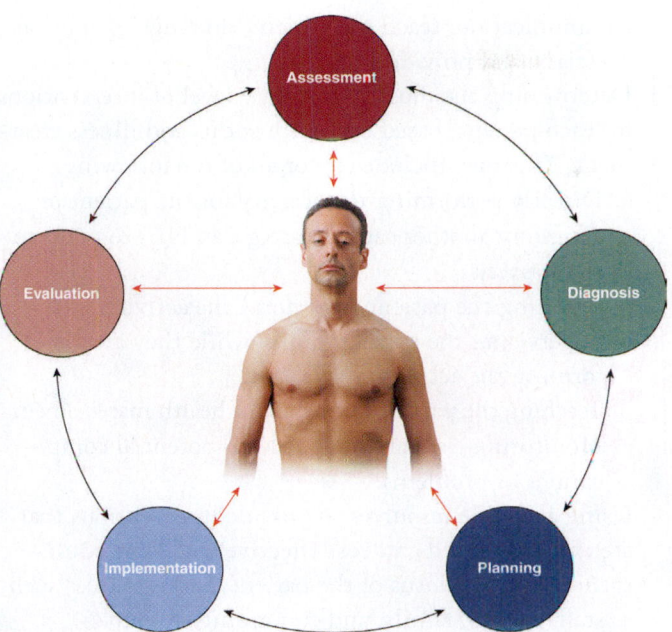

Figure 1-3. ■ Phases of the nursing process. Notice that the phases are interrelated and interdependent, with the patient central throughout. For example, evaluation of the patient might reveal the need for further assessment, additional nursing diagnoses, and/or a revision of the plan of care. (Source: Patrick Watson, Pearson Education.)

and continues as long as the patient requires care. During assessment, the nurse collects *data* (pieces of information) about the patient's health status. Both *subjective* (reported by the patient) and *objective* (obtained through observation or measurement) data are obtained. Accurate assessments are essential for identifying patient responses to health problems, for planning and implementing individualized care, and for evaluating the care that is given. (See guidelines for collecting data in Chapter 5 and the assessment chapters that begin each disorders unit.)

Nurses assess patients in two ways:

1. The *initial assessment* includes a thorough history and physical assessment. It provides comprehensive data about health responses. It identifies factors that contribute to these responses in a specific individual. It begins the mutual process of establishing goals and outcomes of care with the patient. An initial assessment is most often done when a patient enters a health care setting, although it may be deferred if the patient enters with urgent needs.

2. *Focused assessments* occur whenever the nurse interacts with the patient (e.g., at the beginning of each shift in the hospital and during patient care activities). They enable the nurse to evaluate responses to nursing actions and to determine whether interventions should continue or change to meet outcomes. They provide structure for documenting nursing care. They also allow the nurse to identify changes in responses to health

problems or treatments and responses not previously identified (e.g., a patient who previously appeared calm now has signs of anxiety; a reddened area is noted on a patient's heel when none was noted on admission).

To make accurate assessments, nurses must have the knowledge and skills to assess the physical and mental status of the patient. Nurses must know and understand anatomy, physiology, pathophysiology, and pharmacology, as well as the expected course of the disease or recovery process. The nurse must use effective communication to obtain information and establish a relationship of trust with the patient.

Diagnosis

The nurse uses clinical judgment (or clinical reasoning) to interpret assessment data and its meaning. The American Nurses Association (ANA) has defined nursing as the "diagnosis and treatment of human response" to protect, promote, and optimize health; to prevent illness and injury; and to alleviate suffering (2010, p. 1). The nurse identifies these human responses in a **nursing diagnosis**, defined as "a clinical judgment about . . . experiences/responses to actual or potential health problems/life processes . . . [that] provides the basis for selection of nursing interventions to achieve outcomes for which the nurse has responsibility" (Herdman, 2012, p. 515). Although no one list of nursing diagnoses is universally accepted, in 1988 the work of NANDA was accepted by the ANA as the official system of diagnosis for the United States. Nursing diagnoses within the NANDA system are used as appropriate in this book. (See also Appendix II, NANDA International Nursing Diagnoses: Definitions and Classification 2012–2014 on the companion website.)

Once nursing diagnoses are identified, nurses develop and implement a plan of care for actual responses; they also plan interventions to support health and prevent illness for potential human responses.

Clinical reasoning, described in the next section, is used to decide which label (or diagnosis) best describes the patterns of patient data and to plan, develop, and evaluate nursing interventions.

Planning

During the **planning** phase, the nurse identifies patient **outcomes** (achievable, measurable goals) to promote healthy responses to illness and prevent, reverse, or decrease unhealthy responses. The nurse then identifies nursing interventions (activities) to achieve desired outcomes. Both outcomes and nursing interventions are documented in a written plan of care that directs nursing activities, nursing documentation, and appropriate evaluation.

Nurses plan interventions for two types of patient problems: those that nurses manage independently (stated as nursing diagnoses) and those that require interdisciplinary management (clinical problems). In *nursing management*, the nurses develop the diagnosis, plan and initiate selected interventions, and are accountable for achieving outcomes. In *interdisciplinary management* (pathophysiologic, illness, or treatment-related problems), nurses monitor for onset or changes in status and work with other members of the health care team to plan and implement interventions to treat health problems and minimize complications. Examples of nursing activities related to the interdisciplinary management of patients include monitoring a postoperative patient for signs of hemorrhage and administering an antibiotic to prevent or treat an infection.

EXPECTED OUTCOMES   Outcomes are mutually established by the patient and the nurse working together. Expected outcomes for nursing interventions are patient centered, time specific, and measurable (e.g., "The patient will demonstrate the ability to self-administer insulin injections by discharge"). Outcomes are classified into three domains: cognitive ("knowing"), affective ("feeling"), and psychomotor ("doing"). The nurse considers all three domains to ensure achievement of the desired therapeutic outcomes.

In contrast, expected outcomes for interdisciplinary problems are goals for the nurse, generally written, that describe patient responses indicating normal functioning or the absence of a complication or problem. For example, "breath sounds will remain clear," or "postoperative bleeding will remain within expected parameters." In many instances, these goals are not written down as part of the plan of care.

Implementation

Implementation is the "doing" phase of the nursing process, during which the nurse carries out planned activities (*interventions*). Ongoing assessment of the patient before, during, and after the intervention is essential. Although a plan may be appropriate, many variables may occur that make a change of plan necessary. For example, the nurse is not able to force fluids if the patient is nauseated or vomiting.

When implementing the planned interventions, the nurse follows several important principles:

1. Setting priorities, based on initial and focused assessments, the patient's condition, and expected or unexpected changes in the patient's health status. Critical assessments take first priority. These include the ABCs (*a*irway, *b*reathing, and *c*irculation), the status of invasive lines and infusing fluids, or changes in health status during the preceding shift.
2. Being aware of how nursing interventions interrelate. For example, while giving a bath, the nurse can also assess physical and psychological status, use therapeutic

communication, teach the patient, do range-of-motion exercises, and provide skin care.
3. Determining the most appropriate level of interventions for each patient, based on health status and illness treatment. This may include any or all of the following:
   a. Directly performing the activity for the patient or assigning another caregiver (e.g., an NA) to perform the activity.
   b. Assisting the patient to perform the activity.
   c. Supervising the patient/family while they are performing the activity.
   d. Teaching the patient/family about health management.
   e. Monitoring the patient at risk for potential complications or problems.
4. Using available resources to provide interventions that are evidence based and cost effective (available equipment; financial status of the patient; and resources such as staff, agency, family, and community resources).
5. Documenting nursing interventions. This final part of implementation *is a legal requirement.* There are many different ways of documenting care, some of which are narrative or focused charting, charting by exception, and use of EMRs.

Evaluation

The **evaluation** phase of the nursing process is the phase in which the nurse determines if the plan has been effective and whether to continue, revise, or terminate the plan. Evaluation is based on the expected outcomes that were established during the planning step. Though listed as the last phase of the nursing process, evaluation actually takes place continuously throughout patient care.

To evaluate a plan, the nurse assesses the patient and compares the patient's status with the expected outcomes. If the outcomes are being met, the nurse may continue or terminate the plan. If the outcomes have not been accomplished, the nurse must determine if the outcomes or planned interventions should continue or be revised. The LPN has a major role in evaluating the effectiveness of planned nursing care and contributing to revisions when necessary.

APPLYING THE NURSING PROCESS

In the clinical setting, the nursing process creates a structure for planned, individualized interventions. It ensures continuity of care through the written care plan. With experience, the nursing process becomes an integral part of providing care, and the nurse does not consciously stop and consider each step. For example, when caring for a patient who is hemorrhaging, the nurse uses all five steps simultaneously to meet critical, life-threatening needs. In contrast, when considering the long-term needs of a patient with a chronic illness or disability, the nurse makes in-depth assessments, determines goals jointly with the patient, and documents care through a written plan that is revised as necessary by all nurses providing care.

Critical Thinking and Clinical Judgment

Key Concept Clinical judgment is an essential component of safe and effective nursing practice. It is used with critical thinking and the nursing process to identify patient needs and prioritize nursing interventions.

Critical thinking is goal-directed thinking in which a person attempts to use knowledge and skills (rather than habits or assumptions) to determine the best overall result or choose the best action, given the particular circumstances. **Clinical judgment** is the process used by nurses and other health care professionals to determine a patient's needs, to identify appropriate interventions to address those needs, and to use patient responses to determine whether new approaches are appropriate (Tanner, 2006). The terms *critical thinking, clinical reasoning, clinical judgment*, and *problem solving* are used to describe the thinking processes of nurses and other health care professionals.

As you practice critical thinking and develop clinical judgment, you will use:

- Knowledge gained through your studies in the classroom, reading textbooks and current resources, and interacting with experienced nurses and other health care professionals.
- Experience gained by working with patients experiencing similar problems or disorders.
- Your understanding of the patient as an individual and his or her current and previous illness experiences.
- The values that drive your beliefs about what is good and right.
- The ability to identify and consider possible options, evaluate the alternatives, and reach a conclusion.

As a beginning nurse, you will use a deliberate process of collecting data; considering possible causes, meanings, and responses; and choosing the most appropriate action. As you gain knowledge and experience, it will become easier to recognize expected patterns of response, deviations from the expected, and probable meaning of the deviation (often referred to as *intuition*). Clinical reasoning becomes more internalized; you begin "thinking like a nurse." Box 1-3■ highlights some attitudes and habits that critical thinkers develop for clinical reasoning.

Critical thinking and clinical judgment, in conjunction with the nursing process, allow the nurse to provide safe, effective, and patient-centered care. This is an expected ability of all nurses and requires practice. This book offers exercises, titled *Clinical Reasoning Care Maps*, to provide that practice as you study nursing care of adult patients

with a variety of disorders (Figure 1-4■). Care map answers on the companion website will allow you to check the progress of your clinical reasoning skills. In addition, each unit of this book concludes with unit wrap-up activities called Thinking Strategically About. . . , which provide additional clinical reasoning opportunities.

| BOX 1-3 | ATTITUDES AND HABITS FOR CRITICAL THINKING AND CLINICAL REASONING |

Critical thinking and clinical reasoning or judgment are strongly influenced by personal attitudes and mental habits. Effective critical thinking and clinical judgment can occur when the nurse has the following attitudes and mental habits:

- *Thinking independently* so that you make decisions based on sound thinking and reasoning. This means, for example, you are not influenced by negative comments from other health care providers about a patient.
- Using *analytic processes* to sort out the relevant data from data that are not relevant to reach a conclusion. Abnormal data (e.g., a fever or a rapid pulse) are usually considered relevant, and normal data are helpful but may not change the care you provide.
- Using *intuition*—recognizing a pattern or clinical situation and connecting it with knowledge and previous experiences. For example, when you take a pulse you know the normal pulse rate and pattern for a person of this age, medications the patient is taking that may alter the pulse, and the patient's emotional and physical state. On the basis of this knowledge, you recognize whether the pulse rate is as expected or varies from the expected rate and pattern.
- Having *intellectual courage* to listen to and be fair in your evaluation of others' ideas and beliefs. This involves listening carefully to others' ideas and thoughts, making a decision based on what you learn instead of how you feel, and being ready to stand up for what you think.
- Having *empathy* by being able to put yourself in the place of another and taking time to think about the illness experience from the patient's perspective. For example, you consider the meaning of the illness to the patient, the patient's experience and ways of coping, and possible effects of the illness and its treatment on the future of the patient and family (Tanner, 2006).
- *Being fair-minded and considering all viewpoints* before making a decision. This means you consider viewpoints that may be different from yours before reaching a conclusion. You also realize that you are constantly learning and are not afraid to say, "I don't know the answer to that question, but I will find out and let you know."
- Being *disciplined* so that you do not stop at easy answers but continue to consider alternatives.
- Being *creative* and *confident in self*. Nurses often need to consider different ways of providing care and constantly look for better, more cost-effective methods. Confidence in one's decisions is gained through critical thinking.

This line provides an appropriate nursing diagnosis.

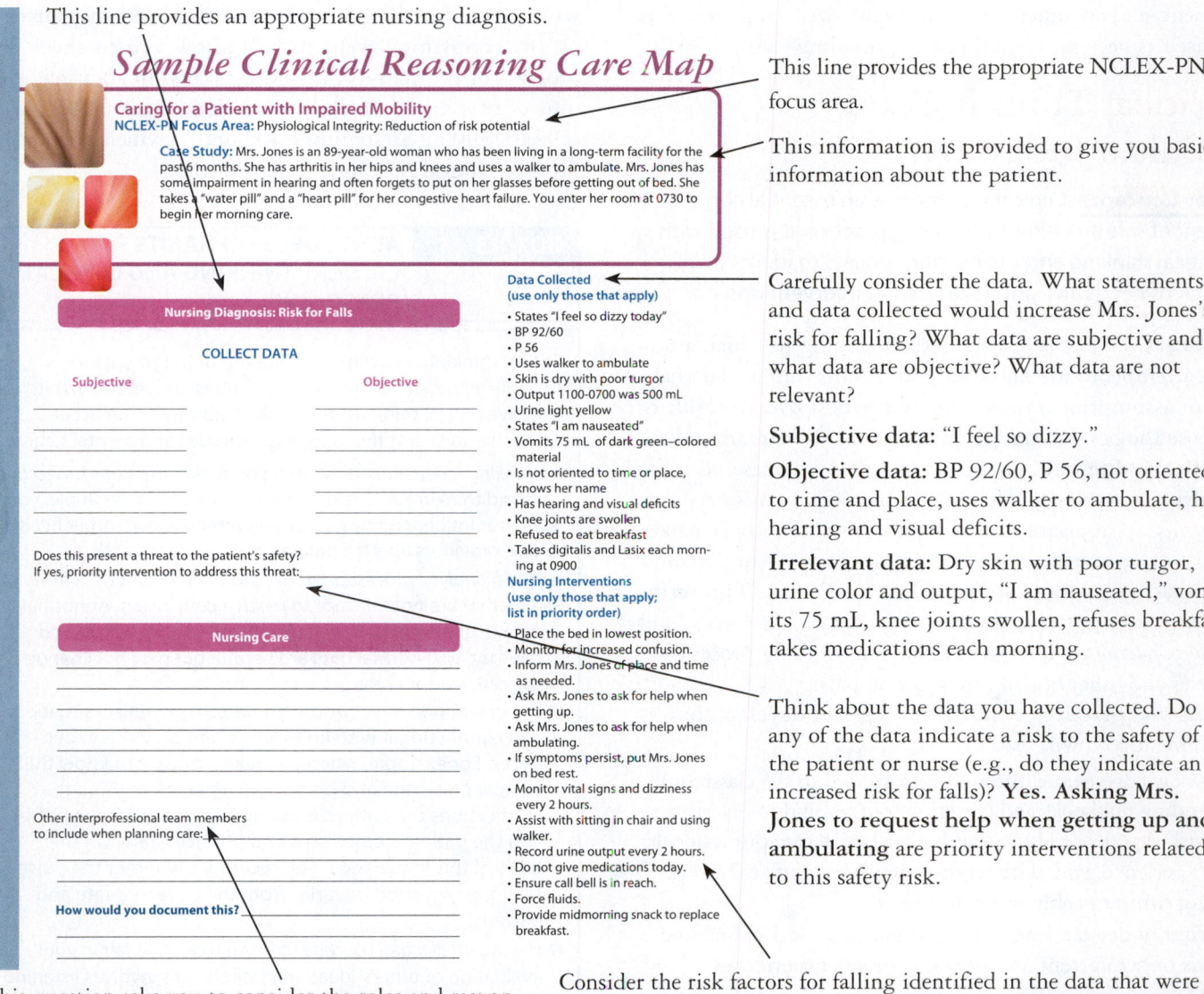

Sample Clinical Reasoning Care Map

Caring for a Patient with Impaired Mobility
NCLEX-PN Focus Area: Physiological Integrity: Reduction of risk potential

Case Study: Mrs. Jones is an 89-year-old woman who has been living in a long-term facility for the past 6 months. She has arthritis in her hips and knees and uses a walker to ambulate. Mrs. Jones has some impairment in hearing and often forgets to put on her glasses before getting out of bed. She takes a "water pill" and a "heart pill" for her congestive heart failure. You enter her room at 0730 to begin her morning care.

Nursing Diagnosis: Risk for Falls

COLLECT DATA

Subjective | Objective
_____ | _____
_____ | _____
_____ | _____
_____ | _____

Does this present a threat to the patient's safety? If yes, priority intervention to address this threat:
_____

Nursing Care
_____
_____
_____
_____
_____
_____
_____

Other interprofessional team members to include when planning care:
_____
_____

How would you document this?
_____
_____
_____

Data Collected
(use only those that apply)
- States "I feel so dizzy today"
- BP 92/60
- P 56
- Uses walker to ambulate
- Skin is dry with poor turgor
- Output 1100–0700 was 500 mL
- Urine light yellow
- States "I am nauseated"
- Vomits 75 mL of dark green–colored material
- Is not oriented to time or place, knows her name
- Has hearing and visual deficits
- Knee joints are swollen
- Refused to eat breakfast
- Takes digitalis and Lasix each morning at 0900

Nursing Interventions
(use only those that apply; list in priority order)
- Place the bed in lowest position.
- Monitor for increased confusion.
- Inform Mrs. Jones of place and time as needed.
- Ask Mrs. Jones to ask for help when getting up.
- Ask Mrs. Jones to ask for help when ambulating.
- If symptoms persist, put Mrs. Jones on bed rest.
- Monitor vital signs and dizziness every 2 hours.
- Assist with sitting in chair and using walker.
- Record urine output every 2 hours.
- Do not give medications today.
- Ensure call bell is in reach.
- Force fluids.
- Provide midmorning snack to replace breakfast.

This line provides the appropriate NCLEX-PN® focus area.

This information is provided to give you basic information about the patient.

Carefully consider the data. What statements and data collected would increase Mrs. Jones's risk for falling? What data are subjective and what data are objective? What data are not relevant?

Subjective data: "I feel so dizzy."

Objective data: BP 92/60, P 56, not oriented to time and place, uses walker to ambulate, has hearing and visual deficits.

Irrelevant data: Dry skin with poor turgor, urine color and output, "I am nauseated," vomits 75 mL, knee joints swollen, refuses breakfast, takes medications each morning.

Think about the data you have collected. Do any of the data indicate a risk to the safety of the patient or nurse (e.g., do they indicate an increased risk for falls)? **Yes. Asking Mrs. Jones to request help when getting up and ambulating** are priority interventions related to this safety risk.

This question asks you to consider the roles and responsibilities of other members of the interprofessional care team, such as the physician (who may re-evaluate Mrs. Jones's medications), physical therapist, and dietitian.

How would you document this? allows you to practice your documentation. It is not necessary to document all the data or interventions for this exercise. For example, the assessment documentation might be:

730 States "I am dizzy" BP 92/60, P 56. Is not oriented to time and place, is oriented to person.

Mr. James, nurse manager notified.

J. Gomez, LVN

Consider the risk factors for falling identified in the data that were collected. Review the effect of dizziness, confusion, and hypotension on the ability to safely get out of bed and ambulate. Review the policy on fall-prevention programs in your health care clinical setting or in a current journal article. Make a decision about which interventions are relevant and which are not relevant.

Relevant interventions: Place bed in lowest position, monitor for increased confusion, inform patient of place and time, ask patient to ask for help when getting up and ambulating, put patient on bed rest if symptoms persist, monitor vital signs and dizziness, assist with sitting in chair and using walker, ensure call bell is within reach.

Irrelevant interventions: Record urine output every 2 hours, do not give medications, provide midmorning snack.

Note:

This sample is provided for the beginning student in medical–surgical nursing. As you learn more about pathophysiology, medications, and nursing care, you will find there are more alternatives for consideration in this sample. For example, the medications Mrs. Jones is taking may cause dehydration and loss of potassium. These conditions may cause nausea, vomiting, and confusion. In turn, there would be an increased risk for falls. These data should be reported to the nurse in charge, who would report the data to the physician. The physician may order the medications to be held. The nurse would not omit the medications without a physician's order.

Figure 1-4. ■ A sample Clinical Reasoning Care Map with guidelines for its use and completion.

Legal and Ethical Aspects of Nursing Practice

Key Concept   Nursing regulations (practice acts) and standards guide nursing practice and protect the public.

Nurses often work with patients who are in vulnerable positions. The nursing profession is highly regulated and has high ethical standards for practice. It is important for every nurse to have a good understanding not only of the laws regulating nursing and the legal system within which nurses practice but also of the ethical principles that guide nursing practice.

NURSING REGULATION

Nursing is governed by nurse practice acts in every state in the United States. Nurse practice acts are made up of both statutory law and administrative law. **Statutory law** is the law created by federal and state legislatures. Statutory law includes regulatory law, civil laws, and criminal laws. *Civil law* protects individual rights (e.g., the right to freedom from harm), whereas *criminal law* protects public welfare.

Nurse practice acts are a type of *regulatory law* enacted by state legislatures. The statutory portion of the nurse practice act empowers a regulatory board (such as the Board of Nursing) to develop and enact *administrative laws* to administer the statute. For example, the statute in a state's nurse practice act may empower the Board of Nursing to regulate nursing education within the state. Then the board determines what to regulate (e.g., who may establish a nursing program, faculty qualifications, and curriculum) and enacts administrative rules or codes to carry out its responsibilities. Although nurse practice acts differ from state to state, all include standards for nursing education, licensure, scope of practice, and disciplinary action.

In general, licensure is required by individual states to practice as an RN or LPN/LVN. Licensing standards specify requirements for preparation for entry into the profession, as well as for maintaining and renewing nursing licenses. Some states have entered into the *Nurse Licensure Compact*, an agreement that allows the nurse to hold a license in his or her state of residency and to practice in other states. In all cases, nurses are subject to the standards and scope of practice where they practice, as well as where they reside.

SCOPE AND STANDARDS OF PRACTICE

Scope of practice laws identify the breadth and limits of nursing practice for those licensed and practicing as nurses within a state. Scope of practice laws often are written in broad, general terms. Although the scopes of practice for RNs and LPNs/LVNs generally are very similar, most practice acts specify that the LPN/LVN must work under the direction or supervision of an RN, physician, or dentist. Other common areas in which RN and LPN/LVN responsibilities differ include patient assessment, delegation of nursing activities, supervision, and clinical decision making (Seago et al., 2004). Institutions may further restrict the scope of practice of LPNs/LVNs they employ, so LPNs/LVNs must know both state regulation and facility policies. The scope and standards for LPN/LVN nursing practice (adapted from the National Council of State Boards of Nursing [NCSBN] model nurse practice act) are outlined in Box 1-4■.

BOX 1-4   LPN/LVN SCOPE OF PRACTICE

The LPN/LVN, practicing under the supervision of an RN, advanced practice registered nurse (APRN), licensed physician, or other authorized licensed health care provider:

A. Participates in nursing care, health maintenance, patient teaching, counseling, collaborative planning and rehabilitation, to the extent of his or her education and experience.
B. Conducts focused nursing assessments.
C. Plans for patient care, including assisting in identification of patient needs and goals, and determining priorities of care.
D. Attends to and monitors patient responses and progress.
E. Contributes to evaluation of the patient-centered health care plan.
F. Implements nursing interventions and prescribed medical regimens in a timely and safe manner.
G. Documents nursing care provided accurately and timely.
H. Collaborates and communicates relevant and timely patient information with patients and other health team members, including status and progress, response (or lack thereof) to therapies, changes in condition, needs, and special requests.
I. Takes measures to promote an environment that is conducive to safety and health.
J. Respects diversity and advocates for the patient's rights, concerns, decisions, and dignity.
K. Maintains appropriate professional boundaries.
L. Participates in performance improvement efforts to improve patient outcomes.
M. Assigns nursing care within the LPN/VN scope of practice to other LPN/VNs; delegates to assistive personnel only those nursing measures for which that person has the necessary skills and competence to accomplish safely, maintaining accountability for the delegation.
N. Functions as a member of the health care team, contributing to implementation of a patient-centered health care plan.
O. Acts as an advocate for the patient.
P. Assumes responsibility for own decisions and actions.
Q. Attends to the patient's concerns or requests.

Source: Adapted from "3.1.2. Standards Related to LPN/VN Scope of Practice" from the NCSBN Model Rules. Copyright © 2012. Used by permission of National Council of State Boards of Nursing (NCSBN).

Scope of practice laws in state nurse practice acts are used together with national, community, and institutional standards to guide nursing practice. A **standard** is a statement or criterion that can be used to measure quality of practice. Professional nursing organizations develop and implement standards of practice to identify clearly the nurse's responsibilities to society. The ANA standards of nursing practice (2010) outline standards for care and professional performance, including ethics, quality of care, education, evidence-based practice, communication, collaboration, leadership, and use of resources. The National Association for Practical Nurse Education and Service (NAPNES) has developed national standards of practice and educational competencies for LPNs/LVNs (Box 1-5■). Scope of practice laws and established standards hold each individual nurse accountable for his or her own practice.

BOX 1-5	STANDARDS OF PRACTICE AND COMPETENCIES OF LPNS/LVNS

Professional Behaviors: Demonstrate professional behaviors of accountability and professionalism according to the legal and ethical standards for a competent LPN/LVN.

1. Comply with the ethical, legal, and regulatory frameworks of nursing and scope of practice as outlined in the LPN/LVN nurse practice act of the specific state in which licensed.
2. Utilize educational opportunities for lifelong learning and maintenance of competence.
3. Identify personal capabilities and consider career mobility options.
4. Identify own LPN/LVN strengths and limitations for the purpose of improving nursing performance.
5. Demonstrate accountability for nursing care provided by self and/or directed to others.
6. Function as an advocate for the health care consumer, maintaining confidentiality as required.
7. Identify the impact of economic, political, social, cultural, spiritual, and demographic forces on the role of the LPN/LVN in the delivery of health care.
8. Serve as a positive role model within health care settings and the community.
9. Participate as a member of an LPN/LVN nursing organization.

Communication: Effectively communicate with patients, significant support person(s), and members of the interdisciplinary health care team, incorporating interpersonal and therapeutic communication skills.

1. Utilize effective communication skills when interacting with patients, significant others, and members of the interdisciplinary health care team.
2. Communicate relevant, accurate, and complete information.
3. Report to appropriate health care personnel and document assessments, interventions, and progress or impediments toward achieving patient outcomes.
4. Maintain organizational and patient confidentiality.
5. Utilize information technology to support and communicate the planning and provision of patient care.
6. Utilize appropriate channels of communication.

Assessment: Collect holistic assessment data from multiple sources, communicate the data to appropriate health care providers, and evaluate patient responses to interventions.

1. Assess data related to basic physical, developmental, spiritual, cultural, functional, and psychosocial needs of the patient.
2. Collect data within established protocols and guidelines from various sources, including patient interviews, observations/measurements, health care team members, family, significant other(s), and review of health records.
3. Assess data related to the patient's health status, identify impediments to patient progress, and evaluate response to interventions.
4. Document collected data and assessment and communicate findings to appropriate member(s) of the health care team.

Planning: Collaborate with the RN or other members of the health care team to organize and incorporate assessment data to plan/revise patient care and actions based on established nursing diagnoses, nursing protocols, and assessment and evaluation data.

1. Utilize knowledge of normal values to identify deviation in health status to plan care.
2. Contribute to formulation of a nursing care plan for patients with noncomplex conditions and in a stable state, in consultation with the RN and as appropriate in collaboration with the patient or support person(s) as well as members of the interdisciplinary health care team using established nursing diagnoses and nursing protocols.
3. Prioritize nursing care needs of patients.
4. Assist in the review and revision of nursing care plans with the RN to meet the changing needs of patients.
5. Modify patient care as indicated by the evaluation of stated outcomes.
6. Provide information to the patient about aspects of the care plan within the LPN/LVN scope of practice.
7. Refer the patient as appropriate to other members of the health care team about care outside the scope of practice of the LPN/LVN.

Caring Interventions: Demonstrate a caring and empathic approach to the safe, therapeutic, and individualized care of each patient.

1. Provide and promote the patient's dignity.
2. Identify and honor the emotional, cultural, religious, and spiritual influences on the patient's health.
3. Demonstrate caring behaviors toward the patient and significant support person(s).
4. Provide competent, safe, therapeutic, and individualized nursing care in a variety of settings.
5. Provide a safe physical and psychosocial environment for the patient and significant other(s).
6. Implement the prescribed care regimen within the legal, ethical, and regulatory framework of LPN/LVN nursing practice.

BOX 1-5   **STANDARDS OF PRACTICE AND COMPETENCIES OF LPNS/LVNS—(continued)**

7. Assist the patient and significant support person(s) to cope with and adapt to stressful events and changes in health status.
8. Assist the patient and significant other(s) to achieve optimum comfort and functioning.
9. Instruct the patient regarding individualized health needs in keeping with the LPN/LVN's knowledge, competence, and scope of practice.
10. Recognize the patient's right to access information and refer requests to appropriate person(s).
11. Act in an advocacy role to protect patients' rights.

Managing: Implement patient care, at the direction of an RN, licensed physician, or dentist, through performance of nursing interventions or directing aspects of care, as appropriate, to UAP.

1. Assist in the coordination and implementation of an individualized plan of care for patients and significant support person(s).
2. Direct aspects of patient care to qualified UAP commensurate with abilities and level of preparation and consistent with the state's level and regulatory framework for the scope of practice for the LPN/LVN.

3. Supervise and evaluate the activities of UAP and other personnel as appropriate within the state's legal and regulatory framework for the scope of practice for the LPN/LVN as well as facility policy.
4. Maintain accountability for outcomes of care directed to qualified UAP.
5. Organize nursing activities in a meaningful and cost-effective manner when providing nursing care for individuals or groups.
6. Assist the patient and significant support person(s) to access available resources and services.
7. Demonstrate competence with current technologies.
8. Function within the defined scope of practice for the LPN/LVN in the health care delivery system at the direction of an RN, licensed physician, or dentist.

Source: "Competencies Which Demonstrate this Outcome has been Attained" from the Standards of Practice and Educational Competencies of Graduates of Practical/Vocational Nursing Programs. Copyright © 2007, used by permission of the National Association for Practical Nurse Education and Service, Inc. (NAPNES). All rights reserved.

Nurses whose behavior or practice presents a risk to the safety of patients (and the public) may be subject to discipline. Complaints of unsafe practice are held as confidential while they are thoroughly investigated. If the nurse's actions are found to be inappropriate or unsafe, the nurse may be subject to a fine or disciplinary action on his or her license. Discipline may range from a reprimand to probation (often with restrictions on the nurse's practice), suspension of the license to practice for a defined period, or even revocation of the license.

NURSING LIABILITY

When a nurse's actions fall outside accepted standards *and* the patient is harmed, a civil action or tort may be filed against the nurse. **Tort law** is the set of laws that deals with injuries that occur to one person through the actions (or failure to take action) of another person.

Torts are classified as intentional or unintentional. An *intentional tort* is a deliberate act that infringes on the rights of another person. Examples of intentional torts follow:

- *Assault* (threat of contact without consent or threat of harm, such as a threatening gesture or remark)
- *Battery* (actual physical contact without consent, such as a nurse administering a medication against the will of a mentally competent patient)
- *Invasion of privacy* (releasing information, taking a patient's picture without consent, or allowing the presence of unauthorized people during a procedure)
- *Defamation* (an act that harms a person's reputation and good name, such as alleging that a certain physician is a "quack")

- *False imprisonment* (restraining a person against his or her wishes, such as preventing a mentally competent adult from leaving a hospital or long-term care facility before discharge).

Negligence and malpractice are *unintentional torts.* Any person whose failure to act in a reasonable manner results in harm to another may be charged with *negligence.* **Malpractice** is harm that results through the actions, or failure to act, of a licensed person. When care by a licensed professional falls below accepted standards, a malpractice claim may be filed. The standard used to establish nursing malpractice is the "reasonable and prudent nurse" standard—that is, the action that would be expected of a nurse with similar education and experience. Four essential elements must be established for malpractice: (1) There was harm, (2) there was an established duty of the professional to the individual harmed, (3) there was failure by the professional to act within accepted standards (breach of duty), and (4) there was causation (e.g., the breach of duty resulted in the harm).

LEGAL PROTECTIONS

All nurses can protect themselves from accusations of improper behavior and malpractice through relatively simple actions.

- Adhere to the scope and standards of care.
- Maintain competence through continuing education and staff development activities.
- Accept only assignments for which you are educationally prepared and have demonstrated clinical competence.
- Obtain instruction and supervision as needed to ensure safe care.

- Communicate with other members of the health care team.
- Document assessments, interventions, and responses to care appropriately.

Malpractice insurance provides money to cover legal fees and damages awarded in malpractice suits. Although all health care institutions and most health care agencies carry liability insurance and many include coverage for their employees, all nurses are encouraged to carry individual insurance. Personal malpractice insurance allows the nurse to engage an attorney to work solely on his or her behalf.

HEALTH INFORMATION PRIVACY RULES

The right to privacy of health and other personal information is an accepted ethical principle of nurses and other health care providers. It is also governed by federal rules about what can be shared and with whom. The Health Insurance Portability and Accountability Act and the Standards for Privacy of Individually Identifiable Health Information, commonly referred to together as **HIPAA**, are laws designed to protect individuals' health information while allowing such information to be shared as needed for effective care. The rules apply to those who transmit health information electronically—including nurses and others employed in hospitals, clinics, and other settings.

It is important to stress that HIPAA rules allow disclosure of health information for treatment purposes, even without the patient's explicit consent. Although the patient's privacy is to be protected, safety protections such as posting the patient's name outside his or her room are allowed to help ensure that care is provided to the correct patient (Anderson, 2007). Unless the patient specifically objects, health information also can be shared with family members who are involved in the patient's care. Other state or federal laws may override the patient's right to privacy of health information, for example, laws that require nurses and other health care providers to report evidence of child, elder, or spousal abuse.

Each health care facility or agency has specific guidelines to assist personnel in determining what is and is not allowed under HIPAA rules. It is the nurse's responsibility to understand and follow these guidelines.

NURSING ETHICS

Ethics is a set of principles of conduct that are concerned with moral duty, values, obligations, and the distinction between right and wrong. Having an established code of ethics is one means of defining a profession. Nursing codes of ethics, such as the ANA Code for Nurses and the NAPNES code of ethics for LPN/LVNs (Box 1-6■), provide a framework for nurses to use when making moral and ethical decisions. They help define the roles of nurses.

BOX 1-6	CODE OF ETHICS FOR THE LPN/LVN

The LPN/LVN shall:

1. Consider as a basic obligation the conservation of life and the prevention of disease.
2. Promote and protect the physical, mental, emotional, and spiritual health of the patient and his or her family.
3. Fulfill all duties faithfully and efficiently.
4. Function within established legal guidelines.
5. Accept personal responsibility (for his or her acts) and seek to merit the respect and confidence of all members of the health team.
6. Hold in confidence all matters coming to his or her knowledge, in the practice of his or her profession, and in no way and at no time violate this confidence.
7. Give conscientious service and charge just remuneration.
8. Learn and respect the religious and cultural beliefs of his or her patient and of all people.
9. Meet his or her obligation to the patient by keeping abreast of current trends in health care through reading and continuing education.
10. As a citizen of the United States, uphold the laws of the land and seek to promote legislation that will meet the health needs of its people.

Source: Adapted from the Code of Ethics for the Licensed Practical/Vocational Nurse by the National Association for Practical Nurse Education and Service, Inc. Used by permission of the National Association for Practical Nurse Education and Service, Inc.

Ethical principles that guide nursing practice include the responsibility to treat others with consideration and fairness (*respect for person* and *justice*), to act for the benefit of the patient (*beneficence*), to avoid doing harm (*nonmaleficence*), to be faithful to one's responsibilities (*fidelity*) and accept responsibility for one's actions (*accountability*), to tell the truth (*veracity*), and to preserve the patient's right to make decisions regarding treatment (*autonomy*).

Examples of the ANA code for nurses include the following:

- The nurse's primary commitment is to the patient, whether an individual, family, group, or community.
- The nurse promotes, advocates for, and strives to protect the health, safety, and rights of the patient.
- The nurse is responsible and accountable for his or her nursing practice.
- The nurse owes the same duties to self as to others, including the responsibility to preserve integrity and safety, to maintain competence, and to continue personal and professional growth.

Professional Boundaries

Nurses are expected to act in the best interests of the patient, to avoid use of their position for personal gain, and not to become involved in the patient's personal relationships.

Professional boundaries are the limits maintained between a person who is vulnerable (the patient) and the person with power (the nurse). The nurse's role as care provider and knowledge of private information about the patient create a position of power. It is vital that the nurse recognize this relationship and establish boundaries to meet the patient's needs safely and effectively. Confusion between the needs of the nurse and those of the patient can result in boundary violations (NCSBN, 1996). It is the nurse's responsibility to establish and maintain professional boundaries while retaining an appropriate level of involvement for effective care.

Ethical Issues in Nursing

Although ethical principles appear to be straightforward, applying them in real situations can be difficult. For example:

- When a patient refuses a medication needed to treat a disorder, the nurse is faced with a conflict between the responsibility to "do good" and the need to honor the patient's autonomy and right to refuse treatment.
- When a patient shares information "in confidence" and the nurse knows the information may affect treatment, the nurse may feel a conflict between honoring the patient's privacy and the responsibility to "do good."

A **dilemma** is a choice between two unpleasant alternatives. Nurses providing medical–surgical nursing care face dilemmas almost daily. Although it is not the nurse's responsibility to "solve" the ethical dilemma, each nurse needs an understanding of guiding principles, legal responsibilities, and available resources (such as ethics committees and social or pastoral services).

Note: The references and resources for all chapters have been compiled at the back of the book.

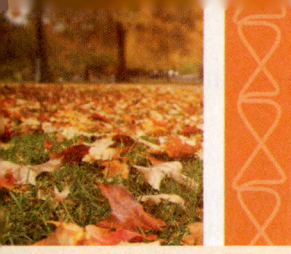

Chapter Review

KEY POINTS

- **Concept:** Medical–surgical nurses promote health and provide care during illness or injury to adult patients. The roles of the medical–surgical nurse include caregiver, manager of care, collaborator, patient advocate, and teacher.
- **Concept:** Nurses, along with other health care providers, are responsible for ensuring the safety of patients and quality of the health care they receive.
- **Concept:** The nursing process is a model of care that differentiates nursing from other health care providers. The five interdependent phases of the nursing process are assessment, diagnosis, planning, implementation, and evaluation.
- **Concept:** Clinical judgment is an essential component of safe and effective nursing practice. It is used with critical thinking and the nursing process to identify patient needs and prioritize nursing interventions.
- Clinical reasoning is the process used to identify a patient's needs and appropriate nursing interventions.

- Critical thinking, necessary for effective clinical reasoning, is goal-directed thinking that applies knowledge and thinking skills to a specific situation. Critical thinking, clinical reasoning, and the nursing process are essential components of nursing practice.
- **Concept:** Nursing regulations (practice acts) and standards guide nursing practice and protect the public.
- Professional boundaries are the borders between the patient's vulnerability and the nurse's power. Nurses must establish boundaries to meet the patient's needs safely and effectively.
- An ethical dilemma is a choice between two unpleasant alternatives. The nurse uses ethical principles and standards (codes of ethics) to guide his or her practice when faced with an ethical dilemma.

PEARSON NURSING STUDENT RESOURCES

Find additional materials at **nursing.pearsonhighered.com**.

NCLEX-PN® Exam Preparation

> **TEST-TAKING TIP**   Data collection is the first step in the nursing process. Select answers that address this step when answering a question about your *initial* nursing action.

1 The nurse who uses the Internet to find national care guidelines for a patient with urinary incontinence is using which of the core competencies identified by the Quality and Safety Education for Nurses project? **Select all that apply.**

1. Providing patient-centered care
2. Using health information technology
3. Practicing evidence-based care
4. Participating in quality improvement
5. Working in an interdisciplinary team

2 The role of the nurse that is most evident when the nurse is protecting the patient's rights is:

1. caregiver.
2. advocate.
3. educator.
4. manager.

3 The nurse is responsible for the *quality* of patient care through a process called:

1. quality improvement.
2. delegation.
3. nursing diagnosis.
4. implementation.

4 During the assessment phase of the nursing process, the LPN/LVN is responsible for obtaining:

1. a complete health history.
2. head-to-toe assessment data.
3. information from the patient's family.
4. a focused assessment.

5 The phase of the nursing process that is complex, involves uncertainty, and requires the nurse to use clinical reasoning and critical thinking is:

1. diagnosis.
2. evaluation.
3. assessment.
4. planning.

6 Planned nursing interventions must be:

1. determined by the nurse alone.
2. specific and individualized.
3. initiated by the physician.
4. based on medical problems.

7 The nurse's role during the implementation phase of the nursing process is to:

1. carry out planned activities.
2. establish outcome criteria.
3. identify patient problems.
4. evaluate the care given.

8 The final component of implementation that the nurse is legally required to complete is:

1. setting priorities.
2. assessing the patient's condition.
3. documenting interventions.
4. teaching the patient.

9 The public is protected and nursing practice is guided by:

1. the nursing process.
2. physicians' oversight.
3. standardized procedures.
4. standards and codes of ethics.

10 The LPN/LVN assigned ADL care for a group of patients to an experienced NA. One of the patients fell while ambulating with the NA. Who is accountable for the care?

1. The unit charge nurse
2. The RN team leader and the LPN/LVN
3. The NA helping the patient ambulate
4. The LPN/LVN and the NA

Answers and rationales for Review Questions appear in Appendix I.

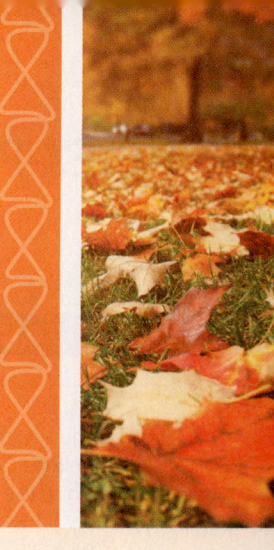

CHAPTER 2
Health, Illness, and Settings of Care

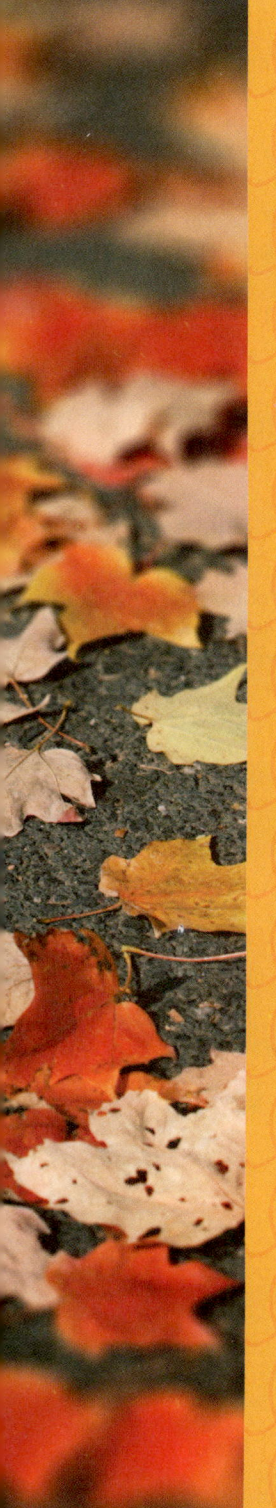

BRIEF OUTLINE

APPLIED LEARNING OUTCOMES

After completing this chapter, you will be able to:

1. Define *health*, the *health–illness continuum*, and *high-level wellness*.
2. Use knowledge of variables affecting health status to promote, maintain, and restore health when providing patient-centered care for adults across the life span.
3. Discuss the purpose and uses of *Healthy People 2020*.
4. Compare and contrast disease and illness and acute illness and chronic illness.
5. Provide safe and effective nursing care and teaching for patients experiencing acute or chronic illness and their families.
6. Describe the focus of various settings of care, including acute, long-term and residential care, and community-based and home care.
7. Discuss the role and responsibilities of the LPN/LVN as a member of the health care team across different settings of care.

KEY TERMS

The key terms are defined on the pages listed below.

Nurses interact with a wide variety of patients who have different health care needs. In primary care settings such as clinics and physicians' offices, the nurse may work with individuals whose goals are to maintain health and wellness. In acute care settings (e.g., hospitals and urgent care), patients may be acutely ill, with critical needs to preserve life and prevent disability. Nurses working in extended care and rehabilitation settings often work with people with multiple chronic conditions, many of whom have little hope of returning home. In community-based care settings and the patient's home, the nurse is meeting the patient in his or her workplace, school, or home.

In this chapter, you will learn about caring for patients in health and illness, as well as providing care across a variety of settings in which LPNs/LVNs work.

Health and Illness in the Adult

> **Key Concept**   Health is a dynamic state influenced by multiple factors, including physical and psychologic characteristics of the individual, as well as social, cultural, and environmental factors.

The World Health Organization (WHO) defines **health** as "a state of complete physical, mental, and social well-being, and not merely the absence of disease or infirmity" (WHO, 1974, p. 1). This is the classic definition of *health*. Even so, it does not take into account the many different levels of health a person may experience or the individual's values and perceptions of health and wellness. These additional factors, which greatly influence nursing care, include the health–illness continuum and high-level wellness.

THE HEALTH–ILLNESS CONTINUUM

The **health–illness continuum** illustrates health as a dynamic process, with high-level wellness at one extreme of the continuum and death at the opposite extreme (Figure 2-1■). Individuals place themselves at different locations on the continuum at specific points in time.

Good health does not necessarily indicate wellness. Good health can be passive, a state of freedom from illness, whereas **high-level wellness** is a way of functioning

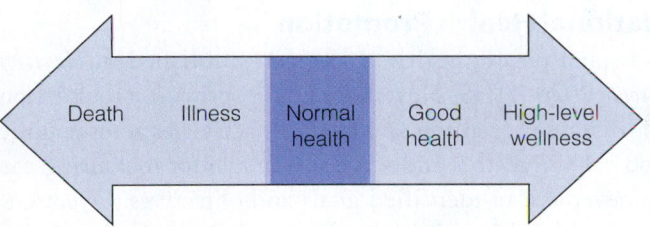

Figure 2-1. ■ The health–illness continuum.

to reach one's maximum potential at a particular point in time (Dunn, 1959).

As commonly illustrated, the health–illness continuum fails to show the complexity and interaction of health and illness. People affected by disease can and do achieve high-level wellness, and people with no evidence of disease can have poor health. It may be more appropriate to consider acute or chronic illnesses as events occurring on a baseline of health status—optimal health, stable health, or poor health. A person who has achieved optimal health can develop an acute or chronic illness. Illness, in turn, can affect the individual's desire and actions to achieve high-level wellness.

A person's self-concept, environment, culture, and spiritual values all influence wellness. Care based on a framework of wellness encourages active involvement by both the nurse and the patient to promote, maintain, or restore health. It also supports the philosophy of *holistic health care*, in which all aspects of a person (physical, psychosocial, cultural, spiritual, and intellectual) are considered as essential components of individualized care.

FACTORS AFFECTING HEALTH

Many different factors affect a person's health or level of wellness. The following factors often interact to promote health or to become risk factors for alterations in health and must be considered when providing patient-centered nursing care.

Genetic Makeup

Each person's genetic makeup influences health status throughout life. Genetic makeup affects personality, temperament, body structure, intellectual potential, and susceptibility to disruptions in health. Heart attack and stroke are examples of acute conditions influenced by genetic makeup. Chronic illnesses that are influenced by genetic makeup include sickle cell disease, hemophilia, diabetes mellitus, and cancer.

Cognitive Abilities and Education

Both cognitive abilities, which are determined before adulthood, and cognitive development (education) affect whether people view themselves as healthy or ill and may affect health practices. Cognitive abilities are influenced by prenatal and developmental factors and may be affected by brain injuries and illnesses. Educational level affects the ability to understand and follow health guidelines. For example, people with some college education are more likely to have regular cancer screening exams.

Ethnicity and Culture

Certain diseases occur at a higher rate in some cultural and ethnic groups than in others. For example, in the United

States, hypertension is more common in African Americans, liver disease and diabetes are among the leading causes of illness in Native Americans, and eye disorders are more prevalent in Chinese Americans. A person's ethnic and cultural background also influences health values and behaviors, lifestyle, and illness behaviors. Every culture defines health and illness in a unique way. In addition, each culture has its own health beliefs and illness treatment practices. (See Chapter 3 for more information about the influence of culture on health and illness behaviors.)

Age and Gender

Age and gender are factors that affect health and the risk for illness. Cardiovascular disorders are uncommon in young adults, but their incidence increases after the age of 40. Heart attacks are more common in men than women until women are past menopause, when their incidence becomes close to equal. Some diseases occur only in one gender or the other, for example, prostate cancer in men and cervical cancer in women. Older adults have an increased incidence of chronic illness and are at greater risk for serious complications of common illnesses such as influenza. The risk for suicide peaks during early adulthood and among older adults.

Lifestyle and Environment

Lifestyle factors that affect health status include diet, use of chemical substances (alcohol, nicotine, caffeine, legal and illegal drugs), exercise and rest habits, and coping methods. The relationship of obesity to hypertension, cigarette smoking to chronic obstructive pulmonary disease, and a sedentary lifestyle to heart disease and certain cancers illustrates lifestyle effects on health.

The environment has a major influence on health. Occupational exposure to toxic substances (e.g., asbestos and coal dust) increases the risk for chronic lung disease. Air, water, and food pollution increases the risk of respiratory disorders, infectious diseases, and cancer. Seasonal temperature variations can result in hypothermia or hyperthermia, especially in the older adult.

Socioeconomic Status

Both lifestyle and environment are affected by one's income level. The culture of poverty, which crosses all racial and ethnic boundaries, negatively influences health status. Living at or below the poverty level may result in crowded, unsanitary living conditions or homelessness. Crowded living conditions increase the risk of transferring communicable diseases. Needed medical care often is omitted or delayed, increasing the risk for more severe illness and complications. Other problems include lack of infant and child care, lack of medical care for injuries or illness, inadequate nutrition, use of addictive substances, and violence.

Geographic Area

The geographic area where one lives influences health status and access to health care. Multiple sclerosis occurs most frequently in the northern United States and Canada. There are more cases of skin cancers in people living in sunny, hot areas and more sinus infections among people living in areas with high humidity.

Where one lives also influences exercise patterns and access to health care. People living in mild climates spend more time outdoors than those who live where the weather is inclement or excessively hot. Clinics and other health care settings not only are more numerous in urban areas than in rural communities, but can also be reached using mass transportation.

HEALTH PROMOTION AND MAINTENANCE

For many years, nursing care focused on the acutely ill patient in the hospital setting. With changes in society and health care, this emphasis has shifted toward preventive community-based care and chronic disease management. Two essential aspects of medical–surgical nursing today are teaching healthy behaviors and health maintenance and providing continuity of care as a patient moves among health care settings.

Certain practices are known to promote health and wellness:

- Eating a balanced diet rich in fruits, vegetables, and whole grains; reducing intake of added sugars, solid and saturated fats, and sodium; and balancing calorie intake to achieve and maintain a healthy weight
- Exercising 30 to 60 minutes a day
- Sleeping 7 to 8 hours each day
- Limiting alcohol consumption, if any, to a moderate amount
- Eliminating smoking and use of other tobacco products
- Keeping sun exposure to a minimum
- Maintaining recommended immunizations (see the Centers for Disease Control [CDC] website for recommended immunizations for adults)

The nurse promotes health by teaching activities to maintain wellness and by providing information about diseases and decreasing identified risk factors for disease. The nurse also promotes health by following healthy practices and serving as a role model.

National Health Promotion

National public health objectives, published in *Healthy People 2020* (HHS, November 2010), provide a foundation for disease prevention and wellness activities across public and private sectors and serve as a model for measuring the achievement of identified goals and objectives. Overarching goals and health indicators for the current decade are described in Box 2-1■.

BOX 2-1	*HEALTHY PEOPLE 2020:* *OVERARCHING GOALS*

Vision

- A society in which all people live long, healthy lives

Overarching Goals

- Attain high-quality, longer lives free of preventable disease, disability, injury, and premature death.
- Achieve health equity, eliminate disparities, and improve the health of all groups.
- Create social and physical environments that promote good health for all.
- Promote quality of life, healthy development, and healthy behaviors across all life stages.

Leading Health Indicators

- Access to health services (including health insurance and primary care provider)
- Clinical preventive services (e.g., cancer screening, hypertension management)
- Environmental quality (e.g., air quality, exposure to second-hand smoke)
- Injury and violence
- Maternal, infant, and child health (e.g., infant deaths, preterm deaths)
- Mental health (e.g., suicides, major depressive episodes in adolescents)
- Nutrition, physical activity, and obesity (e.g., obesity in adults and children, vegetable intake)
- Oral health
- Reproductive and sexual health
- Social determinants (e.g., high school graduation rates)
- Substance abuse (e.g., binge drinking, alcohol or illicit drug use in adolescents)
- Tobacco

Source: U.S. Department of Health and Human Services. (2010, November). *Healthy People 2020.* Washington, DC: Author.

Illness and Disease

Key Concept Medical–surgical nursing focuses on caring for adult patients experiencing acute or chronic illnesses and/or diseases. While physicians focus on treating disease, a disruption of body structure or function, nurses focus on illness, the individual's response to disease.

For optimal health, the body must maintain its internal environment despite constant changes in the external environment. **Homeostasis** is the body's tendency to maintain a dynamic steady state or balance under constantly changing conditions. When this balance is disrupted, the patient may develop a disease or present with symptoms of an illness. The terms *disease* and *illness* are often used with the same meaning, but in fact they are different. In general, nursing is concerned with illness and medicine is concerned with disease.

DISEASE

Disease (literal meaning, "without ease") is defined as any disruption in the structure or function of the body or mind. The cause of many diseases is unknown. The following are known causes of disease:

- Genetic alterations and variations
- Prenatal factors such as exposure to viruses, chemicals, or drugs
- Infectious agents
- Tissue injury due to lack of oxygen, temperature extremes, radiation, or toxins (e.g., alcohol, drugs, cigarette smoke)
- Poor nutrition (obesity, malnutrition)
- Inadequate or disordered immune responses (e.g., allergies, autoimmune disorders), generalized inflammatory or stress responses
- Tumors
- Lifestyle factors (e.g., diet and lack of physical activity)

It is important to remember that disease rarely results from just one cause. Even in an infectious disease such as strep throat, it is not only the infectious agent (streptococcal bacteria) that causes the disease of strep throat but also the responses of the infected tissues and the immune system. Diseases may be classified in a number of ways, for example, acute or chronic, congenital, degenerative, or malignant (Table 2-1■).

TABLE 2-1	Disease Classifications and Definitions
CLASSIFICATION	**DEFINITION**
Acute	A disease that has a rapid onset, lasts a relatively short period of time, and is self-limiting
Chronic	A disease that requires continuing management over a long period, years or even decades
Communicable	A disease that can spread from one person to another
Congenital	A disease or disorder that exists at or before birth
Degenerative	A disease that results from deterioration or impairment of organs or tissues
Functional	A disease that affects function or performance without evidence of organic changes
Malignant	A disease that tends to become worse and cause death
Idiopathic	A disease that has an unknown cause
Iatrogenic	A disease that is caused by medical therapy

In all types of disease, disruptions in structure or function cause **manifestations** (signs and symptoms) that often prompt a person to seek treatment. Both subjective symptoms (e.g., pain, nausea, and anxiety) and objective signs (e.g., bleeding, vomiting, diarrhea, or swelling) commonly appear with disease, although one or the other may predominate. Pain (a subjective symptom) is often the main reason a person seeks health care.

ILLNESS

Illness is the response a person has to a disease. This response is highly individualized, because the person responds not only to his or her own perceptions of the disease but also to the perceptions of others. Illness integrates the structural and biochemical changes associated with the disease; the functional effects of these changes (manifestations); psychologic effects of those alterations; effects on roles, relationships, and values; and cultural and spiritual beliefs. A person may have a disease and not categorize himself or herself as ill or may validate feelings of illness through the comments of others ("You don't look as though you feel well today").

Acute Illness

An **acute illness** is one that occurs rapidly, lasts for a relatively short period of time, and is self-limiting. The condition generally responds to self-treatment or to medical or surgical intervention. Patients with uncomplicated acute illnesses usually have full recovery and return to normal pre-illness functioning.

Illness behaviors are highly individualized and influenced by age, gender, values, culture, socioeconomic status, education, and mental status. Responses to acute illness, however, often follow a predictable sequence:

1. In the first stage of an acute illness, a person *experiences symptoms* or manifestations (e.g., pain, fever, difficulty breathing, or bleeding) that signal a change in normal health. When manifestations are mild or are familiar (e.g., symptoms of the common cold or influenza), the person often uses a traditional remedy or over-the-counter medications for self-treatment. If the symptoms are relieved, no further action is taken. However, if the symptoms are severe or become worse, the person moves to the next stage.
2. In the second stage, the person *assumes the sick role*, accepting the symptoms as evidence of an illness. People at this stage focus on alterations in function resulting from the illness. If the illness is resolved, the person resumes normal activities. If manifestations remain or increase, the person moves to the next stage by seeking care.

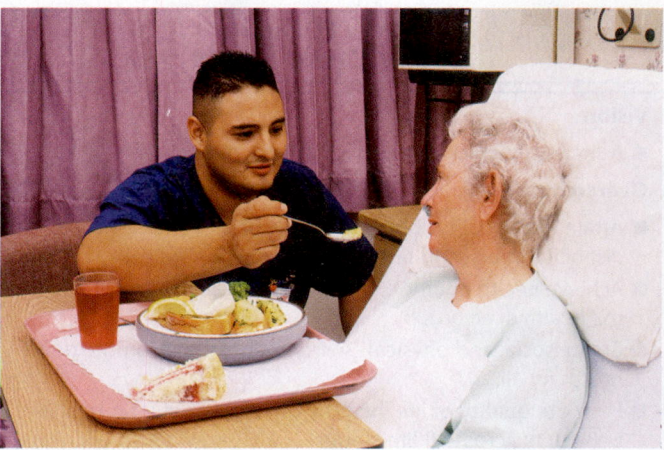

Figure 2-2. ■ A patient with an acute illness assumes the dependent role. (Source: Pearson Education.)

3. The third stage is *seeking medical care*. In our society, a physician or another recognized health care provider usually provides validation of illness. People who believe themselves to be ill (or who are encouraged by others to contact a health care provider) make the medical contact for diagnosis and treatment of the illness. If the medical diagnosis is an illness, the person moves to the next stage.
4. The stage of *assuming a dependent role* begins when a person accepts the diagnosis and planned treatment for the illness (Figure 2-2■). The person's responses to care during this stage depend on many different variables: the severity of the illness, the degree of anxiety or fear about the outcome, the impact on roles, the support systems available, individualized reactions to stress, and previous experiences with illness care. The cause and severity of illness and individual resources affect whether the person moves to the next stage, recovery and rehabilitation, or to chronic illness or even death.
5. The final stage of an acute illness is *recovery and rehabilitation*. The person now gives up the dependent role and resumes normal roles and responsibilities.

Chronic Illness

The term *chronic illness* describes many different long-term pathologic and psychologic alterations in health. A **chronic illness** is a condition that requires continuing management over a long period—years or even decades. Chronic illness is the leading health problem in the world today, accounting for 70% of all deaths in the United States (CDC, 2012a). Current trends affecting an increased incidence of chronic illnesses include an aging population, diseases of lifestyle and behavior (e.g., smoking and obesity), and environmental factors.

Chronic illnesses may be caused by communicable diseases such as tuberculosis or HIV infection and noncommunicable diseases such as heart disease, cancer, asthma, or diabetes mellitus. Long-term mental health disorders such as schizophrenia are chronic as are physical, sensory, or structural conditions such as arthritis or cataracts.

More than one body system often is affected in chronic illness. Sensory perception, self-care abilities, mobility, cognition, and social skills may be affected by chronic illness. The demands on the individual and family as a result of these responses often last across the life span.

The intensity of a chronic illness and its related symptoms ranges from mild to severe. Some chronic illnesses are characterized by periods of remission and exacerbation. During periods of **remission**, the person does not experience symptoms, even though the disease is still clinically present. During periods of **exacerbation**, the symptoms reappear.

Each person with a chronic illness has a unique set of responses and needs. The response of the person to the illness is influenced by many different factors, including the following:

- The point in the life cycle at which the onset of the illness occurs
- The type and degree of limitations caused by the illness
- The effect of the illness on lifestyle
- The pathophysiology causing the illness
- The effect of the illness on functioning in family, occupational, and social roles
- Pain and fear

These factors are complex and interrelated within each person, resulting in individualized illness behaviors and needs. Although the experience of each person with a chronic illness is unique, people with chronic illness face challenges such as the following:

- Recognizing and appropriately responding to symptoms
- Using medications safely and effectively (Figure 2-3■)
- Modifying lifestyle to adapt to and minimize the impact of the illness
- Developing strategies for coping with the psychosocial impact of chronic illness
- Managing an ongoing treatment plan
- Maintaining a feeling of being in control
- Interacting effectively with the health care system on an ongoing basis

Many people with chronic illness successfully manage health-related needs; others do not. Adaptation is influenced by variables such as anger, depression, denial, self-concept, locus of control, hardiness, and disability.

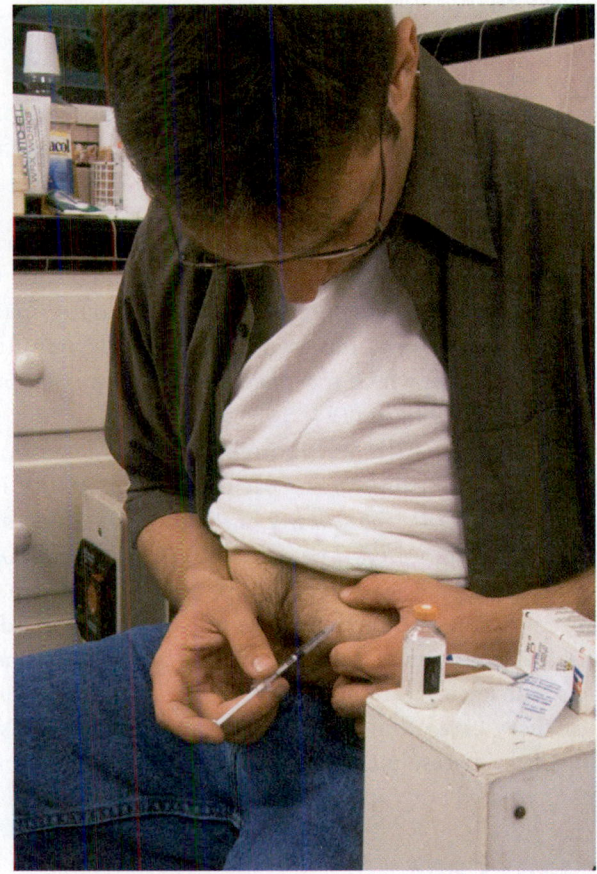

Figure 2-3. ■ In chronic illness, the patient learns how to adapt to and manage the disorder. (Source: Bill Aron / PhotoEdit, Inc.)

Nurses play an important role in promoting independent functioning, reducing health care costs, and improving well-being and quality of life for patients with chronic illness.

Although the patient with a chronic illness may be hospitalized during acute exacerbations, care is primarily managed at home by the patient or family members (such as a spouse). Chronic illness is a major stressor that may cause changes in family structure and function as well as changes in the performance of family roles and tasks.

Family responses to chronic illness are influenced by such factors as personal, social, and economic resources; the nature and course of the disease; and demands of the illness as perceived by family members. Family responses in turn affect the patient's response to, and perception of, the illness.

Patient and family considerations for continuing care are integrated throughout this book. Chronically ill patients and families should be given information about helpful literature, self-help or support groups, and interactions with others with the same illness. Information provided by the nurse must be tailored to specific, current needs.

Health and Illness Care

> **Key Concept**   Most health and illness care occurs outside the acute hospital environment, in primary care and community- based settings such as clinics, residential care, and the patient's home.

In the current health care system, hospitals are primarily acute care providers, focusing on high-technology care for severely ill or injured people or for people having major surgery. Health care is now a managed care, community-based system, in which most health care services are provided outside the hospital.

The setting in which health care is provided depends, in large part, on the acuity of the patient's needs. **Acuity** is a term used to describe the severity of the patient's illness and the level of care required. The Affordable Care Act of 2010 places increasing emphasis on effective patient management to prevent hospital admission or readmission following discharge. Selected models and settings of care follow. These models and settings are not mutually exclusive; for example, primary care often is delivered in community-based settings, and disease management often occurs within programs associated with acute medical centers.

PRIMARY CARE

Primary care is comprehensive first contact health and illness care across the life span. Preventive services as well as care for acute and chronic diseases occur within the primary care model. Primary care occurs in diverse settings such as a doctor's office or clinic, retail walk-in clinics, hospital-affiliated practices, and the workplace. Community centers and clinics under the direction of a physician or nurse practitioner often provide primary care for patients who are unable to get care elsewhere. This group includes the homeless, the poor, those with substance abuse problems, those with sexually transmitted infections, and the victims of violent or abusive behavior. LPN/LVNs are often employed in community centers and clinics to carry out focused assessments (such as current medications, allergies, weights, and vital signs), to assist the physician or advanced practice registered nurse (APRN) with examinations and to teach the patient any needed self-care activities.

The *patient-centered medical home* (*PCMH*, also called a *health care home*) is a primary care model designed to provide accessible, comprehensive, and coordinated patient and family care within the community. For people with chronic illnesses, the goal of the PCMH is to provide comprehensive care with a focus on preventing acute disease crises. In addition to the primary care provider (physician, nurse practitioner, advanced practice nurse), the PCMH team often includes care coordinators or case managers, social workers, and rehabilitation therapists.

Care or disease management models of primary care focus on the needs of patients living with chronic illness. Nurses are an integral part of these models, providing education and instruction about the disease (e.g., heart failure, diabetes mellitus, chronic obstructive pulmonary disease), its management, self-monitoring, and helping the patient and family communicate with providers and navigate the health care system.

TRANSITIONAL CARE

Transitional care focuses on facilitating transitions for chronically ill patients from one health care setting to another or to home. Interventions are typically planned and led by a nurse or advanced practice nurse and include ongoing support for the patient and family. The goal of transitional care is to improve the care and outcomes for chronically ill patients by streamlining plans of care, improving the ability of patients and caregivers to manage care, and interrupting patterns of frequent acute health crises (Naylor et al., 2011).

ACUTE CARE

Patients with highly acute needs often receive care in a hospital as an inpatient. The primary reasons for hospital admission vary by age group: Childbirth and related conditions are the most common reason for hospital admission of young adults (18 to 44 years of age), followed by admission for mood disorders, whereas osteoarthritis and coronary heart disease are the primary diagnoses leading to admission of adults between the ages of 45 and 64 years. Older adults (age 65 years and older) are more likely to be admitted for heart failure (Wier et al., 2011). Table 2-2■ lists the most common diagnoses for adults entering U.S. hospitals in 2009 (excluding those diagnoses associated with childbirth). Commonly performed procedures associated with each diagnosis are listed in the right-hand column.

Patients who are hospitalized often require a high level of professional and technologic care. LPN/LVNs provide care in acute settings under the direction of the registered nurse. Although some hospitals have gone to an all-RN staff, the LPN/LVN is a vital member of the health care team in many others. Hospitals vary in size, the acuity level of patients, and technologic availability, from small, rural hospitals that may have no more than 20 beds and limited technology to large, urban hospitals where the latest technologically advanced care is available.

Acute care nurses must be able to care safely and effectively for patients who are acutely ill and have multiple needs. In addition, the nurse must prioritize the needs of multiple patients, use and manage equipment, communicate effectively with physicians and other members of the health care team, and practice cost-effective care. In this setting, managing and organizing care and patient advocacy

TABLE 2-2	Most Common Diagnoses on Discharge From U.S. Hospitals in 2009*
DIAGNOSIS	**TOP ASSOCIATED PROCEDURES**
Pneumonia	Respiratory intubation and mechanical ventilation
Congestive heart failure	Diagnostic cardiac catheterization, coronary angiography Echocardiogram
Osteoarthritis	Knee arthroplasty
Mood disorders	Psychologic and psychiatric evaluation and therapy
Coronary atherosclerosis	Diagnostic cardiac catheterization, coronary angiography Percutaneous transluminal coronary angioplasty (PTCA)
Septicemia	Enteral and parenteral nutrition
Cardiac dysrhythmias	Insertion of cardiac pacemaker or cardioverter/defibrillator
Chronic obstructive pulmonary disease	Respiratory intubation and mechanical ventilation
Spondylosis; intervertebral disk disorders; other back problems	Laminectomy, excision intervertebral disk

*Excludes diagnoses associated with childbirth.

Source: Data from Wier, L., Pfuntner, A., Maeda, J., Stranges, E., Ryan, K., et al. (2011). *HCUP Facts and Figures: Statistics on Hospital-Based Care in the United States, 2009*. Rockville, MD: Agency for Healthcare Research and Quality.

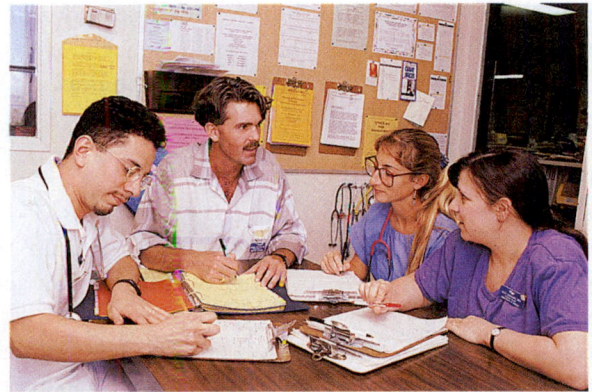

Figure 2-4. ■ The rehabilitation team discusses the patient's plan of care. (Alain McLaughlin, Pearson Education.)

are major nursing roles. The nurse needs to maintain focus on the patient and his or her needs, using technology only as a tool to provide care.

Psychiatric Hospitals

Patients with mental health disorders whose behavior is a risk to themselves or to others may require hospitalization for evaluation and treatment. Acute psychiatric care may be provided in specialized units within a major medical center or may occur in psychiatric hospitals designed and established for that purpose. For safety reasons, acute psychiatric units or hospitals may be locked facilities, although patients may have visitors.

REHABILITATION

Current health care financing has shortened the length of stay in acute care hospitals and increased the needs for rehabilitation care. **Rehabilitation** is the process of achieving one's maximum potential after acute illness (physical or mental), surgery, trauma, or with a chronic impairment

and the resulting functional disability. Rehabilitation nursing is based on a philosophy that each person has a unique set of strengths and abilities that can enable him or her to live with dignity, self-worth, and independence. This philosophy applies to patients with both acute and chronic illnesses. Rehabilitation services are provided in the home, skilled care facilities, and specialty programs (e.g., cardiac rehabilitation programs).

Rehabilitation promotes reintegration into the family and community through a team approach. The plan of care includes many different aspects of the patient's life: physical function, mental health, interpersonal relationships, social interactions, family support, and vocational status. Assessment includes functional status and self-care abilities, educational needs, psychosocial needs, and the home environment. It is critical to determine the priorities of needs from the patient and family perspective before establishing any plan of care. This comprehensive plan requires the expertise of a team of health care providers (Figure 2-4■).

Nursing interventions are revised to meet patient and family needs as the patient progresses. Individualized interventions are planned and implemented to prevent complications, assist in achieving a realistic level of independence, educate the patient and family about home care, and make referrals to community agencies (for nursing care, special equipment or supplies, support groups, counseling, therapy, vocational guidance, and assistance with daily living activities).

LONG-TERM CARE

Extended or long-term care options range from independent senior housing to skilled nursing home care. Increasingly, multiple levels of support and care are available, allowing older adults to remain on the same campus as independence diminishes and increasing levels of care are required (an aging-in-place model). The focus of independent living, residential care, and assisted living facilities is on providing the support necessary to maintain resident function and independence. Residential care and assisted living facilities may or may not provide licensed nursing care. LPN/LVNs working in these settings may provide little direct care to residents; however, their role in planning, directing, and evaluating care is vital.

Skilled Nursing Care Centers

Increasingly, intermediate or skilled care is provided for patients as an alternative to hospitalization (step-up care) or for rehabilitation as the patient transitions from acute care to home (step-down care) (Figure 2-5 ■). Skilled care centers offer care to patients who need short-term nursing or rehabilitation care as well as for patients with long-term disabilities who have significant ongoing care needs (e.g., patients who have had a severe traumatic brain injury or who require a mechanical ventilator to breathe). These patients may remain in skilled care for years or even the remainder of their lives.

Care given to residents in skilled care is performed by or under the direct supervision of a licensed nurse. The LPN/LVN, under the direction of the registered nurse, provides

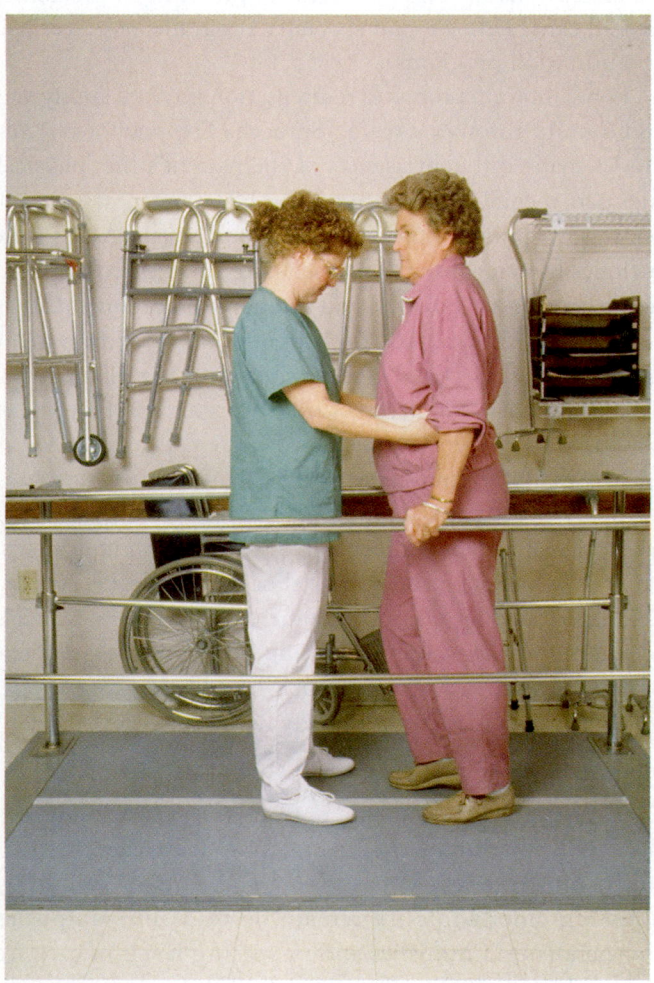

Figure 2-5. ■ A patient receives therapy in a long-term care facility. (Source: Pearson Education.)

direct care, administers medications, and delegates and supervises care administered by nursing assistants. The nurse is responsible for assessing the residents, planning and directing care, and monitoring health care needs.

Assessment of the patient's needs begins with the first contact and continues throughout care. Assessment includes functional and self-care abilities, educational needs, psychosocial needs, and the home environment. It is critical to determine the patient's and family's values, preferences, expressed needs, and priorities before establishing any plan of care. Questions for assessment include the following:

- What is the patient's present level of physical function (mobility, self-care, communication, skin integrity, bowel and bladder function)?
- What are the patient's and family's short-term and long-term goals?
- Are those goals realistic, measurable, and attainable?
- What concerns are verbalized by the patient and family (values, financial, work, housing, school, transportation, sexual activities, social activities, relationships)?
- What stage of grief and loss is present (denial, anger, bargaining, depression, acceptance)?
- To what home environment will the patient be going? Or is discharge from the setting unrealistic?
- What resources are available to assist reintegration (personal, support, community, federal)?

Nursing interventions are revised to meet patient and family needs as the patient progresses, or when recovery is not expected. General areas of intervention and teaching include the following:

- Preventing infection
- Maintaining functional status (mobility, self-care, social interactions)
- Preventing skin breakdown
- Providing adequate nutrition and fluids
- Providing care as necessary and appropriate to achieve a realistic level of independence
- Initiating referrals to community agencies (nursing care, special equipment or supplies, support groups, counseling, physical therapy, occupational therapy, respiratory therapy, vocational guidance, house cleaning, meals) as indicated

Dementia Care

People with progressive dementia (such as Alzheimer disease) often require residential care when families are no longer able to provide home care. In many cases, this occurs when the patient with Alzheimer disease develops wandering behavior (leaving and being unable to find the way home) or becomes unable to assist with activities of daily living such as eating and toileting. Alzheimer care units may exist within a residential treatment facility or community or may be independent. These units, while providing a homelike setting, are secure, with locked doors and fully fenced outdoor areas.

COMMUNITY-BASED NURSING CARE

A community is many things. A community may be a small neighborhood in a major urban city or a large area of rural residents. People who live in a community may share a culture, history, or heritage. Although a community is where people live, have homes, raise families, and carry on daily activities, people often cross community boundaries to work or to seek health care.

In contrast to community health nursing, which focuses on the health of the community as a whole, **community-based nursing** focuses on individual and family health care needs in a community setting. Nurses provide direct services and teaching for individuals to manage acute or chronic health problems and to promote self-care. Nursing care is based on a philosophy that directs culturally competent nursing care for patients wherever they are, including where they live, work, play, worship, and go to school.

Community-based nursing care occurs in many different settings, including community-based health centers and clinics, day care programs, churches, schools, and correctional facilities (Figure 2-6■). Box 2-2■ illustrates the varied settings within the community in which a nurse may provide care.

Parish Nursing

Parish nursing, an example of community-based nursing, is a nontraditional way of promoting health and providing nursing care for a group of people. A parish nurse works with a faith community to promote health and healing through counseling, referrals, teaching, and assessment

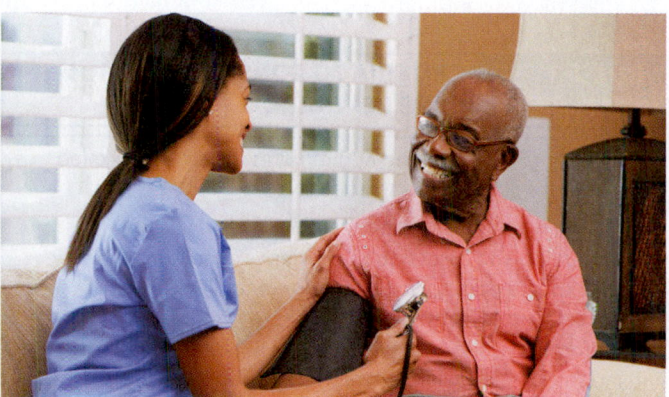

Figure 2-6. ■ Community-based care settings may serve people where they work, worship, or play. (© Monkey Business/Fotolia)

BOX 2-2	COMMUNITY-BASED NURSING CARE SETTINGS

- County health departments
- Senior centers
- Churches
- Adult day care centers
- Homeless shelters
- Mobile vans
- Mental health centers
- Schools
- Crisis intervention centers
- Free clinics
- Urgent care centers
- Rural health centers
- Home care
- Hospice care
- Industry
- Jails and prisons

of health care needs. A parish nurse may be employed by a hospital and contracted by a church, employed directly by a church, or work as a volunteer with the congregation of a church. The parish nurse often helps members of the church or parish navigate the health care system.

HOME HEALTH CARE

Home care is not simply illness care at home, nor is it the act of setting up a hospital room in someone's house. **Home health care** is the delivery of services to restore or maintain the health of individuals and families in the home. Home health care includes a variety of services, including skilled nursing, physical and occupational therapy, pharmacy services, and durable medical equipment such as ventilators and enteral feeding pumps. Home care is also provided as a person nears the end of life, in a program called *hospice* (hospice care is discussed in Chapter 13). Nursing services include acute and chronic illness care and palliative care that reduces hospital admissions or readmissions.

Home health care services must be necessary and medically indicated, and ordered by a physician or primary care provider to qualify for reimbursement by private insurance, Medicare, or Medicaid. Referrals for home care may be made by a physician, nurse, social worker, discharge planner, or family. Among patients who benefit from home health care services are those who:

- Need short-term help at home because of surgery, an injury, or prescribed treatments.
- Have chronic illnesses such as heart failure, heart disease, kidney disease, respiratory diseases, diabetes mellitus, or muscle–nerve disorders.

- Are terminally ill and want to die with comfort and dignity at home.
- Do not need inpatient hospital or nursing home care but require additional assistance.
- Cannot live independently at home because of age, illness, or disability.

Home health agencies are either public or private organizations that provide skilled nursing and other therapeutic services in the patient's home. All home health agencies must meet uniform standards for licensing, certification, and accreditation. Services provided within the home include professional nursing care, home health care assistance, physical therapy, speech therapy, occupational therapy, medical social worker services, and nutritional services.

Patients receiving home health care services are under the care of a physician, with the focus of care being treatment, rehabilitation, or comfort in dying. Nursing care is provided by registered nurses or LPN/LVNs based on a treatment plan developed in conjunction with the physician, other members of the interdisciplinary team, and the patient. These nurses give direct care; supervise other health care providers; coordinate patient care with the physician; advocate for the patient and family; and teach the patient, family members, and friends how to provide care.

Nursing care in the home differs in many ways from nursing care in a hospital setting. Nurses are invited into homes as guests; they cannot assume entry as they do in clinical settings. The environment belongs to the patient, who retains control. Every nursing action must communicate respect for these boundaries. Nurses must establish trust and rapport quickly, because most home health nurses are with each patient for only 1 hour a few times a week.

The patient in home health is both the person receiving care and that person's family. The patient's family is not limited to persons related by birth, adoption, or marriage, but may be significant others, colleagues, other significant people, and even animals. Family dynamics are more visible in the home. As the nurse becomes a familiar presence and the family's behavior relaxes, the nurse can gain a clearer and more complete picture of family issues and relationships, lifestyle choices, and coping patterns.

Caregiver burden is not easily hidden in the home. Millions of Americans are taking care of relatives and friends with disabilities, and many of the caregivers are themselves older adults. When planning for discharge and transition to the home, families may not be asked about their ability to cope with the level of care expected. Caregiving is now recognized as a complex activity that requires adjustment in family living patterns, relationships, and finances. For some families, the crisis of caregiving is short-lived, but for others, it lasts for years. As a result, caregivers are at great risk for both physical and emotional illness. The success of home care heavily depends on the supports in place, so it is crucial to address the needs of the support network.

Referrals for Home Care

The nurse considers making a referral to a home health agency, a hospice, or a community resource if the patient has a need for continuing health care services beyond the present clinical setting. It is vital that nurses talk with patients and their caregivers about their preferences and concerns related to home management. It is quite common for family members to disagree about whether additional help is necessary. In some cases, the family may desire home care assistance, but the patient's needs do not qualify for reimbursement by Medicare or the insurer. Box 2-3 ■ identifies criteria to be considered in referring for home care services. Suggesting services when families have no funds to pay for them only adds to the problem. For patients with limited means, the nurse can identify staff or agencies to provide information about available resources and options. It is always important for the nurse to avoid making assumptions. Intelligent, well-educated, and financially secure patients can be just as overwhelmed by illness as the less educated and the poor. Everyone is a referral candidate. If the patient or family feels that no help is necessary and the nurse believes otherwise, the nurse may suggest an evaluation visit, explaining that the situation may look different once the patient is home.

Once a referral is made and an initial set of physician orders is obtained, a nursing assessment visit is scheduled to identify the patient's needs. If the input of another provider, such as a physical therapist, is necessary to complete the initial assessment, the nurse coordinates this visit.

At the nursing assessment visit, the nurse identifies patient needs, values, and preferences, and begins to formulate the plan of care. Essential components of a home

---

BOX 2-3	CRITERIA TO CONSIDER FOR HOME CARE REFERRAL

The patient is homebound and requires intermittent skilled services of a licensed nurse, such as:

- Managing and evaluating the plan of care.
- Observing and assessing the patient's condition when the skill, knowledge, ability, and judgment of a licensed nurse is necessary to determine status.
- Performing a skilled procedure or a hands-on service requiring the skill, knowledge, ability, and judgment of a licensed nurse.
- Teaching the patient, a family member, or caregiver about a new or acute situation.

care plan include the frequency of visits, types of services needed, functional limitations and permitted activities of the patient, safety measures, and plans for discharge from home care services. The plan of care is reviewed by the physician. The physician's signature on the plan of care authorizes the home health agency's providers to begin with services and also serves as a contract indicating agreement to participate in the care of the patient on an ongoing basis.

Nursing in Community-Based Care

Key Concept Nurses working in community-based settings are important members of the interdisciplinary team, with major responsibility for assessing patient needs, managing and coordinating care, and providing health education and teaching.

In community-based and home care settings, the nursing roles of manager, educator, and advocate are more prominent than the role of provider of care. The licensed nurse often provides only skilled care, delegating direct care activities such as assisting with activities of daily living to assistive personnel or family members. The focus of care may shift from an individual to the family or a group (e.g., the residents of an adult foster home).

CARE PROVIDER

The LPN/LVN working in community-based care settings uses the nursing process to assess, diagnose, plan, and implement care and evaluate patient needs. During the course of this process, nurses frequently perform specific procedures and treatments, such as physical assessments, care of intravenous lines, ostomy care, wound care, and pain assessment and management. The assessments and interventions for each visit are documented.

CARE MANAGER

Care management is a major component of the licensed nurses' role in community-based and home care. Based on the initial and continuing assessment, the nurse formulates a plan of care and communicates this plan with the family and caregivers. In addition, the nurse must ensure that caregivers have the knowledge, skills, and ability to safely perform any required procedures (e.g., dressing changes). The nurse documents his or her instructions and periodically observes the caregiver to ensure that he or she is performing the task appropriately. The nurse also monitors for measures of quality and safety, for example, appropriate wound healing, absence of infection, evidence of nutritional status, and freedom from injury.

As a manager of care, the nurse also identifies when the patient needs or could benefit from services provided by other members of the health care team (e.g., physical or occupational therapists or social services) and recommends or initiates referrals as appropriate.

TEACHER

Teaching patients, families, and caregivers is a major nursing responsibility in home and community-based care. Patients need help understanding their conditions, making health care decisions, and changing health behaviors. It is unrealistic to believe that patients can be taught everything they need to know during a short hospital stay. The nurse should recommend a home health referral for anyone who needs follow-up teaching.

Patients, their families, and their caregivers must have complete information about prescribed medications. They need to know when it is important to contact their doctor. Finally, they must be able to manage any necessary treatments. This means not only performing procedures safely but also knowing how to obtain necessary supplies in the community.

In community settings and the home, most of the nurse's time is spent teaching about illness care and disease prevention. Often, the greatest teaching challenge is to develop a shared understanding of the desired outcomes of care. Patient-centered care and teaching requires the nurse to develop an understanding and acceptance of the patient's culture, values, and preferences. Because the nurse's role as educator is increasingly important, continuing care is included in the discussion of every major disorder in this book.

ADVOCATE

As patient advocate, the nurse explores, informs, supports, and affirms the choices of patients. As a protector of patient rights, the nurse discusses advance medical directives, living wills, durable power of attorney for health care, and patients' rights in that setting or as a patient of the particular agency. Box 2-4■ outlines the rights of long-term care residents as guaranteed by the federal 1987 Nursing Home Reform Law.

During the course of care, patients may need help negotiating the complex medical system (especially in regard to medical insurance), accessing community resources, recognizing and coping with required changes in lifestyle, and making informed decisions. When the family's desires differ from those of the patient, advocacy can be a challenge. If a conflict arises, the nurse must remain the primary patient's advocate, regardless of any negative response from the family.

ETHICAL AND LEGAL GUIDELINES

The legal issues in community-based and home care center on privacy and confidentiality, patient access to health information, freedom from unreasonable restraint, witnessing

---

BOX 2-4   RIGHTS OF LONG-TERM CARE RESIDENTS

The federal Nursing Home Reform Law passed in 1987 requires nursing homes to "promote and protect the rights of each resident." A person residing in long-term care retains the same rights as an individual in the larger community. Care provided should promote and enhance quality of life and ensure dignity, choice, and self-determination. Nursing homes must "provide services and activities to attain or maintain the highest practicable physical, mental, and psychosocial well-being of each resident." The law specifically protects the following residents' rights:

1. Right to Be Fully Informed of
   - Available services and their associated costs
   - Facility rules and regulations
   - Contact information for the State Ombudsman and state regulatory agency
   - Survey reports and plans for corrective actions

2. Right to Complain
   - Present grievances without fear of negative consequences and with actions by the facility to resolve the grievances
   - Complain to the ombudsman and file a complaint with the state regulatory agency

3. Right to Participate in Own Care
   - Receive adequate and appropriate care
   - Be informed about changes in condition and review own medical record
   - Participate in planning care
   - Refuse medication, treatment, and chemical or physical restraints

4. Right to Privacy and Confidentiality
   - Private and unrestricted communication with persons of choice
   - Privacy during treatment and care of personal needs and regarding medical, financial, and personal affairs

5. Rights during Transfers and Discharges
   - Right to remain in facility unless transfer or discharge is necessary for welfare of self or others, resident no longer needs nursing home care, or for failure to meet financial obligations
   - Receive 30-day notice of transfer or discharge with right to appeal

6. Right to Dignity, Respect, and Freedom
   - To self-determination and to be treated with consideration, respect, and dignity
   - To be free from mental or physical abuse, physical or chemical restraints, or involuntary seclusion
   - Security of possessions

7. Right to Visits
   - By relatives, friends, and others of own choosing
   - By personal physician and ombudsman and representatives of regulatory agencies
   - By those providing health, social, legal, or other services
   - To refuse visits

8. Right to Make Independent Choices
   - Personal decisions such as what to wear or how to spend free time
   - Consideration of needs and preferences
   - Participate in activities within and outside of facility
   - Choose a physician and manage own financial affairs

Source: "What are Residents' Rights?" by the The National Long-Term Care Ombudsman Resource Center. Used by permission of The National Long-Term Care Ombudsman Resource Center.

---

of documents, informed consent, and negligence or malpractice. Nurses working in all settings must familiarize themselves with the standards of practice for the setting and patient population being served, providing care that is consistent with standards and with their agency's policies and documenting all care and teaching fully and accurately according to agency guidelines.

HOME AND RESIDENTIAL CARE CONSIDERATIONS

Safety and infection control in the home are priority concerns for the home health nurse. These issues are of equal or greater concern in residential care settings, where the goal is to create a homelike atmosphere for a group or community of residents. Other considerations are outlined in Table 2-3■.

Safety

Safety assessment is a nursing responsibility and a legal requirement. Nurses cannot close their eyes to an unsafe environment. Whenever noted, the nurse must alert the family or caregivers to unsafe and hazardous conditions, suggest remedies, and document measures taken to correct the situation. In particular, nurses must remain alert to the following conditions:

- How patients handle stairs
- How they manage their own care if they are alone
- The presence of a smoke detector in the home
- The presence of bathroom safety equipment (e.g., grab bars, shower chair)
- Electrical, fire, or infection hazards
- Throw rugs, clutter, or furniture arrangements that may cause a fall
- Expired or inappropriately stored medications
- Inappropriate clothing or shoes
- Cooking or smoking habits that may start a fire
- An inadequate food supply
- Poorly functioning utilities
- Signs of abuse or abusive behavior
- Safe handling of medical gases, such as oxygen

TABLE 2-3	Suggestions for Effective Home and Residential Care
WHAT IS IMPORTANT?	**WHAT TO DO**
Making the first contact with the patient	■ Suggest having a family member, friend, or caregiver present during the first visit to help clarify and remember information. ■ Stress important information and repeat it on following visits. ■ Speak clearly and directly to the patient. ■ Allow patient and family time to process the information.
Establishing trust and rapport	■ Find common ground; establish that the nurse is a guest in the patient's home. ■ Offer suggestions that include the patient's right to say "no." ■ Maintain a respectful distance from the patient. ■ Notice and respect family values and customs. ■ Listen carefully to stories.
Assessing the overall environment	■ Note sights, sounds, and smells. ■ Note dress, tone of voice, and body language. ■ Note visiting patterns of family members and significant others. ■ Note the appearance of the living space, yard, sidewalk, and neighborhood.
Promoting the patient's ability to learn	■ Teach and reinforce information needed for safety. ■ Set priorities by a need-to-know, want-to-know, and ought-to-know basis. ■ Teach while providing care whenever possible.
Paying attention to the needs of the patient	■ Limit distractions as much as possible, but ask before turning off music or television. ■ Be honest about allergies to pets or difficulty hearing because of noise.
Being flexible	■ Enter the home with a plan, but be prepared to modify it. ■ Set goals with the patient, not *for* the patient.

Obviously, nurses cannot go into homes or resident apartments and change the living space and lifestyle, but they must register their concern and reactions if the situation could lead to an injury or if they suspect abuse or neglect. Within the home and community setting, ignoring an unsafe environment is considered nursing negligence. Furthermore, in most states, nurses must report signs of abuse of an older adult to an appropriate agency. Documentation should specify nursing actions to address an unsafe situation, what information the nurse has covered in teaching the patient and family or caregivers, the family's or caregiver's response to the teaching, and assessment of their ongoing practice of safety precautions.

Infection Control

Infection control in the home and residential care settings centers on protecting patients, caregivers, and the community from the spread of disease. Within these settings, nurses may encounter patients with infectious or communicable diseases; patients who are immunocompromised; or patients with multiple access devices, drainage tubes, or draining wounds. The home and residential care settings present a challenging environment for infection control. When infectious hazards are noted, it is vital to document them and provide suggestions and teaching for their correction. Nurses must teach the importance of effective hand hygiene, the use of gloves, the disposal of wastes and soiled dressings, the handling of linens, and the practice of standard precautions.

Note: The references and resources for all chapters have been compiled at the back of the book.

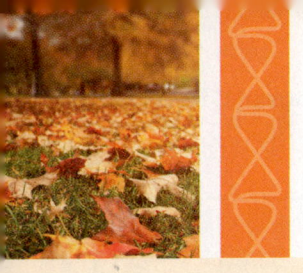

Chapter Review

KEY POINTS

■ **Concept:** Health is a dynamic state influenced by multiple factors, including physical and psychologic characteristics of the individual as well as social, cultural, and environmental factors.

■ Health promotion involves more than simply preventing disease. It also includes a focus on increasing the well-being and maximizing the potential of the individual, family, or community.

■ **Concept:** Medical–surgical nursing focuses on caring for adult patients experiencing acute or chronic illnesses and/or diseases. While physicians focus on treating disease, a disruption of body structure or function, nurses focus on illness, the individual's response to disease.

■ Health and illness are affected by many different factors. Nursing interventions to promote health are essential, no matter the degree of illness or the setting in which care is provided.

■ Disruption of the body's structure and function results in disease; illness is the response of the person to the disease. A person may have a disease without feeling ill.

■ Acute illnesses generally have a rapid onset, last a relatively short period of time, and resolve with a return to normal functioning. Chronic illness, in contrast, often results in a permanent change in structure and function, may require long-term management, and can have significant effects on both the individual and family structure.

■ **Concept:** Most health and illness care occurs outside the acute hospital environment, in primary care and community-based settings such as clinics, residential care, and the patient's home.

■ Health care financing in the United States has caused a shift of illness care away from acute care facilities, such as hospitals, toward rehabilitation, long-term care, community-based care, and home care.

■ Long-term care facilities provide health care and activities of daily living for people who are mentally or physically unable to care for themselves.

■ Rehabilitation nursing care is often provided in community-based settings. The goal of rehabilitation nurses is to assist patients to again become a part of their family and community.

■ **Concept:** Nurses working in community-based settings are important members of the interdisciplinary team, with major responsibility for assessing patient needs, managing and coordinating care, and providing health education and teaching.

■ Community-based nursing care focuses on individual and family health care needs, with nurses providing care in a variety of community settings, including community centers and clinics, day care programs, churches, and homes.

■ Home health agencies are organizations that provide skilled nursing and other therapeutic services in the patient's home. The plan of care is implemented and evaluated within the special characteristics of the home as a nursing care setting.

PEARSON NURSING STUDENT RESOURCES

Find additional materials at **nursing.pearsonhighered.com**.

NCLEX-PN® Exam Preparation

TEST-TAKING TIP Evaluate each question for safety needs and *always* remember the importance of hand washing.

1. A person actively using available personal, physical, and social resources to deal with challenges within the environment where he or she is functioning could be said to have achieved:
   1. health.
   2. high-level wellness.
   3. balance.
   4. homeostasis.

2. The nurse assessing a patient's health teaching needs to understand that health is influenced by which of the following factors? **Select all that apply.**
   1. Culture and ethnicity
   2. Educational level
   3. Choice of health care provider
   4. Lifestyle
   5. Socioeconomic background

3. National health objectives, known as *Healthy People 2020*, are used to:
   1. provide continuity of care across public and private sectors.
   2. provide a standard by which an individual can measure health.
   3. promote health of the public nationwide.
   4. identify risk factors for disease.

4. The response a person has to disease is called:
   1. illness.
   2. biologic.
   3. normative.
   4. developmental.

5. A person experiencing an acute illness can reasonably expect which of the following?
   1. A long period of recovery and rehabilitation
   2. That the disease will be transmitted to others in close contact
   3. Periods of few or no symptoms alternating with periods during which symptoms are acute
   4. That recovery will occur within a relatively short period of time

6. Nearly all people with a chronic illness need:
   1. to manage their disease on a day-to-day basis.
   2. to live in a health care facility.
   3. to be assisted with activities of daily living.
   4. large doses of pain relief medication.

7. Nursing care provided directly to patients wherever they are, including where they live, work, play, worship, and go to school, is known as:
   1. home health nursing.
   2. community health nursing.
   3. community-based nursing.
   4. parish nursing.

8. When the family's desires differ from those of the patient, the home care nurse must:
   1. remain the primary patient's advocate.
   2. try to please everyone.
   3. avoid negative responses from the family.
   4. call the physician to resolve the conflict.

9. In order for home care to receive Medicare reimbursement, certain criteria must be met. Which of the following are necessary? **Select all that apply.**
   1. The patient must need help with cooking and cleaning.
   2. The patient must have a "skilled nursing need."
   3. The patient must have an income below poverty level.
   4. The patient must be essentially homebound.
   5. The patient must have a plan of care.

10. Rehabilitation includes many different aspects of the patient's life, such as physical, mental, social, and vocational status. This comprehensive consideration of the patient requires:
    1. an interdisciplinary approach to care.
    2. primarily nursing care.
    3. focusing on the physical disability.
    4. short-term care.

Answers and rationales for Review Questions appear in Appendix I.

CHAPTER 3
Cultural and Developmental Considerations for Adults

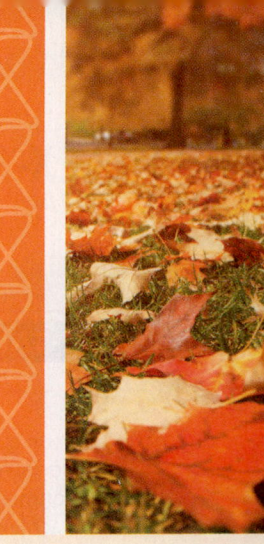

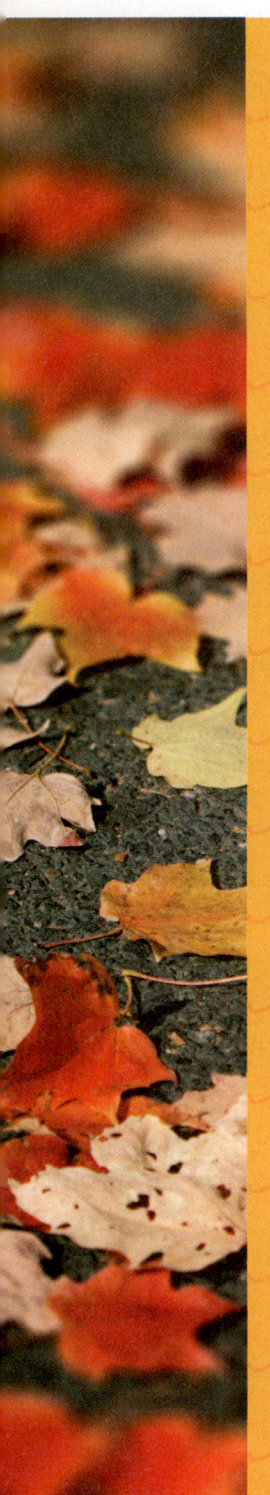

BRIEF OUTLINE

Cultural Considerations in the Adult Patient
Communication
Space
Social Orientation
Time
Environmental Control

Biologic Variations
Adult Development
The Young Adult
The Middle Adult
The Family of the Adult Patient

Family Definitions and Functions
Developmental Stages and Tasks of the Family
Nursing Care to Promote Health in the Adult Patient

APPLIED LEARNING OUTCOMES

After completing this chapter, you will be able to:

1. Recognize and consider cultural differences in contributing to patient assessment, care planning, and implementation.
2. Demonstrate respect for the patient's values and cultural background.
3. Recognize cultural differences that may affect the patient's response to illness, preferences, and plan of treatment.
4. Compare and contrast the physical status, risks for alterations in health, values, and health behaviors of the young adult and middle adult.
5. Provide teaching to reduce high-risk behaviors, such as risks associated with obesity, smoking, or drug use.
6. Describe the functions and developmental stages and tasks of the family.
7. Participate in health screening or health promotion activities for the young or middle adult.

KEY TERMS

The key terms are defined on the pages listed below.

SPECIAL FEATURES

Key Concept The diverse and multicultural nature of the population in the United States requires nurses to provide care that is culturally sensitive while avoiding stereotyping.

Gordon Hight, a 21-year-old African American college student, is admitted to the emergency room with multiple injuries and head trauma after a motorcycle crash. Teresa Guetterez, a 38-year-old Mexican American homemaker, arrives at an ambulatory surgery center for biopsy of a tumor in her left breast. Sam Rosengarten, a 55-year-old Jewish American attorney, is in the intensive care unit for treatment of an acute myocardial infarction. Yui Mae Fang, age 82, recently emigrated from Beijing to live with her adult son and his family. She is receiving home health care after a fall that fractured her right hip. These examples demonstrate the striking variety among adult patients and the settings for their care—the focus of medical–surgical nursing.

The United States is a multicultural society that is becoming ever more diverse. People who identified themselves as Hispanic or Latina accounted for more than half of the total population growth that occurred in the United States between 2000 and 2010. During that same period, the Asian population grew faster than any other major racial group (Humes et al., 2011). As society becomes more diverse, it becomes ever more important and challenging to provide nursing care that is culturally appropriate. The first part of this chapter introduces concepts of transcultural nursing care. These concepts and strategies to provide culturally appropriate care are further expanded in the Cultural Care Strategies features found throughout this book.

In addition to considering the patient's culture when planning and implementing individualized nursing care for adults, the nurse also considers the patient's stage of development. Although growth and development are continuous processes throughout life, the adult years commonly are divided into three stages: the young adult (age 18 to 40 years), the middle adult (age 40 to 65 years), and the older adult (age older than 65 years). With aging, specific changes occur in intellectual, psychosocial, and spiritual development, as well as in physical structures and functions. The second half of this chapter discusses the young and middle adults. (See Chapter 4 for developmental changes and health risks of older adults.) Each chapter concludes with health promotion activities for adult patients.

Cultural Considerations in the Adult Patient

Cultural awareness has become an increasingly important consideration in recent years as nurses and other health care providers work to achieve one of the overarching goals of Healthy People 2020: Achieve health equity and elimi-

nate disparities (U.S. Department of Health and Human Services, 2010). **Health disparities** are differences in health outcomes that occur among specific population groups in the United States and that reflect social inequities (CDC, 2011). By a number of measures, the health of minorities, the poor, and other disadvantaged people in the United States is worse than that of the population as a whole. Culture is recognized as a contributing factor to disparities in health care, along with gender, education, geographic location, and sexual orientation. Furthermore, patient-centered care is identified as an essential quality for all health care personnel, including nurses. **Patient-centered care** means the patient is an active partner in care that respects the patient's values, preferences, and expressed needs (Sherwood & Barnsteiner, 2012). Providing culturally appropriate care is a vital responsibility if a nurse is to be effective in promoting the health of patients (Figure 3-1■).

Culture is the learned behavior, values, beliefs, norms, and practices shared by a particular group of people that guide their thinking, decisions, and actions. People learn beliefs, practices, habits, likes, dislikes, customs, and rituals from their families and cultural group and pass them on to their children (Spector, 2013). Culture gives shape and personal meaning to health or illness events. It also affects how the patient relates to others within the health care environment.

It is important to differentiate culture from race or ethnicity. **Race** is a term used to identify differences in physical characteristics, such as skin color, eye shape, and bone structure. The use of race as an identifying characteristic is becoming less common as people from many cultures mix and as there is increased recognition of the impact of culture and environment on health. Furthermore, use of a concept such as race to identify an individual can lead to stereotyping.

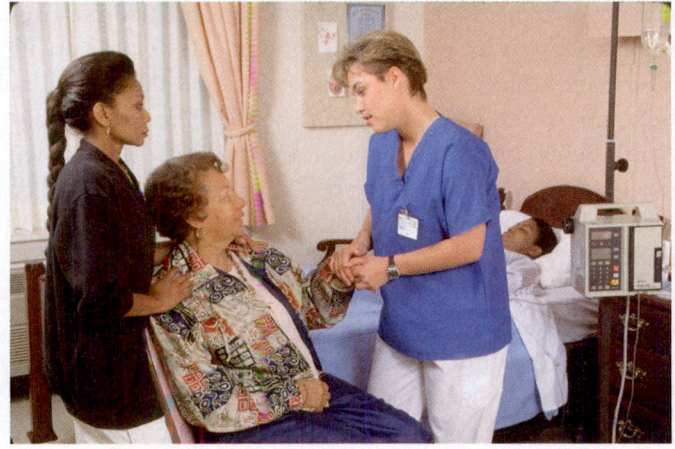

Figure 3-1. ■ The LPN/LVN cares for culturally diverse patients and their families. (Source: Pearson Education.)

A person's **ethnic group** is a group of people who share and are unified by experiences and backgrounds based on such factors as race, nationality, religion, language, ancestry, and culture (Spector, 2013). For example, a person's ethnic identity may be Irish Catholic; the person's culture might be American.

The health care system serves patients who are culturally diverse in their country of origin, health beliefs, sexual orientation, race, socioeconomic level, and age. However, nursing has been slow to address the need for culturally sensitive care. This is partly because the health care system is itself a culture with a shared set of values. Prejudice and *ethnocentrism* (people's belief that their own cultural group's beliefs and values are the only acceptable ones) have often created barriers to culturally sensitive care.

Culturally sensitive care is important for nurses for the following reasons:

- The demographic and ethnic composition of the world, and the United States in particular, has changed markedly, but ethnic groups are not well represented among health care professionals.
- There is a growing awareness and acceptance of diversity and an increased willingness to maintain and support ethnic and cultural heritage.
- People of color and immigrants face limited access to health care.
- Nurses make up the largest force in health care delivery and therefore have tremendous potential to push for fairness and accessibility.
- Consumers are becoming increasingly aware of what constitutes competent and sensitive health care.

People of every culture have the right to have their cultural values known, respected, and addressed appropriately in nursing and other health care services. To provide effective nursing care, the nurse must understand the importance of culturally appropriate nursing care. To provide nursing care that is culturally appropriate, nurses must develop a sensitivity to personal fundamental values about health and illness. Nurses must understand their own beliefs and values, be aware when these differ from the patient's beliefs and values, and accept this difference. They must be respectful of, interested in, and understanding of other cultures without being judgmental. Culturally appropriate caring requires that the nurse understand, or at least accept, the factors that influence an individual's health and illness behavior.

It would be difficult, if not impossible, for the nurse to have in-depth knowledge and understanding of the culture of every person for whom he or she cares. Think about caring for the following group of patients on an acute medical unit: a 22-year-old woman whose parents were born

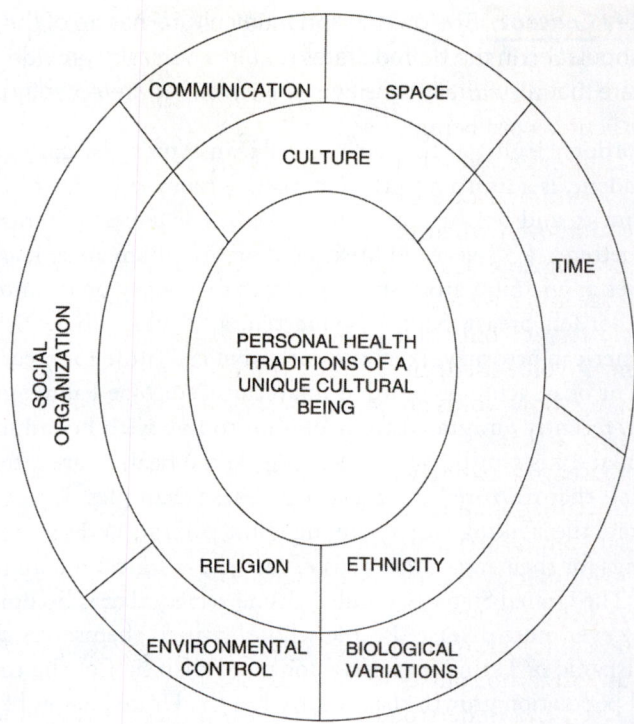

Figure 3-2. ■ Personal health traditions of a unique individual. (Source: "Figure 2.07 - Personal Health Traditions of a Unique Cultural Being" from Cultural Diversity in Health and Illness, 8e by Rachel E. Spector. Published by Pearson Education, © 2013.)

in China; a 60-year-old African American businessman admitted with chest pain; a Native American woman with diabetes; and a homeless man with possible tuberculosis. Culturally appropriate nursing care does not require the nurse to have a detailed understanding of the beliefs and values of each of these individuals; it does, however, require the nurse to accept and respect these differences and not allow his or her personal beliefs to have an undue influence when assessing, planning, and implementing individualized nursing care.

Giger (2013) identifies six cultural characteristics that can help the nurse provide culturally appropriate nursing care. These characteristics, which include communication, space, social orientation, time, environmental control, and biologic variations, affect individual responses to health and health care, as illustrated in Figure 3-2■.

COMMUNICATION

Communication is an essential part of nurses' interactions with their patients. Communication occurs through verbal exchanges, nonverbal expressions, touch, and other behaviors. Language provides just one way of communicating, although it is clearly an important component in health care communications.

Every communication requires a sender, a way of transmitting the message (words, touch, nonverbal expressions), the receiver, and feedback about the message. Think about seeing a cute baby: You catch the mother's eye, look at the baby, and smile; the mother receives the message ("Cute baby!") and smiles in return. Communication occurred without a word being spoken.

Language, which is basic to effective communication, can facilitate or interfere with effective communication even when the nurse and the patient speak the same language. Culture affects vocabulary, grammar, and the meaning we attach to words. Verbal communication includes not only the words that are used but also the tone of voice used; the intonation, rhythm, and speed of talking; how words are pronounced; and the use of silence (Giger, 2013).

Listening attentively and communicating in a nonthreatening manner are vital nursing skills. The nurse must communicate at the patient's level of understanding and modify communication strategies to meet the patient's cultural needs. The nurse should be alert to signs of confusion, fear, or anxiety in the patient and respond. It is important for nurses to avoid assuming that the patient received and understood what the nurse said in the same way as was intended. When communicating with patients of any culture, the nurse needs to be alert for feedback that the patient either is or is not understanding the message. When the feedback is unclear, the nurse should ask the patient what his or her understanding is.

Although language is important, nonverbal communication accounts for a large portion of our understanding of the message being sent. Communication is most effective when the verbal and nonverbal messages "match" or are congruent with each other. Culture affects not only our use of language but also the way we use and interpret nonverbal communication conveyed through touch, facial expression, eye contact, and posture.

Touch is a powerful communication strategy. Depending on how it is used and the situation, touch can communicate caring, understanding, power, or threat. The nurse must be alert to the meaning of touch to the patient and use this to guide the use of touch. It is important that touch be used in a deliberate, empathetic manner, based on the patient's cultural preferences and needs. All cultural groups have rules about touching, including when, where, and between whom touch is acceptable. The nurse must be aware of the patient's reaction to touch to avoid communicating the wrong message (Giger, 2013).

Facial expression, eye contact, and posture are important components of nonverbal communication. The amount and openness of facial expression varies among cultural groups. A lack of expression may communicate disinterest or inattentiveness or may simply reflect a cultural variation in communicating. Although eye contact is seen as a way of communicating openness and attentiveness in the dominant American culture, in some groups it may be seen as impolite or disrespectful. Leaning toward a person or assuming a posture similar to the other person communicates attention and being open to the message, whereas a rigid body posture may communicate disagreement with the message or pain. Standing when the patient is seated or lying in bed may communicate power or dominance on the nurse's part, whereas sitting at the same level as the patient communicates attention and acceptance.

Nonverbal communication becomes even more vital when the patient's primary language differs from that of the nurse. Use of interpreters who are able to translate not only the words used by the nurse but also the underlying message is important. Other strategies for communicating with patients who speak a different language include use of a caring tone of voice and facial expressions, speaking slowly and distinctly (but not loudly—hearing is not the problem, understanding the words and message is), using gestures and pictures to help convey the message, and keeping the message simple. Avoid using medical terms—although the patient may understand basic English, medical terms and abbreviations may be unfamiliar. In all cases, seek feedback from the patient to confirm understanding.

For additional information about communicating with culturally diverse patients, see Cultural Care Strategies: Appreciating Variations in Facial Expression Across Cultures, page 84, and Cultural Care Strategies: Assessing Communication Variables from a Cultural Perspective, page 862.

SPACE

Each person has *personal space*, the area surrounding one's body. As individuals, we need and value territory, or an area that we can call our own. Personal space provides security and privacy; it supports our autonomy, or control over the situation, and our self-identify. As individuals, we each have a comfort zone of social and personal space that is culturally learned. The distance we maintain between ourselves and others varies with the setting. The nurse must be aware of the patient's response to the use of space. A patient who leans or steps back or who turns away from the nurse may be communicating discomfort with the nurse's proximity. It is important that the nurse be sensitive to the patient's need for personal space and territory. Likewise, the nurse must also be aware of his or her own spatial needs. Americans and Canadians tend to require more personal space than do people from Latin America (Giger, 2013).

Patients tend to be more comfortable and feel safer in their own territory, whether that is a home or a room in a long-term care setting that is furnished with the patient's belongings. This personal space also provides privacy and the ability to communicate more freely. It is important that the nurse respect the patient's personal space, not only in the distance maintained when communicating, but also in allowing, to the extent possible, the patient to control his or her own territory. For more information about space as a cultural variable, see Cultural Care Strategies: Considering Cultural Variations Related to Space, page 347.

SOCIAL ORIENTATION

Cultural behavior and practices are learned or acquired as children observe adults and internalize socially acceptable ways of behaving. The *social orientation* of a group includes beliefs, values, and attitudes about important life events such as birth, death, puberty, childbearing, raising children, illness, and disease. The rituals of a culture (weddings, funerals, holiday celebrations) also reflect its social structure. Social organizations include a variety of groups, such as family, religious, and ethnic groups. It is important that the nurse recognize the value of social organizations and their importance to the overall well-being of the patient (Giger, 2013).

As noted earlier in this chapter, although the definition of *family* has evolved over time, the family remains the basic unit of society. Although the *nuclear family*, consisting of a man, woman, and their biologic children, remains the primary family unit in the United States, increasing diversity in family structure is occurring. *Extended families* are multigenerational, including all relatives by birth, marriage, or adoption. In a *skip-generation family*, children are being reared by their grandparents. Other common family structures include *alternative families*, consisting of unmarried partners who may be heterosexual or homosexual and who live together (with or without children), and *blended families*, in which two previous family units join to become a new nuclear family.

The social organization of a cultural group also includes its religious practices and beliefs. Religious beliefs and practices develop within the context of culture and, in turn, influence the sense of identity and purpose of people within that culture. Worldwide, Christianity, Islam, and Hinduism are the religions with the greatest number of followers. Table 3-1 ■ lists the major religions of the world. Most people in the United States identify themselves as Christians; of Christian denominations, the Roman Catholic Church has the most members. Even among Christians, there are significant differences in beliefs and practices (Table 3-2 ■).

The nurse should not make assumptions about the patient's religion and beliefs. Even if the patient's religious affiliation is noted, it is vital that the nurse ask about

TABLE 3-1	Major Religions of the United States	
RELIGION MAJOR DIVISIONS	**ESTIMATED MEMBERS WORLDWIDE**	**POSSIBLE CARE CONSIDERATIONS**
Christianity ■ Roman Catholic ■ Orthodox Eastern ■ Protestant denominations	2.1 billion	■ Vary significantly: See Table 3-2 ■ for care considerations for selected denominations
Islam ■ Sunni ■ Shiite	1.5 billion	■ May request assistance with washing before prayers ■ Provide privacy during prayer ■ May request caregiver of the same gender ■ Do not eat pork or consume alcoholic beverages ■ May fast from sunrise to sunset during Ramadan (9th month of Muslim year)
Judaism ■ Orthodox ■ Reform ■ Conservative	14 million	■ May avoid driving, scheduling surgery, or treatment during Sabbath ■ May refuse meat unless Kosher; avoid having meat and milk in same meal ■ May refuse donor organ transplants
Hinduism (multiple sects)	900 million	■ May be vegetarian ■ Cows are considered sacred; do not eat beef
Buddhism	376 million	■ May appear stoic, not expressing pain outwardly ■ Dietary practices vary; ask patient preferences

TABLE 3-2	Care Considerations for Selected Denominations
DENOMINATION	**POSSIBLE CARE CONSIDERATIONS**
Roman Catholic	▪ Anointment may be desired for healing and strength; also when death is imminent ▪ May abstain from eating meat on Fridays during Lent ▪ Take care to prevent loss or damage to rosary, medals, statues, and other religious objects
Methodist/Wesleyan	▪ On request, clergy may anoint with oil
Lutheran	▪ May request anointing and blessing from clergy
Church of Jesus Christ of Latter-Day Saints (LDS; Mormon)	▪ Avoid caffeinated beverages and alcohol ▪ May wear a sacred undergarment
Assemblies of God	▪ May seek divine healing through prayer and laying on of hands
Episcopal	▪ Anointment may be performed when death is imminent ▪ May avoid eating meat on Fridays
Jehovah's Witnesses	▪ Blood transfusions not allowed but will accept transfusion alternatives; may accept autologous blood transfusion ▪ Avoid foods to which blood has been added (some sausages and lunchmeats) ▪ Do not observe national or religious holidays
Seventh-Day Adventist	▪ Abstain from beverages containing caffeine and eating pork; may avoid lobster, crab, or scavenger fish ▪ May request vegetarian diet ▪ Sabbath is on Saturday
Orthodox Church in America	▪ Abstain from meat and dairy products on Wednesdays and Fridays during Lent and on holy days ▪ Last rites are administered before death
Christian Science	▪ Generally do not seek traditional medical treatment ▪ Avoid immunizations on religious grounds

specific religious practices or preferences. For example, a member of the Church of Jesus Christ of Latter-Day Saints (also known as the Mormon Church) may wear a sacred undergarment that is to be removed only in case of emergencies. Seventh-Day Adventists celebrate the Sabbath on Saturday and may request a vegetarian diet. Women of the Mennonite faith may wear head coverings during hospitalization.

It is always appropriate to offer to contact clergy or church members as desired, to keep religious objects (e.g., a Bible or rosary) within the patient's reach, and to provide privacy for prayers. For more information, see Cultural Care Strategies: Assessing the Patient from Another Culture in a Social Context, page 476.

TIME

The concept of time is learned so early and becomes so integrated into our being that it can be difficult to recognize and understand that the perception of time and its meaning vary among people of different cultures. According to Giger (2013), time and its meaning develop out of the social structure of a cultural group. Because the concept

and measurement of time develop within a culture, clear differences exist among cultures.

There are two different but related meanings of time. The first meaning is measurement of an interval or duration (e.g., think about setting a timer when baking cookies or cake; we measure the amount of time required to fully bake the pastry without burning it). The second meaning is a specified point in time (e.g., my favorite program begins at 9 P.M.). Timers measure intervals of time, whereas clocks identify points in time. Clocks also are used, in our society, to determine the interval since a given event or until an event (e.g., my appointment is at 4 P.M.; because it is now 1:30, I have $2\frac{1}{2}$ hours to wait). A calendar is another device used to measure time (5 days until the weekend!).

Social time is distinctly different from *clock time* (as described earlier). *Social time* develops out of the social patterns and processes of a culture. Even in American culture, which tends to emphasize clock time, many behavior patterns follow social time. Think about phenomena such as "school shopping" in August, sports seasons (football in Fall, basketball in Winter, and baseball in Spring), and the kinds of activities that revolve around family members getting ready for and returning home from school and work. These events are not structured as much by time as they are by the social aspects of the event.

The meaning of time differs between cultures that primarily measure time by social events and those that predominantly measure time using the clock. Groups with a social time focus construct time according to group activities. Those with a clock time focus schedule activities according to the clock (Giger, 2013).

Cultural groups also differ in their orientation in time, or *temporal orientation*. Most Americans of the predominant culture tend to be future-oriented, for example, saving for retirement or deferring childbearing until a career is established. A future orientation leads to engaging in health promotion activities such as health screening examinations, obtaining immunizations, using a seat belt and life preservers, and eating a healthy diet. Other groups, such as Native Americans and Mexican Americans, tend to be more present-oriented. Patients with a present orientation are less likely to value and engage in preventive actions such as changing their diet to reduce their risk for heart disease.

As a nurse working with people from other cultures, it is important to be aware of differences in time orientation and to avoid labeling of patients as ignorant, lazy, or disrespectful if they arrive late for appointments or do not follow through on recommended health promotion activities. The nurse caring for a patient from a present-oriented culture needs to be flexible in scheduling treatments and activities. Adapting care within a range of time, rather than adhering to a fixed schedule, can facilitate the therapeutic relationship between the patient and the nurse. For more information about cultural variations related to time, see Cultural Care Strategies: Considering Cultural Variations Related to Time, page 527.

ENVIRONMENTAL CONTROL

Environmental control refers to the perceived ability of individuals or members of a cultural group to control or affect factors related to the environment (including people). According to Giger (2013), health may be seen as a balance between the individual and the environment. People's perception of their ability to control their environment affects their responses to illness and disease.

The concept of locus of control is used to describe individuals' perception of their ability to control the environment. People who believe that their actions affect the outcomes (e.g., avoiding red meat will help prevent a heart attack) are said to have an internal locus of control. These individuals are more likely to adopt behaviors that are seen as having positive outcomes (e.g., exercising daily). People with an external locus of control have more difficulty seeing the relationship between their actions and future

events. These individuals may perceive illness and disease more as a result of fate or bad luck than of behaviors.

The environmental control concept includes the systems and processes that affect individuals within a culture. Systems of health beliefs and practices vary among cultures. Although the biomedical model of health care, which emphasizes the effects of disease and treatment on the structure and function of the body, is prevalent in the United States, other cultures may view illness and disease as the result of magic or forces of evil.

It is important for the nurse to respect such beliefs and accommodate folk practices whenever possible, for example, encouraging the patient to use prayer in addition to medication in treating a disease. In cultures where supernatural forces are believed to cause illness and disease, it may be appropriate to allow the presence of a healer. However, it is also vital that the nurse recognize that some folk remedies are harmful and inquire of patients what treatment has been tried before seeking care. For more information about environmental control variables, see Cultural Care Strategies: Considering Cultural Variations Related to Environmental Control on page 300.

BIOLOGIC VARIATIONS

As genetic science and our understanding of disease causes and pathology have advanced, there is increasing recognition that differences between peoples of the world are more than skin deep. Certain diseases and conditions are much more likely to develop in some groups than in others; for example, sickle cell disease occurs more frequently in people whose ancestors are from central Africa, the Near East, the Mediterranean region, and parts of India; Caucasian women of small stature of Scandinavian heritage have a higher risk of developing osteoporosis. Biologic variations also may affect the way the body metabolizes drugs, leading to an effect that is either less than or greater than anticipated. In other cases, select drugs may be found to be effective for people of one race but not another.

Biologic differences among people of various cultural groups also affect both food preferences and food tolerance. Most Mexican Americans, African Americans, Native Americans, and Asians are lactose intolerant; that is, they do not produce enough lactose to tolerate large amounts of milk and milk products. If too much milk (or yogurt or milk chocolate) is eaten, undigested lactose in the intestine causes manifestations such as cramping, flatulence, abdominal bloating, and diarrhea.

Although known biologic variables among people of different races and cultures can be helpful in providing individualized health education, it is important to avoid stereotyping based on racial and cultural differences. For example, a person who appears to be African American may actually identify with Native American culture as a result of having a Native American parent; a recent immigrant from Ethiopia has a significantly different cultural background than a Black person who is a descendent of U.S. slaves. Making assumptions about health risk factors and preferences could lead to inappropriate care planning for these individuals.

Food preferences must be included in any discussion of biologic variables among people. Nurses should work with patients to identify and provide preferred foods whenever possible. Doing so not only shows consideration for the patient's culture and traditions, but also supports the patient's nutritional status. For more information about biologic variations among cultures, see Cultural Care Strategies: Recognizing Biologic Variations Among Cultures, on page 49 at the end of this chapter.

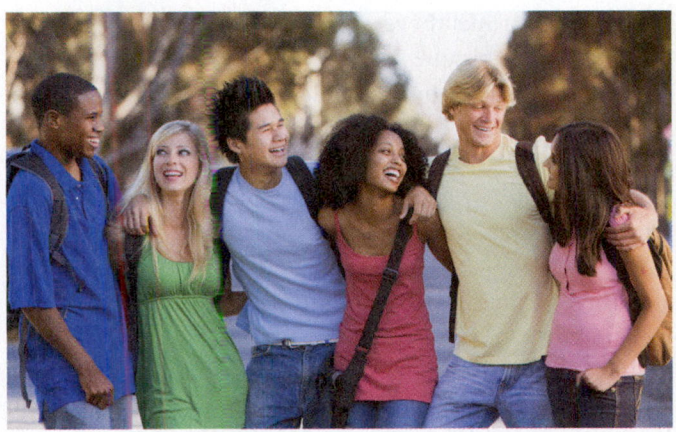

Figure 3-3. ■ Young adults are at the peak of physical development and health. (© Monkey Business Images/Shutterstock)

Adult Development

> **Key Concept** The primary health concerns and risks differ for adults at various times of their lives. As a result, the focus for teaching and health promotion activities differs for young adults and for adults in their middle years.

The developmental tasks of young and middle adults differ. From ages 18 to 40, most young adults have a job, establish a social group, select and learn to live with a mate, have and raise children, manage a home, and take on civic responsibility. From ages 40 to 65, middle adults establish and maintain an economic standard of living, help adolescent children learn to become responsible adults, develop leisure activities, accept and adjust to the physical changes of middle age, and adjust to aging parents.

THE YOUNG ADULT

From age 18 to 25, the healthy young adult is at the peak of physical development (Figure 3-3 ■). All body systems function at maximum efficiency. During the 30s, some normal physiologic changes begin to occur in body systems. The impact of these changes on the cardiovascular, respiratory, and musculoskeletal systems can be minimized by maintaining physical activity and a diet rich in fruits and vegetables with calories balanced to activity. The expected physical status of young adults is shown in Table 3-3 ■.

Health Risks

The young adult is at risk for **alterations in health** (a change from the normal health state) from unintentional and intentional injuries, sexually transmitted infections (STIs), substance abuse, and physical or psychosocial stressors. The Centers for Disease Control and Prevention identifies inadequate physical activity and obesity as major health risks for the young adult (National Center for Health Statistics [NCHS], 2012). These risk factors often are interrelated.

Accidents are the leading cause of injury and death in people between ages 15 and 44 (NCHS, 2012). Most injuries and fatalities occur as the result of motor vehicle crashes, but injuries and death also result from drowning, fire, use of firearms, occupational accidents, and exposure to environmental hazards. Accidental injury or death is often associated with the use of alcohol or other chemical substances or with psychologic stress. Lack of sleep and drowsy driving are increasingly recognized as major risks for accidents, motor vehicle crashes in particular.

Substance abuse is a major cause for concern in the young adult population. Alcohol is the most widely used drug among young adults. Although alcohol abuse occurs at all ages, it is greater in the 20s than during any other decade of the life span, with nearly two-thirds of young adults consuming alcohol. Binge drinking, consuming five or more drinks on one occasion, is common among young adults, particularly among those who consume alcohol

TABLE 3-3	Physical Status in the Young Adult Years
ASSESSMENT	**STATUS IN THE YOUNG ADULT**
Skin	Smooth, even temperature
Hair	Slightly oily, shiny Balding may begin
Vision	Snellen 20/20 (distant vision) Rosenbaum 14/14 (near vision)
Musculoskeletal	Strong, coordinated Skeletal growth complete by age 25–30
Cardiovascular	Maximum cardiac output 60–90 beats/min Mean BP: Less than 120/80
Respiratory	Rate: 12–20 Full vital capacity

with energy drinks (beverages that contain caffeine, other stimulants, and simple sugars). Alcohol contributes to motor vehicle crashes, physical violence, STIs, and unintended pregnancy. Excessive alcohol consumption also contributes to cardiovascular diseases (including high blood pressure and stroke), liver disease, and neurologic damage, and is damaging to the developing fetus in pregnant women (CDC, 2012a).

Other substances that are commonly abused include nicotine, marijuana, amphetamines (including methamphetamine), cocaine, and crack. Marijuana can affect memory and learning for days to weeks after its use; these effects can be significant with heavy use. Methamphetamine, a highly addictive substance of abuse, can lead to structural and functional changes in the areas of the brain associated with emotion and memory. Cocaine and crack can cause death from cardiovascular effects and can lead to addiction and health problems in the baby born to an addicted mother. Smoking increases the risk of respiratory and cardiovascular diseases.

STIs include genital herpes, chlamydia, human papillomavirus (HPV), gonorrhea, syphilis, and human immunodeficiency virus (HIV). The young adult who is sexually active with a variety of partners and who does not use condoms is at greatest risk for the development of these diseases.

The young adult is subjected to a wide variety of physical and psychosocial stressors. Physical stressors that increase the risk of illness include environmental pollutants and work-related risks (e.g., electrical hazards, mechanical injuries, or exposure to toxins or infectious agents). Other physical stressors include exposure to the sun, ingestion of chemical substances (e.g., caffeine, alcohol, nicotine), inadequate sleep, and pregnancy. Rates of obesity are increasing among young adults, possibly related to increased consumption of meals outside the home and lack of physical activity.

PSYCHOSOCIAL FACTORS Many different and individualized psychosocial stressors may affect the young adult. Choices must be made about education, occupation, relationships, independence, and lifestyle. The young adult without an adequate education or job skills may face unemployment, poverty, homelessness, and limited access to health care. Young adults are at significant risk for failed relationships and single parenthood, increasing the potential for loneliness, feelings of failure, financial difficulties, domestic violence, and child abuse. The inability of the young adult to cope with these stressors may result in suicide, which ranks next to accidents as a major cause of death in this age group. Although difficult to prove, it is believed that some accidental deaths, especially when associated with substance abuse, are actually suicides.

THE MIDDLE ADULT

The middle adult, age 40 to 65, has physical status and function similar to that of adults in their 20s and 30s (Figure 3-4■). However, many changes take place between ages 40 and 65 (Table 3-4■). The middle adult is at risk for alterations in health from lack of physical activity, obesity, cancer, cardiovascular disease, substance abuse, and psychosocial stressors. These factors may be interrelated.

Health Risks

The middle adult often has a problem maintaining a healthy weight. Weight gain in middle adulthood is usually the result of continuing to consume the same number of calories while physical activity and basal metabolic rate decrease. Obesity affects all the major organ systems of the body, increasing the risk of atherosclerosis, hypertension, elevated cholesterol and triglyceride levels, and diabetes. Obesity is also associated with heart disease, osteoarthritis, and gallbladder disease.

Cancer is the leading cause of death in adults between ages 45 and 64 in the United States. Cancers of the breast, colon, lung, and reproductive system are common in the middle years. Evidence suggests that approximately one-third of cancer deaths are related to physical inactivity, obesity, and poor nutritional status (American Cancer Society, 2012a). Exposure

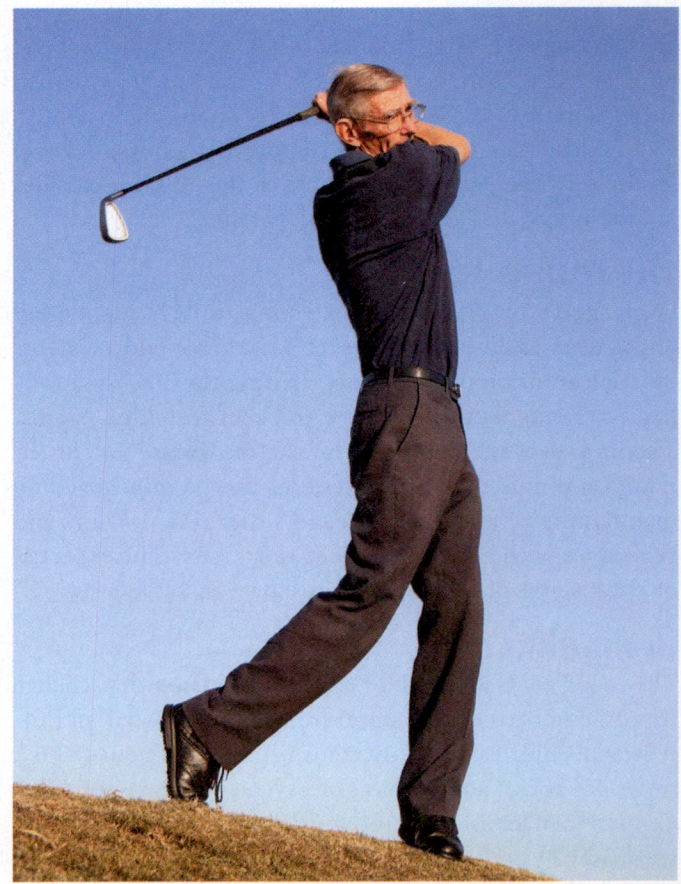

Figure 3-4. ■ In the middle adult, physical activity contributes to good health. (© Duncan Noakes/Fotolia)

TABLE 3-4	Physical Changes in the Middle Adult Years (40 to 65 Years)
ASSESSMENT	**CHANGES**
Skin	Decreased turgor, moisture, and subcutaneous fat result in wrinkles. Fat is deposited in the abdominal and hip areas.
Hair	Loss of melanin in hair shaft causes graying. Hairline recedes in males.
Sensory	Visual acuity for near vision decreases (presbyopia) during the 40s. Auditory acuity for high-frequency sounds decreases (presbycusis). Sense of taste diminishes.
Musculoskeletal	Skeletal muscle mass decreases by about age 60. Thinning of intervertebral disks results in loss of height (about 1 in. [2.5 cm]). Postmenopausal women may lose bone density and have an increased risk for developing osteoporosis.
Cardiovascular	Blood vessels lose elasticity. Systolic blood pressure may increase.
Respiratory	Loss of vital capacity (about 1 L from age 20 to 60) occurs.
Gastrointestinal	Large intestine gradually loses muscle tone; constipation may result. Gastric secretions are decreased.
Genitourinary	Hormonal changes occur: menopause, women (↓estrogen); andropause, men (↓ testosterone).
Endocrine	Gradual decrease in glucose tolerance occurs.

to environmental toxins and the use of nicotine and alcohol also are significant risk factors for cancer in the middle adult.

The major risk factors for cardiovascular diseases, especially for coronary heart disease, include age, cigarette smoking, hypertension, elevated blood cholesterol levels, and diabetes. Other contributing factors include obesity, stress, and lack of exercise. The middle adult is at risk for disorders related to peripheral vascular, cerebrovascular, and cardiovascular diseases.

Although the middle adult may use a variety of substances, the most commonly abused are alcohol, nicotine, and prescription drugs. Excess alcohol use in the middle adult contributes to an increased risk of liver cancer, cirrhosis, pancreatitis, hyperlipidemia, and anemia. Alcoholism also increases the risk of accidental injury or death and disrupts careers and relationships. Cigarette smoking increases the risk for cancer (particularly cancers involving the respiratory tract, upper gastrointestinal tract, urinary system, and pancreas), chronic obstructive lung disorders, and cardiovascular disease. Prescription drug abuse is increasing in the United States. Pain relievers are the most commonly abused class of prescription drugs among adults, followed by tranquilizers.

PSYCHOSOCIAL FACTORS The middle adult years are ones of change and transition, frequently resulting in stress. Both men and women must adapt to changes in physical appearance and function and accept their own mortality. Children may leave home or, as is becoming more common, choose to remain at home. Parents are aging, with illness and death probable. The middle adult thus becomes what has been called "the sandwich generation," caught between the need to care for both children and aging parents. Both men and women may make career changes, and approaching retirement becomes a reality. Divorce in the middle years is a major emotional, social, and financial stressor.

The Family of the Adult Patient

Key Concept All families have structure and function. The nurse must consider the needs of the patient and the needs of the family when providing care.

Although some patients are totally alone in the world, most have significant people in their lives. These significant others may be bonded to the patient by birth, adoption, marriage, or friendship. Although not always meeting traditional definitions, people (or even pets) significant to the patient are the patient's family. Families are integrated systems in which the health and illness of family members are managed. An illness in one family member can disrupt the entire family unit. The nurse includes the family as an integral component of care in all health care settings.

FAMILY DEFINITIONS AND FUNCTIONS

What is a family? The definition of a *family* changes as society changes. According to one definition, a **family** is a unit of people related by marriage, birth, or adoption (Duvall, 1977). An expanded definition states that a family is two or more people who are emotionally involved with each other and live close to each other. In a global society, it may not be possible for family members to live nearby, but they do remain emotionally involved.

Although every family is unique, all families have certain structural and functional features in common. *Family structure* (family roles and relationships) and *family function* (interactions among family members and with the community) provide support, guidance, and stability. The family carries out the tasks that are necessary for its survival and continuity:

■ Providing shelter, food, clothing, and health care
■ Sharing money, time, and space according to each member's needs

- Determining the roles and responsibilities of each member for the support, management, and care of the home and other family members
- Ensuring the socialization of members by raising them to take on increasingly responsible roles in the family and in society
- Establishing socially acceptable ways to interact with others through communication and the expression of feelings in areas such as love, anger, and sexuality
- Rearing and releasing children appropriately
- Relating to the community (neighborhood, school, church, work) and establishing rules for relatives, guests, and friends
- Maintaining morale and motivation, rewarding achievement, dealing with personal and family crises, setting attainable goals, and developing family loyalties and values

DEVELOPMENTAL STAGES AND TASKS OF THE FAMILY

The family, just like the individual, has developmental stages and tasks. Each stage brings change and requires adaptation. Each new stage also brings family-related risk factors for alterations in health. The nurse must consider both the needs of the patient at a specific developmental stage and the needs of the patient within a family with specific developmental tasks:

1. *A couple.* Two people, living together with or without being married, are in a period of establishing themselves as a couple. Their tasks are to adjust to living together as a couple, establish a mutually satisfying relationship, relate to kin, and decide whether or not to have children.
2. *The family with infants and preschoolers.* The young family must adjust to being more than a couple. Family members must now support the needs and economic costs of more than two members. They must develop an attachment between parents and children, cope with lack of energy and privacy, and carry out activities that promote growth and development of the children.
3. *Family with school-age children.* The family with school-age children must adjust to the expanded world of children in school, encourage educational achievement, and promote joint decision making between children and parents.
4. *Family with adolescents and young adults.* The developmental tasks of this family unit focus on transition. Parents must provide a supportive home base and maintain open communications. They must balance freedom with responsibility and encourage adult children to become independent.
5. *Family with middle adults.* When the parents are middle aged and children are no longer at home, the parents' tasks are to maintain ties with older and younger generations, to plan for retirement, to reestablish their relationship, and (if necessary) to acquire the role of grandparents.
6. *Family with older adults.* The older adult family must adjust to retirement and aging. If a spouse dies, the surviving spouse must cope with the loss, adjust to living alone, or close the family home.

The nurse promotes and supports family function and integrity through simple, yet deliberate, actions. In doing so, the nurse also prepares family members to assume a caregiving role:

- Provide for visitation by family members. Numerous studies support the positive effects of open visitation on the ill patient and on family members. Although highly anxious family members can increase patient agitation, supportive family members provide emotional support for the patient. Open visitation also reduces anxiety among family members and increases their knowledge and understanding of the patient's illness.
- As authorized by the patient, provide information to family members. Families need and desire current information about the patient's condition and care. Information not only decreases anxiety but also allows families to make informed decisions about care. Nurses are in a key position to ensure that families have the accurate and up-to-date information they need.
- Provide for family caregiving. Supporting the provision of care by family members is not only beneficial for the patient but also helps prepare family members to assume care after discharge from the care setting. It is important to consider preferences of the patient and family members in the care provided. In many cases, care provided by family members may be limited to emotional support and encouragement of the patient; in others, the family member may assist with direct care needs such as feeding or bathing.
- Address feelings of guilt or anger. Although often unexpressed, the patient and/or family members may have feelings of guilt or anger about the patient's illness. These feelings can have a negative impact on coping and preparations for assuming caregiving. The nurse facilitates discussions by open and active listening and by avoiding minimizing or negating feelings expressed by the patient or family.

Nursing Care to Promote Health in the Adult Patient

The nurse promotes health in adult patients by teaching the activities that maintain wellness (Box 3-1■). The nurse also provides information about known risk factors and recommended screening for early detection of disease, adapting teaching to at-risk cultural variations (Table 3-5■). Supplying specific information about decreasing risk factors, such as recommended immunizations (see Table 11-3), is an important nursing activity. The nurse also promotes health by following healthy practices and serving as a role model.

Note: The references and resources for all chapters have been compiled at the back of the book.

BOX 3-1	**PATIENT TEACHING**

Health Promotion for the Adult

- Choose foods from all food groups and eat a variety of foods. Balance food and calorie intake with physical activity to maintain an appropriate weight.
- Choose a diet that includes at least seven servings of fruits and vegetables and six servings of whole grains daily.
- Choose a diet low in fat (30% or less of total calories), saturated fat (less than 10% of calories), and cholesterol (less than 300 mg daily).
- Use sugar in moderation, and limit sodium intake to less than 1,500 mg daily (Appel et al., 2011). Limit intake of refined grains, and prepared and processed foods.
- Consume at least 1,000 mg of calcium and 600 mg of vitamin D daily.
- For females of childbearing age, maintain iron intake and adequate folate (a B vitamin) daily in the diet.
- Limit alcohol consumption, if any, to no more than one drink per day for women and two drinks per day for men.
- Engage in at least 30 minutes of continuous moderate-intensity physical activity, above usual activity at work or home, 5 or more days per week. Reduce sedentary behaviors.
- Achieve and maintain physical fitness by including aerobic exercises, stretching exercises for flexibility, and weight training or resistance exercises for muscle strength and endurance.
- If weight loss is needed, aim for a slow, steady loss by decreasing caloric intake while maintaining a balanced nutrient intake and increasing physical activity.
- Practice good oral hygiene with teeth brushing and flossing and have an annual dental checkup.
- Sleep 7 to 8 hours each day.
- Eliminate smoking and use of other tobacco products.
- Minimize sun exposure and use sunscreen, hats, and loose, protective clothing.
- Maintain recommended immunizations.

TABLE 3-5	**Recommended Health Screening for Healthy Adults (Without Specific Risk Factors)**	
	RECOMMENDED FREQUENCY	
EXAMINATION	**YOUNG ADULTS (18–40)**	**MIDDLE ADULTS (40–65)**
Health maintenance examination - Height, weight, body mass index - Risk evaluation and counseling - Safety - Behavioral assessment	Every 1 to 5 years	Every 1 to 3 years
Blood pressure	Every 2 years; annually if 120–139/80–89	Every 2 years; annually if 120–139/80–89
Breast cancer - Clinical breast exam - Mammography	Every 3 years	Annually Annually
Cervical cancer (Pap test)	Every 3 years until age 30 Age 30–65, Pap test plus HPV test every 5 years	Pap test plus HPV test every 5 years
Cholesterol and lipid profile	Every 5 years for men over age 34	Every 5 years for men and women
Chlamydia	All sexually active women under age 26	Women with new or multiple partners
Colorectal cancer - Fecal occult blood test (FOBT) or fecal immunochemical test (FIT) or stool DNA (sDNA) test - Flexible sigmoidoscopy *or* double contrast barium enema *or* CT colonography (virtual colonoscopy) *or* - Colonoscopy		Annually beginning age 50 Every 5 years beginning age 50 Every 10 years beginning age 50
Prostate cancer		Individual decision; if testing is done, prostate-specific antigen (PSA) blood test beginning age 50 (age 45 for African American men and men with a strong family history of prostate cancer)

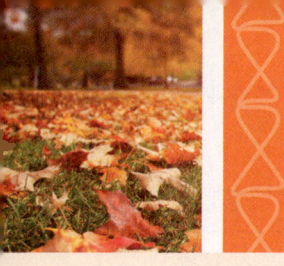

Chapter Review

KEY POINTS

- **Concept:** The diverse and multicultural nature of the population in the United States requires nurses to provide care that is culturally sensitive while avoiding stereotyping.
- When assessing and planning care for culturally diverse patients, the nurse should consider cultural differences in communication, facial expression (including eye contact), personal space and touch, environmental control, social structures (such as family and religion), and biologic variations.
- It is always appropriate for the nurse to ask the patient about specific beliefs or practices that may be related to the patient's culture, avoiding making assumptions.
- **Concept:** The primary health concerns and risks differ for adults at various times of their lives. As a result, the focus for teaching and health promotion activities differs for young adults and for adults in their middle years.
- The young adult is at the peak of physical development. Risks for alterations in health include physical inactivity,

obesity, accidents, sexually transmitted infections, substance abuse, and physical or psychosocial stressors.
- The middle adult, although physically similar to the young adult, does have age-related changes. Risks for alterations in health include physical inactivity, obesity, cardiovascular disease, cancer, substance abuse, and psychosocial stressors.
- **Concept:** All families have structure and function. The nurse must consider the needs of the patient and the needs of the patient's family when providing care.
- Health promotion activities for adults include maintaining physical activity; consuming a diet balanced in nutrients and calories, rich in fruits, vegetables, and whole grains, and with limited sugar, sodium, and fats; getting adequate sleep; maintaining oral health; limiting sun exposure; and maintaining recommended immunizations.

PEARSON NURSING STUDENT RESOURCES

Find additional materials at **nursing.pearsonhighered.com**.

Clinical Reasoning Care Map

Caring for a Patient With Type 1 Diabetes
NCLEX-PN® Focus Area: Psychosocial Adaptation

Case Study: Alexis Burd has had the chronic illness diabetes mellitus (requiring daily insulin injections) since she was 4 years old. She is now 36 years old, is married, and has two teenage children. While you are weighing Alexis during her regular appointment at the diabetes clinic, she begins to cry and says, "I think this disease controls me more than I control it."

Nursing Diagnosis: Powerlessness

COLLECT DATA

Subjective	Objective
_____	_____
_____	_____
_____	_____
_____	_____
_____	_____
_____	_____

Does this present a threat to the patient's safety?

If yes, the priority intervention to address this threat would be:

_____

Nursing Care

_____
_____
_____
_____
_____
_____
_____

Interprofessional team members to include when planning care:

_____
_____

How would you document this?_____
_____
_____

Compare your answers and documentation to those provided on the companion website.

Data Collected (use only those that apply)

- Height: 5'3"
- Weight: 156 lbs
- Blood pressure: 126/64
- Fasting blood glucose: 180 (normal 70–110)
- States "I'm not a good mother anymore."
- States "I have done everything I was told to do."
- States "I think I will just stop taking my insulin."

Nursing Interventions (use only those that apply; list in priority order)

- Discuss weight-reduction diet.
- Discuss exercise plan.
- Listen carefully to Alexis's concerns.
- State "Tell me more about how you think diabetes controls you."
- Suggest that Alexis join a diabetes support group.
- Ask Alexis to keep a daily diary of self-management activities.

NCLEX-PN® Exam Preparation

1 The LPN/LVN is demonstrating cultural sensitivity when he or she:
1. asks the patient about specific food preferences.
2. contacts the hospital chaplain to comfort the patient.
3. uses touch to convey empathy and caring.
4. uses the patient's child to interpret when providing health teaching.

2 The nurse is communicating effectively when he or she:
1. speaks slowly and loudly.
2. uses verbal and nonverbal expressions to convey the message.
3. asks the patient to repeat the message in his or her own words.
4. uses gestures and demonstration to teach the patient.

3 The practical nurse assisting with admission of a seriously injured patient to the emergency department notices a MedicAlert bracelet indicating that the patient is a Jehovah's Witness. The nurse should:
1. notify the emergency physician and the surgeon.
2. contact the patient's family for permission to treat.
3. note the information in the patient's medical record.
4. suggest that legal proceedings to allow blood administration be started.

4 When the nurse is teaching about a medication prescribed to treat high blood pressure, the patient responds, "Why should I take that drug? I feel OK now and everybody has to die of something anyway." The nurse recognizes the patient's response as indicative of:
1. denial of the seriousness of hypertension.
2. a present orientation to time.
3. fear of the adverse effects of the prescribed medication.
4. an internal locus of control.

5 The young adult is at risk for alterations in health from:
1. accidents, STIs, and substance abuse.
2. obesity, cardiovascular disease, and cancer.
3. chronic illness, stroke, and substance abuse.
4. injuries, pharmacologic therapy, and obesity.

6 What factor often causes the middle adult to gain weight?
1. Maintaining calorie intake while decreasing physical activity
2. Physical and psychosocial stressors
3. Chronic illness such as arthritis and hypertension
4. Normal physiologic changes of aging

7 In comparison with young adults, health promotion behaviors in middle adults include:
1. men no longer needing to do a testicular self-exam.
2. women having a mammogram at age 50.
3. having a vision examination every 4 years.
4. carrying out regular exercise that is strenuous.

8 The nurse promotes health in the young adult by encouraging which of the following behaviors? **Select all that apply**.
1. Use of condoms when engaging in sexual activity
2. Visiting a tanning salon regularly during winter months
3. Having an annual clinical breast exam and mammography
4. Participating in physical exercise 5 or more days a week
5. Limiting consumption of processed foods

9 The nurse promotes health in the adult patient when he or she:
1. refers the patient who is overweight to a commercial weight loss program.
2. encourages a young adult to have annual blood cholesterol screening tests.
3. asks when the patient had the most recent tetanus and whooping cough boosters.
4. advises the patient to have annual pneumococcal pneumonia immunizations.

10 Significant others related or bonded to the patient by birth, adoption, marriage, or friendship are the patient's family, and the nurse should:
1. ask them to step out when giving nursing care.
2. expect them to assist with care of the patient.
3. speak with them regarding confidential patient matters.
4. include them as an integral component of health care.

Answers and rationales for Review Questions appear in Appendix I.

CULTURAL CARE STRATEGIES

RECOGNIZING BIOLOGIC VARIATIONS AMONG CULTURES

Mrs. Jamie Jean Johnson is a 38-year-old African American woman who was diagnosed at age 6 with sickle cell disease. She has had few symptoms in recent years, but now has developed unbearable pain and is in sickle cell crisis. When she arrives at the hospital, the admitting nurse notes that Mrs. Johnson's complaints include severe joint pains in both the upper and lower extremities, a temperature of 101.8°F, and shortness of breath. On physical examination, Mrs. Johnson has coarse crackles in the base of both lungs and her lips are cyanotic and dry. Her nail beds are cyanotic, and capillary refill is slow. Initial laboratory examination reveals a hemoglobin of 8 g/dL.

During the past three decades, a field of study about biocultural differences (*biocultural ecology*) has developed. Scientific facts about biologic variations can aid the nurse in giving culturally appropriate health care.

Biologic Variables Examples

Body weight
- African American men average 166.1 lb, and White men average 170.6 lb.
- African American women from 35 to 65 years of age are an average of 20 lb heavier than White women.
- Mexican Americans, on average, weigh more than Whites due to truncal fat.

clinicalALERT
Standardized height/weight charts may be inappropriate, because they are based on standard White measurements.

Skin color
- Assessing skin color is more difficult with darker skin. Assess skin color using daylight or a 60-watt bulb. Examine least pigmented areas: palms, soles, abdomen, volar surfaces of forearms, and buttocks. Also assess nail beds, conjunctiva, and mouth. Oral hyperpigmentation occurs in 50% to 90% of African Americans and in 10% to 50% of Whites. The lips of some Blacks have a natural bluish hue.

Other visible physical characteristics
- Mongolian spots are more common in African Americans, Asian Americans, Native Americans, and Mexican Americans.
- Keloids (scar tissue that extends beyond the original injury) are more common in African Americans.

Drug interactions and metabolism
- Isoniazid (antituberculosis drug)—Up to 60% of Whites, 40% of African Americans, 10% to 40% of Native Americans, and 10% to 15% of Asians inactivate this drug slowly and are at increased risk for toxicity.
- Propranolol (Inderal, an antihypertensive drug)—African Americans often require higher doses of the beta blocker propranolol to achieve the desired effect, whereas Chinese men are more sensitive to its cardiovascular effects than Whites are (Giger, 2013).

Disease incidence
- Tuberculosis—The incidence of tuberculosis is higher among African Americans, Asians and Pacific Islanders, and Native Americans than it is among non-Hispanic Whites; in children, ethnic minorities account for almost 83% of reported tuberculosis. The incidence of HIV disease among ethnic groups with higher rates of tuberculosis may account from some of the difference (Giger, 2013).
- Diabetes has a high incidence among Seminoles, Pimas, and Papagos but is rare among Native Alaskans. Diabetes is the seventh leading cause of death in U.S. Whites, whereas it is the fourth leading cause among Native Americans and the fifth leading cause in Blacks, Asians, and Hispanics or Latinos.

Hypertension
- Among African Americans, hypertension has an earlier onset, is more severe, and has a higher mortality than among Whites; 44% of African Americans over 40 years of age are hypertensive.

Sickle cell disease
- This common genetic disorder primarily affects African Americans. It also occurs in people from Asia Minor, India, the Mediterranean, and the Caribbean.

clinicalALERT
Early recognition and treatment of crisis symptoms are essential. Mrs. Johnson is in sickle cell crisis and needs immediate hospitalization.

HIV/AIDS
- The incidence of HIV/AIDS among African Americans is nearly 8 times as high as it is in Whites. HIV disease is the tenth leading cause of death in African Americans.

Lactose intolerance
- Intolerance affects 66% of Mexican Americans and 90% of African Americans, Asians, and Ashkenazi Jews.
- Most affected patients only need to restrict, not eliminate, lactose-containing foods.

Nursing implications
- Be aware that people differ in their susceptibility to disease because of biologic variations.
- Remember that a relationship exists between culture and body weight, skin color, other visible physical characteristics, enzymatic and genetic variations, and risk for certain diseases.
- Many diseases can be linked to a genetic influence. People of certain cultures may be more susceptible to some diseases or conditions.

Self-Reflection Questions
1. What is your understanding of the role that biologic variations play in susceptibility to disease by culture?
2. Have you been educated in a system that acknowledges biologic variation among cultural groups?
3. How can you provide culturally competent care without overgeneralizing or stereotyping?

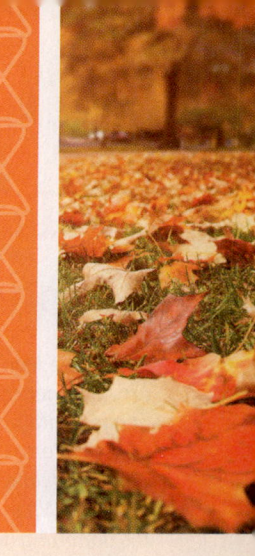

CHAPTER 4
The Older Adult in Health and Illness

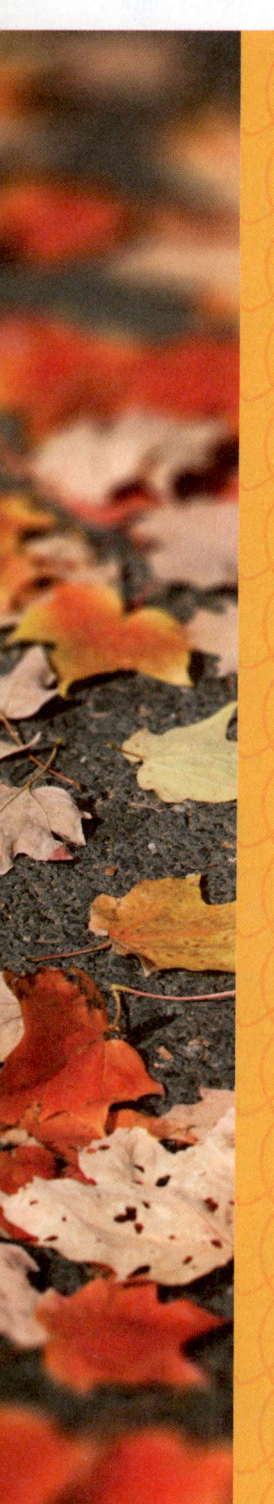

BRIEF OUTLINE

What Is Old?

Why Do People Age?

Ageism and Stereotypes About Older Adults

Developmental Aspects of Aging

Experiencing and Adapting to Change

Health of the Older Adult

Nursing Care to Promote Health

APPLIED LEARNING OUTCOMES

After completing this chapter, you will be able to:

1. Describe what is meant by the term *old*, including who is considered an *older adult*.
2. Discuss selected theories of aging, including those involving genetics, immunity, free radicals, and apoptosis.
3. Define *ageism*, incorporating common myths of older adults.
4. Apply an understanding of cognitive, psychosocial, moral, and spiritual development when caring for the older adult.
5. Consider age-related physical and psychosocial changes common to older adults when assessing, planning, and implementing care.
6. Describe common threats to the health of the older adult, including chronic illness, accidental injuries, medication management, and dementia and confusion.
7. Incorporate actions to promote health and quality of life into nursing care of older adults.

KEY TERMS

The key terms are defined on the pages listed below.

ageism 53

cognition 53

dementia 59

geriatrics 51

gerontologic nursing 51

reminiscence 54

senescence 53

sundowning syndrome 59

widowhood 57

Key Concept   The population of older adults in the United States is growing more rapidly than any other age group. Nurses need a good understanding of the unique needs and health issues affecting older adults.

Growing older is not always easy, but it happens to everyone who lives long enough. As one ages, physical and psychosocial processes are altered; developmental tasks continue to influence choices and behaviors; and changes may occur in living arrangements, employment, and income. Added to those areas of adjustment are the very real possibility of loss of a spouse and significant others, changes in role and status, and disruptions in health.

The older adult population (those age 65 years and older) is increasing more rapidly than any other age group. In the last century, the number of adults in the United States living to age 65 or older more than tripled. That percentage is projected to be about 19% by the year 2030, with the largest increase occurring in adults over the age of 75 years (Figure 4-1■). At that time, the life expectancy is projected to be 78.5 years. Currently, the life expectancy in North America is 78.7 years, with the White population living about 4 years longer than Black Americans (National Center for Health Statistics, 2013).

The increase in the number of older adults has important implications for nursing. The aging of America will result in a huge demand for health care and social services. Patients needing health care in all settings will be older. They will require nursing interventions and teaching designed specifically to meet their needs. **Geriatrics** is the area of health care that focuses on the holistic care of older adults, including physiologic, psychologic, and socioeconomic aspects of aging. Although **gerontologic nursing**

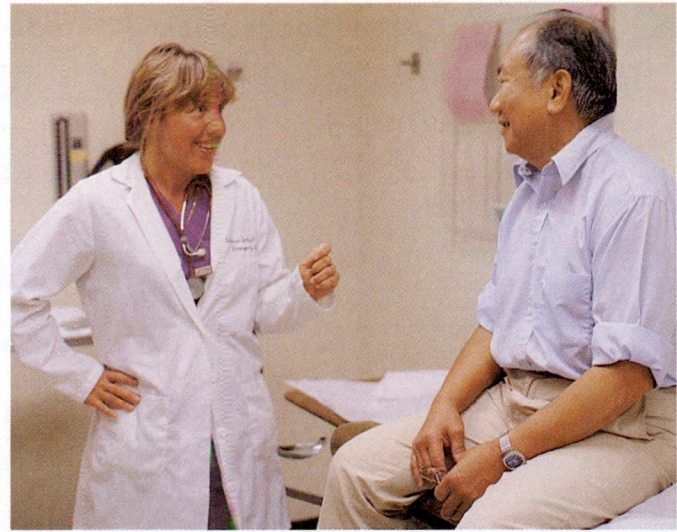

Figure 4-2. ■ The older population is increasing more rapidly than any other age group, making gerontologic nursing a major part of medical–surgical nursing. (Photographer: Richard Tauber, Pearson Education.)

(nursing care of the older adult) is a nursing specialty area, it is also an integral component of medical–surgical nursing (Figure 4-2■).

What Is Old?

Aging is defined in a number of ways. To some, aging is seen as a universal process beginning at birth. To others, aging is viewed as being "old" or reaching "older adulthood," with people defining *aging* in terms of personal meaning and experience. On the basis of the 1935 Social Security Act, reaching the age of 65 years has been established as the criterion for retirement and eligibility for economic and health care benefits. However, most experts in gerontology agree that there is no one age that defines a person as "old."

The older adult period begins at age 65, but it can be further divided into three periods: the "young-old" (age 65 to 74 years), the "middle-old" (age 75 to 84 years), and the "old-old" (age 85 years and older). The rapid increase projected in the aging population by the 2030s is largely the result of the "baby boom," which refers to the increased number of people born in the post–World War II period from 1946 to 1964. People in this generation began turning 65 years old in 2011; by 2030, the projected number of people 65 and older is expected to reach nearly 72.8 million (U.S. Census Bureau, 2012).

In addition to the effect of the baby boom, the United States has experienced growth in migration from other countries. As a result, minority older adults comprise 20% of all older Americans, and their numbers are expected to increase even more dramatically than the older non-Hispanic White population. By the year 2050, it is projected that 58% of

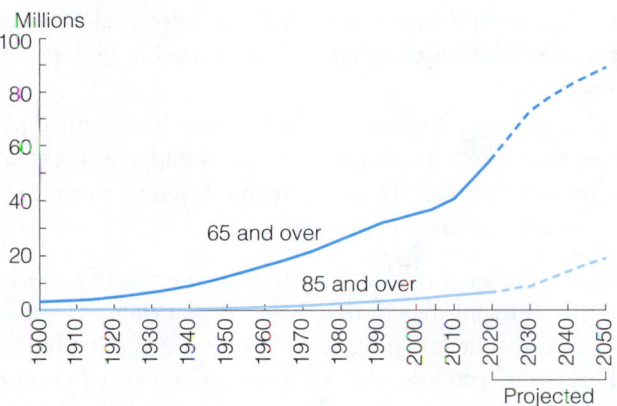

Note: These projections are based on Census 2000 and are not consistent with the 2010 Census results. Projections based on the 2010 Census will be released in late 2012.
Reference population: These data refer to the resident population.

Figure 4-1. ■ Number of people age 65 years and older, by age group, for selected years 1900–2010 and projected 2020–2050.
(Source: Federal Interagency Forum on Aging-Related Statistics. [2012]. *Older Americans 2012: Key Indicators of Well-Being*, p. 2. Federal Interagency Forum on Aging-Related Statistics. Washington, DC: U.S. Government Printing Office. June 2012.)

TABLE 4-1	Age and Socioeconomic Characteristics of Older Adults
CHARACTERISTIC	**INFORMATION**
Average life expectancy remaining on reaching one's 65th birthday	Men: 17.3 years Women: 20.0 years
Number of older adults	Men: 17.5 million Women: 23 million
Married	Men: 74.2% Women: 44.5%
Live alone	Men: 19% Women: 37.3%
Median income per year	$31,408/year
Sources of income	Social Security: 37% Assets: 11% Pensions: 19% Earnings: 30%
Living below the poverty line	Total: 9% Non-Hispanic White: 6.8% Black: 18% Asian: 14.6% Hispanic: 18%
Completed high school education	80%
Bachelor's degree or higher	23%
Living with a chronic disease	Heart disease: 30.4% Hypertension: 55.9% Any cancer: 24% Asthma: 11.3% Chronic bronchitis or emphysema: 10.3% Diabetes: 20.5% Arthritis: 51.2%

Source: Federal Interagency Forum on Aging-Related Statistics. (2012). Older Americans 2012: Key Indicators of Well-Being.

older adults will be non-Hispanic Caucasians, with 20% of older adults Hispanic, 12% Black, and 9% Asian. The older Hispanic population is expected to grow the most rapidly, surpassing the population of older Black adults to reach 17.5 million in 2050 (Federal Interagency Forum on Aging-Related Statistics, 2012). These numbers have major implications for nurses in providing culturally competent care to an older, increasingly diverse population.

In addition to characteristics unique to age, the older population also has socioeconomic characteristics that differ from those of younger adults, as well as gender and racial group differences. Age and socioeconomic characteristics are outlined in Table 4-1 ■.

Why Do People Age?

Although there is no one answer to this question, different theories (best guesses by experts in an area) have been developed to try to find the cause of aging. It is known that aging is a complex process with great individual variation. The major theories of aging are categorized as biologic and senescence.

Biologic aging theories examine the basic aging processes that affect all living organisms and try to explain age-related changes. There are many different theories; selected ones include the following:

- *Genetic/biologic clock theories* emphasize the role of genes in aging. A major idea in this theory is that there is a programmed code for aging stored in the DNA of body cells. This theory proposes that each person's inherited genetic code predicts physical condition, risk for certain diseases, and, to a certain extent, the age and cause of death.

- *Immunity theories* are based on the knowledge that components of the immune system are affected by aging. Because of this effect, called *immunosenescence*, a person has fewer defenses against foreign organisms with aging. Therefore, the older adult is more susceptible to chronic illnesses such as cancer, arthritis, cardiovascular disease, and Alzheimer disease.

- In the *free-radical theory* (free radicals are very unstable and reactive molecules, formed during metabolism and in response to environmental pollutants), free radicals interact with and damage cellular components, such as lipids and proteins. Antioxidants are among the major protective mechanisms of the body; however, these may become less effective with aging.

- The *programmed aging theory* proposes that cells stop dividing as they age, resulting in cell death, or *apoptosis*. Apoptosis is a normal process that occurs throughout life, regulated by opposing genes. With aging, the process becomes imbalanced or ineffective, and the disability and degeneration common to increasing age are seen.

- The *wear and tear theory* holds that over time, aging cells lose their ability to repair damage due to injury, inflammation, or other causes. Tissues of vital organs are unable to regenerate, leading to impaired organ function.

Longevity and **senescence** (aging) theories focus on why people live as long as they do. Studies have found that the factors that influence a long and healthy life include genetic factors, physical environment, physical activity throughout life, consumption of alcohol, sexual activity persisting into advanced years, dietary factors, and social environment. Other theories have been developed to explain the relationships between aging and health behaviors and to design interventions to delay the onset of senescence and chronic illness.

Ageism and Stereotypes About Older Adults

Ageism is a form of prejudice (like racism) in which older adults are stereotyped by characteristics found only in a small number of their age group. Basic to the prejudice of ageism is the belief that all older people are different and will remain different; as a result, they do not experience the same needs, desires, and concerns. In an industrial society that values productivity, retired people may be considered to have "outlived their usefulness." In addition, younger generations often lose ties with the older generation because of increased mobility of the family, so many young adults lack experiences with older relatives.

Older adults may be incorrectly pictured as being rigid and narrow-minded, unable to learn, unreliable because of memory problems, too old to enjoy sexual pleasure, or childlike and dependent. Many older adults dread growing older because they believe others will see them as poor, lonely, in frail health, and housed in a nursing home during their final years. These characteristics and descriptions are not true of most older adults. Myths about older adults, compared with the realities of aging, are outlined in Table 4-2■. Health care workers may have negative perceptions of older adults and need to understand that most older adults are healthy and want to maintain their level of health and function as long as possible.

Most older people are satisfied with their lives, enjoying retirement and the time to do more of the things they have not had time to do before. The majority have adequate incomes, live in their own homes, maintain close ties with their families, and maintain an interest in community activities.

Developmental Aspects of Aging

Although older adults do not continue to grow and develop physically, they do develop in other areas of life and have well-defined stages and tasks.

COGNITIVE DEVELOPMENT

Cognition is a term used to mean the ability to perceive and understand one's world. Cognitive function does not normally change with aging. Intelligence continues to

TABLE 4-2	Common Myths About Older Adults
MYTH	**REALITY**
Families do not care for older members.	Their families provide 80% of the care needed by older adults.
Most older adults live in nursing homes.	Less than 5% of older adults live in nursing homes and other institutional settings.
Most older adults are sick.	Almost half of all older adults rate their health as good or excellent.
Older adults are incapable of learning new knowledge and skills.	Although the speed that new information is processed becomes slower with age, older adults are capable of learning new things.
Older adults are not interested in sex.	Although sexual activity may be less frequent, the ability to perform and enjoy sexual activity lasts well into the 90s in healthy older adults.
All older adults have problems with constipation and incontinence.	Constipation results from inactivity and diet, not aging. Incontinence is not a normal part of aging and requires medical attention.
Older adults require fewer hours of sleep.	The amount of sleep needed does not change with aging; maintaining sleep quality and quantity becomes more difficult, however.

develop and increase well into the 60s, and learning continues throughout life. Older adults do often take longer to process information and to respond, especially in new environments. Nurses should allow extra time when teaching older adults and should slow the pace of care for those who are ill. Mild short-term memory loss is often experienced, but is managed with lists and calendars. Long-term memory usually remains intact. Dementing diseases do occur and cause cognitive impairment, as stated later in this chapter and discussed in Chapter 48.

PSYCHOSOCIAL DEVELOPMENT

Although a person's self-concept and sense of identity remain relatively stable throughout the life span, the way in which the older adult feels about self is often the result of the type of person he or she was before reaching later years. For example, the person who successfully met challenges and made adjustments will be more likely to consider himself or herself healthy and remain socially active. On the other hand, a person who has had difficulty coping with life may find retirement, loss of a spouse, or an illness to be devastating. An early psychosocial theory, called *disengagement theory*, proposed that as people age they become more introspective and focused on self, withdrawing from usual roles and interactions with others. This has been proven untrue; rather as societal interactions decrease (e.g., as a result of retirement), older adults increase their close relationships with family and friends.

Erikson (1963) identified ego integrity versus despair and disgust as the last stage of human development. During this stage, which begins at about 60 years of age, adults begin to reflect on their lives. If they are satisfied, they accept the past as a part of the present and accept physiologic decline without fear of death. In the process, older adults often tell stories of their past in what is called *life review* or **reminiscence**. This allows the older adult to relive and restructure life experiences and is part of achieving ego integrity. The same process can be used therapeutically to facilitate coping with change, such as treatment for an illness or moving to a residential care facility. Examples of activities to facilitate reminiscence are listed in Box 4-1 ■.

Havighurst (1972) believed the major tasks of old age centered on maintaining social contacts and relationships, with successful aging depending on one's ability to adapt to age-related roles. He described the developmental tasks for later maturity as adjusting to decreasing physical strength and health, adjusting to retirement and reduced income, adjusting to death of a spouse, establishing an affiliation with one's age group, adjusting and adapting social roles in a flexible way, and establishing a satisfactory physical living arrangement.

BOX 4-1	**EXAMPLES OF ACTIVITIES TO ENCOURAGE REMINISCENCE**

- Choose a comfortable place to sit and talk.
- Use open-ended questions to encourage the person to talk about both negative and positive life events.
- Encourage the person to write about his or her life and share it with family and friends.
- Record the person telling the stories and play this oral history back as appropriate.
- Ask the person to write about significant events on or near the year they occurred (forming a time line of his or her life).
- Ask family members to bring in pictures or scrapbooks that depict events in the person's life.
- Encourage the person to develop a family tree. Many sources are now available on the Internet about genealogy.

MORAL AND SPIRITUAL DEVELOPMENT

According to Kohlberg (1969), older adults have completed the stages of moral development and are at the conventional level, following society's rules and meeting the expectations of others. Spiritually, most older adults integrate faith and truth to see the reality of their own beliefs, trusting in a greater power and believing in the future. By integrating the past and future into the present, the older adult can more easily accept where he or she is in life without regretting past mistakes or fearing the future, in a process called self-transcendence (Reed, 1996). With aging, spirituality and transcendence are sources of strength when faced with inevitable changes and loss. Many older adults openly express their spiritual beliefs with pictures, bibles, and religious items such as rosaries or crucifixes. It is very important for health care providers to respect the older adult's views and take proper care of these items if the older adult is not able to do so.

Experiencing and Adapting to Change

Key Concept Older adults must adapt not only to physiologic changes of aging but also to psychosocial, socioeconomic, and environmental changes.

The older adult is a member of a unique population in the world today. Older adults have lived the longest and experienced the most change, both in themselves and in the society in which they live. Adaptation is necessary with advancing age because of limitations involving one's spouse, loss of health, or changing economic ability and living arrangement. Numerous role changes are necessary, and lost roles must be replaced with those that are satisfying to the person. Depending on the ability to adapt to change, older adults may live out their remaining years happy and at peace or in a state of conflict and confusion.

AGE-RELATED PHYSICAL CHANGES

As we age, the number of cells of the body is gradually reduced. Lean body mass decreases, but fat tissue increases until one is in one's 60s. Bone mass and intracellular fluids tend to decrease. As a result, older adults are at increased risk for bone fractures from falls and trauma and for dehydration in response to illness or environmental heat.

Many physical changes are obvious, including hair graying and loss, wrinkled skin, baggy eyelids, facial hair in women, and a reduction in height by about 2 in. by age 80 years. These changes are gradual over time and are highly individualized. Some people look old at 50, whereas others still retain a youthful appearance when they are 70. Other age-related changes affect specific body systems, as illustrated in Figure 4-3 ■ and summarized in Table 4-3 ■. More detailed information is provided in each assessment chapter of this book, and nursing actions specific to age-related physical changes are integrated throughout the text.

Most older adults adjust their lifestyle over time to accommodate age-related changes. Although continued physical activity and exercise are important, regular periods of rest are also needed. With decreasing body reserves, the older adult is at increased risk for both acute and chronic illnesses. As a result, diet modifications and prescribed medications may be necessary, as well as learning to live with some pain from common chronic illnesses such as arthritis. The older adult is at greater risk for injuries from accidents and falls and may need to curtail driving or use some type of assistive device to remain mobile. All of these factors cause some loss of independence.

AGE-RELATED SLEEP CHANGES

Age-related changes in the nervous and other body systems contribute to changes in the quality and quantity of sleep in the older adult. Older adults tend to have more difficulty falling asleep, experience more frequent awakenings during sleep, and sleep fewer hours at night with more frequent daytime napping (Tabloski, 2014). Other health problems commonly associated with aging also can affect sleep. People with heart or lung disease may have difficulty breathing when recumbent, making it necessary to sleep in an upright position. Chronic pain associated with arthritis can interfere with finding a comfortable sleeping position and maintaining sleep. Depression commonly leads to sleep

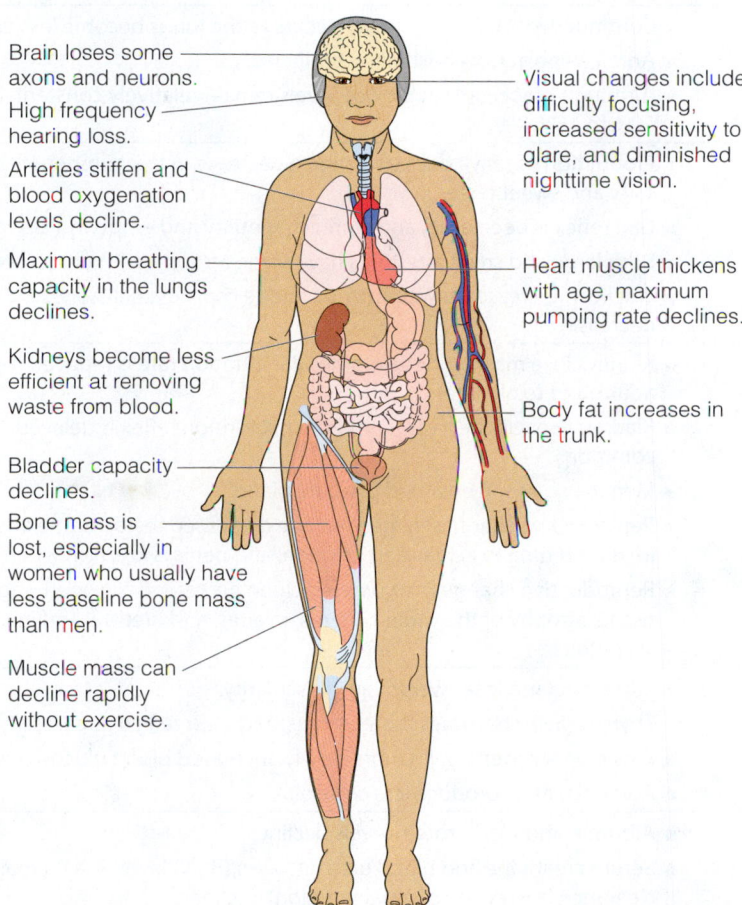

Brain loses some axons and neurons.

High frequency hearing loss.

Arteries stiffen and blood oxygenation levels decline.

Maximum breathing capacity in the lungs declines.

Kidneys become less efficient at removing waste from blood.

Bladder capacity declines.

Bone mass is lost, especially in women who usually have less baseline bone mass than men.

Muscle mass can decline rapidly without exercise.

Visual changes include difficulty focusing, increased sensitivity to glare, and diminished nighttime vision.

Heart muscle thickens with age, maximum pumping rate declines.

Body fat increases in the trunk.

Figure 4-3. ■ Multisystem changes associated with aging. (Source: "Figure 1.08 - Normal Changes of Aging" from Gerontological Nursing, 2e by Patricia A Tabloski. Published by Pearson Education, © 2010.)

TABLE 4-3	Age-Related Physical Changes in Older Adults
ASSESSMENT	**CHANGES**
Skin	■ Decreased subcutaneous tissue and sebaceous gland activity results in dry, wrinkled skin. ■ Melanocytes cluster, causing "age spots" or "liver spots."
Hair and nails	■ Scalp, axillary, and pubic hair thins; nose and ear hair thickens. ■ Women may develop facial hair. ■ Nails grow more slowly and may become thick and brittle.
Sensory	■ Visual field narrows, and depth perception is distorted. ■ Pupils are smaller, reducing night vision. ■ Lenses yellow and become opaque, resulting in distortion of green, blue, and violet tones and increased sensitivity to glare. ■ Production of tears decreases. ■ Sense of smell decreases. ■ Age-related hearing loss progresses, involving middle- and low-frequency sounds. ■ Threshold for pain and touch increases. ■ Alterations in proprioception (sense of physical position) may occur.
Musculoskeletal	■ Loss of overall mass, strength, and movement of muscles occurs; tremors may occur. ■ Loss of bone structure and deterioration of cartilage in joints result in increased risk of fractures and limitation of range of motion.
Cardiovascular	■ Systolic blood pressure increases. ■ Cardiac output decreases. ■ Peripheral resistance increases, and capillary walls thicken.
Respiratory	■ Continued loss of vital capacity occurs as the lungs become less elastic and more rigid. ■ Anterior–posterior chest diameter increases. ■ Although blood carbon dioxide levels remain relatively constant, blood oxygen levels decrease by 10% to 15%.
Gastrointestinal	■ Production of saliva decreases, and a decrease in the number of taste buds reduces perception of salty and sweet tastes. ■ Gag reflex is decreased, and stomach motility and emptying are reduced. ■ Both large and small intestines have some atrophy, with decreased peristalsis. ■ The liver decreases in weight and storage capacity; gallstones increase; pancreatic enzymes decrease.
Genitourinary	■ Kidneys lose mass, and the glomerular filtration rate is reduced (by nearly 50% from young adulthood to old age). ■ Bladder capacity decreases, and the micturition reflex is delayed. Urinary retention is more common. ■ Men may have an enlarged prostate gland. ■ Reproductive changes in men include decreased testosterone and sperm count, smaller testes, and increased time to achieve an erection, and penis is less firm when erect. ■ Reproductive changes in women include decreased estrogen, vaginal lubrication, and breast tissue; atrophy of the vagina, uterus, ovaries, and urethra; and increased alkalinity of vaginal secretions.
Endocrine	■ Pituitary gland loses weight and vascularity. ■ Thyroid gland becomes more fibrous, and plasma T_3 decreases. ■ Pancreas releases insulin more slowly; increased blood glucose levels are common. ■ Adrenal glands produce less cortisol.
Laboratory values	■ Albumin and total protein levels decline. ■ Serum creatinine and blood urea nitrogen (BUN) levels may remain within normal limits; creatinine clearance (a measure of renal function) declines. ■ Serum cholesterol, high-density lipoprotein (HDL), and triglyceride levels increase with aging. ■ Blood glucose levels increase slightly.

problems, including difficulty falling asleep, early awakening, and frequent daytime napping. Dementia-related sleep problems include disruption of the normal sleep–wake cycle, less REM sleep (also called "dream sleep"), and little or no deep sleep.

AGE-RELATED PSYCHOSOCIAL CHANGES

Psychosocial changes for the older adult include the illness or death of a spouse, decreased or limited income, retirement, and isolation from friends and family because of distance, lack of transportation, or relocation to a long-term care facility. A further change may be role loss or reversal, for example, when a wife who has been considered the dependent one becomes the caregiver of her chronically ill husband.

Widowhood

Life changes immeasurably when a spouse dies, even though it is a common event. Suddenly the remaining spouse is faced with not only adjusting to the loss of the loved person but also to living alone. **Widowhood** (loss of a spouse) affects more women than men, primarily because women tend to live longer than men. Many older women find that income from the husband's pension or retirement is discontinued or reduced after his death, necessitating living on a sharply reduced income. Sexual desires are unfulfilled, and the number of single friends is limited. However, after the initial grief diminishes (see Chapter 13), most widows adjust well.

Retirement

The loss of one's role as a worker through retirement is a major adjustment for aging adults. When one's work is the primary interest and focus of life, activities, and social contacts, separation from employment leaves a large void. In addition, income may be significantly reduced, despite pensions and Social Security benefits, with retirement income often being only half of the income earned when employed. However, many retirees take advantage of more free time to become more active in volunteer activities, to join senior citizen groups for socialization, and to do things they enjoy but have not previously had time to do (Figure 4-4■).

Living Arrangements

Although almost all older adults would prefer to live in their own homes, and more than 90% do, it is not always possible. The ability to function safely and independently at home depends on one's functional health, transportation, income, and family or support systems. Many older adults, even though in poor health, can continue living at home with some assistance through home health services, home-delivered meals, and senior transportation. Assisted-living housing for older adults is becoming more common, providing housekeeping, meals, and health care

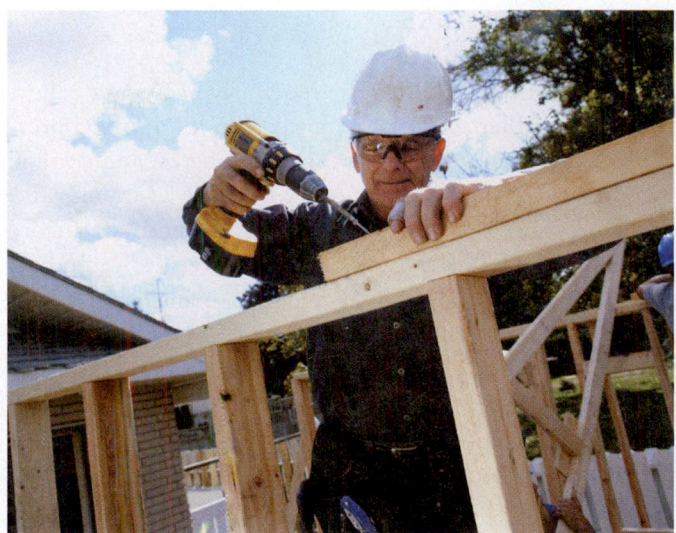

Figure 4-4. ■ Many older adults find creative outlets during retirement. (Source: © Radius Images/Alamy.)

services. Some areas now provide "aging-in-place" models, where people are provided the care needed as they advance in age. There are many different types of housing options for older adults; a selected few are described as follows:

- Home modification, such as replacing door knobs with handles, replacing faucet handles with levers, and installing grab bars in bathrooms, may allow older adults to remain in their own home.
- Senior retirement communities offer rental apartments or houses for people who are mobile and can care for themselves. Meals may be available, housekeeping services may be provided (at additional cost), social and recreational activities are carried out, and transportation is provided.
- Residential care facilities provide services that include room, meals, personal care, and medical care.
- Long-term care facilities provide skilled nursing care, including meals, personal care, and medical care. Bedrooms and bathrooms may be shared.

Health of the Older Adult

Key Concept   Although most older adults rate their health as good, the incidence of chronic diseases, sensory and cognitive deficits, and activity limitations is higher in older adults. Older adults also use more medications and are at high risk for injury due to falls, fire, and motor vehicle crashes.

The older adult is at risk for alterations in health from a variety of causes, including chronic illnesses, accidental injuries, medication management, and dementia. This section provides a broad overview of the health care problems and needs of the older adult; more specific information is found throughout the book.

CHRONIC ILLNESS

More than 50% of all older adults are affected by at least one chronic illness. The most frequently occurring conditions in the older adult are hypertension (high blood pressure), arthritis, heart disease, cancer, diabetes, and chronic lung disease. These conditions can cause years of pain, disability, and loss of function and independence before resulting in death. Daily functional activities, including such activities as shopping and meal preparation, are limited for just over 40% of older adults (Federal Interagency Forum on Aging-Related Statistics, 2012). The leading causes of death for older adults are heart disease (Chapter 16), cancer (Chapter 12), chronic lower respiratory disease (Chapter 23), stroke (Chapter 38), and Alzheimer disease (Chapter 48) (NCHS, 2012).

Like the general population of the United States, the older adult population is becoming more culturally diverse. The health status of racial and ethnic minority populations lags behind that of the White majority; while 78% of non-Hispanic White older adults rate their health as good to excellent, 63% of African Americans and Hispanics age 65 and older give a comparable health rating. Chronic conditions such as high blood pressure, diabetes, and cancer affect a disproportionate number of ethnic minorities.

In the older adult, the accumulation of years of exposure to environmental hazards such as sun and noise may be manifested by skin cancer, cataracts, or impaired hearing. The older adult may develop chronic respiratory disorders from years of smoking or from exposure to pollutants in the environment. Socioeconomic status affects the health of older adults in a variety of ways. Behaviors such as smoking and physical inactivity are more common in people with lower socioeconomic status. Predominantly low socioeconomic neighborhoods tend to be less safe and have fewer available health-related resources (NCHS, 2012).

New challenges have been created by the increase in life span and the increasing incidence of chronic illness in older adults. Medicare spending increased rapidly in the 1990s and early part of the twenty-first century. By 2030, health care spending is predicted to increase by 25% simply because the population will be older. Most people with significant limitations in activities of daily living (ADLs) live at home or in a community setting rather than an institution. Many of these older adults rely on a family caregiver, often an aging spouse or adult child. The value of family caregivers, considered "free," is estimated to be $257 billion a year.

Some suggested areas for teaching older adults how to cope with chronic illness follow. Encourage patients to:
- Assume responsibility for their own health care by getting as much information from as many sources as possible.
- Define what has been lost, so as to develop alternate ways to regain those lost functional abilities.
- Recognize that behavior that is appropriate for acute illness may not be adaptive when a person is chronically ill.
- Deal with emotional realities and go forward with life.
- Develop coping strategies for adapting to the way things are at this moment in time.
- Be positive.

ACCIDENTAL INJURIES

Injuries in the older adult cause many different problems: illness, financial burden, hospitalization, self-care deficits, loss of independence, and even death. The risk of injury is increased by normal physical changes that accompany aging, by changes in health, by environmental hazards, and by lack of support systems. The three major causes of injury in the older adult are falls, fires, and motor vehicle crashes. Of these causes, falls that result in hip fractures are the most significant in terms of long-term disability and death.

Older adults should practice the following to avoid injury:
- Have adequate lighting in all rooms of the house including stairs, basements, and bedrooms. Use night-lights in bedrooms, bathrooms, and halls.
- Avoid sitting or standing rapidly; if dizziness occurs, remain in one position until dizziness is gone.
- Have handrails installed by the toilet and in the shower or bathtub.
- Do not use throw rugs.
- Install smoke alarms.
- Never step into a tub or shower without checking the temperature of the water.
- Always wear corrective lenses and/or hearing aids when driving.
- Do not drive a car after taking medications that cause drowsiness or dizziness.

clinicalALERT

Elder abuse and neglect further increase the risk of injury or illness.

MEDICATION MANAGEMENT

The majority of community-dwelling older adults take at least one prescription medication; 40% or more take five medications every week (Tabloski, 2014). Older adults spend an average of about $660 out of pocket annually on prescribed medications, which represents less than one-fourth the actual cost (the remainder is paid by private insurance or by Medicare). Older adults also consume over-the-counter medications such as nonsteroidal anti-inflammatory drugs and analgesics, multivitamins, and other supplements. Consumption of multiple medications, while often necessary to treat chronic conditions, carries a risk of adverse drug reactions, drug–drug and drug–food interactions, and decreased ability of the liver and kidneys to detoxify and excrete substances. Age-related changes in body tissues (decreased lean body mass and increased adipose tissue) also increase the older adult's risk for toxic and adverse drug responses. In older adults, adverse effects such as dizziness, numbness, dehydration, anorexia, nausea, and diarrhea can have more serious consequences than in younger adults. These consequences include falls, depression, confusion, hallucinations, and malnutrition. Factors contributing to problems with medication management in this age group include visual deficits, memory changes, cost, transportation difficulties, and noncompliance.

Nurses must have knowledge of medications and how their effects may differ for older adults. For example, caution must be used when giving benzodiazepines such as *lorazepam* (Ativan) and *clonazepam* (Klonopin), which increase the risk of impaired cognition, delirium, falls, and fractures in older adults. Long-acting oral antidiabetic agents in the sulfonylurea class such as *glyburide* (DiaBeta) are avoided as they place the older adult at risk for severe prolonged hypoglycemia. Other drugs to avoid because of their toxic effects include the antidepressant *amitriptyline* (Elavil), the antihypertensive methyldopa (Aldomet), the nonsteroidal anti-inflammatory drug indomethacin (Indocin), and gastrointestinal antispasmodics hyoscyamine (Anaspaz) and propantheline (Pro-Banthine). *Digoxin* is commonly prescribed for older adults with heart failure, but carries a high risk of toxicity (American Geriatrics Society, 2012). (Note: Italicized medications are among the 200 most frequently prescribed drugs in the United States.)

DEMENTIA AND CONFUSION

Although growing older is often associated with becoming demented, this is not true. **Dementia** is a term used to refer to different kinds of organic disorders that progressively affect cognitive function, and it is **not** a part of the normal aging process. Although there are various dementias, the one most devastating to the older population, as well as society as a whole, is Alzheimer disease (AD). AD is the most common degenerative neurologic illness and the most common cause of cognitive impairment (Grossman & Porth, 2014). Scientists do not know what causes AD, but they do know that age is the most important risk factor, with the number of people with AD doubling every 5 years after age 65. It is believed that as many as 5.1 million Americans have AD, with the highest prevalence among people 90 years and older (National Institute on Aging [NIA], 2012). The early symptoms of AD, such as loss of concentration and forgetfulness, are frequently missed because the same

symptoms are common with aging. However, it is important to note that AD is not considered a normal part of aging and the majority of people with mild cognitive impairment do not progress to dementia; some even improve (NIA, 2012). AD is discussed in detail in Chapter 48.

Confusion and depression in an older adult can be mistaken for true dementia. It is important to assess for other causes, including circulatory or metabolic problems, electrolyte imbalances, effects of medications, or nutritional deficiencies. Depression commonly affects older adults: 12% of people age 65 and older have clinical symptoms of depression, while 18% of those 85 years and older are affected (Federal Interagency Forum on Aging-Related Statistics, 2012). An older adult may also become confused when too many changes or losses occur at one time or when he or she is moved to a different environment. A type of confusion called **sundowning syndrome** may also occur, in which the older adult becomes confused and agitated after dark.

clinical**ALERT**

A new onset of confusion in an older adult may indicate an acute disease (such as an infection) or an adverse drug response. A sudden change in mental status (over hours, days, or even a week) should prompt notification of the RN or physician and a focused assessment of possible causes.

Nursing Care to Promote Health

Key Concept   Nurses promote health in older adults by teaching healthy behaviors and encouraging healthy lifestyles, preventive medicine (including screening examinations and immunizations), injury prevention, and self-management of illness.

Older adults get the same benefits from health teaching that young adults and middle adults do. They should never be viewed as being "too old" to learn healthy living practices. However, nurses should adapt teaching methods to this age group, such as by providing written material, using charts and literature with large print. Hospitals, long-term care facilities, retirement centers, outpatient clinics, senior citizen centers, and other community settings all provide health education for the older adult. Many older adults are computer and Internet literate, and can be referred to appropriate Web resources for health information, support, and additional information. The nurse provides nursing care as outlined in Table 4-4■. The nurse also promotes health in the older adult by teaching and encouraging the behaviors listed in Box 4-2■ and by providing information about known risk factors and recommended screening for early detection of disease.

TABLE 4-4	Nursing Care to Promote Health in Older Adults
FUNCTIONAL AREA	Nursing Actions
Physiologic function	■ Assess current status, including functional ADLs, and monitor for changes on an ongoing basis. ■ Review beliefs about current health status and health problems. ■ Maintain a list and periodically review use of prescribed and over-the-counter medications and supplements. ■ Provide nursing care to maintain physical status, such as skin care and assisting with ADLs.
Psychosocial function	■ Discuss major stressors, such as illness, injury, hospitalization, or change in living arrangements. ■ Ask preferred name. ■ Respect belongings. ■ Assess and encourage use of sources of support and strength, including family, friends, pets, community resources, and cultural and spiritual values and rituals. ■ Encourage independent decision making about care. ■ Encourage life review and reminiscence. ■ Encourage self-care. ■ Develop plans of care that are patient-centered and individualized to the patient's background, interests, capabilities, values, culture, and lifestyle.
Cognitive function	■ Ensure eyeglasses and hearing devices are used; ensure lenses are clean and batteries are good. ■ Slow pace of activities. ■ Wait for responses during conversations. ■ Encourage interaction with other people.
Sleep and rest	■ Discourage excessive napping. ■ Assess and use information about normal bedtime, time for rising, and bedtime rituals. ■ Assess effects of pain, medications, and anxiety on sleep.
Nutrition	■ Assess for lost or damaged teeth and state of dentures if present. ■ Assist with oral care as necessary. ■ Provide food that the patient is able to chew and swallow. ■ Assess height, weight, eating patterns, and food choices. ■ Suggest programs such as Meals-on-Wheels if appropriate.
Elimination	■ Assess frequency of urinary elimination, including problems with urinary incontinence. ■ Assess usual times for bowel movements. ■ Monitor frequency and consistency of bowel movements, and if a problem is present, consider effects of diet, activity, and medications. ■ Review diet for fiber and fluid intake.
Activity and exercise	■ Assess mobility; ensure assistive devices (e.g., a cane or walker) are available. ■ Consider effects of illness, surgery, medications, and changes in diet and fluid intake on strength and motor function. ■ Recommend moderate exercise 30 minutes each day.
Safety	■ Assess ability to swallow. ■ Review medications with the patient, including type, dosage, times of administration, and precautions (e.g., interactions, adverse effects). ■ Ensure an environment that is free of clutter and well lit. Suggest removing throw rugs and using night-lights. ■ Discuss safety of neighborhood and community.
Sexuality	■ Assist as necessary with hygiene, hair care, clean clothing, makeup, and shaving. ■ Maintain a clean, odor-free environment. ■ Discuss safer sex if appropriate. ■ Discuss vaginal lubricants with women; refer men for evaluation of erectile dysfunction if appropriate.

BOX 4-2   PATIENT TEACHING

Health Promotion for the Older Adult

- Choose foods from all food groups, and eat a variety of foods. Balance food and calorie intake with physical activity to maintain an appropriate weight.
- Choose a diet that includes at least seven servings of fruits and vegetables and six servings of whole grains daily.
- Choose a diet low in fat (30% or less of total calories), saturated fat (less than 10% of calories), and cholesterol (less than 300 mg daily).
- Use sugar in moderation, and limit sodium intake to less than 1,500 mg daily. Limit intake of refined grains and prepared and processed foods.
- If possible, obtain at least 30 minutes of exposure to sunlight daily. Use sunscreen and avoid sunburn.
- Increase calcium intake to 1,200 mg and consume 600 mg of vitamin D daily.
- Limit alcohol consumption, if any, to no more than one drink per day.
- If weight loss is needed, aim for a slow, steady loss by decreasing caloric intake while maintaining a balanced nutrient intake and increasing physical activity.
- Make exercise a part of life, carrying out regular exercise that is moderately strenuous, is consistent, and avoids overexertion. Include stretching, aerobic exercise, and weight training or resistance exercises for 30 minutes or longer five or more days per week.
- Sleep 7 to 8 hours each day.
- Eliminate smoking and use of other tobacco products.
- Maintain recommended immunizations.

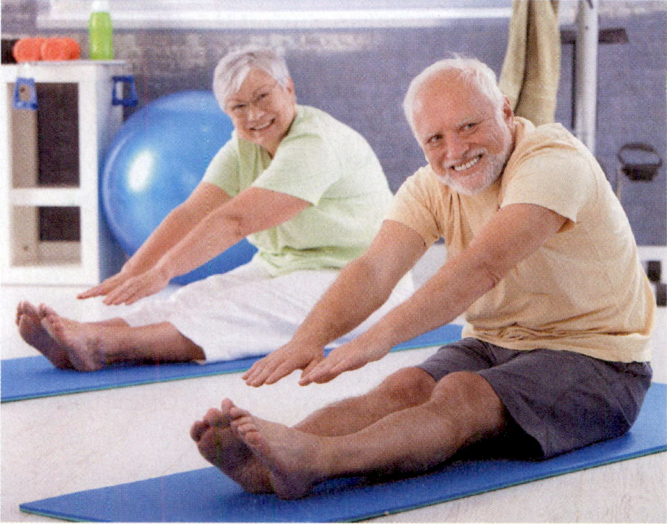

Figure 4-5. ■ A regular program of exercise is important for maintenance of joint mobility and muscle tone. Participation in exercise classes or groups also can promote socialization. (Source: © nyul/Fotolia.)

It is important to remember that illness and loss of independence are not inevitable consequences of aging. In fact, three behaviors—smoking, poor diet, and physical inactivity—are major risk factors for the leading causes of death and disability in the United States: heart disease, cancer, stroke, and diabetes. These behaviors, all of which are modifiable through health promotion teaching and programs, are the root cause in one-third of deaths in the United States. Actions to improve older Americans' health and quality of life are the following:

- **Addressing health disparities:** Providing health care services and support for older adults who are chronically ill, of low socioeconomic status, and members of an ethnic minority is an increasingly urgent goal to improve the overall health of the nation.
- **Healthy lifestyles:** People who are physically active, eat a healthy diet, do not use tobacco, and practice other healthy behaviors reduce their risk for chronic illnesses

and have half the rate of disability as those who do not (Figure 4-5 ■).

- **Early detection of diseases:** Screening to detect chronic diseases (with examinations such as mammograms and colonoscopies) when they are early in their course and most treatable can save many lives (Table 4-5 ■).
- **Immunizations:** Immunizations for influenza and pneumonia reduce the risk of hospitalization and death. More than 40,000 people age 65 and older die each year of influenza and pneumonia.
- **Oral health:** Maintaining oral health through regular dental care and prevention of dental disease is an important strategy for promoting good nutritional status and overall health.
- **Injury prevention:** Falls are the most common cause of injuries to older adults. More than one-third of adults age 65 and older fall each year, and of that number, 20% to 30% have moderate to severe injury that reduces mobility and independence.
- **Self-management techniques:** Programs to teach older Americans self-management techniques for illnesses such as diabetes and arthritis can reduce both the pain and the costs of chronic disease.
- **Communicating end-of-life wishes:** Talking with family members and health providers about end-of-life decision making, preferably before the onset of serious illness, promotes the older adult's autonomy and control, particularly when unanticipated crises occur.

TABLE 4-5	Recommended Health Screening and Immunizations for Older Adults
EXAMINATION	**FREQUENCY**
Health maintenance exam ■ Height, weight, body mass index (BMI) ■ Risk evaluation and counseling (including alcohol and tobacco use) ■ Safety ■ Behavioral assessment (including depression screening)	Every 1 to 2 years
Blood pressure measurement	At least every 2 years; annually if 120–139/80–89
Breast cancer screening	Clinical breast exam annually Mammogram every 1 to 2 years for women to age 75
Cervical cancer (Pap smear)	May discontinue if no abnormal results in 10 years; resume if has new sexual partner
Cholesterol and lipid profile	Every 5 years
Chlamydia	Women with new or multiple partners
Colorectal cancer	Fecal occult blood test *or* fecal immunochemical test (FIT) annually; and/or Flexible sigmoidoscopy *or* double contrast barium enema every 5 years; or Colonoscopy every 10 years to age 80
Glaucoma	Every 2 years
Osteoporosis	Bone mineral density at least once; may repeat every 2 years for those at risk
Prostate cancer	Prostate-specific antigen (PSA) as determined by risk
Vision and hearing	Objective vision and hearing screening
RECOMMENDED IMMUNIZATIONS	**FREQUENCY**
Tetanus, diphtheria	1 dose every 10 years; substitute 1-time dose of Tdap (includes pertussis) for Td booster
Varicella	2 doses, 4 to 8 weeks apart
Influenza	1 dose annually
Pneumococcal	1 dose
Zoster	1 dose

Note: The references and resources for all chapters have been compiled at the back of the book.

Chapter Review

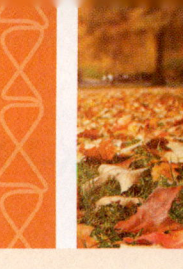

KEY POINTS

- **Concept:** The population of older adults in the United States is growing more rapidly than any other age group. Nurses need a good understanding of the unique needs of and health issues affecting older adults.
- Aging may be defined in many ways, including age in years as well as by personal definition. Older adulthood may be divided into three periods: "young-old" (ages 65 to 74 years), "middle-old" (ages 75 to 84 years), and "old-old" (ages 85 years and older). The rapid increase in older adults in the United States is the result of the baby boom and increased growth of minority populations.
- The theories of why people age include genetic/biologic clock, immune factors, free radicals, programmed aging (apoptosis), and wear and tear. Scientists also study the factors that influence having a long and healthy life, which include genetic inheritance, physical environment, physical activity, and diet.
- Ageism is a form of prejudice in which older adults are stereotyped by characteristics found in only a small number of their age group. Most older adults are satisfied with their lives, have adequate income, live in their own homes, are close to family and friends, and take part in community activities.
- Older adults continue to have developmental tasks. Cognition does not normally change with age. As people

age it is important for them to review their lives through reminiscence in order to achieve ego integrity. Most older adults are at the moral development stage of the conventional level, and find strength in spirituality and transcendence.
- **Concept:** Older adults must adapt not only to physiologic changes of aging but also to psychosocial, socioeconomic, and environmental changes.
- Aging does bring physical changes as well as the strong probability of psychosocial changes, involving widowhood, retirement, and changes in living arrangements.
- **Concept:** Although most older adults rate their health as good, the incidence of chronic diseases, sensory and cognitive deficits, and activity limitations is higher in older adults. Older adults also use many medications and are at high risk for injury due to falls, fire, and motor vehicle crashes.
- The older adult is at risk for alterations in health from chronic illnesses, accidental injuries, medication management, and dementia.
- **Concept:** Nurses promote health in older adults by teaching healthy behaviors and encouraging healthy lifestyles, preventive medicine (including screening examinations and immunizations), injury prevention, and self-management of illness.

PEARSON NURSING STUDENT RESOURCES

Find additional materials at **nursing.pearsonhighered.com.**

NCLEX-PN® Exam Preparation

1 You are assigned to care for Mr. Sanchez, an 84-year-old Hispanic American. Which term might you use to describe Mr. Sanchez's age group accurately?

1. Very old
2. Elderly
3. Middle-old
4. Older adult

2 The immunity theory of aging supports the idea of immunosenescence, meaning people have fewer defenses against foreign organisms with aging. What results from this?

1. Increased risk of chronic illnesses
2. People living a predetermined life span
3. Decreased tolerance of environmental pollutants
4. An imbalance in cell regeneration and cell death

3 A member of your health team says, "Oh, that old lady in Room 232 won't be able to learn how to take her own pulse." What is this an example of?

1. Reality
2. Ageism
3. Critical thinking
4. Nursing process

4 Which of the following statements is true of cognitive function in the older adult?

1. The ability to learn new skills ends at about age 45.
2. Dementia is inevitable as one reaches the 70s.
3. Long-term memory loss interferes with learning.
4. Cognitive function normally does not change.

5 You are caring for an older woman in a long-term care facility. She says, "When I was 10 years old, my parents took me to the circus and I had such a good time." What does this statement facilitate?

1. Problems with short-term memory
2. Achievement of ego integrity
3. Inability to cope with change
4. Increasingly living in the past

6 What two terms might best describe the time after widowhood?

1. Loss, loneliness
2. Bitterness, sadness
3. Peace, strength
4. Friends, family

7 You are caring for an older man who has been hospitalized for treatment of pneumonia. He says, "I want to be able to live in my own home, but I don't know if I can." What topic would you discuss with him?

1. Need for nursing home care
2. Services of the local community center
3. Educational opportunities at a local college
4. Assistance from home health services

8 Which of the following chronic diseases is a leading cause of death in older adults?

1. Pneumonia
2. Influenza
3. Stroke
4. Arthritis

9 You are caring for an older adult who is caring for herself at home alone. What would you assess on a regular basis to facilitate safety?

1. Her temperature, pulse, and respirations
2. Prescribed and over-the-counter medications
3. Amount of food in her refrigerator
4. Condition of the windows in her house

10 Which of the following nursing actions will facilitate cognitive function in an older adult?

1. Giving a complete bed bath
2. Ensuring the television is on
3. Monitoring ability to use walker or cane
4. Ensuring hearing aid battery strength

Answers and rationales for Review Questions appear in Appendix I.

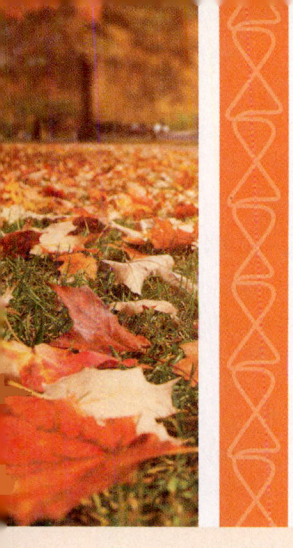

CHAPTER 5
Guidelines for Patient Assessment

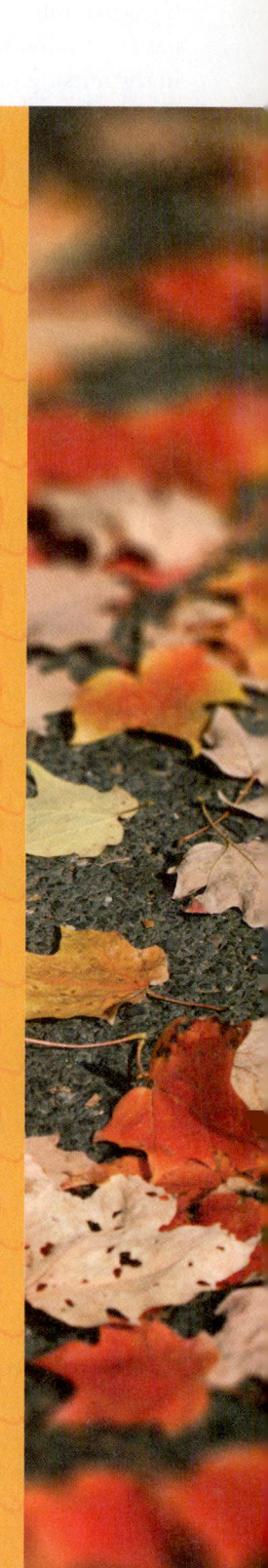

BRIEF OUTLINE

Purposes of a Patient Assessment

Types of Assessment

Sources and Accuracy of Assessment Data

Obtaining a Health History

Methods of Physical Examination

Preparation for a Physical Examination

The Physical Examination

Documentation

APPLIED LEARNING OUTCOMES

After completing this chapter, you will be able to:

1. Discuss the purposes of a patient assessment.
2. Understand and use the types of patient assessment appropriately.
3. Compare sources and accuracy of assessment data.
4. Effectively collect a health history, demonstrating consideration and respect for the patient's culture, ethnicity, values, and health beliefs.
5. Demonstrate the methods of physical examination.
6. Prepare a patient for a physical examination.
7. Perform a physical examination, identifying expected and unexpected findings.
8. Document a health assessment using a written narrative or electronic medical record.

KEY TERMS

The key terms are defined on the pages listed below.

assessment 66	manifestations 66	orthopnea 75
auscultation 69	miosis 74	palpation 68
dyspnea 75	mydriasis 73	percussion 68
inspection 67	objective data 66	subjective data 66

SPECIAL FEATURES

CLINICAL REASONING CARE MAP: Caring for a Patient With Risk for Excess Fluid Volume, 82

CULTURAL CARE STRATEGIES: Appreciating Variations in Facial Expression Across Cultures, 84

> **Key Concept**   Assessment is a critical element of nursing care. Depending on the situation and setting, the nursing assessment may be comprehensive and holistic or focused on a specific event, body system, or problem.

One of the most important aspects of nursing care is assessment. **Assessment** is the process of collecting data (pieces of information) that provide information about the patient's individualized health care needs. It is the first step in the nursing process, providing the base for the planning, implementation, and evaluation of patient care. Assessment by nurses is mandated by nursing standards, nurse practice acts, accrediting bodies, and institutional policies. Depending on state nurse practice acts and agency or institutional protocol, licensed practical or vocational nurses may do most components of the physical assessment, or they may do only selected parts that are within the scope of their defined practice. This chapter provides information about all components of a physical assessment to serve as a knowledge base.

Purposes of a Patient Assessment

The purposes of a patient assessment are to:

- Collect objective data about the patient. **Objective data** (also called *signs*) are observable and/or measurable pieces of information. Objective data can be seen, heard, touched, or smelled. Examples of objective data are the color of urine, vital signs, discoloration of the skin, and breath odor. Laboratory results are also objective data.
- Collect subjective data from the patient. **Subjective data** (also called *symptoms*) are experiences only the patient can describe. Examples of subjective data are nausea, pain, itching, and fatigue.
- Collect information about the patient's family, community, culture, ethnicity, and spiritual factors.
- Identify past and present patient behaviors that support health or increase the risk of illness.
- Identify data that suggest risk for actual health problems.

This chapter provides guidelines for conducting the two components of a health assessment: a health history and a physical examination. Information about health assessments is included in the first chapter of each unit that discusses a disrupted body system function. The term **manifestations** is used throughout this book to refer to objective and subjective data that are associated with specific illnesses. It is essential to remember that documenting (recording) the patient assessment is as important as conducting it.

Types of Assessment

The type of assessment varies depending on the setting, the situation, and the needs of the patient. The types of assessment are an initial comprehensive assessment, an ongoing partial assessment, and a focused assessment.

COMPREHENSIVE ASSESSMENT

When a patient first enters a health care setting, a comprehensive assessment of the patient's health history and physical status is conducted. This provides a baseline for comparing later assessments. The comprehensive assessment may be the responsibility of one health care professional or of different members of the health care team. For example, when a patient enters the hospital setting for inpatient care and receives a comprehensive assessment, a nurse may collect data about the patient's health history, the physician may perform a complete physical examination, and a nursing technician may take vital signs and weight. In a community or home setting, the nurse usually collects all of the assessment data.

PARTIAL ASSESSMENT

An ongoing partial assessment is one that is conducted on a regular basis throughout the patient's care. It usually reviews any problems that have been identified to determine whether changes have occurred or whether new problems are present. A partial assessment is conducted in any type of setting, although the timing may differ. In the hospital, the nurse conducts a partial assessment at the beginning of each shift. In the home, a partial assessment is conducted at each visit (which may vary from daily to once a week).

FOCUSED ASSESSMENT

A focused assessment (through both a focused interview and a focused physical examination) is one that is conducted to assess a specific patient problem. For example, assessment for a patient who has abdominal pain includes assessing body temperature; frequency of bowel movements; pain with urination; any associated trauma; menstrual history (for women); and the location, duration, and type of pain experienced. It does not include assessment of musculoskeletal function or visual acuity. A focused assessment is also a part of other nursing responsibilities, such as when the nurse takes an apical pulse before administering a drug that affects the heart rate. An *emergency assessment* is a special type of focused assessment. It is a very rapid assessment to determine life-threatening situations. The practice of assessing the ABCs (*a*irway, *b*reathing, *c*irculation) before beginning cardiopulmonary resuscitation is an example of an emergency assessment.

Sources and Accuracy of Assessment Data

Data may be collected from primary or secondary sources. The patient is the best source of data and is the primary source. However, if the patient is very young, very ill, unconscious, or confused, data may be collected from secondary sources. Secondary sources include the patient's family or friends, the patient records (such as medical records and laboratory data), and other health care professionals.

Data that are collected must be accurate and factual. General guidelines for ensuring this include the following:

- Compare subjective and objective data. If the patient says, "I feel like I have a fever," compare the statement to an actual measurement of body temperature.
- Consider factors that may interfere with accurate measurements. The patient who has just walked up three flights of stairs may have an increased pulse rate or respiratory rate that is unrelated to a disease process.
- Clarify statements made by the patient. If the patient says, "I have this terrible pain in my stomach," ask the patient to point to the area of pain (which may be abdominal rather than gastric).
- Double-check data that are very high or low. A pulse of 120 or a blood pressure of 70/30 would need verification.
- Do not leap to conclusions. The older patient's dry skin with decreased turgor may be a result of aging; it may not mean the patient is dehydrated.

Obtaining a Health History

> **Key Concept** The health history is a comprehensive record of the patient's past and current health. This information provides valuable cues about the patient's health status and responses to health.

The health history is a collection of subjective and objective data that provide an overall picture of the patient's health status. The data are collected through an interview with the patient and often from secondary sources such as a family member. Many health care institutions and agencies have specific forms with standardized questions to use in obtaining the health history. Although these may vary, most contain the data listed in Table 5-1■.

During the health history, principles of therapeutic communication help you collect accurate data. Most important, use words the patient can understand and listen carefully. Sit in a relaxed posture and maintain eye contact. This open body language tells the patient that you are interested in what is being said. Barriers to collecting accurate data include offering advice, acting disgusted or defensive, disagreeing, offering false assurance, and jumping to conclusions.

Open-ended questions ("Tell me the reason you are here at the clinic today") give the patient the chance to provide more information than closed-ended questions ("Did you come here today because of your back pain?"). Closed-ended questions allow for a "yes" or "no" answer and do not allow the nurse to gather meaningful assessment data. Avoid "why" questions ("Why didn't you come last week when you first noticed this problem?"). "Why" questions often make the patient feel threatened or intimidated. Closed-ended questions are appropriate in emergency situations, when specific information must be collected quickly.

It is very important to be sensitive to cultural differences between you and the patient. Cultural differences influence how both verbal and nonverbal communications are interpreted. Culture and ethnicity, as well as the family in which one grew up and the community in which one lives, also influence health beliefs, health behaviors, and health treatments.

If the patient does not speak the same language as the nurse, a translator is necessary to assist with the interview. The room should be arranged so the patient can see both the nurse and the translator at the same time. Look at the patient, not the translator, and ask questions one at a time in clear, concise terms. It is best to use a facility translator as using the family to translate may often lead to miscommunicated information as well as the patient being uncomfortable sharing information with family members.

Methods of Physical Examination

> **Key Concept** The ability to perform an accurate physical examination and to differentiate normal from abnormal findings is one of the most important roles of today's nurse.

Physical examination is a skill that takes practice. The four basic methods of physical examination are inspection, palpation, percussion, and auscultation. The methods of physical examination used depend on the nurse's level of education, knowledge, and skill acquired through clinical practice and on institutional or agency policy. The four basic methods of physical examination are introduced next.

INSPECTION

Inspection is the method of observing the patient in a careful and deliberate manner, using the senses of seeing, smelling, and hearing to observe abnormal findings. Some body systems are inspected with special equipment; for example, an otoscope is used to inspect the ear canal and

TABLE 5-1	**Information Included in a Health History**
COMPONENT	**INFORMATION**
Biographical data	Name, address, age, gender, marital status, occupation, religious preference, health care financing, usual source of medical care (primary health care provider)
Reason for health care visit (chief complaint)	Documented in patient's own words
History of present illness	When symptoms began Whether onset was sudden or gradual Exact location of the problem Character of the problem (e.g., type of discharge or intensity of pain) Other associated symptoms Type of self-treatment
Past medical history	Childhood illnesses Childhood immunizations Allergies Accidents and injuries Hospitalizations All current adult vaccinations and/or immunizations, such as influenza vaccine All current prescribed and over-the-counter medications, including nutritional supplements and herbal preparations
Family history of health and illness	Ages of brothers/sisters, parents, and grandparents Health status of living relatives and cause of death if no longer living
Lifestyle	Amount, frequency, and use of tobacco, alcohol, and street drugs Type and amount of foods eaten each day Sleep patterns Any difficulty with activities of daily living Type and amount of exercise Education and occupation Support systems (family, friends, community) Expectations of treatment and care

tympanic membrane. Inspection is the first method used in an assessment of the whole body and of each body system. The guidelines for inspection are as follows:

- The room temperature should be comfortable. If the room is too hot or too cold, it may alter the appearance of the patient's skin and change his or her behavior.
- Use good lighting. Dim light can obscure abnormalities, and fluorescent lights can change the perception of skin color.
- Look before touching.
- Completely expose the body part being inspected.
- Compare symmetric (matching) parts (e.g., eyes, ears, arms, legs).
- Inspect for these characteristics: color, size, symmetry, patterns, location, consistency of tissue, movement, behavior, odors, sounds.

PALPATION

Palpation is the method of using hands to touch and feel. Light and moderate palpation is used most often by nurses. Light palpation is performed by placing the hand lightly

on the surface to palpate for pulses, tenderness, skin texture, skin temperature, and skin moisture. To perform moderate palpation (Figure 5-1 ■), the hand is placed on the skin surface and the surface is depressed 1 to 2 cm (1/2 to 3/4 in.). A circular motion is used to feel for the size, shape, or mobility of underlying structures such as masses or body organs. A distended urinary bladder may be assessed with moderate palpation. The guidelines for palpation are as follows:

- Make sure hands are clean and warm and fingernails are short.
- Follow Standard Precautions as appropriate.
- Use the pads of the fingers to palpate pulses, texture, size, shape, and *crepitus* (air in subcutaneous tissue).
- Assess for the characteristics listed in Table 5-2 ■.

PERCUSSION

Percussion is a method of tapping the body to produce sound waves. The sounds produced are used to assess underlying structures. Although percussion can be used

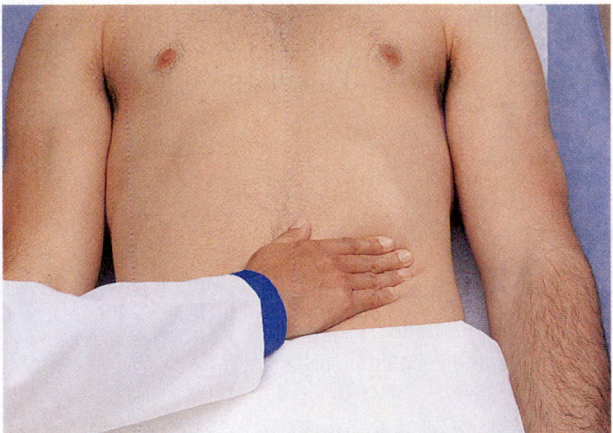

Figure 5-1. ■ The position of the hand for moderate palpation. (Photographer: Richard Tauber, Pearson Education.)

to assess the density of tissue and the size and shape of organs, it is used most often to assess abdominal structures. *Tympany* is a characteristic loud, drumlike sound heard over an organ that is filled with air, such as the intestines. Percussion is a more advanced assessment skill and may not often be used by the LPN/LVN. It can, however, be very useful when trying to determine whether abdominal distention may be due to flatus (tympany) or when assessing a distended bladder (which produces a dull sound).

The guidelines for percussion are as follows:

- Make sure hands are clean and warm and fingernails are short.
- Follow Standard Precautions as appropriate.
- To use direct percussion, use one or more fingertips to tap over the area being assessed.
- To use indirect percussion (Figure 5-2■):
  - Place the middle finger of your nondominant hand over the area to be percussed.

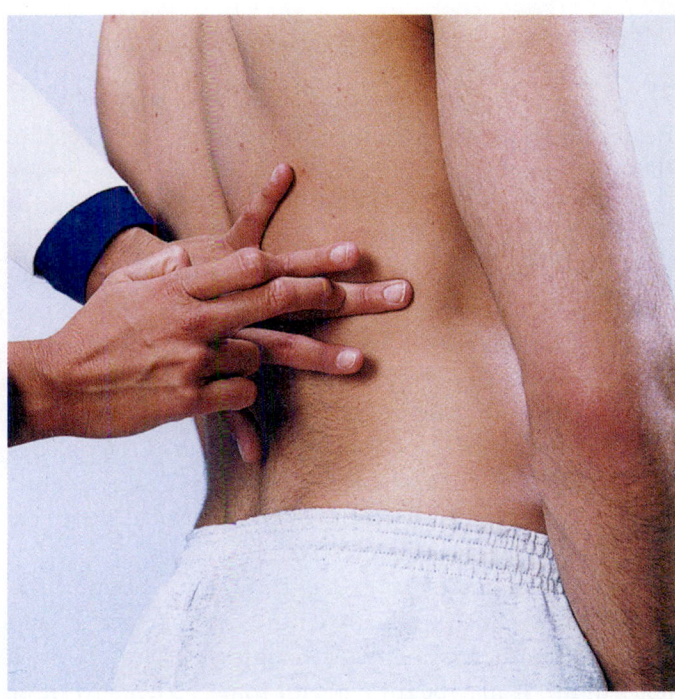

Figure 5-2. ■ Indirect percussion. Use the finger of one hand to tap the finger of the other. (Photographer: Richard Tauber, Pearson Education.)

- Use the pad of the middle finger of your dominant hand to strike the area between the knuckle and the fingernail of the hand over the body part.
- Deliver two quick taps by flexing your wrist and listen to the tone.

AUSCULTATION

Auscultation is the method that uses a stethoscope to listen for body sounds, including those of the heart, bowel, and lungs.

Sounds are described in a variety of ways, depending on the body part being assessed. Sounds are generally classified according to intensity (loud/soft), pitch (high/low), duration, and quality (crackles, wheezes, etc.). Auscultation is also used to assess the apical pulse.

General guidelines for auscultation are as follows:

- Make sure hands are clean and warm and fingernails are short.
- Follow Standard Precautions as appropriate.
- Make the environment as quiet as possible.
- Auscultate over bare skin.
- Press the diaphragm of the stethoscope firmly on the body part being assessed to listen to high-pitched sounds, such as normal heart sounds, breath sounds, and bowel sounds.
- Hold the bell of the stethoscope lightly on the body part being assessed to listen to low-pitched sounds, such as abnormal heart sounds and vascular sounds.

TABLE 5-2	Characteristics Assessed by Palpation
CHARACTERISTIC	**DESCRIPTORS**
Consistency	Soft, hard, filled with fluid
Mobility	Movable, fixed
Moisture	Wet, dry
Pulse strength	Strong, weak, full, bounding, thready
Shape	Regular, irregular
Size	Small, medium, large
Temperature	Warm, cold
Texture	Rough, smooth

Preparation for a Physical Examination

Before beginning the examination, the nurse should ensure that the room temperature is comfortable, that the area is quiet, and that adequate lighting is available. All equipment that will be used should be clean and in good working order. The nurse should wash his or her hands before and after the assessment. Gloves should be worn and Standard Precautions should be followed if either the nurse or the patient has an open cut or abrasion; if the patient has drainage from a cut or wound; if body fluids or excretions are being collected; and for any examination of the mucous membranes, genitalia, or rectum. If there is any possibility of being splashed with fluids or secretions, the nurse should wear a mask and protective eye goggles.

The purpose and techniques of the physical examination should be explained to the patient to decrease anxiety and feelings of embarrassment. Although the examination is not painful, it may be difficult for some patients to sit or lie in a position necessary for a specific assessment, especially if the patient is in pain or is older. The length of the examination should be adjusted to the physical condition and age of each patient. The nurse should be aware of normal changes in structure and function that occur with aging because they can affect patient tolerance and the data that are collected. Normal age-related changes in the older adult are outlined in Box 5-1■ and are further described in each assessment chapter.

If at all possible, the nurse should conduct the physical examination in a private location at a time agreeable to the patient. For a complete physical examination, the nurse should (if needed) assist the patient in removing clothing and putting on a gown. The patient should empty the bladder before the examination to facilitate abdominal assessment. A drape should be placed over the patient so that only the body part being assessed is exposed. The nurse should also determine whether any positions are contraindicated during the examination.

The Physical Examination

Key Concept A physical examination will involve particular equipment and the senses of the nurse in order to measure, observe, touch, and listen to the sounds of the body. This examination should be performed in a safe, comfortable environment that allows for the comfort, privacy, and dignity of the patient.

A comprehensive physical examination (Table 5-3■) can be conducted in a system-by-system or head-to-toe sequence. Some parts of the examination, such as a rectal examination, male and female genitalia with a pelvic examination, internal

| BOX 5-1 | FOCUS ON OLDER ADULTS |

Age-Related Assessment Findings in the Older Adult

Skin, Hair, and Nails
- Dry and wrinkled skin
- Thin scalp and body hair (men may be bald)
- Facial hair in women
- Loss of hair pigment
- Areas of pigmentation and moles
- Thickened and yellowed nails

Eyes and Ears
- Cataracts (opacity of the lens)
- Decreased visual acuity (*presbyopia*)
- Decreased hearing acuity (*presbycusis*)

Mouth
- Loss of teeth
- Presence of dentures

Heart and Lungs
- Increased respiratory rate
- Increased blood pressure

Abdomen
- Decreased frequency of bowel sounds
- More frequent voiding, including at night

Extremities
- Blood vessels more prominent and less straight
- Peripheral pulses sometimes more difficult to palpate
- Decreased muscle mass and strength
- Decreased range of motion
- Stooped posture

Mental Status
- Slower response to questions
- Occasional confusion in unfamiliar surroundings

eye examination, and external ear canal examination, are most often conducted by an advanced practice nurse or physician and are not included here. The following discussion of a basic physical examination provides structure for a head-to-toe assessment.

GENERAL SURVEY

The general survey provides the nurse with information about the patient's overall appearance and behavior, as well as vital signs and height and weight. Data for the general survey are collected from the first meeting with the patient and continue through the physical examination or during nursing care. The following information is assessed:

- Facial expressions, mood, speech patterns
- Hygiene, grooming, odors
- Posture, physical deformities, ability to move and walk
- Manifestations of illness, such as difficulty breathing, pain, swelling

TABLE 5-3	Guidelines for a Physical Examination
COMPONENT	**METHODS AND AREAS OF ASSESSMENT**
General survey	Inspection, auscultation ■ General appearance, posture, gait, thought process, speech patterns ■ Vital signs ■ Height and weight
Integument	Inspection, palpation ■ Skin: Color, moisture, temperature, turgor, lesions (color, size, shape) ■ Hair: Distribution, texture, condition of scalp, presence of lice or nits ■ Nails: Shape, angle at nail bed, color, texture
Eyes	Inspection, palpation ■ Eyebrows: Hair distribution, alignment, movement, symmetry ■ Eyelashes: Distribution, direction of curl ■ Eyelids: Skin texture, symmetrical closure, ability to blink ■ Conjunctiva: Color, texture, lesions ■ Lacrimal glands: Tenderness, redness, edema, tearing ■ Cornea: Transparency, reflex ■ Pupils: Color, shape, size, symmetry, reaction to light, accommodation, convergence ■ Extraocular muscles: Coordination ■ Visual acuity: Near and distance vision (normal visual acuity = 20/20)
Ears	Inspection, palpation ■ Auricles: Color, symmetrical size, position, texture, tenderness ■ External ear canal: Cerumen (wax), blood, redness, lesions ■ Hearing acuity: Voice tones, watch tick
Nose/sinuses	Inspection, palpation ■ External nose: Shape, size, color, discharge, tenderness ■ Nasal cavities: Patency, mucosa, discharge, lesions, location of septum ■ Sinuses: Tenderness, drainage
Mouth/oropharynx	Inspection, palpation ■ Lips/buccal mucosa: Symmetrical, color, moisture, lesions ■ Teeth/gums: Number of teeth; dental care, caries; gum color, adherence of gums to teeth ■ Tongue: Position, color, texture, movement, moisture, swelling, ulceration, masses, lesions ■ Palate/uvula: Color, shape, bony growth, lesions; position of uvula ■ Oropharynx/tonsils: Color, size, discharge
Neck	Inspection, palpation, auscultation ■ Neck: Movement, range of motion, pain, swelling, masses ■ Lymph nodes: Size, pain ■ Carotid arteries, thyroid: Presence of *bruits* (soft rushing sound heard through bell of stethoscope)
Breasts/axillae	Inspection, palpation ■ Breasts: Size, shape, symmetrical, color, swelling, tenderness, masses, lesions ■ Areola: Size, shape, symmetrical, color, masses, lesions ■ Nipples: Size, shape, position, color, discharge, lesions, masses, retraction ■ Axillary lymph nodes: Size, tenderness, nodules
Thorax/lungs	Inspection, palpation, auscultation ■ Thorax: Shape, symmetrical, spinal curves, skin lesions, tenderness, masses, expansion ■ Lungs: Breath sounds, respiratory patterns (normal adult respiratory rate = 12–20 breaths/min)

(continued)

TABLE 5-3	Guidelines for a Physical Examination *(continued)*
COMPONENT	**METHODS AND AREAS OF ASSESSMENT**
Cardiovascular	Inspection, palpation, auscultation ■ Precordium: Location of point of maximum impulse, pulsations ■ Heart: Heart sounds, rate and rhythm of contractions (normal adult heart rate = 60–100 bpm) ■ Peripheral pulses: Strength, symmetrical, volume ■ Peripheral veins: Visibility, symmetrical, tenderness ■ Circulation: Skin color, temperature, skin changes, nail changes, lesions, edema, capillary refill
Abdomen	Inspection, auscultation, percussion, palpation ■ Skin: Lesions, color ■ Abdomen: Contour, distention, movements ■ Bowel sounds: Audible, timing (normal bowel sounds every 5–20 sec = 3–12/min) ■ Percussion tone: Tympany, dullness ■ Light palpation: Local or generalized tenderness, bladder distention
Musculoskeletal	Inspection, palpation ■ Muscles: Symmetrical, size, tone, movement, contractures, tenderness, masses ■ Bones: Symmetrical, alignment, tenderness ■ Spine: Curves
Neurologic	Inspection, palpation, percussion ■ Motor function/balance: Gait, ability to stand on one foot and walk heel to toe ■ Fine motor movement: Ability to repeatedly touch nose with hand, pat knees with palms and backs of hands, run heel down opposite shin ■ Sensory/light touch: Ability to distinguish between sharp and dull touch ■ Cranial nerves: Ability to smell, see, clench teeth, move eyes, have facial expressions, hear, taste, feel touch, swallow, shrug shoulders against resistance, protrude tongue ■ Reflexes: Type of response (using percussion hammer)

■ Vital signs (temperature, pulse, respirations, blood pressure)
■ Height and weight

SKIN, HAIR, AND NAILS

The skin, hair, and nails make up the integumentary system and often provide a general indication of the patient's overall health. These structures are assessed by inspection and palpation in conjunction with other body parts during a head-to-toe physical examination.

The skin varies in color from pale white to dark brown, depending on race and individual characteristics. It is normally warm, smooth, dry, and intact. Various diseases and injuries or environmental exposure may change the color, moisture, or continuity of the patient's skin (see Chapters 44 and 45). Changes in color are more difficult to assess in dark-skinned individuals (such as Native Americans, African Americans, Hispanics, those of Mediterranean descent, and Caucasians who are deeply suntanned). Abnormal assessments are described as follows:

■ *Cyanosis*. Cyanosis is a blue or gray discoloration of the skin that is the result of a decreased level of oxygen in the blood. Cyanosis in people with dark skin is often seen as a dullness in color.

■ *Pallor*. Pallor, or paleness of the skin, is most often the result of a loss of blood. Pallor may be assessed over the entire body or only in the lips, nail beds, and conjunctiva of the eyes. People with dark skin often are ashen gray or appear slightly yellowish when pallor is present.

■ *Jaundice*. Jaundice is a yellow color of the skin and mucous membranes. It is caused by liver or gallbladder disease or by an excessive breakdown of red blood cells. Jaundice is usually seen first in the eyes and then in the skin and mucous membranes. Darker skin does not show jaundice, but it can be seen in the eyes, oral mucous membranes, and palms and soles.

■ *Erythema*. Erythema is redness of the skin. It may appear during a fever, in response to inflammation or allergy, or from a sunburn.

■ *Ecchymosis*. Ecchymosis is a purple discoloration resulting from a collection of blood in the subcutaneous tissues.

■ *Petechiae*. Petechiae are small red spots caused by capillary bleeding. The location and size of the discolorations should be documented.

TABLE 5-4	**Evaluating Edema**

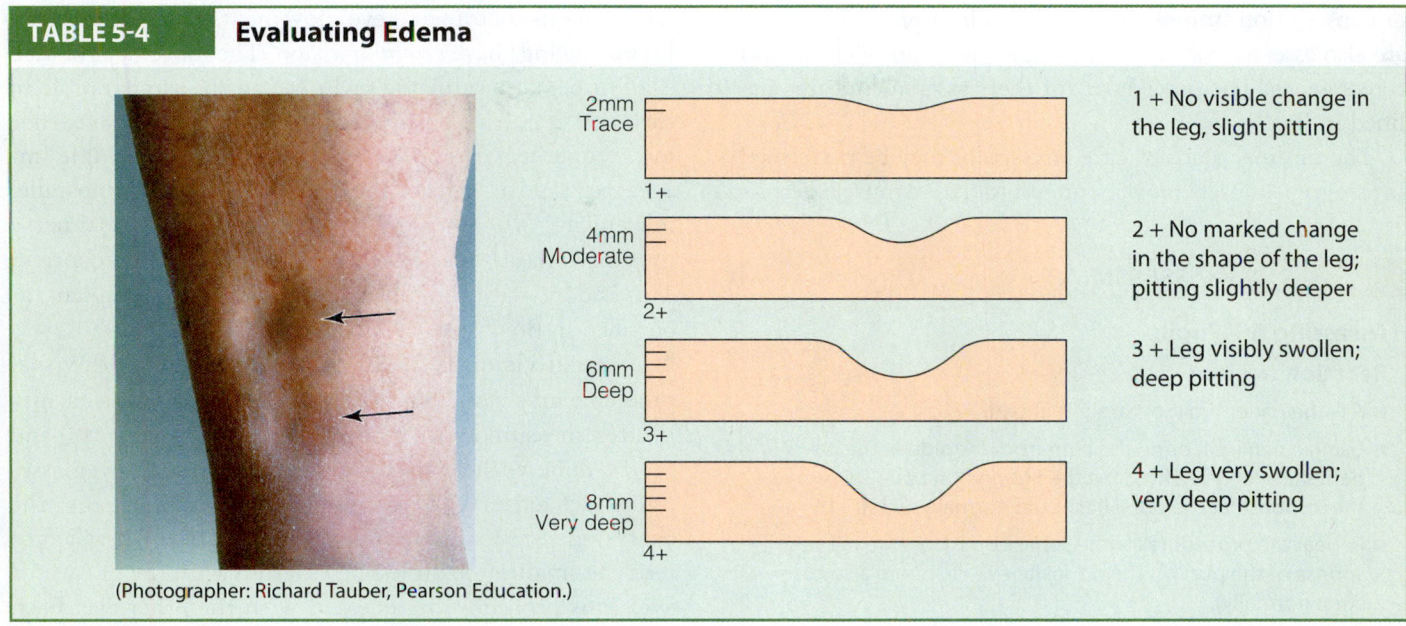

2mm Trace 1+		1 + No visible change in the leg, slight pitting
4mm Moderate 2+		2 + No marked change in the shape of the leg; pitting slightly deeper
6mm Deep 3+		3 + Leg visibly swollen; deep pitting
8mm Very deep 4+		4 + Leg very swollen; very deep pitting

(Photographer: Richard Tauber, Pearson Education.)

■ *Lesions.* Lesions are alterations in the surface of the skin. *Wounds* may be the result of an injury or a surgical incision. A *scar* is a healed wound. Other types of lesions are bites, scratches, blisters, warts, moles, acne, burns, and rashes. When assessing lesions, document the size, shape, location, drainage, odors, and associated pain or itching.

■ *Turgor.* This term refers to the fullness or elasticity of the skin. With normal turgor, skin can be pinched up in a fold, and when released it immediately returns to its previous shape. *Dehydration* decreases the skin's turgor, so that skin folds remain elevated (like a tent) or return to shape very slowly.

■ *Edema,* or excess fluid in tissues, is manifested by swelling covered by tight, shiny skin. Edema may be caused by trauma, heart disease, peripheral vascular disease, kidney disease, or overhydration. Edema is often measured by palpating with the fingers; if the skin remains indented, the term *pitting edema* is used. The scale used to describe the levels of edema is shown in Table 5-4■.

The nails are inspected for shape, color, and consistency. The hair is inspected for color, texture, and distribution. *Alopecia* (loss of hair on the head or all of the body) may result from hereditary factors (specific to the hair on the head in men), infection, inadequate nutrition, or treatment of cancer with chemotherapy or radiation therapy. *Hirsutism* (excessive hair) is often caused by hormone disorders.

HEAD AND NECK

A basic physical examination of the head and neck includes assessing the skull, face, eyes, ears, nose and sinuses, mouth, and lymph nodes. These structures are assessed by inspection and palpation. More advanced physical assessment techniques, not discussed here, use the ophthalmoscope to

examine the internal eye and the otoscope to examine the tympanic membrane and internal nasal structures.

Skull and Face

The skull and face are inspected for shape and proportion and should be symmetrical. If the skull appears abnormally large, its circumference should be measured with a tape measure. The face is inspected for color, symmetry, and distribution of hair. The facial muscles and nerves are assessed by asking the patient to raise the eyebrows, puff out the cheeks, smile, and show the teeth. Abnormal findings that should be documented are edema around the eyes (*periorbital edema*), inability to move a part of the face, and any abnormal movements such as *tremors* (involuntary quivering) and *tics* (spastic muscle contraction usually involving the muscles above the shoulders).

Eyes

The external structures of the eyes (including the eyebrows, eyelids, eyelashes, and lacrimal glands) are inspected. The eyes and eyebrows should be in alignment, the eyelashes should curl outward, and the eyelids should cover the eyes equally. The lacrimal gland is palpated for tenderness. The conjunctiva should be pink and the sclera white. The pupils are normally black and round and equal in size (Figure 5-3■). When a patient has a cataract, the pupil appears white or cloudy. Other abnormal findings are dilation (**mydriasis**)

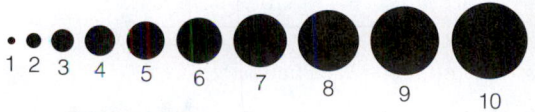

Figure 5-3. ■ Size of pupil in millimeters.

or constriction (**miosis**) of one or both pupils. The pupils are also assessed for reaction to light, accommodation, and convergence. The procedures for these assessments are outlined in Box 5-2■.

The cardinal fields of gaze assessment may be performed to assess eye muscle movement and to detect muscle defects

---

BOX 5-2　ASSESSMENT

Assessing the Pupils

Reaction to Light

■ Ask the patient to look straight ahead.

■ Using a penlight, bring the light from the side of the patient's face and briefly shine the light on one pupil. Observe the response of the pupil (it should normally constrict).

■ Repeat the procedure for the same pupil. Observe the response of the pupil in the opposite eye (it should also constrict normally).

■ Repeat the above two procedures with the other eye.

Accommodation

■ Hold your finger about 10 to 15 cm (4 to 6 in.) from the bridge of the patient's nose.

■ Ask the patient to look at your finger, then at a distant object, and then back at your finger. Observe the response of the pupils. They should normally constrict when looking at your finger (a near object) and dilate when looking at the distant object.

Convergence

■ Move your finger toward the patient's nose from a distance of about 15 cm (6 in.) and observe the eyes. Normally, the pupils move toward the nose, assuming a cross-eyed appearance (convergence).

Cardinal Fields of Gaze Assessment

■ With the head held steady, ask the patient to follow the movement of an object (your finger, pen, or penlight) with their eyes only. Hold the object 12 to 18 in. away, allowing the patient to focus on it comfortably.

■ Move the object to each of the cardinal positions of gaze, holding it momentarily and then returning it to the center (see diagram).

■ Progress clockwise.

The eyes should move together (*parallel tracking*). Inability to follow in any direction indicates weakness of an extraocular muscle or cranial nerve dysfunction. Mild nystagmus at extreme lateral gaze (positions 2 and 5) is normal; nystagmus at any other position is not.

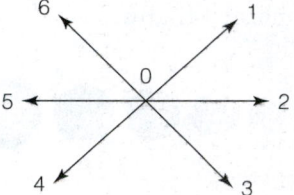

---

that cause uncoordinated eye movements or misalignment. Human beings have *binocular* vision. The movement of each eye muscle is coordinated or linked to the same muscle in the other eye. This ensures that when the eyes move, they move together (*conjugate movement*) to deliver a single image. Extra movements of the eyes (*nystagmus*) or nonparallel movements (*strabismus*) may indicate disease, cranial nerve dysfunction, or muscle weakness and should be reported. This is done with the cardinal fields of gaze assessment, as outlined in Box 5-2■.

Normal vision is 20/20, whereas a person with visual problems may have a visual acuity of 20/100. Visual acuity is often measured with a Snellen chart (Figure 5-4■) and can be done with or without corrective lenses (eyeglasses or contact lenses). The patient is placed 20 feet from the chart and asked to cover one eye. The patient is asked to read the smallest possible line of letters with the uncovered eye. This procedure is repeated with the other eye. Each line on the chart has a fraction on the side, with the top number always being 20 (the distance at which a person with normal vision can read the line of letters). The bottom number indicates the vision of the person being tested, and larger numbers represent poorer vision. Visual acuity is documented as the smallest line of letters that can be read with only two errors. The visual acuity for each eye is documented, and use of corrective lenses is noted. (See Chapter 40 for disorders of the eye and ear.)

Ears

Inspect the external ears for location, symmetry, lesions, redness, and drainage. Gently palpate the external ears for tenderness and swelling. An estimate of hearing may be made by asking the patient to cover one ear as you whisper

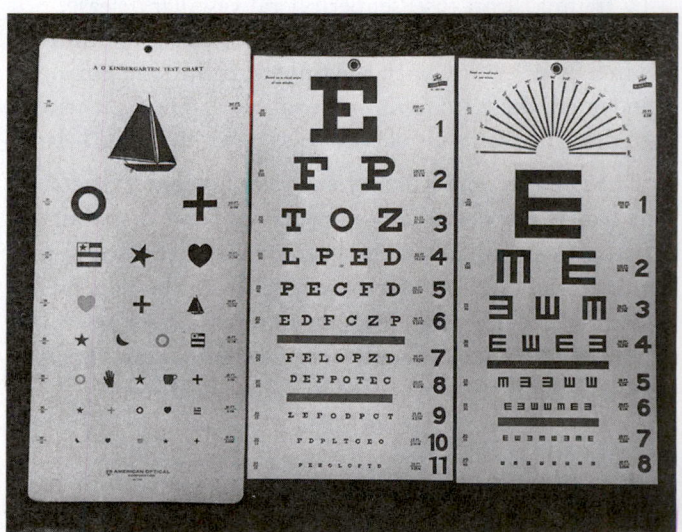

Figure 5-4. ■ Types of eye charts: the preschool children's chart (left), Snellen standard chart (center), and the Snellen E chart for patients who are unable to read (right). (Pearson Education.)

a word while standing about 1 to 2 feet away out of the patient's line of vision (to prevent lip-reading). Repeat with the other ear.

Nose and Sinuses

To test the patency of the patient's nostrils, have the patient occlude one side at a time and then inhale and exhale. A penlight can be used to assess the mucous membranes in the lower nasal passages. Abnormal findings include swelling, bleeding, discharge, and a crooked (deviated) septum. The sinuses are assessed by gentle palpation over the frontal and maxillary sinuses, noting any tenderness or pain.

Mouth

Ask the patient to open the mouth widely. Inspect the lips, the oral mucous membranes, the tongue, the teeth, and the gums. Palpate the lips. The lips, mucous membranes, gums, and tongue should be pink, smooth, and moist. The teeth should be in good repair. There should be no bad odors. Abnormal findings are swelling, redness, pallor, drainage, lesions, or poor dental hygiene.

Lymph Nodes

Palpate the lymph nodes of the head and neck (Figure 5-5 ■). The lymph nodes normally are not palpable. If they are palpable, assess for size, location, consistency, and tenderness.

THORAX

Assessment of the thorax in a head-to-toe examination includes the chest and back, the lungs, the heart, and the breasts. The assessment techniques most often used are inspection and auscultation, with palpation also used to assess the breasts and lymph nodes in the axilla.

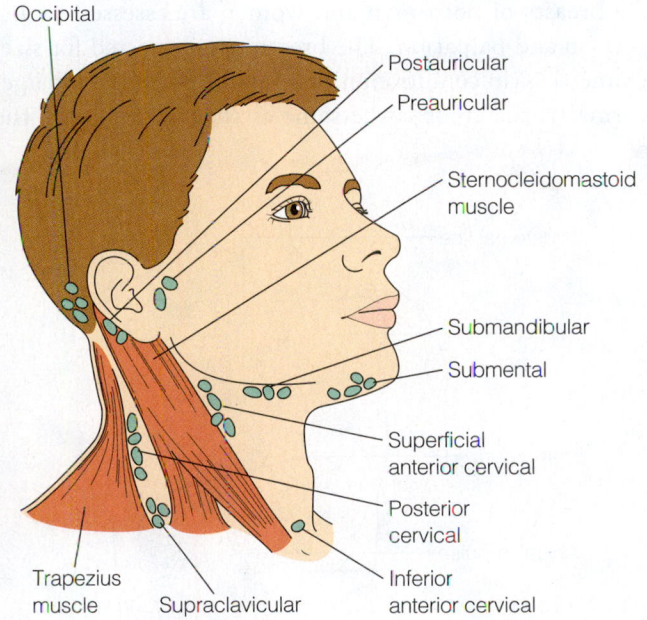

Figure 5-5. ■ Lymph nodes of the head and neck.

Chest and Back

The color, size, shape, muscles, and breathing movements of the chest and back are inspected. The color should be the same as the face and neck. Bilateral sides of the chest and back should be symmetrical, with equal expansion and relaxation during respirations. The thorax should have a greater transverse (side-to-side) diameter than anteroposterior (front-to-back) diameter. The reverse (referred to as a *barrel chest*) is seen in patients with chronic obstructive pulmonary diseases. The scapulae should be equal in height, and the spine should be aligned midline with normal curves (concave cervical and convex thoracic). Abnormal findings of the thoracic spine include *kyphosis* (increased thoracic curve) and *scoliosis* (lateral deviation). In patients with respiratory difficulty, the intercostal and upper thoracic muscles may *retract* (pull in) on inhalation.

Lungs

The lungs are assessed by inspection of the external thorax and by auscultation with a stethoscope (both anteriorly and posteriorly). Inspection can be used to determine respiratory rate, depth, and rhythm. **The normal respiratory rate for an adult is 12 to 20 regular breaths per minute** (known as *eupnea*). Respiratory rates may increase to more than 24 breaths per minute (*tachypnea*) in response to exercise, fever, pain, and illnesses that cause an increase in the amount of carbon dioxide or a decrease of oxygen in the blood. Respiratory rates may decrease to less than 10 breaths per minute (*bradypnea*) in a patient with an increase in intracranial pressure or in response to certain narcotic drugs.

The normal depth and rhythm of respirations is about equal during inspiration and expiration, but may abnormally be very deep or shallow. A patient may also have increased respiratory rate and depth (*hyperventilation*) or decreased respiratory rate and depth (*hypoventilation*) in response to factors such as respiratory disorders, metabolic disorders, fear, pain, and drug overdose. *Cheyne–Stokes respirations*, a response to organ failure, drug overdose, or increased intracranial pressure, are manifested by a pattern of increasing respiratory rate and depth followed by *apnea* (periods in which there is no breathing). Other abnormal respiratory findings are **dyspnea** (difficulty breathing), **orthopnea** (breathing more easily in an upright position), and apnea.

Auscultation is used to assess normal and abnormal (or *adventitious*) breath sounds. To auscultate the chest, the patient should be in a sitting position. Warm the stethoscope diaphragm before placing it on the patient's chest and ask the patient to breathe slowly and deeply through the mouth. It may be necessary to wet the patient's chest hair with a little warm water to decrease the sounds caused by friction of hair against the stethoscope. A regular pattern of auscultation should be used, beginning above the clavicle or scapula and moving the diaphragm down at regular intervals to the bottom of the ribs (see Figure 21-7). Compare and document sounds for both the right and left lungs. If adventitious sounds are heard, verify sounds by encouraging the patient to deep breathe and cough. Auscultate again. Note and document remaining adventitious sounds and where in the respiratory cycle they are heard (beginning of inspiration, end of expiration).

There are several different types of abnormal breath sounds. Noisy respirations are often labeled *stertorous*. *Crackles*, heard most often during inspiration, are crackling sounds made as air moves through secretions in the airways. *Wheezes* are high-pitched continuous sounds heard on both inspiration and expiration. Wheezes are heard when secretions, swelling, or tumors narrow the airways. A grating sound indicates a *pleural friction rub*, resulting from an inflamed pleura rubbing against the chest wall.

While assessing the lungs, it is important to note whether the patient has a cough and to ask whether and when sputum is coughed up. If the cough is productive of sputum, note the color, amount, and consistency. Depending on the cause, sputum may be clear, yellow, green, or blood-tinged and may be thin or thick. Additional documentation is necessary if the patient is receiving oxygen. Record how it is administered (i.e., by mask or nasal cannula) and at what rate (in liters per minute). (See also Chapters 22 and 23.)

Heart

The heart is assessed by auscultation for heart sounds and to take an apical pulse. **The normal pulse rate in an adult ranges from 60 to 100 beats per minute.** A rapid heart rate (greater than 100 beats per minute) is labeled *tachycardia*. Tachycardia can be caused by many different factors, including pain, anxiety, fever, and heart disease. A slow heart rate (less than 60 beats per minute) is labeled *bradycardia*. Bradycardia can be caused by medications, increasing age, or disorders of the cardiac conduction system. The equipment used to take an apical pulse is a stethoscope with a diaphragm. The diaphragm should be warmed before placement on the patient's chest, and the room should be quiet so sounds can be heard without difficulty. The nurse assesses the rate and rhythm of the heart and the normal heart sounds. Assessing abnormal heart sounds is an advanced assessment technique. It may be helpful to have the patient briefly hold his or her breath when auscultating heart sounds in order to decrease respiratory sounds that could interfere with the assessment.

The apical impulse is used as a landmark for taking an apical pulse. This landmark is located at the fourth or fifth left intercostal space at or medial to the midclavicular line (Figure 5-6 ■). It may often be palpated as a slight tap against the fingers. The apical pulse is the most accurate pulse measurement. It should be taken if there is any question about the peripheral pulse or if the patient is taking a medication that affects heart rate. The apical pulse is taken for one full minute.

The first heart sound heard (S_1) is the "lub" of "lub-dub." This is a single low-pitched sound that occurs as the mitral and tricuspid valves close at the same time. The second heart sound (S_2) is the "dub" of "lub-dub." This sound is not as low-pitched and is shorter than the first heart sound. It occurs as the aortic and pulmonic valves close in unison. Both sounds normally occur within 1 second or less and are counted together to determine the heart rate.

clinicalALERT

Remember to count only once for each two sounds that are heard and to count for one full minute when taking an apical pulse. It is helpful to always begin counting when the second hand of your watch is on 12 (to avoid forgetting when you began counting).

While assessing the heart rate, it is important to note whether the rhythm is regular or irregular, whether there are extra heart sounds (S_3 or S_4), and whether the sounds are strong or weak. The rhythm should be regular. An irregular pattern of heartbeats is called a *dysrhythmia* (see Chapter 16). The patient should also be asked about any other symptoms that might indicate heart disease, such as swelling of the feet, pain in the chest, difficulty breathing, fatigue, and dizziness. During an assessment for a patient who complains of chest pain, also assess skin color for cyanosis or pallor; pulse, blood pressure, and respirations; location, duration, and intensity of the pain; and any other accompanying manifestations such as nausea or loss of consciousness.

Breasts and Axillary Lymph Nodes

The breasts of both men and women are assessed by inspection and palpation. The breasts are inspected for size, symmetry, skin condition, nipple condition, and discharge. Normally, the color is the same as that of the chest, the

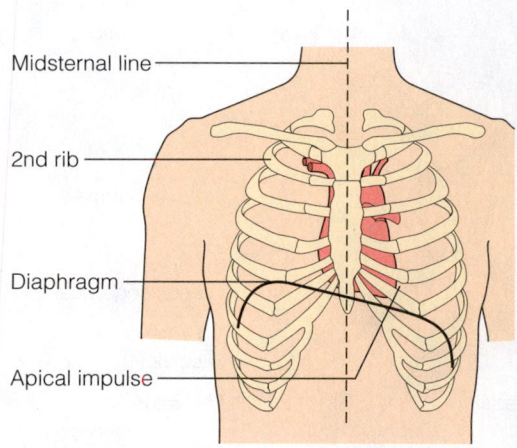

Midsternal line

2nd rib

Diaphragm

Apical impulse

Figure 5-6. ■ Location of the apical impulse.

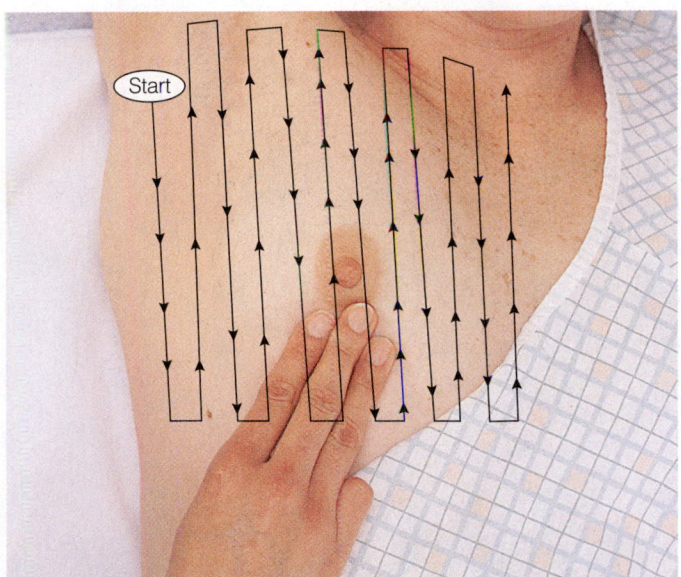

Figure 5-7. ■ Possible pattern for palpation of the breast.
(Photographer: Richard Tauber, Pearson Education.)

breasts are bilaterally symmetrical (although slight variations are normal), the areola and nipples are bilaterally equal in size and color, and there is no sign of skin dimpling or redness or discharge from the nipples.

The breasts are gently palpated by using the pads of the first three fingers to compress the breast tissue against the chest wall (Figure 5-7■). Breast tissue normally is firm with a granular consistency. Assess for tenderness or pain,

abnormal consistency, or the presence of a mass. If the breasts feel nodular, ask the woman about a diagnosis of fibrocystic breast disease as well as the time of her last period (if she is still menstruating). While palpating the breasts, also palpate well into the axilla for the presence of pain and enlarged lymph nodes. If a mass or enlarged lymph node is palpated, document size and consistency. Any abnormal findings are documented by quadrant (upper inner, upper outer, lower inner, lower outer). Ask women about a history of breast cancer, self-breast examinations, and mammograms (if age appropriate) (see Chapter 30).

ABDOMEN

Abdominal assessment includes inspecting the exterior abdomen, auscultating bowel sounds to determine intestinal function, and lightly palpating all abdominal quadrants for tenderness and *guarding* (muscle tension). Because palpation may alter bowel sounds, the sequence of examination is inspection, auscultation, and palpation. Percussion and moderate to deep palpation of the abdomen are more advanced assessments and are not discussed here. Before beginning an abdominal assessment, be sure your hands are warm. For documentation purposes, mentally divide the abdomen into four quadrants (right upper, right lower, left upper, left lower) and know the underlying organs of each quadrant (Figure 5-8■).

Exterior Abdomen

The abdomen is normally slightly rounded, with the umbilicus midline. Fine white or silver-colored lines (*striae*) may

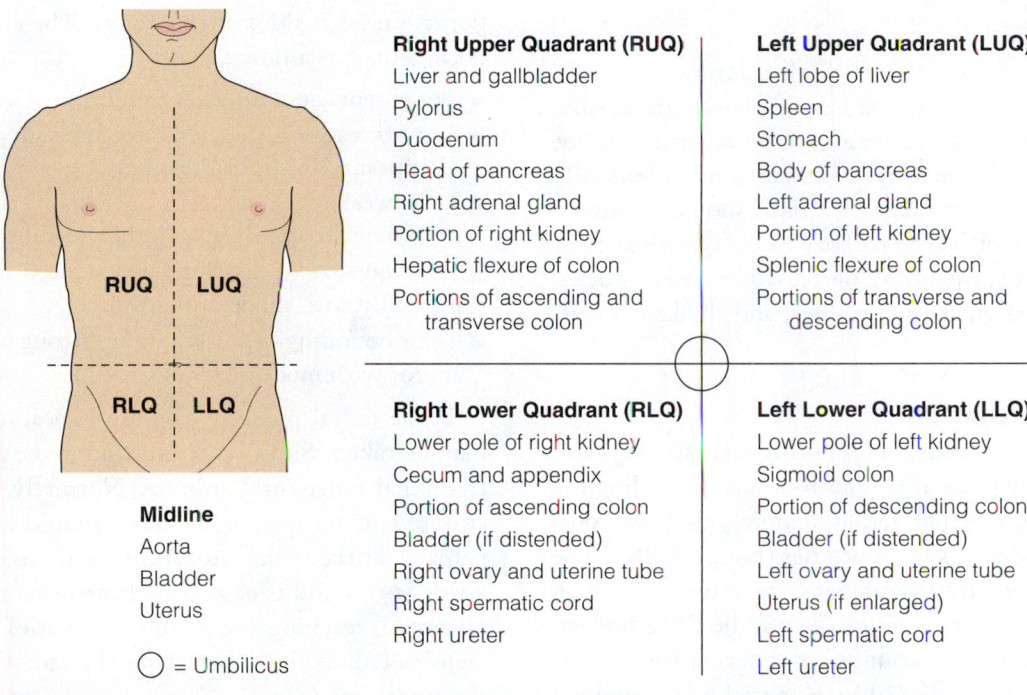

Right Upper Quadrant (RUQ)	Left Upper Quadrant (LUQ)
Liver and gallbladder	Left lobe of liver
Pylorus	Spleen
Duodenum	Stomach
Head of pancreas	Body of pancreas
Right adrenal gland	Left adrenal gland
Portion of right kidney	Portion of left kidney
Hepatic flexure of colon	Splenic flexure of colon
Portions of ascending and transverse colon	Portions of transverse and descending colon

Midline
Aorta
Bladder
Uterus

◯ = Umbilicus

Right Lower Quadrant (RLQ)	Left Lower Quadrant (LLQ)
Lower pole of right kidney	Lower pole of left kidney
Cecum and appendix	Sigmoid colon
Portion of ascending colon	Portion of descending colon
Bladder (if distended)	Bladder (if distended)
Right ovary and uterine tube	Left ovary and uterine tube
Right spermatic cord	Uterus (if enlarged)
Right ureter	Left spermatic cord
	Left ureter

Figure 5-8. ■ The four quadrants of the abdomen, with anatomic location of organs within each quadrant.

be visible; they result from skin being stretched by weight gain or pregnancy. There should be no visible masses. If the abdomen is distended, ask questions about any changes in usual patterns of bowel movements and urination.

Bowel Sounds

Bowel sounds are auscultated to assess intestinal function. Warm the diaphragm of the stethoscope and gently place it on the abdominal skin, listening in all four quadrants. Bowel sounds are clicks and gurgles made as intestinal contents move through bowel and should always be present. **Bowel sounds normally occur every 5 to 20 seconds (3 to 12 per minute).** Those that occur less often are referred to as *hypoactive*, and those that occur more often are referred to as *hyperactive*. Hypoactive or absent bowel sounds may result from abdominal surgery, paralysis of the intestinal wall (*paralytic ileus*), or advanced intestinal obstruction. Hyperactive bowel sounds are heard during diarrhea and in the early stage of intestinal obstruction (see Chapter 24).

Urinary Bladder

Normal urine output is at least 30 to 50 mL/hr, approximately 1,200 to 1,500 mL/day. The urinary bladder, if distended with urine, may be gently palpated in the midline of the abdomen above the symphysis pubis. If a patient has not voided for 8 to 10 hours, or if the voidings are frequent and in small amounts, palpating a distended urinary bladder is essential to identify the need for further interventions to empty the bladder (see Chapter 28).

EXTREMITIES

The extremities are assessed for color, temperature, lesions, condition of hair and nails, peripheral circulation, and muscle strength. Skin color and temperature should be similar to that of the face. Hair distribution is normally symmetrical on arms and legs, and nails should be intact. Patients with peripheral vascular disease often have abnormal assessments, including decreased or absent pulses; cool, pale, shiny skin; absence of hair; and thickened nails (see Chapter 19).

Peripheral Circulation

Peripheral pulses are assessed by noting the rate, rhythm, and strength of the pulse at various locations, including the temporal, carotid, brachial, radial, femoral, popliteal, posterior tibial, and dorsalis pedis arteries (Figure 5-9■). The pulse is taken by gently compressing the artery against an underlying bone with the tips of the middle three fingers. During a physical examination, or if abnormalities are assessed, bilateral pulses should be palpated and compared

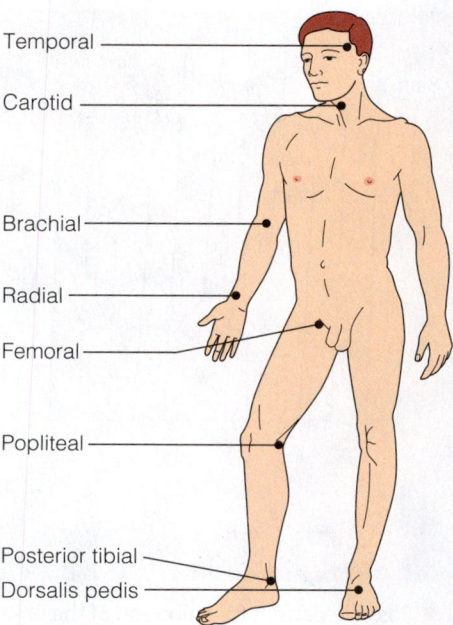

Figure 5-9. ■ Body sites at which peripheral pulses are most easily palpated.

(although both carotid arteries should never be palpated at the same time). If peripheral pulses are abnormal or cannot be palpated, a Doppler ultrasound can be used to determine the rate.

The rhythm of the heartbeat (the pattern of pulsations and pauses) should be regular. An abnormal rhythm should be reported. The *amplitude* is normally strong. Pulse amplitude should be bilaterally equal (at corresponding pulse points on both sides of the body). The amplitude can be documented as follows:

- 0 or absent—no pulsation is felt.
- 1+ or thready—pulsations are not easily palpated and disappear with slight pressure.
- 2+ or weak—although stronger than a thready pulse, pulsations disappear with light pressure.
- 3+ or normal—pulsations are palpated easily and disappear only with moderate pressure.
- 4+ or bounding—pulsations are strong and do not disappear with moderate pressure.

If the radial pulse is irregular, an apical–radial pulse may be taken. Simultaneously count the apical pulse and the radial pulse for 1 minute. Normally, every beat auscultated at the apex of the heart should be perfusing and palpable at the radial site. A difference in the rate is called a *pulse deficit* and is caused by heartbeats that are weak or are not all reaching the peripheral arteries. The pulse deficit is calculated by subtracting the radial pulse rate from the apical rate.

Capillary refill also provides information about peripheral circulation. To assess capillary refill, the nurse squeezes the patient's fingernail or toenail until it turns white, then releases the pressure, and observes the time for normal color to return. The return is normally immediate.

Musculoskeletal Function

Musculoskeletal function is initially assessed by observing the patient's posture and ability to move, walk, and carry out activities of daily living. Range of motion of joints may be observed during the physical examination. Muscle strength is often assessed through hand grips and feet pushes. The nurse asks the patient to grasp the nurse's index and middle fingers and squeeze, and to push the soles of the feet against the nurse's hands. Muscle strength should be bilaterally equal.

MENTAL STATUS

Mental status is most often assessed by determining the patient's level of awareness (*orientation*) and degree of wakefulness or ability to be aroused (*level of consciousness*). These are not the same conditions; a patient may be conscious but disoriented.

The patient's level of awareness is assessed by orientation to time, place, and person. When awareness is lost, the usual sequence of loss is time orientation, followed by place orientation, and then person orientation. It is important to remember that pain, trauma, illness, and a change in surroundings may make it difficult for patients to know the exact day and date. The following questions can be used to assess orientation:

- *Time*—What is the date today? What day of the week is today? What was our last holiday?
- *Place*—Where are you now? What state do we live in?
- *Person*—What is your name? How old are you?

Level of consciousness can be assessed and labeled as follows:

- *Awake and alert*. Patient is fully awake; responds to verbal requests; and is oriented to time, place, and person.
- *Lethargic*. Patient appears drowsy or asleep but can be awakened by calling his or her name and gently shaking.
- *Stuporous*. Patient is deeply asleep most of the time and can be awakened only by shouting and shaking, responds to painful stimuli by making purposeful movements, and verbally responds but may make inappropriate responses.
- *Comatose*. Patient cannot be aroused, even with painful stimuli; some reflexes (such as the gag reflex) may still be present.

Documentation

Key Concept   Accurate documentation of initial and ongoing assessment data is critical for effective nursing care planning and for guiding treatment decisions.

Data from the initial comprehensive assessment provide a foundation for the development and application of the nursing process. Documentation of ongoing focused assessments identifies improvement or worsening of identified health problems, provides information to help diagnose new problems, and serves as a means of communication among all members of the health care team. In addition, documentation of assessments provides the base for evaluation of health care outcomes, provides evidence to support health care cost reimbursements, and is legal evidence of the health status of the patient at that point in time.

Each institution or agency has its own requirements for the timing and method of documentation. The types seen most often are the traditional narrative form, the checklist or standardized form (ranging from an initial admission record to a flow sheet for vital signs), and the nursing minimum data set (used in long-term care facilities). Increasingly, documentation is entered into a computer, where it becomes part of a database or an electronic medical record that is shared within and between health care settings. With this method, for example, a nurse caring for a patient in the home would have access to previous assessment data and would not have to repeat the entire procedure, nor would the patient have to repeat all the information.

To document factually and accurately, follow these principles:

- *Document as soon as possible.* It is difficult to remember information accurately for long periods of time.
- *Document legibly or make computer entries accurately.* Errors in documentation must legally be corrected in the format approved by the health care institution or agency. Check the policy of your institution.
- *Organize the data in a logical way.* The health history is generally documented before the physical examination. If the health care setting uses a specific framework for organizing the data, data are documented within this framework. When documenting the health history, present health problems are described beginning with the onset of the problem.
- *Avoid inferences, judgments, and biases.* An inference is a statement about something unknown based on observation. For example, the nurse should not write "Obesity and body odor indicate little knowledge of nutrition and hygiene" or "Requests pain medication although obviously is not in pain."

■ *Record findings rather than methods of assessment.* A detailed description of the method of assessment is unnecessary. For example, when recording a blood pressure, the nurse writes "BP 120/70," not "The diaphragm of the stethoscope was placed over the brachial artery and the sounds were auscultated."

■ *Write concisely, using approved abbreviations and grammar.* It is not necessary to use entire sentences or to begin the narrative with the words "the patient." Group phrases, such as "Bowel sounds heard in all four quadrants," rather than "The patient has bowel sounds in the right upper and lower quadrants and left upper and lower quadrants." Use only those abbreviations approved by policy in the setting. Avoid jargon and slang words unless they are direct quotes.

■ *Do not use the word* normal *for normal findings.* It is better to write what was assessed, such as "Breath sounds clear in both lower lungs," rather than "Breath sounds normal."

■ If the agency uses documents called "charting by exception," document only abnormal findings.

Note: The references and resources for all chapters have been compiled at the back of the book.

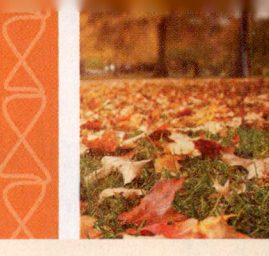

Chapter Review

KEY POINTS

- **Concept:** Assessment is a critical element of nursing care. Depending on the situation and setting, the nursing assessment may be comprehensive and holistic or focused on a specific event, body system, or problem.
- Assessment is the process of collecting data that provide information about the patient's individualized health care needs. Nurses collect these data through the patient assessment, comprised of a health history and a physical examination.
- The primary source of data is the patient.
- **Concept:** The health history is a comprehensive record of the patient's past and current health. This information provides valuable cues about the patient's health status and responses to health.
- The health history, collected through an interview of the patient, provides subjective data.
- **Concept:** The ability to perform an accurate physical examination and to differentiate normal from abnormal findings is one of the most important roles of today's nurse.

- The four methods of physical examination are inspection, palpation, percussion, and auscultation. The skills of physical examination take practice.
- **Concept:** A physical examination will involve particular equipment and the senses of the nurse in order to measure, observe, touch, and listen to the sounds of the body. This examination should be performed in a safe, comfortable environment that allows for the comfort, privacy, and dignity of the patient.
- A comprehensive physical examination is conducted in a head-to-toe sequence. If a focused or emergency assessment is being conducted, the nurse assesses only the specific patient problem.
- **Concept:** Accurate documentation of initial and ongoing assessment data is critical for effective nursing care planning and for guiding treatment decisions.
- Documenting assessments factually and accurately provides the base for evaluation of health care outcomes, provides evidence to support health care cost reimbursements, and is legal evidence of the health status of the patient at that point in time.

PEARSON NURSING STUDENT RESOURCES

Find additional materials at **nursing.pearsonhighered.com**.

Clinical Reasoning Care Map

Caring for a Patient With Risk for Excess Fluid Volume

NCLEX-PN® Focus Area: Coordinated Care

Case Study: Cath Cole, age 62, has a long history of congestive heart failure. She lives in a small apartment with her cat, Tom. She states, "You know, I have had many problems with water in my lungs and my legs swell something awful." Cath is supposed to take her "heart pill" and "water pill" every day, but she ran out of money and couldn't buy any this month. Although a low-sodium diet has been prescribed, Cath eats anything she wants.

Nursing Diagnosis: Excess Fluid Volume

COLLECT DATA

Subjective	Objective
_____	_____
_____	_____
_____	_____
_____	_____
_____	_____
_____	_____

Does this present a risk to the patient's safety?

If yes, the priority intervention to address this threat would be:

_____

Nursing Care

_____
_____
_____
_____
_____
_____
_____

Interprofessional team members to include when planning care:

_____

How would you document this? _____

_____
_____

Compare your answers and documentation to those provided on the companion website.

Data Collected
(use only those that apply)

- Height: 5'5"
- Weight: 125 lbs
- Blood pressure: 180/96
- Pupils cloudy, conjunctiva red
- States she has chronic infection in her sinuses
- Kyphosis present
- R = 30, crackles and wheezes present
- Apical pulse = 108, irregular
- Bowel sounds present in all four quadrants
- 4+ edema from toes to knees in both legs
- Has not taken medications for more than a week
- Does not follow prescribed diet

Nursing Interventions
(use only those that apply; list in priority order)

- State "Why didn't you ask for help with your medicines?"
- Ask Cath if she would consider being seen by a social worker.
- Monitor vital signs on a regular basis.
- State "You need to follow your diet."
- Monitor breath sounds, apical pulse, and peripheral pulses.
- Measure circumference of lower legs.

NCLEX-PN® Exam Preparation

1. When the nurse collects a urine specimen and notes the color of the urine, this assessment data is referred to as:
   1. comprehensive.
   2. objective.
   3. subjective.
   4. secondary.

2. A focused assessment for a patient complaining of abdominal pain would include assessing the patient's:
   1. legs.
   2. vision.
   3. bowel movements.
   4. blood pressure.

3. It is preferable to collect assessment data from secondary sources instead of directly from the patient when the:
   1. patient is irritable or agitated.
   2. patient is very young, unconscious, or confused.
   3. patient's family prefers to speak for him or her.
   4. patient's medical records are available.

4. The health history data are collected through an interview with the patient. Questions that give the patient a chance to provide more information are called:
   1. "yes" or "no."
   2. "why."
   3. closed-ended.
   4. open-ended.

5. A basic method of physical examination that uses the hands to touch and feel is called:
   1. inspection.
   2. auscultation.
   3. palpation.
   4. percussion.

6. The first thing that the nurse should do in preparing for a physical examination is:
   1. wash his or her hands.
   2. don gloves and mask.
   3. set up the equipment.
   4. position the patient.

7. Two nurses are checking a patient's pulse for a pulse deficit. The nurse taking the apical pulse counts the pulse as 100. The nurse taking the radial pulse counts the pulse as 85. What is the pulse deficit? _____

8. Mrs. Haynes developed a bowel obstruction after abdominal surgery 3 days ago. To monitor peristalsis, the nurse would:
   1. inspect the abdomen.
   2. auscultate the abdomen.
   3. percuss the abdomen.
   4. palpate the abdomen.

9. Mr. Scott has a history of alcohol abuse and has developed cirrhosis of the liver. His conjunctivae are yellow, and he is complaining of abdominal tenderness in the upper right quadrant. The nurse might expect to observe what change in skin color?
   1. Mottling
   2. Erythema
   3. Jaundice
   4. Cyanosis

10. Documenting the patient assessment is as important as the actual assessment. Identify the documentation that is most correctly stated.
    1. Breath sounds normal
    2. The patient had bowel sounds in the right upper and lower quadrants and the left upper and lower quadrants.
    3. BP 120/70
    4. Patient obese, indicating lack of knowledge about nutrition

Answers and rationales for Review Questions appear in Appendix I.

CULTURAL CARE STRATEGIES

APPRECIATING VARIATIONS IN FACIAL EXPRESSION ACROSS CULTURES

The home health care supervisor received an angry call from Mrs. Espanito, a Mexican American woman who had been the recipient of a home health care visit that day by a nurse. Mrs. Espanito explained that her infant was crying and feverish today, and it was undoubtedly because the nurse had complimented the baby but had not touched the infant during the compliment. Mrs. Espanito felt the nurse had given the infant the evil eye. Mrs. Espanito explained that in Mexican culture, babies are considered very weak and susceptible to the power of an envious glance. A simple compliment without touching a child can bring on the evil eye. While touching a child during a compliment can neutralize the power of the evil eye, no touch had occurred, and therefore she felt her child had become sick from the glance of the nurse.

Throughout the world, facial expression and eye contact are considered an important part of the communication message (Giger, 2013). From birth, individuals learn how to communicate nonverbally and how to interpret different facial expressions and eye behaviors. Because nursing occurs in an interpersonal arena, nurses need to be aware of facial expression and eye behavior and the meaning that different cultures may associate with facial expressions.

Facial Expression

Facial expression is commonly used as a guide to a person's feelings. A constant stare with immobile facial muscles is generally an indication of coldness. However, it can also be an indication of shock, guardedness, or fear. In an individual with schizophrenia or Parkinson's disease, it may be a symptom of the disease process. Facial expression is usually only one part of the total verbal and nonverbal communication that an individual provides. It is important to use facial expression in conjunction with other information to draw conclusions about another's feelings.

The meanings of facial expression vary among persons from different cultures. For example, Italian, Jewish, African American, and Hispanic persons tend to smile readily and use many facial expressions, gestures, and words to communicate feelings. Persons in other cultures (including the Irish, the English, and northern Europeans) tend to use less facial expression and to be less responsive. Facial expression can also convey the opposite meaning from the one that is felt; for example, Asian people may conceal negative emotions with a smile (Sue & Sue, 2012).

Eye Behavior

Eye contact is a valuable source of information. Typically, individuals look at each other for 3 to 10 seconds in a glance. For many people, longer contact may arouse anxiety or a feeling of confrontation (Sue & Sue, 2012). Most Caucasians value eye contact. They may equate avoidance of eye contact with rudeness, disrespect, or lack of attention. Fleeting eye contact may suggest insecurity, shyness, anxiety, or, in some cases, rejection. Embarrassment, guilt, fear, or anger may be interpreted from eye contact.

Because eye contact is learned in a family and cultural context, patterns of eye behavior can sometimes be related to cultural groups. For example, most Mexican American and African American people are comfortable with eye contact (Giger, 2013). Asian people and some Native Americans tend to have difficulty with eye contact; they may relate eye contact to impoliteness and an invasion of privacy. Some Filipinos may interpret eye contact that is diverted as a sign of a witch. Some cultures may associate eye contact with the "evil eye" (Spector, 2013).

Nursing Implications

- Assess facial expression for possible cultural significance. Most individuals use facial expression to reveal feelings. However, because facial expression is learned in a cultural context, the nurse should use an understanding of the individual's culture when interpreting the meaning of a facial expression.
- Assess eye behavior for possible cultural significance. Because individuals are unique, nurses should interpret eye behavior in the context of other available interpersonal information. Because eye behavior is learned in a cultural context, the cultural significance of eye behavior should also be considered.
- Be aware that your health care team members may use culturally oriented communication behaviors that make others uncomfortable. When the communication of a coworker makes you uncomfortable, it is important to assess whether the communication difference is related to cultural behavior.

Self-Reflection Questions

1. What facial expression and eye behavior do you use in communicating with others?
2. What eye behavior of others makes you uncomfortable?
3. What facial expression and eye behavior in patients or staff would you interpret as negative or hostile?

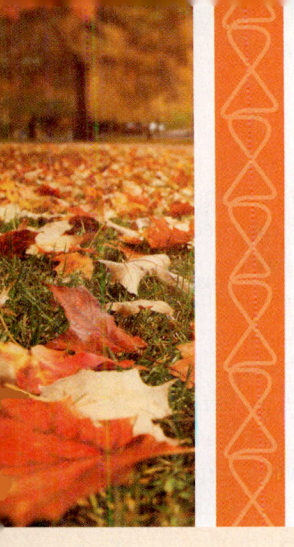

CHAPTER 6
Essential Nursing Pharmacology

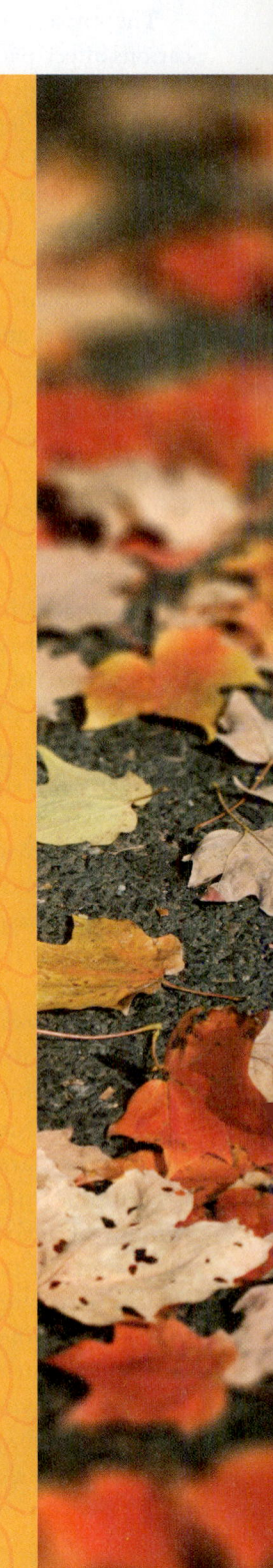

BRIEF OUTLINE

Drug Sources and Names
Drug Legislation and Resources
Pharmacokinetics
Absorption
Distribution
Metabolism (Biotransformation)
Excretion
Pharmacokinetics in Older Adults

Pharmacodynamics
Drug Effectiveness
Dose–Response Relationship
Variables in Drug Response
Drug Interactions
Adverse Drug Reactions

APPLIED LEARNING OUTCOMES

After completing this chapter, you will be able to:

1. Describe the naming of drugs and the laws that govern the prescription, storage, and administration of drugs.
2. Describe the processes of pharmacokinetics: absorption, distribution, metabolism, and excretion.
3. Explain factors that affect pharmacokinetics in older adults.
4. Identify how pharmacodynamics affects drug action.
5. Apply the nursing process to administering medications.
6. Practice the six rights of medication administration and the nursing implications of each right.
7. Use nursing strategies to reduce medication errors.

KEY TERMS

The key terms are defined on the pages listed below.

SPECIAL FEATURES

The study of drugs and their uses in the body is called **pharmacology**. Drugs can be used to prevent disease, aid in the diagnosis and treatment of disease, and restore or maintain body system function. For many disease conditions, drug therapy is the only treatment available to control or cure the disease. In other disease processes, the goal may be relief of symptoms in order to increase the patient's quality of life.

The nurse is responsible for understanding how medications affect patients, as well as the legal implications for administering medications. This chapter focuses on drug standards and legislation, pharmacokinetics, and pharmacodynamics. The nurse's role in applying the nursing process during medication administration is also presented.

Drug Sources and Names

Drugs are made from natural resources, including plants, animal tissue, and minerals. Some drugs are produced synthetically in the laboratory, whereas others are developed through genetic engineering. Synthetic drugs have the advantage of being made in large quantities, possibly reducing the cost when compared with that of natural drugs. Genetic engineering uses recombinant DNA techniques to put together DNA material from different organisms to form new drugs. An example of a product of this process is Humulin, which is used to manage diabetes mellitus.

All drugs have four names: chemical, generic, trade, and official. The *chemical name* describes the chemical compounds and molecular structure of the drug. Chemical names are long and seldom used, for example, acetylsalicylic acid. For this reason, drugs are given a shorter name called a nonproprietary or *generic name*. The nonproprietary name is approved by the United States Adopted Names (USAN) Council. Thus acetylsalicylic acid is known by its generic name aspirin. The *trade name*, sometimes called a brand name, identifies drugs sold by a specific manufacturer. The symbols ® or ™ (trademark) after the drug signify that the *trade name is registered*. A common trade name for aspirin is Bufferin®. The *official name* is usually the trade name. Official names are listed in the *United States Pharmacopeia–National Formulary (USP–NF)*.

Laws regulate generic and nongeneric drugs with respect to the amount and purity of each drug. Only a small amount of active ingredient is in every tablet, leaving the rest of the tablet to be filled with nonmedicinal substances. Although a generic drug is therapeutically equal to its trade name drug, some patients may not receive the same therapeutic effect. It is unclear why a few patients may not receive the same effect. In many states, the law requires pharmacists to fill prescriptions with the generic form. However, a prescriber can direct the pharmacist to fill a prescription with a specific trade name drug. Some prescription drug plans have a higher co-pay amount when generic drugs are not prescribed. Patients may request the generic form in order to decrease their co-pay amount. Prescriptions may not be listed on an insurance company's formulary, resulting in additional costs to the patient.

Nurses must be familiar with both the generic and trade names for a drug in order to prevent potential errors. Physicians are encouraged to write prescriptions by using both names. To recognize the difference between generic and trade names, the generic name is listed first in small letters with the trade name capitalized and placed in parentheses after it, for example, digoxin (Lanoxin).

Drug Legislation and Resources

Key Concept The Food and Drug Administration is responsible for approving drugs for clinical safety before they are sold on the market. The Controlled Substances Act passed in 1970 set rules for the manufacture and administration of narcotics and dangerous drugs.

Several drug laws are important in nursing practice. In 1906, the Pure Food and Drug Act was passed to protect the public by restricting the manufacture and sale of drugs. This act was replaced in 1938 by the Food, Drug, and Cosmetic Act, which added new regulations regarding labeling and packaging of drugs, as well as requiring drug companies to perform toxicity tests on lab animals. Under the U.S. Department of Health and Human Services, the Food and Drug Administration (FDA) enforces this legislation.

The Controlled Substances Act identifies and regulates the manufacture and sale of narcotics and dangerous drugs. Under this law, five schedules (Table 6-1 ■) of drugs based on abuse potential and medical effectiveness have been developed. For instance, Schedule I drugs (e.g., heroin, peyote) have the highest abuse potential without any proven medical use in the United States. This act is administered by the Drug Enforcement Administration (DEA), under the Department of Justice. Anyone who possesses a controlled substance without a prescription is subject to fines, imprisonment, or both. In addition, special DEA duplicate prescription pads must be used when a prescriber prescribes certain controlled substances.

All health care facilities are required to have narcotic control systems in place. Policies must be in place regarding use, drug wastage, and documentation. Narcotics are always locked up, and only authorized persons have access to them.

Nurses require reliable and up-to-date drug information to give medications safely and accurately. Given that numerous new drugs and medicinal agents are approved and marketed each year, textbooks quickly become outdated. In the acute care setting, *Micromedex*, an Internet site, and the

TABLE 6-1	Schedule for Controlled Substances	
SCHEDULE	**DEFINITION**	**EXAMPLES**
Schedule I	Drugs with high abuse potential and no accepted medical use	Heroin, peyote
Schedule II	Drugs with high abuse potential and accepted medical use	Opioid analgesics (morphine, codeine, meperidine); cocaine; amphetamines
Schedule III	Drugs with moderate abuse potential and accepted medical use	Drugs containing an opioid plus a nonnarcotic (Vicodin, Lortab)
Schedule IV	Drugs with low abuse potential and accepted medical use	Benzodiazepines (diazepam [Valium], chloral hydrate, phenobarbital)
Schedule V	Drugs with limited abuse potential and accepted medical use	Narcotics used in small amounts for antitussive and antidiarrheal

Hospital Formulary are the most readily available and accurate sources of drug information. Two additional references are *Facts and Comparisons*, a loose-leaf notebook, containing drug information that is updated monthly and the *Physicians' Desk Reference* (PDR). Package inserts that accompany drugs are another resource to check. The FDA and RxMed have websites that provide drug information.

Pharmacokinetics

Key Concept Medications are substances that alter body function to prevent or treat disease, aid in diagnosis, and restore or maintain function. The goal of drug therapy is to provide maximum therapeutic benefit with minimal side effects.

Pharmacokinetics is the study of how drugs are processed by the body. It describes the steps that occur from the time a patient is administered a drug until it is eliminated from the body. Specific processes that make up pharmacokinetics include absorption, distribution, metabolism (or biotransformation), and excretion (Figure 6-1■).

ABSORPTION

Absorption is the first step in the passage of a drug through the body. The absorption process occurs from the time a drug enters the body until it enters the body fluids that carry the drug to its site(s) of action. A drug's absorption rate is important in identifying how soon the drug becomes available to exert its action. If the drug is not absorbed properly, it may not reach its targeted organs or tissues.

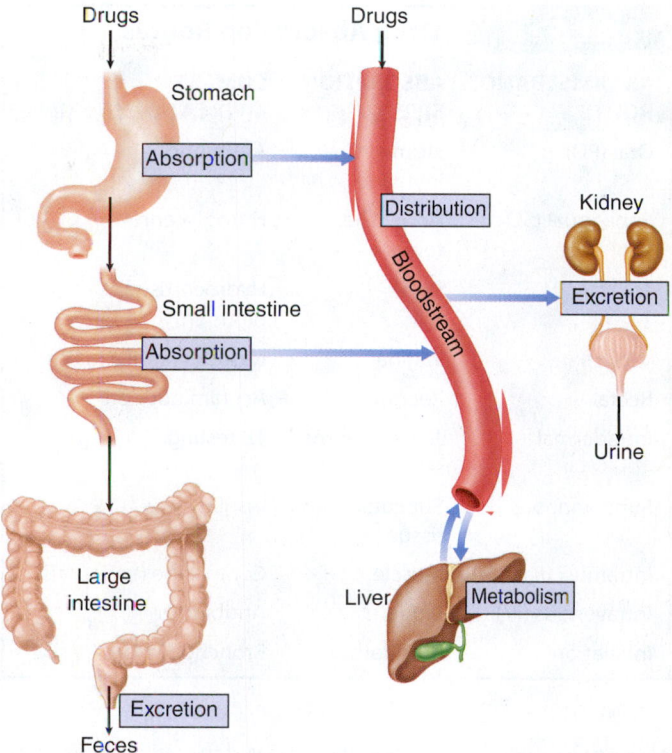

Figure 6-1. ■ The four processes of drug movement (pharmacokinetics): absorption, distribution, metabolism, and excretion. (Source: "Figure 4.01 - The Four Processes of Drug Movement (Pharmacokinetics): Absorption, Distribution, Metabolism, and Excretion" from *Core Concepts in Pharmacology*, 4e by Leland Norman Holland; Michael Patrick Adams; and Jeanine Lynn Brice. Published by Pearson Education, © 2014.)

Oral preparations are swallowed and dissolved by gastric juices before they reach the small intestine. They must pass through the gastrointestinal (GI) lining and blood vessels before they gain access to the blood. *Sublingual* (under the tongue) or *buccal* (placed in the inner lining of the cheeks) drugs enter the bloodstream through the lining of the mouth. Topical ointments enter through the skin, and rectal suppositories are absorbed through the mucous membranes into the blood. Transdermal (applied to the skin) patches absorb drugs slowly into the body and usually have a longer duration of action.

Parenteral (injectable) drugs, such as *subcutaneous* (below the skin) and *intramuscular* (IM; into a muscle) drugs, are absorbed faster than oral drugs. Drugs given via the *intradermal* route (injection into dermis) are also absorbed faster than oral drugs and are used to test for diseases (e.g., tuberculosis) and allergies. Intravenous (IV) drugs have the fastest absorption rate because they are delivered directly into the bloodstream. Other medication routes include ear, eye, nose, and inhalation. Common routes and drug examples are listed in Table 6-2■.

DISTRIBUTION

After a drug is absorbed, it is distributed to various organs and tissues. Several factors affecting *drug distribution* include blood flow, plasma protein binding, and the blood–brain barrier. Within minutes after

TABLE 6-2		Drug Absorption Routes
ADMINISTRATION ROUTE	ABSORPTION SITE	COMMON MEDICATION EXAMPLE
Oral (PO)	Stomach/intestine	Antibiotics
Sublingual (SL)	Under the tongue	Nitroglycerin
Topical	Skin	Hydrocortisone ointment
Vaginal	Vagina	Nystatin (antifungal)
Rectal	Rectum	Acetaminophen
Intradermal	Just under the skin	TB testing
Subcutaneous	Subcutaneous tissue	Insulin
Intramuscular (IM)	Muscle	Compazine (antiemetic)
Intravenous (IV)	Blood	Antibiotics
Inhalation	Respiratory	Bronchodilators

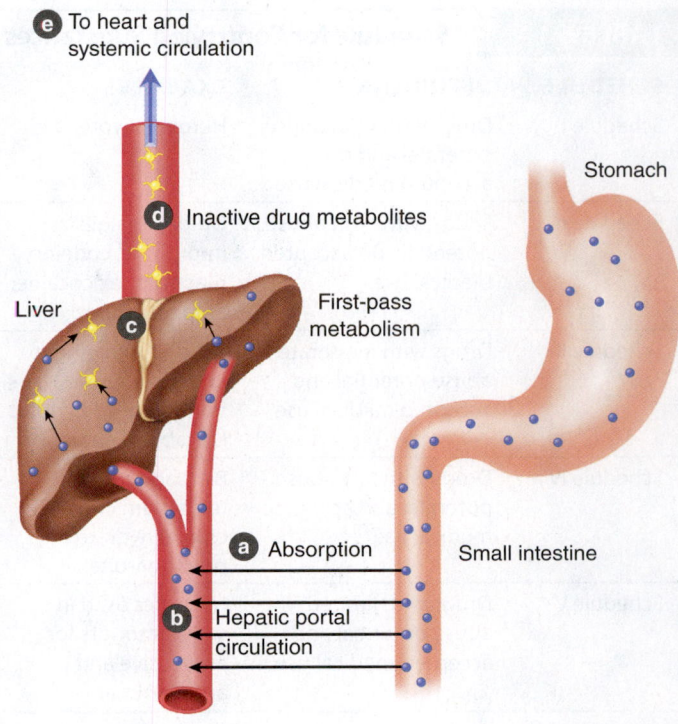

Figure 6-2. ■ First-pass effect. (Source: "Figure 4.02 - First-Pass Effect" from *Core Concepts in Pharmacology* 4e by Leland Norman Holland; Michael Patrick Adams; and Jeanine Lynn Brice. Published by Pearson Education, © 2014.)

absorption into the bloodstream, a drug is delivered to those organs (heart, liver, kidney, and brain) with the largest blood supply. When blood supply from the heart is reduced, adequate tissue levels of a drug are difficult to attain. Drug delivery to other internal organs, muscle, skin, and fat is slower and may take from minutes to hours.

After absorption into the bloodstream, most drugs bind with the plasma proteins, especially albumin, which transports the drug to its site of action. However, because the albumin molecule is too large to pass through the capillary wall, the drug must be released from the albumin molecule to be available to the tissues. Thus drugs bound to albumin have slower absorption, resulting in a longer duration of action. For example, warfarin (Coumadin), an anticoagulant, lasts longer and can accumulate, increasing the patient's risk for bleeding.

Drug distribution to the brain is limited because of the blood–brain barrier. The blood–brain barrier protects the central nervous system (CNS) against severe toxic drug effects by preventing access to the cerebrospinal fluid. However, some drugs, such as anesthetics, can cross the blood–brain barrier.

METABOLISM (BIOTRANSFORMATION)

Drug metabolism (also called **biotransformation**) refers to the process by which the body changes a drug from its original chemical structure into a form that can be readily eliminated or excreted. The metabolism of most drugs takes place in the liver. Microsomal enzymes

(drug-metabolizing enzymes) in the liver break down the drug and also detoxify any potentially harmful substances to the body. Liver diseases such as hepatitis and cirrhosis inhibit the enzyme action, resulting in excess drug accumulation in the body.

Oral drugs, absorbed from the GI tract, move from the intestine into the liver before passing into the systemic circulation. This means that for drugs metabolized extensively in the liver, only a portion of the drug dose will ever reach its action site. This is referred to as a *first-pass effect* (Figure 6-2■). In order for a patient to receive a therapeutic effect, the oral dose is often much greater than a parenteral dose (e.g., an IM or IV dose), which bypasses the liver.

EXCRETION

The common routes of *drug excretion* are the kidneys, lungs, and the large intestine (in feces). The kidney is the most important organ of drug excretion. Drugs are eliminated either unchanged or as metabolites in urine. Kidney disease may impair excretion, lead to drug accumulation, and increase the potential for severe adverse reactions. The respiratory system is involved with excretion only when a drug changes into a gaseous form, as do, for example, anesthetics. Biliary excretion involves the drug being taken up by the liver, released into the bile, and eliminated in the feces. Drugs excreted by this process remain in the body longer than those excreted by other means.

PHARMACOKINETICS IN OLDER ADULTS

Older adults, aged 65 years or older, often have at least one chronic health problem such as arthritis, diabetes, heart failure, and hypertension for which they take medications. Many take at least four or more prescription drugs daily as well as about 40% of the over-the-counter (OTC) drugs sold. Physiologic changes occur in the older adult that affect the normal pharmacokinetic processes (Box 6-1■). The practice of *polypharmacy* (use of many prescribed and OTC drugs at the same time), along with pharmacokinetic changes, increases the risks of adverse drug reactions (ADRs) and drug toxicity in the older adult. For example, an older adult may take aspirin to prevent myocardial infarction, but physiologic changes increase the risk for aspirin toxicity. Studies indicate that up to 30% of hospital admissions of older adults are related to ADRs. To help reduce ADRs, the Beers Criteria has been developed, which lists medications that are inappropriate for older adults. Also, it is recommended that new medication dosages should be started at a lower dose with the dose increased slowly over time.

clinicalALERT

Changes in mental status and falls may mistakenly be associated with aging rather than the use of multiple drugs or from psychotropic medications.

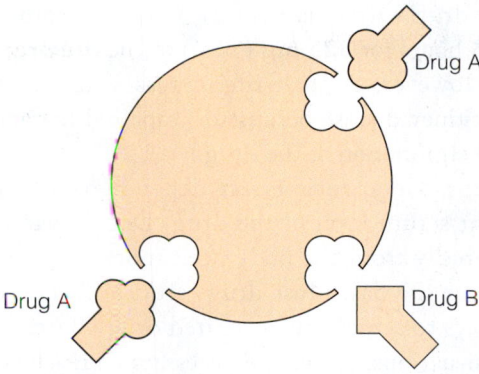

Figure 6-3. ■ Receptor site action: Drug A fits into the receptor site like a key into a lock to initiate a drug reaction. Drug B does not fit into this receptor site; therefore, no drug action occurs at this site.

Pharmacodynamics

Pharmacodynamics is the study of how drugs produce their effects in the body to result in a pharmacologic response. Drug action begins after a drug attaches itself to a specific area on the cell, called a *receptor site* (Figure 6-3■). By binding to the receptor, a drug can either initiate or block a cell response. Drugs that combine with a specific receptor to cause a pharmacologic response are called **agonists**. For example, morphine is an agonist, binding to receptors in the CNS to decrease pain. **Antagonists** are drugs that prevent a receptor response or block a normal cellular response. Naloxone (Narcan) blocks the depression of the CNS caused by narcotic agonists such as morphine. Antihistamines block the normal release of histamine to stop allergy symptoms.

Drugs can have a *local* or *systemic* effect, depending on the location and action on the cell receptors. Examples of drugs with a local effect include eye, ear, and nose drops; lozenges; skin ointments; and suppositories. Systemic drugs, such as narcotics for pain relief, must travel through the bloodstream to affect cells or tissues.

DRUG EFFECTIVENESS

The effectiveness of a drug depends on its action and dose. Each drug has an onset, peak, and duration of action. *Onset of action* is the time it takes for a drug to reach an effective blood level and to initiate a body response. The onset can be slow, intermediate, or rapid depending on the route of administration and pharmacokinetic principles. *Peak action* occurs when the drug achieves its highest blood concentration. The length of time that a drug has a pharmacologic effect is called its *duration of action*.

The length of time that a drug remains effective depends on its half-life. **Half-life** is the amount of time needed for elimination processes to decrease the original blood concentration by 50% (one-half). For example, if a 650-mg dose of a drug with a half-life of 3 hours is administered, it takes 3 hours for 325 mg (50%) of the drug to be eliminated. However, the half-life increases in patients with liver or kidney disease because of impaired metabolism or impaired elimination of the drug.

A drug's therapeutic effect depends on maintaining a constant serum level of the drug. Drugs that are eliminated rapidly from the body need more frequent dosing throughout the day. Most drugs require several doses or several days to achieve their desired drug effect. In certain clinical situations, it may be necessary to reach therapeutic drug levels rapidly. In these cases, a **loading dose** (an initial higher-than-normal dose of drug) is given, usually intravenously, to produce the desired result quickly. After the loading dose, smaller *maintenance* doses are given to maintain the drug level within a therapeutic range. A common example of this practice is the administration of digoxin (Lanoxin) to a patient in acute heart failure. (Refer to Chapter 16 for more information on heart failure.)

DOSE–RESPONSE RELATIONSHIP

The response to any drug depends on the amount of drug given. As the dose increases, so does the response, until a maximum response is attained. Potency and efficacy are two factors used to determine dose responsiveness. *Potency* is the relationship between the dose of the drug and the intensity of its effect. A more potent drug will achieve effects similar to another drug. However, the more potent drug can be administered in a smaller dose. For example, 10 mg of morphine equals 1 mg of hydromorphone (Dilaudid). It is clear that hydromorphone is more potent; however, the doses are equally effective. A dose–response curve is used to plot the potency of drugs (Figure 6-4A■).

Efficacy refers to a drug's maximum effect. The efficacy of a drug is seen on the dose–response curve when it reaches a plateau (Figure 6-4B■). For example, acetaminophen effectively controls mild to moderate pain; morphine effectively controls all levels of pain. This makes morphine a more effective pain reliever than acetaminophen. Once a

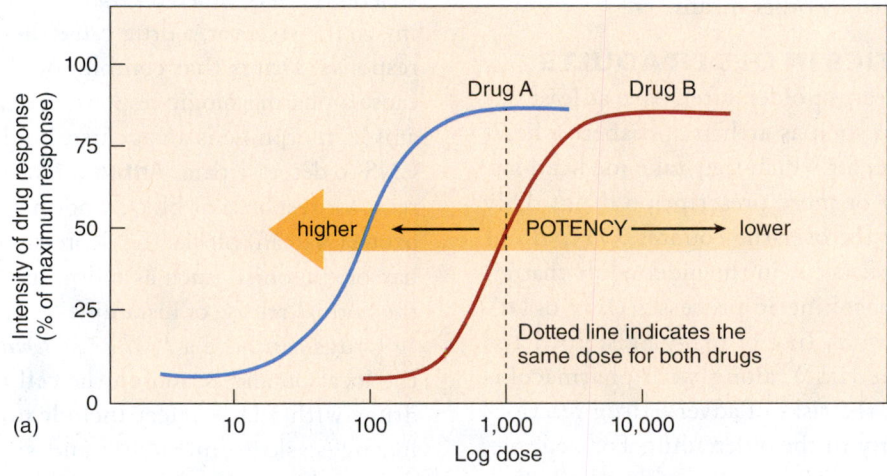

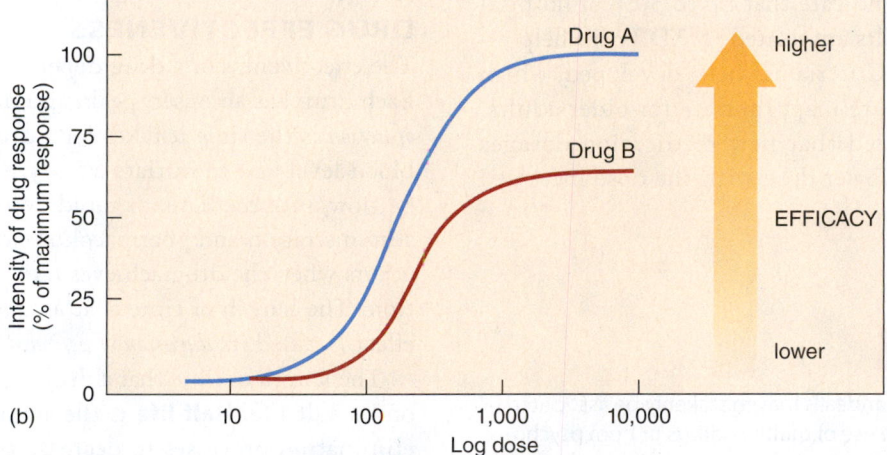

Figure 6-4. ■ Potency and efficacy. (A) Drug A has a higher potency than drug B. (B) Drug A has a higher efficacy than drug B. (Source: "Figure 4.06 - Potency and Efficacy. (a) Drug A has a Higher Potency than Drug B. (b) Drug A has a higher efficacy than Drug B" from *Core Concepts in Pharmacology*, 4e by Leland Norman Holland; Michael Patrick Adams; and Jeanine Lynn Brice. Published by Pearson Education, © 2014.)

drug is at its plateau, a further increase in dose will not increase its effectiveness.

Some drugs have a **ceiling effect**, which means that there is a dose limit to produce a specific effect. For instance, acetaminophen (Tylenol) has a ceiling effect of 3,200 mg/day. Doses exceeding the ceiling effect usually cause undesirable results, such as liver toxicity with acetaminophen.

VARIABLES IN DRUG RESPONSE

Drug response varies in each patient, even when the same dose and dosage regimen are followed. Factors that contribute to this variation include age, body weight, genetics, ethnicity, disease conditions, and psychosocial influences.

Age

Infants, children, and older adults are more sensitive to drug actions than middle-aged adults. The very young have an immature liver and kidneys, which slow drug metabolism and excretion. Altered pharmacokinetics in older adults increases and prolongs the effects of drugs.

Body Weight

Dosage is often prescribed in relation to a patient's weight. Patients who are underweight or overweight may require different doses. The usual adult dose of a drug is based on individuals between 18 and 65 years old and weighing 150 pounds (70 kg). Some drug doses are calculated on body weight (milligrams per kilograms), such as drugs given to pediatric patients.

Genetics

Drugs are expected to have predictable results. However, in some patients given the same drug in the same dose, the results vary. Some may not achieve the therapeutic effect, whereas others experience adverse effects. In the new field of *pharmacogenetics*, the relationship between a person's genetic makeup and response to medication is being studied. To date it has shown that some people lack certain drug-metabolizing enzymes as a result of their genetic makeup. When an enzyme is missing, drug metabolism slows, increasing the risk for prolonged drug effects and possible serious consequences. Other patients do not lack enzymes but rather have an increased metabolic rate. They may need higher doses or more frequent drug administration to overcome the rapid metabolism of the drug.

Ethnicity

Ethnicity also plays a role in drug response. For example, in African Americans, some antihypertensive drugs are less effective than in Caucasians. Asian patients may need lower doses of the antianxiety drug alprazolam (Xanax), the antipsychotic agent haloperidol (Haldol), and the analgesics codeine and morphine.

Disease Conditions

Liver disease alters metabolism, whereas kidney disease decreases excretion. Cardiac conditions, such as heart failure, reduce the heart's pumping ability, decreasing all pharmacokinetic processes. Inflammatory bowel disorders (Crohn's disease, ulcerative colitis) can either increase or decrease absorption. Hyperthyroidism and fever increase metabolism, causing a shorter duration and faster elimination. Hypothyroidism slows a person's metabolic rate, which prolongs drug action. Malnutrition lowers the concentration of albumin, which is necessary for plasma protein binding.

Psychosocial Influences

Patients' living arrangements, family involvement and interactions, financial resources, emotional state, and cognitive function can affect the outcome of their drug therapy. For example, a patient who is homeless or unemployed often lacks adequate resources to follow through with drug therapy. A person who is grieving may lack the motivation to follow a therapeutic drug regimen. Usually individuals with a positive attitude and supportive environment respond better to drug therapy. In contrast, patients who are depressed may not respond as well.

DRUG INTERACTIONS

Drug interaction refers to the effects that occur when the actions of one drug are affected by another drug. The most common types of interactions are called additive, synergism, and potentiation. An **additive** effect develops when two drugs with similar actions are taken. Additive effects increase the sum of the effects of the two drugs. Combining aspirin with codeine increases pain relief and usually lowers the dose of each drug, resulting in fewer toxic effects. However, a dangerous situation occurs when alcohol is consumed with sedative drugs, because the combination increases their sedative effect.

When two drugs given together cause a greater response than each drug given separately, it is called **synergism**. A patient may receive two different drugs for hypertension, lowering blood pressure in two different ways. The combined effect of these two drugs more effectively lowers the blood pressure than either one by itself.

Potentiation is the process by which the action of one drug increases the effect of the second drug. Patients who take anticoagulants are advised against taking aspirin because the two drugs together increase the risk for bleeding.

Other drug interactions develop during the pharmacokinetic process. For instance, antacids decrease the absorption of drugs in the GI tract. This action affects such drugs as digoxin (cardiac drug), isoniazid (antitubercular drug), and tetracycline (antibiotic). Another interaction occurs in smokers. Nicotine increases the action of the drug-metabolizing enzymes, causing rapid metabolism of medications.

Drug dosages in smokers would have to be increased to obtain therapeutic results similar to those for nonsmokers.

Drug incompatibilities can occur while preparing or administering intramuscular or intravenous medications. A drug *incompatibility* is defined as a chemical or physical reaction between two drugs. This reaction can either inactivate one of the drugs or form a precipitate (discoloration or particles). For example, Lantus insulin (antidiabetic) forms a precipitate when mixed with regular insulin.

clinical**ALERT**

Before combining or administering two drugs together, consult with a pharmacist or a drug compatibility chart.

Food–Drug Interactions

Food can increase, decrease, or delay drug absorption. Box 6-2■ lists some food–drug interactions that may occur.

clinical**ALERT**

Before administering oral medications, determine whether they should be given before, with, or after meals.

Over-the-Counter Drugs

OTC drugs can be purchased without a prescription. About 60% of all medications are classified as OTCs. The FDA is responsible for maintaining the safety of this drug class. Common OTCs include analgesics for pain, antacids, antihistamines, cough and cold medications, eyedrops, hemorrhoid products, herbal supplements, laxatives, sleep aids, vitamin supplements, and weight loss aids. Some OTCs such as ibuprofen and famotidine (Pepcid) were once prescription drugs.

OTCs allow the consumer to treat minor illnesses. Usually they are an effective, inexpensive way to manage common health problems for a short period of time. However, OTCs are not without potential problems. Patients may delay seeking medical care, resulting in serious or life-threatening consequences. Drug interactions can occur with prescription drugs, herbal therapies, or other OTCs. Individuals with liver and kidney disease should avoid OTCs unless recommended by their health care provider.

Herbal Therapy

The practice of using herbal therapy has existed for thousands of years. Many cultures believe that herbs can prevent or cure health problems. For the past two decades, there has been increased interest in products without preservatives or additives, resulting in greater use of herbal therapy and other nontraditional remedies.

In the early 1990s, the FDA threatened to ban all herbal remedies. As a result of public outcry, Congress passed the Dietary Supplement Health and Education Act of 1994. It reclassified herbal remedies as dietary supplements. However, the safety and effectiveness of herbal therapies are not regulated and manufacturing regulations are not standardized. Allergic, adverse, and toxic reactions can develop from herbal remedies, just like with OTC and prescription drugs. To help protect the public, Congress passed the Dietary Supplement and Nonprescription Drug Consumer Protection Act in 2007, which mandates reporting of serious adverse events to dietary supplements and nonprescription drugs.

Herbal therapies are available in a variety of forms, including dried or fresh herbs, teas, ointments, oils, syrups, and tinctures. The most common herbal therapies are listed in Box 6-3■. Their uses can be found throughout this textbook as they relate to specific disease conditions.

Patients should be taught to avoid taking herbal therapies if pregnant or nursing. Herbal therapies should not be given to infants or children. Older adults with renal or hepatic impairment have a higher risk for drug interactions with herbal therapies. All patients are advised to contact their health care provider before substituting an herb for a

---

BOX 6-2	SELECTED FOOD–DRUG INTERACTIONS

- Vitamin K (dark-green leafy vegetables) reduces the absorption of warfarin (anticoagulant).
- Calcium in milk and milk products binds with tetracycline (antibiotic), reducing its absorption.
- Caffeine can increase the action and adverse effects of theophylline (bronchodilator).
- Protein delays the absorption of levodopa.
- Grapefruit juice can increase drug levels, especially calcium channel blockers, caffeine, cyclosporine (immunosuppressant), and cholesterol-lowering drugs.
- Foods with tyramine (aged cheeses, fermented meats, bean curd, aged beer, and Chianti wine) can create a toxic reaction if consumed while taking monoamine oxidase (MAO) inhibitors. Combining tyramine foods with the MAO inhibitor can cause a hypertensive crisis or stroke.

BOX 6-3	COMPLEMENTARY THERAPIES

Common Herbal Therapies

- Black cohosh
- Echinacea
- Feverfew
- Flaxseed
- Garlic
- Ginger
- Ginkgo
- Ginseng
- Green tea
- Saw palmetto
- St. John's wort
- Valerian

prescription drug. Herbal therapies should be considered medicines and, therefore, used cautiously.

ADVERSE DRUG REACTIONS

The desired action of all drugs is achievement of a *therapeutic effect*. However, drugs are not without the potential to cause harm. ADRs can develop that range from mild to severe—even death. The most frequent ADRs include side effects, allergies, idiosyncratic effects, and toxic effects.

Side effects are anticipated effects from a therapeutic drug dose. Most often they are mild. For example, opioid analgesics may cause nausea and constipation, whereas antihistamines are known to cause drowsiness and dry mouth. Gastric irritation is a common side effect after the administration of corticosteroids and aspirin. Side effects can develop within a few hours of starting a new drug or can be delayed for weeks.

Drug *allergy* occurs when an individual becomes sensitized to a specific drug, producing antibodies against the drug (antigen). Subsequent administration of the drug leads to an antigen–antibody reaction. Reaction between the antibody and the antigen causes damage to body tissues. The injured cells release histamine that generates the characteristic symptoms of an allergy. These include hives, rashes, itching, and nasal secretion. Severe allergic reactions, called *anaphylaxis*, begin within minutes of exposure. They produce hypotension, tachycardia, and bronchoconstriction; without immediate treatment, death may result. (See Chapter 14 for further information about anaphylaxis and anaphylactic shock.)

When a very small percentage of the population develops an unusual or unexpected response, the reaction is termed an *idiosyncratic effect*. The response may be opposite the desired effect, such as agitation from a sedative drug. Often idiosyncrasy is triggered by a genetic difference not found in most individuals.

Toxic effects denote harmful, undesired effects (e.g., persistent vomiting) or the possibility of organ damage. Most drugs are capable of producing toxic effects when administered in high doses. For example, patients taking excessive amounts of opioid narcotics are at risk for severe respira-

tory depression and possibly death. Toxicity can also develop when serum drug levels exceed the therapeutic range. Drugs with a narrow therapeutic range, such as digitalis, aminoglycoside antibiotics, and anticonvulsants, are monitored through serum blood levels to prevent toxic effects.

Because most drugs are metabolized in the liver and excreted in the kidneys, these organs can suffer potential damage. Liver damage (*hepatotoxicity*) results from an overdose of acetaminophen. Aminoglycosides can damage the kidneys (*nephrotoxicity*) as well as the eighth cranial nerve, causing *ototoxicity*.

Other *systems* most often affected include the blood, GI tract, skin, and lungs. Bone marrow suppression (anemia, thrombocytopenia, and leukopenia) results from chemotherapy agents. Gastrointestinal toxicity includes GI ulceration, bleeding, or pseudomembranous colitis (a severe form of colitis). Severe skin reactions such as exfoliative dermatitis and Stevens–Johnson syndrome can develop. Some antibiotics and chemotherapy drugs may cause drug-induced asthma or pneumonitis.

Drugs that cause birth defects are known to have a *teratogenic effect*. They must be avoided in pregnant women. Other drugs with a *carcinogenic effect* may promote the growth of cancerous tumors.

NURSING CARE

The nursing care process is a systematic process for providing care to patients. The nursing process, when correctly applied to drug therapy, reduces the potential for errors and promotes sound decision making.

PRIORITIZING NURSING CARE

Before administering any medication, the nurse must determine that the patient does not have allergies to the medication and that the medication is appropriate for the patient's age and diagnosis. Vital signs must be within safe limits, especially if the medication affects blood pressure, pulse, or respiratory rate. The dose also must be within safe limits.

ASSESSING

Assessment begins by collecting data on the patient's medication history. When first meeting the patient, assess weight, age, health status, and symptoms for any disease conditions. The nurse conducts a nonjudgmental interview about medication use and any factors that could affect the patient's adherence with a medication schedule (Box 6-4 ■). When information cannot be obtained from the patient, contact family members and check the chart for the patient's history. The patient's level of education and understanding is included during assessment.

BOX 6-4	MEDICATION HISTORY

- Use of prescription and OTC drugs and herbal remedies
- Purpose of and response to current drugs
- Types of allergies—drugs, food, animal, dust, plants
- Allergic reactions, side effects, or toxic effects to current or past drugs
- Use of alcohol, nicotine, caffeine, contraceptives, or street drugs
- Presence of liver, kidney, GI, or heart diseases
- Attitude about taking medications
- Adherence to drug therapy
- Financial resources
- Access to family, friends, or neighbors
- Dietary habits and cultural influences

A physical examination is performed to determine whether the patient has physical or mental problems that could affect his or her ability to take any medication. The nurse assesses for hearing and visual deficits, swallowing difficulty, tremors, motor weakness, and manual dexterity. Patients with mental disorders may have difficulty remembering or understanding how to take their medications. Those with reading deficits may be unable to follow the directions on a drug label. The nurse should review pertinent laboratory test values such as liver and kidney function studies, white blood cell (WBC) count, hemoglobin, hematocrit, electrolytes, and albumin levels.

DIAGNOSING, PLANNING, AND IMPLEMENTING

Diagnosing focuses on identifying the patient's actual and potential health problems based on the assessment data. The LPN contributes to the development of the nursing diagnosis. Several nursing diagnoses can be selected for patients receiving drug therapy. The following are examples of appropriate nursing diagnoses:

- Deficient Knowledge
- Ineffective Health Maintenance
- Noncompliance
- Risk for Injury Related to Side Effects

During the planning step, the nurse reviews the drug's purpose, recommended dose, potential side effects, and therapeutic effects. The nurse plans when medications are scheduled according to the physician's orders. Factors to consider include drug–food or drug–drug interactions and frequency of dosing. In addition, the nurse plans patient teaching about taking medications at home.

The implementing step involves the actual nursing interventions used to administer drug therapy. Before giving any medication, an authorized health care pro-

vider must either write or verbally state an order. It is recommended that verbal orders be used only during emergency situations to reduce the potential for errors occurring. When a verbal order is given for a medication, ask the prescriber to spell out the drug name and dosage. To further reduce error potential, the Joint Commission requires nurses to read back all orders to the health care provider. All medication orders must include the following information:

- Patient's name
- Date and time order was written
- Drug with dose, route, and frequency
- Any special instruction for administration
- Physician's or health care provider's signature

clinicalALERT

Never implement an order that is incomplete, unclear, or written illegibly.

Different types of drug orders are used to direct when the nurse should administer drugs. *Routine orders* are applied until a discontinuation order is written. Some agencies have an automatic stop date, which encourages the physician to reevaluate the patient's condition and reorder, change, or stop the drug. A *standing order* is used for a specific condition in which a drug is to be given. For example, "Give acetaminophen (Tylenol) 650 mg suppository for temperature above 101.6°F." *Stat orders* are to be done immediately, and *prn orders* are to be implemented when the patient needs them.

The nurse is responsible for carrying out an order as it is written, but only after determining that the medication is appropriate for the patient. The nurse cannot change an order without clarifying it with the health care provider who wrote the order. It is the nurse's duty to clarify any unclear orders. In addition, the nurse must know that medication reconciliation has occurred not only on admission to or discharge from a health care facility but also when the patient is transferred from one unit to another. Medication reconciliation involves verifying and clarifying all of the patient's medications and reconciling any discrepancies in the current orders.

To administer drugs safely, the nurse is expected to follow the "Six Rights" so that the potential for errors is reduced:

- Right drug
- Right patient
- Right time
- Right route
- Right dose
- Right documentation

Right Drug

Before administering any medication, always compare the drug label to the medication administration record (MAR) three times: (1) Compare the drug before taking it from the shelf or drawer. (2) Compare on removing the ordered amount of drug from the container. (3) Compare again before returning the container to the shelf or drawer, or with unit-dose packaging, as the drug is placed into the patient's hand.

clinicalALERT

Never administer medications that someone else has prepared.

Right Patient

Check the patient's name against an identification (ID) bracelet (in the hospital setting) and the MAR. Be sure that the ID bracelet is on the correct patient. When the ID bracelet is unclear or missing, ask the patient for identifying data such as first, middle, and last name and date of birth. For health care facilities that use bar coding, the nurse scans the bar code on the drug label, on the patient's ID band, and on the nurse's personal ID badge. An error message or alarm sounds if the nurse is about to make an error.

Right Time

Check the time for giving the drug with the MAR and check that the medication time is appropriate for the patient. Follow the routine times according to the facility's policies. Know patient-specific situations when it is inappropriate to administer a drug. For example, the indications for holding digoxin (Lanoxin) would be a pulse rate less than 60. Failure to administer drugs at the correct time is a medication error.

Right Route

Check the physician's order and the MAR to verify the correct route for administering the drug. Be aware of changes in the patient's health that could alter the route; for instance, a patient who is vomiting probably cannot take oral medications. The physician must be notified to change the route. Before crushing any medications, refer to a "do not crush" list supplied by the Institute for Safe Medical Practices (ISMP), or check with the pharmacist.

clinicalALERT

Do not crush enteric-coated and controlled-, extended-, or sustained-release medications because the patient could receive an overdose.

Right Dose

Be sure the dose matches the amount stated on the MAR, falls within the usual dose range for the drug, and is appropriate for the patient's condition. The *unit-dose system* (individually packaged drugs) has helped to reduce medication errors. If dose calculations are necessary, have another licensed nurse check them. Double-check all high-alert medications, such as insulin and heparin, with another nurse.

Right Documentation

Chart medications immediately after giving them, including drug, dose, route, date and time, and nurse's initials. Record and report immediately any unusual patient reaction to a medication or inability or refusal to take the prescribed drug.

clinicalALERT

Never chart a medication before giving it because it increases the risk of missing a dose.

Medication Errors

Key Concept Medication errors are preventable events that can greatly affect the patient's treatment or outcome. The nurse is the patient's last line of defense against medication errors.

Medication errors occur in all health care facilities. The National Coordinating Council for Medication Error Reporting and Prevention (NCC MERP) defines a medication error as "any preventable event that may cause or lead to inappropriate medication use or patient harm while the medication is in the control of the health care professional, patient, or consumer." Although nurses are the primary individuals administering medications, errors can occur at any point in the process. The most common types of errors causing patient death include the wrong dose, wrong drug, and wrong route. When the error involves a high-alert medication, it is considered a **sentinel event**. A sentinel event is any unexpected event in a health care facility that causes death or serious injury to a patient.

Numerous factors can contribute to medication errors. Most errors are due to communication failures such as poor handwriting, incomplete or verbal orders, and look-alike or sound-alike drugs. Human factors include miscalculation of doses and misuse of zeroes in decimal points (e.g., a dose written as .2 mg instead 0.2 mg).

Any medication error must be reported immediately to the nurse in charge. The next steps are to assess the patient, followed by notification of the patient's physician. Many health care facilities require the physician to make a follow-up visit to see the patient. The nurse who made the error is expected to complete an incident report. This is an objective, factual account of how the error occurred so that future errors can be prevented.

In addition to always following the Six Rights of medication administration, nurses can implement other strategies to prevent errors. For instance, an unfamiliar abbreviation, unusual drug name or dose, confusing drug name, or ambiguous drug order should signal a need for follow-up with the prescriber. When transcribing medication orders to the MAR, use only acceptable abbreviations and symbols as compiled by the ISMP and required by Joint Commission–accredited health care facilities.

While the nurse prepares the patient's medications, it is essential to think about why each drug is prescribed. The nurse should ask the following questions: "Does the drug, dose, and route seem appropriate for the patient's diagnosis? Has the patient achieved the desired therapeutic effect? Is the patient experiencing any drug side effects or adverse reactions?"

During drug preparation, several principles should be followed. The nurse should reduce distractions such as noise or talking with coworkers as much as possible while performing a medication-related task. It is unacceptable to use the dropper of one medication to administer another drug. When the pharmacy has dispensed multiple tablets, ampules, or vials to provide a single dose, the nurse should question the dose. If a dose seems unusually small or large, ask the pharmacist or physician for a clarification. As a final safety check, the MAR is either taken into the patient's room or accessed on the computer and the drug is compared with the MAR before administering it to the patient.

Patients can also assist in preventing errors. When a patient questions the color of a tablet or capsule, the number of pills, or an injection instead of a pill, recheck the MAR and physician orders. If a patient reports an allergy to a medication, do not give it, and verify the order with the patient's physician.

Acute health care facilities are implementing new strategies to reduce medication errors. Computerized provider order entry (CPOE) is becoming the standard to eliminate errors from illegible writing. A high-alert drug list developed by the ISMP includes the following medications: anticoagulants, insulin, opioids, oral hypoglycemics, injectable potassium chloride, neuromuscular blocking agents, paren-teral nutrition preparations, and chemotherapy. To further reduce potential medication errors, the ISMP recommends using capital letters for the part of the drug name that might be misread as another drug (e.g., glyBURIDE). Hospitals are expected to develop safety measures to reduce errors in administering these high-alert drugs. The Joint Commission's annual National Patient Safety Goals (The Joint Commission, 2013) continue to require interventions that can decrease errors.

The overall goal of medication administration is patient safety. To accomplish this goal, everyone involved in writing medication prescriptions, dispensing, and administering must make a conscious effort to prevent medication errors.

EVALUATING

The success of the nursing interventions is measured by evaluating the patient's outcomes. The patient should exhibit manifestations that the medication is effective. For example, pain should decrease after analgesic therapy. The nurse determines whether the patient has developed side effects or any drug interactions. The nurse should also evaluate the success of the teaching session with the patient.

CONTINUITY OF CARE

Another important aspect of medication administration is patient teaching. The patient should know the following information: name, dose, route, and purpose of the drug; special storage; preparation or disposal directions; and any expected or unusual side effects. It is essential that the patient realize the importance of not crushing or chewing long-acting oral medications, because this could result in an overdose. Teach patients to use an acceptable commercial device to crush or split appropriate medications. Patients must also understand the need for follow-up tests or evaluation related to their drug therapy and the duration of drug use. For example, patients taking analgesics for pain must know to discontinue the drug when the pain subsides. On the other hand, patients who take thyroid medications for hypothyroidism must understand the need to continue the medication lifelong. Remind the patient to not share medications with others. To ensure accurate drug information is provided, give the patient approved, preprinted drug information sheets. After patient teaching, the information presented must be documented in the chart.

Note: The references and resources for all chapters have been compiled at the back of the book.

Chapter Review

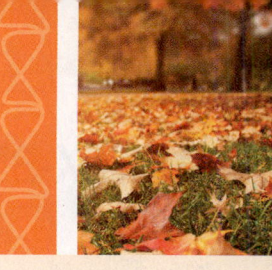

KEY POINTS

- **Concept:** The Food and Drug Administration is responsible for approving drugs for clinical safety before they are sold on the market. The Controlled Substances Act passed in 1970 set rules for the manufacture and administration of narcotics and dangerous drugs.
- Drugs have three basic names: chemical, generic, and trade. Each drug has only one generic name but may have several trade names.
- The administration of narcotics is strictly regulated. All narcotics are kept in locked cabinets or drawers and can be accessed only by authorized health care personnel.
- **Concept:** Medications are substances that alter body function to prevent or treat disease, aid in diagnosis, and restore or maintain function. The goal of drug therapy is to provide maximum therapeutic benefit with minimal side effects.
- Pharmacokinetics focuses on "what the body does to a drug" through the processes of absorption, distribution, metabolism, and excretion. Pharmacodynamics focuses on "what the drug does to the body."
- Older adults experience age-related decline in organ function that can change absorption, distribution, metabolism, and especially excretion of medications. Because older adults may have several disease conditions and take multiple medications, polypharmacy becomes a significant concern. To prevent possible drug interactions and adverse reactions, older adults should have a current list of all medications with them at all times.
- Common herbal therapies include echinacea, ginkgo, ginseng, and St. John's wort. Patients taking herbal therapies should notify their health care provider before taking them with prescribed medications.
- Adverse drug reactions (ADRs) range from expected side effects to toxic effects. The most common toxic effects include liver and kidney damage. Older adults have a higher risk for ADRs. To minimize this risk the principle of drug dosing is to "start low and go slow."
- **Concept:** Medication errors are preventable events that can greatly affect the patient's treatment or outcome. The nurse is the patient's last line of defense against medication errors.
- Nurses are responsible for safe and correct decision making in the administration of medications. Safe medication administration means implementing the "Six Rights" in order to prevent a medication error.
- The most common causes of fatal medication errors are miscommunication, performance or knowledge deficits, and confusion between sound-alike and look-alike drugs.
- Preventing medication errors requires everyone to make a commitment to patient safety.

PEARSON NURSING STUDENT RESOURCES

Find additional materials at **nursing.pearsonhighered.com**.

NCLEX-PN® Exam Preparation

1 Decreased serum albumin levels in the older adult would affect which part of the pharmacokinetic process?

1. Excretion
2. Metabolism
3. Distribution
4. Absorption

2 The nurse receives the following order: Lasix 40 PO BID. Dr. Lowe. What action should the nurse take?

1. Call the physician for a complete dosage.
2. Give the medication as ordered.
3. Wait until the physician calls the unit.
4. Call the physician for a time to start the drug.

3 Which of the following drug examples indicates a synergistic drug response?

1. Aspirin and an anticoagulant drug
2. Two different antihypertensive drugs
3. Nicotine and an anticonvulsant drug
4. Alcohol and a sedative drug

4 To prevent a medication error, the nurse should:

1. check illegible handwriting with another nurse.
2. accept atypical drug names as a new medication.
3. use the dropper of one medication to administer another.
4. question the use of multiple tablets to provide a single dose.

5 In which of the following patients is an adverse drug reaction most likely to occur?

1. A 4-year-old with croup
2. A 35-year-old with pneumonia
3. A 50-year-old with kidney disease
4. A 60-year-old with osteoarthritis

6 List the order of drug absorption from the most rapid route to the least rapid route.

1. Subcutaneous
2. Oral (PO)
3. Transdermal
4. Intravenous (IV)
5. Sublingual
6. Intramuscular (IM)

7 The physician prescribes Vicodin for a patient experiencing pain. Under what category of controlled substances is this drug found?

1. Schedule V
2. Schedule IV
3. Schedule III
4. Schedule II

8 What is the most important factor in administering medications to a 1-year-old infant?

1. Weight
2. Age
3. Ethnicity
4. Sex

9 When digoxin (Lanoxin) is started, a larger-than-normal dose may be given. This is called a:

1. scheduled dose.
2. maintenance dose.
3. therapeutic dose.
4. loading dose.

10 The nurse is reviewing information on a medication in a drug handbook and notices that the drug is teratogenic. Which of the following patients should not receive this medication?

1. Patients with renal failure
2. Pregnant patients
3. Children younger than 10 years
4. Patients older than 65 years

Answers and rationales for Review Questions appear in Appendix I.

CULTURAL CARE STRATEGIES

Integrating Cultural Diversity in Patient Education

Judith Lightfoot, a 29-year-old Native American, comes in to see the nurse about her diet for diabetes. While the nurse and Judith are talking, Judith says, "I really can't follow the diabetic diet you gave me. You see, on our Indian reservation, everybody shares what we have. We don't have much food at our house, so if I have special food I can't save it for the week. I need to share it with anybody in the house who is hungry. Of course, that means that some days we don't have anything to eat. But things usually work out. It is part of our culture to be generous with what we have and we will worry about tomorrow when the time comes."

When a patient is from a different culture, the nurse should be alert for cultural barriers that may interfere with the treatment regimen or effective patient education. Initial and ongoing assessments are essential to determine whether the patient understands the language being spoken and the care being provided. Health care facilities are expected to institute the National Standards for Culturally and Linguistically Appropriate Services (CLAS). Part of the CLAS standards includes providing an interpreter to limited English-proficient patients. When interpreters are not available at an agency, a telephone translator service may be an option. Unless an interpreter or bilingual staff member is unavailable, family (including children and friends) should not be used as interpreters, because they may be unable to translate medical information correctly.

Differences in Dialect

It is important for nurses to be aware that there can be significant contrasts within cultural groups. For example, there are 10 Hispanic/Latino groups, more than 20 Asian American/Pacific Islander groups, and more than 500 Native American tribal groups. In addition, census-defined African Americans may come

from non-African countries such as Haiti, Jamaica, and Panama. Significant differences in language and dialects within a culture may exist. Thus even though an interpreter may speak the language of the patient—for example, Spanish—communication may be unclear.

Differences in Communication Variables

It is important to assess not only language, but also the essential elements of communication of the language, including dialect, style (language and social situations), volume (silence), use of touch, context of speech (emotional tone), and kinetics (gesture, stance, and eye behavior). If the nurse always associates a soft voice with timidity, lack of assertiveness, and incompetence, the cultural reasons for this behavior may be ignored. If the nurse associates loudness with aggressiveness, while in the patient's culture loudness has a different meaning, behavior may be misinterpreted.

Even when individuals speak the same language, communication may be difficult. The meaning of words and how facts are presented may vary based on life experiences and cultural context.

Differences in Gender and Family Member Roles

Gender and gender roles can significantly influence attitudes about health and health education. Taboos related to sexual behavior have special significance for patient education. In male-dominated societies (Arab, Hispanic, and many Asian societies), information and decision-making responsibility must be given to the male. Women are expected to be modest and submissive. Thus education about sexual matters needs to

take into account who should be present in the room and who is appropriate (Giger & Davidhizar, 2012).

Literacy/Educational Handouts

Many English-speaking people have difficulty understanding medical terminology. If English is a second language, medical terminology is even more challenging. When written instructions are used, the language, the literacy, and the reading level of the patient should be evaluated. Written handouts should match the patient's reading level.

Nursing Implications

- *Before teaching, assess the patient's understanding of English.* If the nurse and the patient do not speak the same language, an interpreter may be necessary in order to provide effective teaching. If the patient and family can speak English but either speaks English as a second language or is from another culture, the nurse should be aware that there may be obstacles to communication.
- *Match patient education materials to the literacy level of the patient.* If a patient is from another culture, both literacy level and understanding of medical terminology should be assessed. Select appropriate educational materials that can be understood.

Self-Reflection Questions

1. What strategies could increase your effectiveness in teaching patients and their significant others?

2. If your patient cannot understand English, what translating services are available to assist in patient teaching?

3. What teaching materials are available that can assist in patient education?

You are a newly graduated LPN working in a long-term care facility. Because you have been employed here only 3 days, you are assigned to the following three patients. An LPN medication nurse will administer all routine medications, but you are to administer any PRN medications.

- James, an 83-year-old widower, has a diagnosis of peripheral vascular disease. He is a retired farmer. He is alert and oriented but forgetful. He enjoys most activities in the facility. He is ambulatory with a walker and can feed himself but needs reminding to use the toilet. He has an open sore on his right shin. The dressing needs changing daily.

- Margarita, a 92-year-old Spanish-speaking widow, has many chronic diseases that are stable with medication. She understands only a few words of English. Three months ago she fractured her left hip and underwent surgery to replace the femoral head. After surgery, she was admitted to the nursing home. She is alert but has become increasingly confused. She enjoys some activities, especially church service on Sunday. She is able to walk only a few steps. She needs assistance with all ADLs. She is incontinent of both bowel and bladder.

- Joseph, a 75-year-old married man, was injured in a car accident 15 years ago. He sustained a spinal cord injury and is a quadriplegic. Because of his increased weight, his 73-year-old wife was unable to care for him at home. She visits daily and enjoys helping him with his meals. Joseph is cheerful and enjoys attending activities. Because of his spinal cord injury, daily bowel care is critical. He has a suprapubic urinary catheter.

CRITICAL THINKING

- What activities will you plan to assist James with reminiscence of his farming career?

- Margarita takes many medications to treat her chronic diseases. How might this polypharmacy have affected Margarita's health status?

- What will be the safest method of transferring Joseph from the bed to the wheelchair?

PRIORITIES IN NURSING CARE

- In what order will you assess your patients?

- What is your rationale for your prioritization of care?

MANAGEMENT OF CARE

- Identify the nursing care needed for each patient over an 8-hour shift using a timeline format.

- If Margarita is able to return to her home, what interprofessional team members would be involved in planning her discharge?

DELEGATING

- If a CNA is available to assist with your assignment, what care would you delegate?

- What supervision and follow-up would be needed?

PATIENT TEACHING

- You are preparing to change the dressing on James's leg. What patient teaching should you provide before the dressing change?

- What teaching will you provide to Margarita?

- Joseph has been a quadriplegic for 15 years and understands his disorder and care. What teaching techniques might be beneficial when providing Joseph's care?

CULTURAL CARE STRATEGIES

- Has Margarita's language barrier (Spanish with limited English) had an impact on her confusion?

- How has Joseph's stage of psychosocial development impacted his acceptance of his quadriplegia?

DOCUMENTING AND REPORTING

- For each patient, what observations should be reported to the RN?

- Document the dressing change on James's right shin.

Note: Discussion of Unit Wrap-Up questions appears on the companion website.

UNIT II
Foundations of Medical–Surgical Nursing

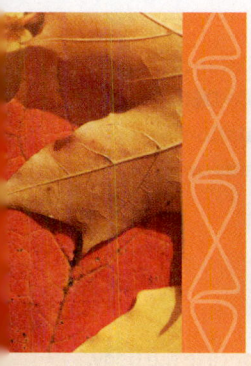 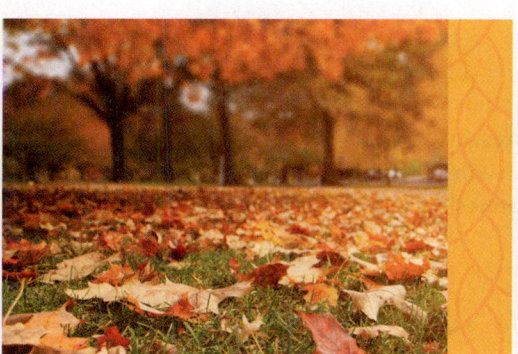 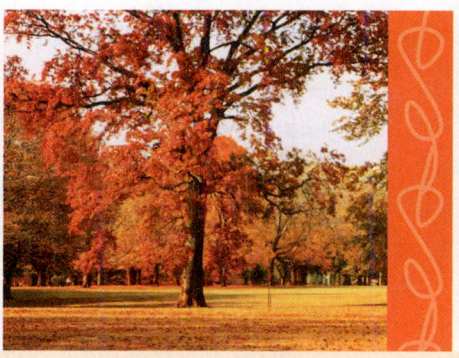 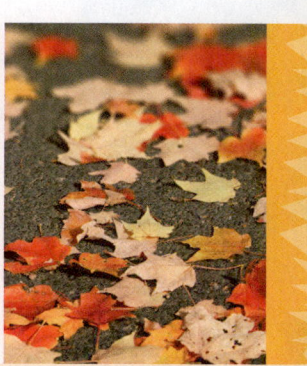

Cultural Care Strategies:

Unit II Wrap-Up

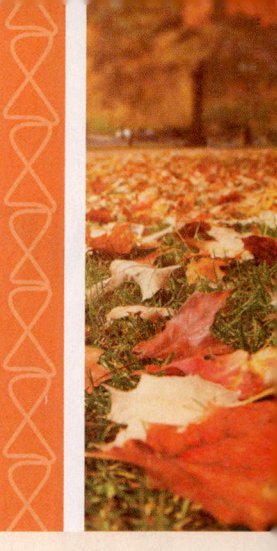

CHAPTER 7

Caring for Patients With Altered Fluid, Electrolyte, or Acid–Base Balance

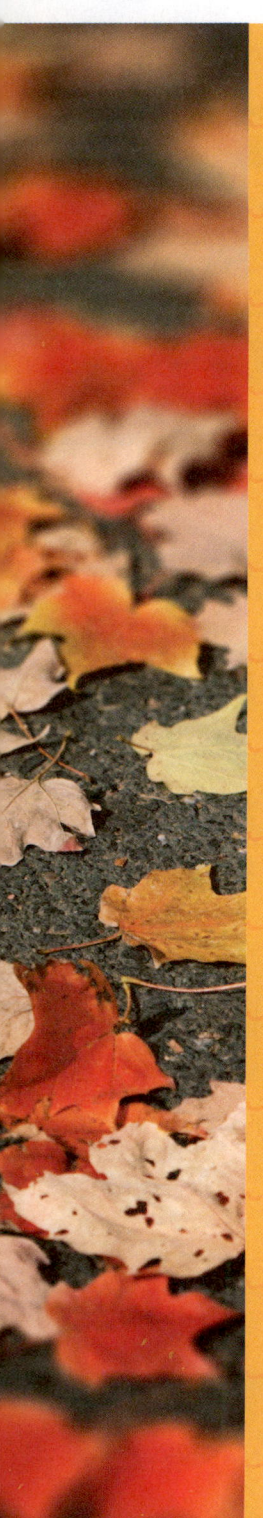

BRIEF OUTLINE

FLUID AND ELECTROLYTE BALANCE

Body Fluids: Composition and Regulation

Fluid Volume Deficit

Fluid Volume Excess

Sodium Imbalance

Potassium Imbalance

Calcium Imbalance

Magnesium Imbalance

Phosphorus Imbalance

ACID–BASE DISORDERS

Acid–Base Regulation

Acid–Base Imbalances

APPLIED LEARNING OUTCOMES

After completing this chapter, you will be able to:

1. Identify the functions and regulatory mechanisms that maintain water and electrolyte balance in the body.
2. Identify patients at risk and assess appropriately for effects of fluid volume deficit and excess.
3. Identify tests used to diagnose and monitor treatment of fluid and electrolyte imbalances.
4. Recognize normal and abnormal serum electrolyte values, appropriately reporting abnormal or unexpected values.
5. Use arterial blood gas results to identify acid–base imbalance in a patient and report findings to the interprofessional team.
6. Implement nursing measures to reduce patients' risk for fluid, electrolyte, or acid–base imbalances.
7. Provide appropriate evidence-based and patient-centered nursing care and teaching for patients with fluid, electrolyte, or acid–base disorders.

KEY TERMS

The key terms are defined on the pages listed below.

SPECIAL FEATURES

Key Concept A balance of body fluids, electrolytes, and acids and bases is normally maintained through processes that regulate the intake, output, and distribution of fluids and the solutes they contain.

Normal life processes depend on a relatively stable state within the body. **Homeostasis** is the body's tendency to maintain a state of physiologic balance in constantly changing conditions. For the body to function and survive, the volume, electrolyte composition, and pH of body fluids all must remain within a relatively narrow and constant range. Disorders in fluid volumes, electrolyte concentrations, and hydrogen ion concentration (pH) often occur in response to illness and trauma. Furthermore, disruptions in fluid, electrolyte, and acid–base balance affect the ability to maintain activities of daily living (ADLs), to think clearly, and to provide self-care.

Nursing care related to homeostasis focuses on identifying patients at risk for developing imbalances, monitoring for early signs of imbalance, assessing for their manifestations,

and intervening to prevent or correct imbalances. Although all patients are at risk for fluid, electrolyte, and acid–base disorders, some people have a greater risk for some imbalances as a result of age or condition. For example:

- Older adults are at risk for dehydration.
- People with heart failure are at risk for fluid volume excess and edema.
- Kidney failure increases the risk for potassium imbalance.
- Patients with type 1 diabetes are at risk for metabolic acidosis.
- Alcoholic patients often have low magnesium levels.
- Long-term bed rest increases the risk for calcium imbalance.

Normal fluid and electrolyte balance and the mechanisms that maintain this balance are discussed first, followed by sections on common imbalances. A discussion of normal acid–base balance precedes the discussion of acid–base imbalances.

FLUID AND ELECTROLYTE BALANCE

Key Concept Fluid and electrolyte imbalances occur when the intake, output, or distribution of water or electrolytes is altered. Age, lifestyle, and environmental factors affect fluid and electrolyte balance, as can disease processes or manifestations and treatment.

Body Fluids: Composition and Regulation

COMPOSITION

Water is the primary component of body fluids. Water has a number of vital functions in the body:

- It transports nutrients and oxygen to the cells and transports waste products, such as carbon dioxide, away from the cells.
- It provides a medium for metabolic reactions within cells.
- It insulates and helps regulate and maintain body temperature.
- It provides form for body structure and acts as a shock absorber.
- It acts as a lubricant.

About 50% to 60% of total body weight is water; this amount varies with age, gender, and body fat. In people older than 65 years, body water decreases to about 45% of total body weight. The proportion of water to total body weight is smaller in an obese person, because fat cells

contain comparatively little water. Adult females have a higher percentage of body fat and a lower percentage of body water than males.

To maintain normal fluid balance, water intake and output (I&O) should be approximately equal. The average daily fluid I&O usually is about 2,500 mL. Water enters the body through ingested fluids and foods. It also is produced by the cells during metabolism. Water is lost in urine, feces, and sweat and when we exhale air from the lungs (Table 7-1 ▪).

TABLE 7-1	Average Fluid Intake and Output in Adults	
	SOURCE	**AMOUNT**
Intake	Oral fluid intake	1,500
	Water in food	750
	Water from metabolism	250
		↓
	Total	2,500
Output		↑
	Urine	1,500
	Feces	100
	Perspiration	200
	Respiration	700

Besides water, body fluids contain solutes such as oxygen, dissolved nutrients, waste products of metabolism such as carbon dioxide, and electrolytes.

Electrolytes are substances that *dissociate* (separate) in solution to form *ions* (electrically charged particles). *Cations* are positively charged electrolytes; *anions* are negatively charged electrolytes. Electrolytes have many functions:

■ They help regulate water and acid–base balance.
■ They contribute to enzyme reactions.
■ They are essential to neuromuscular activity.

The concentration of most electrolytes in body fluids is measured in milliequivalents per liter of water (mEq/L). A *milliequivalent* is a measure of the combining power of the ion. For example, 100 mEq of sodium (Na^+) can combine with 100 mEq of chloride (Cl^-) to form sodium chloride (NaCl), or table salt. Some electrolytes (e.g., calcium and magnesium) may be measured by weight, in milligrams per deciliter of water (mg/dL). Table 7-2■ lists normal laboratory values for electrolytes.

DISTRIBUTION

Body fluid is classified by its location. Membranes such as the cell membrane and capillary walls separate the body fluid compartments. **Intracellular fluid (ICF)** is that which is within the cells; it contains solutes such as electrolytes, glucose, and oxygen. ICF is essential for normal cell function. **Extracellular fluid (ECF)** is outside cells, distributed within three compartments:

■ *Interstitial fluid*, which accounts for the majority of ECF, is in the spaces between most of the cells of the body.
■ *Intravascular fluid* or *plasma* is in the arteries, veins, and capillaries.

TABLE 7-2	Normal Laboratory Values for Electrolytes, Osmolality, and Urine Specific Gravity
ELECTROLYTES	**NORMAL VALUE**
Sodium (Na)	135–145 mEq/L
Potassium (K^+)	3.5–5.3 mEq/L
Calcium (Ca^{2+}), total	4.5–5.5 mEq/L or 9–11 mg/dL
Magnesium (Mg^{2+})	1.5–2.5 mEq/L or 1.8–3.0 mg/dL
Chloride (Cl^-)	95–105 mEq/L
Bicarbonate (HCO_3^-, total carbon dioxide)	22–30 mEq/L
Phosphate/phosphorus (PO_4^{2-})	1.7–2.6 mEq/L or 2.5–4.5 mg/dL
Serum osmolality	280–300 mOsm/kg
Urine specific gravity	1.005–1.030

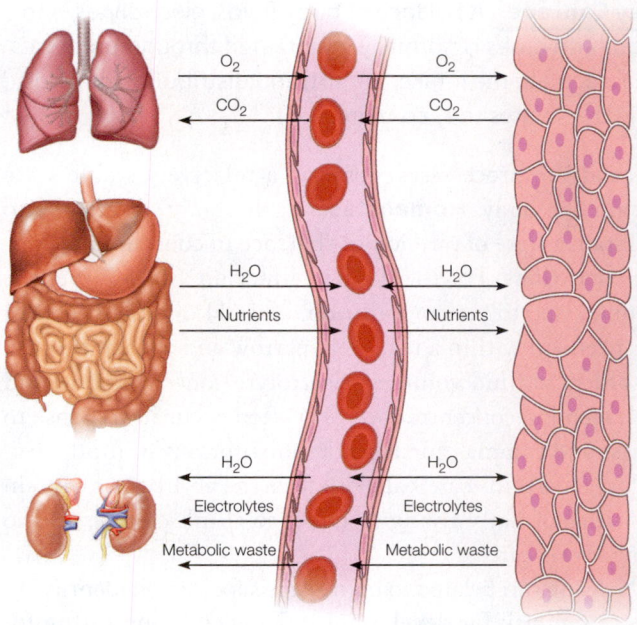

Figure 7-1. ■ Exchange of gases, nutrients, water, and wastes between the fluid compartments of the body. (Source: "Figure 10.03–Exchange of Gases, Nutrients, Water, and Wastes between the Fluid Compartments of the Body" from Medical Surgical Nursing: Critical Thinking in Patient Care, 6e by Priscilla LeMone; Karen Burke; and Gerene Bauldoff. Published by Pearson Education, © 2015.)

■ *Transcellular fluid* includes cerebrospinal fluid, urine, digestive secretions, perspiration, and small amounts of fluid found within organs and joints.

ECF transports oxygen and nutrients to cells and waste products away from the cells (Figure 7-1■). For example, plasma transports oxygen from the lungs and glucose from the gastrointestinal tract to the tissues. Waste products of metabolism such as carbon dioxide are carried away from the tissues to the lungs and the kidneys for elimination.

Electrolytes are found in both fluid compartments, but the concentration or amount of individual electrolytes in ICF and ECF differs (Figure 7-2■). Sodium (Na^+), chloride (Cl^-), and bicarbonate (HCO_3^-) are plentiful in ECF. The principal intracellular electrolytes are potassium (K^+), magnesium (Mg^{2+}), and phosphate (PO_4^{2-}).

MOVEMENT

Membranes separating body fluid compartments are *selectively permeable*; that is, they allow water and some solutes (e.g., oxygen, carbon dioxide, electrolytes, and glucose) to cross, but block proteins and other large molecules. Water and solutes move across these membranes by the processes of osmosis, diffusion, filtration, and active transport.

Osmosis

In the process of **osmosis**, water moves across a membrane from an area of lower solute concentration to an area of higher solute concentration (Figure 7-3■). Osmosis

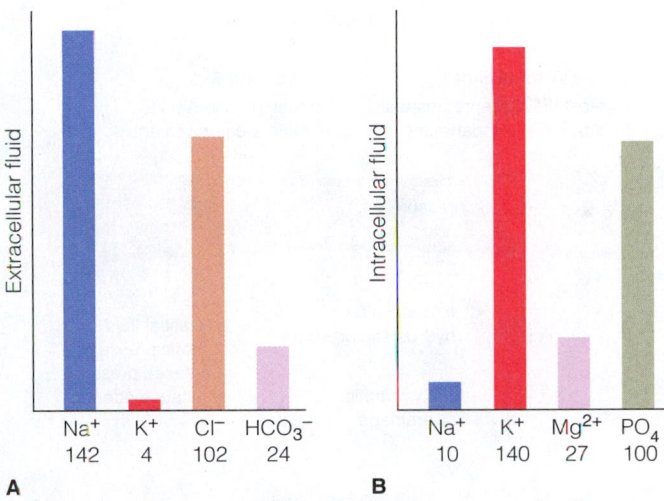

Figure 7-2. ■ The principal electrolytes (in milliequivalents) of (**A**) extracellular fluid and (**B**) intracellular fluid.

continues until the solute concentration on both sides of the membrane is equal. For example, if a selectively permeable membrane separates pure water from a salt solution, water moves into the salt solution. Osmosis is responsible for water movement between the ICF and ECF compartments.

Osmolality is the concentration of all solutes within a body fluid compartment. It is measured in milliosmoles per kilogram (mOsm/kg). The osmolality of ECF is primarily determined by sodium. The normal osmolality of both ICF and ECF ranges between 280 and 300 mOsm/kg (see Table 7-2).

The power of a solution to draw water across a membrane is known as the *osmotic pressure* of the solution. All solutes in a solution contribute to its osmotic pressure. While the composition of interstitial fluid and plasma is essentially the same, plasma proteins in the blood (albumin, in particular) exert osmotic pressure, helping to hold water within the blood vessels. The draw exerted by plasma proteins is usually referred to as the *oncotic pressure* of plasma.

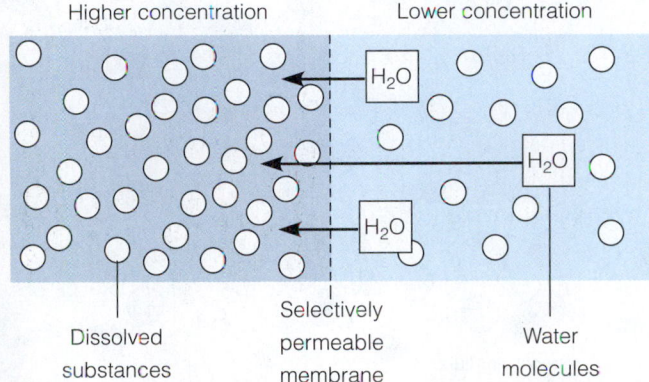

Figure 7-3. ■ Osmosis. Water moves across a selectively permeable membrane from an area of low-solute concentration to an area of high-solute concentration.

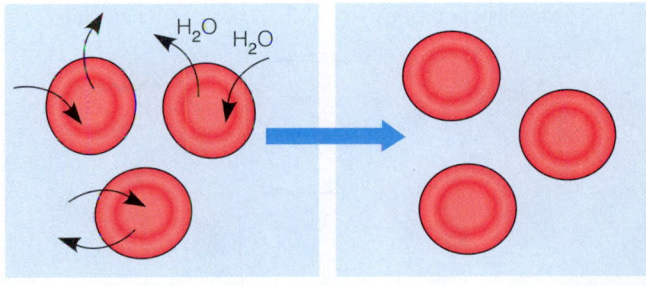

A Isotonic solution

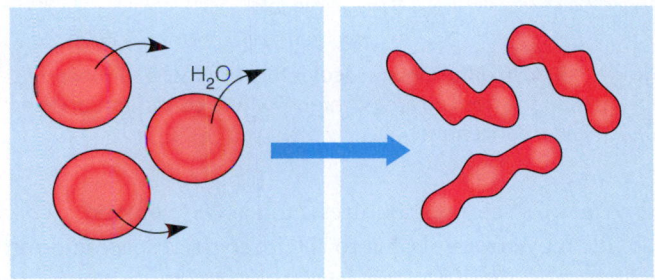

B Hypertonic solution

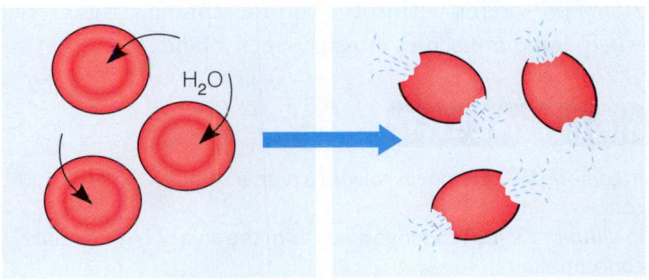

C Hypotonic solution

Figure 7-4. ■ The effect of changes in the concentration of solutions on red blood cells. (**A**) Cells neither gain nor lose water, size, or shape in isotonic solutions. (**B**) Cells lose water and shrink in hypertonic solutions. (**C**) Cells absorb water, swell, and burst in hypotonic solutions.

Tonicity refers to the effect of the osmotic pressure of a solution on cells within that solution. *Isotonic* solutions (such as normal saline, 0.9% sodium chloride solution) have the same concentration of solutes as plasma. Cells placed in an isotonic solution do not gain or lose water (Figure 7-4■). *Hypertonic* solutions (e.g., 3% sodium chloride solution) have a greater concentration of solutes than plasma. A cell placed in a hypertonic solution shrinks as water is drawn out of it into the solution. *Hypotonic* solutions (such as 0.45% sodium chloride) have a lower solute concentration than plasma. A cell placed in a hypotonic solution swells as water moves into it. The cell may burst.

Diffusion

Diffusion is the process in which solutes move from an area of high solute concentration to an area of low concentration to become evenly distributed (Figure 7-5■). There are two types of diffusion. *Simple diffusion* occurs by the random

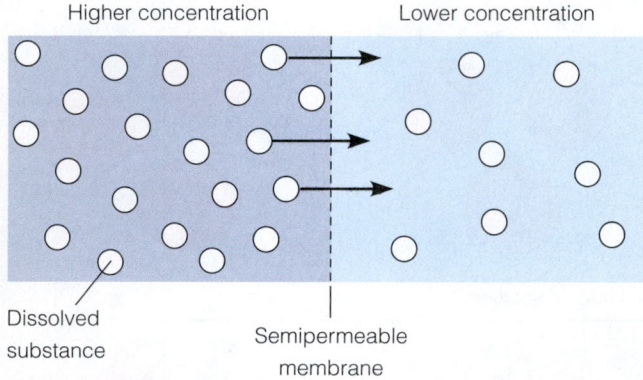

Higher concentration   Lower concentration

Dissolved substance

Semipermeable membrane

Figure 7-5. ■ In diffusion, molecules move across a semipermeable membrane from an area of higher solute concentration to an area of lower concentration.

movement of solutes. Solutes such as oxygen and carbon dioxide move from plasma to the interstitial space and into cells by simple diffusion. Large water-soluble molecules such as glucose move into cells by a process of *facilitated diffusion*. Proteins within the cell membrane act as carriers to help large molecules cross the membrane.

memory**ALERT**

In *osmosis*, WATER moves *toward* a higher solute concentration.
In *diffusion*, SOLUTES move *away from* the area of higher solute concentration.

Filtration

Filtration is the process in which water and solutes move across capillary membranes driven by fluid pressure. Fluid (or *hydrostatic*) pressure is created by the pumping action of the heart and by gravity. At the arterial end of capillaries, this pressure pushes water and solutes into the interstitial space, an area of lower fluid pressure. At the venous end of the capillary, the osmotic force of plasma proteins draws fluid back into the capillary. A balance of filtration and osmosis regulates the movement of water between the intravascular and interstitial spaces in the capillary beds of the body (Figure 7-6■).

Active Transport

Active transport allows molecules to move across cell membranes into an area of higher solute concentration. This movement requires cellular energy (adenosine triphosphate, or ATP) and a carrier mechanism. The sodium–potassium pump is an important example of active transport (Figure 7-7■). High concentrations of potassium within cells are maintained because cells actively move potassium from interstitial fluid (where the potassium concentration is only about 5 mEq/L) into ICF (K^+ concentration about 150 mEq/L). Sodium is "pumped" from ICF into ECF.

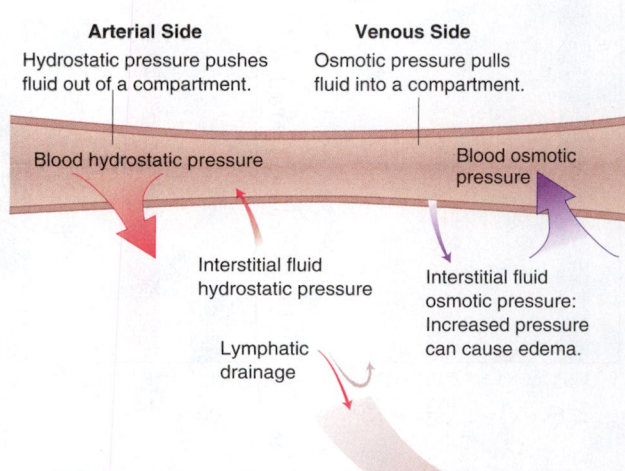

FILTRATION

Arterial Side
Hydrostatic pressure pushes fluid out of a compartment.

Venous Side
Osmotic pressure pulls fluid into a compartment.

Blood hydrostatic pressure

Blood osmotic pressure

Interstitial fluid hydrostatic pressure

Interstitial fluid osmotic pressure: Increased pressure can cause edema.

Lymphatic drainage

Normally, lymphatic drainage removes small proteins and excess interstitial fluid. Blocked lymphatic drainage can cause edema.

Figure 7-6. ■ Fluid balance between the intravascular and interstitial spaces is maintained in the capillary beds by a balance of filtration at the arterial end and osmotic draw at the venous end.

REGULATION

Homeostasis depends on a number of mechanisms and processes that regulate the balance between fluid intake, output, and distribution. These regulatory mechanisms include thirst, the kidneys, the renin–angiotensin–aldosterone mechanism, antidiuretic hormone, and atrial natriuretic peptide.

Thirst

Thirst is the primary regulator of water intake. It plays an important role in maintaining fluid balance and preventing dehydration. The thirst center in the brain is

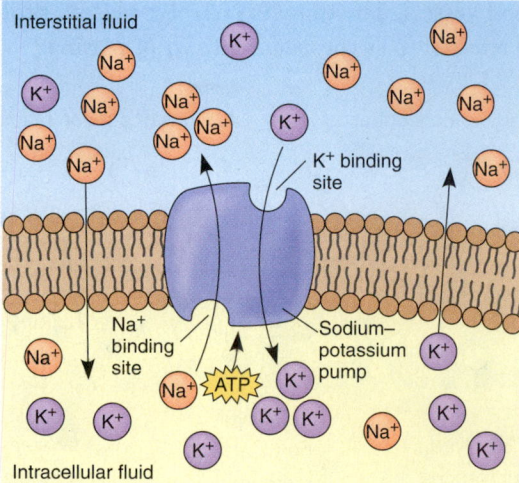

ACTIVE TRANSPORT

Interstitial fluid

K^+ binding site

Na^+ binding site

Sodium–potassium pump

ATP

Intracellular fluid

Figure 7-7. ■ The sodium–potassium pump. Active transport moves sodium and potassium ions across cell membranes against their concentration gradients.

stimulated when the blood volume drops because of water losses or when the solute content (osmolality) of body fluids increases (Figure 7-8■).

Kidneys

The kidneys are primarily responsible for regulating fluid volume and electrolyte balance in the body. In adults, about 170 L of plasma is filtered by the kidneys every day. About 99% of this filtrate is reabsorbed, and only about 1,500 mL of urine is produced. By selectively reabsorbing water and electrolytes, the kidneys maintain the volume and osmolality of body fluids.

Renin–Angiotensin–Aldosterone System

The *renin–angiotensin–aldosterone system* helps maintain intravascular fluid balance and blood pressure (BP)

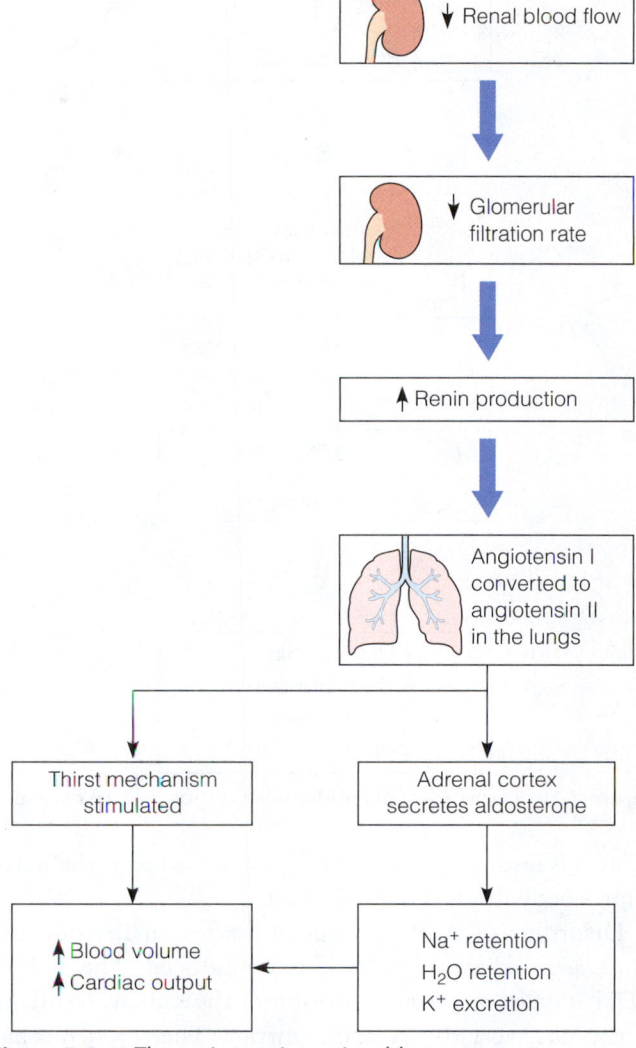

Figure 7-9. ■ The renin–angiotensin–aldosterone system.

(Figure 7-9■). A fall in blood flow to the kidneys stimulates specialized receptors in the kidney to produce renin (an enzyme). Renin converts angiotensinogen (a plasma protein) in the blood to angiotensin I. In the lungs, angiotensin I is converted to angiotensin II by angiotensin-converting enzyme (ACE). Angiotensin II constricts blood vessels, which raises BP. It also stimulates thirst, releases aldosterone (a hormone) from the adrenal cortex, and acts directly on the kidneys, causing them to retain sodium and water. Aldosterone also promotes sodium and water retention by the kidneys, restoring blood volume.

Antidiuretic Hormone

Antidiuretic hormone (ADH) regulates water excretion from the kidneys. Receptors in the hypothalamus detect changes in osmolality and blood volume, stimulating ADH production and release as needed. When ADH is present, more water is reabsorbed in the kidney. Urine output falls, blood

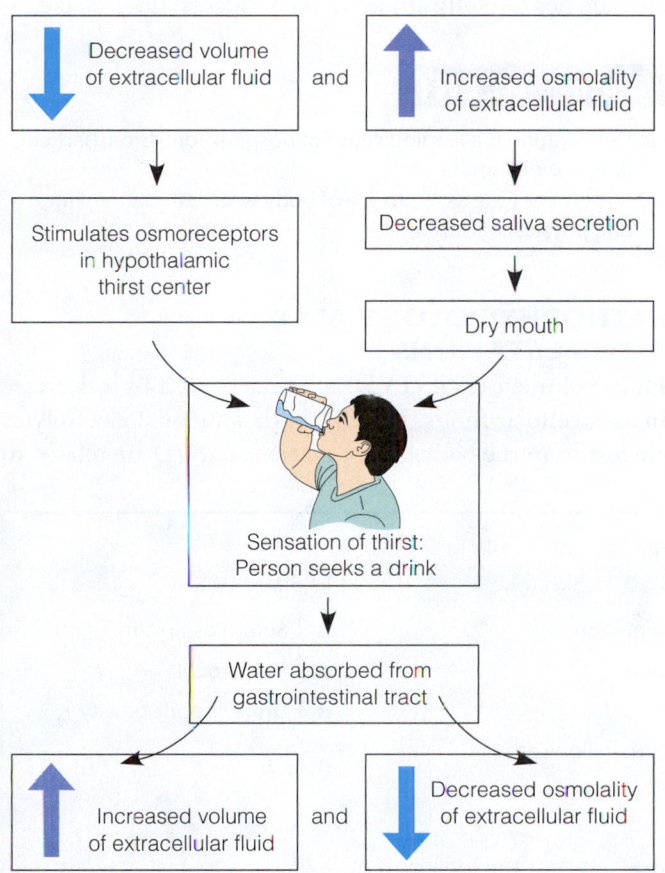

Figure 7-8. ■ Factors stimulating water intake through the thirst mechanism.

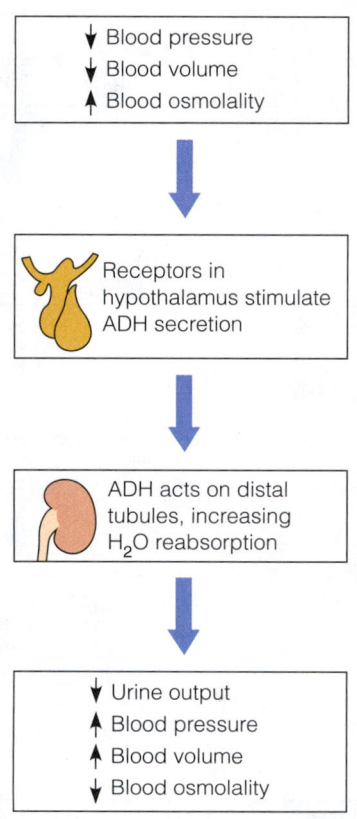

↓ Blood pressure
↓ Blood volume
↑ Blood osmolality

Receptors in hypothalamus stimulate ADH secretion

ADH acts on distal tubules, increasing H₂O reabsorption

↓ Urine output
↑ Blood pressure
↑ Blood volume
↓ Blood osmolality

Figure 7-10. ■ The effect of antidiuretic hormone (ADH) release.

volume is restored, and serum osmolality drops as the water dilutes body fluids (Figure 7-10■).

Disorders of ADH production affect urine output. In *diabetes insipidus*, ADH is not produced. The lack of ADH impairs water reabsorption in the kidney, resulting in copious, very dilute urine output. The thirst mechanism is stimulated, and the patient drinks additional fluids, maintaining high urine output. In the *syndrome of inappropriate ADH secretion (SIADH)*, excess ADH is released. More water is reabsorbed, fluid volume increases, and urine output is scant and concentrated. (See Chapter 35 for more information about diabetes insipidus and SIADH.)

Atrial Natriuretic Peptide

Atrial natriuretic peptide (ANP) is a hormone released by cells in the atria of the heart in response to stretching from fluid overload. ANP inhibits renin secretion and blocks the secretion and effects of aldosterone. In doing so, it promotes sodium and water loss and causes blood vessels to dilate.

memory**ALERT**

- ADH and aldosterone → ↑ blood volume, ↓ urine output
- ANP → ↓ blood volume, ↑ urine output

Fluid Volume Deficit

Fluid volume deficit (FVD) or **dehydration** may occur due to excessive fluid losses, insufficient fluid intake, or both. The most common causes are vomiting, diarrhea, or gastrointestinal suctioning. Other common causes are listed in Table 7-3■. Inadequate fluid intake may result from decreased thirst sensation, limited access to fluids, difficulty swallowing, or lack of awareness of the need to replace fluids. Older adults are at particular risk for fluid volume deficits (Box 7-1■). Nursing home residents have an even higher risk of becoming dehydrated when nurses and nursing assistants do not carefully attend to the residents' fluid intake.

memory**ALERT**

- Dehydration is a leading cause of hospital admission, particularly in older adults.
- A loss of as little as 1% to 2% of body water affects thinking and physical performance.

PATHOPHYSIOLOGY AND MANIFESTATIONS

Fluid volume deficit (FVD) is characterized by a decrease in extracellular fluids. Usually, both water and electrolytes are lost from the body. Manifestations of FVD are related to

TABLE 7-3	Fluid Volume Deficit	
CAUSES	**MANIFESTATIONS**	**LAB VALUES**
■ Inadequate fluid intake	■ Fatigue, altered mentation	■ ↑ Serum osmolality
■ GI fluid losses: vomiting, suction, diarrhea	■ Postural hypotension	■ ↑ Hematocrit
■ Excess urine output: diuretics, diabetes	■ Tachycardia	■ ↑ Urine specific gravity
■ Hemorrhage	■ Weak, thready peripheral pulses	
■ Sweating	■ Weight loss	
■ Fever	■ Flat neck veins	
■ Draining wounds, burns	■ Dry skin, poor turgor	
■ Fluid shifts (third spacing)	■ Decreased urine output, concentrated urine	

| BOX 7-1 | FOCUS ON OLDER ADULTS |

Fluid Volume Deficit in Older Adults

The older adult is at risk for fluid volume deficit from a variety of factors:

- Decreased thirst perception
- Decreased total body water
- Age-related changes in kidney function and the ability to regulate body temperature
- Self-limiting of fluids due to fear of incontinence
- Self-care deficits or disabilities that limit access to fluids
- Cognitive impairments (confusion, dementia, depression)
- Medications such as diuretics and sedatives

the cause and severity of the imbalance. With rapid fluid losses, manifestations of *hypovolemia*, or decreased circulating blood volume, may be seen within minutes or hours. These may include anxiety, rapid heart rate, and difficulty thinking. With gradual losses, interstitial fluid shifts into the vascular space to maintain blood volume. A significant amount of ECF may be lost by the time symptoms develop (see Table 7-3). In many cases, the extent of fluid loss can be estimated by the amount of total body weight lost:

- Mild FVD—2% to 4% weight loss
- Moderate FVD—5% to 7% loss
- Severe FVD—8% or greater loss

Third Spacing

Third spacing is a shift of fluid from the vascular space into an area where it is not available to support normal physiologic processes (e.g., within the bowel or the peritoneal cavity). Fluid may also become trapped within soft tissues after trauma or burns. Fluid loss due to third spacing can be difficult to detect, because the weight may remain stable, and I&O records may not show the loss.

COLLABORATIVE CARE

In addition to the history and physical examination, laboratory tests and invasive monitoring help determine and monitor fluid status.

Diagnostic Tests

- *Serum electrolytes* may show increased or decreased sodium levels, depending on the cause of the FVD. Serum potassium levels often are low.
- *Serum osmolality* is high when primarily water has been lost; if both water and sodium are lost, it may be normal.
- The *hematocrit* may be elevated due to loss of intravascular fluid volume and concentration of the blood cells.
- *Urine specific gravity* and *osmolality* are high due to increased concentration of the urine as the kidneys attempt to conserve water.

- *Hemodynamic monitoring* may be necessary to monitor fluid volume status in critically ill patients. Patients requiring hemodynamic monitoring usually are placed in intensive or coronary care units. See Chapter 17 for more information about hemodynamic monitoring.

Fluid Management

Depending on the severity of the deficit, fluids and electrolytes may be replaced orally, *enterally* (into the gastrointestinal tract), or intravenously. Whenever possible, oral or enteral (nasogastric or gastrostomy tube) fluid replacement is preferred. The patient is encouraged to drink increased amounts of fluid. Box 7-2■ lists suggested measures to increase fluid intake in hospitalized older adults and residents of nursing homes. Whenever possible, fluids that also contain electrolytes (e.g., commercial products such as sports drinks or Pedialyte) are preferred for fluid replacement to avoid potential electrolyte imbalances resulting from pure water intake.

Intravenous Therapy

In acute FVD, intravenous (IV) fluids are necessary. IV delivery effectively supplies fluids directly into the blood and can be used to replace electrolytes as well. Although IV fluids generally require a physician's order, the nurse is responsible for initiating, monitoring, and maintaining *parenteral* (administered by a route other than the GI tract) fluid replacement. Box 7-3■ outlines nursing care for the patient receiving IV fluids.

The fluid administered depends on the type and rapidity of the fluid loss. Isotonic electrolyte solutions (0.9% NaCl or Lactated Ringer solution) are used to expand blood volume or to replace abnormal losses (e.g., loss of gastric fluid via nasogastric suction). Hypotonic saline solution (0.45% NaCl), often with dextrose added (D_5/0.45% NaCl), or mixed solutions are used as maintenance solutions to provide electrolytes and water. (See Table 7-4■.)

| BOX 7-2 | FOCUS ON OLDER ADULTS |

Increasing Fluid Intake in Older Adults

- Provide a variety of preferred fluids with and between meals.
- Frequently offer freshly prepared fluids at preferred temperature.
- Use glasses and cups that are not too large, heavy, or difficult to grip.
- Keep frozen juice bars readily available to patients, residents, and families.
- Remind nursing assistants to offer fluids whenever they interact with the patient or resident.

BOX 7-3	**NURSING CARE CHECKLIST**

Intravenous Infusion

☑ Identify the type, amount, and duration of the infusion from the physician's order.

☑ Calculate the flow rate or infusion pump settings for the type of infusion set used.

- To determine the amount to infuse each hour, divide the total amount of fluid to be infused by the number of hours over which the infusion is to run.
- To determine the amount to infuse per minute, divide the total amount to be infused by the number of minutes over which the infusion is to run (e.g., an 8-hour infusion runs over 480 minutes).
- To determine the number of drops per minute, use the following formula:

$$\frac{\text{Amount to be infused} \times \text{Drop factor of infusion set}}{\text{Total time of infusion in minutes}}$$

For example

$$\frac{1,000 \text{ mL} \times 10 \text{ drops/mL}}{480 \text{ minutes}} = 21 \text{ drops/min}$$

☑ Perform hand hygiene and observe standard precautions.

☑ Identify the patient, introduce self, provide for privacy, and explain the purpose of your visit.

☑ Verify that the correct solution is being infused. If the solution in incorrect, slow the rate of flow and change the solution to the correct one. Document and report the error per agency protocol.

☑ Observe the rate of flow every hour. Slow an infusion that is too fast; report an infusion that is running too slow. Notify the charge nurse or follow agency protocol for adjusting the rate.

☑ Check the patency and integrity of the system:

- Check solution container position; increase its height as needed to maintain gravity flow.
- Check fluid level in the drip chamber; if less than half full, squeeze the chamber to add fluid. If too full, invert the solution container and squeeze the chamber to empty fluid.

- Inspect tubing for kinks or obstructions. Position tubing to avoid tension on the intravenous catheter, dangling below the insertion site, and occlusion by the patient's weight.
- Check for catheter patency: Lower the solution container below the infusion site, and observe for blood return. Lack of blood return may indicate partial occlusion or catheter dislodgement from the vein.
- If the tip of the catheter is against the vein wall or a valve, reposition it slightly, using care to avoid contamination or dislodging of the catheter.
- Check for leaks in the system. Tighten connections. If unable to repair a leak or if the connection has become contaminated, replace the infusion set. Estimate the amount of fluid lost if significant.

☑ Inspect the insertion site for infiltration, inflammation, or bleeding.

- Infiltration, fluid flow into interstitial tissues when the catheter is outside the vein, causes local swelling, coolness, pallor, and discomfort at the IV site. If present, stop the infusion and remove the catheter. Restart the infusion at another site. Apply a warm compress to the site to promote reabsorption of the fluid.
- Phlebitis, inflammation of a vein, results from mechanical trauma or chemical irritation of the vein. It is characterized by redness, warmth, and swelling at the insertion site and burning pain along the vein. If detected, discontinue the infusion and apply a warm compress to the site.
- Oozing or bleeding into the surrounding tissues can occur while the infusion is in place, but usually occurs after the needle has been removed. Apply a sterile pressure dressing and inspect frequently for continued bleeding.

☑ Instruct the patient to avoid stress or tension on the tubing or infusion site and to notify the nurse if the solution container is nearly empty, the flow rate changes, there is blood in the tubing, or the infusion site is painful or swollen.

☑ Document the solution infusion, its flow rate, assessment data, and any measures taken to correct problems.

IV solutions usually are supplied in plastic bags of various sizes from 50 to 1,000 mL. Glass containers may be used for solutions or medications that are incompatible with plastic. Glass containers require an air vent to allow air to enter the bottle as the fluid flows into the patient. Plastic bags collapse as the fluid flows out, making an air vent unnecessary. IV fluids must be sterile and free from contamination. Before administering, inspect the container and solution for evidence of tampering, clarity, and expiration date. Do not administer any solution that is expired, is questionable, or may have been contaminated. IV bottles or bags are changed before they are completely empty to prevent air from entering the IV line. All IV bags are changed at least every 24 hours, regardless of how much solution remains, to reduce the risk of bacterial growth.

IV poles are used to hang the solution container. They may be free-standing, attached to the bed, or hanging from the ceiling. The pole height is adjustable to promote gravity flow of the IV solution.

An infusion set is used to connect the solution container to the IV catheter or needle. This equipment varies by manufacturer, so the nurse must become familiar with that used by the agency. Infusion sets usually include an insertion spike, a drip chamber, a roller valve or screw clamp, tubing with secondary ports, and a protective cap over the needle adapter (Figure 7-11 ■). The sterile insertion spike is inserted into the solution container. The drip chamber allows the nurse to observe the amount of fluid being administered. Administration sets commonly deliver 10 to 20 drops/mL of solution. This information is found on the

TABLE 7-4	Commonly Administered Intravenous Fluids	
FLUID	**TONICITY**	**USES**
0.9% NaCl (Normal saline)	Isotonic	Restore intravascular volume Replace extracellular fluid Replace sodium losses
0.45% NaCl (1/2 normal saline)	Hypotonic	Replace water losses Maintain sodium and chloride levels
3% NaCl	Hypertonic	Correct sodium depletion
5% dextrose in water (D_5W)	Isotonic	Replace water losses Correct hypernatremia (excess sodium)
10% dextrose in water ($D_{10}W$)	Hypertonic	Replace water losses Provide calories (340 kcal/L)
20% dextrose in water ($D_{20}W$)	Hypertonic	Promote diuresis Provide calories (680 kcal/L)
50% dextrose in water ($D_{50}W$)	Hypertonic	Treat severe hypoglycemia Provide calories (1,700 kcal/L)
5% dextrose in 0.45% NaCl (D_5 1/2 NS)	Hypertonic	Maintain fluid level Replace water losses Maintain sodium and chloride levels
Ringer solution (balanced electrolyte solution)	Isotonic	Replace fluid losses Maintain intravascular volume
Lactated Ringer solution (electrolyte solution with buffer)	Isotonic	Replace fluid losses Prevent acidosis

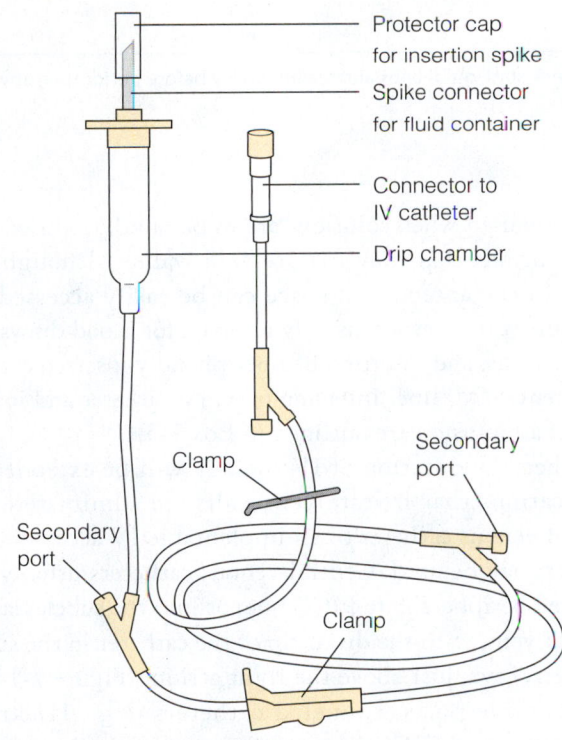

- Protector cap for insertion spike
- Spike connector for fluid container
- Connector to IV catheter
- Drip chamber
- Secondary port
- Clamp
- Secondary port
- Clamp

Figure 7-11. ■ A standard IV administration set.

package. When smaller amounts of solution are given (e.g., less than 50 mL/hr), a microdrip set that delivers 60 drops/mL of solution is used. The rate of flow is controlled by a roller valve or screw clamp, which compresses the lumen of the tubing. A protective cap over the needle adapter maintains sterility of the end of the tubing until it is attached to the IV needle, catheter, or venous access device. A special infusion set may be required when an infusion pump or controller is used. IV tubing and the site dressing are changed every 24 to 72 hours. Box 7-4■ outlines the process for changing an IV solution container, tubing, and the IV site dressing.

Infusion pumps or devices control the rate of an infusion. They also have alarms that are triggered by air in the tubing or low solution levels in the IV bag. Infusion pumps reduce the risk of administering fluids too rapidly or too slowly. It is vital to use an infusion pump when medications such as heparin are added to the IV solution. Infusion control devices vary by manufacturer; the nurse must become familiar with the devices used within each agency.

Catheters and needles are used to administer IV infusions. Over-the-needle catheters are commonly used. The plastic catheter fits over a needle used to pierce the skin and vein wall (Figure 7-12■). Once in the vein, the needle is withdrawn, leaving the catheter in place. IV catheters promote comfort, allow more mobility, and are less likely to become dislodged from the vein, allowing fluid to flow into interstitial spaces (*infiltrate*). Butterfly, or wing-tipped, needles with plastic flaps attached to the shaft may

---

BOX 7-4 | **PROCEDURE CHECKLIST**

Changing an Intravenous Bag, Tubing, and Site Dressing

Before the Procedure

☑ Verify the order or agency protocol for bag, tubing, and dressing changes.

☑ Gather equipment: IV container with correct type and amount of solution, fluid administration set, timing label, appropriate antiseptic for cleansing site, transparent dressing, tape.

During the Procedure

☑ Use Standard Precautions throughout the procedure.

☑ Verify the physician's order for solution type, added medications, and infusion rate.

☑ Select the appropriate solution (generally supplied by the pharmacy); verify that it is the correct solution (and medication, if appropriate) and amount for the patient.

☑ Calculate the drip rate.

☑ Mark the timing strip with start time, appropriate amount to be delivered per hour, and end time; apply the strip to the container, taking care to avoid covering the label.

☑ Open the infusion set (see Figure 7-11). Maintaining sterility of the spike and IV solution, insert the spike into the solution container.

☑ Prime the tubing, keeping the IV catheter connection sterile. Close the drip regulator.

☑ Identify the patient and explain the procedure.

☑ Assess the IV site for infiltration, bleeding, and phlebitis; appearance of the dressing; and date and time of previous dressing change.

☑ Prepare dressing supplies. Prepare transparent dressing for application, tear two or more strips of tape for securing tubing, and open antiseptic swabs.

☑ Place a towel or clean absorbent pad under the extremity to prevent soiling bed linens. Be sure the IV and tubing and all dressing supplies are within easy reach.

☑ Remove soiled dressing and tape to expose catheter connection.

☑ Clamp the tubing on the existing infusion and carefully loosen the tubing from the IV catheter or needle, securing the catheter with the nondominant hand.

☑ Remove the used IV tubing and securely attach the new tubing to the IV catheter or needle; open the regulator clamp to restart the infusion.

☑ Continuing to hold the IV catheter or needle, clean the IV site, following agency protocol.

☑ Apply transparent dressing to the IV insertion site. Secure tubing with tape to prevent inadvertent tension on the catheter or needle with movement.

☑ Label the dressing with the date and time of the dressing change and your initials.

☑ Regulate the IV flow rate as ordered.

☑ Chart assessment findings and any pertinent data.

Note: Refer to a nursing fundamentals or skills text for more detailed instruction. Check state guidelines and facility policy before performing any procedure.

---

be used, particularly for very small veins. The flaps are used to direct the needle during insertion. Once in place, the flaps are flattened against the skin and secured with tape.

The type of IV access device and insertion site depend on a number of factors: patient age and condition of veins, duration of the infusion, and type of solution to be infused. For adults, veins in the hand and arm (the metacarpal, basilic, and cephalic veins) are commonly used (Figure 7-13■). The radius and ulna splint the veins of the arm, reducing catheter movement during activities such as eating. Larger

veins are used when solutions are to be rapidly infused and for solutions that may irritate vein walls. Although the veins in the antecubital space can be easily accessed for venipuncture, they are usually reserved for blood draws, IV medications, and insertion of a peripherally inserted central catheter (PICC) line. Insertion of an IV catheter and initiation of an infusion are outlined in Box 7-5■.

When the duration of IV therapy will be extended or medications that irritate vein walls are administered, a central venous catheter or an implantable IV access device or port may be used. Central venous catheters usually are inserted peripherally (a PICC line) or into the subclavian or jugular vein, with the distal tip of the catheter in the superior vena cava, just above the right atrium (Figure 7-14■). Implantable ports, tunneled catheters (e.g., Hickman catheters), and PICC lines often are used for long-term intravenous access, for example, when a patient is receiving chemotherapy. Because these devices remain in place for long periods of time, there is a risk of infection and occlusion.

Introducer needle | Cannula | Translucent catheter hub | Preview chamber | Flashback chamber | Filter vent

Tapered catheter tip | Luer lock tabs | Finger guard | Needle bevel position indicator

Short bevel introducer needle | Needle heel

Figure 7-12. ■ An over-the-needle IV catheter.

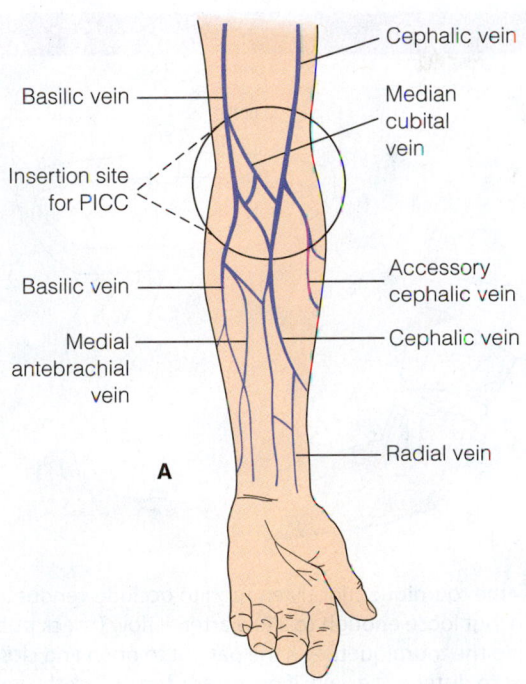

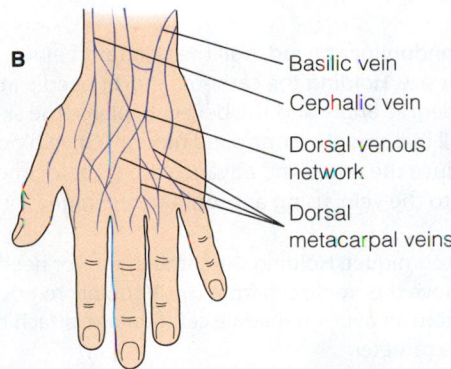

Figure 7-13. ■ Commonly used venipuncture sites of the (**A**) arm and (**B**) hand. A also shows the site used for a peripherally inserted central catheter (PICC).

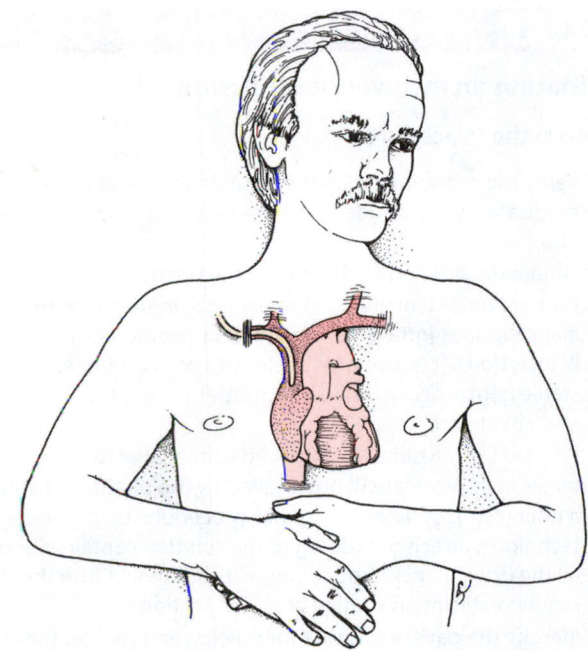

Figure 7-14. ■ A central venous catheter inserted via the right subclavian vein.

NURSING CARE

PRIORITIZING NURSING CARE

Restoring blood and fluid volume is the priority of care for the patient with fluid volume deficit. Low blood volume, usually due to a total body fluid volume deficit, increases the patient's risk for injury due to falls, impaired mental status, and kidney failure.

HEALTH PROMOTION

The nurse promotes health for the patient at risk for fluid volume deficit by teaching patients and their caregivers how to prevent dehydration. Discuss the importance of maintaining adequate fluid intake, particularly during hot weather, when exercising, and when ill. Advise patients to use noncaffeinated sports drinks and water drinks that contain electrolytes to replace fluid losses associated with exercise, heat, or GI losses. Instruct caregivers to frequently offer a variety of fluids to patients at risk for developing fluid volume deficit.

ASSESSING

When assessing the patient with fluid volume deficit, the nurse focuses on possible causes and the effects of dehydration (Table 7-3). Ask about weakness or lightheadedness (particularly on standing), thirst, and recent weight loss. Inquire about risk factors such as strenuous exercise (particularly in warm weather); acute illness (e.g., fever, nausea, vomiting, diarrhea); and chronic diseases such as diabetes and use of medications such as diuretics.

Obtain vital signs, including orthostatic vitals (see Box 7-6■), and weight. Palpate peripheral pulses and capillary refill. Assess skin and mucous membrane color, temperature, and moisture and skin turgor; auscultate breath and bowel sounds. Note mental status, including level of consciousness.

Monitor serum electrolytes and osmolality, the hematocrit, and urine specific gravity. As the fluid deficit is corrected, expected findings include a slight drop in these values. Report values that fall outside the normal or expected range.

clinical**ALERT**

Assess skin turgor over the sternum in older adults. Loss of subcutaneous tissue in aging makes the skin of the arms a less reliable indicator of fluid status.

BOX 7-5   PROCEDURE CHECKLIST

Initiating an Intravenous Infusion

Before the Procedure

☑ Verify the order, including the solution to be used, any medications to be added, and the time and the rate of the infusion.

☑ Obtain the ordered solution from the pharmacy.

☑ Gather equipment: Infusion set, IV pole, infusion controller if appropriate, intravenous catheter or needle, clean gloves, IV insertion set (tourniquet, cleansing pads and/or solutions, sterile gauze, occlusive dressing, tape), clean protective absorbent pad.

☑ Prepare the infusion: Apply a medication label to the container as appropriate (if not applied by the pharmacy) and a timing strip or label per agency procedure. Using sterile technique, attach the tubing to the solution container and fill the drip chamber and tubing with solution. Close the drip regulator. Maintain sterility of all connections.

☑ Identify the patient, provide for privacy, and explain the procedure. Allow time for questions.

During the Procedure

☑ Use Standard Precautions throughout the procedure.

☑ Select the insertion site. If possible use the nondominant arm, selecting a vein that is relatively straight (see Figure 7-13). Choose a site that allows normal arm movement to the extent possible and where the tip of the catheter will not be at a joint.

☑ Place a clean protective pad or towel under the arm to protect linens or furniture.

☑ If necessary, apply heat to the extremity (using a heating pad or hot, damp towel) for 10 to 15 minutes to promote blood flow and venous distention.

☑ Cleanse the site according to agency protocol. Use a circular motion, starting at the insertion site and working outward for several inches. Allow the site to dry. Do not touch the site once it has been cleansed.

☑ Prepare IV catheter/needle, dressing, and tape while the site dries.

☑ Apply tourniquet firmly approximately 12 cm (5 in.) or more above (proximal to) the site (see accompanying figure).

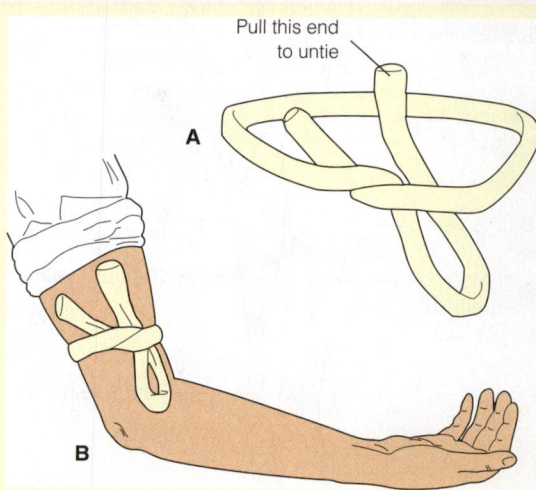

Pull this end to untie

A

B

Apply the tourniquet tightly enough to occlude venous return, but loose enough to allow arterial flow (check pulse distal to the tourniquet). Ask the patient to open and close the fist to distend the vein; if necessary, tap or flick the vein above or below the cleansed site to promote distention.

☑ Using the nondominant hand, pull the skin taut below the insertion site. Holding the catheter and/or needle at a 10- to 15-degree angle and the bevel up, pierce the skin and vein wall in a smooth, controlled motion. Once blood appears, reduce the angle and advance the catheter and/or needle into the vein, using appropriate technique for the device.

☑ Release the tourniquet. Holding the catheter and/or needle in place, remove the sterile cap from the IV tubing; remove the needle from an over-the-needle catheter and attach the tubing to the catheter.

☑ Open the drip regulator and adjust to maintain flow.

☑ Apply dressing to the site per agency protocol. Secure IV tubing to prevent tension on the IV catheter or on connections. Label the dressing with the time, date, type of infusion device or catheter, and your initials.

☑ Adjust flow rate to maintain ordered rate of infusion.

☑ Document the procedure and patient responses.

Note: Refer to a nursing fundamentals or skills text for more detailed instruction. Check state guidelines and facility policy before performing any procedure.

IDENTIFYING POTENTIAL COMPLICATIONS

Tachycardia, hypotension, decreased level of consciousness, and a drop in urine output (to less than 30 mL/hr) indicate decreased cardiac output. Immediately report these symptoms to the registered nurse or physician. Without prompt intervention, the patient is at risk for developing shock or kidney failure.

DIAGNOSING, PLANNING, AND IMPLEMENTING

Deficient Fluid Volume

Expected outcome: Will have a balanced I&O over 24 hours and demonstrate hydration by moist mucous membranes; warm, moist skin; and good skin turgor.

BOX 7-6	OBTAINING ORTHOSTATIC VITAL SIGNS

- Measure BP and pulse with patient supine; leave cuff in place and allow to remain flat for 3 to 5 minutes.
- Have the patient sit up; immediately measure BP and pulse.
- After another 3 to 5 minutes, have the patient stand; measure BP and pulse.
- A BP drop of 10 to 15 mm Hg and increase in pulse of 10 beats per minute indicates orthostatic or postural hypotension (an indicator of hypovolemia).
- Allow the older adult to sit or stand quietly for 3 to 5 minutes after changing positions to ensure accurate measurements.

- Monitor I&O. Report a urine output of less than 30 mL/hr for 2 or more hours to the charge nurse or primary care provider. *Urine output of less than 30 mL/hr indicates poor kidney perfusion and a risk for kidney failure.*
- Measure urine specific gravity. *Urine specific gravity is normally 1.010 to 1.035. A reading higher than 1.025 may indicate fluid volume deficit.*
- Assess vital signs and peripheral pulses every 4 hours. *Hypotension, tachycardia, and weak peripheral pulses indicate hypovolemia.*
- Weigh daily with standard conditions (same time of day, approximately the same clothing, balanced scale). *Rapid weight changes often reflect changes in fluid balance. Weight is a more accurate indicator of overall fluid volume status than I&O records.*
- If a fluid challenge is ordered, assess vital signs, urine output, breath sounds, and mental status before fluid administration and every 10 to 15 minutes during the challenge. *A large amount of fluid may be given very rapidly in a fluid challenge. Patients with impaired cardiac or renal status may develop signs of a fluid overload during the challenge.*
- Provide oral fluids as ordered. Identify the patient's beverage preferences; monitor fluid intake. *Oral fluids are used to replace lost fluids and relieve thirst.*
- Administer intravenous fluids as ordered. *Patients with severe fluid volume deficit or who are unable to tolerate oral fluids may require intravenous fluid replacement to restore blood volume.*

Risk for Injury

Expected outcome: Will remain free of physical injury.

- Institute safety precautions, including keeping the bed in a low position, using side rails, and raising the patient slowly from the supine to sitting or sitting to standing position. *The patient with orthostatic hypotension is at risk for dizziness, fainting, or falling with rapid position changes.*
- Teach patient to get up slowly, sitting on the side of the bed for several minutes before standing. *These measures reduce orthostatic hypotension and the patient's risk for injury.*

MANAGING NURSING CARE

Nursing care activities such as assisting with fluid intake, transfers and ambulation, hygiene and toileting, and measuring I&O for the patient with fluid volume deficit are appropriate to assign to assistive personnel.

EVALUATING

Monitor the patient's I&O records to evaluate short-term goals of increasing fluid intake. Assess for measures of fluid volume status such as stable vital signs and weight and safety to evaluate the effectiveness of nursing measures to maintain or restore fluid balance. Assess the patient's and caregivers' knowledge about and participation in measures to improve fluid intake to evaluate progress toward maintaining fluid balance.

DOCUMENTING

Document continuing assessment data as well as the effectiveness of interventions. Note the patient's ability and willingness to take oral fluids, as well as the amount of fluids consumed. Monitor for, document, and report possible adverse effects of treatment, such as shortness of breath or abnormal breath sounds.

CONTINUITY OF CARE

For the patient being discharged to home, assess the patient's ability to perform ADLs and access fluids, as well as the availability and knowledge of caregivers as needed.

Provide verbal and written instructions:

- Recommended fluid intake and suggestions for obtaining fluids.
- Early manifestations of dehydration and measures to prevent or correct it.
- Avoid overexposure to heat and exercise (adjust activity level and fluid intake in hot weather).
- If vomiting, take small, frequent amounts of ice chips or clear liquids (weak tea, flat cola, or ginger ale).
- Avoid beverages containing caffeine or large amounts of sugar and alcohol, which can increase urine output.
- Replace fluids lost through diarrhea with fruit juices or bouillon rather than large amounts of tap water.
- Monitor weight, reporting changes of more than 3 to 5 lb in a week to primary care provider.

Teach older adults and their caregivers to prevent fluid volume deficit by offering preferred fluids on a regular basis throughout the day and using alternative sources of liquid (e.g., gelatin, broth, or ice cream).

For the patient being discharged to a long-term care or residential facility, provide verbal and written information to caregivers about the patient's preferred type and temperature of fluids and other measures to maintain fluid intake.

Be sure to note any prescribed medications likely to affect fluid intake or balance. Discuss the importance of providing additional water to patients who are receiving enteral nutrition via tube feedings.

Fluid Volume Excess

Fluid volume excess usually results from sodium and water retention. It is rarely a problem in healthy adults. However, older adults, people with chronic or debilitating illnesses, and patients receiving intravenous therapy are at risk.

PATHOPHYSIOLOGY

Fluid volume excess usually is caused by retention of both sodium and water. Conditions that can lead to sodium and water retention include heart, liver, or kidney failure and endocrine conditions that affect ADH and aldosterone release. Sodium and water are retained in approximately the same proportion as is present in ECF. Other causes of fluid volume excess include an excessive intake of sodium-containing foods, drugs that cause sodium retention, and administration of intravenous fluids containing sodium.

MANIFESTATIONS AND COMPLICATIONS

Excess fluid tends to remain within the extracellular space, leading to manifestations of **hypervolemia** (excess intravascular fluid) and **edema** (excess fluid in body tissues). Manifestations of hypervolemia include tachycardia and bounding peripheral pulses, increased respiratory rate with crackles on auscultation, and distended neck veins. The BP often is elevated. Interstitial fluid causes weight gain and edema of dependent tissues (the lower extremities in ambulatory patients and the back and sacrum in bedridden patients). When fluid volume excess is associated with kidney disease, edema may be generalized, affecting soft tissues around the eyes and the upper extremities as well.

Causes and manifestations of fluid volume excess are listed in Table 7-5■.

Heart failure not only is a potential cause of fluid volume excess, but may be a complication of the problem. The heart may be unable to handle the workload caused by excess fluid, leading to failure. See Chapter 17 for more information about heart failure.

COLLABORATIVE CARE
Diagnostic Tests

Diagnostic tests to determine the severity and possible causes of fluid volume excess may include the following:

- *Serum electrolytes* and *serum osmolality* often remain within normal limits in fluid volume excess.
- *Hemoglobin* and *hematocrit* levels may be reduced as a result of dilution of the blood by excess fluid.
- *Liver* and *kidney function tests*, such as serum ALT, AST, BUN, and creatinine, may be done to help determine the cause of fluid volume excess.

Medications

Diuretics, which promote sodium and water excretion, may be prescribed. Three classes of diuretics are commonly used: loop diuretics, thiazide diuretics, and potassium-sparing diuretics (Table 7-6■).

Diet and Fluid Management

Because sodium retention is a primary cause of fluid volume excess, a sodium-restricted diet often is prescribed. People require about 500 mg of sodium per day, but Americans typically consume about 4 to 5 grams daily, mostly from salt, processed foods, and foods themselves. A mild sodium restriction can be achieved by reducing the amount of salt in recipes by half, by not using the salt shaker at the table, and by avoiding foods that contain high levels of sodium either naturally or because of processing

TABLE 7-5	Fluid Volume Excess	
CAUSES	**MANIFESTATIONS**	**LAB VALUES**
■ Kidney failure	■ Hypertension	■ ↓ Serum osmolality
■ Heart failure	■ Tachycardia	■ ↓ Hematocrit
■ Cirrhosis of the liver	■ Full, bounding peripheral pulses	■ ↓ Urine specific gravity
■ Medications	■ ↑ Respiratory rate	
■ Excess fluid intake	■ Cough, **dyspnea** (difficult or labored breathing), **orthopnea** (difficulty breathing when supine)	
■ Excess sodium intake	■ Moist respiratory crackles, wheezes	
	■ Weight gain	
	■ Distended neck veins	
	■ Dependent edema	

TABLE 7-6	Giving Medications Safely: Fluid Volume Excess		
CLASS/DRUGS	**PURPOSE**	**NURSING RESPONSIBILITIES** *(FOR ALL DRUG GROUPS)*	**PATIENT TEACHING** *(FOR ALL DRUG GROUPS)*
Loop diuretics ■ *Furosemide* (Lasix) ■ Ethacrynic acid (Edecrin) ■ Bumetanide (Bumex) ■ Torsemide (Demadex)	Loop diuretics inhibit sodium and water reabsorption in the loop of Henle and increase potassium loss in the distal tubule. As a result, loop diuretics promote sodium, chloride, potassium, and water excretion.	Obtain baseline weight and vital signs. Monitor I&O, weight, vital signs (VS), skin turgor, and edema. Report manifestations of volume depletion: dizziness, orthostatic hypotension, tachycardia, muscle cramping. Loop and thiazide diuretics cause potassium wasting. Monitor serum electrolytes (especially potassium) and blood glucose. Notify physician of abnormal values. Notify the physician if the patient is receiving a loop diuretic with another ototoxic drug such as an aminoglycoside antibiotic.	The drug will increase the amount and frequency of urination. Take the drugs in the morning and afternoon to avoid having to get up at night to urinate. Change position slowly to avoid dizziness. Report the following to your primary health care provider: flulike symptoms, weakness, dehydration, thirst, dizziness; trouble breathing; or swelling of face, hands, or feet. Weigh yourself at the same time every day and report sudden gains or losses. Try to avoid using the salt shaker when eating. If the drug increases potassium loss, eat foods high in potassium, such as orange juice and bananas. Unless restricted, drink six to eight glasses of water daily.
Thiazide diuretics ■ Chlorothiazide (Diuril) ■ Chlorthalidone (Hygroton) ■ *Hydrochlorothiazide* (HydroDiuril) ■ Methyclothiazide (Enduron) ■ Metolazone (Zaroxolyn) ■ Others	Thiazide diuretics promote the excretion of sodium, chloride, potassium, and water by decreasing their reabsorption in the distal tubule.		
Potassium-sparing diuretics ■ Spironolactone (Aldactone) ■ Amiloride HCl (Midamor) ■ *Triamterene* (Dyrenium)	Potassium-sparing diuretics promote excretion of sodium and water by inhibiting sodium–potassium exchange in the distal tubule.		

Note: Medications identified in *italics* are among the 200 most frequently prescribed drugs in the United States.

(Box 7-7■). In moderate and severely sodium-restricted diets, salt and all foods containing significant amounts of sodium are avoided altogether.

Fluid intake also may be restricted in patients who have fluid volume excess. The amount of fluid allowed per day is prescribed by the care provider. All fluid intake must be calculated, including fluid provided with meals and fluid used to administer medications orally or intravenously. Box 7-8■ provides guidelines for patients on a fluid restriction.

NURSING CARE

PRIORITIZING NURSING CARE

Preventing fluid volume excess and identifying its manifestations are important nursing responsibilities. Excess fluid volume and hypervolemia can have serious consequences for patients, particularly older adults. The heart may not be able to adapt to increased blood volume, leading to heart

BOX 7-7	FOODS HIGH IN SODIUM

High in Added Sodium
■ *Processed meat and fish*—bacon, sausage, smoked fish, luncheon meat, and other cold cuts
■ *Selected dairy products*—buttermilk, cottage cheese, cheeses, ice cream
■ *Processed grains*—graham crackers, most dry cereals
■ *Canned goods*—meats, vegetables, soups
■ *Snack foods*—salted popcorn, nuts, potato chips/pretzels, gelatin desserts
■ *Condiments and food additives*—barbecue sauce, saccharin, catsup, pickles, chili sauce, soy sauce, meat tenderizers, salted margarine, Worcestershire sauce, salad dressings

Naturally High in Sodium
■ Kidney, oysters, shrimp, clams, crab, lobster
■ Dried fruit
■ Spinach, carrots

BOX 7-8	NURSING CARE CHECKLIST

Fluid Restriction Guidelines

☑ Subtract requisite fluids (e.g., ordered IV fluids, fluids in which IV medications are mixed) from total daily allowance.

☑ Divide remaining fluid allowance:
  - Day shift (0700 to 1500): 1/2 of total
  - Evening shift (1500 to 2300): 1/4 to 1/3 of total
  - Nights (2300 to 0700): Remainder

☑ Explain the fluid restriction to the patient, family members, and caregivers.

☑ With the patient, determine preferred fluids and intake pattern.

☑ Offer fluids in small glasses (allows perception of a full glass).

☑ Offer ice chips (which, when melted, are approximately half of the frozen volume).

☑ Provide frequent mouth care and opportunities to rinse mouth.

☑ Provide sugarless chewing gum or hard candy (if allowed) to reduce thirst.

failure. Congestion of pulmonary vessels can impair gas exchange, affecting tissue oxygenation. For this reason, the excess fluid volume is the priority nursing care focus.

HEALTH PROMOTION

Teach patients at risk for excess fluid volume and edema (e.g., patients with heart, liver, or kidney failure) about the relationship between sodium intake and water retention. Instruct about a low-sodium diet, teaching the patient to identify "hidden" sodium in foods as well as ways to reduce salt intake. Facilitate referral to a dietitian for additional teaching as appropriate.

ASSESSING

Assess for subjective complaints of cough, shortness of breath, and difficulty sleeping or breathing when lying down; ask about the number of pillows used to sleep. Inquire about recent changes in fluid intake, output, or weight and risk factors such as kidney or heart failure, cirrhosis of the liver, or an endocrine disorder. Ask about use of medications such as corticosteroids (e.g., prednisone) or nonsteroidal anti-inflammatory drugs (NSAIDs).

Obtain vital signs, peripheral pulses, oxygen saturation, and weight; evaluate color and moisture of skin and mucous membranes, and assess for distended neck veins and edema. Auscultate breath sounds for crackles or wheezes and heart sounds for S_3 (heard immediately after S_2) and/or S_4 (heard immediately before S_1). Evaluate mental status and level of consciousness.

Monitor laboratory values, including serum electrolytes and osmolality, reporting abnormal or unexpected findings.

IDENTIFYING POTENTIAL COMPLICATIONS

Patients with heart disease are at greatest risk for the effects of excess fluid volume. Tachycardia, acute dyspnea, orthopnea, anxiety, cough (which may be productive of pink, frothy sputum), and a decrease in oxygen saturation levels may indicate acute pulmonary edema, a medical emergency.

clinicalALERT

Elevate the patient's head, start oxygen, and immediately notify the registered nurse or physician if the patient with fluid volume excess develops acute respiratory distress.

DIAGNOSING, PLANNING, AND IMPLEMENTING

Nursing care for the patient with excess fluid volume is directed at the multisystem effects of the excess fluid.

Excess Fluid Volume

Expected outcome: Will exhibit fluid balance: stable vital signs, clear breath sounds, balanced I&O, weight within expected range, and decreasing edema.

- Monitor daily weights and I&O. Report weight or fluid gain to the charge nurse or physician. *Daily weights are one of the most important gauges of fluid balance. Two kilograms (approximately 5 lb) of weight gain is equivalent to 2 L of fluid gain.*

- Monitor edema, particularly in the lower extremities and the sacral and periorbital areas. *Localized edema tends to occur in dependent tissues such as the lower extremities of ambulatory patients and the sacrum in bedridden patients. Periorbital edema indicates generalized edema.*

- If fluid is restricted, carefully monitor record intake. Instruct the patient, family, and caregivers about the restriction and how to accurately measure fluid intake. *All sources of fluid intake, including ice chips, should be strictly monitored to avoid excess fluid.*

- Provide frequent oral hygiene. *Oral hygiene contributes to patient comfort and keeps mucous membranes intact; it also helps relieve thirst if fluids are restricted.*

- Encourage the patient to rest frequently in bed or a recliner with the feet elevated. *Bed rest promotes excretion of excess fluid by promoting its reabsorption into blood vessels and excretion by the kidneys.*

- Place in Fowler's position if dyspnea is present. *Fowler's position improves lung expansion and promotes fluid excretion.*

Risk for Impaired Skin Integrity

Expected outcome: Skin will remain intact with no evidence of breakdown.

Edema, which results from excess fluid in the interstitial spaces, decreases the delivery of nutrients to tissues and increases their susceptibility to injury.

■ Reposition at least every 2 hours. *Frequent position changes minimize tissue pressure.*
■ Assess pressure areas—particularly tissues over bony prominences—with each position change, and provide appropriate skin care. *Edematous tissue over bony prominences is more prone to tissue breakdown.*
■ Minimize tissue pressure by providing an alternating pressure mattress, foot cradles, and other devices. *An alternating pressure mattress distributes pressure over a wider area of the body surface and reduces pressure over bony prominences. A foot cradle minimizes the pressure that bedding can exert on the feet and lower extremities.*

MANAGING NURSING CARE

Nursing care activities for the patient with fluid volume excess such as measuring I&O, toileting assistance, hygiene measures, and assisting with position changes are appropriate to assign to assistive personnel.

EVALUATING

To evaluate the effectiveness of nursing care for patients with fluid volume excess, assess for changes in vital signs, weight, ease of breathing, and relief of edema. Monitor skin integrity and the need for additional measures to protect skin and underlying tissues from injury.

DOCUMENTING

Document continuing assessment data and the patient's response to treatment. Document teaching about fluid and sodium restrictions and the patient's understanding of foods to eat and those to avoid.

CONTINUITY OF CARE

Assess the patient's and family's readiness and ability to provide home care prior to discharge. Focus on prevention of future episodes of excess fluid volume in teaching. Emphasize the importance of taking medications as prescribed and avoiding foods that are high in sodium. Instructions for a low-sodium diet are found in Box 7-9■. Provide verbal and written instructions:

■ Amount and type of fluids allowed, including a specific plan if fluids are restricted.
■ Ways to reduce sodium intake when buying and preparing foods.
■ Elevate feet and legs when sitting, avoid crossing legs, change positions often, and wear support hose and clothing that do not impair circulation.
■ To reduce the risk of damage to edematous tissue, wear well-fitting shoes that do not bind feet or ankles.

BOX 7-9   PATIENT TEACHING

Low-Sodium Diet

■ The body needs less than 1 teaspoon (about 500 mg) of salt per day. About one-third of sodium intake comes from adding salt during cooking and at the table, about one-third from processed foods, and the remainder from food and fluids naturally high in sodium.
■ In place of salt, use herbs, spices, lemon juice, vinegar, and wine as flavoring when cooking. The taste for salt will eventually diminish.
■ Use salt substitutes sparingly if at all; they often taste bitter in large amounts and contain significant amounts of potassium.
■ Low-sodium salt substitutes may contain half the sodium of regular salt.
■ Read labels. Salt, monosodium glutamate, baking soda, and baking powder contain significant amounts of sodium. Processed foods list the sodium content. Some nonprescription drugs (e.g., laxatives and antacids) contain high amounts of sodium.

■ Use more than one pillow or a recliner chair for sleeping if orthopnea is a problem.
■ Weigh daily and report sudden increases of more than 2 lb to your doctor.

If the patient is being discharged to a long-term care or residential care facility, review the patient's medications, prescribed diet, and fluid restrictions with caregivers. Discuss potential adverse medication effects (e.g., potassium depletion if taking a diuretic) and early manifestations of fluid retention and excess.

NURSING CARE PLAN
Patient With Fluid Volume Excess

Dorothy Rainwater is a 45-year-old former high school principal hospitalized with acute kidney injury. She is expected to recover from this acute illness, but she currently has very little urine output.

Assessment
Mike Penning, Ms. Rainwater's nurse, notes that her output for the previous 24 hours is 250 mL; this low output has been constant for the past 8 days. She has gained 1 lb (0.45 kg) in the past 24 hours. Ms. Rainwater is on a fluid restriction of 500 mL plus the amount of her output for the previous day.

Mr. Penning assesses the following: T 98.6°F, BP 160/92, P 102, with obvious neck vein distention, R 28, with crackles and wheezes; SaO$_2$ 95%; head of bed elevated 30 degrees; periorbital and sacral edema noted, 3+ pitting edema in feet bilaterally; skin pale and shiny. Alert and oriented; responds appropriately to questions; states she is thirsty, slightly nauseated, and extremely tired.

Nursing Diagnosis

The following priority nursing diagnoses are established for Ms. Rainwater:

■ *Excess Fluid Volume* related to acute kidney injury
■ *Risk for Impaired Skin Integrity* related to edema
■ *Risk for Impaired Gas Exchange* related to pulmonary congestion
■ *Activity Intolerance* related to fluid volume excess, fatigue, and weakness

Expected Outcomes

The expected outcomes specify that Ms. Rainwater will:

■ Regain fluid balance, as evidenced by weight loss, decreasing edema, and normal vital signs.
■ Experience decreased dyspnea.
■ Maintain intact skin and mucous membranes.
■ Increase activity levels as prescribed.

Planning and Implementation

The following nursing interventions are planned and implemented:

■ Weigh q12hr at 0600 and 1800.
■ Monitor vital signs and breath sounds q4hr.
■ Intake and output q4hr.
■ Restrict fluids as follows: 375 mL, 0700 to 1500; 275 mL, 1500 to 2300; 100 mL, 2300 to 0700. Prefers water or apple juice.
■ Turn every 2 hours, following posted schedule. Inspect skin, and provide skin care when turned.
■ Assist with oral care every 2 to 4 hours (caution not to swallow water).
■ Elevate head of bed to 30 to 40 degrees; prefers two small soft pillows under her head.
■ Up at bedside in recliner as tolerated. Monitor carefully for fatigue and weakness as activity level increases.

Evaluation

At the end of the shift, Mr. Penning notes that Ms. Rainwater gained no weight, and her urinary output during his shift is 300 mL. Her vital signs remain unchanged, but her crackles and wheezes have decreased, and she states that she can breathe more easily. Her skin and mucous membranes are intact. She enjoyed sitting in the chair at her bedside and did not experience any shortness of breath.

Critical Thinking in the Nursing Process

1. Why are Ms. Rainwater's respiratory rate, blood pressure, and pulse elevated?

2. Explain how elevating the head of the bed 30 degrees makes breathing easier.
3. Outline a plan for teaching Ms. Rainwater about diuretics.
4. Suppose Ms. Rainwater says, "I would really like to have all my fluids at once instead of spreading them out." What would be your reply, and why?

Note: Discussion of Critical Thinking questions appears on the companion website.

Sodium Imbalance

Key Concept Manifestations of electrolyte imbalances can be vague and nonspecific. Monitoring and tracking changes in laboratory values is critical in patients who have or are at risk for electrolyte imbalance.

Sodium (Na^+), the most plentiful electrolyte in ECF, has a normal serum range of 135 to 145 mEq/L. Sodium regulates ECF volume and distribution and contributes to neuromuscular activity and acid–base balance. Because of the close relationship between sodium and water balance, disorders of fluid volume and sodium balance often occur together. Sodium imbalances affect the osmolality of ECF. When sodium levels are low (*hyponatremia*), water is drawn into the cells of the body, causing them to swell. In contrast, high sodium levels in ECF (*hypernatremia*) draw water out of body cells, causing them to shrink (see Figure 7-4).

Although the body requires only about 500 mg of sodium per day, the average intake is significantly higher. Sodium excretion is controlled by the kidneys. The kidneys work together with the renin–angiotensin–aldosterone system and ANP to regulate sodium levels. A fall in blood volume stimulates the renin–angiotensin–aldosterone system, prompting reabsorption of sodium and water by the kidneys. Urine output falls, and blood volume increases. In contrast, when blood volume increases, ANP is released by cells in the heart. ANP increases sodium excretion by the kidneys. These mechanisms usually maintain ECF sodium concentration within its usual range despite variations in daily intake.

HYPONATREMIA

Hyponatremia (serum sodium less than 135 mEq/L) usually results from excess sodium loss. It may also be caused by excess water that dilutes ECF. Hyponatremia affects the function of voluntary and involuntary muscles. Brain cells swell, leading to neurologic manifestations such as headache and possible brain damage. The causes, manifestations, and laboratory values of hyponatremia are shown in Table 7-7 ■. Serum sodium levels of less than 110 to 120 mEq/L are considered critical, necessitating immediate intervention.

TABLE 7-7	Sodium Imbalances	
IMBALANCE	**CAUSES**	**MANIFESTATIONS**
Hyponatremia ■ Serum sodium less than 135 mEq/L ■ Critical value: less than 110–120 mEq/L *Other lab values* ■ Serum osmolality less than 280 mOsm/kg	■ Excess sodium loss through kidneys, skin, or GI tract (vomiting, diarrhea, gastric suctioning or irrigation, enemas with water) ■ Excess sodium excretion due to diuretic medications or kidney or endocrine disorders ■ Water gains related to kidney disease, heart failure, or cirrhosis of the liver ■ Syndrome of inappropriate secretion of antidiuretic hormone (SIADH) ■ Excessive hypotonic IV fluids	■ Anorexia, nausea, vomiting, abdominal cramping, and diarrhea ■ Headache ■ Mental status changes ■ Hyperreflexia, muscle twitching, and tremors ■ Convulsions and coma
Hypernatremia ■ Serum sodium greater than 145 mEq/L ■ Critical value: greater than 160 mEq/L *Other lab values* ■ Serum osmolality greater than 300 mOsm/kg	■ Altered thirst or inability to respond to thirst ■ Hyperventilation ■ Profuse sweating ■ Diarrhea ■ Diabetes insipidus ■ Oral electrolyte solutions or hyperosmolar enteral formulas ■ Excess IV fluids such as normal saline, 3% or 5% sodium chloride, or sodium bicarbonate	■ Thirst ■ Restlessness, weakness ■ Altered mental status, decreasing level of consciousness, seizures ■ Muscle irritability ■ Dry, sticky mucous membranes ■ Postural hypotension ■ Hot, dry skin, fever, and decreased sweating

Collaborative Care

The following laboratory tests may be done to determine the extent and cause of hyponatremia:

■ *Serum electrolytes* and *serum osmolality* levels are drawn. Values for sodium and osmolality are low, reflecting an excess of water in relation to the amount of sodium in the body.

■ A *24-hour urine specimen* may be ordered to evaluate sodium excretion and help identify the cause of hyponatremia.

If hyponatremia is mild, increased intake of foods high in sodium may restore normal sodium balance (see Box 7-7). Oral fluids often are restricted. If the patient is unable to eat or drink, or if hyponatremia is severe, sodium-containing intravenous fluids may be administered. Normal saline (0.9% NaCl) may be given, or a 3% or 5% NaCl solution may be used cautiously to replace sodium and draw fluid out of the intracellular compartment. A loop diuretic such as furosemide (see Table 7-6) may be given along with sodium replacements to remove excess water.

HYPERNATREMIA

Hypernatremia (serum sodium concentration greater than 145 mEq/L) almost never occurs in people with an intact thirst mechanism and access to water. Hypernatremia results either from a gain of sodium in excess of water or from a loss of water in excess of sodium. Patients receiving concentrated enteral feeding formulas are at risk for hypernatremia if additional water is not provided.

With hypernatremia, excess sodium in the ECF draws water out of cells, causing them to shrink. Dehydration of brain cells causes manifestations such as confusion and a decreasing level of consciousness. Cellular dehydration also causes dry, sticky mucous membranes. Causes of excess water loss or excess sodium intake, as well as manifestations and laboratory values of hypernatremia, are summarized in Table 7-7. Serum sodium levels greater than 160 mEq/L are considered critical, requiring immediate intervention.

Collaborative Care

Hypernatremia is treated by correcting any water deficit with oral or hypotonic intravenous solutions such as D_5W or 0.45% NaCl. Diuretics may be given to increase sodium excretion, and a low-sodium diet may be prescribed. Hypernatremia is corrected slowly (over a 48-hour period) to avoid rebound cerebral edema as water shifts back into the dehydrated brain cells.

NURSING CARE

Nurses need to identify and monitor patients at risk for sodium imbalances. Treatments such as gastrointestinal suction and administering IV fluids or diuretics such as furosemide and thiazide diuretics increase the risk for hyponatremia.

Hypernatremia, on the other hand, usually is associated with an inability to access fluids or to respond to the thirst sensation. Patients who are elderly, debilitated, or confused are at highest risk for hypernatremia.

PRIORITIZING NURSING CARE

Sodium levels in the body have a significant role in regulating water balance; therefore, a risk for imbalanced fluid volume and its consequences are the highest priority nursing diagnoses.

HEALTH PROMOTION

Identifying patients at risk for sodium imbalance and teaching ways to prevent problems are primary health promotion activities. Athletes, people who do heavy labor in a hot environment, and older adults without access to air conditioning during hot weather are at risk for developing sodium imbalances. Teach people who frequently labor or strenuously exercise in hot weather to replace fluid losses with sodium-containing fluids (e.g., sports drinks, Pedialyte), not pure water. When teaching, remind patients that some sports drinks also contain caffeine, which may have a diuretic effect.

To prevent hypernatremia, instruct caregivers of older adults and debilitated patients to provide fluids at regular intervals. Carefully monitor patients receiving enteral nutrition for adequate fluid intake, and provide additional water as needed.

ASSESSING

Ask about manifestations such as thirst, nausea, vomiting, abdominal cramps, muscle weakness, headache and their duration. Inquire about precipitating factors such as heavy perspiration, vomiting, diarrhea, or water deprivation. Identify current medications and any chronic diseases such as heart, kidney, liver, or endocrine disorders.

Evaluate mental status, obtain vital signs including temperature and orthostatic vitals, palpate peripheral pulses, and assess for manifestations of fluid volume excess or deficit. Monitor serum sodium levels and serum osmolality, as well as levels of other serum electrolytes such as potassium; report changes outside the expected or normal range.

IDENTIFYING POTENTIAL COMPLICATIONS

A very low or very high sodium level can have significant neurologic effects. With very low levels, brain cells swell and cerebral edema develops, affecting mental status and potentially causing convulsions and coma. Very high serum sodium levels can cause brain cells to shrink, leading to changes in mental status and potential seizures and coma.

DIAGNOSING, PLANNING, AND IMPLEMENTING

Risk for Imbalanced Fluid Volume

Expected outcome: Will have balanced I&O over 24 hours.

- Monitor I&O, and weigh daily. *Fluid excess or deficit may occur in patients with sodium disorders.*
- Maintain oral and intravenous fluid intake as prescribed. Monitor serum sodium levels and osmolality. Report rapid changes in laboratory values. *Body water and sodium are replaced gradually to prevent cerebral edema or fluid volume excess.*

clinical**ALERT**

Promptly report changes in mental status or decreasing levels of consciousness to the registered nurse or physician.

- In patients who are receiving IV solutions containing sodium, monitor for signs of hypervolemia (increased BP, tachypnea, tachycardia, gallop rhythm, shortness of breath, crackles). *Hypertonic saline solutions may cause fluid retention and lead to heart failure, particularly in older adults or people with preexisting heart problems.*
- Explain ordered fluid restrictions, how much fluid is allowed over 24 hours, and how to measure fluid volumes. *Fluid intake may be restricted in patients with a sodium imbalance; teaching increases understanding and compliance.*

Risk for Injury

Expected outcome: Will remain free of injury.

- Assess muscle strength and tone by asking the patient to move upper and lower extremities against resistance. *Muscle weakness resulting from sodium imbalance increases the risk for falling.*
- Assess for mental status changes, such as altered level of consciousness, confusion, and seizures. Monitor behavior, mental status, and orientation. *Baseline data and ongoing assessments are critical because changes in serum sodium and serum osmolality may affect neurologic status and safety.*
- Maintain a quiet environment, and institute seizure precautions as indicated: Keep the bed in its lowest position, side rails up and padded, and airway at the bedside. *A quiet environment reduces neurologic stimulation. Seizures often occur unexpectedly. Safety precautions reduce the risk of injury from seizure.*

MANAGING NURSING CARE

Nursing care activities such as measuring vital signs and I&O, obtaining daily weights, and providing assistance with ADLs are appropriate to assign to assistive personnel helping care for the patient with sodium imbalance.

EVALUATING

To evaluate the effectiveness of nursing care for patients with sodium imbalances, collect data related to fluid balance, serum sodium level, and freedom from injury. Monitor laboratory values, reporting lack of response to treatment or overcorrection of the imbalance.

DOCUMENTING

Document continuing assessment data throughout treatment, including mental status and any changes that occur. Document teaching provided to help prevent future episodes of sodium imbalance.

CONTINUITY OF CARE

Teach patients and caregivers about risk factors for and manifestations of sodium imbalances.

Emphasize the importance of adequate water intake and discuss ways to ensure that water needs are met. Suggest drinking liquids containing sodium and other electrolytes (e.g., Gatorade and other sports drinks) at frequent intervals when perspiring heavily, when environmental temperatures are high, or if experiencing prolonged watery diarrhea.

Teach patients and caregivers about a low-sodium diet if prescribed (see Box 7-9). When helping the patient plan a low-sodium diet, include cultural foods and identify nondietary sources of sodium, such as softened water or over-the-counter medications.

Potassium Imbalance

Potassium (K^+), the primary intracellular cation, is vital for cell metabolism and for cardiac and neuromuscular function. The normal serum (ECF) potassium level is 3.5 to 5.3 mEq/L, while the potassium concentration of ICF is 140 to 150 mEq/L. The sodium–potassium pump maintains this significant difference in concentrations between ICF and ECF.

To maintain normal potassium levels in the body, potassium must be replaced every day. Virtually all foods contain potassium, although some foods and fluids are richer sources than others. The kidneys eliminate potassium very efficiently; even when potassium intake is stopped, the kidneys continue to excrete potassium. The hormone aldosterone contributes to potassium regulation by the kidneys. When aldosterone is present, more potassium is excreted; when it is absent, potassium is retained.

Potassium shifts into and out of the cells constantly. For example, it shifts into or out of the cells in response to changes in hydrogen ion concentration (pH, discussed later in this chapter), as the body strives to maintain a stable acid–base balance. This movement can significantly affect the serum potassium level.

HYPOKALEMIA

Hypokalemia (abnormally low serum potassium, less than 3.5 mEq/L) usually results from excess loss of potassium. However, hospitalized patients are at risk for hypokalemia because of inadequate intake. Patients who are NPO for extended periods, as well as patients with nausea and anorexia, are at risk for inadequate intake of potassium.

Excess potassium may be lost through the kidneys or the gastrointestinal (GI) tract (Table 7-8■). Drugs such as diuretics and corticosteroids are a major cause of excess potassium loss from the kidneys. GI losses may be caused

TABLE 7-8	Potassium Imbalances		
IMBALANCE	**CAUSES**		**MANIFESTATIONS**
Hypokalemia ■ Serum potassium less than 3.5 mEq/L ■ Critical value: less than 2.5 mEq/L	■ Excess GI losses: vomiting, gastric suction, diarrhea, ileostomy drainage ■ Kidney losses: diuretics, corticosteroids; hyperaldosteronism ■ Inadequate intake (NPO, anorexia nervosa) ■ K^+ shift into cells (alkalosis, tissue repair)		■ Muscle weakness or leg cramps ■ Nausea and vomiting ■ Anorexia ■ Decreased bowel sounds or ileus ■ Dysrhythmias and ECG changes ■ Polyuria
Hyperkalemia ■ Serum potassium greater than 5.3 mEq/L ■ Critical value: greater than 6.5 mEq/L	■ Kidney failure ■ Medications: Potassium-sparing diuretics, ACE inhibitors, angiotensin-receptor blockers (ARBs) ■ Adrenal insufficiency ■ Excess potassium intake (e.g., excess potassium replacement) ■ Administering aged blood ■ K^+ shift out of cells (acidosis, tissue damage)		■ ECG changes, dysrhythmias, heart block, cardiac arrest ■ Nausea, abdominal cramping, diarrhea ■ Muscle weakness, paresthesias, flaccid paralysis

by severe vomiting, prolonged gastric suction, diarrhea, or excessive ileostomy drainage.

A temporary shift of potassium into the intracellular space may occur because of alkalosis, rapid tissue repair (e.g., after a burn or trauma), or high blood insulin levels.

Hypokalemia affects the transmission of nerve impulses and the contractility of smooth, skeletal, and cardiac muscle. All patients with serum potassium values of 3.5 mEq/L or lower should be closely monitored. Manifestations of hypokalemia generally are not seen until the serum K^+ falls below 3.0 mEq/L. Values lower than 2.5 mEq/L are considered to be critical. Serious and potentially life-threatening cardiac *dysrhythmias* (abnormal heart rhythms) are a major concern, particularly in patients who are receiving digitalis to treat heart failure (see Chapter 17). The manifestations of hypokalemia are summarized in Table 7-8 and illustrated in Figure 7-15■.

Collaborative Care

Diagnostic Tests The following diagnostic tests are done to determine potassium levels and their effect:

- *Serum potassium levels* are drawn; results show a serum K^+ of less than 3.5 mEq/L.
- *Arterial blood gases (ABGs)* may be ordered to determine acid–base status, because hydrogen ion balance (pH) and serum potassium levels are linked.
- An *electrocardiogram (ECG)* is done to evaluate cardiac rhythm and assess for characteristic changes associated with hypokalemia, such as flattened T waves and dysrhythmias.

Additional diagnostic tests such as serum electrolyte levels and kidney function studies (blood urea nitrogen and serum creatinine levels, creatinine clearance) may be ordered to help determine the cause of the electrolyte imbalance.

Potassium Replacement Potassium replacement therapy (by mouth or intravenously) is implemented both to prevent and to treat hypokalemia. Commonly prescribed potassium supplements, their actions, and nursing implications are described in Table 7-9■. Several days of therapy may be required to correct hypokalemia.

Increased intake of foods high in potassium may be recommended for patients at risk for hypokalemia, either to prevent its occurrence or to supplement pharmacologic

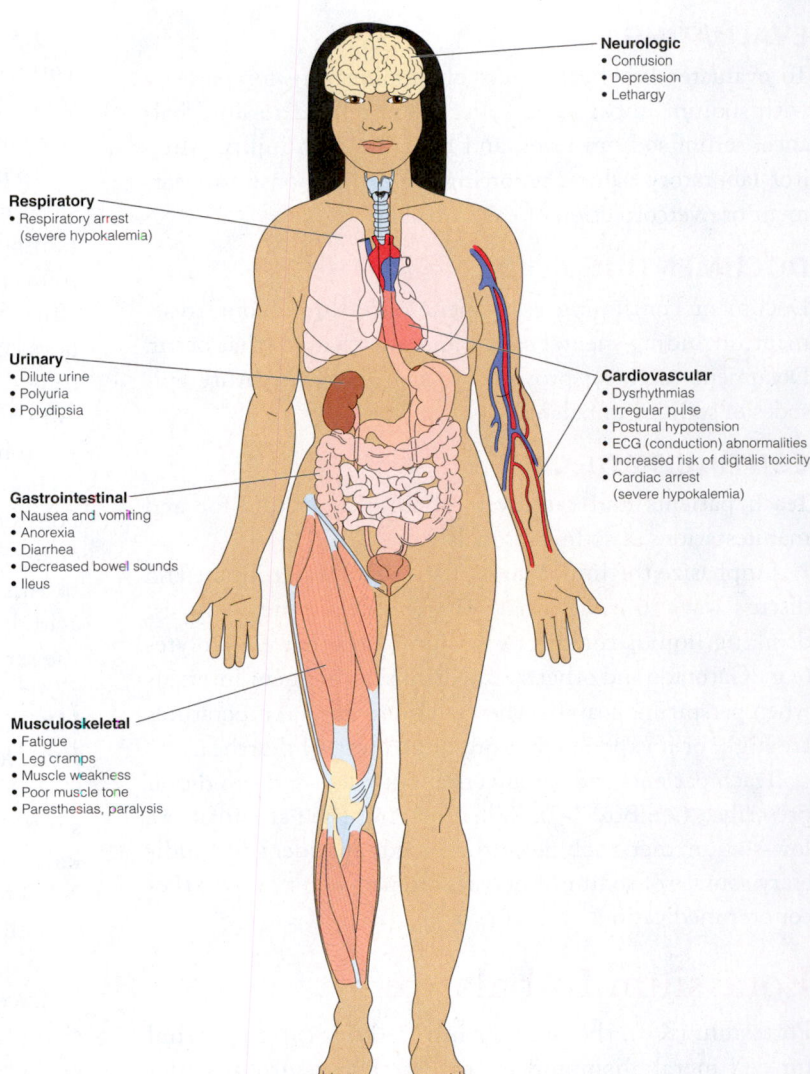

Neurologic
- Confusion
- Depression
- Lethargy

Respiratory
- Respiratory arrest (severe hypokalemia)

Urinary
- Dilute urine
- Polyuria
- Polydipsia

Gastrointestinal
- Nausea and vomiting
- Anorexia
- Diarrhea
- Decreased bowel sounds
- Ileus

Cardiovascular
- Dysrhythmias
- Irregular pulse
- Postural hypotension
- ECG (conduction) abnormalities
- Increased risk of digitalis toxicity
- Cardiac arrest (severe hypokalemia)

Musculoskeletal
- Fatigue
- Leg cramps
- Muscle weakness
- Poor muscle tone
- Paresthesias, paralysis

Figure 7-15. ■ The multisystem effects of hypokalemia. (Source: "The Multisystem Effects of Hypokalemia" from Medical Surgical Nursing: Critical Thinking in Patient Care, 5e by Priscilla LeMone; Karen Burke; and Gerene Bauldoff. Published by Pearson Education, © 2011.)

therapy. Box 7-10■ lists foods and fluids that are high in potassium.

HYPERKALEMIA

Hyperkalemia (abnormally high serum potassium, greater than 5.3 mEq/L) results from inadequate potassium excretion, excessive potassium intake, or a shift of potassium from the ICF to the ECF. The major cause of hyperkalemia is impaired kidney excretion (see Table 7-8). Excess potassium intake often occurs when people use potassium-based salt substitutes while taking medications that affect potassium excretion. Administration of aged blood from a blood bank can also lead to hyperkalemia, because the potassium concentration of blood increases during storage. Burns and crushing injuries release potassium from cells into ECF. In

TABLE 7-9	**Giving Medications Safely: Potassium Replacement**		
CLASS/DRUGS	**PURPOSE**	**NURSING IMPLICATIONS**	**PATIENT TEACHING**
Potassium sources ■ Potassium acetate (Tri-K) ■ Potassium citrate (K-Lyte) ■ *Potassium chloride* (Klor-Con, K-lease, Micro-K10, Apo-K, others) ■ Potassium gluconate (Kaon Elixir, Royonate)	Potassium is used to prevent and treat hypokalemia. It is rapidly absorbed from the gastrointestinal tract. Potassium chloride is the agent of choice, because low chloride levels often accompany low potassium.	**When giving oral potassium:** 1. Position patient upright (sitting or standing). 2. Administer tablets whole with a full glass of water or juice. 3. Dilute or dissolve soluble or liquid potassium in fruit or vegetable juice or cold water. **When giving parenteral potassium:** 1. Administer slowly. 2. Never administer undiluted. 3. Assess injection site frequently for pain and inflammation. 4. Use an infusion control device. Monitor I&O Monitor serum potassium levels; do not administer if serum K^+ is greater than 5.0 mEq/L.	Take as prescribed; do not skip a dose or double your prescribed dose unless instructed to do so by your physician. Take potassium supplements with meals to reduce gastric irritation. Do not chew enteric-coated tablets or allow them to dissolve in the mouth; this may affect the potency and action of the medications. Do not use salt substitutes when taking potassium (most salt substitutes are potassium-based). Do not take potassium supplements if you are also taking a potassium-sparing diuretic.

Note: Medications identified in *italics* are among the 200 most frequently prescribed drugs in the United States.

BOX 7-10	**FOODS HIGH IN POTASSIUM**

■ *Fruits*—apricots, avocados, bananas, cantaloupe, dates, oranges, raisins
■ *Vegetables*—carrots, cauliflower, mushrooms, peas, potatoes, spinach, tomatoes
■ *Meat and fish*
■ *Milk and milk products*

acidosis, hydrogen ion moves into the cells and potassium shifts out into ECF as the body attempts to maintain a normal pH.

memoryALERT

■ In acidosis, potassium shifts out of cells into ECF → increased serum potassium and hyperkalemia.
■ In alkalosis, potassium shifts into cells from ECF → decreased serum potassium and hypokalemia.

Hyperkalemia alters nerve and muscle function. Its most harmful effects are on the heart, with a risk for dysrhythmias, heart block, and cardiac arrest. The strength of cardiac contractions decreases as the potassium level increases. Hyperkalemia also affects skeletal and smooth muscle, causing weakness and GI symptoms. Levels higher than 6.5 mEq/L are considered critical, carrying a high risk for cardiac arrest.

clinicalALERT

Remember: Both *hypo*kalemia and *hyper*kalemia affect heart function and can result in serious, even fatal, dysrhythmias.

Collaborative Care

Managing hyperkalemia focuses on returning the serum potassium level to normal by treating the underlying cause, promoting potassium excretion, and avoiding additional potassium intake.

Diagnostic Tests The following diagnostic tests are ordered to determine the extent of hyperkalemia and its effects:

■ *Serum electrolytes* are monitored, because low calcium and sodium levels may increase the effects of hyperkalemia.
■ *ABGs* are measured to determine whether acidosis is present.
■ *ECG monitoring* is performed to evaluate the effects of hyperkalemia on cardiac function.
■ *Kidney function tests*, including BUN, serum creatinine, and creatinine clearance, may be done to help determine the cause of hyperkalemia.

Medications Mild hyperkalemia may be reversed by treating the cause (e.g., correcting acidosis) or by discontinuing drugs that caused it. Loop diuretics such as furosemide (Lasix) promote excretion of potassium by the kidneys and may be administered (see Table 7-6 for nursing care related to diuretic therapy). A cation-exchange resin, sodium polystyrene sulfonate (Kayexalate), may be given orally or rectally (by enema) to remove excess potassium by exchanging sodium for potassium in the intestinal tract. In the patient with kidney failure, hemodialysis and peritoneal dialysis are used to manage hyperkalemia (see Chapter 29).

For moderate to severe hyperkalemia, intravenous insulin and glucose may be given to drive potassium into the cells. Intravenous sodium bicarbonate has a similar effect. Calcium gluconate may also be given to block the effects of hyperkalemia on the heart.

NURSING CARE

PRIORITIZING NURSING CARE

Nursing care focuses on early identification and reporting of abnormal serum potassium levels and monitoring cardiac status.

HEALTH PROMOTION

Health promotion related to potassium imbalances starts with identifying patients at risk (e.g., patients taking diuretics; those who are on a severely restricted diet; people with kidney disorders, anorexia nervosa, or who are using anabolic steroids for body building) and teaching measures to prevent an imbalance. Teach patients at risk for hypokalemia about including foods high in potassium in the diet and the importance of regular monitoring of potassium levels (e.g., for people taking a diuretic). Teach patients at risk for hyperkalemia to carefully read food and dietary supplement labels and to avoid salt substitutes that contain potassium.

ASSESSING

Ask about symptoms such as anorexia, nausea, vomiting, abdominal discomfort, muscle weakness, or heart palpitations and their duration. Inquire about medications such as diuretics (see Table 7-4) and other antihypertensives, drugs associated with potassium loss (e.g., corticosteroids), and compliance with prescribed potassium supplements if ordered. Ask about usual diet, including use of salt substitutes.

Obtain vital signs including apical pulse and orthostatic vitals, and assess abdomen, including bowel sounds. Test muscle strength and tone, and evaluate mental status. Review serum potassium, electrolyte, and glucose levels and ABG results, as indicated.

IDENTIFYING POTENTIAL COMPLICATIONS

Place patients with significant potassium imbalances on a cardiac monitor. Carefully observe the ECG pattern for changes in waveforms, the T wave in particular, and dysrhythmias. Promptly report changes or abnormal rhythms.

DIAGNOSING, PLANNING, AND IMPLEMENTING

The patient with a potassium imbalance is at risk for injury because of its potential effects on the heart, as well as muscle weakness resulting from the imbalance.

Risk for Injury

Expected outcome: Will avoid adverse effects of potassium imbalance and physical injury.

■ Carefully monitor serum potassium levels in patients at risk for imbalances and notify the charge nurse or physician of abnormal levels (less than 3.5 mEq/L or greater than 5.3 mEq/L). *Early identification of a potassium imbalance allows prompt treatment and reduces the risk for injury from very high or very low potassium levels.*

clinicalALERT

Immediately report critical values (less than 2.5 mEq/L or greater than 6.5 mEq/L). Critical values are associated with a high risk of cardiac dysrhythmias and cardiac arrest.

■ Monitor for manifestations of potassium imbalance, such as muscle weakness, nausea and anorexia, abdominal cramping, or decreased bowel sounds. *Weakness and GI manifestations of potassium imbalance increase the risk for injury from falls or aspiration of vomitus.*

■ Closely monitor patients receiving sodium bicarbonate or sodium polystyrene sulfonate (Kayexalate) for fluid volume excess. *Increased sodium levels can cause water retention.*

■ Closely monitor the ECG of patients receiving calcium gluconate, particularly if the patient also is on digitalis. *Digitalis toxicity may develop when calcium gluconate and digitalis are given concurrently.*

Decreased Cardiac Output

Expected outcome: Vital signs and heart rhythm will remain stable within expected parameters.

■ Monitor vital signs, including apical pulse. Chart and report any irregularities. *Disruptions of heart rhythm are more easily detected by listening to the apical pulse than by palpating peripheral pulses.*

■ Place on a cardiac monitor and observe for changes in heart rhythm or pattern (e.g., prolonged PR interval, ST-segment and T-wave changes, and the presence of U waves). (See Chapter 16 for more explanation of ECG waveforms.) Notify the physician of changes. *A monitor allows early identification of and intervention for life-threatening dysrhythmias.*

■ Monitor patients taking digitalis for signs of digitalis toxicity, such as anorexia, nausea, headache, confusion, and blurred vision. *Hypokalemia increases the risk for digitalis toxicity.*

■ Monitor intravenous potassium infusions closely. Dilute intravenous potassium as recommended and administer using an electronic infusion device. *Administering more than 40 mEq of potassium per hour is not safe.*

■ Promote comfort by slowing the intravenous infusion rate or applying an ice pack to the IV site if necessary. *Potassium may cause local irritation of the vein wall.*

clinical**ALERT**

Do not administer undiluted potassium directly into the vein. Potassium usually is mixed to a concentration of 20 to 40 mEq/L of solution and should not exceed 60 mEq/L. The rate of infusion should not exceed 20 to 40 mEq of potassium per hour. Evaluate the serum potassium level during therapy. In patients requiring rapid potassium replacement, monitor the ECG. Too rapid administration of intravenous potassium may cause cardiac dysrhythmias and death.

EVALUATING

Collect data related to the patient's serum potassium level, safety, and cardiovascular status to evaluate the effectiveness of nursing interventions for patients with potassium imbalances.

DOCUMENTING

Document continuing assessment data, including laboratory test results, and the patient's compliance with and response to treatment. Document teaching provided and the patient's and family's understanding of instructions.

CONTINUITY OF CARE

Discharge planning for patients with potassium imbalances focuses on teaching about prescribed medications (potassium supplements or diuretics), diet, and the importance of regular follow-up assessments. Include the family, a significant other, or a caregiver in teaching as indicated. Provide both written and verbal instructions. Provide a list of salt substitutes and foods high in potassium, with instructions for their use (see Box 7-10). Instruct patients taking supplemental forms of potassium and potassium-sparing diuretics to avoid salt substitutes that contain potassium. Instruct patients with chronic renal failure to avoid foods high in potassium. Discuss measures to make potassium supplements more palatable: Dilute liquid potassium supplements with water or juices, or mix with sherbet or gelatin. Emphasize the importance of regular laboratory tests as ordered by the physician. Teach the patient taking digitalis to count the pulse before taking the medication. Report a rate of less than 60 to the primary health care provider.

When the patient is being discharged to a long-term care or residential care facility, communicate with caregivers about any drugs that affect potassium balance, ordered potassium replacement therapy, any dietary restrictions, and the recommended frequency of follow-up laboratory tests.

NURSING CARE PLAN
Patient With Hypokalemia

Rose Ortiz is a 72-year-old woman who is being treated for mild heart failure with digoxin (Lanoxin) 0.125 mg, hydrochlorothiazide (Oretic) 75 mg orally (PO) daily, and a mildly sodium-restricted diet (2 g daily). For the last several weeks, Ms. Ortiz has been feeling weak and sometimes faint, light-headed, and dizzy. Her physician ordered serum electrolytes drawn, which showed a potassium level of 2.4 mEq/L. Potassium chloride 20 mEq (Klor-ConM20) PO twice daily is prescribed, and the clinic nurse does a nursing assessment before teaching Ms. Ortiz about her care.

Assessment
Ms. Ortiz has adhered to her sodium-restricted diet and has been taking her prescribed medications. She occasionally takes an additional "water pill" when her ankles swell. She says she is reluctant to take the potassium the doctor has ordered because her neighbor says it causes "heartburn." Physical assessment findings include T 98.4, P 70, R 20, and BP 138/84.

Nursing Diagnosis
The following priority nursing diagnosis is identified for Ms. Ortiz:

■ *Risk for Ineffective Health Maintenance* related to lack of knowledge of side effects of diuretic therapy and of foods high in potassium

Expected Outcomes
The expected outcomes specify that Ms. Ortiz will:

■ Have a potassium level within normal limits (3.5 to 5.3 mEq/L).
■ Verbalize understanding of the side effects of diuretic therapy.
■ State measures to avoid gastrointestinal irritation when taking oral potassium.
■ Identify potassium-rich foods.

Planning and Implementation
The following nursing interventions are planned and implemented:

■ Discuss the side effects of diuretic therapy, and explain how taking additional diuretics may have contributed to her hypokalemia.

- Explain the need for the prescribed potassium and its role in reversing her muscle weakness.
- Instruct to take the potassium supplement after breakfast and supper, with a full glass of juice or water. Instruct her to call if gastric irritation occurs.
- Discuss dietary sources of potassium, and provide a list of potassium-rich foods (see Box 7-10).

Evaluation

On a follow-up visit 1 week later, Ms. Ortiz says that her symptoms have been resolved. She is taking her prescribed drugs as directed. She also reports that she has increased her intake of potassium-rich foods. Her potassium level is within normal limits.

Critical Thinking in the Nursing Process

1. What did Ms. Ortiz do that contributed to her hypokalemia?
2. What additional teaching at the time that digitalis and hydrochlorothiazide were prescribed might have prevented Ms. Ortiz from developing hypokalemia? How could the nurse reinforce this teaching?
3. Ms. Ortiz states that she gets "terrible stomach cramps" from eating fresh fruits and vegetables. What suggestions could the nurse provide to increase her potassium intake?

Note: Discussion of Critical Thinking questions appears on the companion website.

Calcium Imbalance

Calcium (Ca^{2+}) is one of the most abundant ions in the body. Most of it is in the bones and teeth; only a small amount is found in the ECF. The normal adult total serum calcium concentration is 4.5 to 5.5 mEq/L or 9 to 11 mg/dL. About half of this extracellular calcium is ionized; the rest is bound to protein, phosphate, or other ions.

Ionized calcium is essential to a number of body processes. It affects neuromuscular irritability, nerve impulse transmission, muscle contraction and relaxation, blood clotting, and hormone secretion. It is vital in maintaining heart rhythm and contraction.

Three hormones interact to regulate serum calcium levels: parathyroid hormone (PTH), calcitriol (a metabolite of vitamin D), and calcitonin. When serum calcium levels fall, the parathyroid glands secrete PTH. PTH mobilizes calcium from the bones, increases calcium absorption in the intestines, and promotes calcium reabsorption by the kidneys (Figure 7-16■). Calcitriol assists these processes.

Calcitonin is secreted by the thyroid gland in response to high serum calcium levels. Calcitonin has the opposite effect of PTH: It inhibits the movement of calcium

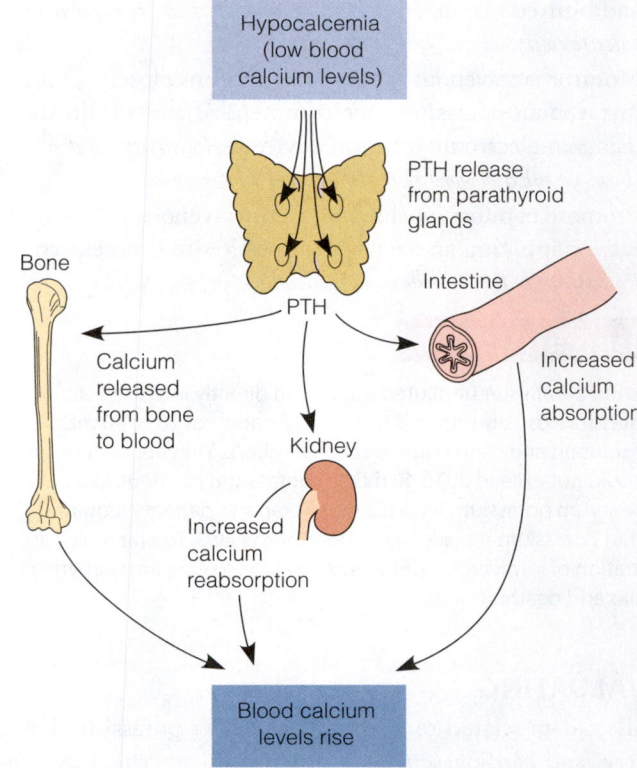

Figure 7-16. ■ Low serum calcium levels stimulate the parathyroid glands to release parathyroid hormone, which increases serum calcium levels by triggering three processes: release of calcium from the bone, calcium absorption in the intestine, and calcium reabsorption in the kidneys.

out of bone, reduces intestinal absorption of calcium, and promotes urinary calcium excretion.

memoryALERT

- PTH and calcitriol → ↑ serum calcium levels
- Calcitonin → ↓ serum calcium levels

HYPOCALCEMIA

Hypocalcemia is serum calcium lower than 9 mg/dL (or 4.5 mEq/L). People at risk for hypocalcemia include those who have undergone bariatric surgery for weight loss, older adults (especially women), and alcoholics. Bariatric surgery increases the risk for hypocalcemia due to reduced food intake and malabsorption. Older adults often consume less milk and milk products (good sources of calcium) and may have less exposure to the sun (a source of vitamin D). They may be less active, leading to loss of calcium from bones. They are more likely to be taking drugs that interfere with calcium absorption or promote calcium excretion (e.g., furosemide). Older women are at particular risk after menopause because of estrogen deficiency. Alcohol consumption reduces intestinal absorption of calcium and interferes with other processes that help maintain serum calcium levels.

Hypocalcemia can result from decreased total body calcium or low levels of calcium in ECF with normal amounts of calcium stored in bone. Many disorders can cause hypocalcemia (Table 7-10■). *Hypoparathyroidism*, usually due to surgical removal of the parathyroid glands, is the most common cause. Hypoparathyroidism also may result from total thyroidectomy or radical neck surgery (see Chapter 35). Hypocalcemia is common in patients with acute pancreatitis (see Chapter 27), often accompanies hypomagnesemia, and is common in malnourished alcoholics.

The manifestations of hypocalcemia are caused by insufficient ionized calcium in ECF. Calcium has a sedative effect on neuromuscular transmission. When calcium levels are low, neuromuscular excitability increases. **Tetany** (a group of symptoms caused by this increased excitability) is the most characteristic and serious consequence of hypocalcemia. Manifestations of tetany are *paresthesias* (numbness and tingling around the mouth and in the hands and feet) and muscle spasms. Chvostek sign (facial muscle spasm when the facial nerve is tapped in front of the ear) and Trousseau sign (carpal spasm that occurs when blood flow to the lower arm is restricted) also may be present (Figure 7-17■). Other manifestations are listed in Table 7-10. Critically low values, less than 6 mg/dL, may lead to respiratory or cardiac arrest or convulsions.

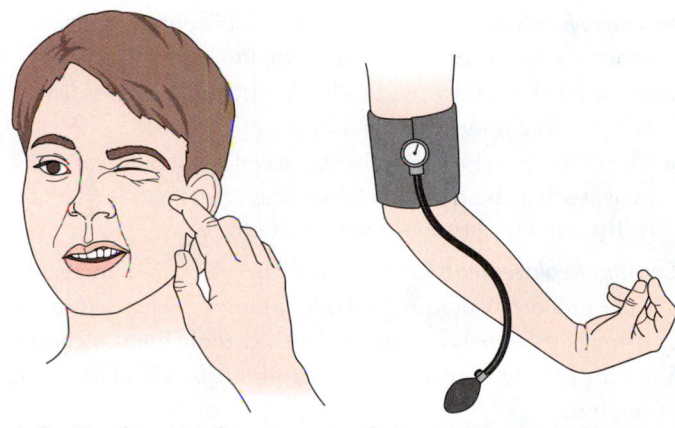

A Positive Chvostek Sign   **B** Positive Trousseau Sign

Figure 7-17. ■ **(A)** Positive Chvostek sign and **(B)** positive Trousseau sign.

Collaborative Care

Diagnostic Tests The following diagnostic tests may be performed to evaluate calcium levels and possible causes of calcium imbalance:

■ The *total serum calcium* will be less than 9 mg/dL (less than 4.5 mEq/L), and ionized calcium (the active form) generally is about 50% of that.

■ *Serum magnesium* is measured because hypocalcemia is often associated with hypomagnesemia.

TABLE 7-10	Calcium Imbalances	
IMBALANCE	**CAUSES**	**MANIFESTATIONS**
Hypocalcemia ■ Serum calcium less than 9 mg/dL (less than 4.5 mEq/L) ■ Critical value: less than 6 mg/dL	■ Parathyroidectomy or neck surgery ■ Bariatric surgery ■ Acute pancreatitis ■ Inadequate dietary intake ■ Lack of sun exposure (vitamin D) ■ Lack of weight-bearing exercise ■ Drugs: loop diuretics (e.g., furosemide), calcitonin ■ Hypomagnesemia (alcohol abuse, some chemotherapy)	■ Numbness and tingling ■ Tetany: paresthesias, muscle spasms, laryngospasm, seizures ■ Positive Chvostek and Trousseau signs ■ Anxiety and confusion ■ ↓ BP ■ Dysrhythmias ■ Abdominal cramping ■ Diarrhea
Hypercalcemia ■ Serum calcium greater than 11 mg/dL (greater than 5.5 mEq/L) ■ Critical value: greater than 13 mg/dL	■ Hyperparathyroidism ■ Some cancers (lung, breast, multiple myeloma) ■ Prolonged immobilization ■ Paget's disease ■ Excess milk or antacid intake ■ Kidney failure	■ Muscle weakness ■ ↓ Deep tendon reflexes ■ Confusion, impaired memory, behavior changes ■ Dysrhythmias ■ ↑ BP ■ ↑ Urine output, thirst ■ Constipation ■ Anorexia, nausea, vomiting

- *Serum phosphate* is measured because phosphate levels generally rise as calcium levels fall and vice versa.
- *Serum PTH* is measured to identify hypoparathyroidism as a possible underlying cause.
- The *ECG* shows changes in the waveforms and dysrhythmias, such as bradycardia (slow heart rate) or ventricular tachycardia (a very rapid ventricular rate).

Calcium Replacement Oral calcium preparations, increased dietary intake of calcium, and oral vitamin D are used to increase calcium levels in patients with chronic hypocalcemia. Vitamin D may be given as well to increase GI absorption of calcium.

In acute hypocalcemia, intravenous calcium (calcium chloride, calcium gluconate, or calcium glucceptate) is given to prevent or treat tetany. Calcium may be given by slow IV push or by infusion. It is given with caution to patients taking digitalis, because it increases the risk of digitalis toxicity. (See Table 7-11■.)

HYPERCALCEMIA

Hypercalcemia (serum calcium greater than 11.0 mg/dL) usually results from increased calcium release (*resorption*) from the bones. Increased calcium intake and decreased renal excretion of calcium are other causes.

Increased resorption of calcium from the bones may result from *hyperparathyroidism* and excess PTH secretion, prolonged immobilization, or certain malignancies (such as lung and breast cancers and multiple myeloma). Excess PTH also impairs renal excretion of calcium, as does

kidney failure. Other causes of hypercalcemia are listed in Table 7-10.

The effects of hypercalcemia largely depend on the extent and rapidity of calcium level increase. The primary effects are neuromuscular. Calcium has a sedative effect on neuromuscular transmission, which affects skeletal, smooth, and cardiac muscle. Excess calcium in cerebrospinal fluid affects behavior, and excess calcium in the urine can lead to kidney stones. Review Table 7-10 for the manifestations of hypercalcemia.

memory**ALERT**

Remember, calcium has a sedative effect on neuromuscular transmission. Therefore:

- Hypocalcemia → *Increased* neuromuscular excitability, muscle twitching, spasms, and possible tetany
- Hypercalcemia → *Decreased* neuromuscular excitability, muscle weakness, and fatigue

Hypercalcemia can lead to complications such as peptic ulcer disease and pancreatitis. Critically high serum calcium levels, greater than 13 mg/dL, may cause complete heart block and cardiac arrest.

Collaborative Care

Diagnostic Tests

- Hypercalcemia is diagnosed by measuring *serum calcium levels*.

TABLE 7-11	Giving Medications Safely: Calcium Preparations		
CLASS/DRUGS	**ACTION/USES**	**NURSING IMPLICATIONS**	**PATIENT TEACHING (*FOR ALL DRUG GROUPS*)**
Oral calcium ■ Calcium carbonate (BioCal, Calsam, Caltrate, OsCal, Tums) ■ Calcium gluconate ■ Calcium lactate	Oral calcium preparations are used to increase calcium levels in the body.	Administer oral calcium 1–1.5 hours after meals. Calcium absorption is improved by concurrent administration of vitamin D.	A daily intake of 1,000–1,200 mg of calcium is recommended for adults. Older adults should consume 1,200 mg/day. Milk and milk products are a good source of calcium.
Intravenous calcium ■ Calcium gluconate ■ Calcium chloride	Intravenous calcium is used to treat acute hypocalcemia. It also may be ordered postoperatively for patients who have had neck surgery such as parathyroidectomy, thyroidectomy, or radical neck surgery.	Administer into a central line or large peripheral vein. Dilute calcium solutions with normal saline or administer by infusion to reduce irritation of the vein. Monitor IV site closely; stop the infusion if infiltration occurs. Closely monitor ECG and serum calcium levels.	If you have a history of kidney stones, talk to your doctor before taking calcium supplements. Smoking and alcohol consumption interfere with calcium absorption. Regular weight-bearing exercise (walking, bicycling, weight training) helps maintain calcium in the bone and can help prevent osteoporosis.

■ *Serum PTH* is measured to identify possible hyperpara-thyroidism. Levels are increased in hyperparathyroidism but may be low in other cases of hypercalcemia.

■ An *ECG* is done to identify changes in impulse trans-mission and rhythm related to hypercalcemia.

Medications In acute hypercalcemia, intravenous normal saline solution (0.9% NaCl) is given to restore fluid volume and dilute plasma calcium. Diuretics such as furosemide (Lasix) may be given to promote calcium excretion by the kidneys.

When hypercalcemia is due to excess bone resorption, *bisphosphonates* may be used. This group of drugs, includ-ing *alendronate* (Fosamax), ibandronate (Boniva), risedro-nate (Actonel), and related drugs inhibit bone resorption and can reduce serum calcium levels with few side effects. Phosphates may be prescribed to inhibit bone resorption and reduce intestinal absorption of calcium. Other drugs used to treat hypercalcemia include calcitonin or intrave-nous plicamycin (Mithracin) to inhibit bone resorption and glucocorticoids to decrease GI absorption of calcium and increase its excretion.

NURSING CARE

PRIORITIZING NURSING CARE

The mental and neuromuscular effects of calcium imbal-ances place the patient at significant risk for injury due to falls, airway impairment, dysrhythmias, or seizures. Ensur-ing patient safety is a nursing care priority.

HEALTH PROMOTION

Health promotion activities related to calcium balance include teaching to promote bone health: discussing the importance of maintaining adequate calcium intake, including calcium supplements as indicated; encouraging all patients to obtain at least 15 minutes of daily exposure to sunlight; and teach-ing about the relationship between weight-bearing activities (walking, running, weight training) and maintaining bone calcium. Incorporate early and continued ambulation into nursing care plans whenever possible.

ASSESSING

Patients who have or are at risk for calcium imbalance are assessed for the following:

■ Heart rate and rhythm
■ Respiratory rate and effort; laryngeal *stridor* (a high-pitched, harsh sound heard during inspiration)
■ Mental status and neuromuscular function
■ Manifestations of tetany (tingling around the mouth and fingers, muscle twitching or cramps, hyperactive reflexes)
■ Serum calcium, magnesium, phosphate, and albumin levels

IDENTIFYING POTENTIAL COMPLICATIONS

Manifestations such as respiratory distress, muscle twitch-ing, flaccid and weak muscles, changes in mental status or alertness, or irregular heart rhythms may indicate critical blood calcium levels and should be immediately reported. Patients on long-term activity restrictions or bed rest may develop kidney stones due to shifts of calcium out of bones. Symptoms such as flank pain or *hematuria* (blood in the urine) may indicate kidney stones and should be reported to the registered nurse or physician.

DIAGNOSING, PLANNING, AND IMPLEMENTING

Risk for Injury

Expected outcome: Will remain free of adverse effects of electrolyte imbalance.

■ Institute safety precautions for patients who have mental changes resulting from hypercalcemia. *Changes in mental status may impair the patient's judgment and ability to main-tain his or her own safety.*

clinicalALERT

Frequently monitor airway and respiratory status. Report any changes, such as respiratory stridor or increased respiratory rate and effort. These may indicate laryngeal spasm, a respiratory emergency that requires immediate intervention to maintain ade-quate ventilation of the lungs.

■ Monitor cardiovascular status, including heart rate and rhythm and BP. *Calcium imbalances can affect heart contrac-tility, leading to decreased cardiac output, dysrhythmias, and hypotension.*

■ Place patients receiving intravenous calcium replace-ment on a cardiac monitor. *Patients receiving intravenous calcium may develop dysrhythmias.*

■ Provide a quiet environment. Institute seizure precautions: Raise padded side rails and keep an airway at the bedside. *A quiet environment reduces central nervous system stimuli. The patient with tetany is at risk for developing seizures.*

■ If excess bone resorption has occurred, use caution when turning, transferring, or ambulating the patient. *Bone may fracture more easily if excess calcium has been lost.*

■ Ambulate patients as soon as allowed and encourage weight-bearing activity. *These measures help move calcium into bone, lowering serum calcium levels and reducing the risk of fracture.*

■ Promote fluid intake to keep the patient well hydrated and maintain dilute urine. Encourage fluids such as prune or cranberry juice. *The patient is at risk for devel-oping calcium kidney stones. These juices help maintain acid urine, which inhibits calcium stone formation.*

■ Keep emergency resuscitation equipment available. *Cardiac arrest may occur with extremely high serum calcium levels.*

MANAGING NURSING CARE

Instruct assistive personnel to promptly report changes in patient behavior and symptoms of muscle weakness or tremor in the patient at risk for calcium imbalances.

EVALUATING

In addition to monitoring serum calcium levels, collect assessment data such as mental status, muscle strength, deep tendon reflexes, and cardiovascular status to evaluate the effectiveness of interventions for patients with calcium imbalances. Monitor laboratory results to evaluate the effectiveness of interdisciplinary interventions.

DOCUMENTING

Document continuing assessment data, as well as nursing and medical interventions implemented to restore calcium balance. Document the patient's understanding of the condition, teaching provided, and compliance with treatment measures.

CONTINUITY OF CARE

Assess risk factors for future episodes of calcium imbalance, such as poor dietary intake, cigarette smoking, alcohol consumption, lack of exposure to sunlight, and lack of weight-bearing exercise. Evaluate the patient's knowledge and understanding of measures to prevent calcium imbalances. Discuss dietary sources of calcium and vitamin D; provide a list of foods that are high in calcium (Box 7-11 ■).

Encourage taking prescribed oral calcium and vitamin D replacements as directed; caution to avoid excess doses of vitamin D supplements. Advise the patient to increase fluid intake to at least 2,000 to 3,000 mL/day. Instruct patients who are at high risk for kidney stones to increase their fluid intake. Discuss the relationship between weight-bearing activities and maintaining bone calcium. Help the patient identify activities that fit with his or her lifestyle. Finally, instruct the patient to increase dietary fiber and fluid to maintain normal bowel function and avoid constipation.

BOX 7-11 **FOODS HIGH IN CALCIUM**

■ Milk and milk products
■ Canned salmon and sardines
■ Rhubarb
■ Broccoli, collard greens, spinach
■ Soy flour, tofu

For patients being discharged to long-term care or residential care facilities, communicate the patient's increased risk for calcium imbalance with caregivers. Discuss measures implemented and recommended to maintain bone health and calcium balance and to prevent kidney stones.

Magnesium Imbalance

Only about 1% of the magnesium (Mg^{2+}) in the body is in ECF; the rest is in bone and the cells. The normal serum magnesium is 1.5 to 2.5 mEq/L or 1.8 to 3.0 mg/dL. Magnesium affects neuromuscular irritability and contractility. Excess magnesium depresses skeletal muscle contraction and central nervous system activity, whereas a deficit causes increased neuromuscular irritability, cardiac dysrhythmias, and peripheral vasodilation. Serum magnesium values less than 1 mg/dL or higher than 4.7 mg/dL are considered to be critical.

Magnesium enters the body in the foods we eat. It is abundant in green vegetables, grains, nuts, meats, and seafood. The kidneys regulate extracellular magnesium levels by conserving or excreting it as needed.

HYPOMAGNESEMIA

Hypomagnesemia (serum magnesium less than 1.5 mEq/L or 1.8 mg/dL) is usually due to a total body deficit of magnesium. In fact, body stores of magnesium may be depleted even when the serum magnesium level is within normal limits. Chronic alcoholism is one of the most common causes of hypomagnesemia (Table 7-12 ■). Low serum potassium and calcium levels usually accompany hypomagnesemia, contributing to its effects.

Manifestations of hypomagnesemia, which usually do not occur until the serum level drops below 1 mEq/L, include increased neuromuscular excitability with muscle weakness and tremors. Electrical conduction in the heart is affected, as is central nervous system function. The manifestations of hypomagnesemia are also listed in Table 7-12.

HYPERMAGNESEMIA

Hypermagnesemia (serum magnesium level greater than 2.5 mEq/L or 3.0 mg/dL) can occur in patients with kidney disease. Older adults who use magnesium-containing antacids or laxatives are at risk as kidney function declines with aging. Hypermagnesemia also may develop when magnesium solutions are given to treat complications of pregnancy.

Elevated magnesium levels interfere with neuromuscular transmission and depress the central nervous system. Hypermagnesemia also affects the cardiovascular system and respiratory function. With mild hypermagnesemia, nausea and vomiting, hypotension, facial flushing, sweating, and a feeling of warmth occur. Table 7-12 summarizes the manifestations of hypermagnesemia.

TABLE 7-12	Magnesium Imbalances	
IMBALANCE	**CAUSES**	**MANIFESTATIONS**
Hypomagnesemia ■ Serum magnesium less than 1.8 mg/dL (1.5 mEq/L) ■ Critical value: less than 1 mg/dL	■ Chronic alcoholism ■ GI losses (intestinal suction, vomiting and diarrhea, ileostomy) ■ Impaired intestinal absorption ■ Increased excretion: drugs (loop diuretics, aminoglycoside antibiotics), kidney disease	*(Generally seen with serum levels less than 1 mEq/L)* ■ Muscle weakness, tremors ■ Positive Chvostek and Trousseau signs ■ Personality changes, possible seizures ■ ↑ BP, tachycardia ■ ECG changes, dysrhythmias
Hypermagnesemia ■ Serum magnesium greater than 3.0 mg/dL (2.5 mEq/L) ■ Critical value: greater than 4.7 mg/dL	■ Kidney disease or failure ■ Excess intake of antacids, laxatives ■ Excess magnesium administration	■ Muscle weakness, decreased reflexes ■ Confusion and lethargy ■ Flushing, sweating, feeling of warmth ■ ↓ BP, bradycardia ■ Cardiac arrest ■ Respiratory depression, paralysis ■ Coma

COLLABORATIVE CARE

Identifying patients at risk for magnesium imbalances and treatments that increase this risk can prevent the adverse effects of imbalance.

In patients who are able to eat, a mild deficiency may be corrected by increasing the intake of magnesium-rich foods (Box 7-12 ■) or by using oral magnesium supplements (e.g., magnesium-containing antacids). The use of these supplements is limited by their tendency to cause diarrhea.

Magnesium also can be given intravenously or by deep intramuscular injection. Serum magnesium levels and deep tendon reflexes are monitored frequently during treatment. Depressed deep tendon reflexes indicate high serum magnesium levels and a need to stop treatment.

Hypermagnesemia is treated by withholding all medications and solutions that contain magnesium. In patients with kidney failure, excess magnesium is removed by dialysis treatments (see Chapter 36). When magnesium levels are extremely high, intravenous calcium is given to protect heart function. Some patients may require mechanical ventilation to maintain respirations.

NURSING CARE

Nursing interventions for patients with magnesium imbalances focus on carefully monitoring individuals at risk, assessing signs and symptoms, implementing safety measures, teaching the patient and family, and administering prescribed medications.

Monitor patients at risk for magnesium imbalances for:

■ Serum magnesium and other electrolyte levels.
■ Manifestations such as muscle twitching, tremors, grimaces, paresthesias, leg cramps, and hyperactive reflexes.
■ Changes in GI function, such as nausea, vomiting, anorexia, diarrhea, and abdominal distention.
■ Changes in BP or heart rate or rhythm. In patients receiving digitalis, monitor for digitalis toxicity.

Closely monitor serum magnesium levels and deep tendon reflexes in patients receiving intravenous magnesium solutions. Refer to the section on calcium imbalances for measures to reduce the risk of injury related to increased neuromuscular excitability.

CONTINUITY OF CARE

Teach patients about foods that are high in magnesium (see Box 7-12) and provide information about magnesium supplements. Teach patients who have high magnesium levels to avoid magnesium-containing medications, such as

BOX 7-12	FOODS HIGH IN MAGNESIUM

■ Green, leafy vegetables
■ Legumes
■ Whole grains
■ Bananas, oranges, grapefruit
■ Dairy products
■ Meat
■ Seafood

antacids, mineral supplements, and laxatives. Refer patients for whom alcohol abuse is a problem to a treatment program. Discuss support systems for alcoholics such as Alcoholics Anonymous, Al-Anon, and/or Al-a-Teen.

Phosphorus Imbalance

The normal serum phosphorus level in adults is 2.5 to 4.5 mg/dL (1.7 to 2.6 mEq/L). Phosphorus is found in all body tissues, but most of it is in body cells or combined with calcium in bones and teeth. Although only about 1% of phosphorus is in ECF, it is essential for normal neuromuscular activity. Phosphate, the ionized form of phosphorus, is responsible for its physiologic effects. Phosphate is abundant in many foods, including meat, fish, poultry, eggs, milk products, and legumes. The kidneys regulate serum phosphorus levels, excreting excess phosphorus or retaining it if phosphate intake is low. An inverse relationship exists between phosphorus and calcium levels: When one increases, the other decreases. Thus regulatory mechanisms that maintain calcium levels in the body also affect phosphorus levels.

Hypophosphatemia (serum phosphorus less than 2.5 mg/dL) may indicate a phosphorus deficit, or it may occur when phosphate shifts from ECF into the cells. Decreased phosphate absorption in the GI tract or increased phosphate excretion by the kidneys can lead to a deficit.

Hypophosphatemia also may occur as an effect of certain medications (Table 7-13■). Alcoholism can cause severe hypophosphatemia.

The manifestations of hypophosphatemia are caused by a lack of intracellular phosphate. Cellular energy resources for vital processes are depleted. The ability of red blood cells to transport oxygen is affected, resulting in tissue hypoxia.

Hyperphosphatemia (serum phosphate greater than 4.5 mg/dL) usually results from kidney failure and impaired phosphorus excretion. It also may be caused by increased phosphate intake or when phosphate is released from damaged cells (see Table 7-13).

When serum phosphate levels are high, the excess phosphate combines with calcium. The primary manifestations of hyperphosphatemia relate to the resulting hypocalcemia rather than to high phosphate levels themselves.

COLLABORATIVE CARE

Care focuses on preventing a phosphate imbalance in patients at risk and treating any underlying disorder causing the imbalance.

For mild hypophosphatemia, improved intake may be enough. Unless contraindicated, milk may be recommended because it supplies phosphate, calcium, and potassium. Oral phosphorus supplements may be prescribed, but

TABLE 7-13	Phosphorus Imbalances	
IMBALANCE	**CAUSES**	**MANIFESTATIONS**
Hypophosphatemia ■ Serum phosphorus less than 2.5 mg/dL ■ Critical value: less than 1 mg/dL	■ Decreased GI absorption or increased renal excretion ■ Shift from ECF into cells ■ Alcoholism ■ Iatrogenic causes: 　■ IV glucose administration 　■ Total parenteral nutrition without phosphorus 　■ Aluminum- or magnesium-based antacids 　■ Insulin administration 　■ Diuretic therapy	■ Tremor, paresthesias ■ Irritability, confusion ■ Impaired coordination ■ Seizures, coma ■ Bone and joint pain ■ Anemia, ↑ risk of infection, bleeding ■ ↓ BP, tachycardia
Hyperphosphatemia ■ Serum phosphate greater than 4.5 mg/dL	■ Kidney failure ■ Increased phosphate intake or absorption ■ Chemotherapy ■ Muscle tissue trauma ■ Sepsis ■ Severe hypothermia ■ Heat stroke	■ Circumoral and peripheral numbness and tingling ■ Muscle spasms ■ Tetany ■ Nausea and vomiting

common adverse effects (nausea and diarrhea) may limit their effectiveness. For severe hypophosphatemia, intravenous phosphate solutions may be ordered.

For hyperphosphatemia, agents such as aluminum hydroxide (Amphojel) that bind with phosphate may be used to lower serum phosphate levels. Dialysis may be used to remove excess phosphate. In patients with adequate kidney function, intravenous normal saline may promote phosphate excretion. In severe hyperphosphatemia, glucose and insulin may be given to drive phosphate into the cells, lowering the serum phosphate level.

NURSING CARE

Identifying patients at risk for phosphate imbalances is an important nursing responsibility. Monitor serum phosphorus levels in malnourished patients, alcoholics, patients with kidney failure, and patients being treated for diabetic ketoacidosis. Assess for and report manifestations of phosphate imbalance (paresthesias, muscle weakness and pain, or changes in mental status). Protect patients with severe hypophosphatemia from infection. Administer intravenous phosphate solutions carefully, observing for signs of hyperphosphatemia or other electrolyte imbalances (particularly potassium and calcium).

Teach at-risk patients and their families how to prevent and recognize manifestations of phosphate imbalance. Discuss the effects of phosphorus-binding antacids and phosphate-containing laxatives and enemas. Provide information about appropriate alternatives to these products and directions for their use. Teach patients that a well-balanced diet provides adequate phosphate. Milk and milk products, meats, and legumes (e.g., dried beans) are particularly rich in phosphate. Stress the importance of good nutrition, particularly with patients for whom alcohol is a problem. Provide information about alcohol treatment programs such as Alcoholics Anonymous. Instruct patients to mix powdered oral phosphorus supplements with very cold water or juice to make them more palatable.

ACID–BASE DISORDERS

Key Concept   Acid–base disorders usually occur due to disrupted metabolic processes or impaired respiratory or kidney function. The nurse provides teaching to prevent imbalances, monitors the effects of treatment, and provides care to reduce the risk of harm associated with these disorders.

For optimal cell function, the concentration of hydrogen ions (H^+) in body fluids must remain relatively constant. Hydrogen ions determine the relative acidity of body fluids. Acids release hydrogen ions in solution; bases (or alkalis) accept hydrogen ions in solution. The hydrogen ion concentration of a solution is measured as its **pH**, from 0 to 14, with 7 being neutral. The relationship between hydrogen ion concentration and pH is inverse; that is, as hydrogen ion concentration increases, the pH falls, and the solution becomes more acidic. As hydrogen ion concentration falls, the pH rises, and the solution becomes more alkaline or basic. The normal pH of body fluids is slightly basic, ranging from 7.35 to 7.45.

Acid–Base Regulation

Acids are continually produced by metabolic processes in the body. Carbonic acid (H_2CO_3) is an acid that dissociates into carbon dioxide (CO_2) and water (H_2O). The carbon dioxide is eliminated from the body through the lungs. All other acids produced in the body (e.g., lactic acid, hydrochloric acid, phosphoric acid, and sulfuric acid) must be metabolized or excreted from the body in fluid. Most acids and bases in the body are weak (close to a pH of 7).

Three systems work together in the body to maintain a normal pH despite continuous production of acid waste products: buffers, the respiratory system, and the kidneys.

BUFFER SYSTEMS
Buffers prevent major changes in pH by attaching to or releasing hydrogen ion. When body fluid becomes excessively acid, buffers bind with hydrogen ions to minimize the change in pH. If body fluids become too basic or alkaline, buffers release hydrogen ion, restoring the pH. Although buffers act within a fraction of a second, their capacity to maintain pH is limited. The major buffer systems of the body are the bicarbonate–carbonic acid buffer system, phosphate buffer system, and protein buffers.

Bicarbonate is a weak base; when an acid is added to the system, it combines with bicarbonate, and the pH changes only slightly. Carbonic acid is a weak acid produced when carbon dioxide dissolves in water. If a base is added to the system, it combines with carbonic acid, and the pH remains within the normal range. The normal serum bicarbonate level is 24 mEq/L, and that of carbonic acid is 1.2 mEq/L. Thus the ratio of bicarbonate to carbonic acid is 20:1. As long as this ratio is maintained, the pH remains within the 7.35 to 7.45 range (Figure 7-18■). When a strong acid is

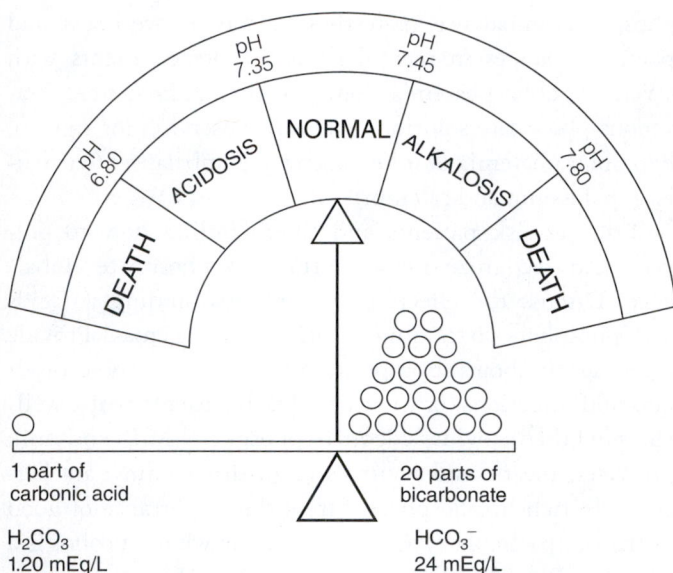

H₂CO₃
1.20 mEq/L
HCO₃⁻
24 mEq/L

Figure 7-18. ■ As long as the ratio of bicarbonate to carbonic acid is 20:1, the pH remains within the normal range of 7.35 to 7.45.

added to ECF, bicarbonate is depleted, changing the 20:1 ratio. The pH then drops below 7.35. If a strong base is added, carbonic acid is depleted, the 20:1 ratio is altered, and the pH rises above 7.45.

Inorganic phosphates and plasma proteins serve a lesser role as buffers in ECF, although they are important intracellular buffers. Within red blood cells, hemoglobin also acts as a buffer.

RESPIRATORY SYSTEM

The respiratory system (including the respiratory center of the brain) regulates carbonic acid in the body by eliminating or retaining carbon dioxide. Carbon dioxide is a potential acid; when combined with water, it forms carbonic acid. Acute increases in either carbon dioxide or hydrogen ions in the blood stimulate the respiratory center in the brain to increase the rate and depth of respirations. This eliminates carbon dioxide from the body; carbonic acid levels fall, bringing the pH to a more normal range. This compensation for increased hydrogen ion concentration

occurs within minutes. It becomes less effective over time, however. Patients with chronic lung disease may have consistently high carbon dioxide levels in their blood.

Alkalosis, by contrast, depresses the respiratory center. The rate and depth of respirations decrease, and carbon dioxide is retained. The retained carbon dioxide then combines with water to restore carbonic acid levels and bring the pH back within the normal range.

KIDNEYS

The kidneys respond more slowly to changes in pH (within hours to days). They are responsible for the long-term regulation of acid–base balance in the body. The kidneys regulate bicarbonate levels in ECF and can either excrete or retain hydrogen ion as needed. When excess hydrogen ions are present and the pH falls, the kidneys excrete hydrogen ions and retain bicarbonate. When bicarbonate levels are high, the kidneys retain hydrogen ion and excrete bicarbonate to restore acid–base balance.

ASSESSMENT OF ACID–BASE BALANCE

Acid–base balance is evaluated by measuring *arterial blood gases* (*ABGs*). The elements measured are the PaCO₂, the PaO₂, bicarbonate, and pH. Normal ABG values are listed in Table 7-14■. Arterial blood is used because it reflects acid–base balance throughout the entire body and allows evaluation of oxygenation.

safety**ALERT**

In contrast to veins, arteries are high-pressure vessels. ABGs are drawn by a registered nurse, respiratory therapist, or laboratory technician who has had specialized training. After the sample has been drawn, apply firm pressure to the puncture site for at least 5 minutes to prevent bleeding into the surrounding tissues.

The *PaCO₂* measures the amount of dissolved carbon dioxide in the blood. The PaCO₂ is regulated by the lungs. The normal value is 35 to 45 mm Hg. A PaCO₂ of less than 35 mm Hg is known as *hypocapnia*; a PaCO₂ greater than 45 mm Hg is *hypercapnia*.

TABLE 7-14	Normal Arterial Blood Gas Values		
COMPONENT	**NORMAL VALUE**	**SIGNIFICANCE**	**CRITICAL VALUES**
pH	7.35–7.45	Relative acidity or alkalinity of the blood; hydrogen ion concentration	Less than 7.20 or greater than 7.60
PaCO₂	35–45 mm Hg	Amount of carbon dioxide dissolved in the blood	Less than 20 or greater than 70 mm Hg
PaO₂	75–100 mm Hg	Amount of oxygen dissolved in the blood	Less than 40 mm Hg
SaO₂	Greater than 95%	Percentage of hemoglobin combined with oxygen	
HCO₃⁻	24–28 mEq/L	Bicarbonate concentration in the blood	
Base excess (BE)	−2.0 to +2.0 mEq/L	Buffering capacity of the blood	

The abbreviations $PaCO_2$ and PaO_2 often are used interchangeably with PCO_2 and PO_2. The "P" stands for partial pressure: the pressure exerted by the gas dissolved in the blood. The "a" indicates that the sample is arterial blood. Because these measurements rarely are done on venous blood, the "a" often is deleted from the abbreviation.

The PaO_2 measures the amount of oxygen dissolved in the plasma. Only about 3% of oxygen in the blood is in solution; most oxygen is carried by hemoglobin, as measured by the SaO_2, the percentage of hemoglobin combined with oxygen. Together, the PaO_2 and the SaO_2 indicate the oxygen content of the blood. The dissolved oxygen (as indicated by the PaO_2) is available to the cells for metabolism. As dissolved oxygen diffuses out of plasma into the tissues, more is released from hemoglobin. The normal PaO_2 is 75 to 100 mm Hg; the normal SaO_2 reading is greater than 95%. A PaO_2 of less than 75 mm Hg

indicates **hypoxemia**. The PaO_2 level and SaO_2 are valuable for evaluating respiratory function, but are not used as primary measurements in determining acid–base status.

The serum bicarbonate (HCO_3^-) reflects the kidneys' regulation of acid–base balance. It often is referred to as the *metabolic component* of ABGs. The normal HCO_3^- is 24 to 28 mEq/L.

The *base excess (BE)* also may be reported on ABGs. It reflects the degree of acid–base imbalance; it represents the amount of acid or base that must be added to a blood sample to achieve a pH of 7.4. The normal base excess is -2.0 to $+2.0$.

ABGs are analyzed to identify acid–base disorders and their probable cause, determine the extent of the imbalance, and monitor treatment. When analyzing ABG results, it is important to use a systematic approach (see Box 7-13 ■). First, evaluate each individual measurement and then look at relationships among the values to determine the patient's acid–base status.

BOX 7-13   **NURSING CARE CHECKLIST**

Interpreting Arterial Blood Gases

1. Look at the pH.
   - ☑ pH less than 7.35 = acidosis.
   - ☑ pH greater than 7.45 = alkalosis.
2. Look at the $PaCO_2$.
   - ☑ $PaCO_2$ less than 35 mm Hg = hypocapnia; more carbon dioxide is being exhaled than normal.
   - ☑ $PaCO_2$ greater than 45 mm Hg = hypercapnia; carbon dioxide is being retained.
3. Evaluate the pH–$PaCO_2$ relationship for a possible respiratory problem.
   - ☑ If the pH is less than 7.35 (acidosis) and the $PaCO_2$ is greater than 45 mm Hg (hypercapnia), retained carbon dioxide is causing *respiratory acidosis*.
   - ☑ If the pH is greater than 7.45 (alkalosis) and the $PaCO_2$ is less than 35 mm Hg (hypocapnia), low carbon dioxide levels are causing *respiratory alkalosis*.
4. Look at the bicarbonate.
   - ☑ If the HCO_3^- is less than 24 mEq/L, bicarbonate levels are lower than normal.
   - ☑ If the HCO_3^- is greater than 28 mEq/L, bicarbonate levels are higher than normal.
5. Evaluate the pH, HCO_3^-, and BE for a possible metabolic problem.
   - ☑ If the pH is less than 7.35 (acidosis), the HCO_3^- is less than 24 mEq/L, and the BE is less than -2 mEq/L, low bicarbonate levels are causing *metabolic acidosis*.

- ☑ If the pH is greater than 7.45 (alkalosis), the HCO_3^- is greater than 28 mEq/L, and the BE is greater than $+2$ mEq/L, high bicarbonate levels are causing *metabolic alkalosis*.

IMBALANCE	pH	$PaCO_2$	HCO_3	BE
Metabolic acidosis	↓	Normal	↓	↓
Metabolic alkalosis	↑	Normal	↑	↑
Respiratory acidosis	↓	↑	Normal	Normal
Respiratory alkalosis	↑	↓	Normal	Normal

6. Look for compensation.
   - ■ *Renal compensation:*
     - ☑ In respiratory acidosis (pH less than 7.35, $PaCO_2$ greater than 45 mm Hg), the kidneys retain HCO_3^- to buffer the excess acid, so the HCO_3^- is greater than 28 mEq/L.
     - ☑ In respiratory alkalosis (pH greater than 7.45, $PaCO_2$ less than 35 mm Hg), the kidneys excrete HCO_3^- to minimize the alkalosis, so the HCO_3^- is less than 24 mEq/L.
   - ■ *Respiratory compensation:*
     - ☑ In metabolic acidosis (pH less than 7.35, HCO_3^- less than 24 mEq/L), the rate and depth of respirations increase, increasing carbon dioxide elimination, so the $PaCO_2$ is less than 35 mm Hg.
     - ☑ In metabolic alkalosis (pH greater than 7.45, HCO_3^- greater than 28 mEq/L), respirations slow, and carbon dioxide is retained, so the $PaCO_2$ is greater than 45 mm Hg.

Acid–Base Imbalances

Acid–base imbalances fall into two major categories: *acidosis* and *alkalosis*. **Acidosis** occurs when the hydrogen ion (H^+) concentration increases above normal and the pH falls below 7.35. **Alkalosis** occurs when the hydrogen ion concentration decreases below normal and the pH rises above 7.45.

memory**ALERT**

- $\uparrow H^+$ concentration = $\downarrow$ pH = acidosis
- $\downarrow H^+$ concentration = $\uparrow$ pH = alkalosis

Acid–base imbalances are further classified as *metabolic* or *respiratory* disorders. In *metabolic disorders*, the primary change is in bicarbonate concentration. In *metabolic acidosis*, the amount of bicarbonate is decreased in relation to the amount of acid in the body (Figure 7-19A ■). *Metabolic alkalosis*, by contrast, occurs when there is an excess of bicarbonate (Figure 7-19B). In *respiratory disorders*, the primary change is in carbon dioxide elimination and the concentration of carbonic acid. *Respiratory acidosis* occurs when carbon dioxide is retained, increasing the amount of carbonic acid in the body (Figure 7-19C). When too much carbon dioxide is "blown off," carbonic acid levels fall, and *respiratory alkalosis* develops (Figure 7-19D).

Acid–base disorders are further classified as primary (simple) and mixed. *Primary* or *simple disorders* usually are due to one cause. For example, respiratory failure often causes respiratory acidosis; kidney failure usually causes metabolic acidosis. With primary disorders, the amount of change in pH may be minimized by *compensatory* responses by the acid–base regulatory system. The kidneys compensate for simple respiratory imbalances by altering bicarbonate production and hydrogen ion excretion; the lungs compensate for simple metabolic imbalances by changing the rate and depth of respirations. *Mixed disorders* occur when both metabolic and respiratory imbalances are present. For example, a patient in cardiac arrest develops a mixed respiratory and metabolic acidosis due to respiratory arrest and hypoxia of body tissues that affects normal cell metabolism.

METABOLIC ACIDOSIS

Metabolic acidosis may be caused by excess acid or inadequate bicarbonate in the body. It is characterized by a low pH (less than 7.35) and a low bicarbonate level (less than 24 mEq/L). When metabolic acidosis develops, the respiratory system attempts to return the pH to normal (compensate) by increasing the rate and depth of respirations. Carbon dioxide elimination increases, and the $PaCO_2$ falls (less than 35 mm Hg).

Pathophysiology and Manifestations

Metabolic acidosis rarely is a primary disorder; it usually develops during the course of another disease (Table 7-15 ■):

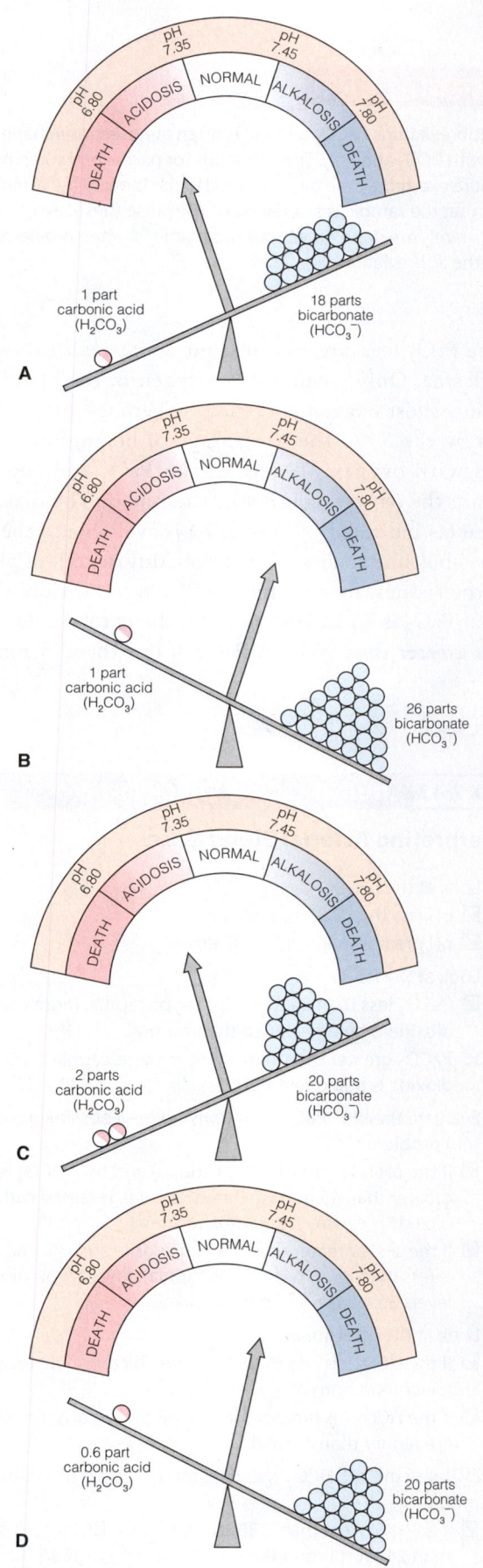

Figure 7-19. ■ Acid–base imbalances. (**A**) Metabolic acidosis. (**B**) Metabolic alkalosis. (**C**) Respiratory acidosis. (**D**) Respiratory alkalosis.

TABLE 7-15	Primary Acid–Base Imbalances		
IMBALANCE	**LAB VALUES**	**COMMON CAUSES**	**MANIFESTATIONS**
Metabolic acidosis	■ pH less than 7.35 ■ HCO_3^- less than 24 mEq/L ■ Compensation: $PaCO_2$ less than 35 mm Hg ■ Serum K^+ usually greater than 5.3 mEq/L	Increased acid production ■ Lactic acidosis ■ Ketoacidosis (diabetes mellitus, starvation, or alcoholism) Decreased acid excretion ■ Kidney failure Increased bicarbonate loss ■ Diarrhea, ileostomy drainage, intestinal fistula	■ Headache ■ Confusion ■ Decreased level of consciousness ■ Anorexia ■ Nausea and vomiting ■ Warm, flushed skin ■ ↓ BP, tachycardia ■ Increased respiratory rate and depth (hyperventilation)
Metabolic alkalosis	■ pH greater than 7.45 ■ HCO_3^- greater than 28 mEq/L ■ Compensation: $PaCO_2$ greater than 45 mm Hg ■ Serum potassium often less than 3.5 mEq/L	Increased acid loss or excretion ■ Vomiting, gastric suction ■ Hypokalemia Increased bicarbonate ■ Alkali ingestion (bicarbonate of soda) ■ Excess bicarbonate administration	■ Dizziness ■ Numbness and tingling (around the mouth and fingers and toes) ■ + Trousseau sign ■ Hyperactive deep tendon reflexes ■ Depressed respirations (compensatory)
Respiratory acidosis	■ pH less than 7.35 ■ $PaCO_2$ greater than 45 mm Hg ■ Compensation: HCO_3^- greater than 28 mEq/L	Acute respiratory acidosis ■ Acute respiratory conditions (e.g., pneumonia) ■ Narcotic overdose ■ Chest trauma ■ Respiratory arrest Chronic respiratory acidosis ■ Chronic respiratory conditions (e.g., COPD) ■ Multiple sclerosis, other neuromuscular diseases ■ Stroke	Acute respiratory acidosis ■ Feeling of fullness in head ■ Mental cloudiness, decreasing level of consciousness ■ Dizziness, muscle twitching, seizures ■ Warm, flushed skin ■ Cardiac dysrhythmias Chronic respiratory acidosis ■ Dull headache ■ Weakness
Respiratory alkalosis	■ pH greater than 7.45 ■ $PaCO_2$ less than 35 mm Hg ■ Compensation: HCO_3^- less than 24 mEq/L	■ Anxiety-induced hyperventilation ■ Fever ■ Early salicylate intoxication ■ Hyperventilation with mechanical ventilator	■ Light-headedness ■ Inability to concentrate ■ Numbness and tingling around the mouth and distal extremities ■ Palpitations, shortness of breath, chest tightness ■ Tremulousness, sweating, dry mouth ■ Feeling of panic ■ Loss of consciousness, seizures

■ Insufficient oxygen to support cell metabolism leads to the production of lactic acid (lactic acidosis).

■ When glucose is unavailable for cell metabolism (due to starvation or a lack of insulin), the body breaks down fatty tissue to meet its needs. In this process, fatty acids are released. This occurs in diabetic ketoacidosis, a common cause of metabolic acidosis.

■ Kidney failure, which impairs the body's ability to excrete excess hydrogen ion and form bicarbonate, also is a common cause of metabolic acidosis.

■ Bicarbonate-rich fluid from the small intestine can be lost through intestinal suction, severe diarrhea, ileostomy drainage, or fistulas.

- Administering excess chloride solutions (e.g., NaCl or ammonium chloride) also can lead to metabolic acidosis.

Manifestations of acid–base imbalances may be subtle. Metabolic acidosis primarily affects the central nervous system, GI tract, and cardiovascular function. Deep, rapid respirations (*Kussmaul respirations* or hyperventilation) are characteristic of metabolic acidosis, as the body tries to eliminate excess acid by "blowing off" carbon dioxide. See Table 7-15 for the manifestations of metabolic acidosis.

Collaborative Care

The focus of treatment for acute metabolic acidosis is correction of the underlying cause. (See Chapter 36 for treatment of diabetic ketoacidosis and Chapter 29 for treatment of kidney failure.)

In addition to ABGs, *serum electrolytes* are measured. The serum potassium often is high (greater than 5.3 mEq/L) as potassium ions shift out of cells in exchange for hydrogen ions. Serum potassium levels are measured throughout treatment for metabolic acidosis because hypokalemia can develop as the acidosis is corrected. An *ECG* is done to evaluate the effects of metabolic acidosis on heart function.

Bicarbonate or another alkaline solution may be given to correct severe metabolic acidosis, particularly when the pH is less than 7.1. The patient is closely monitored for possible adverse effects during treatment. IV insulin and fluid are given to patients with diabetic ketoacidosis.

clinicalALERT

Closely monitor serum potassium levels during treatment of metabolic acidosis. As the acidosis is corrected, potassium shifts into the cells. This can lead to hypokalemia and cardiac dysrhythmias.

NURSING CARE

PRIORITIZING NURSING CARE

Acidosis affects heart function and the nervous system, increasing the patient's risk for injury. The nursing focus is on maintaining patient safety and monitoring the effects of treatment.

HEALTH PROMOTION

Teaching and advocating for patients at risk for metabolic acidosis (e.g., people with type 1 diabetes or kidney failure) to effectively manage their underlying disorder and prevent complications are important health promotion activities. Because early manifestations of metabolic acidosis are vague and often mistaken for "the flu," stress the importance of seeking medical care if symptoms such as fatigue, malaise, nausea, abdominal pain, and flushing develop.

ASSESSING

Inquire about symptoms of anorexia, nausea, abdominal discomfort, fatigue, or lethargy and their onset and duration. Ask about precipitating factors, such as diarrhea and aspirin ingestion; chronic diseases such as diabetes or kidney failure; and current medications.

Assess mental status and level of consciousness; vital signs including respiratory rate and depth; apical and peripheral pulses; skin color and temperature; and urine output.

Monitor laboratory results, including ABGs and serum electrolytes. Report changes that are not within expected ranges for treatment.

IDENTIFYING POTENTIAL COMPLICATIONS

Promptly obtain and report ABG results and serum electrolyte values. Continue to monitor these and other laboratory reports throughout treatment. Closely monitor mental status, heart rate and rhythm, and urine output.

DIAGNOSING, PLANNING, AND IMPLEMENTING
Decreased Cardiac Output

Expected outcome: Vital signs and heart rhythm will be stable within expected range.

Metabolic acidosis decreases the strength of heart contractions, slows the heart rate, and increases the risk of dysrhythmias.

- Monitor vital signs, peripheral pulses, and capillary refill. *Hypotension, weak pulse strength, and slow capillary refill may indicate decreased cardiac output.*
- Monitor ECG pattern for dysrhythmias. Notify the physician of changes. *Dysrhythmias further decrease cardiac output, which may worsen acidosis.*

Risk for Injury

Expected outcome: Will remain free of adverse consequences and physical injury related to acid–base imbalance or treatment.

- Monitor mental status, level of consciousness, and muscle strength. *As the pH falls, mental function declines, causing confusion and a decreasing level of consciousness. This increases the risk for injury.*
- Institute safety precautions as necessary: Keep the bed in its lowest position with side rails up. *These measures help protect the patient from injury resulting from confusion or disorientation.*
- Keep clocks, calendars, and familiar objects at the bedside. Orient to time, place, and circumstances as needed. Allow significant others to remain with the patient as much as possible. *An unfamiliar environment and altered*

thought processes can further increase the risk for injury. Significant others provide a sense of security and reduce anxiety.

Risk for Excess Fluid Volume

Expected outcome: Intake and output will balance over 24 hours.

Administering bicarbonate to correct acidosis increases the risk for hypernatremia and fluid volume excess.

- Obtain daily weights. *Daily weights are an accurate indicator of fluid balance.*
- Monitor I&O. Obtain hourly urine outputs as indicated, reporting an output of less than 30 mL/hr. *Heart failure and inadequate renal perfusion may lead to decreased urine output.*
- Monitor respiratory status. *Increasing dyspnea and adventitious lung sounds may indicate excess fluid volume. Report to the care provider.*
- Assess for distended neck veins and edema in dependent tissues and periorbital areas. *Distended neck veins and dependent or generalized edema may indicate excess fluid volume.*

Nursing care also includes measures to treat the underlying disorder, such as diabetic ketoacidosis. Refer to the chapters on diabetes (Chapter 36) and kidney failure (Chapter 29) for specific interventions.

EVALUATING

To evaluate the effectiveness of nursing care, monitor the patient's mental status, cardiac output, safety, and fluid balance, as well as laboratory results for ABGs and serum electrolytes.

MANAGING NURSING CARE

Although the patient in metabolic acidosis may be critically ill, nursing care activities such as measuring I&O and assisting with daily living activities such as toileting, ambulating, and hygiene are appropriate to assign to assistive personnel. Alert caregivers to promptly report changes in the patient's behavior, level of consciousness, breathing, or vital signs to the nurse.

DOCUMENTING

Document the care and interventions provided and the patient's response (e.g., improved mental functioning, fewer cardiac dysrhythmias) to interventions. Document continuing assessments, including assessments of fluid balance.

CONTINUITY OF CARE

Discharge planning focuses on the underlying cause of the metabolic acidosis. Teach the patient who has developed ketoacidosis as a result of diabetes mellitus, starvation, or alcoholism about diet and medications. Refer for treatment of alcoholism and to a support group such as Alcoholics Anonymous. Discuss the importance of day-to-day management of kidney failure (e.g., diet and dialysis) to prevent future problems with metabolic acidosis. With patients who developed acidosis as a result of diarrhea or ileostomy drainage, provide information about strategies to prevent or treat diarrhea, and when to call their primary care provider.

When discharge to a long-term care or residential care facility is planned, provide information to caregivers about the underlying disorder and measures to prevent future episodes of metabolic acidosis. Discuss ways to identify and potentially correct the disorder early in its course.

METABOLIC ALKALOSIS

Metabolic alkalosis may be caused by loss of acid or excess bicarbonate in the body. It is characterized by a high pH (greater than 7.45) and a high bicarbonate level (greater than 28 mEq/L). When metabolic alkalosis develops, the respiratory system attempts to restore acid–base balance by slowing the respiratory rate. Carbon dioxide is retained, and the $PaCO_2$ increases (greater than 45 mm Hg).

Pathophysiology and Manifestations

Vomiting or gastric suction often leads to loss of hydrogen ions from the body. Gastric secretions are highly acidic (pH 1–3). Hypokalemia also reduces hydrogen ion concentration, as the kidneys excrete hydrogen ion in exchange for potassium. In addition, when potassium shifts out of the cells to maintain potassium levels in ECF, hydrogen ion shifts into the cells.

Excess bicarbonate usually results from ingestion of antacids that contain bicarbonate (such as soda bicarbonate or Alka-Seltzer) or when bicarbonate is administered to treat metabolic acidosis. Review Table 7-15 for common causes of metabolic alkalosis.

Alkalosis affects calcium ionization in ECF. Because of this, the manifestations of both metabolic and respiratory alkalosis are similar to those of hypocalcemia. As the respiratory system compensates for metabolic alkalosis, respirations are depressed (see Table 7-15).

Collaborative Care

Treatment of metabolic alkalosis focuses on identifying and correcting the underlying cause. Serum electrolytes are monitored; hypokalemia (K^+ less than 3.5 mEq/L) and hypochloremia (Cl^- less than 95 mEq/L) are often present. The potassium level is closely monitored during treatment, because correcting the alkalosis may affect serum potassium.

Treatment includes restoring normal fluid volume and administering potassium chloride and sodium chloride solutions. Chloride is necessary for the kidneys to excrete excess bicarbonate. Potassium helps restore intra- and extracellular potassium levels, allowing the kidneys to more effectively retain hydrogen ion. Sodium chloride is given to treat accompanying fluid volume deficits. When the pH is critically high (greater than 7.6), an acidifying solution such as dilute hydrochloric acid or ammonium chloride may be given.

NURSING CARE

PRIORITIZING NURSING CARE

Metabolic alkalosis inhibits the respiratory center of the brain, slowing respirations as the body attempts to retain carbonic acid to balance the excess of bicarbonate. This places the patient at risk for impaired gas exchange, the priority for nursing care.

HEALTH PROMOTION

Because ingestion of bicarbonate of soda is a common cause of metabolic alkalosis, teaching patients to use other effective antacid preparations is a primary prevention strategy. For patients undergoing gastric suction, carefully monitor laboratory values to promptly identify patients at risk for developing metabolic alkalosis.

ASSESSING

Ask about current symptoms, such as numbness and tingling, muscle spasms, or dizziness; and any precipitating factors such as bicarbonate ingestion or vomiting, and current medications. Obtain vital signs including apical pulse, rate and depth of respirations; and assess muscle strength and deep tendon reflexes. Monitor and report laboratory data, including ABGs and serum electrolytes.

IDENTIFYING POTENTIAL COMPLICATIONS

Respiratory depression is a major potential complication of metabolic alkalosis. Frequently monitor the respiratory rate and depth, as well as oxygen saturation levels (SaO_2). Promptly report *bradypnea* (respiratory rate less than 12) or a drop in SaO_2 levels (less than 95%) to the nurse or physician.

DIAGNOSING, PLANNING, AND IMPLEMENTING
Risk for Impaired Gas Exchange

Expected outcome: Color, level of consciousness, and SaO_2 will remain within expected parameters.

- Monitor respiratory rate, depth, and effort. Monitor oxygen saturation continuously; report an SaO_2 of less than 95% (or as ordered). *Depressed respirations can lead to hypoxemia and impaired tissue oxygenation. An SaO_2 of less than 90% indicates significant problems.*
- Monitor mental status and level of consciousness (LOC). Report decreasing LOC or behavior changes such as

restlessness, agitation, or confusion. *Changes in mental status or behavior may be early signs of hypoxia.*
- Place in semi-Fowler's or Fowler's position as tolerated. *Elevating the head of the bed improves ventilation and gas exchange.*
- Schedule nursing care activities to allow rest periods. *The hypoxemic patient has limited energy reserves, requiring frequent rest and limited activities.*
- Administer oxygen as ordered or necessary to maintain SaO_2 levels. *Supplemental oxygen can help maintain blood and tissue oxygenation despite depressed respirations.*

Deficient Fluid Volume

Expected outcome: Will have balanced I&O, moist mucous membranes, and stable vital signs.

Patients with metabolic alkalosis often have an accompanying fluid volume deficit.

- Assess I&O; monitor hourly if indicated. *Urine output of less than 30 mL/hr for 2 or more hours indicates inadequate kidney perfusion and an increased risk for acute kidney injury and impaired tissue perfusion.*
- Monitor vital signs and peripheral pulses at least every 4 hours. *Hypotension, tachycardia, and weak, easily obliterated peripheral pulses indicate hypovolemia.*
- Weigh daily. *Rapid weight changes accurately reflect changes in fluid balance.*
- Administer intravenous fluids as ordered using an infusion pump. Monitor for dyspnea, tachypnea, tachycardia, neck vein distention, and edema. *Rapid fluid replacement may lead to hypervolemia.*
- Monitor serum electrolytes, osmolality, and ABG values. *Rehydration and administration of potassium chloride will affect both acid–base and fluid and electrolyte balance. Careful monitoring is important to identify changes.*

EVALUATING

Collect data related to the patient's respiratory status, tissue oxygenation, and fluid balance to evaluate the effectiveness of nursing interventions for patients with metabolic alkalosis.

DOCUMENTING

Document nursing and interdisciplinary care provided, continuing assessment data, and the patient's and family's understanding of the condition and its causes.

CONTINUITY OF CARE

Planning and teaching for home or community-based care of the patient who has experienced metabolic alkalosis focus on the underlying cause of the imbalance. Teach patients how to prevent and manage problems such as acute gastroenteritis that can lead to excessive vomiting. Discuss the importance of adequate potassium in the diet, foods high in potassium (see Box 7-10), and potassium supplements with patients for whom hypokalemia contributed to metabolic alkalosis. Explain the need to avoid using bicarbonate-based antacids, and suggest alternatives.

RESPIRATORY ACIDOSIS

Respiratory acidosis is caused by an excess of dissolved carbon dioxide or carbonic acid. It is characterized by a pH of less than 7.35 and a $PaCO_2$ greater than 45 mm Hg. Respiratory acidosis may be either acute or chronic in nature. In chronic respiratory acidosis, the bicarbonate is higher than 28 mEq/L as the kidneys compensate for the imbalance by retaining bicarbonate.

Pathophysiology

Both acute and chronic respiratory acidosis are caused by inadequate ventilation, leading to carbon dioxide retention. Hypoxemia (low oxygen levels in the arterial blood) frequently accompanies respiratory acidosis.

Acute respiratory acidosis occurs due to an acute failure of ventilation. Chest trauma, aspiration of a foreign body, acute pneumonia, and overdoses of narcotic or sedative medications can lead to acute respiratory acidosis. In acute respiratory acidosis, the $PaCO_2$ rises rapidly and the pH falls markedly. The serum bicarbonate initially is unchanged because the compensatory response of the kidneys occurs over hours to days.

Chronic respiratory acidosis is associated with chronic respiratory or neuromuscular conditions such as chronic obstructive pulmonary disease (COPD), asthma, cystic fibrosis, or multiple sclerosis. These conditions affect ventilation of the alveoli because of airway obstruction, structural changes in the lung, or limited chest wall expansion. COPD with chronic bronchitis and emphysema is the most common cause of chronic respiratory acidosis (see Table 7-15). In chronic respiratory acidosis, the $PaCO_2$ increases over time and remains elevated. The kidneys retain bicarbonate, increasing bicarbonate levels, and the pH often remains close to the normal range.

Manifestations

The manifestations of acute and chronic respiratory acidosis differ. An acute rise in $PaCO_2$ causes manifestations of hypercapnia (elevated serum carbon dioxide levels). Carbon dioxide dilates cerebral blood vessels, causing a feeling of fullness in the head and mental cloudiness. Rapid and dramatic changes in ABGs can lead to unconsciousness and cardiac arrest.

Patients with chronic respiratory acidosis may have few symptoms because carbon dioxide levels rise gradually, allowing compensatory changes to occur. See Table 7-15 for other manifestations of acute and chronic respiratory acidosis.

Collaborative Care

Patients with acute respiratory failure usually require treatment in the emergency department or intensive care unit to restore adequate ventilation and gas exchange. Hypoxemia often accompanies acute respiratory acidosis, so oxygen is administered as well. Supplemental oxygen is used with caution for patients with chronic respiratory acidosis.

clinicalALERT

In patients with chronically high blood levels of carbon dioxide, hypoxemia becomes the primary stimulus to breathe. Administering oxygen at a high flow rate may suppress respirations and lead to acute respiratory failure.

Bronchodilator drugs may be given to open the airways. Antibiotics may be ordered to treat respiratory infections. If excess narcotics or anesthetic has caused acute respiratory acidosis, drugs to reverse their effects may be given. Respiratory therapy, such as breathing treatments or percussion and drainage, may be used to clear airways and support ventilation. Adequate hydration is important to promote removal of respiratory secretions. Intubation and mechanical ventilation may be necessary for some patients in respiratory acidosis. (See Chapter 23 for more information about mechanical ventilation and its nursing implications.)

NURSING CARE

PRIORITIZING NURSING CARE

Restoring effective gas exchange in the lungs is the primary focus of interdisciplinary and nursing care for the patient with acute or chronic respiratory acidosis.

HEALTH PROMOTION

Health promotion activities focus on identifying patients at risk for respiratory acidosis (e.g., patients with chronic lung disease or a chronic neuromuscular disorder, people who receive narcotic analgesics or who have experienced chest trauma), monitoring respiratory status carefully, and teaching to prevent respiratory acidosis. Teach patients with chronic lung disease about maintaining good general health and avoiding exposure to respiratory infections or air pollution. Stress the importance of carefully monitoring respiratory status for patients taking narcotic analgesics. Instruct all patients at risk to notify their care provider promptly should respiratory symptoms worsen or manifestations of respiratory acidosis develop.

ASSESSING

Identify current symptoms such as headache, difficulty thinking, blurred vision, and their onset, duration, and precipitating factors such as drug use or infection. Inquire about chronic diseases such as cystic fibrosis or COPD, and current medications. Assess mental status and level of consciousness; vital signs; skin color and temperature; and rate and depth of respirations, and lung sounds. Monitor and report laboratory results, including ABGs and serum electrolytes.

IDENTIFYING POTENTIAL COMPLICATIONS

Frequently monitor respiratory rate, depth, and oxygen saturation levels, as well as mental status and level of consciousness for evidence of declining respiratory status. Monitor serum electrolytes, potassium in particular, as acidosis is being corrected.

DIAGNOSING, PLANNING, AND IMPLEMENTING

Impaired Gas Exchange

Expected outcome: Color, level of consciousness, and oxygen saturation will remain within desired ranges.

■ Frequently assess respiratory status (rate, depth, effort, and SaO_2) and LOC. *Decreasing respiratory rate, effort, oxygen saturation level, and LOC may indicate worsening of the patient's condition.*

■ Promptly report ABG results to the physician and respiratory therapist. *Rapid changes in carbon dioxide or oxygen levels may indicate a need to modify the treatment plan.*

■ Place in semi-Fowler's to Fowler's position as tolerated. *Elevating the head of the bed promotes lung expansion and gas exchange.*

■ Administer oxygen as ordered. Carefully monitor response. Reduce the oxygen flow rate or percentage and immediately report decreased level of consciousness. *Supplemental oxygen can suppress the respiratory drive in patients with chronic respiratory acidosis.*

Ineffective Airway Clearance

Expected outcome: Will have clear breath sounds throughout lung fields.

In some instances, for example, a patient with acute asthma or chronic bronchitis, obstruction of the airways impairs the flow of gases to and from the alveoli, affecting gas exchange.

■ Frequently auscultate breath sounds. *Increasing adventitious sounds or decreasing breath sounds (faint or absent) may indicate worsening airway clearance due to obstruction or fatigue.*

■ Encourage the patient with chronic lung disease to use pursed-lip breathing. *Pursed-lip breathing helps maintain open airways throughout exhalation, promoting carbon dioxide elimination.*

■ Frequently reposition and encourage patient to get out of bed as tolerated. *Movement and ambulation promote airway clearance and lung expansion.*

■ Encourage fluid intake of up to 3,000 mL/day as tolerated or allowed. *Fluids help liquefy secretions and hydrate respiratory mucous membranes, promoting airway clearance.*

■ Administer medications such as inhaled bronchodilators as ordered. *Inhaled bronchodilators help relieve bronchial spasm, dilating airways.*

■ Provide percussion, vibration, and postural drainage as ordered. *Pulmonary hygiene measures such as these help loosen respiratory secretions so they can be coughed out of airways.*

EVALUATING

Collect data such as ABG results, oxygen saturation levels, mental status, skin color, lung sounds, activity tolerance, and ease of respirations to evaluate the effectiveness of nursing interventions for the patient with respiratory acidosis.

DOCUMENTING

Document continuing assessment data, as well as the patient's response to interventions. Document care and teaching provided, as well as the patient's and family's understanding of the disorder and measures to prevent future episodes of respiratory acidosis.

CONTINUITY OF CARE

Planning and teaching for discharge focus on the problem that caused the patient to develop respiratory acidosis. Patients with acute respiratory acidosis resulting from acute pneumonia or chest trauma may need only teaching to prevent future problems. If acute respiratory acidosis was secondary to a narcotic overdose, determine whether the drug was prescribed or an illicit street drug. Provide teaching to the patient who requires narcotic medication on a continuing basis. Refer the patient using illicit drugs or misusing prescription narcotics to a substance abuse counselor, treatment center, or Narcotics Anonymous as appropriate.

For patients with chronic lung disease, discuss ways to avoid future episodes of acute respiratory failure. Encourage the patient to obtain immunization against pneumococcal pneumonia and annual influenza vaccines. Discuss ways to avoid acute respiratory infections and measures to take when respiratory status is further compromised.

RESPIRATORY ALKALOSIS

Respiratory alkalosis is always caused by hyperventilation, leading to a carbon dioxide deficit. It is characterized by a pH greater than 7.45 and a $PaCO_2$ of less than 35 mm Hg.

Pathophysiology and Manifestations

In acute respiratory alkalosis, the pH rises rapidly as the $PaCO_2$ falls. The bicarbonate level remains within normal limits because the kidneys require time to increase bicarbonate elimination. Anxiety-induced hyperventilation is the most common cause of acute respiratory alkalosis.

Other causes are listed in Table 7-15. Low carbon dioxide levels cause cerebral blood vessels to constrict, reducing blood flow. The manifestations of respiratory alkalosis relate to this cerebral vasoconstriction and decreased calcium ionization (which also occurs in metabolic alkalosis). Table 7-15 lists the manifestations of respiratory alkalosis.

Collaborative Care

Anxiety-induced respiratory alkalosis is treated by instructing the patient to breathe slowly into a paper bag or rebreather mask. This allows the patient to rebreathe exhaled carbon dioxide, which increases $PaCO_2$ levels and reduces the pH. A sedative or antianxiety agent may be given. In other cases, such as salicylate intoxication or excessive ventilation by a mechanical ventilator, treatment is aimed at the underlying cause of the hyperventilation.

NURSING CARE

PRIORITIZING NURSING CARE

The priority of care for the patient with respiratory alkalosis is restoring an effective breathing pattern to prevent excess loss of carbon dioxide.

INEFFECTIVE BREATHING PATTERN

Expected outcome: Will resume normal respiratory rate and pattern.

- Assess respiratory rate, depth, and ease. Monitor vital signs (including temperature) and skin color. *Assessment data can help identify the underlying cause, such as a fever or hypoxia.*
- Obtain subjective assessment data, such as circumstances leading up to the current situation, current health, and recent illnesses or medication use, as well as current manifestations. *Subjective data provide clues to the cause and circumstances of hyperventilation.*
- Reassure the patient that he or she is not having a heart attack and that symptoms will resolve when breathing returns to normal. *Manifestations of hyperventilation and respiratory alkalosis, such as dyspnea, chest tightness or pain, and palpitations, can mimic those of a heart attack.*
- Instruct patient to maintain eye contact and breathe with you to slow the respiratory rate. *These measures help make the patient aware of respirations and provide a sense of support and control.*
- Have the patient breathe into a paper bag. *This allows the patient to rebreathe exhaled carbon dioxide, increasing the $PaCO_2$ and decreasing the pH.*
- Protect from injury. *If hyperventilation continues, the patient may lose consciousness, causing respirations and acid–base balance to return to normal.*
- Refer patients with repeated episodes of hyperventilation or a chronic anxiety disorder for counseling. *Counseling can help the patient develop strategies for dealing with anxiety.*

CONTINUITY OF CARE

Planning and teaching for home care are directed toward the underlying cause of hyperventilation. If anxiety precipitated the episode, discuss anxiety management strategies. Refer the patient and family to a counselor if appropriate. Teach how to identify a hyperventilation reaction and breathe into a paper bag to manage it at home.

Note: The references and resources for all chapters have been compiled at the back of the book.

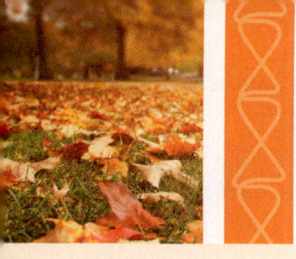

Chapter Review

KEY POINTS

- **Concept:** A balance of body fluids, electrolytes, and acids and bases is normally maintained through processes that regulate the intake, output, and distribution of fluids and the solutes they contain.
- A balance of fluid and electrolyte intake, the elimination of water, electrolytes, and acids by the kidneys and hormonal influences normally maintain the volume and composition of body fluid.
- **Concept:** Fluid and electrolyte imbalances occur when the intake, output, or distribution of water or electrolytes is altered. Age, lifestyle, and environmental factors (such as air temperature) affect fluid and electrolyte balance, as can disease processes or manifestations (e.g., nausea or diarrhea) and treatment measures (e.g. medications, gastric suction).
- Fluid, electrolyte, and acid–base imbalances can affect all body systems, especially the cardiovascular system, the central nervous system, and the transmission of nerve impulses.
- Fluid and sodium imbalances commonly are related; both affect serum osmolality.
- **Concept:** Manifestations of electrolyte imbalances can be vague and nonspecific. Monitoring and tracking changes in laboratory values is critical in patients who have or are at risk for electrolyte imbalance.
- Both hypokalemia and hyperkalemia affect cardiac conduction and function. Carefully monitor cardiac rhythm and status in patients with very low or very high potassium levels.

- Calcium imbalances primarily affect neuromuscular transmission: Too little calcium causes increased neuromuscular irritability; too much calcium depresses neuromuscular transmission. Magnesium imbalances have a similar effect.
- **Concept:** Acid–base disorders (broadly classified as acidosis or alkalosis) usually occur due to disrupted metabolic processes or impaired respiratory or kidney function. The nurse provides teaching to prevent imbalances, monitors the effects of treatment, and provides care to reduce the risk of harm associated with these disorders.
- Buffers, lungs, and kidneys work together to maintain acid–base balance in the body. Buffers respond to changes almost immediately; the lungs respond within minutes; the kidneys, however, require hours to days to restore normal acid–base balance.
- The lungs compensate for metabolic acid–base imbalances by excreting or retaining carbon dioxide. This is accomplished by increasing or decreasing the rate and depth of respirations.
- The kidneys compensate for respiratory acid–base imbalances by producing and retaining or excreting bicarbonate and by retaining or excreting hydrogen ions.
- Careful monitoring of respiratory and cardiovascular status, mental status, neuromuscular function, and laboratory values is an important nursing responsibility for all patients with fluid, electrolyte, or acid–base imbalances.

PEARSON NURSING STUDENT RESOURCES

Find additional materials at **nursing.pearsonhighered.com**.

Clinical Reasoning Care Map

Caring for a Patient With Acute Respiratory Acidosis
NCLEX-PN® Focus Area: Physiologic Adaptation

Case Study: Marlene Hitz, age 76, is eating lunch with her friends when she suddenly begins to choke and is unable to breathe. After several minutes of trying, an attendant at the senior center successfully dislodges some meat caught in Ms. Hitz's throat using the Heimlich maneuver. Ms. Hitz is taken by ambulance to the emergency department for follow-up.

Nursing Diagnosis: Impaired Gas Exchange

COLLECT DATA

Subjective	Objective
_____	_____
_____	_____
_____	_____
_____	_____
_____	_____

Does this present a threat to the patient's safety?

If yes, the priority intervention to address this threat would be:

_____

Nursing Care

_____
_____
_____
_____
_____
_____
_____
_____
_____
_____

Interprofessional team members to include when planning care:

_____
_____

How would you document this? _____
_____

Compare your answers and documentation to those provided on the companion website.

Data Collected
(use only those that apply)

- T 98.2°F, P 102, R 36 and shallow, BP 146/92
- Skin warm and dry
- Alert but not oriented to time or place
- Responds slowly to questions
- Restless
- Oxygen at 4 L/min per nasal cannula

- D_5 1/2 NS running intravenously at 50 mL/hr
- Chest x-ray normal
- ABGs: pH 7.38 (normal 7.35 to 7.45), $PaCO_2$ 48 mm Hg (normal 35 to 45 mm Hg), PaO_2 92 mm Hg (normal 80 to 100 mm Hg), HCO_3^- 24 mEq/dL (normal 22 to 26 mEq/L)

Nursing Interventions
(use only those that apply; list in priority order)

- Monitor ABGs, to be redrawn in 2 hours.
- Monitor respiratory status and vital signs every 15 minutes for the first hour and then hourly.
- Assess mental status, LOC, and color of skin, nail beds, and oral mucous membranes hourly.
- Maintain a calm, quiet environment.
- Reorient to setting and explain all activities.
- Keep side rails in place, and place call bell within reach.

NCLEX-PN® Exam Preparation

1 Which of these patients would most likely develop dehydration after surgery?

1. 24-year-old male diagnosed with an inguinal hernia
2. 70-year-old female with ovarian cancer
3. 65-year-old male with prostate cancer
4. 19-year-old female with a badly fractured leg

2 A patient has been diagnosed with deficient antidiuretic hormone (ADH). Which assessment finding should the nurse anticipate?

1. Increased serum osmolality
2. Dilute urine
3. Decreased thirst
4. Normal blood pressure

3 The nurse assessing a patient in the emergency department notes dry, sticky mucous membranes; weak peripheral pulses; and tachycardia. The primary nursing diagnosis should be:

1. Deficient Fluid Volume.
2. Impaired Skin Integrity.
3. Risk for Injury.
4. Decreased Cardiac Output.

4 A patient admitted to the medical unit has muscle spasms and a positive Chvostek sign. In obtaining the history, the nurse notes that the patient had a thyroidectomy 6 weeks ago. On the basis of this finding, the nurse anticipates that the physician will order a lab test for:

1. sodium.
2. potassium.
3. magnesium.
4. calcium.

5 A patient presents with muscle weakness, tremors, and confusion. Laboratory testing reveals a serum magnesium level of 0.9 mg/dL (normal 1.8 to 3.0 mg/dL). The nurse recalls that a common cause of hypomagnesemia is:

1. kidney failure.
2. excessive antacid use.
3. chronic alcoholism.
4. lack of sun exposure.

6 A patient is hyperventilating due to anxiety. Which of the following lab values indicates an altered acid–base balance?

1. pH 7.51
2. $PaCO_2$ 38 mm Hg
3. HCO_3^- 22 mEq/L
4. PaO_2 95 mm Hg

7 The nurse knows that a patient's low bicarbonate level may be caused by:

1. gastrointestinal suction.
2. constipation.
3. use of baking soda for indigestion.
4. alcohol abuse.

8 A patient with hyperkalemia is admitted to the medical floor. For which of the following complications of this electrolyte imbalance does the nurse monitor most closely?

1. Paralytic ileus
2. Cardiac dysrhythmias
3. Fluid retention and edema
4. Kidney stones

9 The nurse administered the prescribed dose of furosemide (Lasix). To evaluate the effectiveness of the drug, the nurse should assess:

1. weight.
2. apical pulse.
3. breath sounds.
4. fluid intake PO.

10 The nurse is caring for a patient being treated for diabetic ketoacidosis (metabolic acidosis). Which laboratory value should the nurse monitor closely as the acidosis is corrected?

1. Hemoglobin and hematocrit
2. Serum potassium
3. Urine specific gravity
4. Serum magnesium

Answers and rationales for Review Questions appear in Appendix I.

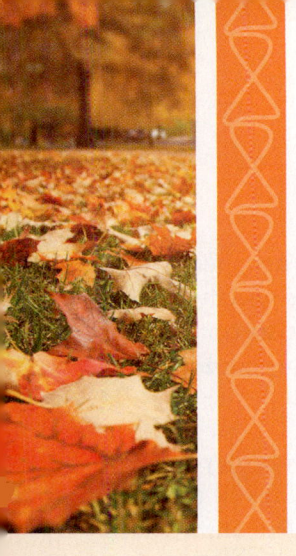

CHAPTER 8
Caring for Patients in Pain

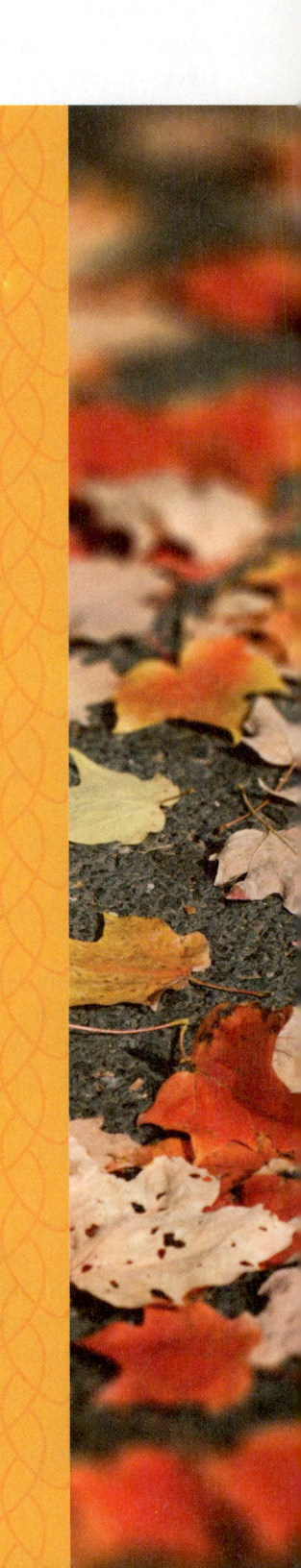

BRIEF OUTLINE

Physiology of Pain
Types of Pain

Factors Affecting Patient
    Response to Pain

Collaborative Care

APPLIED LEARNING OUTCOMES

After completing this chapter, you will be able to:

1. Describe the physiology of pain.
2. Assess patients for the characteristics of acute, chronic, cancer, and neuropathic pain.
3. Identify factors that may affect a patient's response to pain.
4. Discuss collaborative care for the patient in pain, including medications, surgery, and transcutaneous electrical nerve stimulation.
5. Use complementary therapies for patients to reduce or relieve pain.
6. Apply pain rating scales in assessing patients' pain.
7. Use the nursing process in the care of patients experiencing pain.
8. Explain the nurse's role in administering medications to reduce or relieve pain.

KEY TERMS

The key terms are defined on the pages listed below.

SPECIAL FEATURES

Key Concept Pain can be classified in many ways such as acute pain (postoperative pain), cancer pain, and chronic pain (osteoarthritis pain). Assisting patients to manage pain often requires analgesic medications such as nonopioids or opioids and nonpharmacologic measures such as biofeedback or relaxation techniques.

Pain is a subjective response to physical and psychologic stressors. All people feel pain at some point during their lives. An estimated 100 million Americans live with chronic pain. The most common types of chronic pain are low back pain, severe headache and migraine pain, and neck pain (American Academy of Pain Medicine, 2012).

Although pain is usually experienced as uncomfortable and unwelcome, it often serves as a warning of potentially health-threatening conditions. For this reason, pain is referred to a *fifth vital sign*. Because vital signs are routinely monitored, it is felt that by including pain, more patient problems would be addressed. The Joint Commission has established pain standards that identify the relief of pain as a patient right. These standards focus on the patient's right to appropriate pain assessment and intervention and the health care professional's responsibility to treat pain.

Each pain event is a unique, personal experience. It can be affected by biologic, psychologic, cognitive, social, cultural, and spiritual factors. Pain is the most common reason for seeking health care. There are many accepted definitions of pain. McCaffery and Pasero (1999, p. 5) define **pain** as "whatever the person experiencing it says it is, and existing whenever the person says it does." This definition recognizes the patient as the only person who can accurately describe his or her own pain and serves as the basis for nursing assessment and care of patients in pain. It also supports the values and beliefs about pain necessary for holistic nursing care, including the following:

■ If the patient reports pain, the patient is in pain. All pain is real.
■ Pain affects the whole body, usually negatively.
■ Pain may serve as both a response to and a warning of actual or potential trauma.

Because pain is subjective, it challenges nurses to rely on the patient's description and nonverbal cues to determine the type, location, duration, and intensity of pain. Usually nurses assess clear objective manifestations of a disorder, such as skin color or decreased pulse. In addition, many physicians and nurses do not understand the newer concepts of pain management. The public and health care professionals fear addiction. The nurse's own bias can positively or negatively affect how a patient's pain is managed. Because pain is subjective, it is not the nurse's role to judge whether the patient is actually experiencing pain. Nurses have an obligation to react positively to the patient's report of pain and a responsibility to minimize or eliminate pain.

Physiology of Pain

Key Concept Pain is transmitted by the peripheral nervous system (PNS) and central nervous system (CNS) and is perceived in the CNS. Pain impulses are conducted through the four steps of transduction, transmission, perception, and modulation.

The ability of the body to produce pain depends on **nociceptors**. Nociceptors are nerve endings in the skin, viscera, blood vessels, muscles, and joints that are activated when *noxious* (unpleasant) stimuli are applied. Chemical, mechanical, or thermal noxious stimuli start the pain process (Table 8-1 ■). Once tissue damage occurs from the noxious stimuli, inflammation begins. Pain impulses are initiated both by direct tissue damage and by the release of internal chemicals. For example, inflammation causes the release of bradykinin and prostaglandins, which also activate the nociceptors. The intensity and duration of the stimuli determine the sensation. Long-lasting, intense stimulation produces greater pain than does brief, mild stimulation.

PAIN CONDUCTION
The conduction of pain impulses involves four steps: transduction, transmission, perception, and modulation (Figure 8-1 ■).

Transduction
Transduction is the change of a noxious stimulus into an electrical action potential stimulus that sends impulses throughout the CNS. Pain is transmitted through large afferent A-delta and small C nerve fibers to the spinal

TABLE 8-1	Pain Stimuli
STIMULI	**EXAMPLE**
Chemical	■ Ischemia (e.g., angina, bowel infarct) ■ Tissue trauma ■ Inflammation, inflammatory mediators such as histamine, prostaglandins (e.g., sore throat)
Mechanical	■ Spasm (ureteral colic, gallstones, kidney stones) ■ Compression (e.g., invasive tumor, carpal tunnel syndrome, compartment syndrome) ■ Extreme muscle stretch or contraction (e.g., after a sprain or fracture)
Thermal	■ Contact with extreme heat or cold

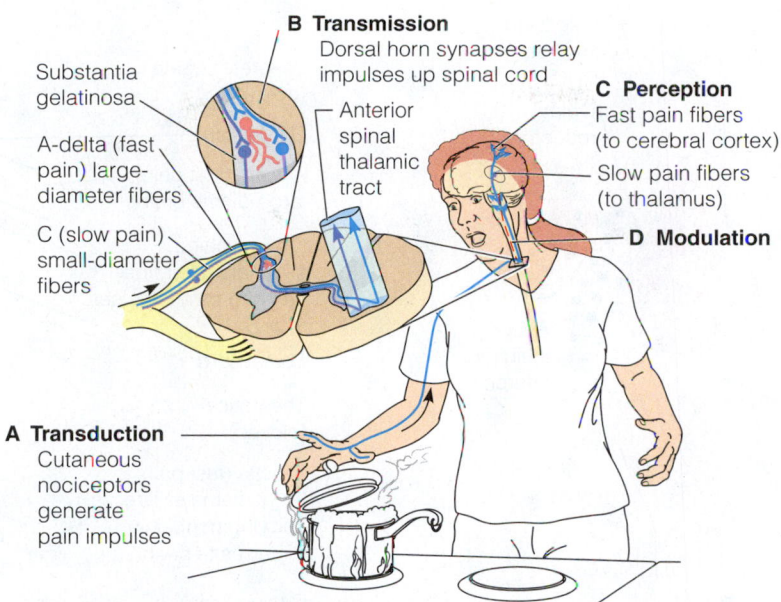

Figure 8-1. ■ Pain conduction. (A) *Transduction*: Cutaneous nociceptors send impulses to spinal cord. (B) *Transmission*: Impulses synapse in the substantia gelatinosa. (C) *Perception*: Pain impulses are processed in the thalamus and cerebral cortex. (D) *Modulation*: Along efferent fibers from cerebral cortex to substantia gelatinosa, pain may be inhibited or modulated.

cord. A-delta fibers are *myelinated* (covered with an insulating sheath). They transmit impulses rapidly and produce sharp, well-defined pain sensations usually associated with acute pain. C fibers are not myelinated and transmit pain impulses more slowly. C-fiber pain is diffuse, usually chronic, and described as dull, burning, or aching.

Both A-delta and C fibers are involved in most injuries. For example, if a person bangs an elbow, A-delta fibers transmit this pain stimulus within 0.1 second. The person feels this pain as a sharp, localized, smarting sensation. One or more seconds after the blow, the person experiences a duller, aching, diffuse sensation of pain impulses carried by the C fibers.

Transmission

Transmission, the second step, involves sending the impulses from the *afferent* (sensory nerve that transmits impulses toward the CNS) neurons to the dorsal horn in the spinal cord, where they *synapse* (transmit an impulse) in the substantia gelatinosa. Substance-P helps send the impulse across the synapse. From here the impulses travel to the spinothalamic tracts and ascend to the thalamus and cerebral cortex.

Perception

Perception is the processing of pain impulses in the thalamus and cerebral cortex. During this step, pain impulses are perceived and interpreted. The patient experiences pain when the sensation reaches a conscious level.

Pain threshold and pain tolerance are part of perception. **Pain threshold** is the point at which each person recognizes pain; it is closely related to actual tissue damage

(Porth, 2011). Research shows that pain threshold varies little among people. If a patient reports more pain than is expected, the nurse should investigate further.

Pain tolerance is the amount (duration, intensity) of pain a person can stand before reporting it and seeking relief. Unlike pain threshold, pain tolerance varies among individuals. It is influenced by culture, expectations, emotions, and psychosocial factors. Pain tolerance may be decreased by repeated episodes of pain, fatigue, anger, anxiety, and sleep deprivation. On the other hand, it may be increased by medications, alcohol, warmth, distraction, and spiritual practices.

Modulation

Modulation is the last step of pain conduction, in which the body attempts to decrease the perception of pain. Descending pathways of efferent fibers run from the cerebral cortex to the substantia gelatinosa in the dorsal horn. Along these fibers, pain may be inhibited or modulated. The body's naturally occurring **endorphins** (endogenous morphines) are released in response to afferent noxious stimuli or from efferent impulses. Endorphins bind with opiate receptors on the neurons and inhibit the release of substance-P. This process stops the pain impulse transmission (Figure 8-2■).

GATE-CONTROL THEORY OF PAIN

In 1965, Melzack and Wall developed the *gate-control theory* of pain. This theory states that when pain impulses travel from the skin to the substantia gelatinosa in the dorsal horn of the spinal cord, the substantia gelatinosa can either open or close the "gate" to transmit pain impulses to the brain.

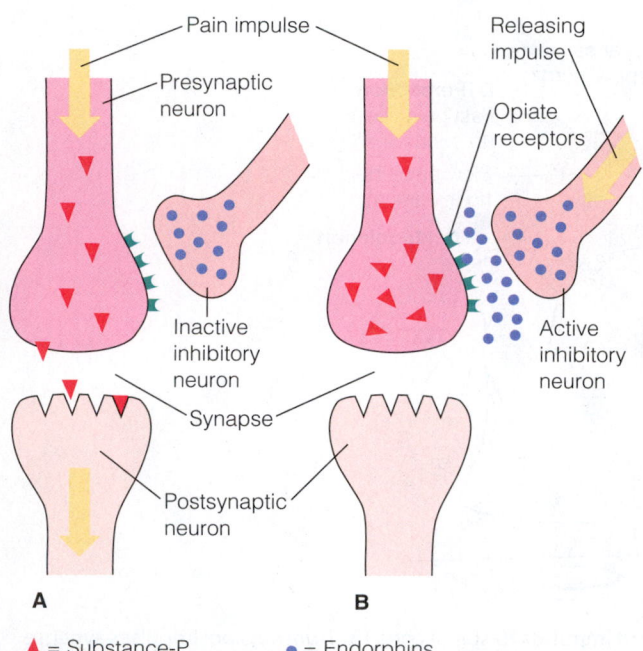

= Substance-P   **= Endorphins**

Figure 8-2. ■ (A) Substance-P transmits pain impulse across synapse between presynaptic neuron and postsynaptic neuron. (B) During modulation, endorphins are released from inhibitory neuron, which prevents the release of substance-P, and pain impulse is inhibited.

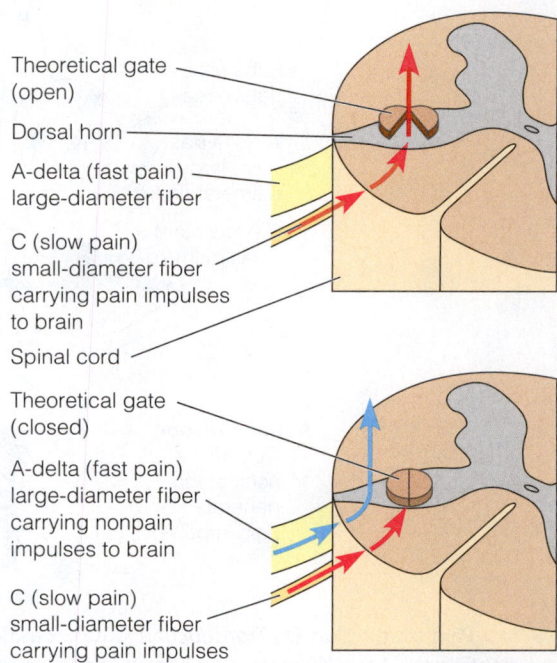

Figure 8-3. ■ Diagram of gate-control theory. When small-diameter C fibers are stimulated, the gate is open and pain is transmitted. When large-diameter A-delta fibers are stimulated, the gate is closed and pain transmission is stopped.

Whether the gate is opened or closed in the substantia gelatinosa depends on the amount of stimulation the large and small nerve fibers receive. If more small-diameter C fibers are stimulated, the gate is open, and pain impulses travel uninhibited to the brain. In contrast, if more large-diameter A-delta fibers are stimulated, the gate is closed and pain is inhibited (Figure 8-3 ■).

Stimulation of the A-beta or touch fibers closes the gate and "turns away" pain impulses. Massaging a stubbed toe activates A-beta fibers, so it reduces intensity and duration of the pain.

Pain impulses may also be inhibited in the brainstem. Opioids or distraction techniques signal receptors in the medulla, which in turn stimulate nerve fibers in the spinal cord to block pain transmission. This regulation process may explain why a patient who experiences severe pain may not feel it under certain circumstances. For example, an athlete often fails to notice an injury until the competition is over.

New research is investigating further the complex relationship between pain and modulation. Possible genetic and sensory influences may play a greater role than previously thought.

Types of Pain

ACUTE PAIN

Acute pain is usually temporary, has a sudden onset, and is localized. It normally lasts for less than 6 months and has an identified cause. Acute pain is caused by tissue injury from trauma, surgery, or inflammation. Examples of acute pain include sprains, toothache, needle sticks, and muscle spasms. Acute pain may warn of actual or potential injury to tissues. As a stressor, it can initiate the fight-or-flight response, triggering tachycardia, rapid and shallow respirations, increased blood pressure, dilated pupils, sweating, and pallor. The person with acute pain may be anxious and fearful. Acute pain is classified into four major types:

1. *Cutaneous somatic pain* arises from the skin, mucous membranes, or subcutaneous tissues that would be caused by sunburn and skin contusions. It is described as sharp, cutting, burning, and well localized. Throbbing pain occurs when blood vessels are involved.

2. *Deep somatic pain* results from injury to deep body structures such as muscles, bones, ligaments, tendons, and joints. This type of pain results from arthritis and tendonitis. It is characterized as dull and diffuse.

3. *Visceral pain* comes from the body organs lined with viscera. Visceral pain is deep, dull, and poorly localized and is associated with nausea and vomiting, hypotension, and weakness. It may radiate or be referred to another area of the body. It is described as deep, cramping, stabbing, colicky, or intermittent. A kidney stone passing through the ureter to the bladder causes severe, acute visceral pain.

4. ***Referred pain*** is an unpleasant sensation that starts in one site but is perceived in another area, distant from

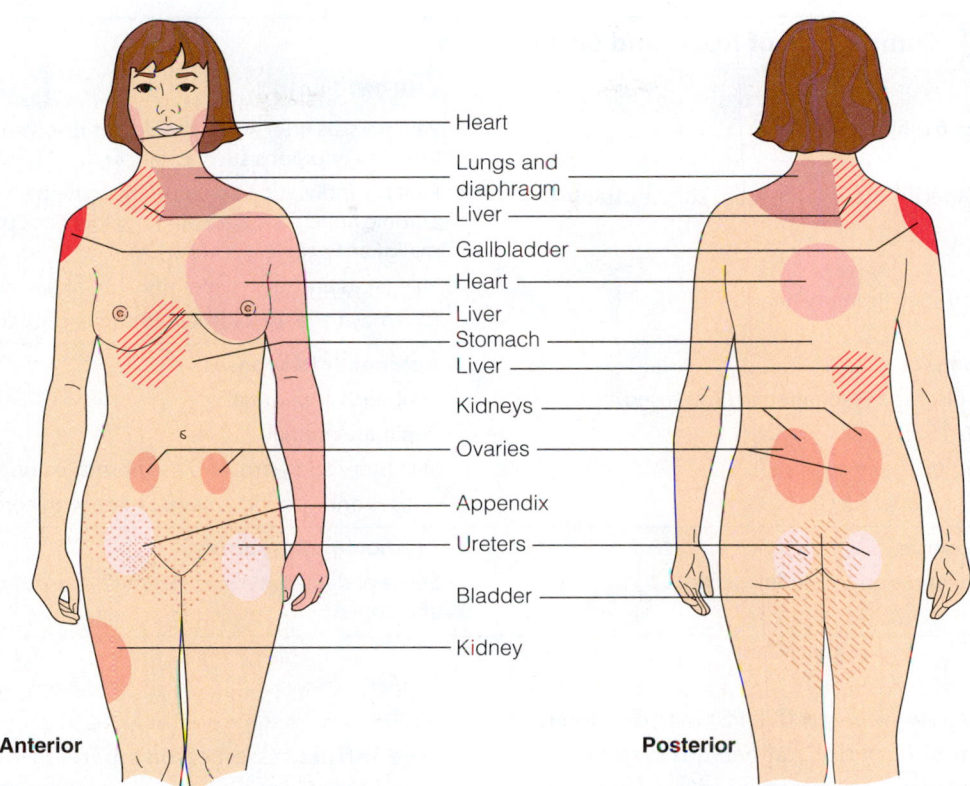

Heart
Lungs and diaphragm
Liver
Gallbladder
Heart
Liver
Stomach
Liver
Kidneys
Ovaries
Appendix
Ureters
Bladder
Kidney

Anterior   **Posterior**

Figure 8-4. ■ Referred pain begins in one site but is felt in another area. For example, pain from an inflamed gallbladder may be felt in the shoulder, or angina from ischemia of the heart muscle may be felt in the left arm or jaw.

the site of the stimuli (Figure 8-4■). It often occurs with pain that starts in the thoracic or abdominal viscera.

CHRONIC PAIN

Chronic pain is prolonged pain or pain that persists after the condition causing it has resolved. There may not be an identifiable cause, and often it is unresponsive to conventional medical treatment. Chronic pain is more complex than acute pain. Patients with chronic pain are often depressed, withdrawn, immobile, irritable, or controlling. They may experience social withdrawal, fatigue, and reduced activity level. The autonomic nervous system is unaffected because the body adapts to the constant presence of pain.

Chronic pain is subdivided into three categories: recurrent acute pain, chronic nonmalignant pain, and chronic malignant pain. *Recurrent acute pain* is characterized by well-defined episodes of pain interspersed with pain-free periods such as migraine headaches. *Chronic nonmalignant pain* is non-life-threatening pain that continues beyond an expected time for healing. Examples include low back pain, arthritis, chronic abdominal pain (Crohn's disease), peripheral neuropathy, and neuralgia. In many instances, chronic pain cannot be eliminated. Treatment focuses on helping the patient cope with the pain and be as functional as possible.

Chronic malignant pain can result from the disease itself (tumor pressing on nerves or other structures, stretching

of viscera, or metastasis to the bones). It may be associated with chemotherapy and radiation therapy. Cancer pain is a type of chronic malignant pain usually requiring multiple pharmacologic and nonpharmacologic approaches, as discussed later. (A comparison of the characteristics of acute and chronic pain is found in Table 8-2■.)

NEUROPATHIC PAIN

Neuropathic pain is pain caused by abnormal impulse processing of sensory input by the central or peripheral nervous system. Although neuropathic pain may be acute (e.g., the pain associated with shingles [herpes zoster]), usually it is chronic. The pain may be described as gnawing, electric shocklike, burning, shooting, or tingling. Pain may occur with a stimulus such as touch that normally does not cause pain (*allodynia*), or its intensity may be greater than the stimulus (*hyperalgesia*). There are four types of neuropathic pain: central pain, complex regional pain syndromes, peripheral neuropathy pain, and phantom limb pain.

Central pain is caused by a lesion or damage in the brain or spinal cord. A brain tumor, stroke, trauma, or disorder such as multiple sclerosis or epilepsy may cause central pain. The location of the pain depends on the area of the CNS affected. The pain may be described as burning, pressing, or aching. Affected areas may have decreased sensation.

TABLE 8-2	Comparison of Acute and Chronic Pain	
ACUTE PAIN		**CHRONIC PAIN**
Pain lasts less than 6 months.		Pain persists after acute problem is resolved or occurs due to disease conditions such as cancer.
Pain results from specific tissue injury (e.g., surgery, trauma).		Pain is subdivided into recurrent acute pain (e.g., headache), chronic nonmalignant pain (e.g., low back pain), and chronic malignant pain (e.g., cancer).
Pain is localized.		Pain areas are hard to identify.
Pain resolves when specific injury heals.		Pain may have no foreseeable end except death.
Autonomic Responses		**Autonomic Responses**
Blood pressure, pulse, and respiration are increased.		Vital signs are normal.
Pupils are dilated.		Pupils are normal.
Skin is diaphoretic, pale, and cool.		Skin is dry and warm and has normal color.
Nausea and vomiting often occur.		Nausea and vomiting may develop with chronic malignant pain.
Psychologic Responses		**Psychologic Responses**
Anxiety, fear, facial grimacing, guarding, crying.		Sense of depression, hopelessness, frustration, decreased sleep and appetite.

Complex regional pain syndromes (CRPS) may develop from damage to the central or peripheral nervous system or possibly an immune process. Extremity pain is severe, diffuse, and burning and is accompanied by vasomotor changes, affecting skin color and temperature. Initially, the affected extremity appears red, warm, and swollen; later it is cool, cyanotic, and edematous.

Peripheral neuropathy pain often accompanies conditions such as neuropathy from diabetes mellitus or long-term alcohol use and postherpetic neuralgia. Peripheral pain is either felt along the distribution of many peripheral nerves, as seen in diabetic neuropathy, or associated with specific peripheral nerve injury, as in trigeminal neuralgia.

Phantom limb pain occurs after surgical or traumatic amputation of a limb. The patient experiences pain in the missing body part even though there is complete awareness that the limb is gone. The pain may be described as burning, cramping, or shooting. It may be due to the stimulation of the severed nerves at the site of the amputation.

Factors Affecting Patient Response to Pain

Responses to pain stimuli are as individualized as the person experiencing the pain stimulus. A person's response is shaped not only by physiologic responses but also by age, sociocultural influences, psychologic influences, the source and meaning of pain, and knowledge base. Pain threshold may be affected by factors such as the presence of chronic pain, which tends to lower the threshold. Pain tolerance varies not only among individuals but also within an individual over time.

AGE

Age influences a person's perception and expression of pain. No scientific evidence proves that age reduces pain perception or sensitivity to pain. Older adults may experience acute and chronic pain due to chronic disorders such as arthritis, osteoporosis with compression fractures, and diabetic neuropathy. Older adults tend to deny pain or self-medicate with over-the-counter medications. They are more likely to report discomfort, aching, or soreness. Patients and health care providers may believe that pain is a part of growing older. They may have misconceptions about using opioids for fear of respiratory depression or drug addiction. Older adults with dementia are less often assessed for pain and less often receive pain medications.

SOCIOCULTURAL INFLUENCES

Family, community, and culture strongly influence a person's response to pain. From childhood, people learn from their families what behavior is expected when they experience pain. Expected behaviors range from being stoic to feeling comfortable reporting pain and requesting pain medication. Pain behaviors are the way a patient expresses his or her pain and can vary greatly within a culture and from generation to generation. Cultural standards teach an individual how much pain an individual should tolerate, what types of pain to report and to whom, and what kind of treatment to seek. In some cultures, one family member or the entire extended family is involved in pain management decisions.

The nurse also has a set sociocultural values and beliefs about pain. If these values and beliefs differ from the patient's, pain assessment and management may be based on the nurse's values rather than the patient's needs. The nurse must remember that pain behaviors are not an objective indicator of the amount of pain an individual patient has. It is important for the nurse to understand how ethnicity and culture affect pain expression and management and to respect cultural differences.

PSYCHOLOGIC INFLUENCES

Pain intensity can be affected by psychologic variables such as attention, expectation, and suggestion. The sensation of pain may be blocked by intense concentration as seen during sports activities or increased by anxiety or fear. Pain is often increased when it occurs along with other illnesses or physical discomforts like nausea or vomiting. The presence or absence of support people or caregivers who genuinely care about pain management also may alter emotional status and how a patient perceives pain.

Anxiety may increase the perception of pain, and pain, in turn, may cause anxiety. In addition, muscle tension is common with anxiety and can add to the pain. This explains why relaxation and guided imagery are helpful in relieving or decreasing pain. Fatigue, lack of sleep, and depression are often related to pain experiences. Pain interferes with a person's ability to sleep, which produces fatigue. In turn, fatigue can lower pain tolerance. In clinically depressed people, serotonin (a neurotransmitter that modulates pain in the CNS) decreases, leading to increased pain sensation.

Previous experiences with pain influence how the person reacts to a current pain episode. If the person's childhood experiences with pain were positive, then the adult usually will have a healthy attitude toward pain. If, however, the person's experiences were unfavorable, then future responses to pain will be negative.

The meaning associated with the pain affects the pain experience. For example, the pain of labor to deliver a baby is experienced differently from the pain after removal of a major organ for cancer. Individuals usually associate pain with the potential for disability, loss of role, and death. Misunderstanding the source, outcome, and meaning of pain can negatively affect the pain experience. For this reason, it is important for patients to understand the *etiology* (source) and *prognosis* (predicted outcome) of their pain.

The patient who perceives advantages from the sick role may be motivated to maintain pain. These advantages may include support from others and avoidance of disagreeable work or stressful social obligations. Such patients may require assistance not only to treat the pain but also to learn new ways for handling personal stresses.

DEFICIENT KNOWLEDGE

When the patient understands pain, it is easier for the nurse to teach the patient about pain management strategies. The nurse must assess the patient's readiness to learn, use teaching methods appropriate for the patient and family,

and evaluate the level of learning. Teaching content should include the pain process and the plan of care. The nurse should encourage patients to describe what pain relief measures work best for them. Patients should learn how to let family know about their pain and how they can help promote effective pain management.

Collaborative Care

Effective pain relief involves collaboration among the patient and all members of the health care team. Acute pain management may be straightforward, accomplished through short-term analgesia and management of the underlying problem. On the other hand, chronic pain usually requires an interprofessional approach. Pain clinics are centers staffed by a team of health care professionals who use a variety of approaches to manage chronic pain. Therapies may include medications, herbs, vitamins, biofeedback, hypnosis, acupuncture, and massage. Hospice provides care and support for terminally ill patients and their families.

MEDICATIONS

Medication is the most common approach to pain management. Acute pain management usually relies on analgesic drugs such as acetaminophen, nonsteroidal anti-inflammatory drugs (NSAIDs) and opioids. Chronic pain presents additional challenges; drugs called adjuvant analgesics, such as anticonvulsants and antidepressants, may be used. In addition to administering the prescribed medications, the nurse is responsible for assessing the side effects of the medications, evaluating the medication's effectiveness, and providing patient teaching. The nurse's role in pain relief includes being a patient advocate as well as a direct caregiver.

Types of Pain Medications

Key Concept Opioid analgesics work at the CNS level; nonopioid analgesics work at the peripheral nervous system level. By using opioid and nonopioid analgesics together, different pain mechanisms are targeted to increase pain medication effectiveness. Often this allows lower doses of each drug and fewer side effects.

Analgesics are pharmacologic agents used to relieve or reduce pain. The pharmacologic agents most commonly ordered to provide *analgesia* (pain relief) are the nonopioids, opioids, and adjuvant analgesics.

NONOPIOIDS **Nonopioids** are drugs used for pain that are not derived from opium. They include acetaminophen (Tylenol) and NSAIDs. Acetaminophen reduces pain and fever but does not have an anti-inflammatory effect. It is often combined with an opioid to provide effective pain relief for patients with mild to moderate pain with a lower opioid dose (e.g., Percocet, Tylenol #3, Vicodin).

Acetaminophen is toxic to the liver; exceeding the daily recommended dose of 3,200 mg/day could result in liver failure. It does not produce adverse effects on the kidney, gastric lining, or platelets.

NSAIDs act on the peripheral nervous system. They reduce pain by interfering with prostaglandin synthesis. Examples are aspirin, ibuprofen, and ketorolac (Toradol). NSAIDs have anti-inflammatory, analgesic, and antipyretic actions. They are the treatment of choice for mild to moderate pain and continue to be effective when combined with opioids for moderate to severe pain. However, they have an *analgesic ceiling*. This means that increasing the dose beyond a certain dosage will not increase its pain relief effect. NSAIDs can cause gastric ulcers and increase the risk of bleeding. This is especially true for aspirin, because aspirin interferes with platelets and blood clotting. (Nursing implications and patient teaching guidelines for acetaminophen and NSAIDs are found in Table 8-3 ■.)

OPIOIDS   **Opioids** are derivatives of the opium plant. These drugs are the most potent pain-relieving drugs available and are the treatment of choice for moderate to severe pain. They produce analgesia by binding to opioid receptors in the CNS, especially the brain and spinal cord. They differ from one another in potency, speed of onset, duration of action, and preferred route of administration. Opioids are subdivided into two groups: opioid agonists (e.g., morphine, hydromorphone, and codeine) and opioid agonist–antagonists (e.g., buprenorphine and nalbuphine). Nursing responsibilities and patient teaching recommendations for opioids are found in Table 8-3.

Opioid analgesics can depress the CNS and respiratory center, causing drowsiness, sedation, dizziness, and respiratory depression. They should be avoided or used with caution in patients with chronic obstructive pulmonary disease (COPD) because they can decrease respirations. Other common side effects include nausea, vomiting, and constipation. All opioids can cause physical and

TABLE 8-3	Giving Medications Safely: Acetaminophen, NSAIDs, and Opioids		
CLASS/DRUGS	**PURPOSE**	**NURSING IMPLICATIONS**	**PATIENT TEACHING**
Acetaminophen (Tylenol)	It is given to decrease pain and fever but not inflammation.	Give with a full glass of water.	Take with a full glass of water.
NSAIDs ■ Aspirin ■ Celecoxib (Celebrex) ■ *Ibuprofen* (Motrin) ■ Ketorolac (Toradol) ■ Naproxen (Naprosyn) ■ Piroxicam (Feldene)	NSAIDs have analgesic, antipyretic, and anti-inflammatory effects.	Give with meals or a full glass of water. Do not give aspirin with other NSAIDs. Monitor for signs of GI bleeding. If given for fever, monitor the patient's temperature. If the patient takes anticoagulants, assess for bleeding; NSAIDs increase this risk.	Take with meals or a full glass of water. Do not take more than the recommended amount. Do not take aspirin or alcohol with other NSAIDs. Monitor for GI bleeding (e.g., black stools, vomiting of blood).
Opioid agonists ■ Codeine ■ Fentanyl ■ Hydrocodone ■ Hydromorphone (Dilaudid) ■ Meperidine (Demerol) ■ Morphine sulfate ■ Oxymorphone (Numorphan) **Opioid agonist–antagonists** ■ Buprenorphine (Buprenex) ■ Butorphanol (Stadol) ■ Nalbuphine (Nubain)	Opioids are used to manage moderate to severe pain. They bind to opiate receptors in the brain to alter the perception of pain. They are addictive, causing psychologic and physical dependence.	Record the date, time, patient name, and type and amount of drug used, and sign the entry on the narcotic inventory sheet. Follow institution policy for wasting any narcotic. Monitor for side effects of sedation, respiratory depression, urinary retention, constipation, nausea, and vomiting. Keep naloxone (Narcan) available to treat respiratory depression.	The use of opioids to treat severe pain is unlikely to cause addiction. Do not drink alcohol. Do not take over-the-counter drugs without health care provider approval. Increase intake of fluids and fiber to prevent constipation. The drugs often cause dizziness, drowsiness, and impaired thinking; use caution when driving or making decisions. Do not increase dosage or take extra doses without discussing with health care provider.

Note: Medications identified in *italics* are among the 200 most frequently prescribed drugs in the United States.

psychologic dependence, especially when taken at high doses for an extended time (Adams & Urban, 2013).

Certain opioids, while still available, have limited use because of toxic effects. For example, meperidine (Demerol) produces a metabolite that is toxic to the CNS. If needed, meperidine should be used for no more than 2 days. It must be avoided in older adults.

ADJUVANT ANALGESICS   Adjuvant analgesics are drugs with other specific uses that can provide analgesia in patients with chronic nonmalignant and cancer pain. They include anticonvulsants, tricyclic and serotonin norepinephrine reuptake inhibitor (SNRI) antidepressants, topical and systemic anesthetics, corticosteroids, CNS stimulants, and bisphosphonates. Anticonvulsants include such drugs as gabapentin (Neurontin) and carbamazepine (Tegretol). Tricyclic antidepressants include amitriptyline (Elavil) and doxepin (Sinequan), and SNRIs include duloxetine (Cymbalta) and venlafaxine (Effexor). Xylocaine (lidocaine) is a topical anesthetic, whereas bupivacaine (Marcaine) is a systemic anesthetic. A common corticosteroid is dexamethasone (Decadron). Methylphenidate (Ritalin) is a useful CNS stimulant. Bisphosphonates include such drugs as etidronate (Didronel) and pamidronate (Aredia).

Anticonvulsants are used for diabetic neuropathy and neuralgia. *Antidepressants* promote normal sleeping patterns in patients with chronic pain and are useful in treating neuropathic pain. Topical anesthetics are used to treat neuropathic pain. *Systemic anesthetics* can be injected into nerves for a nerve block or given via the intraspinal route for cancer pain. Metastatic bone cancer pain may be relieved by using *corticosteroids*. *CNS stimulants* decrease sedation from opioids without decreasing pain relief in persons with cancer. *Bisphosphonates* may decrease bone pain when cancer metastasizes to the bone.

Routes of Administration

The route of administration affects how much of the medication is needed to relieve pain. For example, because of differences in absorption and distribution, oral doses of some opioids may be up to five times greater than parenteral doses to achieve the same degree of pain relief. Of course, different narcotics have different recommended dosages. Consulting an equianalgesic dosage chart when converting from one route of administration to another or from one drug to another helps ensure that **equianalgesic doses** will have an equivalent effect for the patient (Table 8-4■).

ORAL   The simplest route for both patient and nurse is the oral (PO) route. Special nursing care is still required because some medications must be given with food, some irritate the gastrointestinal system, and some patients have trouble swallowing pills. The nurse is responsible for making sure that the medication is actually swallowed.

Of the opioids, only fentanyl is available in alternate oral forms: buccal tablet, lozenge, or microadhesive polymer disk. These products provide a rapid onset of action because the medication is absorbed directly into the circulation via the oral mucosa. They are mainly used to treat breakthrough pain for patients with cancer pain. Special precautions are needed in storing the lozenge to prevent children mistaking it for candy.

RECTAL   The rectal route is useful for patients who cannot swallow, are experiencing nausea and vomiting, or have a mental status change. Acetaminophen, morphine, hydromorphone, and oxymorphone are available in this form. To be effective, any rectal medication must be placed above the rectal sphincter. The rectal route is effective and simple, but the patient and family may not accept it.

TRANSDERMAL   The transdermal ("patch") form of medication is simple and painless and delivers a continuous level of medication (Figure 8-5■). Transdermal medications are easy to store and apply. Fentanyl (Duragesic) patch is the only transdermal opioid. It is used to treat moderate to severe cancer pain and takes approximately 12–24 hours until a therapeutic level is absorbed. Absorption is increased by fever, heating pads, and electric blankets. If breakthrough pain occurs, short-acting medications are added.

Topical analgesic agents such as lidocaine patch 5% and capsaicin (Zostrix) are used to relieve pain related to arthritis, diabetic neuropathy, and neuralgia from herpes zoster infection. Capsaicin is derived from cayenne peppers and acts by depleting substance-P in the nerve endings.

PARENTERAL   The intramuscular (IM) route is no longer preferred for analgesics. Its disadvantages include uneven absorption from the muscle and pain during injection. The subcutaneous route may be used when continuous analgesic administration by the parenteral route is needed.

INTRAVENOUS   The intravenous (IV) route provides the most rapid onset, usually ranging from 1 to 15 minutes. Medication can be given by drip, bolus, or **patient-controlled analgesia (PCA)**, a pump with a handheld button that allows patients to manage their own pain (Figure 8-6■). The medication dose and interval between doses are programmed into the PCA pump so that the patient does not receive an overdose. The PCA pump allows patients to take control of their pain relief. The commonly ordered drugs include morphine, hydromorphone, and fentanyl.

INTRASPINAL   The intraspinal (epidural or intrathecal) route delivers an analgesic or a combination of analgesic and anesthetic drugs directly into the spinal column and then to the brain. This method is invasive and requires experienced nursing care. Patient-controlled epidural analgesia (PCEA) is currently used for patients

TABLE 8-4	Equianalgesic Dosage Chart		
ANALGESIC	**DOSAGE (MG)**	**DURATION (HOURS)**	**NURSING CONSIDERATIONS**
Opioid agonists			
Morphine sulfate	10 IM/IV 30 PO	3–4 IM/IV 3–6 PO	The analgesic effect of parenteral morphine 10 mg is used as the base against which all other opioids and administration routes are compared.
Codeine	130 IM 200 PO	3–4 IM 3–4 PO	Usual dose is 30 mg PO/IM. Higher doses are **not** recommended. Often combined with aspirin or acetaminophen for mild to moderate pain.
Hydrocodone	30 PO	4–6	Usual dose is 5 mg combined with acetaminophen (Vicodin) for mild to moderate pain.
Hydromorphone (Dilaudid)	1.5 IM/IV 7.5 PO	3–4 IM/IV 3–4 PO	More potent than morphine for severe pain; monitor patient closely during first doses.
Meperidine (Demerol)	75 IM/IV 300 PO	3 IM/IV 2–4 PO	Not recommended as first-line opioid for acute or chronic pain. Metabolizes to normeperidine, which is toxic to the CNS. Do **not** give 300 mg PO dose.
Oxycodone	20 PO	3–4	Combined with acetaminophen (Tylox, Percocet) for mild to moderate pain.
Oxymorphone (Numorphan)	1 IM/IV 10 PO/R	3–6 IM/IV 4–6 PO	For moderate to severe noncancer and cancer pain. Rectal suppository (10 mg).
Opioid agonist–antagonists			
Buprenorphine (Buprenex)	0.4 IM/IV	3–6 IM 3–4 IV	For moderate to severe postoperative pain.
Butorphanol (Stadol)	2 IM/IV	3–4	Given preop and postop for moderate to severe pain.
Nalbuphine (Nubain)	10 IM/IV	4–6	Given preop and postop for moderate to severe pain.
Pentazocine (Talwin)	30 IM/IV 50 PO	3–4 IM/IV 3–4 PO	Given preop and postop for moderate to severe pain.

Source: Adapted from Pasero, C., & McCaffery, M. (2011). *Pain Assessment and Pharmacologic Management*. St. Louis, MO: Elsevier.

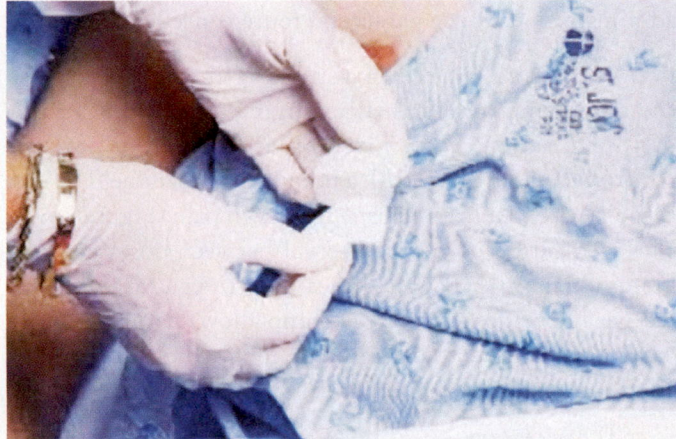

Figure 8-5. ■ Transdermal patch. To apply the patch, clip any hair from the site, clean the site with clear water, and dry it. Apply the patch immediately after opening the package by placing it in the palm and pressing firmly onto the prepared site for 30 seconds. Be sure that contact is complete around the edges. A patch lasts for 72 hours, and the next patch is applied on a different site. (Pearson Education.)

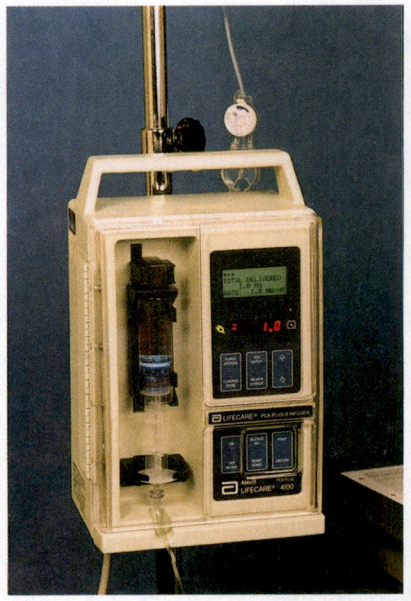

Figure 8-6. ■ PCA unit allows the patient to self-manage severe pain. It can be mounted on an intravenous pole. (Pearson Education.)

who have had major surgery. Box 8-1■ provides nursing implications for patients receiving intraspinal analgesia.

NERVE BLOCKS   In a nerve block, a local anesthetic, sometimes mixed with steroid anti-inflammatory drugs, is injected into or near a nerve to reduce unrelenting pain. Sometimes this procedure is used to locate the source of pain before permanent blocking is done. Temporary nerve blocks may give the patient enough relief to (1) feel hopeful that pain relief is possible, (2) allow local procedures to be done without causing discomfort, or (3) move the affected part.

Permanent nerve blocking is done with a neurolytic agent that destroys the nerve. Neurolytic blocks are reserved for terminally ill patients because of the risks of weakness, paralysis, and bowel and bladder dysfunction.

SURGERY

As a pain relief measure, surgery is performed only after all other methods have failed. Patients need to understand thoroughly the implications of surgery for pain relief. The common surgical procedures (Figure 8-7■) are briefly explained next.

Cordotomy

A *cordotomy* is an incision into the anterolateral tracts of the spinal cord to interrupt the transmission of pain. It is difficult to isolate the nerves responsible for upper body pain, so this surgery is most often performed for pain in the abdominal region and legs, including severe pain from terminal cancer.

BOX 8-1	NURSING CARE CHECKLIST

Patient Receiving Intraspinal Analgesia

Intraspinal analgesia is used to manage severe postoperative and cancer pain. The intraspinal route may be either intrathecal (into the subarachnoid space) or epidural (into the epidural space). Opioids such as morphine and fentanyl and local anesthetics like bupivacaine (Marcaine) are given. Opioids act on the opiate receptors in the CNS; anesthetics block conduction of pain impulses. This method can provide complete pain relief but has some serious adverse effects. The opioids may cause pruritus (itching), urinary retention, nausea, sedation, and respiratory depression. Local anesthetics can cause motor and sensory deficits.

In this procedure, the physician places a catheter into the epidural space. The catheter is attached to infusion tubing and an infusion pump, and the prescribed medication is given. A portable or implantable pump may deliver an opioid infusion for longer term therapy.

☑ Monitor pulse, blood pressure, respirations, and pulse oximetry every 15 minutes for the first 2 to 3 hours and then every hour for the first 24 hours.

☑ Have naloxone, a narcotic antagonist, at bedside to reverse respiratory depression.

☑ Monitor for effectiveness of pain relief.

☑ Monitor intake and output.

☑ Monitor for motor and sensory deficits.

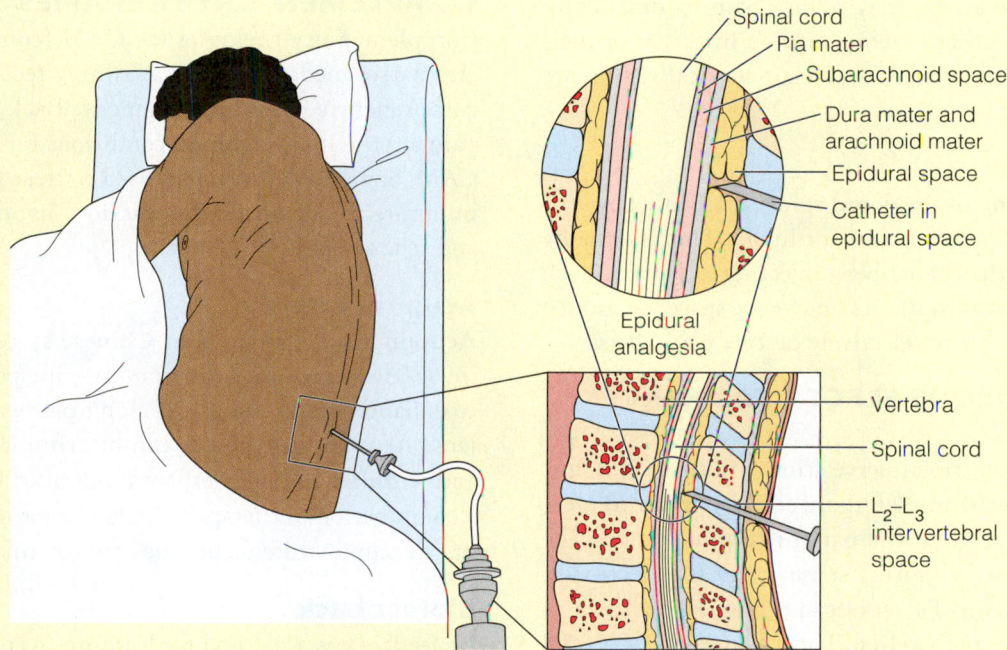

Placement of catheter in the epidural space.

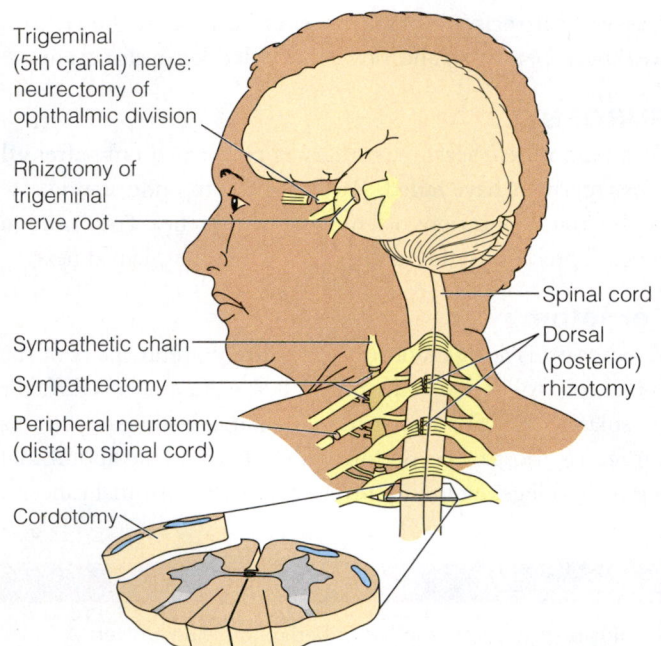

Figure 8-7. ■ Surgical procedures are used to treat severe pain that does not respond to other types of management. They include cordotomy, neurectomy, sympathectomy, and rhizotomy.

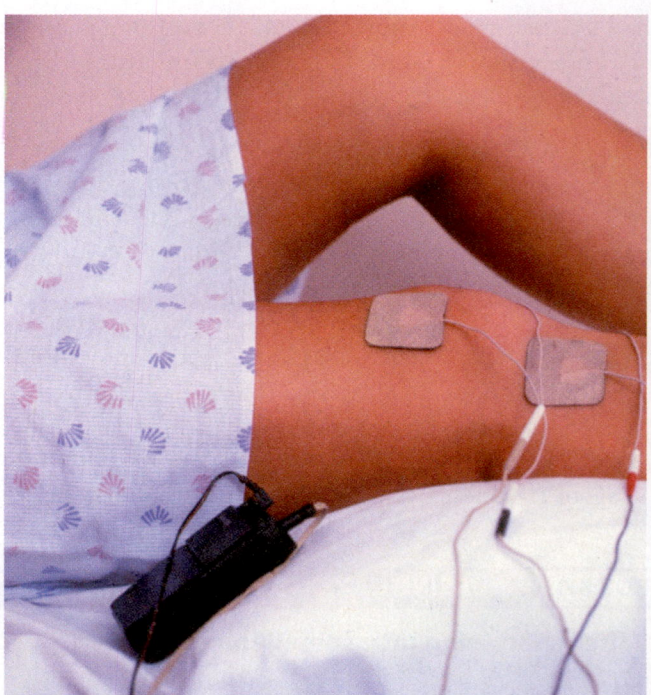

Figure 8-8. ■ TENS unit. Electrodes that deliver low-voltage electrical stimuli are placed directly on the patient over painful areas. (© CMSP/Custom Medical Stock Photo.)

Neurectomy

A *neurectomy* is the removal of a nerve. It is sometimes used for pain relief such as to relieve the pain of trigeminal neuralgia. A peripheral neurectomy is the severing of a nerve at any point distal to the spinal cord.

Sympathectomy

Because sympathetic nerves produce and transmit the pain sensation, a *sympathectomy* may reduce pain by destroying the involved sympathetic nerve with an injection or incision. Usually, nerves in the lumbar or cervical region are considered for this procedure.

Rhizotomy

Rhizotomy is severing of the dorsal spinal roots to relieve the pain of cancer of the head, neck, or lungs. This is done by surgically cutting the nerve fibers, injecting a chemical such as alcohol or phenol into the subarachnoid space, or using a radiofrequency current to selectively destroy pain fibers.

TRANSCUTANEOUS ELECTRICAL NERVE STIMULATION

A transcutaneous electrical nerve stimulation (TENS) unit is a low-voltage transmitter connected by wires to electrodes that are placed on the patient (Figure 8-8 ■). The patient experiences a vibrating sensation at the electrodes, which decreases pain. Patients can adjust the voltage to achieve maximum pain relief. The advantages of TENS units are avoidance of drug side effects and patient control. Disadvantages are its cost and the need for training.

A TENS unit is most commonly used to relieve chronic benign pain and acute postoperative pain. The nurse explains the manufacturer's directions, where to place the electrodes, and the importance of placing the electrodes on clean, unbroken skin. The patient is taught how to assess the skin daily for signs of irritation.

COMPLEMENTARY THERAPIES

Complementary therapies (or CAM [complementary and alternative medicine]) is increasingly recognized as part of comprehensive pain management. Back, neck, and joint pain are the most common conditions for which adults use CAM. Some CAM therapies used to treat pain include acupuncture, biofeedback, distraction, hypnotism, massage, and relaxation.

Acupuncture

Acupuncture is an ancient Chinese system of pain relief involving stimulation of certain specific points on the body to enhance energy flow (Qi) along pathways called meridians. Acupuncture points can be stimulated by inserting and withdrawing needles, applying heat, massage, laser, or a combination of therapies. Only care providers with training in acupuncture techniques can use this method.

Biofeedback

Biofeedback is a method for learning to control physiologic responses of the body. Electronic instruments measure brain waves, muscle contraction, and skin temperature, and then "feed" this information back to the patient. Electrodes are placed on the patient's skin, and an amplification unit transforms data into visual cues, such as colored lights. The patient learns to recognize stress-related responses and to replace them with relaxation responses. The goal is for the patient to initiate those actions that cause relaxation independently.

Distraction

Distraction focuses the patient's attention away from the pain and onto something that the patient finds more pleasant. Examples of distracting activities are practicing focused breathing, listening to music, tapping out a musical rhythm with the fingers or foot, and humor. Humor is known to be highly effective in pain relief. Laughing for 20 minutes or more produces an increase in endorphins that may continue pain relief even after the patient stops laughing.

Hypnotism

Hypnosis is a trancelike state in which the mind becomes extremely suggestible. For this technique to work, the patient must be fully relaxed and believe in the concept. It usually requires a skilled practitioner, but some patients can hypnotize themselves. Hypnosis has been successful in modifying pain.

Massage

Massage therapy is often used as a CAM therapy to relieve pain and provide relaxation. Muscles and soft tissues are manipulated to relax soft tissues; increase warmth, blood flow, and oxygen delivery to the area; and decrease pain. Massage therapy carries very little risk, but should be used appropriately and performed by a licensed or certified massage professional.

Relaxation Techniques

Relaxation involves learning to relax the body and mind deeply. The primary goal of relaxation is to decrease muscle tension and anxiety. Some examples of relaxation activities are as follows:

- **Diaphragmatic breathing.** The patient assumes a comfortable position in a quiet room and keeps the eyelids closed. The patient inhales and exhales slowly, using the diaphragm to help extend the breath. (Diaphragmatic breathing is described and illustrated in Chapter 10.)
- **Progressive muscle relaxation.** The patient is taught to tighten one group of muscles slowly and then relax them completely. The patient should repeat the sequence for all parts of the body. Audiotapes may guide the patient through this process.
- **Guided imagery.** To distract patients from their pain and produce relaxation, patients use their imagination to create a scene that is pleasurable and relaxing. The nurse assists the patient through the steps of imagery. Patients should understand that several sessions may be necessary before they experience some pain relief.

- **Meditation.** The patient empties the mind of all sensory data and may concentrate on a single object, word, or idea. This activity can produce a deeply relaxed state. A variety of exercises can induce the meditative state, and all are relatively easy to learn. Many books and tapes are available commercially.

NURSING CARE

PRIORITIZING NURSING CARE

Nursing care of the patient in pain presents more of a challenge than other illnesses or injuries. Whether pain is acute or chronic, the goal of nursing care is to assist the patient to achieve optimal control of the pain. To accomplish pain control, the nurse uses a combination of medications and complementary therapies.

> **Key Concept** Effective pain management requires an individualized and preventative approach. It is essential for the nurse to assess the patient's pain, work collaboratively with the health care provider in implementing appropriate pain-reducing methods, evaluate the effectiveness of the intervention, and advocate for the patient.

ASSESSING

The first step in relieving the patient's pain is to conduct an accurate, unbiased, and thorough assessment of the patient's pain. A comprehensive pain assessment ensures adequate and appropriate interventions. The nurse should assess the patient's perceptions, physiologic responses, and behavioral responses.

Patient Perceptions

Because pain is subjective, the patient's perceptions provide the most reliable indicator about the type and degree of pain. Remember, the patient's self-report is the standard for assessing the existence and intensity of pain (Pasero & McCaffery, 2011). The McGill Pain Questionnaire is one tool for assessing the patient's pain (Figure 8-9■). A thorough pain assessment will ensure a complete database for pain management (Box 8-2■).

The most common method of assessing the severity of pain is a pain rating scale (several scales are illustrated in Figure 8-10■). For patients who do not understand English or numerals, a scale using colors may be helpful. Another resource is the "Wong–Baker Faces Pain Rating Scale," which ranges from a happy face to one with a huge frown.

To ensure consistent communication, explain the specific pain rating scale being used. If a word descriptor scale is used, verify that the patient can read and understand the language being used. If a numerical scale is used, be

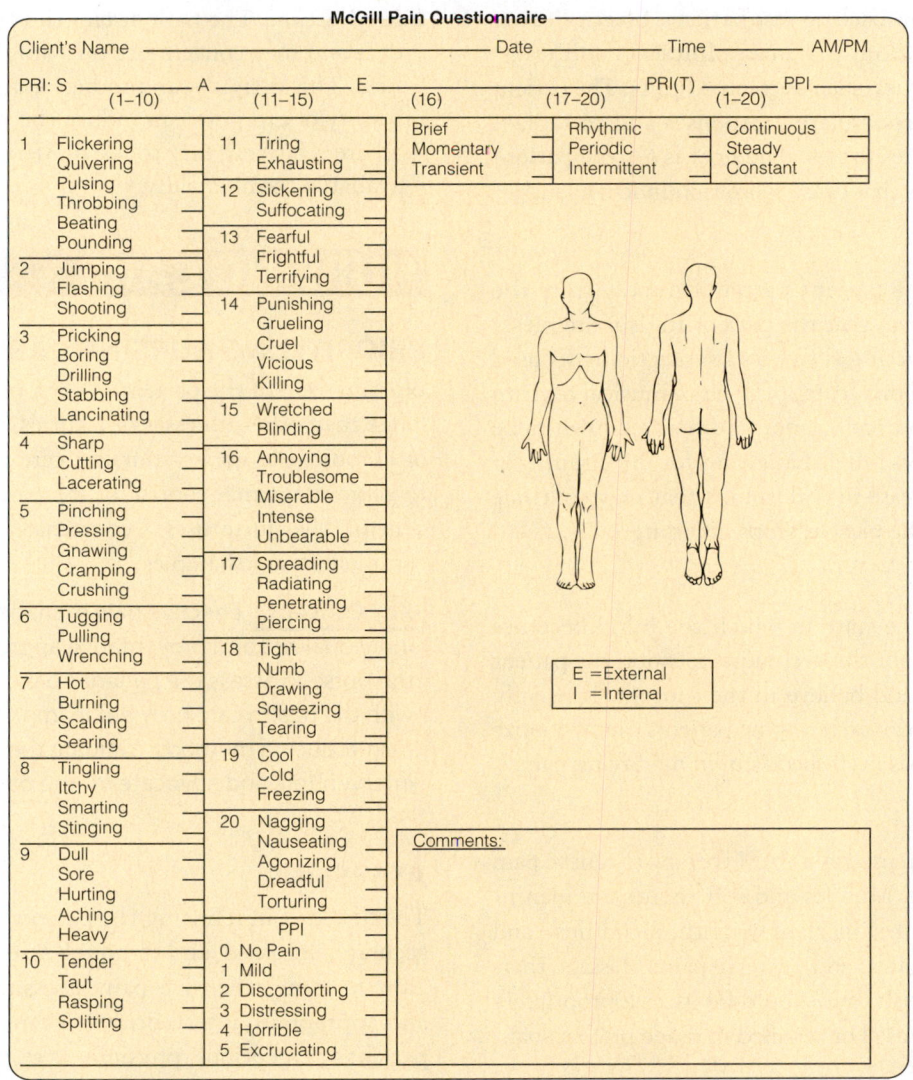

Figure 8-9. ■ The McGill Pain Questionnaire.
(Source: The McGill Pain Questionnaire by Ronald Melzack. Copyright © 1970, 1984, 1987 by Ronald Melzack. Used by permission of Ronald Melzack.)

sure the patient can count to 10. It is often helpful to use the patient's own words when describing the pain. Ask the patient to identify a *comfort-function goal*, that is, a level of pain that does not interfere with or prevent performance of essential activities of living. The patient should understand that reporting pain is important for recovery, not just for achieving temporary comfort.

Physiologic Responses

In the presence of acute pain, physiologic changes can occur from sympathetic nervous system (SNS) stimulation. These include muscle tension; tachycardia; rapid, shallow respirations; increased blood pressure; dilated pupils; sweating; and pallor. Over time, however, the body adapts to the pain stimulus, triggering less SNS response. These physiologic changes may be absent, especially in patients with chronic pain. The patient with chronic pain may have an unexpressive, tired facial appearance.

clinicalALERT

Assess patients for pain every time you check blood pressure, pulse, respirations, and temperature, because pain is the fifth vital sign.

Behavioral Responses

Behavioral responses to pain may or may not match the patient's report of pain. The nurse must accept the patient's pain rating regardless of the patient's behaviors. For example, one patient may rate pain at an 8 on a 0–10 scale while laughing or walking down the hall; another may deny pain completely while tachycardic, hypertensive, and grimacing. Discrepancies between the patient's report of pain and behavioral responses may result from cultural factors, coping skills, fear, denial, or the use of relaxation or distraction techniques.

BOX 8-2	ASSESSMENT

Assessing for Pain

Subjective Data

Location
- Where does it hurt?
- Does the pain radiate?
- Is the pain superficial or deep?

Onset, Pattern, Duration, Quality
- When did the pain start?
- Did it begin gradually or suddenly?
- Is it constant or intermittent?
- Does it occur in cycles (e.g., same time each day)?
- How often does it appear?
- How long does the pain last?
- Is the pain throbbing, dull, aching, sharp, stabbing, prickling, or burning?

Precipitating, Aggravating, and Relieving Factors
- What seems to trigger the pain?
- What seems to make the pain worse (e.g., movement, position changes, coughing, straining, or eating)?
- What seems to make the pain better (e.g., rest, sleep, food, pain medications, standing, or sitting)?

Intensity
- How strong is the pain? (Have the patient rate the pain using a rating scale.)

Other Problems
- Does the pain cause nausea, vomiting, anorexia, or insomnia?
- Does the pain interfere with activities at home, work, or social interactions?
- Are there other diseases or conditions (e.g., arthritis)?

Methods of Pain Relief
- What has helped control pain in the past?
- What has not worked to relieve the pain?

Objective Data
- Vital signs: blood pressure, pulse, respirations.
- Assess skin moisture and color; pupils for dilation.
- Observe appearance for signs of grimacing, clenching jaws or fist, guarding, drawing up into fetal position, lying rigidly, restlessness.
- Observe behavioral responses: moaning, sighing, crying, becomes quiet, withdraws from others, appears frightened, has sad facial expression.
- Gently palpate painful area; identify possible trigger points.

Patients may deny pain for a variety of reasons, including fear of injections, fear of drug addiction, or misunderstanding of terms. For example, patients may think that aching or soreness does not qualify as pain. Some patients believe

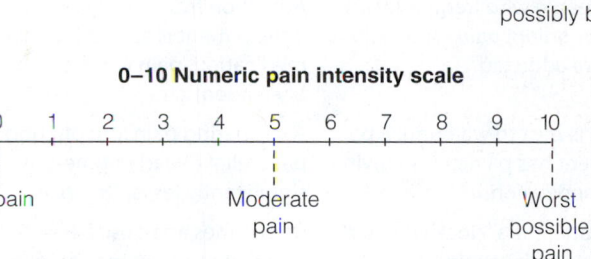

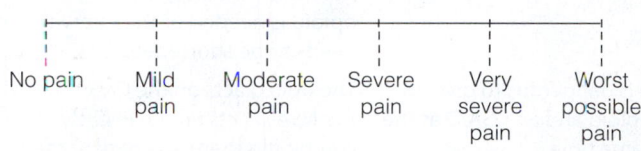

Figure 8-10. ■ Examples of commonly used pain scales. Other examples include pictures of faces (from happy and relaxed to sad and frowning) or colors from bright blue (no pain) to bright red (terrible pain).

they will be labeled as an addict if they ask for analgesics. **Addiction** is a condition of seeking drugs habitually (other than for a medical purpose) and of not being able to give them up without adverse effects.

clinicalALERT

When opioids are used as recommended for pain treatment, there is little to no risk of addiction.

Patients may think that health care providers know when they are experiencing pain. Some patients may deny pain as part of an attempt to deny that anything is wrong with them. Other patients believe that "as-needed" medications are given only if their pain rating is high.

The nurse should not assume that a sleeping patient is without pain. Pain is physically exhausting. Unrelieved pain leaves patients fatigued. Sometimes patients sleep out of fatigue rather than because they are pain free.

Behavioral cues are also essential for assessing pain intensity in patients with advanced dementia (unable to respond to simple yes-or-no questions) or who are nonverbal.

ClinicalALERT

The Pain Assessment in Advanced Dementia (PAINAD) scale uses five behavioral indicators of pain:
- Breathing
- Negative vocalization
- Facial expression
- Body language
- Consolability

BOX 8-3   MISCONCEPTIONS ABOUT PAIN MANAGEMENT

MISCONCEPTION	CORRECTION
People who frequently ask for opioid pain medications are addicted.	Addiction from opioids is rare. If the patient is asking for pain medication, pain relief is probably inadequate.
It is best to wait until a patient has pain before giving medication.	Anticipating pain and offering pain relief ahead of time can significantly lessen the pain.
Patient is a "clock watcher," asking for analgesics before the specified due time.	Sometimes analgesics are ordered at intervals longer than their duration. Investigate to determine if a longer acting opioid is needed or the interval needs to be shortened.
It is dangerous to give an opioid and an NSAID at the same time.	The opioid acts on the CNS; the NSAID acts on the PNS. By combining them, the patient receives better pain management.
Opioid medication is too risky to be used in chronic pain.	Opioid analgesics are now recognized as an appropriate method for managing chronic pain unrelieved by other strategies.

Source: Data adapted from Pasero, C., & McCaffery, M. (2011). *Pain Assessment and Pharmacologic Management*. St. Louis, MO: Elsevier; LeMone, P., & Burke, K. M. (2011). *Medical–Surgical Nursing* (5th ed.). Upper Saddle River, NJ: Prentice Hall Health; and Adams, M. P., & Koch, R. W. (2010). *Pharmacology: Connections to Nursing Practice*. Upper Saddle River, NJ: Pearson.

DIAGNOSING, PLANNING, AND IMPLEMENTING

Numerous misconceptions about pain and its management exist among patients and health care providers. Before appropriate nursing care can be delivered, the nurse must explore these misconceptions and understand the facts. Box 8-3■ lists a few common misconceptions and their corrections.

Managing pain in the older adult requires special considerations. Box 8-4■ lists guidelines and rationale for managing pain in the older adult.

Acute Pain

Expected outcome: Will describe location, quality, pattern, intensity, and precipitating or relieving factors of pain.

Communicate belief in the patient's pain. Acknowledge the presence of pain, listen carefully to the description of pain, and act to help the patient manage the pain. *By conveying belief in the patient's pain, the nurse can reduce anxiety and possibly lessen pain.*

clinicalALERT

Do not assume the older patient or cognitively impaired patient cannot identify the intensity of pain.

- Discuss with the patient his or her desired comfort-function goal and any fears about proposed interventions. *Understanding the patient's goals and fears will help the nurse determine suitable pain relief methods.*
- Individualize the choice of medication, route, dose, and interval between doses. *Because each patient absorbs, metabolizes, and excretes medications differently, the nurse carefully selects an analgesic based on the patient's needs. When frequent injections are needed, consider the intravenous route.*
- Adjust the analgesic regimen by using a flow sheet (Figure 8-11■). The dose can be adjusted within prescribed limits according to the patient's response. Adjustments should be considered:
  - When the patient still feels most of his or her pain an hour after administration (dose is too low).
  - When dose causes significant side effects such as sedation and/or respiratory depression (dose is too high).
  - When most of the pain returns before the next scheduled dose (interval is too long). *The pain flow sheet records the effectiveness of each pain intervention. It is the nurse's role to inform the physician if the prescribed medication, route, dose, and interval do not meet the patient's needs.*
- Use a preventive approach. Administer pain analgesics at regular, scheduled intervals around the clock (ATC) when the patient's pain is expected for at least 12 of the next 24 hours. PRN (as-needed) administration is appropriate for unpredictable pain. It should be administered before the pain becomes severe and before painful procedures such as a dressing change or physical activities. *Preventive approaches allow patients to know that their pain needs will be met. They help reduce anxiety about the return of pain and may result in decreased doses, fewer side effects, and less time in pain. When analgesics are given ATC, the patient's physical activity may increase, lessening the potential for problems from immobility due to pain. Physical activity may increase, so problems caused by immobility can be avoided.*
- Use a multimodal analgesia approach by administering nonopioids and opioids as ordered. *Nonopioids act on the peripheral nervous system; opioids act on the CNS. Combining these medications improves pain relief and lowers the incidence of side effects.*
- Demonstrate use of self-administered PCA. *PCA allows patients more control over their pain relief.*
- Use complementary measures (e.g., relaxation, distraction) as appropriate. *Nondrug measures by the nurse or patient's family can provide pain relief with minimal risk to*

BOX 8-4   **FOCUS ON OLDER ADULTS**

Pain Management Guidelines

GUIDELINE	RATIONALE
■ Reduce initial opioid dose by 25% and then carefully titrate dose based on patient response.	■ Drug absorption, distribution, metabolism, and excretion decrease with age; therefore, monitor dosages carefully.
■ Avoid giving benzodiazepines such as diazepam (Valium) or lorazepam (Ativan).	■ They can alter cognition, increasing the risk for falls.
■ Use all NSAIDs and acetaminophen with caution and monitor for side effects.	■ Older adults have a higher risk for gastric and duodenal ulcers and bleeding. Acetaminophen can accumulate, causing liver toxicity.
■ Choose NSAIDs, for example, ibuprofen (Motrin) and naproxen (Naprosyn) for mild to moderate pain and morphine or hydromorphone for severe pain.	■ Their shorter half-lives will not accumulate and cause toxicity.
■ Avoid using meperidine or propoxyphene (Darvocet).	■ Both produce toxic metabolites with long half-lives, leading to toxicity.
■ Monitor closely for sedation, confusion, and respiratory depression with opioid use.	■ Decreased renal and liver clearance rates increase potential opioid side effects.
■ Monitor for altered voiding patterns and decreased urine output.	■ Older adults are prone to urinary retention.
■ Observe for nonverbal pain-behavior changes in cognitively impaired older adults.	■ Cognitively impaired older adults may be given antipsychotic drugs for aggressive behavior when the underlying problem is pain.
■ Assess frequently for signs of constipation.	■ Older adults are prone to constipation that is increased by opioids.
■ Assess the ability to self-administer pain medications safely.	■ Older adults may have short-term memory loss that may require assistance to take their medications.

the patient. *They should not be substituted for medications but rather combined with them.*

■ Provide comfort measures, such as changing positions, back massage, oral care, skin care, and changing bed linens. *Basic comfort measures for personal cleanliness, skin care, and mobility promote physical and emotional well-being.*

■ Avoid actions that increase pain, for example, jarring the bed or moving the patient too quickly out of bed. *By avoiding actions that increase pain, the nurse shows a caring attitude.*

■ Teach the patient to request pain medication before the pain becomes severe. *This strategy prevents the patient from experiencing highs and lows of pain relief.*

■ Use an equianalgesic dosage chart when changing doses or medications. *If the patient is receiving inadequate pain relief or is being switched from a parenteral to an oral route, an equianalgesic dosage chart helps the patient maintain adequate pain relief.*

■ Monitor effectiveness of pain relief measures at least every 2 hours and ATC. *Planned assessments prevent inconsistent pain relief for the patient.*

Chronic Pain

Expected outcome: Able to perform ADLs with use of analgesics and noninvasive methods of pain relief.

Chronic nonmalignant pain can occur throughout the body. This type of pain may accompany chronic diseases or occur as the result of an injury (e.g., low back pain). Chronic pain can significantly affect the patient's daily life, including the ability to work, maintain relationships, and enjoy life. Because chronic pain is prolonged, different interventions are used by the nurse.

■ Ask the patient to describe the pain and its effects on life style, roles, and relationships. *Pain is a stressor that may affect coping ability. Chronic pain can affect sleep quality, work performance, and personal relationships.*

■ Assess for signs of depression. *Patients with chronic pain may become depressed when they cannot follow a normal daily routine.*

■ Ask the patient to keep a diary of pain ratings, precipitating events, medications, and treatments that help to relieve pain. *Maintaining a diary assists health care providers to plan pain management strategies.*

■ Administer nonopioids, opioids, and adjuvant pain medications ATC and as ordered. When possible, the oral or transdermal routes should be used. *The type of chronic pain determines the combination of analgesics needed by the patient. Giving analgesics ATC helps to maintain pain within an acceptable range. As-needed medications may be required for breakthrough pain.*

PAIN FLOWSHEET

Client: Mrs. J   **Age:** 55   **Physician:** Dr. Masson   **Date:** [date]

Diagnosis: [date] Abdominal hysterectomy

Pain rating scale: 0 to 10 (0 = no pain, 10 = worst pain)

Analgasic ordered: Morphine 6-12 mg. IM q 4 hours

Date and Time	Pain rating	Analgesic	Vital signs R, P, BP	Level of arousal	Other: Nausea and vomiting, bowel function	Initials
[date] 14:00	10	MS 10 mg. IM	24, 90, 138/88	Awake, "I have sharp pain in my stomach. It really hurts to move."	Denies nausea and vomiting. No bowel tones since returning from surgery at 1300.	KC
14:30	8		22			KC
15:00	4		20	"The pain is much less than before."		KC
16:30	4		18	"Pain is about the same."		EB
17:45	7		20	"The pain is coming back."	No nausea or vomiting.	EB
18:10	8	MS 10 mg. IM	20, 88, 130/82	"The pain isn't quite as bad as before, but it still hurts a lot."		EB
18:30	8		20	"Pain is a little less."		EB

Figure 8-11. ■ A flow sheet for nursing documentation of pain management.

clinicalALERT

Older patients who take opioid analgesics for chronic pain have an increased risk for falls from decreased alertness or dizziness.

■ Teach patients not to crush, break, or chew controlled-release oral opioid drugs such as MS Contin. *Crushing, breaking, or chewing controlled-release drugs may lead to overdose.*

■ Teach the patient and family about the nature of chronic pain, various pain relief methods, and how to manage side effects of prescribed medications. *Inclusion of the family enables them to support the patient better. Many analgesics cause side effects that may limit the patient's willingness to continue therapy. Most side effects can be managed, allowing the patient continued use of effective analgesics.*

■ Encourage the patient to use complementary pain management methods, such as relaxation, distraction, and massage. *These techniques are useful in managing chronic pain.*

■ Encourage the patient to plan activities around periods of greatest comfort. *Patients may be able to perform their daily activities and enjoy social interactions when pain is within an acceptable range.*

■ Consult with the health care team about referral to an interprofessional pain management facility. *Patients with unresolved pain problems may need more advanced pain management techniques or referral to a pain clinic.*

Cancer Pain

Patients with cancer usually do not develop pain until the later stages of the disease. Their pain may be acute or chronic. Cancer-related pain requires many different approaches.

Expected outcome: Will use a variety of pain management strategies to reach pain comfort-function goal.

■ Discuss goals of care with the patient. *These goals may include the amount of pain the patient will tolerate in order to participate in activities of daily living. The nurse needs to understand these goals and help the patient meet them.*

- Encourage the patient and family to express concerns about opioid use. *Fears of addiction may prevent the patient from obtaining adequate pain relief.*

- Administer a combination of nonopioid, opioid, and adjuvant analgesics according to evidence-based pain medication recommendations (Figure 8-12■). *As cancer pain becomes more severe, more potent analgesics are used progressively until the cancer pain is relieved or at least reduced to an acceptable level.*

- Give analgesics ATC. *Patients with cancer pain usually have persistent pain. Consistent administration should prevent peaks and valleys of pain relief.*

- Have fast-acting analgesics available for breakthrough pain. *As cancer progresses, patients will experience breakthrough pain. They need fast-acting analgesics to control it.*

- Give analgesics orally. *The oral route is safe and easy to administer. When patients cannot take their medications orally, the transdermal, rectal, intravenous, and intraspinal routes should be used.*

clinicalALERT

For patients with cancer, who need frequent analgesic doses, avoid the IM route because it is painful.

- Teach the patient about **opioid tolerance**—the loss of opioid effectiveness with chronic use. For the patient to receive the same amount of pain relief, increased doses are required. *Patients need to understand why they need increased doses.*

- Aggressively treat adverse effects of analgesics (see the following nursing diagnosis). *Sedation, respiratory*

depression, nausea, and constipation are the common adverse effects of opioids.

- Add noninvasive pain management strategies, such as massage, aromatherapy, or relaxation. *Noninvasive strategies promote short-term psychologic well-being in patients with cancer pain.*

- Refer to support groups and pastoral counseling. *Patients and families need emotional and spiritual resources.*

Risk for Injury: Side Effects of Opioid Analgesics

Expected outcome: Will remain free from injury related to side effects of opioid use.

The four main side effects of opioid therapy are sedation, respiratory depression, constipation, and nausea and vomiting. Usually, side effects develop at the beginning of opioid therapy. Only sedation and respiratory depression may subside with long-term use.

- *Sedation* often occurs at the start of opioid therapy or when the dose is increased. This results from opioids acting on the CNS. Assess the patient's sedation level every hour for the first 12 hours and then every 2 hours for the next 12 hours. *Sedation precedes respiratory depression. Monitor the patient frequently during initial opioid therapy or dosage increases.*

- If pain relief is adequate and sedation is clinically significant, consult with the physician about reducing the dose. *The goal is to decrease sedation, yet maintain pain relief. Often decreasing the dose by 25% to 50% will increase the patient's level of alertness.*

- Add a mild stimulant such as caffeine during the day or discuss with the physician about ordering methylphenidate (Ritalin), a CNS stimulant. *Stimulants may offset the opioid sedative effects.*

- *Respiratory depression.* All opioid analgesics may cause respiratory depression. Monitor respiratory rate and depth and oxygen saturation every hour for the first 12 hours at the beginning of opioid therapy or after increasing dosage and then every 2 hours for the next 12 hours. Listen to the sound of the patient's respiration. *Patients are at risk for respiratory depression when they start on opioids or dosage is increased. Snoring indicates airway obstruction. If snoring occurs, first place the patient in an upright position. If the snoring is severe, the patient may need further evaluation for obstructive sleep apnea (OSA).*

clinicalALERT

Respiratory depression is clinically significant when there is a decrease in the rate and depth of respirations from the patient's baseline.

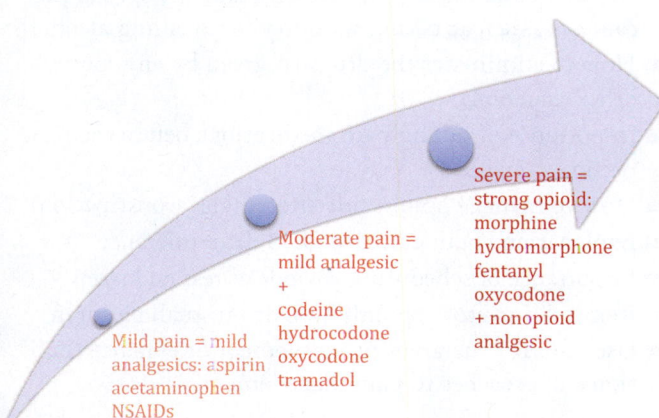

Mild pain = mild analgesics: aspirin acetaminophen NSAIDs

Moderate pain = mild analgesic + codeine hydrocodone oxycodone tramadol

Severe pain = strong opioid: morphine hydromorphone fentanyl oxycodone + nonopioid analgesic

Figure 8-12. ■ As pain level increases, a combination of analgesics must be administered to help manage pain.

- Encourage the patient to take deep breaths every 15 to 30 minutes and use incentive spirometry. *These measures help counteract respiratory depression.*

- When the patient is unresponsive to physical stimulation, has shallow respirations, and has a respiratory rate of less than 8 breaths per minute with pinpoint pupils, naloxone (Narcan) may be required. *Naloxone, an opioid antagonist, reverses the effects of opioids. Give only enough naloxone to reverse respiratory depression. Excess naloxone can cause acute withdrawal and lack of pain relief. Opioids often last longer than naloxone; therefore, continue to monitor for sedation and respiratory depression.*

- *Constipation* is the most common side effect of opioids. Opioids decrease gastric emptying and peristalsis, increasing the patient's risk for constipation. Auscultate the abdomen for presence of bowel tones. *Reduced bowel tones mean decreased peristalsis.*

- Encourage at least eight glasses of water per day and a diet high in bulk and fiber such as beans, carrots, bran cereals and breads, and prunes. *Increased fluid intake promotes moist, soft stool. The high-fiber diet improves stool consistency and promotes passage through the colon.*

- Promote activity and exercise as tolerated. *Increased movement stimulates peristalsis.*

- Give a stool softener and peristaltic stimulant such as docusate and senna (Senokot-S) daily during opioid therapy. *An aggressive bowel regimen is needed to prevent and treat opioid-induced constipation.*

- Monitor the patient's bowel pattern carefully. *Monitoring is essential to prevent further complications of constipation such as ileus, fecal impaction, and obstruction.*

- *Nausea and vomiting* may occur during the beginning of opioid therapy but usually decrease with longer use. They are caused by the stimulation of a trigger zone in the brain and slowed gastric motility. Administer drugs such as ondansetron (Zofran), dexamethasone (Decadron), or prochlorperazine (Compazine). *These medications are the most effective in decreasing nausea and vomiting.*

- Provide a clean-smelling environment and frequent oral care. *Reducing unpleasant odors decreases the potential for nausea. Oral care helps to decrease bad tastes in the mouth.*

- Have the patient try to eat dry toast or crackers. *Dry foods tend to decrease nausea.*

- If nausea continues from opioid use, add a nonopioid or adjuvant medication before reducing opioid dose. *To maintain patient's pain relief while decreasing nausea, add other pain medications.*

- For chronic nausea with advanced cancer, give metoclopramide (Reglan). *This medication increases gastric motility.*

MANAGING NURSING CARE

As appropriate and allowed by the designated duties and responsibilities of assistive personnel, the nurse may delegate nursing care activities such as measuring vital signs, providing oral and skin care, assisting with meals and fluid intake, and helping with activities of daily living. Before assigning tasks such as obtaining vital signs, ensure assistive personnel understand the importance of reporting decreased respiratory rate and altered level of consciousness to the nurse.

EVALUATING

Evaluation focuses on determining the effectiveness of pain management strategies. The nurse collects data on the patient's report of pain relief, physical responses, and emotional behaviors.

DOCUMENTING

The nurse documents subjective and objective assessment findings related to the patient's pain. Document the patient's pain relief in response to pain medications and nonpharmacologic measures. Be sure to include effectiveness of interventions for managing opioid side effects. Record patient teaching about pain medications and nonpharmacologic pain management strategies.

CONTINUITY OF CARE

Patients can learn to manage most types of pain at home. The nurse should explain about expected pain, when it will happen, what it feels like, and what to do to help oneself during the event. Education should decrease anxiety about the unknown and provide the patient with a means of controlling the pain.

All instructions should be in writing so that the patient can take them home. The following teaching points should be included for the patient and family:

- Specific drugs, including the frequency, potential side effects, possible drug interactions, and any special precautions, such as taking with food or avoiding alcohol
- How to administer the drugs (if given by any route other than oral)
- Importance of taking pain medications before the pain becomes severe
- How to manage opioid side effects (e.g., constipation)
- Explanation about addiction and drug tolerance
- Importance of scheduling periods of rest and sleep
- Reminder to store opioids away from small children
- Use of CAM therapies to supplement or enhance traditional approaches to pain management

In addition, suggest the following resources: pain clinics, community support groups, American Cancer Society, and American Pain Society.

NURSING CARE PLAN
Patient With Chronic Pain

Susan Akers, 37 years old, is being seen at an outpatient clinic for a 3-year history of neck and shoulder pain. She believes the pain is caused by lifting heavy objects at work, but she says now household chores make it worse. She misses work about three times a month from her pain. About twice a month the pain becomes so intense that she needs injections for pain at the local emergency department. She takes two Percocet-5 tablets, usually two to three times a day, without complete relief.

Assessment

Ms. Akers rates her pain during an acute episode as a 7 on a 0–10 scale. When she raises her arms above shoulder level, she feels sharp pain. The pain never really goes away, but it does decrease when she rests her arm.

Nursing Diagnosis

The main nursing diagnosis for Ms. Akers is:

- *Chronic pain* related to muscle inflammation

Expected Outcomes

The expected outcomes for the plan of care are that Ms. Akers will:

- Return for follow-up visits with a journal of activities and pain experiences.
- After 3 to 5 days on regularly scheduled doses of analgesics, report a decrease in pain from 7 to 3–4 on a 0–10 scale.
- Decrease number of absences from work.
- Modify activities at work and at home, especially when pain is intense.

Planning and Implementation

The following interventions are implemented for Ms. Akers:

- Encourage discussion of pain, and acknowledge belief in Ms. Akers's report of pain.

- Consult with a physician for an appropriate NSAID analgesic with minimum side effects.
- For episodes of acute pain, take opioid analgesics as soon as the pain begins. Take opioids and NSAIDs at regular intervals.
- Teach Ms. Akers relaxation and distraction techniques.
- Discuss with Ms. Akers and her children ways for dividing the household tasks among everyone.

Evaluation

Ms. Akers reports for scheduled follow-up visits with a completed journal. She reports that the oral opioids have relieved her pain and that within 3 weeks of starting the NSAID, her pain has decreased to 2–3 on a 0–10 scale. She says she has been reassigned to a position that requires no lifting and that her children are helping with the household tasks. She has missed only one day of work in the last 3 months.

Critical Thinking in the Nursing Process

1. Ms. Akers asks you how often she should take her pain medications. You tell her to (a) take them on a regular basis or (b) wait until she experiences pain. Which action would you choose, and why?
2. If Ms. Akers experienced acute pain, what assessment findings would the nurse expect to see?
3. What suggestions should the nurse give to Ms. Akers for treating constipation?

Note: Discussion of Critical Thinking questions appears on the companion website.

Note: The references and resources for all chapters have been compiled at the back of the book.

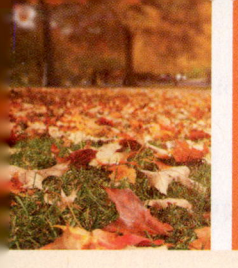
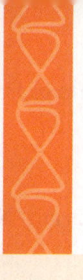

Chapter Review

KEY POINTS

- **Concept.** Pain can be classified in many ways such as acute pain (postoperative pain), cancer pain, and chronic pain (osteoarthritis pain). Assisting patients to manage pain often requires analgesic medications such as nonopioids or opioids and nonpharmacologic measures such as biofeedback or relaxation techniques.
- **Concept:** Pain is transmitted by the peripheral and central nervous systems and is perceived in the CNS. Pain impulses are conducted through the four steps of transduction, transmission, perception, and modulation.
- Acute pain is usually a short-term event, whereas chronic pain is prolonged. Cancer pain may result from the cancer or be associated with chemotherapy or radiation therapy. Neuropathic pain is caused by damage to the central or peripheral nervous system.
- Culture, patient's emotional state, past experiences with pain, the underlying cause, and the meaning of the painful experience can affect pain perception and behavior.
- Tolerance can develop with long-term use of opioids, necessitating larger doses of medication to achieve the same effect.
- **Concept:** Opioid analgesics work at the central nervous system level; nonopioid analgesics work at the peripheral nervous system level. By using opioids and nonopioids together, different pain mechanisms are targeted to increase pain medication effectiveness. Often this allows lower doses of each drug and fewer side effects.
- Pharmacologic pain management includes nonopioids, opioids, and adjuvant analgesics. Surgical procedures such as cordotomy and neurectomy and nonsurgical methods such as TENS can be used to manage pain. Complementary therapies include biofeedback, distraction, massage, and relaxation.

- Nonopioids such as NSAIDs are used to manage mild to moderate pain. Frequently used opioids to manage moderate to severe pain include morphine, hydromorphone, hydrocodone, and oxycodone.
- Adjuvant analgesics such as anticonvulsants and antidepressants are used to manage chronic, cancer, and neuropathic pain.
- **Concept:** Effective pain management requires an individualized and preventative approach. It is essential for the nurse to assess the patient's pain, work collaboratively with the physician in implementing appropriate pain-reducing methods, evaluate effectiveness of the intervention, and advocate for the patient.
- Assessment tools such as the McGill Pain Questionnaire are useful in identifying new or ongoing pain problems. Assessment should include the location, intensity, and quality of the pain; its onset, duration, and timing; factors that aggravate or relieve the pain; and measures taken to treat the pain or its cause. The nurse must listen to the patient's description of his or her pain.
- Pain intensity can be assessed by the visual analog, numeric, or simple descriptive pain rating scale. The Wong–Baker Faces Pain Rating Scale is used for patients who do not understand English or numbers. For patients with advanced dementia who are nonverbal, the nurse can use the Pain Assessment in Advanced Dementia (PAINAD) scale.
- For patients receiving opioids the nurse must not only monitor for side effects of sedation, respiratory depression, nausea, and constipation but also implement strategies to minimize these side effects.

PEARSON NURSING STUDENT RESOURCES

Find additional materials at **nursing.pearsonhighered.com**.

Clinical Reasoning Care Map

Caring for a Patient With Acute Pain
NCLEX-PN® Focus Area: Physiologic Adaptation

Case Study: Mrs. Bruski, 98 years old, has returned to her room after a colon resection. Four hours later, the nurse enters Mrs. Bruski's room and finds her lying on her right side with her eyes closed. When the nurse asks about her pain, she says, "It hurts right here," as she points to her lower abdomen. She describes the pain as dull and rates it at a 7 on a 0–10 scale. She complains of feeling thirsty and cold. She says, "I just wish I could sleep. I feel so tired."

Nursing Diagnosis: Acute Pain

COLLECT DATA

Subjective	Objective
_____	_____
_____	_____
_____	_____
_____	_____
_____	_____
_____	_____

Does this present a threat to the patient's safety?

If yes, priority intervention to address the threat:

_____

Nursing Care

_____
_____
_____
_____
_____
_____
_____

Interprofessional team members to include when planning care:

_____
_____

How would you document this?_____

_____
_____

Data Collected
(use only those that apply)

- Says she feels cold
- Pulse 100
- Dull pain in lower abdomen
- Temperature 99°F
- "It hurts right here."
- Blood pressure 150/92
- Rates pain at a 7
- Lying on her right side with eyes closed
- Complains of being thirsty
- "I'm tired. I wish I could sleep."

Nursing Interventions (use only those that apply; list in priority order)

- Teach Mrs. Bruski to use the incentive spirometer.
- Give acetaminophen (Tylenol) 650 mg PO q 4 hours PRN.
- Offer a back massage at HS.
- Give morphine sulfate 8 mg IM q 4 hours PRN.
- Listen attentively to Mrs. Bruski.
- Teach Mrs. Bruski a relaxation technique.

Compare your answers and documentation to those provided on the companion website.

NCLEX-PN® Exam Preparation

1 Which one of the following patients has the greatest risk of developing pain tolerance?

1. Patient who receives morphine after a hip replacement
2. Patient who takes codeine for chronic low back pain
3. Patient who uses a PCA pump after major abdominal surgery
4. Patient who takes antidepressants for neuropathic pain

2 A patient is admitted to the hospital with complaints of abdominal pain that radiates to the left shoulder. What type of pain is this patient experiencing?

1. Referred pain
2. Deep somatic pain
3. Visceral pain
4. Cutaneous somatic pain

3 Which of the following complementary approaches would be appropriate for a patient hospitalized with a malignant brain tumor and reports a pain rating of 4 out of 10? **Select all that apply**.

1. Offer a back and shoulder massage.
2. Have the patient keep a diary of pain ratings and interventions.
3. Encourage the patient to use guided imagery.
4. Give hydromorphone (Dilaudid).
5. Teach the patient muscle relaxation techniques.
6. Administer controlled-release morphine such as MS Contin.

4 A patient has a below-the-knee amputation of the right leg. The patient reports pain in the right foot and requests pain medication. What is the appropriate nursing intervention?

1. Report the symptoms to the charge nurse.
2. Remind the patient that the foot has been amputated.
3. Administer pain medication.
4. Elevate the patient's right stump.

5 For a patient with a history of gastric ulcer, which of the following analgesics should the patient avoid?

1. Ibuprofen (Motrin)
2. Acetaminophen (Tylenol)
3. Meperidine (Demerol)
4. Codeine sulfate (Codeine)

6 A patient complains of surgical incision pain. To assess the severity of the patient's pain, which of the following would be most effective?

1. Observe the patient's facial expressions.
2. Assess the patient's vital signs.
3. Ask if the pain is mild, moderate, or severe.
4. Ask the patient to describe the pain using a scale of 0 to 10.

7 A nurse is caring for a Japanese American patient, age 75, after surgery. Which of the following points should the nurse consider when assessing this patient's pain?

1. All cultures respond to pain in the same way.
2. Older adults tend to underreport pain.
3. Patients having acute pain tend to be less anxious.
4. It is important to use a visual pain scale in an older adult patient.

8 A patient receives morphine sulfate 10 mg intravenously for severe abdominal pain. Thirty minutes later the patient is unresponsive to physical stimulation with shallow breathing and a respiratory rate of 8. What intervention should the nurse implement first?

1. Encourage patient to take deep breaths.
2. Ask the health care provider for an NSAID order.
3. Notify the patient's health care provider.
4. Administer naloxone (Narcan).

9 A patient is prescribed acetaminophen with hydrocodone (Vicodin) to manage pain from a fractured wrist. What teaching point should the nurse reinforce to this patient for home care?

1. Discontinue the medication after 1 week.
2. Avoid alcohol while taking this medication.
3. Take with meals three times a day.
4. Take additional acetaminophen if the pain is unrelieved.

10 A patient, age 67, is started on morphine sulfate via PCA pump for pain. What is the highest priority nursing intervention for this patient?

1. Assess bowel sounds every 4 hours.
2. Increase fluids to 1,500 mL/day.
3. Assess respiratory rate every 1 to 2 hours.
4. Monitor for manifestations of gastrointestinal bleeding.

Answers and rationales for Review Questions appear in Appendix I.

CULTURAL CARE STRATEGIES

RESPONDING TO PAIN AS A CROSS-CULTURAL VARIABLE

Mr. Chu, a 48-year-old Chinese patient, refused pain medication after surgery. When asked by the nurse about whether he needed pain medication, he said his discomfort was bearable and he could survive without any medication. Later, the nurse noticed he was restless and perspiring. Again, the nurse offered pain medication. Again, he refused, saying her responsibilities were far more important than his discomfort and he did not want to impose. In the Chinese culture the needs of the group are more important than individual needs. Chinese individuals are taught it is polite to say no the first time an offer is extended. The nurse said, "Mr. Chu, it will help you recover sooner if you are able to relax. I have time to get it for you and would like to do that. If I bring you some medication, will you take it?" Mr. Chu smiled, looked relieved, and said, "Yes, you are very kind."

Pain is a universal experience of human existence, but it is not a concrete entity. McCaffery and Pasero (2011) stated: "Pain is whatever the experiencing person says it is, existing whenever the experiencing person says it does." Today, this phrase is often quoted when holistic pain management is discussed.

Holistic pain management involves consideration of the physical, emotional, social, and spiritual components of pain. It also includes consideration of the patient in the context of family, culture, past experiences, and the meaning of the event being experienced (Giger, 2013). Culture shapes beliefs and behaviors related to pain and influences the way pain is expressed.

Affective Response to Pain

Cultural responses to pain are varied, ranging from stoic to emotional. Stoic patients are those who tend to "grin and bear it" by refusing pain relief measures. Emotional people are more likely to verbalize their feelings of pain out loud. They may moan and describe their pain as unbearable. An African American patient may react to a physical injury stoically, saying, "It does not hurt much," whereas a Hispanic patient may react to the same injury very demonstratively. In the Jewish culture, a family member, rather than the patient, may report the patient's pain (Giger, 2013).

Communication of Pain

Words used to describe symptoms differ among cultures. A nurse may understand what is said by a patient from the same cultural background, but have less understanding of a patient from another culture who uses different terms, is less fluent in English, or speaks another language.

Nonverbal communication also differs among cultures. A patient may feel that he or she is communicating the level of pain nonverbally and does not need to describe it. However, the nurse may not recognize culturally unique communications of pain (Giger, 2013).

Biologic Variations and Cultural Reaction to Pain

People within cultural groups may differ biologically in their reaction to pain and to pain medication. For example, when White patients and Chinese patients are compared for reactions to analgesics, Chinese patients reported more pain but greater incidence of drug-induced gastrointestinal effects (Aschenbrenner & Venable, 2009).

Nursing Implications

- *Assess individuals in pain from a holistic and cultural perspective.* A "meaning-centered" approach must be used when assessing the patient in pain. This approach includes an assessment not only of what the patient is saying verbally and nonverbally, but also of personal meanings that pain may have for that person.
- *Avoid reacting judgmentally to the patient who is demonstrative about pain.* When a patient's reaction to pain appears excessive, the nurse should appreciate that the behavior may be customary in the patient's culture and that any other behavior would be considered abnormal. The nurse should react with sensitivity and provide emotional support.
- *Provide appropriate care to promote health in a patient who may have a stoic reaction to pain.* When the patient is stoic, the nurse may need to be more directive in controlling pain. The nurse should assess for physiologic symptoms of pain and tell the patient why intervention will help recovery.
- *Recognize differences in responses to pain among health team members.* If team members are stoic themselves, they may be less responsive to complaints of pain by patients.

Self-Reflection Questions

1. What is your attitude toward pain—your own and others'?

2. How do you think your family has shaped your attitude toward pain?

3. How do you react when you are around people who have different reactions to pain than yours?

CHAPTER 9
Caring for Patients With Inflammation and Infection

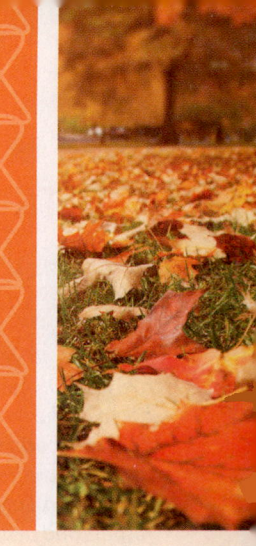

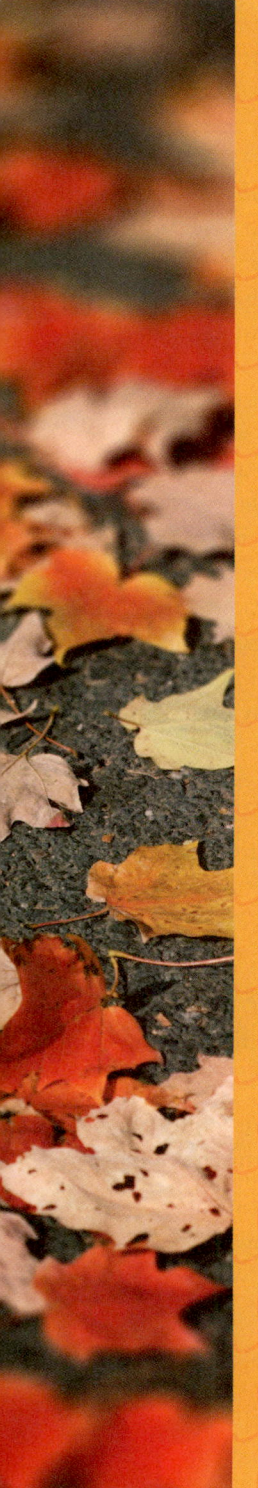

BRIEF OUTLINE

Inflammation
Pathophysiology
Collaborative Care
Nursing Care

Infection
Pathophysiology
Collaborative Care
Nursing Care

APPLIED LEARNING OUTCOMES

After completing this chapter, you will be able to:

1. Differentiate between the local and systemic manifestations of acute inflammation.
2. Describe diagnostic tests used to identify inflammation and infection.
3. Explain treatments and implement nursing actions to manage patients with inflammation.
4. Review the mechanisms by which infection occurs and progresses.
5. Identify common health care–associated (nosocomial) infections.
6. Explain the types and spread of common multidrug-resistant organisms, emerging infectious diseases, and biologic threats.
7. Explain age-related changes and other factors in older adults that increase their risk for infection, and apply nursing implications for these infections.
8. Implement common antimicrobial medications, nursing implications, and patient teaching guidelines for patients with infectious diseases.
9. Apply the guidelines for Standard and Transmission-Based Precautions to patients with infectious diseases.
10. Use the nursing process to collect data, establish outcomes, provide individualized care, and evaluate responses for patients with inflammation and infections.

KEY TERMS

The key terms are defined on the pages listed below.

abscesses, 176
anabolism, 179
antibiotics, 190
bactericidal, 190
bacteriostatic, 190
broad-spectrum antibiotics, 190
carriers, 184
catabolism, 179
cellulitis, 176
chain of infection, 182

colonization, 184
endogenous pyrogens, 176
fistula, 176
health care–associated infections, 185
immunosuppression, 182
incision and drainage, 176
infection, 182

infectious disease, 184
inflammation, 175
invasiveness, 183
leukocytosis, 176
leukopenia, 177
lymphadenopathy, 176
macrophages, 175
mutation, 185
narrow-spectrum antibiotics, 190

pathogens, 183
phagocytosis, 175
prophylactic, 190
Standard Precautions, 194
superinfection, 190
Transmission-Based Precautions, 194
virulence, 183

SPECIAL FEATURES

NURSING CARE PLAN: Patient With MRSA Infection, 197
CLINICAL REASONING CARE MAP: Caring for a Patient Exposed to *Staphylococcus aureus*, 200

In recent years, more multidrug-resistant organisms (MDROs), such as community-acquired and hospital-acquired methicillin-resistant *Staphylococcus aureus*, have emerged. It is important to understand local and systemic inflammation and the infectious disease process in order to provide effective nursing care. This foundation can help the nurse teach patients and families to follow recommended treatments, to promote and maintain health, and to prevent disease.

Inflammation

> **Key Concept** Inflammation is the body's protective response when injured by factors such as abrasions, chemicals, pathogenic organisms, overuse, or extreme temperatures. While the acute inflammatory response is usually short term; chronic inflammation is often long term.

Inflammation is a "nonspecific" response to an injury, meaning the same sequence of events occurs regardless of the cause. Inflammation brings fluid, dissolved substances, and blood cells into the interstitial tissues where an injury has occurred. Its purpose is to destroy the harmful agent, limit spread to other tissues, and begin the healing process. Inflammation develops as soon as one or more harmful invaders injure the body's cells.

PATHOPHYSIOLOGY

Normally, the skin and mucous membranes act as the body's first line of defense, preventing an invasion by external organisms. Mucous membranes lining the inner surfaces of the body trap microorganisms and other foreign substances. These foreign elements are removed by other protective mechanisms, such as ciliary movement in the respiratory tract or the washing action of tears and urine. Many body fluids contain bactericidal substances that provide barrier protection. These include acid in the gastric fluid and lysosomes in tears, nasal secretions, and saliva.

External or internal agents can destroy the body's defense mechanisms and trigger the inflammatory process. Inflammation can be caused by the following factors:

- Mechanical injuries, such as cuts or surgical incisions
- Physical damage, such as burns
- Chemical injury from toxins or poisons
- Microorganisms, such as bacteria, viruses, or fungi
- Extremes of heat or cold
- Immunologic responses, such as hypersensitivity reactions
- Ischemic damage or trauma, such as a stroke or myocardial infarction

The inflammatory response involves three steps:

1. *Vascular response.* Initially, the blood vessels around the injured area constrict briefly. Then they dilate as chemical mediators, such as histamine, bradykinin, and prostaglandins, are released. Blood flow to the injured area increases, causing redness and warmth. It also raises local *hydrostatic pressure* (pressure within the capillary), which causes capillaries to leak fluid into surrounding tissues. The increased permeability results in edema at the injury site and dilution of the organisms or toxins in the area. The chemical mediators and edema are responsible for pain and impaired function.

2. *Cellular response.* As blood flow increases to the injured tissues, white blood cells (WBCs) move into the area. *Neutrophils*, the first WBCs to respond, usually arrive within 90 minutes. The process by which neutrophils move from inside the capillary to the injured tissue is known as *diapedesis* (Figure 9-1■).

   Neutrophils and **macrophages** (large WBCs that develop from monocytes) ingest harmful bacteria and dead tissue cells in a process called **phagocytosis** (see Figure 9-2■). Once neutrophils have ingested their full capacity of bacteria, they die. The accumulation of dead neutrophils, dead bacteria, and tissue debris forms pus. Bacteria such as staphylococci, streptococci, and *Neisseria* often cause purulent drainage.

3. *Healing and tissue repair.* After neutrophils die, macrophages clean up the site for healing. In minor injuries, the inflammatory process and healing restore normal structure and function. If the injury is more

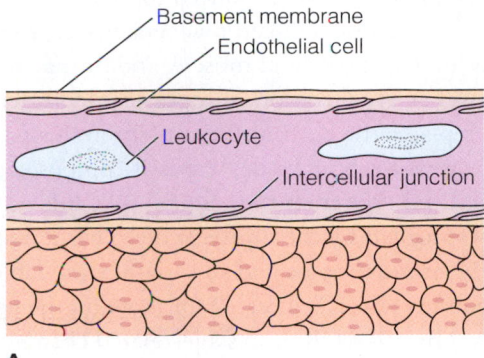

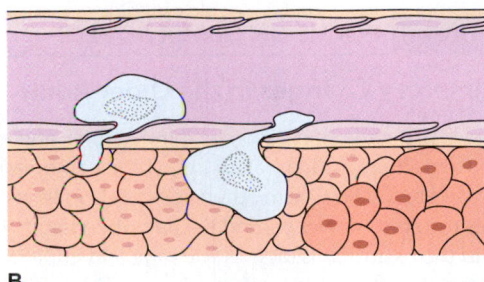

Figure 9-1. ■ (A) Leukocytes in the circulation. **(B)** Diapedesis, the process of leukocytes moving from inside the capillary to injured tissue.

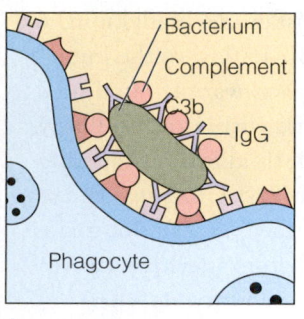
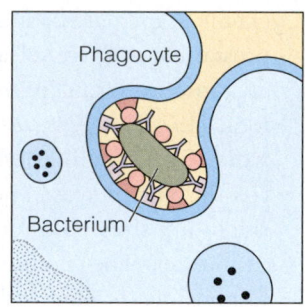
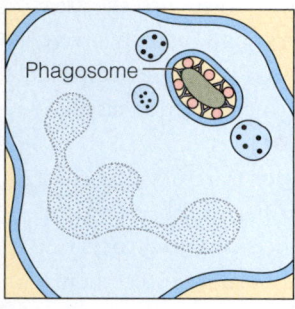
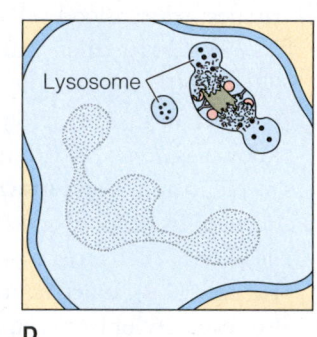

Figure 9-2. ■ The process of phagocytosis.(**A**) Opsonization coats the surface of the bacterium with immunoglobulin G (an antibody) and complement. (**B**) The bacterium is bound to and engulfed by the phagocyte. (**C**) The phagosome is ingested into the cytoplasm of the phagocyte. (**D**) Lysosomes fuse with the phagosome, releasing digestive enzymes and destroying the antigen.

extensive, new cells are produced to replace the functional tissue. Most cells can regenerate or reproduce (except for nerve, skeletal muscle, and cardiac muscle cells). When regeneration is impossible, collagen scar tissue replaces the destroyed tissue through a process known as *repair*. Scar tissue, which is composed of a different cell type from the original cell, fills in the empty space left by the injury. It often has less strength than the original tissue and so is more vulnerable to future injury. (See Chapter 10 for more on the healing process.) Box 9-1■ discusses age-related changes related to inflammation in the older adult.

BOX 9-1	FOCUS ON OLDER ADULTS

Inflammatory Changes in the Older Adult

In the older adult, the skin becomes thinner, drier, and more fragile, increasing the potential for injury. The combination of decreased blood flow from atherosclerosis and fewer macrophages results in slower wound healing. The phagocytic activity of the neutrophils lessens with age and impairs local resistance to infection. Older adults also take more medications that interfere with inflammation and healing. The cardinal signs of inflammation—redness, heat, and swelling—tend to be diminished or absent in older adults.

Acute Inflammation

Inflammation may be either acute or chronic. *Acute inflammation* is a short-term reaction of the body to any tissue damage. It is immediate and aimed at protecting the body and preventing further invasion or injury. It usually lasts less than 1 to 2 weeks. Once the harmful agent is removed, the inflammation subsides. Healing and tissue repair occur, and the body returns to normal or near-normal function. Acute inflammation produces local and systemic manifestations.

LOCAL MANIFESTATIONS Local manifestations develop at and around the site of injury. The degree of functional loss depends on the location and extent of the injury. Increased tissue damage results in more swelling, pain, and functional impairment. The amount of prostaglandin release determines whether pain is immediate or delayed.

Sometimes the inflammatory process does not end immediately with healing and tissue repair. **Cellulitis** is an infection that develops when inflammation spreads to the surrounding connective tissues. In other circumstances, pus develops and accumulates in pockets called **abscesses**. Abscesses are the body's way of walling off the infection. Abscesses may need to be artificially drained with a procedure called **incision and drainage** (I&D). Inflammation may also cause the formation of a **fistula** (an abnormal tubelike passage from one body cavity to another cavity). More extensive treatment is necessary to manage a fistula.

Patients with diabetes mellitus are at an increased risk for poor wound healing and cellulitis. High blood glucose levels alter phagocytic function and damage the capillaries. Both of these changes impair wound healing. Once a wound heals, it loses some of its original strength, so the diabetic patient has a higher incidence of leg and foot ulcers.

SYSTEMIC MANIFESTATIONS One systemic response to inflammation is enlargement of the lymph nodes (**lymphadenopathy**). This process occurs when bacteria, phagocytes, and destroyed lymph tissue accumulate in the affected lymph node. Enlarged lymph nodes are palpable in the groin, axillae, and neck (Figure 9-3■). Loss of appetite and fatigue develop as the body tries to conserve energy during the inflammatory process. **Leukocytosis** (increased WBC production) supports inflammation and phagocytosis.

Another systemic manifestation is fever. Fever inhibits the growth of many microorganisms and may increase tissue repair. Macrophages release chemicals called **endogenous pyrogens** that act on the temperature control center in the

memory**ALERT**

Lymphadenopathy is seen in nodes that are involved in local, regional, or systemic inflammation. When it occurs with metastatic cancer, the nodes are hard, enlarged, and immobile.

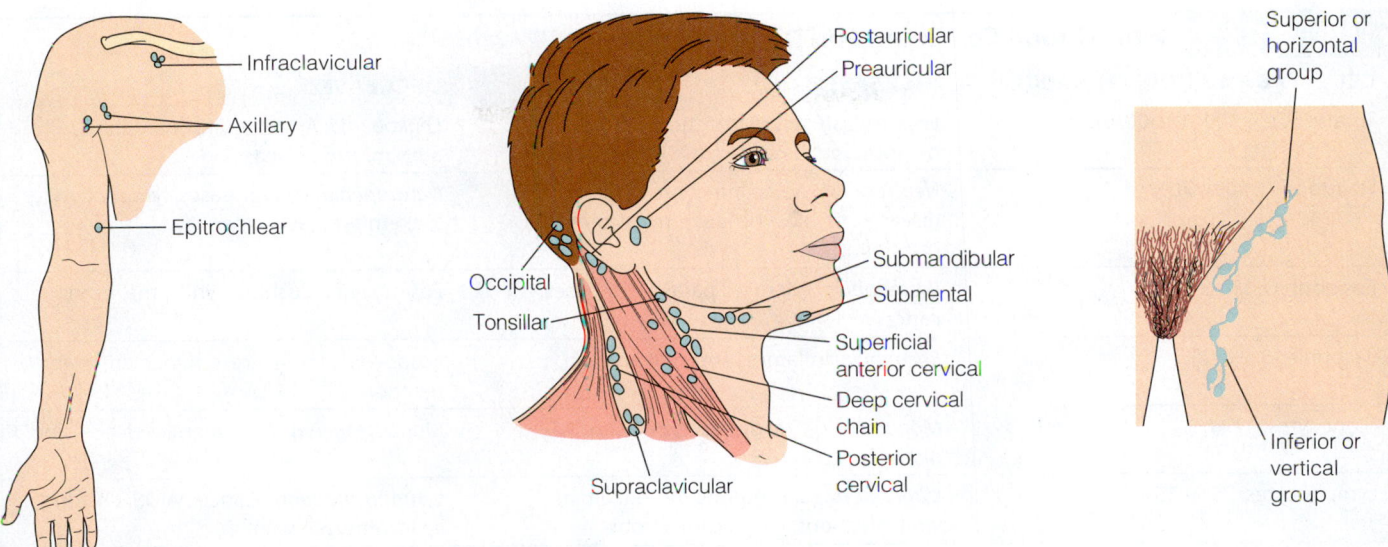

Figure 9-3. ■ Lymph nodes that may be assessed by palpation.

hypothalamus to elevate the temperature set point. As the temperature rises, the patient complains of being cold and shivers because the blood vessels constrict to conserve heat. Once the new set point is reached, the body attempts to cool itself by vasodilation and sweating. Fever should end when the microorganism is destroyed or antibiotics or antipyretics are given. Patients who are immunosuppressed may not experience a fever. Local and systemic manifestations of inflammation are summarized in Box 9-2■.

Chronic Inflammation

Chronic inflammation is slower in onset and lasts for weeks to months or years. It may develop when the acute inflammatory process has been ineffective in removing the offending agent. For example, in tuberculosis (TB), the mycobacteria resist phagocytosis. *Mycobacterium tuberculosis* can survive for many years and emerge only when the patient's immune system is compromised. Rheumatoid arthritis is another condition characterized by chronic inflammation. Inflammatory changes in the joints make joint movement very painful.

COLLABORATIVE CARE

Management of the patient with an inflammation focuses on promoting healing. Care is generally supportive, allowing the patient's own physiologic processes to remove

BOX 9-2	MANIFESTATIONS OF INFLAMMATION
Local Manifestations	**Systemic Manifestations**
■ Redness	■ Fever
■ Warmth	■ Tachycardia
■ Edema	■ Increased respiratory rate
■ Pain	■ Loss of appetite
■ Loss of function	■ Fatigue
	■ Enlarged lymph nodes
	■ WBC count > 10,000/mm^3

foreign matter and damaged cells. The patient is encouraged to rest, increase fluid intake, and eat a well-balanced nutritious diet. Antibiotics may be prescribed to help eliminate an infection.

Diagnostic Tests

Diagnostic tests can identify the source and extent of inflammation. The following diagnostic tests may be ordered:

■ *WBC count with differential* provides information about five leukocytes: neutrophils, eosinophils, basophils, monocytes, and lymphocytes. It measures the percentage of the total WBC made up of each type of leukocyte and provides clues about the type of inflammation (Table 9-1■). With inflammation, leukocytosis (a WBC count of greater than 10,000/mm^3) typically occurs. **Leukopenia** (a WBC count of less than 4,500 mm^3) may indicate a viral infection.

■ *Erythrocyte sedimentation rate* (ESR or sed rate) is a nonspecific test that can detect generalized inflammation.

TABLE 9-1	White Blood Cell Count and Differential	
CELL TYPE AND NORMAL VALUE	**INCREASED**	**DECREASED**
Total WBCs: 4,500–10,000/mm^3	*Leukocytosis:* Acute infection, tissue necrosis, leukemia, stress	*Leukopenia:* Anemia, viral infections, autoimmune diseases
Neutrophils: 50%–70%	*Neutrophilia:* Acute infection, inflammatory diseases, myelocytic leukemia, acute pancreatitis	*Neutropenia:* Viral diseases, lymphocytic leukemia, aplastic anemia
Eosinophils: 1%–3%	*Eosinophilia:* Allergies, parasitic diseases, cancer	*Eosinopenia:* Cushing syndrome, burns
Basophils: 0.4%–1%	*Basophilia:* Inflammation, leukemia	*Basopenia:* Acute stress, hypersensitivity reactions
Monocytes: 4%–6%	*Monocytosis:* Viral diseases, parasitic diseases	*Monocytopenia:* Bone marrow depression
Lymphocytes: 25%–35%	*Lymphocytosis:* Lymphocytic leukemia, viral infections, chronic infections	*Lymphocytopenia:* Cancer, AIDS, Cushing syndrome, renal failure

Source: Data from Kee, J. L. (2013). *Laboratory and Diagnostic Tests With Nursing Implications* (8th ed.). Upper Saddle River, NJ: Prentice Hall.

Normal levels are less than 20 mm/hr; significant increases may be seen in both acute and chronic inflammation.

■ *C-reactive protein* (CRP) is produced by the liver and excreted into the bloodstream during the acute inflammation. A positive result indicates acute or chronic inflammation.

■ *Cultures* of the blood and other body fluids are also ordered to determine whether infection is the cause of inflammation.

Medications

The medications prescribed to relieve the effects of inflammation include acetaminophen, antibiotics, anti-inflammatory agents, and corticosteroids.

Acetaminophen (Tylenol) may be given to reduce the fever and pain associated with inflammation. It does not have an anti-inflammatory effect. Acetaminophen decreases fever by acting directly on the hypothalamic heat-regulating center. It also works on the central nervous system to relieve pain sensation.

Antibiotics are used to treat infection and prevent infection from interfering with the healing process. If an infection is present, a culture and sensitivity (C&S) test is done to determine the most effective antibiotic. Anti-infective therapy is discussed in greater depth later in the chapter under infectious diseases.

Although inflammation is a beneficial process to prepare injured tissue for healing, it can have harmful effects. When inflammation presents a danger to the patient, anti-inflammatory medications are prescribed. Anti-inflammatory medications fall into four broad groups: salicylates, other nonsteroidal anti-inflammatory drugs (NSAIDs), cyclooxygenase-2 (COX-2) inhibitors, and corticosteroids.

Aspirin (acetylsalicylic acid, or ASA) and NSAIDs have a similar action. They produce anti-inflammatory, antipyretic, and analgesic effects. Patients receive varying degrees of relief with aspirin and different NSAIDs. Sometimes several different drugs are tried before the patient reports any relief. All of these medications can produce gastrointestinal (GI) irritation and the possibility of bleeding. COX-2 inhibitor blocks the production of prostaglandins and is used to manage pain and inflammation (see Table 9-2■).

clinicalALERT

Aspirin should not be given to children with chickenpox or influenza, because it can cause Reye syndrome, which is characterized by increased intracranial pressure and seizures.

Corticosteroid therapy is prescribed for acute hypersensitivity reactions, such as poison oak rash, or for inflammation unrelieved by aspirin or NSAIDs. Corticosteroids are also used to manage chronic inflammatory diseases such as arthritis, but they do not cure disease. They suppress the immune and inflammatory responses as well as delay healing; therefore, they should be used cautiously. Remember the following principles when administering corticosteroids:

■ Use the smallest effective dose.

■ An alternate-day dose schedule may decrease suppression of adrenal gland activity.

■ Never stop steroid therapy abruptly. Taper the dose gradually so that adrenal gland function can return to normal.

■ Harmful side effects increase with higher doses and prolonged therapy.

TABLE 9-2	Giving Medications Safely: Anti-Inflammatory Drugs		
CLASS/DRUGS	**PURPOSE**	**NURSING IMPLICATIONS**	**PATIENT TEACHING**
Salicylates			
■ Aspirin (acetylsalicylic acid)	Aspirin is a nonsteroidal anti-inflammatory drug with analgesic, antipyretic, and antiplatelet effects.	Do not give to patients with peptic ulcers, with gastritis, or taking anticoagulants. Give with food or full glass of water to prevent gastric irritation. Monitor for GI bleeding (black or bloody stools, vomiting blood) or tinnitus.	Take with food or full glass of water to avoid gastric irritation. Report GI bleeding (dark stools, vomiting of blood), unusual bleeding, bruising, or ringing in the ears. Do not use with other drugs containing aspirin.
Nonsteroidal anti-inflammatory drugs (NSAIDs)			
■ Fenoprofen calcium (Nalfon) ■ *Ibuprofen* (Motrin, Advil) ■ Indomethacin (Indocin) ■ Ketoprofen (Orudis) ■ Ketorolac (Toradol) ■ Naproxen (Aleve, Naprosyn) ■ Piroxicam (Feldene)	NSAIDs are used to reduce pain and inflammation.	Give cautiously to patients with a history of GI bleeding, peptic ulcers, or renal disease. Give with food or full glass of water. Monitor for GI bleeding, decreased urine output, or rash.	Take with food or full glass of water. Report GI bleeding (coffee-ground emesis or dark stool); rash; or changes in urination, vision, or hearing. *Do not take with alcohol, aspirin, or other NSAIDs.*
Cyclooxygenase-2 inhibitor			
■ Celecoxib (Celebrex)	COX-2 inhibitor is used to decrease pain and inflammation.	Assess patients for sulfa, aspirin, or NSAID allergy. Monitor for GI bleeding.	Take with full glass of water. Report GI bleeding. Do not take with warfarin (Coumadin) or aspirin.

Note: Medications identified in *italics* are among the 200 most frequently prescribed drugs in the United States.

The nursing implications of caring for a patient receiving corticosteroid medications are presented in Chapter 35 (see Table 35-3).

Wound Care

Minor wounds may require no more than gentle cleansing with soap and water. If wounds are more extensive, wound care may involve irrigations and debridement of the necrotic tissue. To prevent additional wound damage, the nurse cleanses the site with sterile normal saline or commercially prepared nontoxic wound cleansers such as Comfeel (Coloplast Corporation) or ClinisWound (Sage Laboratories). Hydrogen peroxide, povidone–iodine (Betadine), and sodium hypochlorite (Dakin solution) have a drying effect on the tissue. They can also inhibit the healing process. They should be used as a last resort. Because granulation tissue in a healing wound is fragile and bleeds easily, wound care must be performed gently. (See Chapter 10 for wound care.)

Nutrition

Inflammation and wound healing require adequate nutrition, blood supply, and oxygenation. *Malnutrition* makes the phagocytes ineffective so that there is a delayed inflammatory response. The macrophages cannot prepare the wound site for healing. If an infection develops, it interferes with effective wound healing. Oxygen is an essential element in healing. Arterial and venous disorders reduce available oxygen to peripheral tissues. Also, inadequate circulation cannot deliver sufficient nutrients or remove waste products. Without normal circulation, the injury site cannot heal properly.

The patient with an inflammation or wound requires a well-balanced diet to promote healing. Protein deficiency and weight loss increase the risk for poor wound healing and wound complications. Inflammation produces **catabolism**, a condition in which body tissues are broken down. During healing, the desired result is tissue building (**anabolism**). Diets low in calories and essential nutrients lead to catabolism and impaired healing.

Encourage the patient to eat a diet high in carbohydrates, protein, and vitamins. Carbohydrates are important to meet energy demands and to support leukocyte function. Protein is necessary for tissue healing and the production of antibodies and WBCs. Some vitamins and minerals are also important. Vitamin A fosters capillary formation and tissue growth. B-complex vitamins promote wound healing.

Vitamin C is necessary for collagen synthesis. Vitamin K is essential for blood clotting. Minerals, especially zinc, are important for tissue growth, skin integrity, and immune function.

Complementary Therapies

Aloe gel from the aloe vera plant is applied topically to treat minor skin irritations such as sunburns. Topical camphor is used to provide pain relief from cold sores and warts. To reduce the inflammation of bruises and strains, comfrey may be used topically.

NURSING CARE

PRIORITIZING NURSING CARE

The nursing care needs of the patient with an inflammatory process are related to the manifestations of inflammation and altered tissue integrity. Priority nursing diagnoses include Pain, Impaired Tissue Integrity, and Risk for Infection.

HEALTH PROMOTION

Health promotion activities to prevent inflammation focus on decreasing the risk for accidents and exposure to harmful agents that can result in injury. Discuss safety guidelines such as not drinking and driving, wearing a protective helmet when riding a bicycle, and using a seat belt in the car. Because most injuries occur at home, it is important to discuss ways to make the home safer.

ASSESSING

The nurse must collect assessment data to help determine the extent to which the inflammatory process is interfering with the patient's life. Data can also identify risk factors for complications and can determine the type of medical intervention (Box 9-3■).

IDENTIFYING POTENTIAL COMPLICATIONS

Inadequate nutrition, blood supply, and oxygenation can prolong inflammation and tissue healing. When inflamed tissue becomes infected, the inflammatory process is extended. Chronic diseases such as diabetes mellitus impair healing because the high blood glucose level impairs neutrophil action. Corticosteroid medications suppress the immune and inflammatory processes, delaying healing.

DIAGNOSING, PLANNING, AND IMPLEMENTING

When caring for a patient with inflammation, it is important for the nurse to monitor for increased temperature, pulse, and respiratory rate. It is essential to observe the color, consistency, and odor of any wound drainage and to report any abnormal findings.

BOX 9-3	ASSESSMENT

Patients With Inflammation

Subjective Data

Ask the patient about:

- General health and nutritional status.
- Any injuries; redness, warmth, swelling, or pain.
- Any drainage associated with current injury or previous procedure? Is drainage clear or purulent?
- Changes in appetite or energy level.
- Any frequent infections?
- Past or present use of anti-inflammatory medications, corticosteroids, or antibiotics.

Objective Data

- Measure vital signs: blood pressure, pulse, respirations, temperature.
- Observe the patient for fatigue and listlessness.
- Observe the ability to move injured area and indications of pain.
- Assess circulation to the affected area.
- Inspect the skin and surrounding area of injury for redness and warmth, purulent drainage, odor, and poor healing.
- Measure the size (depth and width) of wounds.
- Palpate the skin for the presence of edema.
- Palpate for enlarged lymph nodes.
- Monitor and report abnormal results of WBC count with differential, ESR, CRP.

Acute Pain

Along with redness, warmth, swelling, and impaired function, pain is one of the cardinal manifestations of inflammation. Depending on the cause, affected area, and degree of inflammation, pain may be acute and immobilizing or chronic.

Expected outcome:

Will report pain level on a scale of 0 to 10.

- Assess pain using a scale of 0 to 10; note the character, location, and duration of pain. *Only the patient can provide the most accurate intensity rating and description of the pain.*
- Give anti-inflammatory medications as prescribed. *These medications can lessen the pain resulting from inflammation.*
- Give mild analgesic medications as prescribed. *Although most analgesics do not reduce inflammation, they may decrease pain perception.*
- Encourage rest. *Strenuous activity or exercising an inflamed body part may increase discomfort and cause tissue damage.*
- Apply cold or heat therapy as ordered. Ensure there is a covering between the patient and the application. Remove ice pack or heating pad after 10 minutes and check the patient's skin. (For cold, note bluish color or a feeling of numbness; for heat, observe for redness.) *For an acute injury, cold reduces swelling and relieves pain. After the initial stage, heat increases blood flow to the affected tissue*

and promotes absorption of edema. It is important to monitor the patient's skin for untoward effects and to prevent injury to the skin.

clinical**ALERT**

Use heat or cold application cautiously in older adults who have fragile skin and are at risk for tissue injury.

■ Elevate the inflamed area if possible. *Elevation promotes venous return and reduces swelling.*

Impaired Tissue Integrity

Both an injury and the inflammatory response to it can lead to impaired skin integrity. The nurse must prevent any additional skin problems.

Expected outcome

Will maintain tissue integrity without any signs of skin breakdown.

■ Assess general health, nutrition status, and circulation to the affected area. *Poor general health or chronic diseases such as diabetes mellitus or renal failure interfere with healing. Adequate tissue perfusion is essential for healing.*

■ Clean the inflamed tissue gently; use water or normal saline only. *Soap and harsh cleansing agents can cause drying and further tissue damage.*

■ Balance rest with activity. *Rest decreases metabolic demands and promotes cell growth. Activity promotes oxygenation and circulation.*

■ Provide a well-balanced diet with adequate carbohydrates, protein, vitamins, and minerals. If the patient is NPO or unable to eat an adequate diet, suggest parenteral nutrition, between-meal supplements, or multivitamin supplements. *A well-balanced diet promotes immune function and healing and helps to prevent catabolism.*

Risk for Infection

The inflammatory response is meant to protect the patient against microorganisms. However, when the intact skin is broken (as in a healing wound) the risk for infection increases.

Expected outcome

Will remain free from infection.

■ Monitor the patient's temperature, pulse, respirations, and pain at least every 4 hours. *Increased vital signs usually indicate inflammation. A temperature of 101°F (38.3°C) or above indicates infection.*

■ Assess the wound for manifestations of infection such as purulent drainage, foul odor, and delayed healing. Culture purulent or odorous wound drainage. The normal inflammatory response can indicate infection. *Wound*

culture is used to determine the infectious organism and appropriate antibiotic therapy.

■ Provide fluid intake of 2,500 mL/day unless otherwise contraindicated. *Adequate hydration helps maintain blood flow and nutrient supply to the tissues. Fluids may be limited for the patient with heart or renal failure.*

■ Use proper hand-washing techniques (including at least 15 seconds of friction). *Hand washing is the fundamental tool for preventing the spread of infection to a susceptible person.*

■ Wear sterile gloves when providing wound care. *Sterile gloves prevent further wound contamination and the spread of infection to other patients.*

MANAGING NURSING CARE

As appropriate and allowed by the designated duties and responsibilities of assistive personnel, the nurse may assign nursing care activities such as taking vital signs, recording intake and output and assisting with providing diet and fluids for the patient with inflammation. The nurse retains responsibility for providing wound care.

EVALUATING

To evaluate the effectiveness of care for a patient with acute inflammation, collect data about the presence of redness, heat, swelling, and loss of function. For the patient with systemic inflammation, note vital signs, appetite, energy level, and lymph nodes.

DOCUMENTING

The nurse should document the patient's vital signs; type and location of pain; and the color, consistency, and odor of any wound drainage. In addition, describe the patient's response to any heat or cold therapy ordered. Document teaching related to prescribed medications, fluid intake, well-balanced diet, and wound care at home.

CONTINUITY OF CARE

Patient and family teaching should focus on understanding the inflammatory process, its cause, and its management. When planning for home care, assess the patient's ability to perform self-care at home. Remind the patient to avoid other members of the household with infections. Teach the patient about potential hazards in the home and at work that could cause injury and possibly lead to infection.

Provide the patient with the following verbal and written instructions:

■ Increase fluid intake to 2,500 mL/day (approximately 2.5 quarts), unless contraindicated.

■ Eat a well-balanced diet that is high in carbohydrates, protein, vitamins, and minerals.

■ Use good hand-washing techniques when caring for wounds and after using the bathroom.

- Elevate the inflamed area to reduce swelling and pain.
- Apply heat or cold for no longer than 20 minutes at a time to reduce the risk of tissue damage from burns or frostbite, respectively.
- Take all medications as prescribed. Review the use, expected effects, and side effects of anti-inflammatory medications. Notify the physician if adverse effects occur.
- Rest acutely inflamed tissue. Do not engage in strenuous activity until the inflammation has subsided.

Infection

Key Concept Microorganisms are able to cause disease due to their ability to invade tissues or secrete toxins. Loss of the body's defense mechanisms increases the risk of infection. Hospitalized patients have an increased risk for developing health care–associated infections.

Microorganisms invade humans in order to grow and reproduce. Contact between humans and microorganisms is often beneficial to both. For example, the normal flora of the skin, mucous membranes, and gastrointestinal tract plays an important part in the body's defense system. However, all microorganisms are capable of producing **infection** (growth and invasion of microorganisms that leads to disease), especially when an individual is in poor health.

Infectious diseases have existed throughout history. Modern medicine, antibiotic therapy, immunizations, and public health measures that protect food and water supplies have significantly reduced the prevalence of infectious diseases in many parts of the world. Although smallpox has been eliminated, malaria, typhoid, and TB are still common in many developing nations (Box 9-4■). In spite of vaccines and anti-infective drugs, new strains of bacteria for sexually transmitted infections (STIs) and TB and multidrug-resistant strains of *Staphylococcus* and *Streptococcus* such as MRSA have emerged. Tuberculosis is on the rise in the United States because organisms are resistant to antitubercular medications. New strains of human immunodeficiency virus (HIV) and newer diseases such as *Hantavirus* pulmonary syndrome and Avian influenza challenge modern medicine to find new treatments. Even diseases that once were unrelated to microorganisms now have an infectious disease connection; for example, *Helicobacter pylori* is the underlying cause of chronic gastritis.

To a certain extent, modern medicine has contributed to the development of infectious diseases caused by antibiotic-resistant strains of microorganisms. Invasive procedures that use metal and plastic prosthetic devices provide potential sites for infection. **Immunosuppression** (inability of the immune system to provide adequate immunity) is part

of the medical consequence for organ recipients. Patients who receive immunosuppressive therapy after organ transplantation or chemotherapy are, therefore, more susceptible to infection.

PATHOPHYSIOLOGY

Chain of Infection

For an individual to develop an infection, the **chain of infection** must be in place. Key elements of the chain include (1) a microorganism, (2) a reservoir, (3) a portal of exit from the reservoir, (4) a mode of transmission from the reservoir to the host, and (5) an entry point into a (6) susceptible host (Figure 9-4■). Each element is presented in more detail in the following discussion.

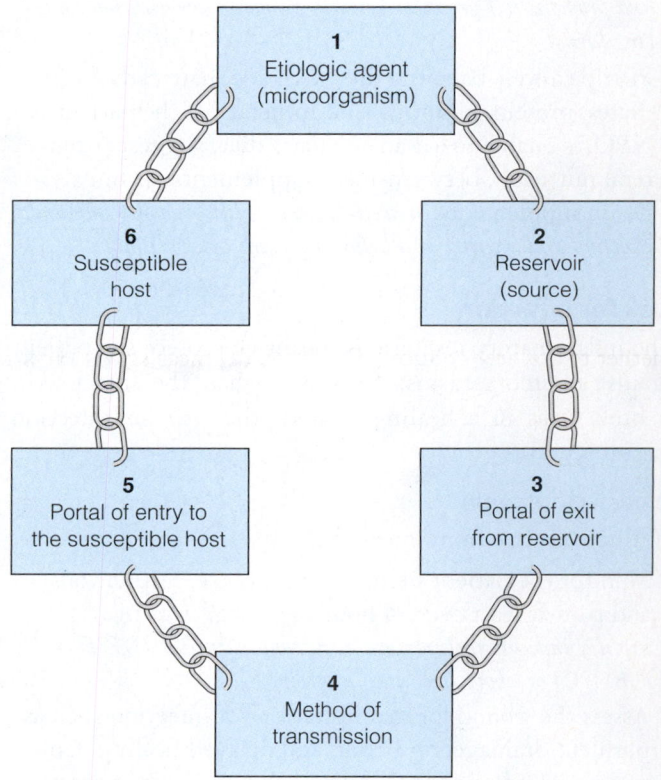

Figure 9-4. ■ The chain of infection.

BOX 9-5	PATHOGENIC ORGANISMS

Bacteria

Bacteria are single-celled organisms. They have different shapes: round (*cocci*), rod shaped (*bacilli*), or spiral (*spirochete*). Bacteria can adapt to different environments: *Aerobes* require oxygen for survival; *anaerobes* survive without oxygen. In the laboratory, they are classified by staining properties: *Gram-positive* bacteria stain purple and *gram-negative* bacteria stain red. Common bacteria that cause infections include *Streptococcus pneumoniae*, *Staphylococcus aureus*, and *Escherichia coli*.

Viruses

Viruses are the smallest pathogens. They are incapable of reproducing outside a living cell. They use the host's metabolic and reproductive materials to multiply. Viruses consist of a protein shell around a DNA or RNA core. Some viruses are short-lived, such as rhinovirus (the common cold). Latent viruses remain dormant in the host until they are reactivated, for example, herpes zoster (shingles) and fever blisters (cold sores). HIV is classed as a retrovirus because of the way it reproduces (see Chapter 11). Oncogenic viruses are so named because they may be able to transform normal cells into cancer cells (onco + gene).

Fungi

Fungi are prevalent throughout the world, but few are capable of causing disease in humans. They grow in two forms: yeasts and molds. Fungal infections can be mild, affecting the skin and subcutaneous tissue. Some fungi, such as *Pneumocystis jiroveci*, can cause life-threatening opportunistic infections in an immunocompromised host.

Mycoplasma

Although similar to bacteria, mycoplasmas are smaller. They are more resistant to antibiotics such as penicillins and cephalosporins.

Rickettsia and Chlamydia

Rickettsia and chlamydia have some features similar to bacteria and viruses. Rickettsia infects the cells of arthropods (e.g., fleas, ticks, and lice) without causing disease. When they are transmitted from these vectors to humans, they cause diseases such as typhus. Chlamydia are transmitted by direct contact and can cause STIs.

Parasites

Protozoa, helminths, and arthropods are considered parasites. Protozoa are single-celled organisms transmitted via direct or indirect contact or an arthropod vector. Helminths are wormlike parasites (e.g., roundworms, tapeworms, and flukes). They gain entry into humans primarily through the ingestion of fertilized eggs or penetration of larvae through the skin or mucous membranes. Arthropod parasites, such as scabies (mites), lice, and fleas, typically infest external body surfaces, causing localized tissue damage and inflammation. Transmission is by direct contact with the arthropod or its eggs.

PATHOGENS   **Pathogens** capable of infecting and causing disease include bacteria; viruses; fungi; mycoplasmas; rickettsiae; chlamydiae; and parasites such as protozoans, helminths, and arthropods (Box 9-5 ■). Each organism causes a different reaction in the host.

For microorganisms to result in disease, several factors are required, including virulence and invasiveness. **Virulence** is the power of a microorganism to cause infection. It is affected by the number of organisms, the host's health, and whether toxins are produced. For example, measles has a low virulence, but rabies has a high virulence. An organism's ability to invade and multiply in a host determines its **invasiveness**. Microorganisms that produce enzymes or toxins are better able to resist the host's defenses and can easily invade the body. For example, *Staphylococcus aureus* releases an enzyme that increases its resistance to certain antibiotics.

Bacteria may release *exotoxins* (from *Staphylococcus*, *Streptococcus*, or tetanus bacteria) or *endotoxins* (from gram-negative bacteria). Also, bacteria that cause botulism and cholera release deadly bacterial exotoxins. Gram-negative organisms that produce endotoxins can cause septic shock. (Common infections and their causative organisms are noted in Table 9-3 ■.)

TABLE 9-3	Common Infectious Diseases and Causative Organisms
DISEASE	**CAUSATIVE ORGANISM**
Chickenpox	Varicella zoster
Gonorrhea	*Neisseria gonorrhoeae*
Foodborne hepatitis	Hepatitis A virus
Bloodborne hepatitis	Hepatitis B, C, or D
Herpes simplex	Human herpes virus 1 and 2
Influenza	Influenza virus A, B, or C
Lyme disease	*Borrelia burgdorferi*
Meningitis	*Haemophilus influenzae*
Meningococcal meningitis	*Neisseria meningitidis*
Pneumococcal pneumonia	*Streptococcus pneumoniae*
Rabies	Rabies virus
Ringworm	*Microsporum* species
Rubella	Rubella virus
Streptococcal pharyngitis	*Streptococcus pyogens*, group A
Syphilis	*Treponema pallidum*
Tetanus	*Clostridium tetani*
Tuberculosis	*Mycobacterium tuberculosis*

RESERVOIR AND PORTAL OF EXIT The reservoir is where the pathogen lives and multiplies. Humans, animals, insects, and nonliving or inanimate objects such as equipment, needles, and utensils act as reservoirs. Infectious diseases are usually transmitted from human sources who have the clinical disease. People who have the disease but do not show any clinical manifestations are called **carriers**. For a pathogen to escape its reservoir, it must have a portal of exit. Pathogens exit humans through respiratory secretions, gastrointestinal and genitourinary body fluids, skin or mucous membrane lesions, or the blood.

MODE OF TRANSMISSION Pathogens move from their reservoir to a susceptible host by several routes: direct or indirect contact, droplet or airborne transmission, or a vector. *Direct contact* includes person-to-person spread or contact with infected body fluids as well as contact with contaminated food or water. *Indirect contact* occurs when the infectious agent is carried on inanimate objects, such as dirty eating utensils.

Droplet transmission involves large, moist droplets released during sneezing, talking, and coughing. Contaminated droplets can be sprayed to another person within a 2- to 3-foot radius. In *airborne transmission*, small respiratory particles that stay suspended in air are carried by air currents and then inhaled by the host. For example, TB is spread by airborne transmission. *Vectors* are insects and animals (e.g., flies, mosquitoes, or rodents) that act as intermediate hosts between the source and the host.

Pathogenic organisms must be able to survive their transport from the reservoir to a host. Over time, they have developed mechanisms to resist drying and unfavorable temperatures (e.g., tetanus bacteria produce spores).

PORTAL OF ENTRY An organism needs a portal of entry to gain access into the host. Portals of entry include eyes; mouth; respiratory, gastrointestinal, and genitourinary tracts; broken skin; and blood.

SUSCEPTIBLE HOST The susceptible host is the final link in the chain of infection. The concepts of normal flora, colonization, infection, and disease are important to how bacteria can affect a host. Normal flora (resident bacteria) works in harmony with the host and provides benefits, for example, the normal flora in the intestinal tract. **Colonization** occurs when pathogenic microorganisms live in the host but do not cause injury or initiate the inflammatory response. For example, *S. aureus* may colonize on the skin. Infection indicates that pathogenic bacteria have triggered the inflammatory process, such as when *S. aureus* enters a surgical wound, causing redness, heat, and pain. **Infectious disease** is the illness that results from an infection.

Whether an infection develops depends on microbe virulence and host resistance. The following factors help the host resist infection:

- Physical barriers, such as the skin and mucous membranes
- Chemical barriers created by stomach acid secretions, urine, and vaginal secretions
- Antimicrobial factors in saliva, tears, and prostatic fluid
- Coughing, sneezing, and the cilia in the respiratory tract
- Neutrophils and macrophages

When host resistance is compromised, the host becomes *susceptible* to infection. Invasive procedures (urinary catheters, chest tubes, IV lines) penetrate the body's physical barriers. The very young and very old may have underdeveloped or failing immune systems, respectively. Patients who are malnourished, have AIDS, or have cancer and are being treated with chemotherapy or radiation therapy have increased susceptibility. Susceptibility is lowered when a person receives an immunization or has previously developed the disease.

Stages of the Infectious Process

Infectious disease usually follows a predictable course through five stages as it develops in the host:

1. The *initial stage* is the incubation period. The pathogen actively reproduces but does not cause symptoms. Some diseases have short incubation periods (e.g., food poisoning caused by *Salmonella*). On the other hand, HIV infection has an incubation period of months to years.

2. In the *prodromal stage*, symptoms begin to appear, although they are often vague and nonspecific. The patient will report general malaise, fever, muscle aches and pains, headache, and fatigue.

3. During the *acute stage*, the pathogen continues reproducing and disperses rapidly. Manifestations become obvious and reflect the specific organism and site. Usually, the patient develops a fever, chills, tachycardia, and tachypnea. Infections of an internal organ cause an inflammatory response. The patient may have tenderness over the site or show signs of altered function, such as hematuria in kidney infections. If the infectious process continues over an extended period, patients show signs of increased catabolism and malnutrition. They lose weight, and their muscles become weak. Sometimes products of the immune process, formed in other sites than the primary infection site, cause an inflammatory reaction. For example, a sore throat caused by a streptococcal infection may result in glomerulonephritis.

4. In the *convalescent stage*, the infection is contained and the pathogen is continually destroyed. At this point, affected tissues are repaired and symptoms disappear.

5. During the last stage, *resolution*, the infection is totally eliminated from the body without residual manifestations. Patients with chronic infections never reach the convalescent and resolution stages.

Complications

Complications may be associated with the type of infecting organism and its virulence. They also may be related to the physical condition of the host. As discussed earlier, if the host is immunosuppressed, the body's normal defenses are missing. Immunosuppression causes not only poor wound healing but also slower disease resolution.

Microorganisms such as bacteria, fungi, and viruses can enter the bloodstream, causing *bacteremia*, *fungemia*, or *viremia*, respectively. If gram-negative organisms release their toxins into the bloodstream, the patient develops *septicemia* (infection in the blood). Septicemia in an immunosuppressed host can lead to septic shock. Septic shock is a systemic inflammatory response to infection resulting in inadequate blood flow to the internal organs; unless treated aggressively, it can lead to widespread cell and tissue injury, organ failure, and death. (See Chapter 14 for an in-depth discussion.)

HEALTH CARE–ASSOCIATED INFECTIONS   **Health care–associated infections** (HAI; formerly *nosocomial* infections) refer to infections associated with health care delivery in any setting (CDC, 2012b). More than 1.7 million patients a year develop HAIs while hospitalized. HAIs add hospital days and are costly in terms of diagnosis and treatment. The frequency of HAIs varies according to the type of patient, the severity of illness, and the number of health care workers within each facility.

Patients entering hospitals are often the least able to resist infection. Invasive procedures and altered immune defenses are the main factors contributing to infection. Catheter-associated urinary tract infections (CAUTIs), central line–associated bloodstream infections (CLABSIs), and ventilator-associated pneumonia (VAP) are the most prevalent types of HAIs (CDC, 2012b). CAUTIs are often caused by inappropriate use of urinary catheters such as being inserted when the only indication is incontinence. CLABSIs can develop from improper skin cleansing technique and inadequate barrier precautions. VAP is related to being in the intensive care unit and having mechanical ventilation.

Numerous other factors can affect whether the hospitalized patient develops an HAI (Box 9-6■). Surgical site infections, another type of HAI, may result from wound contamination during surgery, for example, when *E. coli*, normally found in the colon, is accidentally transferred to another site via contaminated instruments. Health care personnel may transmit microorganisms between patients due to poor hand hygiene. Visitors who might carry infectious diseases can unknowingly transmit infections to patients. Even health care equipment such as stethoscopes and blood pressure cuffs can carry nosocomial organisms. The most common pathogens that cause HAIs include *E. coli*, *S. aureus*, group A streptococci, and *Enterococcus*.

BOX 9-6	RISK FACTORS FOR HEALTH CARE–ASSOCIATED INFECTIONS

- Chronic diseases (e.g., renal disease, lung disease, cancer, AIDS, diabetes, pressure ulcers)
- Morbid obesity
- Long-term use of corticosteroids, chemotherapy, radiation therapy
- History of frequent antibiotic use
- Major surgery (e.g., heart, lung, or intra-abdominal surgeries, or organ transplantation)
- Invasive procedures (e.g., urinary catheter, peripheral and central IV lines, respiratory care procedures, percutaneous endoscopic gastrostomy [PEG] feeding tube, dialysis)
- Prosthetic devices: vascular grafts, heart valves, orthopedic joints
- Burns
- Very young and very old age

Another contributing factor is the alarming rise in antibiotic-resistant microorganisms due to prolonged or inappropriate use of antibiotics. Although antibiotics are expected to eliminate targeted microorganisms, sometimes a few hardy bacteria survive. When these bacteria reproduce, they pass along their antibiotic resistance. Other bacteria produce enzymes that inactivate drugs or change drug-binding sites.

Patients' expectations regarding when to receive antibiotic therapy and how to take an antibiotic can contribute to drug resistance. When antibiotics are given for viral infections, bacteria learn to thrive in an antibiotic environment. The use of broad-spectrum rather than narrow-spectrum drugs can lead to multidrug-resistant strains of bacteria. When a patient fails to complete the prescribed doses, the pathogen is inadequately destroyed and new microbe **mutation** (minute alterations in the genetic structure) can arise. Then, when a new infection occurs, the patient may need a stronger antibiotic. This process, if repeated frequently enough, can establish a pattern of *multidrug resistance*. The nurse must teach patients the importance of completing their drug prescriptions.

The most common MDROs include methicillin-resistant *S. aureus* (MRSA), vancomycin-resistant *Enterococcus* (VRE), and *Clostridium difficile*–associated diarrhea (CDAD). MRSA, VRE, and CDAD are discussed in the following subsections.

Methicillin-Resistant Staphylococcus aureus   Staphylococci normally live in the mucous membranes of the respiratory tract and on the skin. MRSA infection is a type of staphylococcal infection that resists broad-spectrum antibiotics such as methicillin, amoxicillin, and penicillin. This potentially fatal disease is divided into two types: health care–acquired MRSA (HA-MRSA; acquired in hospitals and health care settings) and community-acquired MRSA (CA-MRSA) infections. HA-MRSA infection in hospitalized patients may lead to infections of wounds, skin around invasive tubes or catheters, the lungs, the blood, or the urinary system. In the community setting where young people such as children in day care or amateur athletes share equipment, CA-MRSA infection is more prevalent. The general population and health care workers can be silent carriers, because the colonized bacteria grow in the anterior part of the nose.

In health care facilities, MRSA is transmitted on the hands of health care workers. After exposure, it can live on a person's hands for more than 3 hours. Patients with MRSA infections may be isolated using Contact Precautions (see Table 9-4■ for further guidelines). When providing direct care, gowns and gloves must be worn. HA-MRSA infections are treated with vancomycin or linezolid (Zyvox).

CA-MRSA infections may present as abscesses or cellulitis and may be mistaken for a spider bite. The first choice of treatment is incision and drainage of the lesion when possible. When systemic antibiotics are needed, the preferred antibiotic treatment includes trimethoprim-sulfamethoxazole (Bactrim), doxycycline (Vibramycin), or clindamycin (Cleocin).

Resistance to vancomycin has led to the development of *vancomycin-intermediate S. aureus (VISA)* and *vancomycin-resistant S. aureus (VRSA)*. Currently, VISA and VRSA

infections have been successfully treated with other antibiotics, but new, totally antibiotic-resistant organisms may emerge in the future. The Joint Commission's 2012 National Patient Safety Goals are focused on strategies to prevent further increase in HAIs.

Vancomycin-Resistant Enterococcus   Enterococci are primarily found in the GI and female genital tracts as part of the normal flora. VRE develops from overuse of vancomycin and can cause infections of the urinary tract, bloodstream, or wounds. It is spread by direct contact from patient to patient or health care worker to patient. VRE can live on equipment or environmental surfaces such as over-bed tables. Patients and health care workers can carry the colonized bacteria into a health care facility.

Once VRE is confirmed, Contact Precautions are instituted (see Table 9-4), which includes wearing gloves and gowns when providing direct care and dedicating essential equipment (thermometer, blood pressure cuff, and stethoscope) to the affected patient. VRE is treated with linezolid (Zyvox).

Clostridium difficile–Associated Diarrhea   *Clostridium difficile* is an anaerobic gram-positive bacillus producing two endotoxins that cause damage to the mucosal lining of the bowel. Because the organism forms spores, it can live for months on environmental sources. Antibiotics such as penicillins,

TABLE 9-4	Transmission-Based Precautions		
CATEGORY	**INFECTIOUS DISEASES**	**PURPOSE**	**PRECAUTIONS**
Airborne Precautions	Pulmonary TB, varicella (chickenpox) until lesions are crusted over, rubeola (measles), widespread herpes zoster (until lesions are crusted over)	Reduce transmission of airborne droplets or dust particles containing the infectious agent.	Private room with hand-washing and toilet facilities. Use airborne infection isolation room (AIIR) (negative pressure pulls air from hall inward when someone enters the room); and keep the door closed. Don N95 disposable respirator when entering the room and remove after exiting the room. Place mask on the patient if transport is needed.
Droplet Precautions	Meningitis, pneumonia, influenza, mumps, pertussis, diphtheria, adenovirus, rhinovirus	Reduce transmission of large droplets generated during coughing, sneezing, talking, or procedures such as suctioning. Can infect others if droplets land on conjunctivae, nasal mucosa, or mouth.	Private room with hand-washing and toilet facilities; mask, eye protection, and/or face shields worn by everyone entering the room. Place mask on the patient if transport is required.
Contact Precautions	Acute diarrhea herpes simplex; respiratory syncytial virus; skin, wound, or urinary tract infection with multidrug-resistant organisms; *S. aureus* infections; hepatitis; norovirus in incontinent patients	Reduce transmission by direct skin-to-skin contact or indirect contact with a contaminated object. Direct contact may occur between patients or during direct care activities such as bathing or turning patients.	Private room with hand-washing and toilet facilities; gowns and protective apparel to provide barrier protection; disposable supplies or decontamination of all articles upon leaving the room.

cephalosporins, and fluoroquinolones reduce the bowel's normal flora, allowing the growth of *C. difficile*. It is the most common cause of health care–associated diarrhea.

Manifestations may range from foul-smelling, watery diarrhea and lower abdominal pain to the life-threatening condition of pseudomembranous colitis, peritonitis, and toxic megacolon. The patient is placed in a private room with Contact Precautions (see Table 9-4). Alcohol-based gels do not destroy *C. difficile* spores. Therefore, health care providers must wash their hands with antimicrobial soap and water before and after patient contact and after glove removal. Management includes discontinuing any antibiotic therapy, giving fluids and electrolytes lost with the diarrhea, and providing nutritional support. Loperamide (Imodium), an antidiarrheal drug, is avoided because it may cause toxic megacolon. Patients with severe cases usually receive oral metronidazole (Flagyl) or vancomycin (Vancocin). A new, highly virulent strain is showing resistance to metronidazole and vancomycin.

COMMUNITY-ACQUIRED INFECTIONS   Community-acquired infections are usually referred to as *communicable diseases*, because they can be transmitted to other people. Smallpox, diphtheria, polio, mumps, measles, rubella, pertussis, and tetanus are long-standing communicable diseases. Other community-acquired infections include influenza, community-acquired pneumonia, MRSA infection, hepatitis A, and TB. Smallpox is the only communicable disease to have been completely eradicated. In the United States, most of these communicable diseases are under control through immunization programs. (See Chapter 11 for more information on immunizations.)

Communicable diseases are monitored from an international to a local level. The World Health Organization (WHO) focuses on controlling diseases throughout the world. In Atlanta, Georgia, the Centers for Disease Control and Prevention (CDC) (a federal government agency) is responsible for monitoring, controlling, and preventing infectious diseases. It routinely publishes guidelines and recommendations to use in caring for patients with infections. State and local health departments work cooperatively with the CDC to manage diseases in their area. Physicians and health care facilities are expected to report any communicable disease to their local health department.

Emerging Infectious Diseases   Emerging infectious diseases are defined as diseases that have increased in the past 20 years or threaten to increase in the near future. Worldwide food supply and distribution, increased international travel and crowding in cities, resistant microorganisms, and poor sanitation are contributing to this threat.

Public health officials remain concerned about multidrug-resistant TB and HIV, West Nile virus, avian influenza, and noroviruses. Diarrheal diseases are increasing throughout the world and the United States. Infectious diarrhea results from organisms such as *E. coli*, *Salmonella*, *Shigella*, *Campylobacter*, and *Giardia*, which are transmitted by contaminated food or water.

The WHO and CDC are responsible for protecting the public from infectious diseases. The role of the nurse is education and prevention of the spread of infectious diseases. Through the efforts of the health care community, the battle against these new infections may be won.

Biologic Threat Infections   After the terrorist attacks on September 11, 2001, and the development of anthrax cases in the United States, the possible use of biologic weapons still remains. The most likely pathogens to be used for this purpose include the causative agents of anthrax, smallpox, botulism, plague, and viral hemorrhagic fevers.

Anthrax is an acute bacterial infection caused by *Bacillus anthracis*, a gram-positive, spore-producing organism. It can be contracted by inhalation, ingestion, and skin contact. The spores cannot be destroyed by sunlight or temperature and remain viable for years.

Inhalation anthrax carries the highest mortality rate. At first, the patient exhibits flu-like symptoms that progress to respiratory failure and shock. Patients who ingest the spores develop fever, nausea, vomiting, abdominal pain, and bloody diarrhea. Skin contact produces an itching papule progressing to a painless fluid-filled vesicle. Those exposed to aerosolized *B. anthracis* spores should be treated prophylactically with oral ciprofloxacin (Cipro) or doxycycline (Vibramycin) for 60 days. In addition, the CDC recommends three subcutaneous doses of anthrax vaccine adsorbed (AVA) over a 4-week period (CDC, 2010b).

In 1980, WHO certified that smallpox had been eradicated. Routine smallpox vaccination was discontinued in 1972, leaving people under the age of 39 at risk for the disease if it reappears or is used as a weapon. Smallpox spreads by direct contact or by inhalation of respiratory droplets. Symptoms include a high fever, malaise, and headache, followed by a vesicular/pustular rash, which appears simultaneously on the face and extremities. Anyone exposed to smallpox should be vaccinated and monitored closely. Vaccination up to 4 days after exposure and before a rash appears provides almost complete protection (WHO, 2009).

Health care providers should be alert to unusual illness patterns that could indicate an unusual infectious disease outbreak. Indicators of a biologic agent release include the following: Increased disease occurrence is found among people in the same geographic area (e.g., people who attended the same event); the disease is unusual for the patient's age, such as chickenpox in adults; and a patient presents with symptoms of a rare disease. Any one of these factors should be reported to the public health authorities to identify the infectious disease source and to prevent further exposure.

INFECTIOUS PROCESS IN OLDER ADULTS Infections are a leading cause of disease and death in older adults. Those older than 75 years of age have a higher rate of infections. The geriatric patient is especially prone to several infectious diseases. Part of their increased risk is related to the physiologic changes of aging. (Common infections in older adults, as well as associated factors, are outlined in Table 9-5■.)

In addition to physiologic changes, the following factors can increase the risk for infectious diseases:

- Lower activity level related to musculoskeletal, neurologic, or balance problems
- Poor nutrition and an increased risk of dehydration
- Chronic diseases, such as diabetes mellitus, cardiac disease, and renal disease
- Use of multiple medications
- Lack of recent influenza and pneumococcal vaccinations
- Altered mental status and dementias
- Hospitalization or residence in a long-term care facility

The older adult is not only at increased risk for infection, but also may not exhibit the classic manifestations of infection. Many older adults take NSAIDs and corticosteroids that interfere with inflammation and healing. The cardinal signs of inflammation—redness, warmth, and swelling—

TABLE 9-5 **Common Infectious Diseases in Older Adults, Age-Related Changes, and Nursing Implications**

DISEASE WITH CONTRIBUTING FACTORS	AGE-RELATED CHANGES	NURSING IMPLICATIONS
Urinary tract infections (UTIs) UTIs are a leading cause of bacteremia and sepsis. UTIs often result from poor hygiene, incomplete bladder emptying, inadequate fluid intake, and long-term urinary catheters.	Loss of bladder tone, reduced bladder contractility, altered bladder reflexes, and prostatic hypertrophy in men lead to reduced bladder capacity and incomplete emptying.	Monitor for burning and urgency. Increase fluids to increase urinary output unless contraindicated by cardiac status. Cranberry juice may prevent recurrent UTIs. Give antibiotics as ordered.
Pneumonia and influenza The leading causes of pneumonia in older adults are *S. pneumoniae, Haemophilus influenzae,* and *Klebsiella pneumoniae.* Influenza A and B are common in older adults and can be deadly to those with chronic cardiac and respiratory diseases. Pneumonia and influenza have high mortality rates in older adults.	Decreased ciliary action, poor chest expansion, shallow breathing, and reduced cough inhibit removal of inhaled organisms. Impaired swallow reflex from CVA increases the risk for aspiration pneumonia.	Monitor for increased respiratory rate, listlessness, anorexia, and confusion. (Cough and pleuritic chest pain are often absent.) Recommend annual influenza vaccine and pneumococcal vaccine in those 65 and older. Give antibiotics as ordered.
Tuberculosis Increased incidence, especially in long-term care facilities. Usually recurs from a previous infection.	Decreased phagocytosis reduces the ability to resist TB infection. See other respiratory changes above.	Monitor for weight loss and confusion. (Classic signs of night sweats and fever are absent.) Give anti-TB drugs and monitor closely for side effects.
Skin infections Caused by *S. aureus* and *Streptococcus* group A.	Thinning of skin, loss of elasticity, and decreased sensation increase susceptibility to injury, tissue breakdown, and decubitus ulcers.	Wash hands for 15 seconds with friction to reduce disease transmission. Give antibiotics as ordered. Maintain skin integrity by frequent turning and using pressure mattresses. Perform wound care as indicated.
Herpes zoster or shingles Reactivation of a latent varicella (chickenpox) virus.	Altered immune system function reduces the ability to prevent virus reactivation.	Give analgesics, steroids, antivirals, and topical ointments to alleviate symptoms.

are often absent in older adults. Fever and chills that signal infection may be mild or absent. It is not unusual for an older patient's normal temperature to range from 96 to 98°F. The WBC count may be only slightly elevated.

clinicalALERT

Confusion is a frequent atypical sign of infection in older adults, along with restlessness, fatigue, and mild behavioral changes. Even older adults with sepsis may appear only slightly disoriented and tachypneic.

If an infection is suspected, the physician will order a chest x-ray, urinalysis and culture, and complete blood count. The nurse must complete a baseline assessment and be alert for subtle changes in the patient's mental status or behavior. Other important data to collect include fluid and diet intake, urinary output, respiratory and cardiovascular assessment, and activity level. Early diagnosis and prompt treatment will improve outcomes for the older adult. Nursing implications for common infectious diseases in older adults are provided in Table 9-5.

Collaborative Care

For the patient with an infection, it is important to identify the organ system affected by the infection; to identify the causative agent; and to achieve a cure by the least toxic, least expensive, and most effective means.

Most infectious diseases are self-limiting and will resolve with little or no medical care. However, medical treatment can be lifesaving in case of an overwhelming infection or in an immunocompromised host.

The body part or organ system affected by the infection is often obvious from the patient's history and manifestations. This usually can limit the number of possible infectious agents. Asking about recent activities may provide the necessary clues. For instance, family members who all developed vomiting and diarrhea within 12 hours after a picnic probably do not have the flu.

Once the infecting agent and disease are identified, the type of therapy is selected for each patient. Viral infections may resolve without treatment other than supportive care, such as providing rest and fluids. Skin infections may respond to a topical agent. Severe systemic infections may require long-term intravenous antibiotic therapy.

Diagnostic Tests

Diagnostic tests assess the patient's response to infection, identify the infecting organism, and monitor progress of the medical intervention. The following laboratory tests may be ordered:

- *WBC count* provides clues about the infecting organism and the body's immune response to it (see Table 9-1). The normal WBC count ranges from 4,500 to 10,000/mm^3.
- *WBC differential* is also ordered. During acute infections, more mature neutrophils are produced. If the infection is severe, the body may require more neutrophils than are made. The bone marrow responds by releasing immature neutrophils called *bands*. This condition is termed a *shift to the left* (Figure 9-5 ■). Eventually the band cells mature and assist in fighting the infection.
- *Cultures of the wound, blood, or other infected body fluids* may be obtained. Using sterile technique, a specimen is collected and immediately taken to the laboratory. There, it

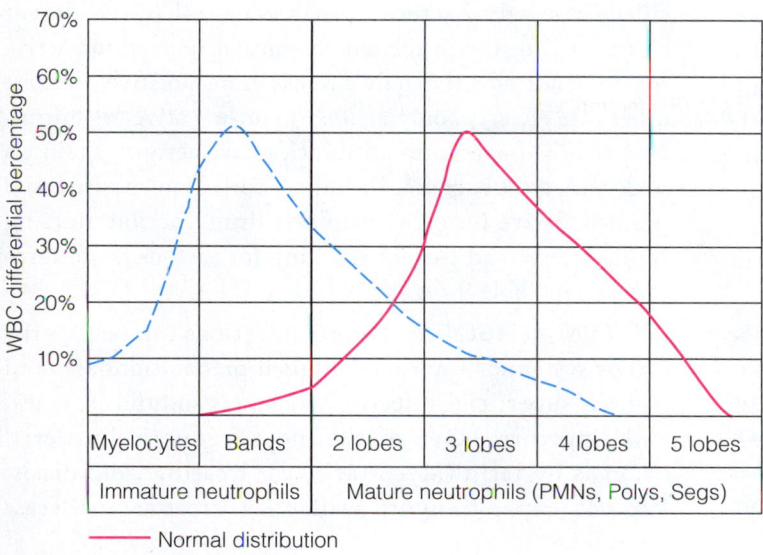

Type of WBC	Normal differential	Shift to left
Myelocytes	0%	Present
Band neutrophils (Bands)	3% to 5%	Increased
Mature neutrophils (Segs, Polys, PMNs)	55% to 70%	May be stable, increased, or decreased

Figure 9-5. ■ Neutrophils by stage of maturity and normal distribution in the blood versus shift to left caused by severe infection.

is placed in or on a special culture medium. The culture is placed in an incubator to encourage the growth of the organism outside the body. Most cultures take 24 to 48 hours to grow. Then the culture is examined under the microscope to identify the offending microorganism.

■ *Sensitivity studies* determine which antibiotics are most effective against the identified pathogen. Often, several antibiotics are listed. The health care professional selects the appropriate drug based on host and pathogen factors. (See Medications section for additional information.)

■ *Antibiotic peak and trough levels* monitor therapeutic blood levels of a prescribed medication, especially aminoglycosides. It is important to maintain drug levels within a *therapeutic range*, the amount of the drug that will effectively destroy pathogens while producing few toxic effects. By measuring blood levels at the predicted *peak* (1 hour after IM injection and 30 minutes after IV infusion) and *trough* (lowest level, usually just before the next scheduled dose), the physician can determine whether the patient is maintaining a level within the therapeutic range.

Other diagnostic tests may confirm an infectious diagnosis in a specific organ. Two of the common tests are as follows:

■ *Lumbar puncture* is done to obtain cerebrospinal fluid (CSF) for examination and culture if meningitis or encephalitis is suspected. (See Box 38-2 for nursing responsibilities related to lumbar puncture.)

■ *Ultrasound examination* is a noninvasive diagnostic test, such as an echocardiogram or renal ultrasonogram, to identify an infectious site or evaluate the effects of infection on organ function.

Medications

After identifying the infecting organism and affected body part or organ, *antimicrobials* (drugs capable of killing or incapacitating pathogens) can be started. Antimicrobial therapy includes antibiotic, antifungal, antiviral, or antiparasitic drugs. Antibiotics are classified according to the way they interfere with the bacterial growth. **Bacteriostatic** agents inhibit the growth of microorganisms. Tetracycline and erythromycin are bacteriostatic preparations.

Bactericidal agents kill the microorganism and include penicillin, cephalosporin, and aminoglycoside antibiotics. In addition, antibiotics have either a narrow spectrum or broad spectrum of action. **Narrow-spectrum antibiotics** are drugs that act against a limited number of pathogens, whereas **broad-spectrum antibiotics** are those that inhibit a wide variety of microbes.

Antimicrobials can be applied topically or administered by oral, intramuscular, intravenous, intraperitoneal, or intrathecal routes. Oral and intravenous routes are most commonly used.

A C&S test should be done before antimicrobial therapy is started. If antibiotics are started before the culture is collected, they could interfere with the organism growth on the culture medium. When patients are scheduled for surgery or invasive procedures that could cause an infection, they are started on **prophylactic** (preventive) anti-infective therapy.

Selection of an appropriate antimicrobial is based on its effectiveness, level of toxicity, ease of administration, and cost-effectiveness. The health care professional must also consider several factors about the patient, such as the following:

■ History of allergic reactions
■ Patient's age and childbearing status
■ Patient's present health status; presence of malnutrition, cancer, or AIDS
■ Renal and hepatic function
■ Site and extent of the infection
■ History of chronic diseases and other drug therapy

As with all drug therapy, antimicrobials can cause adverse reactions. Allergic responses can range from mild itching to anaphylaxis (See Chapter 14 for further discussion about anaphylaxis and anaphylactic shock.) Toxicity to the liver, kidneys, ears, and bone marrow and superinfections may develop. A **superinfection** is a new infection that appears because the antibiotic has eliminated normal bacterial flora. For example, yeast infections called candidiasis (or *thrush*) will appear in the mouth or vaginal area.

ANTIBIOTIC DRUGS Medications used to treat bacterial infections are generally known as **antibiotics**. New antibiotics are constantly being developed to overcome multidrug-resistant bacteria. Antibiotics fall into different classes of drugs with related chemical structure and activity. Some are effective only against gram-positive bacteria; others are effective only against gram-negative organisms. Newer broad-spectrum antibiotics have activity against a wide variety of bacteria, including both gram-positive and gram-negative forms. (Antibiotic drugs, action, nursing implications, and patient teaching for each class are summarized in Table 9-6■.)

ANTIFUNGAL AGENTS Fungal infections can be superficial or systemic. Topical antifungal preparations are used to treat superficial infections such as candidiasis, tinea, and ringworm. One of the most frequently ordered drugs is nystatin (Mycostatin) for treating candidiasis. Vaginal preparations are available to treat vaginal yeast infections.

Amphotericin B (Fungizone) is a systemic antifungal agent for parenteral administration. It is used to

TABLE 9-6 Giving Medications Safely: Antibiotic Therapy

CLASS/DRUGS	PURPOSE	NURSING IMPLICATIONS	PATIENT TEACHING
Penicillins ■ Penicillin G ■ *Penicillin V* ■ *Amoxicillin* (Amoxil) ■ Nafcillin (Unipen) ■ Ampicillin (Polycillin) ■ Carbenicillin (Geocillin) ■ Dicloxacillin (Dynapen) ■ Mezlocillin (Mezlin) ■ Oxacillin (Prostaphlin) ■ Piperacillin (Pipracil) ■ Ticarcillin (Ticar) *Penicillin/beta-lactamase inhibitors* ■ *Amoxicillin/clavulanate* (Augmentin) ■ Piperacillin/tazobactam (Zosyn)	Penicillins are bactericidal and effective against streptococci, staphylococci, meningococci, and gonococci. They are safe, effective, and have a low toxicity. Penicillin is ordered in units or milligrams. They are available in PO, IM, and IV forms.	Check for allergies to penicillins or cephalosporins before giving the first dose. Monitor the patient for an allergic response: rashes, hives, itching, and anaphylaxis. Notify the health care provider immediately. Observe patients for 30 minutes after an IM injection. Monitor for white patches in mouth or a vaginal discharge due to candidiasis.	Take as ordered with a full glass of water 1 hour before or 2 hours after meals. If an allergic reaction occurs, stop the drug and contact the physician. Notify the physician if white patches occur on the oral mucosa or if vaginitis develops. Eating yogurt or buttermilk may prevent fungal infection but do not take these products within 1 hour of taking the drug.
Cephalosporins *First generation* ■ *Cephalexin* (Keflex) ■ Cefazolin (Ancef) *Second generation* ■ Cefaclor (Ceclor) ■ Cefoxitin (Mefoxin) ■ Cefuroxime (Ceftin) *Third generation* ■ Cefoperazone (Cefobid) ■ Ceftazidime (Fortaz) ■ Ceftriaxone (Rocephin) *Fourth generation* ■ Cefepime (Maxipime)	Cephalosporins are related structurally to the penicillins, so there may be a cross-sensitivity between them. First generation acts against gram-positive organisms; second and third generations are more effective against gram-negative organisms; fourth generation acts against gram-positive and gram-negative organisms.	Monitor for previous allergic response to cephalosporins or penicillins. Monitor IV site for phlebitis or local pain at IM site. Monitor for decreased output and elevated blood urea nitrogen (BUN) in older patients. Monitor for diarrhea; if blood or mucus appears, notify the health care provider immediately.	Take the medications as ordered on an empty stomach, 1 hour before or 2 hours after meals. Eat yogurt or drink buttermilk to prevent oral or vaginal infections. Notify the health care provider if skin develops rashes, hives, or itching, or if white patches develop on the oral mucosa or vaginitis.
Aminoglycosides ■ Amikacin (Amikin) ■ Gentamicin (Garamycin) ■ Streptomycin ■ Tobramycin (Nebcin)	Aminoglycosides are bactericidal against serious gram-negative organisms: *Pseudomonas, E. coli, Klebsiella*. They may be combined with penicillins to provide a greater effect.	Monitor for ototoxicity (ringing in the ears) and nephrotoxicity (decreased urine output, elevated BUN and serum creatinine). Monitor peak and trough levels. Increase fluid intake to 2,000–3,000 mL/day. Give IV drugs 1 hour apart from other IV antibiotics.	If adverse effects occur, stop the drug and notify the health care provider. Monitor for sudden weight gain that may indicate adverse effects on the kidney and report it to the health care provider.
Fluoroquinolones ■ *Ciprofloxacin* (Cipro) ■ Levofloxacin (Levaquin) ■ Moxifloxacin (Avelox)	Fluoroquinolones are bactericidal against gram-positive and gram-negative organisms to treat respiratory, GI, GU, and soft tissue infections.	Increase fluid intake to 2,000–3,000 mL/day. Monitor for decreased urine output. Monitor laboratory results for hepatotoxicity (increased ALT, AST).	Check label before taking with food. Drink six to eight glasses of water per day. Avoid exposure to sunlight; notify the health care provider if skin rashes or redness occur.

(continued)

TABLE 9-6	Giving Medications Safely: Antibiotic Therapy *(continued)*		
CLASS/DRUGS	**PURPOSE**	**NURSING IMPLICATIONS**	**PATIENT TEACHING**
Tetracyclines ■ Tetracycline (Sumycin) ■ *Minocycline* (Minocin) ■ *Doxycycline* (Vibramycin)	Tetracyclines act against gram-positive and gram-negative bacteria such as *Mycoplasma* and *Chlamydia*. Tetracyclines are not used during pregnancy or in children under 8 years to prevent tooth discoloration.	Give 1 hour before or 2 hours after meals. Do not give with milk, dairy products, or antacids. Monitor for thrush or vaginal itching. Report signs to the physician.	Take 1 hour before or 2 hours after meals. Do not take with milk, dairy products, or antacids. Avoid sun exposure and wear protective clothing to reduce photosensitivity reactions.
Sulfonamides ■ Sulfamethizole (Thiosulfil Forte) ■ Sulfamethoxazole (Gantanol) ■ Trimethoprim-sulfamethoxazole (Bactrim, Septra) ■ Sulfisoxazole (Gantrisin)	Oral sulfonamides treat UTIs by bacteriostatic action. Trimethoprim-sulfamethoxazole is used for *Pneumocystis jiroveci* pneumonia (PJP).	Give with a full glass of water. Increase fluid intake to 2,000–3,000 mL/day. Monitor for skin rash, itching, easy bruising, or bleeding gums and notify the physician.	Take the drug with full glass of water. Drink 2–3 quarts of fluids per day. Avoid sun exposure to reduce sunburn. Notify the physician if skin develops rash, itching, hives, easy bruising, or if bleeding gums develop.
Macrolides ■ Erythromycin (E-Mycin) ■ *Azithromycin* (Zithromax) ■ *Clarithromycin* (Biaxin)	Macrolides are used for gram-positive and gram-negative organisms in patients allergic to penicillin. Zithromax causes less nausea.	Give with a full glass of water. Check whether to give with or without food. Monitor for nausea, vomiting, diarrhea, dark urine, jaundice.	Take with a full glass of water. Check label for taking with or without food. Notify the physician if GI upset is severe or if dark urine or yellowish-tinge of eyes appears.
Miscellaneous drugs ■ Metronidazole (Flagyl) ■ Vancomycin (Vancocin)	Flagyl is effective against anaerobic gram-negative bacteria and protozoan infection caused by amebiasis, giardiasis, and trichomoniasis. It is used to prevent and treat infections after intestinal surgery. It is the first-choice drug for *C. difficile*. Vancocin is used for serious gram-positive infections such as MRSA infection.	*Flagyl:* Give with meals to decrease GI upset and metallic taste. Increase fluid intake to 2,000–3,000 mL/day. Notify the physician if dizziness, headache, tingling of extremities, or seizures occur. *Vancocin:* Give IV dose over 1 hour to avoid Red Man syndrome—red rash, flushing, and hypotension. Monitor for ototoxicity and nephrotoxicity. Draw peak and trough levels with IV route.	*Flagyl:* Take with meals to decrease GI upset. Drink 2–3 quarts of water daily. Avoid alcohol during therapy to prevent flushing, nausea, vomiting, and headache. Notify the physician if dizziness, headache, tingling of extremities, or seizures occur. *Vancocin:* Report tinnitus, hearing loss, or decreased urine output immediately.

Note: Medications identified in *italics* are among the 200 most frequently prescribed drugs in the United States.

TABLE 9-7	Giving Medications Safely: Antifungal and Antiviral Drugs		
CLASS/DRUGS	**PURPOSE**	**NURSING IMPLICATIONS**	**PATIENT TEACHING**
Antifungal drugs			
■ Amphotericin B (Fungizone) ■ Clotrimazole (Lotrimin) ■ *Fluconazole* (Diflucan) ■ *Ketoconazole* (Nizoral) ■ Miconazole (Monistat) ■ *Nystatin* (Mycostatin)	Antifungals treat oral and vaginal candidiasis, ringworm histoplasmosis, and cryptococcosis. May be applied topically or given PO and IV.	Use Standard Precautions when cleaning skin lesions and applying topical medications. Have patient swish nystatin suspension in mouth for 2–3 minutes before swallowing. Premedicate with Tylenol and/or Demerol to prevent rigors with amphotericin B.	For topical agents, wash and dry the area before applying the medication. Swish nystatin suspension in mouth for 2–3 minutes before swallowing. Follow instructions for using vaginal preparations.
Antiviral drugs			
■ Amantadine (Symmetrel) ■ *Acyclovir* (Zovirax) ■ Ganciclovir (Cytovene) ■ Vidarabine (Vira-A) ■ Zidovudine (AZT, Retrovir)	Antivirals treat influenza A, herpes virus, and opportunistic viral infections in patients with AIDS. Specific antiretroviral drugs reduce viral loads in HIV infection. May be given PO, IV, or topical.	Apply topical agents with gloves. For IV acyclovir: increase fluid intake to 2,000–3,000 mL/day and monitor for dizziness and headache. Monitor for signs of bone marrow suppression with zidovudine. See Chapter 11 for discussion of antiretroviral drugs.	Take drugs as prescribed. Cleanse area and apply topical ointment with gloves. Report unusual dizziness or headache. Discuss sexual abstinence during active herpes infection.

Note: Medications identified in *italics* are among the 200 most frequently prescribed drugs in the United States.

treat severe, life-threatening fungal infections, including histoplasmosis, coccidioidomycosis, and candidiasis. Fluconazole (Diflucan) is preferred over amphotericin B because it is less toxic and is available in oral and parenteral forms. (Nursing responsibilities are listed in Table 9-7 ■.)

Antiviral Drugs   Viral infections can be as mild as the common cold, chronic like herpes infections, or life threatening like acquired immunodeficiency syndrome (AIDS). Antiviral therapy is relatively new and quite limited because new viruses can reproduce before a drug is developed. The drugs in this class are expensive and fairly toxic to the patient. Common antiviral agents are summarized in Table 9-7.

Antiparasitic Agents   Drugs used to treat parasitic infections are as varied as the organisms that cause them. Generally, these drugs are expensive and often toxic. Quinine was one of the first antiparasitic drugs developed to treat malaria. Quinine is very toxic, but newer forms such as chloroquine (Aralen), primaquine, and hydroxychloroquine (Plaquenil) are widely used as antimalarial drugs. Metronidazole (Flagyl) is used to treat protozoan infections and is discussed in Table 9-6.

INFECTION PREVENTION AND CONTROL TECHNIQUES

Prevention is the most important control measure for HAIs and begins with health care workers. Health care personnel should wear clean clothing and follow good hygiene practices. Most infectious organisms are spread by direct contact with health care workers. *Effective hand washing (at least 15 seconds, using friction and antimicrobial soap) is the single most important measure in infection control.*

It is the nurse's responsibility to adhere to the principles of medical and surgical asepsis and to assist other health care personnel to follow these principles when caring for patients. Health care workers must keep immunizations current and should not care for patients when ill with an infectious disease or open skin lesions.

clinicalALERT

Since October 2002, alcohol-based hand rub is recommended by the CDC as the preferred method of hand hygiene. Antiseptic soaps and detergents are the next most effective agents, and nonantiseptic soaps are the least effective. A soap and water wash is recommended for visibly soiled hands. Wearing gloves does not eliminate the need for hand washing.

Controlling the spread of infectious diseases in the hospital or long-term care setting is essential. Each health care facility follows infection control guidelines developed by the CDC. Each institution also develops its own specific policies for handling biologic waste disposal, housekeeping and sterilization procedures, and employee health standards. Other policies outline the frequency for changing urinary drainage bags or intravenous bags and tubing. For instance, intravenous bags are changed every 24 hours and tubing every 24 to 72 hours.

The Occupational Safety and Health Administration (OSHA) is responsible for reducing the risk of exposure to infectious diseases. It publishes mandatory guidelines about routine training to prevent bloodborne pathogens and TB. Institutions that do not follow OSHA standards face penalties and fines.

Isolation Precautions The CDC developed and implemented two tiers of isolation precautions to be used in health care facilities. These two tiers are Standard Precautions and Transmission-Based Precautions. To determine the need for isolation precautions, the nurse must consider the source of the microorganism, the mode of transmission, and susceptibility of hospital staff and other patients. For example, patients with active TB are highly contagious and must be placed in Airborne Precautions.

Standard Precautions **Standard Precautions** are guidelines for the handling of blood and other body fluids to protect the health care worker as well as prevent transmission to other patients. These guidelines are used with all patients, whether they are known to have an infectious disease or not. All health care workers who have direct contact with patients or with their body fluids or who have indirect contact, such as by emptying trash, changing linens, or cleaning the room, must use Standard Precautions. Standard Precautions apply to (1) blood; (2) all body fluids, secretions, and excretions regardless of whether they contain visible blood; (3) nonintact skin; and (4) mucous membranes.

Personal protective equipment (PPE) is the use of a barrier protection to prevent exposure of skin and mucous membranes to blood and body fluids. PPE involves using gloves, gowns, masks, goggles, or respirator masks as appropriate. The CDC has added a new guideline for Standard Precautions, which is called respiratory hygiene/cough etiquette. Because respiratory infections can be spread by droplets, it is important for health care providers and the public to follow respiratory hygiene/cough etiquette. Standard Precautions are outlined in Box 9-7■.

Transmission-Based Precautions In addition to hand hygiene and Standard Precautions, some infectious diseases require special techniques. The CDC identifies three types of **Transmission-Based Precautions** are Airborne, Droplet, and Contact Precautions. Transmission-Based Precautions may be combined for diseases that have multiple routes of

BOX 9-7	STANDARD PRECAUTIONS GUIDELINES

- Perform hand hygiene: (a) immediately after touching blood, body fluids, secretions and excretions, and contaminated items, whether or not gloves were worn; (b) immediately after removing gloves; and (c) between contacts with patients.
- Wear clean, nonsterile gloves when touching blood, body fluids, secretions and excretions, and contaminated items. Don clean gloves just before touching mucous membranes and nonintact skin.
- Change gloves between tasks on the same patient to prevent cross-contaminating different body sites.
- If hands are not visibly soiled, use an alcohol-based hand rub for routine hand decontamination in all other situations.
- Wear PPE (mask, eye protection, face shield, gown, or plastic apron) to avoid being splashed or sprayed with blood, body fluids, secretions, and excretions. Remove soiled gown promptly and wash hands immediately after gown removal.
- Do not recap or break needles; dispose of needles and other sharp objects in puncture-proof containers. Use one-handed "scoop" technique or a special needle-recapping device.
- Clean spills immediately with 1:10 bleach solution or facility-recommended germicide.
- Handle used patient equipment and linen carefully to prevent self- and clothing contamination and transfer of organisms to other patients. Place in leak-proof bags and follow institution's policies regarding double-bagging.
- Place the patient who may contaminate the environment in a private room with a private bathroom.

Respiratory Hygiene/Cough Etiquette

- Cover the mouth and nose with a tissue when coughing or sneezing and dispose of soiled tissues into a no-touch waste container.
- Perform hand hygiene immediately after disposal of the soiled tissue.
- Turn the head away from others to avoid coughing in their face.

Source: Adapted from CDC (2007). Guideline for isolation precautions: Preventing transmission of infectious agents in health care settings. Available at CDC website.

transmission. (Specific guidelines for Transmission-Based Precautions were outlined earlier in Table 9-4.)

Complementary Therapies
Oral echinacea is taken to decrease inflammation and to prevent the common cold and influenza. It should be used for less than 8 weeks at a time. Anyone who is currently taking immunosuppressants (see Table 11-7) should not take echinacea because it stimulates immune function.

NURSING CARE

Key Concept   As members of the health care team, nurses play a key role in reducing the potential for infection. Basic prevention strategies include practicing and promoting hand hygiene, using Standard Precautions, assessing patients for possible signs and symptoms of infection, and teaching patients about preventive strategies.

PRIORITIZING NURSING CARE

Priority nursing management related to an infection or infectious disease focuses on prevention, health promotion, and health maintenance. Prevention includes assessing the patient's risk for infection, based on underlying conditions, immune response, and the need for immunizations. Health promotion and maintenance activities include monitoring vital signs; administering prescribed antibiotics; using aseptic technique and infection control measures; and promoting rest, activity, and nutritional intake.

HEALTH PROMOTION

Preventing infection requires understanding the importance of immunizations, the guidelines for using antibiotics to prevent multidrug-resistant microorganisms, and the ways to prevent the spread of infection. Encourage all family members to keep immunizations current. If they are not up to date, discuss where immunizations can be obtained. Increase public awareness regarding appropriate antibiotic use.

Prevent the spread of infection to others by avoiding crowds and contact with infectious persons and using disposable tissues when coughing or sneezing. Cough into the elbow or upper arm instead of the hand if disposable tissues are unavailable. Use appropriate food-handling precautions for diseases spread by the oral–fecal route, such as hepatitis A. Avoid contact with or sharing of body fluids. For example, do not share needles or razors. Practice safe sex practices by using a condom during sexual activity. Keep the home clean by disinfecting with 1:10 bleach solution for blood spills.

ASSESSING

Before implementing nursing care, the nurse must collect assessment data. These data can help determine the extent to which an infection or infectious disease is interfering with the patient's life, can identify risk factors for complications, and can be used by the physician to determine the type of medical intervention needed (Box 9-8■). The nurse must also assess for risks of HAI from invasive procedures and therapies.

BOX 9-8   **ASSESSMENT**

Patients With Infection

Subjective Data

Ask the patient about:

- General health and nutritional status.
- Fever: How long has the fever existed? Has patient had chills?
- Describe cough and/or sputum; sore throat, congestion, runny or stuffy nose.
- Anorexia, nausea, vomiting, abdominal pain, diarrhea.
- Weakness, malaise, muscle aches, joint pains, headache.
- Pain on urination, odor, urgency, frequency, flank pain.
- Vaginal discharge—color, odor, itching.
- Describe any rash or presence of animal or insect bite.
- Any prior infections or exposure to infectious person.
- Treatment for TB or sexually transmitted disease.
- Has the patient been tested for HIV?
- Use of antipyretics and antimicrobials; immunization history.
- Any travel overseas?

Objective Data

- Measure vital signs: blood pressure, pulse, respirations, temperature.
- Record height and weight.
- Observe for fatigue, shortness of breath, and altered mental status.
- Assess for dehydration: increased thirst, dry mucous membranes, decreased skin turgor.
- Auscultate chest for crackles and wheezes.
- Inspect sputum, stool, genitourinary excretions for amount, color, consistency, and odor.
- Inspect throat for redness.
- Palpate the skin for the presence of any rash, warmth, or tenderness.
- Palpate for enlarged lymph nodes and tenderness.
- Monitor WBC and C&S report; report abnormal findings.

IDENTIFYING POTENTIAL COMPLICATIONS

Complications are varied and are usually specific to the infecting organism and the body system affected. Acute invasion of the blood by certain microorganisms or their toxins can result in septicemia and septic shock. See Chapter 14 for an in-depth discussion of septic shock.

DIAGNOSING, PLANNING, AND IMPLEMENTING

Individuals with an acute infection or infectious disease may require hospitalization until the crisis is resolved. Those with chronic infections or side effects from the infectious disease process may need care in long-term care facilities or at home. Infections of each body system are discussed in the unit related to that system. Priority nursing diagnoses are Risk for Infection, Imbalanced Nutrition, and Ineffective Thermoregulation.

Risk for Infection

Expected outcome

Will remain free from infection.

The spread of infection is a risk in any facility that houses many people. There is increased risk in hospitals, where many patients may have some degree of immunosuppression and many drug-resistant microorganisms exist. It is vital that nurses use good hand hygiene techniques at all times, implement Standard Precautions with all patients, and use Transmission-Based Precautions as indicated.

■ Admit patients with known or suspected infections to a private room. *This minimizes risk to other patients.*
■ Perform hand hygiene using hand sanitizer on entering and leaving the patient's room. *Hand hygiene removes microorganisms from the skin and helps prevent transmission of infection to or from the patient.*
■ Use Standard Precautions with all patients and PPE as indicated. *Standard Precautions and PPE significantly reduce the risk of disease transmission during patient care.*
■ Use Transmission-Based Precautions when appropriate. *Transmission-Based Precautions reduce the spread of disease by airborne, droplet, or direct and indirect methods.*
■ Explain to the patient and family the reasons for isolation precautions. *Patients with isolation precautions may feel neglected or dirty. Explaining the reasons and procedures can enhance understanding and acceptance.*
■ Place a mask on the patient or cover all infectious lesions or wounds completely when transporting the patient to other parts of the facility for diagnostic or treatment procedures. *These measures minimize air contamination and the risk to visitors and personnel.*
■ Collect a C&S specimen as ordered. *C&S can identify infectious organisms and determine the most effective antibiotics.*

clinicalALERT

Collect the specimen for C&S before administering the first dose of antibiotics to ensure adequate organisms for culture.

■ Administer prescribed antimicrobial agents. *Antimicrobial agents are given to destroy invading microorganisms.*
■ Notify all personnel who have contact with the patient about the diagnosis. *Personnel must take appropriate precautions, particularly for patients with diseases requiring category-specific isolation.*

■ Ensure that visitors wear appropriate protective garments before they enter the patient's room. *Protective wear reduces visitors' risk of infection.*
■ Follow facility guidelines for disposal of contaminated tissues, dressings, or other material and for removal of soiled linens and equipment from the patient's room. *These measures prevent the transmission of pathogenic organisms.*

Imbalanced Nutrition

Fever, especially prolonged high fever, increases the body's metabolism. Inadequate nutrition may prolong the infectious process.

Expected outcome

Will maintain adequate nutrition to promote healing.

■ Encourage a high-calorie, high-protein diet. *Increased calories and protein are needed to meet increased metabolic demands.*
■ Provide liquid or soft, easily digested foods. *Difficult-to-digest foods increase heat production. If the patient has a sore throat, liquids and soft food are easier to swallow.*
■ Encourage patient to choose appealing foods. *Patients with a systemic infection often lose their appetite. An inadequate diet can prolong the infectious process. If they can choose foods they like, it may stimulate their appetite.*
■ Minimize offensive odors from draining wounds. *Decreasing odors may increase the patient's appetite.*

Ineffective Thermoregulation

Patients with an infectious disease usually develop a fever. Although fever serves a useful purpose, abnormally high fevers can put the patient at risk for other complications.

Expected outcome

Fever will be reduced to normal limits.

■ Monitor temperature, pulse, and respirations at regular intervals and especially during episodes of chills. Monitor heart rate and respirations. *Chills indicate a rising temperature. Hyperthermia can cause an irregular heart rate and increased respiratory rate.*

clinicalALERT

Monitor temperature between 5 pm and 7 pm because the body's temperature cycle peaks during these hours.

■ Monitor intake and output at least every 8 hours and increase oral fluid intake to 2,500 mL/day, as appropriate, for the patient's cardiopulmonary status. *Fever can cause dehydration as indicated by decreased urine output; increased fluid intake reduces this risk. Fluids are given cautiously to patients with cardiopulmonary disease to prevent fluid overload.*

- Administer IV fluid and electrolytes as ordered. *If fluid loss is severe, patient will need IV electrolyte solutions.*
- Give prescribed antipyretics as ordered for an elevated temperature. *Antipyretics lower the body's temperature; however, they decrease WBC activity, especially phagocytosis. Some microorganisms can be destroyed when the body reaches a certain temperature.*
- Promote body cooling through lowering the room temperature. Use tepid baths, ice packs in the groin and axilla, or a hypothermia blanket only if temperature is greater than 104°F. *These methods can reduce fever too rapidly, causing more shivering and increased temperature. Be sure to wrap ice bags in a towel to prevent tissue damage.*

clinicalALERT

Use ice packs, cool/tepid baths, or hypothermia blanket cautiously to prevent unnecessary shivering.

- Maintain bed rest. *Bed rest conserves energy and reduces metabolic demands.*
- Bathe the patient and provide dry clothing and bedding if the patient is diaphoretic; replace wet gowns and linen. *Personal hygiene promotes patient comfort and reduces further water evaporation.*
- Monitor the patient for decreased level of consciousness and seizures. *High fevers can cause dehydration, leading to an altered mental status and seizures.*

MANAGING NURSING CARE

As appropriate and allowed by the designated duties and responsibilities of assistive personnel, the nurse may assign nursing care activities such as monitoring vital signs and intake and output and assisting with providing diet and fluids for the patient with an infection. The nurse retains responsibility for overseeing the use of Transmission-Based Precautions and collecting any ordered C&S specimens.

EVALUATING

Evaluate the effectiveness of nursing care for the patient with an infection by collecting the following data: temperature remains normal for 24 hours, no signs of dehydration, clear breath sounds, and cultures negative for pathogens. Also, evaluate whether the patient takes precautions to prevent the spread of an infection and is completing any ordered antibiotics.

DOCUMENTING

Document assessment findings related to increased temperature, pulse and respiratory rates, and the presence of dehydration. Note the relationship between any changes in assessment findings and treatments provided, such as changes in temperature after receiving antipyretics. Document

whether the patient has increased oral fluid intake and is eating a high-calorie, high-protein diet.

CONTINUITY OF CARE

Patient and family teaching focuses on promoting patient recovery, preventing the spread of infection to others and preventing potential complications. Instructions should include the following points:

- Use good hand hygiene, especially after touching infected wounds or lesions, coughing, sneezing, blowing the nose, and using the bathroom; before preparing food or eating; or before wound care. Do not share eating utensils.
- Take all prescribed antibiotics until the prescription is completed, even after symptoms are relieved. Take the prescription at intervals around the clock as directed.
- Never allow anyone else to take your medications and never use anyone else's prescription even if they appear to be the same.
- Notify your health care provider if any of the following occurs:
  - Symptoms do not improve within 24 to 48 hours after antibiotic therapy is started, they worsen, or symptoms reappear after completing antibiotic therapy.
  - Signs of antibiotic allergy (itching, rash, difficulty breathing or swallowing; swelling of face or tongue). Discontinue medication and contact prescriber.
  - Adverse reactions, such as gastrointestinal distress or diarrhea, that interfere with completion of the prescription.
  - Redness, swelling, or drainage around wounds; persistent high fever or chills; vaginal discharge or itching (vaginitis); white plaques in mouth or on tongue (oral candidiasis); loose, watery, and foul-smelling diarrhea; blood in urine; or unusual cough.
- Wear MedicAlert bracelet noting medication allergies.
- Increase fluid intake to at least 2.5 quarts/day and eat a well-balanced diet.
- Suggest the following resources: county or public health department; CDC.

NURSING CARE PLAN
Patient With MRSA Infection

Mr. Frank Kendall, 87 years old, is transferred from a nearby long-term care facility to the medical unit of the community hospital. Mr. Kendall has been in the long-term care facility for 6 months after a cerebrovascular accident (CVA). Two months ago he was in the hospital for urosepsis. He has been widowed for 9 months. One daughter lives

1,000 miles away and has visited him only once in the past 6 months.

The nurse from the long-term care facility reports that he is too weak to get out of bed by himself. He has a poor appetite and seems frail. About 1 month ago he developed a large decubitus ulcer on the sacral area that is not healing.

Assessment

On admission, vital signs are BP 150/84, P 92, R 24, T 100°F (37.7°C), weight 165 lb, and height 5'10". He is listless, with decreased right arm and leg movement, thin extremities, and poor skin turgor. He answers the nurse's questions without looking at her. The decubitus ulcer on the sacral area measures 7 cm long, 4 cm wide, and 1.5 cm deep, with yellowish-green drainage. The wound edges are red and tender. He grimaces as the nurse assesses the wound. An intravenous line is inserted, and 5% dextrose/0.45 normal saline is started at 75 mL/hr. After 24 hours a preliminary culture report shows MRSA in the decubitus ulcer. The nurse implements Contact Precautions for Mr. Kendall.

Nursing Diagnosis

The following nursing diagnoses (among others) are developed for Mr. Kendall:

- *Imbalanced Nutrition: Less Than Body Requirements* related to poor appetite
- *Impaired Skin Integrity* related to large decubitus ulcer
- *Acute Pain* related to decubitus ulcer
- *Hopelessness* related to recent widowhood and CVA

Expected Outcomes

The expected outcomes established in the plan of care specify that:

- Mr. Kendall will increase dietary intake.
- Wound will show signs of healing.
- Wound cultures will no longer show a MRSA infection.
- Mr. Kendall will report that pain is decreased.
- He will communicate feelings about his situation.

Planning and Implementation

Ms. Thompson, RN, implements the following interventions:

- Monitor daily weight, intake and output, and hydration status.
- Assess for risk of aspiration during eating and drinking.
- Identify foods Mr. Kendall likes and dislikes.
- Provide small, frequent, high-protein meals.
- Consult with a dietitian regarding supplemental foods such as Ensure.
- Monitor serum albumin levels.
- Assess the skin every 8 hours; keep clean and dry.
- Turn at least every 2 hours; minimize time Mr. Kendall lies on his back; and prevent shearing.

- Consult with the physician for an air/water mattress or specialized bed (e.g., Clinitron Bed).
- Follow Contact Precautions; perform meticulous hand hygiene before and after care.
- Premedicate before dressing changes or wound care.
- Use aseptic technique to provide wound care to decubitus ulcer.
- Administer antibiotics as ordered.
- Determine the level of pain using a 0–10 pain scale.
- Administer pain medications PRN.
- Encourage Mr. Kendall to discuss his feelings and concerns.
- Arrange for social services to talk to his daughter.

Evaluation

After a month in the hospital Mr. Kendall's wound culture is negative for MRSA. The wound is showing signs of healing. His daughter has visited him twice. He smiles occasionally and interacts with the staff more positively. Mr. Kendall's appetite has improved, and he no longer needs supplemental feedings. He reports that his pain is tolerable. He understands that he has to return to the long-term care facility until his wound heals completely. His daughter plans to move him to her home sometime in the near future.

Critical Thinking in the Nursing Process

1. What type of isolation garments should the nurse wear while providing care to Mr. Kendall?
2. How did Mr. Kendall contract MRSA?
3. How does the diagnosis of MRSA in one patient affect the care of other patients on the nursing unit? What strategies should the nurse employ to prevent the transmission of MRSA to other patients?

Note: Discussion of Critical Thinking questions appears on the companion website.

Note: The references and resources for all chapters have been compiled at the back of the book.

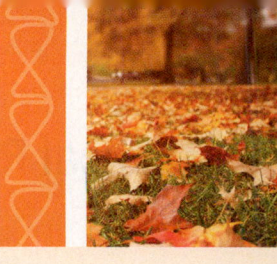

Chapter Review

KEY POINTS

- **Concept:** Inflammation is the body's protective response when injured by factors such as abrasions, chemicals, pathogenic organisms, overuse, or extreme temperatures. While the acute inflammatory response is usually short term, chronic inflammation is often long term.
- The body is protected from microorganisms by the skin, physical barriers such as coughing, and chemical defenses such as stomach acid secretion, urine, and vaginal secretions.
- Cardinal manifestations of local inflammation are redness, warmth, pain, edema, and loss of function.
- **Concept:** Microorganisms are able to cause disease due to their ability to invade tissues or secrete toxins. Loss of the body's defense mechanisms increases the risk for infection. Hospitalized patients have an increased risk of developing health care–associated infections.
- The chain of infection includes a microorganism, a reservoir, a portal of exit from the reservoir, a mode of transmission from the reservoir, and an entry point into a susceptible host.
- Localized infections may damage tissue and cause pain, but systemic infections are life threatening if they progress to septic shock. Fever, tachycardia, increased respiratory rate, lymphadenopathy, and WBC count greater than 10,000/mm^3 may indicate a systemic infection.
- Health care–associated infections are often caused by multidrug-resistant organisms such as methicillin-resistant

Staphylococcus aureus (MRSA), vancomycin-resistant *Enterococcus* (VRE), and *Clostridium difficile*–associated diarrhea (CDAD).
- Aging causes a decline in the immune system's responsiveness to harmful invading pathogens. This increases older adults' risk for developing pneumonia, influenza, and urinary tract and skin infections.
- Antibiotic, antiviral, antifungal, and antiparasitic medications are the common medications used to manage infections.
- **Concept:** Nurses as members of the health care team play a key role in reducing the potential for infection. Basic prevention strategies include practicing and promoting hand hygiene, using Standard Precautions, assessing patients for possible signs and symptoms of infection, and teaching patients about preventative strategies.
- Health care environments often harbor numerous pathogens. Consistent use of Standard Precautions and aseptic technique can limit the development of HAIs during medical procedures.
- Hand hygiene is the most important measure in preventing HAIs.
- Standard Precautions include respiratory and cough etiquette guidelines. Transmission-Based Precautions focus on pathogens spread by the airborne, droplet, or contact route.

PEARSON NURSING STUDENT RESOURCES

Find additional materials at **nursing.pearsonhighered.com**.

Clinical Reasoning Care Map

Caring for a Patient Exposed to *Staphylococcus aureus*
NCLEX-PN® Focus Area: Reduction of Risk Potential

Case Study: Mr. Fields, age 76, was transferred from a long-term nursing care facility for a mild left-side stroke. He has an intravenous line and Foley catheter in place. Mr. Fields weighs 140 lb and is 6' tall. He shares a hospital room with another patient who is diagnosed with *Staphylococcus aureus* pneumonia. Mr. Fields's vital signs are BP 158/90, P 88, R 24, T 99°F.

Nursing Diagnosis: Risk for Infection

COLLECT DATA

Subjective	Objective
_____	_____
_____	_____
_____	_____
_____	_____
_____	_____
_____	_____

Does this present a threat to the patient's safety?

If yes, the priority intervention to address this threat would be:
_____

Nursing Care

_____
_____
_____
_____
_____
_____
_____
_____
_____

Interprofessional team members to include when planning care:
_____
_____

How would you document this?_____
_____
_____

Data Collected
(use only those that apply)

- Roommate with *S. aureus* pneumonia
- Pale coloring
- Weight 140 lb
- Urine output 200 mL for shift
- Temperature 99°F
- Dislikes being in the nursing home
- Pressure ulcer on right great toe
- History of type 2 diabetes

Nursing Interventions
(use only those that apply; list in priority order)

- Monitor the skin for further breakdown.
- Place in protective isolation.
- Monitor vital signs every 4 hours.
- Increase fluid intake as tolerated.
- Provide a diet high in protein.
- Prevent food from pocketing on the right side of his mouth.

Compare your answers and documentation to those provided on the companion website.

NCLEX-PN® Exam Preparation

1. A patient, age 82, is admitted to the surgical unit after 3 days in the intensive care unit after a colon resection. His vital signs are stable, and his urinary drainage bag contains 300 mL of clear yellow urine. Which of the following information is most important to determine whether the patient is at risk for developing a health care–associated infection?
   1. Foley catheter insertion during surgery
   2. Use of an antibiotic for 1 week before surgery
   3. Weight of 150 lb
   4. Poor venous circulation in the left leg

2. A patient is scheduled for a left knee replacement. Which of the following lab values should the nurse report to the physician immediately?
   1. Erythrocyte sedimentation level is decreased.
   2. WBC differential shows the absence of bands.
   3. WBC count is 15,000/mm^3.
   4. C-reactive protein result is negative.

3. A patient is in an outpatient clinic for a severe sprain to the left ankle. Which of the following interventions should the nurse anticipate implementing?
   1. Apply a heating pad to the ankle for 1 hour daily.
   2. Start corticosteroid therapy immediately.
   3. Measure the circumference of the ankle.
   4. Elevate the ankle on pillows when the patient is sitting in a chair.

4. Three days after starting ampicillin therapy for a staphylococcal infection, the patient returns to the clinic, complaining of vaginal itchiness and redness. The nurse suspects that the patient has developed vaginitis. What response should the nurse make to the patient?
   1. "Oh, don't worry about that. It will go away after you finish the medication."
   2. "I will let the doctor know right away."
   3. "It's just vaginitis. We'll give you something for it."
   4. "Okay. Are you having any other problems?"

5. The nurse is planning discharge care for a patient who has suffered numerous abrasions sustained in a motor vehicle crash. Which of the following should be included in the discharge instructions?
   1. "Discontinue the antibiotics once the redness has subsided."
   2. "A slight fever is common and should not be reported."
   3. "Drink at least 2 quarts of water per day."
   4. "Wash your hands carefully before changing the wound dressings."

6. Which medication treatment should the nurse anticipate administering for the patient with a diagnosis of MRSA infection?
   1. Vancomycin (Vancocin)
   2. Azithromycin (Zithromax)
   3. Gentamicin (Garamycin)
   4. Cephalexin (Keflex)

7. A 70-year-old male patient was admitted to the medical floor with a diagnosis of left periorbital cellulitis. Based on this diagnosis, which of the following interventions would the nurse anticipate as part of the patient's care plan in order to promote the healing process?
   1. Administer IV antibiotics as ordered.
   2. Maintain bed rest.
   3. Medicate the patient around the clock with IM morphine.
   4. Monitor the WBC count.

8. A patient is hospitalized with an open wound on the lower leg that is draining yellow-colored fluid. Which of the following clinical manifestations could indicate an infection has become systemic?
   1. The patient reports tenderness around the wound.
   2. The nurse palpates enlarged lymph nodes in the groin.
   3. The patient reports pain when ambulating.
   4. The nurse notes cellulitis of the patient's lower leg.

9. Which one of the following patients has the highest risk for developing herpes zoster or shingles?
   1. A 48-year-old with rheumatoid arthritis
   2. A 58-year-old recovering from surgery
   3. A 60-year-old with diabetes mellitus
   4. A 75-year-old woman

10. Which of the following isolation precautions should the nurse implement for a patient admitted with a diagnosis of varicella? **Select all that apply.**
    1. Don mask and face shield when caring for the patient.
    2. Use alcohol-based hand rub before and after leaving the patient's room.
    3. Wear an N95 disposable respirator when entering the patient's room.
    4. Remind the family to wear a gown and mask when visiting the patient.
    5. Wear sterile gloves when providing care to the patient.
    6. Place mask on the patient when transporting to another department.

Answers and rationales for Review Questions appear in Appendix I.

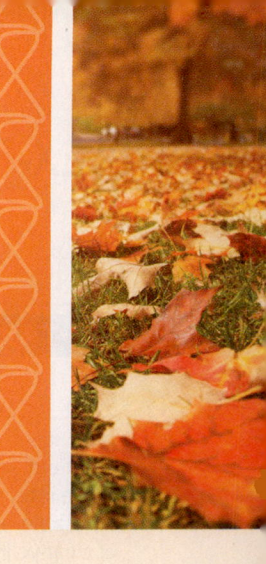

CHAPTER 10
Caring for Patients Having Surgery

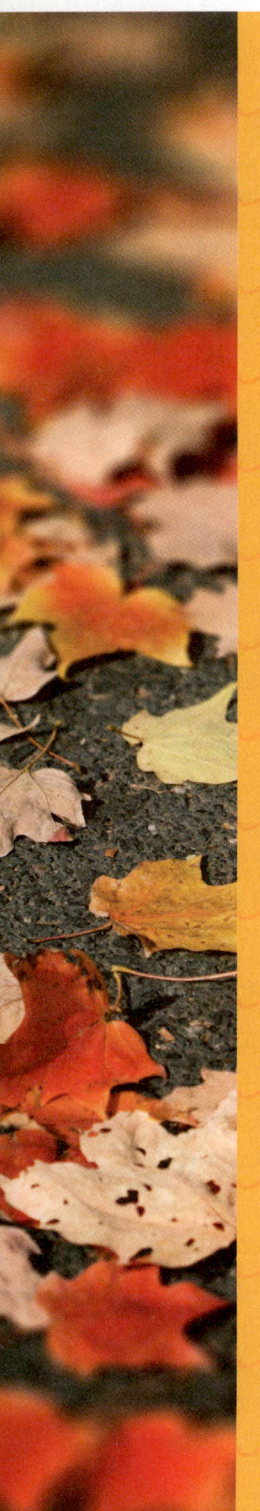

BRIEF OUTLINE

Informed Consent   **PHASES OF THE SURGICAL EXPERIENCE**   Intraoperative Phase

Safety in Perioperative Care   Preoperative Phase   Postoperative Phase

APPLIED LEARNING OUTCOMES

After completing this chapter, you will be able to:

1. Describe how surgical procedures are classified.

2. Discuss roles and responsibilities of nurses and interdisciplinary team members in ensuring patient safety during the perioperative experience.

3. Identify and use specific communication techniques and protocols to promote safety in the perioperative setting.

4. Assess stated needs, values, and expectations of the preoperative patient; planning and implementing patient-centered care; and teaching in collaboration with the interdisciplinary team.

5. Plan for and provide appropriate evidence-based nursing care for the patient in the preoperative, intraoperative, and postoperative phases of surgery.

6. Adapt perioperative care for the older adult as appropriate.

7. Apply principles of pain management for the postoperative patient.

8. Compare and contrast patient needs and nursing responsibilities related to outpatient and inpatient surgery.

KEY TERMS

The key terms are defined on the pages listed below.

SPECIAL FEATURES

Surgery is an invasive medical procedure used to diagnose and treat disease, repair injury, or correct deformity. Surgical procedures can be further classified by surgical technique, risk, and urgency (Table 10-1 ■). The nurse assumes an active role in caring for the patient before, during, and after surgery. The LPN/LVN collaborates with the health care team to prepare the patient before surgery, prevent injury and complications, and promote optimal recovery after surgery.

Perioperative nursing care (care provided immediately before, during, and after surgery) requires knowledge and understanding of many factors, including the following:

■ Surgical anatomy
■ Anticipated physiologic disruptions related to the surgery and their potential consequences
■ Potential injuries to the patient and their prevention
■ Risk factors and potential complications of the surgery
■ Evidence-based nursing care to promote optimal recovery
■ The emotional and psychosocial effects of the surgery on the patient and family

Surgery may be performed in a hospital or in an ambulatory care setting. **Inpatient surgery** requires admission to a hospital before the procedure and inpatient nursing care after the procedure. Inpatient surgery may be planned (e.g., a joint replacement) or an emergency situation (e.g., an appendectomy). Major surgical procedures may require inpatient care for 3 or more days after surgery.

Ambulatory surgery (or *outpatient surgery*) is a surgical procedure performed in a physician's office, free-standing ambulatory surgery center, or hospital facility, depending on the complexity of the procedure and required anesthesia. After the procedure and anesthesia recovery, the patient may be immediately discharged or remain for a short period of postoperative recovery and observation. Surgeries such as cataract removal, hernia repair, vasectomy, and biopsy are routinely performed in an ambulatory surgery setting, as well as more complicated procedures such as laparoscopic gallbladder removal and simple mastectomy. The patient's responses after surgery drive the decision for discharge or admission to a short-stay unit (less than 24 hours) or an inpatient facility for further observation.

Ambulatory surgery has advantages and disadvantages. Advantages are that the patient recovers more quickly in the home and is less likely to be exposed to pathogens that could lead to a wound infection. Disadvantages include limited time and opportunity for assessment of patient needs and teaching for home care. The increased number and complexity of procedures and patient acuity present a challenge to the perioperative nurse.

Many similarities exist in nursing care of the inpatient and ambulatory surgical patient. The focus of collaborative and nursing care during the preoperative, intraoperative, and postoperative phases of surgery is much the same. The major differences are in the time for patient teaching and emotional support. The need to learn a great deal of information in a short span of time is an additional stressor for the ambulatory surgical patient. The nurse teaches self-care to the patient and family in both the preoperative and postoperative periods. Patients with complicated health problems or who are undergoing complex surgical procedures require more extensive teaching and emotional support.

TABLE 10-1	Classification of Surgical Procedures	
	CLASSIFICATION	**PURPOSE**
Purpose	Diagnostic	Establish a diagnosis
	Ablative	Remove diseased tissue
	Reconstructive	Rebuild damaged tissues
	Palliative	Alleviate symptoms (not curative)
	Transplant	Replace organs or tissue
Technique	Minimally invasive surgery (MIS)	Minimize incision and tissue disruption
	Laser surgery	Minimize tissue damage
Risk	Minor	Minimal physical assault and risk
	Major	Extensive physical assault and/or serious risk
Urgency	Elective	No foreseen ill effects if postponed
	Urgent	Necessary within 1–2 days
	Emergency	Performed immediately

Informed Consent

Informed consent is an agreement by the patient to accept treatment or undergo a procedure after receiving complete information, including risks of the procedure and those associated with failing to undergo the procedure (Blais & Hayes, 2011; Guido, 2010). Informed consent includes the following information:

- An explanation of the proposed procedure, its purpose, and expected outcome
- Who will perform the procedure, including name and qualifications of those involved
- Potential risks and harm that may occur, including pain
- Alternative treatments or procedures, including the risk of no treatment at all
- The right to refuse the proposed procedure, while alternative care or support is continued
- The right to refuse treatment or withdraw consent after treatment has begun (Guido, 2010)

The physician who performs the procedure is responsible for providing the information necessary to obtain the patient's informed consent. The nurse may clarify information as needed. If the patient has questions or concerns or the nurse questions the patient's understanding, the physician should be contacted to provide further information. After a thorough discussion of the treatment or procedure, the nurse may witness the patient's signature on the form. The nurse also signs the form, indicating that the correct person signed the form and that the patient was alert and aware of what was being signed.

clinicalALERT

Although the nurse may witness the patient's signature on an informed consent form, it is the physician's responsibility to explain the planned procedure and associated risks and benefits, and to obtain the patient's consent.

Hospital policies specify circumstances in which consent may be given by someone other than the patient and the procedure to follow if consent cannot be obtained. Most states require patients ages 18 and over to sign their own consent and a parent or legal guardian to sign for patients under age 18. **Emancipated minors** (persons under age 18 who are responsible for their own welfare, who live independently from their parents, and those who are married or are parents) also sign their own consent. The signature of a legal guardian is required for adults who are mentally challenged or who have been determined by the courts to be incompetent to make their own medical decisions. In life-threatening situations when surgery is required but the patient is unable to sign the consent, every effort is made to contact *next of kin* (as specified by facility policy)

for consent. If next of kin cannot be located and continued delay would be life threatening, a court order may be obtained, or the surgeon may assume responsibility for proceeding without consent. The nurse carefully documents the steps taken to obtain consent and the circumstances dictating the need for surgery.

When obtaining informed consent from older adults, allow adequate time for the patient to process information, ask questions, and make decisions with the assistance of professionals and family members.

Safety in Perioperative Care

Maintaining patient safety is a concern of nurses in all settings of care. The role that established health care systems, practices, and protocols play in promoting or threatening patient safety has recently gained attention. In response, organizations such as the Joint Commission (TJC), the World Health Organization (WHO), and the Association of periOperative Registered Nurses (AORN) have published patient safety guidelines focused on preventing errors and unintentional injury during the perioperative period. In addition, Centers for Medicare & Medicaid Services (CMS), the federal agency that administers Medicare, Medicaid, and other health-related federal programs, no longer pays the cost of treating selected negative outcomes resulting from unsafe patient care (e.g., wrong site surgery, surgical site infection after certain surgeries). Box 10-1■ summarizes TJC 2013 National Patient Safety Goals for hospitals. Those for ambulatory care and office-based surgeries are similar. The WHO Surgical Safety Checklist is shown in Figure 10-1■.

Effective communication with the patient and among all members of the health care team is an essential element of perioperative patient safety. Both documentation in the clinical record and focused, purposeful verbal communication among team members are critical. Documentation of perioperative nursing care includes the nursing assessment, plan of care for the individual patient, and implementation and evaluation of planned outcomes of care.

Effective communication of information must occur during a **handoff** (or *handover*), when responsibility for care is transferred from one individual or care unit to another. Handoff reports provide essential, up-to-date, and specific patient information. Handoffs also must include an opportunity to ask and respond to questions (Rothrock, 2011). Timely, accurate, complete, and clear information that is understood by the recipient is necessary for effective communication (Amato-Vealey et al., 2008). Use effective communication strategies and techniques such as SBAR (situation, background, assessment, and recommendations) to help ensure clarity and reduce the risk for error.

BOX 10-1	HOSPITAL NATIONAL PATIENT SAFETY GOALS

The purpose of the National Patient Safety Goals is to improve patient safety. The goals focus on problems in health care safety and how to solve them.

1. Identify patients correctly.
   - Use at least two ways to identify patients (e.g., name and date of birth).
   - Make sure the correct patient gets the correct blood when they receive a transfusion.
2. Improve staff communication.
   - Report test and diagnostic procedure results to the appropriate person in a timely manner.
3. Use medications safely.
   - Label medications and solutions that are not given immediately.
   - Use additional precautions with anticoagulant medicines.
   - Maintain and communicate accurate information about the patient's current medications. Compare current medications with those taken by the patient

before admission. Make sure the patient knows which medications to take at home.

4. Prevent infection.
   - Use current CDC or WHO guidelines for hand hygiene.
   - Use evidence-based practices to prevent health care–associated infections (HAIs), including those that are difficult to treat, bloodstream infections, surgical site infection, and catheter-associated urinary tract infections.
5. Prevent mistakes in surgery.
   - Make sure the correct surgery is done on the correct body part of the correct patient.
   - Mark the correct place on the patient's body where the surgery is to be done.
   - Pause before surgery to make sure a mistake is not being made.

Source: Adapted from the 2014 Hospital National Patient Safety Goals by The Joint Commission. Copyright © 2013 by The Joint Commission. Used by permission of The Joint Commission.

Surgical Safety Checklist

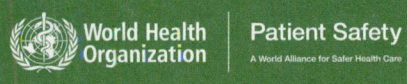 World Health Organization | Patient Safety
A World Alliance for Safer Health Care

Before induction of anaesthesia	Before skin incision	Before patient leaves operating room
(with at least nurse and anaesthetist)	(with nurse, anaesthetist and surgeon)	(with nurse, anaesthetist and surgeon)

Before induction of anaesthesia

Has the patient confirmed his/her identity, site, procedure, and consent?
- ☐ Yes

Is the site marked?
- ☐ Yes
- ☐ Not applicable

Is the anaesthesia machine and medication check complete?
- ☐ Yes

Is the pulse oximeter on the patient and functioning?
- ☐ Yes

Does the patient have a:

Known allergy?
- ☐ No
- ☐ Yes

Difficult airway or aspiration risk?
- ☐ No
- ☐ Yes, and equipment/assistance available

Risk of >500ml blood loss (7ml/kg in children)?
- ☐ No
- ☐ Yes, and two IVs/central access and fluids planned

Before skin incision

- ☐ **Confirm all team members have introduced themselves by name and role.**
- ☐ **Confirm the patient's name, procedure, and where the incision will be made.**

Has antibiotic prophylaxis been given within the last 60 minutes?
- ☐ Yes
- ☐ Not applicable

Anticipated Critical Events

To Surgeon:
- ☐ What are the critical or non-routine steps?
- ☐ How long will the case take?
- ☐ What is the anticipated blood loss?

To Anaesthetist:
- ☐ Are there any patient-specific concerns?

To Nursing Team:
- ☐ Has sterility (including indicator results) been confirmed?
- ☐ Are there equipment issues or any concerns?

Is essential imaging displayed?
- ☐ Yes
- ☐ Not applicable

Before patient leaves operating room

Nurse Verbally Confirms:
- ☐ The name of the procedure
- ☐ Completion of instrument, sponge and needle counts
- ☐ Specimen labelling (read specimen labels aloud, including patient name)
- ☐ Whether there are any equipment problems to be addressed

To Surgeon, Anaesthetist and Nurse:
- ☐ What are the key concerns for recovery and management of this patient?

This checklist is not intended to be comprehensive. Additions and modifications to fit local practice are encouraged.

Revised 1 / 2009   © WHO, 2009

Figure 10-1. ■ WHO Surgical Safety Checklist. (Source: WHO *Surgical Safety Checklist*, http://whqlibdoc.who.int/publications/2009/ 9789241598590_eng_Checklist.pdf, by the World Health Organization. Copyright © 2009. Used by permission of the World Health Organization. All rights reserved.)

PHASES OF THE SURGICAL EXPERIENCE

Perioperative nursing care incorporates the three phases of the surgical experience: preoperative, intraoperative, and postoperative. The **preoperative phase** begins when the decision for surgery is made and ends when the patient is transferred to the surgical suite. The **intraoperative phase** begins with the patient's entry into the surgical suite and ends with transfer to the postanesthesia care unit (PACU, or recovery room). The **postoperative phase** begins when the patient is admitted to the PACU and ends when recovery from the surgical intervention is complete.

Preoperative Phase

> **Key Concept** Assessing, coordinating, and implementing preoperative preparation and patient teaching are key nursing roles during the preoperative phase.

The focus of the preoperative phase of the surgical experience is on:

- Obtaining informed consent for surgery.
- Identifying patient risk factors and needs before and during surgery.
- Physical and psychologic preparation of the patient.
- Educating the patient and family about the surgery, expected outcomes, and the recovery process.
- Teaching postoperative measures to promote recovery and prevent complications, for example, pain management, using an incentive spirometer, and techniques for changing positions.

Surgery is a physical stressor that evokes the general stress response. Three major organ systems are involved in the stress response: the nervous system, endocrine system, and immune system.

The sympathetic nervous system is activated and norepinephrine is released from sympathetic nerve endings. Norepinephrine, together with epinephrine from the adrenal glands, increases the heart rate and improves cardiac output and blood flow to skeletal muscles. Gastrointestinal tract motility and secretions decrease in response to these substances. Hormones such as cortisol, glucagon, and growth hormone help maintain blood glucose levels, providing fuel to the cells. However, cortisol also suppresses the immune response and healing processes.

Surgery also presents significant psychosocial stress for the patient and family. Anxiety is a common response to impending surgery. The level of anxiety the patient and family experiences is unique and depends on the significance of the underlying diagnosis and procedure to the individuals. For example, a patient scheduled to have a biopsy to rule out cancer may be more anxious than a patient undergoing gallbladder removal. Previous experiences with surgery and hospitalization also affect anxiety levels. The level of anxiety affects the ability to learn new information and understand instructions, as well as physical responses to anesthetics and postoperative pain.

SURGICAL RISK ASSESSMENT

Preoperative assessment of the patient's overall health status and specific risk factors for surgery is vital. This information helps determine the type and extent of surgery and the most appropriate anesthetic. The preoperative assessment is used in planning nursing care during all phases of the surgical experience. Table 10-2■ identifies selected surgical risk factors and their nursing implications.

COLLABORATIVE CARE

The **Universal Protocol** (Box 10-2■) is an important safety initiative established by TJC in 2003 to reduce the "wrong site, wrong procedure, wrong person" surgery risk. All members of the health care team, including the patient

---

BOX 10-2   THE UNIVERSAL PROTOCOL

The Universal Protocol to reduce wrong site, wrong procedure, and wrong person surgery includes a preprocedure verification, site marking, and a time-out.

1. *Conduct a preprocedure verification process* when the procedure is scheduled, during preadmission testing, on admission to the facility, before entering the procedure room, and whenever the patient is transferred to another caregiver during the procedure. This process addresses missing information or discrepancies before the procedure and includes verifying:

   - ✓ The procedure, the patient, and the site. Whenever possible, the patient should be involved in the verification process.
   - ✓ Availability of relevant documents, such as the history and physical, signed consent form and preanesthesia assessment.
   - ✓ Correct and accurately labeled diagnostic test results, including x-rays.
   - ✓ Any required blood products, implants, devices, or special equipment.

2. *Mark the procedure site* when there is more than one possible location for the procedure. The site is to be marked by the licensed health care provider performing the procedure and while the patient is awake. In some cases, site marking may be delegated to an advanced practice RN or a physician's assistant.

3. *"Time-out" before starting the procedure* to conduct a final verification that the correct patient, site, positioning, and procedure are identified and that all relevant documents, information, and equipment are available.

TABLE 10-2	Nursing Implications for Surgical Risk Factors	
FACTOR	**ASSOCIATED RISK**	**NURSING IMPLICATIONS**
Advanced age	■ Age-related changes affect physiologic, cognitive, and psychosocial responses to surgery; increase risk for adverse responses to anesthesia and postoperative medications; impair immune defenses; and delay wound healing.	■ Closely monitor vital signs, level of consciousness and mental status, response to anesthesia and medications, kidney function, and wound healing. ■ Promptly report signs of infection (temperature may remain within normal range), changes in vital signs or mental status, or low urinary output.
Obesity	■ Increased risk for delayed wound healing, wound dehiscence, infection, pneumonia, atelectasis, thrombophlebitis, dysrhythmias, and heart failure.	■ Promote weight reduction if time permits. ■ Monitor closely for wound, pulmonary, and cardiovascular complications postoperatively. ■ Encourage coughing, turning, and diaphragmatic breathing exercises and early ambulation.
Malnutrition	■ Increased risk for adverse outcomes of surgery (shock, organ system failure). ■ Increased risk for impaired wound healing, infection, and sepsis.	■ Minimize duration of fasting or diet restriction associated with surgery. ■ With the physician and dietitian, promote a well-balanced, high-calorie, high-protein diet. ■ Weigh daily. ■ Monitor wound healing and for signs of infection. ■ Monitor WBC, hemoglobin, hematocrit, and serum albumin.
Dehydration/electrolyte imbalance	■ Increased risk for cardiovascular instability, dysrhythmias, and heart failure. ■ Increased risk for acute kidney injury, paralytic ileus, impaired wound healing, pressure ulcers, and venous thrombosis (see Chapter 18).	■ Administer intravenous fluids as ordered. ■ Monitor vital signs, intake, and output. ■ Monitor serum electrolytes, osmolality, and hematocrit. ■ Restore oral intake as soon as possible. ■ Ensure safety when ambulating.
Cardiovascular disorders	■ Increased risk of cardiovascular instability, shock, hypotension, venous thrombosis, pulmonary embolism, stroke, and fluid volume overload.	■ Monitor vital signs, including apical pulse rate, regularity, and rhythm; respiratory rate and ease; oxygen saturation levels; and general condition. ■ Assess skin color. ■ Assess for chest pain, lung congestion, and peripheral edema. ■ Provide early postoperative ambulation.
Respiratory disorders	■ Increased risk for respiratory complications such as atelectasis and pneumonia. ■ Respiratory depression from general anesthesia and acid–base imbalance may also occur.	■ Closely monitor respirations, pulse, oxygen saturation, and breath sounds. ■ Encourage use of incentive spirometer and early mobilization and ambulation.
Diabetes mellitus	■ Increased risk for cardiovascular disease, delayed wound healing, and wound infection; unstable blood glucose levels during and after surgery.	■ Monitor blood glucose and electrolyte levels. ■ Assess for and report signs of hypoglycemia and hyperglycemia.

(continued)

TABLE 10-2	Nursing Implications for Surgical Risk Factors *(continued)*	
FACTOR	**ASSOCIATED RISK**	**NURSING IMPLICATIONS**
Kidney and liver dysfunction	■ Poor tolerance of general anesthesia; increased risk for fluid and electrolyte imbalances and adverse drug reactions.	■ Monitor intake and output. ■ Weigh daily. ■ Monitor response to drugs. ■ Assess pulse strength, skin turgor, and for edema. ■ Monitor laboratory values for kidney and liver function (BUN, creatinine, bilirubin, liver enzymes).
Alcoholism	■ Often associated with malnourished status; may require more anesthesia; at risk for hemorrhage and delayed wound healing.	■ Monitor for signs of delirium tremens. ■ Monitor diet. ■ Assess for evidence of bleeding. ■ Monitor serum electrolytes, hemoglobin, and hematocrit.
Smoking	■ Increased risk for respiratory complications such as pneumonia, atelectasis, and bronchitis because of increased mucous secretions and a decreased ability to expel them.	■ Encourage to quit smoking. ■ Monitor oxygen saturation levels and respiratory status. ■ Encourage coughing and breathing exercises. ■ Promote early ambulation.
Medications	■ Interaction between anesthetics and some medications increases risk for impaired mentation, respiratory complications, bleeding, hypotension, and circulatory collapse.	■ Inform the anesthesiologist and surgeon of all prescribed and over-the-counter medications, including herbal preparations.
Anticoagulants	■ Increased risk for intraoperative and postoperative bleeding.	■ Monitor for bleeding. ■ Assess prothrombin time (PT)/partial thromboplastin time (PTT) values, hemoglobin, and hematocrit.
Diuretics	■ Increased risk for fluid and electrolyte imbalances and cardiovascular instability. ■ Some affect blood glucose levels.	■ Monitor intake and output and serum electrolytes. ■ Assess cardiovascular and respiratory status. ■ Monitor blood glucose.
Antihypertensives/antidepressants	■ Increase the hypotensive effects of anesthesia.	■ Closely monitor blood pressure.

whenever possible, are involved in carrying out the protocol, which starts when the decision to schedule surgery is made and continues into the intraoperative phase.

Diagnostic Tests

Preoperative laboratory and diagnostic tests provide baseline data and help identify surgical risk factors. These studies are performed within a week before elective surgery and immediately before surgery in emergency situations.

Commonly performed preoperative laboratory and diagnostic tests include *complete blood count* (CBC), *serum electrolytes* (Na^+, K^+, Cl^-), *coagulation studies* (prothrombin time [PT or INR], partial thromboplastin time [PTT]), *urinalysis*, *chest x-ray*, and *electrocardiogram* (ECG) (Table 10-3 ■). The urinalysis is obtained to evaluate kidney function and to rule out urinary tract infection and pregnancy. Additional laboratory tests are performed as needed. For example, if the patient has a history of diabetes mellitus, blood glucose levels are monitored before, during, and after surgery.

The chest x-ray provides baseline information about the size, shape, and condition of the heart and lungs. Pulmonary complications, such as chronic lung disease or pneumonia, may require postponement of surgery for further evaluation or treatment.

The ECG is ordered for patients who are undergoing general anesthesia, are older than age 40, or have a history

clinical**ALERT**

Monitor
Monitor laboratory test values and diagnostic test results for the preoperative patient.

Report
Report abnormal values to the charge nurse or physician.

TABLE 10-3	Laboratory Tests for Perioperative Assessment			
TEST	**NORMAL VALUE**	**SIGNIFICANCE OF INCREASED VALUES**	**SIGNIFICANCE OF DECREASED VALUES**	**NURSING IMPLICATIONS**
■ Hemoglobin (Hgb) ■ Hematocrit (Hct)	12–15 g/dL Females 13.5–18 g/dL Males 36%–46% Females 40%–54% Males	Dehydration, excessive plasma loss Polycythemia	Fluid overload, excessive blood loss, anemia	Monitor intake and output and vital signs; assess for bleeding.
■ White blood cell count (WBC)	4,500–10,000 μL	Infection/inflammation process	Immune deficiencies	Monitor for signs of inflammation and infection.
■ Platelet count	150,000–400,000 μL	Malignancies	Clotting disorders, chemotherapy	Assess for signs of bleeding at the incision site and drainage tubes. Assess for hematoma.
■ Potassium (K^+)	3.5–5.3 mEq/L	Kidney failure, dehydration, cell damage	Diuretics, malnutrition, gastric **suction** (process of promoting drainage)	Monitor cardiac and GI status; monitor intake and output.
■ Chloride (Cl^-)	95–105 mEq/L	Dehydration, kidney dysfunction	Diuretics, vomiting, gastric suction	Monitor lab values; monitor intake and output.
■ Sodium (Na^+)	135–145 mEq/L	Kidney dysfunction, IV fluids containing sodium chloride	Diuretics, vomiting, gastric suction	Monitor lab values; monitor intake and output and mental status.
■ Prothrombin time (protime, INR) ■ Partial thromboplastin time (PTT or APTT)	11–13 seconds 60–70 seconds (PTT) 20–35 seconds (APTT)	Clotting disorders, anticoagulant therapy, side effects of other drugs affecting clotting time	Increased risk for deep venous thrombosis (DVT)	Monitor lab values. Assess for bleeding from incision, urine, and hematoma formation. Encourage leg exercises and ambulation.
■ Urinalysis	Glucose negative Protein negative WBC negative RBC negative Bacteria negative Ketones negative	May indicate urinary tract infection, impaired kidney function, malnutrition, or diabetes mellitus.		Monitor and report abnormal values.

of cardiovascular disease. The ECG is used to evaluate the cardiac status of the patient and identify new or preexisting cardiac conditions.

Medications

Preoperative medications, which may be administered before the patient is transferred to the surgical suite, are used for sedation and to reduce anxiety, enhance anesthesia, and reduce the risk of intraoperative or postoperative complications. Table 10-4■ outlines selected commonly prescribed preoperative medications. The nurse is responsible for administering these drugs before surgery. Antibiotic therapy also may be initiated before surgery to reduce the risk for infection.

Any final questions by or of the patient should be addressed before administering preoperative medications. In addition, members of the surgical team verify the patient's identity, the planned procedure, and the side and site of surgery before premedication. Marking the surgical site (see later) also is completed before premedication.

Preoperative medications may be given orally with a small sip of water to facilitate swallowing or parenterally. Intravenous medications often are administered within the surgical suite.

Physical Preparation

Physical preparation of the patient for surgery may include the following:

■ *Marking the operative site* is done while the patient is awake and before any sedation is given. The site is clearly and unambiguously identified with an indelible marker that will remain visible after the skin preparation (e.g., do not use an X because it could be interpreted to mean "not this one"). When marking, specific attention is paid to the incision site; to the specific extremity, digit, or lesion to be treated; for spinal surgery,

TABLE 10-4	Giving Medications Safely: Preoperative Medications		
CLASS/DRUGS	**DOSE AND ROUTE**	**PURPOSE**	**NURSING IMPLICATIONS**
Antibiotics			
■ Cefazolin	1–2 g IV	Prevent surgical site infections	Report known allergy to penicillin or other antibiotics.
Benzodiazepines			
■ Midazolam (Versed)	3–5 mg IM, IV	Decrease anxiety and produce sedation	Monitor for respiratory depression, hypotension, drowsiness, confusion, and lack of coordination.
■ *Lorazepam* (Ativan)	1–4 mg IM, IV	May induce substantial amnesia	
Opioid analgesics			
■ Morphine	5–15 mg IM, IV	Decrease anxiety, provide analgesia, allow reduced anesthetic dose	Monitor for respiratory depression, nausea, vomiting, orthostatic hypotension, and pruritus.
■ Fentanyl (Sublimaze)	25–50 mcg IV, IM		
■ *Oxycodone* (OxyFast, Roxicodone)	5–10 mg PO		
■ *Tramadol* (Ultram)	50–100 mg PO		
H₂ receptor antagonists			
■ *Famotidine* (Pepcid)	20 mg IV	Reduce gastric acid volume and concentration	Monitor for confusion and dizziness in older adults.
■ *Ranitidine* (Zantac)	50 mg IV, IM, PO		
Proton-pump inhibitors			
■ Lansoprazole (Prevacid)	15–60 mg PO	Suppress gastric acid secretion	Monitor for dizziness and headache, rash, or thirst.
■ *Omeprazole* (Prilosec)	20–40 mg PO		
Antiemetics			
■ Metoclopramide (Reglan)	10 mg IV	Enhance gastric emptying	Monitor for sedation and extrapyramidal reaction (involuntary movement, muscle tone changes, and abnormal posture).
■ Droperidol (Inapsine)	2.5–10 mg IM	Reduce anxiety	
Anticholinergics			
■ Atropine sulfate	0.4–0.6 mg IM, IV	Reduce oral and respiratory secretions to decrease risk of aspiration; decrease risk of vomiting and laryngospasm	Monitor for confusion, restlessness, and tachycardia. Prepare the patient to expect a dry mouth.
■ Glycopyrrolate (Robinul)	0.1–0.3 mg IM, IV		

Note: Medications identified in *italics* are among the 200 most frequently prescribed drugs in the United States.

to the level of the spine; for procedures involving paired organs (e.g., the lungs, kidneys, ovaries), to the affected side (even if the incision is to be made at midline). When a stoma is to be created during surgery, an enterostomal therapist works with the patient and surgeon to identify and mark the appropriate stoma location.

■ *Skin preparation* to reduce the number of bacteria on the skin in the surgical area is often performed in the surgical suite immediately before the procedure. However, any body jewelry should be removed and safeguarded before transfer to the surgical suite. The areas to be prepped are determined by the type and location of surgery to be performed. Patient allergies to iodine, seafood (which may indicate an iodine allergy), or other topical agents are determined before skin preparation to reduce the risk of reactions.

■ Any moles, warts, rashes, or lesions within the surgical site are noted and documented.

■ The patient is instructed to shower and shampoo, often prior to arrival at the facility. The choice of cleansing agent may be determined by agency policy or the surgeon.

■ When necessary, hair is removed from the surgical site immediately before surgery by trained personnel using clippers or depilatory cream or lotion. Clippers are the safest for removing hair and are associated with lower postoperative infection rates than other methods. Razors, which can damage skin and increase the risk for infection, generally are avoided.

■ *An indwelling (Foley) catheter* may be inserted to reduce the risk of injury to the bladder during abdominal surgery. It also provides a means to assess urinary output accurately during extensive surgery.

- *Bowel preparation* may be necessary to prevent introduction of bacteria into the peritoneum during surgery on the bowel. Bowel prep may be initiated by the patient using a stimulant laxative before admission to the hospital or by the nurse for inpatients. Oral antibiotics also may be ordered to reduce resident bacteria in the bowel. The nurse should explain the procedures thoroughly to the patient and document evaluation of patient understanding. See Table 26-4 for nursing responsibilities related to medications used for bowel preparation.
- *Withholding of food and fluids* may be part of preparation for surgery. Patients are instructed to withhold all food and fluids for a specific period of time before surgery, generally 6 or more hours. Current evidence supports allowing intake of clear liquids up until about 2 hours before surgery and fasting for the remaining time. The surgeon and the anesthesiologist determine the exact amount of time the patient should be fasting (nothing by mouth or NPO status). Fasting reduces the risk of aspiration of stomach contents during surgery, especially if the patient receives general anesthesia. The nurse should explain the rationale for and importance of following these instructions. Patients with a history of chronic medical problems such as diabetes mellitus, hypertension, or heart disease often are allowed to take their oral medications before surgery. The nurse must verify this with the physician and instruct the patient to take the medications with a minimal amount of water.

NURSING CARE

The LPN/LVN assesses, plans, and implements care with the registered nurse to identify and meet the individualized needs of the preoperative patient.

PRIORITIZING NURSING CARE

Priorities in the preoperative phase are to accurately identify the patient and procedure, to evaluate and enhance the patient's understanding, to manage anxiety, and to assess and prepare the patient before surgery. A nursing care checklist for the day of surgery is provided in Box 10-3■.

HEALTH PROMOTION

Patient teaching is an essential health promotion activity in the preoperative period. Patient education combined with emotional support has been shown to reduce pain and anxiety; reduce complications; and facilitate early discharge, patient satisfaction, and the patient's return to normal activities. These positive outcomes may be attributed in part to the perceived sense of control gained through education.

Teaching should begin as soon as the patient is aware of the upcoming surgery. The amount and type of information

BOX 10-3   NURSING CARE CHECKLIST

Day of Surgery

Verify Medical Record includes the following:
- ☑ Completed, signed, and witnessed consent for the procedure
- ☑ Completed history and physical exam
- ☑ Laboratory and diagnostic test results
- ☑ Current vital signs
- ☑ Documentation of preoperative care and all medications administered

Patient Preparation
- ☑ Identification, blood, and allergy bands are correct, legible, and secure.
- ☑ The operative site is accurately and appropriately marked.
- ☑ Reinforce and clarify teaching. Provide support for the patient and family.
- ☑ Remove and secure jewelry, hair pins, glasses, contact lenses, and prostheses. Remove nail polish per policy.
- ☑ Remove and secure dentures unless instructed to do otherwise.
- ☑ Leave a hearing aid in place if the patient cannot hear without it, and notify the surgical team.
- ☑ Assist with bathing, hygiene, and changing into operating room gown as needed.
- ☑ Verify NPO status for the prescribed period. Notify the anesthesiologist if fasting orders have not been followed.
- ☑ Complete skin or bowel preparation as ordered.
- ☑ Instruct to empty the bladder before the preoperative sedation is given.
- ☑ Insert an indwelling catheter, intravenous line, or nasogastric tube as ordered.
- ☑ Administer preoperative medication as scheduled (see Table 10-4).
- ☑ Ensure safety after medication administration with side rails up and call light within reach.

Transferring Care to Surgical Team
- ☑ Verify the patient's identity, the procedure to be performed, and surgical site.
- ☑ Report pertinent information including vital signs, pain level, allergies, medications taken or administered, and specific laboratory data or medical history as appropriate.
- ☑ Assist with patient transfer as needed.

provided is determined by the surgical procedure being performed. To be effective, patient education must be based on the patient's needs, preferences, and values. Essential patient teaching includes the following:

- Information about the procedure and what to expect before, during, and after the procedure. Discuss anticipated sensations, including pain. Explain the importance of effective pain management to surgical recovery, and explain the patient's role in managing pain.

- Expected timetable for surgery and recovery
- Ordered laboratory and diagnostic tests, including the reason for the tests, when they are to be done, and any required preparations for the tests
- Required preoperative preparations, such as any prescribed medications, shower with antibacterial soap, bowel preparation
- Specific instructions regarding current medications, including drugs that should be discontinued before surgery (e.g., avoid aspirin, even low-dose aspirin, for 7 days prior to surgery) and whether to take regularly scheduled medications the morning of the surgery
- Preparations for the day of surgery: NPO as instructed, preoperative medication, and handling of valuables (e.g., rings, watch, money)

- Time the patient and/or family should arrive at the facility
- Location of the surgical waiting area
- Anticipated postoperative routine and devices or equipment (e.g., drains, tubes, equipment for intravenous infusions, oxygen or humidifying mask, dressings, splints, casts)

Patient teaching that helps to reduce postsurgical risk for most patients is included in Box 10-4■.

ASSESSING

Thorough nursing assessment is critical for the preoperative patient. The LPN/LVN contributes to the assessment by collecting focused assessment data to identify physiologic and psychologic alterations that require nursing and/or medical intervention.

- *Subjective data:* reason for surgery and understanding of the procedure to be done; current complaints or

---

BOX 10-4	PATIENT TEACHING

Preoperative Exercise Instructions

Breathing and Coughing Exercises

Deep-breathing and coughing exercises help to prevent pulmonary complications like atelectasis or pneumonia following surgery. Risk factors include general anesthesia, abdominal or thoracic surgery, prolonged immobility, history of smoking, chronic lung disease, obesity, and advanced age. Deep breathing opens distal airways, while coughing helps loosen, mobilize, and remove pulmonary secretions.

1. Assist the patient, as needed, to a sitting position.
2. Have the patient place hands lightly on the lower rib cage (see Figure A).

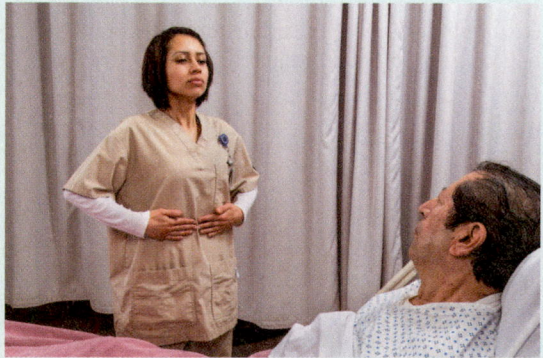

Figure A Demonstrating deep-breathing exercise. (Rick Brady, Pearson Education.)

3. Instruct to breathe in deeply through the nose, allowing the chest and abdomen to expand.
4. Have the patient hold the breath for a count of 5.

5. Instruct to exhale completely through pursed (puckered) lips, allowing the chest and abdomen to deflate.
6. After five deep breaths, instruct the patient to inhale deeply, hold breath briefly, and then cough once or twice while contracting abdominal muscles.
7. Instruct the patient for whom coughing is painful to splint the incision with interlocked hands or a pillow (see Figure B).

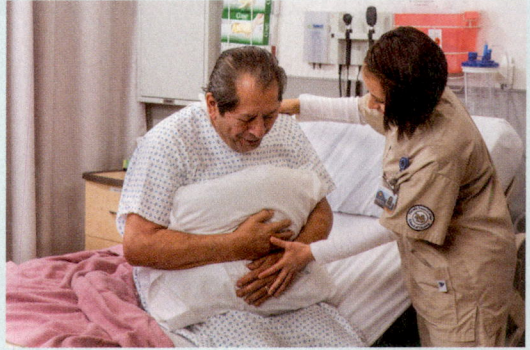

Figure B Splinting abdomen while coughing. (Rick Brady, Pearson Education.)

8. Instruct or remind the patient to repeat deep-breathing and coughing exercises every 1 to 2 hours while awake, taking short rest periods between coughs, if necessary.

clinicalALERT

Coughing may be contraindicated after some surgeries (e.g., neurosurgery). Pay close attention to orders and protocols for postoperative care as they relate to specific surgeries.

BOX 10-4   **PATIENT TEACHING (continued)**

Leg, Ankle, and Foot Exercises

Leg exercises are taught to reduce the risk for developing deep venous thrombosis (DVT, blood clot formation in a vein). Risk factors for DVT include decreased mobility; a history of circulatory disorders; and cardiovascular, pelvic, or lower extremity surgeries.

As the leg muscles contract and relax, blood is pumped back to the heart, promoting cardiac output and reducing venous stasis. Leg exercises also maintain muscle tone and range of motion, which facilitates early ambulation.

Teach the patient to perform the following exercises while lying in bed (see drawings):

1. *Muscle pumping exercise:* Contract and relax calf and thigh muscles at least 10 times in a row.
2. *Leg exercises:*
   a. Bend the knee and raise it toward the chest (Figure C).

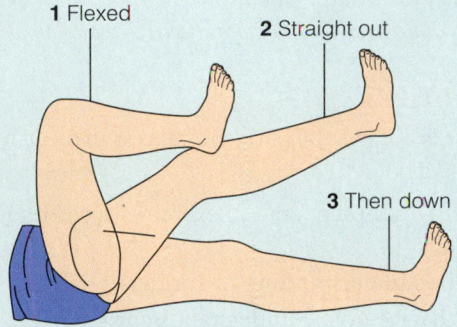

1 Flexed   2 Straight out   3 Then down

Figure C Leg exercises.

   b. Straighten out the leg and hold for a few seconds before lowering the leg back to the bed.
   c. Repeat the exercise five times with one leg and then do them with the other leg.
3. *Ankle and foot exercises:*
   a. Rotate both ankles by making complete circles, first to the right and then to the left (Figure D). Repeat five times and then relax.

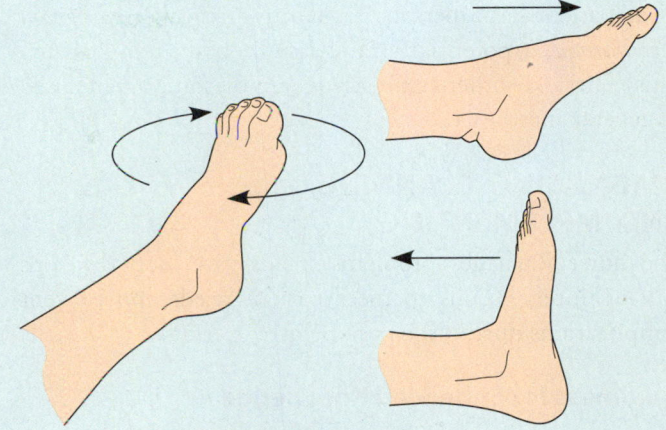

Figure D Ankle and foot exercises.

   b. With feet together, point toes toward the head and then to the foot of the bed. Repeat this pumping action 10 times and then relax.

Encourage to perform leg, ankle, and foot exercises every 1 to 2 hours while awake, depending on the patient's needs and ambulatory status, the physician's preference, and institutional protocol.

Turning in Bed

Patients may need to be taught how to minimize discomfort when turning in bed. Appropriate analgesia and splinting the incision with the hand and a small pillow or blanket reduce discomfort while turning. Encourage the patient to turn at least every 2 hours while awake.

1. Instruct to grasp the side rail toward the direction to be turned, to rest the opposite foot on the mattress, and to bend the knee.
2. Instruct to roll over in one smooth motion by pulling on the side rail while pushing off with the bent knee.
3. Pillows may need to be positioned behind the patient's back to help maintain side-lying position. The older adult may also need padding over pressure points between the knees and ankles to prevent pressure ulcer formation.

symptoms; reaction or feelings about proposed surgery; completion of prescribed preoperative preparation (e.g., bowel preparation, shower, last food and fluid intake); current health status; chronic diseases or conditions; current medications (including herbal and other complementary or alternative therapies); allergies to medications, topical agents, and other substances (e.g., latex, iodine, seafood); smoking history, alcohol intake, and use of recreational or street drugs; and previous surgeries and their outcomes and any problems experienced during or after previous surgeries

- *Objective data:* apparent general health and nutritional status, mobility, mental status and level of consciousness, and ability to communicate; skin color, warmth, and condition; vital signs including apical and peripheral pulses, respiratory rate and depth, oxygen saturation, and temperature; weight; lung sounds; abdominal assessment including bowel sounds, distention, and tenderness to palpation; and urine color and clarity.

IDENTIFYING POTENTIAL COMPLICATIONS

Document and report as appropriate the presence of risk factors such as chronic respiratory or heart disease; malnutrition or obesity; diabetes mellitus; kidney or liver disease; or use of substances such as tobacco, alcohol, or recreational or street drugs. Note when medications such as aspirin, anticoagulants, diuretics, or other prescribed drugs were last taken by the patient. Notify the surgeon and anesthetist if the patient has a personal or family history of *malignant hyperthermia*, a potentially fatal rise in body temperature. This genetic disorder can be triggered by some agents used in general anesthesia.

DIAGNOSING, PLANNING, AND IMPLEMENTING

The nurse identifies problems, plans care, and develops nursing interventions to meet patient needs and prevent complications during the perioperative period.

Readiness for Enhanced Knowledge

Expected outcome: Will demonstrate appropriate understanding of the planned procedure and expected postoperative course.

- Assess the patient's current level of knowledge. *This allows the nurse to prioritize teaching, provide new information, and reinforce prior knowledge about the surgical procedure and postoperative course of treatment.*
- Assist the patient to obtain information about expectations during the intraoperative and postoperative phase. Refer to the physician for detailed information about the surgical procedure. *The physician provides information so the patient can make an informed decision about care. The nurse clarifies information as necessary and reinforces teaching to promote understanding and reduce anxiety.*
- Teach postoperative breathing and coughing exercises, turning techniques, and leg exercises. (See Box 10-4.) *This knowledge helps prevent postoperative complications.*
- Discuss postoperative pain management with the patient. Explain the pain scale to be used and the importance of adequate pain management in the recovery process. *This assures the patient that pain will be managed and makes the patient an integral member of the pain management process.*

Anxiety

Expected outcome: Will communicate specific concerns and needs appropriately.

The nurse's ability to listen actively to both verbal and nonverbal messages is essential to establishing a trusting relationship with the patient and family. Therapeutic communication can help the patient and family identify fears and concerns. The nurse plans interventions and supportive care to reduce the patient's anxiety level and assist the patient to cope successfully with the stressors encountered during the perioperative period.

- Assess specific source(s) of anxiety. *Common fears include loss of control, pain, death, disfigurement, disability, and disturbing diagnosis and prognosis. The unfamiliar environment*

increases anxiety. Assessment provides the basis for planning specific nursing interventions.

- Answer all questions thoroughly and honestly. Refer to appropriate resources as needed. *Honesty establishes trust and helps relieve anxiety.*
- Allow expression of fears. Use active listening. *Listening helps the patient identify fears and clarify concerns.*
- Refer to clergy or spiritual support of the patient's choice. *Spiritual support provides comfort to most patients.*

Disturbed Sleep Pattern

Expected outcome: Will obtain adequate sleep.

- Assess usual sleep pattern. *This identifies alterations in pattern. Anxiety before surgery often results in sleep disturbance.*
- Provide an environment with minimal stimuli before surgery. *A relaxing environment encourages sleep.*
- Collaborate with the physician to obtain sleep medication as appropriate. *Adequate rest reduces the risk of complications and contributes to more effective induction of anesthesia.*

EVALUATING

The nurse evaluates the patient's success in meeting expected outcomes. The patient:

- Demonstrates preoperative exercises according to teaching plan.
- Verbalizes understanding of surgical procedure.
- States that he or she understands anticipated pain management techniques.
- States that anxiety is decreased.
- Sleeps 8 hours without interruption the night before surgery.

MANAGING NURSING CARE

As appropriate and allowed within the designated duties and responsibilities of assistive personnel, the nurse may assign nursing care activities such as assisting with preoperative hygiene measures (e.g., shower and shampoo with antibacterial soap) and daily living activities as required by the patient.

DOCUMENTING

Document the patient's and family's understanding of, and emotional response to, the planned procedure. Fully document all assessment data and preoperative preparation, including teaching provided, skin marking and preparation, bowel preparation and results, medications administered, and other procedures.

CONTINUITY OF CARE

Patient handoffs, when responsibility for care of the patient is transferred from one caregiver or unit to another, are identified as opportunities for errors to occur. To provide for continuing care of the patient during the intraoperative and postoperative periods, communicate with the surgical nursing team and, as appropriate, nurses on the unit to which the patient will be returning. Use a systematic communication format, such as SBAR:

- **Situation:** Patient name and date of birth; procedure to be performed, including specifics as appropriate (e.g., which extremity, which kidney); and the presence (or absence) of pertinent documents
- **Background:** Relevant information from the patient's history (e.g., chronic diseases, medications, alcohol use, or smoking); allergies; NPO status; vital signs and pain level; medications taken or administered before surgery; specific laboratory results; code status of the patient
- **Assessment:** Patient's level of understanding about and psychologic response to the surgery; specific patient needs or precautions; relevant cultural and spiritual or religious implications; special needs related to communication, sensory perception, ambulation, or daily living activities
- **Recommendations:** Most recent interaction with the physician and anesthetist; readiness for surgery; contact information for the family; specific patient or family requests

Allow time and opportunity to clarify information and address questions or concerns (Amato-Vealey et al., 2008).

NURSING CARE PLAN
Preoperative Care for a Patient Having Inpatient Surgery

Martha Overbeck is a 74-year-old widow who lives in a senior citizens' housing complex. She is in good health and is independent; however, she has become progressively less active as a result of arthritic pain and stiffness. Mrs. Overbeck has degenerative joint changes that have particularly affected her right hip. On the recommendation of her physician, Mrs. Overbeck has been admitted to the hospital for an elective right total hip replacement. Her surgery has been scheduled for 0800 the following day.

Mrs. Eva Jackson, a close friend and neighbor, accompanies Mrs. Overbeck to the hospital. Mrs. Overbeck explains that her friend will help in her home and assist her with the wound care and prescribed exercises.

Assessment
Gloria Nobis, LVN, completes the admission assessment for Mrs. Overbeck. Mrs. Overbeck appears to be an alert, oriented, healthy 74-year-old patient. She is 30 pounds over her ideal weight. Mrs. Overbeck states she has pain and some stiffness in her weight-bearing joints, particularly her right hip. Enteric-coated aspirin 650 mg four times daily is the only medication she has been taking. Preadmission laboratory tests are normal except for a slightly elevated clotting time (which suggests an increased risk for bleeding). The x-ray of her right hip reveals degenerative joint changes indicative of osteoarthritis.

Mrs. Overbeck confides that although she has faith that her surgery will be successful, she feels uneasy. She cannot identify exactly why she is apprehensive. She states she has had a number of restless nights since her decision to have surgery. She has never had major surgery and is not familiar with the hospital routine.

Nursing Diagnosis
The following nursing diagnoses are identified for Mrs. Overbeck and are included in her preoperative plan of care:

- *Anxiety* related to unfamiliar environment (hospital) and upcoming surgery
- *Readiness for Enhanced Knowledge* about the perioperative surgical experience
- *Disturbed Sleep Pattern* related to environmental changes (hospitalization) and anxiety response

Expected Outcomes
The expected outcomes established in the plan of care specify that Mrs. Overbeck will:

- Describe an increase in psychologic and physiologic comfort.
- Verbalize an understanding of perioperative events to occur.
- Demonstrate turning, coughing, deep-breathing exercise, and leg exercises.
- Report sleeping soundly from 2200 to 0700.

Planning and Implementation
Ms. Nobis plans and implements the following interventions to assist Mrs. Overbeck in the preoperative surgical phase:

- Establish a therapeutic relationship with Mrs. Overbeck and her friend.
- Provide reassurance and comfort by acknowledging concerns and conveying understanding.
- Familiarize Mrs. Overbeck with hospital routines.
- Initiate perioperative teaching to include:
  - Preparation for surgery.
  - A visit from the operating room nurse and anesthesiologist.
  - Coughing, turning, deep-breathing, and leg exercises.
  - Postoperative pain management.
  - Written materials describing total hip replacements.

- Help Mrs. Overbeck identify factors that interfere with her ability to sleep.
- Decrease noise, lighting, and disturbances between 2200 and 0700.
- Encourage the use of prescribed hypnotic/sedative medications to assist in sleep before surgery.

Evaluation

By the end of the shift, Ms. Nobis assesses that Mrs. Overbeck's anxiety has diminished. Mrs. Overbeck confirms that she feels more comfortable about the upcoming surgery. She is able to describe the preoperative preparations that will occur the following morning, events that are most likely to occur in surgery and the recovery room, and routine postoperative nursing care after her total hip replacement. She expresses an understanding of her role in assessing and managing postoperative pain. She states that she will take the hypnotic/sedative prescribed to help her sleep. She asks Ms. Nobis to convey to the evening and night nurses that she would like to have her door closed and lights off except for the one in the bathroom.

Critical Thinking in the Nursing Process

1. What teaching would you implement with Mrs. Overbeck and her friend to prepare them for the first 72 hours of postoperative recovery?
2. What consultations may be appropriate for you to make to other health care providers to assist Mrs. Overbeck before and after surgery?
3. Develop a care plan for Mrs. Overbeck for the nursing diagnosis "Deficient knowledge related to lack of information about preoperative care."

Note: Discussion of Critical Thinking questions appears on the companion website.

Intraoperative Phase

Key Concept The nurse's focus during the intraoperative phase is on maintaining patient safety. Patient advocacy is a critical nursing role during this phase, as the patient is unable to speak for or meet his or her own needs.

The intraoperative phase begins when the patient is admitted to the operating room and ends when the patient is admitted to the PACU. The duration of the intraoperative phase depends on the type and extent of the surgery being performed, as well as any problems or complications that develop during surgery.

On entry into the surgical suite and while the patient is awake (if possible), the Universal Protocol for preventing surgery on the wrong person, the wrong site, or performing the wrong procedure is followed (see Box 10-2). During this preprocedure check, availability of relevant chart documents, laboratory and diagnostic test results, and any required blood products, implants, or special equipment is verified. A "time-out" is taken immediately before starting the procedure to conduct a final verification of the correct patient, procedure, and site. This is a process of active communication among surgical team members. The surgery itself does not begin until all questions or concerns are resolved and all team members agree (The Joint Commission, 2010).

COLLABORATIVE CARE
The Surgical Team

The surgeon, surgical assistant(s), anesthesiologist and/or certified registered nurse anesthetist (CRNA), circulating nurse, scrub nurse, and certified surgical technologist (CST) constitute the surgical team. Because the intraoperative environment is so complex, members must function as a coordinated unit. The surgeon and anesthesiologist maintain primary roles in managing the patient physiologically; nurses are responsible for maintaining the safety of the patient and the environment, monitoring patient status, and providing psychologic support.

The *surgeon* is the physician performing the procedure and the head of the surgical team. All medical actions and judgments are the surgeon's responsibility.

The *surgical assistant* works closely with the surgeon in performing the operation. The number of assistants varies according to the complexity of the procedure. The assistant may be another physician, a nurse, a physician's assistant, or other trained personnel. RNs may become certified to function as a first assistant (RN first assistant or RNFA) through academic education and clinical training (AORN, 2013). The assistant performs such duties as exposing the operative site, retracting nearby tissue, sponging or suctioning the wound, tying off bleeding vessels, and suturing or assisting with suturing of the surgical wound.

The *anesthesiologist* (a physician) or *certified registered nurse anesthetist (CRNA)* (an advanced practice nurse) administers anesthesia and assumes responsibility for the patient's general well-being during surgery. The anesthesiologist or CRNA evaluates the patient preoperatively, administers medications, transfuses blood or blood products, infuses intravenous fluids, continuously monitors physiologic status, alerts the surgeon to developing problems and treats problems as they arise, and supervises the patient's recovery in the PACU.

The *circulating nurse* is a registered nurse who coordinates and manages a wide range of activities before, during, and after the surgical procedure. The circulating nurse oversees the physical aspects of the operating room and its equipment. The circulating nurse assists with transferring and positioning the patient, preparing the surgical site, ensuring that no break in aseptic technique occurs, and counting all sponges and instruments. The circulating nurse assists other team members and documents intraoperative nursing activities, medications, blood administration, placement of drains and catheters, and length of the procedure. The circulating nurse is at all times an advocate for the safety and well-being of the patient.

The *scrub nurse* (or *certified surgical technologist*) handles sutures, instruments, and other equipment immediately adjacent to the sterile field (Figure 10-2■). This role requires technical skills, manual dexterity, and in-depth knowledge of the anatomic and mechanical aspects of a particular surgery. LPNs/LVNs often assume the role of scrub nurse, acquiring skills through facility training programs or a formal surgical technology program.

All members of the surgical team are responsible for managing noise and other distractions during the intraoperative phase. Patients are particularly vulnerable to noise stress during induction and emergence from anesthesia. Measures to reduce noise during the intraoperative phase include minimizing the number of people present, reducing voice volume, and minimizing conversations among surgical team members or using the telephone.

Medications

Anesthesia is the use of chemical substances to produce loss of sensation and reflexes and muscle relaxation during a surgical procedure, with or without the loss of consciousness. Factors that influence the type of anesthesia used include the surgery to be performed and the patient's medical and surgical history, age and health status, and preferences.

GENERAL ANESTHESIA *General anesthesia* produces a state in which the patient is unconscious and does not respond to painful stimuli. Intravenous injection of a rapid-acting drug is usually used to induce general anesthesia; drugs are then given by inhalation or intravenous injection to maintain anesthesia.

General anesthesia depresses the central nervous system, resulting in loss of consciousness and amnesia. The patient perceives no pain, skeletal muscles relax, and reflexes diminish. Advantages of general anesthesia include rapid excretion of the anesthetic agent and prompt reversal of its effects when desired. In addition, general anesthesia can be used with all age groups and most surgical procedures.

Its disadvantages include risks associated with circulatory and respiratory depression. Patients with serious respiratory or circulatory diseases, such as emphysema or heart failure (see Chapter 17), are at greater risk for these complications.

The phases of general anesthesia are as follows:

1. The *induction phase* begins when the anesthetic agent is administered and ends when the patient is ready for the surgical procedure to begin. During this phase, airway patency is achieved with endotracheal intubation (Figure 10-3■). The patient is positioned and the skin is prepared during this phase.

2. The *maintenance phase* begins with surgical incision and continues until the procedure nears completion. The anesthesiologist maintains the proper depth of anesthesia using inhaled agents or intravenous medications, while constantly monitoring such parameters as heart rate, blood pressure, respiratory rate, temperature, and oxygen and carbon dioxide levels.

3. The *emergence phase* begins as the patient "emerges" from the anesthetic agents and continues until the patient is ready to leave the operating room. The endotracheal

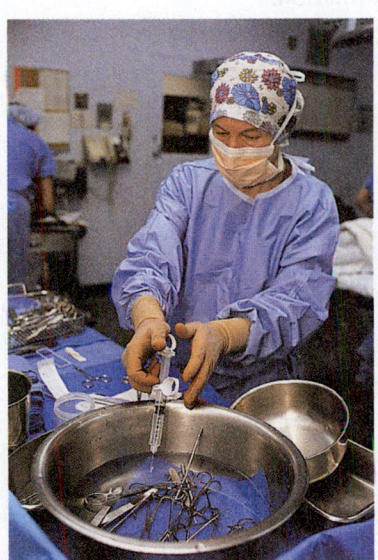

Figure 10-2. ■ A scrub nurse in the surgery suite.
(Alain McLaughlin, Pearson Education.)

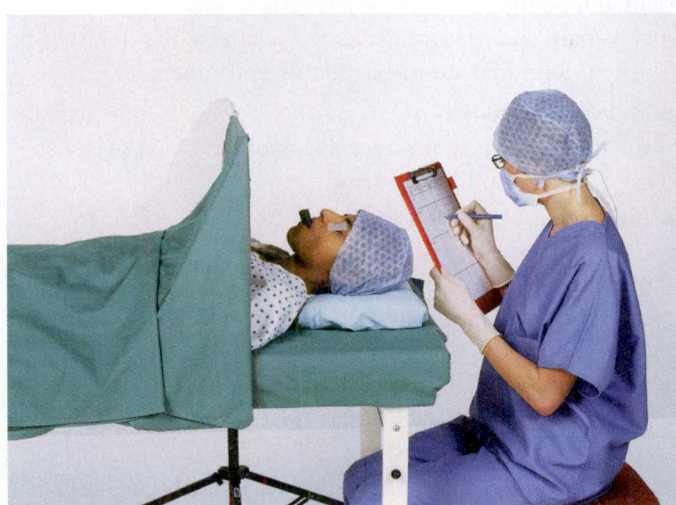

Figure 10-3. ■ The anesthesiologist monitors the status of an anesthetized patient ready to undergo surgery. Note the endotracheal tube to maintain airway patency. (Source: Dorling Kindersley Media Library.)

tube is removed (*extubation*) once the patient has reestablished voluntary breathing. Airway patency is critical during this period, because extubation may cause bronchospasm or laryngospasm.

MODERATE SEDATION/ANALGESIA **Moderate** (or **conscious**) **sedation/analgesia** provides analgesia, amnesia, and depressed consciousness but allows the patient to independently maintain airway and respirations and to respond to verbal commands and physical stimulation (Rothrock, 2011). An increasing number of surgical and diagnostic procedures are performed using moderate sedation/analgesia. Moderate sedation/analgesia may be administered in the absence of an anesthesia provider by an RN with specific training and demonstrated competency. A combination of opioids and sedative intravenous medications produces the pharmacologic effects. Opioids include morphine sulfate and fentanyl (Sublimaze). Sedatives include *diazepam* (Valium) and midazolam (Versed). Propofol (Diprivan) is an anesthetic agent commonly used for moderate sedation/analgesia.

The patient's respiratory rate, heart rate and rhythm, blood pressures, oxygen saturation, level of consciousness, and skin color, temperature, and moisture must be continuously monitored during moderate sedation/analgesia. Resuscitation medications and equipment should be immediately available (Rothrock, 2011).

REGIONAL ANESTHESIA In *regional anesthesia*, medication is instilled around the peripheral nerves to block transmission of nerve impulses in a particular area. Regional anesthesia produces analgesia, relaxation, and reduced reflexes. The patient is awake and conscious during the surgical procedure but does not perceive pain. Careful positioning of the patient undergoing regional anesthesia is vital to prevent injury as pain and sensory input to the affected region will be blocked. Regional anesthesia has several subclassifications:

- *Peripheral nerve blocks:* An anesthetic agent is injected at the nerve trunk to produce a lack of sensation over a specific body area, like the hand.
- *Epidural and caudal anesthesia:* Local anesthetic agents are injected into the epidural space, outside the dura mater of the spinal cord. Access usually is achieved through the intervertebral spaces in the lumbar region of the spine or the caudal canal in the sacrum. This may be used for surgeries of the abdomen and lower extremities.
- *Spinal anesthesia:* A local anesthetic is injected into the cerebrospinal fluid (CSF) in the subarachnoid space via a lower lumbar intervertebral space. The patient is positioned to allow the anesthesia to settle into the desired region. Surgeries of the abdomen, perineum, and lower extremities are likely to use this type of regional anesthesia. Hypotension and respiratory muscle paralysis are

potential risks during spinal anesthesia, necessitating close monitoring. Leakage of CSF from the needle insertion site may reduce CSF pressure and cause postoperative headaches. Bed rest, maintaining hydration, and applying pressure to the infusion site combat this common side effect.

LOCAL ANESTHESIA **Local anesthesia** is administration of an anesthetic to a specific area of the body. The anesthetic may be applied topically or injected directly into the area (infiltrated) to block nerve impulses at that site. Drugs such as cocaine hydrochloride, tetracaine, or lidocaine may be applied topically to mucous membranes of the nose, throat, or urethra. Lidocaine and bupivacaine (Marcaine) are commonly used to infiltrate the skin (e.g., around a wound to be sutured or before a procedure). Epinephrine may be added to the anesthetic solution to constrict local blood vessels and control bleeding.

Infection Control

Surgery disrupts a major defense system, the skin. In addition, hormones released during the general stress response suppress the immune system. As a result, procedures used to prevent contamination of the surgical site are vital to prevent infection. *Surgical asepsis* is followed to prevent introduction of all microbes that can cause disease into the surgical wound.

SURGICAL ATTIRE Strict dress codes in the surgical department facilitate infection control, reduce cross-contamination between the surgery department and other patient care areas, and promote the health and safety of patients and personnel. All personnel in the surgical department wear surgical attire to minimize bacterial shedding and reduce wound contamination.

The surgical department is divided into three zones:

1. Unrestricted zones permit access by persons in hospital uniforms or street clothes and allow limited access for communicating with operating room personnel.
2. Semirestricted zones require scrub attire, including a scrub suit, shoe covers, and a cap or hood (Figure 10-4A■). Hallways, work areas, and storage areas are semirestricted.
3. Restricted zones, within operating rooms, require personnel to wear masks, sterile gowns, and gloves in addition to appropriate scrub attire (see Figure 10-4B). The entire surgical attire is changed between procedures and whenever soiled or wet.

SURGICAL HAND HYGIENE Surgical hand hygiene, using a sponge or brush and an antimicrobial agent or an FDA-approved alcohol-based antiseptic surgical hand rub, is required for all personnel who participate directly in the

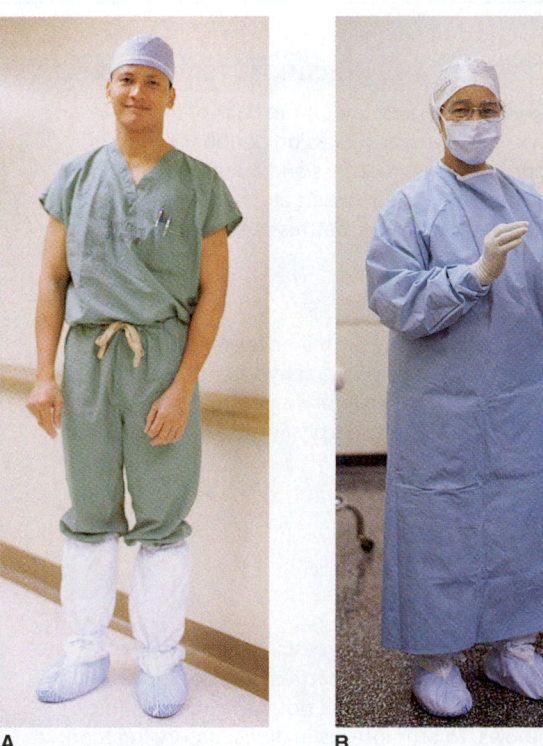

Figure 10-4. ■ (**A**) Surgical attire. (**B**) Sterile surgical attire. (Photo: Richard Tauber, Pearson Education.)

procedure. Skin cannot be sterilized, but it is considered "surgically clean" after surgical hand hygiene. The purposes of surgical hand hygiene are to:

- Remove dirt, skin oils, and transient microorganisms from nails, hands, and forearms.
- Reduce the number of resident microorganisms on surgical personnel.
- Leave an antimicrobial residue on the skin to inhibit the growth of microbes for several hours.

SITE PREPARATION   The patient's skin is cleansed in the surgical department to decrease microorganisms on the skin and reduce the possibility of wound infection. The surgeon also may order hair removed from the proposed incision area. Clippers, which pose less risk of injury to the skin, are preferred for hair removal. The site is then cleansed with an antimicrobial agent, starting at the point where the incision will be made and continuing outward (Figure 10-5■). Hospital policy and surgeon preference should be followed.

Positioning

The patient is positioned on the operating table for exposure of the operative site and access for administration of anesthesia (Table 10-5■). Careful positioning is crucial to

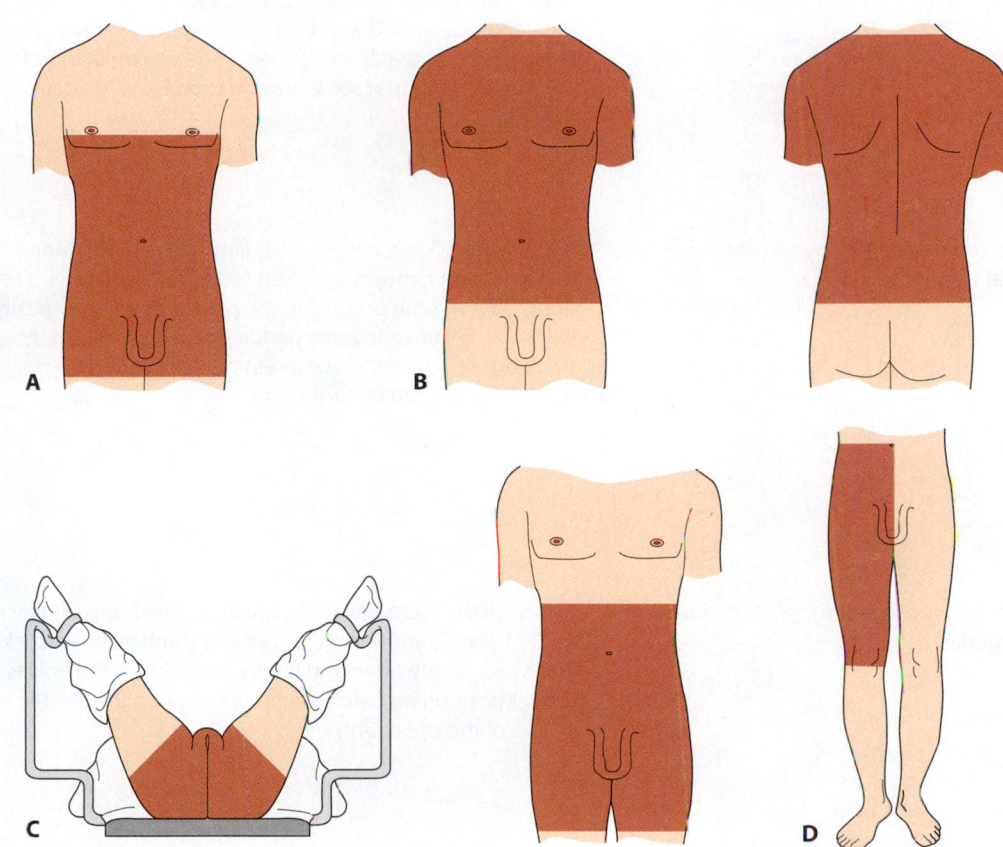

Figure 10-5. ■ Surgical site preparation. (**A**) Abdominal surgery. (**B**) Thoracoabdominal surgery. (**C**) Genitourinary surgery. (**D**) Hip surgery.

TABLE 10-5	Common Surgical Positions

POSITION AND USE	POSSIBLE ADVERSE EFFECTS AND NURSING INTERVENTIONS
(a) The *supine position* is used for abdominal surgeries, some thoracic surgeries, and some surgeries on the extremities. 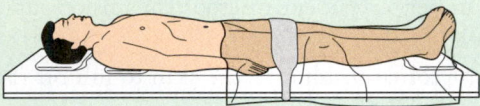	This position may cause excessive pressure on the back of the head, scapulae, sacrum, coccyx, and heels, as well as on peripheral vessels and nerves. Use a pressure-reducing mattress and additional padding as needed. To avoid compressing blood vessels and nerve damage, ensure that armboards are level with the mattress and the ankles are not crossed.
(b) The *semisitting position* may be used for surgeries on the head, face, neck, or shoulders. 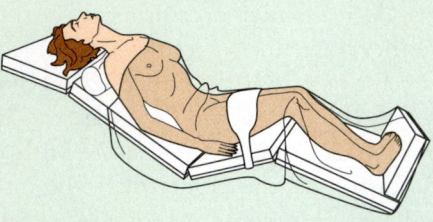	In addition to placing pressure on bony prominences of the back and buttocks, this position can lead to postural hypotension and venous pooling in the legs. Sciatic nerve injury is possible. Assess for hypotension. Ensure that knees are not sharply flexed. Use soft padding to prevent nerve compression.
(c) The *prone position* may be used for spinal fusion and rectal surgeries. 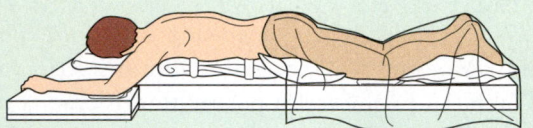	This position causes pressure on the face, breasts, genitalia, knees, thighs, and toes. Use a pressure-reducing mattress and additional padding as needed. Support arms in a flexed position with padding above and below the elbows. To promote optimal respiratory function, use chest rolls and closely monitor respiratory status.
(d) The *lateral position* is used for some thoracic surgeries, kidney surgeries, as well as hip replacements. 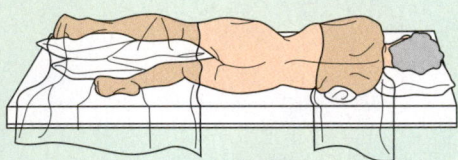	This may cause excessive pressure on the bony prominences on the dependent side. Ensure adequate padding and support, especially on the downside arm. The weight of the upper leg may cause peroneal nerve injury on the downside leg. Both legs must therefore be padded. Cardiovascular and respiratory compromise may occur; monitor carefully.
(e) The *lithotomy position* is used for gynecologic, perineal, or rectal surgeries. 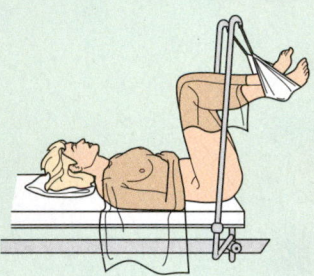	This position decreases vital capacity of the lungs. Monitor respirations, and assess for hypoxia and dyspnea. Hip dislocations, fracture, and nerve damage can occur, and the risk for deep venous thrombosis (DVT) increases. Ensure adequate padding and support; apply antiembolic stockings or sequential compression devices (SCDs); closely monitor respiratory and circulatory status.
(f) The *jackknife position* is used for rectal surgeries and some spinal surgeries. 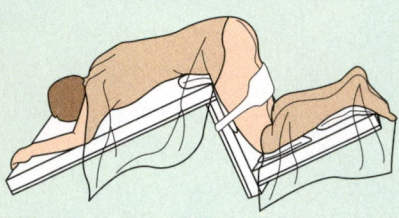	This position decreases vital capacity of the lungs and increases the risk for DVT. Monitor respirations and apply antiembolic stockings or SCDs. Place pads at the groin and knees, as well as at the ankles. Padding and proper positioning help prevent pressure on the ear, the neck, and the nerves of the upper arm.

The Older Adult Undergoing Surgery

Age-related changes increase the risk for complications when the older adult undergoes surgery. Organ systems such as the respiratory system, cardiovascular system, and the kidneys have fewer reserves for adjusting to the physiologic stress associated with surgery. The older adult is more prone to hypotension, hypothermia, and hypoxemia resulting from anesthesia and the cool temperature in the operating room.

Intraoperative positioning of arthritic joints can result in postoperative joint pain that is unrelated to the surgical procedure. The older patient is at increased risk for skin breakdown and delayed wound healing because of decreased subcutaneous tissue and reduced peripheral circulation. Older patients undergoing lengthy surgeries have increased risk for this complication.

Some older adults have hearing or visual impairments. Sensory impairments, coupled with an unfamiliar environment, can make the operating room a frightening, disorienting place. By effectively communicating with the patient, the nurse can provide support and reassurance to minimize these factors.

prevent injury to the patient. Pressure, rubbing, or shearing forces can damage the tissue over bony prominences. If normal joint range of motion is exceeded, muscle and joint injuries can occur. Improper positioning also can lead to sensory and motor dysfunction and nerve damage. Pressure on peripheral blood vessels can decrease venous return to the heart and negatively affect the blood pressure. Oxygenation of the blood can be decreased if lung expansion is impaired.

The anesthetized patient cannot respond to discomfort. It is the surgical team's responsibility to position the patient for the best surgical advantage and for safety and comfort. The circulating nurse follows agency policy, the surgeon's preference, and the patient's history to ensure optimal positioning. The circulating nurse continuously assesses the patient. Box 10-5 ■ lists special considerations for the older adult undergoing surgery.

NURSING CARE

Nurses assume many roles in caring for the patient during the intraoperative phase. Depending on the setting, the LPN/LVN may assist with obtaining necessary supplies and equipment, safely transferring and positioning the patient, prepping and draping for the procedure, serving as the scrub nurse, and monitoring the patient throughout the procedure.

PRIORITIZING NURSING CARE

Maintaining the patient's physiologic and psychologic safety is the priority of nursing care during the intraoperative period.

HEALTH PROMOTION

Protecting the patient's rights and safety during the intraoperative phase is critical to health promotion. As a member of the health care and surgical team, the LPN/LVN protects the patient's rights to privacy and confidentiality of information. On admission to the surgical suite, the nurse verifies the patient's identity, the procedure to be done, the operative site, and the presence of necessary documents such as the signed consent, history and physical, and relevant laboratory and diagnostic test results.

clinical**ALERT**

Carefully identify the patient on admission to the surgical suite. Ensure that verbal report and written documentation of the procedure to be done is congruent. Immediately inform all surgical personnel of any discrepancies.

Other patient safety measures include:

- Verifying any allergies to medications or medical products (e.g., latex) and specific patient needs or precautions such as chronic diseases (e.g., diabetes) that may affect patient responses during the procedure.
- Noting pertinent religious or cultural preferences (see Chapter 3) and the presence of any relevant advance directive.
- Observing the six rights of medication administration during the intraoperative phase; meticulously documenting medications, fluids, blood, or blood products administered.
- Maintaining a quiet environment with an appropriate temperature.
- Locking wheels and stabilizing stretchers and/or procedure tables when moving patients from one to the other.

ASSESSING

The nurse verifies identity, the type and site of surgery, and previously obtained assessment data on receiving the patient in the surgical suite. During the procedure, the nurse collaborates with the anesthesiologist or CRNA to collect and relate objective assessment data such as vital signs and peripheral pulses to the surgical team.

DIAGNOSING, PLANNING, AND IMPLEMENTING

Risk for Perioperative Positioning Injury

Expected outcome: Will have no evidence of injury resulting from positioning during surgery.

- Assess for potential risk factors, including history of arthritis or other musculoskeletal disorders and loss of subcutaneous tissue and skin elasticity due to aging or nutritional status. *Information provides a basis for planning and may direct modification of planned positioning.*

- Notify the surgeon if the planned position must be adjusted. *This ensures patient safety yet provides the means to accomplish the surgical procedure.*
- Use safety belts to secure the patient to stretcher and operating table, ensuring that distal circulation is unimpaired. *Belts reduce the risk of falls when the patient's awareness is decreased.*
- Support and pad tissues and areas at risk for tissue breakdown due to prolonged pressure. *Padding prevents excessive pressure on body parts.*

Risk for Infection

Expected outcome: Will remain free of evidence of wound infection.

- Assess sterility of all instruments and supplies used in the operating room. *Surgical asepsis decreases the risk of introducing pathogens during the surgical procedure.*
- Report results of lab studies that may indicate systemic infection or altered immune status. *Patient may require prophylactic antibiotics.*
- Follow instructions and established protocols related to skin prep. *Preparation reduces bacteria at the surgical site, but, if done improperly, may damage the skin, increasing the risk for infection.*
- Observe for and verbally report breaks or potential breaks in asepsis (e.g., tears in sterile gloves, contamination of equipment or surgical instruments). *The circulating nurse is responsible for ensuring strict aseptic technique is followed in the operating room.*

Risk for Imbalanced Body Temperature

Expected outcome: Will maintain body temperature within expected range during and after surgery.

Surgical patients are at risk for hypothermia from the cool environment, the effects of anesthesia, administration of cool intravenous fluids, or medications used during the intraoperative phase. Rarely, hyperthermia may occur in response to anesthesia.

- Assess temperature before induction of anesthesia. *This provides baseline data.*
- Assess environmental temperature and patient response. *Temperature can be modified to maintain the patient's body temperature.*
- Notify the anesthetist and surgeon if a personal or family history of malignant hyperthermia is reported. *Malignant hyperthermia is a genetic disorder that can cause potentially fatal hyperthermia in response to some anesthetic agents. Patients with a personal or family history of malignant hyperthermia must be closely monitored for muscle*

tension and rapidly increasing temperature during anesthesia and surgery.

- Note changes in temperature, and intervene as soon as possible (e.g., provide cooling or warming blanket or gown). *Prompt response reduces the risk of injury.*

Risk for Aspiration

Expected outcome: Will have clear lung sounds and a patent airway.

- Assess for and report consumption of food or fluids during the prescribed fasting period to the surgeon and anesthesiologist. *Surgery may be delayed or canceled.*
- Insert nasogastric tube if ordered. *Patients requiring emergency surgery may have eaten. Anesthetic agents may also contribute to aspiration risk. Removal of stomach contents reduces the risk for aspiration.*

EVALUATING

The nurse evaluates whether or not expected outcomes are met. Validation includes the following:

- Patient is free from intraoperative injury: Skin is intact with no evidence of underlying tissue damage; peripheral circulation and sensation are intact; lungs are clear with good breath sounds throughout.
- Patient's body temperature remains within normal limits during the intraoperative period.
- No evidence of breaks in aseptic technique is observed during the intraoperative period.

DOCUMENTING

Document assessment data, care provided, sponge and instrument counts (as appropriate), and any adverse events that occur during surgery using the appropriate forms. Document any unexpected incidents or events occurring during the intraoperative phase.

CONTINUITY OF CARE

Using SBAR or another systematic communication protocol, report pertinent information to nursing staff in the recovery area or on the postoperative unit, including:

- **Situation:** patient name and date of birth; the surgery or procedure done, including any modifiers (e.g., right hip arthroplasty).
- **Background:** name of anesthetist and type of anesthesia used; all medications, fluids, blood, or blood products administered during surgery; estimated blood loss during surgery; presence of any drains or devices; any significant events during surgery.
- **Assessment:** Respiratory and circulatory status; temperature; urine output; pain level and management; any surgical complications.

■ **Recommendations:** Immediate postoperative orders; any specific conditions for discharge from the recovery unit (Amato-Vealey et al., 2008).

Provide an opportunity to address any questions or concerns when handing off the patient to PACU or unit staff.

Postoperative Phase

Key Concept During the postoperative phase, nurses are instrumental in promoting the patient's comfort and initial recovery, identifying and preventing potential complications, and teaching the patient and family or caregivers about continuing care needs.

The postoperative phase of the surgical experience begins in the PACU and ends when wound healing and functional recovery are complete.

POSTANESTHESIA RECOVERY

Postanesthesia recovery begins when the patient is transferred from the surgical suite to the PACU or patient care unit. The nurse immediately assesses the patient's airway, breathing, and circulatory status (the ABCs) on admission to the PACU. After assessing the ABCs, receiving report, and clarifying information as needed, the nurse completes an initial assessment that includes vital signs and pain; level of consciousness; condition of dressings and the surgical site, including the amount and type of drainage; and presence and location of intravenous lines and type of fluid infusing. The nurse may use a head-to-toe or major body systems approach to organize the initial assessment.

During this critical period, the patient is carefully monitored to determine the response to anesthesia and the surgical procedure and to detect significant changes. Hydration status is carefully assessed and maintained to prevent cardiovascular and renal complications. Assessing mental status and level of consciousness are ongoing nursing responsibilities in the PACU. Pain level is assessed and managed through careful analgesic administration to promote comfort. The patient may require repeated orientation to time, place, and person. Emotional support is essential during this vulnerable period.

Discharge from the PACU often is ordered by the anesthesiologist. A recovery score system such as the *Aldrete score* may be used to determine when discharge from PACU is appropriate. Score systems use factors such as ability to move, cough, and deep breathe to command; blood pressure; consciousness; and oxygen saturation levels.

WOUND HEALING

Healing varies, depending on factors such as age, nutritional status, general health, and the type and location of the wound.

Some tissues heal by cell regeneration, called primary intention; in others, connective scar tissue fills the wound to restore the structural integrity of the surgical site, a process known as secondary intention (Figure 10-6■):

1. Healing by **primary intention** occurs when the wound is uncomplicated and clean and has sustained little tissue loss. The edges of the wound or incision are well *approximated* (have come together well) with sutures or staples. This type of incision heals quickly with very little scarring.
2. Healing by **secondary intention** occurs when the wound is large, gaping, and irregular. Tissue loss prevents approximation of wound edges, so the wound fills by granulation. This type of wound takes longer to heal, is more prone to infection, and develops more scar tissue.

Wound healing occurs in three phases: the inflammatory phase, the proliferative phase, and the remodeling phase.

The *inflammatory phase* begins with the surgical incision. Physiologic mechanisms to maintain hemostasis and promote blood clotting are activated. (See Chapter 19 for more information about clotting processes.) Blood vessels initially constrict and then dilate and become more permeable to bring plasma and blood cells to the site. Phagocytic WBCs remove invading organisms and debris from the area. These cells also release growth factors to stimulate tissue repair.

The *proliferative phase* begins within 2 to 3 days after surgery. Fibroblasts (connective tissue cells that synthesize collagen, growth factors, and other wound healing elements) and vascular endothelial cells proliferate to form granulation tissue. This tissue initially is fragile and bleeds easily.

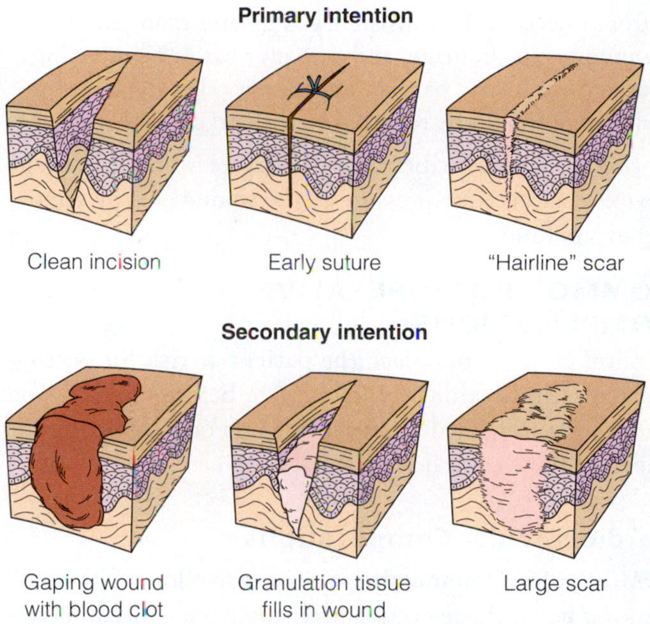

Figure 10-6. ■ Wound healing by primary and secondary intention.

Epithelial cells proliferate at the wound edges to form a new surface.

Sutures or staples are removed during this phase of wound healing. Wound strength is only about 10% of normal tissue strength at the time of their removal, but increases significantly during the next 4 weeks (Grossman & Porth, 2014). Sutures or staples may be removed over a period of several days, with initial removal of every third suture/staple, then half of the remaining sutures/staples, and finally all remaining. Wound closure strips (e.g., Steri-Strips) or surgical adhesives may be used to maintain approximation of wound edges that are not fully healed.

During the *remodeling phase*, scar tissue is remodeled by a process of collagen synthesis and breakdown to increase its strength. This phase begins about 3 weeks after surgery and can continue for 6 or more months.

WOUND DRAINAGE

Wound drainage (*exudate*) results from the inflammatory process that occurs during initial wound healing. (See Chapter 9 for more information about the inflammatory process.) The drainage is composed of escaped fluid and cells from the rich blood supply that surrounds the wound. Drainage is described as serous, sanguineous, or purulent:

- *Serous drainage* contains mostly the clear portion of the blood (serum). The drainage appears clear or slightly yellow and is thin in consistency.
- *Sanguineous drainage* contains both serum and red blood cells and has a thick, reddish appearance. This is the most common drainage from an uncomplicated surgical wound.
- *Purulent drainage* is composed of white blood cells, tissue debris, and bacteria. Purulent drainage results from infection. Its consistency is greater than serous or sanguineous drainage, and the color varies by infecting organism. It may have an unpleasant odor. Purulent drainage should be reported to the surgeon.

Box 10-6■ describes and illustrates wound drainage devices that decrease pressure in the wound area by removing excess fluid.

COMMON POSTOPERATIVE COMPLICATIONS

A number of factors place the patient at risk for postoperative complications. Nursing care before, during, and after surgery is aimed at preventing and/or minimizing the effects of these complications.

Cardiovascular Complications

HEMORRHAGE **Hemorrhage** is excessive loss of blood. A *concealed* hemorrhage occurs internally from a bleeding vessel that is not sealed or ligated (tied off) or that has been eroded by a drainage tube. An *obvious* hemorrhage occurs externally from a dislodged or ill-formed clot at the wound. Hemorrhage also may result from clotting abnormalities due to a coagulation disorder or medications.

A *venous* hemorrhage oozes out quickly and is dark red. An *arterial* hemorrhage is bright red blood that flows freely. Either type of hemorrhage will cause hypovolemic shock if a significant amount of blood is lost from the circulation.

Assessment findings depend on the amount and rate of blood loss. Restlessness and anxiety are observed in the early stage of hemorrhage. The heart rate is increased, but the blood pressure may remain normal. Frank bleeding may be obvious or may only be noted by turning or repositioning the patient if blood pools under the back or buttocks. Manifestations of hypovolemic shock may be noted (see Box 14-2).

SHOCK **Shock** is a life-threatening postoperative complication that results from insufficient blood flow to vital organs. *Hypovolemic shock*, the most common type in the postoperative patient, results from decreased circulating fluid volume from blood loss, severe vomiting, or prolonged diarrhea. The greater the loss of fluid volume, the more severe the symptoms. Manifestations of hypovolemic shock may include altered level of consciousness, confusion and restlessness; tachycardia and tachypnea, weak, thready pulses, and possible hypotension; decreased urine output; and cool, clammy, pale, or cyanotic skin. Chapter 14 provides a full discussion about shock, its manifestations, and treatment.

DEEP VENOUS THROMBOSIS DVT is the formation of a *thrombus* (blood clot) in the deep veins, usually of the lower extremities or pelvis. It may result from a combination of factors, including vessel trauma during surgery, pressure applied under the knees, and sluggish blood flow during and after surgery. Risk factors for DVT include:

- Orthopedic surgery of lower extremities; urologic, gynecologic, or obstetric surgeries; or neurosurgery
- History of previous DVT or pulmonary emboli
- Age over 40
- Extended bed rest or activity limitation
- Obesity
- Malignancy

Common assessment findings of DVT reveal pain or cramping in the involved calf or thigh. Redness, edema, and warmth of the entire extremity may be present. DVT also may be asymptomatic. A positive *Homans' sign* (pain in the calf on dorsiflexion of the affected foot; see Box 18-14) may be noted.

PULMONARY EMBOLISM A *pulmonary embolism* is a blood clot or other foreign substance that lodges in a pulmonary

BOX 10-6 WOUND DRAINAGE DEVICES

A **drain** is a device that promotes drainage of wound debris and healing from the inside to the outside. Use of a drain decreases the risk of abscess formation. The safety pin in the Penrose drain shown in Figure A prevents the exposed end from slipping down into the wound.

Wound care focuses on cleaning around the drain with a prescribed solution, such as sterile normal saline, and replacing the dressings as necessary to keep the surrounding skin dry and to encourage further drainage. An absorbent dressing is placed over the drain and gauze (not shown).

Wound suction devices promote drainage of fluid from the wound, decreasing pressure on healing tissues and reducing hematoma or abscess formation. Shown are the Jackson Pratt (Figure B) and Hemovac (Figure C) wound suction devices.

The frequency with which the device is emptied depends on the time elapsed since surgery, type of surgery, amount of drainage, and agency policy. For example, immediately after surgery, the nurse may empty the device every 15 to 60 minutes. As drainage decreases, the device is emptied every 2 to 4 hours (per policy). Amount, color, consistency, and odor of drainage are documented. Care is taken to maintain asepsis when emptying suction devices, avoiding contamination of the drain or the drain plug.

Drains and suction devices usually are removed on the second to fourth day after surgery. Removal causes minor discomfort. After removal, the drain site is cleaned, and a sterile dressing is applied.

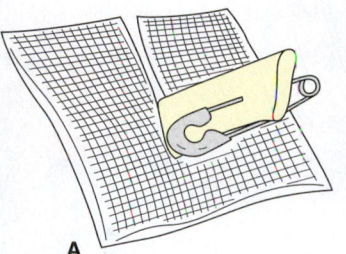

A

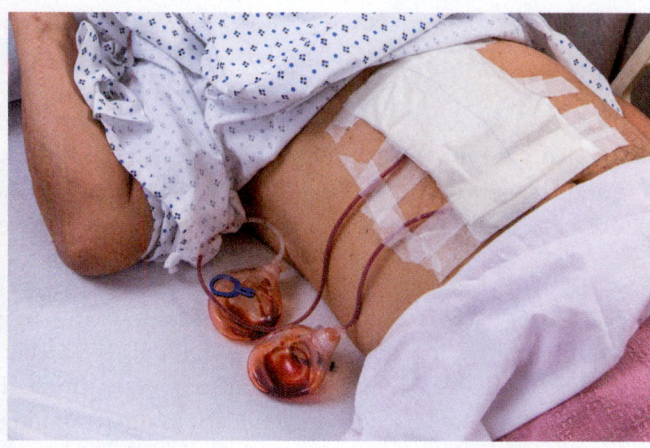

B (Rick Brady, Pearson Education.)

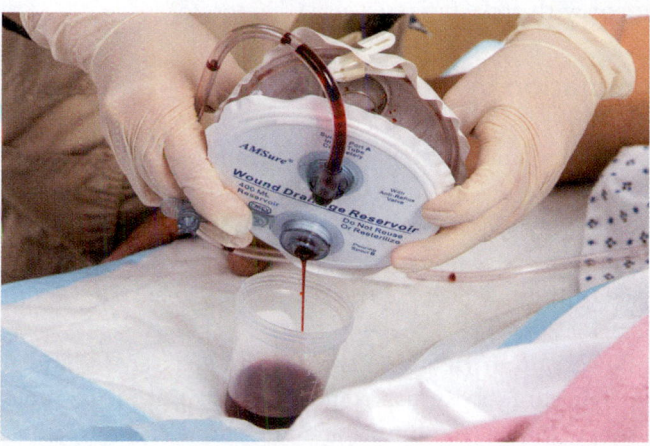

C (Rick Brady, Pearson Education.)

---

artery. It usually occurs as a consequence of DVT, when a portion of the thrombus dislodges and travels through the venous system to the right side of the heart, and from there, to the lung. Pulmonary emboli also may result from fat emboli (which may complicate large bone fracture or orthopedic surgeries) and amniotic fluid emboli, an obstetric complication.

Signs and symptoms of a pulmonary embolism include mild to moderate or severe dyspnea, chest pain, diaphoresis, anxiety, restlessness, rapid respirations and pulse, dysrhythmias, cough, and cyanosis. Sudden death can occur if a major pulmonary artery is completely blocked.

Respiratory Complications

Common postoperative respiratory complications include pneumonia and atelectasis.

PNEUMONIA Pneumonia (inflammation of lung tissue) is caused by infection or inflammation due to a foreign substance in the lung. Retained pulmonary secretions due to an ineffective cough and decreased mobility are the most common risk factor in surgical patients. Other risk factors include aspiration of oral or gastric secretions and an impaired cough reflex due to endotracheal intubation or anesthetic drugs.

Manifestations of pneumonia include (see also Table 23-1):

- Moderate to high fever
- Rapid pulse and respirations
- Chills (may be present initially)
- Productive cough (depending on the type of pneumonia)
- Dyspnea
- Decreased oxygen saturation levels
- Chest pain
- Crackles and wheezes

Treating the infection, supporting respiratory efforts, promoting lung expansion, and preventing the organisms' spread are the goals in caring for the patient with pneumonia.

ATELECTASIS **Atelectasis** is incomplete expansion or collapse of lung tissue. It results from inadequate ventilation and retained pulmonary secretions. Assessment findings commonly include dyspnea, diminished breath sounds over the affected area, reduced oxygen saturation, anxiety, restlessness, crackles, and cyanosis. Promoting lung expansion and systemic tissue oxygenation is a goal in the care of the patient with atelectasis (see also Chapter 23).

Elimination Complications

Common postoperative complications associated with elimination include urinary retention (see Chapter 29) and altered bowel elimination (see Chapter 26). Urinary retention may occur because of pain, postoperative positioning, the effects of anesthesia and narcotics, inactivity, altered fluid balance, anxiety, or surgical manipulation in the pelvic area.

Bowel elimination frequently is altered after abdominal or pelvic surgery. Return to normal gastrointestinal function may be delayed by general anesthesia, narcotic analgesia, decreased mobility, or altered fluid and food intake during the perioperative period. It is important to frequently assess bowel sounds and abdominal distention and to ambulate the patient as early as possible to encourage normal gastrointestinal function.

Wound Complications

INFECTION Despite all the measures designed to prevent contamination of the surgical wound, infection is a common surgical complication. Common assessment findings of an infected wound include redness, warmth, and edema around the edges of the incision. Purulent drainage may be noted inside or from the wound. The patient may have a fever, chills, and increased respiratory and pulse rates.

DEHISCENCE **Dehiscence** is separation of the incision (Figure 10-7A■). When dehiscence occurs, the wound should be covered immediately with a sterile dressing

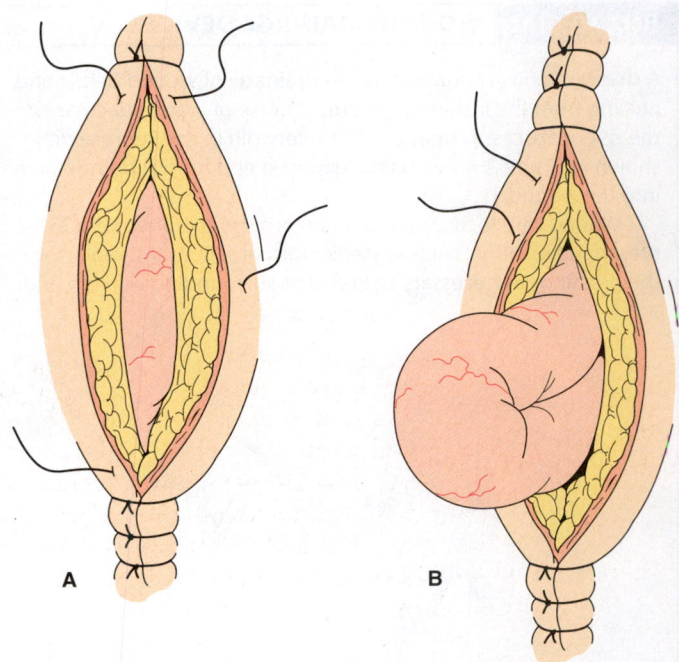

Figure 10-7. ■ Wound complications. (**A**) Dehiscence. (**B**) Evisceration.

moistened with normal saline. The patient is placed on bed rest and the surgeon is notified. Treatment depends on the extent of wound disruption. If the dehiscence is extensive, the patient returns to surgery for wound closure.

EVISCERATION **Evisceration** is the protrusion of body organs from a wound dehiscence (see Figure 10-7B). Like dehiscence, this serious complication may occur immediately after surgery or after forceful straining (coughing, sneezing, or vomiting) or may result from delayed wound healing. Protruding organs are covered with moist sterile dressings or towels. The patient is placed on bed rest and the surgeon is notified. Emergency surgery is necessary to repair evisceration.

SPECIAL CONSIDERATIONS FOR OLDER ADULTS

The older adult is at increased risk for postoperative complications because of physiologic, cognitive, and psychosocial changes associated with aging. The nursing care plan is modified to account for these normal changes and provide for safe, supportive care. Sensory deprivation is responsible for much of the confusion experienced by the hospitalized older adult. Eyeglasses and hearing aids should be returned to the patient as soon as possible after surgery. Early ambulation is vital to prevent complications associated with immobility (pneumonia, skin and tissue breakdown). The older adult's nutritional status often is compromised before surgery; prompt reinstitution of feeding is vital to promote wound healing, immune function, and recovery.

clinicalALERT

Monitor older adults for response to medication and treatment. The older patient is at higher risk for cardiovascular problems and fluid overload. Adverse medication responses occur more frequently because of changes in drug metabolism, distribution, and elimination. Promptly report symptoms such as acute confusion, restlessness, changes in level of consciousness, and withdrawal from the environment.

COLLABORATIVE CARE

Diagnostic Tests

Diagnostic tests commonly ordered during the postoperative period include the following:

- *Hemoglobin* and *hematocrit* to monitor for undetected bleeding
- *Serum osmolarity* and *electrolytes* to evaluate fluid volume status and electrolyte balance
- *Blood glucose levels*, particularly in diabetic patients, to monitor the effects of stress and blood glucose management
- *Therapeutic drug levels* if antibiotic therapy is ordered
- *Chest x-ray* if manifestations of pneumonia, atelectasis, or heart failure develop
- *Oxygen saturation levels*, monitored continuously in the initial postoperative period to ensure adequate tissue oxygenation

Pain Management

Management of acute postoperative pain is of primary concern to the patient, surgeon, and nurse. Established, severe pain is more difficult to treat than pain that is at its onset. Furthermore, pain stimulates the stress response and actually slows healing and recovery. For more in-depth information about acute pain and its management, see Chapter 8.

Initially, postoperative analgesics are administered at regular intervals or using patient-controlled analgesia (PCA) to maintain a therapeutic blood level. As-needed (PRN) administration allows blood levels to fall below the therapeutic range; delays in medication administration further increase pain intensity and make its management more difficult.

Nonsteroidal anti-inflammatory drugs (NSAIDs) (e.g., *ibuprofen*, ketorolac tromethamine [Acular, Toradol]) are administered to treat mild to moderate postoperative pain and as adjuncts to opioid analgesics. They should be given soon after surgery (orally, parenterally, or rectally) along with opioids unless contraindicated. NSAIDs allow for lower dosages of opioid analgesics and, therefore, fewer side effects. Certain NSAIDs, such as ketorolac, when given in higher doses after surgery, may only be administered safely for 2 to 3 days before the dosage must be reduced. NSAIDs can be given safely to older patients, but the nurse should observe closely for side effects, especially gastric, liver, and kidney toxicity.

Opioid analgesics, such as morphine and its derivatives, are the foundation for managing moderate to severe postoperative pain. Opioid dosage requirements vary greatly from one patient to another, so the dosage must be individually tailored.

Contrary to the belief of many patients, physical dependence and tolerance to opioid analgesics are uncommon in short-term postoperative use. Also, when opioid analgesics are used to treat acute pain, they rarely lead to psychologic dependence and addiction.

Older patients tend to experience a higher peak effect and longer duration of pain control with opioids; therefore, the older patient should be monitored closely for signs of respiratory depression and decreased responsiveness.

Food and Fluid Management

Fluids commonly are administered intravenously until the patient is fully awake and bowel sounds are present. Balanced electrolyte solutions are often used to prevent electrolyte imbalance related to fasting. Potassium chloride may be added to the intravenous solution if nasogastric suction is in place or fasting will be prolonged. (See Chapter 7 for more information about intravenous fluid management.)

Oral fluids and feeding are resumed as soon as possible, based on the type of surgery performed, the patient's mental status, and resumption of peristalsis. Recent studies have shown a significant risk for protein-calorie malnutrition (PCM) in the postoperative patient when fasting is prolonged for 12 or more hours. PCM slows wound healing and impairs immune defenses, increasing the risk for postoperative complications. Parenteral nutrition may be required for patients who are unable to resume oral intake for several days or more. See Chapter 25 for more information about PCM, total parenteral nutrition, and the nurse's role in caring for patients with nutritional disorders.

Other Therapies

Oxygen may be administered during the initial postoperative period to support tissue oxygenation and healing. Use of the incentive spirometer often is prescribed hourly (during waking hours) for the first 24 hours and then at least every 2 hours until discharge. The incentive spirometer promotes deep breathing and lung expansion, helping prevent pneumonia and atelectasis.

NURSING CARE

Nursing care of the postoperative patient focuses on promoting comfort and healing and preventing and monitoring for wound complications, as well as complications involving other organ systems. Once stable and awake, the patient is transferred from the PACU to the care unit or discharged home. The PACU nurse communicates information about the patient's surgery, current status, and postoperative care to the unit nurse using the format and information in the Continuity of Care section on page 222 as a guide.

PRIORITIZING NURSING CARE

Nursing care priorities during the postoperative phase are pain management, prevention of postoperative complications, and teaching the patient and family about postdischarge care.

HEALTH PROMOTION

The nurse promotes health for the postoperative patient by managing pain, assisting with early ambulation, and instituting measures to prevent complications and promote recovery. Teaching for health is an important nursing role during the recovery process. Education helps the patient become an active partner in promoting healing and recovery from surgery.

ASSESSING

After major surgery, the patient is assessed every 15 minutes during the first hour and, if stable, every 30 minutes for the next 2 hours, and then every hour during the subsequent 4 hours. Then focused assessments are carried out every 4 hours, unless the patient's condition changes or protocol dictates a more frequent schedule.

■ *Subjective data:* pain (location, intensity, duration, character); effect of analgesia; presence of nausea or other noxious sensations; ability to deep breathe, use incentive spirometer, move in bed or from bed to chair; other concerns

■ *Objective data:* level of consciousness and mental status; skin color, temperature, and moisture; vital signs including temperature and oxygen saturation; breath sounds and depth; bowel sounds, abdominal distention, and tenderness; operative site, including condition of wound and dressings, surrounding tissues, presence of drainage, and evidence of active bleeding (may require checking under the back or buttocks); peripheral vascular assessment as indicated, including pulse strength and equality, capillary refill, color and temperature, presence of edema, movement, and sensation

■ *Laboratory results:* hemoglobin and hematocrit; serum glucose, electrolytes, and osmolality; any abnormal values or significant changes from preoperative or expected results

IDENTIFYING POTENTIAL COMPLICATIONS

A change in mental status (restlessness, agitation, confusion) often is the first indication of a complication such as hemorrhage or an infection. Other assessment data that may indicate a postoperative complication and should be reported include the following:

■ A change in vital signs (tachycardia, hypotension, tachypnea)
■ Decreased urinary output
■ Inadequate pain control with previously effective medications and doses; complaints of pain unrelated to the operative site
■ A decrease in oxygen saturation levels
■ Diminished breath sounds or adventitious breath sounds (crackles)
■ Increased wound drainage or a change in the appearance or odor of wound drainage

clinical**ALERT**

Promptly report assessment data that are inconsistent with expected findings. Carefully document data, measures taken to verify findings, and the person to whom the assessment is reported.

DIAGNOSING, PLANNING, AND IMPLEMENTING

After the initial assessment and ensuring the patient's safety (lowering the bed and placing the call light within reach), the nurse reviews the postoperative orders. Specific orders to be noted include the following: activity level, diet, medications for pain and nausea, antibiotics (if ordered), continuation of preoperative medications, frequency of vital sign assessments, administration of intravenous fluids, and laboratory tests. In most institutions, preoperative orders must be specifically reordered after surgery because the patient's condition is assumed to have changed. If a previously ordered drug for a chronic condition (such as a cardiac drug or insulin) is not included in the postoperative orders, it is the nurse's responsibility to contact the physician to ensure that discontinuation of the drug was intended, not unintentional.

Acute Pain

Expected outcome: Will report pain at a level of 2 or lower on a standard pain scale of 0 to 10.

Pain is expected after surgery. Pain management involves the interprofessional care team, including the patient, physician, and nurse. Managing acute postoperative pain is an important nursing role and responsibility. The patient should be made aware of how much pain to anticipate, the importance of comfort to recovery, and his or her role in pain management (see Chapter 8). After discussing options with the patient, health care providers must respect the patient's personal preferences.

- Assess level of pain at least hourly during the initial postoperative period and then at least every 4 hours or whenever vital signs are obtained. Use a standard pain scale, such as having the patient rate pain on a scale of 0 to 10 (where 0 is no pain and 10 is the worst pain). *Controlling postoperative pain not only promotes comfort, but also facilitates coughing, turning, deep-breathing exercises, early ambulation, and healing. Rating the pain provides a more objective description and helps the nurse to choose pain medication appropriate to the severity of the pain.*

- Identify the location and type of pain. *Assessment data are used to plan interventions. Identifying the location of the pain is important to distinguish between expected pain related to the surgery and pain associated with potential complications such as pneumonia or angina.*

- Administer and document pain medication as prescribed. *Medication provides comfort and allows the patient to rest. Regular analgesic administration maintains a therapeutic blood level for more effective pain relief. Documentation and communication ensure continuity of care.*

- Initiate nonpharmacologic approaches to pain management, such as relaxation, distraction, and imagery techniques. *These techniques complement pain medication.*

- Evaluate and document the effectiveness of pain medication within 30 to 45 minutes of administration. *Ineffective relief may indicate a need for change of dosage or medication.*

Risk for Bleeding

Expected outcome: Color, vital signs, peripheral pulses, urine output, and laboratory data will remain within expected ranges.

- Apply one or more sterile gauze pads and a snug pressure dressing to the area. If external bleeding is severe, apply mechanical pressure with gloved hands. *Pressure assists the coagulation process. Increased pressure may be necessary to achieve coagulation.*

- Notify the physician of excessive bleeding or a decrease in hemoglobin or hematocrit levels. *Medical intervention is needed to correct the complication.*

- Monitor vital signs, level of consciousness, skin color, and temperature frequently. *Data are used to assess physiologic response to the event.*

clinicalALERT

Promptly report a change in mental status or vital signs outside the patient's normal or expected range. Restlessness, anxiety, and tachycardia may be early signs of internal hemorrhage.

- Establish or maintain intravenous access. *Rapid infusion of fluids may be necessary to maintain or replace fluid volume.*

- Monitor urine output. Report output less than 30 mL/hr to the charge nurse or physician. *Low urine output may be an early sign of decreased cardiac output due to blood loss.*

- Prepare the patient and family for emergency surgery. *Surgery may be necessary to locate and repair the source of bleeding.*

Ineffective Peripheral Tissue Perfusion

Expected outcome: Will remain free of evidence of venous thrombosis.

DVT in the postoperative patient usually results from venous stasis related to immobility. Nursing care focuses on preventing this potentially life-threatening complication.

- Assess peripheral pulses and color and temperature of extremities at least every 4 hours. Report changes or abnormal findings to the physician. *This provides early detection of signs of DVT.*

- Encourage postoperative leg exercises at least every 2 hours. Encourage early ambulation. *Exercise prevents venous stasis and enhances venous return.*

- Administer anticoagulants as prescribed. *Anticoagulants prevent platelet aggregation and decrease the risk of clot formation.*

- Monitor laboratory values for clotting times. *This information is used to determine the dosage of anticoagulant medications.*

- Apply thigh-high antiembolism stockings or pneumatic compression devices as ordered. *Antiembolism stockings and pneumatic compression devices promote venous return.*

Impaired Gas Exchange (Pulmonary Embolus)

Expected outcome: Will not experience chest pain or shortness of breath.

- Frequently assess and record general condition and vital signs. *Frequent assessment allows early detection of manifestations of respiratory complications.*

- Immediately notify the charge nurse and physician if manifestations of impaired gas exchange or pulmonary embolism develop. *Stabilizing respiratory and cardiovascular functioning is vital to protect physiologic function. Intensive care and monitoring are critical.*

- Maintain bed rest, with the head of the bed elevated. *This position facilitates breathing and promotes gas exchange.*

- Provide oxygen as ordered and monitor oxygen saturation. *This supports respiratory status and detects a deteriorating condition early.*
- Administer prescribed intravenous fluids. *Circulating volume must be maintained.*

Ineffective Breathing Pattern

Expected outcome: Lung sounds will remain clear with breath sounds throughout all lung fields.

- Assess vital signs, breath sounds, and general condition. *Patients who are chronically ill or malnourished, those who have a history of chronic lung disease, and older adults are at increased risk for these complications. Data allow early detection and evaluation of treatment.*
- Elevate the head of the bed. *This facilitates lung expansion.*
- Encourage the patient to turn and perform deep-breathing and coughing exercises at least every 2 hours. *This mobilizes secretions and supports airway clearance.*
- Assist with and encourage incentive spirometry and nebulizer treatments as ordered. *These expand alveoli and facilitate airway clearance.*
- Ambulate as condition permits and as prescribed. *Ambulation reduces the risk of complications related to immobility.*
- Maintain fluid intake to at least 2,000 mL/day if condition permits. *Fluid liquefies secretions for easier clearance.*

Risk for Infection (Surgical Incision)

Expected outcome: Will remain free of signs of infection.

- Assess vital signs, including temperature. *Elevated pulse, respirations, or temperature may indicate infection.*
- Assess the incision (approximation of the edges, sutures, staples, or drains) and surrounding tissue. *Integrity of the incision site reduces the risk of infection. Redness, warmth, or edema of the incision or surrounding tissue may indicate infection.*
- Evaluate wound discharge (color, odor, and amount). *Purulent wound drainage may indicate the presence of wound infection.*
- Maintain medical asepsis (use effective hand hygiene) and Standard Precautions. Use aseptic technique during dressing changes and handling of tubes and drains. *Asepsis reduces the risk of introducing microorganisms into surgical wounds.*
- Maintain hydration and nutritional status. *Nutrition facilitates healing.*

Risk for Urinary Retention

Expected outcome: Will experience no difficulty voiding and emptying bladder completely.

- Assess for bladder distention if the patient has not voided within 7 to 8 hours after surgery or if the patient is urinating small amounts frequently. Obtain a bladder scan to verify retained urine. *Early detection of urinary retention provides information for intervention.*
- Increase daily oral fluid intake to 2,500 to 3,000 mL as condition permits. *This facilitates renal function.*
- Assist the patient to void by:
  - Assisting and providing privacy when the patient uses a bedpan.
  - Helping the patient to use the bedside commode or to walk to the bathroom.
  - Assisting male patients to stand to void.
  These measures help promote normal urinary elimination.
- As necessary and ordered, empty the bladder using straight catheterization and aseptic technique. *Emptying the bladder promotes comfort. Straight catheterization using aseptic technique carries a lower risk for urinary tract infection than insertion of an indwelling urinary catheter.*

Risk for Constipation

Expected outcome: Will resume normal pattern of bowel elimination after surgery.

- Auscultate bowel sounds every 4 hours while the patient is awake. Assess the abdomen for distention. Determine whether the patient is passing flatus. Monitor for passage of stool, including amount and consistency. *A distended abdomen with absent bowel sounds may indicate paralytic ileus. These measures evaluate the presence or absence of peristalsis.*
- Encourage early ambulation within prescribed limits. *Mobility stimulates peristalsis.*
- Facilitate a daily fluid intake of 2,500 to 3,000 mL unless contraindicated. *Fluids provide moisture and facilitate passage of stool.*
- Provide privacy when the patient is using the bedpan, bedside commode, or bathroom. *Privacy provides relaxation and facilitates bowel elimination.*

EVALUATING

Careful evaluation of the postoperative patient's progress is essential to prevent development of complications and prompt intervention should they occur. Expected outcomes include the following:

- Patient is free of wound or systemic infection.
- Patient remains free of manifestations of venous thrombosis.
- Oxygen saturation remains above 92%.
- Patient voids within 6 hours of return from surgery and at least 1,000 mL in 24 hours.
- Breath sounds are audible throughout lung fields and remain clear.
- Patient performs incentive spirometry exercises at least every 4 hours.
- Bowel sounds are active in all four quadrants within 24 hours of abdominal surgery.

MANAGING NURSING CARE

As appropriate and allowed by the designated duties and responsibilities of assistive personnel, the nurse may delegate nursing care activities such as obtaining vital signs, measuring intake and output, and assisting with ambulation and hygiene for the postoperative patient.

DOCUMENTING

Document initial postoperative and continuing assessments, including any abnormal or unexpected data. When the physician or charge nurse is notified of abnormal or unexpected data, document notification and the care provider's response. Document pain level with vital signs, noting the effectiveness of analgesia and other pain relief measures. Note appearance of the surgical wound, including the presence of any bleeding or drainage on the dressing or within the wound. Document intake and output, including intravenous fluids, oral intake, urinary output, drainage from wound suction devices, and any emesis or abnormal fluid losses. Note ability and willingness to ambulate and assume self-care activities. Document all teaching and the patient's and family's understanding and ability to demonstrate care.

CONTINUITY OF CARE

Because the postoperative phase does not end until recovery is complete, the nurse's role is vital as the patient nears discharge. To prepare the patient to recuperate at home, provide information and support as needed for self-care. Written guidelines, directions, and information should accompany all aspects of teaching. The most common teaching needs are as follows:

- *Wound care.* Demonstrate and explain the procedure and then ask the patient and family to participate in care. As time allows, have the patient or caregiver demonstrate the procedure in return. Ideally, teaching is carried out over several days, evaluated, and reinforced.
- *Manifestations of a wound infection.* Teach the patient what is normal and what should be reported to the physician.
- *How and when to take a temperature.*
- *Limitations or restrictions on activities* (lifting, driving, bathing, sexual activity, return to work or school, and other physical activities).
- *Control of pain.* If analgesics are prescribed, discuss the dosage, frequency, purpose, common side effects, and symptoms to report to the physician. Reinforce effective analgesic use, and provide information on managing side effects such as gastric upset or constipation.

When the patient is discharged to a rehabilitation or skilled-care facility for additional recovery before returning home, it is important to convey information both verbally and in writing. Using the SBAR technique, include the following information:

- **Situation:** patient name and date of birth; the surgery or procedure done, including any modifiers (e.g., right hip arthroplasty)
- **Background:** wound management, current medications and their purpose, prescribed activity and any limitations (e.g., limited weight bearing or restricted joint flexion)
- **Assessment:** vital signs including temperature; respiratory and circulatory status; pain level and management; fluid balance and nutrition; skin status; current activity level and degree of independence; pertinent cultural, emotional, psychosocial, or spiritual care needs
- **Recommendations:** specific rehabilitation orders; conditions for discharge from rehabilitation or skilled care (Amato-Vealey et al., 2008)

Provide an opportunity to address any questions or concerns when handing off the patient to facility staff.

Note: The references and resources for all chapters have been compiled at the back of the book.

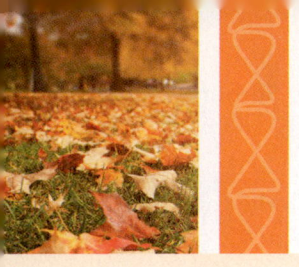

Chapter Review

KEY POINTS

- **Concept:** The nurse plays an important role in protecting the safety and promoting the recovery of the patient undergoing surgery.
- Perioperative nursing includes care of the patient through three phases: preoperative, intraoperative, postoperative.
- Maintaining patient safety through effective communication with the patient and the interprofessional team is a critical nursing responsibility during the perioperative period.
- **Concept:** Assessing, coordinating, and implementing preoperative preparation and patient teaching are key nursing roles during the preoperative phase.
- Care of the surgical patient should focus on psychologic as well as physiologic risk factors and patient needs.
- Thorough nursing assessment is key to identifying potential risk factors that may lead to perioperative complications.
- **Concept:** The nurses' focus during the intraoperative phase is on maintaining patient safety. Patient advocacy is a critical nursing role during this phase, as the patient is unable to speak for or meet his or her own needs.

- Nursing interventions are planned and implemented to prevent the development of perioperative complications such as wrong site surgery, injuries due to positioning or retained objects, and infection.
- **Concept:** During the postoperative phase, nurses are instrumental in promoting the patient's comfort and initial recovery, identifying and preventing potential complications, and teaching the patient and family or caregivers about continuing care needs.
- Control of postoperative pain is a major concern of the surgical patient.
- Patient education is a critical tool to prepare the patient for the perioperative experience. Inclusion of family members and caregivers is essential for success of the nursing plan of care.
- Major postoperative complications include respiratory and cardiovascular disorders, infection, hemorrhage, and elimination disorders.
- Collaboration of all members of the health care team is essential to achieve an optimal outcome for the surgical patient.

PEARSON NURSING STUDENT RESOURCES

Find additional materials at **nursing.pearsonhighered.com**.

Clinical Reasoning Care Map

Caring for a Patient After Surgery
NCLEX-PN® Focus Area: Safety and Infection Control

Case Study: Mrs. Wilson, age 80, is 3 days post right total hip replacement. Daniel Moore, LPN, is assigned to her care. Mr. Moore performs a focused assessment and finds that Mrs. Wilson is alert and oriented. Her skin is warm and moist. Mrs. Wilson rates her pain as 3 on a scale of 0 to 10. She complains of feeling alternately warm and chilled. Vital signs are T 101°F, P 100, R 24, BP 134/82. She states she is "drinking lots of fluids." Mrs. Wilson is receiving ciprofloxacin hydrochloride (Cipro) PO every 8 hours. The surgical incision is red and edematous with a 2-cm opening. Mr. Moore empties 25 mL of dark red drainage from the Jackson Pratt drain.

Mrs. Wilson's feet are pink and warm with rapid capillary refill. Distal pulses, movement, and sensation are strong and equal bilaterally. Review of lab work reveals Hgb 11.3 g, Hct 38.4%, WBC 13,000 mm^3.

Nursing Diagnosis: Infection

COLLECT DATA

Subjective	Objective
_____	_____
_____	_____
_____	_____
_____	_____
_____	_____
_____	_____

Does this present a threat to the patient's safety?

If yes, the priority intervention to address this threat would be:

_____

Nursing Care

_____
_____
_____
_____
_____
_____
_____

Interprofessional team members to include when planning care:

_____
_____

How would you document this? _____

_____
_____

Data Collected
(use only those that apply)

- Alert and oriented
- Incisional pain
- T 101°F, P 100
- Jackson Pratt drain in place
- WBC 13,000 mm^3
- IV infusing at 100 mL/hr
- Pedal pulses strong
- Light-brown drainage on dressing
- Incision red, edematous, 2-cm opening
- Complains of feeling warm and has chills
- Cipro 250 mg q8h
- States she is "drinking lots of fluids"

Nursing Interventions
(use only those that apply; list in priority order)

- Provide extra blankets for warmth.
- Monitor vital signs, especially temperature and pulse, q4h. Report temperature above 100°F to charge nurse.
- Cleanse wound with normal saline qd, per physician's order.
- Assess pedal pulses q8h.
- Empty Jackson Pratt drain q4h.
- Assess wound status with each dressing change.
- Tylenol 325 mg PO q4h for temperature above 100°F.
- Administer antibiotics as ordered.
- Monitor urinary output.
- Change dressing, using aseptic technique, twice per day.
- Administer pain medications as needed.
- Maintain fluid intake at least 2,000 mL/day.
- Collect sample of wound drainage, send to lab for culture and sensitivity.

Compare your answers and documentation to those provided on the companion website.

NCLEX-PN® Exam Preparation

1 A patient is scheduled for a thyroidectomy. Which of the following terms may be used to describe this type of surgery?

1. Reconstructive
2. Emergency
3. Ablative
4. Minor

2 A man is admitted to the ambulatory surgery unit in preparation for a hernia repair. Which of the following lab results noted by the nurse may require medical intervention?

1. Hemoglobin 13.4, hematocrit 44
2. Potassium 2.8
3. Platelets 280,000
4. Blood urea nitrogen (BUN) 10

3 A patient asks the nurse to explain possible complications she might experience as a result of her total abdominal hysterectomy. The most appropriate response by the nurse would be:

1. "I will contact your physician to discuss this with you."
2. "Let's not worry about complications. You will be just fine."
3. "Why are you worried about complications?"
4. "There are many potential complications. Let's discuss them."

4 A patient is 5 hours postoperative. He has an IV infusing at 125 mL/hr. He has not voided and complains of pain in his lower abdomen. All of the following are appropriate nursing actions. Place them in the order in which the nurse would perform them.

1. Assist Mr. Harris to stand to void.
2. Assess the bladder for distention.
3. Notify the physician of inability to void.
4. Prepare to perform a straight catheterization.
5. Run water in the sink.

5 A patient has been taught about pain management, coughing, and leg exercises before surgery. Which one of the following actions indicates a need for further teaching?

1. The patient splints the incision with a pillow.
2. The patient contracts and relaxes calf and thigh muscles frequently while awake.
3. The patient rests quietly when the pain is significant.
4. The patient coughs forcefully after taking a deep breath.

6 The patient's surgical incision is healing by primary intention. Which assessment finding should the nurse expect?

1. Wound edges are approximated.
2. Wound exudate is present.
3. The wound is large, gaping, and irregular.
4. Granulation tissue is evident.

7 Immediately after the patient has been admitted to the surgical suite, the circulating nurse calls for a time-out. The LPN/LVN recognizes the primary purpose of the time-out is to:

1. allow additional time to obtain necessary equipment.
2. prevent wrong patient, wrong site, or wrong procedure surgery.
3. reduce patient anxiety by orienting to the operating room.
4. allow the anesthetist to induce anesthesia.

8 The nurse assesses a postoperative patient on return to the nursing unit. The following data are collected:

1313: T 99°F, P 92, R 20, BP 120/80, alert, oriented
1330: T 98°F, P 100, R 24, BP 116/68, sleeping
1345: T 98°F, P 116, R 28, BP 100/54, restless
1400: T 97°F, P 130, R 32, BP 90/50, restless, drowsy

The appropriate INITIAL nursing action at 1400 would be to:

1. assess the surgical dressing.
2. notify the physician.
3. position the patient flat with the feet elevated 8 to 12 in.
4. increase the IV infusion rate.

9 A older adult patient had a right total hip replacement 1 day ago. The LPN/LVN notes that the patient is now slightly confused and disoriented. The MOST important action by the nurse at this time would be to:

1. document the findings.
2. notify the physician.
3. keep the patient on complete bed rest.
4. assist the patient to put on his glasses and hearing aids.

10 A patient scheduled for cataract removal in an ambulatory care center asks how long she should expect to remain in the facility after the procedure. The MOST appropriate response by the nurse would be:

1. "You will remain here overnight to make sure the implanted lens remains in position."
2. "Although you will be admitted the morning of surgery, expect to stay for several days afterward."
3. "You should plan to have someone available to take you home the day of surgery."
4. "I will clarify this with your physician."

Answers and rationales for Review Questions appear in Appendix I.

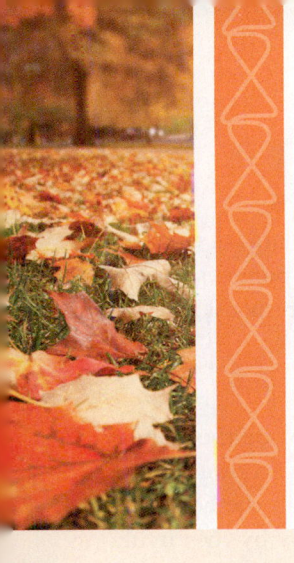

CHAPTER 11
Caring for Patients With Altered Immunity

BRIEF OUTLINE

Overview of the Immune
   System
Natural and Acquired
   Immunity

Altered Immune Responses
Autoimmune Disorders
Organ/Tissue Transplantation

Impaired Immune Responses
and the Patient With HIV
Infection

APPLIED LEARNING OUTCOMES

After completing this chapter, you will be able to:

1. Implement nursing interventions used to promote active and passive immunity in adult patients.
2. Identify laboratory tests used to diagnose and monitor immune response.
3. Apply nursing implications for medications given to patients with altered immunity.
4. Teach patients with altered immune responses and their families the importance of care and follow-up.
5. Use the nursing process to collect data, establish outcomes, provide individualized care, and evaluate responses for the patient experiencing altered immunity.
6. Implement ways to prevent the transmission of HIV infection.
7. Use the nursing process to collect data, establish outcomes, provide individualized care, and evaluate responses for the patient with AIDS.

KEY TERMS

The key terms are defined on the pages listed below.

SPECIAL FEATURES

Key Concept Normal immune function is essential to protect the body from internal and external threats. Immunity begins when the body recognizes foreign antigens as "nonself." This stimulates nonspecific inflammatory responses and specific cellular responses to the foreign antigen.

The human body is constantly threatened by infectious agents such as bacteria, viruses, parasites, foreign substances, and abnormal or damaged cells. Because the body provides the perfect host environment, microbes try to break through the skin and mucous membrane barriers. The role of the immune system is either to keep out the foreign substances or, once they break through the defenses, to inactivate or destroy them.

The immune system can malfunction, causing mild allergic reactions to more complex systemic involvement that is seen with autoimmune diseases such as rheumatoid arthritis. Transplanted organs or tissues can trigger a rejection response by the immune system. Significant immunodeficiency caused by the human immunodeficiency virus can result in the development of acquired immunodeficiency syndrome and its numerous opportunistic infections and cancers.

Overview of the Immune System

The immune system is a complex network of cells and organs that protect the body against infection-causing microorganisms, foreign substances, and cancerous cells. Three defense mechanisms provide this protection. The first line of defense involves the skin, mucous membranes, and body secretions. If these defenses are penetrated, the body's inflammatory response is activated within seconds as the second line of defense. It is a nonspecific response in which white blood cells engulf and neutralize any harmful invaders. (See Chapter 9 on inflammation.) A much slower response involves the third line of defense: immunity. The immune response provides specific immunity with T lymphocytes and B lymphocytes.

The immune system can recognize the body's own cells (self) and foreign cells (nonself). Normally, the body's immune defenses coexist peacefully with any cell marked as "self." When any nonself substance (**antigen**) invades the body, the immune system responds. Antigens can be bacteria, viruses, or tissues transplanted from another person (including blood). If the immune system perceives transplanted tissues or organs as nonself, they may be rejected. Sometimes, harmless substances such as dog hair or pollen set up an allergic response. This kind of antigen is called an *allergen*. In other circumstances, the immune system mistakes self for nonself and attacks it, resulting in autoimmune diseases.

IMMUNE SYSTEM COMPONENTS

The immune system consists of cells and organs that produce the immune response. These components may be involved in the nonspecific inflammatory response, the specific immunologic response, or both.

Leukocytes

Leukocytes, or white blood cells (WBCs), are the primary cells involved in nonspecific and specific immune system responses. Leukocytes start as stem cells in the bone marrow. They are moved throughout the body by the circulatory system. This mobility allows them to detect, attack, and destroy any foreign invaders at the site of involvement.

The normal number of circulating leukocytes is 4,500 to 10,000 cells/mm^3 of blood as indicated on the WBC count. If an infection develops, additional WBCs are released from the bone marrow, leading to *leukocytosis* (increased WBC count). When bone marrow activity is suppressed, such as during cancer treatments with chemotherapy, *leukopenia* (decreased WBC count) can occur. The WBC differential test identifies the percent of the total number of WBCs for each type of leukocyte.

From the original stem cells, leukocytes develop into three major groups of WBCs: granulocytes, monocytes, and lymphocytes (Table 11-1■). Granulocytes make up the greatest number of normal blood leukocytes. Monocytes are the largest leukocyte. Lymphocytes are subdivided into B-cell lymphocytes, T-cell lymphocytes, and natural killer cells (Figure 11-1■). T cells and B cells are the basis for the specific immune response and are discussed further in this chapter.

Natural killer (NK) cells are those cells that survey the body for potential foreign invaders such as viruses, fungi, and malignant cells. Unlike B and T cells, which attack only specific infected cells or malignant cells, NK cells can attack any target identified as foreign. They assume a key role in destroying early malignant cells. The functions of all leukocytes are closely interrelated.

Lymphoid Organs and Tissues

The organs and tissues of the immune system are found throughout the body. They are called lymphoid organs because they are home to the lymphocytes. The *lymphoid system* consists of the bone marrow, thymus, spleen, lymph nodes, and lymphoid tissue scattered in the connective tissues and mucosa (Figure 11-2■). The bone marrow and thymus are considered primary or central lymphoid organs. The spleen, lymph nodes, and other peripheral lymphoid tissue (e.g., the tonsils and appendix) are secondary lymphoid organs.

Bone marrow is the soft tissue in the hollow center of all bones. Red bone marrow produces blood cells from the

TABLE 11-1	Cells of the Immune System
TYPE OF LEUKOCYTE	**FUNCTION**
Granulocytes	Involved in inflammatory response; make up 60%–80% of normal blood leukocytes
■ Neutrophils	First to appear after an injury; involved in phagocytosis
■ Eosinophils	Involved in phagocytosis; protect against parasites; part of allergic response
■ Basophils	Protect mucosal surfaces; secrete histamine during allergic reactions
Monocytes	Involved in inflammatory response; mature into macrophages
	Trap and phagocytize foreign substances and cellular debris
Lymphocytes	Involved in specific immune response; make up 20%–40% of circulating leukocytes
■ T lymphocytes	Provide cell-mediated immunity; mature in thymus gland
■ Helper T cells (T4)	Turn on immune system function:
	Stimulate B cells to produce antibodies
	Release lymphokines to destroy viral infections and cancer cells
	Involved in hypersensitivity reactions (e.g., blood transfusion reaction) and graft tissue rejection
■ Suppressor T cells (T8)	Turn off immune system function
■ Cytotoxic T cells	Kill tumor cells, viral-infected cells, and foreign tissue
■ B lymphocytes	Responsible for humoral immunity; mature in bone marrow
■ Plasma cells	Produce antibodies (immunoglobulins) to specific antigens
■ Memory cells	Produce specific antibody when reexposed to a specific antigen
■ Natural killer cells	Kill virus-infected and tumor cells

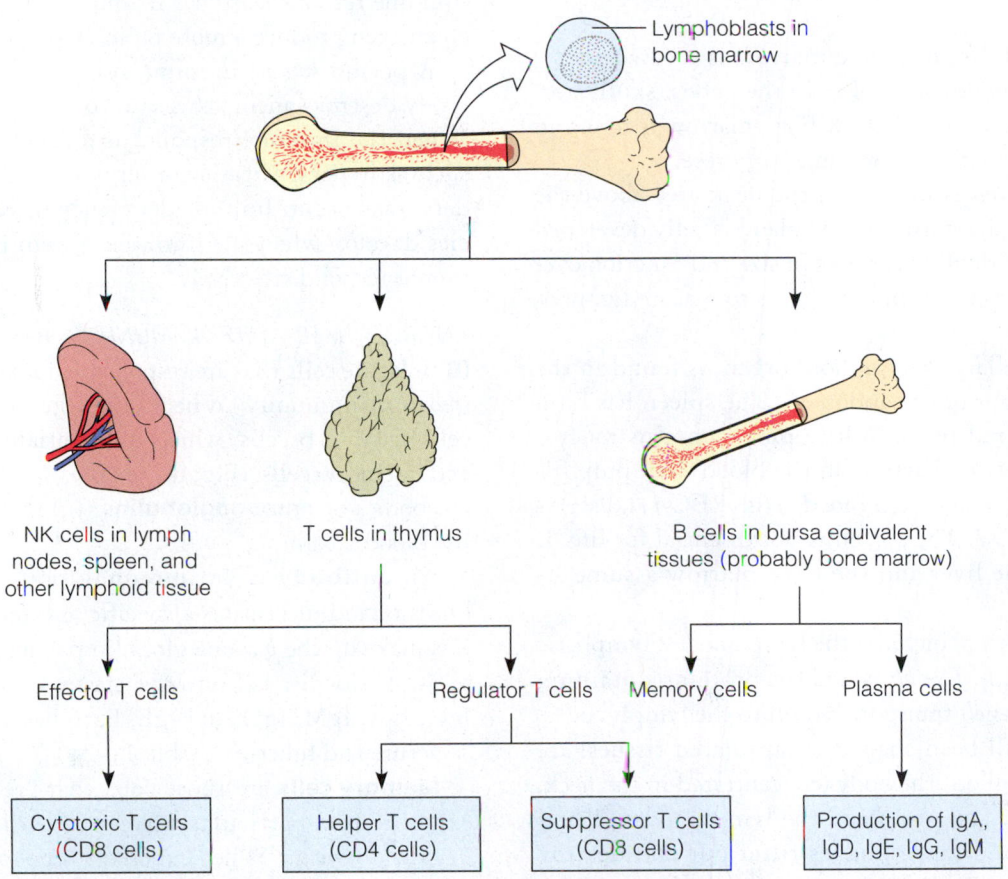

Figure 11-1. ■ The development and differentiation of lymphocytes from the lymphoid stem cell (lymphoblasts).

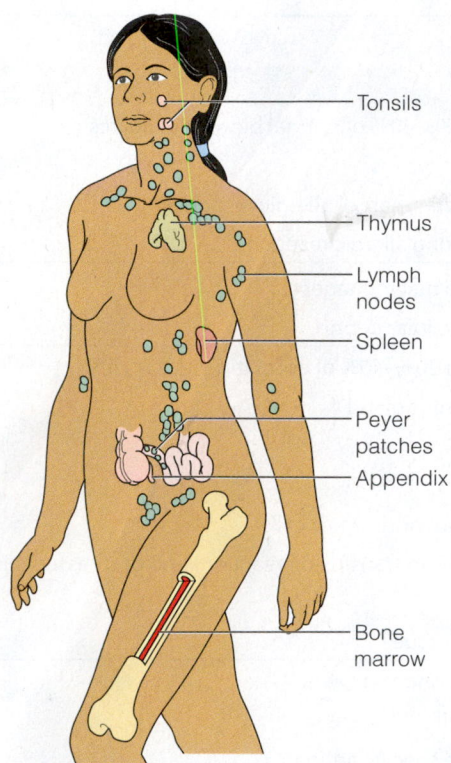

Figure 11-2. ■ The lymphoid system: the central organs of the thymus and bone marrow and the peripheral organs, including the spleen, tonsils, lymph nodes, and Peyer patches.

Labels: Tonsils, Thymus, Lymph nodes, Spleen, Peyer patches, Appendix, Bone marrow

stem cells. In adults, red bone marrow is located in the ends of the long bones, as well as in the pelvis, skull, sternum, ribs, and vertebrae. Yellow bone marrow is found in the other bones; it stores fat for an energy reserve.

The *thymus gland* is located in the neck area above the heart and behind the sternum. The gland is fully developed at puberty and gradually decreases in size and function over a person's life span. Its main function is to mature lymphocytes into T cells.

The *spleen*, the largest lymphoid organ, is found in the upper-left quadrant of the abdomen. The spleen has both white pulp and red pulp. White pulp contains macrophages, which destroy bacteria in the blood. Red pulp filters out damaged or aged red blood cells (RBCs) and stores blood for future use. The spleen is not essential for life. If it is removed, the liver and the bone marrow assume its functions.

The *lymphatic system* includes the lymph nodes, lymphatic vessels, and lymph. *Lymph* is a clear, protein-containing fluid. *Lymphatic vessels* transport lymph to the lymph nodes. *Lymph nodes*, small bean-shaped encapsulated tissues, are distributed throughout the body (concentrated in the neck, axillae, abdomen, and groin). In the lymph nodes, T and B lymphocytes and macrophages filter out and destroy foreign products. The lymph nodes can become tender and palpable when a person develops a systemic infection.

Clumps of specialized lymphoid tissue are also located in the tonsils, adenoids, appendix, and Peyer patches in the intestines. They protect the body from inhaled foreign agents or ingested pathogens.

Recognition of Self

The effectiveness of the immune system depends on whether it can differentiate normal body tissue (self) from foreign tissue (nonself). Each body cell has cell surface markers that are unique to each person. These are known as *human leukocyte antigens (HLAs)*. A person's HLA characteristics are coded within a large cluster of genes known as the *major histocompatibility complex (MHC)*. The possibility of two people having the same HLA is rare except in identical twins. Some siblings may have similar HLA. In organ transplantation, matching the HLA as closely as possible tends to decrease rejection.

Antibody-Mediated Immunity and Cell-Mediated Immunity

When antigens enter the body, a specific immune response occurs. The immune system recognizes the particular antigens (viruses, bacteria, or transplanted tissue) and destroys them without harming itself. Unlike a localized inflammatory response, the immune response is systemic. The immune response also has memory. Repeated exposures to an antigen produce a more rapid response.

A person whose immune system identifies and effectively destroys antigens is said to be **immunocompetent**. When the immune response is altered, health problems such as hypersensitivity (allergy and autoimmune disorders) may occur. Immunodeficiency diseases or malignancies develop when the immune system is incompetent or cannot respond effectively.

ANTIBODY-MEDIATED IMMUNITY **B-cell lymphocytes (B cells)** are cells that are responsible for antibody-mediated (*humoral*) immunity. When an antigen enters the body, T cells activate B cells, which differentiate into plasma cells and memory cells (Figure 11-3■). Plasma cells produce antibodies or **immunoglobulins** (Ig) that are released into the bloodstream.

An **antibody** is an immunoglobulin molecule that binds to and inactivates a specific antigen. Immunoglobulins make up the gamma globulin portion of the blood proteins. Antibodies fall into five classes of immunoglobulins: IgG, IgA, IgM, IgD, and IgE. Each has a slightly different structure and function (Table 11-2■).

Memory cells are those cells that "remember" a prior exposure to a particular antigen, even if they have been inactive for years. When exposed to the same antigen, they convert into plasma cells and inactivate the antigen. This rapid response means that either the person avoids the

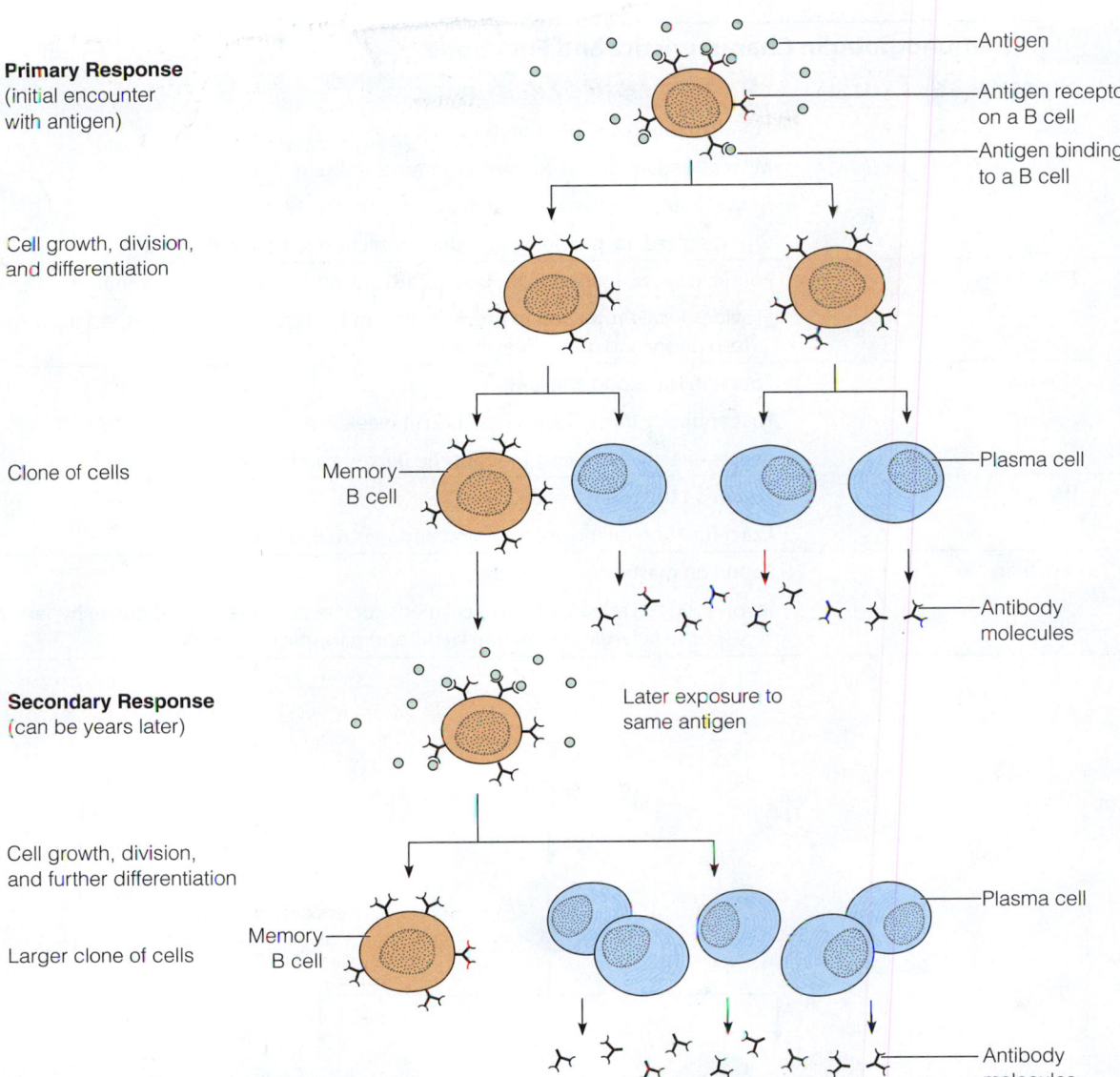

Figure 11-3. ■ Humoral immunity. *Primary response:* During first exposure to an antigen, B cells are stimulated to become plasma cells and produce antibodies or memory cells. *Secondary response:* With reexposure to the same antigen, the memory cells respond rapidly with antibody production.

disease or the second infection is milder. Memory cells are responsible for acquired immunity against diseases such as measles or chickenpox.

CELL-MEDIATED IMMUNITY   **T-cell lymphocytes (T cells)** are the foundation for *cell-mediated* (or cellular) immunity (Figure 11-4■). There are three types of T cells: (1) helper T cells, (2) suppressor T cells, and (3) cytotoxic T cells.

Helper T cells, also known as CD4+ cells, are cells responsible for switching on the immune system. They also recognize antigens such as a virus or transplanted tissue. **Suppressor T cells** (CD8 cells) are the cells that limit the immune response so that the body does not destroy itself. These cells are important in preventing autoimmune disorders. **Cytotoxic T cells** are cells that can destroy cancer

cells, cells of transplanted organs, and grafted tissues. They are vital in the control of viral and bacterial infections.

IMMUNE FUNCTION IN THE OLDER ADULT

As immune function declines with aging, there is an increased susceptibility to infections and a diminished immune response in older adults. The thymus gland atrophies and, by age 60, it no longer is functional. Although the total number of T cells remains the same, T-cell function and reproduction decrease. T lymphocytes cannot eliminate foreign invaders as well as when the person was younger.

With these changes, cell-mediated immune function declines. Immune memory against such diseases as chickenpox and tuberculosis weakens. In the older person, reactivation of the chickenpox virus leads to herpes zoster

TABLE 11-2	Immunoglobulin Characteristics and Functions	
CLASS	**PERCENTAGE OF TOTAL**	**CHARACTERISTICS AND FUNCTION**
IgG	75%	Found in blood, lymph, and intestines
		Most abundant Ig; also known as gamma globulin
		Active against bacteria, bacterial toxins, and viruses
		Crosses placenta, providing immune protection to neonate
IgA	10%–15%	Found in saliva, tears, mucus, bile, colostrum, and prostatic and vaginal secretions
		Provides local protection to prevent entry of bacteria and viruses, especially through the respiratory and gastrointestinal tracts
IgM	5%–10%	Found in the blood and lymph
		First antibody formed and lasts about 1 week
		Reacts effectively against bloodborne bacteria and viruses
IgD	1%	Found on the surface of B cells
		Exact function unknown; may bind antigens to B-cell surface
IgE	Less than 1%	Found on mast cells and basophils
		Involved in the release of chemical mediators responsible for immediate hypersensitivity response (allergic and anaphylactic) and parasitic infections

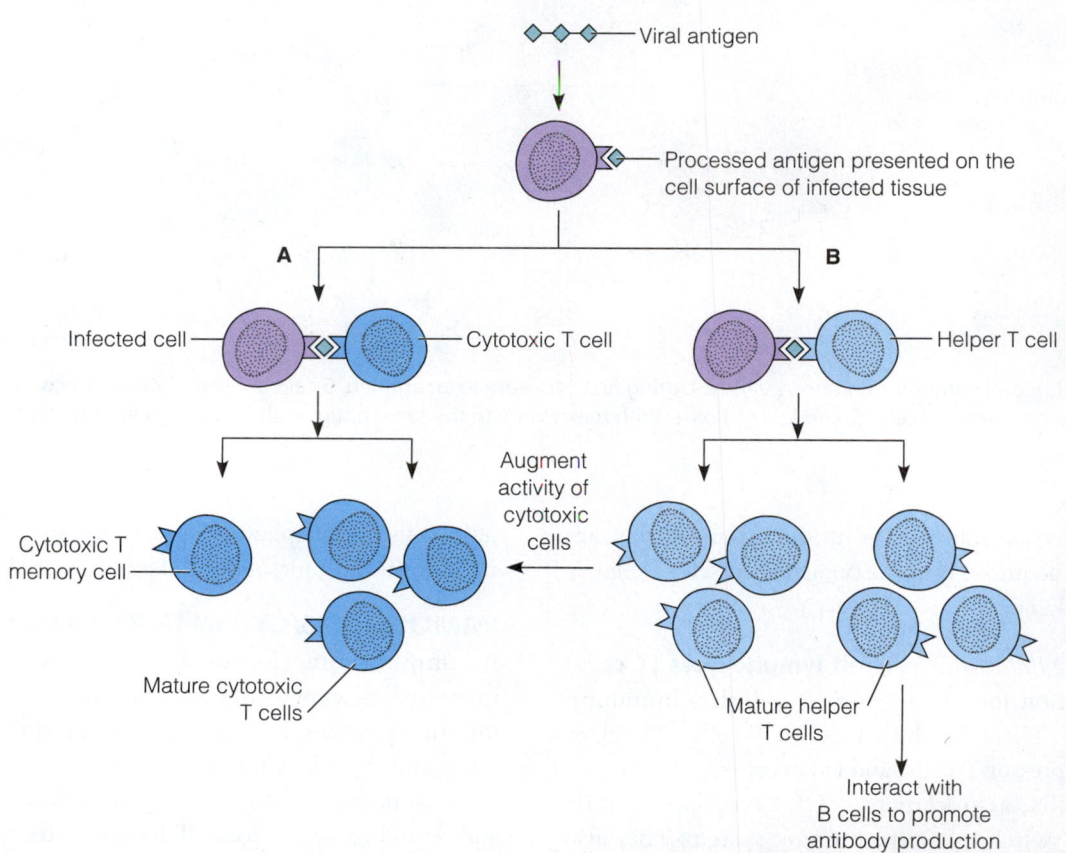

Figure 11-4. ■ Cell-mediated immunity. (**A**) An infected cell with an antigen on its surface binds with a receptor site on a cytotoxic T or a helper T cell. The cytotoxic T cell produces memory cells or mature cytotoxic cells. (**B**) The helper T cell assists the cytotoxic activity of the cytotoxic cells and stimulates B cells to produce antibodies.

(shingles). Immunoglobulins, especially IgG, decrease, followed by a reduced antibody response to influenza, tetanus, and pneumococcal immunizations.

There is also an increase in autoantibody production that may increase the potential for autoimmune diseases. Some autoimmune diseases (e.g., myasthenia gravis, rheumatoid arthritis, and multiple sclerosis) start in young adulthood or middle age and cause progressive damage as the person ages. External factors such as nutritional status and the effects of chemical exposure, ultraviolet radiation, and environmental pollution affect the older person's immune status. Internal factors including genetics, the function of the neurologic and endocrine systems, and chronic and past illnesses may alter immune system function. Even with all of these influences, some older individuals have an immune system as effective as that of a younger person.

Natural and Acquired Immunity

Immunity refers to the protection of the body from disease. Immunity may be natural or acquired, active or passive. Immunity results from activation of antibody-mediated or cell-mediated responses. In the immunocompetent patient, these immune responses inactivate and remove the antigen, allowing recovery or preventing development of the disease.

PATHOPHYSIOLOGY

Innate immunity is a person's resistance to foreign substances that occurs because of gender, race, heredity, age, or health status. Innate immunity does not produce an immune response. Individuals are naturally protected because of their physical and chemical barriers.

Active immunity is resistance that can be *naturally acquired* by actually developing the disease or *artificially acquired* through an immunization. Either way, the body produces plasma and memory cells against specific antigens. Children may naturally acquire active immunity when exposed to mumps or measles. If reexposed later in life, the memory cells should protect them against these diseases. Active immunity can last from years to a lifetime, depending on the disease.

Immunization or vaccination against highly contagious diseases such as influenza provides artificially acquired active immunity. Immunizations require the body to actively initiate an immune response. This process can take days to weeks to complete. Vaccines do not produce disease but rather stimulate the B cells to remember a specific disease.

Passive immunity provides temporary protection against disease-producing antigens. It is obtained by injection of serum with ready-made antibodies produced by other people or animals. Once these antibodies are used up (after a few weeks or months), their protection is lost. For example, human immune globulin or gamma globulin is given to

patients when they are exposed to hepatitis A. This is known as *artificially acquired* passive immunity. *Naturally acquired* passive immunity occurs when neonates receive antibodies from their mothers via the placenta and breast milk.

COLLABORATIVE CARE

Collaborative care focuses on assessing the patient's immune status and promoting acquired immunity to prevent disease.

Diagnostic Tests

- *Serum immunoglobulins* measure the level of IgG, IgA, IgM, IgD, and IgE (see Table 11-2). IgG levels are increased during acute infections. Decreased levels of IgG, IgA, and IgM are found in malignancies.
- *Antibody titer testing* may determine whether a patient has developed antibodies in response to an infection or immunization. Antibodies for hepatitis, rubella, HIV, and toxoplasmosis can be identified. An elevated titer level indicates the presence of antibodies.
- *Skin testing* can detect impaired cell-mediated immunity. A known antigen such as streptokinase, tuberculin purified protein derivative (PPD), or *Candida albicans* is injected intradermally. The site is assessed in 24 to 48 hours for signs of *induration* (hardening of skin) and redness. An induration of 10 mm in diameter is a positive reaction (Figure 11-5■), indicating previous exposure and sensitization to the antigen. Lack of reaction, or **anergy**, indicates depressed cell-mediated immunity.

Immunizations

Immunizations or *vaccines* are suspensions of live, *attenuated* (weakened), or killed microorganisms that promote active immunity against a specific organism. Special treatment makes them incapable of causing disease. Some vaccinations

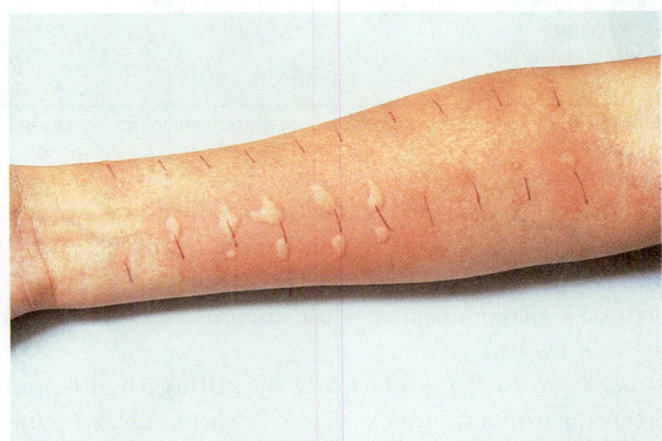

Figure 11-5. ■ Skin testing on the forearm showing induration (hardness) and erythema (redness) typical of a positive response to an antigen. (Source: Southern Illinois University / Science Source.)

	TABLE 11-3		Recommended Immunizations for Adults	
VACCINE	**TYPE**	**DOSE**	**INDICATIONS**	**PRECAUTIONS AND NURSING IMPLICATIONS**
■ Human papillomavirus (HPV)	Not a live virus	0.5 mL IM	Prior exposure to HPV through sexual activity	Three doses for females ≤26 years; IM in deltoid.
■ Measles–mumps–rubella (MMR)	Live, attenuated virus	0.5 mL subcutaneously	All adults born after 1956. Measles and mumps vaccines recommended for males without history of previous infection; rubella vaccine recommended for seronegative females	Do not administer to pregnant females or immunocompromised patients (AIDS, cancer) or those with a history of anaphylaxis or allergy to eggs. Give subcutaneously in fatty tissue over triceps.
■ Tetanus and diphtheria toxoids (Td)	Attenuated toxoid	0.5 mL IM	If never immunized, give series of three injections; give booster every 10 years, and after a contaminated wound	Do not give in the first trimester of pregnancy or to a patient with a history of anaphylactic reaction to horse serum. Give deep IM in deltoid of dominant arm.
■ Hepatitis A		1 mL IM	Persons with chronic liver disease; who travel to endemic areas; with illicit drug use; or men who have sex with men	Give IM in deltoid.
■ Hepatitis B (recombinant) (Recombivax B)	Inactivated viral antigen	1 mL IM	Series of three doses; initial and at 1 and 6 months	Use with caution in pregnant or lactating females or older patients. Give in deltoid site only.
■ Influenza (Fluzone)	Inactivated virus	0.5 mL IM	Yearly for adults over age 19; and especially patients over age 65 and in nursing homes; or patients with chronic pulmonary, renal, or cardiovascular diseases or diabetes	Do not give to patients with a history of anaphylactic reaction to eggs or to acutely ill patients.
■ Pneumococcal (Pneumovax-23)	Bacterial	0.5 mL IM	Adults over age 65 and those at risk for pneumococcal pneumonia, including those with chronic lung disease or other chronic diseases	Do not give to those with a history of anaphylactic reactions.
■ Herpes zoster (shingles)	Live attenuated virus	0.65 mL subcutaneously	Adults ≥60 years of age including those who report having had shingles	Do not give to immunocompromised or HIV-infected persons. Give in fatty tissue over triceps.
■ Meningococcal vaccine (Menactra)		0.5 mL IM	Two doses two months apart; recommended for college students living in dormitories and military recruits	Give in deltoid muscle.

Note: For pediatric patients, please consult a pediatric textbook for recommended immunizations.

are combined to protect against several diseases. The most common combinations in the United States are MMR (measles–mumps–rubella) and DTP (diphtheria–tetanus–pertussis). (Recommended adult immunizations are found in Table 11-3■.)

Inactivated vaccines are made by killing the disease-producing microorganism with heat or chemicals. For example, each year a new influenza vaccine is made, containing the three strains of influenza most likely to occur in the upcoming winter. These vaccines stimulate a weaker immune response, so yearly influenza immunizations are required.

Live, attenuated vaccines (e.g., the MMR) are made by growing the disease-producing organism under special laboratory conditions. The process causes the organisms to lose their virulence or disease-producing power.

Toxoids are substances that contain an inactivated toxin that is produced by a microbe. They are made harmless by exposing them to chemicals or heat. Diphtheria and tetanus toxoids are combined into a single immunization (Td for adults, DT for children). Vaccines such as hepatitis B have been developed by using recombinant genetic engineering. Some vaccines are made from portions or subunits of the antigen; one such vaccine protects patients against pneumonia caused by *Streptococcus pneumoniae*.

Hepatitis B vaccine is recommended for everyone at high risk for exposure to blood or other body fluids. It is mandated by the Occupational Safety and Health Administration (OSHA) for all health care workers. Other high-risk populations include intravenous drug users, sexual partners of infected individuals, patients on hemodialysis, prison guards, and athletic coaches.

People traveling outside the United States and Canada should receive vaccines against diseases that are found in certain regions of the world. Additional vaccines might include cholera, yellow fever, and typhoid vaccines.

When a patient has been exposed to a specific disease, immune globulins made from human or animal sources are given to provide passive immunity. Human sources carry less risk for an allergic reaction and are available for hepatitis A and B, tetanus, varicella, rabies, measles, and rubella.

Animal immune serums are made by injecting an antitoxin into an animal, allowing antibodies to develop, and then withdrawing blood and preparing a serum for human injection. Antitoxins are used against diphtheria, tetanus, rabies, and botulism. Antivenins, another form of passive immunization, are given after a patient has been bitten by potentially lethal snakes or spiders.

For most vaccines, a *sensitivity test* should be done before the first immunization to determine allergy to horse serum or eggs. The test dose is injected intradermally; if no hives appear after 20 minutes, the selected vaccine can be given.

Immunization side effects can range from mild local reactions to **anaphylaxis** (an acute, immediate allergic reaction). Local reactions at the injection site include redness, swelling, tenderness, and muscle ache. Giving the vaccine in the dominant arm of the patient reduces the local discomfort, because arm movement helps to increase absorption of the solution. Warm compresses may also be beneficial. Sometimes the patient may experience systemic manifestations such as fever or malaise. Anaphylaxis most likely occurs with horse serum injections.

NURSING CARE

Nurses have an important role in preventing the spread of communicable diseases. This includes encouraging immunizations. Factors that may prevent active use of immunization programs are religious beliefs, poverty, and unfamiliarity with the health care system (e.g., among immigrants). Also, many people simply neglect routine immunization in adulthood. The result is increased risk for infectious diseases among all people.

BOX 11-1	ASSESSMENT

Assessing Patients' Immune Status

Subjective Data
- History of infectious diseases or exposure to any infections
- Fever; swollen glands in neck, axilla, or groin
- Pregnancy status
- Any immunosuppressive diseases (e.g., AIDS, cancer), chemotherapy, or radiation therapy
- Chronic pulmonary, cardiac, or renal disorders or diabetes
- Immunization history; last tetanus injection; any adverse effects or allergy to horse serum or eggs

Objective Data
- Vital signs: blood pressure, pulse, respirations, temperature
- Height and weight
- Observe the patient for any signs of infection
- Assess for any skin lesion, rashes, or impaired healing
- Monitor and report antibody titer and skin testing results

Before immunizations are given, the nurse should collect assessment data to determine whether immunization is appropriate (Box 11-1■).

Nursing care focuses on preventing injury from the vaccination and on providing patient education.

Risk for Injury

Expected outcome: Will not experience any injury from immunization.

- Check the expiration date and the manufacturer's instructions for administration guidelines, dosage, routes, sites, precautions, and contraindications. *Outdated vaccines may not provide protection against the specific disease. Some sites have better absorption than others.*
- Do not administer any immunization to a patient with an upper respiratory infection (URI) or other infection. *Infections can increase the inflammatory reaction from an immunization.*
- Do not administer oral polio vaccines (OPVs) or MMR to immunosuppressed patients or to patients who are in close household contact with an immunosuppressed person. *Live virus vaccines can cause disease in the immunosuppressed patient or can transmit disease to close household contacts during the initial postvaccination period.*

clinicalALERT

Observe the patient for 20 to 30 minutes after vaccination, because allergic reactions usually occur within this time frame.

- Keep epinephrine 1:1,000 readily available when administering immunizations. *Epinephrine causes vasoconstriction and reduces laryngospasm; in acute anaphylaxis, it can be lifesaving.*

CONTINUITY OF CARE

Provide instructions in the following areas:

- Appropriate immunizations and recommended schedules for initial vaccination and boosters
- How and where to obtain immunizations (County or public health departments may offer immunization clinics at a lower cost than private physicians or urgent care clinics.)
- Possible side effects of the immunization as well as the need to observe the patient for up to 30 minutes after a vaccine for possible adverse reactions
- Self-care measures for side effects, such as warm compresses over the injection site and taking acetaminophen (Tylenol) for fever
- The need to report immediately any adverse reactions such as fever, rash, itching, or shortness of breath
- Importance of maintaining permanent immunization records

Altered Immune Responses

Key Concept A hyper-responsive immune system can overreact to antigens, causing hypersensitivities. When the immune system targets normal cells and tissues, either auto immune disorders (e.g., rheumatoid arthritis) can develop or transplanted tissue or organs can be destroyed.

HYPERSENSITIVITY REACTIONS

Normally, the immune system protects humans against foreign substances, but sometimes it overreacts. **Hypersensitivity** is an altered immune response in which the body overreacts to an antigen, resulting in harm to the patient.

The tissue response to a hypersensitivity reaction may be simply a runny nose or itchy eyes, or it may be life threatening, leading to blood cell hemolysis or anaphylaxis. Hypersensitivity responses include hay fever, blood transfusion reactions, and organ transplant rejections.

Hypersensitivity responses are usually classified by the type of immune response but also may be classified by whether the tissue response is immediate or delayed. There are four types of hypersensitivity reactions (Table 11-4■). Types I, II, and III have an immediate tissue response and are caused by the humoral system. Type IV has a delayed response and results from the cell-mediated system. Anaphylaxis is an immediate hypersensitivity response, whereas contact dermatitis is a delayed response.

Anaphylaxis is an acute response that develops in highly sensitive persons after exposure to a specific antigen. Common causes include seafood, eggs, antibiotics, bee stings, and latex. (See Chapter 14 for other substances that may cause anaphylaxis.) The reaction often begins within minutes of exposure to the antigen. Initially, itchy palms, swollen eyelids, and hives may be found. As the response progresses, laryngospasm and difficulty breathing occur. Without immediate treatment, the patient could develop anaphylactic shock. (See Chapter 14 for anaphylactic shock.)

LATEX ALLERGY

Although protective against infection, the repeated use of latex gloves causes a consistent exposure to latex for health care workers. An estimated 5% to 15% of health care workers are allergic to latex, but less than 1% of the general population has this allergy (AAAAI, 2012). When gloves are powdered with cornstarch to ease donning and

TABLE 11-4	Types of Hypersensitivity Reactions			
TYPE	**CAUSES**	**PATHOPHYSIOLOGY**		**EXAMPLES**
I—Immediate hypersensitivity	Pollens, foods, insect bites, animal dander, and drugs	Allergen binds to IgE antibodies that are attached to mast cells in connective tissue, skin, and mucous membranes, where they release histamine. Histamine constricts smooth muscle and causes peripheral vasodilation, leading to watery, itchy eyes; runny nose; rash; hives; or anaphylaxis.		Allergic asthma, hay fever, insect sting reactions, food allergies, anaphylaxis
II—Cytotoxic hypersensitivity	Incompatible blood	IgG or IgM antibodies bind with an antigen such as ABO or Rh. This triggers an autoimmune destruction of the target cell, causing a systemic reaction.		Blood transfusion reactions, hemolytic disease of the newborn
III—Immune hypersensitivity	Extracellular bacteria; viruses, mold	IgG or IgM antibody–antigen complexes form in the circulation and begin the inflammatory process.		Serum sickness, systemic lupus erythematosus, rheumatoid arthritis
IV—Delayed hypersensitivity	Chemicals or plants; skin tests with fungi or mycobacteria; foreign tissues	T lymphocytes interact with an antigen and activate the inflammatory response. Reactions may be delayed for 24–72 hours after exposure.		Contact dermatitis, tuberculin skin test; graft or tissue transplant reaction

BOX 11-2	NATURAL RUBBER LATEX PRODUCTS

Home
- Balloons, Band-Aids, rubber bands
- Condoms, diaphragms

Health Care Setting
- Ace bandages (brown); Jobst elastic stockings
- Gloves
- Blood pressure cuffs and tubing; stethoscopes
- Tourniquets; intravenous tubing; bulb syringes
- Urinary catheters; wound drains
- Rubber stoppers in medication vials
- Rubber dams used in dental work

removing, the cornstarch particles aerosolize when the gloves are removed. The cornstarch contains latex particles that can enter the body through the skin and mucous membranes or by inhalation. Also, chemicals used in manufacturing latex products may be irritating. Box 11-2■ lists common products of natural rubber latex.

Sensitivity to latex develops without the user being aware until a rash appears on the hands. Type IV response (contact dermatitis) results from an allergic reaction to the processing chemicals. Manifestations develop 24 to 48 hours later and include local redness and itching. Type IV hypersensitivity can progress to type I systemic response within minutes of exposure. Symptoms range from hives and itching to wheezing, dyspnea, laryngospasm, and cardiac arrest. Prevention of adverse reactions is essential. Ask patients about their allergy history, including food allergies. Some patients have a cross-sensitivity between latex allergy and certain foods such as avocados, bananas, kiwi, and pineapples. Instruct patients with known latex sensitivity to wear a MedicAlert bracelet. Hospitals should use latex-free carts for patients with identified latex allergies and select products free of latex. Health care workers with latex allergies should use nonlatex gloves when handling noninfectious material. Hand hygiene should be performed after using latex products to limit exposure (NIOSH, 2012).

COLLABORATIVE CARE

Key aspects of care for patients with allergies are to identify the allergen, minimize exposure, prevent the hypersensitivity response, and provide prompt interventions. A complete history of all of the patient's allergies is obtained, including medications, foods, animals, plants, and other materials. The type of hypersensitivity response is documented, as are onset, manifestations, and usual treatment. Several tests may be ordered:

- A *radioallergosorbent test (RAST)* measures the amount of IgE to specific allergens. This test is very expensive and is time consuming, but poses no risk for an anaphylactic reaction.
- *Skin tests* are used to identify specific allergens to which a person may be sensitive. Allergens used for testing are based on the patient's history. Test solutions are injected intradermally or by a prick or patch on the back or arms.
- The *prick test* may be done first to avoid a systemic reaction. A drop of allergenic solution is placed on the skin, and the skin is punctured through the drop. A positive test yields a wheal and redness within 15 to 20 minutes.
- An *intradermal test* involves a small amount of allergen being injected on the forearm or intrascapular area. If several allergens are being tested, injections are spaced 0.25 to 0.5 in. apart. As a control measure, plain diluent is injected opposite the test site. A positive test yields a wheal and redness within 15 to 20 minutes (see Figure 11-5).
- In a *patch test*, a 1-in. patch impregnated with the allergen, for example, cosmetics, perfume, or detergents, is applied to the skin for 48 hours. Positive responses range from mild redness to severe redness, papules, or vesicles.

Medications

Treatment focuses on avoiding the offending allergen, but sometimes medications provide symptomatic relief. Antihistamines, nasal and oral decongestants, and corticosteroids are usually ordered. Epinephrine is given during an acute anaphylactic reaction (see Chapter 14).

Antihistamines are the major class of drugs for treating symptoms of hypersensitivity responses. (Nursing care for the patient receiving antihistamines is outlined in Table 11-5■.)

Nasal decongestants such as oxymetazoline (Afrin) and oral decongestants such as pseudoephedrine (Sudafed) may relieve allergy symptoms. As of 2006 all medications containing pseudoephedrine must be kept in a locked box behind the pharmacy counter. Purchase does not require a prescription, but pharmacists must keep a log of sales. Overuse of Afrin may result in decreased effectiveness and rebound nasal congestion. Remind patients to see their health care provider if symptoms last longer than a week. Decongestants should be used for less than 5 days.

Glucocorticoids are used in both systemic and topical forms for many types of hypersensitivity responses. They have an anti-inflammatory effect. Short-term corticosteroid therapy is used for severe asthma, allergic contact dermatitis, and some immune-complex disorders. Corticosteroids in topical forms or delivered by inhaler may be used for longer periods of time with few side effects.

TABLE 11-5	Giving Medications Safely: Antihistamines		
CLASS/DRUGS	**PURPOSE**	**NURSING IMPLICATIONS**	**PATIENT TEACHING**
Antihistamines			
■ Diphenhydramine (Benadryl) ■ Chlorpheniramine (Chlor-Trimeton) ■ Hydroxyzine (Vistaril)	Antihistamines block H₁ histamine receptors to relieve allergic rhinitis and anaphylactic reactions such as urticaria and angioedema.	Give cautiously to older adults who are taking other medications. Monitor for side effects: excessive sedation, dizziness, or palpitations. Encourage a fluid intake of 2,500–3,000 mL/day unless contraindicated. Give Benadryl diagnostic tests that use contrast media as ordered.	If drowsiness occurs, do not drive or operate machinery while taking this medication. Do not drink alcohol. Use hard candy, gum, ice chips, or mouth rinses to relieve dryness. Stop the drug and notify the physician if excessive sedation, dizziness, or palpitations occur.

Another option is **desensitization**, a form of immunotherapy that involves injecting small doses of the allergen weekly. Over time, antibodies develop to block the allergic IgE response. This process can take years to accomplish symptomatic relief.

NURSING CARE

Nursing care is directed toward prevention of adverse effects and providing prompt, effective treatment. Prior to administering any medication, ask the patient's allergy history, including the allergic response and its treatment. If the patient experienced rash, hives, or difficulty breathing, check with the physician before giving the drug.

clinicalALERT

When a patient receives a new medication, observe closely. Even without any past allergic reaction, the patient is still at risk for anaphylaxis.

A second exposure increases the risk for a reaction and increases the severity of the reaction. While the patient is hospitalized, ask about allergies to latex, skin cleansers, and radiopaque dyes. When a suspected hypersensitivity reaction occurs, stop the intravenous medication or transfusion immediately.

With a type I hypersensitivity response, the first priority is managing the patient's airway. The patient with a type II hypersensitivity reaction may need aggressive treatment to control bleeding. A type III reaction is treated by removing the antigen and stopping the inflammatory response. Treatment of type IV reactions includes eliminating the antigen and giving anti-inflammatory drugs. Antihistamines may relieve the patient's discomfort. (See Chapter 14 for a discussion on the management of anaphylaxis and transfusion reactions.)

CONTINUITY OF CARE

Most hypersensitivity responses can be treated by the patient or family with little or no medical intervention. Teaching should include the following points:

■ Tell patients to inform health care personnel of all allergens.
■ Encourage patients to wear a MedicAlert bracelet or tag identifying allergies.
■ Discuss when to seek medical attention.
■ Instruct the patient and family members on when and how to use an anaphylaxis kit that contains epinephrine and antihistamines in injectable, oral, or inhaler forms.
■ Teach patients to use prescribed and over-the-counter medications as recommended.
■ For the patient with contact dermatitis, discuss appropriate skin care.

Resources: ALERT, Inc., Allergy to Latex Education and Resource Team.

Autoimmune Disorders

In *autoimmune disorders*, the immune system mistakes self for nonself, and the body reacts against its own cells. **Autoantibodies** (antibodies made against self-antigens) attack various body tissues, leading to tissue damage and chronic inflammation. Autoimmune disorders can affect any tissue, cell group, or organ. When the inflammatory process involves multiple organs, the patient is said to have a systemic autoimmune disorder. Selected autoimmune disorders are listed in Box 11-3■.

Certain families have a greater incidence of autoimmunity. Autoimmune disorders are more common in females and older adults. Patients may develop more than one autoimmune disorder. The onset of an autoimmune disorder is frequently associated with a severe physical or psychologic stressor.

BOX 11-3	AUTOIMMUNE DISORDERS

CELL OR ORGAN SPECIFIC	SYSTEMIC

Blood
Idiopathic thrombocytopenia
  purpura
	Rheumatoid arthritis
	Systemic lupus
	  erythematosus

Other Organs Thyrotoxicosis (Graves disease) Type 1 diabetes mellitus Addison disease Multiple sclerosis Myasthenia gravis Pernicious anemia Ulcerative colitis	

PATHOPHYSIOLOGY

It is unclear exactly how autoimmune disorders develop. Several theories have been proposed:

- Trauma, drugs, radiation, and infections alter body tissues so that the body no longer recognizes itself, and autoantibodies are produced.
- Bacteria such as group A beta-hemolytic *Streptococcus* may cross-react with the heart muscle, causing heart damage.
- Viruses may alter tissues that are not usually antigenic. This may be the cause of multiple sclerosis and type 1 diabetes mellitus.

Manifestations vary according to the tissues or organs affected. Most often, the patient shows signs and symptoms of the inflammatory process (pain, fatigue, and fever). Autoimmune disorders are characterized by periods of acute flare-ups followed by no symptoms. As these diseases progress, remission periods become less frequent.

COLLABORATIVE CARE

Diagnostic Tests

Diagnosis of an autoimmune disorder is usually based on the patient's clinical manifestations. Serum assays are helpful to identify increased levels of antibodies. Other laboratory and diagnostic tests more specific to the suspected disorder are ordered. Symptoms can be managed, but a cure is unlikely.

- *Antinuclear antibody (ANA)* test is used to screen for systemic lupus erythematosus (SLE). *Lupus erythematosus (LE) cell prep* is also used to detect SLE and monitor its treatment. Like the ANA, the LE cell prep is nonspecific for SLE. Positive results may be seen in rheumatoid arthritis or drug-induced lupus from penicillin, tetracycline, phenytoin, and oral contraceptives.
- *Rheumatoid factor (RF)* is an immunoglobulin present in the serum of approximately 80% of patients with rheumatoid arthritis.

Medications

Treatment of autoimmune disorders focuses on relieving symptoms. Because there is chronic inflammation, anti-inflammatory medications such as aspirin, nonsteroidal anti-inflammatory drugs (NSAIDs), COX-2 inhibitors, and corticosteroids may be prescribed (see the Chapters 9 and Chapter 35).

Disease-modifying antirheumatic drugs (DMARDs) such as methotrexate (Rheumatrex) and hydroxychloroquine (Plaquenil) are given to patients with rheumatoid arthritis. They are discussed further in Chapter 43. Immunosuppressive drugs such as azathioprine (Imuran) may be used along with plasmapheresis in treating some autoimmune disorders. Slow-acting anti-inflammatory drugs such as gold salts and penicillamine may be used when other treatments are ineffective. However, these drugs are relatively toxic and less frequently used.

NURSING CARE

Nursing care is individualized for the patient with an autoimmune disorder. Patients are taught stress reduction techniques, good nutrition, and medication uses and side effects. Most patients can be managed in outpatient settings. Interventions for the following nursing diagnoses should be included in the nursing care plan:

- *Activity Intolerance* related to inflammatory effects of autoimmune disorder
- *Acute Pain* and *Chronic Pain* related to inflammation
- *Ineffective Coping* related to chronic disease process
- *Disturbed Body Image* related to joint deformity, rashes, and altered body function
- *Ineffective Protection* related to immune disorder

CONTINUITY OF CARE

Because autoimmune disorders are chronic, the patient and family need to understand their long-term effects. They must learn about medications and possible side effects. During periods of remission, patients may not appear ill, and it may be difficult for the family to understand their needs. Often, these patients are at risk for unproven remedies and quackery. Nurses can provide psychologic support, listening, teaching, and referral to local support groups and state or national agencies, such as the American Autoimmune Related Diseases Association.

Organ/Tissue Transplantation

Transplantation has become fairly common. Skin, cornea, bone, and heart valve transplant are done more frequently and require less extensive tissue matching. Transplants of organs (e.g., kidney, heart, heart and lung, liver, pancreas, and bone marrow) are increasingly common. However, these surgeries cannot be considered lightly. Not only are they expensive in terms of the surgical procedure but also the patient must be able to afford the yearly cost of medications.

Organ and tissue transplantation is used when patients with cancer need healthy cells; for example, those with leukemia may need stem cells. It is also used when an organ is about to fail or has irreversible disease, or when part of the body is destroyed, as in transplantation of skin to a burn victim.

Transplantation success is closely tied to obtaining an organ with tissue antigens as close to those of the recipient as possible. Every body cell has HLA antigens that are unique to the individual. Even though identical twins may have the same HLA type, a few of their antigens may be unlike enough to cause rejection of transplantation. Matching the HLA type of the donor and recipient as closely as possible decreases, but does not eliminate, the potential for transplant rejection. Combining multiple organs for transplant such as liver–kidney seems to have less rejection.

PATHOPHYSIOLOGY

An **autograft** (transplantation of the patient's own tissue) is the most successful type of tissue transplantation. Skin grafts are the most common examples of autografts. Increasingly, **autologous** (self) bone marrow transplantation and blood transfusions are being used to reduce the immune response. When the donor and recipient are identical twins, the term *isograft* is used. These grafts are usually successful, with only mild rejection episodes.

Most often, an organ and tissue transplantation is an **allograft** (graft between members of the same species). Because of the growing number of transplantation candidates, allografts from living donors are needed to fill the shortage of organs. Living donors do not have to be blood relatives. Whole or partial organs are donated (one kidney, the lobe of the liver or lung, and part of the pancreas tail). Bone marrow transplantation (BMT) is exclusively from a living donor.

Organs are obtained most often from cadavers. Donors must meet the criteria for brain death; are less than 65 years old; and are free from diabetes, hypertension, cancer, HIV, hepatitis B, and hepatitis C. The organ is removed immediately before or after cardiac arrest and is preserved until transplanted into the waiting recipient. Organ donation is coordinated by the United Network for Organ Donation, a federally funded organization (see also Chapter 14).

A *xenograft* (transplantation from an animal species to a human) is the least successful type of transplantation and is seldom used. The one exception is the use of pig skin as a temporary covering for a massive burn.

Tissue typing determines the **histocompatibility** (the ability of cells and tissues to survive transplantation without rejection). Tissue typing identifies HLA type and blood types (ABO, Rh) of the donor and recipient, as well as any preformed antibodies to the donor's HLA antigens.

Transplant rejection is stimulated by antibody-mediated and cell-mediated immune responses. It typically begins 24 hours after the transplantation procedure, although it may develop immediately. Rejection episodes are characterized as follows (Table 11-6■):

1. *Hyperacute rejection:* The grafted organ initially appears pink and healthy, but then turns soft and white and is usually lost.
2. *Acute rejection:* The patient shows signs of inflammation such as fever, redness, tenderness, and swelling over the graft site. Manifestations are related to the specific organ, for example, elevated blood urea nitrogen

TABLE 11-6	Transplant Rejection Episodes		
TYPE	**CAUSE**	**PRESENTATION**	**TREATMENT**
Hyperacute	Preexisting antibodies immediately react against donor ABO and HLA antigens	Occurs within minutes to hours or days of the transplantation / Rapid deterioration of organ function	Transplant cannot usually be saved. Prevent with cross-match and use antimetabolite and anti-inflammatory drugs before surgery.
Acute	Antigens on the donor organ (usually from a cadaver) trigger the release of cytotoxic T cells that attack the foreign organ	Occurs within days to months after the transplantation / Signs of inflammation and impaired organ function	Most common and treatable type of rejection. Increase immunosuppression using steroids, cyclosporine, monoclonal antibodies, or antilymphocyte globulins.
Chronic	Probably antibody-mediated response; may involve inflammatory damage to vessel endothelium	Occurs 4 months to years after the transplantation / Gradual deterioration of organ function	None. Loss of graft will occur, requiring retransplantation.

(BUN) and creatinine; liver enzyme and bilirubin elevations; or elevated cardiac enzymes and signs of heart failure.

3. *Chronic rejection:* This results from antibodies and complement being deposited in the transplant vessel walls. Narrowing of the vessels causes decreased blood flow and ischemia. The organ eventually fails.

Graft-versus-host disease (GVHD) is a frequent and potentially fatal complication of bone marrow transplant and some liver transplants. When there is no close match between donor and recipient HLA antigen, immunocompetent cells in the grafted tissue attack other body tissues, especially the skin, liver, and intestine. Acute GVHD occurs within the first 100 days after transplantation. A maculopapular rash begins on the palms of the hands and soles of the feet. The rash may spread over the entire body, eventually causing the epidermis to shed. Intestinal symptoms are abdominal pain, nausea, and bloody diarrhea. Chronic GVHD has a poor prognosis.

COLLABORATIVE CARE

Pre- and post-transplantation care focuses on reducing the risk of tissue rejection. Laboratory tests are used to identify a suitable donor and to monitor the immune response to the transplant. Immunosuppressive medications are often the key to successful organ transplantation.

Diagnostic Tests

Basic diagnostic tests are done before surgery (complete blood count [CBC] and differential, urinalysis, chemistry panel, coagulation studies, arterial blood gases, an electrocardiogram, and chest x-ray). Other laboratory studies are ordered specifically before organ or tissue transplantation:

- *Blood type* and *Rh factor* of both the donor and the recipient must match.
- *Cross-matching* of the patient's serum against the donor's lymphocytes to identify preformed antibodies against antigens on donor tissues.
- *HLA histocompatibility testing* to identify donors with an HLA type close to that of the recipient.
- *Mixed lymphocyte culture (MLC) assay tests* to determine histocompatibility between the donor and the recipient.
- *Ultrasonography* or *magnetic resonance imaging (MRI)* of the transplanted organ to evaluate its size, perfusion, and function.
- *Tissue biopsies* of the transplanted organ are done routinely to assess for evidence of tissue rejection.

Medications

Preoperatively, antibiotic and antiviral drugs may be prescribed, such as trimethoprim–sulfamethoxazole (Septra, Bactrim), acyclovir (Zovirax), and ganciclovir (Cytovene).

Postoperatively, a combination of immunosuppressive drugs is given to prevent tissue rejection. Drug selection is based on the transplanted tissue or organ and the preference of the medical center.

Corticosteroids, prednisone (Deltasone), and methylprednisolone (Solu-Medrol) reduce the inflammatory response and decrease the production of T-helper cells and cytotoxic cells. Although beneficial, corticosteroids have numerous side effects: poor wound healing, fluid retention, hypertension, gastrointestinal (GI) distress, increased sodium and glucose levels, and muscle weakness. (See Chapter 35.)

Cytotoxic agents such as azathioprine (Imuran) and cyclosporine (Sandimmune) have been used as immunosuppressants for more than 30 years. *Monoclonal antibodies* and *antilymphocyte globulins* are newer agents. (Nursing responsibilities and patient teaching for immunosuppressive agents are outlined in Table 11-7 ■.)

NURSING CARE

The patient who has undergone an organ or tissue transplantation procedure has immediate and long-term nursing care needs. Immediately after transplantation, the patient is transferred to the critical care or transplant unit and is monitored closely. Both the physical and psychosocial needs of the patient and family must be considered. Priority nursing diagnoses include Ineffective Protection, Risk for Impaired Tissue Integrity: Allograft, and Anxiety.

Ineffective Protection

Expected outcome: Will remain free of any infection.

- Monitor vital signs and temperature every 4 hours. Assess for signs of inflammation, abnormal wound drainage, changes in urine or body secretions, complaints of pain, or behavior changes that may indicate infection. Culture abnormal wound drainage. *Incisions, invasive lines and tubes, nutritional deficits, immunosuppressive drugs, and chronic disease all increase the potential for infection. The patient on immunosuppressive therapy is more susceptible to infection, but the usual signs and symptoms may be absent. To prevent life-threatening complications, assess the patient constantly and start appropriate interventions immediately.*
- Wash hands and use hand sanitizer on entering the room and before providing direct care. *Hand hygiene provides first-line defense against infection and cross-contamination.*

clinicalALERT

Use strict aseptic technique in changing dressings and caring for invasive catheters, such as intravenous lines and indwelling urinary catheters, to reduce the risk of transferring microorganisms to the patient.

TABLE 11-7	Giving Medications Safely: Immunosuppressive Agents		
CLASS/DRUGS	**PURPOSE**	**NURSING IMPLICATIONS**	**PATIENT TEACHING**
Cytotoxic agents ■ Azathioprine (Imuran) ■ Cyclophosphamide (Cytoxan) ■ Cyclosporine (Sandimmune) ■ *Methotrexate* (Rheumatrex) ■ *Mycophenolate* (CellCept) ■ *Tacrolimus* (Prograf)	Cytotoxic agents are used to prevent tissue or organ rejection reactions.	Use meticulous hand hygiene. Notify the physician if WBCs fall below 4,000 or platelets below 75,000. Monitor BUN, creatinine, and liver enzymes. Increase fluids to maintain output. Monitor for bleeding gums, bruising, petechiae, or tarry stools.	Follow directions for taking the medications. Avoid large crowds and people with infections. Report signs of infection, any bleeding, reduced urine output, and jaundice. Do not take aspirin or ibuprofen. Use contraception to prevent pregnancy; drugs could harm the fetus.
Monoclonal antibody ■ Muromonab-CD3 or (Orthoclone-OKT3) ■ Basiliximab (Simulect) ■ Rituximab (Rituxan) ■ Daclizumab (Zenapax)	A mouse is injected with an antigen that produces a specific monoclonal antibody. The antibody is harvested from the mouse and given by IV route to prevent organ transplant rejection.	Obtain chest x-ray 24 hours before therapy starts. Premedicate the patient as ordered to reduce potential side effects. Monitor closely for infusion reaction of chills, fever, rash, dyspnea, wheezing, or hypotension.	Discuss potential side effects and the need to report symptoms promptly. Explain that side effects may occur during the first two doses, requiring close observation at that time.
Antilymphocyte globulins ■ Antilymphocyte globulin (ALG) ■ Antithymocyte globulin (ATG)	These drugs are given to horses or rabbits to produce antibodies. They are removed from the animal, refined, and given IV to the patient. They are used after an organ transplantation to cause immunosuppression.	Before the initial dose, perform skin test to test for allergy to horse serum. Premedicate as ordered. Monitor for anaphylaxis during the infusion. Monitor patient's WBC and platelet count daily.	Explain the need for special precautions and close monitoring during the IV infusion. Report any side effects to the nurse immediately.

Note: Medications identified in *italics* are among the 200 most frequently prescribed drugs in the United States.

■ Monitor CBC, especially WBC differential; report changes to the physician. *An elevated WBC count with a shift to the left may be an early indication of infection.* (See Chapter 9.)
■ Initiate protective isolation precautions as indicated by facility policy and the patient's immune status. Screen staff, family, and visitors for signs of infection. *These procedures further protect the severely immunocompromised patient from infection.*
■ Encourage deep breathing and coughing. *This mobilizes respiratory secretions and reduces the potential for atelectasis and pneumonia.*
■ Provide adequate nutrition with supplementary feedings or parenteral nutrition if necessary. *Adequate nutrition is important for healing and immune system function.*
■ Provide frequent mouth care. *Meticulous mouth care reduces oral microorganisms and helps maintain an intact mucous membrane lining.*

■ Change intravenous bags and tubing at least every 24 hours and change peripheral intravenous sites every 48 to 72 hours, unless contraindicated. Remove invasive catheters and lines as soon as possible. *Changing lines and sites helps reduce bacterial contamination. Fewer invasive lines mean fewer sites for bacterial invasion.*
■ Monitor for potential adverse effects of medication:
  ■ Bleeding due to thrombocytopenia
  ■ Fluid retention with edema and possible hypertension
  ■ Decreased urine output from renal toxicity
  ■ Jaundice from hepatic toxicity
  ■ Bone or joint pain

Medications used to maintain immunosuppression and to preserve the allograft have many potential adverse effects that can alter normal protective and homeostatic mechanisms.

Risk for Impaired Tissue Integrity: Allograft

Expected outcome: Will not experience any organ/tissue rejection episodes.

- Administer immunosuppressive therapy as ordered. *Agents that suppress the immune response reduce transplant rejection.*
- Assess for signs of graft rejection: tenderness, redness, and swelling over the site; sudden weight gain, edema, and hypertension; chills and fever; malaise; and an increased WBC count and sedimentation rate. Report any changes immediately. *The risk for transplant rejection is highest in the initial postoperative period, but it is never completely eliminated. Early identification allows adjustment of medication regimens and may preserve the graft.*
- Monitor tests of organ function. Report changes to the physician. *A decline in the function of the transplanted organ (e.g., increasing BUN and creatinine in the renal transplant recipient) may be an early indication of transplant rejection.*
- Assess for and report signs of GVHD immediately. Look for maculopapular rash, erythema of the skin and possible desquamation, hair loss, abdominal cramping and diarrhea, and jaundice with elevated bilirubin and liver enzymes (aspartate transaminase [AST], alanine transaminase [ALT]). *GVHD is a potentially lethal complication and requires immediate intervention.*
- Stress the importance of maintaining immunosuppressive therapy and of reporting signs of graft rejection promptly. *The risk for transplant rejection is never completely eliminated.*

Anxiety

Expected outcome: Will verbalize needs, fears, and concerns.

- Assess the level of anxiety by noting restlessness, tension, apprehension, fear, facial expression, and poor eye contact. *Patients may have difficulty talking about their fears and anxieties about organ rejection. When the transplant comes from a living donor, patients may also worry about the condition of the donor. Nonverbal cues help to identify anxiety.*
- Use opening statements such as "Facing an organ transplant must be very stressful." Listen attentively. *Encouragement and active listening help identify issues that can lead to problem solving.*
- Arrange tasks to allow as much time with the patient as possible. When leaving, tell the patient when you will return. Encourage family members to remain with the patient as much as possible. *Time the nurse spends with the patient promotes trust. The presence of family helps reduce anxiety.*
- Provide clear, concise information and directions. *Highly anxious patients have difficulty focusing and retaining information.*
- Encourage the use of coping behaviors that were useful in the past. If necessary, consult with a mental health

specialist. Encourage the patient and family to meet other transplant recipients. *Past coping mechanisms may work again. A specialist can help the patient deal with feelings. Hearing about the success and problems of others can reduce anxiety.*

CONTINUITY OF CARE

Thorough patient and family education is necessary before the transplantation and should continue throughout hospitalization and follow-up treatment. Transplant coordinators are nurses specializing in the transplant process and are excellent resources for patients, families, and nursing staff.

After the transplantation, provide verbal and written instructions about the following points:

- Signs and symptoms of transplant rejection and the importance of notifying the physician
- How to monitor temperature, blood pressure, pulse, and weight
- Immunosuppressive drug therapy regimen and side effects, interactions with other medications, and appropriate OTC drugs; include management techniques for minor side effects; indicate which side effects should be reported to the physician
- Avoiding exposure to infectious diseases, especially URI, influenza, or pneumonia, and wearing a mask when going outside
- Meticulous personal hygiene, hand hygiene technique, and frequent oral hygiene
- Wound care
- Wearing a MedicAlert bracelet or tag
- Follow-up visits to the physician or clinic
- Helpful resources:
  - American Council of Transplantation
  - Local and state support groups related to specific organ transplant, for example, National Kidney Foundation

Impaired Immune Responses and the Patient With HIV Infection

Key Concept Impaired immune function, whether congenital or acquired, threatens health and well being because the patient cannot effectively respond to threats such as infection. Nurses play a key role in teaching not only how to prevent HIV infection but also how to manage the disease in those affected.

When function of either the B cells or T cells is impaired, the result is an immunodeficiency disorder. Immunodeficiency disorders can be inherited, acquired through infection, or produced unintentionally by immunosuppressive drugs.

Primary immunodeficiency is a rare congenital disorder that is usually found in infants and young children. In addition to a higher risk for infection, these children have more autoimmune diseases and cancer.

Secondary immunodeficiency is acquired and results in impaired immune function. One or more factors can cause immunodeficiency: stress, malnutrition, trauma, age, viral infections, cancer, or drugs. Infection with HIV may lead to **acquired immunodeficiency syndrome (AIDS)**, the final, fatal stage of HIV infection and the most well-known secondary immunodeficiency.

AIDS was first identified in 1981 among homosexual males in Los Angeles and New York who had developed an unusual opportunistic infection. By 1982, the Centers for Disease Control (CDC) acknowledged the presence of a new infection involving immune system deficits and associated opportunistic disorders. In 1985, the **human immunodeficiency virus (HIV)** was isolated as the cause of AIDS.

By 2010, the CDC estimated that 1.2 million people in the United States were living with HIV infection, with 20% of them unaware of their HIV status. An estimated 33,000 new HIV infections develop each year in the United States. By 2009, the death rate decreased by 35%, in part due to improved treatment rather than a decrease in the spread of the disease. AIDS is the leading cause of death among African American males ages 25 to 44. Women account for 23% of the AIDS cases, with more than 66% infected through heterosexual contact, and the others were exposed through injection drug use (McPhee, Papadakis, & Rabow, 2012). Other AIDS statistics are found in Table 11-8■, and its incidence in older adults is discussed in Box 11-4■.

In 2011, approximately 34.2 million adults and 2.5 million children under the age of 15 were living with HIV/AIDS worldwide and in nearly every country (UNAIDS, 2012). The highest incidence is in sub-Saharan Africa, Asia, and the Pacific. New cases of HIV/AIDS continue to increase in North Africa, the Middle East, Eastern Europe, and central Asia. By 2011, through a concentrated effort in the developing countries, more than 5 million people were receiving HIV therapy, but this only represents a third of the people who still need HIV therapy (UNAIDS, 2012).

There are three main routes of transmission: (1) direct person to person through sexual contact; (2) direct injection with contaminated blood, blood products, or needles; and (3) mother to fetus. HIV is transmitted through blood, semen, vaginal secretions, the placenta, and breast milk. It can also be found in saliva, but no known cases have been transmitted by saliva.

TABLE 11-8	Persons Living With AIDS at the End of 2009 by Race/Ethnicity, Sex, and Transmission Category		
TRANSMISSION	**WHITE (%)**	**BLACK (%)**	**HISPANIC (%)**
Male adult or adolescent			
Male to male sexual contact	48	30	19
Injection drug user	20	51	27
Heterosexual contact	14	66	18
Female adult or adolescent			
Injection drug user	25	54	17
Heterosexual contact	18	63	17
Child (less than 13 years at diagnosis)			
Perinatal	13	63	22

Source: U.S. Centers for Disease Control and Prevention (2012a).

BOX 11-4	FOCUS ON OLDER ADULTS

The Older Adult With HIV/AIDS

Approximately 29% of persons living with HIV/AIDS in the United States are over age 50. Survival of persons infected earlier in life accounts for a significant portion of these adults. Decline in immune system function in older adults increases their risk for contracting HIV/AIDS. Many older adults mistakenly believe that they cannot be infected with HIV, but they can contract it through heterosexual and homosexual activities. Because older adults are beyond childbearing years, they often fail to use condoms or practice safe sex. Common manifestations such as fatigue, weight loss, and altered memory are overlooked and associated with normal age-related health problems, causing a delayed diagnosis and increased severity of the disease.

Certain behaviors increase the risk for contracting HIV. The most common behavior is intercourse with an infected partner. Sexual relations by anal, oral, or vaginal routes without the use of a condom are the major risk factor. Sharing of needles and other drug paraphernalia is the second leading risk factor for IV drug users. Multiple sexual partners, heterosexual intercourse with an infected drug user, and exchanging sex for drugs or money are major risk factors for women. Hemophiliacs who received intravenous clotting factors and people infected through blood transfusion represent less than 2% of the cases.

Among the general population of the United States, HIV infection is very low. HIV is not transmitted by casual contact such as sneezing, coughing, handshaking, hugging, dry kissing, or sharing eating utensils or linens. There is no evidence that it can be transmitted by mosquitoes. Blood donation also poses no risk, because only new, sterile equipment is used.

A small but real occupational risk exists for health care workers. The main exposure routes are needle-stick injuries or nonintact skin and mucous membranes. A needle-stick injury poses a 0.3% risk of becoming HIV positive. Mucosal exposures, such as splashing in the eyes or mouth, pose a much smaller risk.

PATHOPHYSIOLOGY

HIV is a retrovirus, which means it reproduces in a "backward" manner. Instead of reproducing from deoxyribonucleic acid (DNA) to ribonucleic acid (RNA), it uses RNA to make DNA copies. After the virus enters the bloodstream, it attaches to CD4+ T4 helper lymphocytes. CD4 is a receptor antigen on the T4 helper surface.

Once inside the CD4+ cell, the virus sheds its protein coat and releases an enzyme called *reverse transcriptase* to convert the RNA to DNA (Figure 11-6■). Then the viral DNA inserts itself into the host cell DNA and duplicates

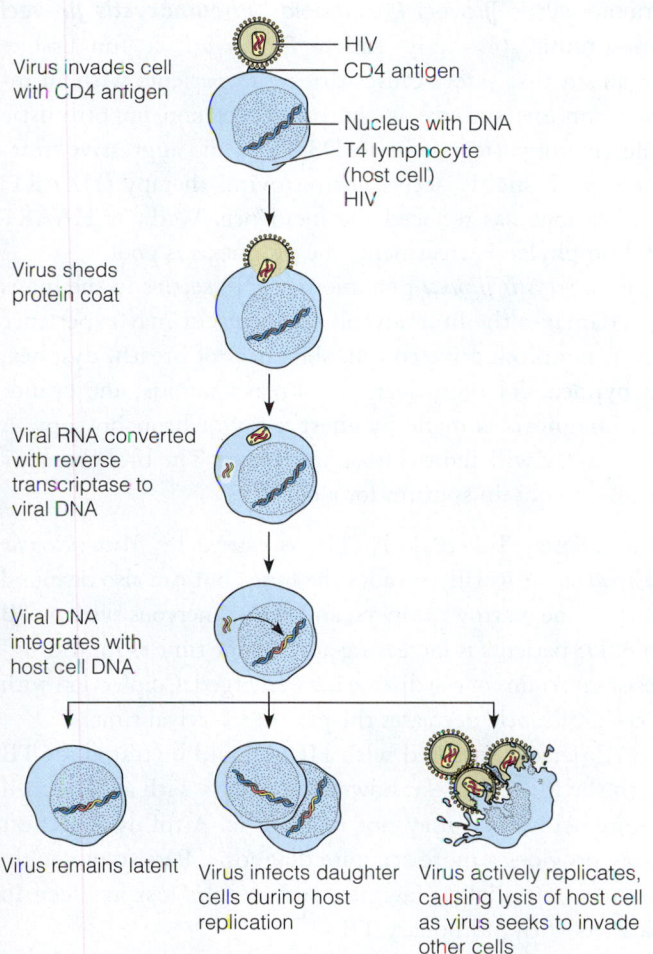

Virus invades cell with CD4 antigen
- HIV
- CD4 antigen
- Nucleus with DNA
- T4 lymphocyte (host cell)
- HIV

Virus sheds protein coat

Viral RNA converted with reverse transcriptase to viral DNA

Viral DNA integrates with host cell DNA

Virus remains latent

Virus infects daughter cells during host replication

Virus actively replicates, causing lysis of host cell as virus seeks to invade other cells

Figure 11-6. ■ The process of HIV infection and CD4 cell destruction.

during normal cell division. At this point, the virus may remain latent or produce new RNA with the assistance of an enzyme called *protease* to form very small virus particles (buds). These buds have the ability to move to other CD4+ cells, where they disrupt and eventually destroy the host cell. Billions of HIV buds are produced and destroyed each day along with CD4+ cells. The loss of helper T cells leads to the immunodeficiencies seen with HIV infection. The infection eventually overwhelms the body's immune system (Figure 11-7■).

The virus may remain inactive in infected cells for years. During this stage, B-cell antibodies are produced in a process known as **seroconversion**. These antibodies can be detected 6 weeks to 6 months after the initial infection.

A diagnosis of HIV infection is based on the patient's history and risk factors, physical examination, laboratory studies, and manifestations. HIV infection and AIDS in adolescents and adults are classified according to the CDC system. This system uses CD4+ T-cell counts and clinical manifestations to diagnose a patient.

Manifestations

Clinical manifestations of HIV infection range from no symptoms to severe immunodeficiency with multiple opportunistic infections and cancers in the late stages (Box 11-5■). Most patients develop an acute mononucleosis-type illness within days to weeks after contracting the virus.

After the primary infection, patients enter a long-lasting asymptomatic period (about 10 years). The virus can be

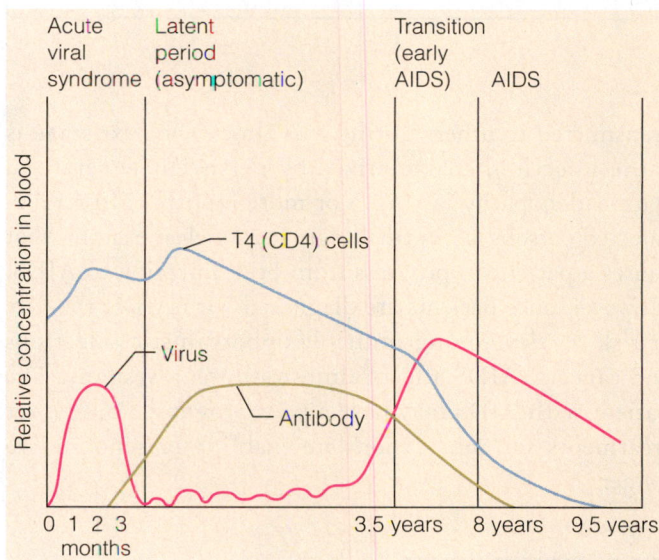

Acute viral syndrome | Latent period (asymptomatic) | Transition (early AIDS) | AIDS

Relative concentration in blood

- T4 (CD4) cells
- Virus
- Antibody

0 1 2 3 months   3.5 years   8 years   9.5 years

Figure 11-7. ■ The progression of HIV infection. The primary infection begins shortly after contracting the virus, corresponding with a rapid increase in viral levels. Antibodies are formed and remain throughout the infection. Late in the disease, viral activity increases, destroying CD4 (T4) cells. Antibody levels gradually decrease as immune function is impaired.

BOX 11-5	MANIFESTATIONS OF HIV INFECTION

1. Acute retroviral syndrome or primary HIV infection
   - Fever, sore throat, general malaise, rash
   - Arthralgias, myalgias, headache
   - Nausea, vomiting, abdominal cramping, diarrhea
   - Night sweats
2. Asymptomatic infection
   - Usually asymptomatic but may develop persistent generalized lymphadenopathy
   - Converts to seropositive status
3. AIDS: HIV-associated neoplasms and opportunistic infections

   A. AIDS dementia complex

   B. Opportunistic infectious diseases
   - *Pneumocystis jiroveci (carinii)* pneumonia
   - *Mycobacterium tuberculosis*
   - *Mycobacterium avium* complex
   - Candidiasis
   - Cryptosporidiosis
   - Wasting syndrome
   - Cryptococcosis
   - Toxoplasmosis
   - Herpes simplex or herpes zoster
   - Cytomegalovirus (CMV)

   C. Secondary cancers
   - Kaposi sarcoma
   - Non-Hodgkin lymphoma
   - Cervical dysplasia and cervical cancer

   D. Other conditions
   - Pelvic inflammatory disease
   - Human papillomavirus

transmitted to others during this time. The next stage is acute infection, characterized by persistent generalized lymphadenopathy lasting 3 or more months. Most HIV-infected persons are in this stage. It is unclear exactly what causes a patient to progress from HIV infection to AIDS. However, once patients are diagnosed with AIDS, they are at risk for developing multiple opportunistic infections and cancers. AIDS affects almost all organ systems. The patient with AIDS may have a poor prognosis, but newer treatments and medications are enabling patients to live longer.

memoryALERT

If HIV testing is done during the "window period" (2 to 4 weeks after exposure), the patient may have a false-negative reading. Retesting should be done 6 to 12 weeks after initial HIV exposure to confirm the initial test results.

AIDS Dementia Complex

AIDS dementia complex is caused by HIV acting directly on the brain. It results in the progressive deterioration of cognitive, motor, and behavioral functioning. Typical manifestations include forgetfulness, difficulty concentrating, confusion, leg weakness, and clumsiness. Patients lose interest in personal hygiene, work, and social activities. In the later stages, the patient may develop tremors, ataxia, incontinence, and paraplegia.

Opportunistic Infections

Opportunistic infections are the most common manifestation of AIDS and often develop simultaneously. The risk for opportunistic infections is predictable by the person's CD4 T-cell count. The normal CD4+ T-cell count is 800 to 1,200 mm^3. When the CD4+ count is less than 500 mm^3, manifestations of immunodeficiency are seen. Opportunistic infections are more likely when the CD4+ count falls below 200 and mostly affect the respiratory, gastrointestinal, and neurologic systems.

RESPIRATORY SYSTEM

Pneumocystis jiroveci Pneumonia **Pneumocystis jiroveci pneumonia** (formerly called *P. carinii*, a fungus-like organism that rarely causes disease in patients with an intact immune system) is the most common opportunistic infection in patients with AIDS. Early and aggressive treatment with highly active antiretroviral therapy (HAART) medications has reduced the incidence. Without HAART and prophylactic treatment, the prognosis is poor.

Pneumocystis jiroveci pneumonia (PJP) settles in the lungs and damages the lung alveoli. The patient may experience fever, nonproductive cough, shortness of breath, dyspnea, tachypnea, crackles, decreased breath sounds, and cyanosis. Diagnosis is made by chest x-ray or bronchoscopy. A chest x-ray will show diffuse infiltrates. The bronchoscopy is used to obtain sputum for a culture.

Tuberculosis   Tuberculosis (TB) is caused by *Mycobacterium tuberculosis*. It usually invades the lungs but can also be found in the bone marrow, kidneys, and central nervous system. TB in AIDS patients is increasing at the same time as multidrug-resistant strains of the disease have emerged. Coinfection with TB significantly decreases the patient's survival time.

All persons infected with HIV should be tested for TB with the Mantoux test; however, patients with a CD4+ cell count below 200 may not react to it. A follow-up chest x-ray provides a more accurate diagnosis. Persistent cough, night sweats, fever, fatigue, and weight loss are seen in patients with pulmonary TB.

Mycobacterium avium Complex   *Mycobacterium avium* complex (MAC) is caused by a bacterial organism found in the food, water, and soil. MAC affects nearly every organ but most often affects the lungs. It has a high mortality rate and occurs late in the disease. The most common manifestations are a high fever and weight loss. The organism is cultured from the blood, liver, lymph nodes, or bone marrow.

GASTROINTESTINAL SYSTEM

Candidiasis   Oral candidiasis or *thrush* (a fungal infection caused by *C. albicans*) occurs in most patients with AIDS. It is characterized by white patches in the mouth that may extend to the esophagus and stomach. Patients may complain of mouth soreness and an unpleasant taste. Esophagitis may lead to painful swallowing, an inability to eat, and malnutrition. In women, vaginal candidiasis is frequent and often recurs.

Cryptosporidiosis   The protozoan *Cryptosporidium* is normally found in birds, fish, reptiles, and humans. Transmission occurs from ingesting contaminated water or food or from human-to-human contact. The organism settles in the small intestine. AIDS patients experience large watery, non-bloody diarrhea that often causes dehydration, electrolyte imbalances, and malnutrition. Diagnosis is made by sending a stool sample for ova and parasites.

Wasting Syndrome   In the later stages of AIDS, most patients develop wasting syndrome. This is described as an unplanned weight loss of 10% along with chronic diarrhea or an unexplained fever. Fatigue, nausea, vomiting, and oral lesions lead to poor food intake, and chronic diarrhea results in malabsorption of nutrients. The patient appears emaciated (Figure 11-8■).

NEUROLOGIC SYSTEM   Toxoplasmosis and cryptococcosis are parasitic infections with *Toxoplasma gondii* and *Cryptococcus neoformans*. Toxoplasmosis can cause encephalitis. Cryptococcosis settles in the lungs but can travel to the brain or meninges, causing meningitis. Symptoms for both conditions include headache, fever, stiff neck, altered mental status, and seizures.

Other Infections

Herpes simplex 1 and 2 frequently develop in patients with AIDS. Type 1 infections involve the oral cavity, whereas type 2 infections develop in the genital and anal regions. Large groups of painful lesions form in the affected areas. When the lesions rupture, the virus is easily transmitted to other parts of the body and to caregivers.

Cytomegalovirus (CMV) is part of the herpes virus family. It can affect the retina, the gastrointestinal tract, or lungs. CMV is the primary cause of blindness in patients with AIDS.

Women with AIDS have a high incidence of pelvic inflammatory disease (PID). They seem to contract the **human papillomavirus** (virus causing genital warts), which increases their risk for cervical *dysplasia* (abnormal tissue development) and cancer. Women with HIV infection and cervical cancer usually die of the cervical cancer, not AIDS. For this reason, women with HIV infection should have a Papanicolaou smear every 6 months and aggressive treatment of cervical dysplasia.

Secondary Cancers

KAPOSI SARCOMA   Kaposi sarcoma (KS) is the most common cancer associated with HIV infection. However, with the use of HAART, the KS occurs less than 1% in patients with HIV. Tumors develop in the lining of small blood vessels, causing reddish-purple lesions on the skin and mucous membranes (see Figure 11-8). Initially, the lesions are painless, but they may become painful as the disease progresses. Tumors within body organs can disrupt function or cause bleeding. Diagnosis is made by tissue biopsy.

LYMPHOMAS   Lymphomas are malignancies of the lymphocytes, lymph nodes, spleen, and bone marrow. AIDS patients develop either non-Hodgkin lymphoma or primary lymphoma of the brain. Symptoms may be vague or reflect brain involvement, such as headache and changes in mental status.

COLLABORATIVE CARE

Although new treatments are continually being investigated, research has not yet found a cure for HIV infection and AIDS. Because an AIDS diagnosis eventually means death, preventive strategies are most important. Patients at risk for HIV infection need help in identifying their HIV status. Once a positive diagnosis is made, they should be taught how to maintain their health and prevent opportunistic infections. Health care workers and support persons play a key role in providing emotional and psychosocial support.

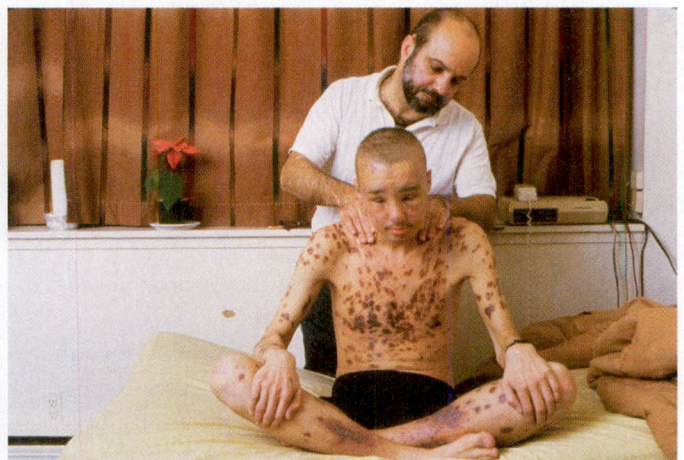

Figure 11-8. ■ A patient with wasting syndrome and Kaposi sarcoma. (Source: Dr. M.A. Ansary/Photo Researchers, Inc.)

Prevention

Vaccines against HIV infection are being investigated, but to date, none have been successfully developed. Education, counseling, and behavior modification are the key elements for HIV prevention.

The nurse first focuses on sex education. All sexually active individuals need to know how HIV is spread. The only totally safe sex practices are (1) no sex, (2) long-term monogamous sexual relations between two uninfected people, and (3) mutual masturbation without direct contact. Patients who engage in sexual activity must understand and practice safer sex (Box 11-6■).

It is often difficult to find and educate injection drug users. People in this group should never share needles, syringes, or other drug paraphernalia. Needle-exchange programs provide a sterile needle and syringe in exchange for a used one. A fresh solution of household bleach and water in a 1:10 ratio is effective to clean injection paraphernalia when sterile supplies are unavailable. This population also should be taught safe sex practices. Most heterosexual HIV transmission occurs between injection drug users and their partners.

Screening of voluntary blood donors and donated blood supplies has reduced the risk of transmission by transfusion. However, it is possible for HIV to be transmitted during the time between contracting the virus and developing detectable antibodies (the *window period*). The window period usually lasts from 6 weeks to 6 months. For this reason, it is important for persons to donate their own blood before an anticipated surgery.

HEALTH CARE EXPOSURE AND PROPHYLAXIS   Health care workers can prevent most exposures to HIV by using Standard Precautions. With Standard Precautions, all body fluids are treated as if they are infectious, and barrier precautions are used to prevent skin, mucous membrane, or percutaneous exposure to them.

Any health care worker who is exposed to blood or receives a needle-stick injury should wash the exposure site with soap and water, or (if mucous membranes) flush with water, and then report it immediately to an employee health department. Treatment must be started *within 1 to 2 hours* after exposure and be continued for 4 weeks. The CDC recommends postexposure prophylaxis with combination therapy such as zidovudine (AZT) and lamivudine (Epivir) after a needle-stick injury from an HIV-positive patient. The exposed person should be tested at regular intervals for a year and receive appropriate counseling. Research confirms that follow-up treatment can reduce the rate of infection.

Diagnostic Tests

- *Rapid HIV antibody test* includes six screening tests that provide HIV results in 20 minutes by obtaining a blood sample from a finger stick. Positive results must be confirmed by the ELISA and Western blot assay.
- *Enzyme-linked immunosorbent assay (ELISA)* is the most widely used screening test to determine the presence of HIV antibodies (not the presence of the virus itself). The patient must give informed consent before the test is performed. An infected patient may test negative during the window period. If the test is positive, a second test is done to confirm it. When the second test is positive, the Western blot assay is done.
- *Western blot assay* is a reliable test that is used to confirm that the patient is HIV seropositive.
- *HIV viral load tests* measure the amount of HIV viral activity. Viral loads are used to monitor disease progression and response to antiretroviral medications. Levels greater than 5,000 to 10,000 copies/mL indicate the need for treatment.

BOX 11-6   GUIDELINES FOR SAFER SEX

- Limit the number of sexual partners, preferably to one.
- Do not engage in unprotected sex, especially if HIV status of the partner is unknown.
- When entering into a new monogamous relationship, both partners should undergo HIV testing initially. If both are negative, practice abstinence or safer sex for 6 months, followed by retesting.
- Use only latex condoms for oral, vaginal, or anal intercourse with a water-soluble lubricant.
- Store condoms in a cool, dry place and prevent damage to condom.
- Apply and remove condom properly; do not reuse condoms.
- Do not swallow urine or semen.
- Women should carry and use a female condom.
- Remember that oral contraceptives provide no protection against HIV.
- Engage in safer sexual practices that are less damaging to sensitive tissues (e.g., mutual masturbation, avoiding anal or oral sex).
- Do not share needles, razors, toothbrushes, sexual toys, or other items that may be contaminated with blood or body fluids.
- If HIV positive:
  a. Do not engage in unprotected sexual activity.
  b. Inform all current and former sexual partners as well as health care personnel—primary care providers, physicians, and dentists, in particular—of HIV status.
  c. Do not donate blood, plasma, blood products, sperm, organs, or tissue.
  d. If female, do not become pregnant.

- *CD4+ cell count* is used to confirm progression from HIV infection to AIDS. The normal range for the CD4+ count is 800 to 1,200 mm^3. AIDS is defined not only by the presence of opportunistic infections but also by a CD4+ count of less than 200/mm^3 or a percentage of CD4 lymphocytes of less than 14%. CD4 counts are recommended every 3 to 6 months for all people with HIV disease.
- *CBC* detects anemia, leukopenia, and thrombocytopenia, which are often present in HIV infection.

Tests may be ordered to diagnose secondary cancers and opportunistic infections. *Tuberculin skin testing* can identify TB infection. *Magnetic resonance imaging* and a *computed tomography (CT) scan* of the brain can identify lymphomas and other opportunistic infections. *Cultures* of urine, blood, stool, spinal fluid, and sputum identify PJP, toxoplasmosis, cryptosporidiosis, and cryptococcosis.

Medications

Antiretroviral medications are given (1) to reduce the patient's viral load, (2) to maintain CD4+ cell counts above 500, and (3) to treat opportunistic infections and malignancies. Five classes of antiretroviral drugs are used: nucleoside reverse transcriptase inhibitors (NRTIs), nonnucleoside reverse transcriptase inhibitors (NNRTIs), protease inhibitors, entry inhibitors, and integrase inhibitors. Drug combinations and simpler dosing schedules are helping patients adhere to their medication schedules. HAART, the standard for treating HIV infection, combines three or more antiretroviral drugs. (Each drug group, with nursing responsibilities, is discussed in Table 11-9■.)

Before patients begin the HAART protocol, they should understand the benefits and risks as well as the effects on their daily life. They will need to take multiple medications at specific times throughout the day, and the HAART drugs cost more than $20,000 per year. This does not include the cost of other medications to treat or prevent opportunistic infections or cancers. Antiretrovirals cause adverse reactions that affect quality of life. For these reasons, patients with HIV must be fully committed to the treatment plan and be partners in their care.

Treatment is started when the patient (1) has CD4+ cell count less than 500, (2) shows symptoms of an AIDS-defining disease, (3) has viral load greater than 100,000 copies, or (4) is pregnant. Usually, the patient is given at least three drugs from two different classes. Single drugs are avoided to prevent drug resistance.

If successful, the drug regimen should reduce the viral load to undetectable levels in 12 to 24 weeks. However, not all patients experience the same results. Some patients cannot tolerate the multiple medications, side effects, or strict dosing schedule. Resulting feelings of despair, depression, and hopelessness may require antidepressants and counseling.

As mentioned earlier, the patient may need medications for opportunistic infections and malignancies associated with HIV infection and AIDS. Many of these disorders cannot be eliminated, but pharmacologic agents attempt to control their devastating effects (Table 11-10■).

Many patients at some point need central venous access devices, such as a Groshong catheter, to draw blood and to give medications, transfusions, and parenteral nutrition. (See Chapters 7 and 20 for nursing care of the patient with an intravenous access device.)

The following immunizations are recommended for all HIV-infected patients: pneumococcal, influenza, hepatitis A and B, and *Haemophilus influenzae b* vaccines. Persons with a positive PPD and negative chest x-ray film are given isoniazid (INH) for 1 year. When the patient's CD4+ cell count falls to less than 200, prophylactic treatment for PJP is begun, usually with TMP-SMX.

Complementary Therapies

Complementary therapies are used primarily to manage patient problems caused by opportunistic infections and cancers. For instance, ginger root may be given to reduce nausea and vomiting from cancer chemotherapy. Goldenseal seems to decrease fungal infections such as those caused by *C. albicans*, but high doses may cause nausea, vomiting, and diarrhea.

Several herbal supplements may decrease the effectiveness of antiretroviral drugs, mainly the NNRTIs and protease inhibitors. Patients with AIDS who are considering herbal therapy must consult their primary care provider before taking St. John's wort or garlic.

NURSING CARE

PRIORITIZING NURSING CARE

Because HIV and AIDS can affect all body systems, the patient needs physical and psychosocial support. Initially, the nurse focuses on prevention, maintaining a healthy lifestyle, education, and coping with a terminal illness. As the disease progresses and the patient develops opportunistic infections and malignancies, direct care becomes more important while continuing psychosocial support. Nursing care focuses on issues such as coping, infection risk, dietary deficiency, fatigue, altered skin integrity, respiratory problems such as pneumonia, and altered mental function.

Nurses provide care for patients with HIV/AIDS infection on medical–surgical, maternal–child, and pediatric

TABLE 11-9	Giving Medications Safely: Antiretroviral Agents		
CLASS/DRUGS	**PURPOSE**	**NURSING IMPLICATIONS**	**PATIENT TEACHING**
Nucleoside reverse transcriptase inhibitors (NRTIs)			
■ Zidovudine (AZT, Retrovir) ■ Abacavir (Ziagen) ■ Didanosine (Videx) ■ Lamivudine (Epivir) ■ Stavudine (Zerit) ■ Tenofovir (Viread) ■ Zalcitabine (Hivid) ■ Zidovudine and lamivudine (Combivir) ■ Tenofovir and emtricitabine (Truvada)	NRTIs inhibit the action of reverse transcriptase to prevent HIV reproduction.	Give at the ordered times around the clock. Monitor the patient's CBC and assess for anemia and leukopenia. Give epoetin (Epogen) or filgrastim (Neupogen) to treat anemia and neutropenia. Monitor CD4+ counts and viral load for drug effectiveness.	Take the drug at ordered times to maintain serum blood levels. Report all side effects. Have regular blood tests: viral load, CD4+ counts, CBC, liver to monitor for drug toxicity. Notify the physician if any signs of infection occur: sore throat, fever, swollen lymph nodes.
Nonnucleoside reverse transcriptase inhibitors (NNRTIs)			
■ Efavirenz (Sustiva) ■ Etravirine (Intelence) ■ Nevirapine (Viramune) ■ Delavirdine (Rescriptor)	NNRTIs block HIV reproduction.	Give at the ordered times around the clock. Monitor for skin rash, dizziness, and headache. Efavirenz side effects include abnormal thinking, confusion, and hallucinations. Monitor CD4+ counts and viral load for drug effectiveness.	Take the drug at ordered times to maintain serum blood levels. Report side effects. Have regular viral load and CD4+ counts. Notify the physician if any signs of infection occur.
Protease inhibitors			
■ Ritonavir (Norvir) ■ Atazanavir (Reyataz) ■ Indinavir (Crixivan) ■ Nelfinavir (Viracept) ■ Saquinavir (Fortovase) ■ Lopinavir/Ritonavir (Kaletra)	Protease inhibitors block the production of the HIV protease enzyme, which is needed to make mature virions.	Assess for cardiovascular or liver disease and diabetes mellitus. Most PIs cause lipodystrophy (enlarged abdomen, loss of tissue from the face, arms, and legs) and elevated blood glucose. Monitor CD4+ counts and viral load for drug effectiveness.	Take the drug at ordered times to maintain serum blood levels. Have regular viral load, CD4+ counts, and liver to monitor for drug toxicity. Notify the physician if any signs of infection occur.
Entry inhibitors			
■ Enfuvirtide (Fuzeon) ■ Maraviroc (Selzentry)	Fusion inhibitors prevent the virus from entering CD4+ cells.	Enfuvirtide is injected; Maraviroc is given orally. Assess for allergy: cough, fever, or rash.	Notify the physician of possible allergic response: cough, fever, or rash.
Integrase inhibitor			
■ Raltegravir (Isentress)	Blocks integrase enzyme needed for the virus to multiply.	Assess for side effects of headache, fever, and diarrhea.	Report side effects of headache, fever, and diarrhea to the physician.

units, as well as in hospices, clinics, and home settings. It is essential to respect the patients' right to confidentiality and never discuss a patient's diagnosis except with the health care team.

ASSESSING

The nurse must collect a database before selecting the appropriate nursing interventions. The database can help determine the extent to which HIV infection and AIDS

is affecting the patient's life and can identify potential complications (Box 11-7■).

IDENTIFYING POTENTIAL COMPLICATIONS

The most common complications develop after the patient has an AIDS diagnosis. These include opportunistic infections such as PJP, TB, candidiasis, and cryptosporidiosis. Late in the disease process, wasting syndrome, AIDS dementia complex, and cancers such as KS occur.

TABLE 11-10	Pharmacologic Treatment of Opportunistic Infections and Malignancies	
CONDITION	**TREATMENT**	**POTENTIAL ADVERSE EFFECTS**
Infections		
Pneumocystis jiroveci pneumonia	Trimethoprim–sulfamethoxazole (TMP-SMX, Bactrim)	Nausea, vomiting, rash, anemia, neutropenia, Stevens–Johnson syndrome
	Pentamidine (Septra)	
Tuberculosis	Antitubercular drugs	See Chapter 23 for the main discussion of TB
Mycobacterium avium complex	Clarithromycin (Biaxin)	Nausea, diarrhea
Candidiasis (oral thrush)	Nystatin suspension (Mycostatin)	Diarrhea, abdominal pain
Candidiasis (vaginal thrush)	Miconazole (Monistat)	Itching
Cryptococcosis	Amphotericin B	Fever, anemia
	Fluconazole (Diflucan)	Jaundice, rash
Herpes simplex	Acyclovir (Zovirax)	Vomiting, diarrhea, headache
Malignancies		
Kaposi sarcoma	Chemotherapy with vinblastine	Nausea, vomiting, bone marrow suppression
Lymphoma	Chemotherapy	Nausea, vomiting, bone marrow suppression

BOX 11-7	ASSESSMENT

Assessing Patients With HIV Infection and AIDS

Subjective Data

- General health status
- Difficulty swallowing, weight loss, anorexia, abdominal pain, or diarrhea
- Rashes or lesions on the skin or in the mouth
- Reports of fatigue, weakness, difficult walking, insomnia, or night sweats
- Headaches, forgetfulness, personality changes, or visual changes
- Fever, nonproductive cough, shortness of breath, or difficulty breathing
- Swollen lumps in neck, axillae, or groin
- Immunosuppressive or recreational drug or alcohol use
- History of TB, STIs, hepatitis; screening tests for TB or HIV
- History of unprotected sex
- Exposure to blood, blood products, or needles

Objective Data

- Obtain vital signs and height and weight.
- Observe for poor nutritional status: thinness, sunken eyes, muscle wasting.
- Observe for lethargy, depression, inability to concentrate, memory loss, tremors, slurred speech, aphasia, ataxia, and poor coordination.
- Inspect oropharynx with penlight and tongue depressor for gray-white patches (*Candida*).
- Inspect the skin for discolorations (KS) and genital area for lesions or discharge from candidiasis or STIs.
- Palpate lymph nodes in neck, axillae, and groin for swelling or tenderness.
- Auscultate lungs for crackles and wheezes.
- Monitor and report results out of expected range for viral load, CD4+ cell count, and CBC.

DIAGNOSING, PLANNING, AND IMPLEMENTING

Early in the disease process, counseling and preventive health care strategies are important. During acute exacerbations of opportunistic infections, individuals with HIV/AIDS may require hospitalization. Long-term physical and emotional support is needed when the patient experiences physical, debilitating symptoms.

Ineffective Coping

Expected outcome: Will demonstrate acceptance of change in health status by taking an active role in health care decisions.

- Assess the patient's support network and usual methods of coping. *This will help the nurse and the patient identify*

people and mechanisms that can help the patient cope more effectively with the disease.

- Provide continuity of care. Spend time actively listening to the patient. *This promotes trust and a caring atmosphere for the patient to express feelings and work through issues related to HIV infection.*
- Support positive coping behaviors, patient decisions, actions, and achievements. *As the patient's self-esteem is enhanced, coping improves.*
- Promote and support the patient's social network. *The patient will need others in order to cope with the diagnosis and disease progression.*
- Provide referral to counselors, support groups, and agencies. Include addresses and phone numbers for local and

national information resources and hotlines. Encourage the patient, family, and significant others to participate in support groups. *Resource persons and groups can provide information and support. Support groups decrease the risk of social isolation and encourage patients to find ways to cope.*

Risk for Infection

Expected outcome: Will remain free from infection.

■ Perform hand hygiene before and after all care. Use Standard Precautions for all patients. Use aseptic technique when performing invasive procedures. *Hand hygiene and Standard Precautions reduce the risk of disease transmission. Asepsis prevents HAI infections in hospitals or long-term care facilities.*

■ Monitor for signs of infection (e.g., chills, sweating; burning on urination; shortness of breath; redness, tenderness, or drainage from wounds) and WBC count. *Remember, immunocompromised patients may not have a fever; the nurse must look for other signs of infection.*

■ Culture lesions, blood, urine, and sputum as ordered. *Cultures may identify infections or determine the effectiveness of medications.*

■ Clean the patient's nails frequently. *Fungal infections are common under the nails.*

■ Administer antiretroviral and other anti-infective drugs as ordered. *These medications help control the HIV infection and may prevent opportunistic infections.*

Imbalanced Nutrition: Less Than Body Requirements

Expected outcome: Will maintain body weight appropriate for height and serum albumin within accepted ranges.

■ Consult with the dietitian to identify the patient's nutritional needs. *The dietitian can plan appropriate meals, supplements, and the need for parenteral nutrition.*

■ Offer small portions of soft foods and avoid hot or spicy foods. Limit fluids before and with meals. *Small portions are more appealing to the patient with anorexia or nausea. Soft foods are easily digested. Very hot or spicy foods can irritate the patient's mouth when lesions are present. Excess fluids decrease appetite and food intake.*

■ Provide a diet high in protein and kilocalories. *A high-protein, high-kilocalorie diet provides nutrients to meet the patient's increased metabolic needs.*

■ Assist with eating as needed. *Fatigue and weakness can prevent the patient from eating an adequate diet.*

■ Provide or assist with oral hygiene. *Oral hygiene improves comfort and appetite and reduces the risk of mucosal lesions.*

■ Provide supplementary vitamins and enteral feedings, such as Ensure. *This improves the patient's nutritional status and caloric intake.*

■ Give appetite stimulants such as megestrol (Megace) and dronabinol (Marinol) as ordered. *Both drugs may increase appetite and promote weight gain.*

■ Offer topical anesthetics such as Xylocaine viscous to patients with mouth lesions. Give antiemetics before meals and antidiarrheals after stools as ordered. *A topical anesthetic may reduce pain and improve oral intake. Antiemetics reduce nausea and improve food intake. Antidiarrheals improve nutrient absorption.*

clinicalALERT

Avoid high-fiber foods that can increase intestinal motility and diarrhea.

■ Monitor weight and albumin levels. *These measures promote early intervention to prevent anemia and wasting syndrome. Albumin levels reflect the patient's nutritional status.*

Impaired Skin Integrity

Expected outcome: Skin will remain intact without areas of skin breakdown.

■ Monitor lesions for signs of infection or impaired healing. *Infection or poor tissue perfusion not only impairs healing, but may lead to further skin breakdown.*

■ Turn the patient at least every 2 hours with a turn sheet. *Turning decreases stress over bony prominences, improves circulation, and promotes healing. A turn sheet prevents skin shearing that can lead to decubitus ulcers.*

■ Use pressure and egg crate mattresses or sheepskin pads for elbows and heels. *These devices reduce pressure on the skin.*

■ Wash the skin with mild, nondrying soaps and pat dry gently. *Clean, dry skin is a barrier to infection. Gentle drying prevents skin tears and reduces the risk of infection.*

clinicalALERT

Apply protective creams to reddened areas in the rectal area to prevent skin damage from diarrhea.

■ If blisters are present, leave intact, and cover with a hydrocolloid (e.g., DuoDERM) dressing. *Covering may prevent bacterial invasion and promote healing.*

■ Trim fingernails regularly. Teach the patient to avoid scratching. If confused, apply mitts or soft restraints to prevent scratching. Check circulation of hands and fingers frequently. *Scratching with long fingernails can damage the skin, increasing the risk of infection. Tight or restrictive restraints or mitts may decrease circulation.*

■ Encourage ambulation. If the patient is confined to bed, encourage active or passive range-of-motion exercises. *Activity increases circulation, decreases pressure and skin breakdown, and maintains muscle tone.*

Fatigue

Expected outcome: Will be able to perform activities of daily living (ADLs).

- Balance activities with rest periods and assist with ADLs if necessary. *Fatigue may be related to low energy levels, medication side effects, or the emotional stress of the disease. Establishing realistic activity goals helps the patient perform activities when energy levels are the highest and gives the patient a sense of accomplishment.*
- Provide supplemental oxygen as ordered. *Anemia and hypoxemia reduce oxygen to the cells, leading to fatigue.*
- Identify energy-saving techniques (e.g., sitting for a shower; using a cane, walker, or wheelchair). *Energy-saving techniques enable the patient to do more activities throughout the day. Assistive devices help conserve energy.*
- Refer to physical or occupational therapist as needed. *Physical therapy and occupational therapy exercises can increase muscle strength and tone.*

Ineffective Breathing Patterns

Expected outcome: Will have clear breath sounds.

- Promote coughing and deep breathing. Instruct the patient to use incentive spirometry. Suction airway as needed. *Thick secretions (as in PJP infection) reduce the flow of oxygen to the tissues. These interventions promote lung expansion and mobilize secretions.*
- Monitor oxygen levels with pulse oximetry. If less than 90%, give supplemental oxygen. *Oxygen levels should be above 90% to provide adequate oxygen to tissues and cells.*
- Increase fluid intake as tolerated. *Increased fluids will thin secretions and make them easier to expectorate.*
- Place the patient in semi- or high Fowler's position. *Elevating the head of the bed reduces abdominal pressure against the diaphragm and prevents aspiration.*
- Give anti-infective medications according to culture and sensitivity tests. *Anti-infective medications help control opportunistic infections.*

Risk for Acute Confusion

Expected outcome: Will maintain orientation to time, place, and person.

- Use simple, short sentences. Always call the patient by name. *Cognitive and neurologic functioning may be altered by brain malignancies and HIV infection of the central nervous system. These measures decrease confusion and help the patient remain oriented.*
- Reorient to time and place frequently. Provide calendar, clock, radio, TV, and a room with a window. *Frequent reorientation may be necessary during acute periods of confusion.*
- Provide quiet room with minimal lights at night. *Excess noise and bright lights confuse the patient between day and night.*

- Apply a bed alarm if the patient tends to get out of bed unassisted. Move the patient closer to the nurses' station or place in a monitored room. *The patient may experience confusion and impaired judgment. Bed alarms alert nursing staff to check on the patient's safety. Staff can monitor the patient more easily if the room is close or is a monitored room.*
- Encourage family and significant others to socialize with the patient. *Contacts with familiar persons can help maintain reality orientation.*
- Maintain safe environment by removing excess furniture, placing call bell within the patient's reach, and padding side rails as needed. *If motor coordination is altered, patients may injure themselves. These measures can decrease the risk for injury.*

Other Nursing Diagnoses

With a disease such as HIV infection, the list of possible nursing diagnoses is long. Some additional nursing diagnoses to consider are as follows:

- *Powerlessness* related to terminal disease
- *Pain* related to KS and peripheral neuropathy
- *Risk for Caregiver Role Strain* related to care needs of the patient with HIV
- *Impaired Home Maintenance* related to fatigue and weakness
- *Ineffective Sexuality Pattern* related to HIV infection

MANAGING NURSING CARE

As appropriate and allowed by the designated duties and responsibilities of assistive personnel, the nurse may assign activities such as measuring vital signs and intake and output, obtaining daily weights, and assisting with activities and hygiene for the patient with HIV infection.

EVALUATING

Evaluate effectiveness of care by collecting data related to the patient's overall health, absence of opportunistic infections, laboratory values (especially CD4+ cell count), and the ability to care for self at home.

DOCUMENTING

Documentation includes the patient's vital signs and the presence of any manifestations, which indicate opportunistic infections or cancers. Record the patient's response to antiretroviral therapy and other interventions for managing opportunistic infections. The nurse documents patient teaching about medications, diet, infection prevention strategies, and safe sex guidelines.

CONTINUITY OF CARE

Most patients with HIV infection and AIDS are cared for in the home. The patient and significant others need thorough teaching. They should understand HIV infection and

AIDS, disease transmission, and the stages of the disease, including opportunistic infections. Provide the patient and family with current factual information so they can plan their future. Discuss the myths, misperceptions, and prejudices that accompany this diagnosis.

The following topics should be discussed with the patient and family to maintain optimal health and to prepare for home care:

- Guidelines for safe sex practices
- Nutrition, rest and exercise, stress reduction, lifestyle changes, and maintaining a positive outlook
- Infection prevention and transmission including hand hygiene; importance of wearing gloves when handling the patient's secretions or excretions
- Importance of cleaning up blood spills with 1:10 dilution of bleach and water (1/2 cup bleach to five cups water)
- Importance of regular medical follow-up and laboratory testing
- Signs and symptoms of opportunistic infections and malignancies plus other symptoms they should report such as sore throat, night sweats, cough, dyspnea, chest pain, swollen glands, diarrhea, headaches, and skin lesions
- Avoid changing cat litter boxes or bird cages because cats and birds can carry toxoplasmosis, cryptosporidiosis, and MAC
- Medications and adverse effects; the importance of adherence to prescribed HAART once started
- Cessation of smoking, alcohol, and recreational or illicit drug use
- Home health, hospice, and respite care services as needed
- Community resources, such as support groups, social agencies, and counselors
- Helpful resources:
  - CDC National AIDS Hotline
  - Gay Men's Health Crisis Network
  - National Association of People With AIDS
  - National Organization on HIV Over Fifty

NURSING CARE PLAN
Patient With HIV Infection

Sara Lu is a 26-year-old elementary schoolteacher who lives with her parents and two younger sisters. During her yearly physical exam, she complains of feeling fatigued, a persistent sore throat, intermittent bouts of diarrhea, and mild shortness of breath for about a month. Normally, she is very physically active. She is planning to be married in 6 months. Ms. Lu states that she has had unprotected sexual relations only with her fiancé. Seven years ago she had open heart surgery to repair a mitral valve defect. The physician orders a mononucleosis test, ELISA, Western blot assay, CD4 T-cell count, and an erythrocyte sedimentation rate (ESR). She is to return to the office in a week.

Assessment
On Ms. Lu's follow-up visit, she tells Carole Kee, RN, that she still has flulike symptoms but has improved somewhat. She is less active than usual and is worried about her health. Her appetite is poor because of a sore mouth, and she has lost 10 lb during the past month. She has noted white patches on her tongue and cheeks.

A chest x-ray is normal. The results of her laboratory tests are as follows:

- ELISA: positive for antibodies against HIV
- Western blot assay: positive for antibodies against HIV
- ESR: increased
- CD4+ T-cell count: $599/mm^3$ (normal range is 800 to $1,200 mm^3$)

Ms. Lu's physical examination reveals that she has enlarged lymph nodes in her neck and white patches on her oral mucosa and is somewhat dehydrated. Vital signs are BP 100/70; R 20; P 90; T 99.9°F (37.7°C).

Ms. Lu is told the results of her laboratory tests and the medical diagnosis of HIV infection. Ms. Lu is distressed and wants to know how this happened, its meaning, whether she has infected her loved ones, and whether she will get better. She is admitted to the hospital for short-term care.

Nursing Diagnosis
The following nursing diagnoses (among others) are developed for Ms. Lu:

- *Imbalanced Nutrition: Less Than Body Requirements* related to mouth soreness
- *Risk for Deficient Fluid Volume* related to decreased fluid intake and diarrhea
- *Risk for Infection* related to altered immune protection
- *Anxiety* related to diagnosis and fear
- *Deficient Knowledge* about the HIV disease process

Expected Outcomes
The expected outcomes established in the plan of care specify that Ms. Lu will:

- Maintain adequate dietary intake.
- Return hydration status to normal.
- Remain free of infections and any complications.
- Verbalize anxiety and fears.
- State ways to prevent HIV transmission to others, including safer sex practices.

Planning and Implementation

Ms. Kee plans the following interventions to be implemented:

- Monitor daily weight, intake and output, hydration status, and serum albumin.
- Suggest strategies for decreasing anorexia and nausea.
- Provide a consult with a dietitian.
- Provide oral care before and after meals.
- Assess bowel sounds and monitor elimination pattern.
- Administer antiemetic and antidiarrheal medications as ordered.
- Increase fluid to 2,500 mL daily.
- Use strict aseptic technique for all invasive procedures.
- Give antiretrovirals and antibiotics as ordered.
- Encourage physical activity as possible.
- Encourage Ms. Lu to discuss her feelings and concerns.
- Avoid false reassurances.
- Suggest testing for her fiancé.
- Teach about HIV/AIDS, a nutritionally balanced diet, adequate fluid intake, avoiding people with infectious diseases, safe sex practices, and ways to prevent HIV transmission.

Evaluation

Ms. Lu is eager to learn about her illness. She also wants her fiancé and family to attend the teaching sessions with her. Ms. Lu is taking home an antifungal medication, diet plans, and a schedule for increased exercise. She will return in 1 month for a follow-up physical.

Critical Thinking in the Nursing Process

1. Are the laboratory results for Ms. Lu a true indication that she is HIV positive? What additional tests might be ordered?
2. What is the most likely source of Ms. Lu's infection?
3. Ms. Lu says that her fiancé would like to have a child. How will you counsel her regarding pregnancy and childbearing?

Note: Discussion of Critical Thinking questions appears on the companion website.

Note: The references and resources for all chapters have been compiled at the back of the book.

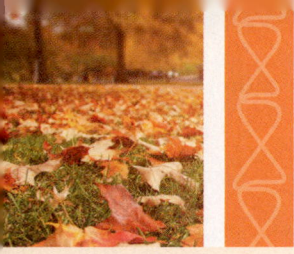

Chapter Review

KEY POINTS

- **Concept:** Normal immune function is essential to protect the body from internal and external threats. Immunity begins when the body recognizes foreign antigens as "nonself." This stimulates nonspecific inflammatory responses and specific cellular responses to the foreign antigen.
- A healthy immune system requires normal functioning leukocytes and lymphoid organs (bone marrow, thymus, spleen, lymph nodes).
- Active immunity provides long-term immunity either by developing the disease or by an immunization. Passive immunity is short term and involves injecting ready-made antibodies from other humans or animals. Patients must be taught the importance of keeping immunizations up to date.
- **Concept:** A hyper-responsive immune system can over-react to antigens, causing hypersensitivities. When the immune system targets normal cells and tissues, either autoimmune disorders (e.g., rheumatoid arthritis) can develop or transplanted tissue or organs can be destroyed.
- Hypersensitivity reactions range from mild, such as hay fever, to severe (e.g., blood transfusion reactions, anaphylaxis, and organ transplant rejections). Allergic reactions are treated with medication to prevent or moderate allergic responses.
- Latex allergy is a problem for health care professionals. Repeated exposure to latex-containing equipment often causes delayed hypersensitivity.
- Any type of allergic reaction can develop into anaphylaxis. Respiratory arrest and shock are the most common complications with major allergic reactions. Nurses must recognize early signs and symptoms and seek medical assistance immediately.

- Patients receiving transplanted organs will be treated with immunosuppressive drugs to maintain the transplant and to prevent the rejection process. Patients will take the antirejection drugs for their lifetime.
- **Concept:** Impaired immune function, whether congenital or acquired, threatens health and well being because the patient cannot effectively respond to threats such as infection. Nurses play a key role in teaching not only how to prevent HIV infection but also how to manage the disease in those affected.
- The human immunodeficiency virus (HIV) causes acquired immunodeficiency syndrome (AIDS). HIV attacks helper T4 lymphocytes, which decreases a person's ability to remain immunocompetent and increases the risk for developing opportunistic infections.
- The ELISA and Western blot tests detect antibodies to identify whether a person is infected with HIV. HIV viral loads are checked constantly to monitor disease progression and response to HAART (highly active antiretroviral therapy).
- Although HIV infection cannot be cured, it can be treated with HAART, a combination of antiretroviral medications that limit viral reproduction and host susceptibility to opportunistic infections and cancers. HAART is expensive and causes numerous adverse effects. However, adherence to the medication regimen is critical to halt viral replication.
- Health teaching focuses on safer sex practices, adverse drug reactions, nutrition, and ways to reduce opportunistic infection, to prevent transmission, and to maintain self-care.

PEARSON NURSING STUDENT RESOURCES

Find additional materials at **nursing.pearsonhighered.com**.

Clinical Reasoning Care Map

Caring for a Patient With *Pneumocystis jiroveci* Pneumonia

NCLEX-PN® Focus Area: Physiologic Integrity

Case Study: A 42-year-old male patient is admitted to the medical floor with *Pneumocystis jiroveci* pneumonia. Two years ago he was diagnosed with AIDS and has "felt good" until last week, when he started to feel tired. His CD4+ T-cell count dropped from 500 to 400/mm³. The nurse notes a dry cough and hears crackles in the bases. He says, "I get really short of breath when I walk." He complains of being cold, yet the room temperature is normal.

Nursing Diagnosis: Ineffective Breathing Pattern

Nursing Diagnosis: Impaired Gas Exchange

Nursing Diagnosis: Imbalanced Nutrition, Less Than Body Requirements

COLLECT DATA

Subjective	Objective
_____	_____
_____	_____
_____	_____
_____	_____
_____	_____

Does this present a threat to the patient's safety?

If yes, the priority intervention to address this threat would be:

_____

Nursing Care

_____
_____
_____
_____
_____
_____
_____

Interprofessional team members to include when planning care:

_____

How would you document this? _____

_____
_____

Data Collected
(use only those that apply)

- States, "Short of breath when I walk."
- BP 140/84
- Crackles in the posterior bases
- T 100.8°F
- Complains of being cold
- Easily fatigued
- Purple spots on both arms
- 4-lb weight loss in last month
- Dry cough
- RR 28, shallow
- Pulse oximetry = 88%
- Night sweats
- CD4+ T-cell count = 400 mm³

Nursing Interventions
(use only those that apply; list in priority order)

- Provide quiet room with minimal lights.
- Collect sputum culture.
- Monitor oxygen levels with pulse oximetry.
- Instruct in use of incentive spirometry.
- Place in semi-Fowler's position.
- Encourage coughing and deep breathing.
- Provide frequent oral hygiene.
- Increase fluid intake as tolerated.
- Monitor weight daily.
- Give nasal oxygen at 3 L/min.

Compare your documentation to the sample provided on the companion website.

NCLEX-PN® Exam Preparation

TEST-TAKING TIP Review therapeutic communication techniques. Communication that contains barriers will not be the correct answer.

1 A patient was given an immunization for influenza 10 minutes ago. Which of these statements made by the patient indicates that the patient has a correct understanding of the discharge instructions?

1. "I must be having a severe reaction; my arm is red."
2. "My ride is here. I have to leave now."
3. "I'll put a heating pad on my arm when I get home."
4. "I'll be back in 2 weeks to get my second shot."

2 A patient diagnosed with AIDS is receiving highly active retroviral therapy (HAART). What laboratory test result would indicate that this therapy is having a therapeutic effect?

1. Positive Western blot assay
2. Negative tuberculin test
3. WBC count of 8,000 mm^3
4. Decreased HIV viral load

3 A patient arrives in the clinic complaining of a swollen lip after being stung by a bee. What is the nurse's first priority action?

1. Assess the respiratory status.
2. Ask the patient about prior episodes with insect bites.
3. Administer epinephrine.
4. Explain the allergic reaction pathophysiology.

4 The physician has ordered azathioprine (Imuran) for a post–kidney transplant recipient. Which of the following teaching instructions should be emphasized to the patient?

1. Restrict PO fluids to 1,000 mL/day.
2. Avoid large crowds.
3. Limit activity to walking.
4. Expect urine output to be increased.

5 The nurse caring for a patient who is HIV positive is stuck with a needle while giving an injection. What action should the nurse implement first?

1. Report to employee health for prophylactic medication.
2. Wash the injection site with soap and water.
3. Notify the charge nurse and complete an incident report.
4. Follow up with the infection control nurse and have lab work drawn.

6 When assessing a patient who was diagnosed with HIV infection 1 month ago, the nurse should expect the patient to have which of these clinical manifestations?

1. White patches in the mouth
2. Shortness of breath
3. Sore throat
4. Difficulty concentrating

7 Which of these safe sex guidelines should be included in teaching a patient who is HIV positive?

1. Apply oil-based lubricants before sexual activity.
2. Females should use oral contraceptives.
3. Anal sex is acceptable if an animal skin condom is used.
4. Do not reuse condoms.

8 A patient reports a persistent cough, night sweats, fever, fatigue, and weight loss. The Mantoux test is assessed at 10 mm. What is the most likely condition that the nurse would expect?

1. *Mycobacterium avium* complex
2. Tuberculosis
3. Kaposi sarcoma
4. Cryptosporidiosis

9 When caring for a patient with AIDS dementia complex, which of these nursing interventions should be given priority?

1. Obtain vital signs every 8 hours.
2. Assess the patient's support system.
3. Serve small portions of soft foods.
4. Remove excess furniture from the room.

10 A patient who is undergoing chemotherapy for Kaposi sarcoma states, "I'm just too sick to eat." Which of these actions should the nurse take first?

1. Remove the tray of food.
2. Administer nausea medication before meals.
3. Encourage fluids with meals.
4. Give appetite stimulants as ordered.

Answers and rationales for Review Questions appear in Appendix I.

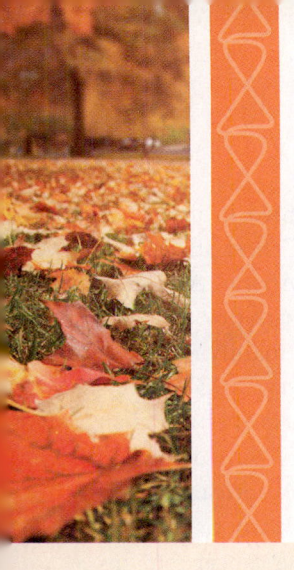

CHAPTER 12
Caring for Patients With Cancer

BRIEF OUTLINE

Cancer

Physiologic Effects and Manifestations of Cancer

Nursing Interventions for Oncologic Emergencies

Long-Term Effects of Cancer and Its Treatment

APPLIED LEARNING OUTCOMES

After completing this chapter, you will be able to:

1. Define cancer and describe its incidence and identified risk factors.
2. Discuss recommended screening procedures and schedules for early cancer detection.
3. Relate the pathophysiology of cancer and its effects on the body to interdisciplinary and nursing care needs of the patient with cancer.
4. Describe diagnostic tests used to diagnose cancer and monitor treatment effectiveness.
5. Discuss the use of surgery, radiation therapy, chemotherapy, and biotherapy in the treatment of cancer.
6. Use the nursing process as a framework for planning and providing holistic and patient-centered care and teaching for the patient with cancer.
7. Discuss nursing care of the patient experiencing an oncologic emergency or long-term effects of cancer and its treatment.

KEY TERMS

The key terms are defined on the pages listed below.

SPECIAL FEATURES

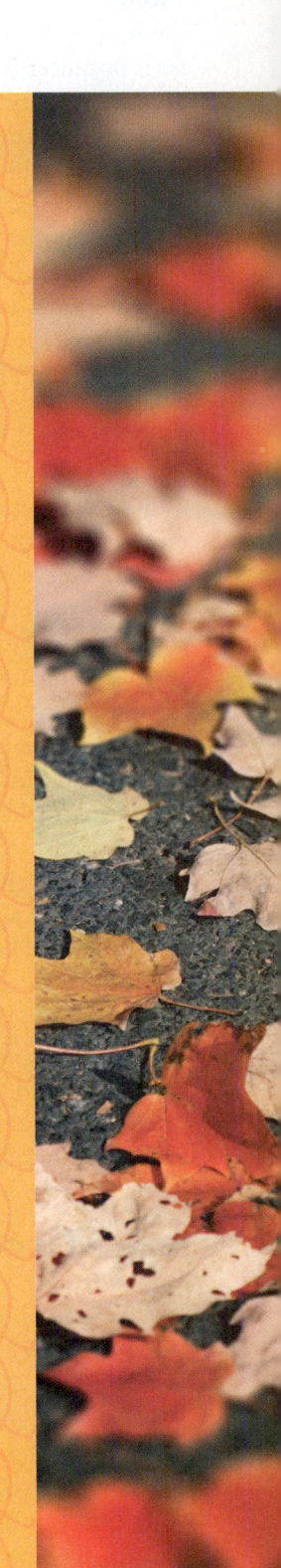

> **Key Concept** Cancer is not one disease, but a number of complex diseases characterized by the uncontrolled growth and spread of abnormal cells.

People of any age, gender, ethnicity, or geographic region can be affected by cancer. Its manifestations vary, depending on the type of cancer and the part of the body that is affected. If the spread of cancer cells is not controlled, it can lead to death. The fear caused by even a possible diagnosis of cancer is considerable. Cancer brings forth feelings of vulnerability and helplessness. However, most people who develop cancer survive; the current 5-year cancer survival rate in the United States is 68% (American Cancer Society [ACS], 2013a).

This chapter focuses on cancer as a disease and its treatment. It discusses nursing care appropriate for most patients with cancer. The care of patients with cancers that affect specific body systems (e.g., breast cancer, lung cancer) is found in corresponding chapters in the text.

Cancer

Cancer develops when normal cells mutate into abnormal cells that grow uncontrollably and spread within the body. Cancer is not one disease, but many diseases. Because cancer can affect any body tissue and has many different effects, patient care can be complex.

Cancer impacts all aspects of life for affected patients and their significant others. This impact is influenced by culture, values, and the unique experiences of the individual. Nursing and interprofessional care, which occurs in varied settings, address the holistic and chronic nature of this disease. Cancer is treated with a combination of therapies, many of which have devastating effects on the patient and family. Nurses are actively involved in cancer care through education, early cancer detection, rehabilitation and long-term follow-up of patients, and palliative care.

Oncology is the study of cancer; *oncologists* are physicians who specialize in caring for patients with cancer. Effective treatment and care for patients with cancer requires collaboration among a team of health care professionals, including physicians, nurses, therapists, social workers and others.

CANCER INCIDENCE AND TRENDS

Approximately 1,660,290 new cancer cases were diagnosed in 2013 according to the American Cancer Society (ACS) (2013a). Cancer is a disease associated with aging; about 77% of cancer diagnoses occur after age 55. Excluding skin cancer, in the United States breast cancer is the most frequently diagnosed cancer in women (232,340 new cases in 2013), and prostate cancer is the most common cancer in men (238,590 new cases during 2013). Lung cancer

and colorectal cancer rank second and third in incidence in both men and women (Table 12-1 ■). Cancer affects different ethnic groups disproportionately. African American men have a significantly higher incidence of prostate cancer than White men, whereas melanoma mainly occurs in White Americans (American Cancer Society, 2013b).

Only heart disease has a higher mortality rate than cancer. Statistics show that one in every four deaths in the United States is caused by cancer (American Cancer Society, 2013a). In 2013, about 580,350 Americans died of cancer—nearly 16 people per day. Lung cancer remains the leading cause of cancer deaths, accounting for approximately 27% of all cancer deaths (American Cancer Society, 2013a). Information about the most recent cancer cases and mortality rates are available on the ACS website.

With advances in cancer prevention, early detection, and treatment, the 5-year survival rate for individuals with cancer continues to improve in the United States. However, minority ethnic groups bear a disproportionate burden of cancer (Box 12-1 ■). African American men are more

TABLE 12-1	Top Ten Cancers and Cancer Deaths in Men and Women in the United States		
CANCER SITES		**CANCER DEATHS**	
MEN	**WOMEN**	**MEN**	**WOMEN**
Prostate	Breast	Lung and bronchus	Lung and bronchus
Lung and bronchus	Lung and bronchus	Prostate	Breast
Colon and rectum	Colon and rectum	Colon and rectum	Colon and rectum
Urinary bladder	Uterus	Pancreas	Pancreas
Skin melanoma	Thyroid	Liver	Ovary
Kidney	Non-Hodgkin lymphoma	Blood (leukemia)	Leukemia
Non-Hodgkin lymphoma	Skin melanoma	Esophagus	Non-Hodgkin lymphoma
Oral cavity and pharynx	Kidney	Urinary bladder	Uterus
Blood (leukemia)	Pancreas	Non-Hodgkin lymphoma	Liver
Pancreas	Ovary	Kidney	Brain

Source: Data from American Cancer Society (2013). *Cancer Facts & Figures 2013.* Atlanta, GA: American Cancer Society.

likely to develop and die from cancer than Caucasian men. Although breast cancer occurs more commonly in White women than in African American women, White women have a higher survival rate for the disease (American Cancer Society, 2013b). Similar disparities are seen in survival rates for colorectal, prostate, and endometrial cancers in these ethnic groups. Hispanics, in contrast, have lower incidence and death rates for the most common cancers as well as for cancer overall (American Cancer Society, 2012a). Although biologic and inherited differences are believed to contribute to these disparities, socioeconomic factors such as access to health care services and information, as well as cultural practices, beliefs, and attitudes, have been identified as contributing factors.

PATHOPHYSIOLOGY

Key Concept   Development of malignancies involves complex interaction of genetic, biologic, and environmental factors.

Mature normal cells of the body are uniform in size and have nuclei characteristic of the tissue to which the cells belong. Within the cell nucleus, chromosomes containing deoxyribonucleic acid (DNA) carry the genetic information that controls protein synthesis. The genetic code in the DNA of every cell is translated into the protein structures that determine the type, maturity, and function of that cell. Any change or disruption in a gene can result in an inaccurate "blueprint" that can produce an abnormal cell, which may then become cancerous.

A **neoplasm** (*neo* = new; *plasm* = tissue) or **tumor** is a mass of abnormal cells that grows independently of its surrounding structures and has no physiologic purpose. Neoplasms grow at a rate unrelated to the needs of the body, do not benefit the host, and in some cases are actively harmful. Neoplasms (or tumors) typically are classified as benign or malignant on the basis of their potential to damage the body and their growth characteristics.

Benign Tumors

Benign tumors are localized growths with well-defined borders; they are frequently encapsulated (Figure 12-1A■). Benign tumors tend to respond to the body's controls. They grow slowly and often remain stable in size. Because they are usually encapsulated, they often are easily removed and tend not to recur. However, they can be destructive if they crowd surrounding tissue and obstruct the function of organs. For example, a benign meningioma (from the meninges of the brain and spinal cord) can increase pressure on structures of the brain and progressively impair the person's neurologic function. Unless the meningioma is successfully removed, increasing intracranial pressure will eventually lead to coma and death.

Malignant Tumors

In contrast, **malignant** tumors grow aggressively and do not respond to the body's controls. They have an irregular shape and cut through surrounding tissues, causing bleeding, inflammation, and *necrosis* (tissue death) as they grow (Figure 12-1B). When health care professionals use the term *cancer,* they are referring to a malignant tumor.

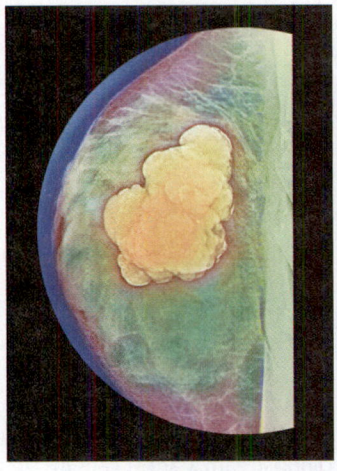 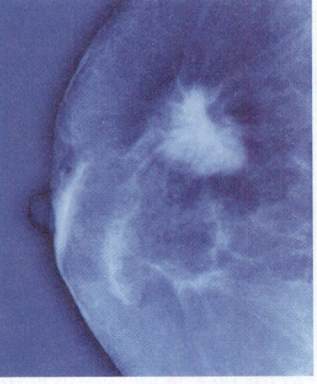

A   B

Figure 12-1. ■ Benign and malignant tumors of the breast as shown on colored mammograms. **(A)** A large benign tumor of the breast. (Source: CNRI /Science Source.) **(B)** A malignant neoplasm of the breast. (Source: Zephyr/Science Source.)

Malignant tumors can recur after surgical removal of the primary tumors and after other treatments. (Table 12-2 ■ compares benign and malignant neoplasms.)

Malignant cells easily separate from the neoplasm, allowing them to move into surrounding body fluids and tissues. Malignant cells may travel through the blood or lymph to invade other tissues and organs of the body (Figure 12-2 ■). The ability of cancer cells to invade adjacent tissues and travel to distant organs is considered their most dangerous characteristic. Both the secondary tumor they form and the process by which malignant neoplasms spread are called **metastasis**.

For metastasis to occur, the cancerous cells must avoid detection by the immune system. Thus impairment or

TABLE 12-3	Selected Cancers and Sites of Metastases
PRIMARY TUMOR	**COMMON METASTATIC SITES**
Bronchogenic (lung)	Spinal cord, brain, liver, bone
Breast	Regional lymph nodes, vertebrae, brain, liver, lung, bone
Colon	Liver, lung, brain, ovary, bone
Prostate	Bladder, bone (especially vertebrae), liver
Malignant melanoma	Lung, liver, spleen, regional lymph nodes, brain

suppression of the immune system is a major factor in the establishment of metastatic lesions. The most common sites of metastasis are the lymph nodes, liver, lungs, bones, and brain (Table 12-3 ■).

It is estimated that 50% of all cancers have metastasized by the time the tumor is identified. This may account for the current 32% death rate and supports the need for patient education to speed early diagnosis. The time it takes for metastasis to occur is extremely variable and often difficult to predict. Some cancers, such as basal-cell carcinomas, do not metastasize. The aggressiveness and location of the tumor, as well as the tumor's ability to escape immune detection, determine whether and how rapidly metastasis takes place.

CARCINOGENESIS

Carcinogenesis is the process in which normal cells are transformed into cancer cells. Cancer begins with transformation of a single normally functioning cell into a cancer cell. No single cause for this transformation can be identified; most cancers are the likely result of the interaction of genetic and internal factors with environmental factors, or **carcinogens** (cancer-causing agents).

Carcinogens damage cellular DNA. It appears that damage to and mutation of multiple genes is necessary to transform a cell into a cancer cell. Six or more gene mutations may be required for a malignant tumor cell to develop. Carcinogenesis occurs in a process of steps, from *initiation* during which cellular DNA is permanently damaged, *promotion* with repeated damage to already abnormal cells, and *progression* of the abnormal, mutant cells to malignancy. As the malignancy continues to progress, its cells become increasingly abnormal, differing significantly from cells of the tissue in which the tumor arose. The period of time between the damage to the DNA and detection of a tumor may be as long as 10 to 20 years.

Specific genes control cell growth, replication, and replacement. All cells in the body have **oncogenes** (genes

TABLE 12-2	Comparison of Benign and Malignant Neoplasms
BENIGN	**MALIGNANT**
Local	Invasive
Cohesive	Noncohesive
Well-defined borders	Does not stop at tissue border
Pushes other tissues out of the way	Invades and destroys surrounding tissues
Slow growth	Rapid growth
Encapsulated	Metastasizes to distant sites
Easily removed	Not always easy to remove
Does not recur	Can recur

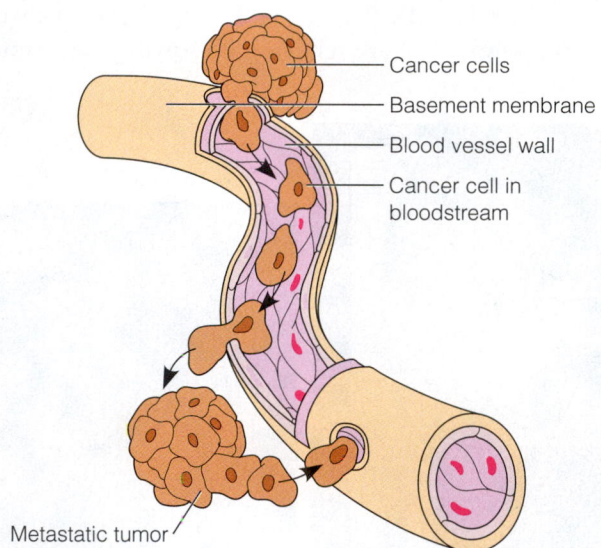

Cancer cells
Basement membrane
Blood vessel wall
Cancer cell in bloodstream
Metastatic tumor

Figure 12-2. ■ Metastasis via the bloodstream. Cancer cells invade the blood vessel, gaining access into the circulation. Once in the blood, most cancerous cells are destroyed by the immune system; however, even one undetected cell can move out of the blood into the tissue. Once in the new site, the malignant cells multiply and establish a metastatic (secondary) tumor.

capable of promoting uncontrolled cellular growth), which normally are repressed. Invading viruses or other carcinogens may "switch on" a cell's oncogenes, causing the cell to replicate (reproduce) faster. Normal inhibitory factors that prevent uncontrolled cell growth are suppressed. This allows the transformed cell to develop into a tumor that invades other body tissues.

Tumor suppressor genes normally inhibit oncogenes and cell growth. When these genes are inactivated, tumor growth is unregulated. Mutations of certain tumor suppressor genes are linked to the leading causes of cancer deaths: lung, breast, and colon cancers. For a tumor to grow, it must be supplied with blood. The growth of new blood vessels (*angiogenesis*) within the tumor also is genetically controlled.

Some researchers suspect that cancerous cells form continuously within the body. The healthy immune system recognizes these cells as "foreign" and destroys them. A tumor takes hold and grows only when it escapes immune surveillance (e.g., people who are immunocompromised). For example, patients with acquired immune deficiency syndrome (AIDS), who have a decreased number of helper T lymphocytes, have a much higher than normal incidence of certain cancers.

Carcinogens

Viruses, drugs, hormones, and chemical and physical agents are known to cause cancer or have strong links to certain kinds of cancers.

Certain *viruses* damage the cells they invade, which in turn can lead to cell mutation and malignancy. Human papillomavirus (HPV) is associated with malignant melanoma and cervical, penile, and laryngeal cancers. Hepatitis B virus is believed to cause primary liver cancer. In addition, certain viruses such as human immunodeficiency virus (HIV) impair immune protection against cancers such as lymphoma and Kaposi sarcoma. Vaccines such as HPV and hepatitis B vaccines are now available to prevent some virus-induced cancers.

Certain *drugs* and *hormones* are also related to the development of cancer. Chemotherapeutic drugs can damage normal cells, increasing the risk of developing new malignancies. Recreational drugs such as heroin and cocaine suppress the immune system. Hormones, such as estrogen, have been linked to cervical, endometrial, and breast cancers. Age-related changes in testosterone may be linked to prostate cancer. Anabolic steroids may promote tumor development.

Many *chemicals* have been identified as carcinogens, including many substances encountered in the workplace. Environmental carcinogens include polycyclic hydrocarbons, found in soot; arsenic, found in pesticides; wood and leather dust; polymer esters, used in plastics and paints; carbon tetrachloride; and asbestos. A number of chemicals found in tobacco are carcinogenic. Some foods also contain carcinogens added during preparation or preservation, such as nitrosamines found in pickled, salted foods. In some cases, food contaminants (e.g., *aspergillus* fungi) produce carcinogenic chemicals.

Excessive *exposure to radiation* causes increased rates of cancer. Both solar radiation from ultraviolet rays and ionizing radiation from industrial or medical sources are carcinogenic. Radon, a naturally formed radioactive gas found in the basements of many homes, is a known carcinogen. People who have lived in areas where nuclear weapons testing has been carried out or whose ground water has been polluted by nuclear wastes are also at increased risk for developing cancers.

Although everyone comes into contact with a vast number of carcinogens, not everyone develops cancer. Other factors, such as genetic predisposition, an impaired immune response, and repeated exposure to the carcinogen, are necessary for a cancer to develop.

RISK FACTORS

Risk factors make an individual or a population vulnerable to a specific disease or other unhealthy outcome. Some risk factors are controllable; others are not. Knowledge and assessment of risk factors are especially important in counseling patients and families regarding cancer prevention.

Uncontrollable Risk Factors

Risk factors over which a person has little or no control include heredity, age, gender, and poverty. Inherited *genetic factors* have been identified in some types of cancer (breast, colorectal, lung, and prostate). About 5% of cancers have a strong hereditary link (American Cancer Society [ACS], 2013a). For example, women who inherit a *BRCA* gene mutation have a high risk of developing breast cancer as well as an increased risk of developing ovarian cancer.

Age is a risk factor, with more than 75% of all cancers diagnosed in people over age 55. One possible factor involved in this increased risk is that at least five cycles of genetic mutations seem to be necessary to cause permanent damage to afflicted cells. Evidence indicates that the immune response is altered with aging, and cells are damaged over time. Also, long-term exposure to carcinogenic agents is usually necessary for cancer to develop. Hormonal changes that occur with aging can be associated with cancer. Postmenopausal women on hormone replacement therapy have an increased risk for breast and uterine cancers. Older men are at risk for prostate cancer, possibly due to breakdown of testosterone into carcinogenic forms. See Box 12-2■ for a discussion about cancer and older adults.

Cancer and the Older Adult

Cancer is the second leading cause of death in people over age 65. The incidence of cancer increases with age, probably as a result of the accumulated exposure to carcinogens and age-related declines in the action of the immune system. Hormonal changes (estrogen, testosterone) may also predispose older adults to cancer. The most commonly seen cancers in older women are breast, lung, colorectal, pancreatic, and ovarian. In older men, prostate, lung, colorectal, pancreatic, and gastric cancers occur most frequently.

The importance of screening and early detection of cancer does not diminish with age. Unfortunately, older adults may be less likely to undergo cancer screening or seek treatment for cancer as a result of fear, depression, cognitive impairments, poor access to health care, or financial constraints. Some older adults (and health care providers) mistake cancer symptoms for normal age-related changes and do not seek appropriate health care. When they do seek treatment, chronic conditions may mask the usual symptoms associated with cancer.

Older adults are at greater risk for side effects associated with cancer treatment (especially chemotherapy) because of age-related physiologic changes and chronic conditions associated with aging. The incidence of toxic effects on the heart and central nervous system is increased. Fatigue, problems related to immobility and functional decline, and risk for infection also occur more frequently in older adults. The nurse needs to monitor the patient closely and consider the effect of aging on responses to the disease and its treatment.

Teach the older patient and family about the warning signs of cancer. Stress the importance of seeking health care if any of the warning signs develop. Encourage all patients to undergo screening for colorectal cancer beginning at age 50. Teach women about the importance of regular mammography after menopause. Teach men the early signs of prostate cancer and discuss the potential benefits of screening.

Gender is a risk factor for certain types of cancer. For example, thyroid cancer and breast cancer occur more commonly among women; bladder cancer and prostate cancer are seen more often among men.

Cancer statistics show that *poverty* is a risk factor for cancer. Inadequate access to health care, especially preventive counseling and screening for early detection, may be a major factor. Some factors that usually come under the category of lifestyle risks, such as diet and stress, may be more prevalent in this population.

Controllable Risk Factors

Controllable or lifestyle risk factors include stress, diet, weight, occupation, infection, tobacco, drug and alcohol use, and sun exposure. Continuous unmanaged *stress* can keep certain hormones (e.g., epinephrine and cortisol) at high levels, leading to systemic "fatigue" and impaired immune surveillance.

A *diet* rich in red and processed meats, potatoes, refined grains, and sugar-sweetened beverages and foods increases cancer risk, whereas foods such as fruits, vegetables, and whole grains may be protective, reducing the risk for cancer. Poor nutrition, physical inactivity, overweight, and obesity account for about one-third of cancer deaths. *Overweight* and *obesity* contribute to up to 20% of cancer-related deaths (American Cancer Society 2013a). Obesity has been linked to malignancies of the breast, bowel, endometrium, esophagus, kidney, and pancreas. Physical activity reduces cancer risk by improving energy metabolism and reducing levels of hormones such as estrogen, insulin, and certain growth factors (American Cancer Society, 2013a).

Occupational risk factors include excessive exposure to solar rays (e.g., farmers, construction workers), chemicals such as benzenes, and particulate matter such as asbestos or coal dust. Health care workers (x-ray technicians, biomedical researchers) are exposed to ionizing radiation and carcinogenic substances. Although federal standards exist to protect workers from hazardous substances, employees may feel they lack the power to prevent violations or worry that reporting violations may cost them their job.

Specific *infections* increase the risk of cancer, but can be avoided through lifestyle modification or, in certain instances, by immunization. For example, genital herpes and human papillomavirus can often be prevented by following safer sex practices (e.g., monogamy, use of condoms) or by HPV vaccine. Hepatitis B virus and hepatitis C virus, which are spread through blood and body fluids, pose a significant risk for liver and pancreatic cancer.

Most lung cancers are preventable because of the relationship to cigarette *smoking*. According to the American Cancer Society (2013a), smoking accounts for at least 30% of all cancer deaths and 87% of lung cancer deaths. The carcinogenic substances in tobacco are weak; prolonged and/or heavy tobacco use increases cancer risk, whereas quitting smoking significantly decreases the risk for cancer and other diseases associated with smoking (e.g., heart disease, chronic lung disease). Tobacco is also related to cancers of the lip, mouth and pharynx, larynx, esophagus, stomach, pancreas, bladder, liver, and kidney and is also related to myeloid leukemia. Secondhand smoke contains at least 69 cancer-causing chemicals, increasing the risk for lung or bladder cancers in nonsmokers.

Alcohol promotes cancer by enhancing the contact between carcinogens such as those in tobacco and the stem cells that line the oral cavity, larynx, and esophagus (Grossman & Porth, 2014). People who both smoke and drink a considerable amount of alcohol daily have an increased risk for oral, esophageal, and laryngeal cancers. *Recreational drugs* suppress the immune system, and drug use often is associated with an unhealthy lifestyle that increases general cancer risk. Marijuana damages lung tissue to a greater extent than tobacco smoke.

As the protective ozone layer thins, more of the sun's damaging *ultraviolet radiation* reaches the earth. The incidence of skin cancers has increased as a result. Sun-related skin cancers are now considered to be a risk for all people, regardless of skin color, but people of Northern European extraction with very fair skin, blue or green eyes, and light-colored hair are most vulnerable. Older adults with decreased pigment are also more at risk, even those with darker skin.

EARLY DETECTION

Early detection and treatment significantly influence the prognosis of people with cancer. Many people do not seek early diagnosis and treatment because of denial, fear and anxiety, stigma, or the absence of specific early signs. Screening procedures (e.g., mammograms, colonoscopy) may be lifesaving.

The ACS promotes early cancer detection by increasing cancer awareness and providing guidelines for screening procedures. Although many cancers produce few manifestations until advanced, often patients relate having experienced common warning signs (Box 12-3■). For people without symptoms, the ACS recommends incorporating a cancer checkup into periodic health examinations. This general cancer checkup includes health counseling, teaching self-awareness, and, depending on age and gender, examination for cancers of the thyroid, oral cavity, skin, lymph nodes, testes, and ovaries. Box 12-4■ lists ACS recommendations for specific screening exams. Nurses should encourage all patients to schedule regular checkups.

Physiologic Effects and Manifestations of Cancer

Although the manifestations and effects of cancer vary with the type and location of the tumor, certain effects are usually observed (Box 12-5■). For manifestations of

BOX 12-3	POSSIBLE CANCER WARNING SIGNS

1. Persistent cough or hoarse voice
2. Unusual bleeding or discharge (rectal, vaginal, from the nipple, or bloody urine)
3. Recent unintended weight loss
4. Recent change in a wart, mole, skin color, or texture
5. Persistent functional change: shortness of breath; difficulty swallowing; indigestion, poor appetite; constipation; difficulty urinating
6. A palpable lump or thickening in breast or other tissue

BOX 12-4	AMERICAN CANCER SOCIETY GUIDELINES FOR CANCER SCREENING

Breast
- Clinical breast examination at least every 3 years from ages 20 to 39 and yearly thereafter
- Annual screening mammography starting at age 40; women at increased risk may have more frequent mammography or other tests such as breast ultrasound exams
- Awareness of how breasts normally feel and prompt reporting of any change in breast tissue to health care provider; routine breast self-examination starting at age 20 is an option
- Screening magnetic resonance imaging (MRI) for women with high risk of developing breast cancer (e.g., strong family history of breast or ovarian cancer, women treated for Hodgkin lymphoma)

Colon and Rectum
Beginning at age 50, a combination of the following exams:
- Annual fecal occult blood test (FOBT) or fecal immuno-chemical test (FIT)
- Flexible sigmoidoscopy every 5 years *or*
- Colonoscopy every 10 years *or*
- Double-contrast barium enema every 5 years *or*
- CT colonography (virtual colonoscopy) every 5 years

Cervix/Uterus
- **Cervix**: Pelvic examination and Pap test:
  - Ages 21–29—Cytology every 3 years
  - Ages 30–65—Cytology and HPV co-testing every 5 years *or* cytology alone every 3 years
  - Ages over 65—Discontinue if 3 negative cytology or 2 negative HPV tests in past 10 years with most recent test in past 5 years
  - Screening exams may stop for women who have undergone total hysterectomy (with cervix removal)
- **Endometrium**: Teaching for all women at menopause about risks and symptoms of endometrial cancer with instructions to report unexpected bleeding or spotting. At age 35, women with risk for hereditary nonpolyposis colon cancer should be offered annual endometrial biopsy to screen for endometrial cancer.

Prostate
Beginning at age 50 (men with average risk) or age 45 (African American men and those with a strong family history), men should receive information about the potential benefits and known limitations of the prostate-specific antigen (PSA) test. There is insufficient evidence for or against routine PSA testing to make a firm recommendation.

Source: American Cancer Society. (2012). *Cancer Prevention & Early Detection: Facts & Figures 2012.* Atlanta, GA: American Cancer Society.

specific cancers, see information about types of cancers in the chapters that follow.

Pain is ranked as one of the most serious concerns of patients, families, and oncology health care professionals.

BOX 12-5 COMMON GENERAL MANIFESTATIONS OF CANCER

- Pain: acute and chronic
- Bone marrow suppression: anemia, leukopenia, thrombocytopenia
  - Fatigue, exercise intolerance
  - Increased incidence of infections
  - Bruising, petechiae, occult or obvious bleeding or hemorrhage
- Anorexia–cachexia syndrome: recent weight loss, poor appetite, early satiety
- Disrupted organ function:
  - Voice hoarseness (laryngeal cancer)
  - Cough, shortness of breath (lung or bronchus cancer)
  - Difficulty eating, swallowing (esophageal or gastric cancer)
  - Jaundice (liver cancer)
  - Constipation, changes in stool diameter, rectal bleeding (colorectal cancer)
  - Hematuria (bladder or kidney cancer)
  - Difficulty urinating (prostate cancer)
  - Abnormal vaginal bleeding (cervical or endometrial cancer)
  - Personality, cognitive, mental status changes (brain tumor)
- Paraneoplastic syndromes: abnormal blood chemistries, manifestations of hormone or electrolyte imbalance

---

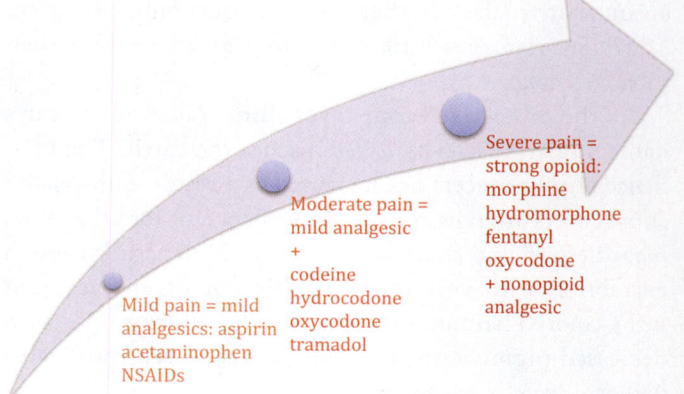

Mild pain = mild analgesics: aspirin acetaminophen NSAIDs

Moderate pain = mild analgesic + codeine hydrocodone oxycodone tramadol

Severe pain = strong opioid: morphine hydromorphone fentanyl oxycodone + nonopioid analgesic

Figure 12-3 ■ As cancer pain becomes more severe, increasingly potent analgesics are used to maintain comfort. Ideally, analgesics are given by mouth, by the clock, and tailored to the pain and to the individual.

Most patients with cancer experience moderate to severe pain associated with their illness. Cancer pain may be *acute,* with a well-defined pattern of onset, and related to the diagnosis or treatment. It may be *chronic,* lasting more than 6 months and frequently lacking the objective manifestations of acute pain. Chronic pain may alter personality, functional abilities, and lifestyle; it may disrupt compliance with treatment and quality of life.

Cancer pain usually is due to the effects of the tumor itself. The tumor may stretch pain-sensitive tissues or press directly on pain receptors. Metastases in other organs or in bone can activate pain and pressure receptors as well. Despite evidence-based pain management recommendations and the availability of treatment, undertreatment of cancer pain is common. The reasons for this vary, but often relate to a lack of understanding of effective cancer pain management by health care providers and institutions, patients, families, and society. Figure 12-3 ■ illustrates a progressive approach to the management of cancer pain.

The *physical stress* of the body's attempt to eliminate abnormal cells requires significant energy. Many patients with cancer experience fatigue, weight loss, anemia, and fluid and electrolyte imbalances as a result of this continuing stress.

Disrupted organ function may result from obstruction or pressure (e.g., urine retention from prostatic tumors obstructing bladder neck or urethra) caused by the tumor. Resulting tissue anoxia and necrosis affect the function of involved organs or tissues. Liver tumors can have significant effects, including impaired production of plasma proteins, altered drug metabolism, and development of ascites (excess fluid in the peritoneal cavity).

Bone marrow suppression is a common effect of cancer and its treatment, leading to anemia, leukopenia (decreased white blood cells), and thrombocytopenia (low platelet levels). Bone marrow function may be suppressed by the invasion of the marrow by malignant cells, poor nutrition, and treatments such as chemotherapy and radiation therapy. Acute or chronic bleeding may contribute to the anemia. Anemia, in turn, contributes to fatigue experienced by the patient. Leukopenia can impair the ability to fight infections. The immune system commonly is suppressed in patients with cancer.

Infection is common due to impaired immune defenses and direct effects of the tumor. Tumors may involve two organs, such as the bowel and bladder, leading to urinary tract infection. They may become necrotic, leading to septicemia. Tumors that grow near the surface of the body can erode through to the surface, providing a site for the entry of microorganisms.

Hemorrhage may be caused by tumor erosion through blood vessels. Thrombocytopenia impairs blood clotting and contributes to the risk for serious bleeding.

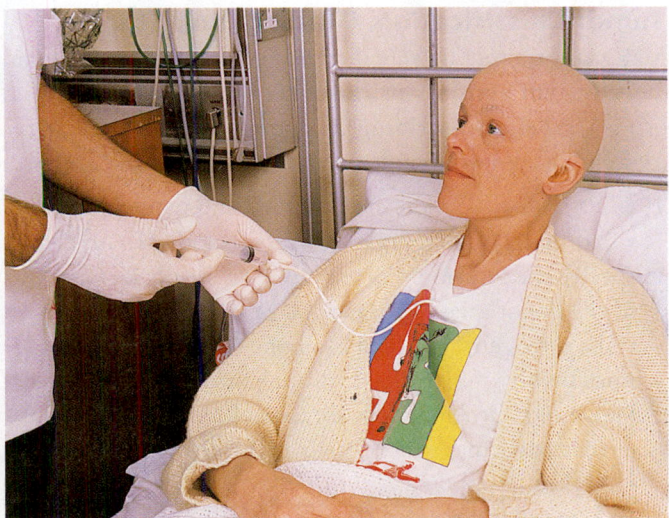

Figure 12-4. ■ Cancer robs its host of nutrients and increases the breakdown of fat and muscle, resulting in a wasted appearance. Also note alopecia (hair loss) related to chemotherapy. (Source: Simon Fraser/Science Source.)

Hemorrhage can be serious enough to cause life-threatening hypovolemic shock.

The **anorexia–cachexia syndrome** is common in patients with cancer. Several factors contribute to the anorexia-cachexia syndrome. The metabolic rate increases as cancer cells reproduce, and the cancer cells divert nutrients from normal cells. The tumor secretes substances that alter taste and smell and produce early satiety (a sensation of fullness). Pain, infection, and depression contribute to anorexia. Cancer cells support their growth processes by breaking down body tissue and muscle proteins, leading to the characteristic wasted appearance (*cachexia*) of many patients with cancer (Figure 12-4■). Unexplained rapid weight loss is often the symptom that brings the patient to a health care provider.

Some cancers produce excessive amounts of hormones and other substances, leading to *paraneoplastic syndromes.* As a result, the patient may develop symptoms of hypoglycemia, abnormal fat deposits, or fluid and electrolyte imbalances. Hypercalcemia is a common manifestation of paraneoplastic syndromes.

Psychologic Responses

People exhibit a variety of psychologic and emotional responses to a diagnosis of cancer. Some see it as a death sentence; they experience overwhelming grief and may give up hope. Others feel guilt and consider cancer a punishment for past behaviors. Fear is common: fear of the outcome, the effects of treatment, pain, and death. Common emotions are grief, anger, powerlessness, isolation, and concern about body image and sexual dysfunction.

COLLABORATIVE CARE

Key Concept The nurse is an important member of the health care team treating the patient with cancer. The nurse advocates for the patient, assists with coordinating care activities, and helps the patient and family manage the effects of the disease and its treatment.

The ACS identifies four major goals of interprofessional care for patients with cancer: (1) to eliminate the tumor or malignant cells (cure), (2) to prevent metastasis (control), (3) to reduce cellular growth and tumor burden, and (4) to promote functional abilities and provide pain relief to those whose disease does not respond to treatment (palliation). These goals may overlap. Cancer may be treated with surgery, radiotherapy, chemotherapy, and biotherapy. Often a combination of several treatment modes is used.

Diagnostic Tests

A number of laboratory and diagnostic tests are used to diagnose cancer and monitor progress and treatment. Abnormal laboratory test results may indicate the possibility of a tumor. These may include the complete blood count (CBC) and specific organ function studies (e.g., liver function tests, renal function tests, pancreatic enzyme levels, thyroid hormone levels). *Tumor markers* are proteins found in the blood that indicate malignancy. High levels of a known tumor marker require follow-up diagnostic studies. The primary use of tumor markers, however, is to determine the patient's response to therapy and to detect residual disease. Table 12-4■ lists selected tumor markers and tumors associated with that marker.

Imaging studies such as x-rays, computed tomography, ultrasonography, magnetic resonance imaging, and nuclear scans are used to locate abnormal tissues or tumors.

■ *X-ray imaging,* the least expensive and least invasive diagnostic procedure, can detect tumors larger than 1 cm in size but cannot distinguish well between cysts and tumors.

TABLE 12-4	Selected Tumor Markers With Associated Tumors
TUMOR MARKER	**SELECTED ASSOCIATED TUMORS**
Alpha-Fetoprotein (AFP)	Hepatocellular (liver) carcinoma, testicular cancer
Carcinoembryonic antigen (CEA)	Adenocarcinoma of the colon, pancreas, lung, breast, ovary
Prostate-specific antigen (PSA)	Prostate cancer
Calcitonin	Thyroid cancer
Immunoglobulin	Myeloma

Source: Data from Grossman, S., & Porth, C. (2014); Kee, J. (2014); Longo D. L. et. al. (2012).

■ *Computed tomography (CT) scans* reveal subtle differences in tissue densities and are much more accurate than x-ray studies for identifying tumors and evaluating for lymph node involvement. Contrast media may be used to enhance the image. Ask the patient about possible allergies to iodine, seafood, or x-ray contrast before the exam.

■ *Ultrasonography* uses reflected sound waves to examine body tissues and structures. Ultrasonography is noninvasive and requires no exposure to radiation. It is increasingly used to detect and monitor tumors in breast tissue, the prostate, and other organs.

■ *MRI* produces images from radio-frequency signals emitted by the body. Because a strong magnet is used, inquire about the presence of a pacemaker or joint prosthesis before the procedure. MRI procedures can produce a feeling of claustrophobia; preparation, support, and reassurance of the patient are important.

■ *Nuclear scans* use a scanner to detect specific radioisotopes administered orally or by injection. In most cases, no special radiation precautions are necessary.

DIRECT VISUALIZATION Direct visualization procedures are invasive but allow inspection of organs and usually permit biopsy of suspicious lesions or masses. Commonly used visualization procedures include sigmoidoscopy (inspection of the sigmoid colon), colonoscopy (inspection of the entire large bowel), cystoscopy (inspection of the urethra and bladder), bronchoscopy (inspection of the bronchial tree), and endoscopy (inspection of the upper gastrointestinal tract).

These procedures require some patient preparation (e.g., food restriction, bowel cleaning), cause discomfort, and may require sedation or anesthesia. Most can be performed in the physician's office or specialty ambulatory clinic.

When the tumor is exposed, a tissue sample (biopsy) is sent to the pathology laboratory for a rapid "frozen-section" histologic examination. If the initial report is negative, the mass is usually removed for further examination and to prevent further symptoms. If the report is positive for cancer, the tumor is resected, often with adjacent lymph nodes and any other suspicious tissue. These tissues are sent to the pathology laboratory for further analysis. The patient then receives the usual postoperative care.

CYTOLOGIC EXAMINATION Microscopic examination of tissue from the tumor is necessary to identify the type of tumor and the tissue of origin and to make a definitive diagnosis. Tissue samples are collected during biopsy, from shedded cells (e.g., Pap smear), collection of secretions (e.g., a sputum or urine sample), or by needle aspiration (solid tumors of breast, lung, or prostate). Lymph nodes are biopsied to determine the presence of metastasis.

Tumor Classification, Grading, and Staging

Malignant tumors are classified using a standardized system. This system consists of *tumor classification* (naming its origin), *grading* (describing its aggressiveness), and *staging* (describing its spread within or beyond the tissue of origin):

1. *Classification.* Tumors are classified and named by the tissue or cell of origin; adjectives are added to further specify the location. For example, an adenocarcinoma of the breast arises in glandular or ductal epithelial cells; osteogenic sarcoma is a bone tumor; and leukemias involve white blood cell precursors (e.g., myeloid leukemia). Other tumors are named for the discoverer of that particular cancer, such as Burkitt lymphoma or Hodgkin lymphoma.

2. *Grading.* Tumor grading evaluates cell differentiation and estimates the rate of growth. Cells that are well differentiated (most closely resemble normal cells of the tissue) are the least malignant and earn a grade of 1. Grade 4 is reserved for the least differentiated (appear significantly different than normal cells) and most aggressively malignant cells. Grading criteria may vary with different locations and types of tumors.

3. *Staging.* Staging refers to the relative size of the tumor and extent of the disease. The TNM classification system is commonly used to stage tumors. T stands for the relative tumor size and invasiveness, N indicates the presence and extent of lymph node involvement, and M denotes distant metastases. Table 12-5 ■ outlines the TNM system. Other systems may be used to differentiate types and locations of tumors (e.g., Hodgkin lymphoma).

TABLE 12-5		TNM Staging Classification System
STAGE		**DESCRIPTION**
Tumor	T_0	**No evidence of primary tumor**
	T_{IS}	**Tumor** *in situ*
	T_1, T_2, T_3, T_4	Ascending degrees of tumor size and involvement
Nodes	N_0	**No abnormal regional nodes**
	N_{1a}, N_{2a}	**Regional nodes—no metastasis**
	N_{1b}, N_{2b}, N_{3b}	**Regional lymph nodes—metastasis suspected**
	N_x	Regional nodes cannot be assessed clinically
Metastasis	M_0	**No evidence of distant metastasis**
	M_1, M_2, M_3	Increasing degrees of metastatic involvement of the host, including distant nodes

Psychologic Support During Diagnosis

Preparing for and awaiting the results of diagnostic tests can be stressful, creating significant anxiety. In addition to coping with the possibility of a life-threatening or life-changing disease, patients often must undergo a series of uncomfortable, even painful, diagnostic procedures. They have important decisions to make that hang on the outcome of those tests. Many unspoken questions may exist:

- Do I have cancer?
- If so, what kind, and how serious?
- Has it spread?
- Will I survive?
- What kind of treatment is needed?
- Are there treatment options?
- How will this affect my lifestyle?
- How will this affect family and friends?

Nurses can provide valuable help during this very difficult time of cancer diagnosis by keeping patients actively involved in managing their life and disease. The LPN can help patients by sitting down with them as soon as they enter the health care system and soliciting questions regarding what the patient already knows about the oncoming diagnostic procedures. Initiating the interaction with objective questions and encouraging patients to share their knowledge and experience are effective strategies to promote their sense of control.

It is essential that patients understand required test preparation, especially when preparation is done at home. Patients also need to know what to expect during the test, such as nausea or flushing from radiopaque dye. A phone call the evening before the procedure to verify the patient's understanding and to answer questions can be very supportive.

As patients begin to feel more comfortable, they may express concerns, fears, and other emotions. The nurse should avoid giving advice and false reassurance, but listen and be supportive, sharing appropriate information when needed. Being nonjudgmental and providing nonverbal support may facilitate more open communication with patients who are not ready to discuss concerns or those who appear angry. An atmosphere of calmness, warmth, caring, and respect can ease the tension and often unspoken terror of this initial period.

Support of and communication with the patient's significant others is extremely important. Family members often try to be strong for the patient and may not feel comfortable expressing their own fears and concerns. The nurse needs to be available to the family without the patient present to allow them to talk without feeling the need to edit for the patient's benefit. This can help family members manage their own difficulties in coping with their loved one's potential cancer diagnosis.

Pain Management

Pain management is a crucial part of care for the patient with cancer. It is estimated that more than 60% of patients with early-stage cancer and up to 95% of patients with advanced cancer experience pain that requires analgesia (Ogboli-Nwasor et al., 2013). Cancer pain falls into two general categories:

- *Pain associated with direct tumor involvement,* for example, metastases to bone, nerve compression, and organ involvement.
- *Pain associated with treatment,* for example, postsurgical incisional or wound pain, ulceration of mucous membranes, and pain resulting from the effects of radiation therapy.

The goal of treatment is to provide pain relief that allows patients to function as they wish and, in the case of terminally ill patients, to die relatively free of pain. Combinations of nonopioid analgesics, opioids, and adjunctive drugs are used to manage acute and chronic cancer pain (see Figure 12-3). Effective pain management requires careful initial and ongoing assessment of the pain as well as the patient's functional goals. When mild analgesics (such as aspirin or ibuprofen) are no longer effective, opioid analgesics are added to the regimen. Combinations of analgesics and increasing dosages are tried, while balancing the patient's functional status and adverse effects of the drugs.

Analgesics are administered orally as long as possible, given on a regular schedule (e.g., every 4 hours) with additional medication prescribed to cover breakthrough pain. When the oral route alone is no longer effective, narcotic analgesics can be administered parenterally (IM or subcutaneously), by transdermal patches, or intravenously, controlled by an infusion pump. When narcotic doses are increased gradually to maintain pain control, there is no dose limit. The body quickly becomes tolerant to the drug's sedative effects, and the dose needed to control pain does not produce excessive sedation or respiratory depression. Adverse effects such as constipation, nausea, and itching, are managed through diet, laxatives, antiemetics, and antihistamines as needed. Adverse drug effects or inadequate pain relief may necessitate use of different narcotics and combinations. Morphine sulfate and transdermal fentanyl are the most commonly used drugs for relief of cancer pain (Ogboli-Nwasor et al., 2013). Opioid analgesics should not be abruptly stopped, because withdrawal symptoms will occur. If the drug needs to be discontinued, it must be tapered gradually.

Surgery

Surgery is used to diagnose and stage more than 90% of all cancers and as a primary treatment for more than 60%. Whenever possible, the tumor is removed entirely, usually with a nonessential portion of organ or tissue to ensure removal of all tumor cells. An organ whose function can be replaced chemically, like the thyroid, may be totally removed. When one of a pair of organs is removed, the unaffected organ can take over (e.g., the lung or kidney).

Tumor-removal surgery sometimes requires creation of new structures to maintain body function. For example, if the sigmoid colon and rectum are removed, the remaining healthy segment of the bowel is brought out through a *stoma* (a created opening) in the abdominal wall, providing a permanent *colostomy* for bowel elimination. Surgery can also alter normal body function by destroying nerves and the lymph system; for example, prostate surgery may lead to incontinence and impotence, and lymph node dissection may lead to lymphedema (swelling) in the affected areas.

If the tumor is *nonresectable* (cannot be removed) or has metastasized, surgery may be used as a palliative measure, to promote function of the involved organs, to relieve pain, or to reduce the bulk of the tumor so that other treatments are more effective. Surgery is often used in combination with radiation therapy, chemotherapy, or biologic therapies. Reconstructive surgery also may be part of the treatment plan (e.g., breast reconstruction after mastectomy).

Radiation Therapy

Radiation therapy is the treatment of choice for some tumors. Radiation causes lethal injury to cellular DNA. It is used to kill the tumor, to reduce its size, to decrease pain, or to relieve obstruction, and when beginning metastases are suspected. *External radiation* (also called teletherapy) places the source of radiation at a distance from the patient and delivers a relatively uniform dose (Figure 12-5 ■). *Brachytherapy* is internal; the radioactive material (*implant*) is placed directly into the tumor site, delivering a high dose to the tumor and a lower dose to the normal tissues around it. It requires special safety measures (Box 12-6 ■). A combination of these two therapies is often used.

In brachytherapy, the radiation source is sealed in tubes, containers, wires, seeds, capsules, or needles that are inserted into the affected tissue or body cavity (Figure 12-6 ■). Internal radiation may also be ingested or injected as a solution or be introduced into the tumor through a catheter. The radioactive substance may transmit rays outside the body or be excreted in body fluids.

External radiation does not place family members at risk because the patient does not emit radioactive particles. Implanted or ingested radiation, however, can be dangerous for those living with, caring for, or treating the patient. Box 12-7 ■ discusses nursing care for the patient receiving radiation therapy.

Potential adverse effects of radiation therapy include skin damage (blanching, erythema, sloughing), ulcerations of mucous membranes, vulnerability to infection, bone

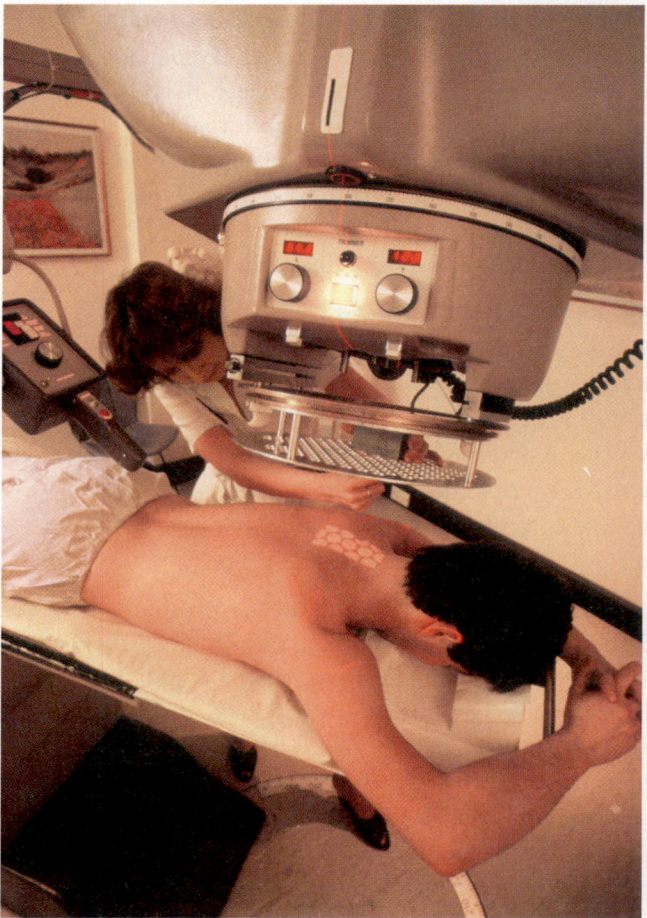

Figure 12-5. ■ A technician adjusts an external radiation machine to focus on the defined area to be treated. (Source: Martin Dohrn/Science Source.)

marrow suppression, gastrointestinal effects (nausea, vomiting, diarrhea, bleeding), exudate in the lungs (called *radiation pneumonia*), and fistulas or necrosis of adjacent tissues.

Chemotherapy

Chemotherapy can cure some cancers (leukemias, lymphomas, some solid tumors). It may be used to decrease tumor size, as an adjunct to surgery or radiation, or to prevent or treat suspected metastases. Chemotherapy disrupts malignant and rapidly dividing cells by interrupting cell metabolism and replication. It reduces the cell's ability to synthesize needed enzymes and chemicals. Some chemotherapy drugs work during specific phases of the cell cycle; others work through the entire cell cycle. Chemotherapy may also be used in conjunction with biotherapy. All chemotherapy has adverse or toxic effects; the type and severity of these effects depend on the drugs and doses used.

Most chemotherapy regimens involve combinations of drugs given over varying periods of time. Treatment is given in cycles with rest periods in between. Treatment is continued until the disease enters remission or until the

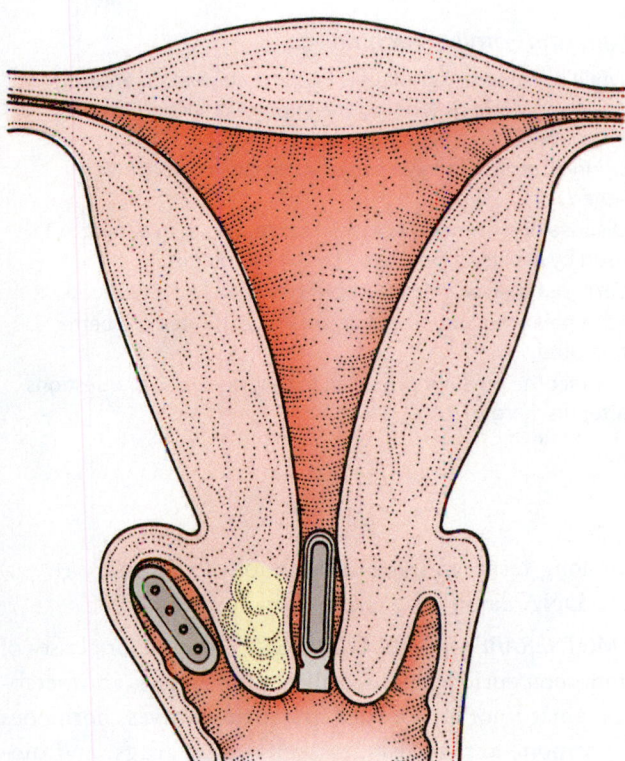

Figure 12-6. ■ A tumor in the wall of the uterus being treated with radioactive implants in the cervix and the vagina. (Source: Dorling Kindersley Media Library.)

particular protocol is abandoned (due to lack of improvement or toxic effects) and a new one is tried.

Several courses of chemotherapy are necessary because a fixed percentage of cells are killed with each course, reducing the tumor burden. The goal is to reduce the number of malignant cells until the body's immune system can finish the job. In general, this involves giving the maximum amount of chemotherapy the patient can tolerate.

During chemotherapy, patients may experience psychologic and emotional distress. The scheduling of chemotherapy treatments and its resulting adverse effects can impair the ability to work, manage a household, function sexually, or participate in social and recreational activities. Weight loss and alopecia affect body image and may prompt feelings of powerlessness and depression. The nurse can assist patients by carefully evaluating symptoms, providing specific interventions as indicated, and providing opportunities to express fears, concerns, and feelings. The nurse should encourage patients to participate in their care and facilitate their sense of control over their life as much as possible. A positive attitude projected by nurses caring for the patient receiving chemotherapy can help the patient cope with its adverse effects. Specific interventions are discussed later in the chapter under the appropriate nursing diagnoses.

COMMON ADVERSE AND TOXIC EFFECTS OF CHEMOTHERAPY
Most drugs used for chemotherapy target cells at a certain point in the cell cycle. Cells that are rapidly dividing are the most vulnerable to damage by these drugs. Cells in certain body tissues such as the bone marrow, gastrointestinal tract, hair follicles, and the testes have rapid growth cycles, making them vulnerable to the effects of chemotherapy.

Bone marrow suppression is common, resulting in reduced numbers of red blood cells (erythrocytes), white blood cells (leukocytes), and platelets (thrombocytes) As a result, patients often become anemic, experiencing fatigue and exercise intolerance. Low white blood cell counts (leukopenia) increase the risk for infection and impair the patient's ability to fight off infections that develop. Thrombocytopenia (low platelet counts) impairs clotting and can result in serious bleeding or hemorrhage.

Colony-stimulating factors (CSFs), or hematopoietic growth factors, often are given to "rescue" the bone marrow after chemotherapy. CSFs regulate the growth and differentiation of blood cells and are used to help reduce bone marrow suppression. Bone pain is a common side effect of these agents. Patients also may experience fevers, chills, anorexia, muscle aches, and lethargy.

Common toxic effects of chemotherapy on the GI tract include *stomatitis* (inflammation of the oral cavity), *nausea* and *vomiting,* and *diarrhea.* Stomatitis interferes with the ability to eat and drink, potentially leading to malnutrition. Nausea

BOX 12-7   NURSING CARE CHECKLIST

Patients Receiving Radiation Therapy

For Both External and Internal Radiation Therapy

Nursing Responsibilities

☑ Working with the patient's health care team, carefully assess for, manage, and document any complications.

☑ Assist in documenting the results of the therapy; for example, patients receiving radiation for a tumor on the spine will show improved neurologic functioning as tumor size diminishes.

☑ Provide emotional support, relief of discomfort, and opportunities to talk about fears and concerns.

☑ Document nursing care and the patient's responses to radiation therapy.

☑ Document teaching, including evaluation and achievement of learning goals, and the need for further patient and family instruction.

For External Radiation

Before the start of treatments, the treatment area is specifically identified by the radiation oncologist and marked with colored semipermanent ink. Treatment is usually given 5 days per week for 15 to 30 minutes per day over 2 to 7 weeks.

Nursing Responsibilities

☑ Monitor for and document adverse effects: skin changes, such as blanching, erythema, sloughing, or hemorrhage; ulcerations of mucous membranes; nausea and vomiting, diarrhea, or gastrointestinal bleeding.

☑ Assess respiratory function, including lung sounds. Document dyspnea, changes in respiratory pattern, or abnormal lung sounds.

☑ Identify and document medications the patient is receiving during radiation therapy.

☑ Monitor white blood cell (WBC) counts and platelet counts for significant decreases. Report changes to the charge nurse or physician.

Patient and Family Teaching

☑ Wash the radiation site with plain water only, no soap; do not apply deodorant, lotions, medications, perfume, or powder to the site during treatment. Do not wash off the treatment marks.

☑ Do not rub, scratch, or scrub treated skin areas. If it is necessary to shave the treated area, use an electric razor.

☑ Apply neither heat nor cold to the treatment site.

☑ Inspect the skin for damage or changes, and report these as well as any mouth sores or pain, difficulty swallowing or breathing, or other problems to the radiologist or physician.

☑ Wear loose, soft clothing over the treated area.

☑ Protect skin from sun exposure during treatment and for at least 1 year after radiation therapy. Wear protective clothing and use sun-blocking agents with an SPF of at least 15.

☑ External radiation poses no risk for radiation exposure to other people, even with intimate physical contact.

☑ Be sure to get plenty of rest and eat a balanced diet.

For Internal Radiation

Nursing Responsibilities

☑ Place the patient in a private room.

☑ Limit family and caregiver visits to 10 to 30 minutes; have visitors sit at least 6 feet from the patient.

☑ Monitor for and document adverse effects such as burning sensations, excessive perspiration, chills and fever, nausea and vomiting, or diarrhea.

☑ Assess for evidence of fistulas or necrosis of adjacent tissues (e.g., cloudy, malodorous urine), documenting and reporting manifestations to the charge nurse or physician.

Patient and Family Teaching

☑ While a temporary implant is in place, stay in bed and rest quietly to avoid dislodging the implant unless otherwise instructed.

☑ During outpatient treatments, avoid close contact with others.

☑ Dispose of excretions in special containers or in a toilet not used by others as instructed by the radiologist.

☑ Carry out daily activities as able; get extra rest if fatigued.

☑ Eat a balanced diet; frequent, small meals often are better tolerated.

☑ Contact the nurse or physician for any concerns or questions after discharge.

---

and vomiting can be severe, resulting from direct effects of the drug on vomiting centers. Administering an antiemetic drug before chemotherapy administration can reduce nausea and vomiting. Diarrhea, which can lead to a fluid volume deficit, often can be managed by including constipating foods (e.g., cheese) and foods high in fiber in the diet.

Other important toxic effects of chemotherapy drugs include *reversible alopecia* (hair loss), *teratogenic* (defect-producing) *effects* on a developing fetus, *irreversible sterility* in males, *hyperuricemia* (high uric acid levels in the blood), and,

in the long term, an increased risk for cancer (*carcinogenesis*) due to DNA damage by chemotherapy agents.

CHEMOTHERAPEUTIC DRUG CLASSES   The major classes of chemotherapeutic agents are alkylating agents, antimetabolites, antitumor antibiotics, plant derivatives, hormones and hormone antagonists, miscellaneous drugs, and biologic response modifiers. Table 12-6■ gives the classifications of chemotherapeutic drugs, common examples, target malignancies, adverse effects and side effects, and nursing implications.

TABLE 12-6	Giving Medications Safely: Selected Chemotherapeutic Drugs		
CLASS/DRUGS	**TARGET MALIGNANCIES**	**ADVERSE EFFECTS**	**NURSING IMPLICATIONS**
Alkylating Agents			
■ Mechlorethamine (Mustargen)	Hodgkin disease Lymphosarcoma Lung cancer Chronic leukemia	Nausea and vomiting Bone marrow depression Hyperuricemia	Maintain good hydration. Administer antiemetics before chemotherapy. Monitor CBC with differential, uric acid. Assess for infection, bleeding.
■ Busulfan (Myleran)	Chronic myelogenous leukemia	Bone marrow depression Kidney failure Pulmonary fibrosis	Monitor CBC, BUN, serum creatinine. Maintain adequate fluid intake. Assess for infection, bleeding. Assess lungs for coarse, loud crackles.
■ Cyclophosphamide (Cytoxan)	Lymphomas Multiple myeloma Leukemias Adenocarcinoma of lung and breast	Hemorrhagic cystitis Kidney failure Alopecia Stomatitis Liver dysfunction	Encourage daily fluid intake of 2–3 L during treatment. Monitor WBCs, BUN, serum creatinine, liver enzymes. Teach ways to manage hair loss.
Antimetabolites			
■ Methotrexate	Acute lymphoblastic leukemia Osteosarcoma Gestational trophoblastic carcinoma	Oral and gastrointestinal ulcerations Anorexia and nausea Bone marrow depression	Monitor CBC with differential, BUN, uric acid, creatinine. Assess oral mucous membranes; treat ulcers as needed (PRN). Assess for infection, bleeding.
■ 5-Fluorouracil (5-FU)	Colon carcinoma Rectal carcinoma Breast carcinoma Gastric carcinoma Pancreatic cancer	Stomatitis Alopecia Nausea and vomiting Gastritis Enteritis Diarrhea Bone marrow depression	Monitor CBC with differential, BUN, uric acid. Administer antiemetics PRN. Assess for infection, bleeding. Evaluate hydration and nutrition status. Teach oral care for stomatitis. Teach care for hair loss.
Antitumor Antibiotics			
■ Doxorubicin (Adriamycin)	Acute lymphoblastic leukemia (ALL) Acute myeloblastic leukemia Neuroblastoma Wilms tumor Breast, ovarian, thyroid, lung cancer	Stomatitis Alopecia Nausea and vomiting Gastritis Enteritis Diarrhea Bone marrow depression Cardiac toxicity Changes in urine color (red or orange)	Monitor ECG for dysrhythmias; assess for abnormal heart sounds, heart failure. Monitor CBC with differential, BUN, uric acid. Administer antiemetics PRN. Assess for infection, bleeding. Evaluate hydration and nutrition. Teach oral care for stomatitis. Teach care for hair loss.
■ Bleomycin (Blenoxane)	Squamous cell carcinoma Lymphosarcoma Reticulum cell sarcoma Testicular carcinoma Hodgkin disease	Mucocutaneous ulcerations Alopecia Nausea and vomiting Chills and fever Pneumonitis and pulmonary fibrosis	Check for fever 3–6 hours after administration. Monitor chest x-ray reports. Assess respiratory status, and report coarse crackles. Evaluate hydration and nutrition status. Teach oral care for stomatitis. Assess for infection. Teach care for hair loss.

(continued)

Table 12-6	Giving Medications Safely: Selected Chemotherapeutic Drugs *(continued)*		
CLASS/DRUGS	**TARGET MALIGNANCIES**	**ADVERSE EFFECTS**	**NURSING IMPLICATIONS**
Plant Alkaloids			
■ Vincristine (Oncovin)	Combination therapy for acute leukemia, Hodgkin and non-Hodgkin lymphomas, rhabdomyosarcoma, neuroblastoma, Wilms tumor	Areflexia Muscle weakness Peripheral neuritis Constipation Paralytic ileus Mild bone marrow depression	Assess neuromuscular function. Monitor CBC with differential. Evaluate gastrointestinal function. Manage constipation.
■ Vinblastine (Velban)	Combination therapy for Hodgkin disease, lymphocytic and histiocytic lymphoma, Kaposi sarcoma, advanced testicular carcinoma, unresponsive breast cancer	Areflexia Alopecia Nausea and vomiting Bone marrow depression	Assess neuromuscular function. Monitor CBC with differential. Administer antiemetics PRN. Teach ways to manage hair loss. Assess for infection, bleeding.
■ Etoposide, also called VP-16 (VePesid)	Nonresponsive testicular tumors Small-cell lung cancer	Alopecia Hypotension with rapid infusion	Hydrate adequately before administration. Administer over 60 minutes. Monitor vital signs every 15 minutes during administration and every 2–4 hours thereafter. Teach ways to manage hair loss.
■ Paclitaxel (Taxol)	Ovarian cancer, breast cancer, non–small-cell lung cancer, head and neck cancer	Hypersensitivity reactions including dyspnea, urticaria, flushing, and hypotension Cardiotoxicity Peripheral neuropathy Alopecia Mucositis Nausea and vomiting	Administer prophylactic histamine blockers. Monitor for dysrhythmias, chest pain, palpitations, and changes in hemodynamic status. Assess neuromuscular function. Teach care for hair loss. Teach oral care for stomatitis. Administer antiemetics PRN.
Hormones			
■ Prednisone	Combination therapy for many tumors Leukemia Lymphoma	Fluid retention Hypertension Steroid diabetes Emotional lability Silent bleeding ulcers Increased risk for infection	Monitor vital signs. Administer diuretics as ordered. Check blood glucose regularly. Evaluate mental status. Administer oral medications with food. Administer proton-pump inhibitors, H_2 blockers, and antacids as ordered. Monitor WBC with differential. Monitor for signs of systemic infection.
■ Diethylstilbestrol (DES)	Advanced breast and prostate cancers	Fluid retention Feminization Uterine bleeding	Monitor vital signs. Administer diuretics PRN as ordered. Explain reason for feminization to men, bleeding to women. Monitor for excessive bleeding.
Hormone Antagonist			
■ Tamoxifen (Nolvadex)	Breast cancer	Hot flashes Nausea and vomiting	Teach ways to manage hot flashes. Explain reason for hot flashes. Administer antiemetics as ordered.

CLASS/DRUGS	TARGET MALIGNANCIES	ADVERSE EFFECTS	NURSING IMPLICATIONS
Table 12-6	**Giving Medications Safely: Selected Chemotherapeutic Drugs** *(continued)*		
Miscellaneous Drugs			
■ Cisplatin (CDDP) (Platinol)	Combination and single therapy for metastatic testicular and ovarian cancers, advanced bladder cancer, head and neck tumors, non–small-cell lung carcinoma, osteogenic sarcoma, neuroblastoma	Bone marrow depression Renal tubular damage Deafness	Monitor WBC with differential and platelets, BUN, creatinine, uric acid. Monitor for signs of infection, bleeding. Evaluate hearing; check for tinnitus. Ensure that patient is well hydrated before administering. Encourage 2–3 L of fluid intake daily.
Biologic Response Modifiers			
■ Interferon-alfa-2 (Roferon-A) ■ Imatinib mesylate (Gleevec)	Leukemia	Nausea and vomiting Fatigue, weakness Anorexia rash Alopecia Hyperlipidemia	Administer prophylactic antiemetics. Explain fatigue and muscle weakness; teach ways to manage activities of daily living (ADLs). Teach oral care for stomatitis. Teach ways to manage hair loss. Instruct to maintain low-fat, low-cholesterol diet.

PREPARATION AND ADMINISTRATION Chemotherapy drugs can be administered orally, intramuscularly, intravenously, intrathecally (into the subarachnoid space), or by direct injection into the tumor itself or body cavities such as the peritoneal space or urinary bladder. They are prepared and given using specific safety guidelines to protect the health care worker.

Vascular access devices (VADs) are commonly used to administer chemotherapy drugs, especially when several cycles of treatment over weeks or months are required. These devices allow the drug to be injected into a large central vein, reducing local irritating effects of the drug on vein walls and the risk of *extravasation* of the drug into subcutaneous tissue. VADs are also used to administer parenteral nutrition, for pain management (see Chapter 8), or for frequent blood draws to monitor blood counts. Types of VADs include peripherally inserted central catheters (PICC lines); tunneled catheters into a major vein, such as a Hickman or Groshong catheter (Figure 12-7■); and surgically implanted ports, such as Mediport.

Chemotherapy generally is administered by RNs who are trained and certified in chemotherapy administration. Practical nurses frequently are responsible for monitoring adverse effects during and after chemotherapy administration. Box 12-8■ discusses chemotherapy and the older adult.

Biotherapy

Biotherapy uses medications to stimulate the patient's immune system to target and destroy cancer cells. Biologic response modifiers and immune therapies are used to treat solid tumors and hematologic cancer and are also used after bone marrow transplants. Biotherapy may be used in combination with chemotherapy. The types of drugs used for biotherapy include *interferons* (natural proteins produced by the immune system), *interleukin-2* (a substance that stimulates killer T cells, the immune cells that normally destroy

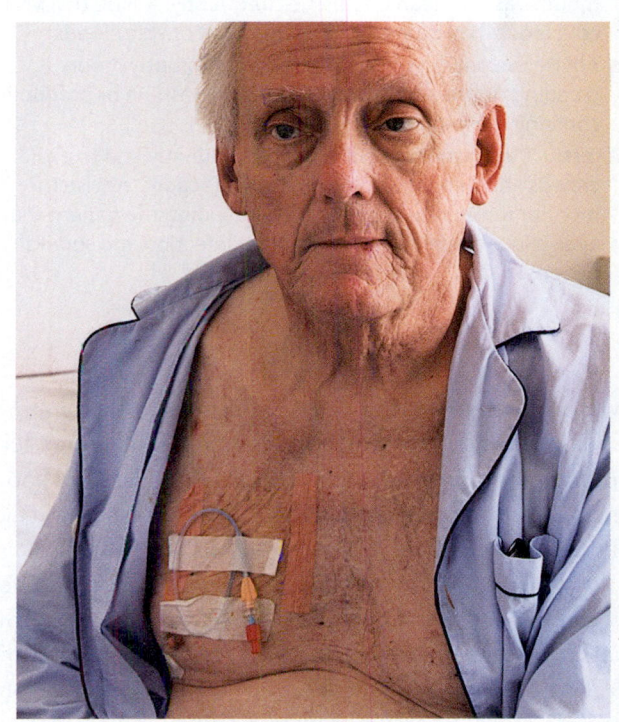

Figure 12-7. ■ A tunneled vascular access device (VAD) for long-term chemotherapy. (Source: Pearson Education.)

Chemotherapy

Physiologic and psychosocial changes commonly associated with aging can affect the older adult's responses to chemotherapy. Older adults may develop toxic effects at drug doses within normal or recommended ranges due to:

- Decreased liver enzyme activity that reduces drug metabolism.
- Lower serum albumin levels resulting in reduced protein binding and more free drug.
- Decreased kidney function and reduced drug elimination.

In addition, the ability of the bone marrow to recover and produce blood cells is reduced, increasing the risk for infection. Older adults are vulnerable to weight loss and poor nutrition due to reduced taste, early sensations of fullness, and lack of social interaction. When these normal factors are combined with the effects of chemotherapy (anorexia, nausea, mucositis, malaise, and fatigue), the older adult is at significant risk for malnutrition.

Psychosocial changes that are often seen with aging include reduced social interaction and increasing isolation. Transportation to a chemotherapy center may present challenges for the older adult who no longer drives. Depression is common in older adults. The older adult who lives alone may have difficulty maintaining activities of daily living (ADLs) while managing the adverse effects of chemotherapy.

Possible nursing interventions to address these problems include the following:

- Instruct the older adult to consume food and fluids throughout the day. Small meals are less fatiguing, easier to manage, and can help reduce nausea.
- Teach the patient to use a soft toothbrush and nondrying mouthwash to clean oral tissues frequently. Advise that very cold foods may be easier to eat than hot or spicy foods.
- Advise the patient to monitor for and promptly report bleeding or bruising and to avoid taking aspirin or products containing aspirin.
- Instruct the patient to wash hands frequently and to avoid crowds and people with respiratory infections. Advise to monitor temperature frequently, reminding the patient that even a low-grade fever may indicate infection and should be reported to the physician.

Biotherapy

Nursing Responsibilities

☑ Monitor for and document adverse effects: mental slowing, confusion, and lethargy; severe flu-like symptoms (chills and fever, nausea, vomiting, diarrhea, anorexia, severe fatigue); stomatitis; acute hypertension.

☑ Monitor and report abnormal results of renal and liver function tests, cardiac enzyme levels (CK, cardiac troponins).

☑ Assess for the desired response to therapy (e.g., reduced tumor manifestations).

☑ Assess coping and teach new strategies as needed.

☑ Monitor and manage fatigue and depression.

☑ Encourage self-care and participation in decision making.

☑ Closely supervise patients with altered mental functioning.

☑ Teach medication administration (subcutaneous injections, ambulatory pumps), equipment care, and site or catheter care to the patient and caregivers.

☑ Document assessments, nursing care, and teaching, including ability to demonstrate medication administration and catheter care.

Patient and Family Teaching

☑ Manage fever and flu-like symptoms: increase fluid intake, take analgesic and antipyretic medications, and maintain bed rest until symptoms abate.

☑ Notify care provider if unable to maintain fluid intake or manage symptoms.

hypersensitivity reactions including anaphylaxis, and acute changes in cardiac, pulmonary, liver, pancreatic, gastrointestinal, and mental functioning. Mental clouding, confusion, and lethargy may develop, particularly when biotherapies are combined with chemotherapy. Nursing care of patients receiving biotherapy is discussed in Box 12-9■.

Photodynamic Therapy

Photodynamic therapy uses light, usually delivered by a laser, to destroy certain superficial tumors (e.g., skin cancer, bladder cancer, and cancers of the lung, colon, and esophagus). A compound that increases the photosensitivity of cells to light is given intravenously 3 days before laser treatment. When subjected to the light, cells containing this compound are destroyed.

Although toxic effects are rare, the drug remains in tissues for 4 to 6 weeks after injection. Any direct or indirect exposure to sunlight activates the drug, resulting in a sunburn. Patients are taught to cover themselves with opaque clothing, including a wide-brimmed hat, gloves, shoes and stockings, as well as sunglasses with 100% ultraviolet block. Moisturizing lotions are used to help protect treated skin from trauma and irritation.

invading and abnormal cells), and *monoclonal antibodies* (proteins designed to target a specific type of tumor cell). Although interferons and interleukins stimulate the body's general immune response, monoclonal antibodies attack only the target cells.

As with other forms of cancer treatment, biotherapy can have serious adverse and toxic effects. Severe flu-like symptoms, with chills and fever of 103 to 106°F (39.4 to 41.1°C), may develop, as well as nausea, vomiting, diarrhea, anorexia, severe fatigue, and stomatitis. Potential toxic effects include bone marrow suppression,

Bone Marrow or Stem Cell Transplant

Bone marrow transplant (BMT) or *stem cell transplant (SCT)* often is used with or after chemotherapy or radiation, particularly in treating hematologic cancers. Hematopoietic stem cells are immature cells that have the ability to become erythrocytes (RBCs), leukocytes (WBCs), or thrombocytes (platelets) and to replace recipient's abnormal blood cells. They are found in bone marrow, umbilical cord blood, amniotic fluid, and in small amounts in peripheral blood. Treatment with hematopoietic growth factors (also called colony-stimulating factors) can boost the number of stem cells in a donor's peripheral blood, allowing stem cells to be collected from peripheral blood for transplantation (Appelbaum, 2012). When donor stem cells are infused intravenously, the cells migrate to the recipient's bone marrow to mature and replace the recipient's WBCs, RBCs, and platelets with cells derived from donor stem cells.

In an *allogeneic* transplant, stem cells of a healthy donor (often a sibling with closely matched tissue) are infused into the patient with the illness. Donor tissue must be closely matched with that of the recipient to prevent reaction between donor cells and the patient's cells. In *autologous* transplant, the patient's own stem cells are aspirated during a period of disease remission, frozen and stored, and then infused if the disease recurs.

Before BMT or SCT, high doses of chemotherapy and/or total-body irradiation are used to destroy malignant cells in the bone marrow. The stem cells are then infused through a central venous line. Before and immediately after BMT or SCT, the patient is critically ill and at significant risk for infection and bleeding due to depletion of WBCs and platelets.

GRAFT-VERSUS-HOST DISEASE   Allogeneic BMT or SCT may precipitate *graft-versus-host disease (GVHD)*, which develops when immune cells of the donated bone marrow identify the recipient's body tissue as foreign (see Chapter 11). Consequently, T cells in the donated marrow attack the liver, skin, and gastrointestinal tract, causing skin rashes and sloughing, diarrhea, gastrointestinal bleeding, and liver damage. *Acute GVHD* develops within days of transplantation, whereas *chronic GVHD* develops later, 100 or more days after transplantation. GVHD is treated with antibiotics and steroids; immunosuppressive drugs also may be used if necessary.

Complementary Therapies

Although advances in cancer treatment have increased the 5-year survival rate, the uncertainty of cure often causes patients to look for complementary and alternative therapies. It is estimated that approximately 30% to 50% of patients with cancer may have used some kind of complementary therapies, which are increasingly accepted as appropriate adjuncts to traditional medical care. Common complementary therapies for cancer include botanicals, nutritional supplements, dietary regimens, mind–body modalities, spiritual approaches, and miscellaneous therapies. Box 12-10■ provides information about commonly used complementary therapies.

Nurses need to understand common complementary therapies because these therapies can affect the patient's response to prescribed treatments. It is also important for nurses to provide truthful, nonjudgmental responses to questions or inquiries about complementary therapies from patients with cancer. Nurses should encourage patients to report the use of any complementary therapies to their primary care provider and oncologist to prevent harmful interactions of the therapies with their medical treatment plan.

NURSING CARE

> **Key Concept**   Nursing care for the patient with cancer is holistic, multidimensional, and ongoing as the patient's and family's needs change over the course of the disease and its treatment.

Nursing care for the patient with cancer occurs in a variety of settings, including ambulatory care, acute and long-term care, the home, and hospice settings. The LPN/LVN is an integral member of the health care team and plays an important role in caring for patients with cancer. Practical nurses are responsible for conducting focused assessments of the patient, contributing to the identification of nursing care problems and care planning, delivering direct care, providing and reinforcing patient and family teaching, and contributing to evaluation of the effectiveness of care.

PRIORITIZING NURSING CARE

Physiologic needs are the priority for nursing care; however, it is important to remember that patients with cancer and their families also have significant psychosocial and emotional needs. Once a cancer diagnosis is established, nurses assist and support patients during their treatment, recovery, and rehabilitation. When cure is not possible, care and comfort for the patient and significant others during the dying process is the priority of care.

HEALTH PROMOTION

Nurses can play an instrumental role in reducing the incidence of cancer. Nurses should educate all patients about cancer risk factors, as well as lifestyle changes to reduce their risk. The risk for some cancers, including those related to the use of tobacco (smoking and smokeless tobacco) and heavy alcohol consumption could be nearly eliminated by avoiding use of these products. Cancers related to infections

BOX 12-10	COMPLEMENTARY THERAPIES

Patients With Cancer

TYPES AND EXAMPLES	DESCRIPTIONS
Botanicals: echinacea, Essiac, ginseng, green tea, pau d'arco, and Hoxsey	Although herbs are believed to be "natural" and safe, the safety of many botanicals hasn't been proved, especially used in conjunction with medical treatment.
Nutritional supplements: vitamins, minerals, enzymes, amino acids, essential fatty acids, and proteins (such as shark cartilage)	Nutritional supplements are believed to promote health and to help cure cancer. The safety of compounds such as vitamins is established; however, in megadoses, many nutritional supplements can be toxic and may interact with therapeutic agents such as chemotherapy.
Dietary regimens: grape diet, carrot juice diet, garlic, onions, and liver	The ingestion of only natural substances is believed to purify the body and slow the growth of cancer. The effectiveness of these dietary regimens still needs to be established.
Mind–body modalities: relaxation, meditation, or imagery	The harmony of mind and body is believed to promote physiologic and psychologic healing. Research has shown that these modalities helped patients adjust to the experience of cancer.
Energy healing: therapeutic touch and healing touch	The human body is believed to be an energy field and cancer the result of a disturbed energy field. Energy therapies promote healing by treating the body's energy field. Clinical practice and research has shown positive effects of energy healing for a variety of patients.
Spiritual approaches: faith healing, prayer, prayer groups or chains	Faith in God or a higher power of the universe is believed to promote healing. Research has shown that faith in God or a higher power also helped people with cancer to adjust to the experience of cancer.
Miscellaneous therapies	Aromatherapy has been used to relieve nausea, vomiting, or retching and to decrease anxiety. Music, art, and humor therapies have also been used to help reduce anxiety, express feelings of loss, and promote optimism.

such as hepatitis B and HPV can be prevented through immunization and lifestyle modifications. An estimated one-third of cancer deaths are believed to be related to overweight or obesity, physical inactivity, and poor nutrition (American Cancer Society, 2013a). The risk for developing skin cancer, including malignant melanoma, can be significantly reduced by protection from the sun's rays (hats, clothing, sunscreen) and avoiding indoor tanning.

The ACS makes specific recommendations for cancer prevention. Based on these recommendations, nurses should provide the following teaching:

- Avoid tobacco use, secondhand smoke, and excessive alcohol use.
- Eat a variety of healthy foods, primarily from plant sources (whole grains, fruits, and vegetables); limit consumption of red meats and processed meats.
- Maintain a healthy weight; if overweight or obese, lose weight.
- Limit exposure to ionizing radiation (x-rays, radon) and ultraviolet (UV) radiation from the sun.

- Whenever possible, avoid exposure to known and potential carcinogenic chemicals such as benzene, asbestos, vinyl chloride, arsenic, and others. If employed in an industry where such chemicals are used, use personal protective equipment and devices to limit exposure.
- Limit exposure to viral diseases associated with certain cancers by using safer sex practices (see Chapter 33) and avoiding use of recreational and illicit drugs.
- Improve immunity by maintaining a healthy lifestyle and managing stress.
- Follow Centers for Disease Control and Prevention (CDC) guidelines for obtaining immunizations for hepatitis B and HPV as appropriate.

Teach patients about cancer screening recommendations for early detection and removal of precancerous and early malignant growths. Tumors of the cervix, colon, and rectum can be prevented by removing precancerous tissue when it is detected. Cancers of the breast, colon, rectum, mouth, and skin can be detected and treated early, increasing chances for cure and reducing mortality (American Cancer Society, 2012b).

ASSESSING

LPNs/LVNs conduct focused assessments to evaluate the responses of patients with cancer to the disease and its treatment. It is important to be alert for evidence of disease progression or complications, adverse effects of treatment, and manifestations of psychosocial or spiritual distress.

Subjective Data

During a focused interview, the nurse collects significant data, including:

- History of the disease, including signs and symptoms that led the patient to seek health care.
- Current symptoms or problems related to the disease or treatment, such as pain, nausea, or constipation.
- Other current or chronic diseases, such as diabetes; current medications.
- Any known allergies to drugs, foods, or other substances.
- Understanding and expectations of the treatment plan.
- Effect of the disease or treatment on current lifestyle and family responsibilities and relationships.
- Support systems or caregivers the patient can rely on.
- Coping strategies and how well they are working; effective coping strategies used in the past.
- The presence of an advance directive and, as appropriate, end-of-life decisions such as designated caregivers, knowledge of hospice care, presence of a will, and desires for a service and burial or cremation.

Objective Data

A complete physical assessment is conducted to establish a baseline against which to evaluate later changes. It is especially important to document current general health status, manifestations, nutritional status, hydration, and laboratory results.

- Apparent state of health, alertness, interaction; voice quality and pattern of speaking; posture, muscle mass, weight for height; ability to move, sit easily; use of any assistive devices
- Vital signs including temperature; current weight; intake and output
- Skin and mucous membranes: color, moisture, temperature and condition; condition of hair and nails; skin turgor; presence of lesions, *petechiae* (small red spots that do not blanch with pressure), bruises, areas of inflammation (red, hot, tender)
- Cardiopulmonary: respiratory pattern and ease, lung sounds; heart rate, rhythm, and sounds; strength and equality of peripheral pulses; color and temperature of extremities, capillary refill; presence of edema
- Abdomen: shape, contour; bowel sounds; presence of tenderness to light palpation; visible or palpable swelling or masses

- Laboratory data: CBC including differential and platelet count; serum electrolytes, osmolality, albumin and total protein, BUN and creatinine, glucose, bilirubin, liver enzymes; urinalysis; specific tests for organ function or cancer markers

IDENTIFYING POTENTIAL COMPLICATIONS

Both cancer and its treatment can lead to complications such as infection, compression of vital structures and organs, and altered homeostasis. See the section on oncologic emergencies at the end of this chapter for more information about potential complications and their manifestations.

DIAGNOSING, PLANNING, AND IMPLEMENTING

The goals of nursing care for patients with cancer focus on providing support and managing specific physical and emotional responses to the disease and its treatment. When cure is not possible, nurses provide care and comfort for the patient and significant others during the dying process. Nursing care includes the whole family from the onset of diagnosis through treatment and the ultimate outcome. Only the most common diagnoses are discussed here.

Acute Pain and Chronic Pain

Expected outcome: Will rate pain at a level of 1 to 2 (on a 0 to 10 scale) on a continual basis.

- Frequently assess comfort and the effectiveness of current measures, using a standardized pain scale (see Chapter 8). *Changes in tumor size with treatment or lack of response to treatment, as well as therapies to treat cancer, can affect the amount and type of pain experienced by the patient. Continuing assessment is necessary to ensure effective pain relief.*
- Administer prescribed medications in combination and to the necessary prescribed dose to maintain comfort, prevent breakthrough pain, and allow desired level of function. *A combination of medications, including nonsteroidal anti-inflammatory drugs and mild (e.g., oxycodone) to potent (e.g., morphine, hydromorphone) narcotic analgesics may be required to manage the patient's pain. Providing pain relief at the level desired allows the patient to maintain control and function at an optimal level.*
- Administer analgesics on a regular schedule (e.g., every 4 hours) with additional medication to cover breakthrough pain. *A regular schedule of medication will provide the patient with more effective pain relief.*
- Closely monitor the patient receiving analgesia per patient-controlled analgesia (PCA), continuous drip, pump, or alternate mechanism for effective pain relief and manifestations of toxicity or overdose. *Although PCA and analgesic pumps are very safe and well controlled, frequent assessment of the drug effects on the patient is necessary to ensure safe and effective care.*

- Teach the patient and family how to effectively manage the prescribed analgesic regimen and potential adverse effects of the drugs (e.g., constipation). Discuss specific precautions, such as removing old transdermal patches before applying new ones and avoiding heat applications over the transdermal patch. *Patients and their families or caregivers will assume primary responsibility for effective analgesic management. They must understand common potential adverse effects and their management, as well as the risks for and manifestations of drug toxicity.*

Ineffective Protection

Expected outcome: Will remain free of signs of infection and hemorrhage.

- Monitor vital signs, including temperature. *Fever and sympathetic nervous system responses, such as increased pulse and respiration, are common early signs of infection.*

clinicalALERT

Severely immunosuppressed patients may have infection without fever.

- Monitor blood cell counts frequently, especially when bone marrow suppression is a risk due to chemotherapy. *Early identification and reporting of decreasing blood cell counts allow institution of infection or bleeding precautions and corrective actions.*
- Teach the patient and significant others to avoid crowds, small children, and people with infections when the WBC count is low and to practice careful personal hygiene. *During periods of leukopenia, even minor infections can be very dangerous. The immunosuppressed patient also is susceptible to opportunistic infections from normal host organisms.*
- Protect skin and mucous membranes from injury. Teach hygiene measures, use of moisturizing lotion to prevent dryness and cracking, frequent position changes, and immediate attention to skin breaks or lesions. *Intact skin is the first line of defense against infection.*
- Encourage a balanced diet high in protein, minerals, and vitamins. *Improved nutrition decreases the risk of infection.*
- Monitor vital signs and assess for obvious or occult bleeding: excessive bruising; bleeding oral mucous membranes; emesis, stool, and urine for visible or occult blood; vaginal bleeding; prolonged bleeding from puncture sites; neurologic or mental status changes; complaints of abdominal pain, diminished bowel sounds. *Early identification of bleeding helps prevent significant blood loss and potential shock.*
- Avoid invasive procedures such as rectal suppositories, urinary catheterization, and parenteral injections if possible. Diagnostic procedures such as biopsy or lumbar puncture should not be done if the platelet count is less than 50,000. *Invasive procedures can cause tissue trauma and bleeding. Procedures that use large-bore needles should be delayed until the platelet count is increased.*
- Apply pressure to injection sites for 3 to 5 minutes, and to arterial punctures for 15 to 20 minutes. *Pressure prevents prolonged bleeding by prompting hemostasis and clot formation.*
- Instruct to avoid picking or forcefully blowing the nose, forceful coughing or sneezing, and straining to have a bowel movement. *These activities can damage mucous membranes, increasing the risk for bleeding.*

Risk for Injury

Expected outcome: Will remain free of injury or adverse effects of treatment.

- Assess frequently for manifestations of obstruction or organ dysfunction (e.g., the brain, lungs, liver, or urinary system). *Early detection allows medical intervention before the problem becomes a crisis.*
- Teach the patient and family to differentiate minor from serious problems. Box 12-11■ provides guidelines to identify problems that must be reported or that require emergency services. *Guidelines for when to call the doctor*

BOX 12-11	PATIENT TEACHING

When to Call for Help

Instruct the patient or family member to call when:

- Oral temperature greater than 101.5°F (38.6°C)
- Severe headache; significant increase in pain at usual site, especially if the pain is not relieved by prescribed medications; or severe pain at a new site
- Difficulty breathing
- New bleeding from any site, such as rectal or vaginal bleeding
- Confusion, irritability, or restlessness
- Withdrawal, greatly decreased activity level, or frequent crying
- Verbalizations of deep sadness or a desire to end life
- Changes in body functioning, such as inability to void or severe diarrhea or constipation
- Changes in eating patterns, such as refusal to eat, extreme hunger, or a significant increase in nausea and vomiting
- Edema in the extremities or significant increase in edema already present

Instruct to call 911 if the patient:

- Is having significant difficulty breathing or if the lips or face has a bluish tinge.
- Becomes unconscious or has a convulsion.
- Exhibits unmanageable behavior, such as being physically abusive, hurting self, or engaging in uncontrollable activity.

provide an anxiety-reducing safety net for the patient and family and promote early detection of complications.

■ Monitor laboratory values; report abnormal findings or significant changes to physicians immediately. *If the cancer impairs organ function or creates ectopic sites of hormone production, laboratory values provide an early indication of this development and are reported so treatment can be instituted to restore homeostasis.*

Imbalanced Nutrition: Less Than Body Requirements

Expected outcome: Will achieve and maintain balanced nutrition.

■ Assess current eating patterns, including likes and dislikes, and identify factors that impair food intake. *This permits an individualized plan based on the patient's needs and preferences.*

■ Evaluate for malnutrition using height–weight charts, skin-fold measurements, body mass (see Chapters 24 and 25), and laboratory values for total serum protein, serum albumin and globins, total lymphocyte count, serum transferrin, hemoglobin, and hematocrit. *These data provide an objective determination of nutritional status.*

■ Teach ways of maintaining good nutrition by using ChooseMyPlate (available at ChooseMyPlate website) and adapting to any medical restrictions and preferences. *Patients comply better with food plans that are tailored to their needs.*

■ Manage problems that interfere with eating:

  ■ Encourage the patient with food aversions to eat whatever is appealing. *It is better for the patient to eat something to maintain calorie intake, even if it is not nutritionally balanced.*

  ■ Eat small, frequent meals. *These are more easily digested and absorbed and usually better tolerated by the patient with anorexia.*

  ■ Encourage to try icy-cold foods (such as ice cream) or more highly seasoned dishes if food has no taste. *Chemotherapy and radiation therapy may harm taste buds. Strong seasonings and coldness make food more enjoyable.*

  ■ Encourage cold, bland, semisoft, and liquid foods for the patient with stomatitis. Have the patient use an anesthetic mouthwash before eating. *These foods are less irritating to sensitive mucous membranes. Reducing discomfort with a local anesthetic can make chewing and swallowing easier.*

  ■ Administer antiemetic medications. Encourage low-fat meals with dry foods such as crackers and toast; to avoid liquids with meals; and to sit upright for an hour after meals. Remove emesis basins and encourage oral hygiene before eating. *Dry, low-fat foods are more readily tolerated by the nauseated patient. Removing odors*

and supplies associated with nausea and vomiting can reduce nausea.

■ Encourage use of nutritional supplements (Ensure, Isocal) and multivitamin and mineral tablets with meals. Suggest increasing calories by adding ice cream or frozen yogurt to the liquid supplement or commercial protein–carbohydrate powders to milk or fruit juice. *Food intake of most cancer patients is less than what is needed to maintain or gain weight. These supplements can add calories and nutrients in a manner often tolerated by the patient.*

■ Teach to keep a food diary to document daily intake. *When patients see how little is being consumed, they may eat more. A food diary also helps the nurse keep a calorie count and alerts the physician if more drastic nutritional measures, such as parenteral nutrition, need to be considered.*

Impaired Oral Mucous Membranes

Expected outcome: Oral mucous membranes will remain intact without evidence of inflammation.

■ Carefully assess and evaluate for manifestations, including: ulcerations on the tongue and oropharyngeal mucosa; herpes simplex type 1 lesions (cold sores); a white, yellow, or tan coating with dry, red, fissured tissue underneath indicative of a fungal infection (*Candida*); red, swollen, gums that bleed with minimal or no trauma; or *xerostomia* (excessive dryness of the oral mucous membranes). *Accurate assessment and documentation are vital for care planning by the interdisciplinary team.*

■ Instruct to clean teeth gently in the morning, after meals, and at bedtime. Use a very soft toothbrush, and obtain a new toothbrush monthly. If gums are bleeding, clean teeth with toothpaste and a soft cloth held over a finger. Floss gently with waxed floss (unless contraindicated by risk for bleeding), and use a non-alcohol-based mouthwash after brushing. Dentures should be soaked nightly in hydrogen peroxide. *Disrupted tissues allow normal oral bacteria into the circulation, potentially leading to sepsis in the immunocompromised person. Reducing oral flora by frequent hygiene decreases the risk of infection.*

■ Culture any oral lesions, and report the problem to physician. *Identifying the cause of the infection, whether viral, fungal, or bacterial, allows appropriate treatment to be initiated.*

■ Advise the patient with xerostomia to use lubricating and moisturizing agents. Avoid putting sharp instruments or utensils in the mouth. Advise to have necessary dental work done by a dental oncologist. Chlorhexidine mouthwash (Peridex) may be used. *These measures protect gums from trauma and decrease risk of hemorrhage.*

■ Administer medications as ordered: acyclovir (viral infections), systemic antibiotics (bacterial infections), Nystatin or clotrimazole solution or lozenges (fungal infections), viscous lidocaine or combination mouthwashes before meals and as needed. *These agents reduce pain and inflammation. Knowing the contents of each mouthwash can prevent hypersensitivity reactions (e.g., to lidocaine).*

Anxiety

Expected outcome: Will report anxiety is within manageable range.

Patients with cancer, especially those with poor coping skills, may exhibit overt signs of anxiety, such as trembling, irritability, increased blood pressure, pallor, or poor eye contact. The patient may report insomnia and feelings of tension, or express concerns about perceived changes caused by the disease and fear of future events.

■ Carefully assess the level of anxiety versus the real threats of the current situation. *A patient in panic may need medical intervention with appropriate medications. Moderate or even severe anxiety often can be managed through listening, counseling, and teaching new skills.*

■ Convey warmth and empathy and listen nonjudgmentally. *A patient who feels safe will more easily express feelings and thoughts and may be more willing to try new behaviors as suggested.*

■ Encourage the patient to acknowledge and express feelings, no matter how inappropriate they may seem. *Acknowledging and expressing feelings help diminish anxiety and direct energy toward healing, as well as lay the groundwork for new coping behaviors.*

■ Review past coping strategies and introduce new strategies as appropriate. Explain why inappropriate strategies (repressing anger, turning to alcohol) are not helpful. *The patient will be more willing to build on strategies that worked in the past and may be more able to reject inappropriate strategies if shown why they did not work in past crises.*

■ Identify community resources, such as crisis hotlines and support groups. *The patient's support systems may be lacking or having their own difficulties dealing with the cancer diagnosis. Programs such as "I Can Cope," sponsored by the ACS, provide education, counseling, and support in a group setting with other cancer patients.*

■ Provide specific information about the disease, treatment, and what may be expected, especially for those patients with obvious misinformation. Avoid advice and false reassurance. *Knowing what to expect gives the patient a sense of control and the ability to make decisions. Discussions about symptom management as part of the treatment plan can significantly relieve anxiety.*

■ Provide a safe, calm, and quiet environment for the patient in panic. Stay with the patient, and administer antianxiety medications as ordered. *Being present and displaying calmness and confidence can protect the patient from injury and prevent further panic. If the panic does not subside, report to the physician for medication management.*

■ Use crisis intervention strategies to promote growth in the patient and significant others, regardless of the outcome of the disease. A referral to a mental health professional may be helpful. *With help, people can transform a major crisis from an experience of defeat and despair to one of personal and spiritual growth.*

Readiness for Enhanced Knowledge

Expected outcome: Will relate an understanding of the disease, treatment options, and anticipated effects.

The nurse plays an important role in preparing patients with cancer and their families for planned cancer treatment strategies such as surgery or chemotherapy.

■ Before surgery, provide the opportunity to ask questions and to discuss concerns and fears. *In some cases, the patient may want to discuss alternative treatment options that are available.*

■ Explain the specific surgical procedure and any anticipated alterations to the patient's body. *Some surgeries will require major lifestyle adjustments, such as a colostomy.*

■ Before surgery, coordinate a conference for the patient with the oncologist and surgeon. *This will provide an opportunity to clarify the planned surgery and follow-up treatment.*

■ When a vascular access device (VAD) is inserted, teach patients and family members to observe for redness, swelling, pain, or exudate at the insertion site and swelling of the neck or skin near the VAD. Teach how to flush catheters and provide site care on a regular basis. *The risk of infection, catheter obstruction, and extravasation of fluid into surrounding tissue are the main problems associated with VADs.*

■ Instruct the patient and family members to assess and monitor for signs and symptoms of toxic side effects of chemotherapy. *This will alert the nurse to the onset of toxicity. Indicators of organ toxicities, such as nephrotoxicity or cardiac toxicity, must be reported immediately to the physician.*

■ Teach patients undergoing chemotherapy to dispose of used equipment and excretions safely. *Excretion of chemotherapy is primarily through the urine.*

Disturbed Body Image

Expected outcome: Will acknowledge impact of disease and change in appearance on personal relationships and roles.

■ Discuss the meaning of the loss or change for the patient. *A seemingly trivial loss may have a big impact on the patient's life. Likewise, a major loss may not be as important as the nurse imagines. The nurse must evaluate each situation in terms of the reactions of the specific patient.*

■ Observe and evaluate the patient's interaction with significant others. *People may unintentionally reinforce negative feelings about body image or the patient may perceive rejection where none exists.*

■ If appropriate, allow the patient to engage in denial, but do not participate in it. (If a patient won't look at the wound, the nurse may say, "I am going to change the dressing to your breast incision now.") *Denial is a protective mechanism and should not be challenged, but it also should not be promoted. A matter-of-fact and empathetic attitude will help the patient accept the change.*

■ Encourage the patient and significant others to express their feelings about the situation and to identify new coping strategies. Give matter-of-fact responses to questions and concerns, and enlist family and friends in reaffirming the patient's worth. *A supportive, safe environment promotes acceptance and encourages new coping strategies. It also reaffirms that the patient's worth is not lessened by physical changes.*

■ Teach the patient or significant others to participate in care of the affected body area. Support and validate their efforts. *Active involvement in providing care empowers the patient and significant others, promotes closeness, and reduces the risk of rejection. Positive reinforcement encourages these behaviors to continue.*

■ Teach specific strategies for minimizing physical changes (skin care during radiation therapy, dressing to enhance appearance and disguise change in a body part). *Early intervention can limit negative effects and promote recovery. Involvement gives the patient some control in a difficult situation.*

■ Teach ways to reduce the *alopecia* (hair loss) from chemotherapy or radiation therapy and to enhance appearance until hair grows back:

  ■ Discuss the pattern and timing of hair loss. *This allows the patient to plan for and cope with changes and incorporate coping strategies into daily activities.*

  ■ Encourage the patient to wear cheerful head coverings, coordinated with usual clothing. *Attractive head coverings protect the head while allowing the patient to feel attractive and well dressed.*

  ■ Advise that hair will grow back after chemotherapy, but that its color and texture may be different. Refer the patient to a good wig shop before hair loss occurs. *Hair color and texture can be matched to minimize obvious changes in appearance. The patient who knows what to expect may experience less anxiety and distress.*

  ■ Refer the patient to support programs such as "Look Good . . . . Feel Better," sponsored by the ACS and the Cosmetic, Toiletry, and Fragrance Association Foundation. *A support group can diminish feelings of isolation and provide practical tips for managing problems. For a list of community resources available to patients with cancer, refer to a local community resource guide or phone book.*

Grieving

Expected outcome: Patient and family demonstrate the ability to make mutual decisions regarding anticipated loss.

■ Use active listening, silence, and nonverbal support to provide an open environment to discuss feelings realistically and to express anger or other negative feelings. *This helps the patient and family members express feelings and confront the possibility of the loss or death. Although 68% of people with cancer recover, facing death and making preparations can be a healthy response that allows the patient and family to work through the dying process and achieve growth (see Chapter 13) or to cope with changes in body image and lifestyle.*

■ Answer questions about illness and prognosis honestly, always encouraging hope. *This allows realistic assessment of and planning for their situation. It also helps combat feelings of hopelessness and depression.*

■ When cure is no longer an option and the disease is terminal, discuss hospice care with the patient and family. *Hospice services provide support and comfort for the patient and family, promoting their sense of control through the dying process.*

■ Encourage the dying patient to make funeral and burial plans ahead of time and to be sure the will is in order. Make sure the necessary phone numbers can be easily located. *This gives the patient a sense of control and frees family members of these concerns when the patient is most in need of their support.*

■ Encourage the patient to continue taking part in activities he or she enjoys, including keeping a job as long as possible. *The patient keeps a sense of continuity of life even in the face of severe losses.*

NURSING CARE MANAGEMENT

Assistive personnel often provide much of the patient's direct care needs when family or significant others are unavailable or unable to provide care. The nurse also may assign nursing care activities such as measuring intake and output, obtaining daily weights, and providing oral and skin care for the patient with cancer.

EVALUATING

Cancer is not a static disease. The patient's nursing care needs change over the course of the disease and its treatment. Evaluate the effectiveness of nursing care for the patient with cancer through ongoing assessment and care planning. Measures that are ineffective, such as pain management, will need to be changed or modified and the effectiveness evaluated over time. The family or significant others can also provide data about the effectiveness of the plan of care.

DOCUMENTING

Cancer is a chronic condition, requiring lengthy treatment. Initial and ongoing documentation of assessment data, plans of care and interdisciplinary interventions, and the effectiveness of these interventions is vital. Carefully document any changes in assessment data and responses to those changes (such as modification of the treatment plan or nursing care plan). Document the patient's and family's psychologic responses and coping strategies throughout the process. Document all teaching provided and the patient's and family's apparent understanding and acceptance of information. Note when reinforcement of teaching is necessary.

CONTINUITY OF CARE

Carefully review home care instructions with the patient and family, making sure they understand medications to be taken, any necessary treatments, and when to see the doctor for follow-up care. Provide or order equipment and supplies needed for home care, especially any special bed or equipment for mobility and safety in the home. Discuss problems that may result from the type of cancer and the treatment received. Provide information on how to manage these problems and when to call the physician. Teach wound care for the patient with an open wound or draining lesion. Explain special diets clearly, or refer the patient to a dietitian before discharge. For the patient with complex care needs, such as parenteral nutrition or continuous medication infusion, provide a referral to a home health nurse before discharge. Because the hospital stay is often short, make follow-up phone calls for several days after discharge, and provide a number to call for concerns and questions.

Rehabilitation

Rehabilitation from cancer involves regaining strength and function, recovering from surgery or chemotherapy, learning to live with an altered body part or appliance, and recovery from associated psychologic and emotional turmoil. Cancer survivors need to learn how to minimize their risk for and identify symptoms of potential long-term effects of cancer and its treatment.

Most patients convalesce at home, with the support of nursing assessment and counseling, direct care, and teaching. Hygiene and home maintenance can be provided by a certified home health aide. Physical and occupational therapists provide muscle strengthening, mobility training (especially with prostheses), and home safety teaching.

Psychologic rehabilitation of cancer survivors addresses quality-of-life issues. Employment and insurance may be difficult to get after a diagnosis of cancer. Relationships may have suffered from the strain the illness placed on significant others and the essential self-focusing required for recovery. In contrast, both the patient and significant others may have undergone personal and spiritual growth leading to a new and enriching period of their lives.

It is important for nurses to remember that patients may have questions about sexual relations during and after cancer treatment, but may not be comfortable asking specific questions. The nurse can raise the topic by asking the patient, "Are you sexually active?" If the response is no, the nurse should follow up by asking, "Is this by choice?" It is important not to assume that because a patient is older, widowed, or single, sexuality is not a concern.

Self-help groups are available in many communities to support people through the cancer experience. Patients and families need to be informed about the many resources that are available through community agencies as well as the survivor support groups.

Hospice Care

Hospice care allows cancer patients with terminal disease to die at home or in a home-like setting. When a patient and family choose hospice care, they are usually deciding against additional hospitalizations, except those required to manage reversible problems. Hospice patients also refuse resuscitation measures (see Chapter 13). The multidisciplinary hospice team usually includes:

- A nurse case manager, who works directly with the patient and family, and coordinates the activities of the other disciplines. The nurse or a designated on-call nurse familiar with the patient is usually available 24 hours a day and makes home visits frequently. The nurse is often with the family when the patient dies.
- A physician, who collaborates with the nurse case manager about medications and treatments and may make periodic home visits.
- An anesthesiologist or pharmacist to manage pain control and watch for drug interactions.
- An infusion therapist, who provides equipment, supplies, solutions, and expertise for intravenous medications or nutrition. This person is usually on call 24 hours a day to troubleshoot equipment problems.
- A social worker, who helps identify resources and who assists with grief work, general support, and counseling as needed.
- A physical therapist, who teaches safe procedures for mobility and moving the patient.
- A home health aide, who provides physical care and assists the family with household chores.
- Volunteers, who provide companionship for the patient and respite to the family for short periods of time.

Many hospice services are connected with an inpatient respite care unit, where the patient can receive 24-hour care for up to several weeks. This source provides the necessary care to the patient if a family member becomes ill or needs to be relieved temporarily of the tremendous burden of caring for a dying loved one. Patients who do not have family available for support during the dying process may be admitted to a "hospice house," a homelike setting in which the patient receives care and hospice support.

NURSING CARE PLAN
Patient With Terminal Cancer

James Casey is a 72-year-old man who has been under medical care for chronic obstructive pulmonary disease, post-myocardial infarction, and type 2 diabetes mellitus for over 15 years. He lost his wife to lung cancer 5 years ago and still "misses her terribly." He reports smoking two packs of cigarettes a day for 52 years and consuming one to two six-packs of beer a week, one "bourbon and water" a night, and "a lot of sugar-free junk food." He quit smoking 2 years ago, when he could no longer walk a block without considerable shortness of breath, and just quit drinking alcohol a few weeks ago at his physician's insistence. About a year ago, he had a basal-cell carcinoma removed from his right ear. Six months ago, he underwent two 6-week courses of chemotherapy for bladder cancer. The latest report indicates that the cancer has returned and no further chemotherapy would be useful. Surgery was considered, but his other medical problems would compromise his chances of survival, so Mr. Casey decided to forgo further treatment and to be managed at home through hospice care. His daughter, Mary Walsh, and her family have moved in with him to provide care and support during his final months. The daughter says she is glad to be able to spend this time with her father. She has been informed of the physical and emotional stress this will entail.

Assessment

The hospice nurse, Ms. Jackson, completes a health history and physical examination during her first two home visits. She gathers this information over 2 days to conserve his strength and allow more time for him and his daughter to talk about their concerns.

During the assessment, Ms. Jackson notes that Mr. Casey is pale and thin, with a wasted appearance and a worried facial expression. His blood pressure is 90/50; apical pulse is 102 and regular; respiratory rate 24; breath sounds are clear but diminished in the bases; and oral temperature is 96.8°F.

Mr. Casey states that he spends most of his time either in bed or sitting up in a chair in his room. He says he has no energy and is unable to walk to the bathroom alone or take care of his own personal hygiene. He complains of severe back pain no longer adequately relieved by alternating Percodan and Vicodin every 2 to 4 hours. The nurse rates Mr. Casey's functional level as capable of only limited self-care, confined to bed or chair 50% or more of waking hours. He tells the nurse that his daughter "is working day and night to help me and is looking awfully tired."

Ms. Walsh reports that Mr. Casey is eating very poorly: He has a small bowl of oatmeal for breakfast, soup and crackers for lunch, and only fruit juice for dinner. Mr. Casey says that he has no appetite and eats just to please his daughter. He does drink at least three to four glasses of water a day plus juice. His finger-stick blood sugars remain within normal range. His current weight is 120 lb, down from 180 lb a year ago. He has lost about 30 lb over the last 2 months.

Laboratory values from his visit with the doctor show the following:

Total protein: 4.1 (normal range: 6.0 to 8.0 g/dL)
Albumin: 2.2 (normal range: 3.5 to 5.0 g/dL)
Hemoglobin: 10.2 (normal range: 13.5 to 18.0 g/dL)
Hematocrit: 30.5 (normal range: 40.0% to 54.0%)
Blood urea nitrogen (BUN): 30 (normal range: 5 to 25 mg/dL, slightly higher in older people)
Creatinine: 2.2 (normal range: 0.5 to 1.5 mg/dL)

Nursing Diagnosis

The nursing diagnoses (among others) for Mr. Casey (and significant others) include the following:

- *Imbalanced Nutrition: Less Than Body Requirements* related to anorexia and fatigue
- *Risk for Caregiver Role Strain* related to severity of her father's illness and lack of help from other family members
- *Chronic Pain* related to progression of disease process
- *Impaired Physical Mobility* related to pain, fatigue, and beginning neuromuscular impairment
- *Risk for Impaired Skin Integrity* related to impaired physical mobility and malnourished state

Expected Outcomes

The expected outcomes established in the plan of care specify that:

- Mr. Casey will increase his oral intake and show improvement in his serum protein values.
- His daughter will be able to maintain her supportive caregiving activities as long as Mr. Casey needs them.
- Mr. Casey will have minimal pain for the rest of his life.
- Mr. Casey will be able to continue his current activity level.
- Mr. Casey will have intact skin.

Planning and Implementation

The following interventions are planned and implemented during Mr. Casey's care:

- Ask Mr. Casey what his favorite foods are, and ask his daughter to offer him a small portion of one of these foods each day.
- Encourage Mr. Casey to drink up to four cans of Ensure Plus with Fiber a day, sipping them throughout the day.
- Talk with the physician about trying a medication to stimulate the appetite.

- Arrange for a home health aide to assist with personal care and some household tasks.
- Request a volunteer to spend up to 4 hours a day, twice a week with Mr. Casey so that Ms. Walsh can attend to outside activities and chores.
- Collaborate with the physician to develop a pain-control program using a fentanyl (Duragesic) patch applied every 3 days and oxycodone (OxyContin) 30 mg p.o. q4h prn for breakthrough pain.
- Leave detailed instructions regarding analgesic regimen, potential adverse effects and how to deal with them, and when to contact the hospice nurse or physician.
- Instruct Ms. Walsh to allow ample rest periods between each activity Mr. Casey must carry out, such as taking a shower or using the commode.
- Order a hospital bed, a special foam pad for Mr. Casey's bed and chair, and a bedside commode from the medical supply house.
- Instruct Ms. Walsh and the home health aide in proper skin care and to report any beginning lesions immediately to the nurse.

Evaluation

Mr. Casey increased his oral intake a little and drank one or two cans of Ensure a day. His weight remained at about 120 lb until his death 2 weeks later. Ms. Walsh was very grateful for the extra help from the home health aide and the volunteer. She did become more rested and reported that "we had some wonderful 3:00 A.M. talks when he couldn't sleep."

Mr. Casey's pain was effectively controlled using the fentanyl patch and oxycodone as needed; after 2 days he was alert enough most of the time to carry on a normal conversation and able to walk to the bathroom with help until 2 days before he died.

The hospital bed simplified Mr. Casey's care and made it much easier for him to rest comfortably and change position. His skin remained intact and in good condition. Mr. Casey died peacefully in his sleep, about 2 weeks after hospice care was started.

Critical Thinking in the Nursing Process

1. What other tests could have been done to evaluate Mr. Casey's nutritional status?
2. Mr. Casey had severe back pain. What were the possible pathophysiologic reasons for his pain?
3. If Mr. Casey's daughter, Ms. Walsh, had a nursing diagnosis of Ineffective Coping, what would you include in a teaching plan to help her learn new coping strategies?

Note: Discussion of Critical Thinking questions appears on the companion website.

Oncologic Emergencies

Key Concept Patients who have cancer are at risk for emergencies related to the size or spread of the tumor or to treatments such as chemotherapy or radiation therapy. Nurses must recognize signs and symptoms of oncologic emergencies, promptly notify the physician, and initiate emergency measures until definitive treatment can be started.

Patients with cancer may experience a number of emergency situations associated with their disease or its treatment. These emergencies require astute observation, accurate judgment, and rapid action once the problem has been identified. In all cases, notifying the physician or emergency team immediately is the first step. A brief description of some of the more common oncologic emergencies follows, with nursing assessment and interventions summarized at the end of the section.

SUPERIOR VENA CAVA SYNDROME

The superior vena cava, which returns blood from the head and upper body to the right heart, can be compressed by mediastinal tumors or adjacent thoracic tumors (Figure 12-8■). The most common cause is lung cancer. Signs and symptoms may develop slowly, with facial and arm edema as early signs. As the problem progresses, pleural effusion and tracheal edema cause respiratory distress, dyspnea, cyanosis, and, eventually, altered consciousness and neurologic deficits. Radiation or chemotherapy is used to reduce the tumor size and relieve superior vena cava syndrome.

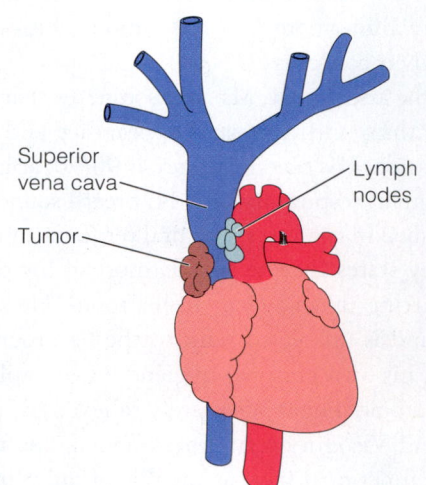

Superior vena cava

Lymph nodes

Tumor

Figure 12-8 ■ A tumor adjacent to the superior vena cava compresses that major blood vessel causing blood to back up into the venous system behind the obstruction. (Source: "Figure 14.07" from Medical Surgical Nursing: Critical Thinking in Patient Care, 5e by Priscilla LeMone; Karen Burke; and Gerene Bauldoff. Published by Pearson Education, © 2011.)

PERICARDIAL EFFUSION AND CARDIAC TAMPONADE

Malignant *pericardial effusion* (a collection of fluid in the potential space between the two layers of the pericardium) compresses the heart, restricts heart movement, and results in cardiac tamponade, a life-threatening emergency. The signs of cardiac tamponade are those of decreased cardiac output and impaired heart function: hypotension, tachycardia, tachypnea, dyspnea, cyanosis, distended neck veins, anxiety, restlessness, and impaired consciousness. Muffled heart sounds may be an early manifestation of cardiac tamponade. Manifestations of cardiac tamponade should immediately be reported to the physician. Hemodynamic monitoring is initiated to monitor cardiovascular function. A pericardial tap (pericardiocentesis) is performed to remove collected fluid and restore cardiac function.

SEPSIS AND SEPTIC SHOCK

Tumor necrosis, immunosuppression, malnutrition, and cancer therapies can result in sepsis. Bacteria enter the blood, grow rapidly, and produce septicemia. The sepsis, which is usually related to gram-negative bacteria, progresses to systemic shock and eventually results in multisystem failure (see Chapter 14). Manifestations appear in two phases. The first phase is characterized by vasodilation and hypovolemia; high fever; peripheral edema; hypotension; tachycardia; tachypnea or Kussmaul respirations; hot, flushed skin with creeping mottling beginning in the lower extremities; and anxiety or restlessness. Without treatment, the shock progresses to the second phase and more classic signs of shock: hypotension; rapid, thready pulse; respiratory distress; cyanosis; subnormal temperature; cold, clammy skin; decreased urinary output; and altered mentation. Identifying the problem early is crucial to the patient's survival.

Cultures are obtained to identify the infecting organism, and aggressive antibiotic therapy is initiated. Hemodynamic monitoring is initiated, and intravenous fluids and volume expanders are given to restore hemodynamic stability.

SPINAL CORD COMPRESSION

Spinal cord compression is usually associated with pressure from expanding tumors of the breast, lung, or prostate; lymphoma; or metastatic disease. Unless relieved, it can lead to irreversible paraplegia. The initial symptom of back pain progresses to include leg pain, numbness, paresthesias, and coldness. Later, bowel and bladder dysfunction occur and, finally, neurologic dysfunction progressing to weakness and paralysis. Treatment often consists of radiation or surgical decompression, but early detection is essential. Corticosteroids (e.g., dexamethasone) are administered to reduce spinal cord edema and protect function.

OBSTRUCTIVE UROPATHY

Patients with intra-abdominal, retroperitoneal, or pelvic malignancies (prostate, cervical, or bladder cancers) may develop obstruction of the bladder neck or the ureters. Bladder neck obstruction usually manifests as urinary retention, flank pain, hematuria, or persistent urinary tract infections. Ureteral obstruction is often not evident until kidney failure develops.

HYPERCALCEMIA

Hypercalcemia is associated with cancers of the breast, lung, head and neck, and with multiple myeloma. Bone metastases may also cause hypercalcemia. (Hypercalcemia is discussed in Chapter 7.) Patients often present with nonspecific symptoms such as fatigue, anorexia, nausea, polyuria, and constipation. Neurologic symptoms include muscle weakness, lethargy, and diminished reflexes. Without treatment, hypercalcemia progresses with alterations in mental status, psychotic behavior, cardiac dysrhythmias, seizures, coma, and death. Emergency treatment includes administration of intravenous normal saline solutions to increase urinary calcium excretion. Corticosteroids and calcitonin are given to reduce serum calcium levels.

TUMOR LYSIS SYNDROME

Tumor lysis syndrome (TLS) is a life-threatening emergency that develops due to massive and rapid destruction of cancer cells. It most commonly is seen in patients undergoing treatment for hematologic cancers such as leukemias or lymphomas. TLS is characterized by hyperuricemia, hyperphosphatemia, hyperkalemia, and hypocalcemia; acidosis may develop (Gucalp & Dutcher, 2012). These metabolic abnormalities increase the risk for cardiac dysfunction and kidney failure. The syndrome develops when the body is unable to excrete the metabolic by-products and intracellular contents from a massive and rapid cell death, resulting in their accumulation in the bloodstream. Manifestations and potential consequences of TLS include nausea, vomiting, lethargy, edema, fluid overload, heart failure, cardiac dysrhythmias, seizures, muscle cramps, tetany, syncope, and possible sudden death.

Aggressive hydration and administration of sodium bicarbonate (to alkalinize the urine) and allopurinol (to reduce serum and urine uric acid levels) are preventive measures for TLS. Patients who develop the syndrome may require dialysis to treat kidney failure.

Nursing Interventions for Oncologic Emergencies

In addition to prompt notification of the physician, and, as appropriate emergency support personnel, nursing interventions for the patient experiencing an oncologic emergency include the following:

- Monitor vital signs and cardiorespiratory status, including apical and peripheral pulses; neck veins; urine output; respiratory effort and lung sounds; mental status and level of consciousness; skin color, temperature, moisture; and presence of edema.

- Thoroughly assess all complaints of back or leg pain or sensory changes. Obtain a neurologic exam, including extremity strength, movement, and sensation.
- Assess for urinary retention in the patient with complaints of flank pain, hematuria, or inability to urinate.
- Start oxygen and alert respiratory therapy for additional respiratory support as needed.
- Insert an intravenous catheter if one is not already in place. Initiate and monitor intravenous infusions and medications as ordered.
- Prepare for hemodynamic monitoring. Once initiated, monitor values and report changes or unexpected findings.
- Assist with obtaining cultures of wound drainage, urine and sputum, and blood cultures.
- Monitor serum electrolytes, BUN, creatinine, uric acid, and alkaline phosphatase, reporting elevated levels.
- Prepare for and assist with emergency measures such as a pericardial tap (pericardiocentesis) or dialysis as indicated.
- Provide a safe environment when mentation and level of consciousness are altered, including initiation of seizure precautions as indicated.
- Provide support and reassurance for the patient and family.

Long-Term Effects of Cancer and Its Treatment

As the population ages and cancer treatment improves, increasing numbers of people are living with the long-term effects of cancer and its treatment. Although most cancer survivors (disease free for 5 or more years) regain their quality of life, many experience long-term effects or *sequelae* (delayed effects) of cancer and its treatment. *Long-term effects* are symptoms that develop during treatment and continue after treatment is completed and the tumor is eradicated. Sequelae, in contrast, may not surface until months or even years after treatment has been completed (American Cancer Society, 2012c).

Both physiologic and psychosocial sequelae of cancer and its treatment have been identified. The physiologic effects of cancer may vary, depending on the body system affected and the treatment undergone. Common effects include:

- Chronic pain related to scarring, disrupted nerve pathways, and other effects such as swelling or edema.
- Fatigue, with tiredness and lack of endurance unrelieved by sleep.
- Changes in mental processing, including difficulty concentrating, poor memory, and inability to perform complex cognitive activities.

- Sexual problems, including decreased libido and erectile dysfunction.
- Cancer treatments that can damage the heart, lungs, lymphatic drainage, and reproductive organs. They can also lead to decreased bone density and possible osteoporosis.
- Increased risk of developing another malignancy unrelated to the initial tumor.

Many cancer survivors report positive outcomes of their experience, including a greater appreciation of life, improved relationships, and a greater sense of meaning and purpose. The experience may lead to more effective coping as well.

Cancer survivors have a risk that the original cancer will recur or metastasis will develop. They also have a somewhat elevated risk of developing a subsequent, different cancer than the original tumor. Factors such as the type and stage of the original tumor, treatment, genetic factors, and continued exposure to substances such as tobacco are thought to influence risk for cancer recurrence or development of more than one cancer.

Nursing measures to promote quality of life and identify possible long-term effects of cancer begin with focused assessment. Inquire about the specific type of cancer and how it was treated. Ask if the patient is experiencing any problems that he or she suspects may be related to the cancer or its treatment. If indicated, follow up with additional questions about current activities of daily living, including any problems with eating and nutrition, energy, exercise and mobility, elimination, and sleep and rest. Ask about any problems with memory or thinking. Inquire about the presence of pain, including its location, character, and intensity, and measures used to manage it. Ask the patient about possible effects of the cancer on his or her lifestyle, work and social relationships, sexuality, and stress and coping.

Acknowledge the validity of the patient's concerns and symptoms. Report any indications of cancer spread or recurrence (e.g., new development of pain, recent weight loss, increasing fatigue) to the patient's primary care provider. Provide referrals to appropriate health care team members, such as social service or a dietitian. Provide information to the patient and family about available community services, such as cancer survivor support groups. Share information about other resources, such as the ACS, the local library, and online resources.

Note: The references and resources for all chapters have been compiled at the back of the book.

Chapter Review

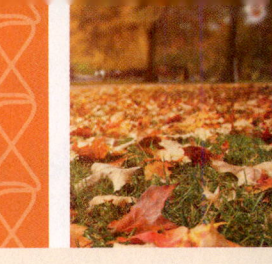

KEY POINTS

- **Concept:** Cancer is not one disease, but a number of complex diseases characterized by the uncontrolled growth and spread of abnormal cells.
- Cancer can affect people of any age, gender, ethnicity, or geographic region.
- **Concept:** Development of malignancies involves complex interaction of genetic, biologic, and environmental factors.
- Many cancer risk factors are controllable; lifestyle changes can significantly reduce the risk of developing cancer.
- Patients with cancer need a great deal of emotional support because fear and anxiety are common responses to a diagnosis of cancer.
- **Concept:** The nurse is an important member of the health care team treating the patient with cancer. The nurse advocates for the patient, assists with coordinating care activities, and helps the patient and family manage the effects of the disease and its treatment.
- Cancer treatment is aimed at cure, control, or palliation of symptoms.
- Cancer may be treated through surgery, radiotherapy, chemotherapy, and biotherapy.
- Early detection and treatment have the greatest influence on the prognosis for people with cancer.
- All people should undergo regular cancer screenings as recommended.
- Cancer pain is the most feared symptom; effective pain management often requires combinations of non-narcotic, opioid, and adjunctive drugs.
- **Concept**: Nursing care for the patient with cancer is holistic, multidimensional, and ongoing as the patient's and family's needs change over the course of the disease and its treatment.
- **Concept**: Patients who have cancer are at risk for emergencies related to the size or spread of the tumor or to treatments such as chemotherapy or radiation therapy. Nurses must recognize signs and symptoms of oncologic emergencies, promptly notify the physician, and initiate emergency measures until definitive treatment can be started.

PEARSON NURSING STUDENT RESOURCES

Find additional materials at **nursing.pearsonhighered.com**.

Clinical Reasoning Care Map

Caring for a Patient Undergoing Chemotherapy
NCLEX-PN® Focus Area: Physiologic Integrity: Reduction of Risk Potential

Case Study: Maria Hernandez, a 78-year-old Hispanic woman, was diagnosed with colon cancer and had a colon resection 6 months ago. When she comes in for chemotherapy, she reports that she has been progressively anorexic and nauseated since beginning chemotherapy of 5-fluoroura-cil (5-FU). She states, "I just can't eat. My mouth is so sore and it hurts to swallow. I've lost so much weight."

Nursing Diagnosis: Imbalanced Nutrition: Less Than Body Requirements

COLLECT DATA

Subjective	Objective
_____	_____
_____	_____
_____	_____
_____	_____
_____	_____
_____	_____

Does this present a threat to the patient's safety?

If yes, the priority intervention to address this threat would be:

_____

_____

Nursing Care

_____
_____
_____
_____
_____
_____
_____
_____

Interprofessional team members to include when planning care:

_____

_____

How would you document this? _____

_____

Compare your answers and documentation to those provided on the companion website.

Data Collected
(use only those that apply)

- Height: 5'4"
- Weight: 102 lb
- Pale skin with poor turgor
- Blood pressure: 134/76
- Apical pulse: 88, regular
- Lungs clear to auscultation
- Pale skin with poor turgor
- Hemoglobin: 13.4
- White blood count: 6,500
- Oral mucous membranes red and swollen
- Bowel sounds present in all four quadrants
- Hair dry and brittle
- Concentrated urine

Nursing Interventions
(use only those that apply; list in priority order)

- Administer pain medications.
- Administer antiemetics.
- Assist Mrs. Hernandez with ambulation.
- Assess hemoglobin and hematocrit.
- Encourage fluid intake.
- Monitor vital signs every 4 hours.
- Suggest referral for counseling.
- Suggest eating soft bland foods at room temperature.
- Offer high-protein drinks.
- Instruct on using soft toothbrush or oral swab (Toothette) for oral hygiene.
- Administer pain medications.

NCLEX-PN® Exam Preparation

1 A patient with a history of lung cancer complains of nausea, anorexia, and upper right quadrant pain. The nurse suspects:

1. an adverse effect of the prescribed chemotherapy.
2. metastasis of the tumor to the liver.
3. superior vena cava syndrome.
4. extension of the tumor to involve the diaphragm.

2 A patient whose father was recently diagnosed with colon cancer asks the nurse what she can do to reduce her risk of developing the disease. The nurse responds that:

1. because colorectal cancer risk is primarily genetically determined, she cannot change her risk.
2. the cause of most cancers, including colon cancer, is unknown, so she should simply maintain a healthy lifestyle.
3. research has shown that a diet rich in whole grains, fruits, and vegetables with limited red meat consumption is associated with a lower risk for colon cancer.
4. it is vital that the patient undergo annual colonoscopy for early detection of precancerous lesions or polyps in the bowel.

3 A male patient asks the office nurse what a PSA test is and why his physician wants him to have one done. What would the nurse's most appropriate answer be?

1. "The PSA test is a general tumor marker for certain types of cancer."
2. "This test will provide information about your general health and risk for cancer."
3. "This is a test for colon cancer, a leading cause of cancer deaths in men."
4. "This is a test to help identify prostate cancer, the most common cancer affecting adult men."

4 After surgery to remove a colon tumor, a patient refuses to care for his colostomy. An appropriate nursing intervention would be to:

1. teach a family member to perform colostomy care.
2. inform the patient that he must learn to change the colostomy bag.
3. tell the patient to turn his head away while colostomy care is performed.
4. refer the patient for psychologic counseling.

5 A patient anticipates alopecia as a result of chemotherapy. The nurse can best assist her to cope with this result by:

1. purchasing a wig for the patient.
2. suggesting that the patient ask her physician about a possible alternative drug regimen.
3. scheduling a consultation with a hairdresser when she loses her hair.
4. encouraging her to choose a wig or other head covering before losing her hair.

6 A patient reports a 15 lb weight loss due to anorexia during a course of chemotherapy. The serum albumin level is 2.0. Which nursing interventions are appropriate? **Select all that apply.**

1. Stress the importance of consuming foods with high nutritional value.
2. Request double portion meals for the patient.
3. Assess food likes and dislikes and encourage small frequent meals.
4. Encourage hot foods such as soup and broth to provide calories.
5. Encourage use of nutritional supplements such as Ensure.

7 A patient is receiving internal radiation to the cervix. The nurse discovers the implant in the patient's bed. The appropriate action would be to:

1. remove the patient from the room.
2. use long-handled forceps to place the implant in a lead container.
3. discard the implant in the trash receptacle.
4. flush the implant in the toilet.

8 A patient is receiving external radiation for treatment of lung cancer. Patient teaching for care of the skin in the marked area includes:

1. applying antibacterial ointment daily.
2. cleansing the skin with mild soap and water.
3. avoiding rubbing or scratching treated skin areas.
4. avoiding contact with others to eliminate radiation risk.

9 A patient complains of nausea and vomiting after her daily chemotherapy treatment. The MOST appropriate nursing intervention would be to:

1. provide antiemetic medication 30 to 40 minutes before each treatment.
2. withhold food and fluids until after each treatment.
3. schedule chemotherapy for bedtime.
4. provide clear liquids until chemotherapy is finished.

10 A patient experiences bone marrow depression as a result of chemotherapy. Which of the following would the nurse expect to find?

1. Nausea and vomiting
2. Alopecia
3. Temperature 102°F
4. Platelet count 200,000

Answers and rationales for Review Questions appear in Appendix I.

CULTURAL CARE STRATEGIES

CONSIDERING CULTURAL VARIATIONS RELATED TO ENVIRONMENTAL CONTROL

Mrs. Jones, 43, a White woman from Appalachia, is admitted to a small Appalachian hospital in respiratory distress and reports she has had difficulty getting her breath for the past 3 days. She has a persistent cough, which she reports having had for 8 months. The nurse doing the admission notes that she is emaciated, has ashen color, tires easily, and has a productive cough. When the nurse asks why she has not sought treatment, she responds, "Sickness is God's will. Whatever will be will be. I have tried some herbal remedies but they have not done much good. It is my time to go. I guess I'm ready, although I wish I could stay and see my children get married."

The term *environmental control* refers to the ability of a person to plan activities that control nature. Environmental control also refers to people's perception that they can direct factors in the environment. Feelings of control are an important part of responding to illness and of taking actions to promote health. Thus it is important to assess each patient for beliefs related to locus of control.

Locus of Control

Individuals may be described as having internal or external locus of control (Rotter, 1966). An individual who feels that actions and outcomes are related to *internal control* feels some power over future behaviors and situations. Personal actions are considered to be important in influencing events.

The term *external control* describes the belief that events are unpredictable and are influenced by outside forces such as luck, change, or fate. Individuals who believe in external feelings of control believe that efforts and rewards are not related to each other.

The locus-of-control construct can be applied to a variety of phenomena including the weather, preventive health, curative actions, and feelings of well-being (Giger, 2013). An individual who believes in internal locus of control is more likely to comply with treatment and to take preventive actions related to future health. On the other hand, an individual who believes that compliance with treatment and health are unrelated will have little motivation to develop behaviors that influence the future or enhance health.

The culturally competent nurse should be aware that people with an Appalachian, Hispanic, or Puerto Rican cultural orientation may have an external locus of control. Northern Europeans or African Americans may have either an internal or external locus of control (Kluckhohn & Strodtbeck, 1961). Many North Americans have a strong internal locus of control and believe they are in control of their own destiny. The beliefs of some Native Americans, Chinese Americans, and Japanese Americans do not include the locus-of-control construct, but focus on harmony with nature.

Folk or traditional medicine beliefs and practices may be part of a person's worldview and belief about what will influence health. Folk medicine beliefs classify illness or diseases as natural or unnatural. Folk medicine differs from Western medicine in the way in which illness is explained and treated. Alternative and traditional therapies provide options for treatment other than relying on medication or surgery.

Nursing Implications

■ *Assess the patient for locus of control.* The nurse needs to appreciate that individuals differ and that actions to seek health care or to promote health may depend on culturally based locus-of-control orientation.

■ *Show respect for folklore and folklore practices.* The nurse should appreciate that persons from diverse cultural backgrounds may have deeply ingrained beliefs about how to attain and maintain health. These beliefs may be linked to the natural and supernatural worlds, may adversely affect the physician–patient or nurse–patient relationship, and may influence the individual's decision to follow or not to follow prescribed treatment recommendations.

■ *Try to incorporate folklore practices with Western medicine.* Rather than disregarding folklore practices, it is important to incorporate beliefs of the patient with practices of Western medicine. When folk beliefs of the patient are respected and incorporated into the nurse's plan of care, the patient may be more cooperative and have a better response to nursing interventions.

Self-Reflection Questions

1. What are your beliefs about internal or external locus of control?

2. Can you relate your beliefs to early parental teaching?

3. Do you have any folk beliefs that are outside the scope of Western medicine?

4. What folk beliefs have you encountered in your patient interactions?

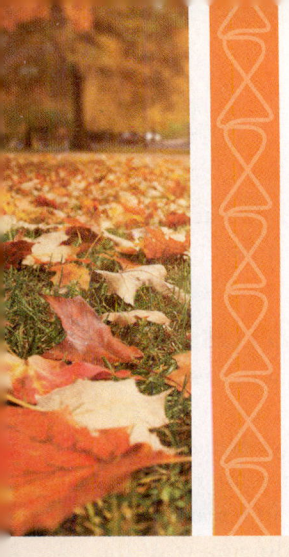

CHAPTER 13
Loss, Grief, and End-of-Life Care

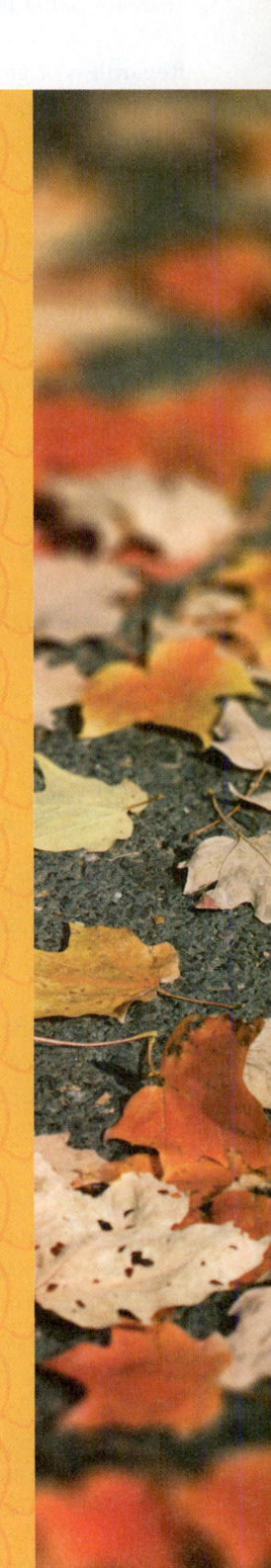

BRIEF OUTLINE

Loss, Grief, and Death
    Experiencing and Resolving Loss
    Family and Other Support Systems
    Spirituality
    Rituals of Mourning

End-of-Life Care
    Legal and Ethical Issues
    Settings and Services for End-of-Life Care
    Physiologic Changes in the Dying Patient
    Support for the Patient and Family
    Death
    Nurses' Grieving

APPLIED LEARNING OUTCOMES

After completing this chapter, you will be able to:

1. Define loss, grief, and death.
2. Recognize commonly experienced emotional responses to each stage of loss.
3. Discuss factors that influence responses to loss.
4. Discuss legal and ethical issues of dying, including advance directives, living wills, do-not-resuscitate orders, and euthanasia.
5. Explain the philosophy and services of hospice and palliative care.
6. Assess physiologic changes as a patient nears end of life and death.
7. Use the nursing process to collect data and provide patient-centered interventions for the patient who is experiencing loss or is at the end of life.

KEY TERMS

The key terms are defined on the pages listed below.

SPECIAL FEATURES

Loss, Grief, and Death

Key Concept Grief is experienced by all individuals in response to loss. The experience of grief and bereavement is unique to each individual and subjective, making it difficult to measure and define. Understanding this unique experience helps the nurse provide sensitive and effective care for patients and families.

Regardless of gender, age, belief system, or culture, all individuals are exposed to grief and loss as well as death and dying. **Loss** occurs when a valued object, person, body part, or situation that was formerly present is lost, potentially lost, or changed and can no longer be seen, felt, heard, known, or experienced. Loss is anything that is perceived as such by the individual. A loss may be temporary or permanent; complete or partial; subjective, physical, or symbolic. Losses that occur in any phase of the life cycle may produce grief responses as intensely painful as those observed in the death experience. Most commonly, people fear losses such as health, a body part, a relationship, a loved one, hopes and dreams, reproductive function, and life itself.

The stress of loss may initiate physical and/or emotional changes in a person or family. To cope adequately with the resulting changes, people must resolve their feelings about the loss through a process called *grief work*. **Grief** is the deep mental and emotional anguish that is a response to the subjective experience of loss, whereas *grieving* may be thought of as the internal process the person uses to work through the response to loss. *Bereavement* is the social experience of processing grief. *Mourning* describes the actions or expressions of that grief. Each person grieves in his or her own unique way. Grief is experienced physically, socially, spiritually, cognitively, and emotionally. It is influenced by factors such as culture and the circumstances surrounding the loss. Grief resolution takes time and goes through a series of highs and lows; it does not fully disappear, but rather the loss becomes integrated into and is a part of one's life. Remembering that grief is individual in nature will assist the nurse in understanding an individual's response to loss and in providing appropriate care.

Death, the most critical loss of all, is defined in a variety of ways. A commonly used definition of death is an irreversible cessation of circulatory and respiratory functions or irreversible cessation of all functions of the entire brain, including the brainstem. Generally, the following characteristics must be present (in some cases for at least 24 hours) for death to be declared: a lack of responsiveness, a lack of movement or breathing, a lack of reflexes, and a flat electroencephalograph (EEG).

Although death is an inevitable part of life, it is often an immensely difficult loss both for the person who is dying and for his or her loved ones. Death may be accidental (trauma), the end of a terminal illness (cancer, AIDS, or heart disease), or purposeful (suicide).

EXPERIENCING AND RESOLVING LOSS

Grief is highly individual. Medical–surgical nurses practicing in all types of settings care for patients who are experiencing loss and are in various stages of the grieving process. The grief process may range from discomforting to debilitating; it may occur in anticipation of, or in response to, a loss; it may last a day or a lifetime, depending on what the loss means to the person experiencing it. For example, one woman with breast cancer may be unaffected by the loss of a breast because the cancer has been removed from her body; another woman with breast cancer may fear that the loss of a breast will make her appear less feminine and unattractive, and these feelings may affect intimate relationships with her significant other.

Kübler-Ross's (1969, 1978) classic research on death and dying provides one framework for understanding the stages of coping with an impending or actual loss. Kübler-Ross identified stages of death and dying, but repeatedly stressed the danger of labeling a "stage" prematurely. She identified five stages and the behaviors associated with each of these stages that can be observed in individuals experiencing the loss of someone or something. The goal was to describe observations of how people come to terms with loss.

Stage I: Denial

A person may have difficulty believing that a loss is real. People may make such statements as "This can't be happening to me" or "This can't be true." This initial stage of denial serves as a buffer and may protect the individual against the psychologic pain of reality. During denial, the person or family mobilizes defenses to cope with the situation.

Stage II: Anger

In the anger stage, reality sets in. Feelings associated with this stage include sadness, guilt, shame, helplessness, and hopelessness. The anger and anxiety may be intense and may be directed toward family and health care providers. Awareness by the health care providers and the family that anger is being displaced may decrease defensive behaviors.

Stage III: Bargaining

The bargaining stage serves as an attempt to delay the reality of the loss. The person makes a secret bargain with whatever God the person believes in, expressing a willingness to do anything to postpone the loss or change the prognosis. This is the individual's plea for an extension of life or the chance to "make everything right" with a dying family member or friend. People facing less serious trauma can bargain or seek to negotiate a compromise (e.g., "Can we still be friends?" when facing a breakup). The individual acknowledges the loss but holds out for hope for additional alternatives.

Stage IV: Depression

Upon realizing the full effect of the actual or perceived loss, the person enters a stage of depression and prepares for the impending loss by working through the struggle of separation. The individual mourns for that which has been or will be lost. While grieving over "what cannot be," the person may either talk freely about the loss or withdraw from others. This is a very painful stage, and therapeutic intervention should be available, but not imposed, after assessing the patient's readiness.

Stage V: Acceptance

The patient has worked through the behaviors associated with the other stages and accepts or is resigned to the loss. Some people who are dying reach a stage of acceptance in which they may appear to be devoid of feelings. They may become withdrawn and quiet as they attempt to facilitate the passage by slowly disengaging from the environment. The dying patient is now ready to die. The struggle is past, and the emotional pain is gone. If the person has experienced the loss of a loved one or other valued object, he or she begins to come to terms with the loss and resumes activities with an air of hopefulness for the future.

Although the theories of Kübler-Ross are widely accepted, other theories provide additional information. Bowlby (1980) developed a model of loss and grief that is based on attachment (or bonding). This model sees grief as a natural response to a loss that continues until the attachment is restored or its loss is accepted. Based on the work of Bowlby, a theory of continuing bonds was designed by Field et al. (2005). In this theory, a continuing bond to the deceased is proposed in which the bereaved continue to maintain a bond by activities such as talking to the deceased, feeling the presence of the deceased, participating in mourning rituals, and visiting the grave of the deceased. A new relationship with the deceased, based on memories, is developed. In this way, the continuity between the past and the present is preserved.

Differences in a person's understanding of and reaction to loss are affected by the individual's developmental stage. In general, as people age and experience life transitions, they are more able to understand and accept the losses associated with those transitions (Table 13-1 ■).

FAMILY AND OTHER SUPPORT SYSTEMS

Grieving is painful and lonely. Reactions to loss are affected by how much social support people feel they have. Lack of a support system has been identified as one factor that may

TABLE 13-1	Development of the Concept of Death
AGE	**BELIEFS/ATTITUDES ABOUT DEATH**
Up to 3 years	Fears separation; lacks comprehension of permanent separation
3–5	Believes death is like sleeping and is reversible
	Expresses curiosity about what happens to the body
6–10	Understands finality of death
	Views own death as avoidable
	Associates death with violence
	Believes wishes can be responsible for death
11–12	Reflects views of death expressed by parents
	Expresses interest in afterlife as an understanding of mortality develops
	Recognizes death as irreversible and inevitable
13–21	May have a religious and philosophic view of death but seldom thinks about it
	Views own death as distant or a challenge, acting out defiance through reckless behavior
	Previously held developmental awareness of death may still be present
22–45	Does not think about death unless confronted with it
	Emotionally distances self from death
	Attitude toward death is influenced by religious and cultural beliefs
46–65	Experiences the death of parents or friends
	Accepts own mortality
	May experience anxiety about death
	Puts life in order to prepare for death and decrease anxiety
66 and older	Fears lingering, incapacitating illness
	Views death as inevitable, but also as freedom from pain and illness or as a spiritual reunion with deceased friends and loved ones

delay grief work. Even if the patient is reacting to the loss in an expected manner, feelings of isolation and withdrawal behaviors are often observed. Patients need encouragement to reestablish contact with significant others in their lives so they may share their grief. If the patient is not making progress in grief work, the nurse may need to explain the benefit of sharing grief with significant others or becoming involved in a local grief support group. Some losses may lead to social isolation, placing patients at high risk for dysfunctional grief reactions. Factors that can interfere with successful grieving include:

- Perceived inability to share the loss.
- Lack of social recognition of the loss.
- Ambivalent relationships before the loss.
- Traumatic circumstances of the loss.

A well-functioning family usually rallies after the initial shock and disbelief, and the family members provide support for each other during all phases of the grieving process. After a loss, the well-functioning family is able to shift roles, levels of responsibility, and ways of communicating.

The nurse needs to be alert for the negative as well as positive effects the family may have on the grieving patient. For example, the dying patient may ask someone the family perceives as an outsider to be near, and the family may respond with anger to this "intrusion." Similarly, certain family members may have hurt feelings or be angry if the patient is unresponsive to them. Well-meaning family members also may try to shield the patient from the pain of grieving. Because no two people grieve alike, the nurse must assess individual family members' reactions to the loss. The family and the patient rarely experience anger, denial, and acceptance in unison. While one member is in denial, another may be angry because "not enough is being done."

SPIRITUALITY

Spiritual beliefs, principles, values, personal philosophy, and meaning of life may be called into question when a patient or family members respond to an actual or perceived loss. Because of a fear of intruding on personal beliefs and practices, the nurse often feels at a loss when implementing interventions that would help the patient respond to a loss and meet spiritual needs.

Developing a trusting relationship with the patient and family helps the nurse overcome his or her discomfort in dealing with the spiritual aspects of care, even when the patient and the nurse have different views. For example, the nurse should be accepting and nonjudgmental if the patient initially expresses a belief that the loss is punishment for some past misdeed or failure "to do right." Even spiritually healthy patients need time to challenge their beliefs and values before moving on to the next stage of grieving.

As the patient becomes aware of the full effect of the loss, spiritual beliefs and rituals often provide comfort and help in finding meaning in the loss. The nurse provides spiritual support by listening as the patient analyzes beliefs

and values, begins to put the loss in perspective, and expresses interest in getting on with life.

RITUALS OF MOURNING

The rituals of mourning are an important part of the work of mourning and grieving a loss. Grief, bereavement, and mourning related to death are concepts common to all cultures. Culture is the primary factor that dictates the rituals of mourning (Table 13-2■). Understanding these cultural differences, as well as religious differences, allows the nurse to provide culturally sensitive care to patients. The funeral ceremony or celebration of life ceremony serves the needs of the bereaved as they gather to share their loss. Through the ceremony, people symbolically express triumph over death and adapt to the loss. This adaptation does not decrease the suffering they will continue to feel, but it does move them toward reinvesting emotionally in the future.

End-of-Life Care

Key Concept Nurses must proactively engage in discussions to elicit and identify patient preferences and concerns regarding end-of-life care, such as management of pain and other symptoms, as well as spiritual needs, to improve the quality of patient care.

People are considered to be dying when they have an illness or injury that is expected to end in death and for which there is no treatment. Dying patients may also be those who choose to have no further treatment to prolong life (e.g., those with end-stage kidney disease who no longer wish to have dialysis).

Nurses care for dying patients in intensive care units, emergency rooms, hospital units, long-term care facilities, hospice facilities, and the home. Regardless of the cause of death or the setting, the patient's wishes about death should be respected.

The statement "Nursing includes the promotion of health, prevention of illness, and the care of ill, disabled, and dying people," in the definition of nursing by the International Council of Nurses (ICN, 2002), promotes end-of-life nursing care that ensures a peaceful death. The importance of quality end-of-life care is further supported in a 2012 ICN position paper stating that "Dying persons and their families have individual cultural beliefs and values. . . . The quality of care during the end stage of life greatly contributes to peaceful and dignified death and provides support to family members in dealing with their loss and grieving process." The importance of quality nursing care for dying patients and their loved ones is further supported by the American Nurses Association's (ANA) *Code of Ethics for Nursing* (2008) and *Nursing's Social Policy Statement* (2010).

TABLE 13-2	Examples of Cultural Responses to Dying and Death
CULTURE/ ETHNICITY	**NURSING IMPLICATIONS**
Native American	Each tribe has its own rituals related to death. Some tribes prefer not to openly discuss terminal prognosis and DNR decisions, as negative thoughts may make inevitable loss occur sooner. Suggest a family meeting to discuss care and end-of-life issues. If the family feels comfortable, all members of the family and close friends may remain 24 hours a day (eating, joking, singing). Mourning is done in private, away from the dying person. After death, the family may hug, touch, sing, and stay close to the deceased. The Navajo of the Southwest do not bury the body for 4 days after death. Beliefs require that a cleansing ceremony take place before burial to prevent the spirit of the dead person from trying to assume control of someone else's spirit.
African American	Traditional African Americans often have a spiritual approach to dying, believing the dying person is "going home" after death. Suggest that the family meet with their own minister or the hospital chaplain early in the dying process. The patient may decide to have an older family member disclose a poor prognosis to the patient. The family feels a strong obligation to gather at the time of death. Elders and family members often gather around the dying person's bed, holding a prayer vigil as they provide spiritual and emotional comfort to the dying person.
Chinese American	Ensure the head of the family is present when terminal illness is discussed. The idea of making end-of-life treatment decisions in advance is not part of the traditional Chinese culture. Men are the primary decision makers, and aggressive life-sustaining treatments are favored. The patient may not want to discuss the approaching death, as this is considered to be disrespectful. Special amulets or cloths may be brought from home. Family members may prefer to bathe the body after death.
Iranian	Information about a terminal illness should be presented by a trusted member of the health care team to the family, never to the patient when he or she is alone. Most Iranians believe in *taqdir* (will of God) in life and death as a predestined journey. When death occurs, notify the head of the family first. DNR decisions are often made by the family. The family may want to bathe the body after death.
Mexican American	Based on the belief that worry may make health worse, the family may want to protect the patient from the seriousness of illness. The information is often handled by an older daughter or son. Extended family members are obligated to pay respects to the sick and dying, although pregnant women do not care for dying persons or attend funerals. May prefer that the patient die at home. Prayers, amulets, and rosary beads are used, and the priest should be notified. Death is seen as an important spiritual event. The family may bathe the body and spend time with the body.

LEGAL AND ETHICAL ISSUES

Nurses are often the health care providers in close contact with dying patients and may have unresolved feelings about the moral, ethical, and legal aspects of their actions. Issues such as those involved in advance directives and living wills, euthanasia, and quality of life are especially important to nurses in upholding the specific care requests of their patients.

Advance Directives

Advance directives are legal documents that enable a person to plan for health care and/or financial affairs in the event of incapacity. (Types of advance directives are defined in Box 13-1■.) A **durable power of attorney for health care** (*health care surrogate or health care proxy*) is a legal document written by a competent (mentally healthy) adult that gives another competent adult the right to make health care decisions on the patient's behalf if he or she cannot. The legal authority is limited to decisions about health care. A **living will** is a legal document that formally expresses a person's wishes regarding life-sustaining treatment in the event of terminal illness or permanent unconsciousness. It

BOX 13-1	TYPES OF ADVANCE DIRECTIVES

- **Living will:** A document that provides written directions about life-prolonging procedures; provides instructions when a person can no longer communicate in a life-threatening situation.
- **Durable power of attorney for health care** (health care surrogate or health care proxy): An individual selected to make medical decisions when a person is no longer able to make them for himself or herself.
- **Durable power of attorney:** A document that can delegate the authority to make financial and/or legal decisions on a person's behalf. It must be in writing and must state that the designated person is authorized to make health care decisions.

is not a type of durable power of attorney and usually does not designate a substitute decision maker. It is the responsibility of the nurse as patient advocate to request and record the patient's preference for care and include it in the plan of care. The nurse's documentation helps communicate these preferences to the other members of the health care team.

All facilities that receive Medicare and Medicaid funds are required to provide patients with written information and counseling about advance directives and the institution's policies governing them. The specific terms of this requirement are found in the Patient Self-Determination Act (PSDA). A copy of the signed advance directive must be kept in the patient's medical record, but patients do not have to sign it in order to be treated. Although advance directives do not ease the pain of seeing patients die, they do help nurses provide patients with the care the patients have chosen.

Do-Not-Resuscitate Orders

A **do-not-resuscitate (DNR) order** (or "no-code") is written by the physician for the patient who is near death. This order is usually based on the wishes of the patient and family that no cardiopulmonary resuscitation be performed for respiratory or cardiac arrest. A **comfort measures only order** is an order that indicates that no further life-sustaining interventions are necessary and that the goal of care is a comfortable, dignified death. Confusing or conflicting DNR orders create dilemmas, because nurses are involved in resuscitation and either begin CPR or ensure that unwanted attempts do not occur. The ANA recommends that guidelines and policies be developed to help resolve conflicts between patients and their families, between patients and health care professionals, and among health care professionals.

Euthanasia

Euthanasia (from the Greek for painless, easy, gentle, or good death) is now commonly used to signify a killing that is prompted by some humanitarian motive. There are many arguments for and against euthanasia, and nurses have often found themselves at the center of the debate. As a result, nurses have pushed for the development of appropriate guidelines and procedures for DNR orders. When no such orders exist, the nurse faces a dilemma. Certainly, there are situations in which the nurse's role is clear. For example, it is considered malpractice to participate in "slow codes" (in which the nurse does not hurry to alert the emergency team when a terminally ill patient without a DNR order stops breathing). It is important to note that euthanasia is different from physician-assisted suicide, which is currently legal in two states (Oregon and Washington).

The natural death laws seek to preserve the notion of voluntary versus involuntary euthanasia. In regard to voluntary euthanasia, the competent adult patient and a physician, nurse, or adult relative make the decision to terminate life (by turning off life-preserving machines, such as mechanical ventilators, or ceasing to provide hydration and tube feedings). Involuntary euthanasia (mercy killing) is performed without the patient's consent. Because care

settings offer many complex and technologic interventions, it is not likely that the ethical aspects of euthanasia will soon be resolved. However, advance directives do give patients a much more active role in decisions about their own care.

SETTINGS AND SERVICES FOR END-OF-LIFE CARE

> **Key Concept** Hospice and palliative care provide physical, psychologic, spiritual, and social care for the dying individual and supportive care to meet the special needs of their families.

Settings and services for end-of-life care range from the critical care unit in a hospital to the patient's own home. Because people are increasingly choosing to die at home, two models of care that focus on the dying patient's quality of life—hospice and palliative care—are described in this section.

Hospice

Hospice is a model of care for patients and their families when patients are faced with a limited life expectancy. It is care provided to meet emotional, spiritual, and comfort needs to ensure death with dignity based on the wishes of the patient and the needs of the family. It is a model rather than a place of care and may be provided in freestanding clinics, hospitals, long-term care facilities, identified hospice facilities, and the home by an interprofessional team that includes physicians, nurses (RNs and LPNs/LVNs), social workers, volunteers, clergy, and any other discipline needed to provide holistic care. Hospice care is initiated for patients as they near the end of life; it emphasizes quality rather than quantity of life. The patient and the family are included in the plan of care. Hospice regards dying as a normal part of life, providing support for a dignified and peaceful death. It is palliative (takes care of the comfort needs of the whole person) rather than curative. Many hospices offer bereavement support groups for family members for up to a year after a patient's death.

Palliative Care

Palliative care is based on the principles of compassionate holistic caring, pain and symptom management, the facilitation of effective communication among health care team members, and provision of bereavement support. It is primarily planned and implemented to alleviate manifestations such as pain, nausea, dyspnea, confusion, anxiety, and depression. It is important to realize that unlike hospice care, palliative care is appropriate for patients in all disease stages, including those undergoing treatment for curable illnesses and those living with chronic diseases, as well as patients who are nearing the end of life.

Although palliative care may be provided by a single person, it (like hospice) usually involves the combined efforts of an interprofessional team. Care is provided in the patient's home, long-term care facility, senior living facility, hospice home, or hospital. The expected outcomes of care are directed by interventions to manage current manifestations of the illness and to prevent new manifestations from occurring.

PHYSIOLOGIC CHANGES IN THE DYING PATIENT

Key Concept   A variety of physiologic changes occur in the last hours and days of life. To effectively manage the dying patient, interprofessional caregivers need to understand these physiologic changes and appropriate actions to promote comfort.

Death may occur rapidly or slowly. Physiologic changes are a part of the dying process. As death nears, these changes result in any or all of the manifestations listed in Box 13-2■.

- *Weakness and fatigue.* Weakness and fatigue cause discomfort, especially in joints, and contribute to an increased risk for pressure ulcers (see Chapter 45).
- *Anorexia and decreased food intake.* Although anorexia and a decrease in food intake are normal in the dying patient, the family often views this as "giving up." Anorexia may be a protective mechanism; the breakdown of body fats results in ketosis, which leads to a sense of well-being and helps decrease pain. Parenteral or enteral feedings do not improve symptoms or prolong life and may actually cause discomfort. As weakness and difficulty in swallowing progress, the gag reflex is decreased and patients are at increased risk for aspiration if oral foods are given.
- *Fluid and electrolyte imbalances.* Decreased oral fluid intake is normal at the end of life and does not cause distress. Parenteral fluids are sometimes given to decrease delirium, but they may cause increased edema, breathlessness, cough, and respiratory secretions. If the patient

has edema or ascites (a collection of fluid in the abdominal cavity), excess body water is present, so dehydration is not a problem.

- *Hypotension and kidney failure.* Cardiac output decreases, so does intravascular blood volume. As a result, renal perfusion decreases and the kidneys cease to function. Urinary output is concentrated and scanty. The patient will have tachycardia, hypotension, cool extremities, and cyanosis with skin mottling.
- *Neurologic dysfunction.* Neurologic dysfunction results from any or all of the following: decreased cerebral perfusion, hypoxemia, metabolic acidosis, sepsis, an accumulation of toxins from liver and kidney failure, the effects of medications, and disease-related factors. These changes may result in a decreased level of consciousness or in agitated delirium. Patients with terminal delirium may be confused, restless, or agitated. Moaning, groaning, and grimacing may accompany the agitation and are often misinterpreted as pain. The level of consciousness may decrease to the point where the patient cannot be aroused. Although decreased consciousness and agitation are both normal states at the end of life, they are very distressing to the patient's family.

clinicalALERT

Hearing is thought to be the last sense a dying patient loses; the nurse should never whisper or engage in conversation with the family as if the patient were not there.

- *Respiratory changes.* Respiratory changes are normal at this time. The patient may have dyspnea, apnea (periods of not breathing), or Cheyne–Stokes respirations (see Chapter 23) and may use accessory muscles to breathe. Fluids accumulated in the lungs and oropharynx may lead to what is sometimes called the *death rattle* (although nurses should not use this term when talking to family members). Oxygen may not relieve these manifestations. Frequent suctioning may add only to the discomfort of the patient and may not eliminate the sound. Family members should be educated on this to prevent increasing anxiety or concern.
- *Bowel and bladder incontinence.* Loss of sphincter control may lead to incontinence of feces, urine, or both.
- *Pain.* Pain is a common problem for patients at the end of life and is what people often say they fear the most. It is of utmost importance to keep the patient comfortable through general comfort measures and by administering ordered medications for pain and anxiety. Be aware that frequent position changes may increase or decrease pain. Assessing this is important in providing adequate end-of-life care.

BOX 13-2	MANIFESTATIONS OF IMPENDING DEATH

- Difficulty talking or swallowing
- Nausea, flatus, abdominal distention
- Urinary and/or bowel incontinence, constipation
- Decreased sensation, taste, and smell
- Weak, slow, and/or irregular pulse
- Decreasing blood pressure
- Decreased, irregular, or Cheyne–Stokes respirations
- Changes in the level of consciousness
- Restlessness, agitation
- Coolness, mottling, and cyanosis of the extremities

SUPPORT FOR THE PATIENT AND FAMILY

As the patient's condition deteriorates, the nurse's knowledge of the patient and family guides the care provided. It may be necessary to provide opportunities for patients to express personal preferences about where they want to die and about funeral and burial arrangements. If the family feels that this is morbid, the nurse explains that it helps patients to keep a sense of control as they approach death.

The patient needs the opportunity to say goodbye to others. The nurse encourages and supports the patient and family as they terminate relationships as a necessary part of the grief process. The nurse acknowledges that termination is painful and, if the patient or family desires, stays with them during this time. Family members are often afraid to be present at the moment of death, yet dying alone is the greatest fear expressed by patients.

DEATH

The manifestations listed in Box 13-3■ are seen after death occurs and are the basis for pronouncing death. They usually appear gradually and not in any special order. Pronouncement of death is legally required by a physician or other health care provider to confirm death. The time of death, with any related data, is documented in the patient's chart.

The nurse may also fear being present at the moment of the patient's death. In fact, Kübler-Ross (1969) noted that the nurse's fear of death may interfere with the ability to provide support for the dying patient and family. Nurses who have worked through their own feelings about death and dying are more at ease in assisting the dying patient toward a peaceful death.

After the death, the family is encouraged to acknowledge the pain of loss. The nurse's presence and support as the bereaved express their sorrow, anger, or guilt can help them resolve their grief. By accepting variations in the expression of grief, the nurse supports the family's grief reactions and helps prevent dysfunctional grieving. Complicated grieving is an extended and unsuccessful resolution of grief.

Resolution of grief begins with the acceptance of the loss. The nurse can encourage this acceptance by maintaining open and honest dialogue and by providing the family with the opportunity to view, touch, hold, and kiss the person's body. As family members realize the finality of the death, they are often comforted by the presence of the nurse who cared for the patient during the final days.

Postmortem Care

The nurse documents the time of death (required for the death certificate and all official records), notifies the physician, and assists the family (if needed) in choice of a funeral home. If the patient dies at home, death must be pronounced before the body is removed. In some states and in some situations, nurses can pronounce death; for specifics, consult state practice acts, laws, and agency policy. All jewelry is removed and given to the family unless they ask that it be left on. The body is kept in place until the family is ready and gives permission. If an autopsy is required or requested, the body must be left undisturbed (e.g., do not remove any tubes) for transportation to the medical examiner. Box 13-4■ provides a nursing checklist for care of the body after death.

Documentation of the death is completed by sending a completed death certificate to the funeral home (for a death in the home) or by completing the required paperwork and sending the body to the morgue or funeral home (for a death in the hospital or long-term care setting).

Interprofessional Care

Interventions for loss and grief may be planned and implemented by any or all members of the health care team. Nurses and social workers may provide interventions to help patients or families adapt to a loss. They may also make referrals to mental health professionals (grief counselors, social services), support groups, chaplains, or legal or financial assistance agencies.

BOX 13-3	MANIFESTATIONS OF DEATH

- Absence of respirations, pulse, and heartbeat
- Fixed and dilated pupils; eyes may stay open
- Release of stool and urine
- Waxen color (pallor) as blood settles to dependent areas
- Drop in body temperature
- Lack of reflexes
- Flat electroencephalograph

BOX 13-4   NURSING CARE CHECKLIST

Postmortem Care

☑ Ensure the patient's death has been pronounced and determine if there is going to be autopsy or a coroner involved.

☑ If the family is not present, ensure they have been notified and if (and when) they will visit the deceased.

☑ If death is in an institution, move other patients from the room and ask family and visitors (if present) to temporarily leave the room.

☑ Straighten the bed linens and raise the head of the bed 30 degrees (to prevent pooling of fluids in the head and face).

☑ Ask the family to return (they should remain as long as they wish).

☑ Provide emotional support for the family as needed.

Care of the Body

☑ Collect necessary equipment, incorporating family wishes, culture, and religion as appropriate.

☑ Don gloves.

☑ Close the eyes, using paper tape and gauze pads if necessary.

☑ Replace dentures and close the mouth.

☑ Remove external objects: oxygen mask, IV lines, catheters, and tubes (unless an autopsy is to be done) per agency policy.

☑ Cleanse the body as needed (i.e., remove body elimination or secretions, wound drainage) (determine whether the family is to provide the postmortem bath).

☑ Place an incontinent pad under the buttocks and pull up between the legs. Place the arms loosely at the sides of the body or on the abdomen.

☑ Place the body in a shroud or morgue bag.

☑ Attach identification tags to the body as directed by agency policy (usually the big toe, wrist, and morgue bag).

☑ Label all personal belongings (if not taken by the family) and put them in the morgue bag.

☑ Remove gloves and perform hand hygiene.

☑ Close the doors to other patient rooms, clear hallway, and place the body on a stretcher for transport to the morgue. Transport the body.

Nurses' Grieving

The nurse who has developed a close relationship with the patient who has died may experience strong feelings of grief. Sharing grief with the family (such as being present, holding a hand, crying) after the death of a loved one helps both the nurse and the family to cope with their feelings about the loss. Taking time to grieve after the death of a patient provides a release that can help prevent "blunting" of feelings, a potential problem often experienced by nurses who care for terminally ill patients. It is important for the nurse to observe boundaries when sharing grief to avoid becoming the individual who requires consoling from the family. Remember that this time belongs to the individuals closest to the deceased.

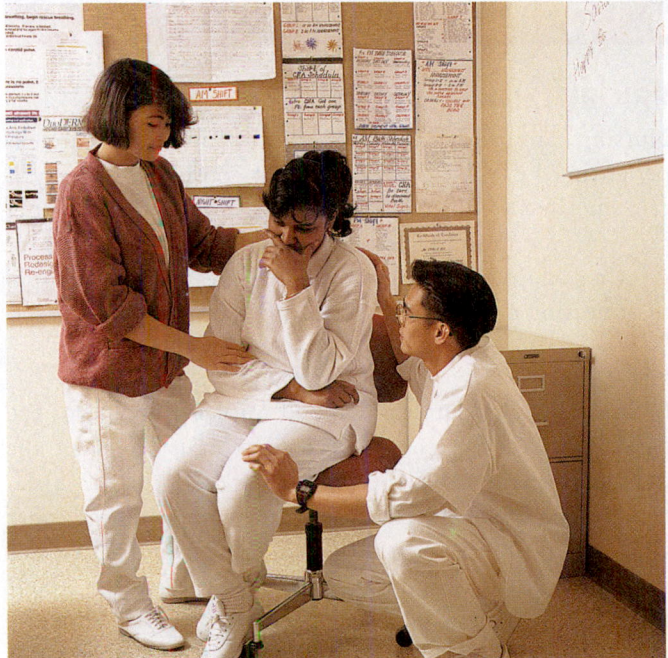

Figure 13-1. ■ Nurses who work with dying patients need support from their colleagues to work through their often overwhelming feelings of grief. (Richard Tauber, Pearson Education.)

Nurses working with critically or terminally ill patients should be aware that witnessing a patient's death and the family's grief may reactivate feelings about some unresolved grief in their own lives. In these cases, nurses may need to reflect on their responses to their own losses. Also, nurses who work with dying patients need support from peers and other professionals to work through the often overwhelming feelings that result from dealing with death, grief, and loss (Figure 13-1 ■). The nurse can promote self-awareness by reflecting on the following questions:

■ What are my personal feelings about how grief should be expressed?

■ Am I making judgments about the meaning of this loss to the patient?

■ Are unresolved losses in my own life preventing me from relating therapeutically to the patient?

A national education program, the End-of-Life Consortium (ELNEC) project, has been created to develop a core of expert academic and clinical staff educators who can better prepare nurses for end-of-life care (American Association of Colleges of Nursing, 2013). The following resources can be accessed via the Internet and may be useful in helping nurses provide care to dying patients:

■ Hospice and Palliative Nurses Association

■ National Hospice and Palliative Care Organization

■ AARP Grief and Loss Program

■ GriefNet

NURSING CARE

PRIORITIZING NURSING CARE

Nursing care of patients and family members who are experiencing loss, grief, or death must consider their physical, emotional, cultural, and spiritual needs. The nursing process is used to provide priority care by interventions for grieving and death anxiety. Comfort measures for the patient nearing death are outlined in Box 13-5 ■.

ASSESSING

Before collecting data to plan and implement care for the patient experiencing a loss, the nurse must consider the individual's response. Approaches for collecting data depend on the age of the patient and the circumstances under which the nurse encounters the patient. The nurse observes for changes in sensory processes and asks questions about the patient's sleeping and eating patterns, activities of daily living, general health status, and pain.

Patients may experience one or more physical reactions as they become aware of a loss. Gastrointestinal symptoms occur frequently (indigestion, nausea or vomiting, anorexia, weight gain or loss, constipation, or diarrhea). The shock and disbelief that accompany a loss may cause shortness of breath, a choking sensation, hyperventilation, or loss of strength. Some patients also report insomnia, preoccupation with sleep, fatigue, and decreased or increased activity level. Crying and sadness are normal during grieving. Crying may make the patient feel exhausted and may interfere with carrying out daily activities. However, a person who is unable to cry may have difficulty completing the mourning process.

The nurse must assess the dying patient's concerns about pain, especially if the patient has cancer or another painful illness. Knowledge of pain theories and pain assessment can help the nurse assess the need for pain medication (see Chapter 8).

It is important for the nurse to explore the patient's spiritual beliefs and practices, because they greatly influence reactions to loss. The spiritually healthy patient has inner resources that help him or her work through the grief process. Faith, prayer, trust in God or a superior being, perception of a purpose in life, or belief in immortality are examples of the inner resources that may sustain the patient during an actual or perceived loss.

Patients often perceive a loss as punishment from God for wrongdoing or for failing to remain faithful to their religious practices. Patients may suddenly turn to religion to seek comfort or to cope with feelings of despair, helplessness, hopelessness, or guilt. They may utter anguished statements such as "Why, God?" or "Please help me, God."

It is more important for the nurse to focus on the meaning of the loss to the patient than to place the patient in a stage or phase of grief. The caring and sensitivity of the nurse's questions will influence the amount of information the patient will be willing to reveal. Asking such questions as "Why do you feel this way?" or "What does this loss mean to you?" is less helpful than making a statement such as "This must be difficult for you." This last sentence conveys the nurse's genuine interest in hearing how the patient feels about the loss.

The nurse may not be able to collect much information during a brief initial contact. However, as trust is built, the patient may reveal the meaning of the relationship and the circumstances surrounding the loss. By establishing trust during the first stages of the nurse–patient relationship, the nurse will be better able to assess the effect of the loss. If the relationship was a significant one, the nurse will observe intense grief. The patient may state, "I know I can't go on without him/her." The patient may even feel anger at the person for having left, whether through death, divorce, or separation. The losses associated with changes in body image or work role may produce similar feelings.

BOX 13-5 **NURSING CARE CHECKLIST**

Providing Physical Comfort for the Patient Nearing Death

☑ Maintain clean skin and bed linens.

☑ Use a draw sheet to turn the patient as often as possible and as is comfortable for the patient.

☑ Position the patient to promote comfort and protect bony areas with padding. Reposition the patient and raise the head of the bed if fluids accumulate in the upper airways and back of the throat.

☑ Use bed pads for urinary incontinence.

☑ Use gentle massage to improve circulation and shift edema.

☑ If patient can swallow, provide small, frequent sips of fluids, ice chips, or Popsicles.

☑ Provide oral care frequently, using a soft moist brush or swab. Avoid lemon and glycerin swabs, as these are drying and may irritate any cracks or open sores. Apply petroleum jelly to lips and anterior nares.

☑ Clean secretions from the eyes and nose. If eyes are open, moisten conjunctiva every 3 to 4 hours with sterile normal saline, artificial tears, or an ophthalmic lubricating gel.

☑ Administer ordered pain medications as needed to maintain comfort.

☑ Administer oxygen as prescribed to relieve dyspnea.

DIAGNOSING, PLANNING, AND IMPLEMENTING

Grieving

Expected outcome: Will express thoughts, feelings, and fears about loss.

"Grieving is a normal complex process that includes emotional, physical, spiritual, social, and intellectual responses and behaviors by which individuals, families, and communities incorporate an actual, anticipated, or perceived loss into their daily lives" (Herdman, 2012, p. 363). Grieving may be a response to one's own future death; to potential loss of body parts or functions; to potential loss of a significant person, animal, or possession; or to the death of a significant other.

- Assess for factors that are causing or contributing to the grief. Ask about support systems, how many losses have occurred, relationship with the lost person, significance of the body part, and previous experiences with loss and grief. *Grief and mourning occur when a person experiences any type of loss.*

- Use open-ended questions to encourage the person to share concerns and the possible effect of the loss on the family unit. *Grief resolution cannot occur until the patient acknowledges the loss.*

- Promote a trusting nurse–patient relationship by:
  - Allowing enough time for communications.
  - Speaking clearly, simply, and to the point.
  - Listening.
  - Being honest in responses to questions, and not giving unrealistic hope.
  - Offering support.
  - Demonstrating respect for the person's age, culture, religion, race, and values.

  An effective nurse–patient relationship begins with acceptance of the patient's feelings, attitudes, and values related to the loss. If the patient is ready to talk, then the nurse's listening and presence are the most appropriate interventions (Figure 13-2■).

- Ask about the patient's strengths and needs in coping with the loss. Current responses are influenced by past experiences with loss, illness, and death. *Socioeconomic and cultural backgrounds, as well as cultural and spiritual beliefs and values, affect a person's ability to adapt to loss.*

- Teach the patient and family the stages of grief. *This helps them to be aware of their emotions in each stage and reassures them that their reactions are normal.*

- Provide time for decision making. *In periods of stress, people may need extra time to make informed decisions.*

- Provide information about appropriate resources, including support from family, friends, and support groups; community resources; and legal/financial aides. *Support*

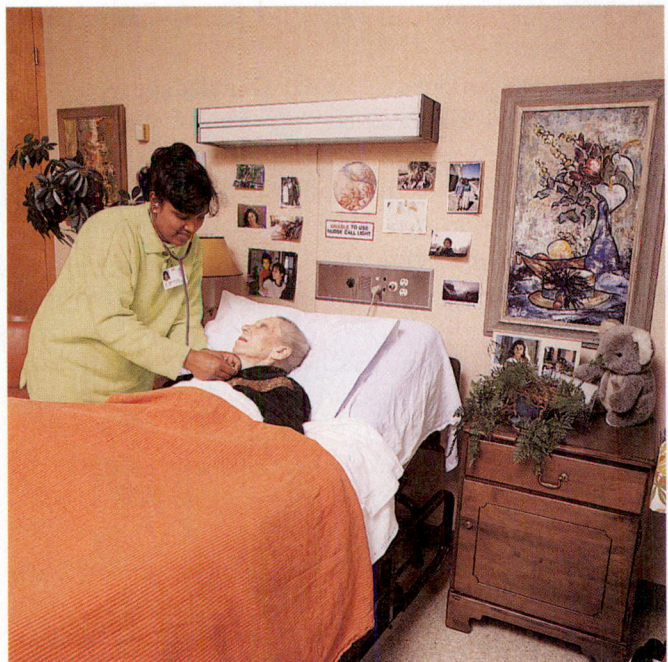

Figure 13-2. ■ The nurse establishes a trusting nurse–patient relationship through therapeutic communications and by demonstrating respect for the person's age, culture, religion, race, and values. (Richard Tauber, Pearson Education.)

from others decreases feelings of loneliness and isolation and facilitates grief work.

Death Anxiety

Expected outcome: Will report feeling less anxious.

Death anxiety is a feeling of dread, apprehension, or anxiety when one thinks of the process of dying, or ceasing to be, or what happens after death. Death anxiety also refers to a morbid, abnormal, or persistent fear of death or dying. It may be present in patients who have an acute life-threatening illness, who have a terminal illness, who have experienced the death of a family member or friend, or who have experienced multiple deaths in the same family.

- Explore the patient's knowledge of the situation. For example, ask, "What has your doctor told you about your condition?" *This informs you about the patient's knowledge base about the condition and about his or her ability to make informed decisions.*

- Ask the patient to identify specific fears about death. *This provides data about any unrealistic expectations or misperceptions.*

- Determine the patient's perceptions of strengths and weakness in coping with death. *Identifying past strengths can help the patient cope with loss, illness, and death.*

- Ask the patient to identify needed help. *This determines whether available resources are adequate.*

- Encourage independence and control in decisions about treatment and care. *This promotes self-esteem, decreases feelings of powerlessness, and allows the patient to retain dignity in dying.*

■ Facilitate the patient's access to culturally appropriate spiritual rituals and practices. *This provides spiritual comfort.*

■ Explain advance directives and assist with them if necessary. *Advance directives ensure that the patient's wishes for end-of-life care are carried out.*

■ Encourage life review and reminiscence. *Life review is self-affirming.*

■ Encourage activities such as listening to music, aromatherapy, massage, or relaxation exercises. *These activities decrease anxiety.*

■ Suggest keeping a journal or leaving a written legacy. *A written document provides continuing support to others after death.*

MANAGING NURSING CARE

Assistive nursing personnel may provide comfort and assistance with activities of daily living and personal hygiene for dying patients as appropriate and allowed by the designated duties and responsibilities. Care of the body after death has occurred also may be provided by assistive personnel.

EVALUATING

Evaluate the effectiveness of nursing care for loss and grief by collecting data from statements by the patient that support grief resolution, such as "I am beginning to accept the fact that my father is gone." The plan of care for the dying patient is effective if the patient has a comfortable and dignified death.

DOCUMENTING

Document the patient's and family's concerns and responses to care. Document referrals made (e.g., social services, clergy, or hospice services) and visits by members of the interdisciplinary care team.

CONTINUITY OF CARE

Nurses teach patients and families to carry out the physical skills that are necessary to the patient's care. They also provide information on identifying signs of deterioration and obtaining additional sources of support (from hospice, home health care agencies, and public health departments). Encourage families to identify friends and other family members who can help out either routinely or occasionally. At discharge, provide the patient or family with information for contacting the appropriate support groups. Box 13-6■ provides a checklist for older adults as they near the end of life, but the information is useful for anyone. Box 13-7■ provides general guidelines for teaching patients and families about grief.

BOX 13-6	PATIENT TEACHING

End-of-Life Checklist

The nurse can help patients who are facing death by providing this list of questions for them to review:

☑ Take time a day or so before appointments with your health care provider to think about the questions you need answered and concerns you want to discuss. It is often a good idea to keep a pad of paper and a pen handy so you can write down things as they come to you.

☑ Do not hesitate to have your doctor explain your diagnosis again if you did not understand the explanation the first time or if you missed some key points. The same goes for details about using medications and possible side effects.

☑ You may wish to have a friend or family member go with you to medical appointments.

☑ When you visit the doctor, take an up-to-date list of all medications (prescribed and over-the-counter) you are currently taking.

☑ If you have physical pain, tell your health care provider. You will probably be asked to rate your pain on a scale of 1 (no pain) to 10 (severe pain). Your rating helps determine what pain-relief measures are appropriate.

☑ It is a good idea to ask your health care provider about hospice services well before you are likely to need them.

☑ Your family and close friends should be aware of your treatment preferences (such as the existence of a do-not-resuscitate order). You might consider documenting your wishes in a living will.

☑ Think about asking and appointing someone you trust to make your health care decisions, in case the moment comes when you can no longer make them yourself.

☑ If you are feeling depressed or anxious or need emotional support, consider talking to a pastor, chaplain, rabbi, or other trusted person in your faith community. If necessary, ask your health care provider to recommend someone to help you sort out your feelings.

☑ Avoid withdrawing from social activities. Keep communicating with your family, friends, and the people who help care for you. If you are open with them, you are more likely to get the care you need.

Source: Adapted from "End of Life Care" by Advanced Senior Solutions, Inc., http://www.advancedseniorsolutions.com. Used by permission of Advanced Senior Solutions, Inc.

NURSING CARE PLAN
Patient Experiencing Loss

Pearl Rogers is a 79-year-old African American woman who is admitted to the Methodist Home Nursing Center. Mrs. Rogers lived with her husband of 58 years until his death 6 months ago. She had one son, who died in an auto accident 2 years ago, and she has one daughter who lives nearby. After her husband's

Patients Experiencing a Loss

- Encourage both children and adults to discuss the expected or impending loss and to express feelings.
- Teach problem-solving skills:
  - Define what the possible changes and problems are related to the predicted loss.
  - Develop potential strategies for dealing with problems.
  - List pros and cons of each strategy.
  - Decide which strategies might be most useful to try first to solve potential problems associated with the loss.
- Identify persons who are at risk for complicated grieving (those at risk are people whose grief resolution does not follow a normal pattern, people with a sudden or unanticipated death of a significant other, emotionally unstable people, or those without social support).
- Teach individuals and families how to support a person who is dealing with an impending loss:
  - Explain what to expect with a loss: sadness, fear, rejection, anger, guilt, and loneliness.
  - Teach signs of grief resolution:
    - No longer living in the past, becoming future-oriented
    - Breaking ties with the lost object or person (acute stages often show signs of resolving in 6 to 12 months)
    - The possibility of having painful "waves" of grief years after the loss, especially on the anniversary of the loss and in response to "triggers" such as pictures, events, songs, or memories
- Identify community agencies that may be helpful to people responding to loss.

death, Mrs. Rogers lived with her daughter until her admission to the nursing center. Mrs. Rogers has become increasingly agitated and helpless, complaining constantly of pain. Her daughter states that Mrs. Rogers is chronically constipated, has difficulty sleeping, and has stopped taking part in all social activities, including weekly church services. She cries frequently. Extensive medical testing before her admission to the nursing center revealed Mrs. Rogers has arthritis but no other pathologic disorder.

Assessment

When Mrs. Rogers arrives at the nursing center, she is admitted by Sandy Sutphin, LPN. Mrs. Rogers tells Ms. Sutphin, "I'm a sick woman, and no one will listen to me! I can't walk, I'm so weak. My head hurts, and I'm always sick at my stomach. I haven't had a bowel movement in a week, and I never sleep more than 3 hours a night." Ms. Sutphin completes data collection and works with her manager to develop a plan of care for Mrs. Rogers.

Nursing Diagnosis

The following nursing diagnoses (among others) are made for Mrs. Rogers:

- *Grieving* related to stress of husband's death
- *Disturbed Sleep Pattern* related to grieving
- *Constipation* related to inactivity

Expected Outcomes

The expected outcomes established in the plan of care are that Mrs. Rogers will:

- Discuss her losses, use constructive coping mechanisms, and discuss positive and negative aspects of the loss.
- Fall asleep within 20 to 30 minutes after retiring and remain asleep for 7 to 8 hours.
- Have a bowel movement at least every other day.

Planning and Implementation

The following interventions are planned and implemented during care of Mrs. Rogers:

- Promote trust: Show empathy and caring, demonstrate respect for her culture and values, offer support and reassurance, be honest, engage in active listening.
- During one-to-one interactions, encourage Mrs. Rogers to recognize normal grieving behavior. Assist her in labeling her feelings: anger, fear, loneliness, guilt, and isolation.
- Explore previous losses and the ways in which Mrs. Rogers has coped.
- Encourage Mrs. Rogers to express her feelings of anger. Do not become defensive, and explain to her family that anger helps her feel as though she has some control over her environment, even though she has no control over her loss.
- Encourage Mrs. Rogers to participate in her spiritual practices.
- Provide afternoon activities for Mrs. Rogers as indicated by the occupational therapist.
- Provide evening care: warm bath; clean, warm bed; night-light; soft music for relaxation; closed door.
- Provide measures that assist in bowel function: Encourage exercise as tolerated, including walks and rocking in a rocking chair. Offer foods that stimulate bowel movements (e.g., fruits, vegetables, and high-fiber cereals). Increase fluid intake. Provide privacy: Close the door, ensuring that the emergency call bell is within reach, and do not interrupt. Assure Mrs. Rogers that a nurse will be there to help her clean herself if she needs one, and have toilet paper, soap, warm water, and a cloth available to promote her dignity.
- Administer a mild laxative and/or stool softener to Mrs. Rogers, if ordered and necessary, but discontinue as soon as possible.

Evaluation

After 4 weeks at the nursing center, Mrs. Rogers states, "I don't feel any better, but I know I have to accept my situation." Although Mrs. Rogers states that she doesn't feel better, she now walks the length of the hall several times a day, is sleeping better, and has regular bowel movements. Mrs. Rogers is also less withdrawn, has greatly reduced the time she spends crying, and has openly discussed her feelings related to her husband's death, including her anger at the loss of her son and her husband less than 2 years apart. She has attended chapel services on Sunday for the past 2 weeks. She plays cards with the other residents two or three afternoons a week.

Critical Thinking in the Nursing Process

1. How might the nursing staff involve Mrs. Rogers's daughter in developing and implementing her mother's plan of care?

2. Suppose Mrs. Rogers said that she did not want any help, that she just wanted to be left alone to die. How would you respond?

3. What factors in Mrs. Rogers's current life would support the nursing diagnosis of Social Isolation?

Note: Discussion of Critical Thinking questions appears on the companion website.

Note: The references and resources for all chapters have been compiled at the back of the book.

Chapter Review

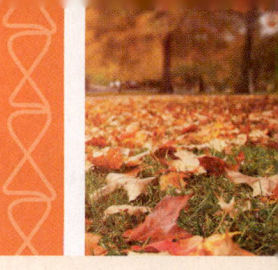

KEY POINTS

- **Concept:** Grief is experienced by all individuals in response to loss. The experience of grief and bereavement is unique to each individual and subjective. Understanding this unique experience helps the nurse provide sensitive and effective care for patients and families.
- When a valued object, person, body part, or situation is lost or changed, the experience of loss occurs. Grief is the emotional response to loss. Grieving responses are individualized to each person but commonly include the stages of denial, anger, bargaining, depression, and acceptance.
- Death is an immensely difficult loss for both the person who is dying and for his or her loved ones. Grief work is often facilitated by family, friends, and spiritual practices.
- **Concept:** Nurses must proactively engage in discussions to elicit and identify patient preferences and concerns regarding end-of-life care, such as management of pain and other symptoms, as well as spiritual needs, to improve the quality of patient care.
- **Concept:** Hospice and palliative care provide physical, psychologic, spiritual, and social care for the dying individual and supportive care to meet the special needs of their families.
- The dying person may control his or her own care through advance directives, living wills, and a durable power of attorney for health care. The patient and family may request that the physician write a do-not-resuscitate (DNR) order.
- **Concept:** A variety of physiologic changes occur in the last hours and days of life. To effectively manage the dying patient, interprofessional caregivers need to understand these physiologic changes and appropriate actions to promote comfort.
- As death nears, specific physiologic changes result in manifestations that indicate impending death. Death is pronounced when respiratory and circulatory functions stop or when all brain function ceases.
- Nursing care for patients who experience loss, grief, or death is implemented to meet the physical, emotional, and spiritual needs of the patient and family. Nurses must also be aware of their own responses to these experiences to provide care more effectively.

PEARSON NURSING STUDENT RESOURCES

Find additional materials at **nursing.pearsonhighered.com**.

Clinical Reasoning Care Map

Caring for a Patient Experiencing a Loss
NCLEX-PN® Focus Area: Psychosocial Adaptation

Case Study: Tom Moore was involved in a serious automobile accident on his way to work and was pronounced dead on arrival at the emergency room. Tom and his wife, Sara, were married for more than 30 years. During that time, Sara did not work outside the home and Tom took care of all the finances. One year after Tom's death, Sara has her annual physical checkup.

Nursing Diagnosis: Grieving

COLLECT DATA

Subjective   Objective

_____   _____

_____   _____

_____   _____

_____   _____

_____   _____

_____   _____

Does this present a risk to the patient's safety?

If yes, the priority intervention to address this threat would be:

_____

Nursing Care

_____

_____

_____

_____

_____

_____

_____

Other interdisciplinary team members to involve when planning care:

_____

_____

How would you document this?_____

_____

Compare your answers and documentation to those provided on the companion website.

Data Collected
(use only those that apply)

- Weight loss of 25 lb
- B/P 110/70
- States, "I can't stand being alone."
- States, "I am still angry at Tom for dying."
- Difficulty sleeping
- States, "My knees sometimes feel like sand-paper inside."
- Unable to continue normal routines
- Has joined a grief support group at her church

Nursing Interventions
(use only those that apply; list in priority order)

- Discuss time needed to resolve a loss.
- Ignore statements and conduct basic physical assessment.
- Explain grief reactions.
- State, "I can't talk about that right now—I'm too busy."
- State, "This must have been very difficult for you."
- Encourage expression of feelings.
- State, "I know it's hard, but you will be okay."

NCLEX-PN® Exam Preparation

1 The grief process may range from discomforting to debilitating, and it may last a day or a lifetime, depending on:
1. whether the loss is temporary or permanent.
2. what the loss means to the person experiencing it.
3. the religion of the person experiencing the loss.
4. the educational level of the person experiencing the loss.

2 A patient has been diagnosed with terminal cancer and is reacting with hostility and abruptness to her family and the hospital staff. She tells them to leave her alone. The patient is most likely in the stage of:
1. denial.
2. anger.
3. bargaining.
4. acceptance.

3 Factors that affect an individual's understanding of and reaction to loss include:
1. age and availability of a support system.
2. income level and age.
3. self-esteem and self-confidence.
4. mental stability and employment status.

4 A do-not-resuscitate order is written for the patient who is near death by the:
1. patient.
2. family.
3. nurse.
4. physician.

5 Regardless of the setting, the patient's wishes about death should:
1. be kept private.
2. be respected.
3. conform to the cultural norm.
4. be the same as his or her family's wishes.

6 A model of care initiated for patients as they near the end of life, emphasizing quality rather than quantity of life, is known as:
1. hospice.
2. euthanasia.
3. advance directive.
4. home-based care.

7 To provide holistic end-of-life care, it is necessary for the nurse to:
1. control his or her own emotions about death.
2. maintain a sense of detachment.
3. agree with the patient's values and beliefs.
4. provide comfort and symptom-management interventions.

8 Respiratory changes to be expected near death include:
1. episodes of tachypnea and coughing.
2. periods of apnea and Cheyne–Stokes respiration.
3. loss of sphincter control and anorexia.
4. emotional distress and crying.

9 Grief before a loss actually occurs is called:
1. complicated.
2. functional.
3. adaptive.
4. normal.

10 The best response of the nurse to help grieving family members express their grief would be:
1. "I know just how you feel."
2. "Things will get better over time."
3. "Tell me how you are feeling."
4. "Let me know if there is anything I can do to help."

Answers and rationales for Review Questions appear in Appendix I.

CULTURAL CARE STRATEGIES

RESPONDING TO BELIEFS RELATED TO DEATH, DYING, AND GRIEF FROM A CULTURAL PERSPECTIVE

Mr. Fazil, 68, a Muslim from Afghanistan, is dying of pancreatic cancer. His brother remains constantly at the bedside where he recites verses from the Koran. When staff offer to sit with Mr. Fazil so the brother can go to the cafeteria, he refuses, saying his voice reciting the Koran must be the last words Mr. Fazil hears before he dies. The nurse offers to bring him some food, and he accepts this offer, provided he is able to perform handwashing rites before eating. The brother requests that a private room be provided for other family members, including the women of the family, where they can meet and grieve together. The brother also requests that he be given all the information concerning Mr. Fazil's status so that he can give this information to the other family members. The women in the family are not permitted in Mr. Fazil's room.

One of the most challenging aspects of providing care for dying people and their families is rendering care that is relevant to cultural, racial, ethnic, and religious needs. There is no universally applicable view of grief. Rather, grief practices and responses to death and dying vary depending on cultural orientation. It is important to determine how the nurse can assist in bereavement and the dying process in a culturally competent manner.

Mourning practices and methods of communicating grief vary across and within cultural groups. For example, for some Chinese individuals, wailing is an essential part of proper mourning. Among African Americans, it has been said that wailing shows how much the family cared about the individual (Perry, 1993). Buddhists use chanting during the dying process. Chanting is thought to facilitate a calm and peaceful atmosphere for the caregivers, thus indirectly helping the dying person. Crying is the most common expression of grief among cultures. Crying serves to

bind individuals who mourn together. In some cultures, grief is expressed through singing and dancing.

Mourning customs related to social organization are important. Individuals may wish to mourn in private, with family members, or with a community group. In some families, such as many Asian families, having the extended family present and involved in decision making is important. This can be problematic when the head of the family group is still resident in Asia. Talamantes et al. (1995) noted that involving Hispanic family members in decision making is important. Issues related to gender role must also be considered. For example, Hispanic, Amish, and Asian American families may have male-dominated decision making. In some cultures, grief expression may be related to the social position, age, and gender of the deceased. In a country with high infant mortality, the death of an infant may not be considered as "important" as it is in Western culture. In Chinese society, husbands require "greater mourning" than wives. Rosenblatt et al. (1976) suggested that this might be a cross-cultural constant, because the average time of mourning by widows was found to be 304 days and by widowers 215 days.

Many cultures are rich in rituals surrounding death. For instance, some Hindus perceive death as a passage from one existence to another. Thus preparation of the body for cremation involves bathing the remains in a milk and yogurt solution, which symbolically cleanses the soul of the deceased. When a married Indian woman dies, she is traditionally placed in a white wedding sari; a man is dressed in a

plain off-white East Indian suit. Religious prayers and chanting are continuous before and after death to promote safe passage of the soul. Russian family members—after washing, dressing, and placing the body in the coffin—may keep vigil over the coffin for hours before the wake and funeral. They may place a black wreath on the door of the deceased person's home. If the individual is Catholic or Russian Orthodox, a priest uses holy oil to anoint the deceased person while making the sign of the cross and saying specific prayers. At the funeral, each member of the Russian Orthodox family may symbolically place a few grains of soil into the coffin.

Nursing Implications

- *Assess individuals for personal beliefs related to death and dying.* Nurses should appreciate that patients' practices related to grief, dying, and death may be significantly different from their own and may be related to cultural practices.

- *Assist the patient and family to grieve and practice death rituals to meet individual needs.* By respecting personal beliefs, the nurse can facilitate grieving in a culturally appropriate manner.

Self-Reflection Questions

1. What beliefs related to grief, death, and dying do you have?

2. Are you flexible in allowing people from different cultures to practice their own traditions in relation to bereavement, the dying process, and death rituals?

3. What can you do to increase your knowledge of bereavement and death practices?

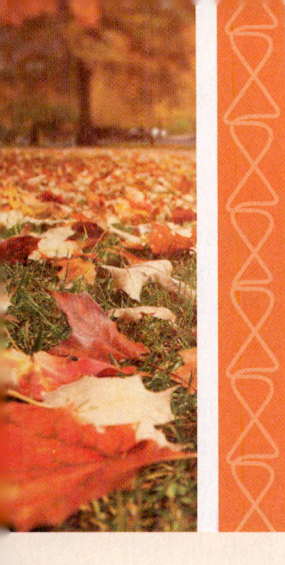

CHAPTER 14

Caring for Patients Experiencing Shock, Trauma, or Disasters

BRIEF OUTLINE

The Patient in Shock
The Patient Experiencing Trauma
The Patient Experiencing a Disaster

APPLIED LEARNING OUTCOMES

After completing this chapter, you will be able to:

1. Describe common causes, pathophysiology, and manifestations for each type of shock: hypovolemic, anaphylactic, cardiogenic, septic, and neurogenic.

2. Apply the medical management and nursing care of the patient in shock.

3. Explain nursing implications for administering fluids, blood products, and medications to patients with shock or trauma.

4. Use the nursing process to collect data, establish outcomes, provide individualized care, and evaluate responses for the patient experiencing shock or trauma.

5. Implement emergency management of patients with trauma, environmental injuries, or poisoning.

6. Describe the effects of a critical care unit on the patient and family.

7. Identify the nurse's role in the care of victims from natural or manmade disasters.

KEY TERMS

The key terms are defined on the pages listed below.

SPECIAL FEATURES

When patients experience shock, trauma, or a manmade or natural disaster, an efficient, knowledgeable response can literally make the difference between life and death. This chapter discusses shock, trauma, and disasters and the roles nurses play in providing care.

The Patient in Shock

Key Concept Shock is characterized by oxygen supply that is less than demand, leading to inadequate tissue perfusion. Without immediate recognition and treatment, shock progresses through the compensatory, progressive, and irreversible stages and can result in death.

Shock is a life-threatening condition, characterized by inadequate blood flow to the tissues and cells. Shock is identified according to its underlying cause. Types of shock are described in Box 14-1■. All types of shock progress through the same stages and exert similar effects on body systems.

BOX 14-1 TYPES OF SHOCK

- **Hypovolemic shock** (low-volume shock)—caused by lack of circulating blood volume, for example, rapid blood loss through hemorrhage.
- **Anaphylactic shock**—caused by immunologic reactions that trigger abnormal dilation of blood vessels, for example, an allergic drug reaction.
- **Cardiogenic shock**—caused by failure of the heart's pumping action, for example, myocardial infarction.
- **Septic shock**—caused by toxins produced from an overwhelming infection, for example, bacterial infection caused by *Pseudomonas*.
- **Neurogenic shock**—caused by changes in the sympathetic tone of blood vessels, for example, spinal cord injury or severe pain.

PATHOPHYSIOLOGY

To maintain homeostasis, all cells require a consistent supply of oxygen and removal of metabolic wastes. The cardiovascular system regulates homeostasis through three basic factors: an adequate blood flow, a correctly functioning heart (pump), and normal blood vessel diameter to maintain tissue perfusion. When one or more of these factors are altered, normal cell function is disrupted. Consequently, tissue perfusion may be inadequate to sustain normal cellular metabolism. The result is the clinical syndrome known as shock. The manifestations of shock result from the body's attempt to maintain vital organ (heart and brain) function. When shock is prolonged or severe, hypoxia occurs and cells die. If shock is not stopped, organs fail and death will result.

Stages of Shock

The three stages of shock are compensatory, progressive, and irreversible. Box 14-2■ lists the fairly distinct manifestations of each stage. Early treatment focuses on preventing the patient from reaching the irreversible stage.

COMPENSATORY STAGE The *compensatory stage* of shock occurs when decreased blood volume significantly reduces the heart's cardiac output, as seen in hypovolemic and cardiogenic shock. In anaphylactic, septic, and neurogenic shock, the blood vessels vasodilate. Vasodilation causes blood to remain in the blood vessels instead of returning to the heart. As a result, blood pressure drops and normal tissue perfusion cannot be maintained. At this point, the body initiates several mechanisms to maintain blood pressure and preserve the vital organs:

1. Baroreceptors in the aortic arch sense the drop in blood pressure and stimulate the sympathetic nervous system (SNS) to release epinephrine and norepinephrine. These "fight-or-flight" hormones constrict arterial blood vessels and increase the heart's rate and strength to

BOX 14-2 MANIFESTATIONS FOUND IN EACH STAGE OF SHOCK

MANIFESTATION	COMPENSATORY STAGE	PROGRESSIVE STAGE	IRREVERSIBLE STAGE
Level of consciousness	Oriented, can follow simple commands; restless	Confused; listless; decreased response to painful stimuli	Lethargy to coma; no reflex response
Speech	Clear	Slurred	Incoherent to absent
Blood pressure	Normal to slightly decreased	Systolic less than 90 mm Hg	Falling to unobtainable
Pulse rate	More than 100 beats/min	More than 150 beats/min, irregular	Slow and irregular
Peripheral pulses	Thready	Weak, thready	Absent
Respirations	More than 20 breaths/min	More than 30 breaths/min; shallow; possible crackles	Slow with Cheyne–Stokes respiration
Skin	Pale, cool, moist	Cold, clammy; possible cyanosis	Cold, cyanotic, mottled
Urinary output	Less than 30 mL/hr	Less than 20 mL/hr	Anuria
Bowel sounds	Decreased	Absent	Absent

contract. Arterial constriction causes the body to *shunt* (push) blood from the kidneys, skin, and gastrointestinal tract to the heart and brain. All of these effects increase venous return to the heart, cardiac output, and oxygen supply to the body's tissues.

2. As blood flow to the kidneys decreases, the **renin–angiotensin–aldosterone system** (a blood pressure regulation system, see also Chapters 7 and 28) is activated. Renin stimulates the production of angiotensin II, a potent vasoconstrictor that raises blood pressure. Angiotensin II signals the adrenal cortex to release aldosterone. Aldosterone causes the kidneys to reabsorb water and sodium, increasing circulating blood volume and also the blood pressure.

3. Low blood volume stimulates the posterior pituitary gland to release antidiuretic hormone (ADH) or vasopressin. ADH increases water reabsorption and helps to increase blood pressure.

If effective treatment is provided during the compensatory stage, the patient should not experience any permanent damage. When the underlying cause cannot be reversed, shock advances to the progressive stage.

PROGRESSIVE STAGE When the compensatory mechanisms fail, the *progressive stage* of shock occurs. Without adequate tissue perfusion, the body's organ functions deteriorate. Unless this stage of shock is treated rapidly, the patient's prognosis is poor.

The progressive stage produces numerous effects on the body's organs (Figure 14-1 ■):

1. *Cardiovascular:* A decrease in cardiac output reduces blood flow to the coronary arteries. The heart muscle receives less oxygen. The imbalance between oxygen supply and demand results in myocardial **ischemia** (reduced blood supply to an organ) that can lead to dysrhythmias and myocardial infarction.

2. *Respiratory:* Decreased pulmonary blood flow alters the exchange of oxygen and carbon dioxide between the alveoli and capillaries. Oxygen levels decrease and carbon dioxide levels increase, leading to respiratory acidosis (see Chapter 7).

3. *Gastrointestinal (GI) and liver:* Blood shunted from the GI tract and liver to the heart and brain causes the GI organs to become ischemic. This results in ulceration of the gastric mucosa and the development of stress ul-

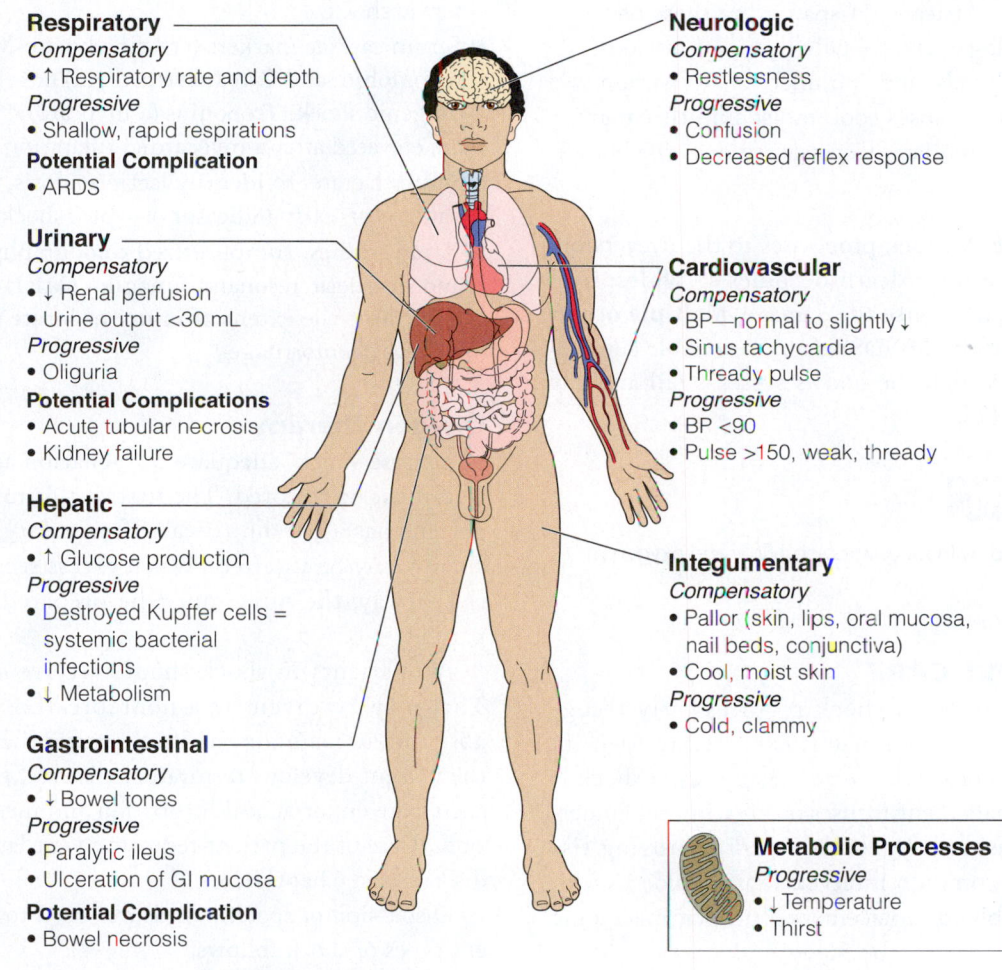

Respiratory
Compensatory
• ↑ Respiratory rate and depth
Progressive
• Shallow, rapid respirations
Potential Complication
• ARDS

Urinary
Compensatory
• ↓ Renal perfusion
• Urine output <30 mL
Progressive
• Oliguria
Potential Complications
• Acute tubular necrosis
• Kidney failure

Hepatic
Compensatory
• ↑ Glucose production
Progressive
• Destroyed Kupffer cells = systemic bacterial infections
• ↓ Metabolism

Gastrointestinal
Compensatory
• ↓ Bowel tones
Progressive
• Paralytic ileus
• Ulceration of GI mucosa
Potential Complication
• Bowel necrosis

Neurologic
Compensatory
• Restlessness
Progressive
• Confusion
• Decreased reflex response

Cardiovascular
Compensatory
• BP—normal to slightly ↓
• Sinus tachycardia
• Thready pulse
Progressive
• BP <90
• Pulse >150, weak, thready

Integumentary
Compensatory
• Pallor (skin, lips, oral mucosa, nail beds, conjunctiva)
• Cool, moist skin
Progressive
• Cold, clammy

Metabolic Processes
Progressive
• ↓ Temperature
• Thirst

Figure 14-1. ■ Multisystem effects of shock.

cers (see Chapter 25). The lining of the small intestine sloughs off, allowing intestinal bacteria to enter the abdominal cavity and move into the circulation, leading to sepsis. Impaired gastric and intestinal motility may cause paralytic ileus.

At first, the liver increases glucose production to compensate for the stress of shock. As shock progresses, the liver fails, leading to hypoglycemia. The liver's *Kupffer cells* (phagocytes that destroy bacteria) cannot function, so bacteria multiply, causing an overwhelming bacterial infection.

4. *Neurologic:* Decreased blood flow to the brain alters mental status and orientation. The patient's level of consciousness deteriorates and may progress to coma. Cerebral edema and irreversible brain cell damage may occur.

5. *Renal:* Blood shunting to the heart and brain reduces flow through the kidneys. Urine output decreases, and the patient develops *oliguria* (low urine output). Prolonged reduced renal blood flow leads to acute renal failure.

6. *Skin and temperature:* In most types of shock, blood vessels in the skin vasoconstrict, leading to skin color changes. Caucasian patients appear pale. Persons with darker skin (e.g., Africans, Hispanics, or those of Mediterranean descent) have pale lips, oral mucous membranes, nail beds, and conjunctiva. Activation of the sweat glands causes cool, moist skin that may become cold. Metabolism decreases, so does the body's temperature.

IRREVERSIBLE STAGE If shock progresses to the irreversible stage, tissue and cellular death becomes so widespread that treatment cannot reverse the damage. **Multiple organ dysfunction syndrome** (MODS) is an irreversible complication of shock in which the body's systems fail and the patient eventually dies.

memory**ALERT**

Shock is characterized by inadequate blood flow and oxygen to cells and tissues.

COLLABORATIVE CARE

Successful management of shock requires early recognition and treatment. The nurse is expected to identify early manifestations of shock. Once a diagnosis of shock is made, medical management focuses on treating the underlying cause, increasing oxygenation, and improving tissue perfusion. The common interventions include oxygen therapy, fluid and blood replacement, and pharmacologic therapy.

Diagnostic Tests

No single diagnostic test can determine shock. However, the following tests may be ordered to help identify the type of shock and to assess the patient's physical status:

- Blood hemoglobin and hematocrit, to detect values that usually occur in hypovolemic shock. Values decrease with hypovolemic shock resulting from hemorrhage. Values may be higher than normal when hypovolemic shock results from the loss of intravascular fluid.
- Arterial blood gases (ABGs), to measure oxygen and carbon dioxide levels and pH. As shock progresses, metabolic acidosis develops from anaerobic metabolism.
- Serum electrolytes and glucose, to monitor the severity and progression of shock. As shock progresses, sodium levels decrease, potassium levels increase, and glucose levels decrease.
- Blood urea nitrogen (BUN) and serum creatinine levels, to check renal function. Decreased renal perfusion reduces renal function; the BUN and creatinine levels increase, as does urine specific gravity.
- Blood cultures, to identify the causative organism in septic shock.
- White blood cell (WBC) count, which is elevated in septic shock.
- Serum cardiac markers (creatine kinase-MB [CK-MB], myoglobin, and C-reactive protein) are elevated in cardiogenic shock. Troponins (a myocardial muscle protein) are elevated after a myocardial infarction.
- Serum lactate, to identify lactic acidosis, that when elevated is an early indicator of septic shock.
- X-ray studies, computerized tomography (CT) scans, and magnetic resonance imaging (MRI) may determine the extent of injury or locate sites of internal hemorrhage.

Oxygen Therapy

To reverse shock, adequate oxygenation and tissue perfusion must be restored. The first step is to ensure that the patient has a patent airway. If necessary, a nasal or oral airway may be inserted. When excess secretions obstruct the airway, the nurse must be prepared to suction the patient.

All patients in shock should receive oxygen therapy. This may be given by a nonrebreather mask at 12 to 15 L/min to maintain the PaO_2 greater than 90 mm Hg. If the patient develops respiratory distress, the nurse should anticipate endotracheal intubation and mechanical ventilation. (Care of the patient requiring ventilation assistance is discussed in Chapter 23.)

Discussion of specific measures used to treat the different types of shock follows.

TYPES OF SHOCK
Hypovolemic Shock

Hypovolemic shock is the most common type. It is caused by a decrease in intravascular volume. Normally, about two-thirds of the body's fluids are found in the intracellular compartment, and the remaining third is in the extracellular compartment. The extracellular compartment is divided into intravascular and interstitial fluids. To remain in balance, each compartment must maintain the correct amount of fluid (see Chapter 7).

The decrease in intravascular volume may result from:

- Loss of blood volume (hemorrhage) as a result of trauma, surgery, GI bleeding, or hemophilia.
- Internal fluid shifts (third spacing) as a result of cirrhosis with ascites, pleural effusion, pancreatitis, or intestinal obstruction.
- Loss of body fluids through persistent and severe vomiting, diarrhea, or continuous nasogastric suctioning and massive diuresis from diuretics or diabetes insipidus.
- Loss of fluids through the skin as a result of profuse diaphoresis or burns.

The pathophysiology of hypovolemic shock as seen in Figure 14-2■ can occur alone or develop along with other types of shock. Manifestations reflect the stage of shock the patient is experiencing (see Box 14-2). They depend on the patient's age, general health, severity of injury or illness, length of time before treatment has started, and the rate of volume loss. Hypovolemic shock caused by fluid losses or internal fluid shifts may have more subtle manifestations than other types of shock (Box 14-3■).

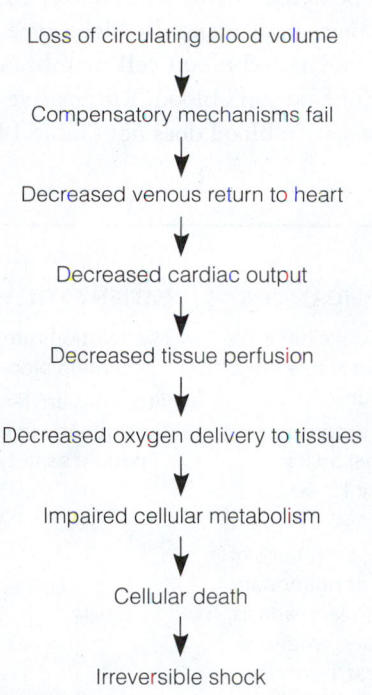

Loss of circulating blood volume

↓

Compensatory mechanisms fail

↓

Decreased venous return to heart

↓

Decreased cardiac output

↓

Decreased tissue perfusion

↓

Decreased oxygen delivery to tissues

↓

Impaired cellular metabolism

↓

Cellular death

↓

Irreversible shock

Figure 14-2. ■ The pathophysiology of hypovolemic shock.

BOX 14-3	INITIAL MANIFESTATIONS OF HYPOVOLEMIC SHOCK

- **Neurologic:** Restlessness and anxiety
- **Cardiovascular:** Decreased blood pressure; rapid, weak pulse
- **Respiratory:** Tachypnea, dyspnea
- **Skin:** Pale, cool, moist
- **Urine output:** Decreased
- **Other:** Thirst, weakness

Hypovolemic shock resulting from trauma or hemorrhage requires immediate emergency care. This care begins as soon as medical rescuers arrive on the accident scene and continues through transport to the emergency department (ED). At the emergency scene, intravenous fluids are started, and pneumatic antishock garments may be applied. Because shock can progress so rapidly, treatment needs to begin within the first hour after an injury if at all possible (the "golden hour" of trauma care). Failure to begin emergency treatment within the first hour increases the patient's risk for death. Box 14-4■ summarizes the prehospital emergency care for a patient in hypovolemic shock.

The **pneumatic antishock garment** (PASG), also called military antishock trousers (MAST), is applied at an accident scene for a patient with a traumatic injury (Figure 14-3■). The device is used to raise blood pressure and can be used

---

BOX 14-4	PREHOSPITAL EMERGENCY CARE OF THE PATIENT EXPERIENCING HEMORRHAGE

1. Scan the area for potential hazards (e.g., fire).
2. Call for help.
3. Ensure adequate airway; assist with ventilation as needed.
4. Assess for the cause of hemorrhage.
5. Control external bleeding by applying direct pressure to the local site. If an extremity is involved, elevate it to stop venous bleeding. When bleeding continues, apply pressure to an arterial pressure point.
6. Apply a tourniquet *only as a last resort.*
7. Assess for manifestations of shock, which may include:
   a. Decreased blood pressure.
   b. Rapid, thready pulse.
   c. Rapid, shallow respirations.
   d. Cool, pale, moist skin.
   e. Thirst.
   f. Restlessness; changes in the level of consciousness.
8. Keep the patient's trunk and head flat and legs slightly elevated. (Use this position *only* when no head injury exists.)
9. Cover the patient to maintain warmth.
10. Do not give the patient anything by mouth.
11. Use touch and verbal communication to reduce apprehension and anxiety.

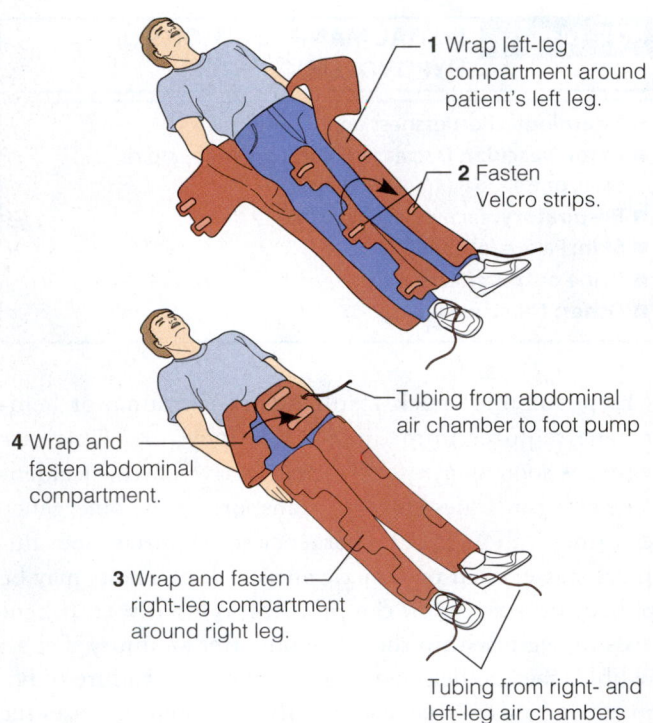

1 Wrap left-leg compartment around patient's left leg.

2 Fasten Velcro strips.

4 Wrap and fasten abdominal compartment.

Tubing from abdominal air chamber to foot pump

3 Wrap and fasten right-leg compartment around right leg.

Tubing from right- and left-leg air chambers

Figure 14-3. ■ Pneumatic antishock garments provide rapid, emergency treatment of shock.

to stabilize pelvic and femoral fractures. Only specially trained personnel can apply or remove the PASG.

FLUID REPLACEMENT The main goal for patients with hypovolemic shock is to restore intravascular volume. Intravenous fluids are used alone or in combination with colloids, blood, or blood products. The type and amount of fluid chosen depends on the type of fluid lost. Usually, fluid replacements are given in a 3:1 ratio (300 mL fluid for every 100 mL of fluid loss).

Crystalloid solutions contain electrolytes dissolved in water. The most commonly ordered intravenous solutions are normal saline (0.9%) and lactated Ringer. Both isotonic solutions increase volume in the intravascular and interstitial spaces. These solutions are given during the emergency phase while the patient's blood is being typed and cross-matched. See Chapter 7 for more information about crystalloid solutions and intravenous therapy.

clinicalALERT

Large infusions of crystalloid solutions can lead to pulmonary edema. Monitor the patient closely for signs of respiratory distress such as dyspnea and crackles.

Colloid solutions contain proteins that increase osmotic pressure. (Osmotic pressure holds fluid within the vessels so that the plasma volume expands.) Colloid solutions include albumin, plasma protein fraction, dextran, and hetastarch. (See how to give medications safely when administering colloids in Table 14-1■.)

Blood and blood products used in treating hemorrhage are obtained from a donor and given as a *transfusion* (an infusion of blood or blood components) to the patient (Table 14-2■). State and institutional policies vary about whether LPNs/LVNs can administer transfusions. Nurses are responsible for knowing their scope of practice.

Each person has one of four blood types: A, B, AB, or O. Blood group antigens A and B form the basis for ABO blood categorization. The presence or absence of these inherited antigens determines one's blood type (type A has A antigen, type B has B antigen, and type AB has both). Persons with neither antigen have blood type O.

A protein on the red blood cell membrane determines the Rh factor of a person's blood. Rh-positive blood has the protein; Rh-negative blood does not (Table 14-3■).

TABLE 14-1	Giving Medications Safely: Colloid Solutions		
CLASS/DRUGS	**PURPOSE**	**NURSING IMPLICATIONS**	**PATIENT TEACHING**
Colloid solutions (plasma expanders) ■ Albumin 5% or 25% (Albuminar, Buminate) ■ Plasma protein fraction (Plasmanate) ■ Dextran 40 or 70 (Gentran 40 or 70) ■ Hetastarch (Hespan)	Colloid solutions expand blood volume and are used to treat hypovolemic shock. Albumin and plasma protein fraction come from healthy human donors. Dextran and hetastarch are made synthetically.	Before infusion, take patient's vital signs and assess lung and heart sounds. Take vital signs according to institutional policy (usually every 15–60 minutes). Monitor for manifestations of heart failure or pulmonary edema (dyspnea, cyanosis, cough, crackles, wheezes). If these appear, notify the physician immediately.	The solutions are helping to maintain blood volume. Vital signs are taken frequently to ensure the patient's safety.

TABLE 14-2	Blood and Blood Products	
TYPE	**COMPOSITION**	**USE**
Whole blood	Contains RBCs, plasma proteins, clotting factors, and plasma.	Replaces blood volume and increases oxygen-carrying capacity in hemorrhage and shock.
Packed red cells	Contains RBCs, some platelets, no clotting factors; very little plasma.	Increases oxygen-carrying capacity of blood.
Platelets	Contains only platelets.	Controls bleeding in patients with platelet deficiencies.
Fresh frozen plasma	Contains all clotting factors except platelets.	Expands blood volume; can be administered to any blood group or type, because it contains no RBCs; takes 30–60 minutes to thaw.
Cryoprecipitate	Contains factor VIII, factor XIII, and fibrinogen.	Treats patients with clotting factor deficiencies.

Note: Each hospital has its own policy about blood transfusions. The nurse must learn and follow those policies.

Before a patient can receive a blood transfusion, a blood **type and cross-match** (test to determine donor and recipient ABO types and Rh groups) must be done. Blood is also tested for hepatitis A, hepatitis B, and human immunodeficiency virus (HIV).

Despite rigorous type and cross-matching procedures, blood transfusion reactions may still occur. The most common is a febrile reaction, which typically begins during the first 15 minutes of the transfusion. In a *febrile reaction*, the patient's antibodies react to the donor's white blood cells, causing fever and chills. (General guidelines for monitoring blood transfusions are found in Table 14-4■.)

When hemorrhage causes hypovolemic shock, the patient may receive whole blood or packed red blood cells (PRBCs). The goal is to increase the patient's hematocrit and hemoglobin levels to near-normal values. Trauma victims may receive a type O blood transfusion while the type and cross-match is done.

Some EDs and trauma centers use autotransfusion for the patient with multiple injuries and/or severe shock. **Autotransfusion** is the collection, filtration, and retransfusion of a patient's own blood. Blood from the chest cavity is the typical source for an autotransfusion.

TABLE 14-3	Blood Group and Rh Types and Compatibilities
BLOOD GROUP	**COMPATIBLE DONOR**
O	O
A	A, O
B	B, O
AB	A, B, AB, O
Rh	
Rh positive	Rh positive, Rh negative
Rh negative	Rh negative

Note: Group O is often called the universal donor, and group AB is called the universal recipient. Do not infuse blood if types are incompatible according to the chart.

Anaphylactic Shock

Anaphylaxis is caused by a severe allergic reaction that can progress to anaphylactic shock. Almost any *antigen* (foreign substance) can trigger an anaphylactic response. Antigens can enter the body by injection, by ingestion, or through the skin or respiratory tract. Some common causes of anaphylactic shock include the following:

TABLE 14-4	Giving Medications Safely: Blood Transfusions	
NURSING IMPLICATIONS		**PATIENT TEACHING**
<ul><li>Take and record baseline vital signs.</li><li>Stay with the patient during the first 15 minutes of the transfusion.</li><li>Monitor for manifestations of a transfusion reaction.</li><li>Take and record vital signs according to institutional policy.</li><li>If a transfusion reaction occurs, take the following actions: a. Stop the transfusion immediately, and notify the charge nurse. b. Disconnect the blood tubing, hang new IV tubing, and start normal saline slowly. c. Take vital signs and assess for manifestations. d. Follow institutional policy for saving the blood bag, returning it to the laboratory, and collecting urine and venous blood samples. e. Continue to monitor the patient and provide prescribed interventions to treat the reaction according to the physician orders.</li></ul>		Immediately report any warm feelings, chills, itching, feelings of weakness or fainting, or difficulty breathing.

- Foods: legumes (nuts, seeds), shellfish, egg whites, milk, chocolate, tomatoes, and strawberries
- Stings and bites of insects and snake venom
- Substances used to diagnose and treat disease: iodine dyes, antibiotics, vaccines, local anesthetics, blood, and narcotics
- Other substances: latex, pollen, and molds or food additives

When a person is first exposed to an antigen, the body produces antibodies against it. The initial antigen–antibody response usually produces no harmful effects, but it may sensitize the person to the antigen. With each future exposure, the antigen reacts with the antibodies, and anaphylaxis may occur.

clinicalALERT

Anaphylactic reactions are more severe when the antigen enters the body by the intravenous route or when a second exposure occurs.

When an antigen–antibody reaction occurs, it stimulates mast cells to release histamine and other chemical mediators into the circulation. These substances cause widespread vasodilation and make capillaries more permeable. The shift of fluids results in hypotension and **relative hypovolemia** (fluid shifts from vascular space into interstitial space, so that blood pools in the tissues). Blood volume is reduced, tissue perfusion is impaired, and cell metabolism is altered. Other effects include inflammation, bronchoconstriction, and cutaneous reactions. Manifestations of anaphylaxis may begin on immediate contact with the antigen. Anaphylactic shock, a severe form of anaphylaxis, is a life-threatening emergency and requires immediate intervention to prevent death within a matter of minutes. People with known allergies should wear a MedicAlert bracelet. Health care providers should carefully assess and document allergies or previous drug reactions. A summary of the manifestations found in anaphylactic shock is listed in Box 14-5.

When an anaphylactic reaction develops, the patient needs immediate intervention. First priorities are a patent airway and supplemental oxygen, followed by drug therapy. Epinephrine, given intramuscularly or intravenously, is the drug of choice to restore arterial blood pressure and promote bronchodilation. Antihistamines such as diphenhydramine (Benadryl) reverse the effects of histamine. Corticosteroids may be given to prevent a delayed reaction to the antigen. If respiratory distress continues, nebulized albuterol (Proventil) is ordered to reverse bronchospasm. Once the patient's condition is stable, the patient must be monitored

---

BOX 14-5 MANIFESTATIONS OF ANAPHYLACTIC SHOCK

- **Skin:** Generalized itching, flushing, sensation of warmth, urticaria (hives), angioedema (edema of eyelids, lips, and tongue)
- **Neurologic:** Restlessness, anxiety, decreased level of consciousness
- **Respiratory:** Difficult breathing, stridor, wheezes, laryngospasm
- **Cardiovascular:** Hypotension, tachycardia
- **Gastrointestinal:** Nausea, vomiting, diarrhea

for reappearance of signs and symptoms of anaphylaxis. The effects of the causative antigen may last for hours.

Cardiogenic Shock

Cardiogenic shock occurs when the heart fails to act as an effective pump, so cardiac output and adequate tissue perfusion cannot be maintained. Myocardial infarction is the most common cause of cardiogenic shock. The amount of myocardial damage determines the severity and progression of shock. (Other cardiac disorders causing cardiogenic shock are discussed more thoroughly in Chapter 17.)

In cardiogenic shock, the ventricles fail to pump blood into the circulatory system. This leads to a decreased *cardiac output* (the amount of blood pumped from the ventricles in 1 minute). Excess blood is left in the ventricle with each beat. This blood backs up into the lungs, leading to pulmonary edema. When cardiac output drops, the patient becomes hypotensive. A compensatory rise in heart rate increases myocardial oxygen consumption and decreases coronary perfusion. This burdens an already overworked myocardium, so eventually it fails. Common manifestations of cardiogenic shock are listed in Box 14-6.

Cardiogenic shock usually results from an acute myocardial infarction. Oxygen is given to prevent further heart muscle damage. Drug therapy and mechanical devices are prescribed to raise blood pressure and improve cardiac output. These patients are acutely ill and are best managed in a critical care unit. Several intravenous medications are used to treat cardiogenic shock. **Vasopressor drugs** such as dopamine (Intropin) and

BOX 14-6 MANIFESTATIONS OF CARDIOGENIC SHOCK

- **Cardiovascular:** Hypotension; rapid, weak, thready pulse; distended neck veins
- **Respiratory:** Rapid, labored respirations; crackles
- **Skin:** Pale, cold, moist
- **Neurologic:** Restlessness, anxiety, lethargy progressing to coma
- **Urine output:** Oliguria to anuria

norepinephrine (Levophed) produce vasoconstriction, which raises the patient's blood pressure. **Positive inotropic drugs**, such as dobutamine (Dobutrex) and amrinone (Inocor), increase the force of myocardial contraction so that cardiac output increases. Nitroglycerin (Tridil) may be used to improve the pumping action of the heart. Diuretics may be given if the patient shows signs of heart failure. Antidysrhythmic drugs regulate the patient's heart rhythm.

In addition to medications, two mechanical devices can also help improve blood circulation: the intra-aortic balloon pump (IABP) and the ventricular assist device (VAD). (See Chapter 16 for further discussion.)

Septic Shock

Septic shock is part of a progressive syndrome called *systemic inflammatory response syndrome* (*SIRS*). It most often results from an overwhelming gram-negative bacterial infection (e.g., *Pseudomonas, Escherichia coli, Klebsiella*) or gram-positive infection (e.g., *Staphylococcus* and *Streptococcus*). Patients at a higher risk for septic shock include those who are older and hospitalized, have chronic debilitating illnesses, and have poor nutritional status. Other risk factors that increase the chance for developing septic shock are the following:

- Extremes of age (less than 1 year, greater than 65 years)
- Chronic debilitating diseases or conditions:
  - Cancer, AIDS, or malnutrition
  - Burns or decubitus ulcers
  - Diabetes mellitus or chronic kidney failure
- Surgery, invasive lines, or tubes (IV or central venous lines, urinary catheters, tracheostomy or endotracheal tube)
- Drug therapy (chemotherapy, corticosteroids, antibiotic therapy)

Septic shock begins with **septicemia** (the presence of pathogens and pathogenic toxins in the blood). The invading bacteria multiply faster than the rate at which the body can kill them. As bacteria are destroyed, endotoxins are released into the bloodstream. The endotoxins damage tissues and starve the cells of oxygen and nutrients. The damaged cells release histamine and other chemicals to dilate peripheral blood vessels and increase capillary permeability. As in anaphylactic shock, fluids shift from intravascular space to interstitial space, resulting in relative hypovolemia. *Microemboli* (tiny blood clots) form in the capillaries, causing further cell damage and death. Early manifestations include weakness; warm, flushed, dry skin; and chills. Other early symptoms often mimic the criteria used to identify SIRS, whereas late manifestations show significant physiologic deterioration. Patients who meet two of more of the SIRS criteria can rapidly progress to septic shock unless treated immediately. Manifestations are summarized in Box 14-7■. Death may result from respiratory, cardiac, or renal failure.

BOX 14-7   MANIFESTATIONS OF SEPTIC SHOCK

SIRS Criteria
- **Cardiovascular:** Heart rate greater than 90 beats per minute
- **Respiratory:** Respiratory rate greater than 20 or PaCO₂ less than 32 mm Hg
- **Temperature:** Below 96.8°F (36°C) or above 100.4°F (38°C)
- **Other:** WBC count less than 4,000 mm³, greater than 12,000 mm³, or greater than 10% immature neutrophils

Late Septic Shock
- **Cardiovascular:** Profound hypotension despite adequate fluid resuscitation; rapid, thready pulse; dysrhythmias
- **Respiratory:** Rapid, shallow with crackles; dyspneic
- **Skin:** Cold, cyanotic extremities
- **Neurologic:** Confused to lethargic to comatose
- **Urine output:** Oliguria to anuria

Toxic shock syndrome (TSS) is caused by a toxin-producing form of *Staphylococcus aureus*. It usually affects menstruating women between 15 and 19 years of age who use tampons. Toxins from the bacteria enter the bloodstream and circulate throughout the body, causing the septic shock process to begin. The manifestations include hypotension, high fever, vomiting, and diarrhea. Without treatment the patient's condition can worsen and be fatal.

For septic shock, rapid interventions are the key to patient survival. A serum lactate level is drawn to determine the presence of anaerobic metabolism from hypoperfusion. Blood cultures are done to identify the causative organism before administering broad-spectrum intravenous antibiotics such as third-generation cephalosporins. Large volumes of intravenous fluids such as 0.9% normal saline are given to counteract the massive vasodilation caused by the release of bacterial endotoxins. Vasopressor drugs are added when the patient continues to be hypotensive. Because these patients are unstable, they must be transferred to the critical care unit for continuous monitoring and treatment.

Neurogenic Shock

Neurogenic shock results from an interruption in the SNS. The problem can result from damage to the vasomotor center in the medulla or from loss of impulse transmission (seen in a spinal cord injury above the T6 level). Other causes include head injury, spinal anesthesia, narcotic overdose, severe pain, and hypoglycemia.

Without SNS impulses, the blood vessels dilate, leading to massive peripheral vasodilation. Blood pools in the venous and capillary beds, leading to inadequate tissue perfusion. Thermoregulation is impaired because the cutaneous blood vessels lose vasomotor tone.

BOX 14-8	MANIFESTATIONS OF NEUROGENIC SHOCK

- **Cardiovascular:** Hypotension, bradycardia
- **Skin:** Warm, dry
- **Neurologic:** Anxiety to restlessness to lethargy
- **Urine output:** Oliguria to anuria
- **Other:** Lowered body temperature

Without appropriate treatment, organ failure and death can occur. Manifestations of neurogenic shock are listed in Box 14-8■.

Treatment of neurogenic shock varies according to its cause. Intravenous fluids are ordered to reverse the peripheral vasodilation, so blood pressure and tissue perfusion are restored. If neurogenic shock is caused by severe pain, appropriate analgesics should be given. Patients receiving spinal anesthesia should have the head of the bed raised to prevent the anesthetic from moving up the spinal cord. (Management of patients with spinal cord injury is presented in Chapter 39.)

COMPLICATIONS OF SHOCK

The two most common complications of shock are **acute respiratory distress syndrome (ARDS)** and **disseminated intravascular coagulation (DIC)**. Both disorders usually develop once the patient has entered the progressive stage of shock.

Acute Respiratory Distress Syndrome

Acute respiratory distress syndrome (ARDS) is characterized by acute respiratory failure due to damage to the alveoli. When alveolar capillaries become more permeable, fluid and proteins leak into the alveoli, causing a type of pulmonary edema. The patient with ARDS may require mechanical ventilation. See Chapter 23 for more information about ARDS and mechanical ventilation.

Disseminated Intravascular Coagulation

Disseminated intravascular coagulation (DIC) is an acute condition characterized by simultaneous bleeding and clotting throughout the body. Tissue damage triggers an abnormal activation of the body's clotting mechanisms. There is widespread, continuous clot formation, which consumes all of the clotting factors, resulting in generalized bleeding. Clots are deposited in the capillaries, reducing blood flow to the skin and causing *mottling* (discoloration). Initially, the patient bleeds from puncture sites and incisions. Treatment is aimed at replacing the platelets and clotting factors while protecting the patient from injury. See Chapter 20 for more information about DIC and its treatment.

NURSING CARE

The nurse assumes an important role in preventing shock as well as potential complications.

PRIORITIZING NURSING CARE

Priorities of nursing care start with maintaining an adequate airway, breathing, and circulation and then focus on replacing fluid volume, restoring and maintaining tissue perfusion, preventing complications, and providing psychosocial support to the patient and family. The highest priority nursing diagnosis appropriate for the patient with any type of shock is ineffective tissue perfusion.

ASSESSING

Assessment data collected by the nurse can determine the severity of the shock condition. The manifestations for each type of shock can be found in the previous discussion. Restlessness, tachycardia, and slight anxiety are common early symptoms, with a fall in blood pressure occurring later. It is important to recognize and notify the physician at this early stage. Frequent assessment of the patient in shock is done at least every hour. When the patient's condition worsens, assessments may be as often as every 5 to 10 minutes.

DIAGNOSING, PLANNING, AND IMPLEMENTING

Ineffective Tissue Perfusion: Cardiac, Peripheral, Cerebral, Renal

Expected outcome: Will have adequate tissue perfusion as evidenced by palpable peripheral pulses, warm and dry skin, and adequate urine output.

- Monitor skin color, temperature, turgor, and moisture. *Decreased tissue perfusion is shown by pale, cool, and moist skin. When hemoglobin levels drop, cyanosis may occur.*
- Monitor cardiopulmonary function every 15 to 30 minutes by assessing blood pressure, heart rate and rhythm, rate and depth of respirations, lung sounds, and peripheral pulses (include presence, equality, rate, rhythm, and quality). If unable to palpate pulses, use a Doppler ultrasound device. If a central line is inserted, measure central venous pressure (CVP). *Vital signs help identify the stage of shock. As shock progresses, BP drops; the pulse becomes rapid, weak, and thready. Decreased lung perfusion causes crackles, wheezes, and dyspnea. Capillary refill is prolonged. Peripheral pulses (dorsalis pedis and posterior tibial) are weak or nonpalpable. CVP measures fluid status; low findings indicate decreased blood volume (normal = 5 to 15 cm).*
- Monitor oxygen saturation by attaching a pulse oximeter to the patient. Start supplemental oxygen as needed. *Oxygen saturation should be maintained between 94% and 100% with oxygen therapy.*

■ Assess for restlessness, confusion, mental status changes, and decreased level of consciousness. *These indicate decreased cerebral perfusion.*

■ Monitor intake and urinary output per Foley catheter hourly, using a urometer. *Urine output is the most reliable indicator of renal perfusion.* Measure daily weight and fluid loss from causes such as emesis and gastric and chest tube drainage. *These measures evaluate fluid status.*

clinicalALERT

Urinary output less than 30 mL/hr indicates reduced renal perfusion and an increased risk for acute renal failure.

■ Monitor bowel sounds, abdominal distention, and abdominal pain. *Decreased gastrointestinal blood flow reduces bowel motility and peristalsis; paralytic ileus may result.*

■ Assess for sudden sharp chest pain, dyspnea, cyanosis, anxiety, and restlessness. *Hemoconcentration and increased platelet aggregation may result in pulmonary emboli.*

clinicalALERT

Assess for irregular heart rate and chest pain because these indicate decreased coronary artery perfusion and increased risk for myocardial infarction.

■ Monitor body temperature and keep the patient comfortably warm without shivering. *An elevated body temperature or shivering caused by hypothermia increases oxygen requirements. Applying warm blankets and keeping room temperature comfortable reduces shivering.*

■ Maintain the patient on bed rest, and provide a calm, quiet environment. Place the patient in a modified Trendelenburg position as tolerated (Figure 14-4■). *Bed rest decreases the workload of the heart. The modified Trendelenburg position increases venous return to the heart. Do not use this position for patients in cardiogenic shock.*

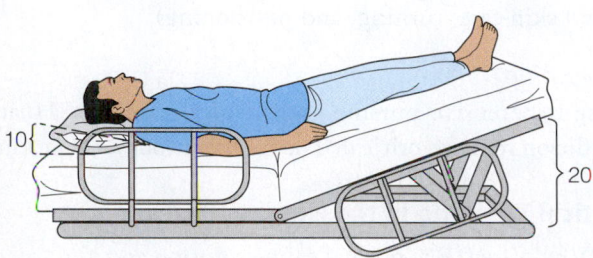

Figure 14-4. ■ Modified Trendelenburg position. Position the patient with the lower extremities elevated approximately 20 degrees (knees straight), trunk horizontal, and the head elevated about 10 degrees.

Anxiety

Expected outcome: Will report that anxiety has been reduced or alleviated.

Many patients in hypovolemic shock have experienced a traumatic injury that has required major surgery and a transfer to a critical care unit. Other types of shock are associated with critical illness or injury, such as acute myocardial infarction, head injury, or spinal cord injury. Throughout these events, the patient and family are frightened, anxious, and often emotionally isolated. Although the nurse's first priority must be to provide emergency care, the psychosocial needs of the patient and family also must be met.

■ Acknowledge the patient's anxiety and fear. *This helps validate the patient's feelings.*

■ Remain with and explain procedures to the patient. Listen carefully to the patient. Speak slowly and calmly, using short sentences. Use touch to provide support. *These measures provide reassurance to the patient and help reduce anxiety.*

■ Provide comfort measures (e.g., calm, quiet environment, back rub). *Comfort measures can reduce the patient's anxiety.*

■ Provide time, space, and privacy for family members. *Allowing the family access to the patient reduces anxiety and gives both the patient and the family some feeling of control.*

■ Provide anticipatory guidance to prepare for recovery or death. *If the prognosis is poor, this helps the family begin the grieving process.*

■ Keep the patient's family informed. *They need information on which to make their decisions.*

MANAGING NURSING CARE

As appropriate and allowed by the designated duties and responsibilities of assistive personnel, the nurse may delegate nursing care activities such as providing personal hygiene and turning and positioning for the patient in shock. Before assigning tasks such as obtaining vital signs, daily weights, pulse oximetry readings, and intake and output, ensure assistive personnel have a clear understanding of the importance of accuracy in measurement.

EVALUATING

Evaluate the effectiveness of care by noting whether the patient's vital signs are stabilized. Also, the nurse notes the patient's tissue perfusion: alert and oriented; warm, dry skin; urine output less than 30 mL/hr; palpable pedal pulses; and oxygen saturation above 94%. Note whether the patient's anxiety is reduced.

DOCUMENTING

Documentation focuses on the patient's vital signs, orientation level, respiratory status, skin temperature and presence of moisture, quality of pedal pulses, urine output, bowel sounds, and level of anxiety. Record the patient's response to acute interventions such as oxygen therapy, fluid replacement, and medications administered.

CONTINUITY OF CARE

Shock must be fully resolved before a patient can be discharged. Although the patient has survived the shock episode, recovery from the original medical problem may be delayed. Teach the family that a lengthy recovery often leads to depression and that the patient will need a supportive and nurturing environment. Teach patients who have experienced an anaphylactic reaction how to prevent a future reaction. Emphasize the following key points in teaching before discharge:

■ Avoid known allergens.
■ Notify health care professionals of allergies.
■ If allergic to insect stings, avoid wearing bright colors, perfumes, and scented hair sprays when outdoors.
■ If allergic to foods, read package labels. When eating out, ask how meals are prepared and what ingredients are used.
■ Wear a MedicAlert bracelet or necklace.
■ Carry an emergency kit for anaphylaxis or an *EpiPen* (epinephrine).
■ Review manifestations of anaphylaxis.
■ Seek medical attention immediately when symptoms occur.

NURSING CARE PLAN
Patient With Septic Shock

Huang Mei Lan is a 43-year-old single woman who had a right mastectomy 4 days ago for recurrent breast cancer. She is underweight, weak, and depressed. Despite her multiple problems, she never complains or asks for pain medication. A central line and a urinary catheter are in place. On her fourth postoperative day, Mrs. Canote, her primary nurse, finds Ms. Huang huddled in the middle of the bed, shivering violently.

Assessment

T 104°F, P 110, R 30, and BP 96/66. Her skin is hot, dry, and flushed with poor turgor. She is nauseated, is oriented to time and place, restless, and appears anxious. Her urine output is 300 mL for the last 12 hours. Her WBC count is elevated. Blood, urine, and wound cultures are collected. She is diagnosed as having septic shock. Intravenous fluids of 0.9% normal saline and of a broad-spectrum antibiotic are begun until the organism and its portal of entry are identified. Ms. Huang's condition worsens. Her blood pressure and urine output continue to drop, her skin becomes

cool and cyanotic, and she has periods of disorientation. She is transferred to the critical care unit. As she is being prepared for the transfer, she begins to cry and asks, "Am I going to die?"

Nursing Diagnosis

The following nursing diagnoses (among others) are established for Ms. Huang:

■ *Deficient Fluid Volume* related to vomiting, high fever, and hypotension
■ *Impaired Gas Exchange* related to rapid respirations
■ *Ineffective Tissue Perfusion* related to hypotension and massive vasodilation
■ *Anxiety* related to feelings that illness is worsening and is potentially life threatening

Expected Outcomes

The expected outcomes for the plan of care are that Ms. Huang will:

■ Maintain adequate circulating blood volume.
■ Regain and maintain ABG parameters within normal limits.
■ Regain and maintain stable hemodynamic levels.
■ State her feelings of fear and anxiety.

Planning and Implementation

The following nursing interventions are implemented for Ms. Huang. Assessments are done frequently to monitor her condition.

■ Monitor mental status and the level of consciousness.
■ Monitor arterial blood pressure; rate, rhythm, and quality of pulses; central venous pressure; pulmonary artery pressure; and cardiac output.
■ Assess color and character of skin.
■ Monitor results of ABGs, blood counts, clotting times, and platelet counts.
■ Monitor respiratory rate, rhythm, and breath sounds.
■ Monitor temperature every 2 hours.
■ Monitor urinary output hourly, reporting any output of less than 30 mL/hr.
■ Explain procedures and provide comfort measures (oral and skin care, turning, and positioning).

Evaluation

Despite intensive nursing and medical care, Ms. Huang's condition remains critical. The interventions are continued.

Critical Thinking in the Nursing Process

1. Why were 0.9% normal saline solution and a broad-spectrum antibiotic started on Ms. Huang?
2. What safety risks are important for the nurse to monitor with Ms. Huang?

3. Why would the nursing diagnosis of Impaired Skin Integrity be appropriate for Ms. Huang?

Note: Discussion of Critical Thinking questions appears on the companion website.

The Patient Experiencing Trauma

Key Concept   Trauma is any life-threatening occurrence, either accidental or intentional, that causes injuries (American Trauma Society, 2012). Leading causes of trauma are falls, motor vehicle crashes, and assaults. Trauma often kills or disables people during their most productive years of life.

Persons who need urgent medical care enter the medical system through the ED. Treatment in the ED is provided by nurses and doctors with special training in emergency care. Emergency nurses take care of patients of all ages with a wide range of medical problems. This type of nursing requires a broad knowledge base, solid observation skills, and the ability to provide care in an unpredictable environment. Severely injured patients may require transport to a regional trauma center.

The goals of emergency care are to stabilize the critically ill, prevent deterioration of a patient's condition, and promote optimal function. To accomplish these goals, patients must be prioritized when they enter the ED. **Triage** systems identify who will receive medical attention first. The most common triage categories are emergent, urgent, and nonurgent. *Emergent* refers to life-threatening conditions that require immediate treatment. *Urgent* means that patients need treatment within at least 2 hours. *Nonurgent* includes patients who would not be adversely affected by a delay in treatment.

CAUSES AND TYPES OF TRAUMA

Trauma is defined as an injury caused by physical force (motor vehicle crashes, falls, drowning, gunshots, burns, stabbing, or other physical assaults). Trauma is the number one cause of death for persons under the age of 44 and is the fifth leading cause of death in the United States for all age groups. At highest risk are males between the ages of 15 and 24 years; geriatric patients are also at risk (Box 14-9 ■). Traumatic injuries can result in temporary physical impairment, permanent disability, or death.

Traumatic injury occurs suddenly, leaving the patient and family with little time to prepare for its consequences. Nurses serve as a vital communication link between the injured patient and the family. They help the patient and family cope with the patient's current injury, as well as understand the potential long-term effects of this injury.

BOX 14-9	FOCUS ON OLDER ADULTS

Geriatric Risks for Trauma

Older adults are hospitalized for trauma twice as often as the general population. Falls resulting in head trauma and fractures are the leading cause of injury in those over age 65. Most falls are caused by preexisting chronic illnesses, environmental factors, medication side effects, or age-related physiologic changes such as diminished vision or hearing, poor balance, and decreased motor strength and coordination. Persons over age 75 experience a high fatality rate after a motor vehicle collision. Older pedestrians have a higher risk for being struck by a motor vehicle because they move less quickly when crossing the street or cannot see traffic lights well.

Minor or Major Trauma

Whether intentional or accidental, trauma causes injury to one or more body parts. *Minor trauma* involves a single body part or system and is usually treated in the ED. A fractured collarbone, a small second-degree burn, and a laceration requiring stitches are all considered minor trauma. *Major trauma* involves serious single-system injury (such as traumatic amputation of a leg). Multiple trauma involves multiple-system injuries. Multiple trauma victims require immediate emergency care.

Blunt or Penetrating Trauma

Trauma also may be classified as blunt or penetrating. *Blunt trauma* does not cause a break in the skin. Common blunt forces are motor vehicle crashes, falls, assaults, and contact sports. *Penetrating trauma* results from foreign objects that pierce the body. The most common sources are knives; bullets; shotgun blast; or impaled, sharp objects. The penetrating object often damages the brain, heart, lungs, intestines, liver, spleen, and vascular system. Both types of trauma can result in greater internal damage than that appears on the surface.

EFFECTS OF TRAUMATIC INJURY

Traumatic injuries have serious consequences that must be identified and treated rapidly. Some common effects of traumatic injury are the following:

- *Airway obstruction* can be caused by blood, teeth, the tongue, or emesis in a patient's airway. Once the cervical spine is immobilized with a cervical collar, oxygen is given. The airway may be cleared by suctioning. Patients with severe airway obstruction may require intubation with an endotracheal tube (Figure 14-5 ■).
- *Pneumothorax* results when air enters the pleural space causing partial or complete lung collapse. Blunt and penetrating injuries to the chest may be the cause. A *tension pneumothorax* develops when air continually enters the chest cavity but cannot exit. In the ED, a chest tube

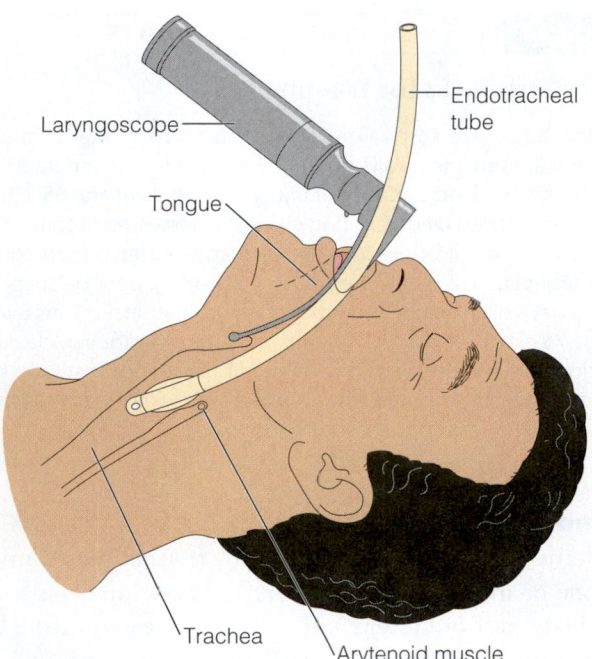

Figure 14-5. ■ Intubation with insertion of an endotracheal tube (ETT). When a patient is experiencing respiratory distress, oxygen can be given into the external opening of the tube.

is inserted to reinflate the lung. See Chapter 23 for more information about pneumothorax.

■ *Hemorrhage* in the trauma patient may be external or internal (see prehospital care in Box 14-4 on page 323). When an artery is severed, the bleeding must be controlled immediately (Figure 14-6■) by placing pressure on it. Internal hemorrhage may lead to blood pooling in several body cavities. For example, chest trauma may cause bleeding into the pleural space. A pelvic fracture may lead to bleeding in the retroperitoneal region. The nurse must identify the cause, location, and extent of blood loss.

■ *Hypovolemic shock* may be caused by hemorrhage from blunt or penetrating injuries, long-bone or pelvic fractures, major vessel injuries, traumatic amputation, or plasma loss from burns or crush injuries (see earlier discussion).

■ *Neurologic injuries* most often include traumatic brain injury (TBI), with spinal cord injury occurring less frequently. Both injuries can have a permanent, devastating outcome. Most head and spinal cord injuries result from motor vehicle crashes; other causes include falls, sports injuries, all terrain vehicle (ATV) crashes when not wearing a helmet, and assault.

■ *Gastrointestinal* and *genitourinary injuries* can be caused by blunt and penetrating injuries. Liver and spleen injuries are the main sources of life-threatening hemorrhage. Peritonitis can occur when damaged intestines leak bile and stool into the peritoneum. Motor vehicle crashes cause most renal injuries.

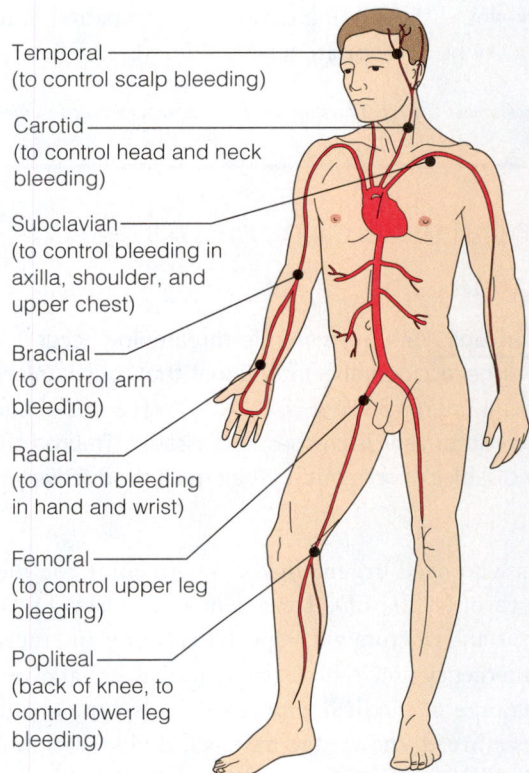

Temporal
(to control scalp bleeding)

Carotid
(to control head and neck bleeding)

Subclavian
(to control bleeding in axilla, shoulder, and upper chest)

Brachial
(to control arm bleeding)

Radial
(to control bleeding in hand and wrist)

Femoral
(to control upper leg bleeding)

Popliteal
(back of knee, to control lower leg bleeding)

Figure 14-6. ■ The major pressure points used to control bleeding.

clinicalALERT

Never remove a penetrating object. Removal may cause internal injuries or possible nerve damage.

■ *Musculoskeletal injuries* are frequently seen in the ED. Injury includes damage to bone, soft tissue, nerves, or blood vessels. Common manifestations of musculoskeletal injuries are swelling, bone protrusion, obvious deformity, abnormal motion, pain, and a pulseless extremity. See Chapter 42 for more information about musculoskeletal injury.

■ *Integumentary injuries* are not usually as serious, except for burns (see Chapter 46). The nurse must assess both the skin and the underlying structures for any sign of injury. Injuries to the integument are often contaminated with dirt, debris, or foreign objects that increase the patient's risk for infection. The four main skin injuries are contusions, abrasions, puncture wounds, and lacerations (Figure 14-7■).

■ *Psychologic effects on the patient* are a consequence of trauma. The patient will feel anxious and insecure in the unfamiliar surroundings. It is important for the nurse to provide explanations about treatment procedures and reassure the patient frequently.

■ *Psychosocial effects on the family* are also a consequence of trauma. Death or serious injury may change family

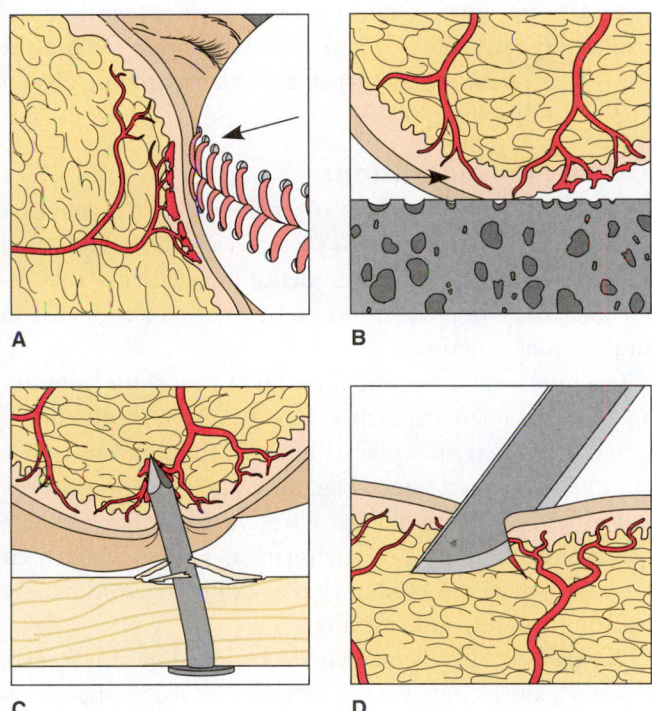

Figure 14-7. ■ (**A**) Contusions (bruises) do not cause a break in the skin. (**B**) Abrasions (scrapes) occur when a partial layer of skin is removed. (**C**) Puncture wounds occur when the integument is penetrated by a sharp or blunt object. (**D**) Lacerations are irregular tears in the skin.

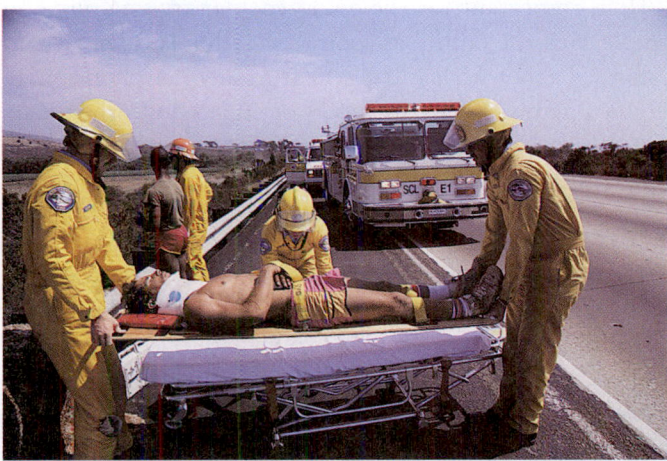

Figure 14-8. ■ Application of a cervical collar at an accident scene immobilizes the cervical spine and prevents further injury to the spinal cord. (Source: Spencer Grant/Science Source.)

dynamics. The suddenness and seriousness of the event predispose families to psychologic crisis. Families may exhibit shock, fear, numbness, anxiety, guilt, hostility, or anger.

COLLABORATIVE CARE

The trauma patient requires collaborative care at the accident scene before arriving in the ED (see Box 14-4, page 323). This type of care may be provided by emergency medical technicians (EMTs), paramedics, flight nurses, or physicians. Flight nurses are educated in trauma care and air transport techniques. They can perform advanced techniques such as intubation or chest tube insertion.

At the accident scene, life-threatening problems must be identified and treated immediately. Before other treatments are started, the patient may require basic life support and advanced cardiac life support. The patient's cervical spine is immobilized at once by placing the patient on a spine board and applying a cervical collar (Figure 14-8■). If the patient's airway is patent, high-flow oxygen is started. Direct pressure may be applied to control active external bleeding. One or two intravenous lines with IV fluids are started.

As soon as the patient's condition is stabilized, the patient is transported rapidly to the ED or trauma center. Ground ambulances and air ambulances (e.g., specially

staffed and equipped helicopters or fixed-wing aircraft) are used. Once the trauma patient arrives at the ED, team members provide medical and nursing care. These team members may include an ED physician, ED nurses, trauma surgeon, anesthesiologist, laboratory technicians, radiologist, and respiratory therapist.

Diagnostic Tests

The diagnostic tests obtained depend on the patient's injuries. Besides the tests used to rule out shock, the following tests may be ordered:

- Blood alcohol levels measure the amount of alcohol in a patient's blood (20% to 50% of people who are injured are intoxicated).
- Urine drug screen determines the presence of cocaine, heroin, or amphetamines.
- Pregnancy test for any woman of childbearing age rules out the potential for pregnancy and fetal injury.
- Diagnostic peritoneal lavage identifies the presence of blood in the peritoneal cavity, which may indicate abdominal injury.
- CT scan locates injuries to the brain, skull, spinal cord, chest, and abdomen.
- MRI identifies brain and spinal cord injuries.

Emergency Surgery

Surgery is indicated when the patient remains in shock despite resuscitation and there is no obvious external sign of blood loss. Nurses prepare the patient for emergency surgery by undressing the patient and removing jewelry, dentures, or other loose objects. Place an identification bracelet on the patient. Report the extent of the injury, allergies and past medical history (if obtainable), and completed nursing interventions to the operating room nurse.

It is important for the emergency or trauma nurse to speak with the family as soon as possible and keep them informed about what is happening to their family member. Unfortunately, family members or significant others may not have time to see their loved one before transfer to the operating room.

Critical Care

Patients with shock or traumatic injuries are best treated in a critical care unit or *intensive care unit (ICU)*. These highly specialized units are designed to provide care to patients in the critical phase of an illness. ICU nurses and physicians have advanced knowledge in the latest medical and technological methods. The critical care nurse constantly monitors the acutely ill patient for life-threatening situations and initiates nursing actions as needed. Because of the critical condition of these patients, the ICU nurse may care for only one or two patients.

Psychosocial Effects

The critical care environment is overwhelming to patients. They are under artificial lighting and are attached to strange machines that make sounds. The environment and the constant nursing care often lead to sensory overload and sleep deprivation. Unfamiliar voices and the lack of personal touch from family members result in sensory deprivation and increase patients' stress levels.

The nurse can reduce sensory overload by monitoring noise levels and limiting conversation directly with the patient. Adding a calendar and clock to the patient's room or playing a favorite radio station or tape may reorient the patient. The patient's psychologic well-being can be increased by encouraging the family to touch the patient. Uninterrupted rest periods are beneficial, but rest must be balanced with the patient's need for family and with the need for hourly monitoring.

ICU psychosis (acute confusion after 2 to 3 days in the ICU) develops rapidly and is generally reversible. Older adults are more prone to this condition. Common features include altered attention span, memory loss, confusion, and visual and auditory hallucinations. Sedatives or psychotropic drugs may be given, but often they can make the condition worse. ICU psychosis usually decreases once the patient's sensory–perceptual problems and sleep deprivation are resolved, but it is distressing to the patient and family.

Although a critical illness affects the patient most, it also affects family roles and functions. The family fears the death of a loved one. They are anxious about all of the equipment surrounding the patient and the potential for pain. They worry about finances and permanent changes in family roles. The nurse can assist the family by giving them a short status report every time they visit. If possible, involve the family in the patient's daily care. Each family member should be assessed for signs of exhaustion. When

necessary, the nurse should consult a social worker and chaplain to help obtain resources for the family. When the family's needs can be met, they are able to provide greater support to the patient.

Forensic Considerations

Sometimes injuries involve criminal activity that requires legal investigation. The nurse's role is to identify, store, and properly transfer potential evidence for medical–legal investigations. All evidence must be marked and sealed in tamper-proof containers.

The nurse must not cut through any clothing containing potential evidence such as blood stains or bullet holes. Each clothing item is placed in an individual breathable container, such as a paper bag, and labeled appropriately. Bullets or knives are labeled with the identifying source and given to the proper authorities. Entrance and exit wounds must be recorded in the chart. Photographs may be needed of wounds and clothing.

The patient's hands may yield important evidence, such as powder burns on the skin or tissue or hair samples beneath the fingernails. Paper bags should be placed over the patient's hands if the presence of evidence is suspected.

ORGAN DONATION

Under the Uniform Anatomical Gift Act, consent for organ donation may be given not only by the donor, but also by a spouse, adult child, parent, adult sibling, or guardian. Most states require health care providers to ask family members about organ donation. Nurses should know their hospital's organ and tissue donation policies. The following organs and tissues can be donated: kidneys, heart, lungs, pancreas, intestines, liver, cornea, bones, bone marrow, and skin.

Before donation is considered, the family is notified of the patient's grave prognosis. They should be given the option of donating the patient's organs, but should realize that organ donation is an option, not an obligation. The family should be encouraged to ask questions and express their feelings in making this difficult decision. A grief counselor or clergy can provide emotional support to the family. Even if the patient carries an organ donor card, many institutions will not remove any organs without a signature from a family member or other authorized person.

Before organs can be removed, the patient must be declared brain dead. **Brain death criteria** are clinical signs used to determine whether a comatose patient is brain dead (Box 14-10■). Once brain death has been confirmed, the family must also agree with the diagnosis and be allowed time to prepare for the patient's death as well as they can.

When the decision has been made to proceed with organ donation, the Organ Procurement Organization is notified (1-800-24-DONOR). Nurses should know the agency in their region that is responsible for organ procurement.

BOX 14-10	BRAIN DEATH CRITERIA

- Irreversible condition
- Unresponsive coma (absence of motor and reflex movements)
- No spontaneous respirations; $PaCO_2$ greater than 60 mm Hg
- Absent brainstem functions (no pupillary, corneal, cough, and gag reflexes)

Confirmatory Testing

- Electroencephalogram (EEG)—no electrical activity for 30 minutes
- Cerebral blood flow study—no intracerebral filling

NURSING CARE

Nursing care of the patient who has suffered a serious injury starts with a primary assessment and includes collaborative interventions to manage any life-threatening injuries.

PRIORITIZING NURSING CARE

The post-trauma patient has many nursing care problems. Two of the most common are actual or potential problems with infection and impaired physical mobility. Other important nursing diagnoses include altered tissue perfusion and anxiety, which were discussed in the section of this chapter on shock. Ineffective airway clearance related to facial fractures, spiritual distress, and post-trauma syndrome from the devastating consequences of a traumatic event should also be considered.

ASSESSING

In the ED, the nurse ensures that the cervical spine is immobilized and then performs a five-step primary assessment: airway, breathing, circulation, disability, and exposure. The ABCs are assessed and managed first. Then the nurse assesses for the degree of disability related to neurologic functioning. A baseline neurologic assessment should include the patient's level of consciousness, pupil reaction to light, and response to verbal or painful stimuli. In the exposure step, the nurse removes the patient's clothes and examines all body surfaces for obvious injuries. The nurse also obtains a brief history, patient allergies, and past medical history.

A Foley catheter is inserted to monitor urinary output. If there is a risk for aspiration, a nasogastric tube is placed. The patient is attached to a cardiac monitor. At least two intravenous lines are used to give IV fluids, blood components, inotropic drugs, and vasopressors as needed to treat hypovolemic shock. The emergency nurse monitors the patient closely for shivering or chills. Warm blankets and warmed IV solutions are used to prevent hypothermia. If the patient has penetrating wounds, a tetanus prophylaxis such as tetanus toxoid or human toxin–antitoxin may be given.

DIAGNOSING, PLANNING, AND IMPLEMENTING

Risk for Infection

Expected outcome: Will remain free from infection.

Traumatic injuries often occur in a dirty environment. Projectiles entering the body carry dirt and debris into the wound. Open fractures provide an entry point for bacteria and dirt. Even after surgery, wounds can remain contaminated.

- Use careful hand hygiene practices. *Hand hygiene remains the single most important factor in preventing infection.*
- Use strict aseptic technique when inserting catheters, suctioning, giving parenteral medications, or changing dressings. *Trauma patients are at a greater risk for infection.*
- Monitor wounds for odor, redness, heat, swelling, purulent drainage, increased pain under casts, and increased drainage over the wound area. Be sure dressings do not restrict circulation. Avoid tape; instead, use mesh or stretch gauze to hold dressings in place. Prevent cross-contamination between wounds. *Because the skin is the first line of defense against infection, the nurse must monitor for signs of infection and prevent any new breaks in the skin.*
- Take vital signs and temperature every 2 to 4 hours. *An elevated body temperature and pulse are indicators of an infection.*
- Provide adequate fluids and nutrition. *Adequate fluids, calories, and protein are essential to wound healing.*
- Monitor for manifestations of sepsis. *Patients with traumatic injuries are at a high risk for developing sepsis and septic shock.*

Impaired Physical Mobility

Expected outcome: Will remain free from complications of impaired mobility.

- Provide active or passive exercises to affected and unaffected extremities at least once every 8 hours. Do not perform exercises if active bleeding or edema is present. *Exercise improves muscle tone, maintains joint mobility, improves circulation, and prevents contractures. Immobility due to trauma increases the risk for complications of the skin, cardiovascular, gastrointestinal, respiratory, musculoskeletal, and renal systems.*
- Assist the patient to turn, cough, and deep breathe, and use the incentive spirometer at least every 2 hours. *Changing positions, coughing, deep breathing, and incentive spirometry reduce the risk of skin and respiratory complications.*
- Monitor the patient's skin for signs of skin breakdown and reposition the patient every two hours. For patients requiring prolonged immobility, consult with the physician regarding the use of a low pressure air mattress or bed (Figure 14-9 ■). *Low-pressure air mattresses and beds can decrease the pressure on bony prominences and skin, but continuous monitoring of skin remains a primary nursing intervention.*

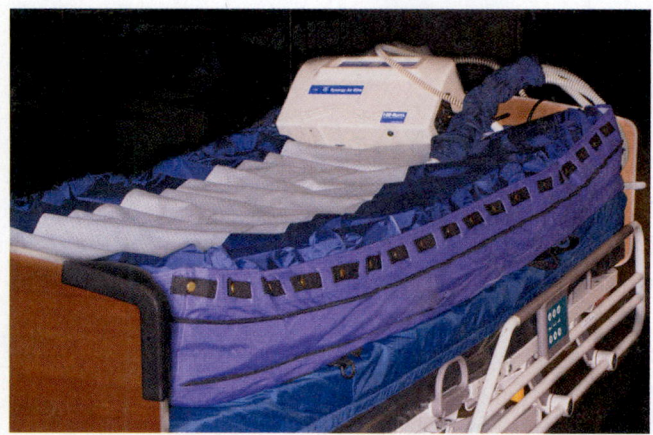

Figure 14-9. ■ A low-pressure bed helps to prevent skin breakdown in patients with restricted mobility. (Source: R.A. Penne-Casanova/Science Source.)

- When the patient cannot be moved and positioned easily, consult with the physician regarding the use of a specialty bed such as the kinetic continuous rotation bed. *The bed helps prevent pneumonia, venous stasis, postural hypotension, urinary stasis, muscle wasting, and bone loss.*
- Monitor the lower extremities every 8 hours for deep venous thrombosis (DVT): heat, swelling, and pain. Measure and record the circumference of the thigh and calf each day. If antiembolism or intermittent compression stockings are used, remove them for 1 hour during each shift and assess the skin for changes. *When injury occurs to the vein and blood flow becomes sluggish, a thrombus (clot) forms. DVT is a major risk for pulmonary embolism.*

MANAGING NURSING CARE

As appropriate and allowed by the designated duties and responsibilities of assistive personnel, the nurse may delegate nursing care activities such as providing oral and skin care and turning and positioning for the patient after a traumatic injury. Before assigning tasks such as obtaining vital signs, daily weights, pulse oximetry readings, and intake and output, ensure assistive personnel have a clear understanding of the importance of accuracy in measurement.

EVALUATING

Evaluate the effectiveness of nursing care by collecting data related to the absence of infection and complications from immobility. As the patient recovers, evaluate the patient's progress toward maximum wellness.

Because the trauma patient is usually managed in the critical care unit, documentation is specific to the patient's injuries. Once transferred to a medical–surgical unit, the nurse documents the patient's progress toward recovery.

CONTINUITY OF CARE

The nurse's main responsibility is to prepare the patient and family for discharge and promote maximum wellness. Before discharge, consult with home health care to determine potential home modifications (e.g., if the patient's bedroom is on an upper floor, first-floor sleeping arrangements may be necessary until healing has occurred). Review when and how to take the medications and their potential side effects. Provide information as needed about special diets. Discuss the patient's rehabilitation plan and identify transportation concerns. Emphasize the need for follow-up appointments with the physician. Discuss with the family emotional changes that the patient may experience (e.g., insomnia, nightmares, and reliving the incident). A resource for patients with neurologic injuries is the National Institute of Neurological Disorders and Stroke. If the family has lost a loved one, provide a referral for grief counseling.

Preventive Health Teaching

Injury is a major health problem in the United States. The nurse is in a unique position to provide preventive education, after assessing for individual risk factors (weakness, poor vision, and risky behaviors). Safety education should be taught in EDs, doctors' offices, clinics, schools, and health fairs. Because many injuries occur at home, individuals should also know how to make their homes safer. Box 14-11■ lists common safety tips.

ENVIRONMENTAL INJURIES

A variety of medical emergencies can result from excessive exposure to heat or cold. This section presents prehospital and basic ED care for patients with environmental emergencies.

Hyperthermia (elevated core body temperature) occurs when the body is exposed to excessive heat. Normally, the body regulates its temperature through sweating and peripheral vasodilation. When the temperature and humidity exceed the body's regulatory mechanisms, heat exhaustion and heat stroke develop. Heat-related illnesses cause more deaths annually in the United States than natural disasters do. *Heat exhaustion* results from increased sweating and electrolyte loss, which causes hypovolemia. It is characterized by profuse sweating, weakness, nausea, and cool skin. Individuals with heat exhaustion should be placed in a cool area and given oral fluids. Loosen clothing and apply cool, wet towels. Victims who are very young or old, or who do not improve within 30 minutes, should be taken to the nearest hospital.

Heat stroke involves a rapid rise in temperature, often above 106°F within 10 to 15 minutes, because the body cannot cool itself. It is not common but is a medical emergency.

BOX 14-11	COMMON SAFETY TIPS

- Be alert in order to avoid potentially harmful conditions or activities.
- Don't drink and drive or use any mechanical/electrical equipment.
- Wear a protective helmet when riding a bicycle, motorcycle, skateboard, or scooter.
- Follow equipment safety precautions when operating power tools.
- Wear safety belts and secure children in a child safety seat or safety belt.

Bathroom
- Use nonskid mats or strips in shower or tub.
- Install handrails in shower or tub and by the toilet as needed.
- Use night-light in the bathroom.
- Use tub bench for unsteady persons.
- Set water heater below 115°F.

Kitchen
- Turn pot handles away from the edge of the stove.
- Keep flammable liquids, paper towels, and pot holders away from the burners.
- Keep a fire extinguisher near the stove.

Floors and Stairways
- Keep entryways, halls, and stairways well lit.
- Remove clutter and trailing cords from pathways inside and outside.
- Install handrails and antiskid strips on stairways.
- Secure or remove scatter rugs.
- Use nonskid shoes on waxed floors.

Other
- Use a stepladder to reach high objects.
- Use good lifting technique when lifting heavy objects.
- Install smoke alarms in the kitchen and on every floor.
- Keep firearms unloaded and locked in a secure place.

Manifestations include altered mental status; hot, dry skin; hypotension; tachycardia; and tachypnea. Heat stroke victims must be cooled immediately. This is done by moving the patient to a shady area, removing the patient's clothes, and misting with cool water. If cold packs are available, place them on the patient's groin, axillae, and back of the neck. The patient is never immersed in icy water (shivering produces more heat). As soon as possible, transport the patient to an ED. If the temperature has not dropped to 102°F, a cooling blanket is used. The patient is given 100% oxygen immediately to compensate for the increased metabolic rate. Monitor the patient closely for acute renal failure and seizures.

Hypothermia (core body temperature is below 95°F) results from exposure to cold temperatures. Infants are at

clinicalALERT

Older adults with diabetes or cardiovascular disease or who take diuretics that alter fluid balance have a higher risk for heat-related illnesses.

higher risk because they have less body fat. Older adults have an increased risk due to a declining basal metabolic rate with age and impaired temperature regulation. Mild hypothermia is characterized by shivering and slowed mental functioning. As the victim's temperature drops, muscle coordination is lost; heart, respiratory, and neurologic functions are slow; and eventually death results.

In cases of mild hypothermia, move the patient to a warm place, remove wet clothing, and cover with warm blankets. Patients with moderate to severe hypothermia should be transported immediately to a nearby hospital. On arrival in the ED, the patient is warmed slowly with blankets, an external warming blanket, or a forced-air blanket system. Warmed intravenous solutions may be given, along with warmed peritoneal lavage. Respiratory therapy includes warmed, humidified oxygen. The patient with moderate to severe hypothermia is at increased risk for cardiac dysrhythmias and arrest. The patient is kept in a horizontal position and moved gently to prevent ventricular fibrillation.

POISONINGS

A *poison* is any chemical substance that damages body structures. Poisons enter the body through ingestion, inhalation, and skin contamination. Common ingested poisons include corrosives such as lye, toilet bowl cleaners, and bleach; plants; and drugs such as aspirin, acetaminophen, antidepressants, and benzodiazepines. Most inhalation injuries occur in the home from carbon monoxide, natural gas, chlorine, and some pesticides. Skin contamination occurs from pesticides and industrial chemicals.

When poisoning is suspected, call 1-800-222-1222 immediately. The call is directed to the appropriate regional poison control center in the United States (McPhee & Papadakis, 2012). They can provide guidelines for appropriate treatment. Some poisonings can be managed at home, but most require treatment in the ED. When the patient arrives in the ED, the first priority is to assess the patient's airway, breathing, and circulation, and then to identify the poison. The medical staff will recommend the appropriate antidote or an elimination method.

Ingested poisons may be treated by giving activated charcoal orally or through a gastric lavage; this binds to the poison for expulsion in the stool. Syrup of ipecac induces

BOX 14-12	GUIDELINES TO PREVENT POISONING

- Use dangerous chemicals only in well-ventilated areas.
- Wear protective clothing such as gloves and goggles.
- Do not mix common household cleaning products.
- Keep all products in their original containers with the label attached.
- Use poison symbols to identify dangerous substances.
- Keep all poisons and medicines locked away.
- Identify poisonous plants and keep them away from children.
- Never call medicine "candy."
- Use childproof safety caps.
- Always take medications in a well-lit room to prevent an error.
- Post the local Poison Control Center telephone number by the phone.

vomiting but is no longer recommended for the treatment of poisoning (McPhee & Papadakis, 2012). Corrosive poisons must be diluted with milk or water. Other elimination methods include gastric lavage, cathartics, whole-bowel irrigation, and hemodialysis. Patients who have inhaled poisonous substances need supplemental oxygen. Contaminated skin must be drenched immediately with running water, and all clothes must be removed. Anyone assisting the patient should wear protective clothing to prevent secondary exposure.

Poisonings can be prevented. Box 14-12■ summarizes prevention tips.

The Patient Experiencing a Disaster

Key Concept Disasters require extraordinary efforts beyond what is needed to respond to everyday emergencies. Nurses play an essential role in knowing how to respond when a disaster occurs and in providing care for disaster victims.

Disasters often occur without warning, making it important for nurses to understand their role ahead of time. Nurses are expected to provide care to disaster victims in a variety of settings, including hospitals, ambulatory clinics, long-term care facilities, or at home. They must be prepared to assist patients, families, and health care workers, in addition to their community.

DISASTER OVERVIEW
There are distinct differences between an emergency and a disaster. Emergencies usually involve a few victims who can be handled immediately by local emergency agencies. For example, care of victims of a motor vehicle crash can be done by local emergency services. In contrast, a disaster often causes multiple deaths, injuries, and property damage. Disasters are of such magnitude that the situation cannot be managed by routine emergency agencies and resources. Examples include Hurricane Katrina in 2005 and Hurricane Sandy in 2012.

Disasters can be natural or manmade. Natural disasters include floods, hurricanes, earthquakes, tornadoes, wildfires, and winter storms. Manmade disasters are accidental or deliberate. Wrecked trains carrying dangerous chemicals or a building collapse are examples of accidental disasters. Deliberate disasters include acts of terrorism, which use biologic, chemical, radiologic, or nuclear weapons. Bioterrorism uses biologic agents in an effort to cause mass casualties by such diseases as anthrax, smallpox, and botulism. (See Chapter 9 for further discussion on biologic threat infections.)

Natural Disasters and Common Injuries
A variety of common injuries take place during disasters. Flood victims may suffer fractures and abrasions from debris in the flood waters, burns from gas leaks that explode, electrocution from fallen power lines, and drowning. Survivors of a hurricane experience similar injuries to those of a flood. In addition, animal, snake, and insect bites; heat-related conditions; and gastrointestinal illness are common. Earthquakes cause bone, joint, and muscle injuries along with gastrointestinal and respiratory problems, and burns from explosions. Victims of tornadoes endure musculoskeletal injuries from flying debris or from being trapped under collapsed buildings. Burns commonly occur during wildfires, in addition to smoke inhalation problems. Winter storms can lead to hypothermia problems such as frostbite and cardiac emergencies from strenuous snow removal. Chronic respiratory disorders frequently worsen during disasters from exposure to the dust-filled air. Health care and emergency service workers in the field are prone to clean-up injuries after a disaster.

Weapons of Mass Destruction Injuries
Chemical and radiation weapons of mass destruction are used to cause significant injury and death. Highly toxic, chemical warfare agents such as phosgene and chlorine produce choking and lung damage. Sarin, a nerve gas, inhibits acetylcholinesterase (AChE), an enzyme that breaks down acetylcholine. Without AChE, normal nerve function is disrupted, causing copious saliva production, seizures, paralysis, and eventual death. Severe respiratory distress results from cyanide poisoning.

Detonation of a dirty bomb or exposure to nuclear or radioactive material can cause extensive injuries. A dirty bomb consists of explosive material and radioactive waste and results in blast injuries. It can cause extensive damage to all body systems, including lung and heart contusions, eardrum rupture, eye injury, and traumatic amputation of extremities. Nuclear exposure can result in thermal burns, flash blindness, and radiation sickness.

Family Disaster Plan

Emergency Meeting Place (outside of the home)_____

Meeting Place (outside of the neighborhood)_____

Family Contact _____ Phone _____

Address _____

Home Disaster Supply Kit

(Prepare enough to last for 3 days.)

- 3 gallons of water per person (1 gallon/person/day)
- 3-day supply of nonperishable food; can opener
- Portable, battery-powdered radio and flashlights with extra, fresh batteries
- First aid kit with prescription medication
- Blankets or sleeping bags; warm clothing; footwear
- Sanitation and hygiene items
- Cash, coins; copies of credit and insurance cards
- Emergency phone numbers
- Set of extra keys and IDs
- Special items for infant, elderly, or disabled family members
- Other essentials: paper, pencil, ABC fire extinguisher, whistle, waterproof matches, work gloves
- Pet food, water, and medications
- Comfort items: Games, books, favorite dolls, or stuffed animals

Figure 14-10. ■ Encourage community members to fill out this form and obtain the supplies listed to have in case of disaster.

DISASTER PLANNING AND RESPONSE

Disaster preparedness is a priority of the U.S. government and military. When disaster strikes, federal, state, and local agencies are activated. Federal agencies include the Federal Emergency Management Agency (FEMA), U.S. Department of Health and Human Services, Office of Emergency Preparedness, American Red Cross, and U.S. Army Corps of Engineers. State and local offices of the national agencies respond to disasters within their area. Disaster Medical Assistance Teams coordinate disaster relief with local fire, police, and public health departments.

Nurses are expected to keep current in new and emerging health care trends. This also includes learning about disaster prevention and participating in the following disaster preparation steps:

- Know how to take care of yourself so that you can help others.
- Take part in disaster training and drills.
- Teach families:
  - To make a disaster plan in advance and work as a team (Figure 14-10■).
  - To make sure everyone knows how to turn off water, gas, and electricity at the main switches.
- To plan for taking care of family pets.

Encourage everyone in the community to assemble a disaster supply kit (see Figure 14-10). There should be

TABLE 14-5	Simple Triage System	
TRIAGE TAG	**TYPICAL INJURIES**	**TREATMENT**
Red	Critical injuries: airway obstruction, hemorrhage, shock, head injuries, full-thickness burns of face and neck	Immediate
Yellow	Major injuries, large wounds, open fractures, burns not involving the head	Treat within 30 minutes to 2 hours
Green	Minor injuries, can walk and care for themselves; contusions, sprains	Have them walk to a safe place
Black	Dead or imminently terminal; multisystem trauma, full-thickness burns over 85% of body	None

sufficient supplies to last at least 3 days. For easier use, store supplies in a sturdy, easy-to-carry container, such as a backpack or duffle bag. Label the supplies and store them in an accessible place. If possible, keep a small disaster kit in the trunk of the car.

Hospitals are the final point of a community response, and health care workers are expected to assist in disaster relief. So that communities are disaster ready, health care facilities should hold routine disaster drills.

Families can cope with disaster by preparing in advance and working together as a team. A family disaster plan should be made, including locations to meet and how to contact family or friends out of the geographic area. After a disaster, it is often easier to call long distance than locally. Each family member should know how and when to turn off water, gas, and electricity at the main switches. In addition, there should be a plan for taking care of family pets.

NURSING CARE

During a disaster, nurses assist in triage, provide physical care and emotional support to the victims, and help to restore normal life routines. Until emergency help arrives, institute basic first aid and assess airway, breathing, and circulation. Once emergency personnel are on the scene, triage is begun. During major disasters, such as earthquakes, plane crashes, or terrorist acts, a tag triage system is used. Patients are tagged as "red" (*emergent*), "yellow" (*urgent*), "green" (*nonurgent*), and "black" (*dead or expected to die*). The goal of disaster medical management is to do the greatest good for the largest number of victims. (See Table 14-5 ■ for further details on triage.)

clinicalALERT

Survey entire disaster area for potential threats before administering first aid or beginning triage to prevent harm to health care workers.

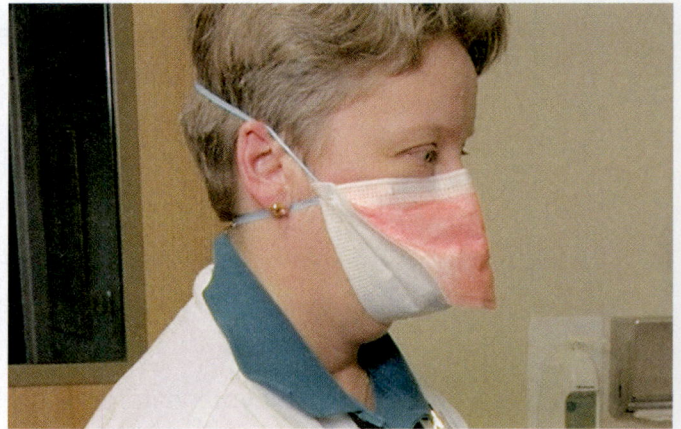

Figure 14-11. ■ When exposed to an unknown biological hazard, use basic protection such as a particulate filter N95 or HEPA filter respirator. (Source: Ronald May, Pearson Education.)

Biologic exposure may require patients to be placed in isolation. Personal protective equipment (PPE) is donned for biologic or hazardous materials such as gas, dust, or other airborne particles (Figure 14-11■). Special decontamination units may be assembled near the disaster site, depending on the contaminant. OSHA provides guidelines for the correct PPE for chemical, biologic, radiologic, and nuclear exposure. Depending on the extent of the disaster, victims may receive care in hospitals or temporary field shelters.

A primary nursing concern is preventing the spread of infection. Sewage and decomposing bodies can contaminate food and water supplies, leading to epidemics of cholera, dysentery, hepatitis A, or typhoid fever. Skin infections develop from open wounds and dirty water. Insect infestation can cause malaria. Crowded shelter conditions often contribute to the infection risk.

Special attention is needed for populations with unique needs, such as older adults, disabled, non-English-speaking, or immunocompromised. Older adults may require eyeglasses, hearing aids, and medical prescriptions for their chronic diseases. Those with mobility problems may require relocation assistance. Visual aids are useful for non-English-speaking patients. Immunocompromised patients require additional protection from infection.

Patients experiencing a disaster have a variety of individual needs. Nursing diagnoses that may be relevant include the following:

- *Anxiety*
- *Coping, Ineffective*
- *Infection, Risk for*
- *Injury, Risk for*
- *Knowledge, Deficient*
- *Powerlessness*

Disasters affect survivors, rescue workers, nurses, first responders, and families and friends. Stress reactions immediately after a disaster are very common; however, most resolve within 10 days. Typical emotional and behavioral responses include poor concentration, memory loss, irritability, depression, and feeling overwhelmed. Physical responses such as nausea, dizziness, tachycardia, insomnia, tremors, and fatigue are noted frequently. For those who develop post-traumatic stress disorder, additional counseling may be needed.

Disasters can affect anyone at any time. Preparation can increase survival and minimize the physical, emotional, and social impact of a disaster. Nurses have a valuable role in disaster planning and disaster relief. They have a responsibility to maintain clinical competency and to be aware of possible public health threats. By knowing the basics of a disaster response, nurses can assist in the workplace, home, or community.

Note: The references and resources for all chapters have been compiled at the back of the book.

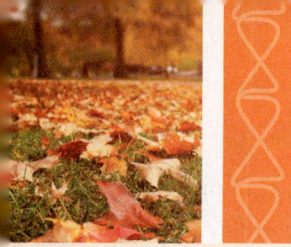

Chapter Review

KEY POINTS

■ **Concept:** Shock is characterized by oxygen supply that is less than demand, leading to inadequate tissue perfusion. Without immediate recognition and treatment, shock progresses through the compensatory, progressive, and irreversible stages and can result in death.

■ Early signs of shock include a change in the level of consciousness and restlessness, indicating decreased blood flow to the brain.

■ Hypovolemic shock, the most common type of shock, is caused by a decrease of 15% or more in circulating blood volume.

■ An allergic reaction to an antigen can progress from a mild to a severe hypersensitivity response, resulting in anaphylactic shock. Anaphylactic shock is caused by blood pooling in the periphery from vasodilation of the blood vessels.

■ Cardiogenic shock is caused by decreased pumping ability of the heart so that the heart cannot maintain adequate cardiac output and tissue perfusion. A serious myocardial infarction can lead to cardiogenic shock.

■ Septic shock is most often caused by gram-negative infections that trigger systemic vasodilation and increased capillary permeability, resulting in relative hypovolemia.

■ Fluid resuscitation and oxygen therapy are the cornerstones for managing patients with shock. Other additional measures include patient support, medications such as epinephrine, antihistamines, diuretics, antibiotics or vasopressors, and blood or blood products. Early recognition and treatment are essential to prevent shock complications such as ARDS, DIC, and renal failure.

■ **Concept:** Trauma is any life-threatening occurrence, either accidental or intentional that causes injuries (American

Trauma Society, 2012). Leading causes of trauma are falls, motor vehicle accidents, and assaults. Trauma kills or disables people often during their most productive years of life.

■ Traumatic injuries can be classified as minor or major, depending on the extent of the damage. Trauma is the leading cause of death in young people. It can be prevented by following common safety guidelines, such as wearing a seat belt when riding in or driving a car or a helmet when riding a bicycle.

■ Airway assessment and management is the highest priority in the trauma patient, followed by assessment of breathing, circulation, disability, and exposure. It is essential to identify all life-threatening injuries and to institute immediate, priority interventions.

■ Nurses in the critical care unit focus not only on the critically ill patient's life-threatening problems but also on basic needs such as comfort, communication, and emotional support. The nurse also plays an important role in providing support, assurance, and information to families of the critically ill patient.

■ **Concept:** Disasters require extraordinary efforts beyond what is needed to respond to everyday emergencies. Nurses play an essential role in knowing how to respond when a disaster occurs and in providing care for disaster victims.

■ Manmade disasters may result from chemical, biologic, radiologic, and nuclear terrorism; food or water contamination; transportation accidents; or building collapses. When disasters occur, a triage system focuses on providing care to those with life-threatening conditions first.

■ Nurses should have their own family disaster plan in place to be able to assist others during a disaster.

PEARSON NURSING STUDENT RESOURCES

Find additional materials at **nursing.pearsonhighered.com**.

Clinical Reasoning Care Map

Caring for a Patient at an Accident Scene
NCLEX-PN® Focus Area: Physiologic Integrity

Case Study: You are driving down a rural road and see a car swerve back and forth across the road. It hits a patch of ice and strikes a utility pole. There is no one else in sight and you stop. You find a young man alone in the car who says his name is Paul Thompson. He is not wearing a seat belt.

Nursing Diagnosis: Risk for Ineffective Tissue Perfusion

COLLECT DATA

Subjective

_____
_____
_____
_____
_____
_____

Objective

_____
_____
_____
_____
_____
_____

Does this present a threat to the patient's safety?

If yes, the priority intervention to address this threat would be:

_____

Nursing Care

_____
_____
_____
_____
_____
_____
_____

Interprofessional team members to include when planning care:

_____

How would you document this? _____

_____

Compare your answers and documentation to those provided on the companion website.

Data Collected
(use only those that apply)

- Scalp is bleeding
- Allergic to penicillin
- Skin slightly pale and dry
- Is awake
- Complains of being thirsty
- Left leg is twisted at an odd angle
- Slow, shallow respirations
- Does not drink alcohol
- Rapid radial pulse rate
- Says his dad will be really mad that he wrecked the car
- Denies any difficulty breathing
- Complains of left leg pain
- Wears glasses

Nursing Interventions
(use only those that apply; list in priority order)

- Splint Paul's left leg.
- Ask how the accident happened.
- Give him a few sips of water.
- Cover scalp wound with a clean cloth.
- Cover the patient with a blanket.
- Keep head and neck in neutral position.
- Assist him out of the car.
- Call for help.
- Lay him on the ground and elevate his feet and legs.
- Look for hazards in the area.

NCLEX-PN® Exam Preparation

1 A patient has an order to receive 2 units of packed red blood cells (PRBCs) for postoperative bleeding. During the transfusion of the first unit, the patient complains of chills. List the actions in the sequence in which the nurse should perform them.

1. Take the patient's vital signs.
2. Notify the charge nurse.
3. Start a normal saline infusion.
4. Stop the infusion.
5. Send the blood bag to the laboratory.

2 A patient is admitted to the surgical unit at 6:00 a.m. after a bicycle crash. One of the nursing diagnoses is hypovolemia due to blood loss. At 10:00 a.m., the nurse finds that the patient's Foley catheter bag has approximately 50 mL of dark, tea-colored urine. Which of the following actions would be the most appropriate at this time?

1. Ask if the patient feels light-headed.
2. Check the patient's CBC results.
3. Assess the patient's pain level.
4. Check the Foley catheter tubing for kinks.

3 A patient is admitted to the critical care unit after surgery for an abdominal aneurysm repair. Vital signs are stable, and the dressing is dry and intact. The patient is restless and repeatedly states, "I know that I might die." Which of the following nursing diagnoses is most appropriate to add to the care plan?

1. Risk for Infection
2. Anxiety
3. Deficient Knowledge
4. Acute Confusion

4 After an industrial explosion in the community, a 50-year-old man with a partial-thickness burn to the left forearm is complaining that he has been waiting to be seen for 3 hours. As the nurse working in the community hospital ED, what is the nurse's best response?

1. "I know; this place has a history of long waiting times."
2. "There are other patients here that are a lot worse than you and they are not fussing."
3. "I understand your concerns. I will check to see how much longer it will be."
4. "The physician doesn't have time for you right now. We'll get to you when we can."

5 The following patients have been injured in a tornado disaster. Which one would receive a red tag by the triage team?

1. 67-year-old male with an open fracture of the femur
2. 16-year-old female with a contusion
3. 45-year-old female with full-thickness burns to the face
4. 30-year-old male with multisystem injuries

6 A 65-year-old man on the medical unit is diagnosed with advanced cirrhosis of the liver. Vital signs: P 130, R 32, BP 110/60, T 100.4°F. The physician states that the patient is in shock. What type of shock is this patient experiencing?

1. Hypovolemic
2. Anaphylactic
3. Septic
4. Cardiogenic

7 Which of the following statements by a patient being treated for a severe reaction to a bee sting indicates that additional teaching might be needed?

1. "I'm going to order a MedicAlert bracelet right away."
2. "My pharmacist can tell me which anti–bee sting medication will be best for me."
3. "I'll just stay away from bees and not worry about them."
4. "I'm going to tell my family what to do if I get stung again."

8 When assessing a patient who has suffered a heat stroke, what clinical manifestations should the nurse expect to find? **Select all that apply.**

1. Cool skin
2. Rapid respirations
3. Nausea and vomiting
4. Severely elevated temperature
5. Rapid pulse
6. Profuse sweating

9 The nurse is caring for a patient with septic shock who is receiving intravenous fluids and antibiotic therapy. Which of the following findings indicates that the intravenous fluids are having a therapeutic effect on the patient?

1. Skin is warm and dry.
2. Blood pressure increases.
3. Respirations are rapid and shallow.
4. Irregular heartbeat has stabilized.

10 An older patient has recovered from a traumatic injury to the right hip from a fall in his bathroom. He will be going home with a walker for ambulation. Which of the following actions is most important to implement before the discharge?

1. Discuss transportation for a follow-up doctor's appointment.
2. Have physical therapy ambulate the patient with a walker.
3. Consult with social services for Meals-on-Wheels.
4. Teach the patient about home safety tips.

Answers and rationales for Review Questions appear in Appendix I.

CULTURAL CARE STRATEGIES

CONSIDERING CULTURAL VARIATIONS RELATED TO SPACE

A 25-year-old male Cuban American patient says to the nurse, "Everybody in this culture is so cold. When I talk up to them they are always backing away. I think the nurses think I'm going to attack them sexually or something. They keep backing away from me. It's especially noticeable if I'm in line waiting for something. I may be standing close to the person in front of me, and they turn around and glare."

All verbal communication occurs in the context of space (Giger & Davidhizar, 2012). *Personal space* is the area needed by an individual to maintain intimacy and safety in relationships. Because health care providers frequently invade a person's space when providing direct care, understanding the cultural perceptions of space is important. For example, among Americans and most Europeans, personal space is highly valued, and an unannounced invasion will often result in the patient becoming suspicious and tense (Bechtel & Davidhizar, 1988).

Proximity to Others

Hall (1966) established three different dimensions of personal space: *intimate zone* (0 to 18 in.), *personal zone* (18 in. to 3 ft), and the *social zone* (3 to 6 ft). The intimate zone is used for close, personal encounters like comforting, counseling, and direct care activities. Invading this area without the patient's acknowledgment may lead to suspicion and hostile feelings.

For most interactions not involving direct care or intimate conversation, the personal zone is considered most appropriate. In presenting patient education and information, a distance of 18 in. to 3 ft is close enough for privacy yet far enough away to avoid intimate

touch. Health care providers who have the respect of their patients and families are often able to interact well in this zone.

Individuals are frequently not conscious of their personal space requirements, although they react to invasion of their territory. The nurse should always be aware of patients' and families' body language during interactions. Signs that suggest the patient's personal space is being invaded include stepping back, looking uncomfortable and tense, and not facing the nurse during communication.

Objects in the Environment

Objects in the environment can have great meaning for patients of different cultures, and the patient may feel uncomfortable when the nurse discards or moves these objects. Objects can also affect patient care and teaching. For example, when the nurse sits behind a desk, a position of authority is assumed. This may be appropriate in some cases, but usually communication is improved by sitting across from or at a 90-degree angle to the patient.

Removal of a patient's personal items can create distrust. For example, it may be necessary to remove a wedding ring before treatment, but the patient may feel this takes away a strong sense of support. Likewise, placing a Roman Catholic person's rosary on a table out of reach can cause anxiety.

Items that may seem worthless to the caregiver can be of great significance to the patient. For example, some patients collect plastic medicine cups to symbolize the adversities overcome in the treatment plan. If the nurse discards

the medicine cups, the patient may lose track of how much success has taken place and may not be as motivated to comply with the treatment.

Nursing Implications

- *Provide information about the need to invade a patient's space.* When it is necessary to invade a patient's space, the nurse should provide information about what will be done and how long it will take. This information will enhance compliance and increase the patient's comfort.

- *Assess the patient for degree of comfort when invading personal space.* Personal space boundaries vary from individual to individual. Although most individuals are comfortable in a conversational space of 3 to 6 ft, some individuals need more space. It is important to be alert for reactions of patients during close physical contact.

- *Provide privacy for patients during close physical care.* Use privacy curtains, keep the patient covered whenever possible, expose only the necessary body part, and ask other persons to leave the room during close physical care. These actions increase feelings of security.

Self-Reflection Questions

1. How much space do you need to feel comfortable during interactions with strangers?

2. How much space do you prefer when you are with friends?

3. What do you do when your personal space is invaded?

4. How can you assist patients to accept your care when you must invade their personal space?

Thinking Strategically About . . .

You are an LPN working the evening shift in a rural 15-bed hospital. The usual staffing pattern is an RN, one or two LPNs depending on the census, and a CNA for each 8-hour shift. Most patients are stable and require routine care. Patients with complex or critical conditions are generally taken to the regional medical center 30 miles away. This evening there is one RN, one LPN, and one CNA to care for the three patients. You will be responsible for the following patients who have been admitted today from the ED. You receive reports on their status.

- Jane Souza, a 25-year-old married woman with two children, was involved in a car crash. Both cars were traveling approximately 35 mph. Ms. Souza was not wearing a seat belt and was thrown forward against the steering wheel. Her lower legs hit the underside of the dashboard. She is conscious, is receiving high-flow oxygen by mask, and has one intravenous line in place. Vital signs are BP 142/76, P 120, R 26. She has multiple bruises and abrasions. She has limited extremity movement because of a broken right arm and an open fracture of the left ankle. There is no active external bleeding. Surgery is planned within the hour to repair the fractured ankle and set her broken arm.

- Howard Still, a 76-year-old widower, has been receiving chemotherapy for recurrent lung cancer. He has been experiencing nausea and vomiting for the past week. His vital signs are BP 102/68, T 102, P 98, R 26. He complains of extreme fatigue and muscle cramps in his legs. His potassium level is 3.0. He has an IV of D5 $\frac{1}{2}$ NS with 20 mEq of KCl at 100 mL/hr. Howard stated, "I am ready to stop this cancer treatment and join my wife in Heaven."

- Juan Martinez, a 28-year-old, came to the emergency room with his third migraine headache in the last 6 weeks. Juan milks cows on a large dairy. He admits to drinking three beers every evening. He smokes one pack of cigarettes a day. His vital signs are stable. He was medicated with 25 mg of Demerol (meperidine) intravenously 30 minutes ago. If his migraine subsides and he does not require further meperidine doses, he will be discharged the next day with instructions to see the doctor in the clinic within 2 days.

CRITICAL THINKING

- What specific observations of Jane must you make to determine whether her condition remains stable and she is not developing further complications?

- What questions should you ask Howard to add clarity to your understanding of his desire to stop cancer treatment and his wish to join his wife in Heaven?

- What questions should you ask Juan to add precision to your assessment of his headache?

PRIORITIES IN NURSING CARE

- In what order will you assess your patients?

- What is your rationale for your prioritization of care?

MANAGEMENT OF CARE

- How frequently should you monitor Jane?

- At 1530 there is 400 mL of fluid in Howard's IV bottle. When will the next bottle need to be hung?

- What nonpharmacologic interventions could you implement for Juan?

DELEGATING

- If a CNA is available to assist with your assignment, what care would you delegate?

- What information must you provide to the RN regarding the care of these patients that was delegated to you?

PATIENT TEACHING

- What preoperative teaching is a priority for Jane?

- What teaching should you provide to Howard about his treatment plan?

- What teaching will Juan require before discharge?

TEAMWORK AND COLLABORATION

- What interprofessional team members should be involved in Howard's discharge planning to address his wishes about his treatment and to "be with his wife in Heaven"?

DOCUMENTING AND REPORTING

- What SBAR report would you give to the operating room nurse regarding Jane's injuries and condition?

- What report would you expect to receive from the nurse caring for Howard during the day shift?

- Write a medical record entry, using the Focus Charting method, regarding Juan's discharge.

Note: Discussion of Unit questions appears on the companion website.

UNIT III
Disrupted Cardiovascular Function

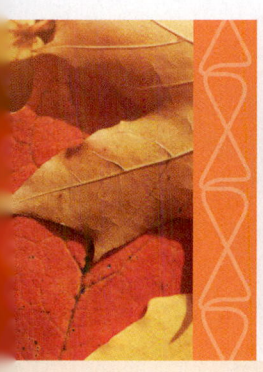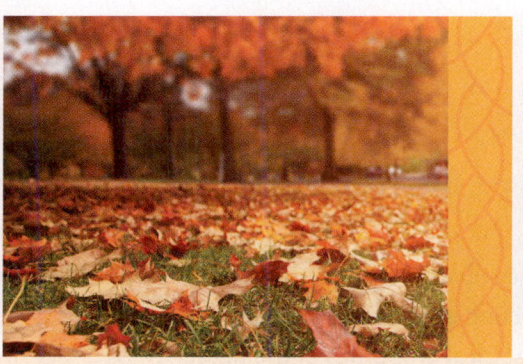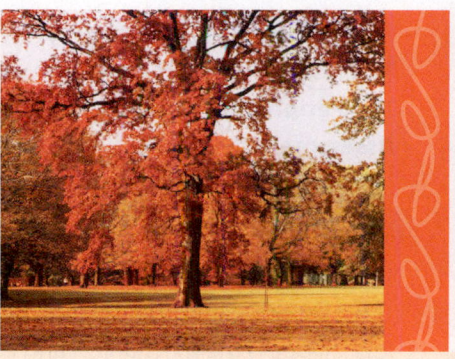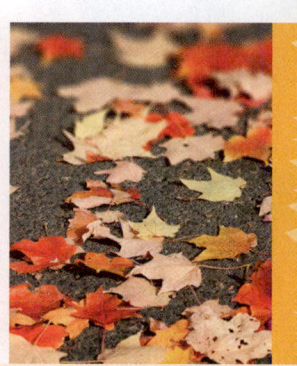

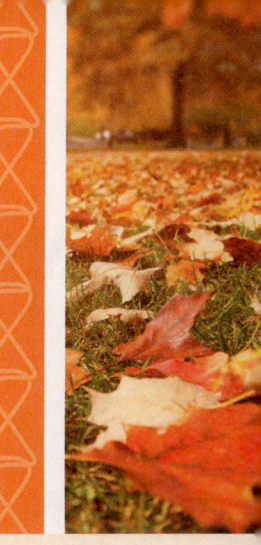

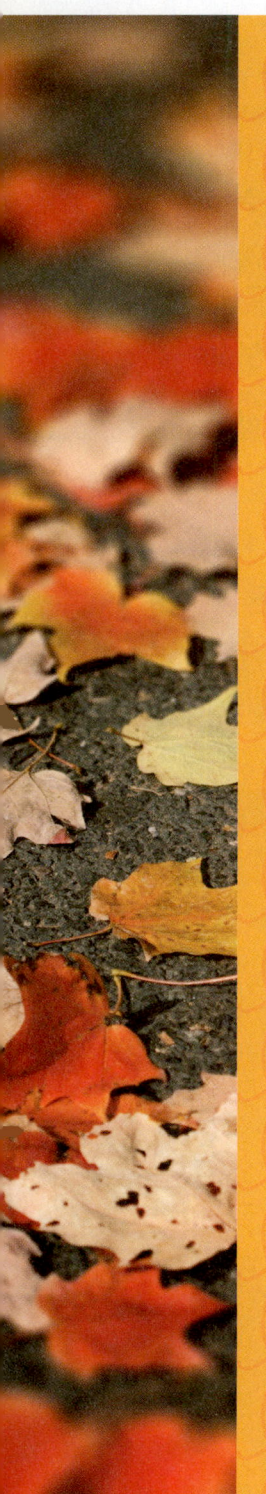

CHAPTER 15
The Cardiovascular System and Assessment

BRIEF OUTLINE

The Heart
The Peripheral Vascular System
Assessment

APPLIED LEARNING OUTCOMES

After completing this chapter, you will be able to:

1. Describe the structure and function of the heart and vascular systems.
2. Discuss the mechanical and electrical properties of the heart.
3. Identify subjective and objective assessment data to collect for patients with cardiovascular disorders.
4. Identify nursing responsibilities for common diagnostic tests and monitor for patients with cardiovascular disorders.

KEY TERMS

The key terms are defined on the pages listed below.

blood pressure, 353
cardiac output, 351
contractility, 352
diastole, 351

electrocardiogram (ECG), 354
peripheral vascular resistance, 352

peripheral vascular system, 352
stroke volume, 351
systole, 351

Key Concept   The heart, blood, and blood vessels—collectively known as the cardiovascular system—work together as a fuel delivery and waste removal system for the body. Cardiovascular disorders affect this distribution system, reducing the fuel available to the cells and leading to accumulated waste products in the tissues.

The heart, a simple pump, pushes blood through a system of blood vessels to deliver oxygen and glucose to the cells and tissues. Waste products such as carbon dioxide and other byproducts of metabolism are, in turn, taken back to the liver, lungs, and kidneys for disposal.

The Heart

The heart, a hollow, cone-shaped organ approximately the size of an adult's fist, weighs less than 1 lb. It is located behind the sternum and between the lungs in the thoracic cavity, slightly to the left of midline (Figure 15-1■). Mechanically, the heart functions as a double pump: The right side receives blood from the body and pumps it to the lungs; the left side receives blood from the lungs and pumps it to the body.

STRUCTURE OF THE HEART

The heart is composed of three layers of tissue covered by a protective sac called the *pericardium*. The pericardium (meaning "around the heart") encases the heart and anchors it to the surrounding structures. It has two layers: The *parietal pericardium* is the outermost layer, and the *visceral pericardium* (also called the *epicardium*) adheres to the heart surface. The small space between these layers contains serous lubricating fluid that cushions the heart as it beats.

The epicardium is the outermost layer of the heart wall. The middle layer is the *myocardium*, or heart muscle, and the innermost layer, the *endocardium*, lines the inside of the heart's chambers and great vessels (Figure 15-2■).

The heart has four hollow chambers: two upper *atria* and two lower *ventricles*. A septum (or wall) separates the two sides of the heart; *atrioventricular (AV) valves* separate the atria from the ventricles. The flaps of these valves are anchored to the muscles of the ventricles by the chordae tendineae. These valves prevent the backflow of blood during contraction of the ventricles.

The *right atrium* receives deoxygenated blood from the veins of the body via the *superior* and *inferior vena cava*. The right atrium is separated from the right ventricle by the *tricuspid valve*. When open, deoxygenated blood flows through this valve into the *right ventricle*, which then pumps it through the *pulmonary artery* to the lungs (Figure 15-3■).

The *left atrium* receives freshly oxygenated blood from the lungs through the *pulmonary veins*. The *left ventricle*, separated from the left atria by the *bicuspid* or *mitral valve*, pumps this freshly oxygenated blood out the *aorta* to the systemic circulation.

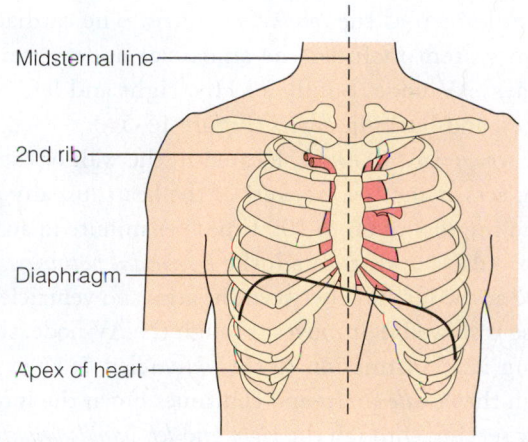

Labels: Midsternal line, 2nd rib, Diaphragm, Apex of heart

Figure 15-1. ■ Location of the heart within the chest cavity.

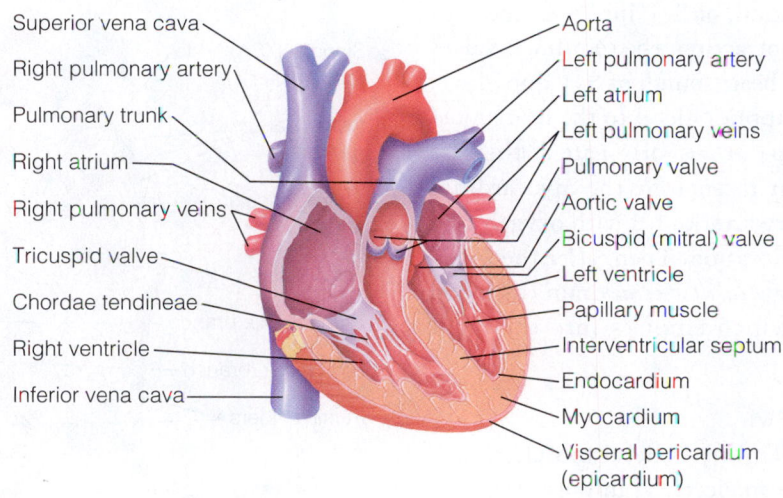

Labels: Superior vena cava, Right pulmonary artery, Pulmonary trunk, Right atrium, Right pulmonary veins, Tricuspid valve, Chordae tendineae, Right ventricle, Inferior vena cava, Aorta, Left pulmonary artery, Left atrium, Left pulmonary veins, Pulmonary valve, Aortic valve, Bicuspid (mitral) valve, Left ventricle, Papillary muscle, Interventricular septum, Endocardium, Myocardium, Visceral pericardium (epicardium)

Figure 15-2. ■ The internal anatomy of the heart.

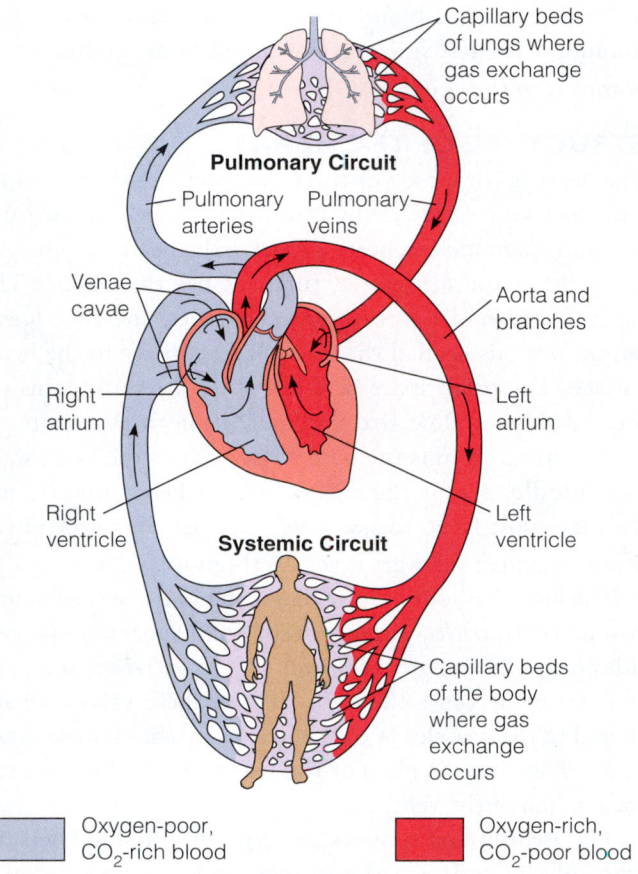

Figure 15-3. ■ Pulmonary and systemic circulation. The right side of the heart receives deoxygenated venous blood from the body and pumps it into the pulmonary circulation. The left side of the heart receives oxygenated blood from the pulmonary system and pumps it out to the peripheral circulation.

The ventricles are connected to their great vessels by the *semilunar valves*. On the right, the *pulmonary valve* joins the right ventricle with the pulmonary artery. On the left, the *aortic valve* joins the left ventricle to the aorta.

The AV valves close as the ventricles start to contract, producing the first heart sound, or S_1 ("lub"). As the ventricles start to relax after contraction, the semilunar valves close, producing the second heart sound, or S_2 ("dup").

The *coronary circulation* supplies blood to the heart muscle. The *left* and *right coronary arteries* originate at the base of the aorta and branch out to encircle the myocardium (Figure 15-4■). The coronary arteries fill with oxygen-rich blood during ventricular relaxation. Then, after the blood perfuses the heart muscle, the *cardiac veins* drain the blood into the coronary sinus, which empties into the right atrium of the heart.

CONDUCTION SYSTEM

Cardiac muscle is unique. Unlike skeletal muscle tissue, cardiac muscle can generate an electrical impulse and contraction without stimulation by the nervous system. The

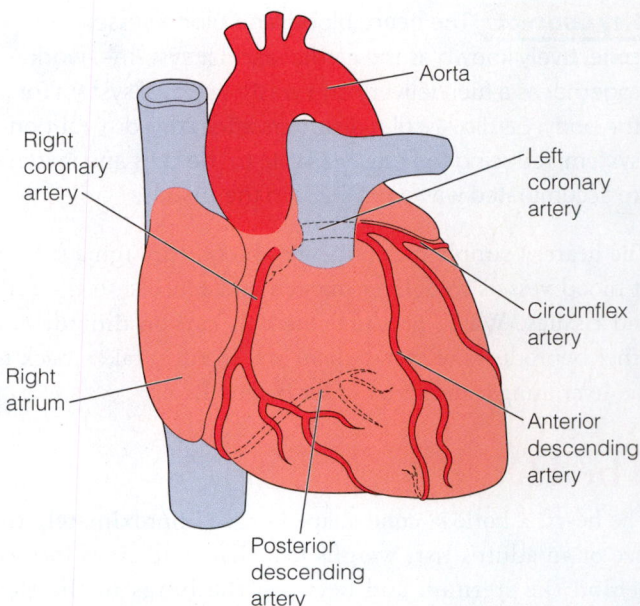

Figure 15-4. ■ The coronary arteries.

heartbeat is controlled by specialized cells within the myocardium known as the *conduction system.* The cardiac conduction system includes the sinoatrial node, internodal pathways, AV node, bundle of His, right and left bundle branches, and Purkinje fibers (Figure 15-5■).

The *sinoatrial (SA) node*, located in the wall of the right atrium, acts as the "pacemaker" of the heart, usually generating an impulse of 60 to 100 times per minute in an adult. This impulse travels through the *internodal pathways* to the *AV node* at the junction between the atria and ventricles. The impulse is slowed as it moves through the AV node, slightly delaying its transmission to the ventricles. It then passes through the *bundle of His* and continues down the interventricular septum through the *right* and *left bundle branches* and out to the *Purkinje fibers* in the ventricular muscle walls.

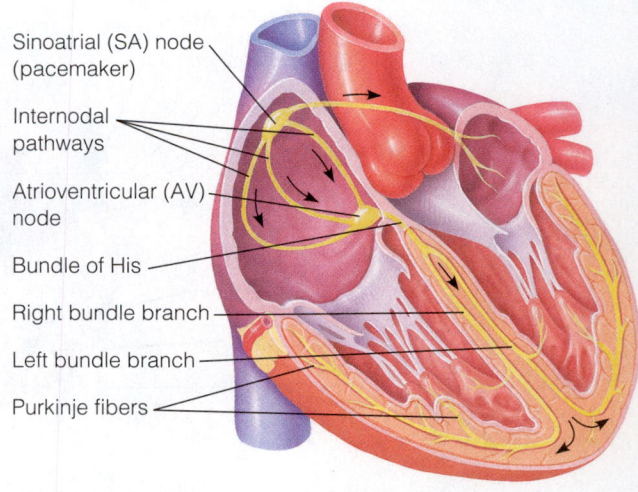

Figure 15-5. ■ The cardiac conduction system.

The electrical impulse, or *action potential*, generated by pacemaker cells is caused by the movement of ions across cell membranes. At rest, myocardial cells are *polarized* or have a negative charge. The action potential causes the cell membrane to become more positive. This is known as *depolarization.* The action potential and depolarization cause the muscle to contract. With each beat, the heart muscle contracts to its fullest potential (the *all-or-nothing response*). *Repolarization* begins immediately after depolarization, returning the cell to its resting state. For a brief period during and after repolarization, the cell resists stimulation. This is known as the *refractory period.* It protects the heart muscle from going into spasm or tetany (continuous contraction). This electrical activity produces the waveforms represented on electrocardiogram (ECG) strips.

CARDIAC CYCLE

The contraction and relaxation of the heart, called the cardiac cycle, constitute one heartbeat (Figure 15-6■). Ventricular filling occurs during **diastole**, when the ventricles are relaxed. Toward the end of diastole, the atria contract, pumping additional blood into the ventricles. During ventricular **systole**, the ventricles contract, ejecting blood into the pulmonary and systemic circuits. In an adult, the complete cardiac cycle normally occurs 60 to 100 times per minute (the *heart rate*).

CARDIAC OUTPUT

With each contraction, a certain volume of blood (approximately 70 mL in an adult), called the **stroke volume** (SV), is ejected from the heart. The **cardiac output** (CO) is the amount of blood pumped by the ventricles in 1 minute. CO indicates how well the heart is functioning as a pump. It is calculated by multiplying the stroke volume by the heart rate (HR):

$$CO = HR \times SV$$

The average adult CO ranges from 4 to 8 liters per minute (L/min).

The heart regulates CO to meet the body's needs. As oxygen demand increases, oxygen supply must also increase. *Cardiac reserve* is the ability of the heart to increase CO and blood pressure to meet the demand. CO is determined by four major factors: heart rate, preload, afterload, and contractility.

Heart rate is affected by the activity level, the autonomic nervous system, and hormones. Increased heart rates increase CO; however, very rapid heart rates allow less time for ventricular filling and may actually reduce the stroke volume and CO. If the heart rate is too slow, cardiac output falls simply because the heart contracts less often.

Preload is the amount of blood in the ventricles before contraction. The blood in the ventricles stretches the muscle fibers, causing them to contract more forcefully. Preload is affected by venous return. If blood volume is low (e.g., due to hemorrhage or dehydration), it falls. To a certain point, the greater the blood volume, the greater the force with which the ventricle contracts. Beyond a certain volume, however, the heart contracts less effectively. This is called *Starling's law of the heart.*

memory**ALERT**

To help remember this concept, think about a new rubber band. The farther you stretch the rubber band (preload), the more forcefully it contracts. However, if you stretch it too far or too often, it loses its stretch and no longer returns to its original shape.

Afterload is the force the ventricles must develop to push blood into the circulation. The right ventricle pushes blood into the low-pressure pulmonary system. The left ventricle ejects its blood into the systemic circulation. Systemic

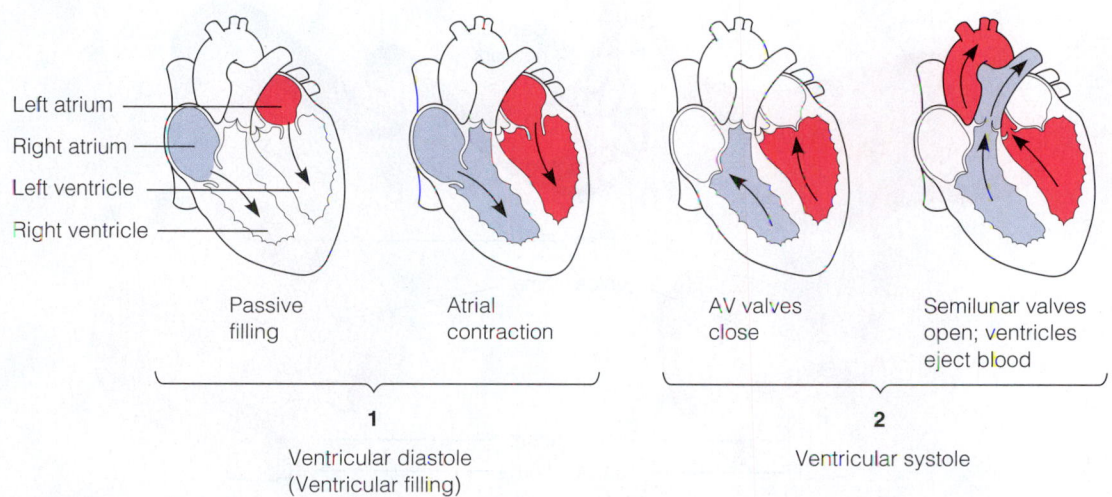

Figure 15-6. ■ The cardiac cycle. **(A)** Ventricular filling occurs during diastole (relaxation); **(B)** blood is pumped out of the heart to the pulmonary and systemic circulation during ventricular systole (contraction).

arterial pressures are much higher than pulmonary pressures; therefore, the left ventricle has to work much harder than the right ventricle.

Contractility is the natural ability of the cardiac muscle fibers to shorten during systole. Contractility is necessary to move blood into the circulation. Poor contractility reduces the ability of the ventricle to eject blood, decreasing the stroke volume. The *ejection fraction*, or the percentage of blood in the ventricle that is ejected with each contraction, is affected by the interaction of preload, afterload, and contractility.

The Peripheral Vascular System

The **peripheral vascular system** is a network of blood vessels that carry blood to peripheral tissues and then return it to the heart. This network includes arteries, veins, and capillaries.

ARTERIES AND VEINS

Arteries carry blood away from the heart. Oxygenated blood leaves the left ventricle via the aorta. Major arteries branch off the aorta and into successively smaller arteries. These eventually divide into *arterioles*. Arterioles feed into beds of hairlike *capillaries* within the organs and tissues.

In the capillary beds, oxygen and nutrients are exchanged for metabolic wastes, and deoxygenated blood begins its journey back to the heart through *venules*. Venules join onto veins, which in turn join larger and larger veins. *Veins* carry blood toward the heart. Peripheral veins empty into the superior and inferior vena cava and then into the right atrium.

Blood Vessel Structure

The structure of blood vessels reflects their different functions within the circulatory system. Except for the capillaries, blood vessel walls have three layers: the tunica intima, the tunica media, and the tunica externa (Figure 15-7 ■).

The innermost layer, the tunica intima, or *endothelium*, has a slick surface to assist blood flow. The middle layer, or tunica media, contains smooth muscle. This layer is thicker and more elastic in arteries than it is in veins. It allows arteries to expand and contract, maintaining blood flow to the capillaries between heartbeats. *Constriction* (narrowing) and *dilation* (widening) of the arterioles is the major factor controlling blood pressure. The tunica externa, or outermost layer, is connective tissue that protects and anchors the vessel. Veins have a thinner tunica media and a thicker tunica externa than do arteries.

The pressure in the veins is much lower than that in the arteries. Veins have thinner walls, a larger lumen, and a greater capacity than arteries. Many have valves that help move blood against gravity back to the heart. Skeletal muscle contraction helps: When skeletal muscles contract against veins, the valves open, and blood is propelled toward the heart. Changes in abdominal and thoracic pressure that occur with breathing also propel blood toward the heart.

The tiny capillaries, which connect the arterioles and venules, contain only one thin layer of tunica intima. This allows gases and nutrients to escape the blood vessels and reach tissue cells. Waste products from metabolism enter the capillaries for elimination. Capillaries are found in interwoven networks called capillary beds.

ARTERIAL CIRCULATION

Arterial circulation is maintained by a balance of blood flow, peripheral vascular resistance, and blood pressure. *Blood flow* is the amount of blood transported.

Peripheral vascular resistance (PVR) is the force opposing blood flow. PVR is determined by three factors:

1. *Blood viscosity (thickness):* The greater the viscosity of the blood, the greater its resistance to moving and flowing.

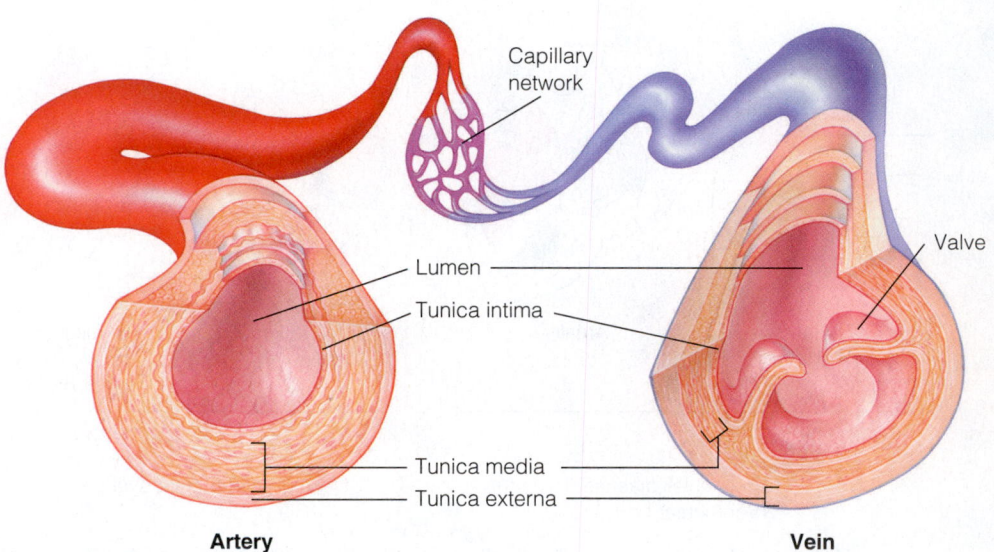

Figure 15-7. ■ Structure of arteries, veins, and capillaries.

2. *Vessel length:* The longer the vessel, the greater the resistance to blood flow.
3. *Vessel diameter:* The smaller a vessel is, the more friction is produced, and the greater the resistance is to blood flow.

Blood pressure (BP) is the force exerted by blood against the walls of the arteries. The *systolic* pressure is the force exerted as the heart contracts (systole). The *diastolic* pressure reflects the force exerted when the heart is filling (diastole). The optimal adult BP is less than 120/80 mm Hg. The blood pressure is regulated mainly by CO and PVR. A number of factors affect CO and PVR:

- Sympathetic nervous system (SNS) stimulation increases CO by increasing the heart rate and contractility and constricting arterioles, thus increasing blood pressure. Pressure-sensitive receptors (*baroreceptors*) and *chemoreceptors* in the aortic arch, carotid sinus, and other large vessels stimulate the SNS.
- Parasympathetic stimulation slows the heart rate and causes dilation of arterioles, lowering the blood pressure.
- The kidneys help regulate BP. A fall in BP stimulates the renin–angiotensin–aldosterone mechanism, causing vasoconstriction and salt and water retention. Antidiuretic hormone (ADH) from the pituitary gland promotes water retention, increasing blood volume, CO, and blood pressure.
- Temperatures affect peripheral resistance: Cold causes vasoconstriction; warmth produces vasodilation.
- Many chemicals, hormones, and drugs affect CO or PVR.

Other factors that affect CO, PVR, and BP include diet (e.g., sodium and calcium intake), race, gender, age, weight, time of day, position, exercise, and emotional state.

Assessment

> **Key Concept**   The patient's general appearance and ability to engage in activities, as well as specific assessment data and diagnostic tests, are used to evaluate the patient's cardiovascular status.

HEALTH HISTORY

Focused assessment of the patient with cardiovascular disease begins by asking about current symptoms. Inquire about the presence of chest pain and its duration.

clinical**ALERT**

If the patient is experiencing acute chest pain or shortness of breath, complete only a brief assessment focused on the acute symptoms. Notify the charge nurse or physician. Complete assessment data collection once the acute symptoms have been relieved and the patient is resting comfortably.

Ask about past episodes of chest or leg pain and their relationship to activity. Inquire about shortness of breath, and determine how many pillows the patient uses to sleep (patients with heart failure may be unable to sleep lying flat). Ask about recent changes in energy level or fatigue, as well as recent weight gain.

Obtain the patient's past medical history and family health history, focusing on previous history of heart disease, circulation problems, or blood disorders. Inquire about a personal or family history of diabetes and high blood pressure.

Ask the patient to identify all medications (including prescription, over-the-counter, and natural or herbal preparations) currently being taken and the purpose of each drug. This information often helps identify the presence of a medical problem not previously mentioned or may help the nurse relate current symptoms to an adverse drug effect or interaction.

Lifestyle factors have a significant effect on the risk for heart disease. Inquire about diet and usual alcohol intake (average number of mixed drinks, beers, or glasses of wine per day). Have the patient describe usual patterns of exercise and physical activity. If the patient smokes, ascertain at what age the patient started smoking and the number of packs of cigarettes per day smoked or type of tobacco product used. Ask about the use of illicit drugs such as cocaine.

PHYSICAL EXAMINATION

The focused physical examination for the patient with cardiovascular disease begins by assessing the patient's general appearance. Observe for apparent general health, facial expression, and body type. Assess skin color and temperature; evaluate hair distribution, particularly on the lower extremities. Observe for taut, shiny, thin-appearing skin and areas of discoloration on the lower extremities as well. Note any wounds or ulcerations, and assess for healing. Evaluate skin turgor. See Box 15-1■ for more information about assessing skin color among people of various cultural backgrounds.

BOX 15-1	**FOCUS ON DIVERSITY**

Assessing Skin Color

Assessing people with darker skin color for the presence of pallor or cyanosis can be challenging.

- Inspect the conjunctiva and oral buccal mucous membrane of very dark skinned Blacks (African Americans or Haitian Americans) for the presence of cyanosis or pallor. Black skin should have a rosy glow; loss of this rosy tone (a dull or "muddy" appearance) may indicate cyanosis.

- The skin of people of Mexican origin ranges from tan to dark brown. Pallor and cyanosis may be seen as an ashen tone, rather than a pale or bluish tint (Giger, 2013).

Obtain the blood pressure on both arms (unless contraindicated), an apical pulse, and the respiratory rate. Note any evidence of neck vein distention. Palpate peripheral pulses on upper and lower extremities, noting their strength and equality. Note capillary refill on both the upper and lower extremities. Observe and palpate the lower extremities for the presence of edema. Measure the circumference of the calves if they appear unequal or if the patient complains of lower extremity pain. Note any heat, tenderness, or redness of the extremities.

Observe the ease of breathing, noting any asymmetry of chest movement or use of accessory muscles of respiration. Auscultate breath sounds throughout all lung fields, noting any diminished or adventitious breath sounds. Note the presence of a cough, and, if present, describe any sputum produced.

Inspect the chest and abdomen for visible pulsations. Palpate for the location of the apical impulse (point of maximal impulse, or PMI). Auscultate the heart, noting the rate and rhythm and any irregularities. Report any abnormal heart sounds such as a gallop or murmur.

For more information about assessment techniques, see Chapter 5. See Box 15-2■ for a documentation example of a cardiovascular assessment.

THE OLDER ADULT

Physical changes commonly associated with aging may affect cardiovascular assessment in the older adult. Subcutaneous tissue is lost with aging, causing the skin to appear paler and thinner. Skin turgor may be more accurately assessed over the sternum than on the arms. Less hair may be noted on the extremities. Thinning of capillary walls and loss of tissue support may lead to easy bruising, petechiae, and bleeding into subcutaneous tissues. Varicose veins and tortuous, irregular veins are more commonly seen in aging.

Many older adults experience occasional early heartbeats, although the rate remains basically regular. Although many older adults become more sedentary, regular exercise such as walking, swimming, and weight training is encouraged. The heart rate does not respond as rapidly to exercise and physical activity, requiring longer warm-up and cool-down periods.

An increased incidence of chronic diseases and medication use in older adults increases the risk of drug interactions that may affect the cardiovascular system. Changes in the heart rate and its regularity may occur in response to medications. Some medications may increase the risk for orthostatic hypotension (a drop in blood pressure occurring with changes in position) and falls.

DIAGNOSTIC TESTS
Laboratory Tests

Several laboratory tests are commonly performed to evaluate the cardiovascular system. Table 15-1■ lists these tests, their normal values, what the test measures and its significance, and any nursing implications for the test.

Electrocardiography

The **electrocardiogram (ECG)** is a record of the heart's electrical activity detected by electrodes placed on the skin (Box 15-3■). ECG waveforms and patterns are used to detect *dysrhythmias* (abnormal heart rhythms), myocardial damage or enlargement, and the effects of drugs.

Electrocardiography may be used on a continual or intermittent basis, depending on the patient's needs. Table 15-2■ summarizes ECG studies used in diagnosing heart problems, along with their nursing implications.

Imaging Techniques

Imaging techniques used to diagnose cardiovascular disease range from noninvasive to very invasive. These diagnostic procedures and their nursing implications are summarized in Table 15-3■.

Electrophysiology Studies

Cardiac electrophysiology (EP) studies are used to diagnose (and sometimes treat) abnormal cardiac rhythms. EP procedures are invasive procedures performed in an electrophysiology laboratory. Electrode catheters inserted into the heart through the brachial or femoral vein are used to evaluate the conduction system of the heart and locate sites where abnormal rhythms originate. Nursing care for the patient undergoing EP studies is similar to that for coronary angiography.

BOX 15-2	DOCUMENTATION OF CARDIOVASCULAR ASSESSMENT

Patient: 72 y.o. Black male admitted to rule out myocardial infarction after acute episode of chest pain. No evidence of infarction; undergoing diagnostic testing. Has type 2 diabetes and peripheral vascular disease.

Assessment note: Alert and oriented. Denies pain, shortness of breath at this time. Appears moderately anxious but in no acute distress. Vital signs stable. Skin color and turgor good; no pallor or cyanosis of oral mucosa or nail beds noted. Skin warm and dry on trunk and upper extremities; cool, dry, and shiny bilaterally below the knees. Several areas of darker pigmentation noted over both shins and medial ankles. No edema or ulcerations noted. Peripheral pulses strong (3+) and equal upper extremities; weak (2+) and equal lower extremities. Upper extremity capillary refill immediate, slower (>3 seconds) lower extremities. Breathing relaxed, chest movement equal. Good breath sounds throughout lung fields with no crackles or rhonchi noted. Apical pulse basically regular with an occasional early beat noted (<1–2 per minute). Clear S_1, S_2.

TABLE 15-1	Common Laboratory Tests for Cardiovascular Disease		
LABORATORY TESTS			
TEST	**NORMAL ADULT VALUES**	**EXPLANATION**	**NURSING IMPLICATIONS**
Lipid profile		Performed to evaluate risk for atherosclerosis and coronary heart disease. Lower levels of total cholesterol and triglycerides are better. Higher levels of HDL help remove excess cholesterol from the blood and are desirable. LDL and VLDL promote cholesterol buildup in arteries; lower levels are better.	These tests should be performed fasting. Instruct the patient to refrain from eating or drinking (sips of water are allowed) for 12 hours before testing and to avoid alcohol intake for 24 hours before testing.
▪ Total cholesterol	150–240 mg/dL; desirable level: less than 200 mg/dL		
▪ Triglycerides	10–190 mg/dL		
▪ High-density lipoproteins (HDLs)	29–77 mg/dL		
▪ Low-density lipoproteins (LDLs)	60–130 mg/dL		
▪ Very low-density lipoproteins (VLDLs)	25%–50% of total triglycerides		
C-reactive protein	Not present	A sensitive measure of inflammation; may help predict coronary heart disease.	Restrict food and fluid intake to water only for 8–12 hours before testing.
Serum cardiac markers		Cardiac markers are proteins released from dead or damaged heart muscle cells. CK is a protein in heart and skeletal muscle; CK-MB is a subset of CK found in heart muscle. Cardiac muscle troponins, cT_nT and cT_n1, are sensitive indicators of heart muscle damage.	Fasting is not required, but intramuscular injections and some drugs may interfere with test results. Serial levels of these enzymes often are obtained, necessitating blood draws every 12 to 24 hours for several days.
▪ Creatine phosphokinase (CK or CPK)	Male: 50–170 IU/L Female: 25–140 IU/L		
▪ CK-MB	0%–6% of total CK		
▪ cT_nT	Less than 0.2 mcg/L (or ng/mL)		
▪ cT_n1	Less than 0.5 mcg/L (or ng/mL)		
Serum cardiac hormones		These hormones are released by the heart muscle in response to changes in blood volume. Increased blood levels indicate heart failure.	These tests are performed fasting. Unless contraindicated, withhold cardiac drugs for 24 hours before testing.
▪ Atrial natriuretic peptide (ANP)	20–77 pg/mL (or ng/L)		
▪ Brain natriuretic peptide (BNP)	Less than 100 pg/mL (or ng/L)		

BOX 15-3   ELECTROCARDIOGRAM

An electrocardiogram (ECG) is a "picture" of the heart's electrical activity. Electrodes placed on different parts of the body enable different views of the heart's electrical activity, much like turning while holding a camera provides different views of the scenery.

A standard 12-lead ECG includes recordings of six limb leads and six precordial leads. The *limb leads* provide a view of the inferior and lateral walls of the heart. The *chest* (or *precordial*) *leads* provide a view of the anterior, septal, lateral, and posterior walls of the heart.

ECG waveforms show the direction of electrical flow. Current moving toward the positive electrode causes an upward (positive) waveform; current moving away from it produces a downward (negative) waveform. When no electrical activity is occurring, a straight line, called the *isoelectric line*, is seen.

ECG waveforms are recorded on paper marked at intervals that represent time and voltage or amplitude (see Figure A). Each small box represents 0.04 second. Five small boxes make one large box, equivalent to 0.20 second. Five large boxes represent 1 full second.

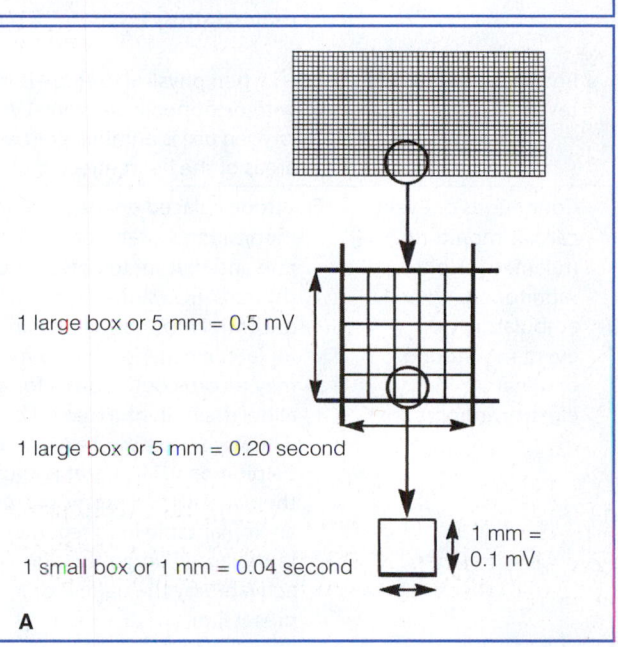

1 large box or 5 mm = 0.5 mV

1 large box or 5 mm = 0.20 second

1 small box or 1 mm = 0.04 second

1 mm = 0.1 mV

A

(continued)

BOX 15-3	ELECTROCARDIOGRAM (continued)

The P, Q, R, S, and T waves represent the cardiac cycle (see Figure B). The *P wave* shows the SA node impulse and atrial depolarization. It precedes the QRS complex and is normally smooth, round, and upright. The *PR interval* is the time required for the impulse to travel to the AV node and the bundle branches. It is measured from the beginning of P wave to the beginning of QRS complex. The PR interval is normally 0.12 to 0.20 second.

The *QRS complex* indicates ventricular depolarization. It occurs rapidly, lasting less than 0.12 second. The *ST segment*, the period from the end of the QRS complex to the beginning of the T wave, is normally isoelectric. The *T wave* represents ventricular repolarization; it is smooth and rounded and points in the same direction as the QRS complex. The *QT interval*, measured from the beginning of the QRS to the end of the T wave, indicates the total time for ventricular depolarization and repolarization. Its duration varies with gender, age, and heart rate; usually, it is 0.36 to 0.44 second long. The *U wave* is not normally seen but may show repolarization of the terminal Purkinje fibers.

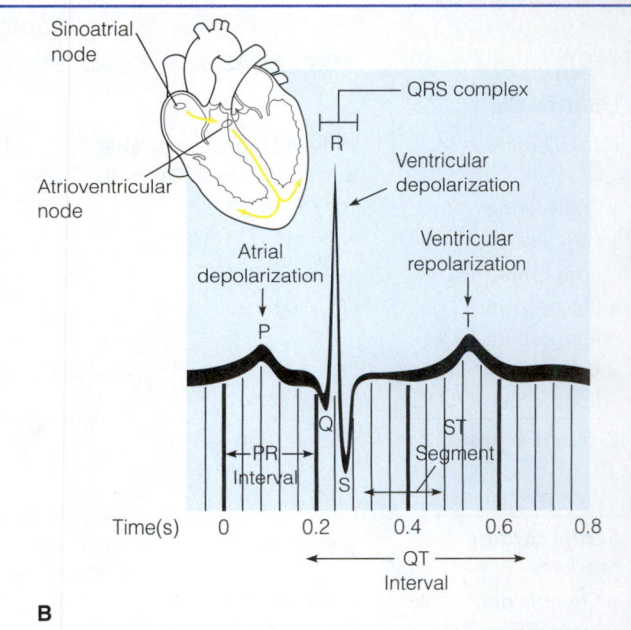

B

TABLE 15-2	Diagnostic Electrocardiographic Studies	
DIAGNOSTIC TEST	**PURPOSE**	**NURSING IMPLICATIONS**
■ 12-Lead ECG (resting ECG)	Used to evaluate the heart rhythm, conduction through the electrical pathways of the heart, and the size and position of the heart in the chest cavity. Can reveal areas of ischemia, injury, or infarction (tissue necrosis).	Noninvasive. Very tense muscles (e.g., a highly anxious patient) and movement can interfere with results. Note current medications because some drugs affect the ECG.
■ Stress electrocardiography (exercise testing)	Monitors the ECG during exercise on a treadmill or stationary bicycle (or, for patients who cannot walk, an arm ergometer) to detect asymptomatic coronary heart disease (CHD). During exercise, the workload of the heart increases; this increased workload may cause myocardial ischemia and angina in patients with CHD. See also Table 15-3 for tests that combine exercise stress testing with perfusion imaging.	Requires informed consent. Smoking and food, alcohol, and caffeine intake should be avoided for 2 to 3 hours before the test. The patient's ECG, heart rate, and blood pressure are monitored continuously during testing. Stress testing may cause a cardiac emergency. A physician is present or immediately available during stress testing, and emergency resuscitation supplies are kept in the immediate area.
■ Pharmacologic stress testing	Used when physical exercise is not possible (e.g., for patients with orthopedic problems). A drug that increases myocardial oxygen use is administered, which may cause ischemia in areas of the heart affected by CHD, much like exercise does.	
■ Continuous or event cardiac monitoring (telemetry, Holter monitoring, ambulatory or event monitoring, or dynamic electrocardiography)	Electrodes placed on the patient's chest are connected to a monitoring system for continuous monitoring of the heart rate and rhythm to detect and diagnose abnormal heart rhythms. ECG signals may be displayed on a bedside monitor or central monitoring station or recorded in a portable unit for later evaluation (*Holter monitoring*). Ambulatory monitors may record continuously for a 24- to 72-hour period or allow the patient to record cardiac activity intermittently when symptoms are experienced (such as chest pain or palpitations). The latter is known as event monitoring. When the patient's symptoms occur only rarely, a device such as an implantable loop recorder (ILR) may be used. The ILR is implanted under the skin of the chest. It records when activated by the patient or if the pulse rate is above or below preset limits.	Provide teaching about the purpose of monitoring. Apply electrodes to clean and dry skin, removing hair as appropriate. Instruct the patient how to replace the electrodes (if appropriate) and about care of the skin and recording or telemetry unit. Caution the patient to avoid getting the telemetry or recording unit wet. Instruct the patient to record activity when symptoms such as chest pain or palpitations are experienced. Instruct when it is appropriate to contact the nurse or physician.

TABLE 15-3	Imaging Studies	
DIAGNOSTIC STUDY	**EXPLANATION AND PURPOSE**	**NURSING IMPLICATIONS**
Sonography (Doppler studies, echocardiography)	Echoes from high-frequency sound waves are used to study the structure and movement of organs (e.g., the heart) and the flow of blood within a vessel.	
■ Echocardiography • M-Mode • Two-dimensional (2-D) • Spectral Doppler • Color Doppler • Contrast	A transducer lubricated with conductive gel held against the chest wall transmits and receives the ultrasonic impulses. A computer converts the impulses to an image of the heart walls, chambers and their movements, heart valves, and, in color Doppler or contrast echocardiography, blood flow through the heart.	Noninvasive unless a contrast agent is injected; performed at the patient's bedside or in an ambulatory care setting. No food or fluid restriction is necessary. Conductive gel may be cold. Provide a washcloth or wash the chest wall after the exam for comfort.
■ Transesophageal echocardiogram (TEE)	A flexible transducer mounted on an endoscope provides a more direct view of the heart by avoiding the interference of chest wall structures.	Requires informed consent. Food and fluid withheld for at least 4 hours before testing. The patient is sedated and the throat anesthetized to allow passage of the endoscope into the esophagus. Monitor breathing, cough, and gag reflexes after the exam. Keep NPO until the gag reflex returns and the patient is fully awake.
■ Stress echocardiogram	This test combines a resting echocardiogram, exercise or administration of a drug to increase myocardial oxygen use with continuous ECG monitoring, and a repeat echocardiogram immediately after exercise to evaluate the effect of exercise on cardiac function.	Requires informed consent, food and fluid restrictions before testing, and monitoring as for a stress ECG (see Table 15-2).
■ Vascular ultrasound (Doppler imaging, duplex scans)	These noninvasive procedures provide information about the structure of and blood flow through major blood vessels. A handheld transducer lubricated with conductive gel is maneuvered over the vessel. Blood pressures at various locations of the extremity are taken when used to evaluate peripheral circulation.	Explain the test and its purpose. Monitor blood pressures as indicated. Wash the extremity after the exam for comfort.
Radiography (x-ray studies)	Used to identify the size and location of structures, and, when combined with use of an injected contrast medium, used to study blood flow through vessels and organs.	If contrast is to be injected, ask about allergies (specifically including contrast media, iodine, or seafood) before the exam; ensure good hydration before and after the exam to reduce the risk of kidney damage.
■ Chest and abdominal x-rays	Used to evaluate the size and position of the heart and to identify abnormalities of major blood vessels such as the aorta (e.g., an abdominal aortic aneurysm).	Although these studies are noninvasive, they expose the patient to potentially damaging radiation. Ask women of childbearing age about possible pregnancy before the exam. Inform the physician and x-ray technician if pregnancy is known or possible.
■ Angiography	Angiography is an invasive procedure that combines x-rays and fluoroscopy (a radiographic image displayed on a screen) with injection of a contrast agent into the vessel to illuminate blood flow through the vessel, and evaluation of its patency and structure. May also be used to treat cardiovascular disease (e.g., insertion of a stent into a partially blocked vessel to restore blood flow).	Requires informed consent. Assess the patient's knowledge and reinforce teaching as needed. Withhold food and fluids as ordered before the procedure, administering ordered cardiac drugs with a small sip of water. Document and report any allergies to iodine, radiographic dyes, or seafood. Document vital signs and strength and equality of peripheral pulses prior to the procedure.
■ Cardiac catheterization	Cardiac catheterization is used to detect abnormalities in the chambers and valves of the heart; often done together with coronary angiography. A catheter inserted into the chambers of the heart (via a large vein to access	Monitor vital signs, distal pulses, temperature, color, capillary refill, movement and sensation of affected extremity as ordered after the procedure. Monitor cardiac rhythm continuously. Maintain activity restriction, position, and pressure

(continued)

TABLE 15-3	Imaging Studies *(continued)*	
DIAGNOSTIC STUDY	**EXPLANATION AND PURPOSE**	**NURSING IMPLICATIONS**
	the right side of the heart, or the radial, brachial, or femoral artery to access the left side of the heart) is used to measure pressures within the chambers of the heart, CO, and the oxygen content and saturation of the blood. Contrast agents injected into the heart outline structures of the heart. Risks associated with insertion of the catheter into a high-pressure artery include (1) bleeding from the insertion site and (2) clot formation at the insertion site and impaired blood flow to the extremity.	dressing as ordered. Check frequently for bleeding. Unless contraindicated, encourage fluids, monitoring intake and output. **clinicalALERT** Closely monitor the patient, the insertion site, and the extremity after the procedure. Immediately report evidence of bleeding, pain, or a pale, pulseless extremity to the charge nurse and physician.
■ *Computed tomography (CT) scans*	Specialized radiographic procedures that produce computer-generated images with significantly more detail than standard x-rays allow. May be done with or without contrast media, although contrast is used when a CT scan is done to identify vessel abnormalities such as an aneurysm. ■ Cardiac CT scan may be done to evaluate the coronary circulation or anatomy of the heart.	Informed consent is required. If contrast is used, inquire about allergies (to iodine and seafood in particular), and ensure that the patient is well hydrated to reduce the risk of kidney damage.
■ Electron beam computed tomography (EBCT)	A noninvasive imaging study that can detect calcium deposits in coronary arteries. Calcium deposits indicate atherosclerosis and can predict coronary heart disease in people with no symptoms. May be used as an alternative to stress testing for diagnosing coronary heart disease.	Ask women of childbearing age about possible pregnancy.
■ *Magnetic resonance imaging (MRI)*	MRI uses a supermagnet and radiofrequency signals to elicit a response from hydrogen nuclei. As a result, blood flow can be studied, and diseased tissue can be differentiated from healthy tissue. ■ Cardiac MRI shows thickness of the heart walls, size of the chambers, valve function, and coronary vessel flow. ■ MRI angiography is noninvasive and is used to evaluate vessel structure and blood flow.	The patient is not exposed to radiation during an MRI. Ask about implanted metal (e.g., a joint prosthesis) or electronic devices such as pacemakers or automatic defibrillators. Provide teaching because the experience can be frightening.
■ *Nuclear scans*	Used to evaluate blood flow to the heart muscle. A radioactive substance is injected intravenously, and the heart is scanned with a radiation detector. Ischemic or infarcted heart muscle cells do not take up the substance normally, creating an image on the scan.	The amount of radioisotope injected is very small; no special radiation precautions are required during or after the scan. Increased fluid intake is encouraged after the scan to speed elimination of the substance from the body.
■ Multigated acquisition (MUGA) scan	Used to evaluate heart size, ventricular wall motion, and ejection fraction. The patient's blood is tagged with a radioactive isotope. Imaging procedures allow visualization of the heart and its function.	Requires informed consent; no food or fluid restriction required. Note patient's current medications as these may interfere with results. Isotope is injected intravenously. The ECG is monitored during scanning.

(continued)

TABLE 15-3	Imaging Studies *(continued)*	
DIAGNOSTIC STUDY	**EXPLANATION AND PURPOSE**	**NURSING IMPLICATIONS**
■ Exercise perfusion imaging or stress tests • Thallium stress test • Technetium stress test	Used to evaluate myocardial perfusion during exercise. A radioisotope such as thallium-201 or technetium-99m is given during exercise stress testing; the heart muscle is scanned for accumulation of the isotope to evaluate perfusion.	Informed consent is required. The patient should withhold medications that may affect heart rate or BP for 24 hours before the test and be NPO for 2 to 3 hours before the test. An IV line is inserted. The isotope is injected before and/or during the test. The patient may need to return for follow-up scanning 3 or more hours after the stress test.
Positron emission tomography (PET)	Used to evaluate coronary blood flow and myocardial oxygen and glucose consumption. Provides information about the presence and severity of coronary heart disease.	Requires informed consent. Instruct patient to avoid using coffee, alcohol, and tobacco for 24 hours prior to the test. Check blood glucose before the test and inform physician or technician of results. Advise patient the test requires 1 to 1.5 hours to complete.

Other Diagnostic Tests

The *ankle-brachial index* is a noninvasive test that has been shown to be highly indicative of atherosclerosis. Blood pressure cuffs (up to four) are placed at intervals on the extremity. Each cuff is inflated, and a Doppler device is used to measure the systolic pressure distal to the cuff, until the entire extremity has been evaluated. The ankle-brachial index is calculated by dividing the systolic pressure at the ankle by the brachial systolic pressure. An index of greater than 1.0 is considered normal.

Note: The references and resources for all chapters have been compiled at the back of the book.

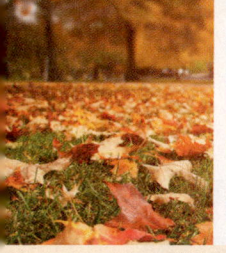
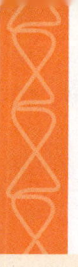

Chapter Review

KEY POINTS

- **Concept:** The heart, blood, and blood vessels—collectively known as the cardiovascular system—work together as a fuel delivery and waste removal system for the body. Cardiovascular disorders affect this distribution system, reducing the fuel available to the cells and leading to accumulated waste products in the tissues.

- The heart is a simple pump: The right side receives blood from the veins and pumps it into the low-pressure pulmonary system; the left side receives blood from the lungs and pumps it to the higher-pressure systemic circulation.

- The coronary arteries supply blood to the myocardium, or heart muscle. The left and right coronary arteries originate at the base of the aorta; the left coronary artery supplies blood to most of the left ventricle.

- Electrical impulses, usually generated by the sinoatrial (SA) node, travel through conduction pathways in the heart, causing the muscle to contract.

- The cardiac output is the amount of blood pumped by the heart in 1 minute; it can be calculated by multiplying the stroke volume (amount ejected during systole) by the heart rate. Cardiac output is affected by heart rate, preload (amount of blood in the ventricles before contraction), afterload (determined primarily by peripheral vascular resistance), and the contractility of the heart muscle.

- **Concept:** The patient's general appearance and ability to engage in activities, as well as specific assessment data and diagnostic tests, are used to evaluate the patient's cardiovascular status.

- Laboratory and diagnostic tests are used to evaluate patients with cardiovascular disease. Laboratory tests include measurements of blood lipids and markers for inflammation and cardiac muscle damage. The electrocardiogram is used to evaluate the heart's rhythm, size, and blood supply. Imaging studies may be either invasive or noninvasive; some require injection of a radiocontrast agent or radioisotope. Nursing care of the patient undergoing diagnostic testing varies, depending on the type of test being performed.

PEARSON NURSING STUDENT RESOURCES

Find additional materials at **nursing.pearsonhighered.com**.

NCLEX-PN® Exam Preparation

TEST-TAKING TIP Knowledge of changes associated with the normal aging process is important for the practical nurse. The NCLEX-PN® test plan reflects this importance in the Health Promotion and Maintenance focus of the exam.

1. The nurse is obtaining a focused assessment of a patient with pericarditis. Which of the following assessment data does the nurse recognize as pertaining to the patient's heart function?
   1. The patient relates having recently been exposed to chickenpox.
   2. Numerous flat moles are noted on the patient's neck and back.
   3. The patient states he takes two extra-strength Tylenol several times a week for headache.
   4. The patient states he often sleeps in a recliner.

2. A patient with mitral valve stenosis is admitted to the medical unit. The nurse knows that this disorder will affect blood flow from the:
   1. right atrium to the right ventricle.
   2. left atrium to the left ventricle.
   3. right ventricle to the lungs.
   4. left ventricle to the body.

3. Ventricular systole corresponds with which waveform on the ECG?
   1. P wave
   2. QRS complex
   3. T wave
   4. ST segment

4. Which of the following factors have a significant effect on peripheral vascular resistance? **Select all that apply.**
   1. The number of capillaries
   2. Length of blood vessels
   3. Blood vessel diameter
   4. The position of the body
   5. Viscosity of the blood
   6. Age of the patient

5. The nurse is teaching a patient about an upcoming echocardiogram. Which information below is accurate?
   1. The test provides information about the size and movement of the heart and its structures.
   2. This test is noninvasive and simply requires external electrodes to be placed on the arms, legs, and chest.
   3. Dye will be injected during this test to illuminate the structures of the heart and blood flow through its chambers and valves.
   4. This test is noninvasive but does expose the patient to a magnetic field.

Answers and rationales for Review Questions appear in Appendix I.

CHAPTER 16
Caring for Patients With Coronary Heart Disease and Dysrhythmias

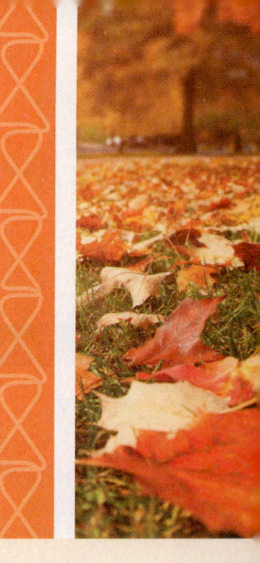

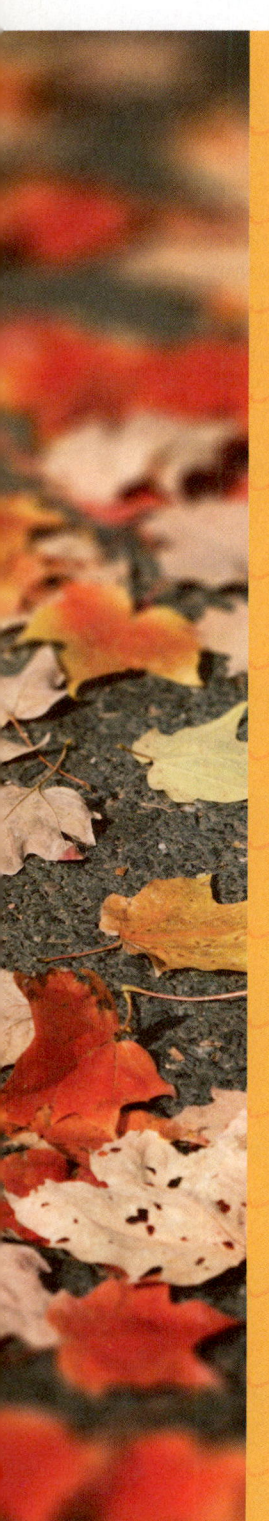

BRIEF OUTLINE

Coronary Heart Disease
Angina Pectoris
Acute Coronary Syndrome

Acute Myocardial Infarction
**CARDIAC RHYTHM
    DISORDERS**

Cardiac Dysrhythmias
Sudden Cardiac Death

APPLIED LEARNING OUTCOMES

After completing this chapter, you will be able to:

1. Describe the causes, pathophysiology, effects, and manifestations of coronary heart disease and heart rhythm disruptions.

2. Differentiate among the effects of coronary heart disease: angina pectoris, acute coronary syndrome, and myocardial infarction.

3. Discuss nursing implications, and safely administer drugs commonly prescribed for patients with coronary heart disease or dysrhythmias.

4. Provide culturally sensitive individualized nursing care for patients undergoing invasive procedures or surgery of the heart.

5. Use the nursing process to conduct a focused assessment, contribute to care planning, and provide nursing care based on patient values, preferences, and expressed needs for patients with coronary heart disease and dysrhythmias.

6. Provide and reinforce appropriate and evidence-based teaching for patients with coronary heart disease or dysrhythmias and their families.

7. Use electronic resources to plan and document nursing care and teaching for patients with coronary heart disease or dysrhythmias.

KEY TERMS

The key terms are defined on the pages listed below.

SPECIAL FEATURES

Key Concept Cardiovascular disease (CVD) is the leading cause of death and disability in the United States, affecting people of all ethnic groups and cultures.

More than 83 million people are affected by CVD, and nearly 788,000 people die from it each year (Go et al., 2013). Public education efforts aimed at reducing fat intake, increasing exercise, and lowering stress levels have made people more aware of risk factors for heart disease, and the incidence of new cases has fallen, as has the number of deaths attributable to heart disease. However, three of the disorders discussed in this unit, namely, heart failure, atherosclerosis, and cardiac dysrhythmias, are in the top 10 diagnoses causing adults to be hospitalized (Wier et al., 2011).

memory**ALERT**

- Heart disease is the leading cause of death in the United States.
- Since 1985, the heart disease death rate has declined in all racial/ethnic groups, with the steepest decline seen in Whites.
- The estimated annual economic cost for cardiovascular disease is approximately $313 billion in 2009 dollars.
- Coronary heart disease is the most common type of heart disease.

Source: National Heart, Lung, and Blood Institute (NHLBI). (2013). *Fact Book Fiscal Year 2012*. Bethesda, MD: National Institutes of Health.

In this chapter, you will learn about the causes and effects of two major heart disorders: impaired blood flow to the heart muscle itself (*coronary heart disease*) and abnormal heart rhythms, or *dysrhythmias*.

Nurses need to know about heart disease and its causes to teach and care for patients appropriately. This chapter provides the beginning nurse with the tools necessary to effectively care for patients with coronary heart disease and dysrhythmias.

Coronary Heart Disease

Key Concept Coronary heart disease (CHD), impaired blood supply to the heart muscle, is the underlying problem in angina pectoris, acute coronary syndrome, and myocardial infarction, and a leading cause of heart failure. Risk factor management is key in reducing mortality and disability associated with CHD.

CHD, or coronary artery disease (CAD), is the leading cause of death for both men and women in the United States. Of the more than 15 million Americans who have CHD, approximately 7.6 million will experience an acute event such as a myocardial infarction (Fihn et al., 2012). Of

these, many will die before reaching the hospital or in an emergency department.

CHD is caused by narrowing of the coronary arteries that supply blood to the heart muscle. *Atherosclerosis* is the primary cause of this narrowing and obstructed blood flow. Patients with CHD may have no symptoms, may experience episodic chest pain (*angina pectoris*), or may experience an acute event such as *acute coronary syndrome (ACS)* or *myocardial infarction (MI)* resulting from complete or nearly complete obstruction of blood flow to part of the heart muscle (Figure 16-1■).

Both men and women are affected by CHD. In women, however, it usually develops later in life because of the heart-protective effects of estrogen. After menopause, women's risk increases, but never becomes equal to that of men. People of all cultural backgrounds are affected by CHD, although the risk varies among ethnic and cultural groups (Box 16-1■).

RISK FACTORS

Although the cause of atherosclerosis is unknown, *risk factors* for CHD have been identified (Table 16-1■). Some risk factors for CHD (*age, gender, race,* and *heredity*) cannot be changed. More than 50% of heart attack victims are age 65 or older. Men are affected at an earlier age than women. Blacks have a higher incidence of high blood pressure and tend to develop atherosclerosis earlier in life. A family history of CHD is a risk factor for both men and women. Educating women about CHD is important, because many do not realize that their risk after menopause increases significantly.

Physiologic Risk Factors

Physiologic risk factors such as high blood pressure (hypertension), diabetes, and elevated blood lipid levels can usually be modified through medication, weight control, and diet. Additional physiologic risk factors include metabolic syndrome, inflammation and clot-promoting factors, and high homocysteine levels.

Hypertension, which affects an estimated 77.9 million people in the United States, is a systolic blood pressure greater than 140 mm Hg or a diastolic blood pressure greater than 90 mm Hg. Controlling blood pressure decreases the risk of heart disease, stroke, and kidney failure. *Diabetes* affects both small and large blood vessels. It is also associated with a higher incidence of high blood lipids, high blood pressure, and obesity—all risk factors in their own right.

High blood lipids (hyperlipidemia) increase the risk for CHD. Lipoproteins carry cholesterol in the blood. Low-density lipoprotein (LDL) is the primary carrier of cholesterol. High levels of LDL promote atherosclerosis because LDL deposits cholesterol on the artery walls. In contrast,

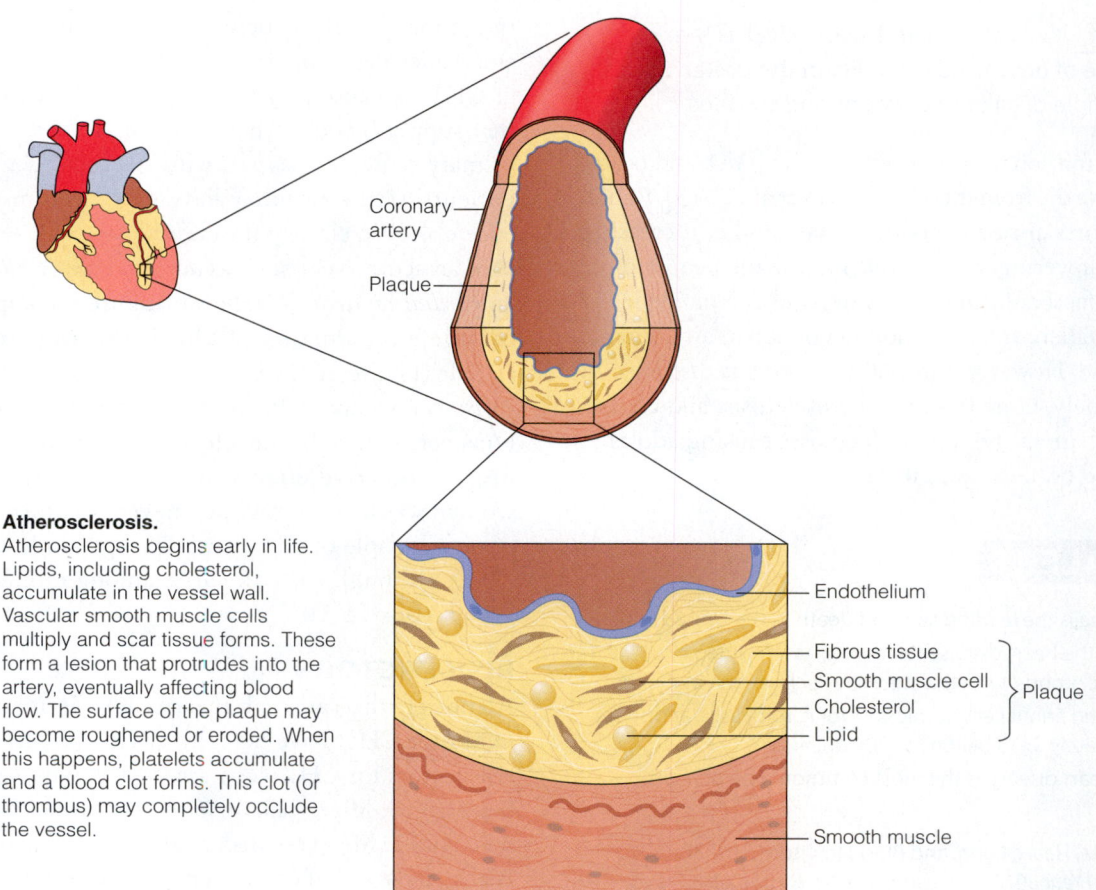

Atherosclerosis.
Atherosclerosis begins early in life. Lipids, including cholesterol, accumulate in the vessel wall. Vascular smooth muscle cells multiply and scar tissue forms. These form a lesion that protrudes into the artery, eventually affecting blood flow. The surface of the plaque may become roughened or eroded. When this happens, platelets accumulate and a blood clot forms. This clot (or thrombus) may completely occlude the vessel.

Angina pectoris.
Angina is characterized by episodes of chest pain. When the heart muscle needs more oxygen than partially occluded vessels can supply, the cells become ischemic. Lactic acid produced by ischemic cells stimulates nerve endings, causing pain. The pain subsides when cells again receive enough oxygen to meet their needs.

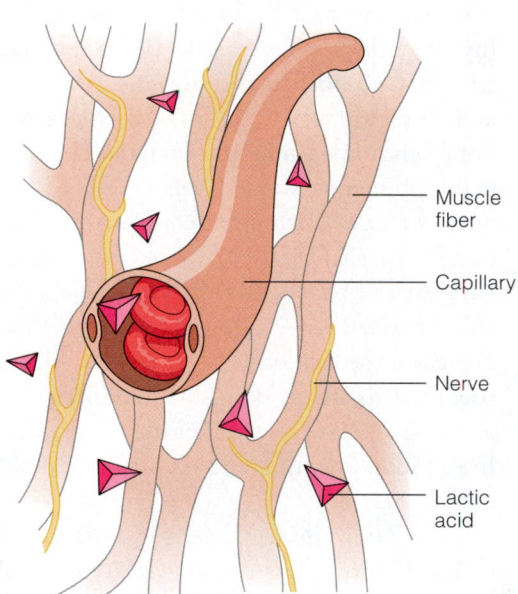

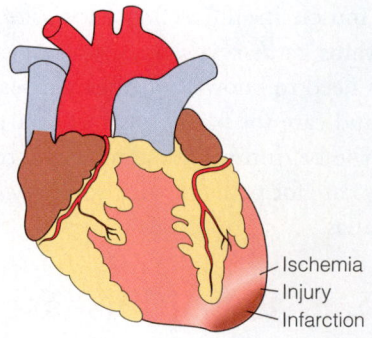

Myocardial infarction.
Myocardial infarction occurs when a coronary artery is completely obstructed, interrupting blood supply to the heart muscle. Affected tissue becomes ischemic and eventually dies (*infarcts*) if the blood supply is not restored. Surrounding the area of infarction, there is an area of tissue injury. Surrounding the injured tissue is an area of ischemic but undamaged tissue.

Figure 16-1. ■ **Coronary heart disease.** Atherosclerosis, occlusion of the coronary arteries by fibrous, fatty plaque, is the leading cause of coronary heart disease (CHD). Patients with CHD may experience angina pectoris or myocardial infarction.

Coronary Heart Disease

- Throughout the adult life span, men are more likely to be affected by CHD than women.
- Deaths associated with CHD are higher for Blacks than for Whites and considerably higher in men than in women.
- Although the CHD death rates are low in most Western and Mountain states, they are significantly higher in a band of states stretching from Oklahoma in the Southwest through Kentucky to New York in the Northeast.
- Heart disease is the leading cause of death for Blacks and Whites in the United States. The number of deaths due to heart disease is second to deaths from cancer in Americans of Hispanic/Latino, Asian or Pacific Island, and American Indian heritage.

TABLE 16-2   Classification of Cholesterol and LDL Levels

	TOTAL CHOLESTEROL (mg/dL)	LDL CHOLESTEROL (mg/dL)	TRIGLYC-ERIDES (mg/dL)
Optimal		Less than 100	
Desirable	Less than 200	Less than 130 (near optimal)	Less than 150
Borderline high	200–239	130–159	150–199
High	240 or higher	160–189	200–499
Very high		190 or higher	Greater than 500

TABLE 16-1   Risk Factors for Coronary Heart Disease

NONMODIFIABLE	MODIFIABLE	
	PHYSIOLOGIC	LIFESTYLE
Age: men ≥45 years; women ≥55 years	High blood pressure	Cigarette smoking
Gender	Diabetes mellitus	Obesity
Race/ethnic background	High blood lipids: high LDL cholesterol, high triglycerides	Physical inactivity
Heredity	Metabolic syndrome: abdominal obesity, hyperlipidemia, hypertension, insulin resistance, clotting, and inflammatory tendencies	Diet high in saturated fats
	High homocysteine levels	Women: oral contraceptive use, hormone replacement therapy
	Women: premature menopause	

National Heart, Lung, and Blood Institute (National Cholesterol Education Program, 2002). Triglycerides, used for fat storage by the body, also contribute to the development of CHD when elevated.

The *metabolic syndrome* is a group of related metabolic risk factors occurring in the same person: hyperlipidemia, hypertension, abdominal obesity, insulin resistance, and a tendency toward clotting and inflammation. High blood levels of *homocysteine,* an amino acid, also have recently been linked with CHD. Stress is a risk factor for CHD, although it is unclear how it contributes to developing CHD.

Lifestyle Risk Factors

Lifestyle risk factors can be controlled or completely eliminated. *Cigarette smoking* is a major risk factor, increasing the risk of heart disease by three to four times that of a nonsmoker. People who quit smoking reduce their risk almost immediately, no matter how long they have smoked.

memoryALERT

Cigarette smoking is the leading independent risk factor for CHD. It is a primary target of risk factor management for people of all age groups.

high-density lipoprotein (HDL) helps clear cholesterol from the arteries, transporting it to the liver for excretion. HDL levels above 35 mg/dL reduce the risk of CHD.

memoryALERT

To help you remember which lipoproteins are "good" or desirable, and which are "bad" or undesirable, use the following:

- **LDL** = *less* desirable lipids
- **HDL** = *highly* desirable lipids

Table 16-2 ■ lists optimal and desired levels of total cholesterol, LDL, and triglycerides as identified by the

Obesity (body weight 30% over ideal) and fat distribution affect the risk for CHD. Central or abdominal obesity is associated with abnormal blood lipids and a higher risk of CHD. People who are obese also have higher rates of high blood pressure, diabetes, and elevated blood cholesterol levels.

Diet is a risk factor independent of fat and cholesterol intake. A diet rich in fruits, vegetables, whole grains, and unsaturated fatty acids (such as olive oil and the fats found in fish like salmon) is associated with a lower risk of CHD.

Physical inactivity, or a sedentary lifestyle, is associated with higher risk. People who maintain a regular program of physical activity are less likely to develop CHD than sedentary people.

PATHOPHYSIOLOGY

Atherosclerosis is the primary cause of CHD. Atherosclerosis is a disease in which lesions called *atheromas* (or *plaque*) develop in the lining of medium and large arteries. These lesions protrude into the artery and may affect blood flow through the artery. The cause of atherosclerosis is unknown. The process of lipid and cholesterol accumulation is thought to start with inflammation of the blood vessel wall. Smooth muscle cells and connective tissue proliferate within the wall of the blood vessel, contributing to plaque growth. As the plaque develops, it gradually occludes the vessel lumen and impairs the vessel's ability to dilate in response to increased oxygen demands. Atheromas often develop where arteries divide, curve, or become narrow.

When a coronary blood vessel is significantly occluded, the cells it supplies become **ischemic**, without enough blood and oxygen to meet their metabolic needs. Ischemic CHD includes stable angina and *acute coronary syndromes* such as unstable angina and myocardial infarction (heart attack).

MANIFESTATIONS

CHD tends to be symptom free until about 75% of the lumen of affected vessels is occluded. When symptoms develop, they are those that indicate myocardial ischemia, in other words, manifestations of angina pectoris or acute myocardial infarction. These disorders are covered in subsequent sections of this chapter.

COLLABORATIVE CARE

Management of CHD focuses on reducing plaque buildup and maintaining adequate coronary blood flow.

Diagnostic Tests

- The total serum cholesterol and a lipid panel are obtained to evaluate serum lipid levels.
- Plasma levels of C-reactive protein, an indicator of inflammation, are measured as well.
- Blood glucose levels are measured to identify presence of or risk for diabetes mellitus.

The ankle-brachial index is a noninvasive test of peripheral vascular disease that also may predict CHD. Other diagnostic tests, such as an ECG stress test and positron emission tomography (PET) scan, also may be done to evaluate the risk for CHD and identify myocardial ischemia.

Risk Factor Management

SMOKING Quitting smoking reduces the risk for CHD within months of stopping. People who quit smoking reduce their risk by 50%, regardless of how many years or how much they smoked before stopping. Additional benefits of smoking cessation include improved blood lipid levels and reduced blood viscosity.

DIET A low-fat, low-cholesterol diet is suggested to help control blood lipid levels and to promote weight loss. The National Cholesterol Education Program recommends reducing total fat intake to 25%–35% of the total daily calories. Saturated fats should make up less than 7% of total calories, with the majority of remaining fat intake comprised of monounsaturated fats. Much saturated fat is found in whole-milk products and in red meats. Eating nonfat dairy products, fish, and poultry as primary protein sources can lower cholesterol levels. Monounsaturated fats, found in olive, canola, and peanut oils, and omega-3 fatty acids found in certain cold-water fish, such as tuna, salmon, and mackerel, help reduce total serum cholesterol, LDL, and triglyceride levels. Several programs that combine diet, exercise, and other therapies have been proven to reduce atherosclerotic deposits. These programs are quite restrictive, however, and require significant commitment to follow (Box 16-2 ■).

EXERCISE Regular exercise (at least 30 minutes of moderate intensity exercise 5 to 6 days per week) has multiple benefits. It improves blood lipid levels, reduces blood pressure and insulin resistance, and promotes weight loss.

BLOOD PRESSURE AND DIABETES Although high blood pressure and diabetes mellitus are chronic diseases that often cannot be cured, they usually can be controlled. Maintaining a blood pressure lower than 140/90 mm Hg is vital, as higher blood pressures promote development of atherosclerosis and plaque buildup. Diabetes also promotes atherosclerosis and CHD. Controlling blood glucose levels helps promote weight loss and the adverse effects of this disorder.

BOX 16-2	COMPLEMENTARY THERAPIES

Coronary Heart Disease (CHD)

The *Pritikin diet* is basically vegetarian, high in complex carbohydrates and fiber, low in cholesterol, and extremely low in fat (10% of daily calories). Egg whites and limited amounts of nonfat dairy or soy products are allowed. The Pritikin program requires 45 minutes of walking daily and recommends multivitamin supplements, including vitamins C and E and folate.

The *Ornish diet* is also vegetarian, although egg whites and a cup of nonfat milk or yogurt per day are allowed. No oil or fat is permitted, even for cooking. Two ounces of alcohol a day are permitted. The Ornish program also calls for stress reduction, emotional social support systems, daily stretching, and walking for an hour three times a week.

Medications

Drug therapy to lower total cholesterol and LDL levels is now the standard of care for patients at risk for CHD. Cholesterol-lowering drugs should be used together with dietary changes to reduce saturated and total fat intake. Statins, such as *atorvastatin (Lipitor), rosuvastatin (Crestor),* and *simvastatin (Zocor),* are widely prescribed for this purpose. These drugs inhibit cholesterol synthesis in the liver. They are very effective in lowering LDL levels; some also reduce serum triglycerides and increase HDL levels. Headache and gastrointestinal (GI) effects are the most common side effects of these drugs. Myalgias (muscle aches) or skin rashes may also develop. *Rhabdomyolysis*, or muscle fiber breakdown, is a possible serious adverse effect of statin therapy that can lead to acute kidney failure. Liver function tests and muscle enzymes are monitored during therapy to assess for possible toxic effects.

If a combination of diet and a statin drug does not lower serum cholesterol and LDL levels to desired goals, a different class of cholesterol-lowering drugs may be added to the treatment plan. Fibric acid agents, including fenofibrate (Tricor) and gemfibrozil (Lopid), may be combined with a statin drug to reduce triglyceride and very-low-density lipoprotein (VLDL) levels to a greater extent than the statin alone. *Ezetimibe (Zetia)* is a unique drug that acts in the small intestine to block cholesterol absorption. It may be used alone or combined with a statin. Although generally well tolerated, ezetimibe may be associated with an increased risk for liver damage and rhabdomyolysis. Niacin or nicotinic acid (Niacor, Nicobid, Nicolar) lowers LDL levels and raises HDL levels. Nicotinic acid is available without a prescription. Flushing, or "hot flashes," and pruritus are common side effects of niacin therapy. Cholestyramine (Questran), colestipol (Colestid), and colesevelam (Welchol) bind with bile acids and cholesterol in the intestine, promoting their excretion in the feces. These drugs may have GI side effects, such as constipation, gas, and abdominal cramping.

Nursing implications for drugs used to lower serum cholesterol levels are summarized in Table 16-3■.

NURSING CARE

Teaching to prevent CHD is a priority of nursing care to promote health for patients of all ages. The LPN/LVN working in an ambulatory care setting is in an ideal position to provide appropriate teaching. Although risk factors such as gender, age, and genetic makeup cannot be changed, lifestyle factors such as smoking, diet, and inactivity can be. Physiologic factors such as high blood pressure, diabetes,

and abnormal blood lipid levels can be managed to reduce this major health and mortality risk.

Strongly encourage all patients to stop all forms of tobacco use. Discuss the effects of smoking on the body and the benefits of quitting. Resource materials to help patients stop smoking are available from the American Heart Association (AHA), the American Lung Association, and the American Cancer Society. Refer to a smoking cessation program to increase the likelihood of success in quitting.

Discuss the role of diet in CHD and obesity. Help assess food intake and patterns of eating to identify areas that can be improved. Refer to a dietitian for diet planning and further teaching. Encourage to make dietary changes gradually but progressively, maintaining a well-balanced low-fat diet. Advise to avoid fad diets for weight loss. Suggest AHA and other cookbooks that offer low-fat recipes to encourage healthier eating.

Discuss the physical and psychosocial benefits of regular exercise. Help the patient identify favorite forms of exercise and schedule exercise periods of 30 to 45 minutes of continuous aerobic activity (i.e., walking, running, bicycling, swimming) five to six times a week. Walking provides many benefits and is an easily accessible and low-cost form of exercise. Encourage identification of an "exercise buddy" to help maintain motivation.

Discuss the importance of controlling high blood pressure, diabetes, and elevated blood lipid levels. Refer patients to their primary care provider for treatment as needed, and provide teaching about specific diseases and/or prescribed treatments.

Stress is a normal part of every person's life. Assist the patient to identify and develop stress-management techniques such as physical exercise or meditation. It is important to emphasize that relaxation techniques require practice.

Angina Pectoris

Angina pectoris is chest pain that occurs when there is a temporary imbalance between myocardial blood supply and demand. Angina often occurs in a pattern: Exercise brings on the pain; rest relieves the pain.

PATHOPHYSIOLOGY

Atherosclerosis and CHD often lead to angina. Obstruction of a coronary artery reduces blood flow to the part of the heart normally supplied by that vessel. Although the heart muscle may still receive enough blood and oxygen to meet its needs at rest, anything that further reduces blood flow or increases the oxygen demand of the heart muscle can cause angina. Exercise increases myocardial oxygen demand. The obstructed vessel is unable to provide an adequate supply, and cells are deprived of oxygen. Inadequate oxygen causes cells to switch from aerobic metabolism (a very efficient

TABLE 16-3	Giving Medications Safely: Cholesterol-Lowering Drugs		
CLASS/DRUGS	**PURPOSE**	**NURSING IMPLICATIONS**	**PATIENT TEACHING**
Statins ■ *Atorvastatin* (Lipitor) ■ Fluvastatin (Lescol) ■ *Lovastatin* (Mevacor) ■ *Pravastatin* (Pravachol) ■ *Rosuvastatin* (Crestor) ■ *Simvastatin* (Zocor)	Lower total serum cholesterol and LDL levels; some also lower triglyceride levels and raise HDL levels.	Monitor serum cholesterol and liver enzyme levels. Report elevated liver enzymes to the physician. Assess for muscle pain and tenderness; report to physician if present. Assess for and report significant alcohol use.	Inform your doctor if you are taking other medications or using natural remedies. Promptly report muscle pain, tenderness, or weakness; skin rash, hives, or color changes; abdominal pain, nausea, vomiting. Do not use these drugs if you are pregnant or intend to become pregnant. Limit your consumption of alcohol and grapefruit juice while taking these drugs.
Fibric acid agents ■ Fenofibrate (Tricor) ■ Gemfibrozil (Lopid)	Lower triglyceride and VLDL levels.	May precipitate gallbladder disease in some patients; report symptoms such as upper abdominal pain, intolerance of fatty foods. Monitor for increased bruising or bleeding. Report symptoms as indicated. Administer with meals to decrease GI distress.	Do not use this medication if you are pregnant, lactating, or may become pregnant. Immediately report unusual bruising or bleeding, right upper abdominal pain, changes in color of stool, or muscle pain or cramping.
Antilipemics ■ *Ezetimibe* (Zetia) ■ *Ezetimibe + simvastatin* (Vytorin)	Act on cells in the small intestine to block cholesterol absorption, thereby reducing levels of total cholesterol, LDL, and triglycerides.	Monitor hemoglobin, hematocrit, and platelet count, liver function tests during treatment. Assess for and report muscle pain, especially when also taking a statin.	Report unexplained muscle pain, weakness, or tenderness. Women of childbearing age should use effective birth control while taking this drug.
Nicotinic acid ■ *Niacin* (Nicobid, Nicolar, Niaspan, others)	Lowers VLDL, LDL, triglyceride, and total cholesterol levels; raises HDL levels.	Give with meals and a cold beverage to minimize GI effects. Monitor blood glucose, uric acid levels, and liver function tests; report abnormal levels to the physician.	This drug often causes flushing of the face, neck, and ears; these effects diminish over time, but are aggravated by alcohol use. Change positions slowly to reduce the risk of injury. Report dizziness or weakness to your doctor.
Bile acid sequestrants ■ Cholestyramine (Questran) ■ Colestipol (Colestid) ■ Colesevelam (Welchol)	Lower LDL levels by binding with bile acids in the intestine. Primarily used in combination drug treatment.	Mix powders with 4 to 6 ounces of water or juice. Administer as ordered with meals.	Drink ample amounts of fluid to reduce the risk of constipation. Do not omit doses. Promptly report back or abdominal pain, nausea/vomiting, or black or bloody stools to your doctor.

Note: Medications identified in *italics* are among the 200 most frequently prescribed drugs in the United States.

process that requires oxygen) to anaerobic metabolism (a very inefficient process that occurs in the absence of oxygen). Lactic acid and other substances that stimulate nerve fibers are released, causing pain.

Three types of angina have been identified:

1. *Stable angina* is the most common and predictable form of angina. It occurs with a known amount of activity or stress. Stable angina is relieved by rest and nitrates.
2. *Unstable angina* occurs with increasing frequency, severity, and duration. Pain is unpredictable and may occur at rest. Patients with unstable angina are at risk for myocardial infarction. Unstable angina is discussed in the section on acute coronary syndromes.
3. *Prinzmetal angina* is atypical angina that occurs without an identified precipitating cause, usually at the same time each day, often waking the patient from sleep. It is caused by coronary artery spasm.

Progression of the disease is marked by decreasing functional capacity or a change from stable angina to unstable angina. This change may herald an impending myocardial infarction. *Silent myocardial ischemia,* or asymptomatic myocardial ischemia, is believed to be common in people with CHD. However, because patients experience no symptoms, its actual incidence is unknown.

MANIFESTATIONS

The cardinal manifestation of angina is chest pain. The pain typically is precipitated by an identifiable event, such as physical activity, strong emotion, stress, eating a heavy meal, or exposure to cold. The classic sequence of angina is activity–pain, rest–relief. Anginal pain usually lasts less than 15 minutes and is relieved by rest. The manifestations of angina are summarized in Box 16-3■.

In women, angina symptoms often are associated with stress or strong emotions instead of physical activity. Women may experience symptoms differently, complaining of sensations of indigestion, nausea, vomiting, and upper back pain.

BOX 16-3	MANIFESTATIONS OF ANGINA

- Chest Pain
  - Substernal or precordial pain (across the chest)
  - Possible radiation to neck, arms, shoulders, or jaw
  - Tight, squeezing, constricting, or heavy sensation
  - Precipitated by exercise or activity, strong emotion, stress, cold, heavy meal
  - Relieved by rest, nitroglycerin
- Shortness of breath, pallor, anxiety

COLLABORATIVE CARE

Angina is diagnosed by the patient's symptoms, past medical history and family history, and physical assessment. Laboratory tests may confirm the presence of risk factors, such as abnormal blood lipids, elevated C-reactive protein levels, or the presence of diabetes mellitus.

Diagnostic Tests

Common diagnostic tests to determine the extent of CHD and angina include electrocardiography, stress testing, nuclear medicine studies, and coronary angiography.

ELECTROCARDIOGRAPHY   A resting ECG may be normal in patients with angina. However, characteristic changes are seen during anginal episodes. During periods of myocardial ischemia, the ST segment is depressed and the T wave may flatten or invert (Figure 16-2■). These changes reverse when adequate blood flow is restored. Stress electrocardiography is also used to help diagnose angina and to identify patients at risk. In CHD, the increased cardiac workload caused by exercise or administration of a vasodilator drug may cause myocardial ischemia, angina, and ECG changes characteristic of ischemia.

IMAGING STUDIES   *Positron emission tomography (PET)* or *electron beam computed tomography (EBCT)* testing often reveals calcium deposits indicative of CHD in the patient

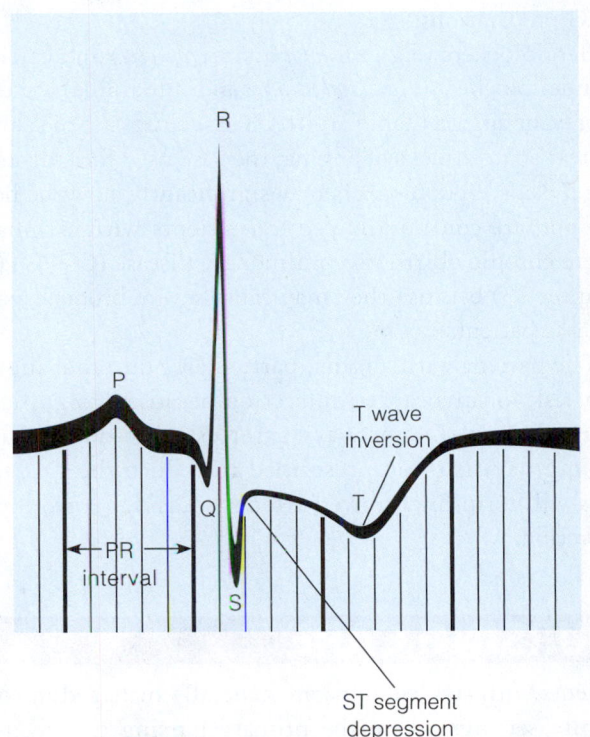

Figure 16-2. ■ ECG changes during an episode of angina. Note the ST segment depression and T wave inversion characteristic of myocardial ischemia.

with angina. An *echocardiogram* may be performed at rest or after exercise stress testing to evaluate heart wall movement. *Transesophageal echocardiography (TEE)* is performed using an endoscope inserted into the esophagus to identify abnormal blood flow to the heart muscle as well as heart structure and function. *Radionuclear scanning* may be performed. Ischemic or infarcted cells of the myocardium may appear as a "cold spot" on the scan. *Coronary angiography* is the "gold standard" for evaluating the coronary arteries. Narrowing of a vessel by more than 50% is considered significant; most lesions that produce symptoms obstruct more than 70% of the vessel. Nursing care of the patient undergoing a coronary angiogram is similar to that provided for patients undergoing percutaneous coronary revascularization procedures (see Box 16-4 on page 377).

Medications

ACUTE CARE Sublingual nitroglycerin (NTG) is the drug of choice to treat acute anginal attacks, acting within 1 to 2 minutes. Rapid-acting NTG is also available as a buccal spray in a metered-dose system.

CHRONIC MANAGEMENT Longer acting NTG preparations include oral tablets, ointment, and transdermal patches. In these forms, NTG is used to prevent attacks of angina, not to treat an acute attack. Headache, nausea, dizziness, and hypotension are common adverse effects of NTG preparations.

Beta blockers (e.g., *atenolol* and *metoprolol*) and calcium channel blockers (e.g., *amlodipine* and nifedipine) are used to prevent angina (Table 16-4 ■). These drugs act too slowly to treat acute attacks of angina; they are used for long-term prophylaxis. Beta blockers may significantly slow the heart rate and are contraindicated for patients with asthma or severe chronic obstructive pulmonary disease (COPD) (see Chapter 23) because they may cause severe bronchospasm in these patients.

The patient with angina, particularly unstable angina, is at risk for myocardial infarction because of significant narrowing of the coronary arteries. Low-dose aspirin (81 mg/day) is often prescribed to reduce the risk that clots will form in narrowed arteries, causing a myocardial infarction.

NURSING CARE

Patients with stable angina are generally managed in community settings where the primary nursing care focus is education. During an acute angina episode, nursing care focuses on reducing the workload of the heart and improving its blood and oxygen supply.

PRIORITIZING NURSING CARE

Maintaining adequate coronary blood flow and perfusion of the heart muscle is the highest priority of care for the patient with CHD and angina. Because physical activity is vital to maintaining heart health, care for the patient with stable angina focuses on improving the supply of blood to the heart instead of reducing the workload of the heart.

HEALTH PROMOTION

In addition to the health promotion measures identified for CHD, emphasize the importance of managing risk factors to slow the progression of the disease. Encourage patients to stop smoking and provide referrals to smoking cessation programs and support groups. Encourage regular exercise, gradually increasing the duration and intensity of the exercise, and resting if pain develops. Provide information about a diet based on AHA or National Cholesterol Education Program guidelines.

ASSESSING

Focused assessment of the patient with angina relates to anginal pain and associated manifestations, as well as measures the patient is currently using to manage this condition. Ask the patient about the following:

- Pain: location, character (heavy, burning, tight, squeezing), intensity, radiation; timing (relationship to activity, meals, or other factors), duration; aggravating and relieving factors; associated manifestations such as nausea or shortness of breath.
- History of angina or other heart disease and treatment measures, including drugs, activity modifications, invasive procedures, or surgery.
- Risk factors for CHD: family history, presence of high blood pressure, diabetes, high blood cholesterol levels, and current treatment of these conditions if present; smoking and alcohol intake, use of other recreational drugs; perceived stress levels, and techniques used to manage stress; if female, age at menopause, use of hormone replacement therapy or oral contraceptives.

Note the frequency and duration of angina episodes and the effectiveness of relief measures (oxygen, NTG, rest). Record the patient's vital signs and ECG tracing during an anginal episode. Monitor cardiac enzyme levels, serum cholesterol, and glucose.

IDENTIFYING POTENTIAL COMPLICATIONS

Angina often is a precursor to an acute cardiac event, such as acute myocardial infarction. Observe for and report increasing frequency, intensity, and duration of anginal episodes, as well as angina occurring with lower levels of physical activity or emotional stress. Promptly report chest

TABLE 16-4	Giving Medications Safely: Antianginal Drugs		
CLASS/DRUGS	**PURPOSE**	**NURSING IMPLICATIONS**	**PATIENT TEACHING**
Nitrates ■ Nitroglycerin (Nitropaste, Nitro-Dur, Nitro-Bid, Nitrol, Transderm-Nitro, Nitrogard, Nitrodisc, Tridil) ■ Isosorbide dinitrate (Isordil) ■ Isosorbide mononitrate (Ismo)	Nitrates dilate blood vessels, increasing blood flow to the myocardium and reducing the workload of the heart. Sublingual nitroglycerin (NTG) tablets and buccal spray are used to prevent and treat acute angina. Oral and transdermal forms are used to reduce the frequency and severity of anginal attacks.	Administer sublingual NTG at the onset of chest pain. In some cases, tablets may be left at the bedside for prompt treatment of angina. Wear gloves when applying NTG ointment to prevent absorbing the drug through your skin. Measure dose carefully and spread evenly in a 2-inch by 3-inch area. Remove NTG patches or ointment at night to help prevent tolerance to the drug. Help the patient identify events that precipitate anginal attacks.	Use only rapid-acting forms to treat acute anginal attacks, taking the drug at the onset of chest pain. Dissolve tablets under the tongue; do not swallow the tablet. If chest pain is not relieved within 5 minutes, take a second dose. After 5 minutes more, a third dose may be taken. If pain continues, seek medical help immediately. Keep NTG tablets in original container and protect them from heat, light, and moisture. Refill your prescription every 6 months and throw away unused tablets. Apply ointment or transdermal patches to a hairless area; spread ointment evenly; do not rub or massage. Remove the old patch or residual ointment before bedtime; apply a fresh dose in the morning. Rotate sites. If you are using long-acting NTG, keep a supply of rapid-acting NTG to treat acute angina.
Beta blockers ■ *Atenolol* (Tenormin) ■ *Metoprolol* (Lopressor) ■ Propranolol (Inderal) ■ Nadolol (Corgard) ■ Timolol maleate (Betimol)	Beta blockers decrease cardiac workload by blocking sympathetic nervous system stimulation. They are frequently used to prevent angina and to treat hypertension.	Record heart rate and BP before giving. Withhold the drug if the heart rate is below 50 beats/min or the BP is below identified levels. Notify the charge nurse or physician. Assess for possible contraindications to beta blockers, such as asthma or COPD. These drugs should not be abruptly discontinued, but gradually withdrawn when necessary.	Beta blockers do not work immediately; keep a supply of fast-acting NTG for acute chest pain. Do not abruptly stop taking this drug. Talk to your doctor about discontinuing its use. Take and record your pulse daily. Do not take the drug, and notify your doctor if your heart rate is below 50 beats/min. Have your BP checked frequently. Report a slow or irregular pulse, swelling or weight gain, or difficulty breathing to your doctor.
Calcium channel blockers ■ *Amlodipine* (Norvasc) ■ Nifedipine (Procardia) ■ Diltiazem (Cardizem) ■ Verapamil (Calan) ■ Bepridil (Vascor) ■ Felodipine (Plendil) ■ Isradipine (DynaCirc) ■ Nicardipine (Cardene) ■ Nimodipine (Nimotop)	Calcium channel blockers are used to control angina, hypertension, and dysrhythmias. They reduce cardiac workload and increase blood flow to the myocardium. They are often ordered for patients with coronary artery spasm (Prinzmetal angina).	Record BP and heart rate before giving the drug. Withhold drug if the heart rate is below 50 beats/min. Notify the charge nurse or physician if withheld. Nifedipine may be given by withdrawing the liquid from the capsule with a syringe and squirting the dose under the tongue (discard the needle first!). Immediately report manifestations of toxicity (nausea, generalized weakness, decreased cardiac output, hypotension, dysrhythmias).	Take your pulse before taking the drug. Do not take the drug, and notify physician if your heart rate drops below 50 beats/min. For acute angina, keep a fresh supply of rapid-acting NTG available (e.g., sublingual tablets). Calcium channel blockers will not work fast enough to relieve an acute attack.

Note: Medications identified in *italics* are among the 200 most frequently prescribed drugs in the United States.

pain unrelieved by rest and rapid-acting NTG and chest pain accompanied by shortness of breath, anxiety, or cool, clammy skin.

DIAGNOSING, PLANNING, AND IMPLEMENTING

Risk for Acute Pain

Expected outcome: Will remain pain free; if angina pain develops, pain will be relieved within 5 minutes of onset.

- If short-acting NTG is ordered, keep it at the bedside so it can be taken at the onset of pain. *Immediate treatment can restore blood flow to the heart muscle and reduce the intensity and duration of anginal pain.*
- Start oxygen at 4 to 6 L/min per nasal cannula unless contraindicated. *Supplemental oxygen reduces myocardial hypoxia.*
- Space activities to allow rest between them. *Activity increases cardiac work and may precipitate angina. Spacing of activities allows the heart to recover.*
- Instruct the patient to take a sublingual NTG tablet before engaging in activities that precipitate angina (e.g., climbing stairs, sexual intercourse). *This prophylactic dose of NTG helps maintain cardiac perfusion when increased work is anticipated, preventing ischemia and chest pain.*
- Encourage risk factor management, for example, losing weight, making dietary changes (reducing fat, cholesterol, and kilocalorie intake), reducing stress, and others as indicated. *Managing risk factors can slow the process of atherosclerosis and preserve myocardial perfusion.*
- Encourage the patient to implement and maintain a progressive exercise program under the supervision of his or her primary care provider. *Exercise slows the atherosclerotic process and helps develop collateral circulation to the heart muscle.*
- Refer the patient who smokes to a smoking cessation program. *Nicotine causes vasoconstriction and increases the heart rate, decreasing myocardial perfusion and increasing cardiac workload.*

Readiness for Enhanced Self-Health Management

Expected outcome: Will express understanding of all components of prescribed regimen and willingness to follow regimen.

- Assess knowledge and understanding of angina. *Assessment allows teaching and interventions to be tailored to the needs of the patient.*
- Teach about angina and atherosclerosis as needed. *Denial or exaggerated fear may be strong in patients with angina pectoris. Teaching helps the patient understand that angina can be managed, pain controlled, and disease progress slowed.*
- Provide written and verbal instructions about prescribed medications and their use. *Written instructions reinforce teaching and are available to the patient for future reference.*

- Stress the importance of taking chest pains seriously while maintaining a positive attitude. *Chest pain is a warning and necessitates appropriate response.*
- Refer to a cardiac rehabilitation program or other organized activities and support groups for patients with coronary artery disease. *Programs such as these help the patient develop strategies for risk factor management, maintain a program of supervised activity, and gain coping skills.*

MANAGING NURSING CARE

As appropriate and allowed by the designated duties and responsibilities of assistive personnel, the nurse may delegate nursing care activities such as measuring intake and output, obtaining daily weights, and providing oral and skin care for the patient with stable angina.

EVALUATING

When evaluating the effectiveness of nursing care for the patient with angina, collect data regarding the onset, duration, and management of anginal episodes. Use subjective and objective data to evaluate knowledge, understanding, and willingness to follow physician's orders and manage risk factors.

DOCUMENTING

Document the frequency and duration of anginal episodes, as well as precipitating factors. Note associated symptoms, such as nausea, shortness of breath, or anxiety. Document teaching provided and the patient's understanding of the disease, risk factors, and the prescribed treatment plan.

CONTINUITY OF CARE

Patients with stable angina often manage their pain effectively, continuing to live active and productive lives. Discuss the relationship between modifiable risk factors and angina. Provide information about risk factor management, as well as the disease process. Emphasize the relationship between reduced blood flow to the heart muscle and pain. Discuss the use of prescribed medications. Instruct to take NTG prophylactically before activities that tend to cause chest pain. Advise taking NTG at the first indication of pain rather than waiting to see whether the pain develops. Emphasize the importance of seeking immediate medical assistance if three NTG tablets over 15 to 20 minutes do not relieve the pain. Instruct to call 911 or go to the emergency department immediately rather than contacting the physician.

Teach safe medication storage, especially for NTG. Because NTG is affected by heat and light and has a short shelf life, instruct the patient to store it in a cool, dry, dark place and to keep no more than a 6-month supply on hand. Advise to always carry a few tablets but not the whole supply, because body warmth (transmitted through a shirt or pants pocket) causes tablets to deteriorate more rapidly. If an NTG patch or ointment is prescribed, teach how to apply it. Explain the rationale for removing the patch or ointment at night.

Stress the importance of not discontinuing medications abruptly, particularly beta blockers. Review their adverse effects, and instruct when to notify the physician.

Acute Coronary Syndrome/ Unstable Angina

Acute coronary syndrome (ACS) is a condition of severe cardiac ischemia. ACS includes **unstable angina (UA)**, angina occurring with increasing frequency, at rest, or unpredictably, and acute myocardial ischemia with or without muscle tissue damage. This section focuses on unstable angina. Acute myocardial infarction is discussed in the next section of this chapter. The diagnosis of ACS is made for up to 25% of the approximately 6 million patients presenting to hospital emergency departments with complaints of chest pain annually. Patients with ACS have a high risk of recurrent ACS or acute myocardial infarction, and a 10% risk of dying within 30 days (Longo et al., 2012).

PATHOPHYSIOLOGY

ACS/UA is generally associated with partial obstruction of one or more coronary arteries. In ACS, blood flow to the myocardium is acutely reduced, but not fully occluded.

The usual cause of this acute reduction in blood flow is rupture or erosion of atherosclerotic plaque. A blood clot forms at the site, significantly impairing blood flow through the damaged vessel. Coronary artery spasm may also cause ACS. Myocardial cells are injured by the resulting acute ischemia. Injured myocardial cells contract less effectively, potentially reducing cardiac output if a large area of the heart is affected. In ACS, the affected myocardium recovers when blood flow is restored.

MANIFESTATIONS

The cardinal symptom of ACS is chest pain, usually substernal or epigastric. The pain often radiates to the neck, left shoulder, or left arm. It may develop at rest and typically lasts longer than angina pain (usually longer than 10 to 20 minutes). The patient may also experience *dyspnea* (difficulty breathing or acute shortness of breath); **diaphoresis** (profuse sweating); pallor; cool, clammy skin; nausea; and light-headedness. *Tachycardia* (rapid heart rate) and *hypotension* (low blood pressure) may occur. Table 16-5■ compares the pathophysiology and manifestations of stable angina, ACS/UA, and acute myocardial infarction.

COLLABORATIVE CARE

The patient with ACS/UA usually presents to the emergency department with chest pain that is more intense or of longer duration than previous episodes of angina. The pain may be unrelieved by NTG.

TABLE 16-5	Comparing Stable Angina, Acute Coronary Syndrome/Unstable Angina, and Acute Myocardial Infarction		
	STABLE ANGINA	**ACUTE CORONARY SYNDROME/UNSTABLE ANGINA (ACS/UA)**	**ACUTE MYOCARDIAL INFARCTION**
Pathophysiology	Myocardial ischemia develops with increased workload (e.g., exercise, stress) due to stable atherosclerotic plaque in coronary arteries.	Unstable plaque and clot formation partially occlude a coronary artery, causing acute myocardial ischemia and tissue injury; often unrelated to activity.	Obstruction of a coronary artery by a clot totally blocks blood flow to a portion of the myocardium resulting in tissue necrosis (cell death).
Chest pain	■ Stable and predictable; precipitated by exertion or emotion, relieved by rest ■ May radiate to neck, shoulder, arms ■ Usually lasts 2 to 5 minutes	■ Often occurs at rest or on arising ■ Increasing frequency and severity ■ Radiates to neck, left shoulder, arm ■ Lasts 10 minutes or longer	■ Begins abruptly, unrelated to rest or exercise ■ Severe, "crushing" ■ Radiates to neck, arms, jaw ■ Unrelieved by rest or nitroglycerin
Other manifestations	■ Indigestion, nausea ■ Possible shortness of breath ■ Anxiety	■ Epigastric pain ■ Dyspnea ■ Tachycardia, hypotension ■ Cool, pale skin	■ Epigastric pain, nausea ■ Dyspnea ■ Pallor, diaphoresis ■ Tachycardia or bradycardia; hyper- or hypotension

TABLE 16-6	Giving Medications Safely: Antiplatelet Drugs		
CLASS/DRUGS	**PURPOSE**	**NURSING IMPLICATIONS**	**PATIENT TEACHING**
Oral antiplatelet drugs ■ Aspirin ■ *Clopidogrel* (Plavix) ■ Prasugrel (Effient) ■ Ticagrelor (Brilinta) ■ Ticlopidine (Ticlid)	Antiplatelet drugs inhibit platelet aggregation in arteries, preventing clot formation.	Ask about a history of intracranial or GI bleeding, peptic ulcer disease, or other abnormal bleeding. Observe for and report increased bruising, petechiae, apparent or occult bleeding. Do not administer concurrently with warfarin (Coumadin).	Take aspirin with milk or food. Do not use NSAIDs or other over-the-counter drugs containing aspirin or an NSAID unless directed to do so by the physician. Check with your doctor before taking any herbal remedies. Report unusual bruising or bleeding to your doctor. Inform all care providers, including dentists, that you are taking these drugs.

Note: Medications identified in *italics* are among the 200 most frequently prescribed drugs in the United States.

Diagnostic Tests

The ECG and serum cardiac markers are the primary diagnostic tests used to differentiate ACS from acute myocardial infarction. *Cardiac muscle troponins* and *creatine kinase* levels may initially be slightly elevated, but usually return to normal ranges within 12 to 24 hours.

When done during the acute episode of chest pain, the ECG shows changes characteristic of acute ischemia and cell injury. An echocardiogram may show abnormal movement of the myocardial wall during an acute episode of ACS. When the patient is pain free and acute myocardial infarction has been ruled out, stress testing is done to evaluate for significant CHD.

Medications

Medications used to treat ACS include drugs to reduce myocardial ischemia and to prevent clotting. Nitrates and beta blockers are given to restore blood flow to the ischemic myocardium and reduce the workload of the heart. NTG is initially administered by sublingual tablet or buccal spray. If chest pain is unrelieved, an intravenous NTG infusion may be started. Beta blockers are generally given orally. See Table 16-4 for the nursing implications and teaching related to these drugs.

Aspirin, antiplatelet drugs, and heparin are given to prevent additional clots from forming. Aspirin, clopidogrel (Plavix), and several related drugs interrupt blood clotting by inhibiting platelet aggregation. Table 16-6■ discusses nursing responsibilities and patient teaching for oral antiplatelet drugs. Intravenous antiplatelet drugs such as abciximab (ReoPro) may be given when an invasive coronary revascularization procedure is anticipated.

Surgery and Revascularization Procedures

Patients with ACS may undergo surgery or a *percutaneous coronary intervention (PCI)* to restore blood flow to the myocardium. In the United States, PCI is the most common

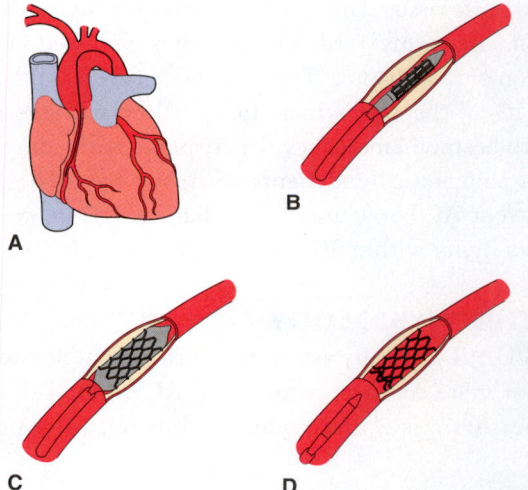

Figure 16-3. ■ Percutaneous coronary intervention (PCI) or balloon angioplasty with stent placement. (**A**) The balloon catheter with the stent is threaded into the affected coronary artery. (**B**) The stent is positioned across the blockage. (**C**) The balloon is inflated, compressing the plaque and expanding the stent. (**D**) The balloon is deflated and removed, leaving the stent in place.

revascularization procedure, performed nearly twice as often as surgical revascularization (Longo et al., 2012).

PCI, or *balloon angioplasty*, is an invasive procedure used to increase blood flow to heart muscle. PCI is performed in the cardiac catheterization laboratory under local anesthesia. Using the femoral or radial artery, a small balloon-tipped catheter is threaded into the obstructed coronary artery. The balloon is positioned across the area of narrowing (Figure 16-3A, 3B■). The balloon is inflated to reduce the narrowing and increase blood flow through the obstructed area. An intracoronary stent usually is inserted at the same time. The stent remains in the artery as a prop after the balloon is deflated (Figure 16-3C, 3D■). *Atherectomy* procedures, another type of PCI, actually remove plaque from an identified blood vessel lesion. Nursing care for the patient having a PCI procedure is outlined in Box 16-4■.

BOX 16-4	NURSING CARE CHECKLIST

Percutaneous Coronary Intervention

Before the Procedure

☑ Assess knowledge and understanding of the procedure. Reinforce teaching and provide additional information as needed.

☑ Provide routine preoperative care as ordered (see Chapter 10).

☑ Administer ordered cardiac medications with a small sip of water before the procedure unless contraindicated.

☑ Document and report any allergies to iodine, radiographic dyes, or seafood.

☑ Record height, weight, and vital signs. Record equality and amplitude of peripheral pulses; mark their locations.

☑ Explain that patient will remain awake during the procedure, which lasts 1 to 2 hours. Sedation may be given, and a local anesthetic will be used where the catheter is inserted. A sensation of warmth (a "hot flash") and a metallic taste may be experienced as the dye is injected. A rapid pulse or a few "skipped beats" are also common during the procedure.

After the Procedure

☑ Provide routine postoperative care (see Chapter 10).

☑ Monitor vital signs, distal pulses, color, movement, sensation, temperature, and capillary refill of affected extremity as ordered, usually every 15 minutes for the first hour, every 30 minutes the next hour, hourly for 8 hours, and then every 4 hours.

☑ Monitor cardiac rhythm continuously. Report dysrhythmias, ECG changes, or chest pain to the charge nurse or physician.

☑ Maintain position and activity limitations as ordered.

☑ Keep a pressure dressing in place over arterial access sites. Check frequently for bleeding (if the access site is in the groin, check for bleeding under the buttocks).

☑ Unless contraindicated, encourage liberal fluid consumption.

☑ Administer medications as ordered.

☑ Monitor intake, output, and laboratory values. Report abnormal values to the physician.

clinicalALERT

Although PCI procedures are common and generally very safe, complications such as myocardial infarction, bleeding, or formation of a hematoma where the catheter is inserted may occur. Closely monitor the patient for complaints of chest or extremity pain. Frequently check color, temperature, and pulses on the affected extremity. Keep pressure dressing in place as ordered, and check for evidence of bleeding (look in the groin and feel under the buttocks if the femoral artery was used for access). Immediately report pain, changes in vital signs or extremity perfusion, or evidence of excessive bleeding to the physician.

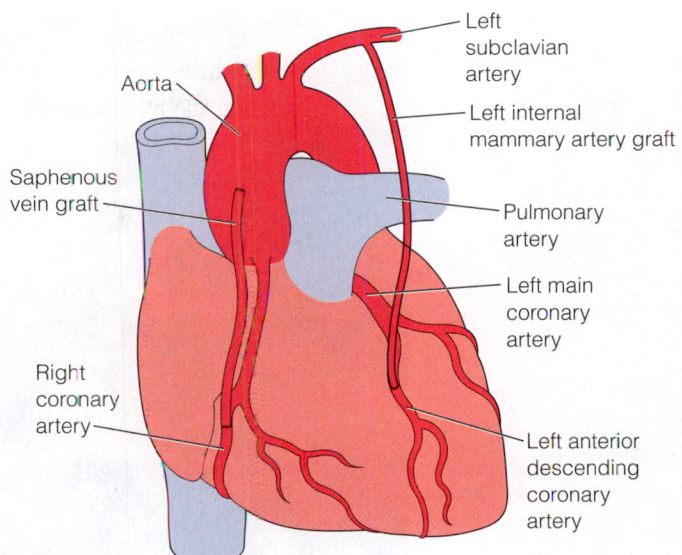

Figure 16-4. ■ Coronary artery bypass graft (CABG) using the internal mammary artery and a saphenous vein graft.

In a *coronary artery bypass graft (CABG)*, a vein or an arterial graft is used to "bypass," or bridge, the coronary artery obstruction and provide blood to the ischemic portion of the heart. The internal mammary artery (IMA) in the chest and the greater saphenous vein from the leg are the most popular vessels used for cardiac bypass grafts. The distal end of the IMA is sutured to the coronary artery distal to the obstruction (Figure 16-4 ■). When the saphenous vein is used, it is removed from the leg, reversed so that its valves do not interfere with blood flow, then grafted to the aorta and the coronary artery, distal to the occlusion. This provides a bridge for blood flow past the obstruction.

Although CABG is a relatively safe procedure, the heart is usually stopped during surgery to make it easier to work on. The *cardiopulmonary bypass pump* is used to maintain blood flow to the rest of the organs during surgery (Figures 16-5 ■ and 16-6 ■). The body temperature is lowered during surgery. Once the procedure has been completed, cardiopulmonary bypass is discontinued and the patient is rewarmed. Nursing care for the patient having cardiac surgery is outlined in Box 16-5 ■.

Minimally invasive coronary artery surgery uses several small incisions to access the affected coronary arteries. Another revascularization procedure, *transmyocardial laser revascularization*, uses a laser to drill tiny holes into the myocardial muscle itself to provide blood to ischemic muscle.

NURSING CARE

Nursing care for the patient with ACS is similar to that provided for patients with acute angina pectoris or myocardial infarction.

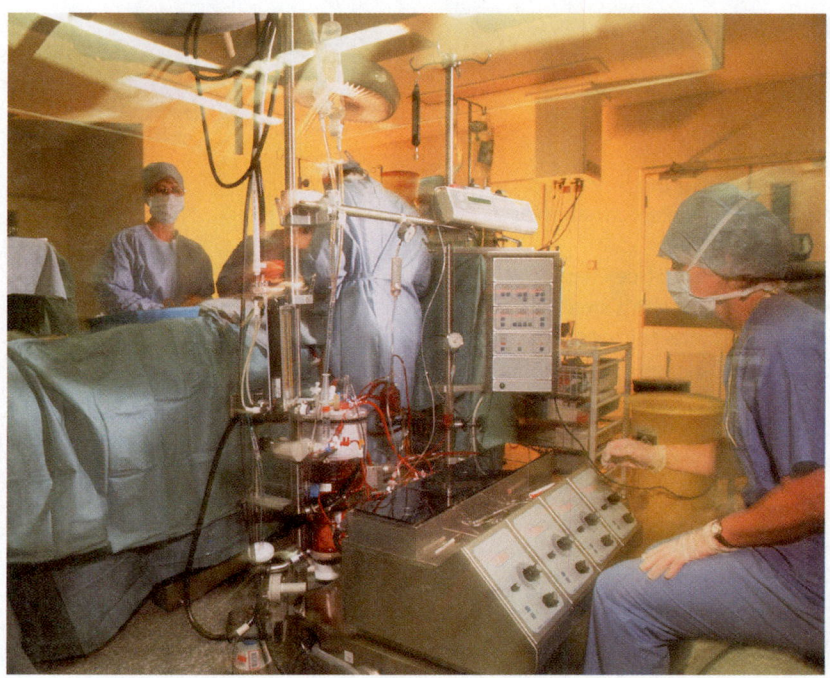

Figure 16-5. ■ Open heart surgery. The cardiopulmonary bypass pump that maintains circulation during the procedure is seen in the foreground. (Source: Deep Light Productions/Science Source)

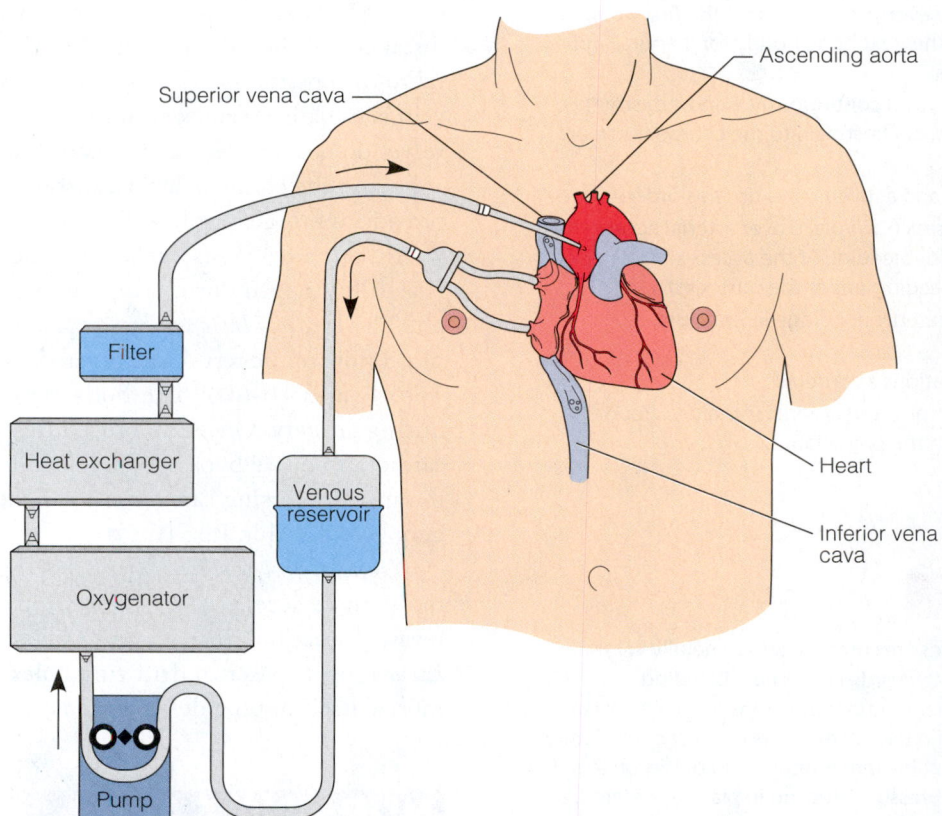

Figure 16-6. ■ A diagram of a cardiopulmonary bypass pump. Venous blood is removed from the vena cava, pumped through the oxygenator, and returned to the body via the ascending aorta.

BOX 16-5   NURSING CARE CHECKLIST

Cardiac Surgery

Before Surgery

☑ Provide preoperative care as ordered or per protocol.

☑ Teach the patient and family what to expect after surgery, including

  ☑ Returning to the cardiac recovery unit

  ☑ Tubes, drains, and general appearance

  ☑ Monitoring equipment (cardiac monitor, hemodynamic monitoring) and alarms

  ☑ Respiratory support (ventilator, endotracheal tube, suctioning, communication while intubated) and exercises

  ☑ Incisions and dressings

  ☑ Activity and diet progression

After Surgery

☑ Provide postoperative care as ordered and per protocol.

☑ Monitor vital signs including temperature, oxygen saturation, and hemodynamic measurements every 15 minutes until stable, then hourly. Report significant changes to the physician.

☑ Assess heart sounds and respiratory status at least every 1 to 4 hours. Monitor arterial blood gas (ABG) results. Report changes.

☑ Assess skin color and temperature, peripheral pulses, and level of consciousness with vital signs. Report changes.

☑ Monitor cardiac rhythm continuously; document rhythm every shift. Document and report any changes as they occur.

☑ Record intake and output hourly. Report urine output of less than 30 mL/hr for 2 consecutive hours.

☑ Record chest tube output hourly. Monitor hemoglobin and hematocrit values. Report excessive blood loss or falling values to the surgeon immediately.

☑ Institute rewarming as needed (per orders or if temperature is below 96.8°F or 36°C), using warmed intravenous fluids or transfusions, warmed blankets, and other prescribed measures.

☑ Manage analgesia (PCA or by schedule) as ordered. Document effectiveness. Report anginal pain immediately to the physician.

☑ Note endotracheal tube (ETT) placement on chest x-ray; secure it in place. Insert an oral airway as needed to prevent biting and obstruction of the ETT.

☑ Maintain ventilator settings as ordered. Suction as needed. Hyperoxygenate before and after suctioning.

☑ After extubation, teach and assist with use of the incentive spirometer. Assist the patient to splint the chest incision when coughing.

☑ Maintain a sterile dressing for the first 48 hours, then leave the incision open to the air. Use Steri-Strips as needed to maintain wound approximation.

☑ Monitor serum electrolytes and other lab values; report significant changes.

☑ Encourage the patient and family to participate in care and decision making.

PRIORITIZING NURSING CARE

The priorities of nursing care for the patient with ACS are restoring blood flow and oxygenation of the heart muscle, assessing for and preventing complications of treatment, and teaching to prevent future episodes of ACS or an acute myocardial infarction.

HEALTH PROMOTION

Health promotion activities related to ACS are those identified to prevent or slow the progression of CHD. This includes reducing or eliminating those risk factors that can be controlled, managing diabetes and high blood pressure, and managing angina. See the previous sections of this chapter on CHD and angina for specific health promotion activities.

ASSESSING

Nursing assessment of the patient with ACS focuses on the onset, duration, and character of chest pain, including its location, radiation, and intensity. Ask about measures undertaken to relieve the pain and their effect. Inquire about associated symptoms, such as nausea, shortness of

breath, or light-headedness. Ask about previous episodes and their treatment, as well as current medications.

Obtain vital signs, including apical pulse and peripheral pulses. Assess skin color, temperature, and moisture. Assess level of anxiety and fear.

IDENTIFYING POTENTIAL COMPLICATIONS

Cardiac dysrhythmias, including sudden cardiac death, are potential complications of ACS. Place the patient on a cardiac monitor for continuous monitoring of heart rhythm. Immediately report and treat abnormal rhythms that affect or potentially can affect hemodynamic status. See the section of this chapter on dysrhythmias for more information about identifying and treating abnormal heart rhythms.

DIAGNOSING, PLANNING, AND IMPLEMENTING

Risk for Acute Pain

Expected outcome: Will experience no further episodes of chest pain.

■ Institute continuous cardiac rhythm monitoring, noting and promptly reporting dysrhythmias. *Myocardial ischemia may affect the conduction system of the heart, resulting in abnormal heart rhythms. A very rapid or irregular rhythm can significantly reduce cardiac output and tissue perfusion unless promptly detected and treated.*

■ Administer nitrates and antiplatelet drugs as ordered. *These drugs are given to improve myocardial perfusion by dilating coronary arteries and inhibiting clot formation.*

■ Monitor for and promptly report complaints of chest pain. Place the patient on bed rest and immediately notify the physician of new complaints of chest pain or pain that is unrelieved with oxygen and medications. *The patient with ACS is at significant risk of acute myocardial infarction. Prompt treatment can limit the extent of heart muscle damage associated with myocardial infarction.*

Risk for Bleeding

Expected outcome: Will remain free of evidence of hemorrhage (vital signs and level of consciousness remain stable; chest tube drainage is within expected limits; no overt bleeding, unusual bruising, or complaints of pain in abdomen or joints).

The patient who has received an antiplatelet drug or an anticoagulant such as heparin is at risk for bleeding. Bleeding may also occur after PCI or CABG procedures.

■ Frequently monitor vital signs and urine output. Report increasing pulse rate, a drop in blood pressure, and/or urine output less than 30 mL/hr. *Tachycardia is an early sign of hypovolemia, as is a fall in urine output. A drop in blood pressure is a later sign of hypovolemia due to bleeding.*

■ As indicated, frequently assess catheter insertion site, incision, or chest tube drainage for evidence of bleeding. Promptly report signs of excessive bleeding. *The patient who has undergone a coronary revascularization procedure, whether surgical or nonsurgical, is at risk for bleeding due to administration of anticoagulant or antiplatelet drugs and disruption of high-pressure arterial vessels.*

■ Monitor skin and mucous membranes for bruising, petechiae, or bleeding. Note the color of urine, stool, and vomitus, and check for occult bleeding as indicated. Promptly report complaints of abdominal pain or changes in neurologic status. *Bleeding may be obvious, evidenced by bruising or overt bleeding from tissues such as mucous membranes, or may be occult. Occult (hidden) bleeding may be detected by the presence of petechiae on skin or mucous membranes, or changes in the color of urine or stool (rust-colored urine or black, tarry stool). Abdominal pain or changes in mental status may indicate internal bleeding into the abdomen or cranial vault.*

■ Protect the patient from injury as indicated. Keep pathways clear, place commonly used objects within reach, and instruct to use an electric shaver instead of a razor. *The patient who is confused or who has sensory impairments such as poor vision may need additional protective measures to prevent injury and bleeding.*

MANAGING NURSING CARE

Nursing care activities such as obtaining vital signs once stable; assisting with hygiene, toileting, and activities as allowed; and measuring oral intake and urinary output for the patient with ACS are appropriate to assign to assistive personnel.

EVALUATING

Assess the patient for relief of chest pain, vital signs within usual ranges, warm and dry skin with good color, and freedom from evidence of complications such as bleeding to evaluate the effectiveness of nursing care.

DOCUMENTING

Document assessment data, nursing care provided, and interdisciplinary treatment measures instituted for the patient with ACS. Document teaching and the patient's and family's response and apparent understanding of information provided and recommended follow-up treatment.

CONTINUITY OF CARE

Teaching to slow the progression of coronary artery disease and prevent future episodes of ACS or development of acute myocardial infarction is the primary focus of continuing care for the patient with ACS. Provide information about and make referrals as appropriate to help the patient manage or reduce risk factors such as smoking, obesity, high blood pressure or diabetes, and inactivity. Refer the patient to a cardiac rehabilitation program for assistance with developing a structured exercise program that is medically supervised.

When cardiac surgery is anticipated, provide general preoperative teaching, as well as specifics related to the planned surgery. Reinforce instructions about respiratory care, activity, and pain management. Reinforce the importance of being an active participant in rehabilitation. Before discharge, teach about ordered medications, the manifestations of an infection, pain management, diet, and activity. Discuss post-hospital cardiac rehabilitation.

See the Clinical Reasoning Care Map at the end of this chapter for an opportunity to apply what you have learned about caring for a patient undergoing cardiac surgery.

Acute Myocardial Infarction

Key Concept Acute myocardial infarction is a medical emergency, requiring prompt intervention to prevent necrosis of cardiac muscle. Timely interventions to restore blood flow to the affected muscle can preserve tissue and heart function.

In an **acute myocardial infarction** (AMI), cells in an area of cardiac muscle *infarct* or *necrose* (die) due to lack of blood and oxygen. It is a life-threatening event: If circulation to the affected cardiac muscle is not restored rapidly, functional muscle is lost and the heart may be unable to maintain an effective cardiac output. This can lead to cardiogenic shock and death. Most deaths from AMI occur within the first hour after the onset of manifestations, often before the patient reaches the hospital.

More than 1 million Americans experience an AMI annually, of which approximately a third are fatal. AMI rarely occurs in patients without preexisting CHD. Although no specific cause has been identified, the risk factors for AMI are those for CHD: age, gender, heredity, smoking, obesity, hyperlipidemia, hypertension, diabetes, stress, and sedentary lifestyle.

PATHOPHYSIOLOGY

AMI occurs when a coronary artery is totally occluded, blocking blood flow to a portion of cardiac muscle for a prolonged period of time. Occlusion is usually caused by ulceration or rupture of atherosclerotic plaque, leading to vessel constriction and development of a *thrombus* (clot) in that area. The occlusion blocks blood flow to myocardium distal to the obstruction.

When the cells are deprived of oxygen and nutrients for more than 20 to 45 minutes, they are irreversibly damaged, leading to cellular death and tissue necrosis. Intracellular enzymes are released as cells die. This necrotic tissue (*infarct*) is surrounded by an area of injured and ischemic tissues. These injured cells often contract ineffectively. Because of this, cardiac output falls.

If blood flow is restored, the injured and ischemic tissue recovers and heals. The infarcted tissue, however, no longer conducts electrical energy and ceases to contract. Collateral vessels connected to the smaller arteries in the coronary system dilate to maintain blood flow to the cardiac muscle when a larger coronary artery is occluded. In patients who remain active, collateral vessels develop and enlarge to meet the demand for blood flow as larger coronary arteries progressively narrow. Good collateral circulation can reduce the size of an infarction.

Myocardial infarction usually affects the left ventricle because it is the major "workhorse" of the heart; its muscle mass is greater, as are its oxygen demands.

AMIs are described according to the area of the heart that is damaged. Occlusion of the left anterior descending (LAD) artery damages the *anterior* portion of the left ventricle; occlusion of the left circumflex artery (LCA) causes *lateral* damage. *Right ventricular, inferior,* and *posterior* AMIs involve occlusions of the right coronary artery (RCA) and posterior descending artery (PDA). (See Figure 15-4.)

AMIs may also be classified as either transmural or subendocardial. A *transmural* infarction affects all layers of the heart (the endocardium, myocardium, and epicardium). A *subendocardial* infarction involves only the inner layer of the heart and does not extend through the myocardium and epicardium.

MANIFESTATIONS

Pain is a classic manifestation of AMI. Chest pain is often described as crushing and severe; the patient may call it a pressure, heavy, or squeezing sensation, or complain of chest tightness or burning. The pain begins in the center of the chest (in the substernal region) and may radiate to the shoulders, neck, jaw, or arms. It lasts more than 15 to 20 minutes and is not relieved by rest or NTG. The patient often experiences a sense of impending doom and death. Typical signs and symptoms of AMI are listed in Box 16-6■.

Women and older adults may not have the "typical" manifestations of AMI, increasing the risk that they will not seek treatment. As with men, the most common symptom of AMI in women is chest pain or discomfort. Upper abdominal pain may also occur. Women and older adults may experience other common manifestations of AMI without chest pain, particularly fatigue, shortness of breath, nausea/vomiting, and back or jaw pain. Box 16-7■ focuses on AMI in women and older adults.

Cocaine-Induced Myocardial Infarction

In recent years, AMI associated with cocaine intoxication has been reported. Cocaine stimulates the heart rate, increases its contractility, and causes vasoconstriction and hypertension. As a result, the workload of the heart increases. Cocaine also increases the risk of dysrhythmias. The patient with cocaine-induced MI may have an altered level of consciousness, confusion and restlessness, seizure activity, tachycardia, hypotension, increased respiratory rate, and respiratory crackles.

COMPLICATIONS

The risk of complications associated with MI is related to the size and location of infarcted tissue.

BOX 16-6	MANIFESTATIONS OF ACUTE MYOCARDIAL INFARCTION

- Chest pain: substernal or precordial; may radiate to neck, shoulder, or arm
- Tachycardia
- Shortness of breath, dyspnea
- Cool, clammy skin
- Diaphoresis
- Anxiety
- Feeling of impending doom
- Nausea and vomiting
- Possible dysrhythmias

Dysrhythmias

Dysrhythmias, disruptions of the electrical conduction system of the heart and/or its rhythm, are the most frequent complication. Sinus tachycardia (heart rate greater than 100 beats/min) is common. The heart rate may slow sufficiently due to bradycardia or heart blocks to produce symptoms such as shortness of breath, dizziness, and altered mental status. Premature atrial contractions (PACs) and atrial fibrillation may occur. Premature ventricular contractions (PVCs) are common, particularly in the first few hours after an AMI. Frequent PVCs (more than six per minute), couplets, short bursts of ventricular tachycardia, and early PVCs (R on T wave) are treated with drugs to reduce the risk of ventricular fibrillation (V-fib). The risk of V-fib is greatest the first hour after AMI; it is a frequent cause of sudden cardiac death associated with AMI. (See the section later in this chapter on dysrhythmias and Table 16-8 on page 391 for more information about dysrhythmias.)

Pump Failure

AMI reduces myocardial contractility and ventricular filling. Heart failure may develop, particularly when large portions of the left ventricle are affected. With loss of 20% to 25% of the left ventricular muscle, the patient may develop manifestations of left-sided heart failure, including dyspnea, fatigue, weakness, and respiratory crackles on auscultation.

If more than 40% of the left ventricle is infarcted, **cardiogenic shock**, impaired tissue perfusion due to pump failure, results. The patient is hypotensive and has signs of impaired tissue perfusion, such as low urinary output, decreased level of consciousness, and cool, clammy skin. Perfusion of the heart muscle itself is also affected, further increasing tissue damage.

Other Complications

Pericarditis (inflammation of the pericardium) may develop after an AMI, usually within 2 to 3 days. Chest pain associated with pericarditis is sharp and stabbing, aggravated by movement or deep breathing. A pericardial friction rub may be noted on auscultation of heart sounds.

Approximately 10% of patients experience *extension* or *expansion* of the MI within 10 to 14 days. The patient may have continuing chest pain, unstable vital signs, or worsening heart failure. Because the scar tissue that replaces necrotic muscle is thinner than the ventricular muscle mass, a *left ventricular aneurysm* may develop or rupture may occur. A ventricular aneurysm is an outpouching of the ventricular wall. Ventricular aneurysm is more likely to affect the left ventricle (because of its significantly greater workload) than the right. *Myocardial rupture* is often fatal and may occur between days 4 and 7 after an AMI, when the injured tissue is soft and weak.

COLLABORATIVE CARE

Rapid assessment and early diagnosis and treatment are vital in an MI. "Time is muscle"—the quicker the artery is reopened (medically or surgically) and blood flow restored, the more myocardium can be saved and fewer complications develop. The AHA recommends definitive treatment be initiated within 1 hour of arrival at the emergency center. Every patient is immediately evaluated for reperfusion therapy using either percutaneous coronary intervention or fibrinolysis.

The major problem is delay in seeking medical care after the onset of chest pain or other cardiac symptoms. Nearly half of patients with symptoms of MI wait more than 4 hours before seeking treatment.

Diagnostic Tests

The principal laboratory tests ordered when an MI is suspected are *serum cardiac markers*. Serum levels of cardiac markers are ordered on admission and at specific intervals thereafter. Serial blood levels are used to establish the diagnosis and to evaluate the extent of myocardial damage. Serum levels of cardiac-specific troponins (cT_nT and cT_n1) are most specific for diagnosis of AMI. These proteins released from necrotic heart muscle are found in the blood within 1 to 3 hours after the onset of symptoms and remain in the blood for 7 to 10 days, so they can help diagnose AMI even when treatment is delayed by several days. Serum creatine phosphokinase (CK) levels rise rapidly after AMI and remain detectable for up to 72 hours. The peak CK level indicates the size of the AMI: The greater the amount of infarcted tissue, the higher the CK level. The CK-MB isoenzyme is a more sensitive indicator of AMI than CK (Table 16-7■).

Electrocardiography, echocardiography, and myocardial nuclear scans are the most common diagnostic tests performed for a suspected AMI. Ischemic or necrotic cardiac cells do not respond normally to electrical stimulation, altering ECG waveforms (Figure 16-7■). The location of myocardial damage can be identified on the 12-lead ECG. ST segment elevation is commonly seen during the acute phase of an MI, although not all patients having an MI develop this characteristic ECG pattern, leading physicians to classify MIs as either ST elevation MI (STEMI) or non-ST elevation MI (NSTEMI). A Q wave may also develop on the ECG tracing.

Echocardiography is used to diagnose AMI and its effect on ventricular function as well as complications such as

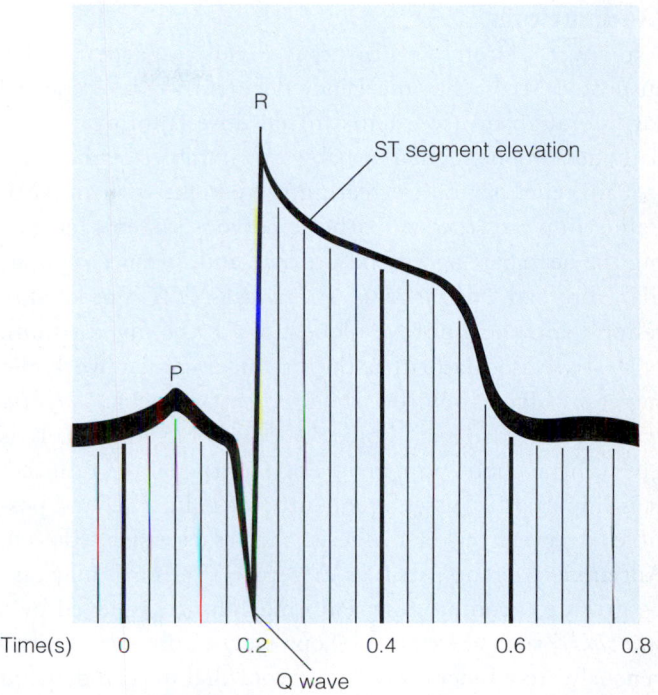

Figure 16-7. ■ ECG changes noted with acute myocardial infarction. Note the deep Q wave and significant elevation of the ST segment, characteristic of AMI.

ventricular aneurysm. *Myocardial perfusion imaging scans* may be done to localize an AMI and evaluate the extent of the infarction.

Medical Management

The focus of medical management for the patient with AMI is on restoring blood flow to the heart muscle, reducing the workload of the heart, and preventing or promptly treating complications. The patient is monitored continuously from entry into the medical system. Care is provided in the intensive coronary care unit (CCU) for the first 24 hours, after which less intensive monitoring (e.g., telemetry) may be appropriate. An intravenous line is established to allow rapid administration of emergency drugs. Oxygen may be administered by nasal cannula at 2 to 6 L/min to improve oxygenation of the myocardium and other tissues.

Bed rest with bedside commode is ordered initially to reduce the cardiac workload. After 12 to 24 hours, activities are gradually increased. A quiet, calm environment with limited outside stimuli, such as television and telephone, is preferred. Visitors are limited to supportive close family members for short periods of time. After an initial period of fasting or clear liquids only to reduce the risk of vomiting, a low-fat, low-cholesterol, reduced-sodium diet is allowed. Small, frequent feedings are often recommended, and foods high in potassium, magnesium, and fiber are encouraged.

TABLE 16-7	Cardiac Marker Changes in Acute Myocardial Infarction		
	CHANGES OCCURRING IN AN MI		
MARKER	**APPEARS**	**PEAKS**	**DURATION**
Creatine phosphokinase (CK or CPK)	4–6 hours	18–24 hours	24–72 hours
CK M-bands (CK-MB)	4–6 hours	18–24 hours	72 hours
Cardiac-specific Troponin T (cT_nT)	1–3 hours	24–36 hours	10–14 days
Cardiac-specific Troponin 1 (cT_n1)	1–3 hours	24–36 hours	5–9 days

Medications

Aspirin, a platelet inhibitor, is given to patients with suspected MI in the emergency department. It is chewed for buccal absorption. This initial dose is followed by a daily dose of one regular or baby aspirin tablet by mouth.

Pain relief is vital in treating the patient with an AMI. Pain stimulates the sympathetic nervous system, increasing the heart rate and blood pressure and, in turn, myocardial workload. *Sublingual* or *intravenous NTG* is ordered to relieve pain and improve blood flow to the myocardium. NTG is a vasodilator that both reduces cardiac work and increases blood flow to ischemic heart muscle. *Morphine sulfate* is the drug of choice for pain and sedation. It is given intravenously in small doses until pain is relieved. It is important to assess frequently for pain relief and possible adverse effects of analgesia, such as excessive sedation. Antianxiety agents, such as diazepam (Valium), may also be given to promote rest. Pain may also be relieved by a *beta blocker* such as *metoprolol* (Lopressor) administered intravenously. Beta blockers reduce myocardial oxygen demand and, more importantly, reduce the risks of reinfarction and dysrhythmias (Longo et al., 2012).

Fibrinolytic agents, drugs that dissolve or break up blood clots, may be used to treat AMI. These drugs activate the *fibrinolytic (fibrin* = a key component of blood clots; *lysis* = break down or destroy) system to destroy the clot, restoring blood flow through the obstructed artery. When given within the first 6 hours of MI symptoms, fibrinolytics limit infarct size, reduce heart damage, and improve the chances of survival. These drugs can also cause multiple complications; up to 5% of patients receiving them experience serious bleeding. Fibrinolytic therapy is contraindicated in patients with known bleeding disorders, history of stroke, uncontrolled hypertension, pregnancy, or recent trauma or surgery. Nursing care of the patient receiving fibrinolytic agents is outlined in Box 16-8■.

In addition to antiplatelet drugs such as aspirin or clopidogrel (Plavix), heparin, an anticoagulant, may also be prescribed during immediate treatment after an MI to prevent further clot development. Antidysrhythmic medications are used as needed to treat or prevent dysrhythmias. Angiotensin-converting enzyme (ACE) inhibitors may also be ordered. These drugs reduce ventricular remodeling after AMI, reducing the risk of heart failure.

Revascularization

For many patients, an immediate or early revascularization intervention (PCI) such as stent placement is performed to restore blood flow to the infarcted section of heart muscle. In some cases, surgery may be performed. These procedures and related nursing care are covered in more depth in the preceding section on ACS.

BOX 16-8   NURSING CARE CHECKLIST

Fibrinolytic Therapy

Before the Infusion

☑ Obtain a focused assessment, including subjective and objective assessment data.

☑ Ask about possible contraindications to fibrinolytic therapy: duration of symptoms, recent surgery or trauma (including prolonged CPR), bleeding disorders or any active bleeding, stroke, peptic ulcer disease, diabetic retinopathy, and uncontrolled hypertension.

☑ Reinforce teaching about the purpose of therapy, bleeding risk, and the need to remain still during and after the infusion.

☑ Initiate at least two intravenous infusion sites as ordered or per facility protocol.

During the Infusion

☑ Assess vital signs, peripheral pulses, and the infusion site every 15 minutes for the first hour, every 30 minutes for the next 2 hours, and then hourly until the intravenous catheter is discontinued. Record all data.

☑ Remind the patient to keep the extremity still and straight.

☑ Maintain continuous cardiac monitoring. Keep antidysrhythmic medications and the emergency cart readily available.

☑ Frequently assess neurologic status. Immediately report changes such as onset of a neurologic deficit, change in level of consciousness, headache, nausea, or vomiting.

After the Infusion

☑ Frequently assess vital signs, distal pulses, and infusion site for bleeding.

☑ Maintain bed rest for 6 hours. Reinforce the need to keep the extremity straight and immobile. Avoid injections for 24 hours after catheter removal.

☑ Assess puncture sites for bleeding. When the intravenous catheter is removed, hold direct pressure over the site for at least 30 minutes. Apply pressure dressings to venous or arterial punctures if needed. Perform routine care in a gentle manner to avoid undue bruising or injury.

☑ Assess body fluids, including urine, vomitus, and feces, for evidence of bleeding. Regularly monitor level of consciousness and neurologic function. Assess surgical sites for bleeding. Monitor hemoglobin and hematocrit levels. Report any bleeding or changes in neurologic status to the physician.

☑ Report manifestations of reocclusion, including ECG changes, chest pain, or dysrhythmias.

Other Invasive Procedures

Patients with large AMIs and pump failure may require invasive devices to temporarily take over the function of the heart, allowing the injured myocardium to heal. The

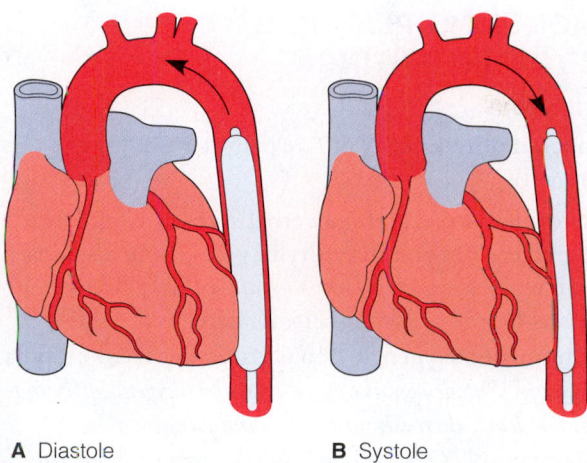

A Diastole   **B** Systole

Figure 16-8. ■ The intra-aortic balloon pump. (**A**) The balloon inflates during diastole to help perfuse coronary, renal, and cerebral arteries. (**B**) During systole, the balloon is deflated, allowing blood to flow past it freely.

intra-aortic balloon pump (IABP) temporarily supports cardiac function by decreasing myocardial workload and oxygen demand and increasing coronary artery perfusion. The balloon inflates during diastole, increasing perfusion of the coronary and renal arteries, and deflates just before and during systole, allowing blood to flow past it (Figure 16-8 ■). The inflation–deflation series is triggered by the ECG pattern. As the heart muscle recovers, IABP is gradually decreased, until the patient no longer requires mechanical assistance.

Ventricular assist devices (VADs) can temporarily take partial or complete control of cardiac function. VADs may be used for patients with AMI and cardiogenic shock, after surgery requiring cardiopulmonary bypass, or while awaiting heart transplant.

Cardiac Rehabilitation

Cardiac rehabilitation is a planned program of activity and exercises, psychologic support, and education for patients who have had an MI. The goal of cardiac rehabilitation is to improve quality of life by reducing risk factors for heart disease. It begins with admission to the hospital. This is followed by a supervised outpatient program focused on education and supervised activity. The final phase of cardiac rehabilitation is a lifetime maintenance program of minimally supervised (or even unsupervised) physical fitness and risk factor reduction.

An interdisciplinary team works with the patient in cardiac rehabilitation to

■ Assess previous activity and exercise habits.
■ Gradually increase activity and exercise in a planned manner.

■ Evaluate and monitor the patient's responses to increasing activity levels.
■ Teach the patient to monitor his or her tolerance of activity.

The initial assessment and teaching may be done while the patient is in the hospital. Activity is gradually increased as tolerated. Subjective complaints of fatigue, shortness of breath, chest pain, and dizziness are used to evaluate the patient's ability to tolerate increased activity, as are objective data including vital signs and ECG changes. The outpatient phase of the program begins after discharge. Teaching emphasizes risk factor reduction and progressive, regular exercise. Issues such as returning to work and resumption of sexual activity are discussed during this phase. Most patients can resume sexual activity within 2 weeks and return to work within 2 to 4 weeks after discharge. The final, maintenance phase of cardiac rehabilitation may be indefinite, continuing for the remainder of the patient's lifetime.

NURSING CARE

PRIORITIZING NURSING CARE

Reducing the workload of the heart to protect injured muscle cells from further damage is a priority of care for the patient with AMI. Pain stimulates the sympathetic nervous system, increasing the heart rate and its contractility—and, consequently, its workload. Eliminating pain and maintaining cardiac output and tissue perfusion are of highest priority in caring for patients with AMI.

HEALTH PROMOTION

Health promotion activities to prevent AMI include risk factor management, promoting healthy lifestyles, and management of diabetes, hypercholesterolemia, obesity, and high blood pressure. Teaching about the importance of promptly seeking medical care for chest pain and other manifestations of AMI is vital to limit the damage of AMI and preserve heart function. For the patient who has experienced an AMI, provide information about cardiac rehabilitation to reduce the risk for complications or future MI.

ASSESSING

The patient who experiences an AMI requires immediate and ongoing focused assessment. Initially, assessments may be done hourly or more frequently as necessary. Once stable, the patient is assessed every 4 hours and when condition changes are noted. Uninterrupted rest periods are important, however, so data are collected when the patient is awake or in conjunction with other procedures. The ECG is continuously monitored, and laboratory results (cardiac markers in particular) are reported to the physician.

Obtain focused subjective assessment data from the patient or significant others as appropriate, including

■ Pain: onset, location, character (heavy, burning, tight, squeezing); intensity (rate on a standardized pain scale); radiation (arms, shoulders, neck, jaw); timing (intermittent or continuous); duration; aggravating and relieving factors; associated manifestations (shortness of breath, nausea, apprehension)

■ Effectiveness of pain relief measures (oxygen, NTG, analgesia, rest)

■ History of angina or other heart disease, previous or current treatment measures

■ Risk factors: family history of CHD; history of hypertension, diabetes, high blood cholesterol levels; smoking and alcohol intake, use of other recreational drugs; activity just before or at onset of pain

■ Expressions of denial or disbelief; acceptance of activity restrictions; readiness for learning and activity progression

Objective data for the patient experiencing AMI include

■ Vital signs; BP, pulse and respiratory rate; changes with activity and during episodes of chest pain

■ Heart and lung sounds; dyspnea and its relationship to activity

■ Skin color, temperature, and moisture; capillary refill; oxygen saturation levels; urinary output

■ Level of consciousness; anxiety or fear

■ Cardiac rhythm; any abnormal rhythms or waveforms and ECG changes that occur during chest pain

■ Hemodynamic pressure measurements, including pulmonary artery pressure, or cardiac output as ordered

■ Laboratory data: cardiac enzyme levels

IDENTIFYING POTENTIAL COMPLICATIONS

The patient with AMI is at risk for a number of complications. Dysrhythmias are the most common complication. Continuously monitor heart rhythm, reporting significant dysrhythmias. See the dysrhythmia section that follows.

Report and document new complaints of chest pain after relief of initial manifestations. Recurrent chest pain may indicate extension of the infarct or reinfarction. Also report changes in the nature of the patient's chest pain, for example, pain that changes in intensity with deep breathing or movement, which may indicate development of pericarditis.

Altered blood flow through the heart and bed rest place the patient at risk for development of a thrombus and resulting neurologic or pulmonary vascular effects. Report a change in neurologic status, complaints of calf pain, or sudden onset of dyspnea, chest pain, and anxiety.

Rupture of the ventricular wall or septum is a potentially lethal complication, often heralded by sudden cardiac death or a sudden deterioration of hemodynamic status with hypotension, heart failure, and development of a new heart murmur.

DIAGNOSING, PLANNING, AND IMPLEMENTING

Acute Pain

Expected outcome: Will rate pain at a 2 or lower on a scale of 0 to 10.

■ Assess for verbal and nonverbal signs of pain. Document characteristics and intensity of pain, using a standard pain scale. *Frequent monitoring allows early intervention and reduces the risk of further tissue damage.*

■ Administer oxygen at 2 to 6 L/min per nasal cannula as ordered. *Supplemental oxygen increases oxygen supply to the myocardium, decreasing ischemia and pain.*

■ Maintain NTG as ordered. *NTG, a vasodilator, reduces the workload of the heart and improves coronary blood flow to the ischemic myocardium.*

■ Provide for physical and psychologic rest. Provide information and emotional support. *Rest decreases cardiac workload and sympathetic nervous system stimulation. Information and emotional support help reduce anxiety and promote psychologic rest.*

■ Administer 2 to 4 mg morphine by intravenous push for chest pain as ordered. *Morphine decreases pain and anxiety and reduces the workload of the heart.*

■ Reassess for relief of chest pain. Report continued pain to the charge nurse or physician. *The goal of pain management in an MI patient is complete relief of pain.*

Decreased Cardiac Output

Expected outcome: Vital signs and cardiovascular assessment data will remain stable within normal range for patient.

■ Report increased heart rate and changes in heart rhythm, blood pressure, and respiratory rate to the charge nurse or physician. *Damage to the heart muscle affects the pumping ability of the ventricles. The heart rate increases when cardiac output falls, increasing the workload of the heart.*

■ Report changes in level of consciousness; decreased urine output; moist, cool, pale, mottled, or cyanotic skin; dusky or cyanotic mucous membranes and nail beds; diminished-to-absent peripheral pulses; or delayed capillary refill. *These are manifestations of decreased tissue perfusion. A change in level of consciousness is often the first manifestation of altered perfusion because brain tissue and cerebral function depend on a continuous supply of oxygen.*

■ Auscultate heart and breath sounds. Note and report abnormal heart sounds (e.g., an S_3 or S_4 gallop or a murmur) or adventitious lung sounds. *Abnormal heart or lung sounds may indicate impaired cardiac function.*

■ Monitor ECG rhythm continuously. Report dysrhythmias. *Dysrhythmias can further impair cardiac output and tissue perfusion.*

■ Administer antidysrhythmic medications as needed. *Dysrhythmias affect tissue perfusion by altering cardiac output.*

clinicalALERT

Dysrhythmias are the most frequent complication after AMI, often developing within the first 24 hours. Prompt recognition and treatment of dysrhythmias is vital; however, remember to treat the patient, not the machine (in this care, the heart monitor). Assess the patient's response to the dysrhythmia before initiating treatment.

Ineffective Coping

Expected outcome: Will demonstrate effective coping, using appropriate behaviors to reduce stress.

- Establish an environment of caring and trust. Encourage the patient to express feelings. *A trusting nurse–patient relationship provides a safe environment for the patient to discuss feelings of helplessness, powerlessness, anxiety, and hopelessness.*
- Accept denial as a coping mechanism, but do not reinforce it. *Denial may initially help decrease anxiety, but, when prolonged, can interfere with acceptance of reality and cooperation, possibly delaying treatment and hindering recovery.*
- Note aggressive behaviors, hostility, or anger. Document any failure to comply with treatments. *These behaviors may indicate anxiety and denial.*
- Help identify positive coping skills used in the past (e.g., problem-solving skills, verbalization of feelings, asking for help, prayer). Reinforce positive coping behaviors. *Previously successful coping behaviors can help the patient deal with the current situation. These familiar methods can decrease feelings of powerlessness.*
- Allow the patient to make decisions about care, as possible. *Participating in care planning gives a sense of control and the opportunity to use positive coping skills.*
- Provide privacy for the patient and significant other to share their questions and concerns. *Privacy allows the patient and partner the opportunity to share their feelings and fears, offer support and encouragement to one another, relieve anxiety, and establish effective coping methods.*

Fear

Expected outcome: Will seek information to reduce fear.

- Acknowledge the patient's perception of the situation. Allow him or her to verbalize concerns. *The sudden change in health status brings on anxiety and fear of the unknown. Verbalizing these fears may help the patient cope with the changes and allow the health care team to provide information and correct misconceptions.*
- Encourage questions, and provide consistent, factual answers. Repeat information as needed. *Accurate and consistent information can reduce fear and help develop realistic expectations. Anxiety and fear decrease the ability to concentrate and retain information; information may need to be repeated.*

- Administer antianxiety medications as ordered. *These medications promote rest and relaxation and decrease feelings of anxiety, which may act as barriers to restoration of health.*
- Teach nonpharmacologic methods of stress reduction (e.g., relaxation methods, mental imagery, music therapy, breathing exercises, meditation, massage). *Stress management techniques may help reduce tension and anxiety, provide the patient with a sense of control, and enhance coping skills.*

MANAGING NURSING CARE

For the patient with AMI, nursing care activities such as assisting with hygiene, toileting, and activities as allowed, and measuring intake and output may be appropriate to assign to assistive personnel.

EVALUATING

To evaluate the effectiveness of nursing care for the patient with an MI, collect data such as the following:

- Pain level and relief with prescribed interventions
- Evidence of adequate tissue perfusion: level of consciousness, urine output, heart and lung sounds, skin color and temperature, peripheral pulses, ECG rhythm
- Acceptance of diagnosis, involvement in care, and participation in care planning
- Expressions or nonverbal evidence of fear and anxiety.

DOCUMENTING

Document the location, frequency, and intensity of pain and the patient's response to pain relief measures. Note level of anxiety. Record vital signs and assessment data, and note any changes that occur with activity. Document ECG rhythm per protocol and when any changes occur. Record any medications given to treat dysrhythmias or other complications of AMI and the response to treatment. Document all teaching with the patient's apparent understanding or acceptance of the information presented.

CONTINUITY OF CARE

Teaching and planning for continuing care in the home and community-based settings begin with admission to the CCU and continue through the hospital stay and after discharge into the rehabilitation period. The emphasis is on restoring optimal health and reducing the risk of future cardiac events.

Assessing readiness to learn is an important first step. The patient in strong denial may not believe that the information being taught has any relevance. Evaluate ability to learn, assessing knowledge base, physiologic and psychologic health, health beliefs, and expectations of the health care system.

Teach about CHD and MI. Explain the purpose of prescribed dietary changes and activity recommendations.

Discuss prescribed medications, including their purposes and side effects. Encourage the patient to ask questions. Reinforce teaching with written materials.

Provide referral to a cardiac rehabilitation program. Emphasize the importance of complying with the medical regimen and cardiac rehabilitation program and of keeping follow-up appointments. Provide telephone numbers of resource personnel who are available to respond to questions and concerns after the patient's discharge.

Provide information about community resources, such as the local chapter of the AHA. Encourage family members to learn CPR in the event of an emergency, and provide information about other community agencies that offer CPR classes.

NURSING CARE PLAN
Patient With Acute Myocardial Infarction

Betty Williams, 62 years old, is admitted to the emergency department complaining of severe substernal chest pain. She initially thought the pain was indigestion, but now describes it "like someone sitting on my chest." The pain radiates to her jaw and left arm, and is accompanied by a "choking feeling," severe shortness of breath, and diaphoresis. The pain is unrelieved by rest, antacids, or three sublingual NTG tablets (0.4 mg).

After administering an aspirin tablet, inserting an intravenous catheter, and beginning oxygen at 6 L/min per nasal cannula, a 12-lead ECG and cardiac troponins are obtained. Mrs. Williams's pain is relieved by intravenous NTG and morphine sulfate. Based on her ECG, an acute anterior wall MI is diagnosed. Intravenous alteplase (t-PA) is administered, followed by intravenous enoxaparin (Lovenox). Mrs. Williams is transferred to the CCU.

Assessment
Mrs. Williams's history includes type 2 diabetes, angina, and hypertension. She has smoked cigarettes for 45 years, averaging 1-1/2 to 2 packs per day. Her father died at age 42 of MI, and her paternal grandfather died at age 65 of MI. Mrs. Williams is currently taking pioglitazone (Actos) and metoprolol (Lopressor).

On admission to the CCU, Mrs. Williams is alert and oriented; P 118; BP 172/92; R 24; T 99.6°F (37.5°C). Auscultation reveals an S_4 and fine crackles in the bases of both lungs. The ECG shows sinus tachycardia with occasional PVCs. Her skin is cool and slightly diaphoretic. Capillary refill is less than 3 seconds, and peripheral pulses are strong and equal. Her nail beds are pink.

A triple-lumen central line is in place, with NTG and t-PA infusions controlled by infusion pumps. A solution of 5% dextrose in 1/4 normal saline solution is infusing in a peripheral intravenous line. Mrs. Williams states, "The pain is better, but it has been coming and going. I would rate it a 4 right now, but it was terrible before. The doctor told me that this drug I'm getting will quickly open up the artery that is blocked. I hope it works! Do many people get this drug?"

Nursing Diagnosis
The CCU nurses formulate the following nursing diagnoses (among others) for Mrs. Williams:

- *Acute Pain* related to cardiac muscle ischemia and infarct
- *Anxiety* related to change in health status
- *Risk for Bleeding* related to fibrinolytic therapy
- *Risk for Injury* related to altered cardiac rate and rhythm

Expected Outcomes
The expected outcomes of the plan of care specify that Mrs. Williams will

- Verbalize relief of chest pain
- Verbalize a reduced anxiety and fear
- Exhibit no signs of internal or external bleeding
- Maintain an adequate cardiac output

Planning and Implementation
The following interventions are planned and implemented:

- Instruct to report any chest pain. Titrate NTG infusion for chest pain; stop infusion if systolic BP drops below 100 mm Hg. Administer 2 to 4 mg morphine intravenously for chest pain unrelieved by NTG infusion.
- Encourage to express fears and concerns. Answer questions honestly, and correct any misconceptions about disease process, its treatment, or prognosis.
- Explain that the t-PA will dissolve the clot that is obstructing blood flow to the heart muscle, thus limiting heart damage.
- Explain the need for frequent assessment.
- Assess for evidence of internal or intracranial bleeding: back or abdominal pain, headache, decreased level of consciousness, dizziness, bloody secretions or excretions, or pallor. Test all stools, urine, and vomitus for occult blood. Notify physician immediately of any abnormal findings.
- Continuously monitor ECG.
- Immediately treat dysrhythmias or other cardiac emergencies per unit protocol.

Evaluation
Mrs. Williams's chest pain is relieved with the morphine, NTG infusion, and fibrinolytic therapy. She states that she feels "much better now that the pain is gone. I was afraid it would just get worse." No indication of bleeding problems

are noted, and while her PVCs increase with reperfusion therapy, she experiences no significant dysrhythmias. Mrs. Williams remains in CCU for 24 hours and is transferred to the progressive cardiac unit.

Critical Thinking in the Nursing Process

1. You are admitting Mrs. Williams to the progressive cardiac unit from CCU. What assessment data will you obtain? What nursing diagnoses and interventions will you anticipate as part of Mrs. Williams's care at this point in her recovery?

2. Two days after her initial therapy, Mrs. Williams complains of palpitations. You notice frequent PVCs on the ECG monitor. What do you do? How does this threaten Mrs. Williams's safety?

3. Mrs. Williams states, "I have been smoking for over 45 years, and I am not going to stop now! Besides, it calms me down when I am feeling anxious." How would you respond to this statement? What evidence can you use to guide your response and teaching?

Note: Discussion of Critical Thinking questions appears on the companion website.

CARDIAC RHYTHM DISORDERS

Cardiac Dysrhythmias

Key Concept   Most cardiac rhythm disruptions (dysrhythmias) are benign, having little effect on cardiovascular function; others are more serious and can affect cardiac output and tissue perfusion. Timely recognition and treatment of these rhythms is vital.

The heart contracts in response to electrical stimulation of its cells. In the normal heart, this produces a coordinated, rhythmic contraction that pushes blood into the circulation. The normal heart rhythm is *normal sinus rhythm (NSR)*. Impulses originate in the sinoatrial (SA or sinus) node and travel through normal conduction pathways without delay. The rate is between 60 and 100 beats per minute in adults. Changes from this rhythm can affect the heart's ability to pump blood effectively to body tissues.

A **cardiac dysrhythmia** (also frequently called *arrhythmia*) is a disturbance or irregularity in the electrical system of the heart. Cardiac dysrhythmias may be benign or life threatening. Changes in heart rhythm occur due to "normal" events, such as exercise or fear, as well as to pathologic changes. Any dysrhythmia can affect cardiac output. The effect of the dysrhythmia determines the need for treatment. Box 16-9■ lists steps for heart rhythm analysis.

PATHOPHYSIOLOGY

Dysrhythmias develop as a result of two mechanisms: altered formation of impulses or altered conduction of the impulse through the heart.

Abnormalities of impulse formation are caused by changes in *automaticity,* the ability of the heart to generate an electrical impulse and contraction without input from the nervous system. Impulses may develop more rapidly or more slowly than normal. Impulses also may originate outside the SA node. These are called *ectopic beats*.

BOX 16-9	ECG RHYTHM ANALYSIS

Interpreting an ECG strip is a skill that takes practice. Use a consistent, systematic method to determine the heart rhythm. A suggested sequence of steps follows:

1. *Determine rate.* Assess the heart rate using one of the following to determine number of beats per minute (beats/min):
   - Count the number of R waves in a 6-second strip and multiply by 10.
   - Count the number of large boxes between two consecutive R waves, and divide 300 (the number of large boxes in 1 minute) by this number. For example, there are six large boxes between two R waves; 300 ÷ 6 = 50 beats/min.
   - Memorize the following sequence: 300, 150, 100, 75, 60, 50. One large box between complexes equals a rate of 300, two = 150, three = 100, and so on.

2. *Determine regularity.* Measure the interval from one R wave to the next R wave, then evaluate successive R to R intervals for their regularity. Irregular rhythms may be *irregularly irregular* (if there is no pattern to the irregularity) or *regularly irregular* (if a consistent pattern can be identified).

3. *Assess P waves.* All the P waves should look alike in size and shape.

4. *Assess P to QRS relationship.* There should be one P wave before every QRS complex and one QRS complex after every P wave.

5. *Measure PR interval and QRS complex.* To determine the duration of any interval, count the number of small boxes from the beginning of the interval to the end and multiply by 0.04 second. The normal PR interval is 0.12 to 0.20 second; the normal QRS complex lasts 0.06 to 0.10 second.

6. *Identify abnormalities.* Note any ectopic (abnormal) beats, deviation of the ST segment above or below the baseline, and abnormalities in waveform shape and duration.

An impulse may be blocked or delayed as it moves through the conduction pathways of the heart. This is known as *heart block*. In some cases, an impulse is delayed in one area of the heart but conducted normally through the rest. This pattern of normal and slow conduction, known as *reentry phenomenon,* is responsible for many dysrhythmias.

Cardiac rhythms are classified according to the site of impulse formation or the site and degree of conduction block (Table 16-8■). In *supraventricular rhythms*, impulses form above the ventricles. *Ventricular rhythms* originate in the ventricles and may be fatal, depending on the heart rate and regularity. *AV conduction blocks* result from impaired impulse transmission from the atria to the ventricles. See Box 16-10■ for a discussion of dysrhythmias in older adults.

Supraventricular Rhythms

Supraventricular (*supra* = above or over) rhythms arise above the ventricles. They may originate in the sinus node, the atria, or within the atrioventricular (AV) node. Conduction of the impulse through the ventricles usually is unaffected, so the QRS complex appears normal.

BOX 16-10   FOCUS ON OLDER ADULTS

Dysrhythmias in Older Adults

Aging affects the heart and the cardiac conduction system, increasing the risk for dysrhythmias, even when no other evidence of heart disease is found. Older adults are more likely to experience ectopic beats during exercise. AV blocks are also more common in people over the age of 65.

Assessing dysrhythmias in older adults focuses on the effect on function.

■ Inquire about episodes of dizziness, light-headedness, fainting, palpitations, chest pain, or shortness of breath.
■ Ask about the relationship of symptoms to food intake and caffeine-containing beverages.
■ Evaluate other contributing factors such as heart disease, medications, smoking, or alcohol intake.
■ Inquire about falls, particularly those occurring without apparent reason.

Teach older adults to reduce their risk for dysrhythmias and their consequences by

■ Taking medications (including over-the-counter drugs) as ordered.
■ Eliminating caffeine intake.
■ Stopping smoking and eliminating alcohol intake if appropriate.
■ Engaging in regular exercise.
■ Contacting their primary care provider for symptoms such as dizziness, fainting, frequent palpitations, shortness of breath, unexplained falls, or chest pain.

SINUS TACHYCARDIA In sinus tachycardia, the heart rate is greater than 100 beats per minute. Tachycardia is a normal response to conditions that increase the body's demand for oxygen and nutrients, such as exercise. Other causes of sinus tachycardia include anxiety, pain, fever, hypoxia, hyperthyroidism, caffeine intake, and some drugs. Sinus tachycardia may be an early warning sign of cardiac problems such as heart failure.

The patient with sinus tachycardia has a rapid pulse rate and may complain of a "racing" heart or shortness of breath. Patients with heart disease may experience chest pain.

SINUS BRADYCARDIA *Sinus bradycardia* is a heart rate less than 60 beats per minute. It may be normal in some patients (e.g., athletes) and during sleep. Bradycardia may also be caused by pain, increased intracranial pressure, hypothermia, heart disease, and certain drugs.

Patients with sinus bradycardia may be asymptomatic or may have manifestations of decreased cardiac output, such as decreased level of consciousness, syncope (faintness), or hypotension.

PREMATURE ATRIAL CONTRACTIONS A *premature atrial contraction (PAC)* is an ectopic atrial beat that occurs earlier than the next expected sinus beat. PACs are *usually* asymptomatic and benign, but they may initiate supraventricular tachycardia in some people. PACs are common in older adults and may occur without an obvious cause. Frequent PACs may cause heart palpitations or a fluttering sensation in the chest.

Supraventricular tachycardia (SVT) is usually characterized by a sudden onset and abrupt cessation. It may be caused by sympathetic nervous system stimulation and stressors such as fever, sepsis, and hyperthyroidism. Manifestations of SVT include complaints of palpitations and a "racing" heart, anxiety, dizziness, dyspnea, chest pain, diaphoresis, and fatigue.

ATRIAL FLUTTER *Atrial flutter* is a very rapid and regular atrial rhythm. Causes include sympathetic nervous system stimulation due to anxiety; caffeine and alcohol intake; thyrotoxicosis; and heart disease.

Patients with atrial flutter may complain of palpitations or a fluttering sensation in the chest or throat. If the ventricular rate is rapid, cardiac output falls, causing decreased level of consciousness, hypotension, decreased urinary output, and cool, clammy skin.

ATRIAL FIBRILLATION *Atrial fibrillation* is a common dysrhythmia characterized by disorganized atrial activity without discrete atrial contractions. Extremely rapid impulses bombard the AV node, causing an irregularly irregular ventricular response. Atrial fibrillation may occur suddenly and

TABLE 16-8	Characteristics, Causes, and Management of Selected Cardiac Rhythms	
RHYTHM/ECG APPEARANCE	**CHARACTERISTICS AND MANIFESTATIONS**	**MANAGEMENT**
Supraventricular rhythms		
Normal sinus rhythm (NSR)	Regular; rate 60–100 beats/min. All waveforms and intervals normal	None; normal heart rhythm
Sinus tachycardia	Regular; rate greater than 100 beats/min. Other characteristics as for NSR	Treated only if symptomatic or if patient at risk for MI. Treat underlying cause
Sinus bradycardia	Regular; rate less than 60 beats/min. Other characteristics as for NSR	Treated only if symptomatic; may give atropine or require pacemaker
Premature atrial contractions (PACs)	Irregular, an ectopic atrial beat occurring earlier than expected	Usually require no treatment; advise smoking cessation, reduced caffeine and alcohol intake
Atrial flutter	Usually regular with sawtooth appearance of P waves. Atrial rate 240+ beats/min; ventricular rate, less than 150 beats/min	Synchronized cardioversion; medication to slow ventricular response
Atrial fibrillation	Irregularly irregular; no identifiable P waves; variable ventricular rate	Synchronized cardioversion; medication to slow ventricular rate; anticoagulants to reduce risk of stroke

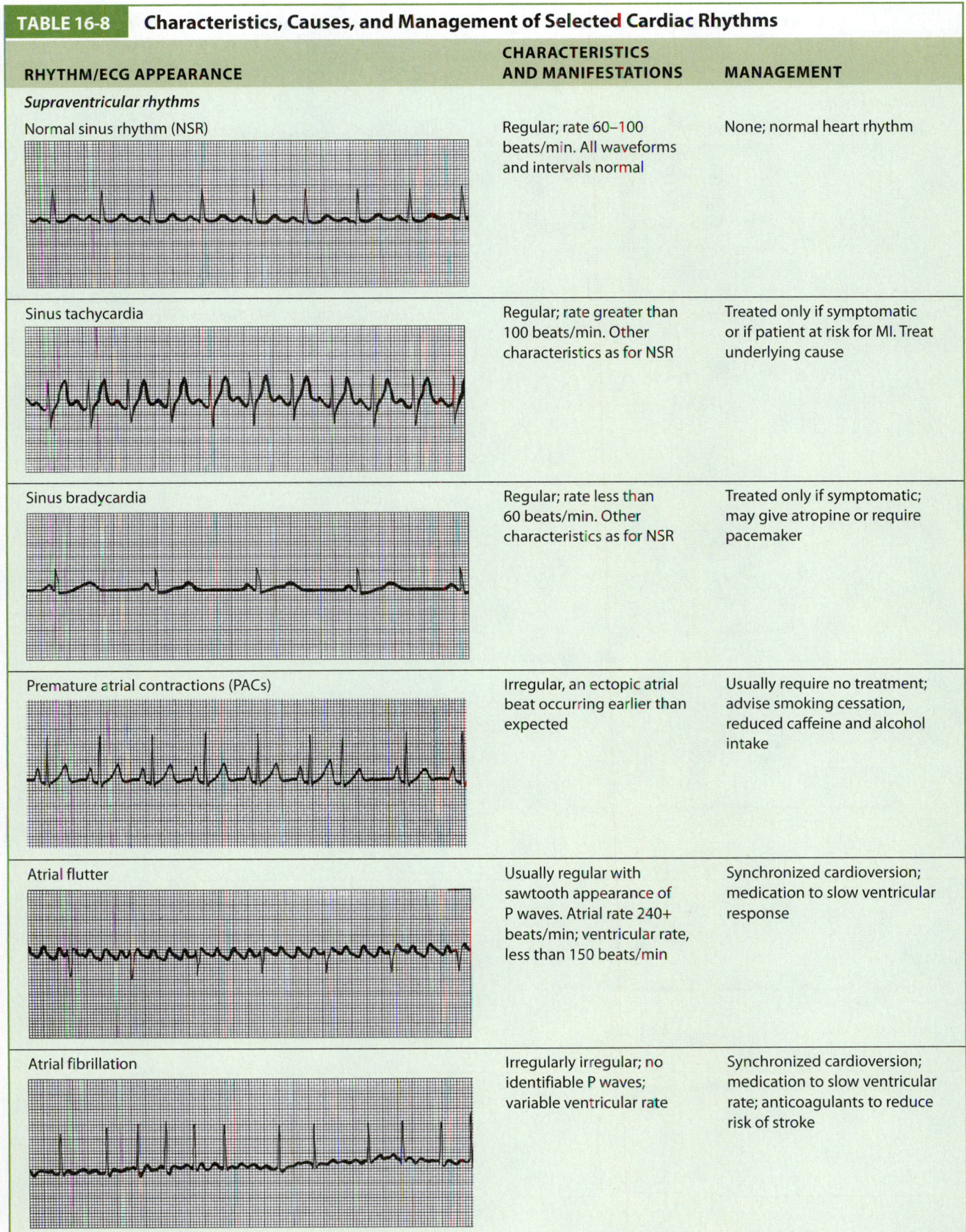

(continued)

TABLE 16-8	Characteristics, Causes, and Management of Selected Cardiac Rhythms *(continued)*	
RHYTHM/ECG APPEARANCE	**CHARACTERISTICS AND MANIFESTATIONS**	**MANAGEMENT**
Ventricular rhythms		
Premature ventricular contractions (PVCs)	Irregular; ectopic ventricular beat interrupts normal rhythm; ectopic QRS wide and bizarre	Abstain from nicotine, caffeine; medication if symptomatic or if result of recent AMI
Ventricular tachycardia (VT or V-tach)	Regular; rate 100–250 beats/min; no identifiable P waves, QRS wide and bizarre	Treated if symptomatic; intravenous drugs; cardioversion or defibrillation if unconscious or unstable
Ventricular fibrillation (V-fib)	Grossly irregular; rate too rapid to count; no P waves, QRS bizarre and variable	Immediate defibrillation necessary to preserve life
AV conduction blocks		
First-degree AV block	Regular; rate usually 60–100 beats/min; PR interval greater than 0.21 sec	No treatment necessary
Second-degree AV block	Atrial rate regular, ventricular rate irregular; some P waves not followed by QRS, PR interval may vary	Monitoring and observation; drug or pacemaker therapy may be required
Third-degree AV block (complete heart block)	Atrial rate regular (60–100 beats/min), ventricular rate regular (30–40 beats/min); no relationship between P waves and QRS complexes	Immediate pacemaker therapy

recur, or it may become chronic. It is common in patients with heart failure.

Manifestations of atrial fibrillation include irregular pulses of variable strength. The patient may have hypotension, shortness of breath, fatigue, and angina. Patients with extensive heart disease may develop syncope or heart failure.

Atrial fibrillation increases the risk of forming thromboemboli (blood clots). Stroke is a risk because these clots may travel to the brain.

AV JUNCTIONAL DYSRHYTHMIAS   *AV junctional dysrhythmias* originate in the AV node or bundle of His. They include escape rhythms, which occur when sinus and atrial pacemakers fail; ectopic beats (premature junctional contractions, or PJCs); and junctional tachycardia. Although the QRS typically appears normal, the P wave may be inverted or occur immediately before, during, or after the QRS complex. AV junctional dysrhythmias may be caused by drug toxicity, hypoxemia, electrolyte imbalance, AMI, or heart failure.

Ventricular Dysrhythmias

Ventricular dysrhythmias originate in the ventricles. Because the ventricles pump blood into the pulmonary and systemic vasculature, any disturbance in their rhythm can affect cardiac output and tissue perfusion. A wide and bizarre QRS complex (greater than 0.12 second) is a characteristic feature of ventricular dysrhythmias.

PREMATURE VENTRICULAR CONTRACTIONS   *Premature ventricular contractions (PVCs)* are ectopic ventricular beats that occur before the next expected beat of the normal rhythm. PVCs may be isolated or occur in patterns such as every other beat, in pairs, or in triplets (three in a row). Isolated PVCs often are benign. They may be triggered by anxiety or stress, tobacco, alcohol, or caffeine. Benign PVCs are common in older adults. In people with heart disease, PVCs are common. Frequent PVCs may signal an increased risk for lethal dysrhythmias.

Patients experiencing PVCs may complain of feeling their hearts "skip a beat" or of palpitations. The early beat may be heard on auscultation; it is felt as a "missed" beat on palpation of peripheral pulses.

VENTRICULAR TACHYCARDIA   *Ventricular tachycardia (VT; V-tach)* is three or more consecutive PVCs. VT may occur in short bursts, or "runs," or it may persist for longer periods. The rate is greater than 100 beats per minute, and the rhythm is usually regular. Myocardial ischemia and infarction are the most common causes of VT, although it may also occur with other heart diseases or in the absence of heart disease. It may be associated with anorexia nervosa, metabolic disorders, and drug toxicity.

Short bursts of VT may cause a sensation of fluttering in the chest, palpitations, and brief shortness of breath. Cardiac output drops with sustained VT, causing severe hypotension, a weak or nonpalpable pulse, and loss of consciousness. Allowed to continue, VT can deteriorate into ventricular fibrillation at any time. Sustained VT is a medical emergency that requires immediate intervention to preserve life.

VENTRICULAR FIBRILLATION   *Ventricular fibrillation (V-fib)* is defined as extremely rapid, chaotic ventricular depolarization that causes the ventricles to quiver and stop contracting; the heart does not pump. This is known as **cardiac arrest**, a medical emergency requiring immediate intervention with cardiopulmonary resuscitation (CPR) measures. Death will follow the onset of V-fib within 4 minutes if the rhythm is not recognized and terminated, with a return to a perfusing rhythm.

V-fib is usually triggered by severe myocardial ischemia or infarction. It occurs without warning 50% of the time. It is the terminal event in many disease processes or traumatic conditions. V-fib may also be caused by digitalis toxicity, electrolyte and acid–base imbalances, certain drugs, mechanical stimulation (as with the insertion of cardiac catheters or pacing wires), and electric shock.

Clinically, loss of ventricular contraction causes the pulse to cease. The patient loses consciousness and stops breathing (*cardiopulmonary arrest*).

Atrioventricular Conduction Blocks

Conduction defects that cause delayed or blocked transmission of sinus impulses through the AV node are called *atrioventricular (AV) conduction blocks*. AV blocks vary from benign to severe.

FIRST-DEGREE AV BLOCK   *First-degree AV block* is a benign conduction delay that poses no immediate threat and requires no treatment. There are no clinical manifestations except a prolonged PR interval. Causes of first-degree block include MI, digitalis therapy or toxicity, complications from cardiac surgery, chronic heart disease, or drug effects.

SECOND-DEGREE AV BLOCK   In *second-degree AV block,* some atrial impulses are totally blocked at the AV node and prevented from reaching the ventricles. Two types of second-degree block are recognized. *Type I,* also known as Mobitz I or Wenckebach, is characterized by a repeating pattern in which PR intervals become progressively longer until one QRS complex is not conducted or is dropped. It is usually asymptomatic, unless the heart rate slows and cardiac output falls.

Type II, also called Mobitz II, is characterized by a regular pattern of nonconducted impulses; usually, two atrial impulses occur for every one that is transmitted to the ventricles. Type II heart block is usually associated with AMI. Its manifestations depend on the ventricular rate and cardiac output.

THIRD-DEGREE AV BLOCK   *Third-degree AV block (complete heart block)* occurs when atrial impulses are completely blocked at the AV node and not conducted to the ventricles. Atrial and ventricular rhythms are completely independent of one another. The ventricular impulse is slow at a rate of 30 to 40 beats per minute, whereas the normal atrial rate of 60 to 100 beats per minute continues.

Third-degree block is frequently caused by an AMI. Other heart diseases, drugs, and electrolyte imbalances can also precipitate it. Cardiac output falls, leading to light-headedness, confusion, and syncope (fainting). Third-degree AV block is life threatening and requires immediate treatment to restore the cardiac output.

COLLABORATIVE CARE

Although many dysrhythmias pose little risk, others, such as ventricular fibrillation, are life threatening and require immediate intervention. Early recognition is vital. Patients at risk for dysrhythmias often are cared for in cardiac intensive care or other specialty units that allow constant monitoring of the ECG and patient's status.

Diagnostic Tests

Diagnostic tests commonly ordered for patients with dysrhythmias include serum cardiac markers (CK, cardiac troponins), serum electrolytes (sodium, potassium, chloride, calcium, and magnesium), and, as appropriate, serum drug levels (e.g., digitalis levels). Cardiac electrophysiology (EP) studies may be done to locate the focus of persistent dysrhythmias. Nursing care of the patient undergoing an EP study is similar to that provided for patients undergoing percutaneous coronary intervention (see Box 16-4).

CARDIAC MONITORING   Cardiac monitoring allows continuous observation of the patient's cardiac rhythm. Different types of ECG monitoring are employed for different situations.

CONTINUOUS CARDIAC MONITORING   Electrodes placed on the patient's chest are connected to a monitoring system. The heart rate and rhythm are visually displayed on a

---

BOX 16-11	PROCEDURE CHECKLIST

Initiating Cardiac Monitoring

☑ Gather supplies.

☑ Provide for privacy.

☑ Explain the reason for ECG monitoring, reassuring the patient that it allows immediate treatment of abnormal rhythms if necessary. Explain alarms, their purpose, and possible causes, such as loose or disconnected lead wires and other mechanical problems. Activity is permitted within ordered restrictions while on the monitor.

☑ Follow standard precautions.

☑ Check equipment for damage (i.e., fraying, bent, or broken wires). Connect lead wires to cable, and secure the connections.

☑ Select electrode sites on the chest wall (see figure), considering lead to be monitored, skin condition, and any incisions or catheters.

☑ Clean sites with soap and water, and dry thoroughly. Alcohol may be used to remove skin oils; allow the skin to dry for 60 seconds after use.

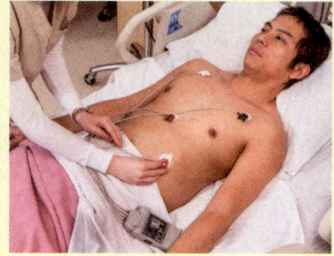

☑ Peel backing from a fresh electrode; check to ensure that the pad is moist with conductive gel.

☑ Apply electrode pads, pressing firmly to ensure contact. Attach leads and position cable with sufficient slack for comfort. Place telemetry unit (if used) in gown pouch or pocket.

☑ Assess ECG tracing on the monitor, adjusting settings as needed.

☑ Set ECG monitor alarm limits as indicated, typically at 20 beats/min higher and lower than the baseline rate. Turn alarms on, and leave on at all times. Assess immediately if an alarm is triggered.

☑ Remove and apply new pads every 24 to 48 hours and as needed. Clean gel residue from previous site, and document skin condition. Use a different site if skin appears irritated or blistered. Initial, time, and date pads with every change.

☑ Save ECG strips according to unit policy and when the rhythm or the patient's condition changes. Note date, time, patient, and monitor lead on each strip. Notify the charge nurse or physician of significant changes in heart rhythm.

Sample Documentation

[date]   Placed on cardiac monitor, lead 2. Monitor shows
1430   NSR at 75/min with no ectopy noted. Resting
        comfortably. S. Craven, LPN.

Note: Refer to a nursing fundamentals or skills text for more detailed instruction. Check state guidelines and facility policy before performing any procedure. (Source: Rick Brady, Pearson Education.)

bedside monitor and a central monitoring station. Alarms on the monitors warn of potential problems, such as very rapid or very slow heart rates. Box 16-11■ describes the steps to initiate cardiac monitoring.

PORTABLE CARDIAC MONITORING Distance ECG monitoring (telemetry) is frequently used on medical–surgical or cardiac units. Telemetry allows the patient to engage in activities while being monitored. Ambulatory or Holter monitoring may be used in community settings to diagnose infrequent dysrhythmias or dysrhythmias associated with activities.

Medications

Antidysrhythmic drugs may be used to treat acute dysrhythmias or to manage chronic conditions. The overall goal of therapy is to maintain an effective cardiac output by stabilizing cardiac rhythm.

Many different classes of drugs are used to treat cardiac dysrhythmias. Table 16-9■ identifies common antidysrhythmic drugs, their class, and the nursing implications in caring for the patient receiving an antidysrhythmic drug.

clinicalALERT

All antidysrhythmic drugs can also *cause* dysrhythmias. Closely monitor all patients receiving cardiac drugs for dysrhythmias.

Cardioversion/Defibrillation

Cardioversion (or defibrillation) is used to treat rhythms that affect cardiac output and the patient's welfare. An electrical shock is administered to depolarize all cells of the heart at the same time. This often stops the abnormal rhythm and allows the sinus node to resume control of the rhythm.

Synchronized cardioversion delivers an electrical current synchronized with the patient's rhythm to prevent ventricular fibrillation. It is used to treat rhythms that are not life-threatening, such as supraventricular tachycardia and atrial fibrillation. It is usually an elective procedure, and the patient is sedated before cardioversion. Anticoagulants may be given before the procedure to reduce the risk of thromboembolism.

Defibrillation is an emergency treatment that delivers an electrical charge without regard to the cardiac cycle. Early defibrillation improves survival of patients experiencing V-fib. External defibrillation may be performed by any health care provider who has been trained in the procedure. Initiate CPR and the cardiac arrest (code) procedure when V-fib is recognized. Remove NTG patches from the patient's chest in preparation for defibrillation, but leave monitor pads in place. Conductive gel pads are applied to the chest wall at the apex and base of the heart, and an

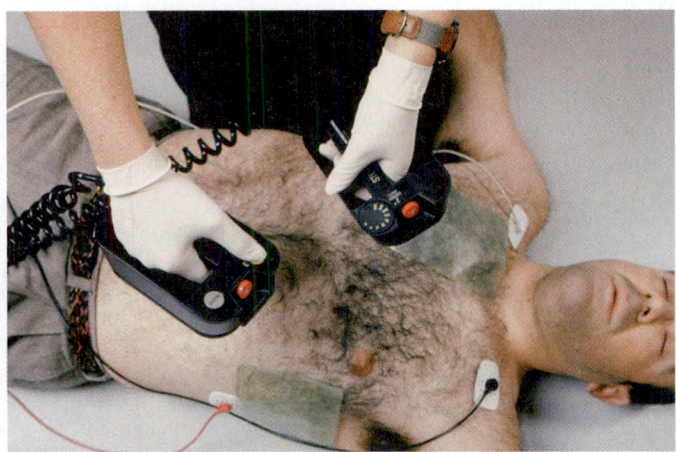

Figure 16-9. ■ Placement of paddles or pads for defibrillation. (Source: Pearson Education)

electrical shock is delivered by *automated external defibrillator (AED)* or manually (Figure 16-9■). The cardiac rhythm is evaluated after each shock is delivered. After successful defibrillation, the patient is transferred to the critical care unit for monitoring and therapy to prevent further episodes of V-fib.

AUTOMATIC IMPLANTABLE CARDIOVERTER–DEFIBRILLATOR The *automatic implantable cardioverter–defibrillator (AICD)* recognizes life-threatening changes in heart rhythm and automatically delivers an electric shock to convert the rhythm back into a normal rhythm. Electrodes surgically placed on the heart are attached to an implanted cardioverter–defibrillator device. The AICD is used for patients with recurrent ventricular tachycardia and people who have survived cardiac arrest not associated with an AMI. When V-tach or V-fib occur, the AICD delivers a shock to convert the rhythm.

Pacemakers

Pacemakers may be used to treat AV blocks. *Temporary pacemakers* have an external generator attached to an electrode threaded intravenously into the right ventricle or to temporary pacing wires implanted during cardiac surgery. *Permanent pacemakers* have an implanted pulse generator attached to electrodes that are sewn directly onto the heart or passed into the heart via the subclavian or jugular vein (Figure 16-10■).

Pacemakers have both sensing and pacing functions. *Sensing* detects the heart's own beats. When the pacemaker senses a heart rate within preset limits, it provides no electrical stimuli. *Pacing,* or the delivery of an electrical pulse to stimulate the heart to contract, occurs when the patient's heart rate falls outside the programmed limits. Pacing is detected on the ECG strip (Figure 16-11■) by the presence of a pacing spike before the P wave (atrial pacing) or QRS

TABLE 16-9	Giving Medications Safely: Antidysrhythmic Drugs		
CLASS/DRUGS	**PURPOSE**	**NURSING IMPLICATIONS**	**PATIENT TEACHING**
Class I: Sodium channel blockers		Obtain baseline vital signs, cardiac rhythm, and physical assessment.	Take the drug exactly as ordered. Do not skip or double doses. Check with your doctor if you miss a dose.
Class IA			
■ Disopyramide (Norpace) ■ Quinidine ■ Procainamide (Procan, Pronestyl)	Used to treat symptomatic or frequent PVCs and supraventricular or ventricular tachycardias, and to prevent ventricular fibrillation	Monitor ECG. Notify the physician of new dysrhythmias. Notify the physician immediately if manifestations of toxicity develop:	Take and record your pulse rate daily before rising. Count pulse for 1 full minute. Bring the record to each office or clinic appointment.
Class IB			
■ Lidocaine ■ Mexiletine (Mexitil) ■ Phenytoin (Dilantin) ■ Tocainide (Tonocard)	Primarily used to treat ventricular dysrhythmias, including PVCs and ventricular tachycardia	Signs of heart failure Changes in ECG complex	Report the following to your doctor: irregular pulse rate or rhythm, dizziness, eye pain, vision changes, skin rashes, wheezing or other respiratory problems, behavior changes.
Class IC		Skin rash or flu-like symptoms	
■ Flecainide (Tambocor) ■ Propafenone (Rythmol)	Usually reserved for serious ventricular dysrhythmias	Urinary retention Neurologic effects such as confusion, dizziness, agitation	
Class II: Beta blockers		Shortness of breath	
■ *Atenolol* (Tenormin) ■ *Carvedilol* (Coreg) ■ Esmolol (Brevibloc) ■ *Metoprolol* (Lopressor, Toprol) ■ *Nadolol* (Corgard) ■ Propranolol (Inderal, others)	Used to prevent SVT and possibly V-fib May cause bronchospasm, so are contraindicated for patients with asthma or COPD	Altered liver function tests Use an infusion pump to administer intravenous infusions. Monitor dose and its effectiveness.	
Class III: Potassium channel blockers			
■ Amiodarone (Cordarone) ■ Bretylium (Bretylol) ■ Dofetilide (Tikosyn) ■ Ibutilide (Corvert) ■ Sotalol (Betapace)	Primarily used to treat V-tach and V-fib		
Class IV: Calcium channel blockers			
■ *Amlodipine* (Norvasc) ■ Diltiazem (Cardizem, Dilacor) ■ Verapamil (Calan, Isoptin)	Used to manage supraventricular tachycardias		
Other drugs			
■ Adenosine (Adenocard) ■ *Digoxin* (Lanoxin)	Used to treat atrial dysrhythmias		

Note: Medications identified in *italics* are among the 200 most frequently prescribed drugs in the United States.

complex (ventricular pacing). Box 16-12■ outlines nursing care for the patient undergoing permanent pacemaker implantation.

Pacemakers and pacing technology have evolved significantly. Some pacemakers pace both the atria and the ventricles (*dual* chamber pacing), more closely simulating the normal sequence of cardiac conduction and contraction. Versatile *cardiac rhythm management (CRM)* devices are capable of pacing when the heart rate is too slow, terminating a potentially fatal ventricular dysrhythmia

(such as ventricular fibrillation) and correcting cardiac conduction abnormalities. Some implanted devices are able to transmit information to health care providers over telephone lines.

Surgery

Surgical *ablation* (removal of a part or pathway) may be used when the site of an ectopic focus can be identified. The affected tissue may be excised (cut out) or destroyed by freezing with liquid nitrogen, laser, or an electric current.

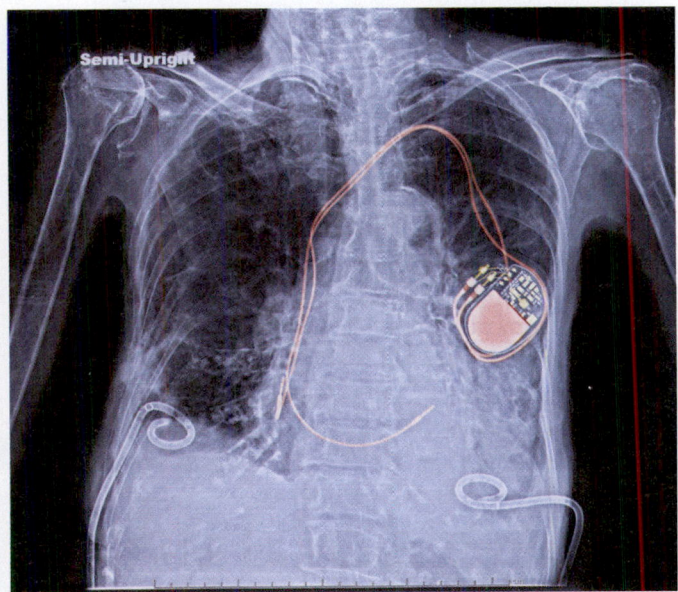

Figure 16-10. ■ A permanent pacemaker with a transvenous electrode into the right ventricle. (Source: Apogee/Science Source.)

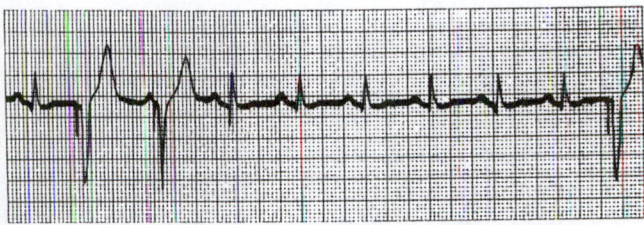

Figure 16-11. ■ Ventricular pacing. Note the presence of pacer spikes before the wide, ventricular QRS complexes and the absence of spikes when the patient's natural rhythm resumes.

BOX 16-12	NURSING CARE CHECKLIST

Permanent Pacemaker Implantation

Before Surgery

☑ Assess knowledge and understanding; reinforce and clarify teaching as needed.

☑ Position ECG monitor electrodes away from potential incision sites.

☑ Provide routine preoperative care and teaching as ordered.

After Surgery

☑ Provide routine postoperative care, including monitoring and incision care.

☑ Obtain a chest x-ray as ordered.

☑ Administer analgesia and position for comfort. Restrict movement of affected arm and shoulder for 24 hours.

☑ After 24 hours, assist with gentle range of motion exercises at least three times a day.

☑ Monitor pacemaker function and cardiac rhythm. Report pacemaker problems, such as failure to pace or hiccups, to the physician.

☑ Report dysrhythmias to the charge nurse or physician.

☑ Document date of insertion, pacemaker model and type, and settings.

☑ Provide a pacemaker identification card that includes manufacturer's name, model number, mode of operation, rate parameters, and expected battery life. Instruct to carry the card at all times and to wear a MedicAlert bracelet or tag.

☑ Teach about the pacemaker, its function, how to take and record the pulse rate, and usual battery replacement procedure.

☑ Instruct to report the following to the physician: pulse rate 5 or more beats/min slower than preset pacemaker rate; fever; signs of pacemaker malfunction, such as dizziness, fainting, fatigue, weakness, chest pain, or palpitations.

☑ Notify all care providers of the pacemaker.

NURSING CARE

PRIORITIZING NURSING CARE

Many dysrhythmias are benign, with no adverse effects. Others, however (such as ventricular tachycardia or ventricular fibrillation), can seriously affect cardiac output. Therefore, the highest priority of care is maintaining adequate cardiac output to ensure delivery of oxygen and nutrients to the body's cells.

HEALTH PROMOTION

Because many dysrhythmias are related to underlying CHD, measures to reduce the risks for CHD also reduce the risk for dysrhythmias. In addition, advise patients who complain of occasional "heart palpitations" or flutters to limit their intake of caffeine, to stop smoking, and to eliminate or limit their intake of other sympathetic nervous system stimulants, such as diet pills or chocolate.

ASSESSING

It is vital to assess the patient before treating any suspected dysrhythmia. What appears to be ventricular tachycardia on the monitor may be a patient brushing the teeth. Apparent asystole on the monitor may be a patient whose electrode patch has come loose. Similarly, a heart rate of 52 beats per minute may be normal for some patients and not affect their functioning at all. Compare the present rhythm with previous rhythm recordings and report significant changes.

Ask about the presence of chest pain, shortness of breath, or palpitations. Inquire about dizziness or feeling lightheaded, faint, or nauseated. Obtain vital signs and an ECG monitor strip. Assess skin color, temperature, and moisture; level of consciousness and mental status; heart sounds and peripheral pulses; respiratory status; and anxiety level. Check electrode placement, leads, the monitor cable, and connections.

clinicalALERT

Remember: Treat the patient, not the monitor!

Monitor laboratory results, including serum electrolytes, hemoglobin and hematocrit, cardiac markers, and drug levels. Report abnormal results to the charge nurse or physician.

IDENTIFYING POTENTIAL COMPLICATIONS

The nurse should be alert for signs that the patient's hemodynamic status is deteriorating. Additionally, the nurse observes for cardiac rhythm changes that may signal increased risk for a potentially fatal rhythm. As noted earlier, having the patient on a cardiac monitor is not a substitute for frequent focused assessment of cardiovascular status. Report changes in vital signs, oxygen saturation, color, and mental status. Report increasing anxiety, as this may be an early sign of impaired oxygenation. Auscultate heart sounds regularly. Frequent PVCs or PVCs occurring in multiples (pairs, three or more in sequence) and PVCs of varied shapes (*morphology*) may signal deteriorating cardiac status and an increased risk of ventricular tachycardia or fibrillation. A patient who develops type II second-degree heart block may require a pacemaker to maintain cardiac output.

DIAGNOSING, PLANNING, AND IMPLEMENTING
Decreased Cardiac Output

Expected outcome: Vital signs and cardiovascular assessments will remain stable and within normal limits for the patient.

■ Assess for manifestations of decreased cardiac output: decreased level of consciousness; tachycardia; tachypnea; hypotension; diaphoresis; decreased urine output; cool, clammy, mottled skin; pallor or cyanosis; decreased peripheral pulses. *Manifestations of decreased cardiac output may indicate the patient is not tolerating the dysrhythmia and needs immediate treatment.*

■ Monitor ECG rhythm and post ECG strip every shift and when rhythm changes occur. *Documenting ECG rhythms helps evaluate status and the effect of treatment.*

■ Frequently monitor vital signs. *Vital signs are an indicator of the effect of the dysrhythmia and treatment on cardiovascular status.*

■ Monitor lab values, especially serum electrolytes and drug levels as ordered. Report abnormal values to the charge nurse and physician. *Electrolyte imbalances can cause*

dysrhythmias. Serum drug levels need to be within the therapeutic range for optimal effectiveness.

■ Maintain intravenous access with an intravenous infusion or saline lock. *Many drugs used to treat dysrhythmias are administered intravenously. In an emergency, an existing intravenous site facilitates rapid treatment of the dysrhythmia.*

■ On recognizing ventricular fibrillation, begin emergency procedures. Call for help. Begin CPR until a defibrillator is available. Initiate advanced cardiac life support (ACLS) protocols. Defibrillate as soon as possible. Assist the code team as needed. *V-fib is a medical emergency requiring immediate treatment to preserve life.*

■ After a cardiac arrest, transfer to critical care. *The period immediately after resuscitation is critical, and the patient needs careful monitoring.*

Risk for Ineffective Cerebral Tissue Perfusion

Expected outcome: Remains alert and oriented, with no evidence of motor or sensory deficits.

■ Monitor level of consciousness and orientation to time, place, and person. *A change in mental status may indicate lack of adequate blood and oxygen supply to cells of the brain.*

■ Assess neurologic status indicators, such as pattern of respirations, movement, grip strength, and pupillary reaction to light. *Changes in neurologic signs may indicate significant ischemia of the brain.*

■ Initiate oxygen therapy if not currently in place. *Supplemental oxygen increases the oxygen saturation of the blood and its delivery to the tissues, including the brain. This helps preserve cellular metabolism and function.*

■ Lower the head of the bed to no greater than 15 degrees if possible. *Lowering the head of the bed supports and improves cerebral blood flow.*

■ Unless contraindicated (e.g., if the patient is vomiting), maintain supine position with the head straight (in alignment with the body). *Alignment of the head and neck with the body facilitates blood flow to and from the brain through major vessels in the neck.*

■ Promote rest with a quiet environment to the extent possible. *Reducing environmental stimuli reduces mental activity and the metabolic needs of brain cells.*

Anxiety

Expected outcome: Family members will verbalize an understanding of the patient's condition and prognosis.

■ Notify family of significant changes in the patient's condition or cardiac arrest, providing up-to-date information. Prepare family members for visits by explaining interventions such as invasive tubes, a ventilator, or additional equipment. *Concern for the family and significant others is part of holistic nursing. Family members need information, honest communication, and compassionate care. Preparing the family for changes in the patient's condition and plan of care helps them to cope with a difficult situation.*

MANAGING NURSING CARE

Nursing care activities such as assisting with personal care and activities as allowed are appropriate to assign to assistive personnel. In some settings, a trained monitor technician may be responsible for continuous cardiac rhythm monitoring, while the nurse retains responsibility for notifying the physician and initiating prescribed treatment.

EVALUATING

To evaluate the effectiveness of care for a patient with a dysrhythmia, collect data related to cardiac output and cerebral perfusion. For example, evaluate level of consciousness and mental status, skin color and temperature, vital signs, oxygen saturation, and urinary output. Monitor cardiac rhythm, promptly reporting increased or significant dysrhythmias or unresponsiveness to treatment measures. Monitor laboratory data such as arterial blood gas results and serum electrolytes.

DOCUMENTING

Document mental status, vital signs, and other assessment data during episodes of dysrhythmia, noting changes from previous status. Document cardiac rhythms, as well as the effect of activities. Record treatment measures and their effects on the dysrhythmia and patient's status. Note the patient's perception of the situation and apparent level of anxiety. If family members are notified of a significant or critical dysrhythmia, document the time and their response or presence.

CONTINUITY OF CARE

Dysrhythmias can have a significant physical and psychologic impact. The patient and family may fear sudden cardiac death. Teaching focuses on coping strategies and specific treatments. Involve both the patient and the family in teaching. Teach about prescribed drugs, including their desired and potential adverse or toxic effects. Stress the importance of follow-up visits with the cardiologist, and schedule them, if possible.

Teach patients with a pacemaker or an AICD about the device and how it works, how to take their pulse, signs of infection or other complications, resumption of and any limitations to activities, and safety issues. Stress the importance of promptly reporting problems to the physician and attending follow-up appointments. In some states, driving is prohibited for patients with AICDs; address the impact of this on lifestyle. Inform the patient that magnetic interference can damage the AICD or cause it to discharge. Procedures such as magnetic resonance imaging (MRI) and equipment such as arc welders, radar, and theft prevention equipment can damage the AICD and should be avoided.

Encourage the patient and family to learn and maintain current training in CPR. Refer to the AHA or the American Red Cross for training.

Sudden Cardiac Death

Key Concept Approximately half of all cardiac deaths are sudden and unexpected, due to cardiac arrest. However, if observed and treated promptly, cardiac arrest may be reversible.

Sudden cardiac death is defined as death occurring within 1 hour of the onset of cardiac symptoms. It usually is caused by ventricular fibrillation and cardiac arrest. Cardiac arrest occurs when effective circulation ceases.

CHD is the most common cause of sudden cardiac deaths in the United States. Other causes include electrocution, pulmonary embolism, and rapid blood loss from a ruptured aortic aneurysm. Ventricular fibrillation is the most common dysrhythmia causing sudden cardiac death; asystole or cardiac standstill also leads to sudden death. The risk of sudden cardiac death is highest in the first 6 to 18 months after an AMI or other major cardiac event.

Effective CPR must be instituted within 2 to 4 minutes of cardiac arrest to prevent permanent brain damage. CPR is a mechanical means of maintaining tissue perfusion and oxygenation using ventilation and external cardiac compressions. All health care providers need to be proficient in CPR or basic life support (BLS). A review of CPR procedures is provided in Box 16-13■. ACLS incorporates drug treatment in addition to mechanical compressions and electrical defibrillation.

CPR can cause traumatic injuries to the skin, thorax, upper airway, abdomen, lungs, heart, and great vessels; however, delaying CPR can be fatal. These complications, which are uncommon, can be minimized by using appropriate CPR techniques.

Because most instances of sudden cardiac death result from ventricular fibrillation, the AHA recommends early defibrillation when appropriate. Automated external defibrillators (AEDs) are easy to use (Figure 16-12■). The device senses the heart rhythm through two electrodes placed on the chest, analyzes the rhythm, and instructs the rescuer to deliver a shock when necessary. A shock can be delivered simply by pressing the "shock" button on the device.

The patient who survives sudden cardiac death and family members have significant teaching needs to recognize and reduce the risk of subsequent events.

If the cause of cardiac arrest is identified, teach risk factor reduction. For example, if an MI precipitated the cardiac arrest, teach the risk factors for MI and ways to

BOX 16-13   PROCEDURE CHECKLIST

Cardiopulmonary Resuscitation (CPR)

☑ Assess for responsiveness and look for no breathing or abnormal breathing.

☑ Call for help. Dial 911 (if outside the health care facility) or initiate the institutional cardiac arrest procedure. Obtain AED if available.

☑ Check for a carotid or femoral pulse. (Take less than 10 seconds to check the pulse.)

☑ If no pulse is felt, begin chest compressions. Place the patient on a firm surface. Place the heel of one hand on the center of the chest between the nipples; place the second hand on top of the first with the fingers either extended or interlocked (see part A of the figure).

☑ With the arms straight, the shoulders directly over the hands, and elbows locked, press straight down to depress the sternum at least 2 in. or 5 cm. (part B of the figure). Release pressure completely between compressions but do not lift the hands from the chest.

☑ Compress the chest hard and fast, at a rate of approximately 100 times per minute.

☑ After 30 compressions, open the airway using the head tilt–chin lift maneuver (part C of the accompanying figure): This involves simultaneously pressing down on the patient's forehead with one hand to tilt the head back and lifting the chin forward using the fingers of the other hand under the bony part of the chin.

☑ Give two full breaths using a pocket mask, mouth shield, or bag-valve mask (see part C of the figure). Observe for chest rise and fall during ventilation. Deliver each breath over 1 second.

☑ If no pulse is detectable, continue cycle of 30 chest compressions followed by two breaths.

☑ When an AED is available: Turn AED on, place pads on chest as indicated, and follow prompts. Resume chest compressions immediately after a shock is delivered.

☑ If pulse is present, continue rescue breathing at 10 to 12 breaths per minute (1 breath every 5 to 6 seconds). Recheck the pulse every 2 minutes.

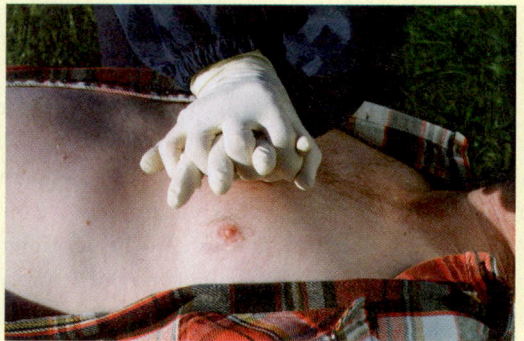 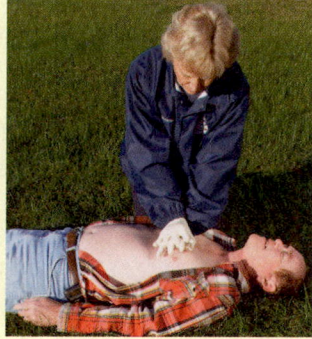  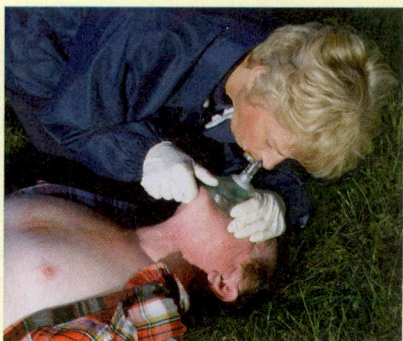

A   B   C

(Source: Michal Heron, Pearson Education.)

Note: Refer to a nursing fundamentals or skills text for more detailed instruction. Check state guidelines and facility policy before performing any procedure.

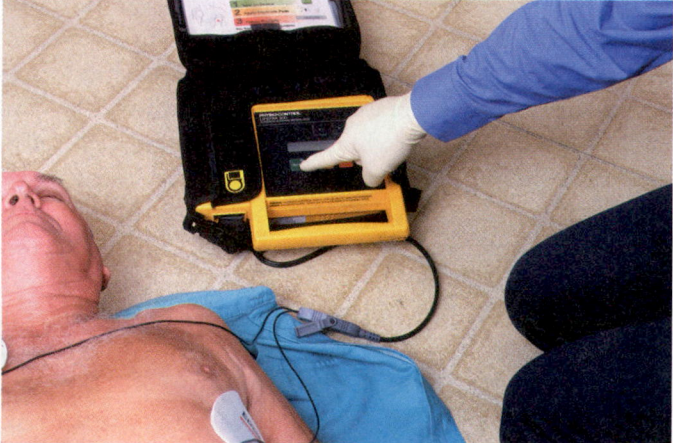

Figure 16-12. ■ Using an automated external defibrillator (AED) for sudden cardiac death. (Source: Pearson Education)

reduce them. If the cause of cardiac arrest is unknown, explain diagnostic studies and discuss possible interventions, such as the AICD. Stress the importance of carrying a card at all times listing all medications and the patient's health care provider. In all cases, teach recognition of early manifestations or warning signs of cardiac arrest. All family members should become proficient in performing CPR.

To reduce death rates from cardiac arrest, teach community members the importance of early intervention and learning how to perform effective CPR. Work with community and emergency services agencies to provide and train community members to use the AED as well.

Note: The references and resources for all chapters have been compiled at the back of the book.

Chapter Review

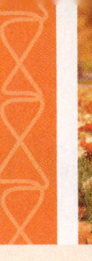
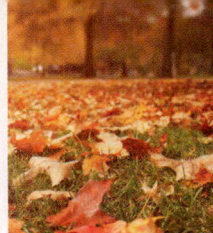

KEY POINTS

- **Concept:** Cardiovascular disease (CVD) is the leading cause of death and disability in the United States, affecting people of all ethnic groups and cultures.
- **Concept:** Coronary heart disease, impaired blood supply to the heart muscle, is the underlying problem in angina pectoris, acute coronary syndrome, and myocardial infarction, and a leading cause of heart failure. Risk factor management is key in reducing mortality and disability associated with CHD.
- The coronary arteries provide the "fuel" for the myocardium. These arteries often are affected by atherosclerosis. Narrowing of the vessel affects myocardial blood supply and can lead to angina, acute coronary syndrome, or myocardial infarction. Early treatment of atherosclerosis and its risk factors is key to preventing coronary heart disease, angina, acute coronary syndrome, and acute myocardial infarction.
- Angina is caused by myocardial ischemia, a temporary imbalance between myocardial oxygen supply and demand. Angina often indicates an increasing risk for myocardial infarction.
- Acute coronary syndrome occurs when a coronary blood flow is acutely restricted, often because atherosclerotic plaque ruptures and a clot forms at the site of this rupture. Resulting ischemia injures myocardial cells; prompt restoration of blood flow will allow these cells to recover.
- **Concept:** Acute myocardial infarction is a medical emergency, requiring prompt intervention to prevent necrosis (death) of cardiac muscle. Timely interventions to restore blood flow to the affected muscle can preserve tissue and heart function.
- Myocardial infarction results from total blockage of the blood supply to a part of the myocardium. Unless blood flow is restored within a few hours, the affected myocardium will infarct and die. This affects function of the heart muscle and cardiac output.
- Health promotion for patients with CHD and its consequences focuses on measures to reduce controllable risk factors, including smoking, diet, obesity, a sedentary lifestyle, and physiologic conditions such as high blood pressure, hypercholesterolemia, and diabetes mellitus.
- Nursing care for patients with CHD and its consequences involves activities to control pain, reduce the workload of the heart, improve oxygenation, and identify and treat complications, and teaching to slow or stop the progression of atherosclerosis.
- **Concept:** Most cardiac rhythm disruptions are benign, having little effect on cardiovascular function; others are more serious and can affect cardiac output and tissue perfusion. Timely recognition and treatment of these rhythms is vital.
- The cardiac conduction system, which controls the heart's rhythm, can be affected by disease, drugs, or electrolyte imbalances, leading to dysrhythmias. Dysrhythmias may originate in the atria, AV nodal tissue, or the ventricles. Disruption of the conduction pathways can lead to heart blocks.
- **Concept:** Approximately half of all cardiac deaths are sudden and unexpected, due to cardiac arrest. However, if observed and treated promptly, cardiac arrest may be reversible.

PEARSON NURSING STUDENT RESOURCES

Find additional materials at **nursing.pearsonhighered.com**.

Clinical Reasoning Care Map

Caring for a Patient After Coronary Artery Bypass Surgery

NCLEX-PN® Focus Area: Coping and Adaptation

Case Study: John Clements, 50 years old, had emergency triple bypass surgery 3 days ago. His initial recovery has been uneventful, and he has been transferred from the cardiac recovery unit to the cardiac unit for the remainder of his hospital stay.

Nursing Diagnosis: Ineffective Role Performance

COLLECT DATA

Subjective	Objective
_____	_____
_____	_____
_____	_____
_____	_____
_____	_____
_____	_____
_____	_____

Does this present a threat to the patient's safety?

If yes, the priority intervention to address this threat would be:

_____
_____

Nursing Care

_____
_____
_____
_____
_____
_____
_____
_____

Interprofessional team members to include when planning care:

_____
_____
_____

How would you document this? _____
_____
_____

Compare your answers and documentation to those provided on the companion website.

Data Collected
(use only those that apply)

- History of progressive angina for 4 years
- Anterior wall myocardial infarction 2 years ago; treated with immediate fibrinolytic therapy and percutaneous balloon angioplasty
- BP 138/72, P 86, regular, R 24, T 99.1°F PO
- Faint crackles left lung base
- Strong family history of CHD (father died age 51, brother died age 48 of myocardial infarctions)
- Does not smoke, uses alcohol occasionally
- Enjoys "good Southern-style cooking" and watching TV; rarely exercises other than dancing with wife and friends about once a month
- Incision clean and dry, healing well
- Color good; O_2 saturation 95% on 4 L O_2 per cannula
- Bowel sounds active, taking regular diet in small amounts
- Usually works 50 to 60 hours per week at own contracting business
- States, "I have got to get back to work! You just can't sit around in my business—you have to make sure that the work is getting done on time."

Nursing Interventions
(use only those that apply; list in priority order)

- Teach about the heart and coronary heart disease; exercise and activities; lifestyle modifications, including diet and stress management.
- Provide analgesics as needed for comfort.
- Ambulate at least four times per day for increasing distances.
- Encourage use of incentive spirometer every 1 to 2 hours.
- Encourage rest before and after activity/exercise.
- Provide information about community resources for emotional support.
- Discuss emotional reactions to CHD and sexual activity after discharge.
- Help identify coping strategies for concerns about role in business.

NCLEX-PN® Exam Preparation

1. The nurse is teaching a patient whose physician has prescribed atorvastatin (Lipitor) to be taken daily. Which of the following is vital to include in the teaching?
   1. "Report any change in the color of your skin or sclera to your doctor."
   2. "Always take this drug with a meal."
   3. "Reduce the amount of fat in your diet to less than 20% of your calories."
   4. "If your muscles become sore, increase the amount of exercise you do."

2. A patient asks the nurse how he can distinguish between angina and chest pain associated with a myocardial infarction. An accurate response by the nurse would be:
   1. "Chest pain associated with myocardial infarction is relieved by nitroglycerin."
   2. "Chest pain associated with angina is unrelieved by nitroglycerin."
   3. "Chest pain associated with angina is relieved by rest."
   4. "Chest pain associated with myocardial infarction is relieved by rest."

3. The nurse caring for a patient who has undergone a percutaneous coronary intervention identifies which of the following as the highest priority nursing diagnosis?
   1. *Ineffective coping* as evidenced by poor compliance with diet and exercise regimen
   2. *Disturbed body image* related to presence of a coronary artery stent
   3. *Impaired tissue integrity* related to catheterization of the brachial artery
   4. *Risk for ineffective peripheral tissue perfusion* related to disruption of the femoral artery

4. A male patient has experienced a myocardial infarction. The nurse assesses him for signs of complications. Which of the following would concern the nurse *most*?
   1. BP 138/84, P 72
   2. BP 90/50, urinary output 20 mL/hr
   3. P 92, urinary output 50 mL/hr
   4. BP 150/70, P 100

5. Which of the following would the nurse identify as an expected finding in a patient who was admitted for an acute myocardial infarction 24 hours ago?
   1. CK 240 U/L
   2. Hct 30%
   3. Blood glucose 210 mg/dL
   4. BUN 45 mg/dL

6. Teaching for a patient with a diagnosis of acute myocardial infarction should include which of the following?
   1. "Take nitroglycerin sublingually every 5 minutes until chest pain disappears."
   2. "Call 911 immediately if chest pain occurs."
   3. "Avoid all stress."
   4. "Adjust diet to low cholesterol, low fat, low sodium."

7. A patient who is being monitored by telemetry has a rhythm in which all ECG waveforms appear normal and have expected relationships to one another. The heart rate is 104 beats per minute. The nurse correctly charts this as:
   1. normal sinus rhythm.
   2. sinus bradycardia.
   3. sinus tachycardia.
   4. sinus arrhythmia.

8. The nurse observing the central monitor in a progressive coronary unit notes that one of the patients has abruptly developed a rhythm that appears to be ventricular tachycardia. What should the nurse do first?
   1. Initiate a cardiac arrest response (Code 99, Code Blue).
   2. Notify the physician.
   3. Assess the patient.
   4. Document the time the dysrhythmia started.

9. In preparing a patient who has experienced dysrhythmias for discharge, the nurse should:
   1. reassure the patient and families that dysrhythmias rarely recur.
   2. encourage the patient and family to become trained in cardiopulmonary resuscitation (CPR).
   3. provide resources for obtaining an automatic external defibrillator unit.
   4. stress the low incidence of adverse effects associated with antidysrhythmic drugs.

10. When initiating cardiac monitoring for a patient on a progressive cardiac unit, the nurse should: (Select all that apply.)
    1. inform the patient of the reason for monitoring.
    2. check equipment, wires, and leads for damage.
    3. apply electrode pads to each shoulder and at the sixth intercostal space, midaxillary line bilaterally.
    4. select electrode sites that are free of irritation or incisions.
    5. discuss reasons for limiting visitors during cardiac monitoring.

Answers and rationales for Review Questions appear in Appendix I.

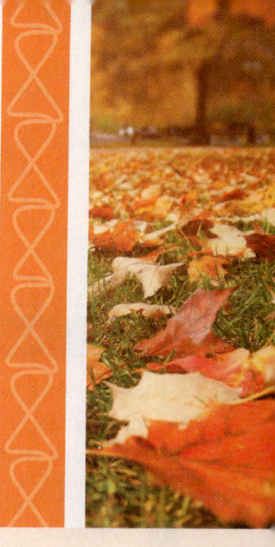

CHAPTER 17
Caring for Patients With Cardiac Disorders

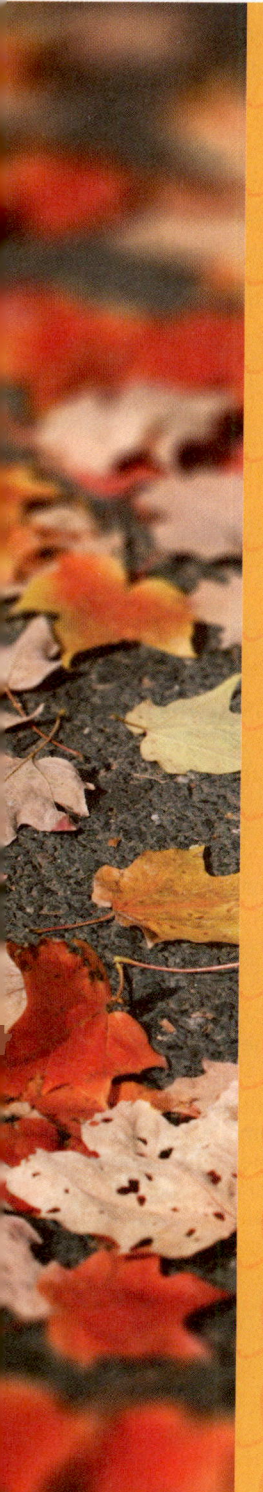

BRIEF OUTLINE

DISORDERS OF CARDIAC FUNCTION
Heart Failure
INFLAMMATORY CARDIAC DISORDERS

Rheumatic Fever and Rheumatic Heart Disease
Infective Endocarditis
Myocarditis
Pericarditis

DISORDERS OF CARDIAC STRUCTURE
Valvular Heart Disease
Cardiomyopathy

APPLIED LEARNING OUTCOMES

After completing this chapter, you will be able to:

1. Compare and contrast the causes, pathophysiology, effects, and manifestations of common cardiac disorders.
2. Safely administer drugs commonly prescribed for patients with heart disease.
3. Provide individualized and evidence-based nursing care for patients undergoing invasive procedures or surgery of the heart.
4. Use clinical judgment and the nursing process to conduct focused assessments, contribute to care planning, and provide individualized nursing care for patients with disorders of the heart.
5. Provide and reinforce appropriate teaching for patients with heart disorders and their families, taking patient values, expressed needs, and preferences into consideration.
6. Use electronic resources for planning and documenting nursing care for patients with heart disorders.

KEY TERMS

The key terms are defined on the pages listed below.

SPECIAL FEATURES

Key Concept　Disorders of the heart muscle or its structures affect its ability to pump blood effectively to meet the needs of the cells of the body. When the heart is unable to function effectively, other organ systems may fail because their fuel supply is impaired.

In this chapter, you will learn about heart failure, a common chronic disease with potentially devastating effects, and about other disorders of the heart that can lead to heart failure. In addition, you will learn how to apply clinical judgment and the nursing process in caring for patients with heart disease.

DISORDERS OF CARDIAC FUNCTION

Heart Failure

Key Concept　Heart failure, the inability of the heart to meet the body's needs for fuel and oxygen, is caused by impaired pumping of the heart. It is usually caused by extensive heart muscle damage from myocardial infarction, but can also result from inflammatory, congenital, or valve disorders.

Heart failure is defined as the inability of the heart to function as a pump to meet the needs of the body. Heart failure is common: It is the fourth leading cause of hospital admissions in the United States, accounting for 970,000 inpatient hospitalizations in 2011 (Pfuntner, Wier, & Stocks, 2013). Heart failure may result from any condition that (1) impairs effective contraction of the heart muscle, (2) chronically increases the workload of the heart, or (3) acutely increases the workload of the heart (Table 17-1■). Hypertension and coronary heart disease with myocardial ischemia and myocardial infarction (MI) are the leading causes of heart failure in the United States.

The incidence of heart failure increases significantly with age, affecting up to 10% of people age 65 and older. African Americans, who have a high incidence of hypertension, also have a significant risk of developing heart failure (see Box 17-1■). Heart failure generally is a chronic progressive disease, with the patient experiencing declining heart function and more frequent episodes of failure. Improved disease management, however, has led to significant declines in hospitalizations among older adults since 1997 (31% in people aged 65–84 and 18% in people aged 85 years and older) (Pfuntner et al., 2013). Box 17-2■ shows the American Heart Association classification for heart failure.

PATHOPHYSIOLOGY

Cardiac output, the amount of blood pumped by the ventricles in 1 minute, is a product of two factors: the amount of blood ejected from the ventricles with each contraction (*stroke volume*) and the heart rate. A change in either the stroke volume or the heart rate affects cardiac output. Damage to the heart muscle, the most common cause of heart failure, affects the ability of the heart to contract effectively and eject blood from the ventricles, reducing stroke volume and cardiac output.

When the cardiac output drops, *compensatory mechanisms* are activated to maintain blood flow to body tissues. The sympathetic nervous system (SNS) is stimulated. As a result, the heart rate and stroke volume increase. SNS stimulation also causes arteries and veins to constrict, increasing venous return to the heart. Increased venous return increases ventricular filling and myocardial stretch (preload), increasing the force of contraction. Blood flow is redistributed to the brain and the heart to maintain perfusion of these vital organs.

TABLE 17-1	Selected Causes of Heart Failure	
IMPAIRED FUNCTION	**INCREASED WORKLOAD**	**NONCARDIAC CONDITIONS**
Coronary heart disease	Hypertension	Pulmonary hypertension
Cardiomyopathies	Valve disorders	Hyperthyroidism
Rheumatic fever	Chronic anemia	
Infective endocarditis	Congenital heart defects	

BOX 17-1	FOCUS ON DIVERSITY

Heart Failure

- Since 1988, the prevalence of heart failure among Blacks has increased, whereas it has slightly decreased among Whites.
- For both men and women, heart failure mortality rates are highest in Blacks and lowest for Asians. Between these extremes, Whites have higher heart failure death rates than American Indians or Hispanics.
- Among all ethnic groups, heart failure death rates are higher in men than in women.

Source: National Heart, Lung, and Blood Institute (NHLBI). (2013). *Fact book. Fiscal year 2012.* Bethesda, MD: National Institutes of Health.

A—At high risk for heart failure, but no structural heart disease or symptoms
B—Structural heart disease, but no symptoms of heart failure
C—Structural heart disease with current or prior symptoms of heart failure
D—Advanced heart disease with symptoms of heart failure at rest despite treatment

A decrease in cardiac output also activates the renin–angiotensin–aldosterone system, which leads to additional vasoconstriction and salt and water retention. Salt and water retention increases the blood volume to help restore cardiac output.

The chambers of the heart dilate to accommodate the additional fluid volume. Initially, this leads to more effective contractions. Cardiac muscle cells enlarge, leading to *ventricular hypertrophy*.

Although all these responses may help maintain cardiac output for a time, their long-term effects hasten the deterioration of cardiac function. Heart failure occurs when these mechanisms no longer maintain a cardiac output that meets the metabolic needs of the body.

The rapid heart rate, salt and water retention, increased preload, and arterial vasoconstriction increase the workload of the heart. The ventricles continue to dilate to accommodate the excess fluid, but the heart eventually loses its ability to contract forcefully. The heart muscle may become so large that the coronary blood supply is inadequate, causing myocardial ischemia.

Cardiac reserve is the ability of the heart to adjust its output to meet the metabolic needs of the body. Patients with heart failure have very little cardiac reserve. At rest, they may be unaffected; however, any stressor (e.g., exercise, illness) taxes their ability to meet the demand for oxygen and nutrients.

Heart failure is often classified by the primary pumping chamber affected. Patients may have manifestations of *left-sided* and/or *right-sided failure*. The effects of heart failure on cardiac output and venous congestion are referred to as *forward* and *backward effects*. Heart failure also may be classified as either *acute* or *chronic*.

Left-Sided Heart Failure

Although either side of the heart can fail, the left ventricle is affected more often than the right because of its high workload and oxygen demand. Left-sided heart failure results from ventricular muscle damage or overloading. As left ventricular function deteriorates, cardiac output falls (*forward effect*). Impaired emptying of the left ventricle leads to increased pressures on the left side of the heart and in

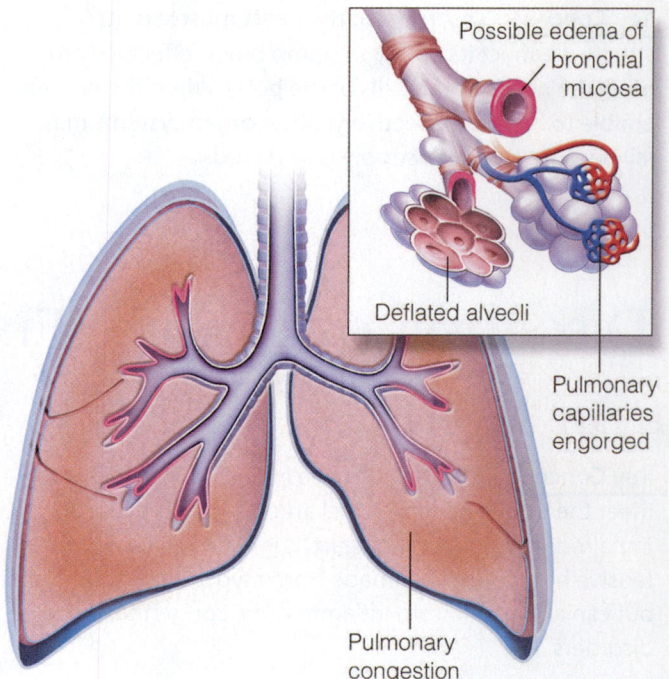

Figure 17-1. ■ Left-sided heart failure causes increased pressure and congestion in the pulmonary vascular system, leading to dyspnea and shortness of breath. (Source: From Pearson Education/ PH College. Published by Pearson Education.)

the pulmonary vascular system (*backward effects*). Increased pressures in this normally low-pressure system push fluid from the blood vessels into interstitial tissues and the alveoli (Figure 17-1■).

The manifestations of left-sided heart failure result from pulmonary congestion and decreased cardiac output (Table 17-2■). Fatigue, activity intolerance, and dyspnea on exertion (DOE) are common early manifestations. **Orthopnea** (breathing difficulty while lying down) may prompt the patient to sleep propped up on two or three pillows or in a recliner. Inspiratory crackles (rales) and wheezes may be heard in lung bases.

TABLE 17-2	Manifestations of Heart Failure	
	LEFT-SIDED FAILURE	**RIGHT-SIDED FAILURE**
Forward effects	Activity intolerance	Fatigue
	Fatigue	Activity intolerance
	Weakness	
	Dizziness and syncope	
Backward effects	Shortness of breath	Jugular vein distention
	Dyspnea, orthopnea	Peripheral edema
	Cough	Anorexia, nausea
	Tachycardia	Abdominal distention, ascites
	Crackles in lung bases	Liver, spleen enlargement, tenderness

ACUTE PULMONARY EDEMA   **Acute pulmonary edema**, accumulation of fluid in the interstitial spaces and alveoli of the lungs, may occur with severe left ventricular failure. The patient in pulmonary edema has acute and severe dyspnea, shortness of breath, and anxiety. The skin is cool, clammy, and cyanotic. A productive cough with pink, frothy sputum is also present. If cerebral hypoxia occurs, the patient may be confused or lethargic. Crackles are heard throughout the lung fields. As the condition worsens, breathing becomes more labored and lung sounds harsher. Pulmonary edema is a medical emergency: The patient is "drowning" as a result of fluid in the alveolar and pulmonary spaces and must be treated immediately.

Right-Sided Heart Failure

The most common cause of right ventricular failure is left ventricular failure. Increased pressures in the pulmonary system or damage to the right ventricle impairs blood flow into the pulmonary circulation. The right ventricle and atrium become distended, and blood accumulates in the systemic venous system. Increased venous pressures lead to abdominal organ congestion and peripheral tissue edema (Figure 17-2■).

Fluid collects in dependent tissues because of the effects of gravity. Edema develops in the feet and legs of an upright patient and in the sacrum of one who is reclining. Congestion of vessels in the abdomen can lead to right upper quadrant pain, anorexia, and nausea. Distended neck veins (Figure 17-3■) may be visible even when the patient is standing (see Table 17-2).

Biventricular Failure

When both ventricles fail to function adequately, the patient has manifestations of both right- and left-sided, or *biventricular,* heart failure. **Paroxysmal nocturnal dyspnea**

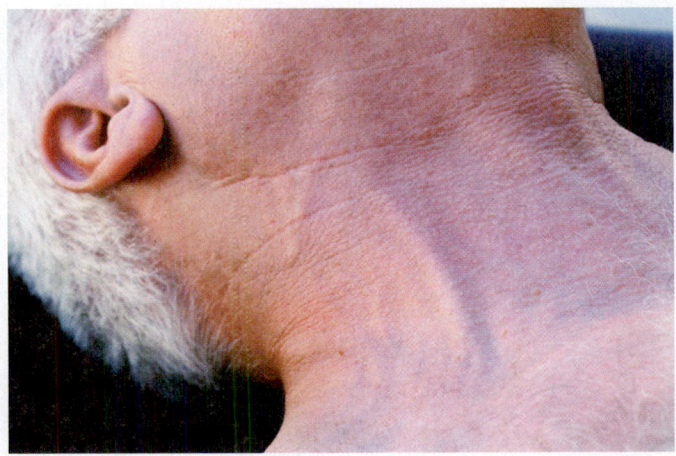

Figure 17-3. ■ Distended neck veins reflecting the backward effects of right-sided and biventricular heart failure. (Source: Pearson Education)

(PND), a frightening condition in which the patient awakens at night acutely short of breath, may occur. PND occurs when edema fluid that has accumulated during the day is reabsorbed into the circulation at night, causing fluid overload and pulmonary congestion. The patient in severe heart failure may be dyspneic at rest as well as with activity, signifying little or no cardiac reserve.

Acute and Chronic Failure

Acute heart failure occurs as a result of acute damage to the heart muscle, for example, resulting from a large acute MI. *Chronic heart failure,* in contrast, develops gradually as the result of a long-standing or progressive condition such as hypertension or valve disease. Figure 17-4■ illustrates the multisystem effects of heart failure.

COLLABORATIVE CARE

The main goals of care for the patient with heart failure are to reduce cardiac workload, improve cardiac pumping ability, and control fluid retention. The focus is on improving activity tolerance and decreasing mortality and morbidity.

Diagnostic Tests

Diagnostic tests are used to identify heart failure and evaluate its effects. *Brain natriuretic peptide (BNP)* is a hormone released from ventricular heart muscle in response to changes in blood volume and pressure overload. BNP levels increase in heart failure but do not change in other cardiac disorders, making it a valuable indicator of heart failure. *Serum electrolytes* are measured to evaluate fluid and electrolyte status, as well as to monitor the effects of treatment. The *chest x-ray* may show pulmonary vascular congestion and cardiomegaly if the heart has hypertrophied or dilated. An *echocardiogram* is done to evaluate left ventricular function and assess for ventricular dilation and hypertrophy. The electrocardiogram (ECG) shows changes associated

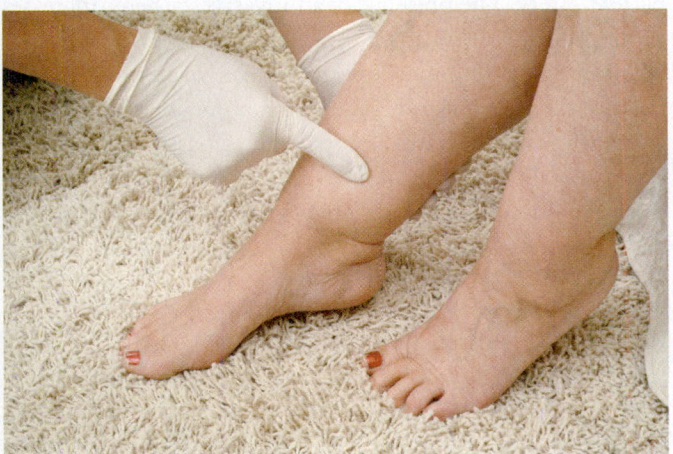

Figure 17-2. ■ Edema of the feet and ankles of a patient with heart failure. (Source: Pearson Education)

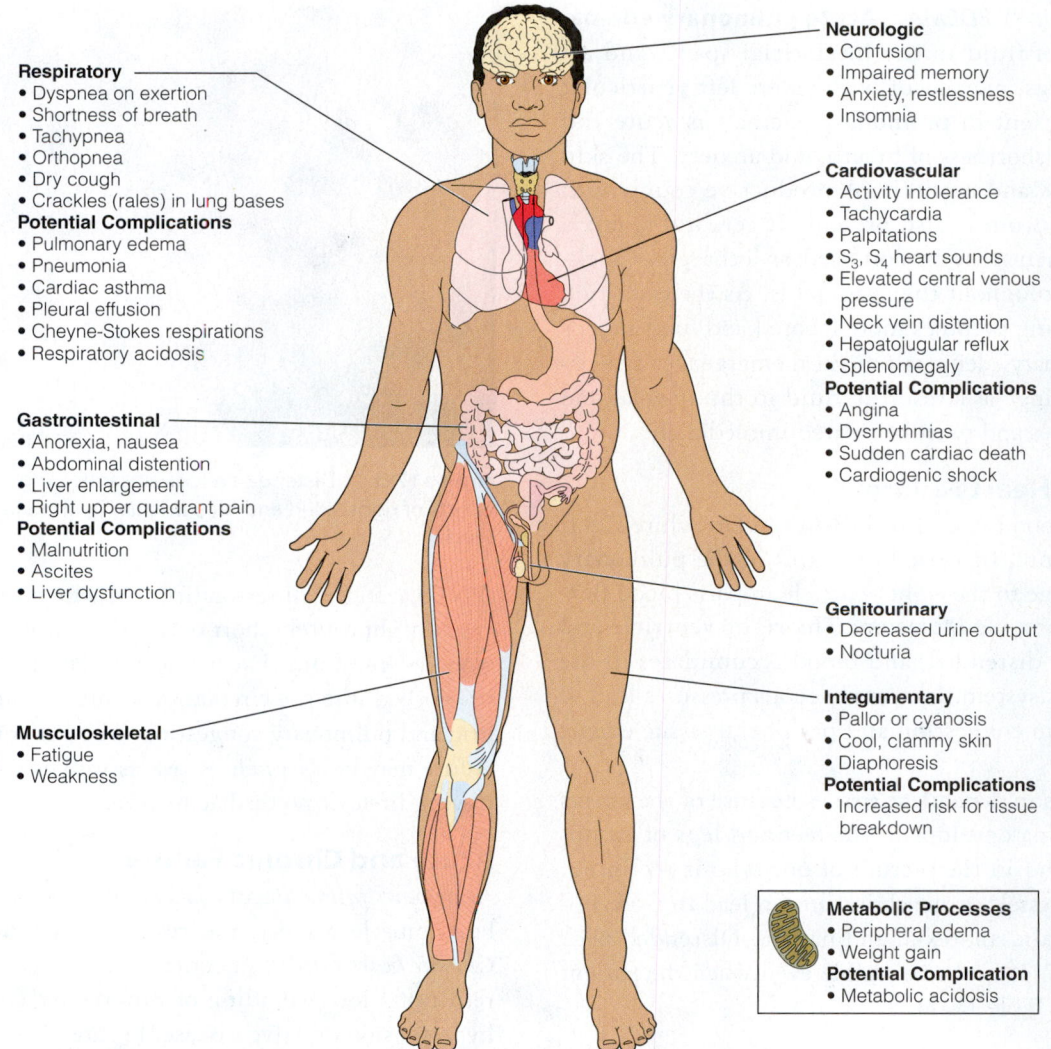

Respiratory
- Dyspnea on exertion
- Shortness of breath
- Tachypnea
- Orthopnea
- Dry cough
- Crackles (rales) in lung bases

Potential Complications
- Pulmonary edema
- Pneumonia
- Cardiac asthma
- Pleural effusion
- Cheyne-Stokes respirations
- Respiratory acidosis

Gastrointestinal
- Anorexia, nausea
- Abdominal distention
- Liver enlargement
- Right upper quadrant pain

Potential Complications
- Malnutrition
- Ascites
- Liver dysfunction

Musculoskeletal
- Fatigue
- Weakness

Neurologic
- Confusion
- Impaired memory
- Anxiety, restlessness
- Insomnia

Cardiovascular
- Activity intolerance
- Tachycardia
- Palpitations
- S_3, S_4 heart sounds
- Elevated central venous pressure
- Neck vein distention
- Hepatojugular reflux
- Splenomegaly

Potential Complications
- Angina
- Dysrhythmias
- Sudden cardiac death
- Cardiogenic shock

Genitourinary
- Decreased urine output
- Nocturia

Integumentary
- Pallor or cyanosis
- Cool, clammy skin
- Diaphoresis

Potential Complications
- Increased risk for tissue breakdown

Metabolic Processes
- Peripheral edema
- Weight gain

Potential Complication
- Metabolic acidosis

Figure 17-4. ■ The multisystem effects of heart failure.

with ventricular enlargement and may show dysrhythmias, myocardial ischemia, or infarction. *Coronary angiography* may be performed in patients who have angina as well as heart failure.

Hemodynamic Monitoring

Hemodynamics is the study of the pressures involved in blood circulation. *Hemodynamic monitoring* may be used to assess cardiovascular function and the patient's response to treatment. A multilumen catheter inserted through a central vein into the right side of the heart and pulmonary artery is used to measure central venous pressure, pulmonary artery pressures, and cardiac output. These pressures and the cardiac output are used to evaluate fluid balance, ventricular function, and the effects of interventions (e.g., drug therapy). The arterial blood pressure can be measured using a peripheral arterial line.

The pressure within a vessel is converted into an electrical signal. The electrical signal is then recorded on

graph paper and displayed on a monitor (Figure 17-5■). Although hemodynamic monitoring provides valuable information to help manage heart failure, it has some risks to patient safety. The presence of an invasive catheter increases the risk of infection, bleeding, and thrombus formation. The lung may be punctured during insertion of the catheter into the subclavian vein, causing a pneumothorax. Dysrhythmias may develop as the catheter passes through the right ventricle. Patients undergoing hemodynamic monitoring require close monitoring and high-level nursing care and therefore usually are placed in an intensive care unit.

Medications

Patients with heart failure typically receive multiple medications to reduce cardiac work and improve cardiac function. The main drug classes used to treat heart failure are the angiotensin-converting enzyme (ACE) inhibitors, angiotensin II receptor blockers (ARBs), beta blockers, diuretics, **inotropic** medications (drugs that increase the

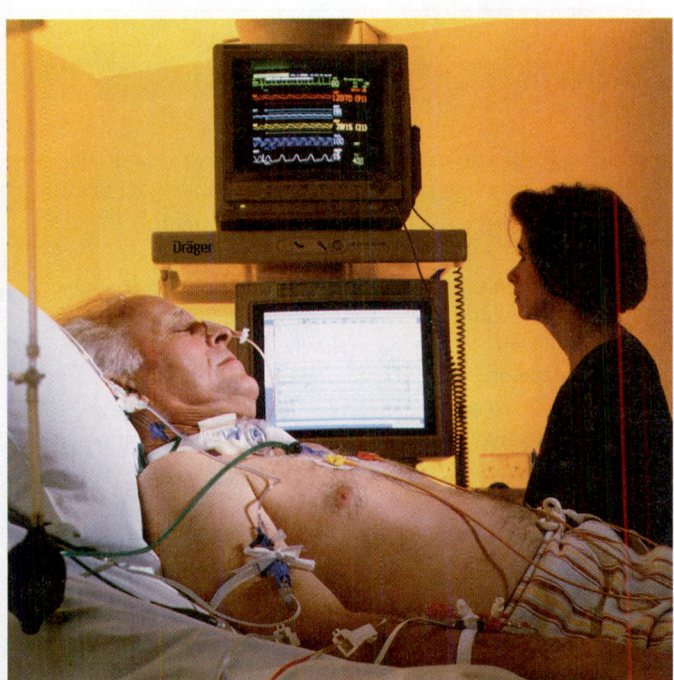

Figure 17-5. ■ The nurse observes tracings of a patient's hemodynamic pressures. The upper screen in the background shows (from top): heart rate (green); arterial blood pressure (red and yellow); central venous pressure (CVP, light blue); blood oxygen (dark blue); respiration rate (white). (Source: James King-Holmes / Science Source.)

strength of the heart's contractions), and direct vasodilators. BiDil, a fixed-dose combination of two vasodilators (hydralazine and isosorbide), is approved by the FDA for treating heart failure in African Americans. Table 17-3■ outlines nursing responsibilities related to several of these drug classes. Complementary treatment with hawthorn is discussed in Box 17-3■.

Acute pulmonary edema is a medical emergency requiring aggressive treatment. A potent loop diuretic such as furosemide is given intravenously. Furosemide is a rapid-acting and very effective diuretic that also acts as a vasodilator. Direct vasodilator drugs such as nitroglycerin, isosorbide, nitroprusside, or nesiritide are also given. Nesiritide (Natrecor), a synthetic form of BNP, is a potent vasodilator that also has diuretic effects. The combination of diuretic and vasodilator drugs can rapidly reduce the workload of the failing heart. Morphine sulfate is also used for treating acute pulmonary edema. Morphine relieves anxiety, improves breathing, and is also a venous vasodilator. It reduces venous return and lowers left atrial pressure.

DIGITALIS   Digitalis (*digoxin*) has a positive inotropic effect on the heart, increasing the strength of myocardial contraction. Digoxin has a *narrow therapeutic index*; in other words, therapeutic levels are very close to toxic levels. Optimal serum digoxin levels are between 0.5 and 0.8 ng/mL; levels

higher than 1.0 ng/mL increase the risk of toxicity. Early manifestations of digitalis toxicity include anorexia, nausea and vomiting, headache, changes in vision, and confusion. A number of dysrhythmias are also associated with digitalis toxicity. Low serum potassium levels increase the risk of digitalis toxicity, as do low magnesium and high calcium levels. Older adults are at particular risk for digitalis toxicity.

clinical**ALERT**

Always take an apical pulse before administering digoxin. If the pulse rate is less than 60 per minute or if the patient has manifestations of digitalis toxicity, hold the drug and notify the charge nurse or physician.

Diet and Activity

Patients in heart failure are generally put on a restricted sodium diet to minimize sodium and water retention. An intake of 2 to 3 g of sodium per day, a moderate restriction, is recommended, although intake of less than 2 g/day may be prescribed for patients with moderate-to-severe heart failure. Activity may be significantly limited during acute episodes of heart failure to reduce cardiac workload. Activity is gradually increased as the patient's condition improves and routine modest exercise is encouraged to improve cardiovascular performance and quality of life (Box 17-4■)

Implanted Devices

An implantable cardiac defibrillator (ICD) to reduce the risk of sudden cardiac death may be prophylactically implanted in patients with mild-to-moderate heart failure. Patients with symptomatic heart failure may benefit from an implanted biventricular pacemaker (also called cardiac resynchronization therapy, or CRT) that coordinates right and left ventricular contraction. CRT improves exercise tolerance and quality of life, and decreases mortality (Longo et al., 2012). Patients with moderate-to-severe heart failure may have a combination ICD/biventricular pacemaker.

Surgery

Heart transplantation is the primary treatment for end-stage heart failure. In most cases, the patient's diseased heart is removed, leaving portions of the atria intact. The donor heart is sutured to the remaining atrial walls (Figure 17-6■). Although cardiac transplantation benefits many patients with end-stage heart disease, it is limited by the availability of donor hearts. Transplanted organs typically are obtained from young accident victims with no evidence of cardiac trauma.

Ventricular assist devices (VADs) are often used as a bridge to transplantation. The VAD is a mechanical pump

TABLE 17-3	Giving Medications Safely: Heart Failure		
CLASS/DRUGS	**PURPOSE**	**NURSING IMPLICATIONS**	**PATIENT TEACHING**
Angiotensin-converting enzyme (ACE) inhibitors ■ Enalapril (Vasotec) ■ *Lisinopril (Prinivil, Zestril)* ■ Captopril (Capoten) ■ Moexipril (Univasc) ■ Ramipril (Altace) ■ Fosinopril (Monopril) ■ Quinapril (Accupril) ■ Trandolapril (Mavik) *Angiotensin II receptor blockers (ARBs)* ■ Candesartan (Atacand) ■ Irbesartan (Avapro) ■ *Losartan (Cozaar)* ■ *Olmesartan medoxomil (Benicar)* ■ Telmisartan (Micardis) ■ *Valsartan (Diovan)*	ACE inhibitors and ARBs block the effect of the renin–angiotensin–aldosterone system, reducing vasoconstriction and sodium and water retention. The result is decreased cardiac workload and reduced edema.	Avoid discontinuing these agents abruptly. Give captopril 1 hour before meals. Maintain bed rest and monitor BP for 3 hours after the initial dose because significant hypotension can develop. Monitor serum potassium levels during treatment because hyperkalemia may develop.	Do not stop taking your drugs without talking to your doctor. Keep follow-up medical appointments. Avoid sudden position changes; for example, rise from bed slowly. Report easy bruising and bleeding, sore throat, fever, weight gain of 2 lb or more per day, edema, dizziness, or skin rash. Immediately report swelling of the face, lips, or eyelids, itching, or breathing problems.
Diuretics ■ *Hydrochlorothiazide (HydroDIURIL)* ■ Chlorothiazide (Diuril) ■ *Furosemide (Lasix)* ■ Ethacrynic acid (Edecrin) ■ Bumetanide (Bumex) ■ Spironolactone (Aldactone) ■ Triamterene (Dyrenium) ■ Amiloride (Midamor) ■ Acetazolamide (Diamox)	Diuretics act on different portions of the kidney tubule to promote sodium and water excretion. With the exception of the potassium-sparing diuretics—spironolactone, triamterene, and amiloride—diuretics also promote potassium excretion, increasing the risk of hypokalemia.	Monitor fluid volume status: BP, intake and output, weight, skin turgor, edema. Assess for volume depletion, particularly with loop diuretics (furosemide, ethacrynic acid, and bumetanide): dizziness, orthostatic hypotension, tachycardia, muscle cramping. Notify the charge nurse or physician of abnormal serum electrolyte values. Administer intravenous furosemide slowly, no more than 20 mg/min. Notify the physician if the patient is on an aminoglycoside antibiotic. When given concurrently with furosemide or ethacrynic acid, there is an increased risk of ototoxicity and hearing loss.	Report abdominal pain, jaundice, dark urine, abnormal bleeding or bruising, flulike symptoms, signs of electrolyte imbalance, or dehydration to your doctor. Monitor your blood pressure, pulse, and weight daily. Report changes in your weight of 2 lb or more per day. Avoid making sudden position changes. You may feel dizzy, light-headed, or faint. Drink at least 6 to 8 glasses of water per day. Take your diuretic when it will be the least disruptive to your lifestyle. Take with meals to decrease GI symptoms. Unless you are taking a potassium-sparing diuretic, increase intake of potassium-rich foods. Limit salt intake.
Positive inotropic agents *Digitalis glycosides* ■ *Digoxin (Lanoxin)*	Improve myocardial contractility, increasing stroke volume and cardiac output. Greater cardiac output improves renal perfusion, decreasing renin secretion and cardiac work. Slow heart rate and reduce oxygen consumption.	Assess apical pulse before giving digitalis. Hold the drug and notify the physician if heart rate is less than 60 beats/min. Record heart rate on medication record. Assess serum electrolytes and digoxin levels. Hypokalemia increases the risk of digitalis toxicity.	Take your pulse before each dose. Do not take the digitalis if your pulse is less than 60. Notify your doctor immediately. Call your doctor if you develop palpitations, weakness, loss of appetite, nausea, vomiting, abdominal pain, blurred or colored vision, double vision.

TABLE 17-3	Giving Medications Safely: Heart Failure *(continued)*		
CLASS/DRUGS	**PURPOSE**	**NURSING IMPLICATIONS**	**PATIENT TEACHING**
		Report manifestations of digitalis toxicity: anorexia, nausea, vomiting, abdominal pain, weakness, vision changes (diplopia, blurred vision, halos seen around objects), and dysrhythmias.	Avoid antacids and laxatives; they decrease the absorption of digoxin. Include high-potassium foods in your diet: orange or tomato juice, bananas, raisins, dates, figs, prunes, apricots, spinach, cauliflower, and potatoes.
Other inotropic agents ■ Dopamine (Intropin) ■ Dobutamine (Dobutrex) ■ Milrinone (Primacor)	These potent inotropic drugs improve the force of ventricular contraction and are used to treat acute pulmonary edema. They are given intravenously, adjusting the dose to obtain maximal effect. Milrinone also causes vasodilation, reducing cardiac workload.	Use an infusion pump to administer these drugs. Frequently monitor vital signs and hemodynamic measurements. Titrate the drug to maintain the BP and heart rate. Avoid discontinuing these agents abruptly. Change solutions and tubing every 24 hours.	Notify the nursing staff if you experience abdominal pain or notice a skin rash or bruising.
Direct vasodilators ■ Nitroglycerin ■ Isosorbide ■ Nitroprusside ■ Nesiritide (Natrecor)	Direct vasodilators act on the blood vessels, causing them to dilate. Venous dilation reduces the amount of blood returning to the right heart, reducing the overall workload of the heart. Arterial dilation reduces afterload, directly reducing the heart's workload. Nitroglycerin primarily affects the veins (venodilation); nitroprusside and nesiritide dilate both arterioles and veins.	These drugs, particularly when given intravenously, can cause significant hypotension. Continuously monitor the blood pressure, promptly reporting a fall below prescribed levels. Reflex tachycardia and cardiac dysrhythmias are a risk. Continuously monitor cardiac rhythm, reporting a heart rate above identified limits or other abnormal rhythms. Nesiritide may cause renal damage. Monitor urine output and renal function studies, reporting an output of less than 30 mL/hr and/or abnormal lab results.	Although these drugs can be very effective in treating acute heart failure, you will be monitored continuously while receiving them because they can have serious adverse effects. Promptly report chest pain, headache, dizziness, or nausea.

Note: Medications identified in *italics* are among the 200 most frequently prescribed drugs in the United States.

connected to the diseased ventricle to reduce its workload and help maintain cardiac output. The VAD usually is used to support the left ventricle (LVAD), although right and biventricular VADs may be used. Blood enters the LVAD through an intake placed in the left ventricle and is pumped into the aorta. Some LVADs pump continuously; others fill to a certain level, then pump a bolus of blood into the circulation, mimicking a normal pulsation. Currently available VADs require an external power source, but portable VADs are small enough to allow the patient to live at home.

Nursing care of the heart transplant patient is similar to the care of any cardiac surgery patient. Bleeding is a major concern in the early postoperative period. Chest tube drainage, urinary output, heart rhythm, and hemodynamic parameters are frequently monitored. Cardiac tamponade (compression of the heart) can develop, interfering with its ability to fill and contract. Care is taken to rewarm the patient gradually and to prevent shivering.

Infection and rejection of the transplanted organ are the leading causes of death in transplant recipients. Rejection of the transplanted heart can occur at any time. Acute

Heart Failure

The dried fruit of the hawthorn (also known as English hawthorn, maybush, or whitethorn) or a tincture or liquid extract of the fruit or leaf may benefit the patient with heart failure. Hawthorn increases coronary blood flow and has positive inotropic effects. Therapeutically, it increases cardiac output; decreases the blood pressure, cardiac workload, and oxygen consumption; and acts similar to an ACE inhibitor. Advise patients to consult their health care provider before taking hawthorn or using it in conjunction with prescribed drugs.

Clinical trials have shown that fish oil supplementation has a beneficial effect in patients with heart failure, reducing both heart-related hospitalizations and mortality. Fish oil supplements improve left ventricular filling and function, and promote vasodilation, reducing cardiac work. Again, patients should be advised to talk with their physician before starting a fish oil supplement.

Mind–body therapy such as mindfulness meditation can improve mental health in patients with a chronic disease such as heart failure. In meditation, the attention is focused on a designated object, such as one's breath. The effect of meditation goes beyond simple relaxation to actually affecting autonomic nervous system responses.

rejection usually occurs within weeks of the transplantation procedure, developing when the immune system identifies the transplanted organ as foreign. Acute rejection is a leading cause of death within the first years after surgery. Immunosuppressive drugs are given to prevent rejection. Although these drugs help prevent rejection, they also leave the patient with impaired defenses against infection.

Aggressive nursing care to prevent infection is vital: limiting visitors with communicable diseases, pulmonary hygiene measures, early ambulation, and strict aseptic technique. Because immunosuppressive drugs may mask symptoms of rejection, patients are routinely monitored with tissue biopsies of the transplanted organ.

NURSING CARE

Heart failure is a chronic disease that impacts quality of life, interfering with such day-to-day activities as self-care and role performance. Patients and their families need a clear understanding of day-to-day management strategies and symptoms that may signal an exacerbation.

PRIORITIZING NURSING CARE

During an acute episode of heart failure, reducing the oxygen demand of the heart is a major nursing care goal. The patient experiencing acute heart failure may be critically ill because the heart is unable to meet the needs of the cells for blood and oxygen. As the heart becomes less effective as a pump, vessels and tissues become congested with fluid. Congestion of the pulmonary circulation can impair gas exchange, compounding the patient's condition. Nursing care for the patient in acute failure is directed toward measures that help reduce the workload of the heart.

HEALTH PROMOTION

Coronary heart disease (CHD) is the major cause of heart failure. Measures to prevent CHD also reduce the incidence of heart failure. Teach all patients about cardiac risk

Activity Guidelines for Patients With Heart Failure

- Perform as many activities as independently as you can.
- Space meals and activities. Eat six small meals a day. Allow rest periods during the day.
- Perform all activities at a comfortable pace; rest for 15 minutes if you get tired.
- Stop any activity that causes chest pain, shortness of breath, dizziness, excessive weakness, or sweating. Rest. Notify your doctor if your activity tolerance changes and if symptoms continue after rest.
- Avoid straining. Do not lift heavy objects. Eat a high-fiber diet and drink plenty of water to prevent constipation. Use bulk-forming laxatives or stool softeners, as allowed, to avoid constipation and straining.
- Begin a graded exercise program. Walking is good exercise. Plan to walk twice a day at a comfortable, slow pace initially, and then gradually increase the distance and pace. Below is a suggested schedule:

Week 1	200 to 400 yards ($\frac{1}{4}$ mile)	Twice a day, slow leisurely pace
Week 2	$\frac{1}{4}$ mile	15 min, minimum of 3 times per week
Week 3	$\frac{1}{2}$ mile	30 min, minimum of 3 times per week
Week 4	1 mile	30 min, minimum of 3 times per week
Week 5	$\frac{1}{2}$ mile	30 min, minimum of 3 times per week
Week 6	2 miles	40 min, minimum of 3 times per week

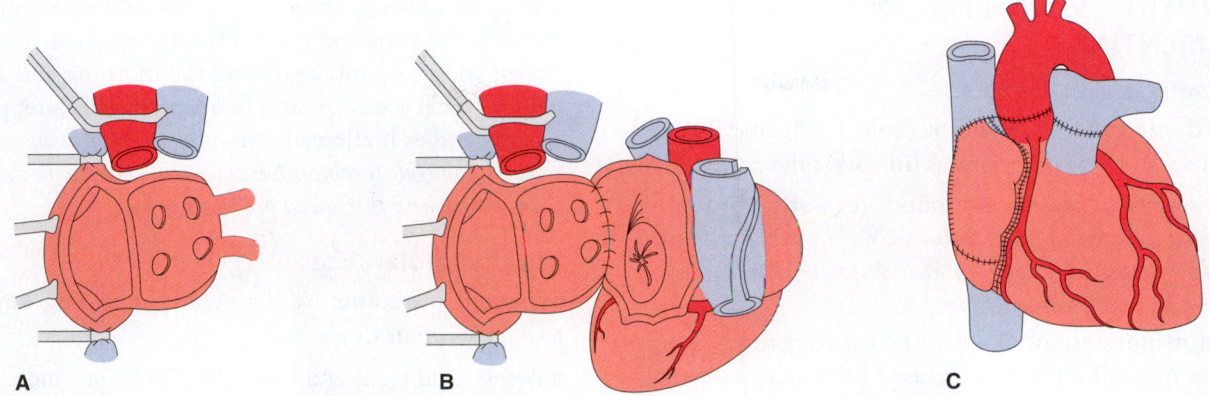

Figure 17-6. ■ Cardiac transplantation. (**A**) The diseased heart is removed, leaving the posterior walls of the atria intact. (**B** and **C**) The donor heart is sutured to the atria and the great vessels.

factors and lifestyle changes to reduce or eliminate controllable risk factors. Emphasize the importance of controlling hypertension, managing diabetes, maintaining a healthy weight, and not starting to smoke or quitting smoking.

For the patient with heart failure, health promotion focuses on teaching measures to maintain cardiac reserve and prevent acute exacerbations: maintaining a progressive exercise program, consuming a diet low in sodium, and avoiding exposure to acute contagious diseases, particularly influenza and other upper respiratory infections.

ASSESSING

Patients with heart failure require frequent and careful nursing assessment. Box 17-5■ outlines initial and ongoing focused assessment for the patient with heart failure.

IDENTIFYING POTENTIAL COMPLICATIONS

Acute pulmonary edema is an acute, emergent complication of heart failure. Report increasing restlessness, anxiety, orthopnea, increased heart and respiratory rates, cough, and dropping oxygen saturation levels, as these may be early manifestations of pulmonary edema. Frequently assess breath sounds for increasing inspiratory crackles. Report cough productive of pink frothy sputum, a hallmark sign of cardiogenic pulmonary edema.

Patients with severe chronic heart failure may develop liver or kidney failure as a result of impaired organ perfusion. Impaired cerebral perfusion can lead to changes in mental status. Report changes in level of consciousness or cognition, skin color, abdominal girth or bowel sounds, or urinary or fecal output. Monitor laboratory values, including liver and renal function tests.

BOX 17-5	ASSESSMENT

Patients With Heart Failure

Subjective Data

- Shortness of breath, level of activity; number of pillows used to sleep; swelling of legs and feet; weight changes; appetite, nausea, abdominal discomfort
- History of MI or other heart disease, recent stressors such as upper respiratory infection; previous or current treatment; current medications
- Risk factors: family history of heart disease; history of hypertension, diabetes, high blood cholesterol levels; smoking, and alcohol intake
- Understanding of disease and treatment, compliance with activity prescriptions; current diet and use of salt

Objective Data

- Vital signs at rest and changes with activity; cardiac rhythm; any dysrhythmias

- Dyspnea and its relationship to activity; oxygen saturation levels
- Skin color, temperature, and moisture; capillary refill; extent and degree of dependent edema; presence of neck vein distention
- Heart and lung sounds; presence of S_3 or S_4 heart sounds; presence and extent of crackles or wheezes on auscultation of lungs
- Intake and output; daily weight
- Level of consciousness; anxiety or fear
- Hemodynamic parameters such as pulmonary artery pressure and cardiac output as ordered
- Laboratory test results: BNP levels; serum electrolytes; serum drug levels (e.g., digitalis levels); arterial blood gases (ABGs)

DIAGNOSING, PLANNING, AND IMPLEMENTING

Decreased Cardiac Output

Expected outcome: Skin will be pink, warm, and dry, and vital signs will be within normal limits for the patient.

■ Auscultate heart and breath sounds regularly. *An S$_3$ or an S$_4$ may be heard in heart failure. Crackles are often heard in the lung bases; increasing crackles, dyspnea, and shortness of breath indicate worsening failure.*

■ Report manifestations of decreased cardiac output: changes in mental status; decreased urine output; cool, clammy skin; low oxygen saturation levels; tachycardia, diminished pulses; pallor or cyanosis; dysrhythmias. *These are manifestations of decreased tissue perfusion.*

■ Administer oxygen as needed. *This improves oxygenation of the blood, decreasing the effects of hypoxia and ischemia.*

■ Administer medications as ordered. *Drugs are used to decrease the cardiac workload and increase the effectiveness of contractions.*

■ Encourage rest, explaining its purpose. Keep the head of the bed elevated to reduce the work of breathing. Provide a bedside commode, and assist with personal needs. *These measures reduce cardiac workload.*

■ Maintain a quiet environment, allow the patient to express fears and feelings, and explain the reasons for medical and nursing care. *These measures reduce anxiety and decrease oxygen consumption.*

Excess Fluid Volume

Expected outcome: Will demonstrate increased ease of breathing and reduced peripheral edema.

■ Immediately notify the physician if the patient develops air hunger, an overwhelming sense of impending doom or panic, tachypnea, orthopnea, or a cough productive of pink, frothy sputum. *Acute pulmonary edema, a medical emergency, can develop rapidly, requiring immediate intervention to preserve life.*

■ Monitor intake and output. Notify the physician if urine output drops to less than 30 mL/hr. *Intake and output records help evaluate the effectiveness of treatment. A drop in urine output may indicate reduced cardiac output.*

■ Weigh daily. *Weight is an accurate measure of fluid status; 1 L of fluid is equal to 1 kg or 2.2 lb of weight.*

■ Place in Fowler's or high Fowler's position, with the head of bed elevated to 45 degrees. *Elevating the head of the bed reduces venous return to the heart, decreasing its work. It also improves lung expansion.*

■ Report vital sign changes, distended neck veins, peripheral edema, weight gain, increased dyspnea, or dysrhythmias to the charge nurse or physician. *These may indicate progressive worsening of the patient's condition.*

■ Administer diuretics and other medications as ordered. *Diuretics increase sodium and water excretion.*

■ Restrict fluids as ordered. Encourage the patient to help choose the time and type of fluid consumed. Schedule the majority of intake during the morning and afternoon. Offer ice chips and frequent mouth care; provide hard candies if allowed. *Involving the patient increases the sense of control. Ice chips, hard candies, and mouth care relieve dry mouth and thirst and promote comfort.*

Activity Intolerance

Expected outcome: Will tolerate increasing amounts of activity without dyspnea.

■ Assess vital signs and heart rhythm before and after activity. *Tachycardia, dysrhythmias, changes in blood pressure, diaphoresis, pallor, or complaints of increasing dyspnea, chest pain, excessive fatigue, or palpitations indicate activity intolerance. Instruct to rest if these manifestations are noted.*

■ Organize nursing care to allow for rest periods. *Grouping care activities as much as possible allows adequate time to "recharge."*

■ Plan and implement progressive activity plan. Employ passive and active range-of-motion (ROM) exercises as appropriate. Consult with physical therapist on activity plan. *Progressive activity slowly increases exercise capacity by strengthening and improving cardiac function without strain. Progressive activity also helps prevent skeletal muscle atrophy. ROM exercises prevent complications of immobility in bedridden or severely compromised patients.*

■ Encourage small, frequent meals rather than three heavy meals per day. *Small, frequent meals provide continuing energy resources and decrease the work required to digest a large meal.*

MANAGING NURSING CARE

As appropriate and allowed by the designated duties and responsibilities of assistive personnel, the nurse may delegate nursing care activities such as assisting with hygiene, toileting, meals, and activities; obtaining vital signs and daily weights; and measuring intake and output for the patient with heart failure.

EVALUATING

Collect data such as the following to evaluate the effectiveness of nursing care:

■ Vital signs, urine output, and degree of dyspnea at rest and during activity

■ Presence or absence of abnormal heart or lung sounds and edema

■ Ability to tolerate gradually increased activity levels

DOCUMENTING

Document assessment findings, noting any changes that occur with activity. Record treatment measures implemented and the patient's response to treatment. Include subjective data such as statements of improved ease of breathing in documentation. Note referrals made (e.g., to a dietitian) and teaching provided, as well as the patient's apparent understanding and acceptance of instruction.

CONTINUITY OF CARE

The chronic and progressive nature of heart failure requires that the patient and family actively participate in managing the disease. When planning for continuing care, carefully assess the patient's and family's understanding of heart failure, prescribed medications, diet and activities, and symptoms to report to the physician. Explain heart failure and its effects on the patient's life. Discuss the warning signs of impending acute failure and when to contact the physician. Teach about prescribed drugs and their potential adverse effects. Stress the importance of the medications in managing heart failure. Provide verbal and written information regarding each specific medication to encourage compliance. Instruct to keep regular follow-up appointments to monitor disease progression and the effects of therapy.

Lifestyle changes are important, although they may be the most difficult to achieve (Box 17-6■). Teach the patient and family about the prescribed diet. Give practical suggestions for reducing salt intake. The American Heart Association (AHA) has written materials and recipes that may make adjusting to a low-sodium diet easier to tolerate. Refer to a dietitian for further teaching and diet planning as needed. Discuss the importance of family support for dietary restrictions and avoiding exposure to cigarette smoke.

Encourage routine exercise within prescribed parameters to strengthen the heart muscle and improve aerobic

capacity. See Box 17-4 for activity guidelines for patients with heart failure.

Provide referrals to a home health agency and community agencies, such as local cardiac rehabilitation programs, heart support groups, or the AHA, as needed for further nursing evaluation and care, education, and psychosocial support.

NURSING CARE PLAN
Patient With Heart Failure

One year ago, Arthur Jackson, 67 years old, had a large anterior MI. On discharge, he was started on furosemide, Coumadin (warfarin), and a potassium chloride supplement. He has now been admitted to the medical intensive care unit (MICU) after developing severe shortness of breath, a productive cough, and no appetite for 1 week. He is diagnosed with heart failure.

Assessment
On entering his room, Mr. Jackson's nurse, Myumi Takashi, notices that he is sitting in the bedside recliner in high Fowler's position. He says, "Lately, this is the only way I feel fairly comfortable." He states that he gets short of breath working in his garden and complains of his shoes and belt being too tight. On questioning, Mr. Jackson insists that he takes his medications regularly. He admits to a fondness for bacon and Chinese food and sheepishly says he snacks between meals "even though I need to lose weight."

Mr. Jackson's vital signs are BP 95/72 mm Hg; AP 124, irregular; R 28 and labored; and T 97.5°F (36.5°C). The ECG shows atrial fibrillation. An S_3 is heard on auscultation. He has crackles and diminished breath sounds in the bases of both lungs. Distended neck veins, 3+ pitting edema of ankles and feet, and abdominal distention are noted. Skin is cool and diaphoretic. Chest x-ray shows cardiomegaly and pulmonary infiltrates.

Nursing Diagnosis
Ms. Takashi identifies the following nursing diagnoses (among others) for Mr. Jackson:

- *Excess Fluid Volume* related to impaired cardiac pump and salt and water retention
- *Activity Intolerance* related to imbalance between oxygen supply and demand
- *Deficient Knowledge* regarding heart failure management

Expected Outcomes
The expected outcomes specify that Mr. Jackson will

- Demonstrate weight loss and decreased edema, jugular venous distention, and abdominal distention.

BOX 17-6	FOCUS ON OLDER ADULTS

Cardiac Function

Aging affects cardiac function. Ventricular walls become thicker and stiffer, affecting filling. Valve leaflets also stiffen with aging, affecting blood flow and ventricular filling as well. The response to exercise and sympathetic stimulation is slowed, and cardiac reserve is reduced. Other health problems (e.g., arthritis) often contribute to a more sedentary lifestyle, further decreasing the heart's ability to respond to stress. Salt intake often increases with aging as taste decreases. Limited mobility or visual acuity may cause the older adult to rely on high-sodium foods like canned soups and frozen meals. Older adults can be taught methods of adapting to changes in cardiovascular function, such as

- Allow longer warm-up and cool-down periods during exercise.
- Engage in regular exercise such as walking 4 to 5 times a week.
- Rest with feet elevated (e.g., in a recliner) when fatigued.
- Maintain adequate fluid intake.
- Reduce sodium intake by using herbs and other flavorings; read food labels for sodium content.

- Achieve improved activity tolerance.
- Verbalize understanding of medications, diet, and exercise recommendations.

Planning and Implementation

Ms. Takashi plans and implements the following interventions for Mr. Jackson:

- Take hourly vital signs until stable.
- Weigh daily. Record intake and output (I&O).
- Auscultate breath and heart sounds every 4 hours and as necessary.
- Monitor oxygen saturation levels. Notify physician if below 94%.
- Teach about all medications.
- Design an activity plan that incorporates preferred activities and scheduled rest periods throughout the day.
- Consult dietitian to assist Mr. and Mrs. Jackson in planning a low-sodium diet.

Evaluation

Mr. Jackson is transferred to the medical unit after 2 days in MICU. He has lost 8 lb. His respirations are unlabored at rest, and his edema is significantly reduced. He is able to sleep in low Fowler's position with only one pillow. The dietitian is helping

Mr. and Mrs. Jackson develop a realistic eating plan to limit sodium, sugar, and fats. Mr. Jackson is relieved to know that he can still enjoy Chinese food that is prepared without monosodium glutamate (MSG) or added salt. The physical therapist has designed a progressive activity plan with Mr. Jackson for both in-hospital and at-home activity. Mr. Jackson's knowledge about his medications is assessed and reinforced. Mr. Jackson is discharged 5 days after his admission.

Critical Thinking in the Nursing Process

1. Design an exercise plan for Mr. Jackson to follow after discharge.
2. Mr. Jackson tells you, "Talk to my wife about my medications—she's Tarzan and I'm Jane now." How would you respond?
3. Nine months later, Mr. Jackson is admitted to the hospital complaining of abdominal pain and weakness. Blood work shows his serum potassium level to be 2.4 mEq/dL. What subjective information will you gather to help determine what has led to this problem?

Note: Discussion of Critical Thinking questions appears on the companion website.

INFLAMMATORY CARDIAC DISORDERS

Key Concept Any layer of heart tissue can be affected by infection or inflammation. Inflammatory disorders can lead to either structural damage or impaired cardiac function. When heart function is compromised, the patient often develops manifestations of heart failure.

Inflammatory disorders of the heart may result from an infection or an abnormal immune response, or may occur as an effect of a systemic disease. The endocardium, myocardium, or pericardium can be affected, damaging the heart valves, heart muscle, or pericardium. Manifestations of inflammation may range from very mild to life threatening. This section discusses rheumatic heart disease, endocarditis, myocarditis, and pericarditis.

Rheumatic Fever and Rheumatic Heart Disease

Rheumatic fever is a systemic inflammatory disease that can develop in response to infection by group A beta-hemolytic streptococci (usually streptococcal pharyngitis or strep throat). Although children between ages 5 and 15 have the highest incidence, rheumatic fever may affect people of any age. Rheumatic fever can damage the heart

valves and often leads to mitral and aortic valve disorders (discussed in the next section of this chapter).

PATHOPHYSIOLOGY

Rheumatic fever results from an abnormal immune response to the *Streptococcus* bacterium or its toxins. Antibodies produced to attack the invading bacteria (the antigen) appear to also attack connective tissues of the heart, blood vessels, joints, and subcutaneous tissues, initiating an inflammatory response.

Carditis, inflammation of the heart, can affect any layer of the heart in acute rheumatic fever; usually all three are involved. The valves become red and swollen, and small inflammatory lesions develop on the leaflets. As the inflammation resolves, scarring occurs, causing deformity. Myocarditis and pericarditis associated with rheumatic fever are generally mild and have no long-term effects.

Rheumatic heart disease (RHD) is slowly progressive valve deformity that can occur after acute or repeated attacks of rheumatic fever. Valve leaflets become rigid and deformed, resulting in stenosis or regurgitation of the valve. In stenosis, the valve leaflets fuse, obstructing forward blood flow. In regurgitation, the valve fails to close properly, allowing

BOX 17-7	MANIFESTATIONS OF RHEUMATIC FEVER

- Fever
- Migratory joint pain and inflammation
- Rash on trunk and proximal extremities
- Chest pain or discomfort
- Tachycardia, shortness of breath
- Cardiac friction rub, S_3, S_4, possible murmur
- Involuntary muscle spasms, difficulty concentrating

blood to flow back through it. Valves on the left side of the heart, the mitral valve in particular, are most often affected.

MANIFESTATIONS

Manifestations of rheumatic fever typically follow the initial streptococcal infection by about 2 to 3 weeks (Box 17-7■). About 60% of patients with rheumatic fever develop RHD.

COLLABORATIVE CARE

The diagnosis of rheumatic fever is based on the patient's history and physical examination. Laboratory testing helps establish the diagnosis.

- The *WBC count* is elevated, as is the *erythrocyte sedimentation rate (ESR)*, a general indicator of inflammation.
- A positive *C-reactive protein (CRP)* indicates active inflammation.
- A *rapid antigen test for group A streptococcus* is positive. The *antistreptolysin-O (ASO)* titer is a streptococcal antibody test that rises within 2 months of the disease's onset and is found in most patients with rheumatic fever.
- In severe carditis associated with rheumatic fever, the *cardiac enzymes* are elevated.

In addition to laboratory testing, an *echocardiogram* is done to evaluate the structures (including valves) and function of the heart.

Management of RHD focuses on treating the primary infection, managing its manifestations, and preventing complications and recurrences of the disease. In patients with acute carditis, treatment focuses on decreasing myocardial work. Activity may be limited, depending on the patient's symptoms.

Antibiotics are prescribed to eliminate the streptococcal infection. Joint pain and fever are treated with aspirin, ibuprofen, or another nonsteroidal anti-inflammatory drug (NSAID); corticosteroids may be used to treat acute carditis.

NURSING CARE

Nurses have a significant role in identifying patients at risk for RHD and teaching for primary prevention. Identify risk factors for streptococcal infections. These include crowded living conditions, poor nutrition, immunodeficiency, and poor access to health care.

PRIORITIZING NURSING CARE

Nursing care for patients with rheumatic fever and carditis generally is supportive, with a focus on teaching for self-care and preventing complications.

HEALTH PROMOTION

Rheumatic fever is preventable. Prompt treatment of streptococcal throat infections helps decrease the spread of this pathogen and the risk of rheumatic fever. Manifestations of strep throat include a red, fiery-looking throat, pain on swallowing, enlarged and tender cervical lymph nodes, fever in the range of 101°F to 104°F (38.3°C to 40.0°C), and headache. Emphasize the importance of finishing the complete course of prescribed antibiotics to eradicate the pathogen.

ASSESSING

Ask about recent sore throat or "strep throat" and treatment. Other subjective data include complaints of chest pain, shortness of breath, fatigue, weakness, fever, or joint pain. Obtain objective data such as heart rate and heart sounds, respiratory rate, and ease of breathing.

clinicalALERT

Auscultate heart sounds every shift and as necessary. Notify the physician if a pericardial friction rub or a new murmur appears. A friction rub may be produced by an inflamed pericardium; it also causes chest pain and discomfort. A change in heart sounds, a newly developed heart murmur in particular, may indicate further valve damage and a risk for complications such as clot formation and embolization or heart failure.

Observe for joint redness, swelling, or heat, and the presence of a rash on trunk or extremities. Note mental status and any abnormal muscle movements. Monitor the results of laboratory and other diagnostic tests, reporting significant changes to the charge nurse or physician.

IDENTIFYING POTENTIAL COMPLICATIONS

Promptly report decreasing activity tolerance, a change in heart sounds (development of a murmur or S_3 or S_4 gallop), or manifestations of heart failure such as increasing dyspnea, tachycardia, respiratory crackles, or cardiac dysrhythmias.

DIAGNOSING, PLANNING, AND IMPLEMENTING

Acute Pain

Expected outcome: Will rate pain as a 2 or lower on a scale of 0 to 10.

- Report increased chest pain to the charge nurse or physician. *Increased chest pain may indicate development of pericarditis or increased carditis.*

■ Administer anti-inflammatory drugs as ordered. Give aspirin and other NSAIDs with food, milk, or antacids to minimize gastric irritation. Report tinnitus (a symptom of aspirin toxicity), vomiting, or GI bleeding. *Anti-inflammatory drugs are given to control inflammation. The dose of aspirin and NSAIDs may be high, and the drugs are given around the clock rather than as needed.*
■ Provide warm, moist compresses for local pain relief. *Direct application of moist heat may help relieve the pain associated with inflamed joints.*

Activity Intolerance

Expected outcome: Will gradually increase levels of activity without evidence of tachycardia or shortness of breath.

■ Monitor activity tolerance (vital signs, fatigue, shortness of breath) as activity is gradually increased. Explain the importance of monitoring response to activity. Instruct to avoid or stop any activity that causes dyspnea or shortness of breath. *Activity intolerance is an indicator of heart failure. While bed rest or severe activity limitations are no longer recommended, the patient needs to be aware of and attend to responses to increasing activity.*

EVALUATING

To evaluate the effectiveness of nursing care, collect data such as the patient's reports of pain and discomfort, vital signs at rest and with activity, and response to increasing activity levels.

DOCUMENTING

Document and notify the physician of any new symptoms or changes in heart or breath sounds. Note the patient's response to activity, as well as teaching about the disorder, activity restrictions, and continuing care.

CONTINUITY OF CARE

To prevent recurrence of rheumatic fever, emphasize the importance of continuing antibiotic prophylaxis as ordered. Teach the patient with chronic RHD about the importance of antibiotic prophylaxis for any invasive procedure (e.g., dental care, endoscopy, or surgery) to prevent bacterial endocarditis. Preventive dental care and good oral hygiene help discourage gingival infections and are important.

clinicalALERT

The patient with chronic RHD is at significant risk for developing infective endocarditis (see the next section of this chapter). Discuss and provide written information about the signs and symptoms of infective endocarditis, and stress the importance of notifying the primary care physician if symptoms develop.

Instruct the patient with rheumatic carditis to limit salt intake to reduce the workload of the heart. A high-carbohydrate, high-protein diet is usually recommended to promote healing and to combat weakness and fatigue. Teach the early manifestations of heart failure. Provide instructions about prescribed medications, including dosage, signs of adverse or allergic reactions, and possible drug interactions. Assess the need for home health care, and provide a referral as needed.

Infective Endocarditis

Endocarditis, inflammation of the endocardium, is an infectious process that usually affects patients with underlying heart disease. Lesions develop on deformed valves, on valve prostheses (artificial valves), or in areas of the heart where tissue has been damaged. Bacteria often enter through invasive procedures or devices, such as intravenous catheters, indwelling urinary catheters, dental procedures, or during heart surgery. The left side of the heart, the mitral valve in particular, is the most common site of infection. Intravenous drug use is also a risk factor; in these individuals, the right side (the tricuspid valve) is often involved.

Endocarditis is frequently classified by its onset and disease course (Table 17-4 ■). *Acute endocarditis* has an abrupt onset and is a rapidly progressive, severe disease. *Staphylococcus aureus* is the usual infective organism in acute endocarditis.

TABLE 17-4	Classifications of Infective Endocarditis	
	ACUTE INFECTIVE ENDOCARDITIS	**SUBACUTE INFECTIVE ENDOCARDITIS**
Onset	Sudden	Gradual
Usual organism	*Staphylococcus aureus*	*Streptococcus viridans;* others
Risk factors	Intravenous drug use, sepsis	Previous heart or valve damage or deformity, intracardiac devices (e.g., implanted pacemaker), invasive procedures
Pathologic processes	Rapid valve destruction	Valve destruction with regurgitation; embolization of fragile vegetations
Presentation	Abrupt onset with spiking fever and chills; manifestations of heart failure	Gradual onset of febrile illness with cough, dyspnea, arthralgias, abdominal pain

In contrast, *subacute endocarditis* has a more gradual onset. It is more likely to occur in patients with preexisting heart disease than in those with healthy hearts. *Streptococcus viridans* is the most common organism causing subacute endocarditis.

Patients who have prosthetic heart valves are at high risk for developing infective endocarditis. Studies indicate that up to 30% of all cases of infective endocarditis involve prosthetic heart valves (Longo et al., 2012). The infection may develop within the first 2 months after valve replacement surgery, often related to contamination of the valve or nosocomial wound infection. Antibiotic-resistant staphylococci organisms are responsible for an increasing number of cases of health care–related endocarditis as well as endocarditis among injection drug users.

PATHOPHYSIOLOGY

The presence of organisms in the bloodstream is necessary before infective endocarditis can develop. Bacteria may enter through oral lesions, during dental work or other invasive procedures, or due to untreated infections such as upper respiratory infection or urinary tract infection. Organisms in the bloodstream attach to the endocardial lining of the heart and become enmeshed in deposits of fibrin and platelets. This covering "protects" the bacteria from quick removal by the immune system. These *vegetations* (wartlike growths) develop on heart valve leaflets, varying in size and shape (Figure 17-7■). *Friable* (easily broken, fragile) vegetations can break off, traveling through the bloodstream to other organs. When they lodge in small vessels, they may cause hemorrhages, infarcts, or abscesses. The vegetations

scar and deform the valves, impairing the valves' ability to open completely or preventing normal closure, causing regurgitation of blood through the valve. The normal flow of blood through the heart chambers is affected, and heart murmurs develop.

MANIFESTATIONS AND COMPLICATIONS

Infective endocarditis generally causes elevated temperature (above 101.5°F, or 39.4°C) and flulike symptoms. The patient may have a cough, shortness of breath, and complain of joint pain. Acute staphylococcal endocarditis presents with sudden and more severe manifestations, including a high fever. Heart murmurs are common.

Peripheral manifestations of endocarditis may include *petechiae* (small, purplish-red spots) on the trunk, conjunctiva, and mucous membranes; *splinter hemorrhages* (Figure 17-8■); small, painful growths on the fingers and toes; or small, purplish-red lesions on the palms of the hands and soles of the feet.

Complications of infective endocarditis include heart failure, stroke, and infarctions of other organs (lungs, kidneys, or bowel) from embolization of vegetative fragments.

clinical**Alert**

Immediately report manifestations of complications of infective endocarditis, such as an abrupt change in mental status, vision, or other neurologic signs; a new heart murmur; or an abrupt onset of a respiratory distress with dyspnea, tachycardia, cough, or cyanosis.

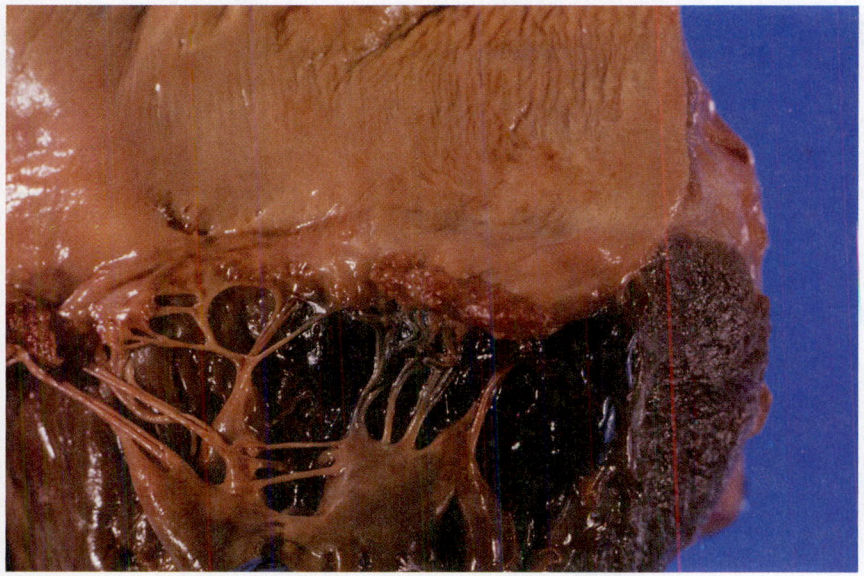

Figure 17-7. ■ Infective endocarditis with colonization of the mitral valve between the left atrium and the left ventricle. (Source: Dr. E. Walker/Science Source)

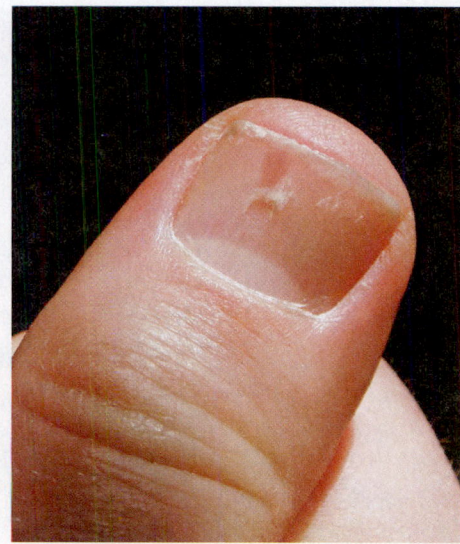

Figure 17-8. ■ Splinter hemorrhage (red streaks under the fingernails or toenails). (Source: Pearson Education)

COLLABORATIVE CARE

Prevention of infective endocarditis is key; educating patients at high risk for the disease is essential. Teaching the public about the risks of injection drug use, including endocarditis, can also help reduce the incidence of this frightening disease. The management priorities for infective endocarditis are to eradicate the infecting organism and minimize valve damage and complications of the disease.

There are no definitive tests for infective endocarditis. A *CBC* and *blood cultures* are done. *Serologic immune testing* for circulating antigens to typical infective organisms may be done. *Echocardiography* is performed to identify vegetations and evaluate valve function.

Medications

To prevent infective endocarditis, antibiotics may be prescribed before high-risk procedures for patients with certain types of preexisting heart disease or damage. Table 17-5 ■ lists conditions and procedures for which prophylactic antibiotic therapy may be prescribed.

After blood cultures, antibiotics are prescribed to eradicate the infecting organism from the blood and heart lesions. Because the fibrin covering that protects organisms from the immune system also protects them from the antibiotic, an extended course of multiple intravenous antibiotics is required. Intravenous drug therapy is continued for 2 to 4 weeks.

Some patients with infective endocarditis require surgery to repair or replace damaged valves. The most common indication for surgery is valvular regurgitation that causes heart failure. When the infection has not responded to antibiotic therapy within 7 to 10 days, the infected valve may be replaced to help eliminate the organism.

NURSING CARE

Nursing care of the patient with infective endocarditis focuses on managing its manifestations, administering antibiotics, and educating the patient and family members.

TABLE 17-5	Indications for Antibiotic Prophylaxis to Prevent Endocarditis
CONDITIONS	**PROCEDURES**
■ Prosthetic heart valves ■ Previous episodes of infective endocarditis ■ Unrepaired cyanotic congenital heart conditions ■ Congenital heart conditions repaired with prosthetic material	■ Dental procedures that involve manipulation of gingival tissue or oral mucosa perforation ■ Surgery on an infected urinary tract ■ Incision and drainage of infected tissue

PRIORITIZING NURSING CARE

Effectively treating the infectious process, maintaining heart function, and preventing complications are the priorities for nursing care of the patient with infective endocarditis.

HEALTH PROMOTION

Teaching is key to preventing endocarditis. Use every opportunity to teach individuals and the public about the risks of injection drug use, including endocarditis. With patients who have known risk factors, such as a congenital heart disease or a prosthetic heart valve, discuss preventive measures such as prophylactic antibiotic therapy. Advise patients at high risk (see Table 17-5) to avoid body piercing because of the possibility of bacteremia.

ASSESSING

Subjective data collected for the patient with infective endocarditis include information about risk factors such as previous heart damage or surgery, recent invasive procedures, and injection drug use. Ask about current symptoms such as persistent fatigue and activity intolerance or shortness of breath. Obtain vital signs, including temperature and apical pulse; observe ease of breathing and auscultate breath sounds; and assess for other manifestations such as petechiae or splinter hemorrhages. Monitor laboratory results, particularly results of blood cultures and serum antibiotic levels. Report results to the physician.

IDENTIFYING POTENTIAL COMPLICATIONS

Monitor patients with infective endocarditis for manifestations of heart failure, including increasing shortness of breath, activity intolerance, tachycardia and tachypnea, respiratory crackles, neck vein distension, and peripheral edema. Embolization of vegetative fragments may be signaled by a sudden change in neurologic, respiratory, cardiovascular, or renal status (see Risk for Ineffective Tissue Perfusion).

DIAGNOSING, PLANNING, AND IMPLEMENTING

Hyperthermia

Expected outcome: Temperature will remain within desired range.

■ Record temperature every 2 to 4 hours. Notify physician if above 101.5°F (39.4°C). *Body temperature usually returns to normal within 1 week of antibiotic therapy. Continuing fever may indicate a need to modify the treatment regimen.*

■ Obtain blood cultures as ordered before giving the first dose of antibiotics. *Blood cultures can identify the causative organism and direct the choice of antibiotic. Initial blood cultures must be obtained before antibiotic therapy is started to obtain enough organisms for culture. Follow-up cultures are used to assess the effectiveness of therapy.*

- Administer anti-inflammatory or antipyretic agents as prescribed. *Fever may be treated with aspirin, ibuprofen, or acetaminophen.*
- Administer antibiotics as ordered; obtain peak and trough drug levels as indicated. *Intravenous antibiotics are given for 4 or more weeks to eradicate the pathogen. Peak and trough levels evaluate the adequacy of the dose to maintain a therapeutic blood level.*

Risk for Ineffective Tissue Perfusion

Expected outcome: Will develop no evidence of organ dysfunction.

- Notify the charge nurse or physician of manifestations of altered organ perfusion:
  - *Brain:* altered level of consciousness, numbness or tingling in extremities, hemiplegia, visual disturbances, or manifestations of stroke
  - *Kidneys:* decreased urine output, hematuria, elevated blood urea nitrogen (BUN) or creatinine
  - *Lungs:* dyspnea, hemoptysis, shortness of breath, diminished breath sounds, restlessness, sudden chest or shoulder pain
  - *Heart:* chest pain radiating to jaw or arms, tachycardia, anxiety, tachypnea, hypotension
  - *Bowel:* abdominal pain, tenderness, guarding, decreased or absent bowel sounds, nausea, vomiting

  Embolization of vegetative lesions can affect tissue perfusion. Vegetations from the left heart may lodge in vessels of the brain, kidneys, or peripheral tissues, causing infarction or abscess. Emboli from the right side of the heart can lead to manifestations of a pulmonary embolism.
- Assess skin color and temperature, quality of peripheral pulses, and capillary refill. *Assessment of peripheral tissue perfusion is important to reduce the risk of tissue necrosis and possible extremity loss.*

MANAGING NURSING CARE

As appropriate and allowed by the designated duties and responsibilities of assistive personnel, the nurse may delegate nursing care activities such as obtaining vital signs, measuring intake and output, and assisting with hygiene and activities as allowed for the patient with infective endocarditis.

EVALUATING

To evaluate care for the patient with infective endocarditis, collect assessment data such as temperature, cardiorespiratory and neurologic status, and comfort.

DOCUMENTING

Document assessment data, including subjective information such as complaints of shortness of breath or fatigue. Note subjective and objective assessments after

activity, as well as the extent of activity tolerated by the patient.

CONTINUITY OF CARE

The patient with infective endocarditis needs education and support throughout the course of the disease, as well as teaching to prevent future recurrences. In basic terms, teach the patient what is happening in the heart and the reasons for the symptoms. Emphasize that infective endocarditis, although serious and frightening, can usually be treated effectively with intravenous antibiotics. Stress the importance of promptly reporting any unusual manifestation, such as a change in vision, sudden pain, or weakness, so that treatment can be promptly implemented. Explain the rationale for all treatments and procedures, including activity restrictions, to reduce anxiety and enhance cooperation. Describe the manifestations of heart failure, and instruct the patient to notify his or her care provider if these manifestations develop.

Patient and family education is also extremely important to prevent recurrences of infective endocarditis. Box 17-8■ outlines a teaching plan for patients at risk.

Patients who acquire infective endocarditis from injection drug use need additional teaching about the risks of drug injections. Refer the patient and significant others as appropriate to a drug or substance abuse treatment program or facility.

Myocarditis

Myocarditis is an inflammatory disorder of the heart muscle that may be caused by infection (viral, bacterial, protozoal), an immune response, radiation, chemical poisons, drugs, or burns. Myocarditis can occur at any age, and it is more common in men than in women. Patients whose immune system is suppressed—those with acquired immunodeficiency syndrome (AIDS) in particular—are at risk. Factors that alter immune response—such as malnutrition,

BOX 17-8	PATIENT TEACHING

Preventing Endocarditis

- Teach the function of the heart valves and the effects of endocarditis. Define endocarditis, and explain why the patient is at risk.
- Stress the importance of notifying care providers of valve disease, heart murmur, or valve replacement before undergoing any invasive procedures.
- Encourage good oral and dental hygiene and regular dental checkups.
- Encourage pneumococcal vaccine and annual influenza immunizations.

alcohol use, immunosuppressive drugs, radiation, stress, and advanced age—increase the risk for myocarditis.

The patient with myocarditis may be asymptomatic or have nonspecific symptoms such as fever, fatigue, general malaise, dyspnea, palpitations, and arthralgias. Often, there is a history of recent nonspecific illness or upper respiratory infection. Manifestations of heart failure, including tachycardia, dysrhythmias, and S_3 and S_4 heart sounds, may be present. A heart murmur, pericardial friction rub, cardiomegaly, and ECG abnormalities may be noted. The long-term effects of the disease depend on the extent of damage to the heart muscle. Although many patients recover fully, others may develop progressive heart failure and cardiomyopathy.

Care for the patient with myocarditis focuses on supporting cardiac function and measures to prevent further damage to the heart muscle. Activity restrictions are ordered during the acute stage to reduce myocardial work. Heart failure and dysrhythmias are treated using standard therapy (see the earlier discussion of heart failure for specific measures). If the cause is infectious, antimicrobial therapy is prescribed. Patients with severe myocarditis may require support measures such as the intra-aortic balloon pump (IABP) or a left ventricular assist device (LVAD).

Nursing care is directed at decreasing myocardial work and increasing oxygen supply. Encourage bed rest to reduce physical activity. Emotional rest also is indicated, because anxiety increases myocardial oxygen demand. Closely monitor vital signs, heart rhythm, and pump effectiveness during the acute phase of the illness. Consider the following nursing diagnoses for the patient with myocarditis:

- *Decreased Cardiac Output* related to impaired cardiac muscle function
- *Fatigue* related to the inflammatory process and inadequate cardiac output
- *Anxiety* related to possible long-term effects of the disorder
- *Excess Fluid Volume* related to compensatory mechanisms for decreased cardiac output

Explain all procedures, tests, and treatments to decrease anxiety and cardiac workload. Teach the early manifestations of heart failure to report to the physician. Stress the importance of following the treatment regimen, including activity restrictions, any dietary modifications (such as a low-salt diet if signs of heart failure are present), and medications. Emphasize that adhering to the treatment plan can reduce the risk of long-term consequences, such as cardiomyopathy.

Pericarditis

Pericarditis is inflammation of the pericardium, the outermost layer of the heart. Acute pericarditis is usually viral in origin. Pericarditis is a frequent complication of end-stage kidney disease. Pericarditis also may follow an MI or open-heart surgery.

PATHOPHYSIOLOGY

Damage to pericardial tissue triggers an inflammatory response. The inflammatory response causes fluid and exudate to collect in the pericardial space, the small potential space between the two layers of the pericardium. Accumulation of a large volume of fluid and exudate may compress the heart and interfere with cardiac filling. The inflammatory process often resolves without long-term consequences. In some cases, scar tissue and adhesions may form between the pericardial layers. Fibrosis and scarring of the pericardium can restrict the heart's ability to function effectively.

MANIFESTATIONS

Classic manifestations of acute pericarditis include chest pain, a pericardial friction rub, and fever. The onset of chest pain is often abrupt. It is usually sharp and may radiate to the back or neck. The pain may be steady or intermittent and is aggravated by deep breathing, coughing, movement, or swallowing. The patient often sits upright and leans forward to reduce the discomfort.

A **pericardial friction rub** is the characteristic sign of pericarditis. It is a leathery, grating sound produced by the inflamed pericardial layers rubbing against the chest wall or pleura. The rub is best heard at the left lower sternal border with the patient sitting up or leaning forward. It may be constant, or it may disappear and then reappear hours later. A low-grade fever (below 100°F [38.4°C]) is often present. Dyspnea and tachycardia are common.

COMPLICATIONS

A **pericardial effusion**, an abnormal collection of fluid between the pericardial layers, may develop in pericarditis. If the fluid collects gradually, the pericardial sac stretches to accommodate it. Heart function is not affected, although heart sounds may be muffled. In contrast, a rapid buildup of pericardial fluid (as little as 100 mL) does not allow the sac to stretch and can compress the heart, interfering with myocardial function. This is known as **cardiac tamponade** (Figure 17-9■). It is a medical emergency that is fatal if it is not aggressively treated.

In cardiac tamponade, cardiac output is critically reduced. The hallmark signs of cardiac tamponade include hypotension, muffled heart sounds, and distended neck veins (increased venous pressure). The increased pressure in the chest cavity during inspiration further interferes with cardiac output, causing a *paradoxical pulse,* in which the systolic blood pressure drops and peripheral pulses weaken or disappear during inspiration. Other manifestations of cardiac tamponade include dyspnea and tachypnea, tachycardia, and a narrowed pulse pressure.

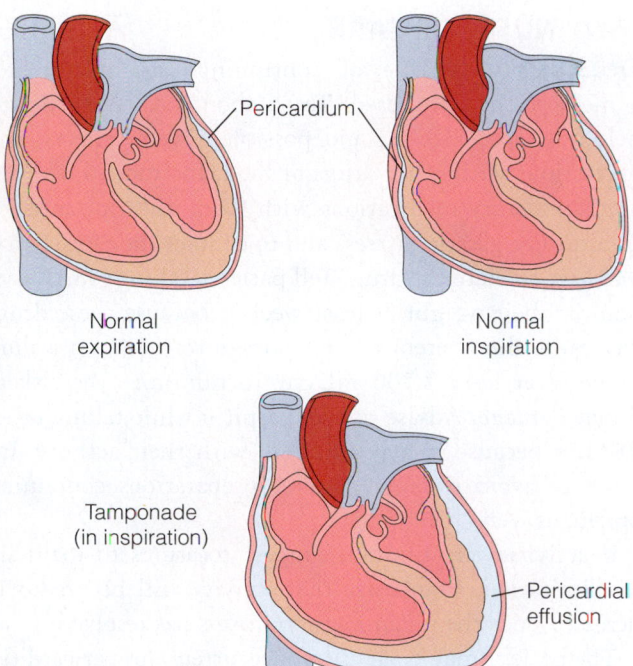

Figure 17-9. ■ Cardiac tamponade. Note the increased volume in the right ventricle during inspiration in both the normal heart and the heart affected by a pericardial effusion. In tamponade, fluid in the pericardial sac and the distended right ventricle restrict filling of the left ventricle and, consequently, cardiac output.

Chronic pericardial inflammation may cause scar tissue to develop, restricting cardiac filling. The patient with constrictive pericarditis experiences progressive dyspnea, fatigue, and weakness. Neck veins are distended, and ascites may develop.

COLLABORATIVE CARE

Although it is uncomfortable, acute pericarditis is usually self-limiting, and will resolve with or without treatment. However, close observation is important to detect early manifestations of increasing effusion or cardiac tamponade.

Echocardiography provides a simple, noninvasive means of diagnosing pericarditis, the extent of pericardial effusion, and, when present, cardiac tamponade. A *computed tomography (CT) scan* or *magnetic resonance imaging (MRI)* may also be used to confirm pericardial effusion or thickening. Acute pericarditis produces characteristic changes on the *ECG.*

Aspirin or NSAIDs are ordered to reduce fever and inflammation and to promote comfort. Corticosteroids may suppress the inflammation and relieve symptoms in pericarditis not due to a bacterial infection.

Pericardiocentesis may be done to remove fluid from the pericardial sac. Guided by fluoroscopy or the ECG, the physician inserts a large (16- to 18-gauge) needle into the pericardial sac and withdraws excess fluid. Pericardiocentesis is done as an emergency procedure for cardiac tamponade.

NURSING CARE

PRIORITIZING NURSING CARE

The nursing care focus for the patient with pericarditis is on promoting comfort and closely monitoring for manifestations of cardiac tamponade or other complications.

Acute Pain

Expected outcome: Will rate pain at a 3 or lower on a pain scale of 0 to 10.

■ Assess chest pain on a standardized scale; note quality and radiation of the pain. Ask about factors that aggravate or relieve the pain. *Assessing the severity, quality, and characteristics of chest pain helps differentiate the pain of pericarditis from angina.*

■ Administer NSAIDs on a regular basis as prescribed with food. *NSAIDs are ordered to reduce fever, inflammation, and pericardial pain. They are most effective when given on a regular schedule. Administering the drugs with food helps decrease GI distress.*

■ Maintain a quiet, calm environment. Provide position changes, back rubs, heat/cold therapy, diversional activity, and emotional support. *Supportive interventions convey caring, enhance the effects of the medication, and decrease the perception of pain.*

Ineffective Breathing Pattern

Expected outcome: Respiratory rate and pattern will be within normal limits; lungs will remain clear to auscultation.

The pain of pericarditis increases with respiratory movement, leading the patient to breathe shallowly.

■ Assess respiratory rate and effort, and auscultate breath sounds every 4 hours. Report adventitious or diminished breath sounds. *Congestion or atelectasis may result from decreased ventilation of peripheral alveoli due to shallow respirations.*

■ Assist to use the incentive spirometer at least every 2 hours. Provide pain medication before respiratory therapy treatments, as needed. *Deep breathing and the incentive spirometer help ensure alveolar ventilation and prevent atelectasis. Analgesia before painful treatments promotes comfort and facilitates participation.*

■ Administer oxygen as needed. *Supplementary oxygen promotes optimal gas exchange and tissue oxygenation.*

■ Place in Fowler's or high Fowler's position. *Elevating the head of the bed reduces the work of breathing and decreases pericardial chest pain.*

Risk for Decreased Cardiac Output

Expected outcome: Vital signs, heart sounds, and peripheral pulses will be within normal range for patient.

- Assess vital signs hourly during acute inflammatory processes. *Frequent assessment allows early identification of manifestations of decreased cardiac output, such as tachycardia, hypotension, or changes in pulse pressure.*
- Assess heart sounds and peripheral pulses, and observe for neck vein distention and pulsus paradoxus every hour.
- If emergency pericardiocentesis and/or surgery is needed to remove pericardial fluid, prepare the patient for the procedure, providing appropriate explanations and reassurance. Observe for adverse effects during pericardiocentesis. *Emotional support and explanations reduce anxiety and promote a caring atmosphere.*

clinicalALERT

Promptly notify the physician of hypotension; distant, muffled heart sounds; new murmurs or extra heart sounds; decreasing quality of peripheral pulses; and distended neck veins. Immediately report altered level of consciousness; decreased urine output; cold, clammy, mottled skin; delayed capillary refill; and weak peripheral pulses. *Acute pericardial effusion and tamponade interfere with cardiac filling and pumping, causing venous congestion, decreased cardiac output, and impaired organ and tissue perfusion.*

CONTINUITY OF CARE

Stress the importance of continuing anti-inflammatory medications as ordered. Teach about prescribed drugs, including dose, desired and possible adverse effects, and interactions with other drugs or food. Instruct to take anti-inflammatory medications with food, milk, or antacids to minimize gastric distress and to contact the physician if unable to tolerate the drug. Tell patients taking NSAIDs to monitor their weight at least weekly, because these drugs may cause fluid retention. Encourage to maintain a fluid intake of at least 2,500 mL/day to minimize the risk of kidney damage. Advise to avoid aspirin while taking other NSAIDs because it may interfere with their activity. Instruct to avoid over-the-counter preparations containing aspirin, as well.

If activities are limited, suggest measures to maintain this limitation. Emphasize that activity will be gradually increased once the inflammatory process has resolved.

The patient may be at risk for recurrence of pericarditis. Teach manifestations that may indicate recurrent pericarditis, and stress the importance of promptly reporting these to the physician.

DISORDERS OF CARDIAC STRUCTURE

Valvular Heart Disease

Key Concept   Properly functioning heart valves allow smooth and unrestricted blood flow through the chambers of the heart. Heart valve disorders interfere with this flow, increasing pressures behind the affected valve and potentially reducing cardiac output.

Rheumatic heart disease is the most common cause of **valvular heart disease**, especially in older adults. Valve disorders also can result from endocarditis or develop after MI, as a result of damaged papillary muscles. Congenital heart defects may affect heart valves, often with no symptoms until adulthood. Changes in the heart valves and supporting structures that occur with normal aging also may lead to symptomatic valvular disease.

PATHOPHYSIOLOGY AND MANIFESTATIONS

There are two major types of heart valve disorders: stenosis and regurgitation. **Stenosis** occurs when valve leaflets fuse together and are unable to open or close fully. The valve opening narrows, impairing the forward flow of blood (Figure 17-10■). *Regurgitant valves* (also called *incompetent*

valves) do not close completely. This allows **regurgitation**, or backflow of blood, through the incompletely closed valve into the area it just left.

Valve disorders affect pressures and blood flow both in front of and behind the affected valve. Stenosis increases the work of the chamber behind the affected valve as the heart attempts to push blood through the narrowed opening.

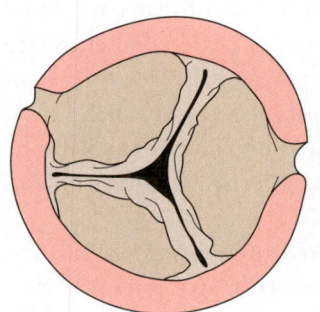 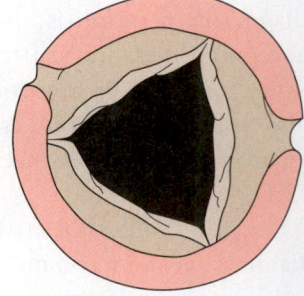

A. Thickened and stenotic valve leaflets

B. Retracted fibrosed valve openings

Figure 17-10. ■ Valvular heart disorders. (**A**) Stenosis restricts opening of the valve and forward blood flow. (**B**) An incompetent or regurgitant heart valve fails to close completely, allowing backflow of blood.

Excess blood volume behind regurgitant valves causes the chamber to dilate. Blood volume and pressures are reduced in front of the diseased valve, because flow is impeded through a stenotic valve and backflow occurs through a regurgitant valve. These changes can lead to pulmonary complications or heart failure. The heart muscle hypertrophies as the heart attempts to maintain cardiac output. Cardiac output falls, and the normal balance of oxygen supply and demand is upset. The increased heart muscle mass and cardiac workload exceed the blood supply, leading to ischemia and chest pain.

The valves on the left side of the heart (mitral and aortic) are subjected to higher pressures, increasing their risk of damage. Blood flow through the heart becomes turbulent as blood moves or attempts to move through damaged valves; the result is a murmur, one of the characteristic manifestations of valvular disease (Table 17-6■).

Mitral Stenosis

Mitral stenosis is narrowing of the mitral valve that obstructs blood flow from the left atrium into the left ventricle during diastole. Mitral stenosis is usually caused by RHD.

The narrowed mitral opening impairs left ventricular filling and cardiac output. It also causes the left atrium to dilate and hypertrophy. High atrial pressures are reflected back into the pulmonary system (Figure 17-11■). Increased pressure in the pulmonary system increases the workload of the right ventricle, causing it also to dilate and hypertrophy. Eventually, right-sided heart failure occurs. Chronic atrial distention often leads to atrial dysrhythmias such as atrial fibrillation. Thrombi may form in the left atrium and become emboli to the brain, coronary arteries, kidney, spleen, and extremities—potentially devastating complications.

Dyspnea on exertion (DOE) is typically the earliest manifestation of mitral stenosis. Others include cough, hemoptysis, frequent respiratory infections such as bronchitis and pneumonia, paroxysmal nocturnal dyspnea, orthopnea, weakness, fatigue, and palpitations. As the stenosis increases, manifestations become more severe. Signs of right heart failure, such as distended neck veins and peripheral edema, may develop. The patient with severe mitral stenosis may be cyanotic.

On auscultation, a diastolic murmur characterized as low pitched and rumbling may be heard in the apical region. It

clinicalALERT

Women with mitral stenosis may be asymptomatic until they become pregnant. The increased circulating volume (30% more in pregnancy) can precipitate sudden pulmonary edema and heart failure, threatening the lives of the mother and fetus.

is heard best with the bell of the stethoscope. The murmur may be accompanied by a palpable *thrill* (a palpable tremor or vibration). Crackles may be noted in the lungs.

Mitral Regurgitation

Mitral regurgitation or *insufficiency* allows blood to flow back into the left atrium during systole because the valve does not close completely. RHD is a common cause of mitral regurgitation. It also may develop as a complication of acute MI, chest wall trauma, or endocarditis.

In mitral regurgitation, only a portion of the blood in the ventricle is ejected into the systemic circulation during systole; the rest returns to the left atrium through the deformed valve. This is added to the blood from the pulmonary system (Figure 17-12■). The left atrium dilates to

TABLE 17-6	Characteristics of Common Heart Murmurs			
MURMUR	**TIMING**	**LOCATION**	**CONFIGURATION**	**QUALITY**
Mitral stenosis	Diastole	Apex—fifth intercostal space (ICS), midclavicular line (MCL)	S_2 — S_1	Continuous rumble, increasing toward end of diastole
Mitral regurgitation	Systole	Apex	S_1 — S_2	Continuous throughout systole (holosystolic)
Aortic stenosis	Systole	Right sternal border, second ICS	S_1 — S_2	Crescendo–decrescendo, continuous
Aortic regurgitation	Early diastole	Third ICS, left sternal border	S_2 — S_1	Decrescendo, continuous

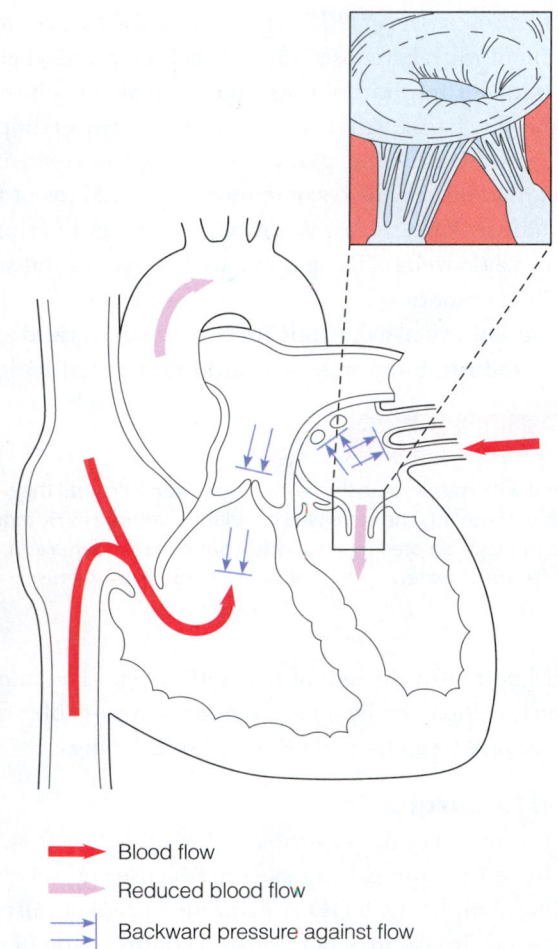

Blood flow

Reduced blood flow

Backward pressure against flow

Figure 17-11. ■ Mitral stenosis.

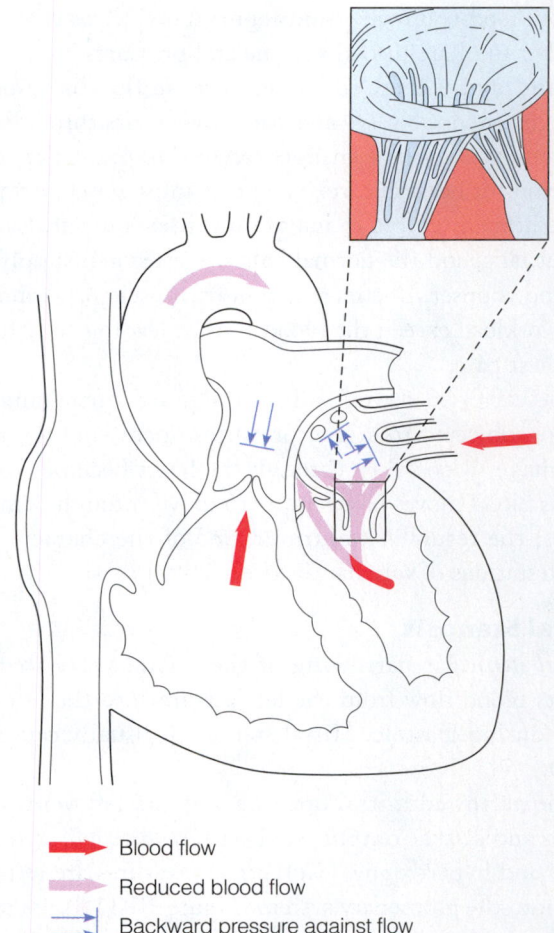

Blood flow

Reduced blood flow

Backward pressure against flow

Figure 17-12. ■ Mitral regurgitation.

accommodate the extra volume; the left ventricle dilates to compensate for increased preload and low cardiac output.

Patients with mitral regurgitation may experience fatigue, weakness, exertional dyspnea, and orthopnea. In severe or acute mitral regurgitation, manifestations of left heart failure may develop, including pulmonary congestion and edema. With high pulmonary pressures, right-sided heart failure may develop as well.

The murmur of mitral regurgitation is usually loud, high pitched, and rumbling. It may be described as "cooing" or "sea gull–like" or have a musical quality. It is heard best at the apex of the heart and often is accompanied by a palpable thrill.

Mitral Valve Prolapse

Mitral valve prolapse (MVP) is a form of mitral insufficiency that occurs when the posterior cusp of the mitral valve flops back into the left atrium during systole. The cause of MVP is unknown although it may be related to an inherited collagen defect in some cases. It is commonly found in young women between the ages of 14 and 30, but also may affect older men. Most patients with MVP are asymptomatic. Chest pain, usually related to fatigue rather than

exertion, is the most common symptom of MVP. Dysrhythmias can cause palpitations, light-headedness, and syncope. A high-pitched late systolic murmur, sometimes described as a "whoop" or "honk," may be present.

Aortic Stenosis

Aortic stenosis obstructs blood flow from the left ventricle into the aorta during systole. Aortic stenosis is more common in males (80%) than in females. It may be *idiopathic* (unknown cause), congenital, or related to RHD. Risk factors typically associated with atherosclerosis and CHD (hyperlipidemia, diabetes, smoking, and the metabolic syndrome) also increase the risk of aortic valve calcification and stenosis in older adults (Longo et al., 2012).

As aortic stenosis progresses, the left ventricle has to work harder to eject blood through the narrowed opening. The ventricle hypertrophies to maintain the cardiac output (Figure 17-13 ■). Because of the extra work, myocardial oxygen needs increase. The increased oxygen consumption can lead to myocardial ischemia. Increased pressures in the left heart are reflected back to the pulmonary vascular system; congestion and pulmonary edema may result.

Manifestations of aortic stenosis usually develop after age 50. They include dyspnea on exertion, angina, and exertional syncope (light-headedness with activity). The pulse pressure narrows as stroke volume and cardiac output fall. Patients with aortic stenosis are at risk for sudden cardiac death.

A harsh systolic murmur can be heard in the second intercostal space to the right of the sternum. A palpable thrill is often noted. As the condition becomes more severe, S_3 and S_4 heart sounds may be heard.

Aortic Regurgitation

In *aortic regurgitation* or *insufficiency,* the aortic valve fails to close completely, allowing blood to flow back into the left ventricle from the aorta during diastole (Figure 17-14■). RHD is the most common cause of aortic regurgitation.

Blood from the aorta causes volume overload of the left ventricle. The ventricle dilates, and stroke volume increases. Over time, the left ventricle hypertrophies, and cardiac output falls. Eventually, pulmonary congestion and possibly right heart failure develop from increased pressures on the left side of the heart. Unlike many other valve disorders, exercise reduces regurgitation and improves heart function in this disorder.

People with mild-to-moderate aortic regurgitation may complain of palpitations, especially when flat or in a left -side-lying position. The heart beat is visible as a throbbing pulse in the arteries of the neck. Sometimes the force of contraction causes a head bob and shakes the whole body. Other manifestations include dizziness, exercise intolerance, fatigue, exertional dyspnea, and angina. Angina often occurs at night and may not respond to common treatments. The pulse pressure often is widened.

The murmur of aortic regurgitation is heard during diastole as blood flows back into the left ventricle from the aorta. It is described as a "blowing," high-pitched sound heard most clearly at the third left intercostal space. It may be associated with a thrill. An S_3 and S_4 may be heard. Because the heart is enlarged, the apical impulse is displaced to the left.

COLLABORATIVE CARE

Valvular disease may be asymptomatic for many years. The initial indication often is a heart murmur heard during a routine physical examination. *Echocardiography* is used to diagnose valvular disease. *Cardiac catheterization* is used to assess the effects of valve disease on heart function.

Asymptomatic patients and those with mild manifestations often require no treatment. They are closely observed for signs of disease progression. Valve damage increases the risk for infective endocarditis because the deformed valve alters blood flow through the heart, damaging the

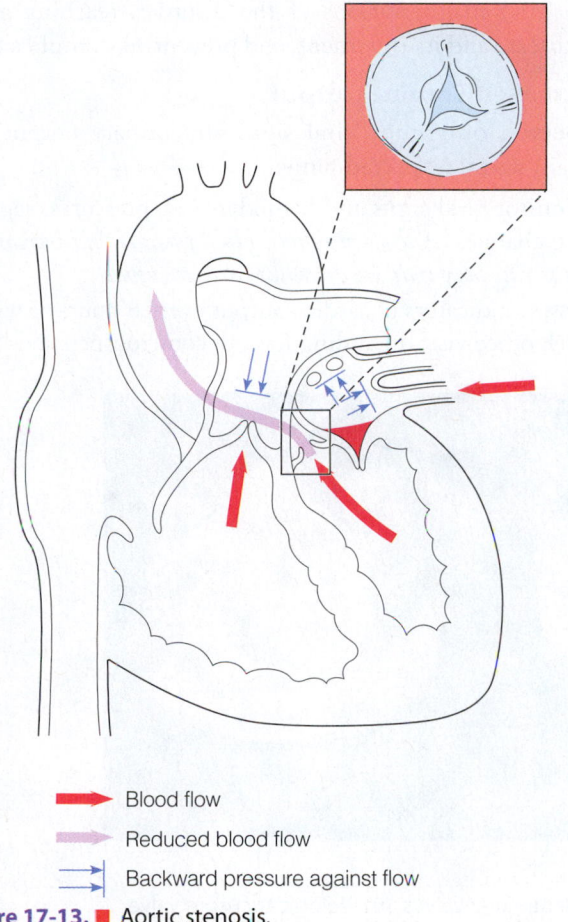

➡️ Blood flow

➡️ Reduced blood flow

➡️ Backward pressure against flow

Figure 17-13. ■ Aortic stenosis.

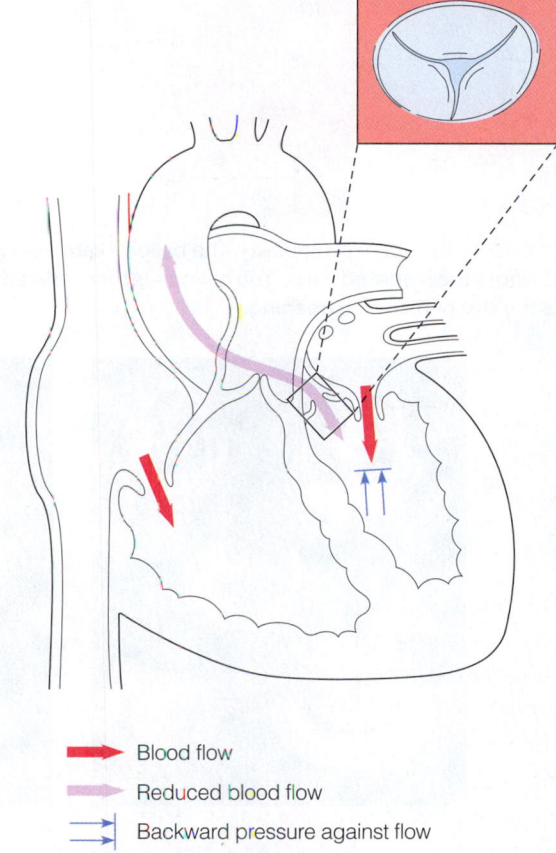

➡️ Blood flow

➡️ Reduced blood flow

➡️ Backward pressure against flow

Figure 17-14. ■ Aortic regurgitation.

endocardium and allowing bacteria to colonize heart tissues. Antibiotics are given prophylactically before some invasive procedures or surgeries (see Table 17-5). Manifestations of heart failure are treated with diet and medications (see the preceding section on heart failure). Surgery is considered before heart failure becomes severe.

Percutaneous Balloon Valvuloplasty

Stenotic valve disease may be treated with *percutaneous balloon valvuloplasty*. A balloon catheter is inserted into the femoral vein or artery and advanced to the stenotic valve. The balloon is then inflated for approximately 90 seconds to divide the fused leaflets and enlarge the valve opening (Figure 17-15 ■). Nursing care of the patient with a balloon valvuloplasty is similar to that of the patient after percutaneous coronary revascularization.

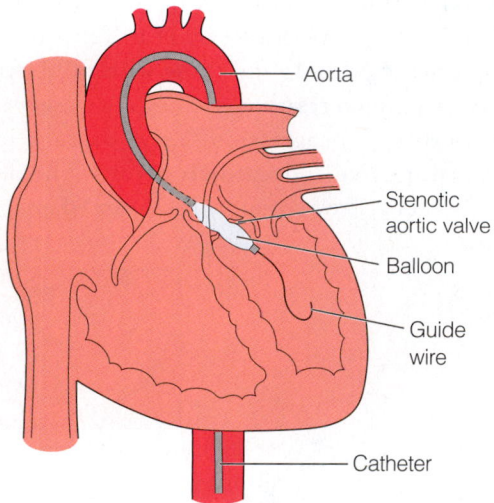

Aorta

Stenotic aortic valve

Balloon

Guide wire

Catheter

Figure 17-15. ■ Balloon valvuloplasty. The balloon catheter is positioned across the stenosed valve. The balloon is then inflated to increase the size of the valve opening.

Surgery

Surgery to repair or replace the diseased valve may be required to restore valve function, relieve symptoms, and prevent complications. *Valvuloplasty* is a general term for reconstruction or repair of a heart valve. Methods include "patching" the perforated portion of the leaflet, resecting excess tissue, removing vegetations or calcification, and other techniques. A *commissurotomy* may be done to open stenotic valves.

Severely damaged valves may be replaced. Many different prosthetic heart valves are available, including mechanical and biologic tissue valves (Figure 17-16 ■). Biologic tissue valves (from animal tissue or a human cadaver) allow more normal blood flow and are less likely to cause clots to form than mechanical ones. Mechanical prosthetic valves are more durable, but require lifetime anticoagulation to prevent clot formation on the valve. Both biologic and mechanical valves increase the risk of emboli and endocarditis, although the incidence of these complications is fairly low. Nursing care of the patient having valve surgery is similar to that for other types of open-heart surgery.

NURSING CARE

PRIORITIZING NURSING CARE

Nursing care focuses on maintaining the cardiac output, managing manifestations of the disorder, teaching about the disease and its treatment, and preventing complications.

Decreased Cardiac Output

Expected outcome: Vital signs and urinary output will remain within expected range.

■ Monitor vital signs and hemodynamic pressures, reporting changes. *A drop in systolic blood pressure and increasing pulse rate may indicate decreased cardiac output.*

■ Assess indicators of cardiac output every 8 hours or with each office visit, including level of consciousness, neck

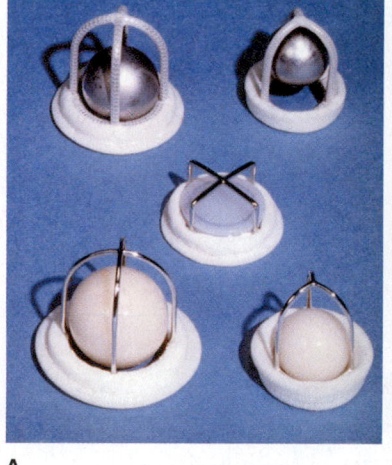

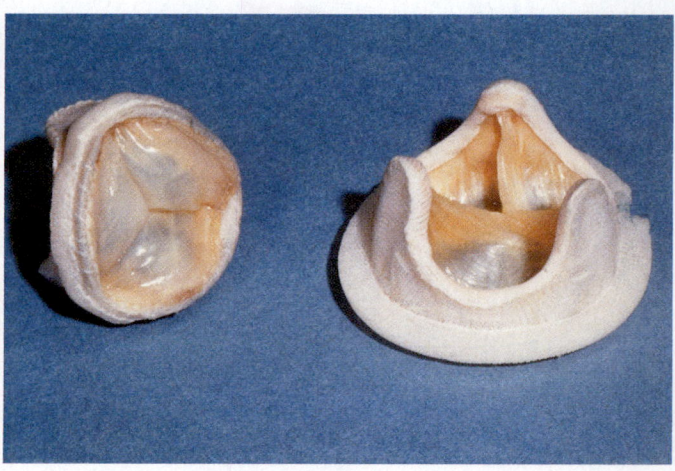

A   B

Figure 17-16. ■ Prosthetic heart valves. (**A**) Mechanical atrioventricular valves. (**B**) Biologic tricuspid valve prostheses. (Source: (A) © Medical-on-Line/Alamy; (B) © Mediscan/Alamy.)

vein distention, respiratory effort and lung sounds, urine output, skin color and temperature, peripheral edema, and peripheral pulses and capillary refill. Notify the physician of significant changes. *Decreased cardiac output impairs tissue and organ perfusion, producing clinical manifestations.*

- Monitor intake and output; weigh daily or with each office visit, reporting any gain of 3 to 5 lb (1 to 2 kg) within 24 hours. *Fluid retention may indicate decreased cardiac output; 2.2 lb (1 kg) of weight is equal to 1 L of retained fluid.*

- Maintain fluid restriction as ordered. *Fluid intake may be restricted to minimize cardiac workload.*

- Elevate head of the bed, and administer oxygen as ordered. *These measures facilitate lung ventilation and improve oxygenation.*

- Monitor pulse oximetry. *Pulse oximetry allows assessment of oxygenation.*

- Promote physical, emotional, and mental rest. *Physical and psychologic rest decrease the cardiac workload.*

- Administer medications as ordered. *Diuretics, ACE inhibitors, and direct vasodilators are often ordered to reduce or redistribute excess fluid volume and reduce the cardiac workload.*

Activity Intolerance

Expected outcome: Will demonstrate gradually increasing activity tolerance.

- Obtain vital signs before and during activities. *An increased heart rate, change in BP, diaphoresis, or complaints of shortness of breath, fatigue, or chest pain may indicate poor tolerance of the level of activity.*

- Encourage gradual increases in activity/self-care as tolerated. *Progressive activity prevents sudden stress on the heart and helps improve exercise tolerance.*

- Provide assistance as needed. Suggest using a shower chair, sitting while brushing hair or teeth, and so on. *Energy-saving techniques reduce cardiac workload.*

Risk for Bleeding

Expected outcome: Will remain free of hemorrhage.

Anticoagulant therapy may be ordered to reduce the risk of clot formation and emboli with valve disorders or an artificial valve. This increases the risk for bleeding and hemorrhage.

- Test stools and emesis for occult blood. *Bleeding in the GI tract may not be visible.*

- Caution to avoid using aspirin or other NSAIDs. Instruct to read ingredient labels on over-the-counter drugs; many contain aspirin. *Aspirin and other NSAIDs interfere with clotting and may increase the risk of bleeding.*

- Instruct to use a soft-bristled toothbrush and an electric razor and to clean fragile skin gently. *These measures reduce the risk of bleeding from skin nicks and cuts or the gums.*

- Monitor hemoglobin, hematocrit, and platelet counts. Notify the charge nurse of significant changes. *Low hemoglobin and hematocrit may indicate blood loss. Platelet counts below 50,000/mm³ significantly increase the risk of bleeding.*

MANAGING NURSING CARE

As appropriate and allowed by the designated duties and responsibilities of assistive personnel, the nurse may delegate nursing care activities such as obtaining vital signs, weight, and oxygen saturation levels; measuring intake and output as ordered; and assisting with hygiene and activities as allowed for the patient with a heart valve disorder.

CONTINUITY OF CARE

Preventing rheumatic fever is important to prevent heart valve disorders. Early treatment of strep throat usually prevents rheumatic fever. Teach individual patients, families, and communities the importance of timely and effective treatment of strep throat. Emphasize the importance of completing the full prescription of antibiotics to prevent development of resistant bacteria. Measures to reduce cardiovascular risk factors such as avoiding smoking and controlling hyperlipidemia and diabetes also appear to reduce the risk for aortic valve disorders associated with aging.

Explain all tests and procedures, including corrective surgery, to increase understanding and decrease anxiety. Discuss symptom management, including activity restrictions or lifestyle changes related to the valve disease. Advise to schedule rest periods to prevent fatigue. Teach about diet restrictions to control heart failure; arrange a consultation with the dietitian for teaching and menu planning. Provide information about prescribed medications, including their purpose, desired and possible adverse effects, scheduling, and possible interactions with other drugs. Refer the patient and family to community resources before discharge. Emphasize the importance of keeping follow-up appointments to monitor the disease and treatment. Emphasize the importance of notifying all health care providers about valve disease or surgery so that antibiotics can be given before any procedure that might cause infection.

Instruct the patient and family to report increasing severity of symptoms, particularly of heart failure and pulmonary edema, to the doctor. The treatment regimen may need to be modified or surgery considered to repair or replace the diseased valve. Advise to report neurologic changes and other symptoms of emboli so anticoagulant therapy can be adjusted. Instruct to notify the physician of manifestations of bleeding, such as joint pain, easy bruising, black and tarry stools, bleeding gums, or blood in the urine or sputum.

Cardiomyopathy

Cardiomyopathy is a disorder that affects the structure and function of the heart muscle. Cardiomyopathies are a diverse group of disorders that affect the filling and output of the heart and often lead to heart failure. In many cases, the

Table 17-7	Classifications and Characteristics of Cardiomyopathy

	DILATED	HYPERTROPHIC	RESTRICTIVE
Description	Ventricles dilate; ventricular contraction is impaired	Left ventricular hypertrophy interferes with filling and outflow	Rigidity of ventricular walls interferes with filling
Manifestations	Heart failure Cardiomegaly Dysrhythmias S_3 and S_4 heard on auscultation	Dyspnea Anginal pain Syncope Dysrhythmias	Dyspnea on exertion Fatigue Heart failure S_3 and S_4 on auscultation

cause is unknown. Cardiomyopathy also may be related to another disease or condition, such as chronic alcohol abuse, myocardial ischemia, or a viral infection. Cardiomyopathies are categorized by their characteristics and effects on the heart (Table 17-7 ■).

Dilated cardiomyopathy is the most common type of cardiomyopathy. Although up to 20% of dilated cardiomyopathy may be genetic in origin, often it is the result of toxins, metabolic conditions, or infection. The heart chambers dilate, and ventricular contraction is impaired. Manifestations develop gradually. Heart failure may develop years after the onset of dilation and pump failure. Dysrhythmias are common, increasing the risk of sudden cardiac death.

Hypertrophic cardiomyopathy is characterized by hypertrophy and decreased compliance of the left ventricle. The interventricular septum tends to hypertrophy to a greater extent than the free wall of the ventricle. This impairs left ventricular filling and outflow. This may be a hereditary disorder, with a family history of the disorder seen in about half of all patients. Sudden cardiac death may be the first sign of the disorder; manifestations can occur suddenly during or after physical activity. Frequent manifestations include dyspnea, angina, and syncope.

Restrictive cardiomyopathy is the least common form of cardiomyopathy. Rigidity of the ventricular walls impairs filling, resulting in decreased ventricular size and decreased cardiac output. The manifestations of restrictive cardiomyopathy are those of heart failure and decreased tissue perfusion.

Medical management of cardiomyopathy focuses on minimizing heart failure, treating dysrhythmias, and

preventing sudden cardiac death. Strenuous physical exertion, which may precipitate dysrhythmias and/or sudden cardiac death, is restricted. Dietary and sodium restrictions may help diminish the manifestations.

Without definitive treatment, patients with cardiomyopathy will develop end-stage heart failure. Cardiac transplant is the definitive treatment for dilated cardiomyopathy; without transplantation, survival time is limited. Transplantation is not used to treat restrictive cardiomyopathy because the underlying disease process will eventually also affect the transplanted organ. Obstructive hypertrophic cardiomyopathy may be surgically treated by resecting excess muscle away from the aortic valve outflow tract.

Nursing goals for patients with cardiomyopathies are to prevent complications, assist the patient to conserve energy while encouraging self-care, and support coping skills. If surgery is done, nursing care is similar to that for any patient undergoing open-heart surgery or heart transplantation.

Patient and family teaching focus on self-care measures such as activity restrictions, dietary changes, and drugs used to reduce symptoms and/or prevent complications. Educate about the disease process, its ultimate outcome, and treatment options. Teach patients who are undergoing invasive procedures for diagnosis or treatment about the procedure, including preparation and care after the procedure. If heart transplant is an option, provide information about the procedure and initiate preoperative teaching.

Note: The references and resources for all chapters have been compiled at the back of the book.

Chapter Review

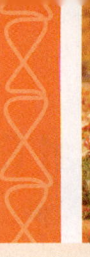
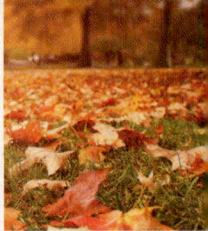

KEY POINTS

- **Concept:** Disorders of the heart muscle or its structures affect its ability to pump blood effectively to meet the needs of the cells of the body. When the heart is unable to function effectively, other organ systems may fail because their fuel supply is impaired.

- **Concept:** Heart failure, inability of the heart to meet the body's needs for fuel and oxygen, is caused by impaired pumping of the heart. It is usually caused by extensive heart muscle damage from myocardial infarction, but can also result from inflammatory, congenital, or valve disorders.

- Heart failure is a chronic condition. Medical management and nursing care focus on promoting effective cardiac output and teaching the patient to manage the disorder.

- **Concept:** Any layer of heart tissue can be affected by infection or inflammation. Inflammatory disorders can lead to either structural damage or impaired cardiac function. When heart function is compromised, the patient often develops manifestations of heart failure.

- Although rheumatic fever, an immune response to streptococcal infection, often affects children, adults may also develop rheumatic fever or may experience long-term effects of rheumatic heart disease. The nursing care focus for a patient with rheumatic fever is on teaching to prevent long-term damage to heart valves and recurrence of the disorder.

- Infective endocarditis, inflammation of the innermost layer of heart tissue, may be acute or subacute in nature. Extended treatment with several antibiotics is usually necessary to eradicate the infection.

- Prophylactic antibiotic therapy is an important measure to prevent infective endocarditis in patients with previous heart damage or deformity.

- Pericarditis generally is a mild, self-limited disorder characterized by chest pain and a pericardial friction rub. It can, however, lead to pericardial effusion and possible cardiac tamponade, a medical emergency. Frequent assessment and prompt intervention for manifestations of muffled heart sounds, hypotension, and pulsus paradoxus are vital to survival of the patient with cardiac tamponade.

- **Concept:** Properly functioning heart valves allow smooth and unrestricted blood flow through the chambers of the heart. Heart valve disorders interfere with this flow, increasing pressures behind the affected valve and potentially reducing cardiac output.

- The aortic and mitral valves are more likely to be affected by valve disorders because of the high pressures on the left side of the heart. When these valves are affected by either stenosis or regurgitation, heart failure is likely to develop.

- Cardiomyopathy, while uncommon, is generally progressive, leading to heart failure. Heart transplant may be required.

PEARSON NURSING STUDENT RESOURCES

Find additional materials at **nursing.pearsonhighered.com**.

Clinical Reasoning Care Map

Caring for a Patient With Infective Endocarditis

NCLEX-PN® Focus Area: Reduction of Risk Potential

Case Study: Larry Schain, 68 years old, saw his physician after experiencing flulike symptoms for 2 weeks, along with increasing fatigue and shortness of breath. Laboratory testing and an echocardiogram confirmed a diagnosis of subacute bacterial endocarditis.

Nursing Diagnosis: Ineffective Health Maintenance

COLLECT DATA

Subjective	Objective
_____	_____
_____	_____
_____	_____
_____	_____
_____	_____
_____	_____

Does this present a threat to the patient's safety?

If yes, the priority intervention to address this threat would be:

_____

Nursing Care

_____
_____
_____
_____
_____
_____

Interprofessional team members to include when planning care:

_____

How would you document this? _____

_____
_____

Compare your answers and documentation to those provided on the companion website.

Data Collected
(use only those that apply)

- History of rheumatic fever as a child
- Has had a heart murmur "for as long as I remember."
- BP 112/68, P 106, regular, R 24, T 102.6°F PO
- Loud (4 to 5/6) rumbling diastolic murmur heard over entire chest wall
- Had oral surgery 2 months ago
- Does not smoke; uses alcohol occasionally
- Retired, but generally very active; enjoys gardening
- Now gets short of breath walking from bedroom to kitchen
- Petechiae noted on trunk and back
- Color gray; O_2 sats 91%
- States he has lost 5 lb during past 2 weeks and has no appetite
- Lives in his own home with his wife; school-age grandchildren live nearby
- Wife seems unconcerned; states, "He just has the flu, nothing serious."

Nursing Interventions
(use only those that apply; list in priority order)

- Provide information about the heart and its structures and about endocarditis.
- Discuss prophylactic antibiotic therapy for patients with valve damage.
- Discuss prescribed outpatient intravenous antibiotic therapy.
- Teach intravenous catheter care.
- Provide analgesics as needed for comfort.
- Encourage gradually increasing activity.
- Discuss symptoms of complications to report to the physician.
- Encourage rest before and after activity/exercise.
- Provide information about community resources for emotional support.
- Help identify coping strategies for concerns about role in business.
- Schedule appointments for intravenous antibiotic infusions.

NCLEX-PN® Exam Preparation

1 A patient develops left-sided heart failure. An appropriate nursing diagnosis is:

1. Activity Intolerance.
2. Ineffective Airway Clearance.
3. Deficient Fluid Volume.
4. Acute Pain.

2 A patient develops right-sided heart failure. Which of the following symptoms would the nurse expect to find?

1. Pulmonary edema
2. Edematous legs and ankles
3. Decreased heart rate
4. Increased urinary output

3 The nurse is to administer digoxin (Lanoxin) 0.25 mg PO. The patient's apical pulse is 48. The appropriate nursing action is to:

1. check the digoxin level and administer the drug if the level is less than 2 ng/mL.
2. hold the drug and recheck the apical pulse in 1 hour.
3. hold the drug and notify the physician.
4. administer the drug and report the apical pulse when the physician makes rounds.

4 A man who has been diagnosed with heart failure is prescribed a low-fat, low-cholesterol, and low-sodium diet. Which of the following food items, if chosen by the patient, indicates a need for further teaching?

1. Baked chicken, green beans, sliced carrots
2. Macaroni and cheese, smoked turkey leg, broccoli
3. Grilled fish, baked potato, tossed salad
4. Turkey bacon, egg white omelet, wheat toast, apple

5 A priority nursing intervention for a patient diagnosed with rheumatic heart disease includes:

1. determining the etiology of the disease.
2. encouraging visits from friends and family.
3. teaching manifestations to report to primary care provider.
4. assessing for signs of recurring streptococcal infection.

6 The nurse caring for a patient with bacterial endocarditis knows that this disease:

1. generally is mild and self-limiting.
2. affects the muscle layer of the heart.
3. often leads to end-stage heart failure requiring cardiac transplant.
4. usually affects patients with previous heart or valve damage.

7 A female patient is diagnosed with pericarditis. The nurse expects which of the following assessment findings?

1. Peripheral edema
2. Wheezing breath sounds
3. Absence of chest pain
4. Pericardial friction rub

8 The nurse caring for a patient with acute pericarditis assesses carefully for manifestations of cardiac tamponade, including:

1. a distinct line of demarcation and pallor of the lower extremities.
2. a loud systolic murmur accompanied by a palpable thrill.
3. muffled heart sounds and a low blood pressure.
4. an irregularly irregular pulse of variable intensity.

9 A patient is diagnosed with mitral stenosis. Discharge teaching should include all but which of the following?

1. How to auscultate heart for murmurs twice per day
2. Signs and symptoms of heart failure
3. The need to notify physician of temperature elevation greater than 100°F for more than 2 days
4. The importance of reporting signs and symptoms of activity intolerance to the physician

10 After replacement of a stenosed mitral valve with a mechanical heart valve, the nurse identifies which of the following as a high-priority nursing diagnosis?

1. Disturbed Sleep Pattern related to sound of mechanical valve
2. Ineffective Protection related to anticoagulant therapy
3. Decreased Cardiac Output related to impaired blood flow through heart valves and chambers
4. Risk for Decreased Cardiac Tissue Perfusion related to disruption of the coronary arteries

Answers and rationales for Review Questions appear in Appendix I.

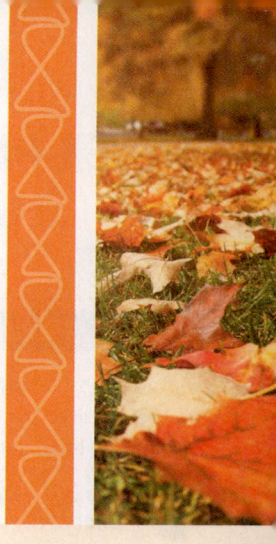

CHAPTER 18
Caring for Patients With Peripheral Vascular Disorders

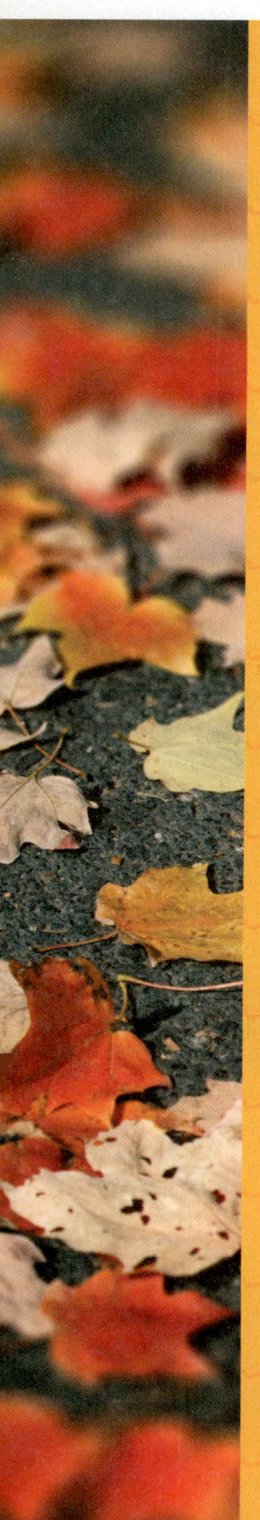

BRIEF OUTLINE

Hypertension
Secondary Hypertension
DISORDERS OF THE AORTA
   AND ITS BRANCHES
Aneurysm

PERIPHERAL ARTERIAL
   DISORDERS
Peripheral Vascular Disease
Other Arterial Disorders

VENOUS DISORDERS
Venous Thrombosis
Varicose Veins

APPLIED LEARNING OUTCOMES

After completing this chapter, you will be able to:

1. Relate physiology of the peripheral vascular system to common disorders affecting the peripheral vascular system.
2. Describe the pathophysiology and manifestations of common peripheral vascular disorders.
3. Conduct focused assessments for patients with peripheral vascular disorders, collecting relevant subjective and objective data.
4. Safely administer drugs used for patients with peripheral vascular disorders.
5. Describe pre- and postoperative nursing care for patients having vascular surgery.
6. Use the nursing process and an evidence base to provide safe and effective care that considers individual expressed values, preferences, and needs for patients with peripheral vascular disorders.
7. Reinforce patient and family teaching to promote and maintain health in patients with common peripheral vascular disorders.
8. Use technology to obtain evidence and guidelines for nursing care and patient teaching and to document care provided.

KEY TERMS

The key terms are defined on the pages listed below.

SPECIAL FEATURES

Key Concept   Processes that affect blood vessels and interfere with peripheral blood flow can impair the delivery of oxygen and nutrients to the tissues, leading to complications such as heart failure, pain, infection, and amputation.

Peripheral vascular disorders, including hypertension, are common health problems in the United States. Many of these disorders are chronic conditions, requiring continuing management by the patient and health care provider. Patients with peripheral vascular disease may have limited mobility and often are affected by other chronic conditions as well, such as diabetes mellitus, obesity, and heart failure. Without appropriate management, peripheral vascular disorders can lead to complications such as kidney failure or amputation.

Nursing care for patients with peripheral vascular disorders focuses on relieving pain, improving peripheral circulation, preventing tissue damage, and promoting healing. A holistic approach to caring is important to address the emotional, social, and economic effects of these often chronic and potentially disabling disorders.

Hypertension

Key Concept   Hypertension is a leading, often undiagnosed, cause of cardiovascular disability and mortality. Few people with hypertension have symptoms of the disorder, yet it can lead to heart failure, stroke, and chronic renal failure.

In adults, **hypertension** is defined as blood pressure higher than 140 mm Hg systolic or 90 mm Hg diastolic on three separate readings several weeks apart. Hypertension is common, affecting nearly one-third of people age 20 and older in the United States. Hypertension primarily affects people older than 40; more than 70% of people age 65 and older are hypertensive (National Heart, Lung, and Blood Institute [NHLBI], 2013). Box 18-1■ discusses hypertension in older adults. Blacks are more commonly affected than Whites: More than 43% of Black adults are hypertensive, whereas less than 33% of Whites and approximately 28% of Hispanics have hypertension (Centers for Disease Control and Prevention [CDC], 2014). The percentage of adults with hypertension in the United States varies by income; people at the lowest income level are more likely to have hypertension than those in the highest income group (National Center for Health Statistics [NCHS], 2013).

Hypertension is often called the "silent killer," because it has few symptoms. Its impact is significant because persistent high blood pressure can lead to stroke, coronary heart disease, and chronic renal failure. The recognition and treatment of hypertension have significantly improved in the past two decades. Approximately 75% of people with hypertension

---

BOX 18-1	**FOCUS ON OLDER ADULTS**

Hypertension

For many years, a gradual increase in blood pressure was thought to be a normal age-related change. It is now recognized that blood pressure control is important in older adults to lower the risk of organ damage and cardiovascular disease (Aronow et al., 2011). Changes associated with aging that can affect older adults' risk for hypertension include the following:

- Isolated systolic hypertension is common. It develops as blood vessels become more rigid, decreasing their ability to expand and contract and increasing peripheral vascular resistance (PVR). The result is increased myocardial oxygen demand and diminished organ perfusion.
- Chronic kidney disease is more common in older adults, contributing to hypertension. Furthermore, hypertension damages small blood vessels in the kidneys, contributing to chronic kidney disease.
- The reflexes that maintain BP with position changes diminish. This can lead to a temporary fall in BP and an increased risk for falls and syncope. When assessing for orthostatic hypotension, allow 2 to 5 minutes after position changes before measuring the blood pressure. Instruct older patients to change positions slowly, especially when rising from bed or a chair.

---

are being treated and more than 50% have achieved effective control of their blood pressure (NHLBI, 2013).

Hypertension is classified both by its cause and by its course. **Primary hypertension** (or *essential hypertension*) has no identified cause, although risk factors have been identified (Box 18-2■). **Secondary hypertension** results from a known cause, such as kidney disease (see the section that follows).

PATHOPHYSIOLOGY

Peripheral vascular resistance is the primary factor in determining the blood pressure. In hypertension, the resistance to blood flow is increased, primarily due to constriction of

---

BOX 18-2	**RISK FACTORS FOR HYPERTENSION**

Risk Factors That Can Be Changed
- Mineral intake
  - High sodium intake
  - Low potassium, calcium, and magnesium intake
- Obesity
- Sedentary lifestyle
- Excess alcohol consumption
- Smoking
- Physical and/or emotional stress

Risk Factors That Cannot Be Changed
- Family history
- Age
- Race

the arterioles. Disruption of the physiologic mechanisms that regulate blood pressure is the underlying cause of hypertension:

- Overactivity of the sympathetic nervous system (SNS) leads to vasoconstriction and increased cardiac output.
- Alterations in the renin–angiotensin–aldosterone system contribute to vasoconstriction and affect the excretion of salt and water. Persistent high levels of angiotensin II can cause permanent changes in the arterioles.
- Other chemical mediators such as atrial natriuretic peptide and hormones secreted by vessel endothelium also affect blood vessel constriction and salt and water excretion.
- Finally, insulin resistance reduces the effects of natural vasodilator substances, affects kidney function, and increases SNS activity.

Blood volume and peripheral resistance increase as a result, leading to increased blood pressure. This increases the workload of the left ventricle. As a result, left ventricular muscle mass increases. More blood flow and oxygen are required to meet the needs of the heart, increasing the risk for coronary heart disease and heart failure. Sustained increases in blood pressure increase the rate of atherosclerosis, also increasing the risk for stroke. Blood vessels in the kidneys are affected, leading to an increased risk for kidney disease.

The classifications of blood pressure (in mm Hg) and stages of hypertension are as follows:

Normal	Less than 120/less than 80
Prehypertension	120–139/80–89
Stage 1	140–159/90–99
Stage 2	160 or higher/100 or higher

MANIFESTATIONS AND COMPLICATIONS

People with hypertension usually have no symptoms other than an increased blood pressure. They may complain of vague headaches or occasional dizziness. Hypertension is usually advanced when symptoms develop. These may include morning headache, fatigue, blurred vision, unsteadiness, depression, and nocturia.

Without treatment, hypertension affects other organs and can lead to premature death (Table 18-1 ■).

Hypertensive Crisis

Patients with hypertension may experience *hypertensive crisis* (also known as *malignant hypertension*), a rapid increase in systolic pressure to greater than 180 mm Hg and/or diastolic pressure to greater than 120 mm Hg. Patients experiencing hypertensive crisis may have manifestations such as headache, confusion, optic nerve swelling, blurred

TABLE 18-1	Effects of Hypertension
ORGAN	**EFFECT**
Eyes	Retinopathy: narrowed blood vessels, hemorrhages, fluid leakage, and swelling of the optic nerve
Heart	Coronary heart disease: angina, acute coronary syndrome, and myocardial infarction
	Left ventricular hypertrophy
	Heart failure
	Dysrhythmias
Vascular system	Peripheral vascular disease
	Aneurysms
Brain	Stroke
	Impaired cognition in older adulthood
	Hypertensive encephalopathy (changes in brain tissue)
Kidneys	Chronic kidney disease
	End-stage renal disease (ESRD)

vision, restlessness, and motor and sensory deficits. Hypertensive crisis requires immediate treatment (within 1 hour) to prevent irreversible damage to the brain, kidneys, and heart.

clinicalALERT

Frequently monitor blood pressure (every 5 to 30 minutes) during a hypertensive emergency.

COLLABORATIVE CARE

Hypertension is diagnosed by blood pressure readings. The BP is measured after resting for at least 5 minutes and avoiding caffeine and smoking for at least 30 minutes.

No specific diagnostic tests are ordered to identify hypertension. Laboratory tests such as urinalysis, blood chemistries (including electrolytes, glucose, and cholesterol levels), and tests of kidney function (serum creatinine and blood urea nitrogen [BUN]) are done to identify secondary hypertension, to evaluate the effects of the hypertension, and to provide baseline data before treatment is started.

Hypertension treatment focuses on lowering the blood pressure to less than 140 mm Hg systolic and 90 mm Hg diastolic. Treatment is directed at reducing the risk of damage to the cardiovascular system and other target organs. Developing a plan of care that the patient can and will follow is vital to prevent long-term complications. Although primary hypertension cannot be cured, it can be controlled with lifestyle management and medications (Table 18-2 ■).

TABLE 18-2	Recommended Follow-Up and Treatment for Hypertension	
STAGE	FOLLOW-UP RECOMMENDATION	TREATMENT RECOMMENDATION
Normal (less than 120/less than 80)	Recheck every 2 years	Lifestyle modification
Pre-hypertension (120–139/80–89)	Recheck every year	Lifestyle modification; medication if diabetes or kidney disease present
Stage 1 (140–159/90–99)	Confirm within 2 months	Medication plus lifestyle modification
Stage 2 (160–179/100–109)	Refer for evaluation and/or treatment within 1 month; evaluate and treat within 1 week if greater than 180/greater than 110	Medication plus lifestyle modification

Source: Adapted from National Institutes of Health, National Heart, Lung, and Blood Institute. (2004). *The seventh report of the Joint National Committee on prevention, detection, evaluation, and treatment of high blood pressure.* NIH Publication No. 04-5230.

Lifestyle Modifications

Lifestyle modifications to reduce blood pressure include weight loss, dietary changes, restricted alcohol use and cigarette smoking, increased physical activity, and stress reduction.

DIET   Dietary changes include limiting sodium and fat in the diet and promoting weight loss if overweight. Foods high in sodium, such as processed foods, canned fruits and vegetables, carbonated beverages, snack foods, and fast foods are avoided. These foods are often high in fats as well, contributing to weight gain. High-sodium, high-fat foods should be replaced with foods higher in potassium and lower in fat (such as fresh fruit and vegetables, freshly cooked meats, and whole grains). The DASH (Dietary Approaches to Stop Hypertension) diet has documented benefits in reducing blood pressure (Box 18-3■). Calories are limited to achieve the goal of weight and body mass within normal limits.

ALCOHOL AND SMOKING   Alcohol intake is limited to no more than 1 ounce of ethanol per day. This translates to 24 ounces of beer, 10 ounces of wine, or 2 ounces of whiskey. Women and lighter-weight people should reduce this limit by half. Because both smoking and hypertension increase the risk of heart disease, patients are strongly urged to quit. Smoking, which constricts the blood vessels and increases peripheral vascular resistance (PVR), reduces the benefits of some antihypertensive medications such as propranolol (Inderal).

PHYSICAL ACTIVITY   Regular exercise (such as walking, cycling, jogging, or swimming) decreases blood pressure and contributes to weight loss, stress reduction, and feelings of overall well-being. At least 30 minutes of continuous aerobic exercise most days of the week (5 or more) is recommended. Exercises that oppose one muscle group to another (isometric), however, can raise systolic blood pressure severely and may not be appropriate.

STRESS REDUCTION   Stress constricts blood vessels, raising the blood pressure. Regular, moderate exercise is the treatment of choice for reducing stress in the hypertensive patient. Other stress reduction techniques may also benefit the patient (Box 18-4■).

Medications

One or more of the following drug classes may be used to treat hypertension: diuretics, beta-adrenergic blockers, centrally acting sympatholytics (drugs that block SNS output), vasodilators, angiotensin-converting enzyme (ACE) inhibitors, angiotensin II receptor blockers (ARBs), and calcium channel blockers. Diuretics, ACE inhibitors, and ARBs reduce circulating blood volume. Diuretics often are used

BOX 18-3	THE DASH DIET

- Whole grains—7 to 8 servings daily
- Vegetables—4 to 5 servings daily
- Fruits—4 to 5 servings daily
- Nonfat/low-fat milk—2 to 3 servings daily
- Lean meat (including fish and poultry)—2 or fewer servings daily
- Nuts, seeds, and dry beans—4 to 5 servings weekly
- Calories—2,000 per day

BOX 18-4	COMPLEMENTARY THERAPIES

Hypertension

Several complementary and alternative therapies have documented benefits for managing hypertension. A number of studies have demonstrated that *garlic* lowers blood pressure in people with hypertension, particularly when combined with antihypertensive therapy. Although the effect is not as significant as is seen with garlic, *fish oil supplements* lower blood pressure as well, particularly when higher doses are used. The antihypertensive effects of *biofeedback*, a mind–body therapy, have been studied for more than 40 years. Its blood-pressure-lowering effects are most significant when combined with *relaxation training* or *cognitive therapy* (Barrows, 2013). Movement therapies such as *yoga* and *t'ai chi* also lower blood pressure and improve overall well-being.

to treat hypertension in older adults, and generally are more effective in treating hypertension in Blacks. Hydrochlorothiazide (HydroDIURIL) has been proven to be effective in treating hypertension in about 50% of patients and has the added benefit of reducing the risk for coronary heart disease. Beta blockers reduce cardiac output. Centrally acting sympatholytics and vasodilators reduce peripheral resistance. Calcium channel blockers produce vasodilation. See Figure 18-1■ for an illustration of the sites of action for various classes of antihypertensive drugs. No one primary antihypertensive drug is used to treat hypertension.

A combination of drugs or a trial with a different category of antihypertensives is often used. Nursing implications for administering antihypertensive drugs (other than diuretics) are outlined in Table 18-3■.

Treatment of patients with other risk factors for coronary heart disease is more aggressive to reduce the risk of an AMI, heart failure, or stroke. When the patient's average blood pressure is greater than 200/120, immediate treatment is vital. Parenteral medications are given to reduce the blood pressure in a rapid but controlled manner and prevent long-term consequences of the emergency.

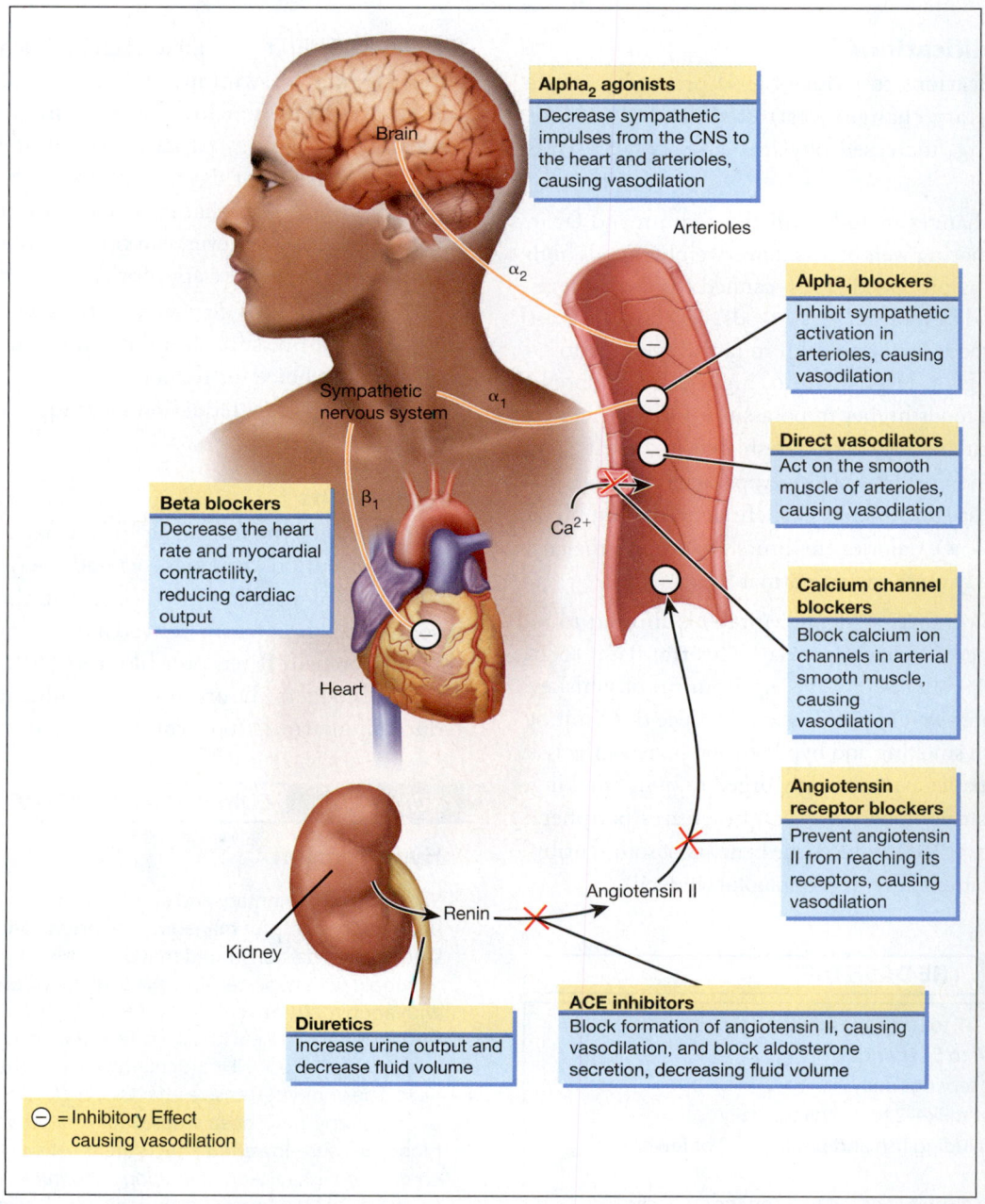

Figure 18-1. ■ Sites and mechanisms of antihypertensive drug action. (Source: "Figure 25.01 - Mechanisms of Action of Antihypertensive Drugs" from Pharmacology for Nurses: A Pathophysiologic Approach, 4e by Michael Patrick Adams; Leland Norman Holland; and Carol Quam Urban. Published by Pearson Education, © 2014.)

TABLE 18-3	**Giving Medications Safely: Hypertension**		
CLASS/DRUGS	**PURPOSE**	**NURSING IMPLICATIONS**	**PATIENT TEACHING**
Angiotensin-converting enzyme (ACE) inhibitors ■ Benazepril (Lotensin) ■ Captopril (Capoten) ■ *Enalapril* (Vasotec) ■ *Lisinopril* (Zestril) ■ Moexipril (Univasc) ■ Ramipril (Altace) ■ Trandolapril (Mavik) ■ Others ***Angiotensin II receptor blockers (ARBs)*** ■ Eprosartan (Teveten) ■ Losartan (Cozaar) ■ *Olmesartan medoxomil* (Benicar) ■ Telmisartan (Micardis) ■ *Valsartan* (Diovan)	ACE inhibitors and ARBs inhibit the renin–angiotensin system, stimulate vasodilation, and may reduce sympathetic nervous system activity. These drugs have relatively few side effects in patients with essential hypertension.	Give 1 hour before meals to increase absorption; tablets may be crushed. Report abnormal laboratory values to the primary care provider. Take blood pressure before each dose. If hypotension occurs, keep flat with legs elevated. Monitor for rash or hives. Report peripheral edema.	Report peripheral edema, infection, persistent cough, or difficulty breathing to your health care provider. Change position (lying to sitting and sitting to standing) slowly to prevent dizziness and possible falls. Do not skip doses or stop taking drugs; this could cause your blood pressure to rise significantly.
Beta-adrenergic blockers ■ *Atenolol* (Tenormin) ■ Bisoprolol (Zebeta) ■ Carteolol (Cartrol) ■ Labetalol (Normodyne) ■ *Metoprolol tartrate* (Lopressor) ■ Propranolol (Inderal) ■ Timolol (Blocadren)	Beta blockers block sympathetic input to the heart. This reduces heart rate and cardiac output. They also interfere with the renin–angiotensin system, blocking vasoconstriction. Beta blockers can have serious side effects and should not be taken by patients with asthma, COPD, or heart block.	Assess blood pressure and apical pulse before giving; notify the charge nurse if they are not within established limits. Monitor for hypotension if patient is also taking a diuretic. Carefully monitor diabetic patients for hypoglycemia.	Take your pulse and blood pressure daily. Change positions slowly to prevent dizziness and possible falls. Report fatigue, lethargy, or impotence to your doctor. If diabetic, check blood glucose more frequently; this medication may block hypoglycemia symptoms. Do not stop taking the drug unless instructed to by your doctor.
Centrally acting sympatholytics ■ Clonidine (Catapres) ■ Guanabenz (Wytensin) ■ Methyldopa (Aldomet)	These drugs slow the heart rate and reduce vasoconstriction, lowering the blood pressure. They may be given in combination with a diuretic.	Administer PO; tablets may be crushed. Methyldopa may be given IV over 30 to 60 minutes; do not give subcutaneously or IM. Apply transdermal forms to dry, hairless, intact skin on the chest or upper arm. Report rash to physician. Report abnormal laboratory values to the primary care provider. Record baseline BP, pulse, and weight; assess vital signs before giving drug. Report peripheral edema or other side effects to the physician.	Relieve dry mouth by sipping water or chewing sugarless gum. Use unsalted crackers, non-cola beverages, or dry toast to relieve nausea. Change positions slowly to prevent dizziness and possible falls. Do not stop taking or skip doses of this drug. The drug may darken your urine. Report depression or difficulty thinking to your doctor. Side effects tend to diminish over time. Do not drive if the drug causes drowsiness.

(continued)

Table 18-3	Giving Medications Safely: Hypertension (continued)		
CLASS/DRUGS	**PURPOSE**	**NURSING IMPLICATIONS**	**PATIENT TEACHING**
Vasodilators ■ Diazoxide (Hyperstat IV) ■ Hydralazine (Apresoline) ■ Minoxidil (Loniten) ■ Nitroprusside (Nitropress)	Vasodilators reduce blood pressure by relaxing vascular smooth muscle and decreasing peripheral vascular resistance.	Administer PO drugs with meals or food; tablets may be crushed. Assess BP and pulse before giving the drug. Monitor BP every 5 to 15 minutes when administering IV. Monitor bowel movements. Monitor for heart failure, fluid retention, and angina.	Change positions slowly to prevent dizziness and possible falls. Eat dry toast or unsalted crackers to relieve nausea. Report muscle, joint aches, and fever to your doctor. Tearing and nasal congestion may occur. Headache, palpitations, and rapid pulse should stop in about 10 days. Do not stop this drug unless your doctor approves. Report black, tarry stools or red blood in stools to your doctor.
Alpha-adrenergic blockers ■ Doxazosin (Cardura) ■ Prazosin (Minipress) ■ Terazosin (Hytrin)	Alpha-adrenergic blockers promote vasodilatation, lowering blood pressure. They also reduce LDL and VLDL levels. Doxazosin and terazosin may cause tachycardia and palpitations and other unwanted side effects. For these reasons, they are primarily used in acute situations.	Maintain safety during position changes; severe hypotension may develop. Give first dose at bedtime to reduce risk of fainting ("first-dose syncope"). Assess apical pulse and BP immediately before each dose and every 15 to 30 minutes thereafter until stable.	Use sips of water or sugarless gum to relieve dry mouth. Eat dry toast or unsalted crackers to relieve nausea. You may experience nasal congestion. Do not expect full benefit for 3 to 4 weeks. Change positions slowly to prevent dizziness and possible falls. Do not stop the drug without contacting your doctor.
Calcium channel blockers ■ *Amlodipine* (Norvasc) ■ Diltiazem (Cardizem) ■ Felodipine (Plendil) ■ Isradipine (DynaCirc) ■ Nicardipine (Cardene) ■ Nifedipine (Procardia) ■ Nisoldipine (Nisocor) ■ Verapamil (Isoptin)	Calcium channel blockers relax arterial smooth muscle, causing vasodilation.	If given parenterally, monitor heart rhythm continuously. Assess apical pulse and BP before giving. Notify charge nurse if outside identified limits. Monitor frequency and consistency of stools. Assess lungs for crackles and wheezes. Monitor intake and output. Assess extremities for peripheral edema.	Take BP and pulse daily. Change positions slowly to prevent dizziness and possible falls. Drink 6 to 8 glasses of water daily, and increase fiber in diet. Do not abruptly stop taking medications. Report difficulty breathing or chest pain to your doctor.

Note: Medications identified in *italics* are among the 200 most frequently prescribed drugs in the United States.

NURSING CARE

PRIORITIZING NURSING CARE

The priority of nursing care for the vast majority of patients with hypertension is teaching. Hypertension is a chronic disease that requires continuing management to prevent its complications. This responsibility falls primarily to the patient.

HEALTH PROMOTION

Nurses promote health in all patients by teaching and discussing the modifiable risk factors for hypertension. Advise all patients to avoid smoking—either to stop or not to start. Provide information about smoking cessation programs as appropriate. Discuss the relationship between obesity, stress, and a sedentary lifestyle and hypertension. Encourage all patients to eat a diet rich in fruits and vegetables and low in fat. Advise all patients to engage in regular physical activity, including at least 30 minutes of continuous aerobic activity such as walking or swimming 5 or more days a week.

ASSESSING

Obtaining accurate blood pressure measurements is key when assessing patients with hypertension. Inaccurate readings often occur because of inappropriate cuff size or incorrect technique. Box 18-5 ■ provides guidelines that help ensure accurate blood pressure readings.

IDENTIFYING POTENTIAL COMPLICATIONS

Hypertension is generally a disease without symptoms. Hypertensive crisis can develop at any time, however. Immediately assess the blood pressure of a patient who complains of headache, blurred vision, anxiety, or new onset of neurologic symptoms. Refer the patient to the primary care provider for follow-up, as appropriate.

DIAGNOSING, PLANNING, AND IMPLEMENTING

Ineffective Health Maintenance

Expected outcome: Will relate an understanding of hypertension as a chronic disease requiring continuing management.

■ Explain the physiology and significance of the blood pressure. *Many people do not understand the significance of the blood pressure and its effects on the body.*

■ Emphasize the importance of adhering to prescribed treatment. *Keeping the blood pressure within normal levels reduces the risk for target organ damage and stroke.*

■ Discuss lifestyle changes with all patients at risk for or with hypertension. *Lifestyle changes may help reduce the risk of hypertension and its consequences. These changes alone will not control stage 2 hypertension, but may lower the amount of medication needed to maintain blood pressure within appropriate levels.*

■ Discuss the relationship between sodium intake and blood pressure. Refer to dietary services for teaching about a low-sodium diet. Provide opportunities to choose low-sodium foods from simulated menus. *Knowledge and practice help patients understand and take control of their disease.*

■ Discuss weight loss strategies and a low-fat diet. If appropriate, refer the patient to an approved weight-loss program (*Weight Watchers, Overeaters Anonymous, Diet Workshop*). *Many overweight patients "diet" frequently without a good understanding of nutrition. Teaching and the support of a weight loss program help the patient learn to make more appropriate food choices.*

■ Help identify realistic and appropriate lifestyle changes such as increasing exercise, stopping smoking, reducing alcohol intake, and controlling stress. *A plan that fits with the patient's lifestyle is more likely to succeed. Family support is vital for maintaining lifestyle changes.*

■ Help identify strengths and weaknesses in maintaining health. *Anticipating potential difficulties allows the patient and family to plan strategies to overcome these hurdles.*

BOX 18-5 NURSING CARE CHECKLIST

Accurate Blood Pressure Measurement

☑ Choose blood pressure cuff that is the correct size: The cuff width should be about 40% of the circumference of the arm (or thigh) (see figure).

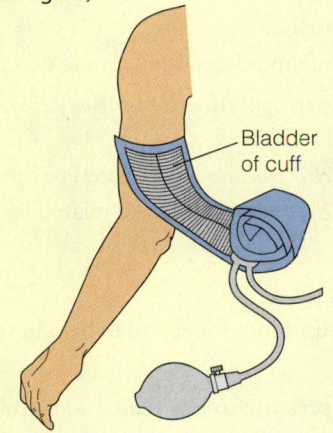

Bladder of cuff

☑ Position the cuff on the extremity with the center of the bladder directly over the artery.

☑ While palpating the artery (brachial if using the upper arm, radial if using the forearm, and popliteal if using the thigh), inflate the cuff until the pulse is no longer felt. Note the pressure and rapidly deflate the cuff. Wait approximately 1 to 2 minutes.

☑ Position the stethoscope over the artery and inflate the cuff to 30 mm Hg above the level at which the pulse was no longer felt. Slowly deflate the cuff at a rate of 2 to 3 mm Hg per second.

☑ Note the systolic reading where the first clear tapping sound (Korotkoff sound) is heard. Note the diastolic reading when the sounds change from distinct, crisp sounds to muffled sounds. In some facilities, a third reading is noted at the point where the last sound is heard.

☑ If possible, measure the pressure on both arms. If there is a difference of more than 5 to 10 mm Hg in the pressures, use the arm with the higher pressure reading for subsequent measurements because it more accurately reflects the systemic blood pressure.

MANAGING NURSING CARE

Obtaining the patient's weight, blood pressure, and other vital signs may be appropriate to assign to unlicensed assistive personnel (nursing assistants, medical assistants) after ensuring use of correct technique and the ability to obtain accurate data.

EVALUATING

When evaluating the effectiveness of nursing care related to hypertension, collect data to assess the patient's knowledge and understanding of the disease and its treatment. Ask about current treatment, including any adverse drug effects if present. Inquire about continued compliance with recommended diet, exercise, smoking cessation, and other lifestyle changes.

DOCUMENTING

Document blood pressure, other vital signs, current medications, and the response to immediate treatment, if provided. Document teaching provided and referrals made (e.g., to a dietitian for dietary teaching, weight management program, or smoking cessation program) and the patient's apparent understanding and acceptance of instructions.

CONTINUITY OF CARE

Hypertension is primarily managed in community settings with regular visits to the primary care provider or hypertension clinic to monitor treatment. Because the patient is ultimately responsible for managing this chronic disease, careful assessment of the patient's knowledge, understanding, and resources for home care is important. Assess the patient's and family's desire and ability to implement and maintain recommended lifestyle changes, adapting recommendations to the individual.

Stress the importance of taking medications as ordered. Discuss common side effects and their management. Inform the patient that some drugs may have unpleasant side effects initially, but these effects diminish within 2 to 3 weeks of starting the medication. Review symptoms that should be reported to the primary care provider.

Help patients, and as appropriate significant others, develop a realistic, regular exercise program that can be continued for life. Aerobic exercise such as walking, swimming, or cycling increases stamina and endurance, reduces stress, and helps manage obesity. Isometric activities (such as weight lifting) should be avoided unless approved by the physician, because they increase blood pressure.

Discuss the impact of stress on blood pressure. Teach stress reduction techniques such as meditation, relaxation, or deep breathing. Discuss the vasoconstrictive effects of anger and hostility, and help identify ways to diffuse these emotions. Explore alternative coping mechanisms to use during stressful situations.

Emphasize the need for regular follow-up care, even if progress is slow or if they have been unable to adhere to the plan. Comparing hypertension to diabetes, another chronic disease that requires lifelong management, may help the patient and family understand the importance of continued care and follow-up.

NURSING CARE PLAN
Patient With Hypertension

Margaret Spezia is a married, 49-year-old Italian American woman with eight children, currently ranging in age from 3 to 18 years. During her annual physical examination 2 months ago, her blood pressure was found to be 146/98. Mrs. Spezia was instructed to reduce her cholesterol intake, to avoid salty foods, and not to add any salt to her foods either at the table or during cooking. An exercise program of short, daily walks was suggested for exercise and to reduce stress. She returns for follow-up.

Assessment

Lisa Christos, the clinic nurse, obtains a nursing history. Mrs. Spezia reveals that between raising their children and working part-time, she rarely gets enough rest. Although her husband has a steady job, money is tight. She admits to a steady weight gain during the past 18 years. There is no known family history of hypertension. Physical assessment data include the following: height 5'3" (160 cm); weight 225 lb (102 kg); T 99°F (37.2°C); P 100, regular; R 16; BP 170/110 (sitting); skin cool and dry; capillary refill 3 seconds in upper extremities. Total serum cholesterol 245 mg/dL (normal adult value less than 200 mg/dL). All other blood and urine studies are within normal limits.

Captopril (Capoten), 25 mg by mouth twice daily, and hydrochlorothiazide, 50 mg by mouth daily, are ordered. She is placed on a low-cholesterol, no-added-salt diet.

Nursing Diagnosis

The following nursing diagnoses (among others) are identified:

- *Imbalanced Nutrition: More Than Body Requirements* related to excess food intake
- *Ineffective Health Maintenance* related to lifestyle behaviors
- *Readiness for Enhanced Knowledge* related to prescribed treatment

Expected Outcomes

The expected outcomes for the plan of care specify that Mrs. Spezia will

- Lower blood pressure to less than 150 systolic and 90 diastolic within 1 week.
- Incorporate in her diet low-sodium and low-fat foods from a list provided.
- Develop a plan for regular exercise.

- Verbalize how prescribed medications, dietary restrictions, exercise, and follow-up visits will help her control her hypertension.

Planning and Implementation

The following nursing interventions are planned and implemented:

- Teach how and when to monitor her blood pressure.
- Instruct to withhold medications and contact the clinic if BP is less than 90 mm Hg systolic or 60 mm Hg diastolic.
- Provide written and verbal instructions including the name, dose, action, and side effects of antihypertensive medications.
- Help develop an exercise plan that includes a daily 15-minute walk and possible swimming classes at local YWCA.
- Discuss a realistic weight loss goal and plan.
- Refer for dietary consultation and teaching about fat and sodium restrictions and weight loss.

Evaluation

When Mrs. Spezia returns to the clinic 1 week later, her blood pressure is 142/88. She has lost 1.5 lb and says her oldest daughter is encouraging her to join a weight-reduction program. Mrs. Spezia is walking about 20 minutes a day at a local mall. She has met with the dietitian to discuss ways to replace salt with herbs and spices. She has a list of low-fat, low-sodium foods and recommended cookbooks. Mrs. Spezia verbalizes the importance of taking her medications as ordered and managing her stress. She tells Ms. Christos, "I just can't believe that I feel better already. I've actually lost some weight—and I want to keep going. I think I can stick with this plan, even though it's like learning to cook all over again."

Critical Thinking in the Nursing Process

1. Identify factors that contributed to Mrs. Spezia's hypertension. Which were modifiable and which were not?
2. What are the reasons for reducing sodium and fat in Mrs. Spezia's diet?

3. When Mrs. Spezia returns to the clinic for a follow-up exam 6 weeks later, she admits to Ms. Christos that she has difficulty remembering to take her blood pressure medications consistently. What suggestions could Ms. Christos provide?

Note: Discussion of Critical Thinking questions appears on the companion website.

Secondary Hypertension

Secondary hypertension is an elevated blood pressure that can be related to an identified disorder. It accounts for only about 5% of all identified cases of high blood pressure. Elevated blood pressure readings in a young patient with few identified risk factors should trigger additional diagnostic testing for unidentified disease processes.

Kidney disease is a leading cause of secondary hypertension. Kidney disease disrupts regulation of the renin–angiotensin–aldosterone system and can lead to salt and water retention. Coarctation (narrowing) of the aorta also is a common cause of secondary hypertension. The aortic narrowing reduces blood flow to the kidneys and peripheral vascular system, triggering responses that raise the blood pressure. Other conditions that can lead to secondary hypertension include pregnancy (about 10% of pregnant women are hypertensive), endocrine or neurologic disorders, or use of stimulant drugs (e.g., cocaine, amphetamines).

Diagnostic testing to identify secondary hypertension includes obtaining blood chemistries (electrolytes, glucose, lipids), urinalysis and renal function studies, and other diagnostic tests as indicated. Secondary hypertension is primarily treated by addressing the underlying disorder. Antihypertensive drugs are prescribed to manage the blood pressure during disease treatment.

Nursing care for the patient with secondary hypertension is the same as that provided to a patient with primary hypertension. In addition, consideration of the underlying disorder is given in planning and implementing nursing care.

DISORDERS OF THE AORTA AND ITS BRANCHES

Key Concept The aorta and its branches can be affected by chronic disorders such as arteriosclerosis, which weakens vessel walls and can result in aneurysm.

Aneurysm

An **aneurysm** is an abnormal dilation of a blood vessel, usually in an area of vessel weakness or vessel wall tear. Aneurysms usually affect the aorta and major arteries, because

of the high pressure within these vessels. Most aneurysms are caused by arteriosclerosis or atherosclerosis. Trauma and congenital weakness of a vessel also may cause an aneurysm to form. Genetics play a role; about 20% of patients with an aortic aneurysm have a family history of the disorder.

PATHOPHYSIOLOGY

Aneurysms are commonly classified by their shape and location (Figure 18-2■). *Fusiform aneurysms* involve the entire

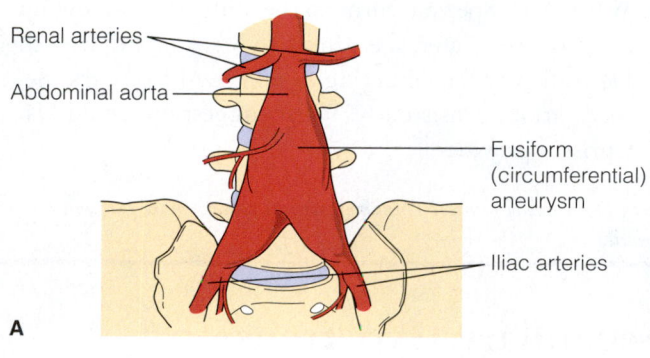

Renal arteries

Abdominal aorta

Fusiform
(circumferential)
aneurysm

Iliac arteries

A

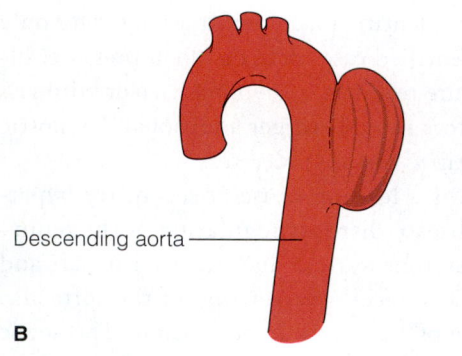

Descending aorta

B

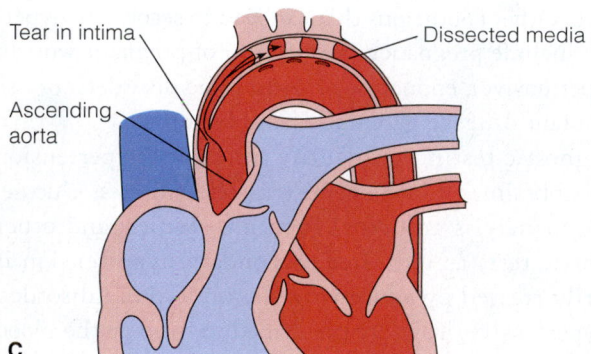

Tear in intima

Dissected media

Ascending
aorta

C

Figure 18-2. ■ Aortic aneurysms.(**A**) Fusiform aneurysm of the abdominal aorta. (**B**) Saccular aneurysm of the descending thoracic aorta. (**C**) Dissection of the ascending thoracic aorta.

circumference of the vessel. They generally grow slowly but progressively. Their length and diameter vary considerably from patient to patient. *Saccular aneurysms* involve only a portion of the vessel. They are more often associated with congenital malformations or syphilis than with arteriosclerosis. *Berry aneurysms* are a common type of congenital saccular aneurysm found in a section of cerebral arteries (the circle of Willis) in the brain. *Aortic dissection* (also called a *dissecting aneurysm*) develops due to weakening of the medial layer of the aorta. Blood leaks into the vessel wall, separating the intimal (innermost) layer of the artery from the externa (outermost layer). Aortic dissection usually occurs in the ascending aorta.

Aneurysms often produce no symptoms and are discovered during a routine physical examination. When manifestations occur, they are due to the pressure of the aneurysm on adjacent tissues and organs (Table 18-4■).

Thoracic Aortic Aneurysms

Thoracic aortic aneurysms frequently cause no symptoms. Substernal (anginal), neck, or back pain may occur. Pressure on the trachea, esophagus, laryngeal nerve, or superior vena cava may cause difficulty breathing, stridor, cough, difficult or painful swallowing, hoarseness, edema of the face and neck, and distended neck veins. Aneurysms of the thoracic aorta tend to enlarge progressively and may rupture, causing death. Blood clots may form within the aneurysm. These clots can become emboli, causing stroke or acute ischemia of the bowel, kidney, or lower extremities.

Abdominal Aortic Aneurysms

Abdominal aortic aneurysms are associated with arteriosclerosis, hypertension, smoking, and increasing age. Most abdominal aortic aneurysms are found in adults older than 70.

Most patients with abdominal aneurysms are asymptomatic, but on examination have a pulsating mass in the mid- and upper abdomen and a bruit over the mass. The patient may complain of mild-to-severe midabdominal or

TABLE 18-4	Manifestations and Complications of Aortic Aneurysms		
	LOCATION		
	THORACIC	**ABDOMINAL**	**DISSECTING**
Manifestations	Chest, back, or neck pain	Pulsating abdominal mass	Sudden, severe chest pain
	Dyspnea, cough	Abdominal or lower back pain	Decreased blood pressure in upper extremities
	Hoarseness, dysphagia		
	Distended neck veins, edema of face and neck	Cool, pale, or cyanotic lower extremities	Absent radial pulses
Complications	Rupture and hemorrhage	Emboli to lower extremities	Hemorrhage
		Rupture and hemorrhage	Kidney failure, cardiac tamponade, sepsis

lower back pain. The degree of pain commonly indicates the severity (and urgency) of the problem. Pain may be an indication of an impending rupture.

Emboli may form due to sluggish blood flow within the aneurysm and travel to the lower extremities. The aneurysm may also rupture and lead to death due to hemorrhage and hypovolemic shock.

Femoral and Popliteal Aneurysms

Femoral and popliteal aneurysms usually are due to arteriosclerosis. They often occur bilaterally. Men are affected more frequently than women. These aneurysms frequently produce no symptoms. A pulsating mass may be detected in the groin (femoral aneurysm) or behind the knee (popliteal aneurysm). Both femoral and popliteal aneurysms can decrease blood flow to the lower extremities, causing cramping and pain in the leg muscles with exercise or at rest, and numbness. Femoral aneurysms may rupture, leading to hemorrhage.

Aortic Dissections

Aortic dissection is a life-threatening emergency caused by a tear in the inner layer of the aorta with bleeding into the middle layer. This *dissects* or splits the vessel wall, forming a blood-filled channel between its layers. Dissection can occur anywhere along the aorta, but is most common in the ascending aorta where pressures are high.

Hypertension is a major risk factor for aortic dissection. Patients with a genetic disorder called **Marfan syndrome** are at risk for aortic dissection (Box 18-6■).

The primary symptom of aortic dissection is sudden, excruciating pain. The pain often is described as a ripping or tearing sensation. It is usually located in the area of dissection (e.g., anterior chest if thoracic, back if abdominal). Blood pressure may initially rise, but then falls rapidly and is often inaudible because the dissection occludes blood flow. Peripheral pulses are also absent.

COLLABORATIVE CARE

The size, location, and type of an aneurysm determines treatment. Small, asymptomatic aneurysms may not be treated or may be managed medically. Large aneurysms that pose a risk of rupture usually are treated surgically.

Diagnostic Tests

Aneurysms often are detected by a *chest* or *abdominal x-ray*. An *abdominal ultrasound* is done when an abdominal aneurysm is suspected. A *CT scan* or an *MRI* may be ordered to measure the aneurysm size. *Angiography*, which requires injection of a contrast solution into the affected vessel, is used to identify the exact size and location of an aneurysm.

Medications

Patients with aortic aneurysms often are treated with beta-adrenergic blocker medications to lower blood pressure. ACE inhibitors or ARBs may benefit patients with Marfan syndrome. Intravenous beta blockers and sodium nitroprusside are administered to patients with aortic dissection to reduce the heart rate and blood pressure.

Surgery

Surgery is done to repair aneurysms that are tender to palpation or enlarging rapidly. The patient's general health and surgical risk are considered, unless immediate surgery is necessary to preserve life. In many cases, patients undergo an open surgical procedure in which the aneurysm is excised and replaced with a synthetic fabric graft (Figure 18-3■). Nursing care of the patient having surgery on the aorta is outlined in Box 18-7■.

BOX 18-6	POPULATION FOCUS

Patients With Marfan Syndrome

Marfan syndrome is a connective tissue disorder with three distinctive features: (1) long, thin extremities, hyperextensible joints, and other skeletal deformities; (2) impaired vision; and (3) cardiovascular defects, including mitral valve prolapse and weakness of the aorta with frequent aortic dissection and rupture. Marfan syndrome affects about 1 in 10,000 people. It is inherited as an autosomal dominant trait.

There is no cure for Marfan syndrome, so teaching is vital. Severe physical and emotional stress and pregnancy increase the risk of aortic dissection and cardiac complications. Encourage to avoid vigorous physical exertion and the physical stress of pregnancy. Teach measures to reduce the risk of endocarditis. Scoliosis and kyphosis are common; refer for physical therapy and bracing as needed. Stress the importance of regular eye examinations and immediate care if visual disturbances develop. Discuss the genetic nature of Marfan syndrome: Each child has a 50% risk of being affected. Encourage consideration of alternatives such as adoption. Make referrals as appropriate.

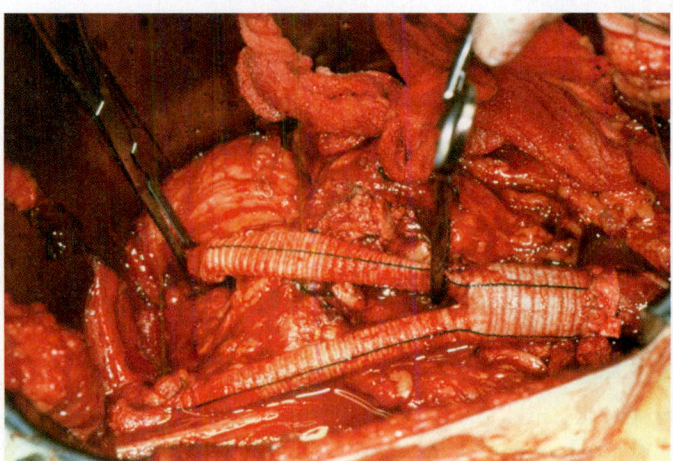

Figure 18-3. ■ Repair of an abdominal aortic aneurysm using a synthetic graft to replace the aneurysm. The aneurysm walls are then sutured around the graft. (Source: Stevie Grand/Science Source.)

BOX 18-7 **NURSING CARE CHECKLIST**

Surgery of the Aorta

Before Surgery

☑ Provide routine preoperative care and teaching.

☑ Orient to intensive care unit. Describe anticipated equipment, tubes, sights and sounds, and postoperative communication. Allow time for questions and to clarify information.

☑ Immediately report changes in blood pressure in upper and lower extremities, peripheral pulses, pain, abdominal girth, and sensation and movement of lower extremities.

☑ Maintain position and activity restrictions as ordered. Instruct to avoid holding breath while moving or defecating.

☑ Report absent peripheral pulses; pale, cyanotic, or cool extremities; diffuse abdominal pain; or an increase in groin, lumbar, or lower extremity pain.

After Surgery

☑ Provide general postoperative care.

☑ Monitor chest tube drainage and status as needed.

☑ Frequently assess for bleeding. Immediately report signs of graft leakage:

a. Bruising of scrotum, perineum, or penis; hematoma at incision

b. Increased abdominal girth

c. Weak or absent peripheral pulses; impaired movement or sensation of extremities

d. Decreased blood pressure, increased pulse; low urine output (30 mL/hr)

e. Increased abdominal, back, or groin pain

f. Drop in hematocrit, hemoglobin, and red blood cell levels

☑ Maintain intravenous fluids and administer blood as ordered.

☑ Report evidence of complications:

a. *Lower extremity embolism:* pain and numbness; diminished pulses; and pale, cool, or cyanotic skin

b. *Bowel ischemia:* blood in stools, diarrhea, severe abdominal pain, and abdominal distention

c. *Impaired renal function:* output less than 30 mL/hr, fixed specific gravity, increasing BUN and serum creatinine levels

d. *Spinal cord ischemia:* lower extremity weakness and paraplegia

---

Endovascular stent grafts (EVSGs) are increasingly used to repair abdominal and thoracic aortic aneurysms. The stent, a metal sheath covered with polyester, is usually placed percutaneously via the femoral artery. This results in a shorter hospital stay and faster recovery for the patient. The patient does, however, require regular follow-up with CT scans to detect possible complications.

NURSING CARE

Nurses may care for a patient with a stable or slowly expanding aneurysm or for patients before and after surgical repair or treatment of an expanding or ruptured aneurysm. Nursing care priorities are on monitoring and maintaining tissue perfusion and, in the surgical patient, relieving pain and reducing anxiety.

DIAGNOSING, PLANNING, AND IMPLEMENTING

Risk for Ineffective Peripheral Tissue Perfusion

Expected outcome: Will remain free of hemorrhage or arterial occlusion as evidenced by stable VS, level of consciousness (LOC), color, and peripheral pulses.

■ As indicated, plan and implement measures to reduce the risk of aneurysm rupture: maintain bed rest in a calm environment, prevent straining during bowel movements and when turning, and administer medications as ordered. *Activity, stress, and straining to have a*

bowel movement raise the blood pressure, increasing the risk of rupture. Medications are given to reduce blood pressure.

clinicalALERT

Immediately report manifestations of impending rupture or other complications, including increasing pain, a discrepancy between pulses and blood pressure on upper and lower extremities, or a change in LOC. Emergency surgery may be required.

■ Monitor for and report manifestations of acute vascular occlusion: absent peripheral pulses, a pale or cyanotic cool extremity, severe abdominal pain, or a change in level of consciousness or neurologic status. *Clots may form within the aneurysm, breaking loose to become arterial emboli. An expanding aneurysm can affect cerebral blood flow or perfusion of the spinal cord, leading to neurologic symptoms.*

Anxiety

Expected outcome: Anxiety will not exceed a mild to moderate level.

Patients with a rapidly expanding aneurysm are often highly anxious. Managing anxiety levels is an important component of nursing care. Establish trust through active listening. Acknowledge the fears and concerns of the patient and family. Use a calm demeanor, appropriate and reassuring manner, and factual explanations to keep patients calm and prevent any additional stress, which might worsen hypertension.

CONTINUITY OF CARE

Small or asymptomatic aneurysms often are managed in the community. Teach measures to control hypertension, discussing diet, stress reduction, alcohol, smoking, and medications. Stress the importance of taking medications as ordered and following the prescribed treatment to prevent complications.

After surgery, provide verbal and written instructions about preventing and recognizing infection, caring for the incision, taking medications to control blood pressure and prevent blood clotting, and recognizing complications. Suggest ways to prevent constipation and straining at stool (such as increasing fluid and fiber in the diet). Instruct to avoid prolonged sitting, lifting heavy objects, exercising strenuously, and having sexual intercourse until approved by the physician (usually 6 to 12 weeks). Provide information about return appointments. Refer to a home health agency or community health service as necessary for continuing care after discharge.

PERIPHERAL ARTERIAL DISORDERS

Key Concept Atherosclerosis, the pathophysiologic process underlying coronary heart disease and stroke, affects peripheral blood vessels as well. Peripheral vascular disease is a leading cause of lower extremity pain, impaired healing, and lower extremity amputation, particularly in older adults.

Adequate blood flow through peripheral arteries is essential to provide oxygen and nutrients to tissues and cells. This blood flow can be affected by arterial wall defects, compression of the blood vessel, or vasospasm. Arterial disorders may be either acute (e.g., arterial embolism or thrombosis) or chronic. Atherosclerosis of the peripheral arteries, known as peripheral vascular disease, is the most common chronic disorder of the peripheral arteries. Other arterial disorders include thromboangiitis obliterans (Buerger disease) and Raynaud phenomenon. The nurse's role in caring for patients with disorders affecting the peripheral arteries focuses on maintaining tissue perfusion and teaching the patient and family about the disorder and its management.

Peripheral Vascular Disease

In the peripheral circulation, arteriosclerosis and atherosclerosis decrease the blood supply to tissues, leading to **peripheral vascular disease (PVD)**, also called *peripheral arterial disease (PAD)*. **Arteriosclerosis** is a common arterial disorder characterized by thickening, loss of elasticity, and calcification of arterial walls. *Atherosclerosis* is a form of arteriosclerosis in which the arterial walls thicken and harden due to deposits of fat and fibrin. PVD usually affects the lower extremities.

Peripheral vascular disease is more common in people over the age of 50 and is seen in men more than in women. Risk factors are similar to those for coronary heart disease, including a high-fat diet, hypertension, diabetes mellitus, smoking, obesity, and stress.

PATHOPHYSIOLOGY

Atherosclerosis is a disease in which lesions called *atheromas* (or *plaque*) develop in the lining of medium and large arteries. Plaque tends to form at arterial *bifurcations* (where the artery divides into two smaller arteries). Peripheral plaque deposits usually affect the femoral arteries, the common iliac arteries, and the abdominal aorta. The cause of atherosclerosis is unknown.

As peripheral arteries thicken and harden because of plaque deposits, the vessel lumen narrows. Furthermore, atherosclerosis impairs the vessel's ability to dilate in response to increased oxygen demands. Blood flow and oxygen delivery to the distal tissues decrease. If the occlusion develops slowly, **collateral circulation** often develops (growth of small blood vessels to maintain tissue perfusion), but it is usually not adequate to supply tissue needs. Few symptoms are seen until 60% or more of the blood supply to the tissues is occluded.

MANIFESTATIONS AND COMPLICATIONS

Pain is the primary symptom of peripheral vascular disease. One type of pain, called **intermittent claudication**, is usually described as a cramping or aching sensation in the calves of the legs or the arch of the foot. It develops with exercise such as walking and is relieved by rest.

Rest pain, in contrast, occurs during periods of inactivity. It is a gnawing, aching, or burning sensation in the lower legs, feet, or toes. Rest pain often occurs at night. It increases when the legs are elevated and decreases when the legs are dependent (e.g., hanging over the side of the bed). Patients often complain that the legs feel cold or numb as well as painful.

The skin is pale when the legs are elevated but often dark red (*dependent rubor*) when the legs are dependent. The skin is often thin and shiny, with areas of discoloration and hair loss. The toenails may be thickened. In addition, areas of skin breakdown may be present. These may lead to ulcerations or gangrene.

Peripheral pulses often are decreased or absent. A **bruit** (a harsh or musical sound caused by turbulent blood flow) may be heard over large affected arteries, such as the femoral artery and the abdominal aorta.

The complications of peripheral arteriosclerosis include gangrene and amputation of one or both lower extremities.

COLLABORATIVE CARE

Management of patients with peripheral vascular disease focuses on slowing the atherosclerotic process, maintaining or improving the blood supply to tissues, and relieving symptoms.

Diagnostic Tests

- The *ankle–brachial index (ABI)* and *segmental blood pressures* are used to compare blood pressure measurements between the upper and lower extremities and within different portions of an extremity (e.g., the ankle and the thigh). Normally, blood pressure readings should be similar when the patient is supine. In PVD, the blood pressure may be lower in the legs than in the arms.
- *Exercise stress testing* can help identify the patient's functional limitations related to PVD.
- *Doppler ultrasound studies* are done to evaluate blood flow. Low-intensity sound waves directed at the affected vessel strike moving RBCs and bounce back to the transducer–

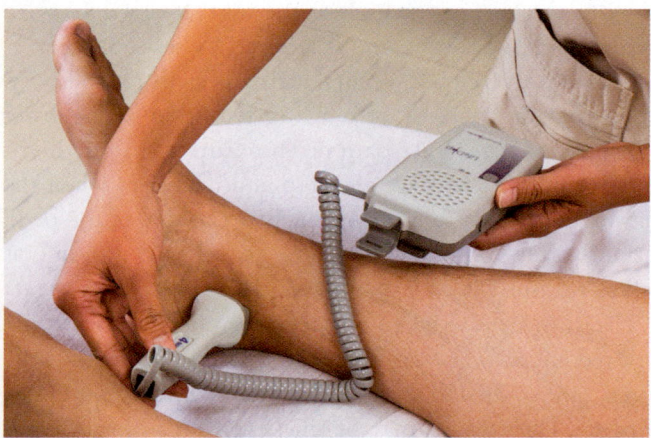

Figure 18-4. ■ A handheld Doppler (ultrasound) device. (Source: Rick Brady, Pearson Education.)

receiver (Figure 18-4■). Blood flow within the vessel can be evaluated by an audible sound or a graphic recording.

- *Transcutaneous oximetry* is performed to evaluate tissue oxygenation.
- *Computed tomography angiography* or *magnetic resonance angiography* is performed if surgery is planned to locate and determine the extent of arterial obstruction.

Medications

Medications may be prescribed to slow the atherosclerotic process and to reduce the risk of clotting in partially obstructed blood vessels. Statin drugs such as *atorvastatin (Lipitor)*, *simvastatin (Zocor)*, or *rosuvastatin (Crestor)* are given to reduce total and LDL cholesterol levels. Aspirin, *clopidogrel (Plavix)*, and cilostazol (Pletal) inhibit platelet aggregation, reducing the risk for clot formation. Cilostazol also acts as a vasodilator, increasing blood flow.

Conservative Therapy

Smoking cessation is vital in managing peripheral vascular disorders. Nicotine promotes atherosclerosis and causes vasospasm, further decreasing blood supply to the extremities. Continued smoking increases the risk for ulcerations, gangrene, and amputation.

Exercise (e.g., walking for 30 to 45 minutes twice a day) is prescribed for patients with PVD. Exercise improves collateral circulation and tissue perfusion distal to the occlusion. The patient is taught to rest when pain develops (intermittent claudication), resuming activity when the pain is relieved.

Weight reduction improves activity tolerance. A low-fat, low-cholesterol diet is prescribed for patients with atherosclerosis.

Meticulous foot care is vital for patients with PVD to prevent ulceration and infection (Box 18-8■). Elastic support hose are avoided, as they reduce circulation to the skin. Rest pain may be relieved by elevating the head of the bed on blocks.

Other measures to prevent vasoconstriction and improve blood flow include keeping extremities warm and protecting them from injury and managing stress. Complementary therapies for PVD are outlined in Box 18-9■.

Revascularization

Patients with severe symptoms that interfere with activities of daily living (ADLs) or who have gangrenous lesions may require a revascularization procedure to restore peripheral blood flow. Nonsurgical procedures include percutaneous transluminal angioplasty, stent placement, and *atherectomy* (removal of the obstructing plaque). Surgical procedures include *endarterectomy* to remove occlusive plaque and bypass grafts. The risks associated with surgery are greater (infection, embolization, acute myocardial infarction, and stroke) than the risks associated with nonsurgical

---

BOX 18-8   **PATIENT TEACHING**

Leg and Foot Care for Patients With Peripheral Vascular Disease

- Keep legs and feet clean, dry, and comfortable.
  - Wash legs and feet daily using a mild soap and warm water.
  - Pat dry with a soft towel; do not rub, and be sure to dry between toes.
  - Apply lotion that does not contain alcohol to dry, scaly skin.
  - Use powder on feet and between toes.
  - Buy shoes in the afternoon (when feet are largest). Never wear or buy shoes that are uncomfortable. Be sure the toes have adequate room.
  - Wear a clean pair of cotton socks each day.
- Prevent accidents and injuries to the feet.
  - Always wear shoes or slippers when getting out of bed.
  - Walk on level ground and avoid crowds, if possible.
  - Do not go barefoot.
  - Inspect legs and feet daily. Use a mirror to examine the backs of your legs and the bottoms of your feet.
  - Have a professional foot care provider (e.g., a podiatrist) trim toenails and care for corns, calluses, ingrown toenails, or athlete's foot.
  - Always check the temperature of bath water before stepping into the tub.
  - Use sunblock on your legs and the tops of your feet.
  - Report increased pain, cuts, bruises, blistering, redness, or open areas on your legs or feet to your health care provider.
- Improve blood supply to the legs and feet.
  - Do not cross your legs when sitting or in bed.
  - Do not wear garters or knee stockings.
  - Do not go swimming in cold water.
  - Do not smoke cigarettes, inhale passive smoke, or use other tobacco products.
  - Walk until you develop pain, stop for 3 minutes, then resume walking until fatigued. Do this eight times a day.
  - Take medications as prescribed.

BOX 18-9   **COMPLEMENTARY THERAPIES**

Peripheral Vascular Disease

Selected complementary and alternative medicine (CAM) therapies may be helpful to slow the atherosclerotic process and improve peripheral circulation. Several studies on the use of garlic have shown slowed plaque development and improved vessel elasticity. Fish oil (either increased fish intake or use of supplements) also slows the progression of atherosclerosis. Ginkgo has been shown to reduce claudication to a modest extent, improve exercise tolerance, and reduce the frequency of vascular surgery and amputation in patients with PVD. Although a benefit is not clear, hypnosis may be helpful for patients who need to quit smoking. Other CAM therapies that may be beneficial to improve circulation include massage, therapeutic touch, and yoga.

HEALTH PROMOTION

Prevention of PVD begins early in life. Discuss healthy lifestyle habits with community groups, schoolchildren, and patients of all ages, including exercising daily; maintaining healthy weight; eating a low-fat, low-cholesterol diet; and avoiding smoking. Encourage patients with cardiovascular risk factors to manage their controllable risks and to undergo regular screening for hypertension, diabetes, and hyperlipidemia.

ASSESSING

Assessment of the peripheral vascular system may focus on the chief complaint (such as swelling or pain in the legs) or may be a part of a full cardiovascular assessment (Box 18-10■).

IDENTIFYING POTENTIAL COMPLICATIONS

Regularly assess skin color, temperature, and condition, sensation, and pulse strength and equality on extremities of the patient with PVD. Promptly report reddened areas, lesions, ulcerations, or sores that are not healing to the primary care provider. Assess color, temperature, and capillary refill of the toes, reporting any toe that is purple or black or that lacks sensation.

DIAGNOSING, PLANNING, AND IMPLEMENTING

Ineffective Peripheral Tissue Perfusion

Expected outcome: Extremity color, temperature, pulses, and skin will remain intact and within expected limits.

- Assess peripheral pulses, color, temperature, and capillary refill at least every 8 hours and on each office or clinic visit. If pulses cannot be felt, use a Doppler device to assess pulses. *Continuing assessment is important to detect changes in blood flow that could affect tissue integrity.*
- Instruct patient to keep extremities in a dependent position. *Gravity helps maintain arterial blood flow to distal tissues.*

---

procedures; however, both short- and long-term outcomes are better after surgery. Nursing care is similar to that provided for patients undergoing surgery of the aorta (see Box 18-7).

NURSING CARE

Peripheral vascular disease impairs peripheral blood flow. Managing the effects of chronic diseases such as atherosclerosis may mean lifetime changes in activities and diet.

PRIORITIZING NURSING CARE

Nursing care priorities for patients with PVD are to help promote blood flow and protect tissues from damage. Because of the chronic nature of this disease, teaching is a major focus of nursing care.

Assessing Patients With Peripheral Vascular Disease

Subjective Data

- Pain: onset, relationship to activities, characteristics, severity, precipitating and relieving factors
- Other symptoms: burning, numbness, or tingling in limbs or digits; leg fatigue or cramps; ankle swelling and when it occurs; effect of temperature or position on symptoms
- Medical and family history of cardiovascular disorders, peripheral vascular disease, stroke, hypertension, hyperlipidemia, blood clots, or other chronic illnesses (e.g., diabetes); previous surgery or evaluation of blood vessels; current medications
- Usual diet, including caffeine and alcohol consumption; smoking history (in pack years) or other tobacco use; activity level, exercise habits and exercise tolerance

Objective Data

- Vital signs
- Capillary refill on upper and lower extremities; strength and equality of peripheral pulses (brachial, radial on upper extremities; femoral, popliteal, posterior tibial, and dorsalis pedis pulses on lower extremities)
- Presence and degree of edema
- Skin color, temperature, texture, and hair distribution on trunk and upper and lower extremities; any skin lesions or ulcers

- Keep extremities warm using lightweight blankets, socks, and slippers. Do not use electric heating pads or hot water bottles. *Warmth helps prevent vasospasm and promotes arterial flow. Sensation of affected extremities may be decreased; avoid electric heating pads and hot water bottles to reduce the risk of burns.*
- Avoid placing pillows under the knees, or positioning with 90-degree hip flexion. *These positions may further impair peripheral blood flow.*
- Encourage frequent position changes and activity as allowed, and remind the patient to avoid crossing legs. *Changing position and activities promote blood flow. Leg crossing may compress arteries, leading to further compromise of circulation.*

clinicalALERT

Immediately report an extremity that has become cool or cold, pale or cyanotic, and in which pulses are very weak or absent. These are signs of complete obstruction of arterial blood flow. Immediate intervention is necessary to save the limb.

Chronic Pain

Expected outcome: Will relate measures to prevent and manage pain associated with PVD.

- Assess pain level using a standard pain scale at least every 4 hours and more often if needed. Immediately report acute or very severe pain accompanied by a pale, cold

extremity. *The pain scale helps evaluate the severity of pain and the effectiveness of relief measures. Very severe acute pain and a pale, cold extremity may indicate an arterial thrombus or embolism. Immediate treatment is vital to save the extremity.*

- Explain the relationship between smoking and pain, and assist the patient in developing a plan for smoking cessation. *Smoking causes vessel constriction and spasm, increasing the pain of PVD.*
- Provide time to discuss issues related to pain. *Allowing time to explore feelings and issues about pain promotes trust. Expressing concerns about pain reduces the patient's anxiety and may help relieve pain.*
- Teach stress reduction and pain relief measures such as relaxation, meditation, and guided imagery. *Stress increases vasoconstriction and pain. Many nonpharmacologic techniques may be used to relieve stress and minimize pain.*

Impaired Skin Integrity

Expected outcome: Will explain importance of leg and foot care to maintain skin integrity.

- Assess skin of extremities at least every 8 hours and with each clinic visit. Report changes to the charge nurse or physician. *Patients may be unaware of accidental injury or skin damage. Early identification helps prevent complications.*
- Provide meticulous leg and foot care daily, using mild soaps and moisturizing lotions (see Box 18-8). *Proper skin care helps prevent drying and cracking, reducing the risk of skin breakdown and infection. Once the skin is broken, the warm, moist, dark tissues of the injured extremity provide an excellent medium for bacterial growth.*
- Use a foot or bed cradle to prevent linens from rubbing against or putting pressure on extremities. *A cradle provides warmth while avoiding pressure on injured or damaged tissues.*

MANAGING NURSING CARE

Nursing care activities such as assessing weight and routine vital signs and assisting with daily living activities may be appropriate to assign to unlicensed assistive personnel. Alert assistive personnel to promptly report any changes in the patient's pain or condition.

EVALUATING

To evaluate the effectiveness of nursing care for a patient with peripheral vascular disease, collect data such as strength and equality of peripheral pulses and capillary refill; skin color, temperature, and condition of extremities; reports of pain and its relief; and evidence of bleeding.

DOCUMENTING

Document subjective data such as complaints of pain, its relationship to position or activity, or unusual sensations in the affected extremity. Regularly document strength and equality of peripheral pulses, color, temperature, and movement of affected extremities, skin condition, and any changes that occur in response to treatment.

CONTINUITY OF CARE

Teach measures such as exercise to help manage peripheral vascular disease. Stress the importance of smoking cessation. Provide a referral to smoking-cessation classes and encourage the patient to discuss alternative treatments for nicotine withdrawal with physicians. Teach care of the legs and feet, as described in Box 18-8.

Provide information about progressive exercise and its benefits for peripheral circulation. Discuss symptom monitoring, medications, and ways to keep the extremities warm. Provide a list of resources such as support groups, public health services, and other community agencies. See Box 18-11■ for continuing care of the older adult with PVD.

If surgery is planned, provide preoperative teaching. Discuss expected postoperative measures such as anticoagulant drugs, diet and activity restrictions, and risk factor reduction strategies. Before discharge, teach the manifestations of postoperative wound infection and other symptoms that should be reported to their physician. Stress the importance of regular follow-up care.

Other Arterial Disorders

Although less common than atherosclerosis, peripheral arteries may be acutely occluded by a thrombus (clot) or embolism, or affected by vessel inflammation or spasm. Acute arterial obstruction can be devastating, resulting in loss of the affected limb unless promptly treated. Chronic intermittent conditions such as thromboangiitis obliterans and Raynaud disease require lifestyle changes to maintain comfort and preserve tissue integrity.

ARTERIAL THROMBUS OR EMBOLUS

Atherosclerotic changes in blood vessels can cause a **thrombus**, or blood clot, to develop. The clot may partially or totally occlude the vessel, acutely obstructing blood flow to the tissues

BOX 18-11	FOCUS ON OLDER ADULTS

Peripheral Vascular Disease

Blood vessels thicken and become less compliant with age. These changes reduce oxygen delivery to tissues and impair the removal of waste products. Impaired vision and arthritis may make it more difficult for an older adult to provide careful and safe foot care. Long-standing smoking addiction is difficult to break. The patient who lives alone may resist walking. It is often helpful to arrange periodic visits by a home health nurse. Encourage the patient to join a support group for stopping smoking, changing eating habits, and taking part in regular activity.

BOX 18-12	MANIFESTATIONS OF ARTERIAL THROMBOSIS OR EMBOLUS

- Pain in the affected area; may be sudden or insidious
- Numbness or tingling of affected extremity
- Coldness of the extremity
- Pallor or mottling of the skin
- Absent pulses distal to the blockage
- Muscle weakness or spasms
- Possible paralysis

it serves. If the blood clot breaks away from the vessel wall and moves, it becomes an **embolus**. Foreign matter such as fat, bacteria, amniotic fluid, and air bubbles also may become emboli. An embolus eventually lodges in a vessel that is too small to allow it to pass through. Both thrombi and emboli block blood flow through the affected vessel to distal tissues. When arterial flow is interrupted, tissue necrosis and gangrene may result. Manifestations of arterial occlusion by a thrombus or embolus are listed in Box 18-12■. A clear line between normal and pale, cold skin may be noted with an embolus.

THROMBOANGIITIS OBLITERANS

Thromboangiitis obliterans (also called *Buerger disease*) is an occlusive disease of small- and medium-sized peripheral arteries. Affected vessels become inflamed, spastic, and thrombotic. It usually affects a leg or foot, although either the upper or the lower extremities can be affected.

Thromboangiitis obliterans primarily (95%) affects men under the age of 40 who smoke. It is more commonly seen in people of Asian or Eastern European descent. Cigarette smoking is the single most significant cause. There also may be a genetic link.

The course of the disease is intermittent, with episodes of pain and impaired blood flow and periods of remission. It may be dormant for weeks, months, or years. As the disease progresses, arteries become more widely involved, and episodes are more intense and longer. The risk of tissue ulceration and gangrene increases.

Manifestations

Pain in the involved extremity is the major symptom of thromboangiitis obliterans. The patient complains of cramping pain in the instep of the foot or the calves of the legs that is relieved by rest (intermittent claudication) or of rest pain in the fingers and toes. Smoking, cold, and emotional distress often trigger burning pain.

The involved digits and/or extremities are pale and cool or cold to the touch. The skin may be shiny and thin, and the nails are often thick and malformed. Distal pulses often are either difficult to locate or absent, even when a Doppler device is used. *Rubor* (redness) is intense when the extremity is dependent.

RAYNAUD PHENOMENON

Raynaud phenomenon is characterized by spasms of the small arteries and arterioles of the extremities. The arterial spasms limit blood flow to the fingers and, on occasion, to the toes, ears, or nose. Raynaud phenomenon is often secondary to another disorder such as rheumatoid arthritis. When the cause is unknown (*idiopathic*), the disorder is known as *Raynaud disease*. In either case, it almost always affects women between the ages of 15 and 45. A genetic predisposition may have some part in this disease.

Manifestations

The manifestations of Raynaud phenomenon occur intermittently, often after exposure to cold or work-related vibration. The attacks tend to become more frequent and prolonged over time. Raynaud phenomenon has been called the blue–white–red disease. Vasospasm causes the fingers to first turn blue, then white as blood flow is severely limited, and finally very red as the fingers are warmed and the spasm resolves (Figure 18-5 ■). Numbness, stiffness, decreased sensation, and aching pain may accompany the color changes.

COLLABORATIVE CARE

Immediate diagnosis and treatment are necessary to save the limb affected by an acute arterial occlusion such as a thrombus or embolus. The diagnosis generally can be made through physical examination; in some cases, angiography may be done to localize the obstruction. Fibrinolytic (thrombolytic) therapy may be administered to break up the clot or embolus, and anticoagulant therapy initiated to prevent further clot formation. Surgery may be done to remove an obstruction, a thrombus, or an embolus. Acute arterial embolus requires emergency surgery to restore blood flow and prevent gangrene.

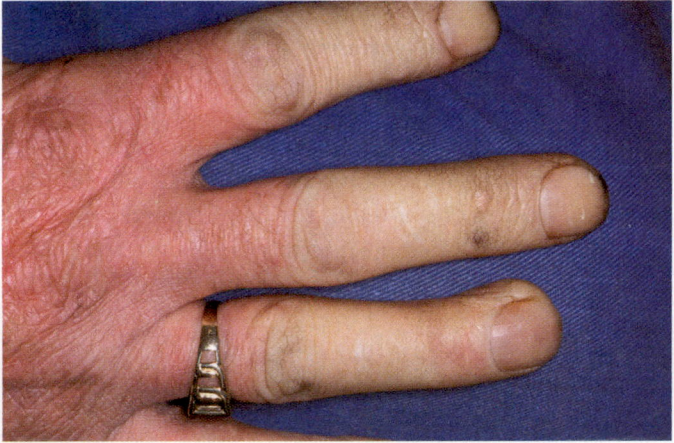

Figure 18-5. ■ Hand of a patient with Raynaud phenomenon. Note extreme pallor of the digits of the right hand. (Source: © Hercules Robinson/Alamy.)

The diagnosis and management of chronic arterial disorders such as thromboangiitis obliterans and Raynaud phenomenon are similar to that for peripheral vascular disease (see the preceding section).

Smoking cessation is vital in all patients affected by a peripheral vascular disease. Attacks of thromboangiitis obliterans increase in severity and duration with continued smoking. Regular exercise is important as well; walking for 30 or more minutes several times a day is recommended. The extremities should be kept warm to reduce the incidence of vasospasm. Patients with Raynaud phenomenon are taught to keep the hands warm, wearing gloves when outside in cold weather and when handling cold items (e.g., frozen foods). Measures to avoid injury to the hands and feet are taught (see Box 18-8 for foot care for patients with PVD).

Amputation is necessary if blood flow cannot be restored and tissue necrosis has occurred. As much healthy tissue as possible is saved, so only part of a limb or digit may be amputated. A below-the-knee amputation may be done for gangrene of the lower leg or for foot pain that cannot be relieved.

NURSING CARE

Nursing assessment for the patient with acute arterial occlusion is highly focused due to the critical nature of the problem. Immediately report assessment findings to the charge nurse and/or primary care provider. Nursing care focuses on protecting the affected extremity before surgery or fibrinolysis. Keep the patient on bed rest, positioning the affected extremity horizontal or lower than the heart. Do not apply heat or cold. Use a cradle and sheepskin or foam pad to protect the extremity from hard or abrasive surfaces. The patient often is highly anxious. Stay with the patient to the extent possible, and allow supportive family members to remain with the patient. Explain procedures, keeping explanations clear and concise. Provide reassurance, focusing on the present. After fibrinolysis to dissolve the clot or embolus, Risk for Bleeding is a priority nursing diagnosis. These drugs interfere with normal clotting; report evidence of bleeding, such as bleeding from incisions or injection sites, bleeding from gums or nose, hematuria, or multiple bruises, petechiae, purpura, or ecchymoses. Rapid identification and treatment of bleeding can prevent significant blood loss.

safety ALERT

Protect the patient receiving fibrinolytic therapy from injury due to falls or inadvertent dislodgment of the intravenous catheter. A minor fall or withdrawal of the IV catheter may lead to serious internal or external bleeding.

Report abnormal hemoglobin and hematocrit levels, which may indicate undetected bleeding. Monitor activated partial thromboplastin time (APTT), prothrombin time (PT), and International Normalized Ratio (INR) values as ordered, reporting those greater than the target therapeutic range.

Nursing assessment and care for the patient with thromboangiitis obliterans or Raynaud phenomenon are similar to that provided for the patient with peripheral atherosclerosis. Assessment data to be collected on a continuing basis include complaints of pain and its relationship to activity or other factors (such as cold or position changes). Regular assessment of the strength and equality of peripheral pulses, color and temperature of the affected extremity, and condition of the skin is vital for patients with acute or chronic peripheral arterial disorders.

Teaching for continuing care is a vital nursing activity for these patients, because the patient is primarily responsible for managing the disorder. Refer to a smoking cessation program or support group. A cardiovascular rehabilitation program may be appropriate to promote physical activity and provide continuing support.

VENOUS DISORDERS

Key Concept   Venous disorders affect the return of blood and waste products from distal tissues, leading to venous congestion and potentially to clotting and inflammation.

In contrast to arterial disorders, which affect the delivery of blood and oxygen *to* body tissues, venous disorders affect the return of blood and waste products *from* distal tissues. Because the pressure is lower and blood flow is slower in the veins than in the arteries, blood can stagnate or pool. As a result, clots may form, leading to inflammation and obstruction of the vessel. Repeated episodes can lead to chronic venous insufficiency. Three of the most common disorders of venous circulation are venous thrombosis, venous insufficiency, and varicose veins.

Venous Thrombosis

Venous thrombosis (or *thrombophlebitis*) occurs when a blood clot (*thrombus*) forms on the wall of a vein and partially or completely blocks blood flow back to the heart. Either deep or superficial veins may be affected. **Deep venous thrombosis (DVT)** is a common complication of immobility or surgery. Superficial venous thrombosis is most frequently associated with the presence of an intravenous catheter.

A number of risk factors are identified for venous thrombosis (Box 18-13■). There is an increased risk in people with impaired heart function, older patients, and people with certain cancers. The major complications of venous thrombosis are chronic venous insufficiency and pulmonary embolism.

PATHOPHYSIOLOGY

Small, localized clots may develop in small veins. In larger veins, extensive thrombi may form. Three pathologic factors, called *Virchow's triad*, are associated with thrombosis: *venous stasis* (sluggish blood flow), increased blood coagulability, and vessel wall injury.

Damage to the lining of a vein attracts platelets to the area, especially if venous stasis is present, and a clot or thrombus develops. The thrombus may partially or totally block blood flow through the vein. Venous blood returns to the heart through collateral vessels. The thrombus may break loose or fragment, becoming an embolus. Emboli from venous clots tend to lodge in the vessels of the pulmonary vascular system.

Deep Venous Thrombosis

The deep veins of the legs, especially in the calf, and of the pelvis provide the best environment for thrombus formation (Figure 18-6■). Most thrombi originate in the vessels of the calf.

MANIFESTATIONS   Deep venous thrombosis (DVT) may cause calf pain and muscle tenderness. The patient may experience dull, aching pain in the leg, particularly when walking. The calf is enlarged and the affected leg may be slightly cyanotic. An elevated temperature and general malaise may be present. A *positive Homans' sign* (pain in the calf when the foot is dorsiflexed) is an unreliable sign of DVT.

COMPLICATIONS   Pulmonary embolism is a serious, potentially fatal complication of DVT. Most pulmonary

BOX 18-13	RISK FACTORS FOR VENOUS THROMBOSIS

- Previous venous thrombosis
- Prolonged immobility, leg paralysis
- Major general surgery or trauma
- Myocardial infarction, heart failure
- Cancer of the breast, pancreas, prostate, or ovary
- Pregnancy or childbirth
- Estrogen therapy, oral contraceptives, especially in women who smoke
- Obesity

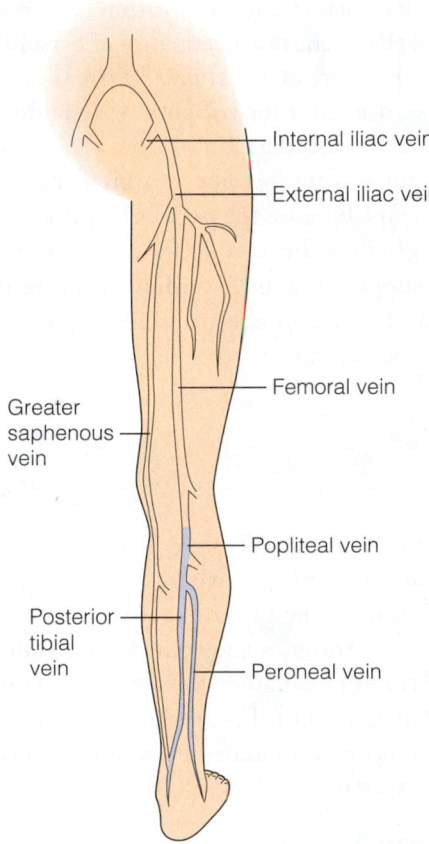

Figure 18-6. ■ Common locations of deep venous thrombosis.

emboli arise in the proximal leg veins (above the knee). When a thrombus breaks loose, it travels through progressively larger vessels until it moves through the right side of the heart into the pulmonary arteries. It becomes trapped in a pulmonary vessel, obstructing blood flow to a portion of the lung. No gas exchange occurs in the affected part of the lung. Occlusion of a large pulmonary artery can cause sudden death. A sudden onset of dyspnea and tachypnea is the most common manifestation of pulmonary embolism; chest pain, hypotension, and cyanosis also may develop. Chronic venous insufficiency, discussed later, is another potential complication of DVT.

Superficial Venous Thrombosis

Thrombophlebitis of the arm veins is a common complication of trauma to the vein wall caused by venous catheters, repeated venous punctures, or intravenous solutions that irritate and inflame the vein. Superficial venous thrombi may also develop in pregnant or postpartum women, but the cause is unknown.

The clinical manifestations of deep and superficial venous thrombosis are listed in Box 18-14■.

VENOUS INSUFFICIENCY

Chronic **venous insufficiency** is *stasis* (stagnation) of venous blood flow in the lower extremities. Chronic venous

insufficiency often results from venous thrombosis and incompetent venous valves.

After DVT, large veins of the legs may remain occluded, increasing pressure in the smaller vessels. This increased pressure distends the veins, preventing closure of the valves. The valves also may be damaged by DVT. When valves in the veins of the legs become *incompetent* and fail to close, the muscle-pumping action on veins during activity cannot move blood back to the heart. The blood collects and stagnates in the lower leg. This further increases pressure in the veins, leading to congestion and edema of leg tissue. Edema develops in the lower leg, and the leg and foot become darkly colored. Subcutaneous tissue changes make the leg and foot feel hard or firm to palpation.

As the congestion worsens, the body is unable to provide adequate oxygen and nutrients to the cells. Eventually, cells begin to die, forming venous stasis ulcers (Figure 18-7■).

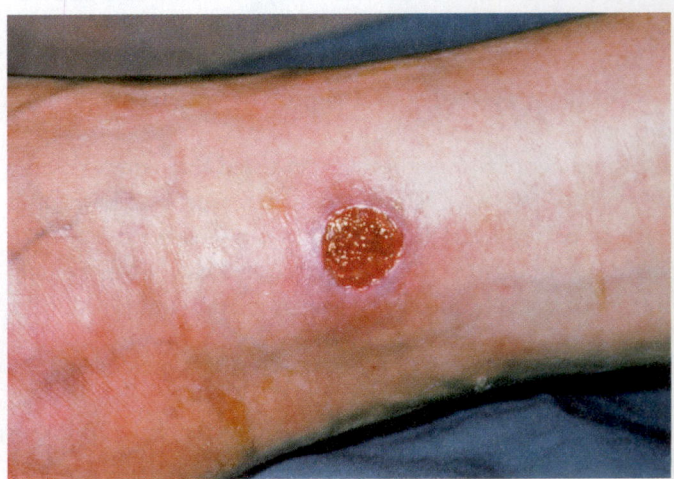

Figure 18-7. ■ Venous ulcer of the ankle. Note discoloration of the tissue surrounding the ulcer.
(Source: Dr. P. Marazzi/Science Source.)

As the condition worsens, the ulcers enlarge. The impaired circulation also increases the risk of wound infection.

Manifestations

Manifestations of chronic venous insufficiency include edema, itching, and discomfort of the affected extremity. These symptoms worsen with prolonged standing. Skin around stasis ulcers appears shiny, atrophic, and brownish. Stasis ulcers heal poorly. Scar tissue commonly forms, causing the affected area of the leg to feel hard and somewhat leathery to the touch, but even minor trauma to the area can lead to serious tissue breakdown.

COLLABORATIVE CARE

Prevention is important to reduce the complications of venous thrombosis. When thrombosis develops, treatment is started to prevent further clots from forming, to treat inflammation, and, in some cases, to dissolve existing clots.

Diagnostic Tests

- *D-dimer*, a fragment released when a clot breaks down, may be measured in patients with symptoms suggestive of DVT.
- *Duplex venous Doppler ultrasonography* is used to visualize the vein and blood flow through it.
- *MRI* may also be used to detect DVT, particularly in the pelvic veins or venae cavae.
- *CT* of the chest is commonly used to identify pulmonary embolism when suspected.

Medications

Anticoagulant therapy is used to prevent and treat DVT. Fibrinolytic drugs may be given to speed the process of clot breakdown; however, they significantly increase the risk for bleeding and hemorrhage.

ANTICOAGULANTS   Anticoagulants are ordered for patients with deep venous thromboses to prevent expansion of the clot and possible pulmonary embolism. Low-molecular-weight (LMW) heparin is given to patients undergoing orthopedic and other surgeries and to people on prolonged bed rest to prevent venous thrombosis.

Anticoagulation generally is started with intravenous or subcutaneous heparin. Anticoagulation is monitored using the *activated partial thromboplastin time (APTT)*. The heparin dosage is adjusted so that the APTT is 1.5 to 2 times the normal value. LMW heparin is administered subcutaneously once or twice per day and does not require the close laboratory monitoring of unfractionated heparins. LMW heparins also are more effective and have lower risk of bleeding, making them the drug of choice.

Fondaparinux sodium (Arixtra) is an alternative to heparin for anticoagulation. It is used to prevent DVT in patients who have had orthopedic or abdominal surgery, as well as to treat DVT and pulmonary embolism. Periodic coagulation tests (e.g., the APTT or INR) are not required during treatment with this drug.

Oral warfarin (Coumadin) is initiated while the patient continues to receive heparin. This overlap of therapy is important because the full anticoagulant effect of warfarin is delayed. The prothrombin time (PT), reported as the *INR*, is used to assess the effect of warfarin on clotting. The dosage is adjusted to achieve an INR of 2.0 to 3.0.

Once this level is achieved, a maintenance dose of warfarin is continued for 3 months. Anticoagulant treatment (Table 18-5 ■) may be extended if a complication such as pulmonary embolus has occurred. Regular follow-up is important to monitor coagulation.

Conservative Therapy

Whenever possible, prevention is key. Elastic stockings and pneumatic compression devices are ordered for postoperative patients, people who are immobile for long periods, and patients who cannot tolerate anticoagulants. Leg exercises and early ambulation are ordered after surgery to minimize venous stasis. Teach patients not to cross their legs, to wear loose-fitting garments, and to incorporate exercise into their daily schedule.

Warm, moist compresses are applied over a superficial venous thrombosis to relieve symptoms. Patients with DVT may be placed on bed rest until the symptoms of tenderness and edema resolve. The legs are elevated, with the knees slightly flexed, above the level of the heart to promote venous return and discourage venous pooling.

Stasis Dermatitis and Stasis Ulcer Care

Stasis dermatitis may be treated with wet compresses with boric acid, Burow solution, or isotonic saline four times daily for 1-hour intervals. After the wet compress, topical ointments (such as 0.5% hydrocortisone cream) are applied. Other topical agents such as zinc oxide ointment or broad-spectrum antifungal agents may also be ordered.

Stasis ulcers may be treated with saline compresses or a semirigid boot applied to the foot and lower leg. This device may be made of Unna paste or Gauzetex bandage. Bony prominences must be well padded. The boot is changed every 1 to 2 weeks, depending on the amount of drainage from the ulcer. This device often allows ambulatory treatment. Once the ulcer is healed, a heavy elastic stocking is worn to promote adequate venous return and to prevent ulcer recurrence.

Surgery

Surgery may be done to remove a venous thrombus or to prevent complications such as a pulmonary embolism. A venous thrombectomy may be done to remove the clot. A

TABLE 18-5	Giving Medications Safely: Anticoagulants		
CLASS/DRUGS	**PURPOSE**	**NURSING IMPLICATIONS**	**PATIENT TEACHING**
■ Heparin sodium	Heparin (also called *unfractionated heparin*) interferes with normal clotting, preventing the formation of new clots and the extension of existing clots. *Heparin-induced thrombocytopenia (HIT)* is a potential complication of treatment with unfractionated heparin.	May be given by intravenous or subcutaneous routes. Check dose with a second licensed person before giving. Subcutaneous: Administer deep into subcutaneous tissue, rotating sites in the lower abdomen. Do not aspirate or massage. IV: Use an infusion pump for continuous infusions; do not mix with other drugs. Report signs of bleeding: bleeding gums, nosebleed, bruising; black, tarry stools; hematuria. Test stools for occult blood. Monitor APTT, platelet count, hemoglobin, and hematocrit. Report results outside the expected range.	Report any unusual bleeding or bruising to your health care provider. Do not take any drugs containing aspirin or NSAIDs while on heparin therapy. Do not smoke or use alcohol while on heparin therapy. Avoid activities that increase your risk of injury. Use a soft toothbrush and electric razor while you are receiving heparin. Tell all health care providers that you are on heparin therapy, and carry an identification card with you at all times.
Low-molecular-weight heparins ■ Dalteparin (Fragmin) ■ Enoxaparin (Lovenox) ■ Tinzaparin (Innohep)	LMW heparins (a shorter form of the heparin molecule) produce the same anticoagulant effect as heparin, with fewer adverse effects. Their response is more predictable, reducing the frequency of laboratory testing.	Assess for and report evidence of active bleeding, history of bleeding disorders, sensitivity to heparin, sulfites, or pork. Administer deep into subcutaneous tissue, rotating sites. Do not aspirate or massage. Monitor for masked or hidden bleeding. Bleeding may occur despite normal APTT results. Teach subcutaneous injection technique. Have patient and family return demonstration of injection.	Take the medication as directed by your physician. Administer subcutaneously, rotating sites. Do not rub the site after the injection. Do not take any over-the-counter drugs unless recommended by your doctor. Promptly report excessive bruising or bleeding, chest pain, difficulty breathing, itching, rash, or swelling to your doctor. Keep appointments with your doctor and for lab testing as scheduled.
■ Fondaparinux (Arixtra)	Selectively inhibits clotting factor Xa. Used to prevent DVT in patients having orthopedic or abdominal surgery, and to treat DVT and pulmonary embolism.	Inject subcutaneously, rotating sites. Do not expel the air bubble from prefilled syringe before injection. Monitor for evidence of bleeding. Monitor baseline and periodic CBC, platelet count, and renal function tests.	Administer subcutaneously as directed, rotating sites. Report signs of unexpected bleeding to your doctor. Check with your doctor before taking any over-the-counter drugs.
■ Warfarin (Coumadin)	Interferes with synthesis of clotting factors, preventing clot formation. Requires 3 to 5 days to provide effective anticoagulation.	Give at the same time each day. Report signs of bleeding: bleeding gums, nosebleed, bruising; black, tarry stools; hematuria. Test stools for occult blood. Monitor INR, CBC, and liver function studies. Report results outside the expected range. Drug interactions are common; monitor carefully when new drugs are added to medication regimen or other drugs are discontinued.	Take the drug as ordered. If you miss a dose, take it as soon as you remember that day. Do not double your dose. Limit your intake of foods rich in vitamin K (asparagus, beans, broccoli, brussels sprouts, cabbage, cheeses, fish, greens, milk, pork, rice, spinach, turnips, yogurt). Report any unusual bleeding or bruising to your doctor. Do not drink alcohol or take drugs containing aspirin or NSAIDs. Use a soft toothbrush and electric razor. Tell all health care providers that you are taking an anticoagulant, and carry an identification card with this information with you at all times. Keep all follow-up appointments for lab work and with your doctor.

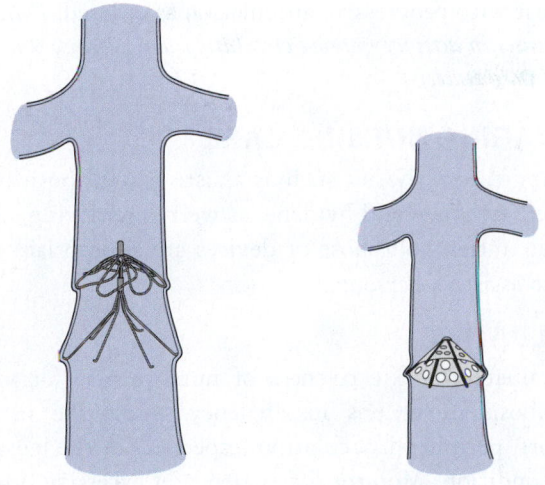

Figure 18-8. ■ A vena cava filter to trap emboli from the pelvis and lower extremities.

filtering device may be inserted into the inferior vena cava via the femoral or jugular vein. This umbrella-like device captures venous thrombi, preventing pulmonary emboli (Figure 18-8■).

NURSING CARE

PRIORITIZING NURSING CARE

Planning and providing care to prevent venous thrombosis is an important nursing responsibility. Early ambulation of postsurgical patients, encouraging frequent leg exercises, positioning, and maintaining ordered devices such as compression hose and pneumatic compression devices are measures that help maintain peripheral circulation and prevent DVT.

HEALTH PROMOTION

Nurses play a vital role in identifying patients at risk for venous thrombosis and implementing preventive measures. Position patients with the feet elevated and the knees slightly bent. Avoid placing pillows under the knees and positioning with the hips and knees sharply flexed. Instruct patients to avoid crossing legs when in bed or sitting. Teach ankle flexion and extension exercises, and remind patients to perform them. Promote ambulation of all patients, particularly those who have undergone surgery. Frequently assess intravenous sites. Change the site and the intravenous catheter per protocol and if signs of inflammation develop.

Discuss measures to prevent DVT in patients with identified risk factors such as use of oral contraceptives or cigarette smoking. Encourage patients to stop frequently and ambulate when traveling for long distances by automobile. Teach patients to perform leg exercises and get up at least every 2 hours when on an extended flight.

ASSESSING

Focused assessment for problems of venous circulation includes patients with diagnosed venous thrombosis as well as those who are at risk. Have the patient describe any lesions or pain, including characteristics, timing, and aggravating and relieving factors. Inquire about ankle swelling, its timing, extent, and the use of support stockings. Ask about a history of cardiovascular disorders, peripheral vascular disease, blood clots, chronic conditions, or cancer. Inquire about the patient's exercise and smoking history, and possible occupational factors, such as prolonged standing or sitting.

Objectively, assess the color, texture, hair distribution, and condition of the skin of legs and feet. Note any lesions, including location, size, characteristics, and evidence of healing. Observe the venous pattern on hands, arms, and legs. Note edema and its extent (feet only, feet and ankles, to mid-calf, etc.); grade as 1+ to 4+ if present. Palpate calves for tenderness, warmth, swelling; presence of cords. Measure leg circumference at forefoot, above ankle, calf, and mid-thigh.

IDENTIFYING POTENTIAL COMPLICATIONS

Rapidly identifying manifestations of pulmonary embolism, a potentially fatal complication of DVT, is critical. Immediately report symptoms such as extreme anxiety, shortness of breath, chest pain, and changes in skin color (cyanosis or a gray tone) or reduced oxygen saturation levels.

clinicalALERT

Remember that DVT may be asymptomatic; symptoms of possible pulmonary embolism may develop in the patient without previously diagnosed DVT.

DIAGNOSING, PLANNING, AND IMPLEMENTING

Ineffective Peripheral Tissue Perfusion

Expected outcome: Will state the reasons for activity restrictions and positioning.

■ Assess peripheral pulses, skin integrity, capillary refill, and color of the extremities at least every 8 hours or with each office visit. Report changes promptly. *Swelling from obstructed venous blood flow can impair arterial circulation to the tissues, increasing the risk for ischemia and necrosis.*

■ Measure calf and thigh diameter on the affected extremity on admission and daily thereafter. Report increases. *As venous thrombosis resolves, the diameter will decrease. Increased diameters may indicate further inflammation.*

- Elevate legs, keeping knees slightly flexed. Avoid flexing hips more than 60 degrees. *Elevation promotes venous return and reduces peripheral edema. Knee flexion promotes comfort.*
- Apply antiembolic stockings or pneumatic compression devices as ordered, removing them for short periods (30 to 60 minutes) during daily hygiene. *Antiembolic stockings and pneumatic compression devices promote venous return to the heart by gently compressing the extremity. The devices are removed daily because they reduce circulation to the skin.*
- Encourage frequent position changes. *Position changes help prevent further venous stasis and other complications of immobility.*
- Administer and monitor the effectiveness of anticoagulants or thrombolytic drugs as ordered. Monitor laboratory values (APTT and INR) before giving prescribed anticoagulants. Promptly report values outside the expected range. *Monitoring is vital to evaluate the effectiveness of therapy and prevent complications of treatment.*

Acute Pain

Expected outcome: Will rate pain as a 3 or lower on a scale of 0 to 10.

- Regularly assess pain. Immediately report increased pain. *Venous thrombosis causes pain that is not affected by exercise or relieved by elevating the leg. Increased pain may indicate extension of the inflammation and clot.*
- Apply warm, moist heat to affected extremity at least four times daily, using warm, moist compresses or an aqua-K pad. *Heat dilates the vessels and promotes the reabsorption of edema fluid, thus improving circulation and reducing pain.*

Impaired Skin Integrity

Expected outcome: Skin will remain intact without evidence of injury or breakdown.

- Assess skin of the affected leg and foot at least every 8 hours and more often as needed. *Careful, frequent assessment allows early detection of signs of potential skin breakdown and early intervention to prevent further problems.*
- Use mild soaps, solutions, and lotions to clean the affected leg and foot daily. Avoid harsh soaps or alcohol-based solutions. Pat dry. *Gentle cleansing with mild agents helps maintain skin integrity, prevent excessive drying and itching, and prevent infection.*
- Use egg crate mattresses or sheepskin as needed. *Egg crate mattresses and sheepskin distribute the weight more equally and prevent skin breakdown and discomfort.*
- Encourage active or perform passive range-of-motion (ROM) exercises at least every 8 hours. *ROM exercises help preserve joint function, promote circulation, and prevent skin breakdown.*

- Assist with progressive ambulation as ordered. *Daily increases in activity improve circulation and increase stamina and endurance.*

MANAGING NURSING CARE

Nursing care activities such as assisting with positioning, allowed activities and hygiene, as well as removing and replacing antiembolic hose or devices are appropriate to assign to assistive personnel.

EVALUATING

To evaluate the effectiveness of nursing care for venous thrombosis or venous insufficiency, assess the patient's comfort, peripheral circulation (especially of the legs), and skin condition. Monitor for evidence of excessive bruising or bleeding (e.g., bleeding gums, occult blood in urine or stool), and monitor laboratory results for the patient receiving anticoagulant therapy.

DOCUMENTING

Document continuing assessment data, care provided, and the patient's responses. Document teaching about the disorder, its prevention, and, if ordered, continuing anticoagulant therapy. Document the patient's (or family's) ability to safely and effectively administer anticoagulant by subcutaneous injection as prescribed.

CONTINUITY OF CARE

Patients who have experienced an episode of venous thrombosis or who have venous insufficiency often will manage their treatment after discharge. Explain the disease process and course of treatment, including

- Ordered laboratory tests, their purposes, and frequency
- Prescribed medications, including dosage, time of day to take the drug, and side effects that should be reported
- Any continuing order for heat application or wound care, including precautions to avoid burns and infection, and symptoms to report to the health care provider
- Activity restrictions and their duration
- The importance of follow-up visits

Reinforce teaching with written instructions, and have the patient demonstrate injection technique or wound care before discharge.

Teach the following measures to reduce the risk of recurrence and complications:

- Elevate legs while resting and during sleep.
- Walk as much as possible, and avoid sitting or standing for long periods of time.
- When sitting, do not cross your legs or put pressure on the back of the knees.

- Do not wear anything that constricts your legs (knee-high hose, garters, or girdles).
- Wear elastic hose as prescribed. Put on the hose after the legs have been elevated. The elastic hose should be tighter over the feet than at the top of the leg, and the tops should not cut into the legs.
- Keep skin on feet and legs clean, soft, and dry. Follow guidelines for care of the legs and feet (see Box 18-8).

Varicose Veins

Varicose veins are irregular, tortuous veins with poorly functioning (incompetent) valves. *Varicosities* may develop in veins anywhere in the body. In the rectum they are called hemorrhoids; when they develop in the esophagus, they are known as varices. They commonly affect the lower extremities (Figure 18-9■). The long saphenous vein of the leg is most often affected by varicosities. Varicose veins affect about one in five people in the world. They are more common in women over the age of 35, perhaps because of venous stasis that occurs during pregnancy.

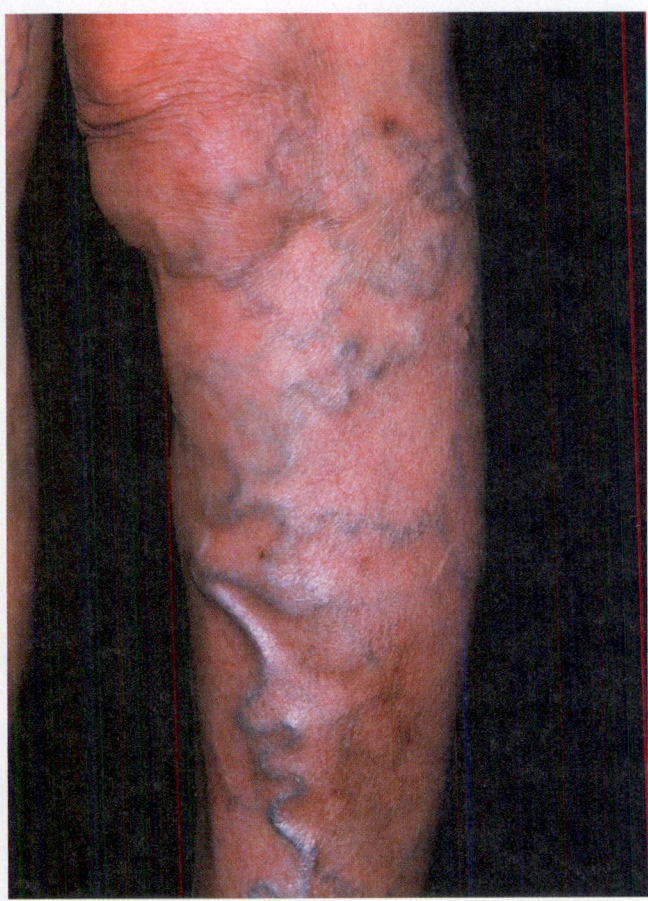

Figure 18-9. ■ A varicose vein in a person's leg.
(Source: Dr. P. Marazzi/Science Source.)

PATHOPHYSIOLOGY

Increased pressure that stretches the vessel wall is the major factor leading to varicose veins. Standing increases pressure in the leg veins and decreases venous return to the heart. Blood collects in the leg veins, stretching the vessel wall. As the vessels stretch, their valves cannot close properly and become incompetent. Prolonged standing, obesity, venous thrombosis, and increased pressure on the veins of the abdomen (from pregnancy or an abdominal tumor) contribute to varicose vein development.

MANIFESTATIONS AND COMPLICATIONS

Some patients are asymptomatic, but most complain of one or more of the manifestations listed in Box 18-15■. The menstrual cycle tends to increase symptoms in women.

Varicose veins can lead to venous insufficiency, stasis dermatitis, and stasis ulcers. The skin above the ankles may be thin and discolored. Venous thrombosis may develop in varicose veins, especially in pregnant or postpartal patients, postoperative patients, or patients taking oral contraceptives.

COLLABORATIVE CARE

Most patients are managed conservatively with measures to improve venous circulation and relieve the pressure on vein walls and valves. Surgery may relieve major symptoms of the disease, but there is no real cure for varicose veins.

Diagnostic Tests

Doppler ultrasonography may be done to identify the location of incompetent valves. The *Trendelenburg test* may be done to differentiate between incompetent valves in the deep veins of the leg and incompetent superficial leg vein valves. For this test, the leg is elevated and a tourniquet is applied just above the knee. The varicosities are then observed while the patient stands. The veins remain flat when the valves of the deep veins are involved, but distend rapidly when the valves of the superficial veins are affected.

Conservative Therapy

Properly fitted antiembolism (elastic) stockings compress veins, helping move blood back to the heart. Regular, daily walking is an important part of treatment. Prolonged

BOX 18-15	MANIFESTATIONS OF VARICOSE VEINS

- Severe, aching leg pain
- Leg fatigue or heaviness
- Itching of the affected leg
- Heat in the affected leg after prolonged standing
- Visibly dilated veins in the leg

sitting and standing are avoided. The legs are elevated for specified periods of time throughout the day.

Surgery

Two surgical techniques are generally used to treat varicose veins: compression sclerotherapy and vein stripping. In *compression sclerotherapy*, a sclerosing (hardening) agent is injected into the varicosed vein. A compression dressing is then applied to compress and obliterate the vein. Venous blood is rerouted through healthy vessels. In *vein stripping*, the varicose veins are surgically removed. Pressure bandages are applied and the legs are elevated to reduce edema. Ambulation is gradually increased, but sitting and standing are forbidden during the recovery period.

NURSING CARE

Nurses in acute care settings rarely interact with patients whose primary diagnosis is varicose veins, except when surgery is planned. Through teaching and referral, however, nurses can be instrumental in helping patients slow their development and minimize the symptoms of varicose veins.

Risk for Ineffective Peripheral Tissue Perfusion

Expected outcome: Will verbalize measures to promote comfort and maintain extremity circulation.

■ Apply properly fitted support or antiembolic stockings. Remove stockings daily for 30 to 60 minutes. Inspect and clean the skin while stockings are off. *Antiembolic stockings exert pressure on the veins of the lower extremities, promoting venous return to the heart. During ambulation, they assist the blood-pumping action of the muscles. Because elastic stockings can impair blood flow through small superficial vessels, they should be removed at least once daily for 30 minutes or more.*

■ Wrap the leg(s) with Ace bandages as directed if sclerotherapy or vein stripping has been done. Assess pulses,

color, temperature, and capillary refill distal to wrappings. Frequently inspect the wrappings, and rewrap as needed to prevent skin irritation or obstruction of blood flow to or from the extremity. *Ace bandages compress the leg from ankle to thigh, obliterating the sclerosed veins and minimizing the risk of bleeding or edema after surgery. Wrinkled or excessively tight bandages can impair skin integrity or interfere with arterial blood flow.*

■ Assist with or instruct to exercise legs at regular intervals. *Exercise promotes normal blood flow and venous return. Walking is excellent exercise and is encouraged.*

■ Position with legs elevated when supine. When sitting, use a recliner-type chair to elevate the legs and reduce the angle of hip flexion. Change position frequently. *Leg elevation and limited hip flexion promote venous return and minimize pressure on lower extremity veins.*

CONTINUITY OF CARE

Most patients with varicose veins provide self-care at home. Emphasize the importance of daily walks. Teach technique for applying antiembolism stockings. Instruct to elevate legs for specified periods of time throughout the day. Help identify strategies to avoid prolonged periods of standing or sitting. If the patient's job requires prolonged standing, encourage to wear elastic stockings. Teach calf and thigh muscle tightening and relaxation exercises to perform while standing. Encourage patients whose job requires extensive sitting to work on incorporating frequent activity into the job.

Provide referrals for home health services as needed for patients recovering from surgery. In some instances, temporary placement in an extended care facility may be necessary before returning home.

Note: The references and resources for all chapters have been compiled at the back of the book.

Chapter Review

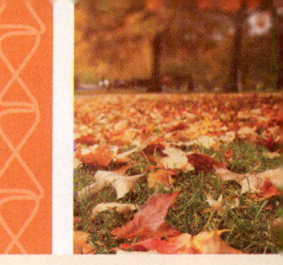

KEY POINTS

- **Concept:** Processes that affect blood vessels and interfere with peripheral blood flow can impair the delivery of oxygen and nutrients to the tissues, leading to complications such as heart failure, pain, infection, and amputation.
- **Concept:** Hypertension is a leading, often undiagnosed, cause of cardiovascular disability and mortality. Few people with hypertension have symptoms of the disorder, yet it can lead to heart failure, stroke, and chronic renal failure.
- Encourage all patients to regularly monitor their blood pressure, reduce their salt and fat intake, stop smoking, limit alcohol intake, exercise regularly, and reduce stress.
- Stress the importance of continuing treatment for hypertension; this disease can be managed but cannot, at this time, be cured.
- **Concept:** The aorta and its branches can be affected by chronic disorders such as arteriosclerosis, weakening vessel walls and resulting in aneurysm.
- **Concept:** Atherosclerosis, the pathophysiologic process underlying coronary heart disease and stroke, affects peripheral blood vessels as well. Peripheral vascular disease is a leading cause of lower extremity pain, impaired healing, and lower extremity amputation, particularly in older adults.
- Arterial disorders are characterized by cool, pale, hairless skin; diminished peripheral pulses; and, often, pain from ischemic tissues. Peripheral vascular disease (PVD) is the most common peripheral arterial disorder.
- **Concept:** Peripheral vascular disorders affecting the arteries interfere with blood flow and oxygen delivery to tissues of the body leading to ischemia. Venous disorders, in contrast, affect the return of blood and waste products from distal tissues, leading to venous congestion and potentially to clotting and inflammation.
- Venous disorders are more often characterized by rubor, edema, and brown, leathery skin. Deep venous thrombosis (DVT) often occurs as a complication of immobility; nursing interventions to promote ambulation in patients are effective preventive measures for DVT.
- Peripheral vascular disorders increase the risk of skin trauma and breakdown. Provide meticulous foot and skin care for patients with peripheral vascular disorders and protect from injury.
- Encourage all patients with peripheral vascular disease to engage in regular activity as approved by their primary care provider.

PEARSON NURSING STUDENT RESOURCES

Find additional materials at **nursing.pearsonhighered.com**.

Clinical Reasoning Care Map

Caring for a Patient With Thromboangiitis Obliterans

NCLEX-PN® Focus Area: Reduction of Risk Potential

Case Study: Jeffrey Fang, a 34-year-old computer programmer, develops leg cramps when he climbs the two flights of stairs to his office each day. The cramps began about 2 months ago and have become so painful during the past week that he cannot walk more than about 50 feet without resting, and he is now taking the elevator to his office. Mr. Fang makes an appointment with his primary care provider.

Nursing Diagnosis: Ineffective Tissue Perfusion: Peripheral

COLLECT DATA

Subjective	Objective
_____	_____
_____	_____
_____	_____
_____	_____
_____	_____

Does this present a threat to the patient's safety?

If yes, the priority intervention to address this threat would be:

_____

Nursing Care

_____
_____
_____
_____
_____
_____
_____

Interprofessional team members to include when planning care:

_____

How would you document this?_____

_____

Compare your answers and documentation to those provided on the companion website.

Data Collected
(use only those that apply)

- Has smoked more than two packs of cigarettes a day for 20 years
- Calf pain with activity progressing during past 2 months
- Must rest frequently when walking
- Anxious about seriousness of symptoms
- Weak peripheral pulses in right leg
- Absent pedal and posterior tibial pulses in left foot
- Third, fourth, and fifth toes of left foot pale
- Relates numbness and tingling of toes of left foot
- Right foot pink and warm; left foot cool to touch
- Skin on left leg shiny and thin; hairless below knee
- Moderate amount of evenly distributed hair on right leg

Nursing Interventions
(use only those that apply; list in priority order)

- Teach the importance of smoking cessation.
- Assess pain at rest and during activity using a scale of 0 to 10.
- Instruct to walk for at least 30 minutes two or three times per day.
- Teach foot care measures.
- Provide time to discuss issues that contribute to anxiety.
- Mutually determine most effective methods of managing pain.
- Encourage questions about the disease and its management.

NCLEX-PN® Exam Preparation

TEST-TAKING TIP Be familiar with the anticoagulant drugs used for various vascular disorders. You will need to know this information in order to answer questions related to the care of patients with vascular disorders.

1. When assessing a bedridden patient with a total arterial occlusion, the nurse can expect to find:
   1. palpable pulses in the area below the occlusion.
   2. cyanosis or mottling of the area above the occlusion.
   3. cyanosis or mottling of the area below the occlusion.
   4. extreme pallor, cold, and pain in the area below the occlusion.

2. When the patient's extremity is affected by peripheral arteriosclerosis, blood flow to the extremity can be enhanced by:
   1. placing the affected extremity in a dependent position.
   2. elevating the affected extremity.
   3. wrapping the affected extremity with an elastic bandage.
   4. range-of-motion exercises to the affected extremity.

3. You are admitting a patient diagnosed with deep venous thrombosis. Which of the following items should you have available for conducting your focused assessment of this patient?
   1. A tape measure
   2. An eye chart
   3. A tuning fork
   4. A pulse oximetry unit

4. The nurse can educate the patient with Raynaud phenomenon by offering the following information:
   1. Elevate the extremities above the heart during an episode.
   2. Wear support hose during cold weather.
   3. Practice relaxation techniques to reduce stress.
   4. Avoid any activities that involve repetitive movement.

5. You are caring for a patient with peripheral vascular disease. The patient complains that his feet are cold. Which of the following are appropriate nursing actions? **Select all that apply.**
   1. Obtain a heating pad for the patient.
   2. Assist the patient to put on cotton socks.
   3. Provide a foot cradle and warmed blanket.
   4. Elevate the foot of the bed.
   5. Provide a heat lamp directed at the feet.

6. The nurse is caring for a patient who has recently been diagnosed with stage 2 hypertension. When educating the patient about hypertension, it is important to emphasize that such patients commonly:
   1. experience severe headaches.
   2. have no symptoms other than an increased blood pressure.
   3. experience symptoms of kidney failure.
   4. experience visual disturbances.

7. When educating a patient with stage 2 hypertension about how to manage the hypertension, the nurse should stress:
   1. adhering to medication schedules.
   2. the short-term aspect of managing hypertension.
   3. making all recommended lifestyle changes.
   4. engaging in range-of-motion exercises.

8. A 70-year-old man comes to the clinic complaining of severe headaches and dizziness and also states that he recently fell and bumped his head. When reviewing the patient's medication history, the nurse should note that the patient is taking:
   1. Cardizem.
   2. Inderal.
   3. Digoxin.
   4. Coumadin.

9. Your 54-year-old female patient has recently been diagnosed with stage 2 hypertension. She states that she cannot understand why smoking is bad for her because it usually helps her to relax. The nurse responds by stating that smoking affects blood pressure because nicotine:
   1. stimulates blood vessels.
   2. increases the pulse rate.
   3. constricts blood vessels.
   4. dilates blood vessels.

10. You are caring for a patient who underwent surgery to repair an abdominal aortic aneurysm 3 days ago. Which of the following findings noted during your focused assessment concerns you?
    1. The right leg is cooler than the left with weak pulses.
    2. The patient complains of abdominal pain when moving from bed to chair.
    3. Bowel sounds are present at about 7 to 8 per minute.
    4. A 2.5-cm spot of dried blood is noted on the abdominal dressing.

Answers and rationales for Review Questions appear in Appendix I.

Thinking Strategically About . . .

You are an LPN/LVN working on a medical unit at a medium-sized hospital. You are assigned to care for the following patients from 1900 to 0700. There is an RN charge nurse available.

- Mrs. Opal Hipps is a 75-year-old widow who lives alone with her dog Chester. She retired from her job as a postal clerk 10 years ago and now spends a lot of time reading and watching television. Over the past week she developed a vague aching pain in her right leg. Last night it became more severe, especially in her right calf. She noticed that her right lower leg seemed larger than the left, and her calf was very tender and felt warm to the touch. Mrs. Hipps was admitted to the hospital this morning with deep venous thrombosis in the right leg. She is on bed rest with her leg elevated, antiembolic stockings, and intravenous heparin. She is to have warm moist compresses to the right leg.

- Hal Williams is a 62-year-old Black man who was admitted 4 days ago with a small myocardial infarction. He was transferred out of the Cardiac Care Unit (CCU) 2 days ago. He has a saline lock for PRN pain medication, but has not needed any for 3 days. He also has hypertension and type 2 diabetes. He is looking forward to going home tomorrow morning. Hap is retired and plans to travel across the country to visit his grandchildren in 2 months. He admits to not managing his diabetes very well.

- Mariah Burgess, a 35-year-old married woman, was admitted 1 week ago with a diagnosis of bacterial endocarditis. She has a history of frequent episodes of sore throat. Sometimes her throat was cultured for beta-hemolytic *Streptococcus*. Other times, she did not seek medical attention, but used over-the-counter gargles and ibuprofen to resolve symptoms. She has been receiving large doses of intravenous antibiotics. Yesterday and today her temperature was normal. She hopes to be discharged in the morning.

CRITICAL THINKING

- What effect does heat have on deep venous thrombosis?
- Could Hap have prevented the MI by controlling his diabetes?
- What is the correlation between beta-hemolytic *Streptococcus* throat infections and bacterial endocarditis?

PRIORITIES IN NURSING CARE

- In what order will you assess these patients?
- What is your rationale for this decision?

- Hap requests a shower before he goes to bed for the night. What are the priorities in helping Hap with this activity?

MANAGEMENT OF CARE

- Knowing that use of the leg muscles will prevent venous stasis, what should Opal do to prevent further episodes of venous thrombosis?
- At 0200 Hap is awake when you check on him. He states he can't sleep because he is concerned he will not be able to visit his grandchildren in 2 months. What therapeutic communication techniques will you use?
- What can the LPN/LVN do between 1900 and 0700 to prepare for Mariah's possible discharge?

DELEGATING

- Can the adjustment of the heparin drip be delegated to you by the RN?
- Can the administration of Mariah's IV antibiotics be delegated to you?

PATIENT TEACHING

- Opal was started on warfarin (Coumadin), an oral anticoagulant, before discharge. What teaching will the nurse provide related to the anticoagulant therapy?
- What teaching can the LPN/LVN provide for Hap?
- What teaching should Mariah receive about repeated strep throat?

DOCUMENTING AND REPORTING

- At 0700 you must provide a report to the next licensed nurse. Besides current vital signs, what should be included in the report for each of your assigned patients?
- Write a focus note documenting Opal's use of antiembolism stockings.

Note: Discussion of Unit questions appears on the companion website.

UNIT IV
Disrupted Hematologic and Lymphatic Function

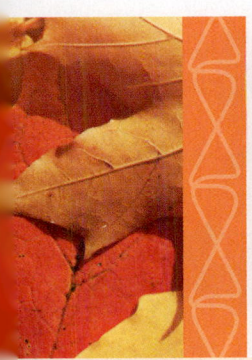 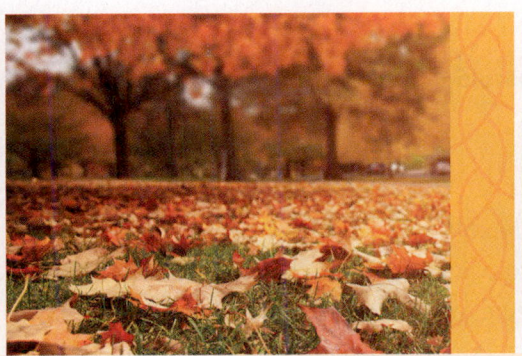 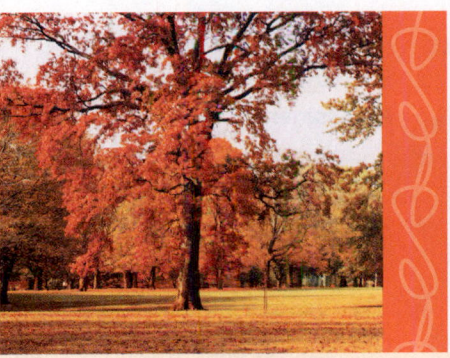 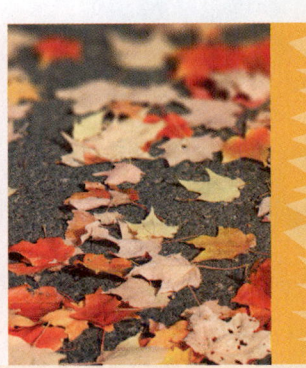

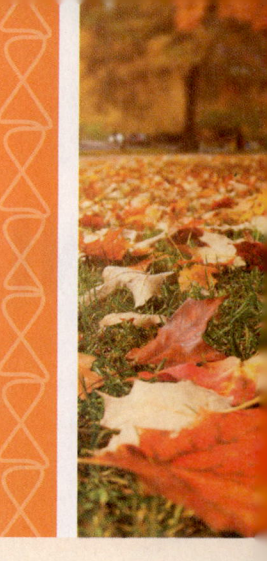

CHAPTER 19

The Hematologic and Lymphatic Systems and Assessment

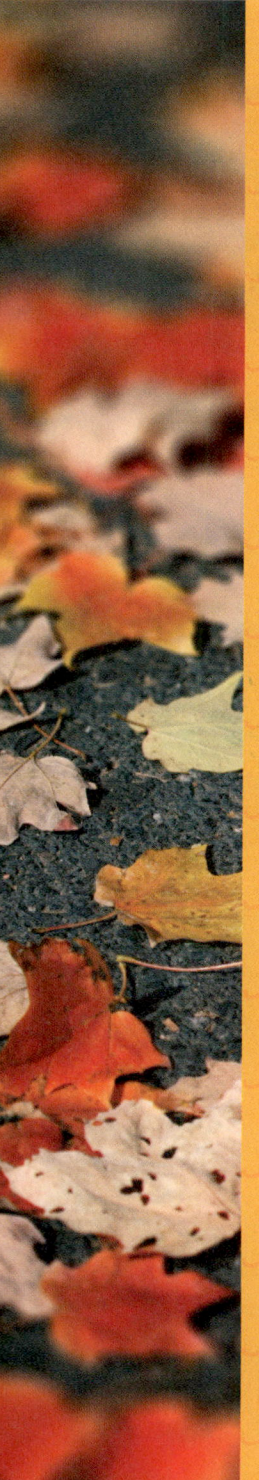

BRIEF OUTLINE

Structure and Function of the Hematologic and Lymphatic Systems
Assessment

APPLIED LEARNING OUTCOMES

After completing this chapter, you will be able to:

1. Describe the cells of the hematologic system with their functions.
2. Identify and describe the structures and functions of the lymphatic system.
3. Collect patient-centered subjective and objective assessment data related to the hematologic and lymphatic systems.
4. Recognize and appropriately respond to abnormal or unexpected assessment findings related to the hematologic and lymphatic systems.
5. Provide safe and effective individualized nursing care for patients undergoing diagnostic tests to evaluate the hematologic and lymphatic systems.

KEY TERMS

The key terms are defined on the pages listed below.

SPECIAL FEATURES

Structure and Function of the Hematologic and Lymphatic Systems

THE BLOOD AND BLOOD CELLS

Key Concept   Blood, the fluid component of the cardiovascular system, carries fuel to body cells and tissues and removes waste products for elimination from the body. Blood cells play essential roles in preventing and eliminating infections and in preventing fluid loss from injured tissues.

Blood transports oxygen, nutrients, and essential substances (such as hormones and other chemical messengers) to cells and tissues, and waste products away from tissues for removal from the body. Blood is made up of **plasma**, a clear yellow, protein-rich fluid, and the cells suspended in it: *red blood cells* (erythrocytes), *white blood cells* (leukocytes), and platelets (or *thrombocytes*).

A number of body systems are involved in forming blood. Many of the plasma proteins are formed in the liver. Blood cells are formed in bone marrow. All blood cells begin as **stem cells**, immature cells known as *hemocytoblasts*. Stem cells differentiate (mature) into the different types of blood cells (red blood cells, platelets, and several kinds of white cells) (Figure 19-1■).

This chapter provides an overview of each type of blood cell and its function, as well as a review of the organs and function of the lymphatic system.

Red Blood Cells

Red blood cells (RBCs) and the hemoglobin they contain are vital for transporting oxygen to body tissues. They also help carry carbon dioxide from the tissues to the lungs for excretion.

RBCs (**erythrocytes**) are shaped like *biconcave disks* (Figure 19-2■). The shape of the RBC maximizes its surface area for gas exchange and allows it to change shape as it moves through very small capillaries. RBCs are formed in bone marrow through a process known as *erythropoiesis*. Tissue *hypoxia* (oxygen deficiency) stimulates the kidneys to release a hormone, *erythropoietin*, that stimulates the bone marrow to produce RBCs. The complete sequence from stem cell to RBC (see Figure 19-1) takes from 3 to 5 days.

RBCs contain **hemoglobin**, an oxygen-carrying protein. Hemoglobin consists of *heme* molecules within a protein structure. Heme contains iron, which binds with oxygen. Hemoglobin molecules are synthesized within the RBC.

RBCs have a life span of less than 120 days. Old or damaged RBCs are destroyed by phagocytes in the spleen, liver, bone marrow, and lymph nodes. The process of RBC destruction is called **hemolysis**. The amino acids and iron from destroyed RBCs are saved and reused by the body. This iron circulates in the bloodstream as *transferrin*. It is not immediately reused; rather it is stored in the liver, spleen, and bone marrow as *ferritin*. Most of the heme unit is converted to *bilirubin*, an orange-yellow pigment that is removed from the blood by the liver and excreted in the bile.

Normal RBC laboratory values often differ by gender (Table 19-1■). Terms used to describe RBCs include *normocytic* (normal size), *microcytic* (smaller than normal), or *macrocytic* (larger than normal), and *normochromic* (normal color) or *hypochromic* (decreased color).

White Blood Cells

White blood cells (WBCs), also called **leukocytes**, are part of the body's defense system against infection and disease. On average, there are 4,500 to 10,000 WBCs per microliter (cubic millimeter) of blood. WBCs make up about 1% of total blood volume. *Leukocytosis* is a higher-than-normal WBC count, whereas *leukopenia* is a lower-than-normal WBC count.

WBCs originate from stem cells in the bone marrow (see Figure 19-1). Unlike RBCs, which remain within blood vessels, WBCs use the circulation to move to where they are needed and can migrate out of blood vessels into other tissues. There are two major types of WBCs: granulocytes and agranular leukocytes.

Granulocytes are the most plentiful WBCs, accounting for 60% to 75% of total leukocytes. Their cytoplasm looks granular, and their nuclei have multiple lobes, giving them a distinctive appearance. Granulocytes also are known as *polymorphonuclear leukocytes* (*PMNs* or *polys*) because of their multilobed nucleus. These cells play a key role in protecting the body from harmful microorganisms during acute inflammation and infection. There are three types of granulocytes:

1. *Neutrophils* make up 50% to 70% of circulating WBCs. Neutrophils are *phagocytic*, that is, responsible for engulfing and destroying foreign matter. They are the first cells to arrive at a site of invasion. Neutrophils have a life span of about 10 hours and must constantly be replaced. *Segmented neutrophils* are mature cells; *bands* are immature neutrophils.
2. *Eosinophils* make up 1% to 3% of WBCs. Their numbers increase during allergic reactions and during infestations with parasites.
3. *Basophils* make up 0.4% to 1% of total WBCs and are believed to be a part of the hypersensitivity and stress responses.

Monocytes are the largest of the WBCs and make up approximately 4% to 6% of the total WBC count. Monocytes

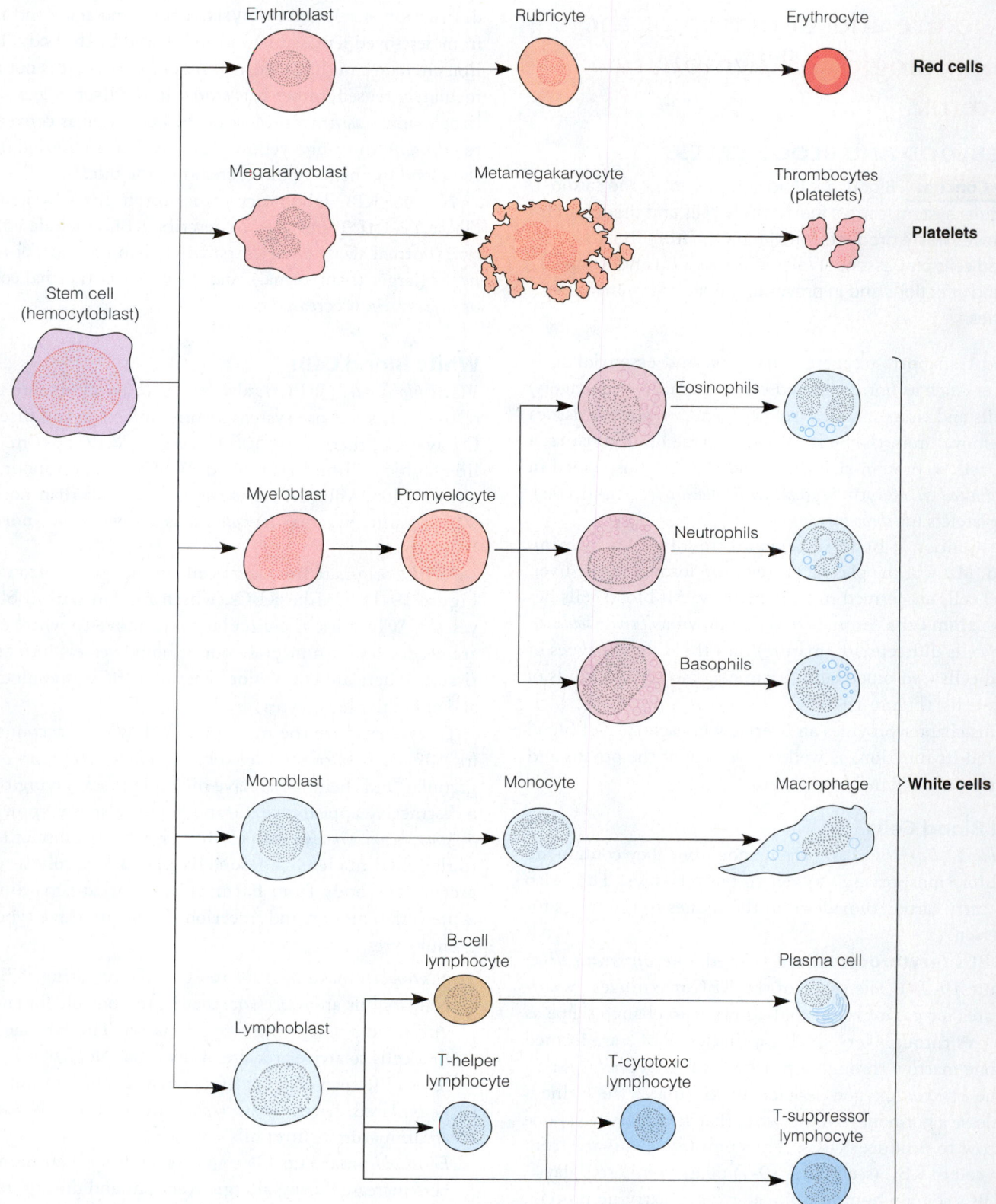

Figure 19-1. ■ The formation of different types of blood cells from the stem cell. Stem cells differentiate into one of five types of blast (immature) cells, which then mature into red blood cells (erythrocytes), platelets (thrombocytes), or white blood cells (leukocytes).

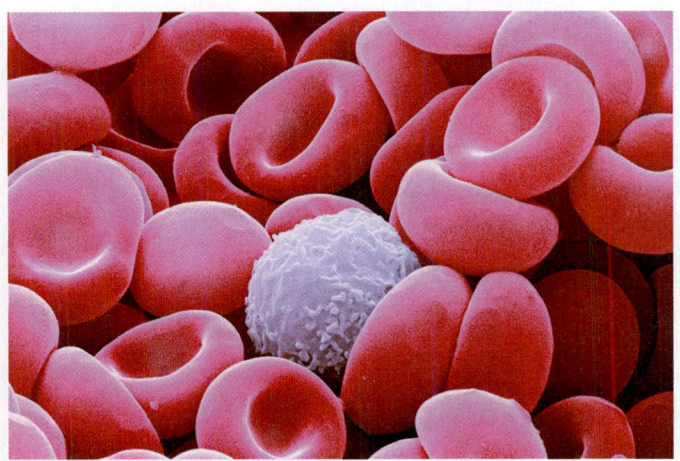

Figure 19-2. ■ Red blood cells. Note the distinctive biconcave shape of the cell that increases its surface area and allows it to flex as it moves through capillaries. (Source: Andrew Syred/ Science Source.)

migrate into body tissues such as the skin, subcutaneous tissue, lungs, and liver. There they mature into *macrophages.* Both monocytes and macrophages are phagocytic cells.

Lymphocytes account for 25% to 35% of WBCs. Although lymphocytes are small and nondescript, they are the primary effectors and regulators of specific immune responses. *B lymphocytes (B cells)* are involved in forming antibodies, whereas *T lymphocytes (T cells)* take part in cell-mediated immunity. A third type of lymphocyte, *natural killer cells (NK cells),* also provides immune surveillance and resistance to infection. Normal laboratory values for WBCs are outlined in Table 19-1.

Platelets

Platelets are an essential part of the body's clotting mechanism. They are small fragments of cytoplasm without nuclei that contain many granules. Most platelets are stored in the spleen before being released into the circulation. There

TABLE 19-1	Common Laboratory Tests for Hematologic and Lymphatic Disorders		
TEST	**NORMAL ADULT VALUES**	**EXPLANATION**	**NURSING IMPLICATIONS**
		Complete Blood Count (CBC)	
Red blood cell (RBC) count ■ Men ■ Women	 4.6–6.0 million/μL (mm³) 4.0–5.0 million/μL (mm³)	Number of circulating RBCs in 1 μL (cubic millimeter, or mm³) of blood Reduced in hemorrhage, anemia, and chronic kidney disease Increased (polycythemia) in high altitude, cardiopulmonary disease	No fasting or special patient preparation is necessary. Explain the test and the reason it is being done. Results may be affected by deficient or excess fluid volume.
Reticulocyte count	0.5%–1.5% of total RBC	Percentage of immature RBCs Used to help diagnose anemias and their underlying cause	No fasting or special patient preparation is necessary. Explain the test and the reason it is being done.
Hemoglobin (Hgb) ■ Men ■ Women	 13.5–18 g/dL 12–15 g/dL	Amount of hemoglobin in 100 mL (1 dL) of blood Used to help diagnose anemias	No fasting or special patient preparation is necessary. Do not draw a sample from an arm in which an IV is infusing.
Hematocrit (Hct) ■ Men ■ Women	 40%–54% 36%–46%	Packed volume of RBCs in 100 mL of blood; reported as a percentage Used to help diagnose acute blood loss and anemias and to monitor chronic diseases	Explain why the test is being done. Results may be affected by deficient or excess fluid volume. No special preparation is required.
Mean corpuscular volume (MCV)	80–98 cuμ (fL)	Average volume of individual RBCs	Explain that these tests are used to help identify the underlying cause or type of anemias.
Mean corpuscular hemoglobin (MCH)	27–31 pg	Weight of the hemoglobin in an average RBC	
Mean corpuscular hemoglobin concentration (MCHC)	32%–36%	Average concentration (percentage) of hemoglobin within RBC	

(continued)

TABLE 19-1	Common Laboratory Tests for Hematologic and Lymphatic Disorders *(continued)*		
TEST	**NORMAL ADULT VALUES**	**EXPLANATION**	**NURSING IMPLICATIONS**
WBC count	4,500–10,000/μL (mm³)	Measures the number of WBCs in circulating blood	No food or fluid restriction is required.
Differential WBC count		Provides more specific information about infections and disease processes	Inquire about manifestations of acute infection or known chronic conditions that may affect WBC count.
▪ Neutrophils	50%–70% (2,500–7,000/μL)	Rapid responders to infection and tissue damage Increase in acute infection and inflammation	Decreased WBCs are seen in disorders affecting blood cell production and some infections.
▪ Eosinophils	1%–3% (100–300/μL)	Increase during allergic and parasitic conditions	Increased WBCs are present in acute infection, leukemias, stress responses, and some acute and chronic diseases.
▪ Basophils	0.4%–1.0% (40–100/μL)	Increase during healing; decrease in stress and allergic reactions	
▪ Lymphocytes	25%–35% (1,700–3,500/μL)	Play a major role in immune response with B lymphocytes and T lymphocytes	
▪ Monocytes	4%–6% (200–600/μL)	Second line of defense against bacterial infection and foreign substances	
Platelets	150,000–400,000/μL (mm³)	The number of circulating platelets in the blood Low platelet count associated with bleeding; increased count may increase risk for abnormal clotting	No patient preparation is required. Observe for manifestations of bleeding. Monitor count in patients undergoing chemotherapy.
Bleeding time	1–9 minutes	Used to screen for disorders caused by platelet dysfunction	Bleeding time is prolonged by ingestion of aspirin and anti-inflammatory drugs.
Coagulation Studies			
Prothrombin time (PT or protime)	10–13 seconds (varies by laboratory)	Evaluates the extrinsic clotting pathway; prolonged in warfarin (Coumadin) therapy	No food or fluid restrictions are necessary.
INR (International Normalized Ratio)	2–3.0	Used to evaluate warfarin (Coumadin) therapy	The INR provides a more standardized measure of warfarin therapy.
Partial thromboplastin time (PTT)	60–70 seconds	Used to evaluate clotting pathways and monitor heparin therapy	No food or fluid restriction is required.
Activated partial thromboplastin time (APTT)	20–35 seconds	More sensitive than PTT; evaluates the intrinsic clotting pathway; prolonged in heparin therapy	Values are increased in clotting factor deficiencies, heparin therapy, and aspirin ingestion.
Coombs test	Negative	Performed to diagnose hemolytic anemias and evaluate transfusion reactions. The expected results are no detected antibodies to RBCs (indirect Coombs) or no detected RBC antigen–antibody complexes (direct Coombs).	No food or fluid restriction is required. Ask about previous transfusions or transfusion reactions. Report manifestations of transfusion reactions.
Hemoglobin electrophoresis	▪ Hb A$_1$ 95%–98% ▪ Hb A$_2$ 1.5%–4% ▪ Hb F less than 2% ▪ Hb C 0% ▪ Hb D 0% ▪ Hb S 0%	Performed to detect abnormal forms of hemoglobin associated with genetic hemolytic anemias (e.g., sickle cell anemia, thalassemia)	No food or fluid restrictions are required. Assess for and report manifestations of hemolytic anemias. Encourage the patient to obtain genetic counseling.

TABLE 19-1	Common Laboratory Tests for Hematologic and Lymphatic Disorders *(continued)*		
TEST	**NORMAL ADULT VALUES**	**EXPLANATION**	**NURSING IMPLICATIONS**
Iron	50–150 mcg/dL (10–27 mol/L)	Serum iron and body iron stores are measured to evaluate iron deficiency anemia.	Antibiotics, estrogen and testosterone, oral contraceptives, aspirin, and ethanol affect results.
Total iron-binding capacity	250–450 µg/dL	Measures the maximum amount of iron that can bind to transferrin, the protein that transports it	
Ferritin	Men: 15–445 ng/mL (15–445 µg/L) Women: 10–310 ng/mL (10–310 µg/L)	A measure of the amount of iron stored in body tissues	No food or fluid restrictions are required. Results in women are affected by age and use of oral contraceptives.
Transferrin	200–430 mg/dL (2.0–4.3 g/L)	Measures the protein that transports iron to the bone marrow for use in synthesizing hemoglobin	Avoid iron supplements for 12 hours before testing. Results are affected by pregnancy and use of oral contraceptives.
D-dimer	Negative	D-dimer is a fragment produced when fibrinolysis occurs. It is used primarily to diagnose disseminated intravascular coagulation.	No food or fluid restriction is required. Report manifestations such as unexplained bleeding. Monitor vital signs.

are about 150,000 to 400,000 platelets in each milliliter of blood. An excess of platelets is *thrombocytosis*. Platelets live approximately 10 days in circulating blood.

HEMOSTASIS

Hemostasis, or blood clotting, is a complex process the body uses to stop bleeding. There are five stages in hemostasis:

1. *Vessel spasm*: Damage to a blood vessel causes it to spasm. This spasm, which lasts more than a minute, constricts the vessel and reduces blood flow.
2. *Formation of the platelet plug*: Platelets adhere to the damaged vessel wall and to one another, forming a platelet plug. Von Willebrand factor is necessary for platelets to adhere to one another. The platelet plug is stabilized by fibrin, which binds the platelets and other blood cells (Figure 19-3■).
3. *Clot formation*: Coagulation occurs as fibrin forms a meshwork that cements blood components together into an insoluble clot. The process involves two different clotting pathways. The *intrinsic pathway* is activated by vessel injury; the *extrinsic pathway* is activated by blood leaking out of the vessel into the tissues (Figure 19-4■). The final outcome is fibrin clot formation. Each clotting factor is activated in sequence; activation of one clotting factor activates another in turn. A deficiency of one or more factors interrupts blood clotting.

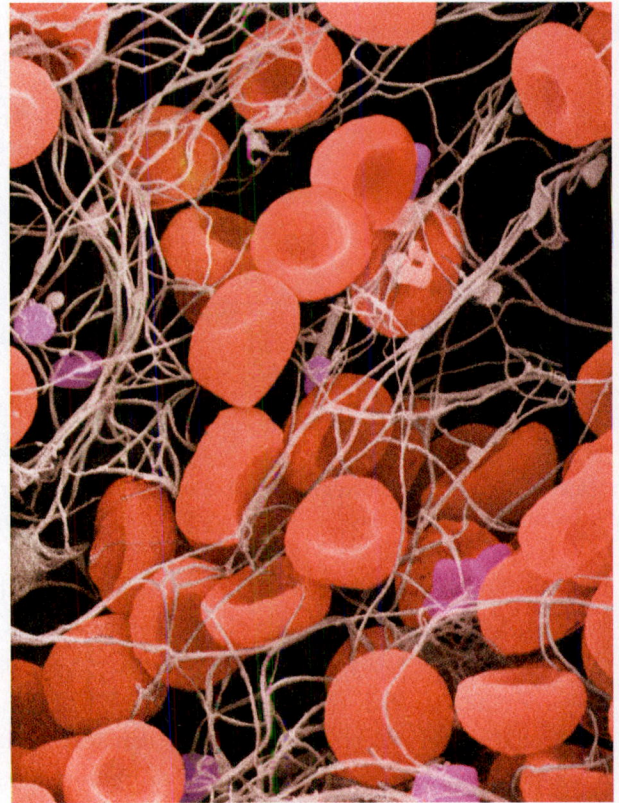

Figure 19-3. ■ Fibrin traps red blood cells and platelets to form a stable clot. (Copyright © Susumu Nishinaga/Science Source.)

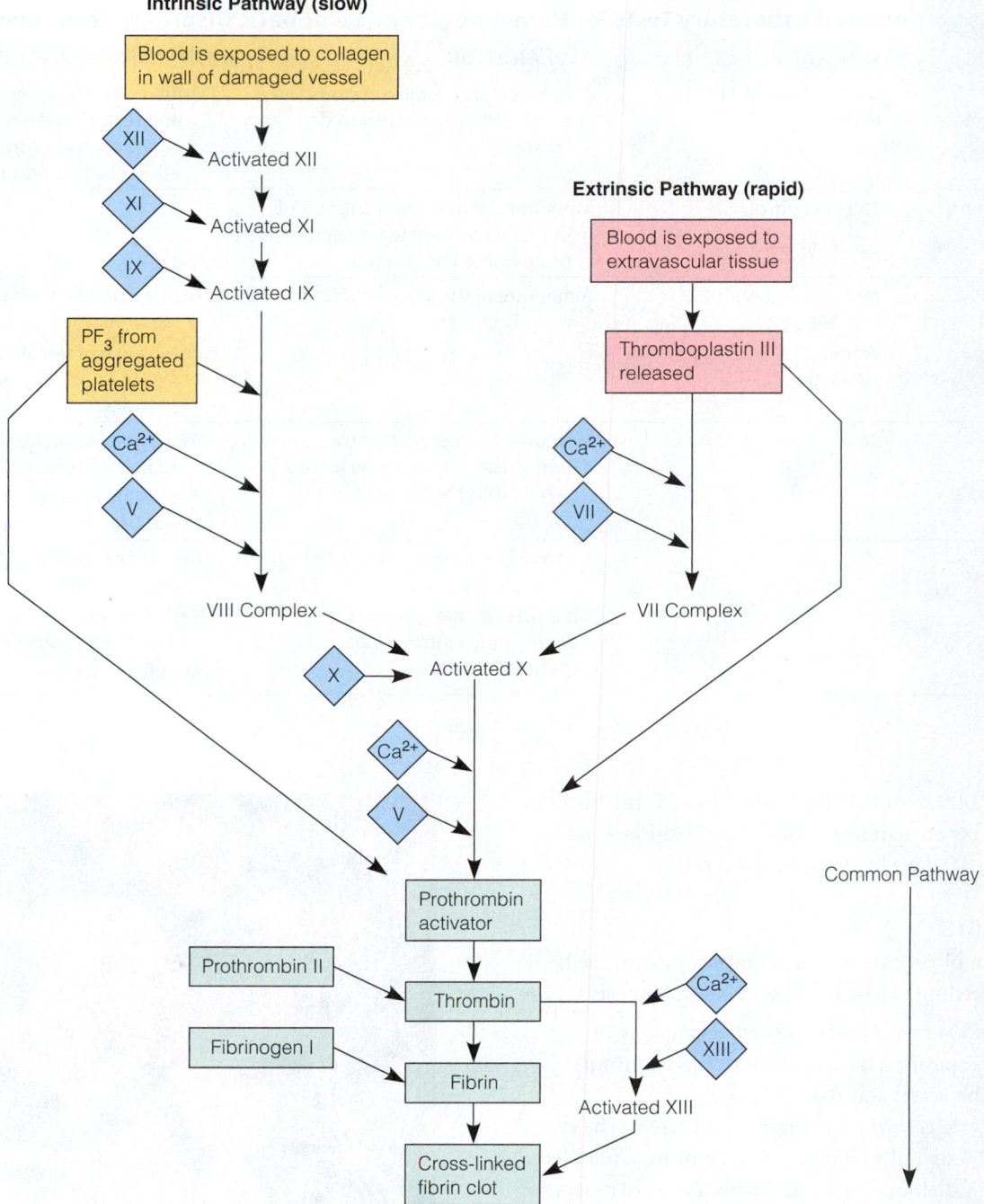

Figure 19-4. ■ Both the slower intrinsic pathway (on the left) and the more rapid extrinsic pathway (on the right) are necessary to form a stable blood clot.

4. *Clot retraction*: After about 30 minutes, platelets trapped within the clot begin to contract. This pulls the broken portions of the ruptured blood vessel closer together. At the same time, platelets release growth factors that stimulate cell division and tissue repair in the damaged vessel.

5. *Clot dissolution*: A process called *fibrinolysis* removes the clot after tissue has been repaired. Fibrinolysis begins within a few days of clot formation and continues until the clot is dissolved.

Normal values for platelets and routinely performed coagulation studies are presented in Table 19-1.

THE LYMPHATIC SYSTEM

Key Concept The tissues and organs of the lymphatic system play an important role in removing damaged and abnormal cells and foreign matter from the body.

The **lymphatic system** (Figure 19-5■), including the lymphatic vessels, lymph nodes, and lymphoid organs such

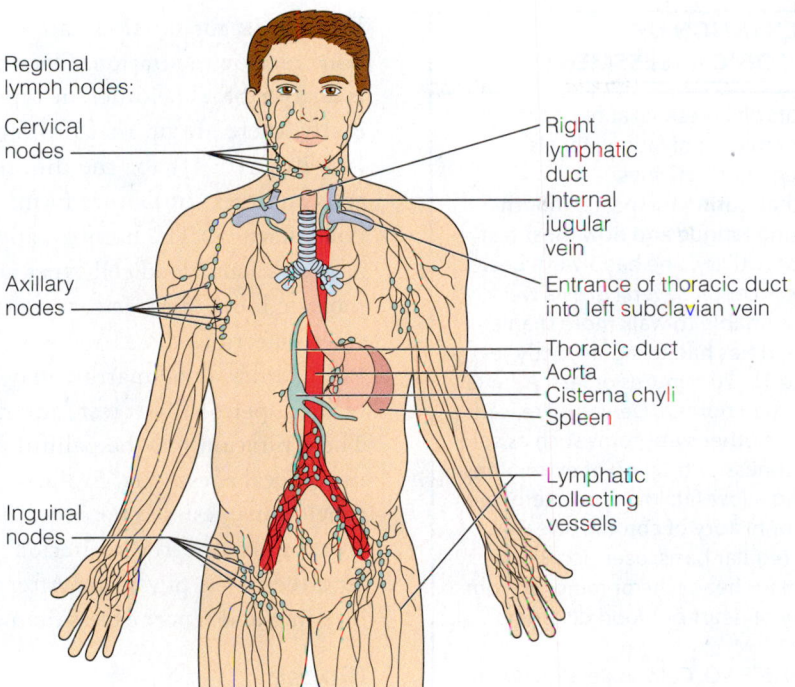

Figure 19-5. ■ The lymphatic system.

as the spleen, has several functions. Excess tissue fluid, called *lymph*, returns to the heart through low-pressure lymphatic vessels. Lymph nodes assist the immune system by removing foreign matter, infectious organisms, and tumor cells from lymph. The largest lymphoid organ is the spleen, located in the upper left quadrant of the abdomen. The spleen filters the blood, produces lymphocytes (a type of WBC active in the immune response), and stores blood and platelets. Other lymphoid organs, such as the thymus and lymphoid tissue in the skin and respiratory and gastrointestinal systems, are important partners in the immune system, helping protect the body from infection.

Assessment

Key Concept Nurses play an important role in identifying manifestations of hematologic and lymphatic system disorders. Effective assessment of these systems requires conscious attention by the nurse.

Assessment of the hematologic and lymphatic systems generally is conducted as part of the general survey of the patient's health or concurrently with focused cardiovascular system assessment.

HEALTH HISTORY

Ask about recent changes in energy level and ability to maintain usual daily activities, including recreational activities and sports. Inquire about any pain, burning or tingling sensations, changes in skin color or temperature, or swelling (edema). Ask about bleeding or easy bruising, dizziness, fatigue, or changes in lymph nodes (swelling, pain or tenderness, warmth). Have the patient relate usual diet, including protein, vitamin, and mineral intake. Ask about current medications and use of tobacco, alcohol, and other recreational drugs.

Obtain the patient's medical history, specifically asking about frequent or recurrent infections, chronic diseases, cancer, kidney disease, or HIV disease. Ask about surgeries, blood transfusions, and exposure to radiation or chemicals (during medical procedures, environmental exposure, or occupational exposure). Inquire about family history of cancer, anemia, or blood disorders.

PHYSICAL EXAMINATION

Assessment of the hematologic and lymphatic systems begins with inspection of the color of the skin and mucous membranes, including observing for pallor or cyanosis. Inspect oral mucous membranes and the skin of the trunk and extremities for erythema, red streaks, or lesions such as petechiae, bruising, or **purpura** (purple rashes caused by blood leaking into the skin). Obtain the vital signs, including temperature and apical pulse. Palpate for skin temperature, capillary refill, and edema of the extremities. Palpate lymph nodes for swelling and tenderness. Lightly palpate the upper left quadrant of the abdomen for tenderness.

Box 19-1 ■ presents an example for documenting assessment of the hematologic system.

Box 19-2■ for nursing care of the patient undergoing a bone marrow aspiration. Once obtained, the bone marrow is analyzed for the different types of cells it contains. Normally, there are up to 15 different types of cells present. (See Figure 19-1 for the different types of mature blood cells and their immature forms that would be expected in bone marrow.) The number, appearance, and development of the various blood cell types are analyzed to diagnose hemolytic blood disorders, tumors, leukemias, and, in some cases, infectious diseases.

In adults, bone marrow may be obtained from the posterior superior iliac crest, anterior iliac crest, or sternum. The aspiration may be painful for the patient, despite the use of local anesthesia. Evaluate pain level after the test and provide analgesics as needed. The site may be sore for up to 3 or 4 days after the aspiration. Continued pain should be reported to the physician. After the aspiration, monitor for bleeding and report excess drainage or bleeding.

Biopsy

When a hematologic or lymphatic malignancy is suspected, bone marrow or tissue from a lymph node is microscopically examined for the presence of abnormal cells. Nursing

---

BOX 19-1	DOCUMENTATION OF HEMATOLOGIC ASSESSMENT

Patient: Janet Hinman, 54 years old, presents at her primary care physician's office with complaints of fatigue that is significantly affecting her usual daily activities.

Assessment Note: States that during the past 3 months she has experienced increasing fatigue and now must rest after only 30 minutes or so of activity. She has always been active, working out at a fitness center several days a week, hiking, and skiing, but now is unable to walk more than a few blocks without resting and has had to significantly reduce her normal workouts to 15–20 minutes or less. Admits that she bruises more easily than normal. Denies increased incidence of infections. Denies other symptoms such as sore mouth, cracking of lips, numbness or tingling of extremities. States she eats well, following a low-fat, low-cholesterol diet, and has no known allergies or history of chronic diseases. Taking no medications on a regular basis; uses occasional acetaminophen or ibuprofen for headache or minor discomfort. No known family history of heart or blood disorders or cancer.

BP 122/64, P 86, R 22, T 97.6°F PO. Color pale; skin warm and dry. Conjunctiva and oral mucous membranes pale and moist. Scattered petechiae noted in oral mucous membranes, on trunk and back. Multiple bruises of varying age noted on extremities. Pulses strong, equal, and regular on all four extremities. Capillary refill approximately 3 seconds. No edema noted. No cervical lymphadenopathy noted. Active bowel sounds heard in all four quadrants; slight tenderness to light palpation noted in upper left quadrant.

DIAGNOSTIC TESTS

A number of laboratory and diagnostic tests can be done to identify disorders of the blood or lymph systems.

Laboratory Tests

- The *complete blood count (CBC)* is often performed as a routine screening examination. The CBC includes the RBC count, the hemoglobin and hematocrit, and RBC indices; the WBC count, and, if ordered, WBC differential; and the platelet count.
- *Clotting studies* or a *coagulation profile* is performed to evaluate clotting and bleeding disorders and are often ordered before major surgeries (such as heart surgery, joint replacements). These tests are also used to monitor thrombolytic (fibrinolytic) and anticoagulant therapy.

These laboratory tests, their normal values, and nursing implications are summarized in Table 19-1, which also includes other laboratory tests that may be done to evaluate hematologic and lymphatic function.

Bone Marrow Aspiration

In many hematologic disorders, it is necessary to aspirate and analyze bone marrow to establish the diagnosis. See

---

BOX 19-2	NURSING CARE CHECKLIST

Bone Marrow Aspiration

Bone marrow studies are used to diagnose aplastic anemia, leukemias, and other cancers. A sample of bone marrow is obtained by inserting a needle or biopsy instrument into a bone (usually the posterior iliac crest or sternum).

Before the Procedure

- ☑ Verify signed consent for the procedure has been obtained.
- ☑ Explain the purpose and procedure of the test.
- ☑ Record vital signs. Have the patient void.
- ☑ Place in supine position if sternum or anterior iliac crest will be used, in prone position if posterior iliac crest is to be used.

After the Procedure

- ☑ Apply pressure to the puncture site for 5 to 10 minutes.
- ☑ Assess vital signs; report changes from baseline.
- ☑ Apply dressing to puncture site. Monitor for bleeding and infection.

Patient and Family Teaching

- ☑ The procedure takes about 20 minutes.
- ☑ A local anesthetic will be used; you will feel some pain during insertion. Take deep breaths to help relieve pain during this time.
- ☑ It is important to remain very still during the procedure.
- ☑ The site of the aspiration may ache for several days.
- ☑ Report any unusual bleeding, drainage, or symptoms of infection immediately.

care for a lymph node biopsy is similar to that provided for the patient undergoing bone marrow aspiration, although the risk of bleeding and discomfort after the procedure generally is less.

Imaging Studies

Computed tomography (CT) scan and magnetic resonance imaging (MRI) may be used to evaluate lymph nodes and when the lymphatic system is suspected as a cause of edema. Informed consent is required for these imaging studies. Inquire about allergies to radiologic contrast media, iodine, or seafood if contrast will be used. When an MRI is planned, ask about implanted metal (e.g., joint prostheses) or electronic devices such as a pacemaker. Provide teaching about the procedure to reduce the patient's anxiety.

Note: The references and resources for all chapters have been compiled at the back of the book.

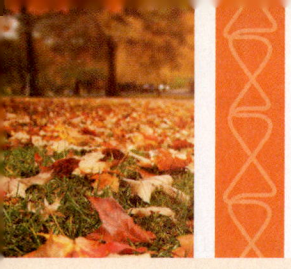

Chapter Review

KEY POINTS

- **Concept:** Blood, the fluid component of the cardiovascular system, carries fuel to body cells and tissues and removes waste products for elimination from the body. Blood cells play essential roles in preventing and eliminating infections and in preventing fluid loss from injured tissues.
- Blood is the transport medium for oxygen, nutrients, and other substances in the body.
- The primary function of RBCs is to transport oxygen to the cells.
- The primary function of WBCs is to fight infection, destroy foreign matter, and eliminate damaged or abnormal cells in the body. WBCs are an integral part of the immune system and necessary for its functioning.
- Platelets and clotting factors work together in the process of blood clotting and the control of bleeding.
- **Concept:** The tissues and organs of the lymphatic system play an important role in removing damaged and abnormal cells and foreign matter from the body.
- The lymphatic system also is involved in the immune response.
- **Concept:** Nurses play an important role in identifying manifestations of hematologic and lymphatic system disorders. Effective assessment of these systems requires conscious attention by the nurse.
- Blood tests to evaluate the number and types of cells present, their size and shape, and the ability of the blood to clot are the primary diagnostic tests used to evaluate the hematologic system. Aspiration of bone marrow may be necessary to provide additional information about blood formation.
- Nursing care of the patient undergoing diagnostic testing for a possible hematologic disorder is both educational, explaining the purpose of tests and any special preparation or expected sensations during the test, and supportive.

PEARSON NURSING STUDENT RESOURCES

Find additional materials at **nursing.pearsonhighered.com**.

NCLEX-PN® Exam Preparation

1. The nurse notes that a patient's hemoglobin is 11.5 g/dL and her hematocrit is 30%. The nurse knows that these levels:
   1. are within normal limits for a woman.
   2. will affect the patient's ability to transport oxygen to her cells.
   3. significantly increase the patient's risk for abnormal clotting.
   4. increase the patient's risk for infection.

2. A patient with kidney failure has low erythropoietin levels. As a result, the nurse would expect which of the following in the CBC? **Select all that apply.**
   1. A low RBC count
   2. A high hemoglobin level
   3. A low hematocrit
   4. A high WBC count
   5. Increased numbers of immature RBCs in the blood

3. On assuming care for a patient who was admitted after a motor vehicle crash, the nurse notes that the patient's spleen was removed to stem abdominal bleeding. The nurse understands that this will affect the patient's:
   1. ability to metabolize drugs.
   2. excretion of toxic waste products.
   3. blood clotting.
   4. immune function.

4. The nurse caring for a patient with a diagnosis of thrombocytopenia knows that this disorder will affect the patient's:
   1. ability to form blood clots.
   2. ability to fight infection.
   3. energy level.
   4. nutritional status.

5. After a bone marrow aspiration, the nurse appropriately plans to:
   1. significantly increase the patient's fluid intake to restore blood volume.
   2. withhold all analgesics to allow accurate assessment of mental status.
   3. carefully monitor the site for signs of excess bleeding.
   4. warn the patient to remain on bed rest for 24 hours after the procedure.

Answers and rationales for Review Questions appear in Appendix I.

CULTURAL CARE STRATEGIES

Assessing the Patient From Another Culture in a Social Context

Mr. Ararnak, 27, a Saudi man, refused to allow a male lab technician to enter his wife's room to draw blood. She had just had a radical mastectomy. The nurse finally convinced the husband of the need for the blood sample, and he reluctantly allowed the technician in the room. However, he made sure his wife was completely covered. Only her arm stuck out from beneath the covers. The nurse was careful to accommodate this request. The nurse knew that for Arab families, honor is one of the highest values. Because family honor is dependent on female purity, many Arabs feel that sexual segregation and extreme modesty must be maintained at all times.

Most patients are part of one or more social organizations, which play an important role in their lives. Thus, the social organizations of which the patient is a part and their effect on the patient need to be assessed so that culturally appropriate and effective care can be delivered to the patient and family.

Family

For many individuals, the most significant social organization influencing behavior is the family. However, the primary responsibility for decision making varies among cultural groups (Giger, 2013). Some individuals, such as those from Appalachia or Mexico, rely heavily on family members for decision making. Some religious groups, such as the Amish, may also want to have the church fellowship involved. On the other hand, many Americans make decisions for themselves without consulting anyone.

The family structure may be male or female dominated. For example, in some Hispanic families, the father is the primary decision maker and controller of the family. The Hispanic female is often submissive and frequently puts the needs and wants of others above her own. In contrast, in many Black American families, the female is dominant and has a greater role in decision making.

The family can be viewed in two separate ways. First, the family is the environment that supports the patient and provides values and practices. Second, in family-centered care, when the patient becomes ill, the nurse is expected to care for the patient and the family. Therefore, it is essential to understand the role family plays in the patient's health.

For some patients, the most important single organization is the nuclear family or the extended family. For others, the family unit may not be composed of blood relatives. The nurse should recognize those individuals who assume the functions customarily provided by blood relatives.

Church or Religious Affiliations

In the United States, there are many church types and many major denominations. This is very different from countries such as Mexico or Spain, where most people belong to one faith and one church. In the United States, some churches are identified with an ethnic group. For example, in the Amish church, religious beliefs are synonymous with the Amish life experience.

Nursing Implications

■ *Assess the patient–family relationship*. Nurses need to assess the patient–family relationship in order to learn their values, the flow of authority, and how decisions are made.

■ *Be aware that unrelated persons may provide the functions of a family*. Rules related to "family members" may need to be interpreted flexibly.

■ *Involve the family as needed to achieve optimal outcomes*. The person with the decision-making power needs to be included in discussions about treatment options. When patient education is done, the individual with the decision-making power should usually be involved. This improves compliance.

■ *Respect religious customs*. Personal articles such as statues, shrines, rosaries, amulets, or pictures may have special religious meaning and should be treated with respect.

■ *Communicate with health team members if they are unfamiliar with the family's decision-making structure*. The nurse may need to provide insight for team members regarding which family members the patient feels need to be included in health care decisions.

Self-Reflection Questions

1. Who made the decisions about health care in your family of origin?

2. When making decisions, do you need or not need input from your family?

3. Do your religious values influence the way you feel about some patients?

4. What conflicts might you have in caring for a patient whose religious values differ from your own?

5. What conflicts might you have in dealing with a male physician who is accustomed to male-dominated relationships with women?

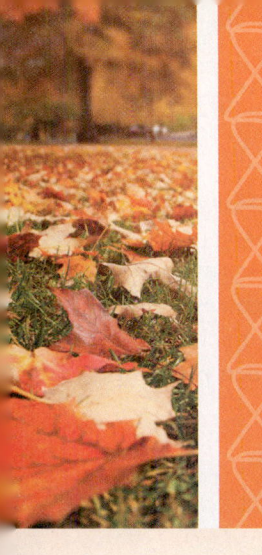

CHAPTER 20
Caring for Patients With Hematologic and Lymphatic Disorders

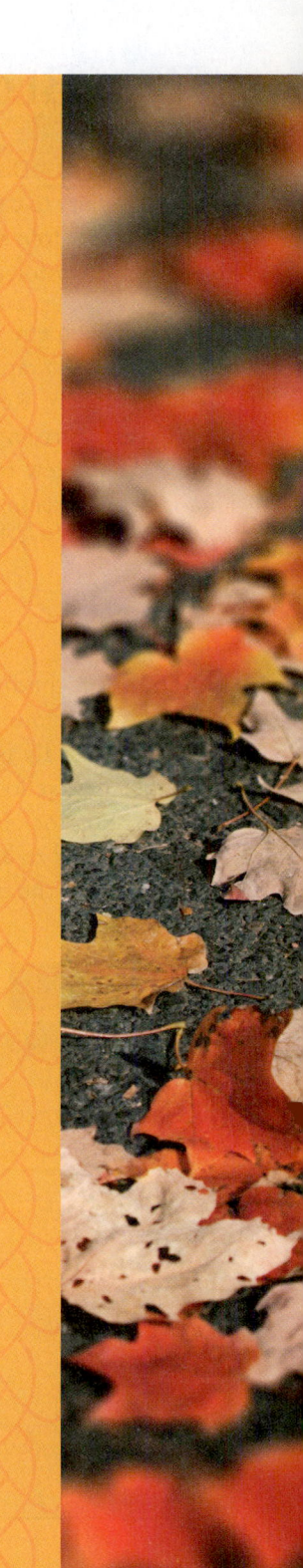

BRIEF OUTLINE

RED BLOOD CELL DISORDERS
Anemia
Polycythemia
WHITE BLOOD CELL DISORDERS
Leukemia
Malignant Lymphoma
Multiple Myeloma
Neutropenia

PLATELET AND COAGULATION DISORDERS
Thrombocytopenia
Hemophilia
Disseminated Intravascular Coagulation
LYMPHATIC SYSTEM DISORDERS
Lymphangitis and Lymphedema
Infectious Mononucleosis

APPLIED LEARNING OUTCOMES

After completing this chapter, you will be able to:

1. Describe the pathophysiology and manifestations of common hematologic and lymphatic disorders.
2. Conduct focused assessments for patients with hematologic or lymphatic disorders, recognizing and responding appropriately to abnormal or unexpected data.
3. Function within the interprofessional team to provide safe and effective care for patients with hematologic or lymphatic disorders.
4. Use the nursing process and current standards of care to provide safe and effective care for patients with hematologic or lymphatic disorders.
5. Provide teaching and nursing care that considers individual expressed values, preferences, and needs for patients with hematologic or lymphatic disorders.

KEY TERMS

The key terms are defined on the pages listed below.

SPECIAL FEATURES

Key Concept   Because of the role the blood plays in transporting oxygen and nutrients to the cells, responding to infection, and preventing significant fluid loss due to injury, hematologic disorders can have wide-ranging effects on patients' daily living activities.

Nurses frequently interact with and provide nursing care for patients with hematologic or lymphatic disorders. This care often occurs in community-based care settings (care providers' offices and clinics), where the nurse's role is primarily one of teaching. In acute and long-term care settings, these disorders frequently are seen as secondary diagnoses: not the primary reason for admission of the patient to the health care setting, but a factor to be considered when planning, implementing, and evaluating nursing care.

RED BLOOD CELL DISORDERS

Key Concept   Disorders of the red blood cells affect the body's ability to carry oxygen to the tissues. As a result, the patient often experiences symptoms such as fatigue and activity intolerance.

When oxygen enters the blood from the lungs, the majority of it (97%) rapidly combines with the hemoglobin in red blood cells. Red blood cell disorders, therefore, affect the oxygen-carrying capacity of the blood. In general, when there are too few red blood cells, the disorder is known as *anemia*. An excess of red blood cells (RBCs) is known as *polycythemia* or erythrocytosis.

Anemia

Anemia is a condition in which the hemoglobin concentration or the number of circulating RBCs is decreased. Anemia typically is caused by either impaired RBC formation or excessive loss or destruction of RBCs (Table 20-1■). Hemorrhage or chronic bleeding (e.g., from a bleeding ulcer) can lead to anemia, as can nutritional problems that interfere with the body's ability to form red blood cells.

PATHOPHYSIOLOGY AND MANIFESTATIONS

Approximately 97% of the oxygen in the blood is carried attached to the hemoglobin molecule in RBCs. Anemia, whether due to decreased RBCs or hemoglobin concentration, reduces the oxygen-carrying capacity of the blood, leading to tissue hypoxia. As tissue oxygenation decreases, the body attempts to restore adequate oxygen delivery. The heart and respiratory rates increase. Blood is redistributed to vital organs, causing pallor of the skin, mucous membranes, nail beds, and conjunctiva (Figure 20-1■). Tissue hypoxia may cause angina, fatigue, dyspnea on exertion, and night cramps. The kidneys release increased amounts of erythropoietin, which stimulates the bone marrow, causing bone pain. Poor oxygen delivery to the brain can cause headache, dizziness, and dim vision. The severity of the manifestations of anemia (Figure 20-2■) depends on the cause and severity of the disorder. For example, rapid blood loss causes immediate symptoms, whereas the person with slowly developing anemia may have no symptoms until the condition is advanced or if the oxygen needs of the body increase (e.g., during exercise or infection).

TABLE 20-1	Selected Types and Causes of Anemia	
CLASSIFICATION	**CAUSE**	**EXAMPLES**
Blood loss	Acute or chronic bleeding	Trauma Internal bleeding Complications of pregnancy
Nutritional	Decreased RBC or hemoglobin production	Iron deficiency anemia Pernicious or vitamin B_{12} deficiency anemia Folic acid deficiency anemia
Hemolytic	Defective hemoglobin synthesis	Sickle cell disease Thalassemia
	Increased hemolysis	Immune reactions Chemical or physical agents
Aplastic (bone marrow failure)	Suppression of bone marrow function	Leukemias Chemical or physical agents

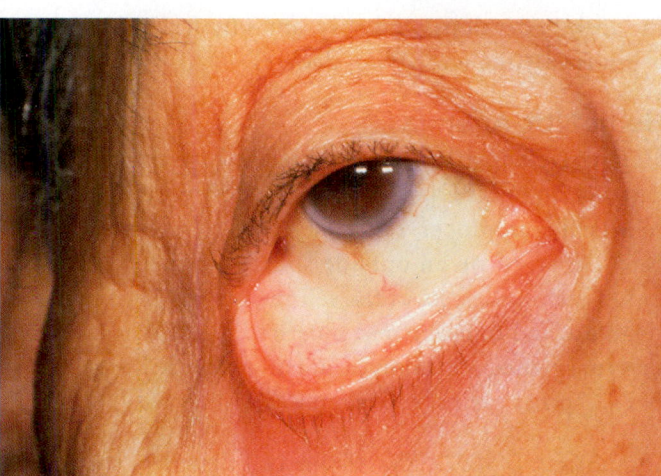

Figure 20-1. ■ Pallor of the conjunctiva and eyelid in a patient with anemia. (Source: Dr. Chris Hale/Science Source.)

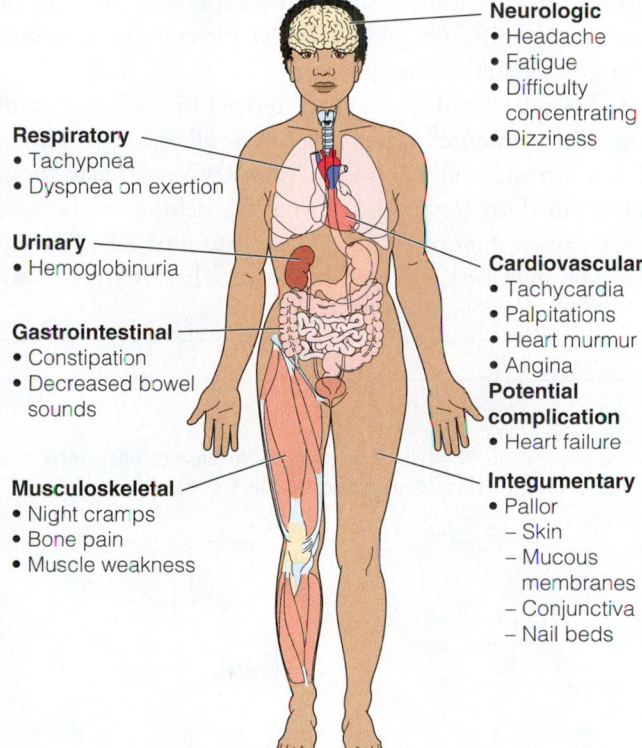

Neurologic
• Headache
• Fatigue
• Difficulty
  concentrating
• Dizziness

Respiratory
• Tachypnea
• Dyspnea on exertion

Urinary
• Hemoglobinuria

Gastrointestinal
• Constipation
• Decreased bowel
  sounds

Cardiovascular
• Tachycardia
• Palpitations
• Heart murmur
• Angina
**Potential
complication**
• Heart failure

Musculoskeletal
• Night cramps
• Bone pain
• Muscle weakness

Integumentary
• Pallor
  – Skin
  – Mucous
    membranes
  – Conjunctiva
  – Nail beds

Figure 20-2. ■ The multisystem effects of anemia.

Blood Loss Anemia

Red blood cells and hemoglobin are lost from the body with acute or chronic bleeding. With acute bleeding, the risk of hypovolemia and shock is greater than the risk of anemia. Chronic bleeding, however, often leads to anemia. Fluids shift into the vascular system to maintain blood volume, but RBC production in the bone marrow cannot keep up with losses. The symptoms of the anemia may actually alert the patient and care provider to the bleeding problem. In blood loss anemia, RBCs are normal in size, shape, and color, but their numbers are reduced. The RBC, hemoglobin, and hematocrit levels fall.

Nutritional Anemias

Nutritional anemias result when a lack of one or more necessary nutrients for RBC formation disrupts RBC development or hemoglobin synthesis. The nutrient deficiency may be due to a poor diet, impaired absorption of the nutrient, or an increased need for the nutrient. The most common nutritional anemias are iron deficiency anemia, vitamin B_{12} deficiency (pernicious) anemia, and folic acid deficiency anemia.

IRON DEFICIENCY ANEMIA   Iron deficiency anemia is caused by an inadequate supply of iron for RBC formation. It is the most common type of anemia. The body cannot make hemoglobin without iron. Iron deficiency leads to fewer RBCs, microcytic (small) RBCs, and hypochromic (pale) RBCs. The RBCs may also be malformed.

In adults, iron loss due to bleeding is the usual cause of iron deficiency anemia. Menstrual blood loss is the common cause in adult females. Chronic, occult (hidden) blood loss may occur from disorders such as bleeding ulcers, gastrointestinal inflammation, hemorrhoids, and cancer.

Inadequate iron intake (less than 1 mg/day) or impaired iron absorption also can lead to iron deficiency anemia. This is common in older adults. Women may develop anemia during pregnancy and lactation because the need for iron is higher.

In addition to the manifestations shown in Figure 20-2, chronic iron deficiency can cause brittle, spoon-shaped nails; *cheilosis* (cracks at the corners of the mouth); a smooth, sore tongue; and *pica* (a craving to eat unusual substances, such as clay or starch).

VITAMIN B_{12} DEFICIENCY (PERNICIOUS) ANEMIA   Vitamin B_{12} is required for RBC formation and maturation. The usual cause of vitamin B_{12} deficiency is impaired absorption of the nutrient from the GI tract. This condition is known as *pernicious anemia. Intrinsic factor*, a substance secreted by the gastric mucosa, binds with dietary vitamin B_{12} so it can be absorbed by the body.

Vitamin B_{12} deficit interferes with the maturation of red blood cells. Great numbers of large, immature RBCs move into the circulation. These cells are fragile and incapable of carrying oxygen in adequate amounts.

Patients with pernicious anemia may develop a smooth, sore, beefy red tongue and diarrhea. Because vitamin B_{12} is important for neurologic function, *paresthesias* (altered sensations, such as numbness or tingling) in the extremities and problems with *proprioception* (the sense of one's position in space) also may develop.

FOLIC ACID DEFICIENCY ANEMIA   Like vitamin B_{12}, folic acid is required for normal production and maturation of red blood cells. Folic acid is absorbed from the intestines and is found in green, leafy vegetables; fruits; cereals; and meats. Folic acid deficiency produces an anemia characterized by fragile, megaloblastic (big and immature) cells.

Folic acid deficiency anemia is more common among people who are chronically malnourished (e.g., older adults, alcoholics, and drug users). People receiving parenteral nutrition (PN) may develop folate deficiency. Pregnant women, whose folic acid requirements are increased, and patients with certain malabsorption disorders also are at risk.

The manifestations of folic acid deficiency anemia develop gradually. In addition to the symptoms common to anemia, gastrointestinal manifestations such as glossitis, cheilosis, and diarrhea often develop. Two serious birth defects, spina bifida and anencephaly, are linked to folic acid deficiency during pregnancy. These birth defects develop very early in pregnancy, before many women realize they are pregnant (CDC, 2012).

Anemia of Chronic Disease

Patients with chronic diseases such as HIV infection, rheumatoid arthritis, inflammatory bowel disease, chronic hepatitis, and chronic kidney disease often have mild to moderate anemia. This type of anemia is common. Its severity often depends on the severity of the underlying disease. Abnormal immune responses with increased RBC destruction and impaired bone marrow function and iron metabolism contribute to the anemia of chronic disease.

Manifestations of this type of anemia are similar to those of iron deficiency anemia. Symptoms often are mild because the anemia develops gradually, and physical activity often is limited by the underlying disease.

Hemolytic Anemias

Hemolytic anemias are characterized by the premature destruction of RBCs. RBCs may be destroyed because the cell itself is improperly formed (*intrinsic*) or because it has been damaged by an outside source (*acquired*). Intrinsic causes include defects in the cell membrane or hemoglobin structure and function and inherited enzyme deficiencies. External causes of hemolytic anemia include drugs, bacterial and other toxins, and trauma.

SICKLE CELL DISORDERS   Sickle cell disorders are genetically transmitted, inherited as an autosomal recessive trait. In disorders with an autosomal recessive inheritance pattern, a person must inherit the abnormal gene from both parents for the disorder to be fully expressed. Box 20-1■ provides more information about sickle cell disorders and their genetic inheritance pattern.

Sickle cell disorders are characterized by the presence of abnormal hemoglobin, hemoglobin S (HbS), in the RBCs. This abnormal hemoglobin affects how RBCs respond to stress. When blood oxygen levels fall, the cells deform and become sickle shaped (Figure 20-3■). These deformed RBCs clump together and obstruct small blood vessels (Figure 20-4■).

BOX 20-1	**POPULATION FOCUS**

Sickle Cell Disease

Inherited sickle cell disorders include sickle cell disease, sickle cell trait, and related disorders. In *sickle cell disease*, abnormal hemoglobin (hemoglobin S) is formed within red blood cells.

Sickle cell disorders usually affect people of African descent. About 8% of African Americans have inherited the HbS gene from a parent. They have *sickle cell trait* and have few symptoms. Each child of a person with sickle cell trait has a 50% risk of inheriting the HbS gene (see figure). If both parents have sickle cell trait, each child has a 25% risk of inheriting the HbS gene from both parents. These children are likely to develop sickle cell disease. Hispanics from the Caribbean and Central and South America and people from the Eastern Mediterranean, Arab regions, and India also may have the HbS gene.

Sickled cells obstruct blood vessels, causing tissue ischemia (see Figure 20-4). Every organ of the body can be damaged, especially the spleen, bone marrow, lung, eye, and head of the femur and humerus. Other acute events may develop in patients with sickle cell disease: sequestration crisis (pooling of blood in the liver or spleen); temporary loss of bone marrow function, leading to aplastic anemia; or hemolytic crisis, a rapid drop in hemoglobin levels (Brown, 2012). Good general health maintenance through nutrition, exercise, and avoiding smoking and excess alcohol intake are important to prevent sickling crises.

Sickle cell disease is chronic, unpredictable, and recurrent, leading to psychosocial stress. Patients with sickle cell disease experience frequent and painful sickling episodes, often leading to hospitalization. The risk of passing the disease to offspring compounds this stress. Genetic counseling is recommended.

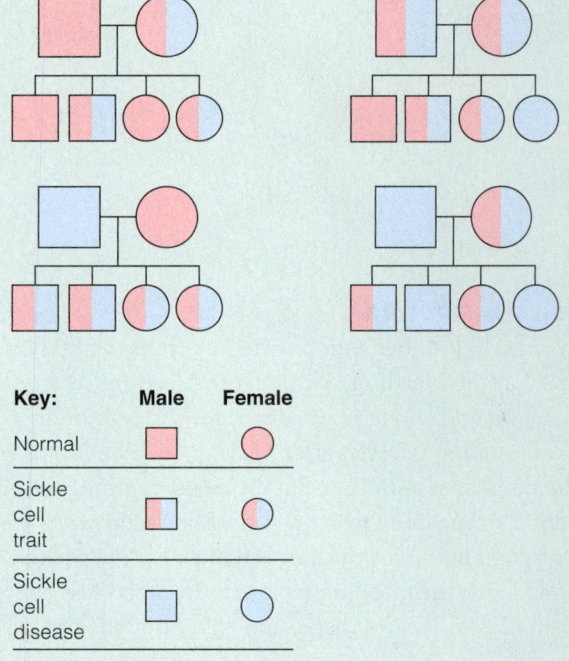

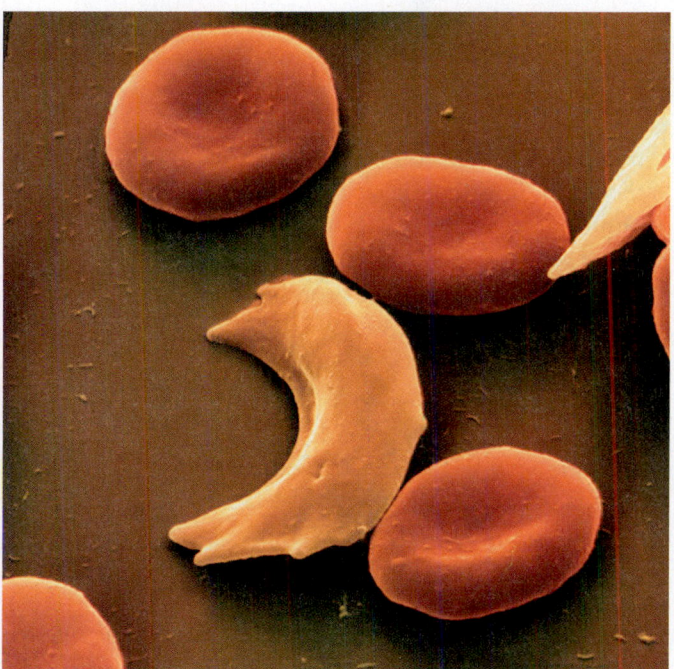

Figure 20-3. ■ A blood smear showing both normal red blood cells and sickle cells. (Source: Eye of Science/Science Source.)

Although the shape returns to normal when normal oxygen levels are restored, repeated episodes of sickling damage RBC membranes. The damaged RBCs break down (hemolysis), leading to anemia. Events likely to trigger a sickling event include hypoxia, low temperatures, excessive exercise, anesthesia, dehydration, infections, or acidosis.

Sickling is usually marked by an abrupt onset of intense pain, often in the abdomen. The acute pain also may occur in the chest, back, or joints. The patient also has manifestations of anemia and may become jaundiced as bilirubin is released when red blood cells are destroyed.

THALASSEMIA   *Thalassemia* is an inherited disorder also caused by abnormal hemoglobin synthesis. It commonly affects people of Mediterranean, Asian, or African descent. Depending on the form of the disorder and whether the person has inherited one or both defective genes, the patient may have few symptoms or severe disease.

Manifestations of thalassemia include liver and spleen enlargement from increased red cell destruction. The RBCs are small and fragile; their distinctive bull's eye appearance has caused them to be called *target cells*. Stress on the bone marrow to produce RBCs can lead to thinning of bones and fractures. People with severe thalassemia may require blood transfusions to sustain life.

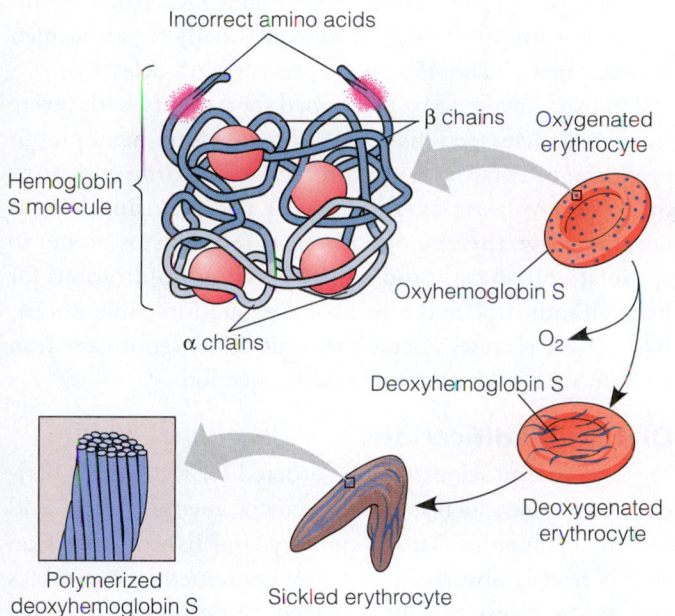

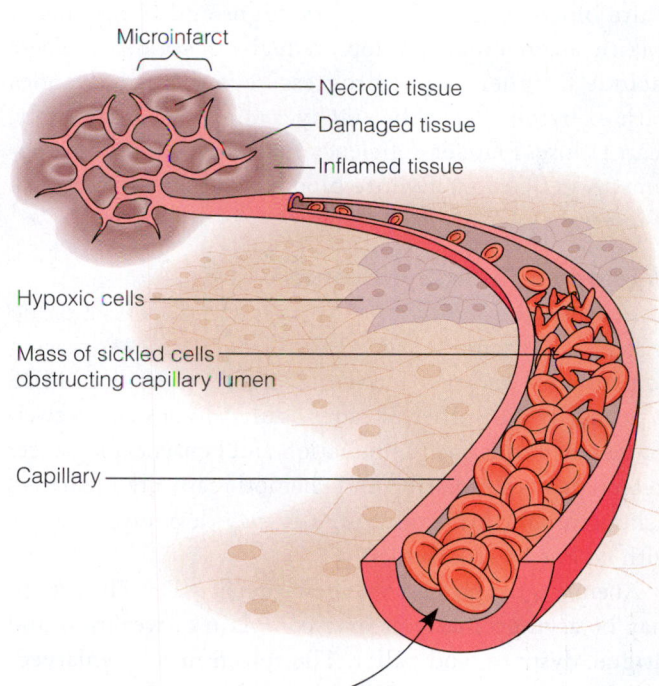

Figure 20-4. ■ Pathophysiology illustrated: sickle cell disease. Sickle cell disease is caused by an inherited defect in hemoglobin (Hb) synthesis. When sickle cell hemoglobin (HbS) is oxygenated, it has the same globular shape as normal hemoglobin. However, when HbS is not bound with oxygen, it becomes insoluble and crystallizes into rodlike structures. Clusters of these rods form long chains that bend the erythrocyte into the characteristic crescent shape of the sickle cell. Sickle cell disease is characterized by episodes of acute painful crises. Sickling crises are triggered by conditions that affect the oxygen supply, increase the oxygen demand, or change the pH. As a sickle cell crisis begins, sickled RBCs cling to capillary walls and each other, obstructing blood flow and causing cellular hypoxia. The crisis accelerates as hypoxia and acidic waste products cause further sickling and cell damage. Sickle cell crises cause small infarctions in joints and organs. Repeated crises slowly destroy organs and tissues. The spleen and kidneys are especially prone to sickling damage.

ACQUIRED HEMOLYTIC ANEMIA *Acquired hemolytic anemia* results when RBCs are damaged by outside factors, such as:

- Mechanical trauma (prosthetic heart valves, severe burns, hemodialysis, or radiation)
- Antibody reactions after infection
- Immune responses (transfusion reactions)
- Drugs, toxins, chemical agents, or venoms

The manifestations of acquired hemolytic anemia depend on the extent of hemolysis. The spleen enlarges as it removes large numbers of damaged or destroyed RBCs. Bilirubin released from the hemoglobin of damaged RBCs can cause jaundice. In severe cases, bones may become deformed or develop pathologic fractures.

Aplastic Anemia

In *aplastic anemia*, the bone marrow fails to produce RBCs. The cause is usually unknown. Aplastic anemia may follow injury to stem cells in bone marrow caused by radiation, certain chemicals, or an immune response. Benzene, arsenic, nitrogen mustard, certain antibiotics (especially chloramphenicol), and chemotherapeutic drugs can cause aplastic anemia. Aplastic anemia also is associated with some viral infections, such as mononucleosis, hepatitis C, and HIV.

People with aplastic anemia usually have *pancytopenia*; that is, they have decreased numbers of red blood cells, white blood cells, and platelets. Signs and symptoms of aplastic anemia may develop gradually or suddenly. These include fatigue, pallor, progressive weakness, dyspnea with exertion, headache, tachycardia, and, ultimately, heart failure. Platelet deficiency may cause bleeding problems. A deficiency of white blood cells increases the risk of infection.

Myelodysplastic Syndrome

Myelodysplastic syndrome (MDS or *myelodysplasia*) is a group of stem cell disorders characterized by abnormal-appearing bone marrow and ineffective blood cell production. MDS is primarily a disorder of older adults. Exposure to environmental toxins such as radiation and benzene and cancer treatment with radiation and chemotherapy are identified risk factors for MDS, although it may develop in people with no known risk factors.

Anemia is the primary manifestation of MDS. The patient may be asymptomatic or may complain of weakness and fatigue, dyspnea, and pallor. The spleen may be enlarged, and some patients with MDS develop skin lesions.

COLLABORATIVE CARE
Diagnostic Tests

When anemia is suspected, the following diagnostic tests may be ordered:

- A *complete blood count (CBC) with RBC indices* to determine the RBC, hemoglobin, and hematocrit levels. The RBC indices provide information about the size, weight, and hemoglobin concentration of RBCs to help determine the type of anemia.
- *Iron levels* and *total iron-binding capacity tests* to identify iron deficiency. If iron deficiency anemia is present, the serum iron concentration will be low, and the total iron-binding capacity will be high.
- *Serum ferritin* to determine deficiency of stored iron. Ferritin is an iron-storage protein produced by the liver, spleen, and bone marrow.
- *Sickle cell screening test* to identify hemoglobin S if sickle cell disease is suspected.
- *Hemoglobin electrophoresis* to identify abnormal forms of hemoglobin when a genetic anemia such as sickle cell anemia or thalassemia is suspected.
- *Bone marrow examination* to diagnose aplastic anemia.

Medications

Drugs used to treat anemia depend on the type of anemia. Iron replacement is prescribed for patients with iron deficiency anemia. Supplemental iron may be given orally or parenterally. Vitamin B_{12} is given orally to patients with nutritional vitamin B_{12} deficiency and by injection to patients with pernicious anemia. Folic acid supplements are ordered for patients with a folic acid deficiency or sickle cell anemia to meet the increased demands of the bone marrow. The Centers for Disease Control and Prevention (CDC, 2012) recommends 0.4 mg (400 mcg) of folic acid daily for all women between ages 15 and 45 years to prevent birth defects.

Hydroxyurea may be prescribed for patients with severe sickle cell disease. This drug promotes fetal hemoglobin production. Fetal hemoglobin reduces sickling and painful crises. Aplastic anemia may be treated using immunosuppressive therapy or androgens (e.g., testosterone) to stimulate blood cell production. Nursing implications for iron, vitamin B_{12}, and folic acid are found in Table 20-2■. Box 20-2■ reviews Z-track technique to administer iron dextran solution by intramuscular injection.

Dietary Modifications

Dietary modifications may be ordered for nutritional deficiency anemias, such as iron deficiency anemia or folic acid deficiency anemia. Meats, poultry, and fish provide iron that is readily absorbed. The iron contained in vegetables and grains is less readily absorbed, but accounts for most of the daily iron intake. Selected dietary sources of iron, vitamin B_{12}, and folic acid are outlined in Box 20-3■.

Blood Transfusion

When anemia is due to a major blood loss, such as from trauma or major surgery, blood transfusions may be given to replace red blood cells. If the bleeding is acute (hemorrhage), whole blood may be given to replace both plasma and blood cells. If the blood loss is chronic, packed

TABLE 20-2	Giving Medications Safely: Anemia		
DRUG/CLASS	**PURPOSE**	**NURSING IMPLICATIONS**	**PATIENT TEACHING**
Iron ■ Ferrous sulfate (Feosol, others) ■ Ferrous gluconate (Fergon, others) ■ Ferrous fumarate (Feostat, others) ■ Carbonyl iron (Feosol-caps, Ferronyl) ■ Iron dextran injection (Imferon) ■ Iron polysaccharide	Iron preparations are used to treat iron deficiency anemia. They are usually taken by mouth and are absorbed from the gastrointestinal tract. Carbonyl iron is a slow-release product.	Assess for drug interactions and GI bleeding. Do not give within 1 hour of bedtime. Give with orange juice to improve absorption. Administer elixirs through a straw to prevent staining of teeth. Avoid infiltration if administering intravenously, as iron is highly irritating to the tissues. Use Z-track technique when administering iron by intramuscular (IM) injection (see Box 20-2). Report manifestations of iron toxicity: nausea, diarrhea, or constipation. Monitor hemoglobin and RBC counts.	Take with food (not milk) to reduce gastric distress. Stools may be dark green or black; this is harmless. Increase fluid and fiber intake to decrease constipation. Carbonyl iron, while more expensive, may be appropriate for use when there are small children in the house. It allows more time for treatment of accidental ingestion. A delayed reaction to iron dextran injection can occur. Report fever, chills, malaise, muscle and joint aches, nausea or vomiting, dizziness, or backache to your primary care provider.
Vitamin B₁₂ ■ Cyanocobalamin (Anacobin, Bedoz, Nascobal, Rubion)	Cyanocobalamin is used to treat vitamin B_{12} deficiencies and pernicious anemia. It is rapidly absorbed and is stored in the liver. Intrinsic factor is required for absorption from the GI tract.	Do not expose injection to light. Do not mix in a syringe with other medications. Administer injections IM or deep subcutaneously to decrease local irritation. Monitor hemoglobin, RBC, reticulocyte counts, and potassium levels.	The burning sensation that may occur with injection is temporary. Avoid alcohol, which interferes with absorption. If used to treat pernicious anemia, the medication must be taken for life.
Folic Acid ■ *Folic acid* (Folvite)	Folic acid is used to treat folic acid deficiency and resulting anemia. Synthetic folic acid is absorbed from the GI tract and stored in the liver.	Do not mix folic acid with other medications in the same syringe. Report hypersensitivity response of skin rash.	Large doses may darken the urine. Excess alcohol intake increases folic acid requirements.

Note: Medications identified in *italics* are among the 200 most frequently prescribed drugs in the United States.

red cells may be given. Patients with severe anemia from other causes (such as sickle cell disease or aplastic anemia) also may require blood transfusions.

clinicalALERT

Members of the Jehovah's Witness faith do not accept blood and blood products. Alternatives to blood transfusion include intravenous solutions to increase blood volume and colony-stimulating factors to increase RBC production. Oxygen-carrying blood substitutes are in the process of being developed.

NURSING CARE

Unless anemia is related to acute blood loss, treatment is usually provided in community-based settings. Nurses in these settings play an important role in identifying patients with anemia, monitoring their status and treatment, and providing appropriate teaching.

PRIORITIZING NURSING CARE

Nursing care priorities for the patient with anemia are determined by the acuity of the situation. When anemia is the result of acute hemorrhage, restoring blood volume

BOX 20-2	PROCEDURE CHECKLIST

Z-Track Technique

Before the Procedure

☑ Verify medication order, including the patient, drug, dose, route, and time.

☑ Gather all supplies. After drawing the correct dosage into the syringe, draw an additional 0.2 mL of air into the syringe and change the needle.

☑ Identify the patient and provide for privacy.

☑ Position appropriately for the site to be used (prone or side-lying).

Procedure

☑ Follow Standard Precautions.

☑ Identify and cleanse the site.

☑ Using the nondominant hand, pull the skin laterally approximately 1–1½ in. (2.5–3 cm).

☑ Holding the skin taut (see figure), administer the medication and withdraw the needle. Release the skin and apply direct pressure to the injection site. Do not massage.

☑ Document the medication administration, site, and patient response.

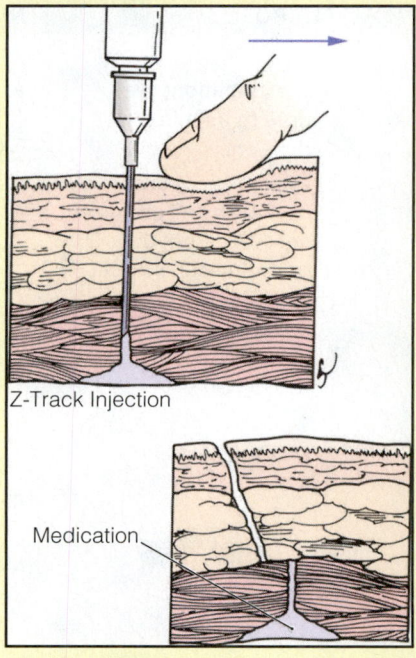

Z-Track Injection

Medication

Note: The skin's return to its normal position forms a seal that prevents medication from seeping into subcutaneous tissue and causing discomfort.

Sample Documentation

[date] 0900   1 mL Imferon given R ventral gluteal site using Z-track technique. Tolerated well.

_____ J. Meyer, LPN

Note: Refer to a nursing fundamentals or skills text for more detailed instruction. Check state guidelines and facility policy before performing any procedure.

BOX 20-3	DIETARY SOURCES OF IRON, FOLIC ACID, AND VITAMIN B$_{12}$

Iron

- Beef, beef liver, pork, ham, chicken, turkey, tuna, shrimp, clams, tofu
- Dried beans, green beans, green peas, spinach, broccoli
- Potatoes, whole grains, brown rice

Folic Acid (Folate)

- Asparagus, okra, spinach and other greens, broccoli
- Green beans and other legumes, dried beans
- Fortified grain products (corn flakes, oatmeal, pasta)

Vitamin B$_{12}$ (Cobalamin)

- Meat, poultry, eggs
- Fish and shellfish
- Milk and cheese

is of highest priority. When anemia develops gradually, its effects on the patient's ability to maintain his or her normal and desired activities are of higher priority.

HEALTH PROMOTION

Teaching good eating habits to people of all ages is the primary nursing intervention to prevent anemia. Provide a list of food sources of iron, folate, and the B vitamins. Discuss alternate sources of iron with patients who are vegetarian, and teach them to include foods high in vitamin C in their diet to improve the absorption of iron from grains, legumes, and other sources. Emphasize the importance of adequate iron and folic acid intake in women of childbearing age and older adults. Monitor eating habits of older adults in long-term care and community-based care settings. Suggest a vitamin supplement when necessary, particularly for women of childbearing age.

Provide information about genetic counseling for patients concerned about passing a genetically linked anemia to their offspring.

ASSESSING

Assessment data can reveal manifestations of anemia as well as provide clues about potential causes of anemia. Collect focused assessment data, including both subjective and objective information.

Health History

Complaints of fatigue, headache, difficulty concentrating, shortness of breath, palpitations, or dizziness; chest pain, muscle cramps, or aching bone pain; sore mouth or tongue, or cracking at corners of lips; reports of obvious bleeding (excessive menstrual flow, rectal bleeding, or vomiting blood) or black or tarry stools. In patients with known or suspected genetically linked anemia, ask about family history, previous episodes, and current complaints of chest, abdominal, joint, or extremity pain.

Physical Examination

Obtain vital signs, including orthostatic blood pressures if bleeding is suspected; inspect skin, mucous membranes, nail beds, and conjunctiva for color, condition, presence of petechiae or ulcers; mouth and lips for *glossitis* (inflammation of the tongue), a beefy red tongue, and *cheilosis* (cracking at the corners); incisions and dressings for acute bleeding; observe for dyspnea or shortness of breath at rest or with activity; auscultate heart, breath, and bowel sounds; if bleeding is suspected, check stool and vomitus for occult blood; evaluate laboratory reports for RBC, hemoglobin, and hematocrit levels.

IDENTIFYING POTENTIAL COMPLICATIONS

Patients with severe anemia are at risk for heart failure due to an increased workload of the heart as it attempts to maintain tissue oxygenation. Report manifestations such as increasing shortness of breath, dyspnea when lying down, increasing fatigue, dizziness or a decline in mental status; tachycardia, tachypnea; respiratory crackles; distended neck veins; or peripheral edema.

Repeated episodes of sickling can lead to tissue damage and organ failure due to ischemia. Monitor level of consciousness (LOC) and mental status; peripheral tissue perfusion (pulses, capillary refill); skin color; and indicators of organ function, such as liver and kidney function tests.

DIAGNOSING, PLANNING, AND IMPLEMENTING

Activity Intolerance

Expected outcome: Will demonstrate a gradual increase in duration and intensity of activity that can be performed without shortness of breath, fatigue, or chest pain.

Inadequate oxygen delivery to the tissues can lead to weakness, fatigue, and shortness of breath with activity.

- Monitor vital signs, especially heart and respiratory rates, before and after activity. *Vital signs are an objective measure of activity tolerance. Heart and respiratory rates should remain within normal limits during and after normal activities.*
- Discontinue activity and allow rest for complaints of chest pain, shortness of breath, palpitations, or dizziness; tachycardia that does not return to normal within 4 minutes of resting; or rapid or labored respirations. *These signs and symptoms indicate intolerance of the activity.*
- Help identify ways to conserve energy during activities of daily living (ADLs), for example, sitting to shower, and spacing activities throughout the day. *Reducing energy use allows greater independence while avoiding excess fatigue or shortness of breath.*
- Help prioritize activities and distribute tasks among family members. *This allows the patient to conserve energy while relieving concerns that necessary tasks are being performed.*
- Help plan a schedule of balanced rest and activity during the day and 8 to 10 hours of sleep at night. *Rest decreases oxygen demand and reduces fatigue.*
- Instruct not to smoke. *Smoking is a vasoconstrictor that further increases the workload of the heart and impairs tissue oxygenation.*

Impaired Oral Mucous Membrane

Expected outcome: Oral mucous membranes will remain intact without lesions.

- Assess condition of lips and tongue daily. *Glossitis and cheilosis increase the risk for bleeding and infection. These conditions also may cause pain and discomfort with eating, interfering with oral intake.*
- Use a mouthwash of saline, saltwater, or half-strength peroxide and water to rinse mouth every 2 to 4 hours. *This cleans and soothes oral mucous membranes.*
- Provide frequent oral hygiene (after meals and at bedtime) with a soft-bristle toothbrush or sponge. *Removing food debris promotes comfort and reduces the risk of infection. A soft toothbrush is less likely to cause irritation or bleeding of the oral mucosa.*
- Instruct to avoid alcohol-based mouthwashes. *Alcohol is drying and will aggravate cracking of the mucous membranes.*
- Apply a petroleum-based lubricating jelly or ointment to lips after oral care. *A lubricating ointment helps to retain moisture, facilitate healing, and protect the lips from other drying agents.*

■ Encourage soft, cool, bland foods and to avoid hot, spicy, or acidic foods. *Foods that are soothing to the mucous membranes promote comfort and help maintain adequate intake.*

Readiness for Enhanced Self-Care

Expected outcome: Will complete ADLs with minimal fatigue and no shortness of breath.

■ Instruct to rest between activities such as bathing and dressing. *Rest reduces oxygen demand and cardiac workload, promoting independence and self-esteem.*

■ Encourage four to six small, high-protein, nutritionally balanced meals daily. *Small, frequent meals reduce fatigue. High-protein, well-balanced meals promote healing.*

■ Listen to and acknowledge concerns about inability to maintain self-care. *Dependence on others for ADLs may signify a loss of control and lead to a loss of self-esteem.*

EVALUATING

To evaluate the effectiveness of nursing care, assess the patient's ability to independently perform ADLs and gradually increase level of activity. Assess the skin and oral mucous membrane condition. Evaluate the patient's knowledge and understanding of dietary changes and recommended treatment.

DOCUMENTING

Document continuing assessment data, as well as teaching provided. Note the patient's apparent understanding of information and willingness to comply with the treatment plan.

CONTINUITY OF CARE

Patients with anemia are primarily managed in the home and community. Assess the patient's ability to independently perform ADLs; to prepare and consume the recommended diet, including financial resources for purchasing recommended foods; and to fill prescriptions and manage ordered medications.

Teach about the type of anemia, its causes, effects, and treatment. Provide a list of foods that should be included in the diet. Refer to a dietitian or nutritionist for further teaching as indicated. Discuss ordered medications, including dose, how and when to take the drug, and anticipated side effects and their management. Stress the importance of keeping scheduled follow-up appointments with the health care provider.

With patients who have sickle cell disease, discuss measures to prevent and treat sickling crises. Provide information about when to contact the primary care provider or seek treatment in the emergency department. Provide contacts for local support groups and national organizations, including the American Sickle Cell Anemia Association and the Sickle Cell Information Center.

Polycythemia

Polycythemia (also called *erythrocytosis*) is an abnormally high red blood cell count with high hematocrit. When the hematocrit is greater than 50%, the blood becomes more viscous or "sticky."

PATHOPHYSIOLOGY AND MANIFESTATIONS

Secondary polycythemia is the most common form of the disorder. It usually develops as a result of chronic hypoxemia or due to excess production of erythropoietin. Decreased tissue oxygenation stimulates erythropoietin production, which in turn stimulates the bone marrow to produce more RBCs. People who live at high altitudes, where low atmospheric oxygen pressures reduce the amount of oxygen available to the tissues, have a gradual increase in RBCs to adapt to the reduced oxygen. People who have chronic lung disease or who are heavy smokers also often develop polycythemia. Excess erythropoietin production may be due to kidney disease or malignancy.

Primary polycythemia, or *polycythemia vera*, is a neoplastic stem cell disorder in which the production of all blood cells (red, white, and platelets) is increased. Its cause is unknown. Polycythemia vera is relatively rare and usually affects people over the age of 50. In polycythemia vera, the RBC count increases. The number of WBCs and platelets also increases, although to a lesser degree than for RBCs. The hematocrit and blood volume increase as well. The liver and spleen become congested with RBCs. The patient is at risk for thrombosis and infarction.

The onset of polycythemia vera is insidious. Its symptoms are related to excess blood volume, increased blood viscosity, and changes in cerebral blood flow. The patient may complain of headaches, dizziness, tinnitus, and blurred vision. Hypertension often develops. Ruddy or dusky cyanosis of the face is common, as is pruritus. The patient may develop heart failure, thrombophlebitis, and thrombosis in distal arteries. Gangrene of fingers or toes is a potential complication.

COLLABORATIVE CARE

The *RBC count* and *hematocrit* are elevated in polycythemia. In polycythemia vera, *WBC* and *platelet counts* also are increased. *Erythropoietin levels* are high in secondary polycythemia, but low in polycythemia vera.

Treatment of polycythemia focuses on reducing blood viscosity and volume and relieving symptoms. Phlebotomy, removal of 300 to 500 mL of blood through a vein, can be done repeatedly to keep blood volume and viscosity within normal levels. In some cases, chemotherapy drugs may be used to suppress the bone marrow in patients with polycythemia vera.

NURSING CARE

Nursing care focuses on teaching the importance of maintaining adequate hydration and preventing blood stasis: elevating the legs when sitting, using support stockings, and complying with treatment measures. To smokers, emphasize the importance of smoking cessation. Instruct to immediately report symptoms of thrombosis such as pallor or pain in an extremity, chest or abdominal pain, and any abnormal bleeding.

WHITE BLOOD CELL DISORDERS

Key Concept The primary function of WBCs is to fight off infection, destroy foreign matter, and eliminate damaged or abnormal cells in the body; WBC disorders affect immune function.

Leukemia

Leukemia (literally, "white blood") is a group of malignant disorders of WBCs. In leukemia, the usual ratio of greater numbers of red blood cells than white blood cells is reversed. Bone marrow is gradually replaced by immature, abnormal cells. Eventually, these abnormal cells spill into the circulation and invade other organs such as the liver, spleen, and lymph nodes. If the disease is not treated, leukemic cells replace all normal blood cells, leading to death.

Although leukemia is often considered a childhood disease, it is diagnosed in 10 times more adults than children each year. It is more common in people over age 50. Leukemia is among the 10 most common types of cancer cases and causes of cancer deaths, accounting for an estimated 48,610 new cases and 23,720 deaths in the United States in 2013 (American Cancer Society [ACS], 2013).

The cause of most leukemias is unknown. Identified risk factors include exposure to chemicals such as benzene, genetic factors, viruses, immune disorders, cigarette smoking, and exposure to large doses of radiation. Its incidence is higher in people who have been treated with radiation or chemotherapy, people living near sites of radiation testing, survivors of atomic bombing sites, radiologists, and people with Down syndrome or other genetic abnormalities.

PATHOPHYSIOLOGY

Leukemia begins with the malignant transformation of a single stem cell. Leukemic cells proliferate slowly, but have an extended life span and are unable to function as normal WBCs. They cannot combat infection or maintain immune function. The bone marrow becomes almost totallly filled with leukemic cells. Because cells that produce RBCs and platelets are crowded out, severe anemia and bleeding result.

Leukemic cells leave the bone marrow and infiltrate other tissues such as the central nervous system, testes, skin, GI tract, the lymph nodes, liver, and spleen. Death usually results from internal hemorrhage and infections.

CLASSIFICATIONS

Leukemias are classified by their onset and duration (acute or chronic) and by the type of abnormal cells (myelogenous or lymphocytic). *Acute leukemia* has an abrupt onset and progresses rapidly. Leukemic cells are immature or undifferentiated. These immature cells are often referred to as *blasts*. The onset and progression of *chronic leukemia* is more gradual. Leukemic cells are abnormal and appear mature. *Myeloid* (also called *myelogenous, myelocytic,* or *myeloblastic*) *leukemias* involve myeloid stem cells in the bone marrow. These are the cells that normally become granulocytes. Myeloid leukemias interfere with the maturation of all blood cells, including RBCs and platelets. *Lymphocytic* or *lymphoblastic leukemias* involve immature lymphocytes in the bone marrow, spleen, lymph nodes, CNS, and other tissues. Acute myeloid and chronic lymphocytic leukemias are the most common types affecting adults; acute lymphoblastic leukemia is the most common childhood type of leukemia. Table 20-3 ■ compares the four major types of leukemia. Some systems also classify leukemia by subtype of the predominant cell.

MANIFESTATIONS

The manifestations of leukemia result from anemia, infection, and bleeding. Anemia causes pallor, fatigue, tachycardia, malaise, lethargy, and dyspnea. Infection, due to impaired WBC function, causes fever; night sweats; ulcers of the mouth and pharynx; and respiratory, urinary

TABLE 20-3	Major Classifications of Leukemia		
CLASSIFICATION	CHARACTERISTICS	MANIFESTATIONS	TREATMENT
Acute myeloid leukemia (AML)	Common in older adults; may affect children and young adults; strongly associated with toxins, genetic disorders, and treatment of other cancers Relative 5-year survival of 25%	Fatigue, weakness; fever; anemia; headache; and bone and joint pain; abnormal bleeding and bruising; recurrent infection; lymph node, liver, and spleen enlargement	Chemotherapy; stem cell transplant (SCT)
Chronic myeloid leukemia (CML)	Primarily affects adults; early course is slow and stable, progressing to aggressive phase in 3–4 years Relative 5-year survival of 56%	Early: weakness, fatigue, dyspnea on exertion; possible spleen enlargement Later: fever, weight loss, night sweats	Interferon-alpha; chemotherapy, SCT
Acute lymphocytic leukemia (ALL)	Primarily affects children and young adults; leukemic cells may infiltrate CNS; 5-year relative survival rate 91% in children, 68% overall	Recurrent infections; bleeding; pallor, bone pain, weight loss, sore throat, fatigue, night sweats, weakness	Chemotherapy; SCT or bone marrow transplant (BMT)
Chronic lymphocytic leukemia (CLL)	Primarily affects older adults; insidious onset and slow, chronic course 5-year relative survival rate 82%	Fatigue; exercise intolerance; enlarged lymph nodes and spleen; recurrent infections, pallor, edema, thrombophlebitis	Often requires no treatment; chemotherapy; BMT

tract, and skin infections. Septicemia may develop. *Thrombocytopenia* (low platelet count) increases the risk of bleeding, leading to bruising, petechiae, and hematomas, as well as overt and hidden bleeding into organs. As leukemic cells infiltrate other organs, pain and other symptoms may occur. The manifestations of leukemia are summarized in Figure 20-5 ■.

COLLABORATIVE CARE

Treatment for leukemia focuses on achieving remission or cure and relieving symptoms. Cure is more likely in children than adults. The prognosis for each type of leukemia differs (see Table 20-3).

Diagnostic Tests

Laboratory tests that may be ordered include:

- *CBC with WBC differential* and *platelet count*. The RBC, hemoglobin, and hematocrit levels typically are low. The platelet count also may be low. The WBC count tends to be high, with abnormal cells.
- The *bone marrow* is examined to look for abnormal cells.

Chemotherapy

Systemic chemotherapy is used to destroy leukemic cells and produce remission. Chemotherapy interferes with the proliferation of cells in the bone marrow. A combination of chemotherapy drugs is usually used to treat leukemia. Combining drugs reduces drug resistance, reduces toxicity

from high doses of single agents, and interrupts cell growth at various stages of the cell cycle.

Therapy generally is divided into two phases, induction and postremission therapy. During *induction*, high drug doses are used to eradicate leukemic cells in the bone marrow. Because these doses also damage stem cells and interfere with the production of other blood cells, the patient is at greater risk for complications during this period. Colony-stimulating factors (discussed later) often are given to "rescue" the bone marrow after induction chemotherapy. Postremission chemotherapy is continued to eradicate any additional leukemic cells after remission is attained.

Radiation Therapy

Radiation therapy may be used to shrink enlarged lymph nodes and destroy leukemic cells in the central nervous system (CNS). Radiation damages the cell DNA so that it is unable to reproduce and multiply. Although normal cells are affected, they are better able to recover from the damage caused by the radiation than are cancer cells.

Biologic Therapy

Biologic agents such as interferons, interleukins, and monoclonal antibodies may be used to treat some leukemias. These agents have multiple effects, including moderating immune function and slowing abnormal cell proliferation and growth. Side effects of interferon therapy include flulike symptoms, persistent fatigue and lethargy, weight loss, and muscle and joint pain.

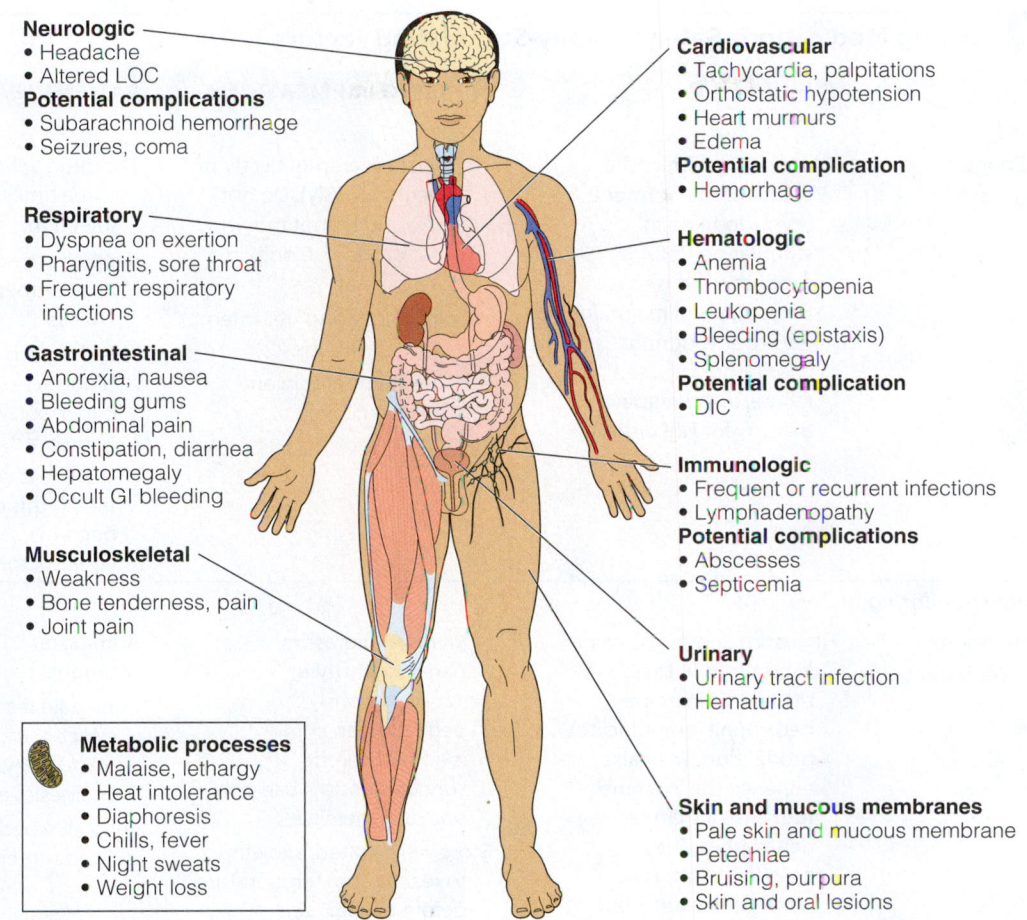

Neurologic
- Headache
- Altered LOC

Potential complications
- Subarachnoid hemorrhage
- Seizures, coma

Respiratory
- Dyspnea on exertion
- Pharyngitis, sore throat
- Frequent respiratory infections

Gastrointestinal
- Anorexia, nausea
- Bleeding gums
- Abdominal pain
- Constipation, diarrhea
- Hepatomegaly
- Occult GI bleeding

Musculoskeletal
- Weakness
- Bone tenderness, pain
- Joint pain

Metabolic processes
- Malaise, lethargy
- Heat intolerance
- Diaphoresis
- Chills, fever
- Night sweats
- Weight loss

Cardiovascular
- Tachycardia, palpitations
- Orthostatic hypotension
- Heart murmurs
- Edema

Potential complication
- Hemorrhage

Hematologic
- Anemia
- Thrombocytopenia
- Leukopenia
- Bleeding (epistaxis)
- Splenomegaly

Potential complication
- DIC

Immunologic
- Frequent or recurrent infections
- Lymphadenopathy

Potential complications
- Abscesses
- Septicemia

Urinary
- Urinary tract infection
- Hematuria

Skin and mucous membranes
- Pale skin and mucous membrane
- Petechiae
- Bruising, purpura
- Skin and oral lesions

Figure 20-5. ■ The multisystem effects of leukemia.

Colony-stimulating factors (CSFs) regulate the growth and differentiation of blood cells. They often are given to patients whose bone marrow function is suppressed due to chemotherapy or leukemic changes. They also are given to stimulate stem cell development before harvesting bone marrow for autologous transplant. Bone pain is a common side effect of these agents. Patients also may experience fevers, chills, anorexia, muscle aches, and lethargy. See Table 20-4■ for the nursing implications for CSFs.

Stem Cell Transplant

Stem cell transplant (SCT) may be used along with chemotherapy or radiation to treat some types of leukemia. Blood (or *hematopoietic*) stem cells are immature cells that mature to become red blood cells, white blood cells, and platelets. Although a few stem cells circulate in peripheral blood, they are concentrated in bone marrow, leading to the frequently used term **bone marrow transplant (BMT)**. Bone marrow containing large concentrations of stem cells typically is aspirated from the anterior and posterior iliac crests, filtered, and infused using a large-bore central venous catheter. When peripheral stem cells are used, the donor is treated with CSFs for several days to increase the concentration of stem cells in circulating blood. During

blood stem cell transplant, the patient is hospitalized in a private room for at least 6 to 8 weeks. The risk of death due to immunosuppression is a major stressor. Complications that may occur are malnutrition, infection, and bleeding.

There are two major categories of SCT. In *allogeneic SCT*, the bone marrow of a healthy donor is infused into the patient with the illness; in *autologous SCT*, the patient is infused with his or her own bone marrow.

ALLOGENEIC SCT   Before an allogeneic SCT, high doses of chemotherapy and/or total body irradiation are given to eliminate leukemic cells. Then new marrow or stem cells from a donor (often a sibling with a closely matched tissue type) are infused (Figure 20-6■). Before SCT and recovery of bone marrow function, the patient is critically ill and at significant risk for infection and bleeding due to inadequate WBCs and platelets.

AUTOLOGOUS SCT   In an autologous stem cell transplant, the patient's own bone marrow is withdrawn, treated to kill any tumor cells, and then frozen for storage (Figure 20-7■). Massive doses of chemotherapy and/or radiation are then given to destroy tumor cells in the patient's body. These high doses destroy any remaining

TABLE 20-4	Giving Medications Safely: Colony-Stimulating Factors		
DRUG/CLASS	**PURPOSE**	**NURSING IMPLICATIONS**	**PATIENT TEACHING**
Erythropoietin ■ Epoetin alfa (Epogen, Procrit)	Epoetin alfa mimics the action of the hormone erythropoietin in stimulating RBC production. It is used to restore and maintain RBC counts during chemotherapy, renal failure, or zidovudine therapy for HIV disease.	Administer parenterally (IV or subcutaneously). Do not shake and do not mix with other drugs. Use only one dose per vial. Monitor BP during treatment; report elevations. Monitor hemoglobin and hematocrit levels.	This drug will be given three times per week by injection. Keep all scheduled appointments and BP checks. This drug can increase your blood pressure; take anti-hypertensive medications as ordered. Headache is common while taking this drug. If it becomes severe, contact your doctor.
Granulocyte colony-stimulating factors ■ Filgrastim (Neupogen) ■ Pegfilgrastim (Neulasta)	Filgrastim and pegfilgrastim act on cells in the bone marrow to increase neutrophil (granulocyte) production. They also enhance the immune function of mature neutrophils. They are used to improve neutrophil counts during chemotherapy, after BMT, and in chronic neutrophilia.	Administer filgrastim parenterally (IV or subcutaneously); pegfilgrastim is administered subcutaneously. Use only one dose per vial. Store refrigerated, allowing it to reach room temperature before giving. Report elevated WBC and neutrophil counts. Monitor temperature every 4 hours.	Administer by injection as taught. Bone pain is a common side effect of these drugs; your doctor may prescribe analgesics as needed. Keep all scheduled appointments.
Granulocyte–macrophage colony-stimulating factor ■ Sargramostim (Leukine)	Sargramostim stimulates bone marrow production of granulocytes and monocytes/macrophages. It also increases the function of mature WBCs. It is given after BMT to stimulate WBC production.	Slow IV infusion to half rate if dyspnea develops. Notify the physician if dyspnea worsens.	Immediately contact the nurse if you develop difficulty breathing or palpitations during the infusion. Keep all scheduled appointments.
Thrombopoietic growth factor ■ Oprelvekin (Neumega)	Oprelvekin (interleukin-11) increases platelet production. It may be given during chemotherapy to treat resulting thrombocytopenia.	Administer by subcutaneous injection. Use reconstituted solution within 3 hours. Causes sodium and water retention; immediately report manifestations of fluid overload. Report hypokalemia and cardiac dysrhythmias.	Keep all scheduled appointments. Administer by injection as taught. Report any of the following to your doctor: shortness of breath, swelling of arms or legs, chest pain, fatigue or weakness, irregular heartbeat, blurred vision.

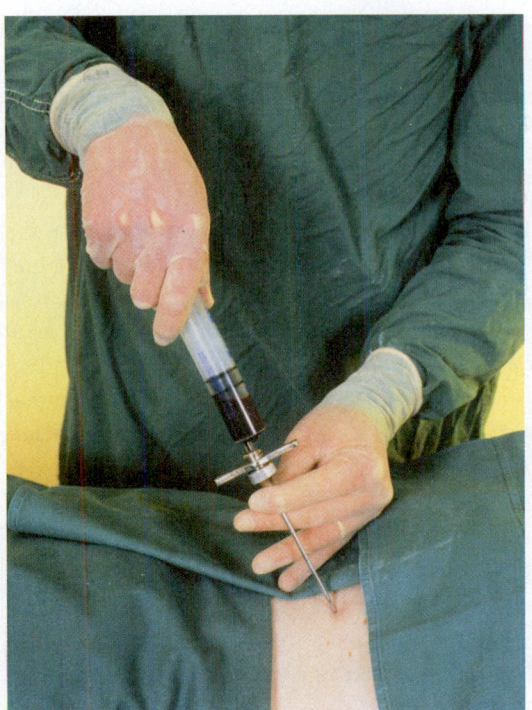

Figure 20-6. ■ Allogeneic stem cell transplant. Bone marrow is removed from the iliac crest of a healthy donor and then infused into the recipient. (Source: Simon Fraser/Science Source.)

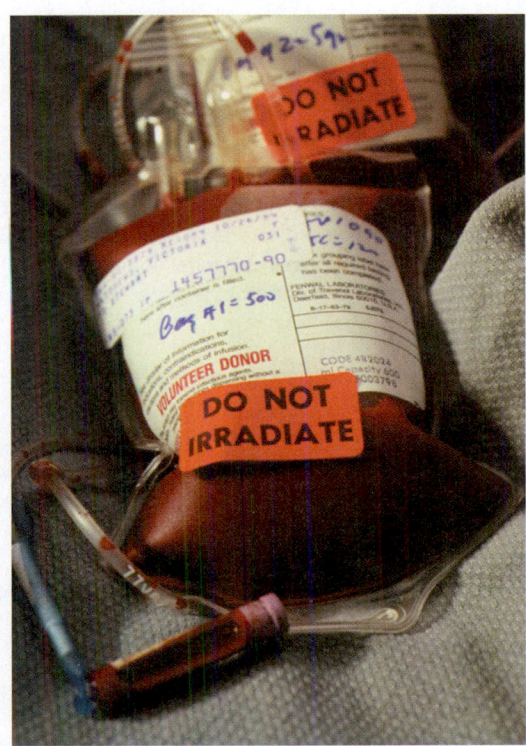

Figure 20-7. ■ Autologous stem cell transplant. Stem cells are collected from the patient's bone marrow or blood, processed, frozen, and later thawed and infused. (Source: Peter Menzel/Science Source.)

bone marrow and the patient's immune system. The stored bone marrow then is thawed and infused. The infused bone marrow gradually restores bone marrow and immune function.

Graft-Versus-Host Disease

After allogeneic SCT, the patient is at risk for *graft-versus-host disease (GvHD)*. In GvHD, immune cells in the donated bone marrow identify the recipient's body tissue as foreign. Consequently, T lymphocytes in the donated marrow attack the liver, skin, and gastrointestinal tract, causing skin rashes and sloughing, diarrhea, gastrointestinal bleeding, and liver damage. Acute GvHD develops within days or weeks of the transplant and is marked by a rash on the palms of the hands and soles of the feet that may extend over the entire body. Chronic GvHD develops 3 or more months after the transplant. GvHD is treated with antibiotics, steroids, and, if necessary, other drugs to suppress the immune response.

NURSING CARE

PRIORITIZING NURSING CARE

Leukemia can be both a chronic and a life-threatening disease. It directly affects a key part of the body's defenses, the immune system. Treatment may require toxic chemotherapy drugs, radiation, or blood stem cell transplant. All of

these therapies have undesirable side effects. Nursing care focuses on the physical and psychosocial effects of the disease and its treatment.

HEALTH PROMOTION

Teaching about the risk factors for leukemia, particularly those risk factors that can be controlled, is the primary health promotion activity. Discuss avoiding exposure to radiation and chemicals such as benzene. For patients living with chronic leukemia, discuss measures to avoid exposure to infection and maintain optimum health, such as consuming a nutritionally balanced diet, engaging in regular exercise, and avoiding crowds and persons with known contagious diseases.

ASSESSING

In all settings, it is important to recognize the manifestations of leukemia. This is particularly important when working with groups at higher risk (e.g., older adults and children). Assessment data related to manifestations of the disease or the current status of the patient with leukemia are outlined in Box 20-4 ■.

IDENTIFYING POTENTIAL COMPLICATIONS

Manifestations of infection (fever, malaise, fatigue, altered mental status), bleeding (abdominal pain, change in LOC, increased bruising, bleeding gums, occult blood

Patients With Leukemia

Subjective Data
- Complaints of general malaise, fatigue, fever, night sweats; sore mouth or throat, bleeding gums; palpitations, shortness of breath with exercise; anorexia, nausea, constipation, or diarrhea; abdominal pain, headache, bone or joint pain; weight loss; changes in mentation.

Objective Data
- Vital signs, including temperature and orthostatic blood pressures.
- Mental status.
- Inspect skin, mucous membranes, nail beds, and conjunctiva for color, condition, petechiae or lesions, excessive or obvious bruising; check mouth for inflammation, lesions, or bleeding gums.
- Respiratory: rate; apparent dyspnea or shortness of breath; lung sounds.
- Cardiac: auscultate for dysrhythmias, abnormal heart sounds.
- Abdomen: bowel sounds; palpate for tenderness (particularly right upper quadrant); check stool and vomitus for occult blood.
- Laboratory reports for CBC (including RBC, WBC and differential, platelets), hemoglobin, and hematocrit levels.

in vomitus, feces, or urine), or nonspecific manifestations such as increased bone pain, tenderness, and pain in the upper abdomen may herald a complication of leukemia or progression of a chronic form of the disease. Report a change in the patient's symptoms to the physician.

DIAGNOSING, PLANNING, AND IMPLEMENTING
Risk for Infection

Expected outcome: Will remain free of infection as demonstrated by absence of fever, malaise, and evidence of inflammation.

- Institute infection precautions, including the following:
  - If prescribed, maintain protective isolation.
  - Use good hand hygiene and remind all care providers and visitors to do the same.
  - Assist to maintain good daily hygiene.
  - Restrict visitors with colds, flu, or infections.
  - As much as possible, avoid invasive procedures such as injections, intravenous catheters, catheterizations, and rectal and vaginal procedures. When necessary to perform these procedures, use strict aseptic technique.

These precautions minimize the patient's exposure to bacterial, viral, and fungal pathogens.

- Promptly report evidence of infection: fever, chills, sore throat, cough, chest pain, burning on urination, purulent drainage, and itching and burning in vaginal or rectal areas. *Early detection of infection allows prompt treatment and is vital when the immune system is suppressed.*
- Monitor vital signs, breath sounds, and oxygen saturation at least every 4 hours, promptly reporting changes. *The patient with leukemia may not show typical manifestations of infection such as fever. It is important to be alert for other manifestations of infection or sepsis.*
- Report decreasing WBC levels to the charge nurse or physician. *The risk for infection increases as the WBC count declines.*
- Explain the precautions and restrictions to the patient and family. Advise that strict precautions are usually temporary. *Understanding increases compliance and thereby lowers the risk of infection.*

Imbalanced Nutrition: Less Than Body Requirements

Expected outcome: Will consume 100% of recommended daily calorie and food intake.

- Regularly monitor weight. *Continued weight loss or a weight below the normal range for height and age may indicate malnutrition. Maintaining adequate nutrition is vital during cancer treatment.*
- Implement measures to promote food and fluid intake, such as:
  - Provide oral hygiene before and after meals.
  - Experiment with food and liquids that have different textures and tastes to identify those best tolerated.
  - Increase liquid intake with meals.
  - Encourage to sit upright when eating.
  - Ensure a clean and odor-free environment.
  - Provide medications for pain or nausea 30 minutes before meals, as needed.
  - Provide rest periods before meals.
  - Offer small, frequent meals six times a day.
  - Use commercial supplements, such as Ensure.
  - Avoid painful or unpleasant procedures immediately before or after meals.

Measures to reduce mouth inflammation, sore throat, nausea, and other effects of the disease and its treatment help promote food and fluid intake. Small, frequent meals are often better tolerated, especially high-protein, high-kilocalorie foods.

Impaired Oral Mucous Membrane

Expected outcome: Oral mucous membranes will remain intact and free of lesions.

- Frequently assess mouth for swelling, lesions, or bleeding. Report complaints of mouth pain or difficulty swallowing to the charge nurse or physician. Culture oral lesions as ordered. *The patient with leukemia is at risk for bacterial, viral (especially herpes simplex), and fungal (especially* Candida*) infections of the oral mucosa.*

- Provide a 1:1 solution of hydrogen peroxide and water or warm saline as a mouth rinse for use every 2 to 4 hours. Apply petroleum jelly to the lips as needed to prevent dryness and cracking. *These measures promote healing and comfort and help prevent infection.*

- Encourage use of a soft-bristle toothbrush or sponge to clean the teeth and gums. *Soft-bristle brushes reduce trauma to the gums and mucous membranes of the mouth.*

- Administer drugs as ordered to treat infections or relieve pain. *Topical antifungal agents such as nystatin may be ordered for* Candida *infections. Topical anesthetics such as lidocaine may be prescribed to promote comfort.*

- Instruct to avoid alcohol-based mouthwashes, citrus fruit juices, spicy foods, foods that are either very hot or very cold, alcohol, and crusty foods. Encourage bland, cool foods and cool liquids. *Avoiding food and liquids that irritate the mucosa increases comfort and oral intake.*

Risk for Bleeding

Expected outcome: Will remain free of signs of hemorrhage or excessive bleeding.

Bleeding due to decreased platelets is a common cause of death in leukemia.

- Monitor LOC and vital signs every 4 hours and report changes such as hypotension or tachycardia to the charge nurse or physician. *A change in LOC or tachycardia can be early signs of bleeding; hypotension is a later sign.*

- Promptly report manifestations of bleeding:

  - Increased petechiae, bruising, or hematoma formation
  - Obvious bleeding from gums, nose; prolonged bleeding from puncture sites
  - Bright red or coffee-grounds emesis; rectal bleeding or tarry stools
  - Hematuria (blood in the urine)
  - Vaginal bleeding
  - Changes in neurologic status: headache, visual changes, altered mental status, decreasing LOC, seizures
  - Complaints of epigastric pain, absent bowel sounds, increasing abdominal girth, abdominal rigidity

Prompt reporting allows early treatment of bleeding or hemorrhage. Bleeding into the abdomen or intracranial bleeding may not be readily apparent and identified only by changes in neurologic status or abdominal assessment data.

- Apply pressure to puncture sites for 3 to 5 minutes; apply pressure to arterial blood gas draw sites for 15 to 20 minutes. *Pressure prevents prolonged bleeding by prompting hemostasis and clot formation.*

- Instruct to avoid straining to have a bowel movement and forceful coughing, sneezing, or blowing of the nose. *Avoiding these activities reduces the risk of external or internal bleeding.*

Grieving

Expected outcome: Will express thoughts and feelings about potential loss.

Grieving is an emotional response to the losses associated with a life-threatening illness such as leukemia.

- Use therapeutic communication skills to allow open discussion of losses as well as permission to grieve. *Encouraging discussion about the meaning of the loss helps to decrease some of the anxiety associated with loss.*

- Accept the patient's and family's responses to the diagnosis without making judgments. *People respond to stress and grieving in many different ways. Denial, anger, bargaining, and depression are common. Demonstrating acceptance of responses and behaviors promotes trust.*

- Assist to identify ways of managing past stressful situations. In addition, help identify effective coping strategies; sources of strength; reactions to changing family roles; and spiritual or cultural influences on grief reactions. *Grieving is a normal response to a real or potential loss that begins at the time of diagnosis. Identifying resources and strategies that have been successfully used in the past helps the patient and family members use these resources during the early crisis of dealing with the diagnosis.*

- Identify agencies, groups, and organizations that may help with the grieving process, and make referrals as indicated. Consider self-help groups, cancer support groups, single-parent groups, and bereavement groups. *A support group that includes others who are anticipating or have experienced a similar loss can decrease the patient's feelings of isolation.*

MANAGING NURSING CARE

Nursing care activities such as obtaining vital signs, assisting as needed with frequent mouth care and hygiene, and promoting food and fluid intake for the patient with leukemia are appropriate to assign to assistive personnel.

EVALUATING

When evaluating the effectiveness of nursing care for the patient with leukemia, look at data that demonstrate freedom from infection (e.g., no fever, vital signs within normal limits). Evaluate weight, food intake, and the integrity of oral mucous membranes. Assess for evidence of bleeding. Finally, look at data that demonstrate coping with the diagnosis, such as talking about the disease and its potential effect on lifestyle and family relationships.

DOCUMENTING

Throughout the patient's care, document continuing assessment data, indicators of complications, and responses to treatment. Document teaching provided to the patient and the family, as well as their apparent understanding and acceptance of information. Note psychologic responses of the patient and family and indicators of their ability or inability to cope with the diagnosis and treatment plan.

CONTINUITY OF CARE

Because leukemia is a chronic disease requiring long-term management, most required care is provided by the patient and family members in the community. Teaching is vital to prepare for discharge.

Reinforce teaching about leukemia and its effects, the function of bone marrow, and potential complications. Discuss cancer as a chronic illness that often can be cured or controlled. Provide information about planned treatment, including chemotherapy, radiation, and/or bone marrow transplant. Discuss the rationale for each type of treatment and techniques to manage the undesirable side effects of the treatment.

Encourage a balance of activity with rest to reduce fatigue. Discuss measures to maintain weight and nutrition: Eat several small, bland meals each day; maintain an ample fluid intake by drinking 4 to 6 glasses of water daily. Instruct to report any continued weight loss, loss of appetite, or an inability to eat for 24 hours. Refer to a dietitian for further teaching and diet planning.

Discuss the importance of measures to prevent infection: Wash hands frequently, especially after using the toilet and before preparing foods or eating; bathe daily; avoid using perineal powders or sprays that could dry mucous membranes; brush teeth using a soft-bristle toothbrush after meals and see a dentist regularly; avoid crowds and contact with people who are ill. Instruct to regularly inspect skin and mucous membranes for signs of bleeding or infection. Instruct to report signs of infection such as fever, chills, burning on urination, foul-smelling urine, vaginal or rectal discharge, or skin lesions to the health care provider. Advise to avoid immunizations unless specifically ordered by the oncologist.

Discuss measures to reduce the risk of bleeding or injury: Avoid contact sports or strenuous exercise if platelet count is low; use an electric razor for shaving; avoid using rectal or vaginal suppositories, vaginal tampons, or enemas to minimize trauma to mucous membranes; increase fiber in the diet, and drink ample water to maintain soft stool and prevent straining. Advise to avoid over-the-counter drugs that increase the risk of bleeding, such as aspirin and preparations containing aspirin, and NSAIDs. Instruct to report

any bleeding (nosebleeds, rectal bleeding, vomiting blood, excessive menstrual periods, blood in the urine, bleeding gums, bruises, or collections of blood under the skin) or changes in behavior to the health care provider.

The patient and family may need help with physical care, finances, and transportation after discharge. Provide referrals to social services, support groups, home care services if needed, and other agencies that can provide needed services (such as local chapters of the American Cancer Society, which can provide hospital beds and transportation for outpatient cancer treatment).

See the Clinical Reasoning Care Map at the end of this chapter for an opportunity to use the nursing process to plan care for a patient with acute myelocytic leukemia.

Malignant Lymphoma

Malignant lymphomas are cancerous tumors of lymphoid tissue. They are characterized by lymphocyte proliferation and progressive, painless enlargement of the lymph nodes. Lymphomas are closely related to lymphocytic leukemias, considered by some experts as different forms or stages of the same disease process.

Malignant lymphomas are common. In the United States, more than 79,000 new cases are estimated to be diagnosed annually; lymphomas are the ninth leading cause of cancer deaths. The incidence of lymphoma has been stable since 2005 (ACS, 2013). In most cases, the cause of lymphoma is unknown. Reduced immune function (e.g., HIV disease, immunosuppression with drug therapy) is a known risk factor. Age plays a role: the incidence of non-Hodgkin lymphoma increases with age, whereas teenagers and young adults are more likely to develop Hodgkin lymphoma. Other potential risk factors include certain viral infections, a family history of lymphoma, and exposure to certain chemicals such as herbicides.

PATHOPHYSIOLOGY AND MANIFESTATIONS

Lymphomas are classified as Hodgkin lymphoma (or Hodgkin disease) and non-Hodgkin lymphomas.

Hodgkin Lymphoma

Hodgkin lymphoma is one of the most curable of all cancers. It is characterized by painless, progressive enlargement of one or more lymph nodes and the presence of *Reed–Sternberg cells* in the affected node. It usually affects people between the ages of 15 and 35 or over age 50. It is slightly more common in men than women. The cause of Hodgkin lymphoma is unknown, but it may be linked to viral infection (Epstein–Barr virus). The lymph nodes of the neck or above the clavicle often are the first affected. If untreated, it spreads via the lymphatic system to nodes throughout the body.

The most common manifestation of Hodgkin lymphoma is an enlarged lymph node that is not painful or tender (Figure 20-8■). The node or nodes are firm but movable. Other common symptoms are listed in Box 20-5■.

Non-Hodgkin Lymphoma

Non-Hodgkin lymphomas are more common than Hodgkin lymphoma, accounting for nearly 90% of new cases of lymphoma. Unlike Hodgkin lymphoma, multiple lymph nodes and lymphoid tissue in other body tissues are involved. Non-Hodgkin lymphomas tend to occur in older adults. They also are more common in people whose immune system has been suppressed by HIV disease or immunosuppressive drugs (e.g., people who have had an organ transplant). Epstein–Barr and other viruses may play a role in their development.

The first symptom of non-Hodgkin lymphoma often is an enlarged lymph node. Other manifestations of non-Hodgkin lymphoma are listed in Box 20-5. Involvement of

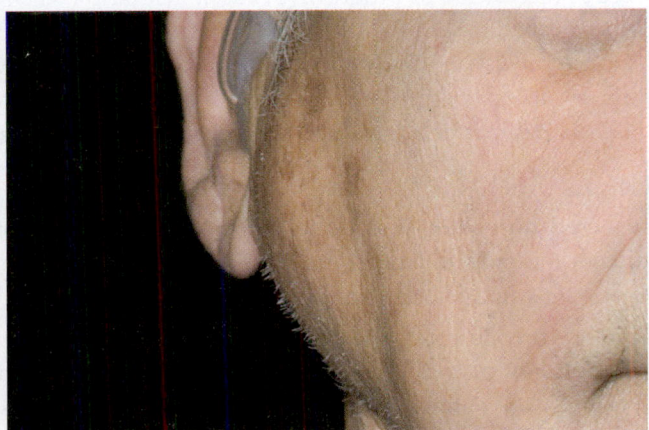

Figure 20-8. ■ Painless, enlarged lymph nodes characteristic of Hodgkin lymphoma. (Source: Dr. P. Marazzi / Science Source.)

BOX 20-5	MANIFESTATIONS OF MALIGNANT LYMPHOMA

Hodgkin lymphoma	Non-Hodgkin lymphoma
■ One or more painless, enlarged lymph nodes	■ Multiple enlarged peripheral or central lymph nodes
■ Fever	■ Abdominal pain
■ Night sweats	■ Nausea, vomiting
■ Pruritus	■ Dyspnea, cough
■ Weight loss	■ Neurologic manifestations
■ Fatigue	■ Weight loss
■ Malaise	■ Fatigue
	■ Night sweats

other organs can lead to symptoms of urinary tract obstruction or infection, neurologic symptoms, shortness of breath, cough, or chest pain. The prognosis for non-Hodgkin lymphoma is not as good as it is for Hodgkin lymphoma.

COLLABORATIVE CARE
Diagnostic Tests and Staging

Laboratory testing includes a *complete blood count*, *erythrocyte sedimentation rate*, and *liver* and *kidney function studies*. *Bone marrow biopsy* is performed. A *chest x-ray* and *chest, abdominal*, and *pelvic CT scans* are done to identify enlarged lymph nodes. *Positron emission tomography* (PET or *gallium scans*) may be performed to diagnose malignant lymphomas or to monitor disease progress.

The diagnosis of lymphoma is made based on *biopsy* of tissue from the enlarged node or tissue mass. If Reed–Sternberg cells are present, the diagnosis of Hodgkin lymphoma is confirmed. For both Hodgkin lymphoma and non-Hodgkin lymphoma, the *Ann Arbor staging system* is used to determine the extent and severity of the disease and to estimate the prognosis. This system uses the number and location of involved lymph nodes to stage the disease:

- Stage I: involvement of a single lymph node region, lymphoid organ, or site outside the lymphatic system
- Stage II: involvement of two or more lymph node regions on the same side of the diaphragm
- Stage III: involvement of additional lymph node regions, organs, or extralymphatic sites
- Stage IV: widely spread disease

An "A" indicates no systemic manifestations; a "B" is used to indicate the presence of systemic symptoms such as fever, night sweats, and weight loss.

Chemotherapy

Combination chemotherapy is used to treat both Hodgkin lymphoma and non-Hodgkin lymphoma. The choice of drug combination depends on the stage of the disease as well as the patient's age and general condition. Chemotherapy results in complete remission in more than 75% of patients with Hodgkin lymphoma who do not have systemic symptoms.

Radiation Therapy

Radiation therapy may be used to treat both Hodgkin lymphoma and non-Hodgkin lymphoma. It may be the initial treatment for early Hodgkin lymphoma; more frequently, it is combined with chemotherapy to treat both Hodgkin and non-Hodgkin lymphomas. Therapy usually involves external radiation of the involved lymph node region.

Stem Cell Transplant

Stem cell transplant may be used to treat patients who experience relapse after remission of malignant lymphoma. Either autologous or allogeneic stem cell transplant may be used. For autologous transplant, stem cells are obtained while the patient is in remission, then frozen and stored. If relapse occurs, chemotherapy and radiation therapy are used to destroy malignant cells and the immune system. The stored stem cells are then infused intravenously. These cells become part of the patient's bone marrow to be formed into new blood cells.

NURSING CARE

PRIORITIZING NURSING CARE

Nursing care of the patient with malignant lymphoma involves providing physical and emotional support throughout the course of treatment. The patient is at risk for infection because cancerous lymphocytes are less effective in mounting an immune response. Nutritional status also must be considered due to the effects of the disease and treatment on appetite and food tolerance.

ASSESSING

Focused assessment of the patient with malignant lymphoma includes obtaining a history of enlarged lymph nodes and inquiring about symptoms such as fatigue, night sweats, abdominal pain, dyspnea and cough, or weight loss. Ask about a known history of infectious mononucleosis, HIV disease, or immunosuppression.

Physical assessment includes inspection and palpation of lymph nodes (cervical, subclavicular, axillary, and inguinal) for enlargement and tenderness; obtaining heart and lung sounds; and inspecting and gently palpating the abdomen for masses, tenderness.

DIAGNOSING, PLANNING, AND IMPLEMENTING

In addition to the nursing diagnoses identified below, see *Risk for Infection and Imbalanced Nutrition*: Less Than Body Requirements in the Nursing Care section for leukemia for nursing activities to address these problems.

Risk for Impaired Skin Integrity

Expected outcome: Skin will remain intact without evidence of lesions or breakdown.

Pruritus and night sweats (symptoms of lymphoma) increase the risk for skin lesions. Radiation therapy also can damage the skin.

- Discuss measures to relieve itching:
  - Use cool water and a mild soap to bathe.
  - Blot (rather than rub) dry skin; apply plain cornstarch or nonperfumed lotion or powder to the skin unless contraindicated (lotions and powders may not be allowed if undergoing radiation therapy).

- Use lightweight cotton blankets and clothing.
- Maintain adequate humidity and a cool room temperature.
- Wash bedding and clothes in mild detergent and put them through a second rinse cycle.

Pruritus is aggravated by excessive warmth, excessive dryness, rough fabrics, fatigue, and stress. These interventions reduce mechanical or chemical irritation of the skin.

Nausea

Expected outcome: Will be able to relate and use appropriate measures to prevent and manage nausea.

- Administer ordered antiemetics before chemotherapy is started. *Premedication with an antiemetic can prevent nausea and reduce the psychological association between chemotherapy and nausea.*
- Teach measures to prevent or relieve nausea and vomiting:
  - Eat soda crackers and suck on hard candy.
  - Eat soft, bland foods that are cold or at room temperature.
  - Avoid unpleasant odors, and get fresh air.
  - Do not eat immediately before chemotherapy.
  - Use distraction or progressive muscle relaxation when nauseated.

Crackers and hard candy often relieve queasiness. Foods that are hot, warm, salty, sweet, or have strong odors often increase nausea. Alternative methods of relieving nausea may be effective.

Fatigue

Expected outcome: Will demonstrate energy conservation through measures to balance rest and activity, using energy-conserving strategies, and adapting lifestyle to energy level.

- Assess complaints of malaise (a vague feeling of body weakness or discomfort) and fatigue (a pervasive, drained feeling that cannot be eliminated). *Malaise and fatigue are subjective experiences.*
- Encourage expression of feelings about the disease and its impact on lifestyle and roles. *Discussion may help the patient identify lifestyle priorities.*
- Encourage enjoyable but quiet activities, such as reading, listening to music, or doing puzzles. *Enjoyable activities such as these help conserve energy and decrease fatigue and can help prevent feelings of helplessness and depression.*
- Help establish priorities, and include rest periods or naps when scheduling daily activities. *This helps the patient maintain control and self-esteem while conserving energy.*
- Encourage patient to delegate some responsibilities to others. *Delegating responsibilities helps conserve energy while allowing others to be more involved in care and decision making.*
- Encourage a diet high in carbohydrates and fluids. *A high-carbohydrate diet helps maintain energy stores, whereas increased fluid intake promotes excretion of waste products that may cause malaise and fatigue.*

Disturbed Body Image

Expected outcome: Will use suggested resources to adapt to change in appearance.

■ Collect subjective data related to body image by asking questions such as these:

- ■ What do you like the most/least about your body?

- ■ What do you understand about your disease?

- ■ How do you feel about this illness?

- ■ How do you think your illness or treatment will affect you?

- ■ Has the illness changed the way you believe others will respond to you?

  A person's image of his or her body is based on past and present experiences. It includes both the physical body and emotional responses to that body. Body image changes constantly.

■ Assess for objective signs of altered body image, such as refusal to touch or look at a body part or to look in a mirror; refusal to discuss body changes; refusal to participate in self-care or rehabilitation; increasing dependence on others; signs of grieving (weeping, despair, anger); hostility toward healthy people; or withdrawal from social contacts. *Although there is no one response to an altered body image, patients may demonstrate any of the above signs.*

■ Teach ways to cope with *alopecia* (hair loss). Discuss using wigs, scarves, hats, and caps during hair loss and regrowth. Teach scalp care using baby shampoo or mild soap, a soft brush, and mineral oil to reduce itching. Emphasize the importance of using sunscreen and covering the head to prevent sunburn. If eyelashes and eyebrows are lost, teach methods of protecting the eyes, such as eyeglasses and caps with wide brims. Discuss and refer to resources (such as the American Cancer Society or insurance) for financial assistance to buy wigs. *Alopecia may range from thinning of hair to total hair loss. Regrowth usually begins 2 to 3 months after treatment ends. New hair may be softer, more curly, and slightly different in color.*

■ Assess knowledge of the effects of illness and treatment on sexuality and reproduction. Provide information and clarify misconceptions as needed. Encourage the patient and significant other to verbalize concerns. Discuss options such as storing sperm in a sperm bank before undergoing radiation therapy. Refer for counseling as indicated. *Sexual function often is altered by the disease and the effects of treatment. This may include temporary or permanent sterility, changes in menstruation, and changes in libido (sexual desire).*

■ Encourage participation in support groups. *Support groups are often effective in helping the patient and family deal with loss and altered body image.*

MANAGING NURSING CARE

Nursing care activities such as obtaining vital signs, assisting with hygiene, skin care and activity for the patient with lymphoma are appropriate to assign to assistive personnel.

CONTINUITY OF CARE

Teach about lymphoma, its treatment, and the side effects of treatments. Topics that are appropriate for the patient with leukemia are also appropriate for the patient with a malignant lymphoma. In addition, teach the patient and family to:

■ Care for the skin and avoid scratching to reduce the risk of infection.

■ Report new or different symptoms that may indicate extension of the disease.

■ Use complementary pain management strategies as well as prescribed drugs to promote comfort.

■ Plan activities of daily living to ensure adequate rest and exercise.

■ Eat a well-balanced diet.

Refer to the local chapter of the American Cancer Society for information, financial assistance, and counseling. Patients with malignant lymphomas may obtain a list of state and local agencies that offer information about the disease and financial assistance from the Leukemia Society of America.

NURSING CARE PLAN
Patient With Hodgkin Lymphoma

Albin Quito, age 28, is a nurse manager in a large hospital. Lately, he has noticed that he is more tired than usual, often wakes up at night covered with sweat, and just does not feel well. He attributed his symptoms to "a touch of the flu" and to his busy work schedule. Yesterday morning, he noticed a large swollen area on the right side of his neck. He made an appointment with his primary health provider. At that appointment, a large cervical lymph node was found, and blood was drawn. A biopsy of the node and a computed tomography (CT) scan of the chest were scheduled.

Assessment

David Herzog, the clinic nurse, obtains a nursing assessment on Mr. Quito. His physical exam is normal, with the exception of the enlarged node, which is not painful to touch. When Mr. Quito is weighed, he says that he has lost 7 lb (3.2 kg) in the past 2 months. Test results include mild anemia and an increased neutrophil count. Reed–Sternberg cells are found in the lymph node biopsy. The physician makes the diagnosis of Hodgkin lymphoma and tells Mr. Quito that his prognosis is very good. After learning about treatment options, Mr. Quito decides to undergo combination chemotherapy.

Nursing Diagnosis

Mr. Herzog identifies the following nursing diagnoses:

- *Anxiety* related to malignancy and uncertainty about ability to continue working in his present position
- *Risk for Infection* related to impaired immunologic function
- *Fatigue* related to the effects of the cancer and planned treatment

Expected Outcomes

The expected outcomes in the plan of care specify that Mr. Quito will:

- Verbalize a decrease in anxiety.
- Remain free of infection.
- Use methods to preserve energy.

Planning and Implementation

The following nursing interventions are planned and implemented:

- Encourage to discuss treatment schedule with supervisor to plan release time.
- Encourage to join a support group for people with cancer.
- Provide information about illness and radiation therapy.
- Discuss ways to decrease the risk of infection.
- Discuss energy management strategies such as:
  - Take a short nap once or twice a day to provide total body rest.
  - Do not overexert during weekends.
  - Maintain a well-balanced diet.

Evaluation

When Mr. Quito returns to begin chemotherapy, he brings his friend Nancy. He asks Mr. Herzog to discuss his treatment with her. Mr. Quito says, "I am still really scared, but being able to talk about this with Nancy will help a lot." Mr. Quito has made arrangements for a leave of absence from work, with the understanding that his job will be held for him. He states that he will have some money problems but is working them out. He also says he feels that taking a nap is silly but he'll try it. They have found a cancer support group and plan to attend the next meeting.

Critical Thinking in the Nursing Process

1. Review cancer treatment with radiation and chemotherapy. How do each of these treatments work to kill malignant cells?
2. What information will you give Mr. Quito about preventing infection while he is at home?
3. How might the psychologic and socioeconomic effect of the diagnosis of cancer differ in a young adult versus an older adult?

Note: Discussion of Critical Thinking questions appears on the companion website.

Multiple Myeloma

Multiple myeloma is a malignancy in which plasma cells multiply uncontrollably and infiltrate bone marrow, lymph nodes, and other tissues. *Plasma cells* are B-cell lymphocytes that develop to produce antibodies (*immunoglobulins*).

The incidence of multiple myeloma is much higher in African Americans than Caucasians. It affects men more often than women, and its incidence increases with age. Multiple myeloma primarily develops in older adults; it rarely occurs before age 40. People of lower socioeconomic groups have a higher rate of multiple myeloma.

PATHOPHYSIOLOGY AND MANIFESTATIONS

Multiple myeloma arises from one abnormal B-cell clone. As myeloma cells proliferate, they replace the bone marrow and infiltrate the bone itself. The bone is weakened by these abnormal cells and may break without trauma (a *pathologic fracture*). Myeloma cells also secrete an abnormal immunoglobulin known as *M protein*. This abnormal protein is ineffective as an antibody to maintain B-cell or humoral immunity. It also increases the viscosity of the blood and damages kidney tubules.

The disease develops slowly and often asymptomatically. Bone or back pain is the most common symptom. As the disease progresses, the pain becomes more severe. Pathologic fractures occur, particularly in weight-bearing bones such as the vertebrae, pelvis, and femur. Vertebral fractures may compress the spinal cord, causing neurologic symptoms. The patient becomes more susceptible to infections and develops signs of anemia and bleeding tendencies. Kidney damage may cause manifestations of renal failure.

COLLABORATIVE CARE

Laboratory and diagnostic tests are ordered to confirm the diagnosis of multiple myeloma.

- Urine samples usually are positive for *Bence Jones protein*, abnormal protein produced by plasma cells in some forms of multiple myeloma.
- The *CBC* reveals moderate to severe anemia.
- *Protein electrophoresis* demonstrates the presence of M protein in the serum of approximately 85% of patients with multiple myeloma.
- *Bone marrow studies* show excessive immature plasma cells.
- *Bone x-rays* reveal punched-out holes in the bone, particularly in the vertebrae, ribs, skull, pelvis, femurs, clavicles, and scapulae.

There is no cure for multiple myeloma. Treatment focuses on slowing progression of the disease and supportive care to manage disease complications and improve quality of life. The disease course typically is chronic and progressive, with the usual survival about 7 to 8 years.

Chemotherapy, radiation therapy, and medications are used to decrease the tumor size and reduce bone pain. Some patients may undergo stem cell transplant. Pain is controlled with analgesics. Blood transfusions are used to treat anemia, and infections are controlled with antibiotics. Braces or splints may be ordered as needed to maintain mobility.

NURSING CARE

Patients with multiple myeloma require nursing care similar to that required by patients with leukemia. Pain and the risk for pathologic fractures are additional nursing care considerations discussed in this section.

Chronic Pain

Expected outcome: Will report pain level of 2 or lower on a scale of 0 to 10.

- Assess pain, including location, onset, duration, precipitating factors, and effective relief measures. *Assessment provides baseline data for evaluating the effectiveness of pain relief measures.*
- Assist into the position of greatest comfort, supporting position as needed. *A patient who is weak and uncomfortable may need assistance with repositioning. Painful bony prominences may require the support of many pillows for comfort.*
- Teach effective use of prescribed analgesics and complementary therapies such as relaxation or guided imagery to control pain. Involve the family as needed to help ensure that pain is relieved. *Taking analgesics on a regular schedule and before pain becomes severe increases their effectiveness. Complementary strategies augment the effectiveness of analgesics.*
- Provide for uninterrupted rest periods. *Rest promotes muscle relaxation and emotional equilibrium, increasing the ability to manage pain.*
- Report unrelieved pain to the physician. *Because of the chronic and increasing nature of cancer pain, different or additional medications may be necessary.*

Impaired Physical Mobility

Expected outcome: Will remain free of complications related to immobility (e.g., skin breakdown, respiratory infection).

- Reposition carefully and gently. *Fractures may occur during common activities such as turning or repositioning. Gentle handling reduces the risk of pathologic fracture.*
- Change position at least every 2 hours; more frequently as needed. *Repositioning promotes comfort and minimizes the risk of skin breakdown.*
- Provide a trapeze to assist in repositioning. *A trapeze enables the patient to assist with repositioning and promotes self-care.*

- Place needed items close at hand. *This reduces the need to reach for objects and the risk of falling.*
- Place bed in low position, use side rails as indicated, and place the call bell within reach. Keep halls and pathways free of clutter; remove scatter rugs; and provide adequate lighting, a nonslippery floor, and nonskid soles on shoes. *These safety measures reduce the risk for falling and injury.*

CONTINUITY OF CARE

As with leukemia, patients with multiple myeloma must be actively involved in their disease management. Teach signs and symptoms that indicate complications and the need to seek medical help. These complications include infection, pathologic fractures, bleeding, and severe anemia. Infection is the leading cause of death for patients with multiple myeloma. Discuss hospice services with the patient and family. Although patients qualify for hospice services during the last 6 months of life, many do not seek services until death is imminent. Hospice services provide pain management, emotional support, and respite services for caregivers.

Neutropenia

Neutropenia is a decrease in the number of circulating neutrophils (the prevalent WBC and an integral component of the immune system). In adults, neutropenia usually develops secondarily to infection, hematologic disorders, a chronic disease, or chemotherapy. *Agranulocytosis* is severe neutropenia. In agranulocytosis, both the total granulocyte count and the number of neutrophils are significantly reduced. It may result from impaired WBC formation in the bone marrow or increased cell destruction.

safety**ALERT**

Decreased neutrophil counts greatly increase the risk of infection. Protect the patient by providing a private room, using excellent hand hygiene, and limiting visitors.

Fatigue, weakness, sore throat, stomatitis, *dysphagia* (difficult or painful swallowing), and fever and chills are the usual symptoms of neutropenia. It is diagnosed by the WBC count. The neutrophil count is less than 1,500 cells/mm^3; it may be less than 500/mm^3 when the condition is severe.

Any drug suspected of causing neutropenia is discontinued and infections are treated. Filgrastim (Neupogen), a drug that stimulates the growth and development of WBCs in bone marrow, may be given, particularly when neutropenia is associated with chemotherapy. This drug, which is given parenterally, is generally safe. Many patients develop bone pain while taking this drug. (See Table 20-4.)

PLATELET AND COAGULATION DISORDERS

Key Concept Adequate numbers of platelets and all of the proteins involved in the clotting cascade are necessary for the body to form stable clots and to achieve hemostasis. Patients with low platelet counts or who are lacking clotting factors are at risk for bleeding and hemorrhage.

In this section, the focus is on three disorders that can interfere with effective clotting and lead to excessive bleeding. In the first, thrombocytopenia, the primary problem is a lack of platelets. In hemophilia, lack of one or more clotting factors interferes with clotting. The third disorder presented, disseminated intravascular coagulation, is characterized by abnormal clotting that depletes both platelets and clotting factors, resulting in bleeding.

Thrombocytopenia

Thrombocytopenia is a platelet count of less than 100,000 platelets/mL of blood. It is the most common cause of abnormal bleeding. If the number of circulating platelets falls below 20,000/mL, spontaneous bleeding (internal and external) is likely. Thrombocytopenia can result from decreased platelet production, increased destruction of platelets, or accumulation of platelets in the spleen. *Immune* (or *idiopathic*) *thrombocytopenia purpura* is the most common form of thrombocytopenia. It typically affects young adults (ages 20 to 40); women are affected more frequently than men. Heparin therapy can lead to drug-induced thrombocytopenia.

PATHOPHYSIOLOGY

In immune thrombocytopenia purpura (ITP), platelets are destroyed much more rapidly than normal. It is an autoimmune disorder in which platelets are destroyed by the body's immune system. Antibodies are developed to proteins in the platelet cell membrane; when these antibodies adhere to the platelet, the spleen identifies the platelet as a foreign cell and destroys it.

Immune thrombocytopenia may be an acute or a chronic condition. Acute ITP is seen in children and is often preceded by a viral infection. Chronic ITP affects adults and may occur secondarily to another autoimmune disorder, such as systemic lupus erythematosus (SLE), or infections, such as HIV and hepatitis C (Konkle, 2012).

Heparin-induced thrombocytopenia (HIT) is an abnormal response to heparin therapy. It occurs more frequently with use of unfractionated heparin than it does when low-molecular-weight heparin is used. In HIT, heparin stimulates an immune response that leads to destruction of platelets.

Thrombocytopenia results; fragments of platelets also can stimulate the clotting cascade, leading to widespread clotting.

MANIFESTATIONS

The manifestations of ITP are caused by abnormal bleeding, particularly into the skin and mucous membranes (Figure 20-9■). **Purpura** (hemorrhage into the tissues), *ecchymoses* (bruises), and **petechiae** (small, flat, purple, or red spots on the skin or mucous membranes) develop on the anterior chest, arms, and neck. Other bleeding may occur as well: *epistaxis* (nosebleed), *menorrhagia* (prolonged and heavy menstrual periods), hematuria, and gastrointestinal bleeding. Spontaneous bleeding into the brain can be fatal. Associated symptoms such as headache, weight loss, and fever also may occur.

COLLABORATIVE CARE
Diagnostic Tests

Thrombocytopenia is diagnosed by its manifestations and diagnostic test results. A *CBC with platelet count* is ordered; the platelet count is less than 100,000/mL. A *bone marrow examination* may be ordered to evaluate platelet production. *Serologic testing* also is performed when HIT is suspected.

Medications

Corticosteroids such as prednisone are given to suppress the immune response and the antibodies targeted for the platelets. Immune globulins (e.g., intravenous gamma globulin) or immunosuppressive drugs such as cyclosporine also may be used.

Prompt withdrawal of heparin therapy is critical in HIT. All sources of heparin are removed, including heparin used to flush intravenous catheters. An alternate anticoagulant drug may be substituted for heparin if anticoagulation must be continued.

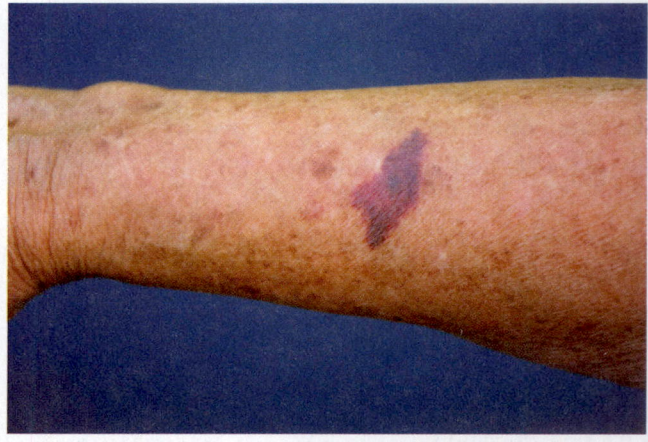

Figure 20-9. ■ Lesions characteristic of thrombocytopenic purpura. (Source: © CMSP/Custom Medical Stock Photo.)

Treatments

Platelet transfusions may be needed to restore the platelet count and prevent bleeding. Platelets are prepared from fresh whole blood; one unit contains 30 to 60 mL of platelet concentrate.

clinicalALERT

Platelets must be administered as soon as they are obtained from the blood bank. As with whole blood, platelets are typed and cross-matched to the individual.

Plasma exchange therapy, also known as plasmapheresis, may be done to remove circulating autoantibodies. In this treatment, the patient's plasma is removed and replaced with fresh-frozen plasma.

Surgery

A *splenectomy* (surgical removal of the spleen) may be necessary. The spleen is the site of platelet destruction and antibody production. This surgery often leads to remission or even cure of the disorder.

NURSING CARE

PRIORITIZING NURSING CARE

Nursing care for the patient with thrombocytopenia focuses on the risk for injury resulting from bleeding. Although the patient faces many challenges related to the disorder and its treatment, protecting the patient from consequences of abnormal bleeding is of highest priority.

Bleeding

Expected outcome: Will remain free of manifestations of abnormal bleeding.

- Monitor LOC and vital signs every 4 hours and report changes such as hypotension or tachycardia to the charge nurse or physician. *A change in LOC or tachycardia can be an early sign of bleeding; hypotension is a later sign.*
- Promptly report manifestations of bleeding:
  - Increased petechiae, bruising, purpura, or hematoma formation
  - Obvious bleeding from gums, nose; prolonged bleeding from puncture sites
  - Bright red or coffee-grounds emesis; rectal bleeding or tarry stools
  - Hematuria (blood in the urine)
  - Vaginal bleeding
  - Changes in neurologic status: headache, visual changes, altered mental status, decreasing LOC, seizures
  - Complaints of epigastric pain, absent bowel sounds, increasing abdominal girth, abdominal rigidity

Prompt reporting allows early treatment of bleeding or hemorrhage. Bleeding into the abdomen or the head may not be readily apparent and identified only by changes in neurologic status or abdominal assessment data.

- Avoid invasive rectal, vaginal, or urinary tract procedures and parenteral injections if possible. *Invasive procedures can damage mucous membranes and tissues, increasing the risk of bleeding.*
- Apply pressure to puncture sites for 3 to 5 minutes; apply pressure to arterial blood gas sites for 15 to 20 minutes. *Pressure prevents prolonged bleeding by prompting hemostasis and clot formation.*
- Instruct to avoid straining to have a bowel movement and forceful coughing, sneezing, and blowing of the nose. *Avoiding these activities reduces the risk of external or internal bleeding.*

CONTINUITY OF CARE

Discuss the need to continue treatment to maintain remission of this chronic disease; also discuss the risks and benefits of long-term corticosteroid or immunosuppressant therapy. Respond to questions about splenectomy. Although surgery is an invasive treatment, most people experience partial or complete remission of the disease after surgery. Teach measures to avoid injury and bleeding.

Hemophilia

Hemophilia is not a single disease but a group of hereditary clotting factor deficiencies. Lack of a clotting factor disrupts blood coagulation, leading to persistent and sometimes severe bleeding. Although it usually is considered a disease of children, hemophilia may be diagnosed in adults.

PATHOPHYSIOLOGY AND MANIFESTATIONS

In hemophilia, the first steps of hemostasis, vasoconstriction and formation of the platelet plug, occur normally. The third step, blood clotting, is disrupted by lack of a specific factor required in the clotting cascade. *Hemophilia A* is the most common type of hemophilia. It is caused by a deficiency in factor VIII. *Hemophilia B* (also called *Christmas disease*) is less common. It is caused by a deficiency in factor IX. The clinical manifestations of hemophilia A and B are the same. Both are transmitted from mother to son as sex-linked recessive disorders on the X chromosome (Figure 20-10■).

People with hemophilia A or B experience hemorrhages into body tissues. Severe clotting factor deficiencies can lead to spontaneous bleeding episodes. Bleeding of the mouth, gums, lips, and tongue are common, as is hematuria. Bleeding into joints (*hemarthrosis*) causes severe pain and can affect joint structure and function.

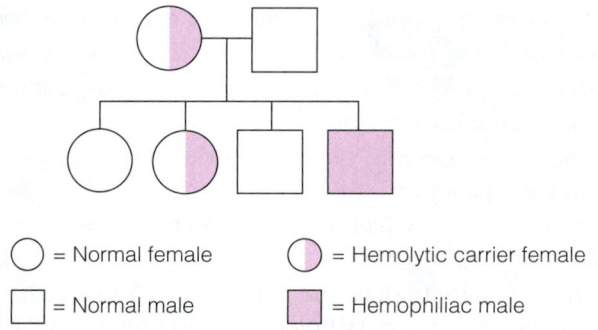

○ = Normal female   ◐ = Hemolytic carrier female

☐ = Normal male   ◼ = Hemophiliac male

Figure 20-10. ◼ The inheritance pattern for hemophilia A and B. Both are X-linked recessive disorders; females may carry the trait, but only males develop the disorder.

Von Willebrand disease is a common hereditary bleeding disorder classified as one of the hemophilias that is usually seen in adults. It is caused by a deficiency of von Willebrand (vW) factor; factor VIII is often lacking as well. This clotting disorder affects both men and women. Von Willebrand disease causes less severe bleeding than hemophilia A or B. It is often diagnosed when surgery or a dental extraction causes prolonged bleeding.

Factor XI deficiency (also called hemophilia C) is usually a mild bleeding disorder. It often is diagnosed only when postoperative bleeding is prolonged. A comparison of the major types of hemophilia is found in Table 20-5 ◼.

COLLABORATIVE CARE

Treatment of hemophilia focuses on preventing and/or treating bleeding, primarily by replacing deficient clotting factors. Treatment varies, depending on the clotting defect and the severity of the illness.

Diagnostic Tests

- The *platelet count* is measured; it frequently is within normal limits.
- Coagulation studies, including the *APTT, bleeding time*, and *prothrombin time*, are done as screening tests for hemophilia. They often demonstrate prolonged bleeding times.
- *Clotting factor assays* are done to identify specific clotting factor deficiencies.

Medications

Replacement of clotting factors is treatment for hemophilia. They may be given on a regular basis, as a prophylactic measure before surgery and dental procedures, and to control bleeding. Clotting factors may be given in the form of fresh-frozen plasma, cryoprecipitates, or concentrates. They may be given intravenously and may be self-administered. Fresh-frozen plasma replaces all clotting factors (including both factor VIII and factor IX) except platelets. People who were treated for hemophilia between 1978 and 1985 have a high incidence of HIV disease, because donated blood was not routinely tested. Rigorous screening of donors, testing of donated blood, and heat treating of blood products have significantly reduced this risk. Factor VIII prepared by recombinant DNA does not contain human plasma, so it carries no risk of infectious disease. It is, however, very expensive.

Desmopressin acetate (DDAVP) also may be used to treat mild hemophilia and von Willebrand disease. This drug stimulates the body to release vW factor, helping promote clotting.

NURSING CARE

PRIORITIZING NURSING CARE

The priority for nursing care for the patient with hemophilia is protection from injury and minimizing the risk for bleeding. Assessment of the patient is similar to that for a patient with leukemia.

Risk for Bleeding

Expected outcome: Will remain free of hemorrhage.

- Monitor for signs of bleeding, including hematomas, ecchymoses, purpura, and obvious oozing or bleeding. *Careful assessment is necessary to identify hidden or occult bleeding. Abdominal pain, joint swelling and pain, or a change in LOC may also be manifestations of occult bleeding.*
- Notify the charge nurse or physician at the first sign of bleeding. *Prompt intervention decreases the risk of hemorrhage.*
- If bleeding occurs, apply gentle pressure until bleeding stops; apply ice; or apply a topical agent to stop bleeding

TABLE 20-5	Comparison of Types of Hemophilia		
TYPE	**DEFICIENCY**	**CHARACTERISTICS**	**TREATMENT**
Hemophilia A (classic hemophilia)	Factor VIII	Most common form of hemophilia; transmitted from mother with defective gene to sons	Factor VIII concentrate or cryoprecipitate
Hemophilia B (Christmas disease)	Factor IX	Less common; transmitted from mother with defective gene to sons	Factor IX concentrate
von Willebrand disease	vW factor	Most common hereditary bleeding disorder; affects both males and females	Cryoprecipitate, factor VIII products, or DDAVP
Factor XI deficiency	Factor XI	Affects both males and females	Fresh-frozen plasma

as ordered. *These measures reduce bleeding until definitive treatment can be given.*

- Avoid giving intramuscular injections, rectal temperatures, and enemas. *These can cause tissue trauma, leading to bleeding.*
- Use safety measures such as a soft-bristle toothbrush and electric razor in personal care. *Use of a soft-bristle toothbrush and electric razor minimize the risk of skin and mucous membrane trauma that may result in bleeding.*
- Protect from injury as needed:
  - Pad side rails of the bed if restless or confused.
  - Assist with ambulation and activities as needed to prevent falling.
  - Provide adequate lighting, especially at night.
  - Keep halls and pathways free of obstruction; make no unnecessary changes in furniture arrangements.
  - Encourage patient to wear shoes with nonskid soles when ambulating.
  These measures help prevent accidental falls or tissue trauma from bumping into objects.

Readiness for Enhanced Self-Health Management

Expected outcome: Will express ability to manage the disorder and demonstrate self-administration of prescribed treatments.

- Assess knowledge and reinforce teaching about disorder and its treatments. *Teaching based on current level of knowledge and understanding is more effective than use of standardized teaching plans.*
- Provide emotional support, and express confidence in self-care abilities. *Support and confidence are necessary to incorporate a care regimen into the patient's lifestyle.*
- Provide opportunities to learn and practice administering clotting factors and topical hemostatic preparations under supervision. *Practice helps with mastery of psychomotor skills and confidence in the ability to perform self-care.*

CONTINUITY OF CARE

Patients with bleeding disorders need to know how to prevent bleeding, how to treat it at home, and how to administer prescribed drugs. Teach to:

- Recognize and immediately report manifestations of internal bleeding: pallor, weakness, restlessness, headache, disorientation, pain, swelling.
- Apply cold packs and immobilize the joint for up to 24 to 48 hours if hemarthrosis occurs.
- Request a prescription for analgesia if pain is severe. Avoid aspirin, which increases the risk of continued bleeding.
- Ensure a safe home environment. For example, pad sharp furniture edges, leave on a light at night, do not use scatter rugs, and wear gloves when working in the house or yard.

- Use only electric razors.
- Wear a MedicAlert bracelet in case of accident.
- Practice good dental hygiene to maintain dental health. If dental procedures are necessary, discuss the need for prophylactic clotting factor with dentist and physician.
- Avoid activities that increase the risk of injury, such as contact sports or racquetball.
- Consider physical demands of the job and risk for injury when planning a career or seeking employment.
- Prepare and administer intravenous medications.

Refer patients with hemophilia or a family history of hemophilia who wish to have a family for genetic counseling.

Disseminated Intravascular Coagulation

Disseminated intravascular coagulation (DIC) is a complex disorder characterized by simultaneous blood clotting and hemorrhage. It is a complication of other disorders, such as shock, sepsis, or other conditions listed in Box 20-6■. Sepsis is the most common cause of DIC.

PATHOPHYSIOLOGY

DIC is a complex process in which the intrinsic and/or extrinsic clotting cascades are activated in response to endothelial damage. Widespread clotting occurs within small blood vessels. Clotting obstructs small blood vessels in the organs, leading to tissue ischemia, infarction, and necrosis. The widespread clotting activates the fibrinolytic pathway that normally breaks down existing clots. Fibrinolytic products interfere with platelet function. Clotting factors are depleted by the abnormal coagulation process, leading to bleeding. Thus, in the patient with DIC, both intravascular clotting and hemorrhage are occurring at the same time.

MANIFESTATIONS

Bleeding is the most obvious manifestation of DIC. The bleeding ranges from oozing blood after an injection to frank hemorrhage from every body orifice. Clotting leads

BOX 20-6	RISK FACTORS FOR DIC

- Hypovolemic or septic shock
- Infection and sepsis
- Drugs
- Malignancy
- Obstetric complications
- Trauma
- Liver disease
- Hematologic or immune disorders
- Acute respiratory distress syndrome
- Venomous snakebite

BOX 20-7	**MANIFESTATIONS OF DIC**

- Petechiae, purpura, ecchymoses
- Bleeding from wounds
- Tachycardia, hypotension
- Cold, mottled fingers and toes
- Tachypnea
- Obvious or occult blood in vomitus and/or stool
- Abdominal distention
- Hematuria
- Oliguria, kidney failure
- Anxiety, confusion
- Decreased LOC

to symptoms of tissue ischemia. The manifestations of DIC are listed in Box 20-7 ■.

clinicalALERT

Promptly report abnormal bleeding (e.g., oozing from injection sites, nosebleed) in critically ill patients because it may be an early sign of DIC.

COLLABORATIVE CARE

Clotting studies are ordered to establish the diagnosis of DIC. *CBC* and *platelet counts* are obtained. The *D-Dimer* test and *fibrin degradation products* are evaluated to confirm the presence of fibrinolysis.

Treatment for DIC focuses on treating the underlying disease and interrupting the clotting/bleeding process. If liver function is intact, it can restore depleted clotting factors in 24 to 48 hours. Patients with severe DIC require hemodynamic monitoring and respiratory support, and may require surgery.

Fresh-frozen plasma and platelet concentrates are given to control bleeding. Heparin also may be ordered. Heparin interferes with the clotting cascade and may prevent depletion of clotting factors due to uncontrolled clotting. In acute DIC, however, heparin may lead to increased bleeding.

NURSING CARE

PRIORITIZING NURSING CARE

The patient with DIC is critically ill. Maintaining vital functions and tissue perfusion are the priorities of nursing care. Managing pain associated with widespread clotting and tissue ischemia is important, as are measures to help relieve the patient's and family's anxiety related to this critical illness.

Ineffective Peripheral Tissue Perfusion

Expected outcome: Peripheral pulses and tissues will remain intact.

Tiny blood clots forming within blood vessels impair perfusion of body tissues.

- Assess peripheral pulses and warmth and capillary refill of extremities. Monitor LOC and mental status. Assess bowel sounds and monitor urine output. Promptly report changes to the charge nurse or physician. *Early treatment of impaired circulation is important to preserve organ function.*
- Carefully turn from side to side at least every 2 hours. *Frequent position changes help relieve pressure, maintain tissue perfusion, and preserve skin integrity. Position changes also provide an opportunity to assess tissue integrity and check for bleeding.*
- Discourage from crossing the legs; do not use the knee gatch on the bed. *These positions can impair blood flow and tissue perfusion of the legs.*

Impaired Gas Exchange

Expected outcome: LOC, breath sounds, and oxygen saturation levels will remain within expected range for patient.

Microclots in the pulmonary vascular system can interfere with gas exchange.

- Report oxygen saturation levels and ABGs outside of established limits to the physician. *Oxygen saturation levels and ABGs are objective measures of gas exchange.*
- Administer oxygen as ordered. *Supplemental oxygen helps maintain adequate gas exchange and relieve dyspnea.*
- Elevate the head of the bed. *Elevating the head of the bed improves lung ventilation and gas exchange.*
- Maintain bed rest. *Bed rest reduces oxygen demands and improves pulmonary circulation for better gas exchange.*
- Encourage deep breathing and coughing. *Coughing and deep breathing help maintain airway patency, facilitating alveolar ventilation.*

Acute Pain

Expected outcome: Will report pain at a level of 2 or lower on a 0 to 10 scale.

- Assess pain using a pain scale. Document location, severity, and character of all reported pain. Promptly notify the charge nurse or physician of new or different pain, or if its intensity changes. *The pain scale provides an objective assessment of pain. Changes in the location or severity of pain may indicate tissue ischemia or bleeding into tissues.*
- Handle extremities gently. *Gentle handling minimizes trauma and pain.*
- Apply cool compresses to painful joints. *Application of cold decreases pain perception and may reduce bleeding into joint tissues.*

Fear

Expected outcome: Will seek information to reduce fear.

DIC is a frightening complication of critical illness.

- Allow patient and family to verbalize concerns. *This helps identify concerns and questions.*
- Answer questions truthfully. *Providing truthful answers establishes trust and helps the patient and family understand what is happening.*
- Help identify coping strategies. *Past effective coping methods may provide skills to manage the current crisis.*
- Provide emotional support. *The presence of a caring nurse may help reduce the fear and anxiety associated with the crisis.*
- Maintain a calm environment. *A calm, quiet environment and evidence that the staff is in control of the situation help relieve fears and promote rest.*
- Respond promptly to calls for help. *Prompt responses help develop a trusting relationship and reduce anxiety.*
- Teach relaxation techniques. *Relaxation techniques can reduce muscle tension and help the patient gain a sense of control.*

CONTINUITY OF CARE

The patient with DIC may have continuing effects of the disorder after the crisis is resolved. Clotting in small peripheral vessels may lead to ulcerations and poor wound healing. Teach the patient and family about proper foot care and any special care needs such as wound care or dressing changes. Teach administration of parenteral medications, if ordered, and provide a referral to home health care or home intravenous management services as appropriate. Discuss manifestations of excessive bleeding or microclotting to be reported to the physician.

LYMPHATIC SYSTEM DISORDERS

Key Concept   The lymphatic system plays an important role in the immune response and in removing damaged and abnormal cells and foreign matter from the body. Lymph nodes often swell during infections, and lymph vessels can become inflamed or obstructed.

Lymphoid tissues are connective tissues that contain many lymphocytes, the WBCs primarily responsible for specific immune responses. **Lymphadenopathy** is swelling and enlargement of the lymph nodes. It may occur in response to infections, inflammation, or cancers.

Lymphangitis and Lymphedema

Lymphangitis is inflammation of the lymph vessels. It is usually caused by a bacterial infection. Patients with lymphangitis develop painful red streaks following the lymph vessels and extending up an arm or leg. If lymph nodes also become inflamed, it is called *lymphadenitis*. The lymph nodes are swollen and may be tender. Fever, malaise, and chills also accompany lymphangitis or lymphadenitis.

Lymphedema is edema caused by obstruction of lymph vessels. Obstruction of the lymph vessels from surgical removal of lymph nodes (as is done in a radical mastectomy), scarring of lymph nodes after radiation, or invasion of lymph nodes by tumor may cause lymphedema. Patients who live in the tropics may develop *elephantiasis*, a type of lymphedema caused by filaria, a nematode worm. *Primary lymphedema* may be congenital in origin or may develop during puberty or adulthood. The cause of primary lymphedema is unknown. It can affect one or all of the limbs, as well as other parts of the body.

The affected extremity is swollen and edematous (Figure 20-11 ■). Early in the course of the disorder, the edema is soft and pitting. With time, the edematous tissue becomes hard to the touch (*brawny edema*). The skin appears thick and hardened and may resemble an orange peel. The edema may worsen in warm weather and (if the legs are affected) after standing for long periods. As the

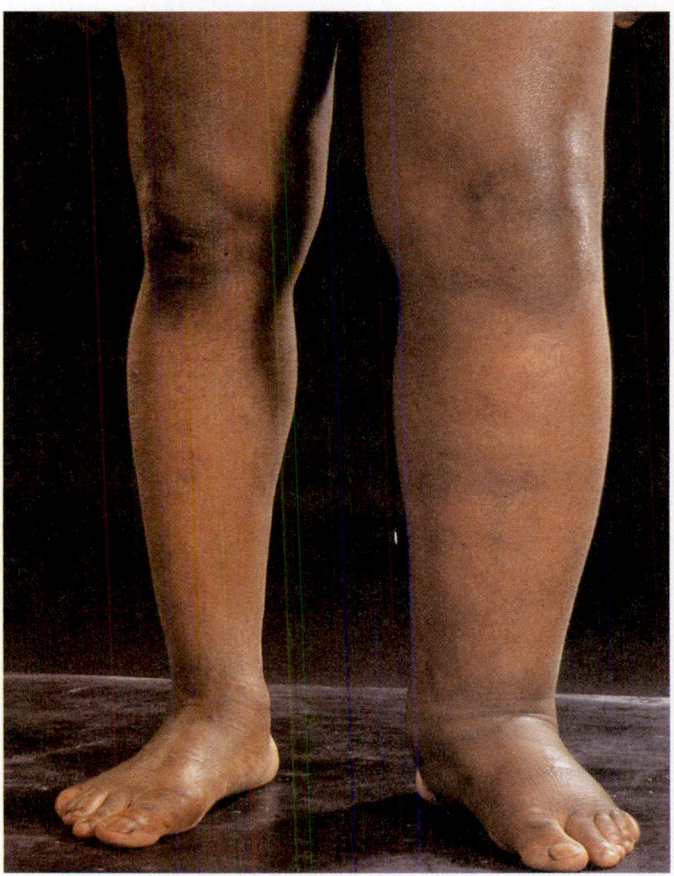

Figure 20-11. ■ Severe lymphedema of the lower extremity. (Source: © Wellcome Image Library/Custom Medical Stock Photo.)

disease progresses, the edema fails to resolve completely with elevation of the limb. Ultimately, the limb becomes grossly enlarged and misshapen. The skin is prone to breakdown and infection.

COLLABORATIVE CARE

Collaborative care for patients with lymphatic system disorders focuses on relieving edema, maintaining skin integrity in the affected extremity, and preventing or treating infection.

For lymphangitis, moist heat is applied, and the affected extremity is elevated and immobilized. Meticulous skin and wound care are vital. Antibiotics are prescribed to treat the infection. Penicillin G is often used because streptococcal bacteria are common causative organisms.

Lymphedema is often chronic and requires longer term treatment. Measures such as the following are ordered:

- Elevate the extremity, especially during sleep.
- Use elastic stockings, elastic bandages, or pneumatic pressure devices.
- Provide meticulous skin hygiene.
- Exercise to stimulate lymph flow.
- Restrict dietary sodium.

Occasionally, surgery may be performed to relieve pain, remove cancerous tissue, or treat repeated episodes of lymphangitis in the affected extremity.

NURSING CARE

The nursing care focus for patients with lymphatic system disorders is on relieving edema, maintaining skin integrity, and preventing infection.

Measure the circumference of the affected extremity daily or as ordered. Mark the position on the extremity where measurements are taken; the use of a consistent location allows accurate comparison of measurements. Maintain intake and output records, and weigh daily or with each clinic visit. Report changes to the charge nurse or physician. Restrict sodium intake and help choose low-sodium foods.

Apply antiembolic stockings and intermittent pressure devices as ordered. Remove stockings and pressure devices at least once each shift to inspect the underlying skin for redness, irritation, dryness, or breakdown. Document findings. Elevate extremities while seated or in bed. Keep skin clean and dry, especially between toes. Use protective devices such as egg crate foam, sheepskin, pillows, or padding to reduce the risk of skin breakdown.

CONTINUITY OF CARE

Teach how to apply and use intermittent pressure devices and/or elastic stockings. Instruct to wear elastic stockings during waking hours and to remove them while sleeping. Emphasize the importance of inspecting the skin at least daily for signs of breakdown or cracking.

Teach skin care to promote its integrity, prevent breakdown, and reduce the risk for infection. Help develop a schedule and plan for elevating the affected extremity that interferes as little as possible with daily schedules. Discuss other prescribed measures such as any activity restriction, dietary sodium restriction, and diuretic therapy. Provide a list of high-sodium foods to avoid, and refer to a dietitian for further teaching about salt-restricted diets. If the patient is taking a potassium-wasting diuretic, provide a list of foods that are high in potassium.

Provide information about contacts for questions, and make referrals as needed. The patient may face long years of self-management and may need assistance with health care management, meals, and housework.

Infectious Mononucleosis

Infectious mononucleosis is an acute infectious disease caused by the Epstein–Barr virus (EBV). This disease, which primarily affects young adults, is usually benign and self-limiting. It appears to be transmitted by saliva; hence, it is often called the "kissing disease."

When the virus enters the body, it invades B cells in the lymphoid tissues of the oropharynx. The infection causes increased lymphocyte production and swelling of lymph glands. The manifestations begin with headache, malaise, and fatigue. Most patients with infectious mononucleosis have fever, sore throat, and enlargement and pain in the cervical lymph nodes. Enlargement of the spleen occurs in about half of all people with the illness.

Laboratory findings include increased lymphocytes and monocytes; about one-fifth of the cells are atypical in form. The WBC count increases and remains high for 4 to 8 weeks. Platelet counts are often low during the illness.

Recovery occurs in 2 to 3 weeks. However, weakness and lethargy may last for up to 3 months. Treatment includes bed rest and analgesics to relieve the symptoms.

Note: The reference and resource listings for all chapters have been compiled at the back of the book.

Chapter Review

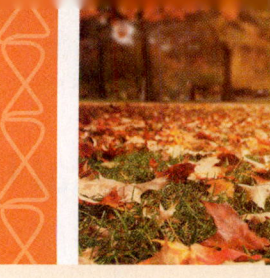

KEY POINTS

- **Concept:** Because of the role the blood plays in transporting oxygen and nutrients to the cells, responding to infection, and preventing significant fluid loss due to injury, hematologic disorders can have wide-ranging effects on patients' daily living activities.
- **Concept:** Disorders of the red blood cells affect the body's ability to carry oxygen to the tissues. As a result, the patient often experiences symptoms such as fatigue and activity intolerance.
- Anemia (lack of RBCs and hemoglobin) is a common disorder that can lead to cellular hypoxia, causing weakness and fatigue. Anemia often is chronic; teaching about its management is a primary nursing intervention.
- Polycythemia (too many RBCs) usually develops secondarily to chronic hypoxia, for example, in patients with chronic lung disease. Too many RBCs increase the viscosity or "stickiness" of the blood.
- **Concept:** The primary function of WBCs is to fight off infection, destroy foreign matter, and eliminate damaged or abnormal cells in the body; WBC disorders affect immune function.
- Leukemia is a malignancy in which abnormal WBCs multiply, gradually replacing normal bone marrow and impairing the ability to form normal blood cells and fight off infection. The risk factors, treatment, and prognosis for different types of leukemia vary. Nursing care focuses on protecting the patient from injury and infection.
- Malignant lymphoma involves lymphoid tissues, including lymph nodes. Hodgkin lymphoma more frequently responds to treatment than non-Hodgkin lymphoma. People whose immune systems are suppressed are at particular risk for developing malignant lymphoma.
- Multiple myeloma is a WBC malignancy that affects B lymphocytes called plasma cells. These cells invade bone marrow, lymph nodes, and other tissues causing bone pain and a high risk for pathologic fractures.
- **Concept:** Adequate numbers of platelets and all of the proteins involved in the clotting cascade are necessary for the body to form stable clots and to achieve hemostasis. Patients with low platelet counts or missing clotting factors are at risk for bleeding and hemorrhage.
- Platelets are vital to the process of blood clotting (coagulation) and control of bleeding. Patients with thrombocytopenia (low platelet count) are at significant risk for bleeding.
- Hemophilia is a clotting disorder that is genetically transmitted. In hemophilia, lack of a specific clotting factor interrupts the clotting cascade, which leads to a significant risk for bleeding with minor injuries.
- **Concept:** The lymphatic system plays an important role in the immune response and in removing damaged and abnormal cells and foreign matter from the body. Lymph nodes often swell during infections, and lymph vessels can become inflamed or obstructed.
- Painless swelling of a lymph node, however, may indicate a malignancy such as Hodgkin lymphoma, non-Hodgkin lymphoma, or others.

PEARSON NURSING STUDENT RESOURCES

Find additional materials at **nursing.pearsonhighered.com**.

Clinical Reasoning Care Map

Caring for a Patient With Acute Myeloid Leukemia
NCLEX-PN® Focus Area: Safe, Effective Care Environment

Case Study: Catherine Cole is a 37-year-old secretary. About 2 months ago, she began to tire easily and experience night sweats and an intermittent fever. She also noticed that her skin was pale, she bruised easily, and she was having heavier menstrual periods. After seeing her primary care physician, Mrs. Cole is admitted to the hospital for a bone marrow biopsy.

Nursing Diagnosis: Ineffective Protection

COLLECT DATA

Subjective	Objective
_____	_____
_____	_____
_____	_____
_____	_____
_____	_____
_____	_____

Does this present a threat to the patient's safety?

If yes, the priority intervention to address this threat would be:

_____

Nursing Care

_____
_____
_____
_____
_____
_____
_____
_____
_____

Interprofessional team members to include when planning care:

_____

How would you document this? _____

_____

Data Collected
(use only those that apply)

- States, "I'm so tired, and I have these bruises all over me. I'm so afraid of the results of the bone marrow test. I don't know what we will do if I have cancer."
- 5'4" (156 cm) tall, weighs 106 lb (48.1 kg)
- Vital signs T 100°F; P 102; R 22; BP 120/82
- Night sweats and intermittent fever for the past 2 months
- Numerous petechiae scattered over trunk and arms
- Ecchymoses on lower right arm and right calf
- Relates menstrual periods heavier than normal
- Oral mucosa red, with several small ulcerations in buccal areas
- Low RBC count; low hemoglobin and hematocrit; low platelets; high WBC count; myeloblasts present

Nursing Interventions
(use only those that apply; list in priority order)

- Frequently assess for and report signs of bleeding such as increased bruising, joint pain, occult blood in body fluids, and menstrual pad count.
- Limit visitors to husband and daughter.
- Teach about the bone marrow biopsy. Allow time for questions.
- Take and record vital signs every 4 hours.
- Assist with oral hygiene every 2 to 4 hours, using a soft-bristle toothbrush or a sponge. Offer warm saline or dilute hydrogen peroxide mouth rinses.
- Place in a private room.
- Encourage to alternate activity with rest.
- Verbally and in writing remind staff, family, and the patient to practice good hand washing. Post a sign in the room as a reminder, and discuss the importance of hand washing with Mrs. Cole and her family.
- Refer to oncology nurse specialist.

Compare your answers and documentation to those provided on the companion website.

NCLEX-PN® Exam Preparation

1 A 19-year-old patient is admitted in sickle cell crisis. The FIRST nursing action would be to:
1. administer pain medications.
2. obtain blood samples for analysis.
3. administer antibiotics.
4. insert a Foley catheter.

2 A patient is admitted with a diagnosis of pernicious anemia. Priority nursing care would include:
1. preventing infection.
2. increasing iron intake.
3. providing rest periods.
4. increasing fluid intake.

3 An LPN/LVN is assigned to a patient with thrombocytopenia. A priority goal of nursing care is:
1. prevention of infection.
2. prevention of injury.
3. prevention of dehydration.
4. prevention of nutritional deficit.

4 A 19-year-old patient with hemophilia A wants to join an athletic team in college. Which of the following sports would be most appropriate?
1. Hockey
2. Golf
3. Basketball
4. Baseball

5 The nurse establishes a nursing diagnosis of Impaired Oral Mucous Membrane for a patient with leukemia who is experiencing stomatitis. Patient teaching would include which of the following interventions? **Select all that apply.**
1. Use of warm saline as a mouth rinse
1. Application of petroleum jelly to the lips
2. Increased intake of citrus fruit juice
3. Intake of cool liquids for hydration
4. Use of viscous lidocaine to relieve discomfort

6 A patient developed disseminated intravascular coagulation (DIC) after injuries sustained in an automobile collision. Which of the following, if observed, requires intervention by the nurse?
1. The patient has two pillows under her knees.
2. The patient is resting on her right side.
3. The patient has oxygen per nasal cannula at 5 L/min.
4. The patient has cool compresses to her knees.

7 A patient diagnosed with multiple myeloma asks the nurse what she should expect when undergoing radiation therapy. The most appropriate response would be that:
1. the skin may look and feel sunburned over the radiated area.
2. radiation therapy is painless and has few side effects.
3. although radiation therapy is painful, it will help reduce the size of the tumor.
4. the patient will need to be careful to avoid exposing the family to the radiation.

8 A patient develops lymphedema of her left arm after a left radical mastectomy. Discharge teaching would include:
1. removing antiembolic stockings or pressure devices daily.
2. elevating the extremity when seated or in bed.
3. inspecting the skin every other day.
4. adding low-potassium foods to the diet.

9 A patient is evaluated for possible Hodgkin lymphoma. Which of the following assessment findings would be expected?
1. Enlarged cervical lymph node
2. Absent Reed–Sternberg cells
3. Negative Epstein–Barr virus
4. Immovable, painful inguinal lymph nodes

10 The nurse develops a nursing diagnosis of Risk for Infection for a patient with leukemia. The best action by the nurse would be to:
1. require visitors with colds or flu to wear masks.
2. wash hands when leaving the room.
3. document signs of infection in the medical record.
4. maintain protective isolation protocols at all times.

Answers and rationales for Review Questions appear in Appendix I.

You are an LPN/LVN working for a group of hematologists in Denver, Colorado. The following patients come to the clinic for diagnostic procedures and follow-up treatment.

Sheri is a 76-year-old widow who lives alone. Sheri has lost 20 lb (9 kg) since her husband died 8 months ago. She says she feels weak and sometimes has heart palpitations. She states she liked to cook when her husband was alive, but preparing a meal for herself seems senseless. She usually has nothing for breakfast; a bologna sandwich and a cup of coffee for lunch; and a hot dog or two, a few cookies, and a glass of milk for dinner. Diagnostic tests indicate folic acid deficiency anemia.

Toby and Victoria, a young married Black couple, hope to become pregnant soon. They are concerned because Victoria's brother has sickle cell disease. They don't want their children to have this disorder. Toby has no family history of sickle cell disease. They have undergone testing and have an appointment today to discuss the results and their options with the doctor.

Ione, a 42-year-old Filipino, has been working in the United States in order to send money to his family in Davao City, Philippines. Ione tells you his home in Davao City is very small and on "stilts" over the ocean. He is a heavy smoker. Ione has developed hypertension and mild heart failure. He has been recently diagnosed with polycythemia. The doctor has ordered a 400-mL phlebotomy.

CRITICAL THINKING

- What psychosocial issue may be affecting Sheri's appetite?

- Because Victoria's brother has sickle cell disease, there is a high probability she is a carrier of the disorder. Using the figure in Box 20-1, explain the probability of their children being carriers of, or having, the disorder.

- What factors contributed to Ione developing polycythemia?

PRIORITIES IN NURSING CARE

- Which has a higher priority in planning Sheri's care: nutrition teaching or helping her understand her depression?

- After the doctor explains to Toby and Victoria their lab results, what is the priority nursing intervention?

- What is the priority nursing intervention in planning care for Ione: providing him with information on smoking cessation or completing the phlebotomy?

MANAGEMENT OF CARE

- Suggest interventions that might assist Sheri to have an improved nutritional intake.

- Do you anticipate Toby and Victoria will need another follow-up appointment?

- What are some possible consequences of removing blood from Ione too rapidly?

DELEGATING

- Can Sheri's nutrition teaching be delegated to the medical assistant, or should the LPN/LVN retain responsibility for it? Why or why not?

- Is performing the phlebotomy within scope of practice for LPN/LVNs in your state? How would you find the answer to this question?

TEACHING

- Why was Sheri placed on a folic acid supplement in addition to dietary modifications?

- In addition to teaching about sickle cell disease, are there any other teaching topics that should be presented to Toby and Victoria at this time?

- What nursing interventions should Ione be taught to prevent further complications of polycythemia?

CULTURAL CARE STRATEGIES

- Because Ione has lived most of his life in the Philippines, what cultural differences may need to be considered before patient teaching?

DOCUMENTING AND REPORTING

- What aspects of care for each patient need to be reported to the RN or doctor?

- Write a focus note documenting the 400-mL phlebotomy you performed on Ione.

Note: Discussion of Unit questions appears on the companion website.

UNIT V
Disrupted Respiratory Function

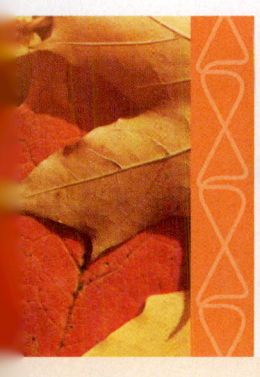
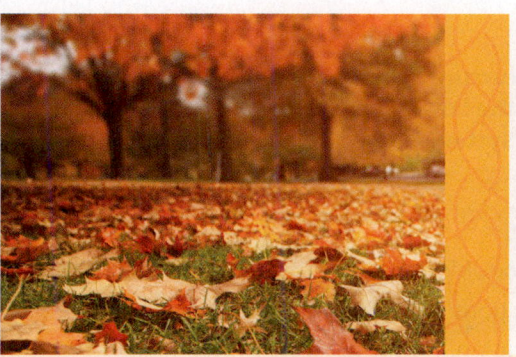
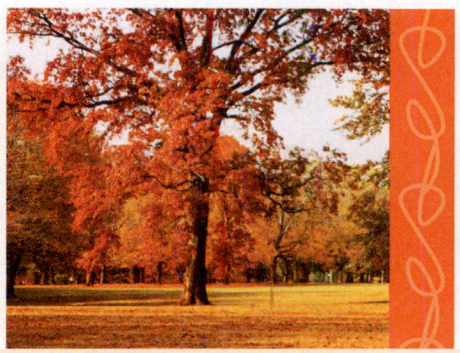
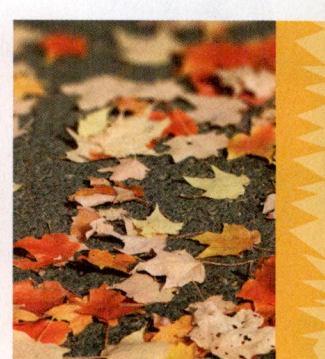

Cultural Care Strategies:

Unit V Wrap-Up

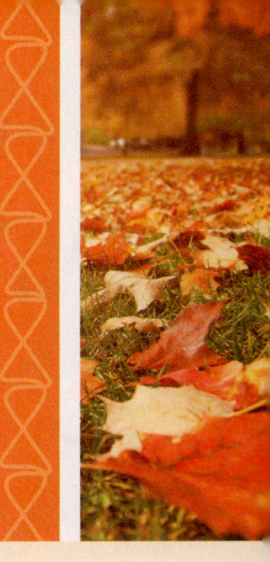

CHAPTER 21
The Respiratory System and Assessment

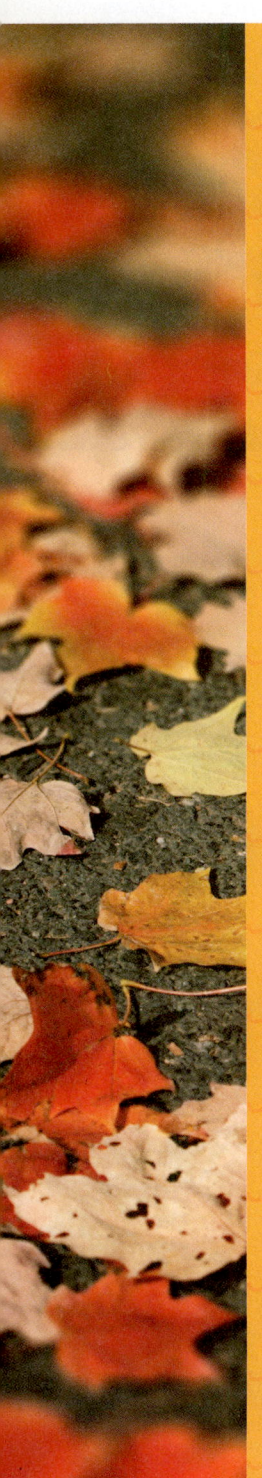

BRIEF OUTLINE

Structure and Function of the Upper Respiratory Tract

Structure and Function of the Lower Respiratory System

Assessment

APPLIED LEARNING OUTCOMES

After completing this chapter, you will be able to:

1. Describe the structure and functions of the respiratory tract.
2. Explain the mechanics of respiration.
3. Conduct and appropriately document a focused assessment of the upper and lower respiratory systems, demonstrating sensitivity and respect for individual concerns, values, and preferences.
4. Provide appropriate nursing care and teaching for patients undergoing diagnostic tests and procedures related to the respiratory system.
5. Monitor diagnostic test results, recognizing and communicating abnormal or unexpected findings within the interprofessional team.

KEY TERMS

The key terms are defined on the pages listed below.

adventitious, 517

barrel chest, 517

compliance, 515

respiration, 513

ventilation, 515

SPECIAL FEATURES

CULTURAL CARE STRATEGIES: Considering Cultural Variations Related to Time, 525

The respiratory system includes the air passages, the lungs, and the structures necessary for effective respiration.

Structure and Function of the Upper Respiratory Tract

Air moves into the lungs and carbon dioxide moves out of the body through the upper respiratory tract. The upper airway cleans, humidifies, and warms air. An open upper airway is needed for effective breathing.

NOSE AND SINUSES

The respiratory system begins at the *nose* (Figure 21-1A■). Cartilage and the facial bones give the nose structure. The nostrils (*nares*) are two cavities in the nose, separated by the *nasal septum*. They open into the nasal portion of the pharynx. Nasal hairs just inside the nares filter air as it enters the nose. The air is warmed by mucous membranes lining the nares. Mucous membranes contain scent receptors and cells that secrete thick mucus. The mucus traps dust and bacteria and contains an enzyme that destroys bacteria. The mucus and trapped debris are moved to the pharynx and then swallowed. Ridges within each nasal cavity help trap heavier particles of debris.

The *sinuses* are openings in the facial bones (Figure 21-1B■). Sinuses lighten the skull, assist in speech, and produce mucus that drains into the nasal cavities and helps trap debris.

PHARYNX

The *pharynx* (throat) is a passageway for both air and food. It is divided into three regions: the nasopharynx, oropharynx, and laryngopharynx.

The *nasopharynx* starts at the nose. Air, mucus, and trapped debris move through the nasopharynx, where the *tonsils* and *adenoids* (masses of lymphoid tissue in the back wall of the nasopharynx) trap and destroy infectious agents. The *auditory tubes* also open into the nasopharynx, connecting it with the middle ear.

The *oropharynx* lies behind the oral cavity. It carries both air and food. During swallowing, the soft palate (see Figure 21-1A) rises to prevent food from entering the nasopharynx. The lining of the oropharynx protects it from damage by friction and from chemicals in food and fluids.

The *laryngopharynx*, a passageway for both food and air, connects the oropharynx to the larynx.

LARYNX

The *larynx* (voice box) connects the laryngopharynx with the trachea and routes air and food into the proper passageway. The larynx is protected by cartilages that help keep it open (see Figure 21-1A). The inlet to the larynx (the *epiglottis*) is open when air is moving through it; during swallowing, the epiglottis tips down to cover the opening of the larynx. The larynx also contains the vocal cords, which help produce speech. If anything other than air enters the larynx, its muscles contract to close the larynx. At the same time, a cough reflex is initiated to expel the foreign substance before it can reach the lungs.

Structure and Function of the Lower Respiratory System

The lower respiratory system includes the lungs and the bronchi. Its function is to provide oxygen to the cells of the body and to eliminate carbon dioxide, a waste product of metabolism. This process, called **respiration**, includes:

■ *Ventilation* (breathing): Air moves into and out of the lungs.

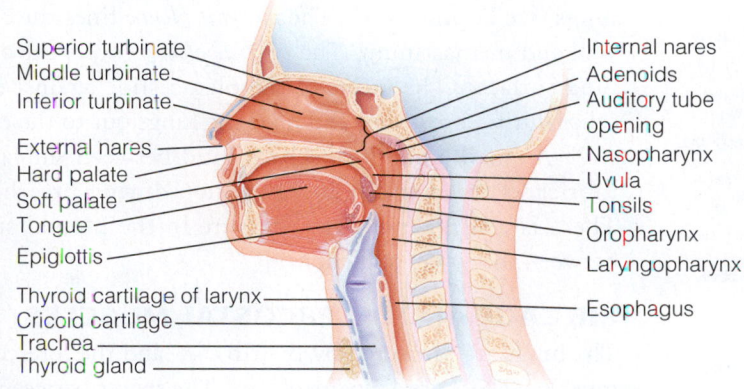

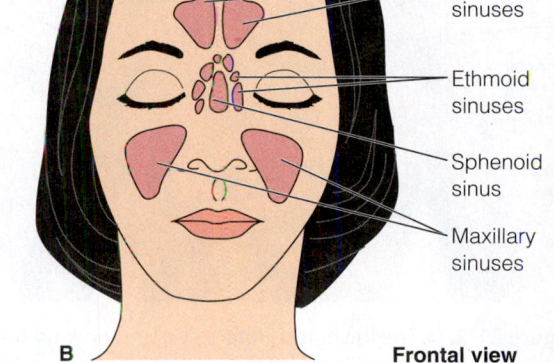

Figure 21-1. ■ (**A**) Structures of the upper respiratory tract. (**B**) The sinuses.

- *External respiration*: Oxygen and carbon dioxide are exchanged between the alveoli and the blood.
- *Gas transport*: Blood transports oxygen and carbon dioxide to and from the lungs and the cells of the body.
- *Internal respiration*: Oxygen and carbon dioxide are exchanged between the blood and the cells.

LUNGS

The lungs fill both sides of the chest, separated by a space called the *mediastinum*. The heart, great blood vessels, bronchi, trachea, and esophagus sit in the mediastinum (Figure 21-2■). The *apex* of each lung lies just below the clavicle, and the *base* of each lung rests on the diaphragm. The lungs are soft and spongy, composed of elastic connective tissue.

The right lung has three lobes; the left is smaller, with only two lobes. Each lobe is further divided into segments.

BRONCHI AND ALVEOLI

The trachea divides into *right* and *left main (or primary) bronchi*. The main bronchi enter the lungs at the *hilus*. The bronchi branch into smaller bronchi and then into smaller and smaller *bronchioles*, ending in the tiny *alveoli* (Figure 21-3■). During inspiration, air moves through these passageways to the alveoli, where gas exchange occurs.

Each lung has millions of alveoli, providing a huge area for gas exchange. Alveoli have extremely thin walls, just a single layer of cells over a very thin connective tissue (basement) membrane. The outer surface of the alveolus is covered with pulmonary capillaries. Oxygen and carbon dioxide

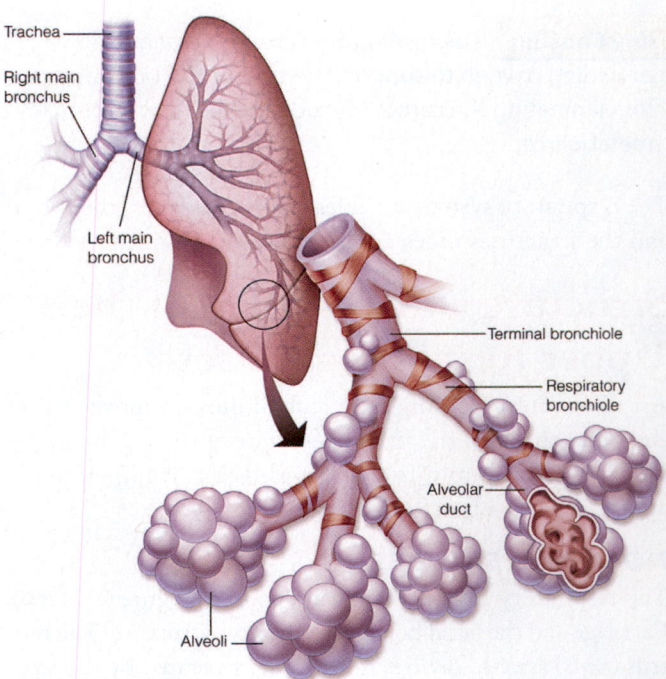

Figure 21-3. ■ The functional tissue of the lungs, including the respiratory bronchioles and alveoli. (Source: Pearson Education.)

easily diffuse between the alveoli and capillaries. The alveoli contain cells that secrete *surfactant*, a detergent-like substance that helps keep the lungs open.

PULMONARY CIRCULATION

The pulmonary circulation includes the pulmonary arteries and pulmonary veins. The pulmonary arteries deliver blood from body tissues via the right heart to the lungs to be oxygenated. The pulmonary veins return oxygenated blood to the left heart, to be pumped out to the rest of the body. In the lungs, the vessels branch into a pulmonary capillary network that surrounds the alveoli. Blood vessels enter and exit the lungs at the hilus.

PLEURA

The *pleura* is a double-layered membrane that covers the lungs (see Figure 21-2). The *parietal pleura* lines the chest wall and mediastinum. The *visceral pleura* covers the outer lung surfaces. The layers of the pleura slide against each other during breathing and hold the lungs out to the chest wall. A small amount of serous fluid between the layers lubricates them and reduces friction during breathing. There is a slight negative pressure in the pleural space between the layers of pleura.

RIB CAGE AND INTERCOSTAL MUSCLES

The lungs are protected by the rib cage and the intercostal muscles. There are 12 pairs of ribs. The spaces between the ribs (the *intercostal spaces*) are named for the rib immediately

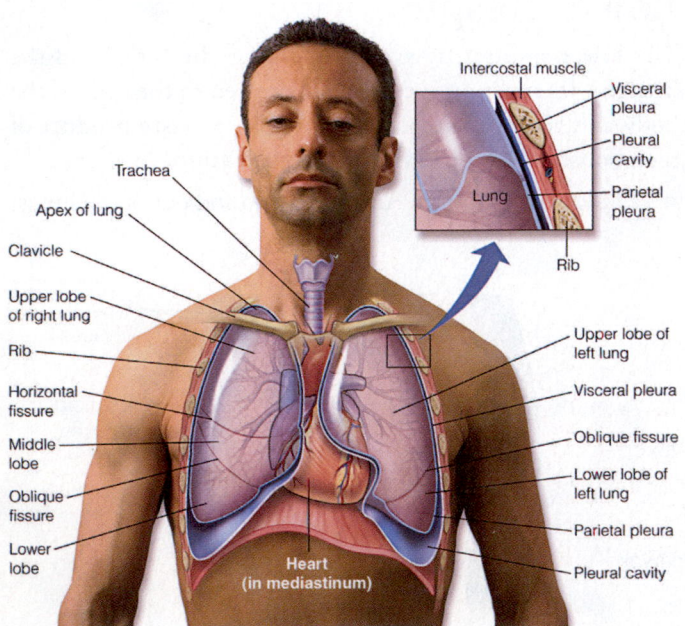

Figure 21-2. ■ The lower respiratory system, showing the lungs, the mediastinum, and layers of the visceral and parietal pleura. (Source: Patrick Watson, Pearson Education.)

above (e.g., the space between the third and fourth ribs is the third intercostal space). The *intercostal muscles* between the ribs, along with the diaphragm, are *inspiratory muscles*.

MECHANICS OF RESPIRATION

Ventilation, air movement into and out of the lungs, has two phases: *inspiration*, as air flows into the lungs, and *expiration*, when gases flow out of the lungs. The two phases make up a breath and normally occur 12 to 20 times per minute. Inspiration lasts about 1 to 1.5 seconds; expiration lasts about 2 to 3 seconds.

During inspiration, the diaphragm contracts and flattens out and the intercostal muscles contract to pull the rib cage up and outward. Together, these movements increase the size of the chest cavity (Figure 21-4A■). The lungs stretch and their volume increases. This reduces the pressure within the lungs to slightly less than atmospheric pressure. As a result, air rushes into the lungs.

Expiration is primarily passive. The inspiratory muscles relax, the diaphragm rises, the ribs descend, and the lungs recoil (Figure 21-4B■). Pressures in the chest cavity increase, compressing the alveoli. The pressure within the lungs is higher than atmospheric pressure, and gases flow out of the lungs.

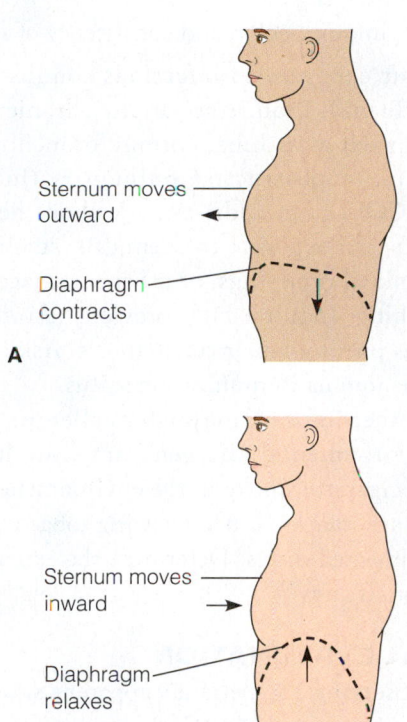

Sternum moves outward

Diaphragm contracts

A

Sternum moves inward

Diaphragm relaxes

B

Figure 21-4. ■ (A) During inspiration, the diaphragm contracts and flattens, and the intercostal muscles contract, moving the chest wall up and outward. This increases the volume of the chest cavity, causing air to enter the lungs. **(B)** During expiration, the muscles relax, the diaphragm rises, and the lungs recoil, causing air to exit the lungs.

FACTORS AFFECTING RESPIRATION

Breathing is controlled by respiratory centers in the brain and by chemoreceptors in the brain, aortic arch, and carotid arteries. These centers and receptors respond to changes in the amount of oxygen, carbon dioxide, and hydrogen ions in arterial blood. For example, increased carbon dioxide or a drop in pH stimulates the respiratory centers, and the respiratory rate increases.

memory**ALERT**

Remember, the relationship between the amount of hydrogen ion in a fluid (e.g., the blood) and its pH is *reciprocal*. This means that as the amount of hydrogen ion increases, the pH falls. On the other hand, as the amount of hydrogen ion decreases, the pH rises.

Other factors that affect ventilation and the work of breathing are the following:

- *Airway resistance* is created by friction as gases move through the airways. Resistance is increased by airway constriction or edema, excess mucus, or tumors that narrow the airways. As resistance increases, gas flow decreases and the work of breathing increases.
- **Compliance** is the *distensibility* (stretchiness) of the lungs. It depends on both the lung tissue and the rib cage.
- *Elasticity* is the tendency of lung tissue to return to its uninflated size and shape.
- Alveoli contain a liquid film that creates *surface tension*, drawing the walls of the alveolus closer together. *Surfactant* reduces this surface tension, prevents the alveoli from collapsing between breaths, and reduces the work of breathing.

memory**ALERT**

A balloon is a good example of compliance and elasticity. When a balloon is brand new, it is very elastic and not very compliant—it takes a lot of work to begin inflating it (poor compliance). When the air is released, the balloon returns to its previous shape (good elasticity). After it has been blown up a few times, it becomes increasingly compliant and easier to inflate. However, it does not return to its original shape, because some of its elasticity has been lost.

RESPIRATORY CHANGES ASSOCIATED WITH AGING

Aging commonly leads to changes in both the structure and function of the respiratory system (Figure 21-5■).

- Cartilage that connects the ribs to the sternum and spinal column calcifies (hardens), decreasing the mobility of the rib cage.
- The anterior–posterior diameter of the chest increases.
- Respiratory muscles become weaker.

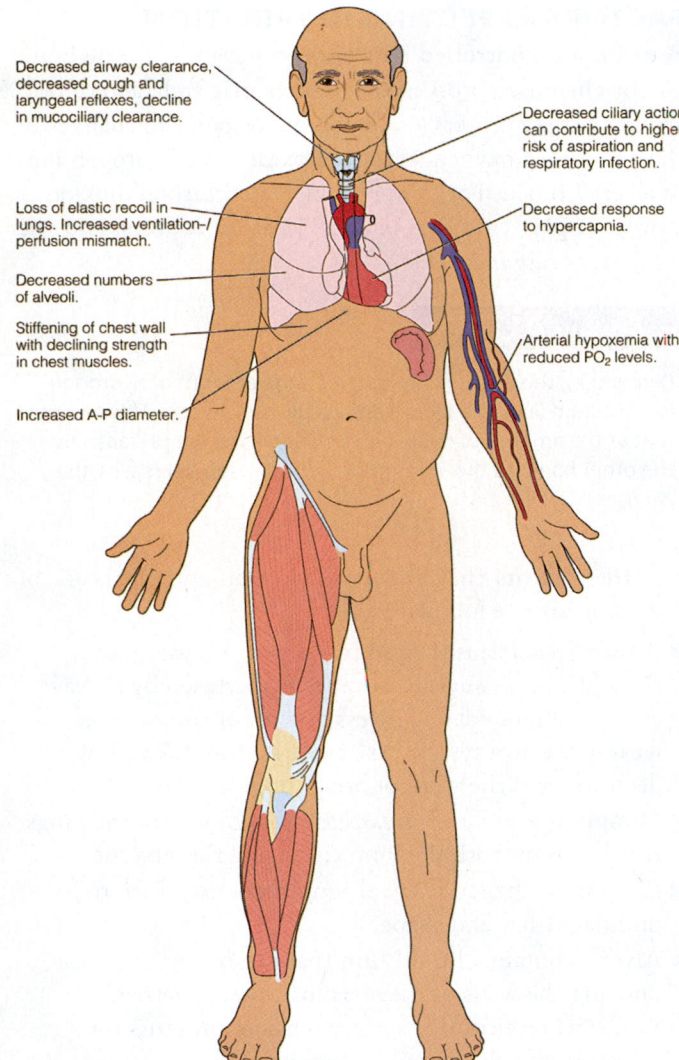

Decreased airway clearance, decreased cough and laryngeal reflexes, decline in mucociliary clearance.

Decreased ciliary action can contribute to higher risk of aspiration and respiratory infection.

Loss of elastic recoil in lungs. Increased ventilation-/perfusion mismatch.

Decreased response to hypercapnia.

Decreased numbers of alveoli.

Stiffening of chest wall with declining strength in chest muscles.

Arterial hypoxemia with reduced PO_2 levels.

Increased A-P diameter.

Figure 21-5. ■ Changes in the respiratory system associated with aging. (Source: Pearson Education.)

- The cough and laryngeal reflexes are less effective.
- The overall size of the lungs is reduced, and alveoli are less elastic (less able to fully recoil on expiration). This loss of elasticity increases the amount of air remaining in the lungs after exhaling (the residual volume) and reduces vital capacity.

As a result of these changes, the patient is at greater risk for developing respiratory infections and being unable to effectively clear secretions from the alveoli and airways.

Assessment

> **Key Concept** The critical role of the respiratory system in supporting body cells, tissues, and organs makes nursing assessment of respiratory function vital in all patients. The nurse needs to be able to recognize and respond appropriately to abnormal or unexpected findings.

Nursing assessment of respiratory function is particularly important when caring for patients with disorders and diseases affecting the respiratory system as well as those who are at risk for respiratory complications of other disorders. It is an especially important component when assessing older adults.

SUBJECTIVE DATA

Collect information from the patient (or family, if necessary) about the current complaint or reason for seeking care. Ask about the onset and duration of symptoms. Address how symptoms have affected the patient's ability to maintain daily living activities. Specifically inquire about the following, as appropriate:

- Nasal congestion, difficulty breathing through one nare, or nosebleeds
- Sore throat or difficult or painful swallowing
- Change in voice quality
- Difficult or painful breathing and ability to breathe when lying down
- Effect of activity on ease of breathing and effect of ability to breathe on activity
- Chest wall pain, effect of deep breathing, coughing, or movement on pain
- Presence of cough, including timing, severity, and production of mucus
- If present, amount, color, and consistency of sputum

Ask about exposure to infectious conditions such as colds or influenza. Inquire about any chronic respiratory conditions, such as asthma, chronic bronchitis, emphysema, or chronic obstructive pulmonary (lung) disease (COPD or COLD). In addition, ask about heart failure. Discuss potential exposure to chemicals, smoke, asbestos, coal dust, animal droppings, or other substances known to affect breathing. Inquire about previous respiratory problems such as pneumonia or tuberculosis. Ask about influenza and pneumonia immunization status.

Obtain other information such as allergies to medications or environmental allergens, smoking history, and exposure to cigarette smoke in the environment. Ask about use of other substances such as chewing tobacco, marijuana, cocaine, or injected drugs. Determine the extent of alcohol consumption, if any.

PHYSICAL EXAMINATION

Begin by observing the patient's apparent state of health, color, and ease of breathing. Note the respiratory rate and pattern. Observe for flaring of the nares, use of accessory muscles of respiration (muscles of the neck, shoulders, abdomen), and any signs of difficult or painful breathing. Listen to the patient's speech for hoarseness or pausing to breathe or cough.

Inspect mucosa of the nares (using an otoscope with a nasal speculum), the mouth, and the oropharynx, being

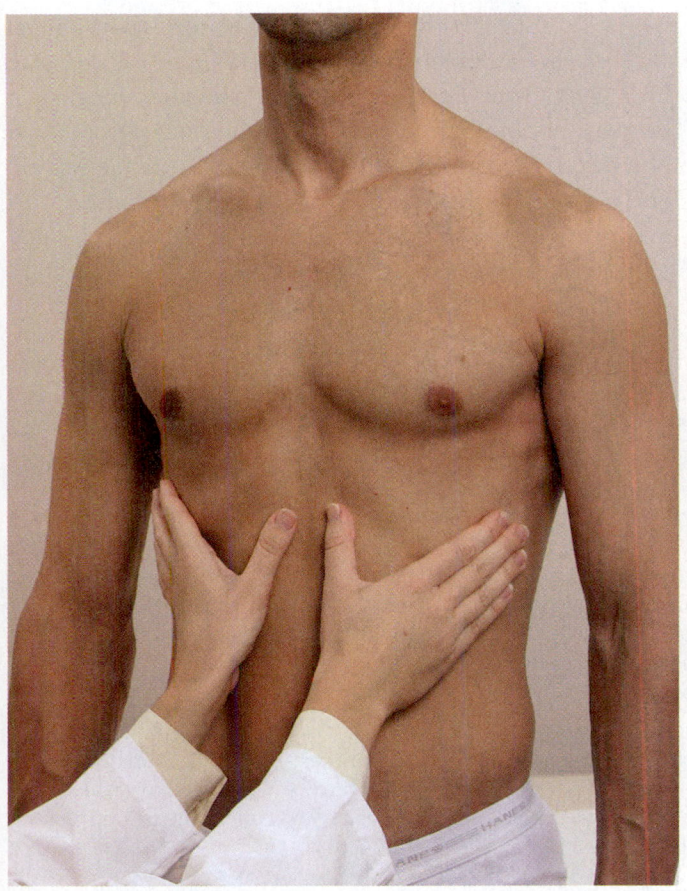
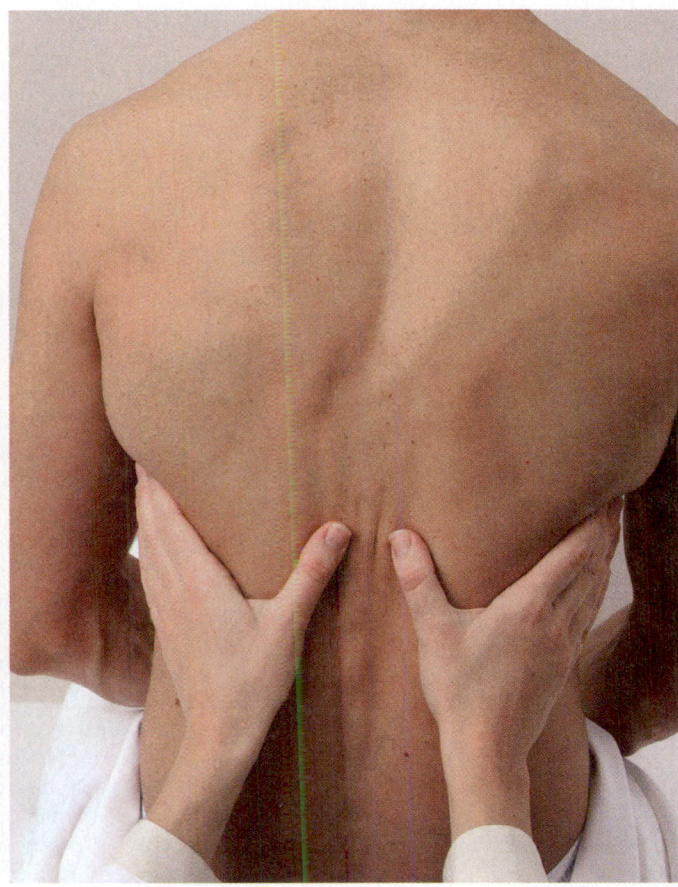

A

B

Figure 21-6. ■ Palpating for equality of chest expansion. (Source: Patrick Watson, Pearson Education.)

sure to check under the tongue and between the cheeks and gums. Inspect the neck for position of the trachea and any apparent swelling. Observe for equal movement of the chest with respirations. Look for **barrel chest**, an increased anterior–posterior (AP) chest diameter.

Palpate the lips for nodules. Assess salivary glands and cervical and supraclavicular lymph nodes for swelling or tenderness. Lightly palpate the chest for tenderness and equality of respiratory movement (Figure 21-6■).

Using the diaphragm of the stethoscope, auscultate the anterior, posterior, and lateral thorax for breath sounds (Figure 21-7■). Note the presence and quality of breath sounds, as well as any abnormal (**adventitious**) breath sounds (e.g., wheezes, crackles) and their location. An example of documentation of a respiratory assessment is presented in Box 21-1■.

DIAGNOSTIC TESTS

A number of diagnostic tests are used to evaluate respiratory function. Some, such as the complete blood count with white blood cell differential (CBC with diff), are not specific to the respiratory system, but provide very useful information. This section focuses on those tests that are used

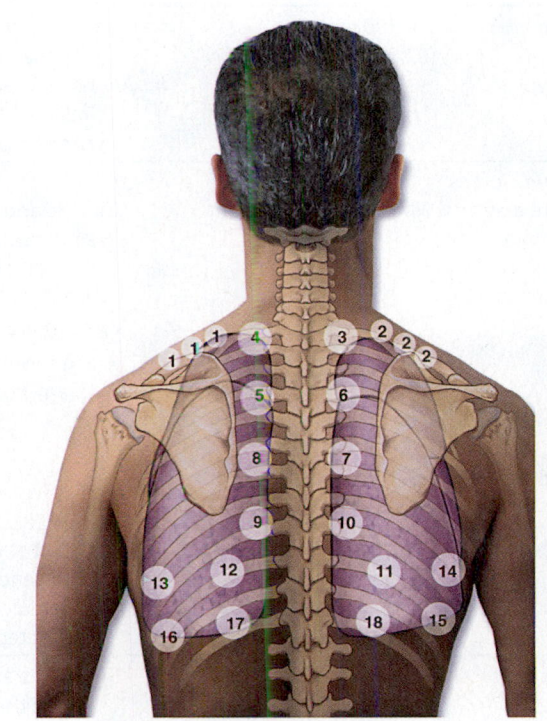

Figure 21-7. ■ Sequence for lung auscultation on the back. (Source: Patrick Watson, Pearson Education.)

primarily to evaluate the respiratory system and diagnose respiratory disorders. Commonly ordered laboratory tests and imaging studies are summarized in Tables 21-1■ and 21-2■. Figure 21-8■ illustrates a pulse oximetry unit to measure oxygen saturation.

Sputum and Tissue Specimens

When infection of the upper or lower respiratory system is suspected, nasal or throat swabs or a sputum specimen is obtained for culture of pathogens. Culture requires 24 to 48 hours for bacterial growth; some pathogens, such as the organism that causes tuberculosis, require longer to grow. For this reason, a sputum smear may be analyzed by Gram staining or for acid-fast bacillus. Nursing responsibilities for obtaining a throat swab are outlined in Box 21-2■; Box 21-3■ details the steps for obtaining a sputum specimen. Tests often performed on sputum specimens are outlined in Table 21-1, along with normal or expected results and specific nursing responsibilities.

TABLE 21-1	Common Laboratory Tests and Studies		
TEST	**NORMAL ADULT VALUES**	**EXPLANATION**	**NURSING RESPONSIBILITIES**
Pulse oximetry	95% or higher	Pulse oximetry is a noninvasive test used to evaluate and monitor oxygen saturation (SaO_2, the percentage of arterial hemoglobin that is combined with oxygen) of blood. The sensor evaluates oxygen saturation by measuring the amount of red and infrared light absorbed by hemoglobin.	The pulse oximeter sensor is applied to a fingertip, the forehead, nose, or earlobe in adults (see Figure 21-8). Lower SaO_2 values indicate impaired lung ventilation and/or gas exchange. Promptly report values of 90% or lower.
Arterial blood gases (ABGs)	pH 7.35–7.45 $PaCO_2$ 35–45 mm Hg PaO_2 75–100 mm Hg HCO_3 24–28 mEq/L Base excess (BE) −2 to +2 mEq/L	ABGs are used to assess acid–base imbalances caused by a respiratory or a metabolic disorder. The $PaCO_2$ reflects air movement into and out of the alveoli. The PaO_2 shows how much oxygen is available to combine with hemoglobin and be transported to the cells. The HCO_3 and BE are used to evaluate bicarbonate, the major buffer in the blood.	Apply pressure to the site for at least 5 minutes after arterial puncture. Arteries are high-pressure vessels that may bleed into the tissue after puncture. Promptly report ABG results to the charge nurse or physician, particularly when values are abnormal or outside the expected range for the patient.
Serum alpha$_1$-antitrypsin (α_1AT)	78–200 mg/dL (0.78–2.0 g/L)	Alpha$_1$-antitrypsin levels are used to determine whether a deficiency of this protein may have caused emphysema and COPD. Inflammatory processes, exercise, and oral contraceptives increase blood levels.	Food and fluids (except water) are restricted for 8 hours before the test. Oral contraceptives are held for 24 hours before testing. Note the name of the oral contraceptive on the lab slip.
Sputum studies Culture and sensitivity (C&S) Gram stain	No pathogens present	Culture and sensitivity testing is done on a single sputum specimen to identify the infecting organism and to help determine which antibiotic will eradicate it. Gram stain may be used to rapidly identify organisms by their staining qualities (gram-positive or gram-negative).	If possible, collect the specimen in the early morning. Use Standard Precautions and sterile technique when collecting the specimen. If the patient is unable to produce sputum, an *induced sputum* specimen may be ordered. The patient inhales a saline mist, which stimulates a cough. Clearly label the specimen as "induced specimen" to alert the laboratory.
Acid-fast stain	Negative for acid-fast bacillus	Acid-fast stain is used to show the presence or absence of acid-fast bacillus (e.g., tuberculosis) when tuberculosis is suspected.	Three sputum specimens, collected in the early morning, are advised when tuberculosis is suspected.
Cytology	No abnormal cells detected	Sputum is examined microscopically to detect the presence of abnormal (cancer) cells.	See above. May require several specimens. Sputum may be collected by bronchoscopy (see Box 21-4 later in the chapter).

<table>
<tr><td>

BOX 21-1   **DOCUMENTING RESPIRATORY ASSESSMENT**

Joanna Speisla, 72 years old, presents with complaints of the flu.

Relates 4-day history of chills, fever, headache, and sore throat. Developed a cough within past 24 hours; initially dry, now productive of thick, yellow-green sputum. States her general health is good. Denies history of serious or chronic heart or lung disease. Allergic to penicillin.

Appears in good general health, although acutely ill at this time. Does not show signs of acute respiratory distress; no nasal flaring or use of accessory muscles noted. Color good, skin very warm and dry. Frequent cough productive of small to moderate amounts of thick yellow sputum. No unusual odor noted. BP 134/86; P 92, reg; R 24, reg; T 101.5°F PO. Nasal mucosa pink and moist. Oropharynx red, no lesions noted. No cervical lymphadenopathy noted. Clear breath sounds noted throughout all lung fields; no adventitious sounds heard.
———————S. Wagner, LPN
</td></tr>
</table>

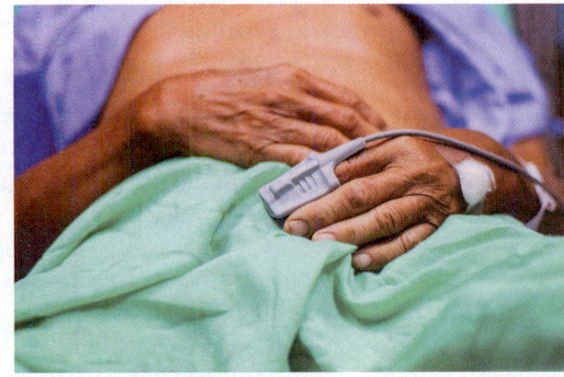

Figure 21-8. ■ Placement of the pulse oximetry sensor on a finger to measure oxygen saturation. (Source: Chaikom / Shutterstock.)

When a tumor is suspected, biopsy (examination of tissue cells) is performed. Tissue for biopsy may be obtained by using a needle to aspirate cells from a lymph node, by using a fiberoptic scope to examine the larynx or bronchi, or during surgery. Tissues are microscopically examined to determine the extent to which tumor cells have changed (differentiated) from normal cells (grading) and to detect whether tumor cells have spread beyond the primary site (staging).

Imaging Techniques

The chest x-ray and other radiologic studies such as CT scans are important diagnostic tools for detecting and evaluating respiratory disorders. Table 21-2 presents imaging studies that may be used to diagnose respiratory conditions.

X-rays and CT scans are used to identify the size and location of structures. They are also used to study blood flow through vessels and organs of the respiratory system. MRI or PET scans provide additional information about lung tissue and abnormalities. *Ventilation–perfusion (V/Q) scans* evaluate both ventilation (air movement) and perfusion

BOX 21-2   **PROCEDURE CHECKLIST**

Obtaining a Throat Swab

- ☑ Obtain a sterile cotton swab or throat swab kit.
- ☑ Identify the patient, explain the procedure, and provide for privacy.
- ☑ Place the patient in a sitting position if possible.
- ☑ Use Standard Precautions.
- ☑ Ask the patient to open the mouth, extend the tongue, and say "ah."
- ☑ Quickly swab the tonsils, reddened areas of the oropharynx, and any exudate (see illustration).
- ☑ Insert the swab into the specimen container. Avoid contaminating the outside of the container or the swab.
- ☑ Label the container.
- ☑ Send the specimen and requisition to the laboratory.

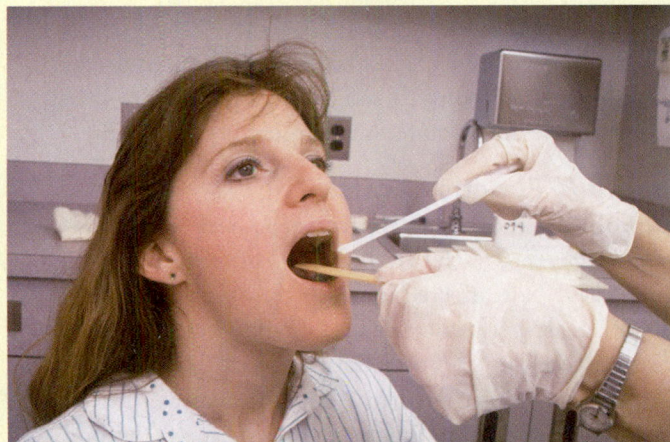

(Source: George Dobson, Pearson Education)

Sample Documentation

[date/time]   Oropharynx red, patches of white exudate noted on tonsils and oropharynx. Throat swab (oropharynx, tonsils, and exudate) obtained and sent to lab for culture.

_____J. Doene, LPN.

Note: Refer to a nursing fundamentals or skills text for more detailed instruction. Check state guidelines and facility policy before performing any procedure.

TABLE 21-2	Imaging Studies	
DIAGNOSTIC STUDY	**EXPLANATION AND PURPOSE**	**NURSING IMPLICATIONS**
X-ray of the head and neck	Used to evaluate the sinuses, larynx, or other tissues of the head and neck.	Have the patient remove jewelry (earrings, necklaces).
Chest x-ray	Used to evaluate the lungs, mediastinum, chest wall, and diaphragm. Detects masses, abscesses, and lung disorders such as pneumonia, obstructive lung disease, and atelectasis.	Although these studies are noninvasive, they expose the patient to potentially damaging radiation. Ask women of childbearing age about possible pregnancy before the exam.
Computed tomography (CT) scan of the head and neck or chest	Provides computer-generated images with more detail than standard x-rays. May be done with or without contrast media.	Ask the patient to remove jewelry. If contrast is used, inquire about allergies (to iodine, seafood or radiologic dye) and ensure that the patient is well hydrated to reduce the risk of kidney damage.
Magnetic resonance imaging (MRI) of the thorax	Used to diagnose lung tissue changes and to identify abnormal masses and fluid accumulation.	Inform the patient of the need to lie still during the examination. Ask about any metallic implants (e.g., pacemakers, joint prostheses, body piercing), notifying the physician if present. Remove transdermal medication patches unless otherwise ordered and replace the patch after the procedure. Patients with claustrophobia may need antianxiety medication before the procedure.
Positron emission tomography (PET)	Relatively noninvasive test; may be performed to identify lung nodules (cancers). The patient is given a radioactive substance, and cross-sectional images are displayed on a computer.	Tell the patient that no alcohol, coffee, or tobacco is allowed for 24 hours prior to the test. Encourage increased fluid intake post-test to help eliminate the radioactive material (LeMone et al., 2015).
Ventilation–perfusion scan (V/Q scan, nuclear medicine scan)	A radioactive gas is inhaled to evaluate lung ventilation; to evaluate blood flow, a radioisotope is injected. This exam is used to detect pulmonary emboli, evaluate chronic lung disease, and assess the function of lung transplants.	Explain the procedure and address fears about exposure to radioactivity (the amount is small and no special precautions are required). Some discomfort may occur during injection of the isotope. Obtain an accurate weight before the procedure.

(blood flow) of the lungs. They are most often used to identify a pulmonary embolus (blood clot in a pulmonary vessel) and may also be done before lung surgery is performed.

Pulmonary Function Tests

Lung volume and capacity are measured with *pulmonary function tests (PFTs)*. Lung volume and capacity (Figure 21-9 ■) are affected by sex, age, weight, and health status. PFTs are performed in a pulmonary function laboratory. After teaching and preparation, a nose clip is applied and the patient breathes into a device for measuring and recording lung volume in liters versus time in seconds. The patient is instructed to breathe in a specific manner for these tests, for example, to inhale as deeply as possible and then exhale as much air as possible. Because bronchodilators, smoking, and caffeine interfere with test results, bronchodilators are withheld for 4 to 6 hours before the test, and the patient is encouraged not to smoke or drink caffeinated beverages before the test.

Lung volume studies include the following:

- *Tidal volume (TV or Vt)*, the amount of air (about 500 mL) exchanged during normal quiet breathing
- *Inspiratory reserve volume (IRV)*, the amount (about 2,100 to 3,100 mL) that can be inhaled over and above a normal inspiration.
- *Expiratory reserve volume (ERV)*, the air (about 1,200 mL) that can be forced out after a normal exhalation
- *Residual volume (RV)*, the air (about 1,200 mL) remaining in the lungs after maximal exhalation

Lung capacities that are calculated include the following:

- *Total lung capacity (TLC)*, the total volume of the lungs at their maximum inflation (about 6,000 mL). It is calculated by adding the TV, IRV, ERV, and RV.
- *Vital capacity (VC)*, about 4,500 to 4,800 mL in healthy adults, is the sum of the TV, IRV, and ERV.

BOX 21-3   PROCEDURE CHECKLIST

Obtaining a Sputum Specimen

Before the Procedure

☑ Gather all supplies.

☑ Unless contraindicated by the patient's condition, obtain specimen before starting oxygen and/or antibiotic therapy.

☑ Unless otherwise specified, obtain specimen early morning, just after awakening.

☑ Increase fluid intake before obtaining specimen to help liquefy secretions.

Procedure

☑ Use Standard Precautions.

☑ Provide for privacy.

☑ Provide mouth care to reduce contamination by oral flora.

☑ Instruct to cough deeply several times, expectorating mucus into container.

☑ To obtain specimen by suctioning:

   ☑ Use aseptic technique.

   ☑ Attach sterile mucus trap between suction catheter and tubing.

   ☑ Perform tracheal suctioning.

☑ Detach and close mucus trap. Clear suction catheter and tubing and dispose of suction equipment appropriately.

☑ Close container securely using aseptic technique.

☑ Label container (name and other identifying data, time and date, and any special conditions).

☑ Enclose container in a clean plastic bag and send to laboratory.

After the Procedure

☑ Provide mouth care.

☑ Document the time and date the specimen was obtained and note its color, consistency, and odor.

Sample Documentation

[date]   Specimen of moderate amount thick green
[time]   odorless sputum obtained by deep coughing. Sent for culture and sensitivity.

_____S. Hamilton, LVN.

Note: Refer to a nursing fundamentals or skills text for more detailed instruction. Check state guidelines and facility policy before performing any procedure.

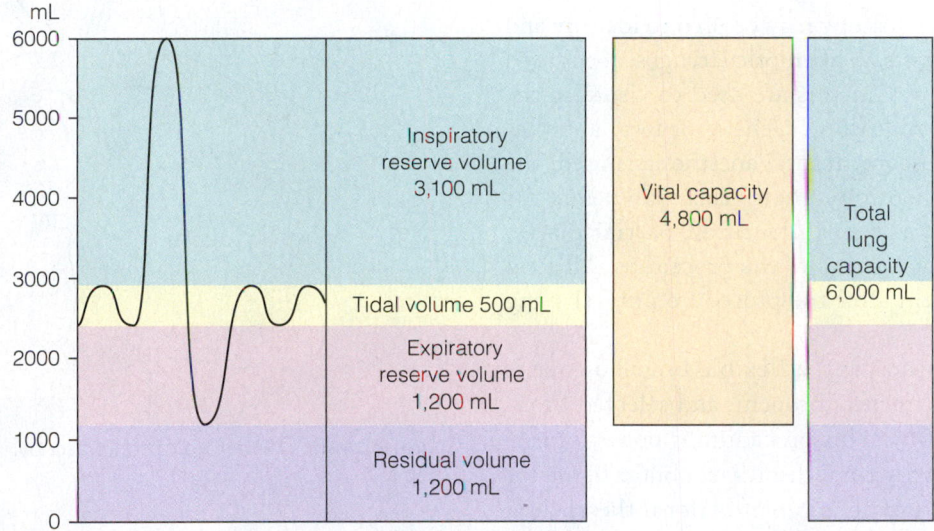

Figure 21-9. ■ The relationship of lung volumes and capacities. Volumes shown are for an average-size adult male.

About 150 mL of air remains in the airways with each breath, never reaching the alveoli. This is called *anatomic dead space volume.*

The rate of airflow during inspiration and expiration also may be measured during PFT:

■ *Peak expiratory flow (PEF),* the highest rate or speed of exhalation achieved after taking in the most air possible

■ *Peak inspiratory flow (PIF),* the highest flow rate achieved when taking in a breath after blowing out the most air possible

■ *Forced expiratory flow (FEF),* the flow rate measured at selected times during exhalation of a maximum breath. The FEF allows evaluation of the airflow through large, medium, and small airways and may be used to evaluate the effectiveness of bronchodilator drugs (Kee, 2014).

BOX 21-4 NURSING CARE CHECKLIST

Bronchoscopy

Before the Procedure

- ☑ Provide routine preoperative care.
- ☑ Reinforce teaching.
- ☑ Remove dentures and partial plates; provide mouth care just before the procedure.

After the Procedure

- ☑ Keep resuscitation and suction equipment at the bedside.
- ☑ Closely monitor vital signs and respiratory status.
- ☑ Maintain NPO status until cough and gag reflexes have returned.
- ☑ Provide emesis basin and tissues for expectorating sputum and saliva.
- ☑ Monitor color and character of respiratory secretions. Sputum may be blood tinged for several hours; notify the physician if sputum is grossly bloody.

Patient and Family Teaching

- ☑ The procedure takes about 30 to 45 minutes and may be done in the patient's room, in a procedure room, or in surgery.
- ☑ There will be little pain or discomfort. An anesthetic will be given. Breathing continues during the procedure, but talking is not possible.
- ☑ A sore throat and hoarse voice are common after the procedure. Throat lozenges or warm saline gargles can help relieve sore throat.
- ☑ A fever may develop during the first 24 hours after the procedure.
- ☑ It is important to report persistent cough, bloody or purulent sputum, wheezing, shortness of breath, difficulty breathing, or chest pain to the doctor.

Patients with asthma or other restrictive lung diseases may use a peak expiratory flow rate (PEFR) meter on a day-to-day basis to monitor airway constriction. These inexpensive meters provide a guide for self-care and use of medications.

Direct Visualization

Direct or indirect laryngoscopy may be used to identify and evaluate laryngeal tumors. A fiberoptic laryngoscope is used for direct laryngoscopy; mirrors are used to visualize the larynx in indirect laryngoscopy. General or local anesthesia is used for laryngoscopy. If local anesthesia is used, the patient receives sedation to promote relaxation before the procedure. Dental prostheses (dentures, partial plates, bridges, etc.) are removed before the procedure. All food and fluids are withheld after the procedure until the gag reflex returns.

In fiberoptic bronchoscopy, a flexible bronchoscope is used to visualize the trachea, bronchi, and selected bronchioles (Figure 21-10■). This procedure is done to identify tumors or other structural disorders, obtain tissue for biopsy or sputum for examination, or perform therapeutic procedures, such as removing a foreign body. Nursing responsibilities related to bronchoscopy are outlined in Box 21-4■.

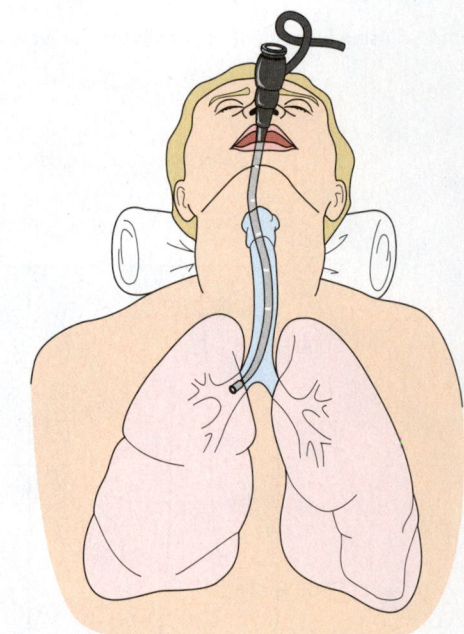

Figure 21-10. ■ Fiberoptic bronchoscopy.

Note: The references and resources for all chapters have been compiled at the back of the book.

Chapter Review

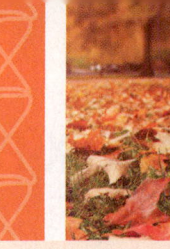

KEY POINTS

- **Concept:** The respiratory system is essential for providing oxygen to support the cells of the body and for eliminating the carbon dioxide formed during cell metabolism.
- A patent airway and unobstructed airflow are vital to sustain life and function.
- The upper respiratory system provides a passageway for air to the lungs, cleaning, humidifying, and warming the air that passes through it. Mucus and lymphoid tissue in the upper airway trap dust and bacteria, reducing the risk of lower airway contamination.
- The lungs and bronchi of the lower respiratory system work together with the pulmonary vessels in the process of respiration, which includes ventilation (breathing) and gas exchange in the alveoli.
- **Concept:** The critical role of the respiratory system in supporting body cells, tissues, and organs makes nursing assessment of respiratory function vital in all patients. The nurse needs to be able to recognize and respond appropriately to abnormal or unexpected findings.
- Respiratory function is evaluated through diagnostic tests such as arterial blood gases, sputum studies, pulmonary function tests, imaging studies, and direct visualization of tissues of the respiratory tract.
- Although specific responsibilities vary, depending on the procedure being performed, nursing care of the patient undergoing diagnostic testing is both supportive and educational. The nurse teaches the patient about the procedure itself and what to expect during and after the procedure. In some cases, such as a throat swab or sputum culture, the nurse is responsible for obtaining the specimen to be examined.

PEARSON NURSING STUDENT RESOURCES

Find additional materials at **nursing.pearsonhighered.com**.

NCLEX-PN® Exam Preparation

TEST-TAKING TIP When preparing for the NCLEX-PN® examination and initial nursing licensure, think about how you will apply knowledge of normal anatomy and physiology to assessing and planning care for your patients. For example, understanding the physiology and mechanics of breathing is important in recognizing how a fractured rib or pneumothorax can affect the patient's ability to breathe and oxygenate the blood and tissues effectively.

1 When caring for a patient admitted after a motor vehicle wreck, the nurse knows that which of the following could interfere with effective respiration? **Select all that apply.**

1. Facial injuries with possible fractures
2. Rib fractures
3. A concussion
4. Torn knee cartilage
5. A cardiac contusion

2 The nurse caring for a patient who is in a coma positions the patient on his or her side with the head elevated to help prevent aspiration because:

1. the esophageal sphincter relaxes in comatose patients.
2. the cough reflex is lost in comatose patients.
3. the patient will gag frequently on oral secretions.
4. this position facilitates mouth care and feeding.

3 A patient scheduled for a ventilation–perfusion scan asks the nurse if this procedure poses a risk of radiation exposure to her children. The nurse's response is based on the knowledge that:

1. special precautions must be taken during and after the procedure to protect others from radiation exposure.
2. no radioactive substances are used in this diagnostic procedure.
3. all radioactivity is internal and excreted via the urine, so double-flushing after urinating is the only precaution necessary.
4. the amount of radioactivity is very small, so no special precautions are required to protect others.

4 When assessing the respiratory status of a 45-year-old man, the nurse observes that the anterior–posterior diameter of the patient's chest is greater than the lateral or side-to-side diameter. The nurse recognizes this finding as:

1. a normal finding.
2. an expected finding due to the patient's age.
3. indicative of a barrel chest, an abnormal finding.
4. of no relevance to the nursing assessment.

5 The nurse is providing instructions to a patient scheduled for pulmonary function tests. Which of the following statements does the nurse include?

1. "Use your bronchodilator inhaler as needed on the day of the test."
2. "Avoid smoking the morning of the test."
3. "Do not eat or drink anything for 12 hours before the test."
4. "This test, although painful, is vital to predict your future care needs."

Answers and rationales for Review Questions appear in Appendix I.

CULTURAL CARE STRATEGIES

CONSIDERING CULTURAL VARIATIONS RELATED TO TIME

Mrs. Torres, 42, a Puerto Rican American, arrived at the doctor's office a half-hour late for her Friday afternoon appointment. When the nurse at the desk asked her about this, she said, "I had a friend stop by who just arrived from Puerto Rico and we got busy talking. Is this a problem? The doctor is usually behind in his appointments." "Yes," the nurse said. "The doctor had an afternoon surgery scheduled and isn't here. He won't be back in the office until Monday. He waited as long as he could for you. You really needed to see him, because he needed to explain these test results for you, decide on a course of action, and give you prescriptions for medication. Now it will be two more days until you can see him and you will miss two days of medication that might have had you feeling better."

Time is an important but seldom recognized aspect of interpersonal communication. Although the phenomenon of time varies among individuals, a person's concept of time is largely the result of experiences within his or her culture of origin (Giger, 2013). Individuals learn the concept of time from persons and events in their environment, and it becomes integrated into every segment of their behavior and thought. Thus it is essential for nurses to understand how perceptions of time vary so culturally competent and sensitive care can be delivered. In the case of Mrs. Torres, the failure to arrive at her appointment on time will delay her recovery. If the nurse had emphasized the need to keep this appointment exactly as scheduled, Mrs. Torres might have made this a higher priority than visiting with her friend.

Temporal Orientation

- Temporal orientation refers to the ordering of past, present, and future events. People who focus on the past have little motivation for formulating future goals that include primary pre-

vention and health promotion activities. For example, Native Americans or the Old Order Amish may be viewed as past-oriented individuals. They hold strongly to traditions and values passed from generation to generation. This belief pattern directly reflects their social order and health care practices (Buccalo, 1997).
- For people whose culture is oriented in the present, the present task is viewed as most important, such as visiting with a friend who has dropped by. These people are unlikely to adhere to rigid time schedules; instead, they focus on the current activity. Present-time orientation may also result in nonadherence to medication regimens, visiting hours at the hospital, and follow-up appointments. For example, a teenager may get caught up in an activity and miss an appointment that required arriving at a precise time.
- People who have a future-time orientation organize and plan their activities to achieve future goals. Many middle-class Americans, regardless of ethnic or cultural origin, tend to be future oriented. They may delay starting a family, purchasing a house, or purchasing an expensive car until education is successfully completed and financial success has been attained. Future-oriented individuals may seem cold and detached and may focus more on tasks to accomplish future goals than on relationships.

Clock Versus Social Time

- Most people in North America organize their activities around the clock, arriving at places or starting behaviors at a very specified time determined by hours and minutes. Some groups, however, initiate activities and behaviors

on the basis of social time. For them, events such as weddings or church services may start when everyone arrives and stop when the event is completed. For these individuals, time is qualitative rather than quantitative (Giger, 2013).

Nursing Implications

- *Assess individuals for time orientation.* The nurse needs to relate health care teaching to the patient's perspective of time. For example, when a patient is present rather than future oriented, the nurse needs to relate present actions to current health status, not to the future.
- *Care planning should be based on cultural orientation.* By acknowledging other time perceptions, the nurse can plan interventions to assist the patient to adapt behavior to meet health needs. For example, stressing the importance of keeping appointments on time, of taking medications as ordered, and of complying with care regimens can increase the patient's compliance.
- *Differences in behavior by health team members may be related to time perception.* Some team members who are social-time rather than clock-time oriented may have difficulty with punctuality and adherence to the time frames for treatments and medication administration.

Self-Reflection Questions

1. What is your predominant time orientation: past, present, or future?
2. Are you predominantly clock-time oriented or social-time oriented?
3. If your patient or coworkers do not share your time orientation, what problems can occur?

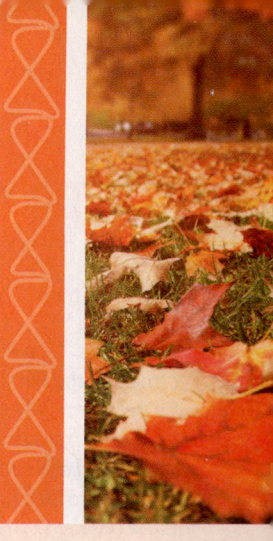

CHAPTER 22
Caring for Patients With Upper Respiratory Disorders

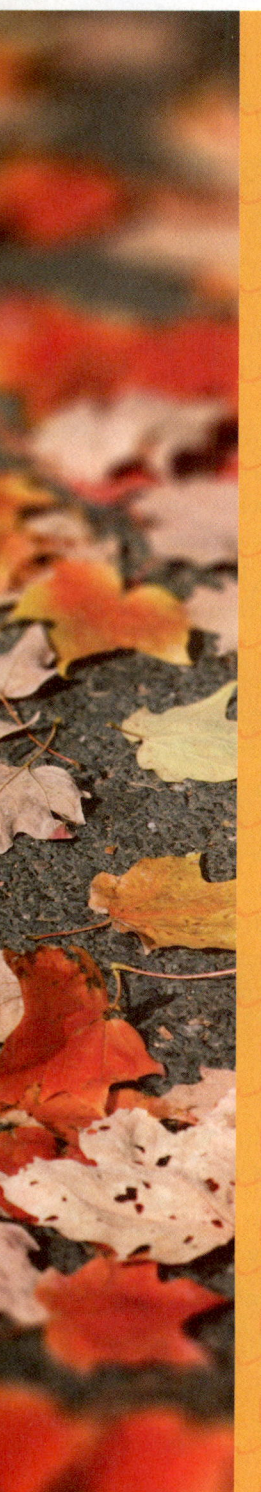

BRIEF OUTLINE

Infections and Inflammations
Pertussis
TRAUMA OR OBSTRUCTION
Epistaxis
Nasal Polyps

Nasal Trauma or Deviated Septum
Laryngeal Obstruction or Trauma
Obstructive Sleep Apnea
Laryngeal Cancer

APPLIED LEARNING OUTCOMES

After completing this chapter, you will be able to:

1. Describe common disorders affecting the upper respiratory tract, their manifestations, and potential impact on the patient.
2. Safely administer medications and treatments ordered for patients with upper respiratory disorders.
3. Plan and provide appropriate individualized nursing care for patients with upper respiratory disorders, showing consideration for expressed values, preferences, and needs.
4. Use technology to identify evidence-based guidelines and document care for patients with upper respiratory system disorders.
5. Provide evidence-based teaching and instructions to ensure continuity of care for patients with upper respiratory system disorders.

KEY TERMS

The key terms are defined on the pages listed below.

SPECIAL FEATURES

Key Concept A patent airway and unobstructed airflow are vital to sustain life and function. Disorders affecting the upper airway range from mild and self-limiting viral infections to acute and life-threatening obstruction.

The upper respiratory tract begins at the nares and extends through the larynx. Common upper respiratory disorders such as viral infections usually are appropriately self-treated by the patient. When swelling, bleeding, or secretions affect breathing, the patient may become frightened and anxious. Emergent intervention may be required to maintain effective respirations. Nursing care for patients with upper respiratory disorders focuses on managing the airway and symptoms, communicating effectively, and providing teaching and psychologic support for the patient and family.

Infections and Inflammations

Key Concept Common upper respiratory tract infections and inflammations generally are mild and appropriate for self-care. Complications such as pneumonia can develop, particularly in older adults and in people who are frail or those with chronic illness.

The upper respiratory tract is constantly exposed to infectious and inflammatory agents in the environment. Upper respiratory infections (URIs) are among the most common illnesses experienced by humans. Most URIs and inflammations are minor illnesses. However, complications may result. In the frail older adult, the risk of serious problems after a URI can be significant. Epiglottitis, an uncommon URI, can severely impair airflow and is a medical emergency.

PATHOPHYSIOLOGY AND MANIFESTATIONS

Most URIs are caused by easily spread viruses. When the virus or an allergen enters the airway, it may cause acute inflammation of the upper airway, including the sinuses, pharynx, or larynx. The airway mucosa swells and secretes clear, yellow, or greenish exudate. A bacterial infection may develop after the viral infection. URIs occur more frequently during the fall and winter.

Rhinitis

Rhinitis, inflammation of the nasal cavities, is the most common upper respiratory disorder.

Acute viral rhinitis (the common cold) is highly contagious. Most adults experience two to four colds each year. More than 200 strains of viruses can cause the common cold, including rhinovirus, respiratory syncytial virus, and adenovirus. These viruses are spread by hand-to-hand contact and by inhaling the virus. The virus can be spread to others for a few days *before* and *after* symptoms appear. Common manifestations of acute viral rhinitis are listed in Table 22-1 ■.

Allergic rhinitis (hay fever) results from an allergic response to substances such as plant pollens, mold, or animal dander. Allergic rhinitis tends to occur seasonally. Histamine and other immune mediators are released in response

TABLE 22-1	Manifestations and Course of Rhinitis and Influenza		
	ACUTE VIRAL RHINITIS	**ALLERGIC RHINITIS**	**INFLUENZA**
Local Manifestations	■ Nasal mucosa red, swollen, and congested ■ Clear, watery secretions with **coryza** (runny nose) ■ Sneezing and coughing	■ Nasal mucosa pale, swollen, and congested ■ Thin, watery nasal discharge ■ Itchy, watery eyes ■ Sneezing	■ Coryza ■ Sore throat ■ Dry, nonproductive cough; may become productive ■ Substernal burning
Systemic manifestations	■ Low-grade fever ■ Headache ■ Malaise ■ Muscle ache	■ Headache	■ Chills and fever ■ Headache ■ Malaise ■ Muscle aches ■ Fatigue and weakness
Course and possible complications	■ Lasts few days to 2 weeks ■ Mild and self-limited ■ Secondary infections (e.g., sinusitis, otitis media) may follow	■ Occurs with exposure to allergens (pollen, mold, animal dander) ■ Chronic congestion may cause snoring and postnasal drip.	■ Abrupt onset ■ 1- to 2-week duration ■ Cough and fatigue may last several weeks. ■ Secondary infections (sinusitis, otitis media, pneumonia, bronchitis) may follow.

to contact with the allergen. This causes vasodilation and increased leakiness of capillaries in the mucosa (Table 22-1). The sinuses may become congested, causing a headache. Chronic allergies may lead to postnasal drip and snoring.

Respiratory Syncytial Virus

Respiratory syncytial virus (RSV) is a common virus that causes the majority of respiratory illnesses in infants and young children. In adults, the virus usually presents as the common cold. Older adults and people who are immunocompromised, however, may develop severe lower respiratory disease when exposed to RSV. The disease is transmitted by direct contact and by droplets spread by coughing and sneezing.

The manifestations of RSV in adults are those of a common URI: *rhinorrhea* (runny nose), sore throat, and cough. Headache, malaise, and low-grade fever may develop. Older adults may present with pneumonia.

Influenza

Influenza (flu) is a highly contagious viral respiratory disease that often occurs in epidemics. Yearly outbreaks of influenza affect about 48 million Americans each winter. Influenza and its complications (primarily bacterial pneumonia) are the ninth leading cause of death in the United States, leading to more than 50,000 deaths yearly (National Center for Health Statistics [NCHS], 2013). The H1N1 strain of influenza virus caused a pandemic (worldwide epidemic) in 2009–2010. While the pandemic is over, H1N1 influenza is expected to continue to spread worldwide along with seasonal influenza (CDC, 2010). Older adults with influenza have an increased risk of complications and a significantly higher risk of death due to influenza and associated complications (Box 22-1■).

memoryALERT

Three major strains of influenza virus have been identified, designated as A, B, and C.

- Influenza A virus is responsible for most infections and the most severe outbreaks (pandemics). This virus is found in birds, pigs, whales, and humans.
- Influenza B virus also is common in humans, but generally causes less severe outbreaks.
- Influenza C virus typically causes mild illness and is often not recognized as influenza.

Influenza viruses are transmitted by airborne droplet and direct contact. The incubation period is short, and the manifestations develop rapidly (see Table 22-1). Fever and acute manifestations last up to a week; cough and fatigue may persist for several weeks.

Sinusitis

Sinusitis is an inflammation of the mucous membranes of the sinuses. Sinusitis may be caused by a viral or bacterial infection and often follows a URI.

When drainage from the sinuses is obstructed, mucous secretions caught in the sinus cavity become a growth medium for pathogens. An inflammatory and immune response leads to more swelling and pressure. Sinusitis may become chronic in some individuals. Patients who smoke, have allergies, or habitually use nasal sprays also may develop chronic sinusitis.

Sinusitis causes pain and tenderness across the affected sinuses, as well as headache, fever, and malaise. The pain usually increases with leaning forward. Pain also may be referred to the upper teeth. The nasal mucous membrane is red and swollen in patients with sinusitis. The patient may complain of nasal congestion, purulent nasal discharge, bad breath, fever, malaise, and fatigue. Symptoms often worsen after awakening and then become less severe in the afternoon and evening as secretions drain.

Sinus infection may spread to surrounding structures, causing complications such as abscess or cellulitis, meningitis, sepsis, or hearing loss.

Pharyngitis and Tonsillitis

Pharyngitis (acute inflammation of the throat) is common. It is usually viral but may also be bacterial. *Group A beta-hemolytic Streptococcus* (strep throat) is the most common bacterial cause. Streptococcal infection also may cause **tonsillitis** (acute inflammation of the tonsils). Streptococcal infections usually occur between late fall and spring, especially in cold climates. Pharyngitis and tonsillitis are contagious and are spread by droplet nuclei. Incubation varies from a few hours to several days.

Pharyngitis causes pain and fever. Throat discomfort may vary from scratchiness to pain and **dysphagia**

BOX 22-1	FOCUS ON OLDER ADULTS

Influenza in Older Adults

Older adults are more susceptible to severe influenza and resulting complications. Unfortunately, influenza vaccine also is less likely to stimulate the kind of immune response that provides protection in older adults and people who are frail or immunosuppressed (Seasonal flu, 2013). Older adults who get influenza have a high risk of developing pneumonia. Respiratory function changes with aging. The cilia become less effective in clearing secretions, chest muscle strength declines, and the chest wall becomes stiffer. The cough is less effective and residual lung volume increases. These changes increase the risk for pneumonia. Pneumonia is a serious complication of influenza that may be fatal. Older adults, particularly those over the age of 75 years, have a higher risk of dying due to influenza and pneumonia.

(difficulty swallowing). The manifestations of acute viral and bacterial pharyngitis are listed in Box 22-2■.

In tonsillitis, the tonsils are bright red and swollen with white exudate. The uvula may also be red and swollen (Figure 22-1■). Cervical lymph nodes are usually tender and enlarged. The patient with tonsillitis complains of a sore throat, difficulty swallowing, general malaise, fever, and *otalgia* (pain in the ear). The infection may extend to the ear through the auditory tubes, causing acute otitis media.

Peritonsillar abscess (*quinsy*) is a potential complication of tonsillitis. In a peritonsillar abscess, pus forms behind the tonsil, causing marked swelling and deviation of the uvula toward one side. The patient may be unable to swallow anything but liquids. Drooling and contraction of the muscles used in chewing may also occur.

Rare but serious complications of streptococcal pharyngitis and tonsillitis include acute glomerulonephritis and rheumatic fever. These potential complications are caused by an abnormal immune response to the bacteria. They can develop 1 to 5 weeks after the acute infection.

Epiglottitis
Acute **epiglottitis** (inflammation of the epiglottis) is uncommon. It is, however, a medical emergency. Patients with epiglottitis have difficulty swallowing food and have manifestations of pharyngitis. The epiglottis appears red, swollen, and edematous.

clinicalALERT

Constantly monitor patients with epiglottitis for signs of respiratory distress: nasal flaring, restlessness, **stridor** (a high-pitched, harsh sound heard during inspiration), use of accessory muscles, and decreased oxygen saturation measurements. Do not insert a nasal or oral airway because this can cause spasm and total airway obstruction. Nasotracheal intubation may be necessary to maintain the airway. Be prepared for emergency intubation of the patient at any time.

Epiglottitis is frightening for both the patient and the nurse. Maintain a calm, reassuring manner to help relieve anxiety.

Laryngitis
Laryngitis (inflammation of the larynx) is common. Laryngitis may occur alone or with other disorders of the upper respiratory tract. It is commonly associated with viral URI and may also occur in patients with bronchitis, pneumonia, or other respiratory infections. Excessive use of the voice, sudden changes in temperature, or exposure to dust or pollutants can also cause laryngitis. It is more common in the winter and in colder climates.

In laryngitis, the mucous membrane lining the larynx becomes inflamed and the vocal cords may be swollen. The primary manifestation of laryngitis is a change in the voice. Hoarseness or *aphonia* (complete loss of the voice) may occur. Patients complain of a sore, scratchy throat and may have a dry, harsh cough.

COLLABORATIVE CARE
Most acute URIs are self-limiting, and patients are encouraged to provide self-care. Rarely is hospitalization required, unless a complication occurs. Medical management focuses on establishing an accurate diagnosis, providing symptomatic relief and preventing complications. Bacterial URIs such as sinusitis and streptococcal pharyngitis

BOX 22-2	MANIFESTATIONS OF ACUTE PHARYNGITIS

Viral Pharyngitis
- Gradual onset
- Low-grade fever
- Sore throat
- Mild hoarseness
- Headache
- Throat bright pink to red

Streptococcal Pharyngitis
- Abrupt onset
- Fever of 101°F (38.3°C) or higher
- Severe sore throat
- Dysphagia
- Malaise, muscle aches
- Tender, enlarged cervical lymph nodes
- Throat bright red
- Patches of creamy exudate may be seen on oropharynx and tonsils.

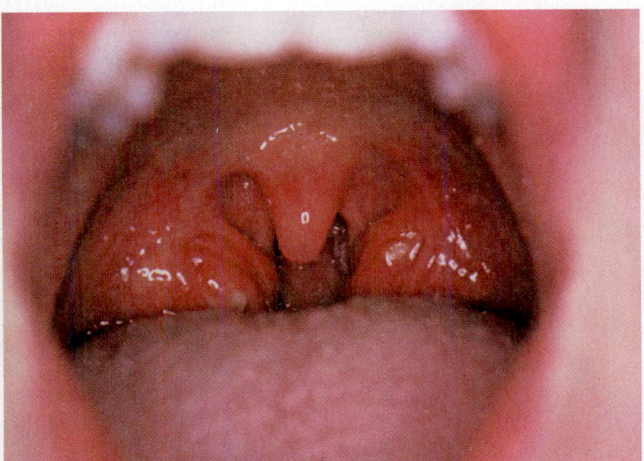

Figure 22-1 ■ Tonsillitis. The tonsils, uvula, and surrounding tissues are red and swollen. (Source: Dr. P. Marazzi/Science Source.)

may be treated to speed recovery and reduce the risk of complications.

In long-term care facilities, URIs can spread rapidly and have devastating effects on the frail older adult population. Box 22-3 ■ outlines measures to help control the spread of influenza in long-term care and other group living facilities.

Diagnostic Tests

A *throat swab* is obtained when streptococcal pharyngitis is suspected. Nurses are often responsible for obtaining the culture. Tests such as the LA antigen and ELISA allow rapid identification of the bacteria (in as little as 10 minutes), but are not highly sensitive. If the test is positive, treatment for strep throat is started. If the test is negative, the swab is cultured to determine whether streptococcus is present.

Rapid influenza diagnostic tests (RIDTs), performed on a nasal, throat, or nasopharyngeal swab, can identify the presence of influenza A or influenza B antigens in as little as 15 minutes. The sensitivity of RIDT to influenza virus is limited, and false negative results can occur (CDC, 2013a).

BOX 22-3	NURSING CARE CHECKLIST

Controlling Influenza in Long-Term Care Settings

- ☑ Provide annual influenza vaccine to all residents and personnel unless contraindicated by allergy or health status.
- ☑ Limit potential exposure to influenza:
  - ☑ Post visual alerts asking people with symptoms of a respiratory infection to notify health care personnel.
  - ☑ Discourage people who are ill from visiting residents.
  - ☑ Exclude or reassign health care personnel with influenza symptoms or confirmed cases to nondirect care activities for 7 days after the onset of symptoms.
  - ☑ Encourage people with upper respiratory symptoms to sit at least 3 feet away from others.
  - ☑ Provide masks to residents with upper respiratory symptoms.
- ☑ Provide hand-hygiene supplies by sinks and in readily accessible locations.
- ☑ Ensure that health care personnel know and follow Standard Precautions.
- ☑ Implement droplet precautions for patients with suspected or confirmed influenza.
- ☑ Move residents with influenza symptoms to a private room.
  - ☑ If private rooms are not available, place residents with similar symptoms in one area (particularly for meals and activities).
- ☑ Provide and instruct all health care personnel to use a facemask when caring for the patient, removing and discarding the mask when leaving the patient's room.

Source: Centers for Disease Control and Prevention, 2013b.

A *complete blood count (CBC)* may be done. The white blood cell (WBC) count is usually normal or low in viral infections and elevated in bacterial infections. A *chest x-ray* may be done to rule out complications such as pneumonia.

Nasal swabs or *radiologic studies* (x-ray or computed tomography [CT] scan) may be ordered if sinusitis is suspected. CT scans are more sensitive than x-rays in detecting the inflammatory changes of sinusitis.

Medications

INFLUENZA   Yearly immunization with influenza vaccine is the most important measure to reduce the risk of influenza (Figure 22-2 ■). *Polyvalent* influenza virus vaccine (containing antigens of several viral strains) is about 62%–85% effective in preventing influenza infection for up to a year. Although the vaccine is readily available and inexpensive, only about a third of people at risk get the vaccine each year. The vaccine should be given annually to all people over 6 months of age who do not have a contraindication to the vaccine. Because the vaccine is produced in eggs, it should not be given to people with an allergy to eggs. About 5% of those vaccinated may develop low-grade fever, malaise, or muscle aches after vaccination. Potential serious adverse reactions include anaphylaxis (an acute allergic response) and Guillain–Barré syndrome, an acute neurologic disorder that can cause temporary paralysis. An intranasal vaccine is available and is recommended as an option for healthy people between the ages of 2 and 49 years. This vaccine, which contains live *attenuated* (weakened) influenza virus, is not recommended for anyone who is immunosuppressed, has a chronic disease, or is pregnant.

Two influenza antiviral drugs are recommended to prevent or shorten the duration of influenza in unvaccinated people who are exposed to the virus. Oseltamivir (Tamiflu),

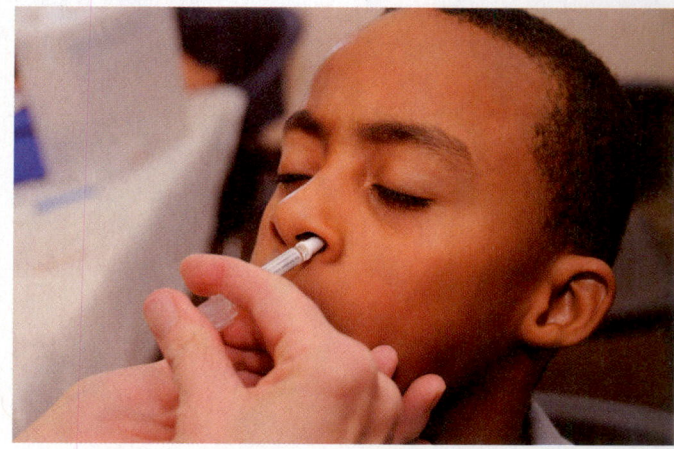

Figure 22-2. ■ The nurse administers intranasal influenza vaccine to a patient. (Source: © Norma Jean Gargasz/Alamy.)

an oral medication, and zanamivir (Relenza), administered by inhalation, reduce the severity and duration of influenza. These drugs attack the virus itself, reducing its spread in the body. Adverse effects are uncommon, but may include nausea, vomiting, or diarrhea. Patients taking zanamivir may experience nasal symptoms, cough, or sinusitis.

BACTERIAL INFECTIONS   Although controversial, bacterial infections such as strep pharyngitis and tonsillitis often are treated with antibiotics. Treatment is continued for at least 10 days. The patient is no longer contagious after 24 hours of antibiotic therapy.

Antibiotics also may be used to treat sinusitis when symptoms are severe or purulent discharge is noted in the pharynx. Antibiotic therapy is continued for a full 2 weeks; a longer course may be prescribed to prevent relapse. If the patient's sinusitis does not improve, he or she is referred to an otolaryngologist for further evaluation.

RHINITIS   A number of drugs, many available without prescription, provide symptomatic relief from viral URIs. Mild decongestants may help relieve the manifestations of coryza and nasal congestion. Oral or topical (nasal spray) decongestants are also prescribed for patients with sinusitis to reduce mucosal edema and promote sinus drainage. See Box 22-4■ for instructions for administering nose drops. Topical nasal steroids may be used, although there is no evidence that they are more effective than placebo in relieving sinusitis symptoms.

Decongestants and antihistamines help relieve the manifestations of allergic rhinitis. Many decongestants and antihistamines are available without a prescription, including long-acting nonsedating antihistamines. Inhaled steroids or cromolyn, a mast cell stabilizer, may be prescribed if nonprescription drugs are ineffective. (See Table 22-2■ on the next page.)

BOX 22-4   NURSING CARE CHECKLIST

Administering Nose Drops

To administer nose drops:

☑ Tilt the patient's head backward and to the side in which the drops are to be instilled.

☑ Have the patient remain in position for 5 minutes to allow the drops to reach the posterior nares.

Warm saltwater gargles, throat lozenges, or mild analgesics may be used for sore throats. Saline nasal irrigation is beneficial in relieving the manifestations of URI and sinusitis. Over-the-counter analgesics such as aspirin, acetaminophen, or NSAIDs help relieve fever and muscle ache. Antitussives may decrease cough and promote rest. Systemic mucolytic agents such as guaifenesin (Anti-Tuss, Mucinex, Robitussin, others) help liquefy secretions and promote sinus drainage.

Complementary Therapies

Complementary therapies and practices are appropriate for treating many URIs. Herbal remedies such as echinacea and garlic have antiviral and antibiotic effects. Garlic supplements have been shown to reduce both the number and duration of URIs (Barrows, 2013). Taken at the first sign of infection, echinacea may reduce the duration and symptoms of a common cold or influenza. The recommended dose of echinacea varies, depending on the part of the plant used in the preparation. It should not be used for longer than 2 weeks. Echinacea is contraindicated for women who are pregnant or lactating. It should not be used by people who have an autoimmune disease such as multiple sclerosis or rheumatoid arthritis.

Aromatherapy with essential oils such as basil, cedarwood, eucalyptus, frankincense, lavender, marjoram, peppermint, or rosemary can reduce congestion, enhance comfort, and promote recovery from a URI. Caution patients that these essential oils should be used only for inhalation and must not be taken internally.

Surgery

Patients with sinusitis, tonsillitis, or peritonsillar abscess may require surgery. *Irrigation* of an infected sinus (*antral lavage*) can be performed in the physician's office under local anesthesia. The sinus is irrigated with saline solution to wash out purulent exudate and promote drainage. *Endoscopic sinus surgery* may be performed to relieve obstruction of the opening to the sinus and restore ventilation and drainage of the sinus. Nasal packing is left in place for 24 to 48 hours after surgery. On discharge, the patient is instructed to:

- Use a humidifier or normal saline spray.
- Avoid blowing the nose, straining, lifting, and strenuous exercise for a week.
- Sneeze with the mouth open.

TABLE 22-2	Giving Medications Safely: Upper Respiratory Infections		
CLASS/DRUGS	**PURPOSE**	**NURSING IMPLICATIONS**	**PATIENT TEACHING**
Decongestants ■ Ephedrine (Pretz-D) ■ Naphazoline (Privine) ■ Oxymetazoline (Afrin 12 Hour, others) ■ Phenylephrine (Neo-Synephrine, others) ■ Pseudoephedrine (Sudafed, Actifed, others) ■ Tetrahydrozoline (Tyzine) ■ Xylometazoline (Otrivin)	Decongestants constrict blood vessels, reducing inflammation and edema of nasal mucosa and relieving nasal congestion. Very effective when applied topically (by nasal spray) due to rapid onset of action. Duration of effect is short, followed by vasodilation and rebound congestion. May be habit forming.	Assess for contraindications such as high blood pressure or chronic heart disease. These drugs constrict blood vessels, increasing the blood pressure and heart rate. Do not give the drug if the patient is taking antihypertensive medications or a monoamine oxidase (MAO) inhibitor.	Do not use more than the recommended dose. Check with your doctor before taking these drugs if you are taking any prescription medications. Do not use nasal sprays for more than 3–5 days. Increase fluid intake to relieve mouth dryness. These drugs may cause nervousness, shakiness, or difficulty sleeping. Stop the drug if these effects occur.
Antihistamines ■ Azatadine (Optimine) ■ Chlorpheniramine (Chlor-Trimeton, others) ■ Clemastine (Tavist) ■ Cyproheptadine (Periactin) ■ Dexbrompheniramine (Drixoral) ■ Diphenhydramine (Benadryl, others) ■ *Promethazine* (Phenergan, Phenazine, others) ■ Others *Nonsedating* ■ Cetirizine (Zyrtec) ■ Desloratadine (Clarinex) ■ Fexofenadine (Allegra) ■ Loratadine (Claritin)	Antihistamines are widely available without prescription. They are frequently combined with decongestants in over-the-counter cold and allergy preparations. Other than the nonsedating forms, most antihistamines cause some drowsiness.	Before giving or recommending these drugs, ask about possible contraindications: a. Acute asthma or chronic respiratory disease b. Glaucoma (increased intraocular pressure) c. Impaired gastrointestinal function or obstruction d. An enlarged prostate gland or other urinary tract obstruction e. Heart disease	Do not drive or operate machinery while taking antihistamines that are known to be sedating. Stop the drug and notify your doctor immediately if you become confused or very drowsy or sleepy, or you experience chest tightness, wheezing, bleeding, or easy bruising. Do not use alcohol or other CNS depressants while taking antihistamines. Hard candy, gum, ice chips, and liquids help relieve mouth dryness caused by antihistamines.

Note: Medications identified in *italics* are among the 200 most frequently prescribed drugs in the United States.

■ Avoid smoking, air pollutants, and nasal trauma.
■ Notify the physician about a temperature greater than 101°F, severe pain, or excessive bleeding.

Tonsillectomy (surgical removal of the tonsils) is done to treat recurrent or chronic infections, enlarged tonsils that may obstruct the airway, peritonsillar abscess, or malignancy. The most significant postoperative complication of tonsillectomy is hemorrhage. If hemorrhage develops, the patient returns to surgery, where the bleeding vessel is *ligated* (tied off). A peritonsillar abscess may be drained by *needle aspiration* or by *incision and drainage (I&D)* under local anesthesia. Tonsillectomy follows the I&D, either immediately or 6 weeks later.

NURSING CARE

Education is the primary nursing role in caring for most patients with URIs. Self-care is appropriate for most patients with viral infections. Patients need to be able to recognize the difference between acute, self-limiting disorders and those that require medical treatment.

PRIORITIZING NURSING CARE

Nursing care for patients with significant manifestations or complications of URI focuses on maintaining airway clearance, breathing patterns, and adequate rest.

HEALTH PROMOTION

Advise all patients about the self-limiting nature of most URIs. Teach the importance of frequent hand washing and other measures to reduce exposure, such as avoiding crowds. Maintaining good general health and controlling stress support the immune system and may reduce the risk of URI.

Inform patients that because most URIs are viral in origin, they do not require or respond to antibiotic treatment. Antibiotic misuse is associated with the development of antibiotic-resistant bacteria. Stress the importance of annual influenza vaccination for all patients, their families, and caregivers.

ASSESSING

Assessment data help determine the effects of an upper respiratory problem on the patient's life, can identify risk factors for complications, and can suggest whether the problem is appropriate for self-care or for medical treatment.

Collect subjective data, such as the presence of pain, including its location (nose, face, throat, or chest), character, timing (frequency, duration), and aggravating factors. Ask about the presence, timing, and productivity of a cough. Inquire about the presence, amount, color, and odor of sputum and/or nasal drainage. Note complaints of shortness of breath, difficult or labored breathing, difficulty swallowing or smelling, or an altered sense of taste. Ask about the patient's past medical history, including known allergies, chronic respiratory problems, surgery or trauma of the upper respiratory tract, and chronic diseases (e.g., diabetes or heart disease). Inquire about the patient's smoking history and/or known exposure to environmental pollutants or allergens.

Observe the patient's general apparent state of health, and note any difficulty breathing, pauses while talking, hoarseness, or cough. Obtain vital signs, including temperature and respiratory rate and depth. Inspect the nares and oropharynx for color; moisture; and the presence of swelling, exudate, or postnasal drainage. Percuss (lightly tap) over frontal and maxillary sinuses for tenderness and auscultate lung sounds.

IDENTIFYING POTENTIAL COMPLICATIONS

Although most URIs are viral in origin, secondary bacterial infections may develop. Report manifestations such as a fever that is higher than 101°F (38°C) or that continues for 5 or more days, cough productive of malodorous green or rust-colored sputum, shortness of breath, or dyspnea. Localized pain and swelling and symptoms such as a change in mental status, hearing, or the ability to swallow may indicate extension of an infection such as sinusitis or pharyngitis into adjacent tissues.

DIAGNOSING, PLANNING, AND IMPLEMENTING

Ineffective Breathing Pattern

Expected outcome: Respiratory rate and pattern will remain within normal or expected limits.

- Monitor respiratory rate and pattern for changes from baseline. *Tachypnea or rapid, shallow respirations may result from fever and muscle ache. Shallow respirations may lead to decreased ventilation of alveoli or to atelectasis (lack of ventilation of an area of the lung).*
- Pace activities to allow rest periods. *Tachypnea increases the work of breathing and is fatiguing.*
- Elevate the head of the bed. *The upright position reduces the work of breathing and improves lung expansion.*

Ineffective Airway Clearance

Expected outcome: Breath sounds will be clear on auscultation; will develop no signs of respiratory distress.

- Monitor the effectiveness of cough and ability to remove airway secretions. *Fatigue and general malaise may decrease the ability to cough effectively and move secretions. Changes in the respiratory system associated with aging also affect the older adult's ability to maintain a clear airway.*
- After tonsillectomy, position the patient with head to the side for drainage of secretions from the mouth and pharynx. Leave the nasopharyngeal airway in place until the patient can swallow and the gag reflex returns. *This prevents aspiration and maintains the airway.*
- Apply an ice collar as ordered. *The ice collar reduces swelling and provides a mild analgesic effect.*
- Immediately report excessive bleeding (large amounts of bright red drainage, choking on drainage, or vomiting of bright red blood) to the charge nurse and physician. *The patient may need to return to surgery to stop the hemorrhage.*
- Maintain adequate hydration. Assess mucous membrane moisture and skin turgor. *Fever, rapid respiratory rate, and decreased fluid intake may lead to dehydration and thick, sticky secretions that are more difficult to expectorate.*
- Increase the humidity of inspired air with a bedside humidifier. *Increasing the water content of inhaled air helps loosen secretions and soothe mucous membranes.*
- Teach the patient how to cough effectively. *The huff technique of coughing increases the cough's effectiveness and spares energy.*
- Administer analgesic medications as ordered. *Relieving muscle ache increases the ability to cough effectively.*

Disturbed Sleep Pattern

Expected outcome: Will obtain adequate sleep.

- Assess sleep using subjective and objective information. *Decreased ability to rest increases fatigue and prolongs recovery time.*

- Provide antipyretic and analgesic medications at bedtime or shortly before. *These medications promote comfort by reducing fever and relieving muscle aches.*
- If necessary, request a cough suppressant medication for nighttime use. *Cough suppressants are not recommended during the day because coughing promotes airway clearance, but at night they may allow the patient to rest.*

Impaired Verbal Communication

Expected outcome: Will communicate needs effectively, minimizing voice use.

- Encourage the patient with laryngitis to rest the voice and to use alternate methods of communicating such as writing. *Resting the voice speeds recovery and decreases throat discomfort.*
- Instruct to use throat lozenges or sprays or to gargle with a warm antiseptic solution. *These measures soothe the throat.*
- If the patient smokes, encourage quitting. *Cigarette smoke is an irritant that increases the risk for laryngitis and delays healing.*

MANAGING NURSING CARE

Nursing care activities such as assisting with positioning and daily living activities, encouraging and monitoring fluid intake, and reminding the patient with URI to cough and deep breathe are appropriate to assign to assistive personnel.

EVALUATING

To evaluate the effectiveness of care for a patient with a URI, collect data such as the rate and ease of breathing, ability to manage symptoms, knowledge of appropriate medication use, and presence or absence of complications.

DOCUMENTING

Document initial assessment data and teaching, as well as follow-up assessments and understanding of information presented.

CONTINUITY OF CARE

Because many URIs are appropriately treated at home, planning and teaching for home care are vital.

Encourage rest during the acute phase of the illness. Stress the importance of staying well hydrated. Teach patients to use disposable tissues to cover the mouth and nose while coughing or sneezing to prevent airborne spread of URIs. Instruct the patient to blow the nose with both nostrils open to prevent infected matter from being forced into the auditory tubes. Remind patients to wash hands frequently, especially after coughing or sneezing, to help prevent spreading the disease to others. Teach the patient that although becoming chilled or going out in the rain does not cause colds and influenza, physical or psychologic stress does make the body more susceptible to URIs. Discuss appropriate use of over-the-counter medications for relief of manifestations (see Table 22-2). Teach patients to limit their use of nasal decongestants to only a few days at a time. Suggest that patients avoid using aspirin or acetaminophen unless needed to relieve muscle aches and promote rest, because these medications may actually prolong acute viral URIs. Encourage warm saline gargles or throat lozenges for symptomatic relief of sore throat.

Help the patient with allergic rhinitis identify possible allergens and strategies to avoid contacting them. Discuss the possible benefits of skin testing to identify allergens and, if necessary, immunotherapy to reduce the allergic response.

Stress the importance of completing the entire course of prescribed antibiotics for bacterial infections. Discuss the prescribed antibiotic and help develop a schedule that helps the patient remember to take all doses. If the course of therapy will be prolonged, discuss measures to prevent superinfections such as vaginitis or oral thrush. Unless contraindicated, suggest that the patient eat 8 ounces daily of yogurt containing live bacterial cultures while on antibiotics.

Teach about possible complications of influenza and other URIs and their manifestations. Emphasize that complications should be reported promptly to the physician.

NURSING CARE PLAN
Patient With Upper Respiratory Infection

Monica Wunderman is a 27-year-old woman who was recently treated for tonsillitis caused by group A *Streptococcus*. She presents to the emergency department (ED) 10 days later appearing acutely ill. She states that her throat is so sore that she has difficulty swallowing even liquids. Barbara Ironhorse, the ED nurse, completes an assessment of Ms. Wunderman.

Assessment

T 102°F (38.8°C). On inspection of her mouth, an acutely swollen and reddened area of the soft palate is noted. Yellow exudate is present. CBC reveals an elevated WBC of 16,000/mm^3. A diagnosis of peritonsillar abscess is made. Needle aspiration of the abscess is performed.

Nursing Diagnosis

The following nursing diagnoses are identified for Ms. Wunderman:

- *Acute Pain* related to swelling
- *Risk for Ineffective Airway Clearance* related to pain and swelling
- *Deficient Fluid Volume* related to fever and difficulty in swallowing fluids

Expected Outcomes

The expected outcomes for the plan of care are that Ms. Wunderman will:

- Experience minimal or no pain.
- Maintain a patent airway as demonstrated by normal respiratory rate and rhythm.
- Maintain optimal fluid intake as evidenced by the ability to consume fluids and semiliquid foods, appearance of moist mucous membranes, normal skin turgor, and a decrease in temperature.

Planning and Implementation

Ms. Ironhorse implements the following interventions to prepare Ms. Wunderman for home care:

- Advise to drink ice-cold fluids, because they may be easier to swallow and may provide a local analgesic effect. Instruct to avoid citrus juices, hot or spicy foods, and rough-textured foods for 1 week.
- Teach pain-relief measures such as applying an ice collar as desired and gargling with warm saline solution every 1 to 2 hours for the first 24 to 48 hours after aspiration of the abscess.
- Instruct to take all medications as prescribed.

Evaluation

When Ms. Ironhorse contacts Ms. Wunderman by telephone 2 days after her visit to the ED, she reports complete relief of symptoms. She is afebrile, takes fluids without difficulty, and has had no problems with her breathing. She has not experienced any pain.

Critical Thinking in the Nursing Process

1. Describe common manifestations of URIs and measures to promote comfort.
2. Describe common pharmacologic interventions for these patients.
3. Although Ms. Wunderman developed a complication that required medical intervention, many patients present in the ED or urgency care clinics with uncomplicated URI. What can nurses do to reduce this unnecessary use of EDs and urgency care clinics?

Note: Discussion of Critical Thinking questions appears on the companion website.

Pertussis

Pertussis, or *whooping cough*, is an acute, highly contagious URI. Although once thought to have been virtually eliminated from the United States, its incidence is increasing among all ages. Infants and children have the highest incidence, but pertussis also affects adults. Infants have the highest risk of complications, including death, related to pertussis (CDC, 2011).

PATHOPHYSIOLOGY AND MANIFESTATIONS

Pertussis is caused by infection with *Bordetella pertussis*, a gram-negative rod that is spread by respiratory droplets. The bacteria attach to cells in the nasopharynx, where they multiply and spread to respiratory tissues. The infection itself is generally symptom free; however, toxins produced by the bacteria damage respiratory mucosa and paralyze the cilia. This impairs respiratory clearance, increasing the risk for pneumonia. These toxins also stimulate an inflammatory response and inhibit immune defenses.

Pertussis often has a predictable pattern, with symptoms of URI beginning 7 to 10 days after exposure. Within 1 to 2 weeks, the cough increases, with frequent *paroxysms* (bursts) of coughing that may end with an audible whoop of rapid inspiration. The whoop occurs less frequently in adolescents and adults than in young children. Coughing episodes may precipitate vomiting and can interfere with eating and sleeping. This stage of the disease can last up to 6 weeks and is followed by gradually decreasing frequency and severity of coughing.

In adults, pertussis usually presents as a simple prolonged cough, although adults may develop the typical disease pattern described earlier. Adults may develop complications such as urinary incontinence, inguinal hernia, pneumothorax, cracked ribs, and pneumonia.

COLLABORATIVE CARE

Nasopharyngeal secretions are cultured to establish the diagnosis of pertussis. Blood tests for antibodies to the bacteria also may be used to identify this disease. The primary preventive strategy for pertussis is active immunization, routinely administered to infants and young children. The Centers for Disease Control and Prevention now recommends that all adults age 19 and older receive a single dose of Tdap (tetanus toxoid, reduced diphtheria toxoid, and acellular pertussis vaccine) (CDC, 2012a).

Adolescents and adults often are treated with erythromycin, traditionally the antibiotic of choice. Recent studies suggest that azithromycin (Zithromax, Zmax) and clarithromycin (Biaxin) are equally effective for treating pertussis. These drugs have fewer adverse effects and may be used as an alternative to erythromycin.

NURSING CARE

Nurses are instrumental in educating patients about pertussis and promoting immunization of vulnerable populations. To reduce the risk for pertussis in infants, people who have or are anticipated to have close contact with the infant (parents, siblings, grandparents, child-care providers) who have not already had a dose of Tdap should receive a dose (CDC, 2011). Nurses also can help identify people with pertussis by recommending that patients with persistent, severe cough that disrupts sleep or causes vomiting have a nasopharyngeal culture.

Patients usually remain in the community during treatment, rarely requiring hospitalization.

clinicalALERT

When hospitalization is required for pertussis, place the patient in respiratory isolation for 5 days after antibiotic therapy is started to prevent spread of the disease to other patients.

The primary nursing role is teaching about pertussis and measures to prevent its spread to others. Advise all adults to have Tdap at their next regularly scheduled tetanus/diphtheria booster. Teach respiratory isolation measures to be used until the patient is no longer communicable (5 days after the start of antibiotic therapy). Discuss control of respiratory secretions and measures to maintain food and fluid intake and rest. Teach about the prescribed antibiotic, its potential adverse effects, and measures to reduce them, such as taking erythromycin with meals to reduce gastric distress. Stress the importance of prophylactic antibiotic therapy for all household contacts of an infected person. Pertussis is a reportable disease; contact the local county health department when a case is identified.

TRAUMA OR OBSTRUCTION

Key Concept Trauma to, or obstruction of, the upper airways can pose a serious threat to respiration and tissue oxygenation. Maintaining and restoring a patent airway are nursing priorities whenever the upper airway is threatened.

Epistaxis

The nose has a rich blood supply. **Epistaxis**, or nosebleed, may result from trauma (picking the nose or getting hit), drying of nasal mucous membranes, local or systemic infection, or substance abuse (e.g., cocaine). Nosebleed may occur secondarily to bleeding disorders, cardiovascular disorders, severe liver disease, or treatment with an anticoagulant or antiplatelet medication. In adults, men have more nosebleeds than women.

PATHOPHYSIOLOGY AND MANIFESTATIONS

Ninety percent of all nosebleeds arise from a rich vascular area in the anterior nasal septum (Figure 22-3■). These vessels are the most susceptible because of their location. Posterior nosebleed may also be caused by trauma but more often occurs secondary to systemic disorders such as hypertension or diabetes. Posterior epistaxis tends to be more severe and occurs more frequently in the older adult.

COLLABORATIVE CARE

The goal of treatment for epistaxis is to identify and control the source of bleeding. Anterior bleeding can usually be managed by simple first-aid measures, such as having the patient sit leaning forward slightly and pinch the nose

toward the septum for 5 to 10 minutes. Instruct the patient to spit out the blood to allow estimation of the amount of bleeding and prevent nausea and vomiting resulting from swallowed blood. If applying pressure does not control the bleeding, pharmacologic interventions, nasal packing, or surgery may be necessary.

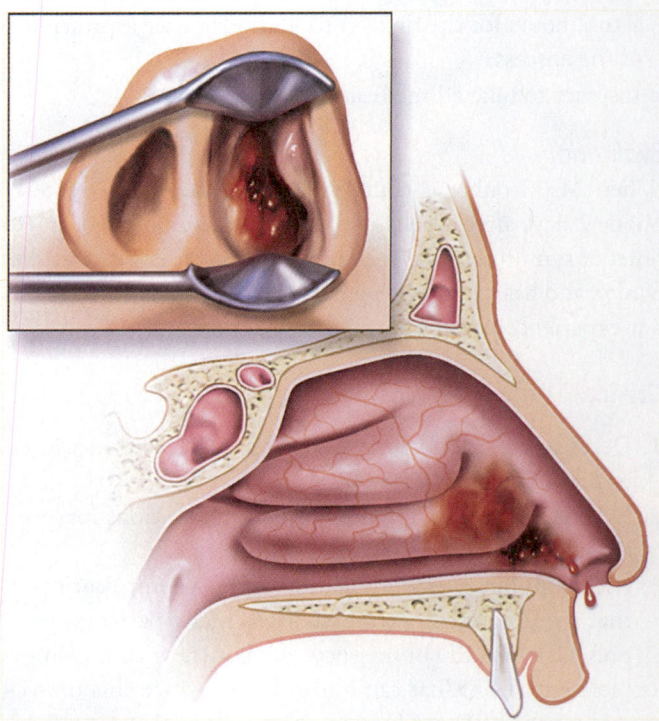

Figure 22-3. ■ Epistaxis. Bleeding usually occurs from the anterior part of the nasal septum. (Source: Pearson Education.)

Medications and Nasal Packing

Topical vasoconstrictors such as cocaine (0.5%), phenylephrine (Neo-Synephrine) (1:1,000), or adrenaline (1:1,000) may be applied by nasal spray or on a cotton swab held against the bleeding site. The bleeding vessel may be cauterized using a chemical such as silver nitrate or Gelfoam.

If bleeding cannot be controlled with pressure and local medications, a nasal tampon or petroleum gauze may be used to pack the nasal cavity. Anterior nasal packs generally are left in place for 24 to 72 hours. Posterior nasal packing (Figure 22-4■) remains in place longer, up to 5 days, and is very uncomfortable for the patient. It can significantly interfere with respirations, leading to hypoxemia. Supplemental oxygen is given while posterior packing is in place. Discomfort is managed with narcotic analgesics. Complications such as dysrhythmias, hypertension, myocardial infarction, and toxic shock syndrome are risks associated with posterior packing. A Foley catheter or inflatable nasal balloon may be used as an alternative to posterior packing.

Surgery

Chemical or surgical cautery procedures may be used to seal bleeding vessels and, in the case of posterior epistaxis, as an alternative to nasal packing. The resulting scab must be left undisturbed until the mucosa has healed, or further bleeding may occur. After surgery, the patient is carefully monitored for bleeding or respiratory complications.

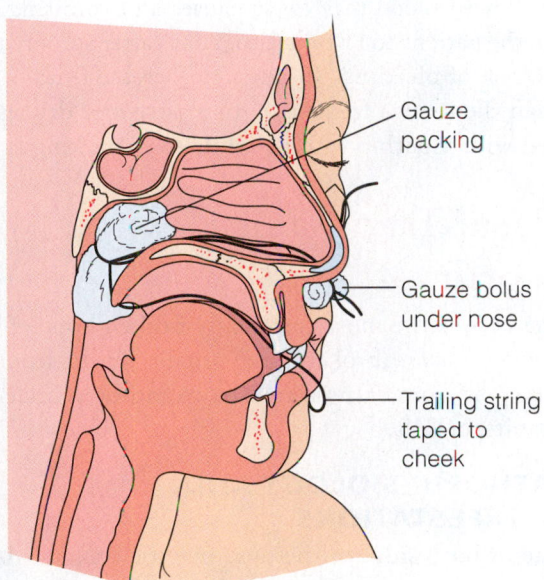

Figure 22-4. ■ Posterior nasal packing. Ties exiting through the nose and mouth are used to stabilize the packing in position and remove it when it is no longer needed.

Gauze packing

Gauze bolus under nose

Trailing string taped to cheek

NURSING CARE

Nosebleeds can be frightening, particularly when they occur spontaneously, without preceding trauma. Support, reassurance, and education are important roles for nurses caring for patients with epistaxis.

PRIORITIZING NURSING CARE

The priorities of nursing care for the patient with epistaxis are reducing the patient's anxiety and helping the patient to maintain an open airway.

HEALTH PROMOTION

Health promotion activities to reduce the incidence and severity of nosebleeds involve teaching children and adults about the importance of appropriate facial protection when engaging in contact sports (e.g., wearing a football helmet, face guards for baseball and softball catchers and hockey goalies). Teach patients how to manage simple nosebleeds and when to contact the physician.

ASSESSING

In patients with epistaxis, data collection occurs while measures to stop the bleeding are implemented. Subjective data include information about when the nosebleed started, how long it has continued, and measures that have been taken to stop the bleeding. The patient's medical history, including chronic diseases and current medications, may provide clues. Objective data to obtain include the patient's vital signs and the extent of bleeding. Inspect the oropharynx using a penlight and tongue depressor for further evidence of bleeding.

DIAGNOSING, PLANNING, AND IMPLEMENTING
Anxiety

Expected outcome: Will follow instructions, demonstrating only mild to moderate anxiety.

- Maintain an attitude of calm encouragement. *This reassures the patient that the nosebleed is not life threatening. If epistaxis has occurred spontaneously, the patient may fear that it indicates a major health problem.*
- Have the patient pinch the nares together at the bridge of the nose. *Most nosebleeds originate in the front of the nose where direct pressure usually stops the bleeding. Having the patient put pressure on the nose provides focus and reduces anxiety.*
- Encourage to breathe slowly and deeply through the mouth. *Controlled mouth breathing maintains lung ventilation and reduces anxiety.*
- Assess the patient with nasal packing frequently for adequate oxygenation (e.g., mental status, oxygen saturation measurements). Maintain supplemental oxygen as ordered. *Cerebral hypoxia produces a sense of apprehension and fear.*

Risk for Aspiration

Expected outcome: Will not aspirate, using appropriate actions to prevent passage of food or fluids into the lungs.

The highly anxious patient who has blood draining into the nasopharynx is at risk for aspirating blood into the trachea. The patient with nasal packing is unable to breathe through the nose, increasing the risk of aspirating food or fluids when eating.

- Position upright with the head forward. Provide a basin into which the patient can expectorate blood. *This reduces the risk of aspiration and nausea from swallowed blood.*
- Apply ice or a cold compress to the nose. *Cold constricts blood vessels and reduces bleeding.*
- Position the patient with nasal packing with the head elevated and on one side when asleep. *This position reduces the risk of aspiration of oral secretions.*

EVALUATING

To evaluate care for the patient with epistaxis, check for additional bleeding (be sure to check the oropharynx for blood running down the throat). Evaluate the patient's understanding of instructions, including when to return for removal of nasal packing and measures to prevent future nosebleeds.

DOCUMENTING

Document the circumstances preceding the nosebleed, assessment data, and the time and measures required to control bleeding. Document teaching provided regarding home care measures, follow-up care, and prevention of future episodes.

CONTINUITY OF CARE

After an episode of epistaxis, teaching focuses on measures to prevent further nosebleeds. Advise the patient to avoid blowing or picking the nose, strenuous exercise, straining, or heavy lifting that could increase pressure and dislodge the crust. Caution to sneeze with the mouth open to avoid increasing pressure in nasal vessels.

Suggest lubricating nasal mucosa with petroleum jelly, a water-soluble lubricant, or antibiotic ointment to reduce the risk of spontaneous bleeding in patients with anterior nose bleeds. Recommend using a humidifier or vaporizer to minimize dryness of the mucous membranes. Encourage the patient who has experienced spontaneous epistaxis to seek medical evaluation for possible underlying problems such as hypertension or bleeding disorder.

Nasal Polyps

Nasal polyps are benign grapelike growths of the mucous membrane lining the nose. These benign tumors are usually bilateral, and can interfere with air movement through nasal passages or obstruct sinus openings, leading to sinusitis. They usually affect people who have chronic allergic rhinitis or asthma. Polyps that develop during an acute URI may regress spontaneously when the infection resolves.

Polyps may be asymptomatic, although large polyps may cause nasal obstruction, rhinorrhea, and loss of sense of smell. Manifestations of sinusitis may develop. The voice may have a nasal tone. Some people with nasal polyps may have an associated aspirin allergy.

Topical corticosteroid nasal sprays or low-dose oral corticosteroids may be prescribed to shrink the polyps and manage allergic symptoms. However, polyps continue to enlarge when corticosteroid therapy is discontinued. Surgery may be required to restore normal breathing. Surgical removal of polyps (*polypectomy*) often is done in the physician's office under local anesthesia. Because polyps tend to recur, repeated surgeries may be necessary.

NURSING CARE

Teaching about home care after polypectomy is a primary nursing responsibility when caring for the patient with nasal polyps. Provide postoperative care instructions and discuss measures to reduce the risk of bleeding:

- Apply ice or cold compresses to the nose to decrease swelling, promote comfort, and prevent bleeding.
- Avoid blowing the nose for 24 to 48 hours after nasal packing is removed.
- Avoid straining at stool, vigorous coughing, and strenuous exercise.

Discuss manifestations of possible bleeding, such as frequent swallowing or visible blood at the back of the throat. Swallowed blood may cause nausea and vomiting. Encourage the patient to rest for 2 to 3 days after surgery to reduce the risk of bleeding. Instruct to increase fluid intake and clean the mouth frequently to reduce oral dryness associated with mouth breathing while nasal packing is in place.

Nasal Trauma or Deviated Septum

The nose is the most commonly broken bone of the face. A *nasal fracture* (broken nose) usually results from a sports injury or from trauma related to motor vehicle crashes, assaults, or falls.

PATHOPHYSIOLOGY AND MANIFESTATIONS

One or both sides of the nose may be broken. A fracture that involves only one side of the nose rarely causes displacement or deformity. It is usually not serious, although swelling can obstruct the airway. Bilateral fractures are more common. Complex fractures may involve other nasal

- Epistaxis
- Deformity (flattening, depression, S or C shape) or displacement to one side
- *Crepitus* (a grating sound or sensation)
- Soft tissue trauma (local swelling, periorbital edema, bruising, black eye)
- Instability of nasal bridge

structures and frontal bones of the face. The manifestations of bilateral nasal fracture are listed in Box 22-5■.

Soft tissue damage nearly always accompanies nasal fracture. Hematoma, infection or abscess, perforation or deviation of the septum, and leakage of cerebrospinal fluid (CSF) may complicate nasal fractures. The patient with a nasal fracture may also have fractures of other facial bones or traumatic brain injury, particularly when facial trauma is severe (e.g., as a result of a motor vehicle crash).

In a *deviated nasal septum*, the septal cartilage bulges or deviates to one side. It causes some degree of nasal obstruction. Few symptoms accompany mild deviation. Partial obstruction of airflow through the affected side may cause noisy breathing or snoring. Pain from sinus obstruction or infection may occur with major deviation. Dry nasal mucosa and nosebleeds may occur. The defect may be severe enough to cause cosmetic deformity.

COLLABORATIVE CARE

The major goals of treatment for nasal fractures are to maintain a patent airway and prevent deformity. CT scans of the head and face are done to identify the fracture and to assess for other facial fractures. The nasal cavity is examined to rule out septal hematoma.

Simple reduction of a nasal fracture may be done in the emergency department using local anesthesia. An external splint may then be applied for 7 to 10 days to maintain proper alignment until healing takes place. Ice may be gently applied to the face and nose to control edema and bleeding. Nasal packing may be used to control epistaxis.

Complex nasal fractures, fractures that do not heal properly, or a persistent CSF leak may require surgical repair of the fracture or realignment of the nasal bones. The most common procedure used is rhinoplasty with concurrent septoplasty.

Rhinoplasty (surgical reconstruction of the nose) is done to relieve airway obstruction and repair visible deformity of the nose after fracture. Using an intranasal incision, the framework of the nose is reshaped. Prosthetic implants may assist in reshaping the nose. Rhinoplasty is usually an outpatient procedure. After surgery, nasal packing is left in place for up to 72 hours to minimize bleeding and provide tissue support. A plastic splint molded to the shape of the nose is removed in 3 to 5 days. The splint protects the reshaped nose and helps to control swelling. Most swelling and bruising subside within 10 to 14 days; normal sensation may take several months to return.

Septoplasty or submucous resection (SMR) may be done to correct septal deviation. The procedures are done using local anesthesia. In these procedures, the deviated portion of nasal cartilage is removed; bone also may be removed if necessary. After the procedure, the nares on both sides are packed to prevent bleeding and provide support to the septum.

NURSING CARE

Nursing care for patients with nasal fracture focuses on airway management; controlling pain, bleeding, and swelling; and providing necessary teaching.

PRIORITIZING NURSING CARE

The primary risk in nasal trauma or with a deviated septum is impaired airway clearance due to swelling or obstruction of the nasal passage.

HEALTH PROMOTION

Teach all people, including children and adolescents and their parents, about the importance of wearing helmets and face protectors when participating in high-risk sports such as football, hockey, and catching baseballs. Promote the use of seat belts with shoulder harnesses and airbags in vehicles to reduce the risk of facial injury in motor vehicle crashes.

ASSESSING

Ask the patient with a suspected nasal fracture how and when the injury occurred. Carefully observe respiratory status and call for help immediately if the airway is compromised. Inquire about pain, bleeding, and difficulty breathing. Inspect the nose and face for apparent deformity, swelling, and *ecchymosis* (bruising). Gently palpate the nose for *crepitus* (a grating sound or sensation). Inspect the oral pharynx for drainage.

DIAGNOSING, PLANNING, AND IMPLEMENTING
Ineffective Airway Clearance

Expected outcome: Airway will remain clear as demonstrated by clear breath sounds and no evidence of respiratory distress.

- Monitor for signs of respiratory distress such as tachypnea, dyspnea, shortness of breath, tachycardia, and use of accessory muscles. Monitor oxygen saturation levels. *Swelling and deformity may obstruct the airway. If the fracture is malpositioned during healing, resulting deformity can also impair nasal airway clearance. Abnormal signs and declining oxygen saturation levels may indicate airway obstruction.*

- Have suction equipment available. *Suctioning of the oropharynx may be necessary to remove blood and secretions and maintain a clear airway. Avoid suctioning the nasopharynx; this could cause additional tissue trauma.*
- Monitor cough effectiveness and ability to manage airway secretions. *Pain, edema, and nasal bleeding may affect the patient's ability to cough effectively.*
- Maintain adequate hydration. *Decreased fluid intake or active bleeding may cause dehydration and increase the viscosity of secretions, making them harder to spit out.*

Risk for Infection

Expected outcome: Will remain free of signs of infection.

- Assess for evidence of a CSF leak (clear fluid leaking from the ear or nose). If noted, test drainage for glucose. CSF will test positive for glucose on a dextrostrip. Report to the charge nurse or physician. *A CSF leak indicates a high risk for ascending infection and meningitis.*
- Avoid suctioning if possible. *Suction catheters could cause additional trauma and introduce microorganisms.*
- Monitor vital signs every 4 hours. *A rise in temperature may indicate infection.*
- Administer antibiotics as ordered. *Antibiotics are often prescribed to prevent infection because the nasal mucosa is populated with many bacteria.*

EVALUATING

Evaluate the effectiveness of nursing care by collecting data related to patency of the airway, comfort, and infection. As the fracture heals, evaluate the position of the nasal septum and appearance of the nose.

DOCUMENTING

Document the circumstances of the injury, initial and continuing assessment data, including the patient's ability to maintain a clear airway, and treatment measures instituted. Document teaching for home care, instructions for follow-up, and the patient's apparent understanding of information.

CONTINUITY OF CARE

When a nasal fracture is suspected, the patient should seek medical evaluation and treatment as soon as possible. Encourage the patient to remain upright and apply ice or cold packs to the nose for 20 minutes four times a day to reduce swelling. Inform the patient that while swelling will subside within days, bruising may persist for several weeks. Reassure that the final cosmetic outcome after a nasal fracture cannot be determined until swelling has subsided.

Instruct the patient who has a CSF leak to rest in bed with the head elevated or in a recliner chair. Fluids may be restricted; with the patient, explore ways to distribute allowed fluids throughout the day. Instruct to avoid straining, blowing the nose, sneezing, or vigorous coughing. Discuss manifestations of infection, including stiff neck,

headache, and fever. Instruct the patient to contact the physician immediately if these manifestations occur.

Laryngeal Obstruction or Trauma

Laryngeal obstruction is a life-threatening emergency. The larynx is the narrowest part of the upper airway. It can be partially or fully obstructed by aspirated food or foreign objects.

PATHOPHYSIOLOGY AND MANIFESTATIONS

The most common cause of obstruction in adults is ingested meat that lodges in the airway (the "café coronary"). Risk factors for food aspiration include ingesting large boluses of food and not chewing them enough, consuming excess alcohol, and wearing dentures. **Laryngospasm** (spasm of the muscles of the larynx) or *laryngeal edema* due to inflammation, injury, or anaphylaxis also can obstruct the larynx. Laryngospasm may be caused by repeated or traumatic attempts at intubation, chemical irritation of the airway, or hypocalcemia. An acute type I allergic response may cause anaphylaxis and severe laryngeal edema.

The manifestations of laryngeal obstruction include coughing, choking, gagging, obvious difficulty breathing with use of accessory muscles, and inspiratory stridor. As the airway is obstructed, signs of asphyxia are seen. Respirations are labored and noisy with wheezing and stridor. The patient may become *cyanotic* (blue). Respiratory arrest and death may result without prompt intervention.

Trauma to the larynx can occur in motor vehicle crashes or assaults (e.g., blows to the neck or attempted strangulation). Trauma may cause laryngeal or tracheal cartilage fractures and loss of airway patency. Soft tissue injuries can cause swelling that impairs the airway further. The patient with laryngeal trauma may have *subcutaneous emphysema* (air under the skin), a change in the voice, dysphagia, inspiratory stridor, *hemoptysis* (bloody sputum), and a cough.

COLLABORATIVE CARE

The goal of treatment is to maintain an open airway. If airway obstruction is partial and the patient is able to cough and breathe, diagnostic tests such as x-rays or ultrasound may be done to locate the foreign body. An endotracheal tube may be inserted to maintain the airway that is in spasm or for laryngeal edema. For the patient in anaphylaxis, epinephrine is given to reduce laryngeal edema and relieve obstruction.

clinicalALERT

When airway obstruction is complete, the Heimlich maneuver must be performed immediately to clear the obstruction. Perform the maneuver by administering forceful thrusts to the upper abdomen or lower chest, continuing until the obstruction is relieved or more definitive care can be given (Figure 22-5■).

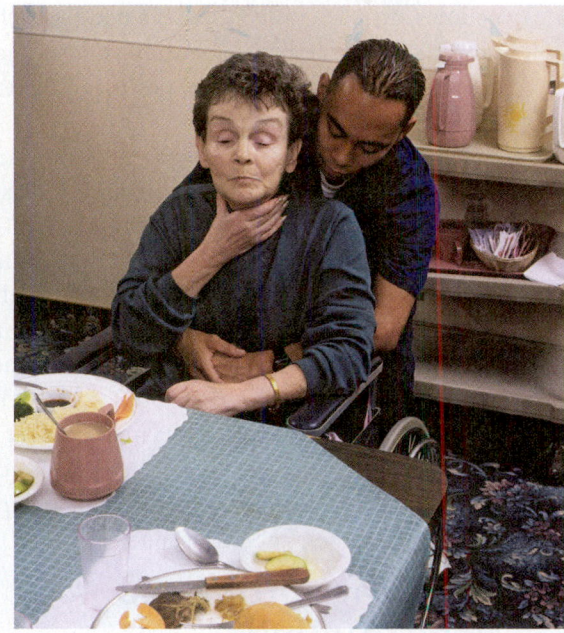
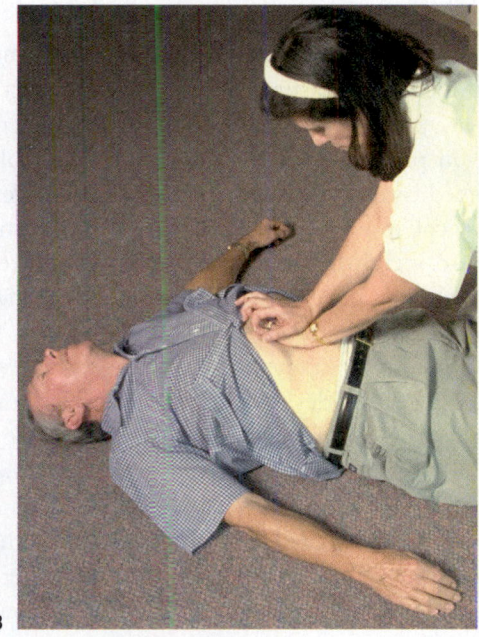

Figure 22-5. ■ Administering abdominal thrusts (the Heimlich maneuver) to (**A**) a conscious victim and (**B**) thrusts to an unconscious victim. (Source: Pearson Education.)

NURSING CARE

Closely monitor patients at risk for laryngeal obstruction (e.g., newly extubated patients and patients receiving medications that may cause anaphylaxis, such as intravenous antibiotics or radiologic dyes) for manifestations such as dyspnea, nasal flaring, tachypnea, anxiety, wheezing, and stridor. Laryngeal obstruction is a medical emergency requiring immediate intervention to open the airway and prevent brain damage or death. Suction the airway as needed; small aspirated foreign bodies may be removed by suctioning. Be prepared to assist with emergency intubation or tracheotomy as needed. If obstruction is complete, initiate a cardiopulmonary arrest procedure (code).

Patient and family teaching focuses on preventing aspiration and teaching techniques to relieve obstruction. Patients who wear dentures should be cautioned to take small bites and to chew carefully before swallowing. Teach patients that excessive alcohol intake increases the risk of food aspiration. Promote training of the general public in cardiopulmonary resuscitation (CPR) and the Heimlich maneuver. The more people who are adequately trained in emergency procedures, the more likely it is that emergency procedures will be initiated in a timely manner. Advise patients with a known risk for anaphylaxis (such as people with a previous anaphylactic response and those allergic to bee venom) to wear a MedicAlert tag and carry a bee-sting kit to prevent severe laryngeal edema.

Obstructive Sleep Apnea

Sleep apnea, the temporary absence of breathing during sleep, is common. Sleep apnea affects men more often than women and is more common in older adults. Obesity, a large neck (a neck circumference of more than 17 in. in men and more than 16 in. in women), and the use of alcohol or sedatives before sleep are risk factors for sleep apnea.

PATHOPHYSIOLOGY AND MANIFESTATIONS

Obstructive sleep apnea is the most common form of sleep apnea. The upper airway is obstructed as muscles of the upper airway relax, allowing it to collapse during inspiration. Gravity pulls the tongue back against the pharynx, causing further obstruction. Airway obstruction causes a fall in oxygen saturation (SaO_2) and brief arousal from sleep, restoring airway patency and breathing. Sleep apnea leads to fragmented sleep and disruption of normal sleep cycles.

Common manifestations of sleep apnea include loud snoring, frequent nighttime waking, daytime sleepiness, headache, and irritability. Other problems may follow, such as hypertension, morning headache, irritability, and impotence. Patients may show personality changes, impaired memory, and inability to concentrate.

Complications such as myocardial ischemia, angina, dysrhythmias, and heart failure may develop. Patients with obstructive sleep apnea experience a higher risk for cardiac or respiratory complications when undergoing surgery.

COLLABORATIVE CARE

Sleep apnea is diagnosed in a sleep laboratory. The treatment plan includes measures to reduce airway obstruction and prevent apneic episodes. Weight loss often is the first intervention prescribed. Strict avoidance of alcohol and hypnotic medications also is vital. Positive pressure to prevent airway collapse is often prescribed for sleep apnea. The patient wears a tightly fitting nasal mask connected to an air compressor that generates positive pressure. In *continuous positive airway pressure (CPAP)*, air is provided at a constant pressure to maintain an open airway. *Bilevel positive airway pressure (BiPAP)* provides a lower level of pressure support during expiration to promote comfort while maintaining an open airway. A more recent development, *automatic positive airway pressure (APAP or AutoPAP)*, automatically adjusts the amount of pressure delivered with each breath to what is required to maintain an unobstructed airway.

Surgical interventions for obstructive sleep apnea may include tonsillectomy and adenoidectomy to relieve upper airway obstruction. In a *uvulopalatopharyngoplasty (UPPP)*, the uvula, soft palate, and pharynx are reconstructed to relieve obstruction. Patients with severe obstructive sleep apnea may require tracheostomy to maintain an open airway.

NURSING CARE

Nursing care for patients with sleep apnea focuses on teaching the patient and family how to manage the disorder. Discuss the relationship of obesity, alcohol, and sedatives to the syndrome. Provide information about ways to promote weight loss. Provide referral to programs such as Weight Watchers and Alcoholics Anonymous as appropriate. When positive pressure airway support (CPAP, BiPAP, or AutoPAP) is prescribed, collaborate with the respiratory therapist in teaching the patient and family about its use and maintenance. Suggest measures to promote comfort and rest and to reduce airway dryness.

Laryngeal Cancer

> **Key Concept** Persistent hoarseness or voice change is a common manifestation of laryngeal cancer. Urge patients to seek medical assessment if this occurs. Stress that with early intervention, laryngeal cancer is curable and the ability to speak is preserved.

Tumors of the upper respiratory tract, although uncommon, can be devastating. Laryngeal tumors may be either benign or malignant. Benign tumors may develop on the vocal cords, particularly in patients who chronically shout, project, or vocalize in a very high or low tone. Vocal cord nodules are often called "singer's nodules"; cheerleaders and public speakers may also develop them. Cigarette smoking and chronic irritation from pollution contribute to their development.

Laryngeal cancer, a malignant tumor, annually affects about 12,260 Americans, resulting in an estimated 3,630 deaths (American Cancer Society [ACS], 2013a). If found early, laryngeal cancer can be cured, especially when it is limited to the vocal cords. The disease usually affects older adults; men are affected nearly four times more often than women. Laryngeal cancer is more common in African Americans than in Whites (Box 22-6■). The two major modifiable risk factors for laryngeal cancer are prolonged use of tobacco and alcohol. Other modifiable risk factors include poor nutrition and occupational exposure to wood dust, paint fumes, chemicals, and asbestos.

PATHOPHYSIOLOGY AND MANIFESTATIONS

Benign Tumors

Benign tumors of the larynx include papillomas, nodules, and polyps. Papillomas are small, wartlike growths, thought to be viral in origin. Polyps and nodules of the vocal cords result from voice abuse. Nodules occur as paired lesions, affecting both sides of the larynx. Hoarseness and a breathy voice are manifestations of vocal cord nodules.

Malignant Tumors

Changes in laryngeal mucosa occur when it is continually subjected to noxious irritants such as cigarette smoke. White, patchy precancerous lesions known as *leukoplakia* develop first, followed by the appearance of red, velvety patches called *erythroplakia*, a later stage of tumor development. Laryngeal cancer spreads both by direct invasion of surrounding tissues and by metastasis.

Laryngeal cancer may occur in any of the three areas of the larynx: the glottis, the supraglottis, and the subglottis. Lesions of the true vocal cords or *glottis* are more common than cancers of other areas of the larynx (Figure 22-6■). Fortunately, these cancers tend to be slow growing.

BOX 22-6	POPULATION FOCUS

Laryngeal Cancer

Laryngeal cancer is about 50% more common in African Americans than it is in Whites (ACS, 2013b). Teach African American patients how to reduce their risk for laryngeal cancer: stopping smoking, abstaining from alcohol or drinking only moderately, and managing other risk factors (exposure to fumes, etc.). Discuss the early manifestations of laryngeal cancer, and stress the importance of seeking treatment promptly.

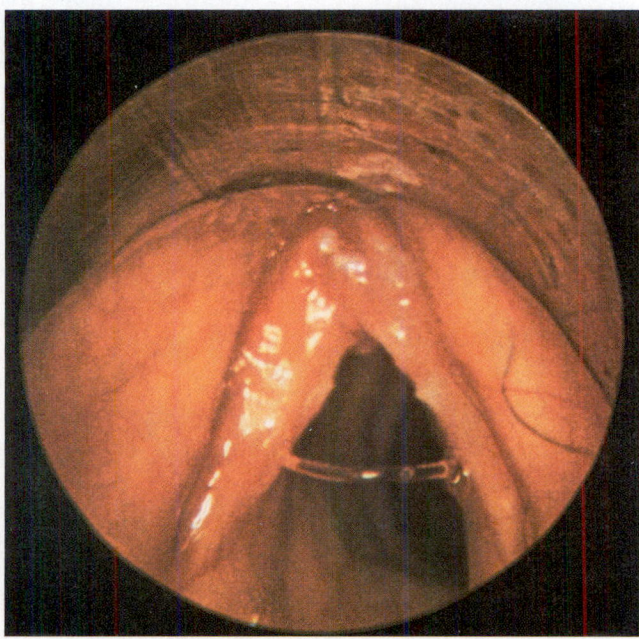

Figure 22-6. ■ Cancer of the larynx (vocal cords). (Source: © Medical-on-Line/Alamy.)

The primary manifestation of cancer of the glottis is a change in the voice; the tumor prevents complete closure of the vocal cords during speech. The *supraglottic* (above the glottis) area includes the epiglottis and false vocal cords. A tumor may be large before manifestations such as painful swallowing, a sore throat, or a feeling of a lump in the throat develop. As the tumor grows, the patient may experience difficulty breathing, foul breath, a palpable lump in the neck, and pain that radiates to the ear. *Subglottic* tumors (below the vocal cords) are the least common laryngeal cancers and often have no early symptoms. As the tumor enlarges, manifestations of airway obstruction develop. Common manifestations of laryngeal cancer are summarized in Box 22-7 ■.

COLLABORATIVE CARE

Most small cord lesions can be cured with early diagnosis and treatment. The rate of cure, however, is significantly

BOX 22-7	MANIFESTATIONS OF LARYNGEAL CANCER

- ■ Hoarseness or voice change that lasts more than 2 weeks
- ■ Persistent cough
- ■ Persistent sore throat
- ■ Difficult or painful swallowing
- ■ Dyspnea
- ■ Foul breath
- ■ Palpable lump in neck
- ■ Persistent earache
- ■ Unintended weight loss

poorer once the tumor has spread to involve lymph nodes or distant metastasis. Treatment (surgical removal, radiation, chemotherapy) is determined by the stage of the cancer.

Diagnostic Tests

Direct or indirect *laryngoscopy* is performed when the patient has manifestations of laryngeal cancer. Suspicious lesions are biopsied. Other diagnostic tests may include CT of the head and neck and chest x-ray or magnetic resonance imaging (MRI) scan. A needle biopsy of enlarged lymph nodes helps confirm the diagnosis.

Radiation

Radiation therapy is often the treatment of choice for localized laryngeal cancer. Radiation disrupts the DNA of the cell, causing it to die. External beam radiation may be used, or implants of radioactive seeds may be inserted directly into the tumor or near the tumor site. Radiation therapy is often combined with surgery or chemotherapy. Radiation preserves the voice, making it a desirable treatment option. It may be used alone in the early stages of laryngeal cancer or when the patient refuses (or is not a candidate for) surgery. In advanced cancer, it may be used in combination with chemotherapy to avoid total laryngectomy, or after laryngectomy to treat cervical lymph nodes.

Chemotherapy

Chemotherapy may be used before surgery or in combination with radiation therapy or excisional surgery. The combination of chemotherapy and radiation therapy results in higher cure rates than radiation alone (Vokes, 2012). Surgery may be avoided in some cases, when the tumor responds well to chemotherapy. Chemotherapy also may be used to treat tumors that have metastasized beyond the head and neck or for tumors that are too large to be surgically removed. A multiple-drug treatment regimen often is used to maximize effectiveness.

Surgery

Surgery may be performed to remove the tumor and maintain an open airway. The type and extent of surgery are determined by the size, site, and invasiveness of the tumor. Carcinoma *in situ*, small localized tumors, and vocal cord polyps may be treated on an outpatient basis, using a laser to vaporize the tumor. The voice is preserved, but total voice rest is prescribed, with only whispering allowed for at least a week after surgery.

Laryngectomy, removal of the larynx, may be necessary for some patients. With a *partial laryngectomy* (removal of one-half or more of the larynx), the patient is able to resume normal speaking, breathing, and swallowing. A **tracheostomy** (a surgical opening into the trachea) tube may be inserted to maintain the airway in the early postoperative period, but it is usually removed within about a week and the stoma is allowed to heal.

In *total laryngectomy*, the entire larynx is removed, along with the surrounding tissues. Normal speech is lost, and a permanent tracheostomy is created. The tracheostomy tube may be removed after healing, leaving a natural stoma, or it may be left in place permanently. Because the trachea and the esophagus are permanently separated by this surgery (Figure 22-7■), there is no risk of aspiration during swallowing.

If cervical lymph nodes contain cancer cells, a *modified* or *radical neck dissection* may be done along with total laryngectomy. In a radical neck dissection, cervical lymph nodes, the sternocleidomastoid muscle, internal jugular vein, cranial nerve XI (spinal accessory), and submaxillary salivary gland are removed on the tumor side of the neck. After surgery, the patient may have difficulty lifting and turning the head because of muscle loss. The shoulder on the affected side drops. Postoperative neck exercises can help reduce shoulder drop and increase range of motion on the affected side. Box 22-8■ outlines nursing care for the patient having a total laryngectomy.

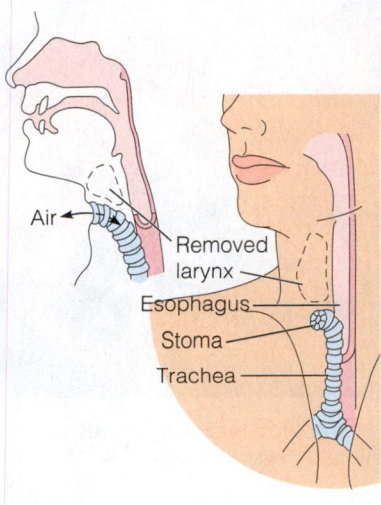

Figure 22-7. ■ After a total laryngectomy, the patient has a permanent tracheostomy. No connection between the trachea and esophagus remains.

BOX 22-8	NURSING CARE CHECKLIST

Total Laryngectomy

Before Surgery

☑ Provide routine preoperative care and teaching.

☑ Assess knowledge and anxiety level of the patient and family members and provide information and psychologic support as indicated.

☑ Discuss postoperative communication strategies. Emphasize that total laryngectomy results in a loss of speech and that the patient will breathe through a permanent stoma in the neck.

☑ Advise the patient that the senses of taste and smell are affected by surgery, which may affect appetite. Reassure the patient that food and fluids will be given by enteral feeding tube until eating can be resumed.

After Surgery

☑ Provide routine postoperative care.

☑ Monitor respiratory status at least every 1 to 2 hours (more frequently in the initial postoperative period), including airway patency; respiratory rate, depth, and pattern; and lung sounds.

☑ Monitor oxygen saturation levels. Report levels of less than 95% (or established parameters) to the charge nurse or physician.

☑ Place the call light within easy reach at all times; answer the call light promptly.

☑ Encourage family members to stay with the patient whenever possible.

☑ Encourage deep breathing and coughing.

☑ Elevate the head of the bed.

☑ Maintain humidification of inspired gases.

☑ Suction tracheostomy using sterile technique as needed.

☑ Provide tracheostomy care per protocol and as needed (see Box 22-9).

☑ Teach to support the head when moving in bed.

☑ Assist out of bed and with ambulation as soon as allowed after surgery.

☑ Teach to protect the stoma from particulate matter in the air with a gauze square or other stoma protector.

☑ Maintain fluid intake with intravenous fluids and/or enteral feedings until able to take adequate amounts of food and fluids orally.

☑ Before initiating feeding, assist to begin performing mouth rinses.

☑ When able to resume oral intake, begin with soft foods, not liquids.

☑ Reassure the patient that choking is not possible, because there is no connection between the esophagus and trachea.

☑ Provide for privacy during initial attempts at eating.

☑ Encourage the patient and family members to express their fears and anxieties.

Speech Rehabilitation

Various techniques may be used to restore speech after a total laryngectomy. A surgical procedure, the *tracheoesophageal puncture (TEP)*, is the usual method used to restore speech. TEP creates a small *fistula* (passage) between the posterior tracheal wall and the anterior esophagus (Figure 22-8■). A small, one-way valve in the fistula allows the patient to force air from the lungs into the mouth by covering the tracheostomy stoma with a finger. The air creates vibration and sound, and the patient uses the tongue, lips, teeth, and palate to articulate the words. The one-way valve prevents food from entering the trachea.

When TEP is not an option, electrolarynx devices can be used to generate speech. These battery-powered devices generate sound vibrations. When placed against the neck or into the corner of the mouth (Figure 22-8 B and C), these vibrations can be formed into words using the muscles of the lips, tongue, and mouth.

Esophageal speech uses swallowed air and controlled belching to create sound and form words. The patient uses muscles of the mouth and tongue normally involved in speech. This form of speech takes practice, and many patients are unable to resume speaking fluently.

NURSING CARE

The diagnosis of cancer is frightening for most patients, no matter what the potential for cure is with treatment. Problems related to communication, nutrition, and anticipatory grieving are included in this section. Nursing care specific to the patient undergoing a laryngectomy is given in Box 22-8. Nursing care of the patient with a tracheostomy is reviewed in Box 22-9■.

PRIORITIZING NURSING CARE

The immediate priority of care for the patient who has undergone a partial or total laryngectomy is maintaining a patent airway. As swelling and tissue edema recede, facilitating communication and promoting nutrition become a priority focus for nursing care.

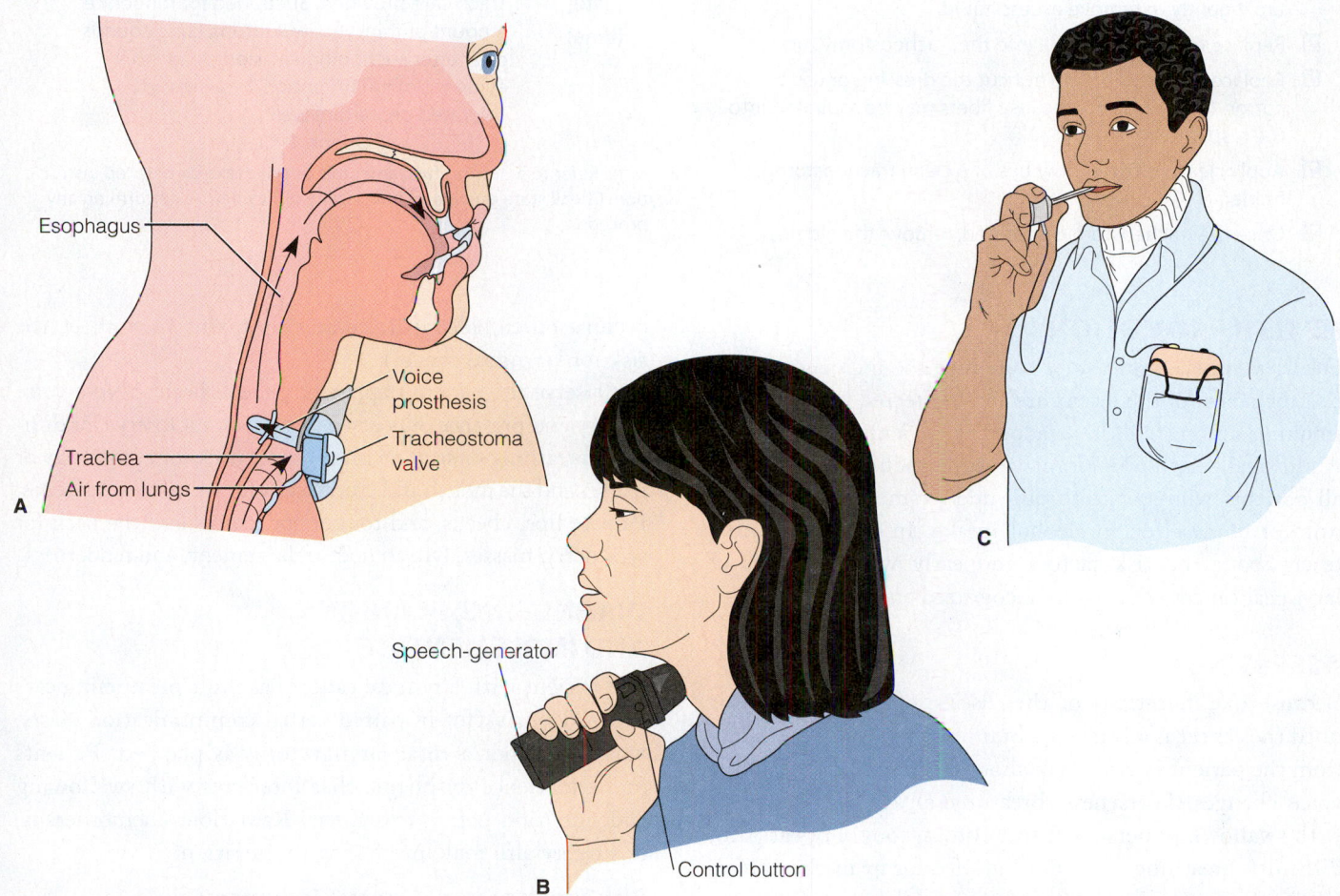

Figure 22-8. ■ (A) The tracheoesophageal puncture (TEP) with voice prosthesis allows air from the trachea to be diverted through the prosthesis into the esophagus and oropharynx, producing speech when the tracheostomy stoma is occluded. A one-way valve prevents food from entering the trachea. **(B** and **C)** The patient holds the vibrating tip of the electrolarynx against the throat or into the corner of the mouth, using the lips, tongue, and mouth to form words.

BOX 22-9	PROCEDURE CHECKLIST

Tracheostomy Care

- ☑ Gather all supplies.
- ☑ Provide for privacy. Explain the procedure and how to communicate (e.g., eye blinking or raising a finger to indicate distress).
- ☑ Place in semi-Fowler's or Fowler's position.
- ☑ Use Standard Precautions and sterile technique as indicated.
- ☑ Assess lung sounds; suction as needed using sterile technique (see figure).
- ☑ Wearing clean gloves, remove the tracheostomy dressing.
- ☑ Wearing sterile gloves, use sterile applicators or gauze 4 × 4s moistened with normal saline to clean the incision.
- ☑ If the tracheostomy tube has an inner cannula that can be removed for cleaning, remove the tube and soak it in sterile saline.
- ☑ Cleanse the tracheostomy tube flange (collar) in the same manner as the incision.
- ☑ Clean the inner cannula using a small brush or cotton-tipped applicators. Rinse thoroughly in normal saline and tap it gently to remove excess liquid.
- ☑ Replace the inner cannula into the tracheostomy tube.
- ☑ Replace the dressing. Do not cut the dressing or use a cotton-filled dressing because fibers may be aspirated into the respiratory tract.
- ☑ Apply clean tracheostomy ties or a clean tracheostomy holder.
- ☑ Once the tracheostomy is secured, remove the old ties.

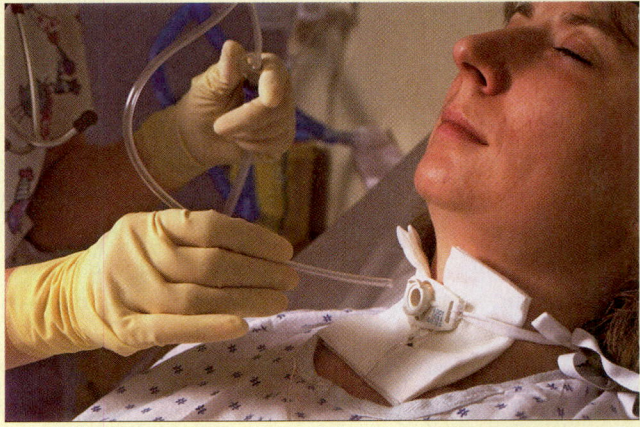

Using sterile technique to suction the tracheostomy during care. (Source: Pearson Education.)

- ☑ Assess breathing and tolerance of the procedure.
- ☑ Dispose of supplies and used solutions. Wash hands.

Sample Documentation

[date]	Trach care provided. Suctioned for moderate
[time]	amount of thin, yellow sputum. Lung sounds clear after suctioning. Incision clean, no evidence of inflammation. Healing well. Tolerated procedure well.
	_____ J. Doene, LPN.

Note: Refer to a nursing fundamentals or skills text for detailed instruction. Check state guidelines and facility policy before performing any procedure.

HEALTH PROMOTION

Health promotion measures to reduce the incidence of and risk for cancer of the larynx are those directed at preventing smoking among children, adolescents, and young adults. Additional health promotion measures include encouraging all patients who smoke to quit and promoting abstinence from or moderation in alcohol intake. In the community, teach about the risk factors and early warning signs of laryngeal cancer so it can be recognized and treated early.

ASSESSING

Because manifestations of the disease often do not occur until the cancer is advanced, obtaining good subjective data from the patient is vital. Ask about recent and/or persistent voice changes (hoarseness, breathiness); difficulty or pain with swallowing; persistent sore throat, cough, or ear pain; difficulty breathing; or sensation of a lump in the throat. Obtain the patient's smoking history: packs smoked per day and number of years of smoking. Inquire about alcohol consumption, noting the amount consumed per day or week, and the number of years of alcohol use. Note the patient's occupation (inhaled particulates or toxins may affect the risk for laryngeal cancer).

Observe the patient's apparent general health. Note voice quality and presence of hoarseness or cough. Observe for difficulty breathing or swallowing. Inspect neck for asymmetry or masses and the mouth and oropharynx for white or red patches. Palpate lips, cheeks, and tongue for masses and the neck for symmetry, masses, lymph node enlargement, and tenderness.

DIAGNOSING, PLANNING, AND IMPLEMENTING

The patient with laryngeal cancer has multiple nursing care needs. The risk for impaired verbal communication exists, whether or not a total laryngectomy is planned. Patients may experience dysphagia that interferes with swallowing and nutrition before treatment. Radiation, chemotherapy, or surgery also may interfere with nutrition.

Risk for Impaired Airway Clearance

Expected outcome: Airway will remain clear as evidenced by clear breath sounds and absence of stridor or respiratory distress.

The larynx is the narrowest portion of the upper airway. Tissue edema after surgery can restrict the airway, interfering with air movement and gas exchange.

clinicalALERT

During the immediate postoperative period, closely monitor for signs of airway obstruction, such as labored breathing, inspiratory stridor, or restlessness and anxiety.

- Apply cold packs to the neck as ordered. *Applying cold constricts blood vessels and reduces edema development.*
- Withhold oral food and fluids until cough and gag reflexes have returned. *Local anesthesia used during removal of benign tumors, nodules, and small malignancies impairs the cough and gag reflexes, increasing the risk for aspiration.*

Impaired Verbal Communication

Expected outcome: Will effectively communicate needs using alternative ways of communicating.

Removing the larynx results in voice loss. Before surgery, discuss alternate methods of communication, both short and long term, with the patient and family members.

- Before surgery, assess for additional obstacles to communication. *Hearing loss, illiteracy, previous stroke, or weakness may affect the ability to use alternate communication strategies.*
- Provide alternate ways to communicate (pencil and paper, Magic Slate, an alphabet board) and encourage practice. *Having the patient choose what to practice helps reduce anxiety and increases the sense of control.*
- Encourage the patient to consult a speech therapist before surgery if possible. *The patient may be a candidate for TEP, or an electrolarynx.*
- Assess frequently. Place the call bell at hand when leaving. *The presence and availability of a caring nurse decrease anxiety and promote communication.*

Imbalanced Nutrition: Less Than Body Requirements

Expected outcome: Will consume 100% of recommended diet once oral intake is allowed. Weight will remain stable.

After surgery, enteral or parenteral feedings often are ordered until the patient is able to eat. After a total laryngectomy, the patient initially loses the senses of taste and smell. The patient may partially recover the sense of taste but may complain that eating no longer holds pleasure.

- Assess nutritional status using height and weight charts, reported weight loss, and body mass indicators such as skin folds. *A complete assessment aids in planning to meet current and anticipated calorie needs.*
- Evaluate current diet, preferred foods, and understanding of nutrition. *Providing a diet that takes the patient's preferences into account will encourage adequate intake.*

- Monitor intake and output and food consumption. *Monitoring food and fluid intake is necessary to determine whether the patient is consuming adequate calories and fluids for healing.*
- Weigh daily. *The daily weight provides a measure of both nutritional status and fluid balance.*
- Contact the dietitian for further evaluation, planning, and education. *A professional can identify nutritional needs and help plan a diet to meet them.*
- Encourage experimentation with foods of different textures and temperatures. *Cold foods or foods with a soft texture are easier to swallow.*
- Encourage frequent, small meals rather than three large meals per day. *The patient who has difficulty swallowing is likely to consume more food this way.*
- Recommend liquid supplements such as Ensure as needed to increase calorie intake. Provide information about where to obtain supplements. *Liquid dietary supplements provide balanced nutrition and added calories. They are available in major supermarkets.*
- Provide mouth care before meals and supplemental feedings. For the patient with stomatitis or esophagitis related to radiation or chemotherapy, provide a topical anesthetic such as viscous lidocaine before eating. *Bad breath or a foul taste in the mouth suppresses appetite. Inflamed mucosa may make eating uncomfortable. A topical anesthetic can relieve discomfort and promote food intake.*
- Provide an antiemetic 30 minutes before eating if nausea is a problem. *An antiemetic can relieve nausea and make eating possible.*

Grieving

Expected outcome: Will express feelings about the diagnosis and effect of treatment on ability to speak.

The patient with laryngeal cancer faces the diagnosis of cancer; the prospect of mutilating surgery; and loss of an important function, speech. Loss of speech affects social interactions, one's career, and the ability to get help when necessary. A radical neck dissection changes the appearance and function of the neck, altering body image and self-concept.

- Provide opportunities for the patient and family members to express feelings of grief, anger, or fear about the diagnosis of cancer, the impending surgery, and the anticipated loss of speech. *The patient needs the opportunity (and permission) to grieve anticipated losses in order to move toward coping and acceptance of the loss.*
- Be calm and supportive. Provide privacy and emotional support for the patient and family to work through the grieving process. *It is important for the patient and family to know that their feelings of loss are real and accepted by caregivers.*
- Encourage the patient and family to discuss the potential impact of the loss on family structure and function. *Discussion helps family members to understand and support one another.*

- Refer the patient and family for counseling as appropriate. *Counseling may be necessary to prevent a sense of defeat and hopelessness.*
- Help the patient and family identify additional resources for coping, such as strategies they have used in the past to deal with crises. *This identifies strengths they can use to deal with the present situation.*

MANAGING NURSING CARE

Nursing care activities such as obtaining daily weights and assisting with hygiene, positioning, and ambulation for the patient with laryngeal cancer are appropriate to assign to assistive personnel. Educate assistive personnel about the importance of responding promptly to the patient's call light, supporting the head and neck when positioning the patient, and immediately reporting respiratory distress.

EVALUATING

Collect the following data to evaluate the effectiveness of nursing interventions for the patient with laryngeal cancer:

- Airway remains patent; experiences no difficulty breathing.
- Communicates care needs effectively.
- Anxiety remains within a manageable level.
- Maintains weight.
- Demonstrates willingness to participate in speech therapy.

DOCUMENTING

Document continuing assessment data, as well as procedures and nursing care performed. Note the patient's and family's responses to the surgery; the resulting voice loss; presence of the tracheostomy (if performed); and, if radical neck surgery was performed, weakness and disfigurement of the neck. Document teaching provided and the patient's and family's ability to demonstrate care measures taught (e.g., protecting the tracheostomy stoma, suctioning and cleaning the tracheostomy, care of the incision).

CONTINUITY OF CARE

For the patient with a benign tumor of the larynx, stress the importance of voice rest. Refer patients, particularly singers and others who must project their voice, to a speech therapist for voice training. Emphasize the need to keep the voice within its normal range to reduce vocal cord stress. Talk about the importance of quitting smoking with all patients.

After diagnosis of laryngeal cancer, provide information and clarify treatment options, discussing the risks and benefits of each. Stress importance of early intervention to reduce the risk of local spread and metastasis. If a total laryngectomy is the treatment of choice, discuss options for communication after surgery. Present the options realistically. Patients may have difficulty manipulating the tracheoesophageal puncture device for speech; only about 30% of patients master esophageal speech.

Teach the patient undergoing radiation therapy about the treatments, care of the skin and secretions during therapy, and expected side effects.

Assess the patient's and family's resources and ability to provide home care after surgery, including activities of daily living, tracheostomy care, and manipulation of TEP or an electrolarynx.

Teach the patient and family members how to care for the tracheostomy and provide the opportunity for practice and feedback. The patient uses clean technique rather than sterile technique in providing stoma care. Once the stoma is fully healed, the tracheostomy tube may no longer be needed. Teach the following:

- Use a humidifier or vaporizer in the home to add humidity to inspired air.
- Increase fluid intake to maintain mucosal moisture and loosen secretions.
- Shield the stoma with a stoma guard (e.g., a gauze square) to prevent particles from entering the lower respiratory tract.
- Promptly remove secretions from the skin surrounding the stoma to prevent irritation and skin breakdown.
- Protect the stoma with a cupped hand or washcloth while showering or bathing; do not submerge the neck or head.
- Do not participate in water sports. All other activities are allowed, but lifting may be more difficult because of the inability to hold the breath (the Valsalva maneuver).

Encourage the patient to work with a physical therapist to regain function and mobility of the neck and shoulder if a radical neck dissection has been done.

Discuss the treatment plan, and suggest measures to deal with adverse effects of radiation or chemotherapy. Address the risk for respiratory infections and measures to reduce exposure, particularly in the patient with a permanent tracheostomy.

Both the patient and family need emotional and motivational support through this trying time. Provide referral to local support groups such as a Laryngectomy Club or Lost Cord Club. Encourage the patient to discontinue the use of cigarettes and alcohol, emphasizing the positive effects of smoking cessation on the potential for cure. Discuss ways to achieve good nutrition. If the patient and family are having difficulty adjusting to the diagnosis of cancer and the effects of treatment, provide referral to counseling. (See the Clinical Reasoning Care Map at the end of this chapter.)

Note: The references and resources for all chapters have been compiled at the back of the book.

Chapter Review

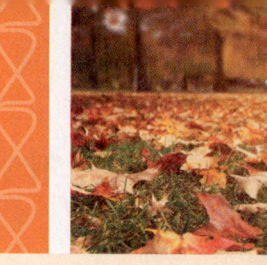

KEY POINTS

- **Concept:** A patent airway and unobstructed airflow are vital to sustain life and function. Disorders affecting the upper airway range from mild and self-limiting viral infections to acute and life-threatening obstruction.
- **Concept:** Common upper respiratory tract infections and inflammations generally are mild and appropriate for self-care. Complications such as pneumonia can develop, particularly in older adults and people who are frail or those with chronic illness.
- Teaching is the primary nursing intervention for patients with upper respiratory infections.
- Although many decongestants and antihistamines are available without a prescription, these drugs are not appropriate for all people. They may cause drowsiness, increased blood pressure, or problems for people who have glaucoma, intestinal problems, or urinary retention.
- Bacterial complications such as pneumonia, sinusitis, and peritonsillar abscess may follow viral URIs. These complications do require medical treatment, often antibiotic therapy.

- **Concept:** Trauma to, or obstruction of, the upper airways can pose a serious threat to respiration and tissue oxygenation. Maintaining and restoring a patent airway are nursing priorities whenever the upper airway is threatened.
- Most nosebleeds occur in the anterior portion of the nose and can be controlled by putting pressure and ice on the nose. Older adults are at risk for posterior nosebleeds. Posterior nosebleeds are more difficult to control and often require medical treatment.
- **Concept:** Persistent hoarseness or voice change is a common manifestation of laryngeal cancer. Urge patients to seek medical assessment if this occurs. Stress that with early intervention, laryngeal cancer is curable and the ability to speak is preserved.
- The primary risk factors for laryngeal cancer are smoking and excess alcohol use. Discuss these lifestyle factors with all patients, especially those who have other risk factors for laryngeal cancer.

PEARSON NURSING STUDENT RESOURCES

Find additional materials at **nursing.pearsonhighered.com**.

Clinical Reasoning Care Map

Caring for a Patient With Total Laryngectomy

NCLEX-PN® Focus Area: Reduction of Risk Potential

Case Study: David Tom is a 61-year-old divorced man with two grown children. He has smoked two packs of cigarettes daily since high school. He drinks three or four cocktails every evening. Mr. Tom was recently diagnosed with advanced laryngeal cancer after he sought care for a sore throat and hoarseness that had persisted for a few months. He has been admitted to the surgical care unit from the intensive care unit (ICU) 2 days post–total laryngectomy.

Nursing Diagnosis: Risk for Ineffective Airway Clearance

COLLECT DATA

Subjective	Objective
_____	_____
_____	_____
_____	_____
_____	_____
_____	_____
_____	_____

Does this present a threat to the patient's safety?

If yes, the priority intervention to address this threat would be:

_____

Nursing Care

_____
_____
_____
_____
_____
_____
_____
_____
_____
_____

Interprofessional team members to include when planning care:

_____

How would you document this? _____

_____

Compare your answers and documentation to those provided on the companion website.

Data Collected
(use only those that apply)

- PB. 146/84; P 92 and regular; R 18; T 100°F (37.7°C) per rectum
- Tracheostomy tube present
- O_2 per tracheostomy collar
- Oxygen saturation 94%
- Rates pain in neck and right shoulder at 6 on a scale of 1 to 10
- Continuous tube feeding per gastrostomy tube
- Two Hemovac wound drains in the right neck draining 15 and 35 mL of serosanguineous fluid
- Complains that head "feels heavy"
- Ambulatory within the room without assistance
- Uses Magic Slate to communicate

Nursing Interventions
(use only those that apply; list in priority order)

- Encourage to deep breathe and cough hourly.
- Assess pain at least every 2 to 3 hours and administer analgesics as ordered.
- Up at bedside and ambulating at least four times per day.
- Provide written information as requested.
- Assess respiratory rate, lung sounds, and cough effectiveness every 2 hours.
- Monitor intake, output, and daily weight.
- Arrange for a dietary consultation to determine calorie needs.
- Monitor quantity, color, and odor of secretions.

NCLEX-PN® Exam Preparation

1 After teaching a patient about the antihistamine Chlor-Trimeton (chlorpheniramine), which statement indicates that further instruction is necessary?
1. "I'm not going to drive today. My sister will pick me up."
2. "I will stop at the grocery store for a bag of hard peppermint candy."
3. "I'm going to a wine-tasting party tonight."
4. "I'll call my doctor if I have trouble breathing."

2 To most effectively anticipate the needs of a patient who has undergone a tonsillectomy, the nurse would plan to:
1. apply a warm compress to the neck.
2. place the patient in a supine position.
3. remove the nasopharyngeal airway immediately.
4. place a humidifier by the bedside.

3 A patient presents at the urgent care clinic with complaints of a severe cough that interferes with her ability to eat and drink and often causes her to vomit. The patient has symptoms of dehydration, and talking stimulates paroxysms of coughing during which she has difficulty catching her breath. Recognizing these as classic manifestations of pertussis, the nurse:
1. administers a narcotic cough suppressant.
2. initiates respiratory isolation precautions.
3. obtains a sputum specimen for culture.
4. alerts coworkers that anyone not vaccinated for pertussis as an infant should avoid contact with the patient.

4 A resident of a nursing home will be receiving an influenza injection. Which information would be most important for the care of this patient?
1. Allergy history
2. Name of insurance company
3. Medical history
4. Respiratory status

5 The nurse understands that the most important intervention for the patient with an uncomplicated upper respiratory viral infection is:
1. obtaining throat cultures.
2. teaching self-care.
3. monitoring vital signs.
4. antibiotic medication teaching.

6 In teaching a patient about laryngitis, it is important to focus on:
1. resting the voice.
2. effective coughing techniques.
3. increasing fluid intake.
4. use of a cough suppressant at bedtime.

7 A patient presents to the emergency department with severe bleeding from the anterior nasal septum. All of the following nursing actions are appropriate. Place them in order of priority.
1. Apply ice packs to the nose.
2. Give the patient an emesis basin into which he or she can spit the blood.
3. Pinch the nose toward the septum.
4. Ask what precipitated the incident.
5. Inquire about current medications.

8 Which of these statements, if made by a patient diagnosed with sleep apnea, would indicate an understanding of this condition?
1. "I'm going to sleep on my back for the next 2 weeks."
2. "I would like to see the dietitian about my weight."
3. "Please ask the doctor to order a sleeping pill for me."
4. "I won't snore so loud if I drink a glass of wine before bedtime."

9 A patient at a blood pressure clinic tells the nurse that his voice has been hoarse for "about a month now." He denies sore throat or difficulty swallowing. The appropriate response by the nurse is:
1. "Since you don't also have a sore throat, it really isn't anything to worry about."
2. "Persistent hoarseness is a sign of voice strain. You should rest your voice for a couple of weeks and see if it improves."
3. "Try using warm saltwater gargles three to four times a day. This sounds like persistent laryngitis."
4. "Persistent hoarseness can be an early sign of laryngeal cancer. Please tell your doctor about this."

10 A patient who has had a total laryngectomy and permanent tracheostomy is afraid to eat for fear of choking. The nurse's response is based on the knowledge that:
1. choking is a significant risk after total laryngectomy.
2. choking can be prevented by closing the tracheostomy stoma with a finger while swallowing.
3. the trachea and esophagus are separate, so choking is not a risk.
4. oral intake should begin with water only until the patient learns to swallow without choking.

Answers and rationales for Review Questions appear in Appendix I.

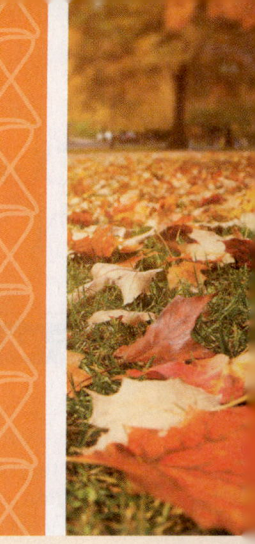

CHAPTER 23

Caring for Patients With Lower Respiratory Disorders

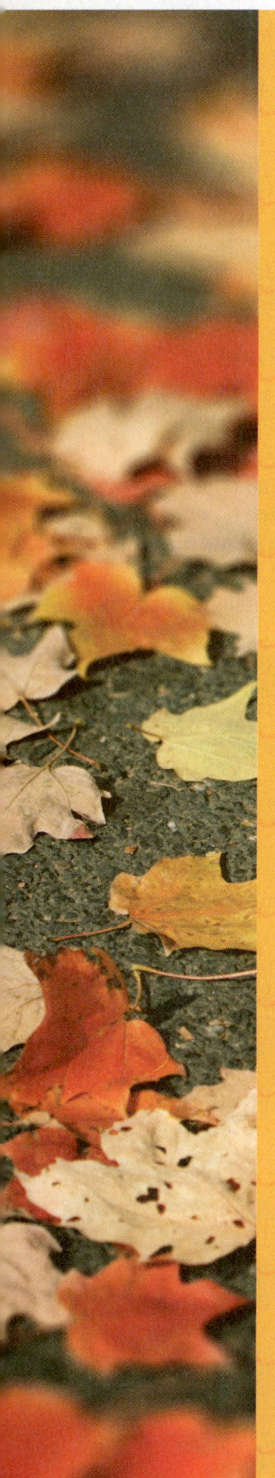

BRIEF OUTLINE

INFECTIOUS AND INFLAMMATORY DISORDERS
Acute Bronchitis
Pneumonia
Tuberculosis
Lung Abscess and Empyema
Emerging Respiratory Infections
OBSTRUCTIVE LUNG DISORDERS
Asthma
Chronic Obstructive Pulmonary Disease

Cystic Fibrosis
Atelectasis
Bronchiectasis
Occupational Lung Diseases
LUNG CANCER
PULMONARY VASCULAR DISORDERS
Pulmonary Embolism
Pulmonary Hypertension
PLEURAL DISORDERS AND TRAUMA

Pleuritis
Pleural Effusion
Pneumothorax
Hemothorax
Chest and Lung Trauma
CRITICAL RESPIRATORY CONDITIONS
Respiratory Failure
Acute Respiratory Distress Syndrome

APPLIED LEARNING OUTCOMES

After completing this chapter, you will be able to:

1. Describe the pathophysiology of common lower respiratory system disorders.

2. Relate manifestations of lower respiratory system disorders to the normal structure and function of the lungs and thoracic cage.

3. Safely administer medications and treatments used for lower respiratory system disorders.

4. Conduct a focused assessment of the patient with a lower respiratory system disorder, identifying and appropriately responding to unexpected or abnormal findings.

5. Relate important concepts of caring for the patient who has had thoracic surgery or who requires airway support and mechanical ventilation.

6. Use current evidence-based guidelines and the nursing process to plan and implement individualized care for patients with lower respiratory system disorders.

7. Reinforce teaching and learning for patients with lower respiratory system disorders and their families, demonstrating consideration for expressed patient values, needs, and preferences.

KEY TERMS

The key terms are defined on the pages listed below.

SPECIAL FEATURES

Key Concept   Effective lung ventilation and gas exchange can be affected by infectious diseases, airway restriction, structural changes of the lung tissue or chest wall, acute or chronic inflammatory disorders, and tumors.

Disorders of the lower respiratory system are common, affecting people in the community and in acute care and long-term care facilities. Lower respiratory disorders are costly. Pneumonia and obstructive lung disease are among the most common diagnoses leading to hospital admission, and the health care costs associated with respiratory failure have increased rapidly in recent years.

Lower respiratory system disorders have both local and systemic effects. Local effects include cough, excess production of mucus, **dyspnea** (difficulty breathing), **hemoptysis** (bloody sputum), and chest pain. Systemic effects may include fever, anorexia and malaise, **cyanosis** (a bluish-gray skin color), edema, clubbing of fingers and toes, and other manifestations of impaired gas exchange.

In this chapter, you will learn about three disorders that are leading causes of death in the United States: pneumonia, chronic obstructive lung disease (COPD), and lung cancer. In addition, you will study about disorders seen across populations: asthma and tuberculosis. A deep understanding of these disorders and the nursing care needs of patients experiencing these problems is important for safe, effective care.

INFECTIOUS AND INFLAMMATORY DISORDERS

Key Concept   Inflammation of lung tissue can interfere with ventilation and gas exchange, affecting tissue oxygenation and carbon dioxide elimination. The nurse must assess for the potential effects of impairment and support and promote effective ventilation and gas exchange in patients with lung infections or inflammation.

The lower respiratory system is protected from infection by a number of defenses. If an organism makes it past the upper respiratory tract, it is usually trapped in the mucus of the lower respiratory tract. *Cilia* (small hairs) that line the airways and the cough reflex then push the mucus-trapped organism out. Organisms that make it past all of these barriers usually are destroyed in the alveolus by the immune defenses of the body. When these defenses are impaired, the risk of infection increases. For example, chronic lung disease impairs the mucus and ciliary responses to invasion. Older adults have a higher risk than others of lower respiratory infections (Box 23-1 ■). Even in healthy patients, pathogens can enter the lungs, causing an infectious or inflammatory response.

Acute Bronchitis

Bronchitis (inflammation of the bronchi) can be either acute or chronic. Acute bronchitis is relatively common among adults. Chronic bronchitis is a component of chronic obstructive pulmonary disease and is discussed in that section of this chapter.

PATHOPHYSIOLOGY AND MANIFESTATIONS

Acute bronchitis typically follows an upper respiratory infection (URI). People with impaired defense mechanisms and smokers have a higher risk for bronchitis. Viruses, bacteria, and toxic gases or chemicals can cause bronchitis. The inflammatory response leads to vasodilation and edema of the bronchial linings. Mucus production increases, stimulating the cough reflex.

The cough is initially nonproductive, but later becomes productive. The cough often occurs in *paroxysms* (uncontrollable bursts) and may be aggravated by cold, dry, or dusty air. Substernal chest pain is common. Other symptoms include fever and general malaise.

COLLABORATIVE CARE

Acute bronchitis usually is diagnosed using the history and examination. A *chest x-ray* may be ordered to rule out pneumonia, because the manifestations can be similar. Treatment includes rest, increased fluid intake, and mild analgesics to relieve fever and malaise. An antibiotic such as erythromycin or penicillin may be prescribed. Because acute bronchitis often is viral in origin, antibiotic therapy is not always appropriate. An expectorant cough

---

BOX 23-1	FOCUS ON OLDER ADULTS

Lower Respiratory Tract Infections

Changes associated with aging and disease affect respiratory function and airway clearance, increasing the risk of infections. The number of cilia decreases, and the cough weakens. Gag and cough reflexes diminish. The chest wall and supportive lung tissue become stiffer (less elastic). Alveoli enlarge, decreasing the surface area for gas exchange. Residual volume increases, and vital capacity decreases. As a result, the older adult is less able to clear respiratory secretions and is at greater risk for complications when an infection develops. The older adult is at risk for dehydration, leading to thick, sticky mucus that is difficult to expectorate. Immune function declines with aging. Limited mobility, a smoking history, surgery, multiple medications, malnutrition, and chronic diseases also may increase older adults' risk for respiratory infections.

medication is recommended for daytime and a cough suppressant at night to facilitate rest.

NURSING CARE

Patients with acute bronchitis are rarely hospitalized, so nursing care focuses on teaching. Advise that bed rest is not often necessary. Daily living activities can be maintained with adequate rest. Instruct the patient to increase fluid intake. Discuss the use and effects of ordered drugs and explain why antibiotic therapy is not always appropriate. Stress the importance of smoking cessation. Instruct to contact primary care provider if symptoms do not improve within a week or if they become worse.

Pneumonia

Pneumonia is inflammation of the respiratory bronchioles and alveoli. It is a leading cause of death in the United States, particularly among older adults and people with debilitating diseases. Pneumonia is a leading cause of hospital admission (Wier et al., 2011). Nurses need a deep understanding of nursing care priorities for patients with pneumonia.

Pneumonia that develops outside of health care settings is known as *community-acquired pneumonia (CAP)*. When the patient has recently received inpatient treatment, it is called *health care–acquired pneumonia*. Pneumonia may be either infectious or noninfectious. Bacteria, viruses, fungi, protozoa, and other microbes can lead to infectious pneumonia. Noninfectious causes include aspiration of gastric contents and inhalation of toxic or irritating gases.

memory**ALERT**

- Pneumonia is the ninth leading cause of death in the United States.
- Older adults have the highest risk of death associated with pneumonia.

Bacterial infection is the leading cause of community-acquired pneumonia. Although anyone may develop pneumonia, certain factors increase the risk. Cigarette smoking interferes with normal defense mechanisms in the lungs. Medications and drugs such as alcohol that impair consciousness also can interfere with normal respiratory defenses. Immune defenses may be impaired in people with chronic diseases such as chronic obstructive pulmonary disease, diabetes, heart failure, or liver or kidney disease.

PATHOPHYSIOLOGY

Community-acquired pneumonia is classified as typical or atypical, depending on the causative organism and presentation. *Typical* pneumonia results from bacterial infection of the alveoli by a pathogen such as *Streptococcus pneumoniae* (pneumococcal pneumonia), *Haemophilus influenzae*, and *Staphylococcus aureus*. *Mycoplasma pneumonia* is the leading cause of *atypical* pneumonia. Influenza and adenovirus, *Chlamydophila pneumoniae*, and *Legionella pneumophila* also may cause atypical pneumonia. Atypical pneumonia generally is less severe than bacterial pneumonia, although older adults and patients with chronic diseases may experience serious effects. *Pneumocystis* pneumonia (PcP) is a pneumonia affecting patients with AIDS. PcP is an opportunistic infection caused by *P. jiroveci*, a common environmental organism that rarely affects patients with intact immune systems.

Pneumonia is further identified by its anatomic location. *Lobar pneumonia* affects all or part of a lung lobe; *bronchopneumonia* leads to a patchy distribution involving more than one lobe. Some pneumonias cause patchy inflammation of supportive lung tissue, including the alveolar septum and interstitial tissue.

In most cases, microbes responsible for infectious pneumonia initially colonize the nasal or oral pharynx. From there, they enter the lungs when secretions from the pharynx are aspirated. Microorganisms released during sneezing, coughing, or talking also may be inhaled. Contaminated water that is aerosolized by air-conditioning units, showers, or respiratory care equipment also may be a source of inhaled pathogens.

When bacteria invade the lungs, an inflammatory response follows. Inflammation causes the alveoli to become edematous and fill with fluid. In some cases, additional damage is caused by toxins released by the infecting organism. Blood cells and bacteria collect in the alveoli and respiratory bronchioles, leading to *consolidation* (solidification) of lung tissue. The lower lobes of the lungs are usually affected because of gravity (Figure 23-1 ■). Edema fluid and collected debris provide a growth medium for bacteria and spread the infection to other parts of the lung. Eventually, macrophages digest and remove the fluid, bacteria, and damaged cells from the infected lung.

Aspiration Pneumonia

Aspiration of gastric contents or material from the oropharynx into the lungs causes a chemical and bacterial pneumonia known as *aspiration pneumonia*. The risk for aspiration pneumonia is highest during emergency surgery and when cough and gag reflexes are depressed or swallowing is impaired. Older adults and patients receiving tube feedings are also at risk for aspiration pneumonia. Vomiting may not be obvious; silent regurgitation of gastric contents may occur if the level of consciousness (LOC) is reduced. The low pH of gastric juice causes severe inflammation in the lungs. Pulmonary edema and respiratory failure may result.

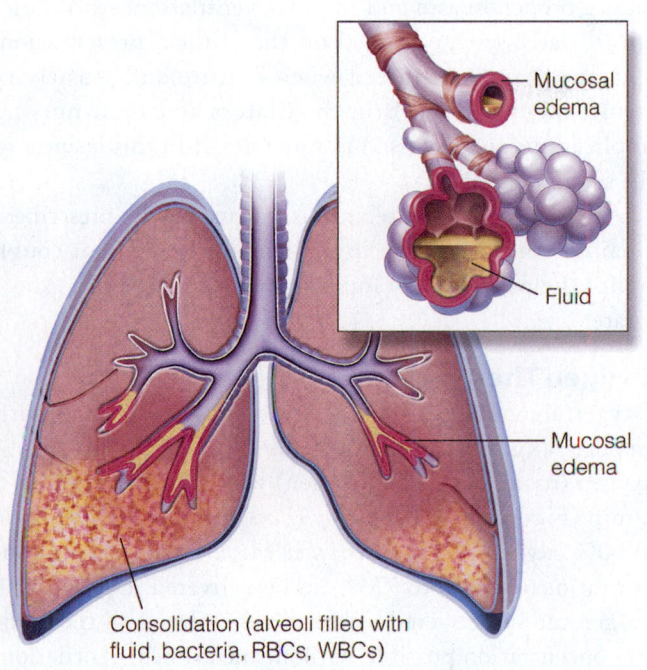

Figure 23-1. ■ Lobar pneumonia with consolidation of the lower lobes of the lungs. (Source: Pearson Education.)

Labels within figure: Mucosal edema; Fluid; Mucosal edema; Consolidation (alveoli filled with fluid, bacteria, RBCs, WBCs)

MANIFESTATIONS AND COMPLICATIONS

The presentation and manifestations of pneumonia vary, depending on the causative organism and patient factors such as age and general health. Common manifestations include fever or hypothermia, chills and diaphoresis, cough, pleuritic chest pain, or dyspnea. Table 23-1 ■ compares the causes, manifestations, and potential complications of typical and atypical pneumonias.

Typical Pneumonia

The onset of bacterial pneumonia usually is acute, with shaking chills, fever, and cough productive of rust-colored or purulent sputum. Chest pain (aching or sharp and localized) is common. Diminished breath sounds and fine crackles are heard over the affected lung area. If the involved area is large, respiratory distress is evident. The older adult may have fewer respiratory symptoms, presenting with fever or hypothermia, tachypnea, and altered mental status (Perry, 2012).

The most common complication of pneumococcal pneumonia is *pleuritis* (pleurisy), painful inflammation of the adjacent pleura. Pneumonias can cause extensive lung damage, leading to necrosis, abscess, and *empyema* (a collection of pus in the pleural cavity).

Atypical Pneumonia

Atypical pneumonia frequently is mild, with symptoms that tend to mimic influenza, leading many people to refer to it as "walking pneumonia." Young adults (college students, military recruits) have the highest incidence of atypical pneumonia. Depending on the organism, it can be highly contagious. Fever, headache, muscle aches, and malaise are common; the cough associated with atypical pneumonia tends to be dry, hacking, and nonproductive. Although atypical pneumonia often is a self-limiting disorder, the cough may persist for up to 6 weeks, usually becoming worse at night.

Complications are rare in atypical pneumonia. Patients with preexisting medical conditions and older adults have the greatest risk of developing complications such as respiratory failure.

TABLE 23-1	Manifestations and Potential Complications of Pneumonia	
	TYPICAL PNEUMONIA	**ATYPICAL PNEUMONIA**
Causes	■ *S. pneumoniae* ■ *S. aureus* ■ *H. influenzae* ■ Others	■ *M. pneumoniae* ■ *C. pneumoniae* ■ *L. pneumophila* ■ Influenza virus ■ Adenovirus
Manifestations	■ Abrupt onset ■ Fever, shaking chills ■ Tachypnea, dyspnea ■ Cough; may be dry or productive of purulent sputum ■ Pleuritic chest pain ■ Diminished breath sounds, crackles	■ Onset usually gradual ■ Fever ■ Headache, malaise ■ Dry, hacking cough ■ Muscle and joint pain ■ Flulike symptoms
Potential complications	■ Pleuritis ■ Lung abscess, empyema ■ Hypoxia, respiratory failure	■ Abnormal immune responses ■ Laryngitis ■ Hypoxia, respiratory failure

COLLABORATIVE CARE

With early diagnosis and treatment, most patients with pneumonia recover fully. However, pneumonia has a significant mortality, especially among the old, weak, and chronically ill.

Diagnostic Tests

The *chest x-ray* is the primary test used to establish the diagnosis of pneumonia. Chest x-ray helps identify the extent and pattern of lung involvement. Fluid, consolidated lung tissue, and *atelectasis* (areas of alveolar collapse) can be identified. Other diagnostic tests may be done to identify the causative organism and effects of the disorder. Before initiation of antibiotic therapy, a *sputum specimen* may be obtained; Gram stain and culture are performed to identify the organism. It is important to obtain sputum for culture from the lower respiratory tract, not the mouth and nasal passages. Other diagnostic tests include:

- *Complete blood count (CBC)* with *white blood cell (WBC) differential* shows an elevated WBC count with more immature WBCs in an acute bacterial pneumonia; the WBC count may be low in atypical pneumonia.
- *Arterial blood gases (ABGs)* may be done to evaluate gas exchange.
- *Pulse oximetry* is used to monitor arterial oxygen saturation. An SaO_2 of less than 95% may indicate impaired gas exchange or ventilation.

Immunization

Pneumococcal vaccine is recommended for people over age 65 and for people with compromised immune function, chronic cardiac or respiratory conditions, diabetes mellitus, alcoholism, or other chronic diseases. Annual influenza vaccine is also recommended for all people who do not have a contraindication to it.

Medications

Medications used to treat pneumonia may include antibiotics to eradicate causative organisms and bronchodilators to reduce bronchospasm and improve ventilation. Antibiotics are initially selected based on the clinical presentation. Therapy may be adjusted when culture and sensitivity results are available. Bronchodilators and their nursing implications are discussed in more detail in this chapter in the section on asthma.

An agent to liquefy tenacious mucus may be prescribed. Guaifenesin, a common ingredient in expectorant cough syrups, helps to liquefy mucus, making it easier to expectorate.

Oxygen Therapy

Oxygen may be ordered when pneumonia interferes with gas exchange. The *nasal cannula* delivers 23% to 45% oxygen (room air is 21% oxygen) with flow rates of 2 to 6 L/min (Figure 23-2■). A *simple face mask* can deliver 40% to 60% oxygen. With a *partial rebreather mask*, oxygen concentrations of 60% to 75% can be delivered. Up to 100% oxygen can be delivered by the *nonrebreather mask*, the highest concentration possible without mechanical ventilation. When the amount of oxygen delivered must be carefully regulated, a *Venturi mask* is used. The percentage of oxygen delivered by Venturi mask can be precisely regulated, from 24% to 50%. A severely hypoxic patient may require intubation and mechanical ventilation. Endotracheal intubation and mechanical ventilation are discussed in the section on respiratory failure.

Other Therapies

Increasing fluid intake to 2,500 to 3,000 mL/day helps liquefy secretions, making them easier to cough up and expectorate. If oral intake is inadequate, intravenous fluids and nutrition may be required.

When mucous secretions are thick and viscous or the cough is weak, percussion, vibration, and postural drainage may be ordered. *Percussion* is done by rhythmically striking or clapping the chest wall with cupped hands (Figure 23-3■). Cupping traps air between the palm and the skin, causing vibrations that loosen respiratory secretions. The trapped air also provides a cushion, preventing

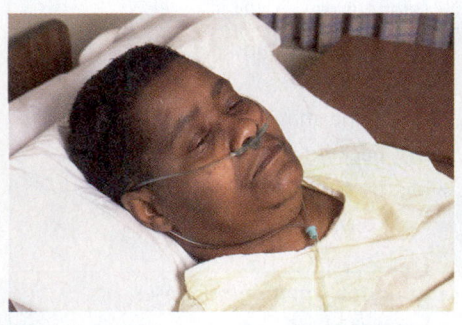
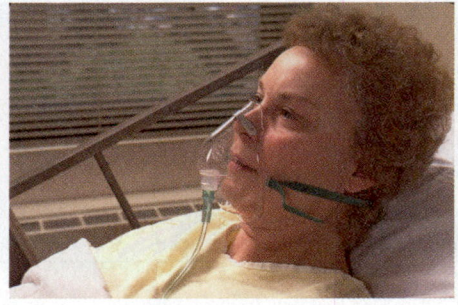
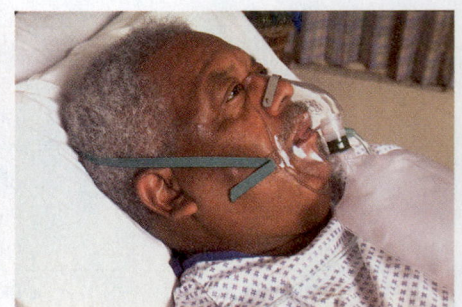

A   B   C

Figure 23-2. ■ Oxygen delivery devices. (**A**) Nasal cannula. (**B**) Simple face mask. (**C**) Partial rebreather mask. (Source: Pearson Education.)

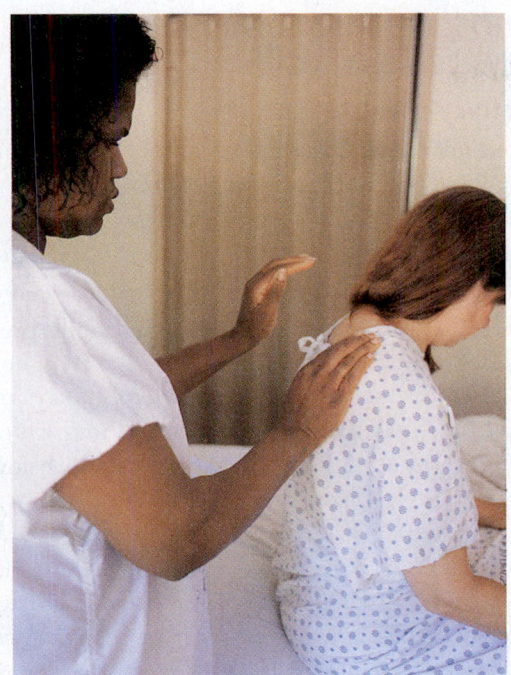

Figure 23-3. ■ Percussing the upper chest. Note the cupped position of the nurse's hands. (Source: Pearson Education.)

injury. A mechanical percussion device also may be used. The breasts, sternum, spinal column, and kidney areas are avoided during percussion.

Vibration helps loosen and move secretions into larger airways. Vibrations are produced by tensing and vibrating the arm muscles while keeping firm pressure on the chest wall with the hands.

Percussion and vibration are performed along with postural drainage. *Postural drainage* uses gravity to help remove secretions from a particular lung segment. The patient is positioned with the lung area to be drained above the trachea or mainstem bronchus. A variety of positions (Figure 23-4■) may be used, depending on the lung segment to be drained. Postural drainage should be done before meals to avoid nausea and vomiting.

Complementary Therapies

Although complementary therapies do not replace conventional treatment for pneumonia, they can promote comfort. The aromas of cedarwood and frankincense or inhaling the steam of water containing eucalyptus or sage may help relieve chest congestion. Massaging the chest with lavender also may help. Licorice root can be used to relieve congestion and as a cough suppressant. Licorice interacts with some drugs used to treat high blood pressure and heart disease and should be used with caution. Its use is contraindicated during pregnancy. Tea tree oil (applied topically or a few drops on a handkerchief) has anti-infective properties and may be used together with conventional treatment of pneumonia.

NURSING CARE

Nurses provide care for patients with pneumonia in a variety of settings. Previously healthy patients with pneumonia usually are cared for in the community. For these patients, the nurse's focus is on assessing and teaching. Patients who require hospitalization often are quite ill, requiring careful monitoring and nursing interventions to support oxygenation and promote comfort.

PRIORITIZING NURSING CARE

The priority of nursing care for patients with pneumonia is monitoring the effects of the disease on the patient's ability to maintain open airways and on the exchange of gases in the alveoli.

HEALTH PROMOTION

Health promotion activities to prevent pneumonia focus on teaching and promoting immunization of vulnerable populations. Encourage patients in high-risk groups to be vaccinated against pneumococcal pneumonia and to obtain annual influenza immunizations.

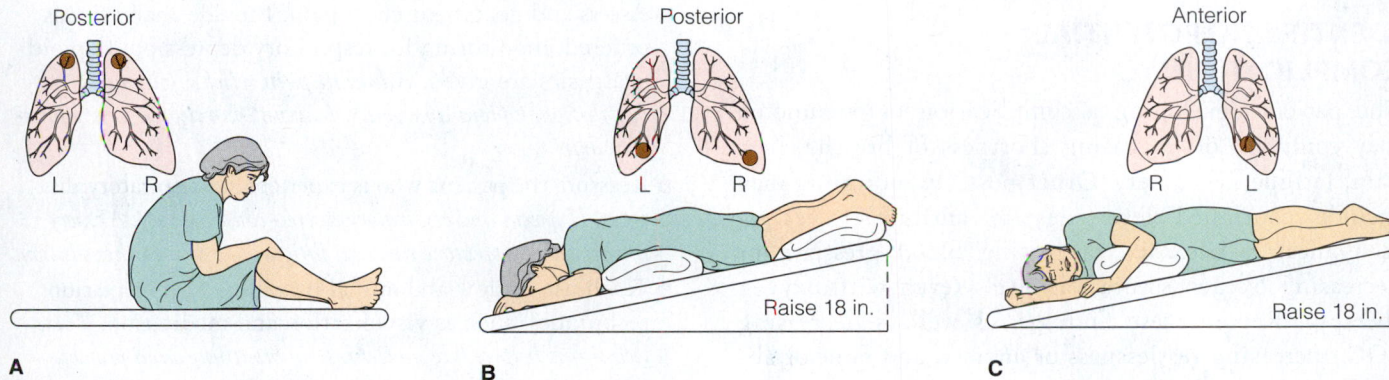

Figure 23-4. ■ Positions for postural drainage of selected specific areas of the lungs.

In older adults, measures to reduce exposure to crowds and ill people are appropriate to help prevent pneumonia. Promoting physical activity helps airway clearance, and measures to support nutrition and rest promote immune function.

ASSESSING

Assessment data is used to identify manifestations of pneumonia and to monitor the progress of patients with pneumonia. Collect subjective data, including complaints of chest pain, shortness of breath or difficulty breathing, and cough. Inquire about the location and severity of pain and changes in the pain associated with breathing or movement. Ask about the timing of a cough and production of sputum. If present, have the patient describe the color and quantity of sputum. Ask about current medications, any chronic diseases, and a history of previous episodes of pneumonia or other respiratory conditions. Inquire about allergies and the patient's history of smoking, use of alcohol or other mind-altering drugs, and known exposure to occupational or environmental pollutants.

Assess vital signs (including temperature and apical pulse), skin color, and mental status. Note respiratory rate and depth, O_2 saturation, and evidence of dyspnea or cough. Auscultate lung sounds, listening for the presence of breath sounds throughout all lung fields and any adventitious sounds, such as the following:

- *Crackles*: short, discrete, crackling, or bubbling sounds
- *Wheezes*: musical sounds caused by narrowed airways due to inflammation, constriction, or excessive mucus
- *Friction rub*: a loud, dry, creaking sound caused by inflammation of the pleura

IDENTIFYING POTENTIAL COMPLICATIONS

The patient developing a complication of pneumonia may complain of increasing shortness of breath, chest pain, fatigue, or anxiety. Other possible indicators may include continued fever despite antibiotic therapy, tachypnea, tachycardia, decreasing blood pressure, or decreasing oxygen saturation levels (even with oxygen therapy). Report these findings, as well as decreasing LOC, increasing restlessness or anxiety, and faint or absent breath sounds.

DIAGNOSING, PLANNING, AND IMPLEMENTING

Ineffective Airway Clearance

Expected outcome: Lung sounds will be present throughout lung fields and clear to auscultation.

Airway inflammation, edema, and secretions interfere with air movement and airway clearance in patients with pneumonia.

- Assess respiratory status, including vital signs, breath sounds, and cough and sputum, at least every 4 hours. *The patient with acute pneumonia can quickly develop respiratory distress; frequent assessment allows early intervention.*
- Notify the physician if oxygen saturation falls below 92% or ordered level. *Airway obstruction can interfere with alveolar ventilation and gas exchange, leading to tissue hypoxia.*
- Elevate the head of the bed and encourage frequent position changes, sitting at the bedside, and ambulation as allowed. *These measures promote lung expansion and facilitate the movement of secretions.*
- Assist to cough, deep breathe, and use the incentive spirometer. *Coughing and deep breathing help clear airways.*
- Provide at least 2,500 to 3,000 mL of fluid per day. *A liberal fluid intake helps liquefy secretions, promoting their clearance.*
- Assist with pulmonary hygiene measures, such as postural drainage, percussion, and vibration. *These techniques help mobilize and clear secretions.*
- Administer ordered medications, and monitor their effects. *If the ordered medications are ineffective or have adverse effects, a different drug may need to be prescribed.*

Ineffective Breathing Pattern

Expected outcome: Respiratory rate and pattern and SaO_2 level will be within normal range for the patient.

Chest pain can lead to rapid and shallow breathing that causes fatigue and does not fully ventilate all areas of the lungs.

- Administer oxygen as ordered. *Oxygen promotes alveolar gas exchange.*
- Assess and document chest pain. Provide analgesics as ordered, monitoring for respiratory depression if opioid analgesics are given. *Adequate pain relief allows better lung ventilation. Opioid analgesics, however, can depress the respiratory drive.*
- Reassure the patient who is experiencing respiratory distress. *Hypoxia and respiratory distress cause anxiety. Anxiety increases the respiratory rate and fatigue and decreases ventilation.*
- Teach use of slow abdominal breathing and relaxation techniques, such as visualization and meditation. *These techniques help reduce anxiety, slow breathing, and promote lung expansion.*

Activity Intolerance

Expected outcome: SaO_2, respiratory rate, and vital signs will remain stable during ADLs.

- Assess for any increase in pulse, respirations, dyspnea, diaphoresis, or cyanosis with activity. *These findings may indicate limited activity tolerance.*
- Assist with activities of daily living (ADLs) as needed. *Assistance with ADLs reduces the patient's energy demands.*
- Schedule activities between rest periods. *Rest periods minimize fatigue and improve activity tolerance.*
- Enlist support persons to help minimize stress and anxiety. *Stress and anxiety increase metabolic demands and can decrease activity tolerance.*
- Provide emotional support and reassurance that strength and activity level will return to normal when pneumonia has resolved. *The patient may be concerned that fatigue will continue after the acute infection is resolved.*

MANAGING NURSING CARE

Activities such as measures to promote fluid intake and assisting with hygiene, toileting, and ambulation are appropriate to assign to assistive nursing personnel. Alert assistive personnel to promptly report increasing respiratory rate, difficulty breathing, inability to tolerate usual activities, or a change in the patient's mental status.

EVALUATING

To evaluate the effectiveness of nursing care, reassess the patient's respiratory status, ability to clear secretions, and ability to gradually increase activity levels.

DOCUMENTING

Document continuing assessment data and the patient's responses to treatment (e.g., improving O_2 saturation levels with decreasing supplemental oxygen, ability to tolerate activities). Note teaching provided to the patient and family, as well as their apparent understanding and acceptance of instructions.

CONTINUITY OF CARE

For patients with pneumonia who are managed in the community, stress the importance of taking ordered medications and completing the entire prescription. Provide information about side effects and their management. Teach to identify adverse effects that should be reported to the primary care provider.

Instruct to limit activities and increase rest to conserve energy. Encourage to maintain fluid intake to keep mucus thin for easier expectoration. Explain that small, frequent meals reduce the energy demand for eating and may be better tolerated. Recommend that the patient and household members avoid smoking to prevent further irritation of the lungs. Complementary therapies may be used to help relieve chest congestion and promote comfort.

Tell the patient and family to report to the physician increasing shortness of breath, difficulty breathing, temperature, fatigue, headache, sleepiness, or confusion, as these may indicate worsening condition. Stress the importance of keeping all follow-up appointments to ensure cure of the disease.

Tuberculosis

Tuberculosis (TB) is a chronic, recurrent infectious disease that usually affects the lungs. Tuberculosis also can involve other organs. This disease, caused by *Mycobacterium tuberculosis*, is an important health problem worldwide, infecting one-third of the world's population (CDC, 2012). It is common in the developing countries of Asia, Africa, the Middle East, and Latin America.

In the United States, TB usually affects immigrants, people with HIV, and disadvantaged populations, such as the homeless (Box 23-2■). People with altered immune function, including older adults, are at particular risk for tuberculosis.

Some strains of tuberculosis have become resistant to the drugs used to treat the disease. *Multiple-drug-resistant tuberculosis* (or *MDR TB*) is resistant to the two primary drugs

BOX 23-2	FOCUS ON DIVERSITY

Tuberculosis

The number and rate of tuberculosis cases in the United States continues to fall steadily, declining nearly 6% between 2010 and 2011. Just over 10,500 TB cases were reported in the United States in 2011, less than half of that reported 15 years earlier.

- In 2011, 62% of the total TB cases reported in the United States occurred in foreign-born persons. Most of these patients came from one of five countries: Mexico, the Philippines, Vietnam, India, or China.
- Of reported TB cases in the United States in 2011, 30% were in Asians, 29% in Hispanics, and approximately 15% in U.S.-born Blacks or African Americans.
- The incidence of MDR TB in the United States is steadily increasing, but still accounts for only 1.3% of cases, nearly 83% of which are in foreign-born patients.
- When obtaining a health history on people within a high-risk group, be sure to ask about known tuberculosis in family members or close contacts; inquire about recent TB testing and the results.

Source: CDC. (2012). *Reported Tuberculosis in the United States, 2011.* Atlanta, GA: U.S. Department of Health and Human Services, CDC.

used, isoniazid (INH) and rifampin (RIF). MDR TB is increasing worldwide. Some strains of tuberculosis (called *extensively drug resistant*, or *XDR TB*) are resistant to INH, RIF, and many of the alternative drugs used to treat tuberculosis.

PATHOPHYSIOLOGY

M. tuberculosis is a slow-growing, slender, rod-shaped, acid-fast organism. It has a waxy outer capsule that increases its resistance to destruction. It is transmitted by *droplet nuclei*, airborne droplets produced when an infected person coughs, sneezes, speaks, or sings. Infection develops when a susceptible host breathes in droplet nuclei and the contaminated particle evades the normal defenses of the upper respiratory tract to reach the alveoli. A small, poorly ventilated or crowded environment and prolonged exposure increase the risk of infection. The risk also is increased by impaired immune function.

Pulmonary Tuberculosis

Droplet nuclei containing the bacillus implant in an alveolus or respiratory bronchiole, usually in an upper lobe. An immune response brings WBCs to the site. These cells phagocytize and isolate the bacteria but cannot destroy them. A sealed-off colony of bacilli, called a *tubercle*, is formed.

Usually, scar tissue forms around the tubercle, and the bacilli remain isolated. These lesions can be seen on x-ray. If the immune system is impaired, primary tuberculosis can progress, destroying lung tissue. A previously healed lesion may be reactivated. This is known as *reactivation tuberculosis*. It occurs when the immune system is suppressed by age (Box 23-3 ■), disease, or immunosuppressive drugs. About 5% of infected people develop active primary disease; another 5% develop reactivation tuberculosis at a later time (Figure 23-5 ■).

MANIFESTATIONS   Manifestations of pulmonary tuberculosis develop gradually. They include fatigue, weight loss, anorexia, low-grade afternoon fever, and night sweats. The cough is dry initially and later becomes productive of

---

| BOX 23-3 | FOCUS ON OLDER ADULTS |

Tuberculosis

Up to 30% of newly diagnosed tuberculosis affects people over age 65. Most cases are due to reactivation of dormant bacilli as cell-mediated immunity declines with aging. Living in long-term care facilities also increases the risk for tuberculosis.

Presenting symptoms of tuberculosis in an older adult may be vague, such as coughing, weight loss, anorexia, or periodic fevers. Yearly tuberculin skin testing with purified protein derivative (PPD) is recommended for long-term care residents.

---

purulent or blood-tinged sputum. It is often at this stage that the patient seeks medical attention.

Extrapulmonary Tuberculosis

Colonies of *M. tuberculosis* can develop in other organs. These distant sites may be active or dormant. The kidney and genitourinary tract are common sites for extrapulmonary tuberculosis. *Tuberculous arthritis* may develop in large, weight-bearing joints, such as the hips and knees. *Miliary tuberculosis* occurs when the bacilli spread throughout the body via the blood. *Tuberculosis meningitis* results when tuberculosis spreads to the subarachnoid space.

The manifestations of extrapulmonary tuberculosis vary, depending on the system affected. Tuberculosis of the genitourinary tract may present with symptoms of a urinary tract infection, prostatitis or epididymitis in men, or pelvic inflammatory disease in women. Headache of increasing severity and behavior changes are early manifestations of tuberculosis meningitis. The symptoms of miliary tuberculosis are generalized, with chills and fever, weakness, malaise, and progressive dyspnea.

COLLABORATIVE CARE

Interprofessional care for tuberculosis focuses on (1) early detection, (2) accurate diagnosis, (3) effective treatment, and (4) preventing its spread to others.

Patients with active tuberculosis rarely need hospitalization. With appropriate treatment, they become noninfective to others fairly rapidly. When a patient with tuberculosis is hospitalized, respiratory isolation is maintained to reduce the risk of infecting other patients and health care workers.

Tuberculosis is a potential threat to public health. As such, it must be reported to local and state public health departments. The patient's contacts are then identified and examined. People who share living or work environments should receive testing and prophylactic treatment.

Screening

The *tuberculin skin test (TST)* is used to screen for tuberculosis in at-risk populations, including:

■ Persons in close contact with someone with active TB.
■ Recent immigrants from a region with a high incidence of TB.
■ Residents and employees in health care facilities, correctional institutions, and homeless shelters.
■ People with conditions that increase their risk of developing active TB: HIV infection, malnutrition, use of injection drugs.

People infected with TB develop an immune response to the bacillus within 3 to 10 weeks after exposure. Injection of a small amount of purified protein derivative (PPD) of

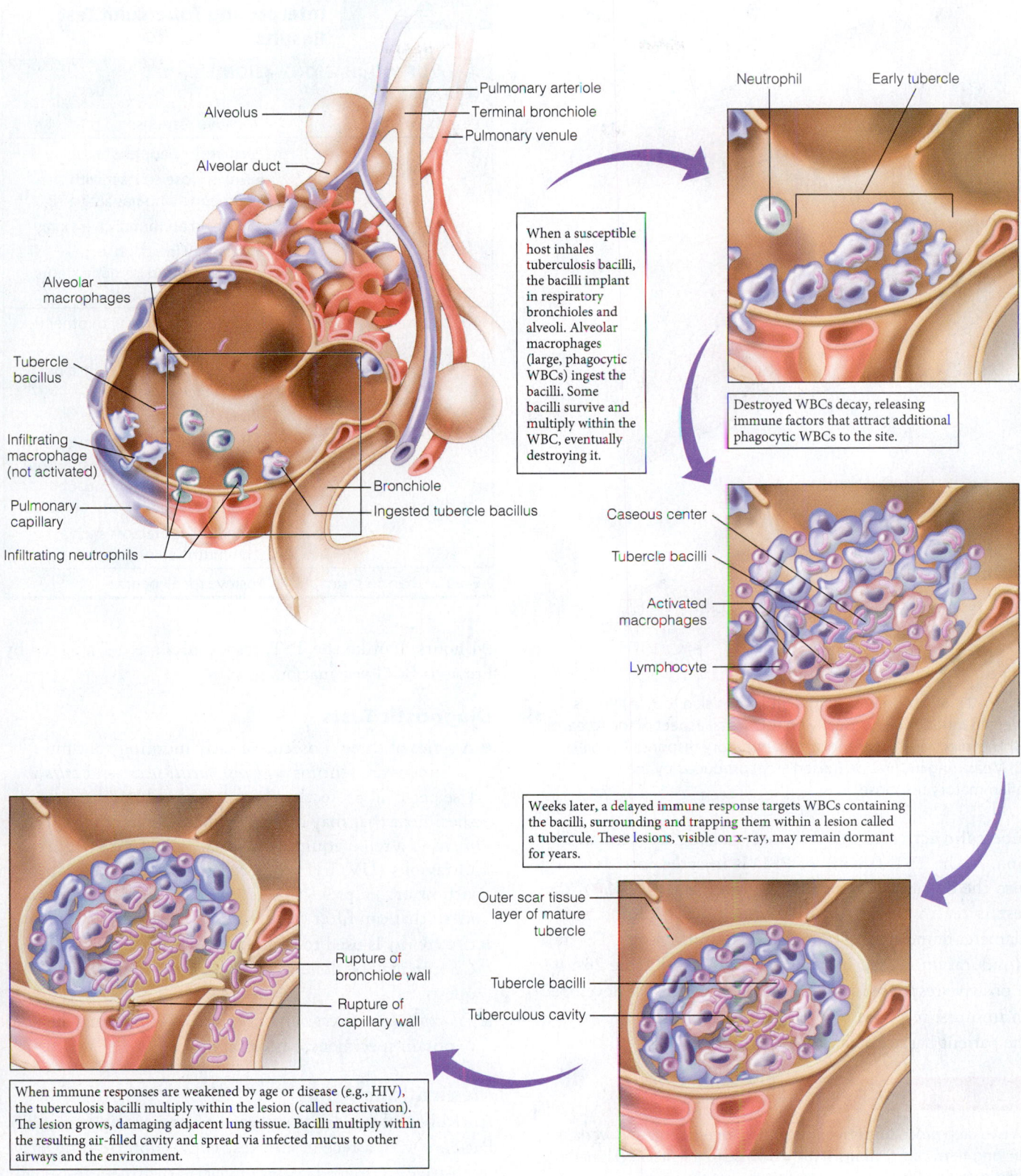

Figure 23-5. ■ The pathophysiology of tuberculosis.

The following labels appear within the figure:

Alveolus
Alveolar duct
Pulmonary arteriole
Terminal bronchiole
Pulmonary venule

Alveolar macrophages
Tubercle bacillus
Infiltrating macrophage (not activated)
Pulmonary capillary
Infiltrating neutrophils
Bronchiole
Ingested tubercle bacillus

Neutrophil
Early tubercle

When a susceptible host inhales tuberculosis bacilli, the bacilli implant in respiratory bronchioles and alveoli. Alveolar macrophages (large, phagocytic WBCs) ingest the bacilli. Some bacilli survive and multiply within the WBC, eventually destroying it.

Destroyed WBCs decay, releasing immune factors that attract additional phagocytic WBCs to the site.

Caseous center
Tubercle bacilli
Activated macrophages
Lymphocyte

Weeks later, a delayed immune response targets WBCs containing the bacilli, surrounding and trapping them within a lesion called a tubercule. These lesions, visible on x-ray, may remain dormant for years.

Outer scar tissue layer of mature tubercle
Tubercle bacilli
Tuberculous cavity

Rupture of bronchiole wall
Rupture of capillary wall

When immune responses are weakened by age or disease (e.g., HIV), the tuberculosis bacilli multiply within the lesion (called reactivation). The lesion grows, damaging adjacent lung tissue. Bacilli multiply within the resulting air-filled cavity and spread via infected mucus to other airways and the environment.

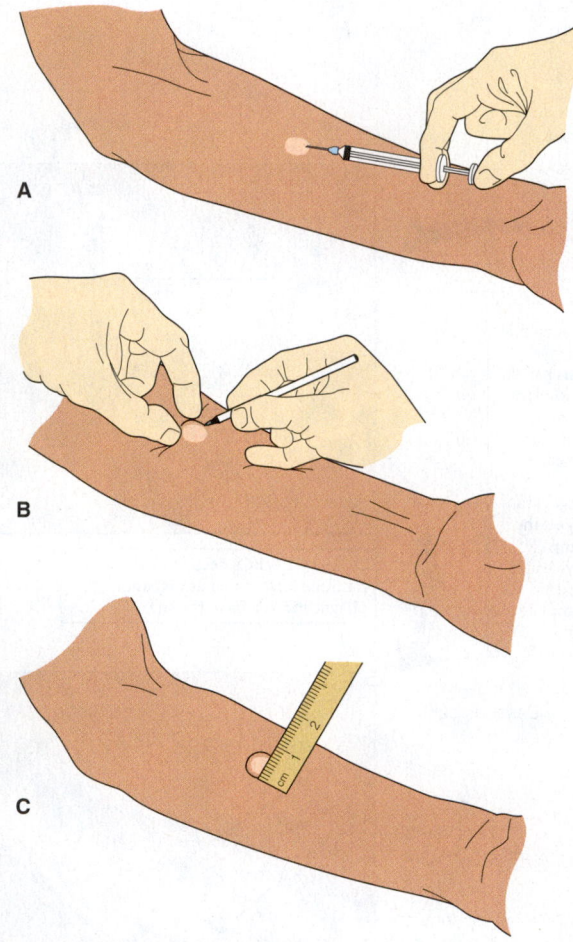

TABLE 23-2	Interpreting Tuberculin Test Results
AREA OF INDURATION (DIAMETER)	**SIGNIFICANCE**
Less than 5 mm	Negative response
5–9 mm	Positive for people who: ▪ Are in close contact with someone who has active TB ▪ Have an abnormal chest x-ray ▪ Have HIV infection, compromised immune status, or organ transplant
10–15 mm	Positive for people with other risk factors: ▪ Recent immigrant from a high-incidence country ▪ Injection drug use ▪ Resident in a long-term care facility, correctional institution, residential care setting, or homeless shelter ▪ Medical risk factors such as malnutrition or diabetes
Greater than 15 mm	Positive for all people

Figure 23-6. ■ Administering a tuberculin skin test. (**A**) PPD is injected intradermally, usually on the dorsal aspect of the forearm. (**B**) The injection causes a local inflammatory response (wheal). (**C**) Measuring induration (raised area) produced by the inflammatory response.

tuberculin activates this response, causing local inflammation. In the TST, 0.1 mL of PPD is injected intradermally into the dorsal aspect of the forearm (Figure 23-6 ■). The test is read within 48 to 72 hours and recorded as the diameter of induration (raised area) in millimeters. The area of induration is used to determine infection (Table 23-2 ■). A positive response indicates that the patient has developed an immune response to the bacillus; it does *not* mean that the patient has active TB or is currently infectious.

<clinical**ALERT**>

A two-step procedure is recommended for residents and workers in long-term care settings. If the response to the first PPD is negative, a second PPD is administered 1 to 3 weeks later.

Blood tests that measure the response of blood cells to TB antigens also are available. These tests, known as IGRAs, have the advantages of providing results within

24 hours. Unlike the TST, test results are not affected by previous BCG vaccination.

Diagnostic Tests

▪ A series of three consecutive early morning sputum specimens are sent for *acid-fast bacilli smear* and *culture*. Use personal protective devices when obtaining sputum specimens that may carry TB bacilli. Collect the specimens in a room equipped with airflow control devices, ultraviolet (UV) light, or a combination of these. If airflow or UV protection is not available, wear a special mask that can filter the droplet nuclei.

▪ *Chest x-ray* is used to diagnose and evaluate TB; *CT scan* may be done when chest x-ray results are questionable.

▪ *Fiberoptic bronchoscopy* and bronchial washing may be used to obtain specimens if necessary.

Medications

Antituberculosis drugs are used to prevent and treat TB. Patients with a recent skin test conversion from negative to positive are started on prophylactic treatment, especially when other risk factors are present. Daily isoniazid (INH) for 6 to 12 months is commonly used to prevent active TB, although 12 weeks of directly observed therapy with INH and rifapentine (RPT) administered weekly has recently been recommended by the CDC (2011).

TABLE 23-3	Giving Medications Safely: Major Antituberculosis Drugs		
CLASS/DRUGS	**PURPOSE**	**NURSING IMPLICATIONS**	**PATIENT TEACHING**
■ Isoniazid (INH, Laniazid, Nydrazid)	Isoniazid is used alone or with rifapentine to prevent tuberculosis, and in combination with rifampin, ethambutol, or both to treat active disease.	Monitor for and report adverse effects: a. Numbness and tingling of the extremities b. Abnormal liver function studies or jaundice c. Rash, drug fever, anemia, or abnormal bleeding. Monitor responses to other medications, because INH may interfere with their metabolism, causing toxicity.	Take as ordered for the entire course of treatment. Avoid alcohol while taking INH, and call your doctor if you develop anorexia and jaundice (yellowing of the skin and eyes). Take pyridoxine as ordered to prevent neurologic effects. Call your doctor if you develop a rash, fever, bruising, bleeding gums, or fatigue. Use birth control while taking INH; this drug may harm the fetus.
■ Rifampin (RMP, Rifadin, Rimactane)	Rifampin is commonly used in combination with INH and other antitubercular drugs. It is relatively low in toxicity. Rifampin increases the rate of metabolism of many drugs, decreasing their effectiveness.	Report abnormal CBC, liver function studies, and renal function studies to the physician. Monitor the effectiveness of drugs administered concurrently.	Rifampin causes sweat, urine, saliva, and tears to turn red-orange. This is not harmful, but may permanently stain soft contact lenses. Report jaundice, fever, flulike symptoms, fatigue, sore throat, or unusual bleeding to your doctor. If you use oral contraceptives, use supplemental birth control while taking this drug.
■ Pyrazinamide (PZA, Tebrazid)	Pyrazinamide often is given during the first 2 months of treatment. It is toxic to the liver. It also increases serum uric acid levels, but rarely causes gout.	Report changes in liver function studies and serum uric acid levels to the physician.	Call your doctor if you develop anorexia, nausea, vomiting, jaundice, difficulty voiding, or a painful, red, hot, swollen joint. Maintain fluid intake of at least 2,000 mL/day while taking this drug.
■ Ethambutol (EMB, Myambutol)	Ethambutol reduces bacterial resistance to other drugs. It is reversibly toxic to the optic nerve. Signs include decreased visual and color acuity. This drug may be safe for use in pregnancy.	Schedule eye exams as recommended before and during treatment. Give with meals to reduce GI effects. Report changes in liver and renal function tests and neurologic status to the physician.	Monitor vision daily by reading newspapers and looking at the same blue object. Notify your doctor if changes in vision or color perception occur.

The tuberculosis bacillus readily becomes drug resistant when only one anti-infective agent is used, so active disease is always treated with at least two antibacterial medications. Because the organism is protected by the tubercle, 6 or more months of treatment generally are required to eliminate it. In the initial treatment stage, four antitubercular drugs may be used for the first 2 months to kill the majority of tubercle bacilli, resolve symptoms, and make the patient noninfectious (Raviglione & O'Brien, 2012). All drugs are given daily or several times a week by mouth. For the remainder of the treatment period, two antitubercular drugs may be given twice weekly (see Table 23-3 ■).

Antitubercular medications have many undesired effects. Most are toxic to the liver; baseline liver function tests are obtained before therapy is started. Warn patients to avoid alcohol and other liver toxins (e.g., acetaminophen) while taking these drugs. Report manifestations of adverse effects to the physician.

Compliance with the prescribed regimen may be a problem. Medications often are given under direct supervision, with a public health nurse watching the patient take and swallow the drug.

When the disease is extensively drug resistant, supplemental or second-line drugs may be used in combination drug therapy. First-line supplemental drugs include rifabutin (Mycobutin) and rifapentine (Priftin), both closely related to rifampin. Second-line drugs include streptomycin, para-aminosalicylic acid (PAS), ethionamide (a drug closely related to isoniazid), cycloserine, capreomycin, or an aminoglycoside or fluoroquinolone antibiotic.

NURSING CARE

Tuberculosis presents a greater threat to public health than it does to the individual. When the treatment regimen is followed, more than 90% of patients become noninfective within 3 months. Relapse is uncommon; the main cause of treatment failure is noncompliance.

PRIORITIZING NURSING CARE

Identifying populations vulnerable to the disease and providing interventions and teaching to reduce the spread of tuberculosis are the priorities of nursing care.

HEALTH PROMOTION

To reduce the incidence of TB, teach people in at-risk populations how to reduce its spread:

- Cover the mouth and nose when coughing or sneezing.
- Use disposable tissues to contain respiratory secretions, promptly discarding tissues.

Because the patient with TB may be infective long before the disease is diagnosed, teach these measures to all people. Encourage people at high risk for TB to have regular screening. Discuss prophylactic treatment for people in close contact with a patient who has active TB.

ASSESSING

Ask the patient at risk for or with symptoms of TB about fatigue, weight loss, night sweats, and respiratory symptoms such as difficulty breathing, cough, bloody sputum, or chest pain. Inquire about known exposure to TB, the most recent tuberculin test and its results, as well as the patient's living circumstances and use of alcohol and/or recreational drugs.

Obtain vital signs, including temperature, and assess the patient's general appearance, respiratory rate, and lung sounds. Monitor laboratory data (including sputum for acid-fast bacillus and liver function tests) and chest x-ray results.

IDENTIFYING POTENTIAL COMPLICATIONS

Bacilli may spread to the pleura when a tuberculosis lesion ruptures, leading to empyema or pleurisy. Report increasing dyspnea, declining SaO_2 levels, complaints of chest pain, a pleural friction rub, or absent breath sounds.

DIAGNOSING, PLANNING, AND IMPLEMENTING

Risk for Infection

Expected outcome: Staff, other patients or residents, and close contacts of the patient will remain free of tuberculosis infection.

- Place in a private room with ventilation that prevents air in the room from circulating into the hallway or other rooms (a negative-flow room). *A negative-flow room with frequent fresh-air exchanges reduces droplet nuclei in the room and prevents their spread to other areas.*
- Use Standard Precautions and TB Isolation as recommended by the Centers for Disease Control and Prevention (CDC). Wear a mask and gown when caring for patients who do not cover the mouth when coughing. *These measures are important to prevent the spread of TB to self and others.*
- Use personal protective devices (HEPA-filtered respirator) during care to protect against occupational exposure to TB. *Surgical masks do not filter droplet nuclei; protective devices capable of filtering bacteria and particles smaller than 1 micron are necessary.*
- Discuss the importance of respiratory precautions during initial treatment. Instruct to avoid crowds and close physical contact and to maintain ventilation in living facilities during the initial phase of treatment. *These measures help protect others when sputum is still likely to contain bacilli.*
- Place a mask on the patient when transporting within the facility. *Covering the mouth during transport reduces air contamination and the risk to visitors and personnel.*
- Communicate the diagnosis to all personnel in contact with the patient. *This allows personnel to take appropriate precautions.*
- Assist visitors to mask before entering the room. *Providing appropriate masks or respirators reduces the risk of infection.*
- Teach to cough and expectorate into tissues and then to personally dispose of tissues in a closed bag. *This reduces potential contact with the bacilli by others.*
- Teach to collect sputum specimens, stepping outside to do so if necessary. *This reduces the risk of exposure to health care personnel, allows rapid dilution of droplet nuclei produced, and exposes them to UV light (which kills the bacteria).*

Deficient Knowledge (Tuberculosis and Treatment Regimen)

Expected outcome: Will verbalize understanding of the treatment regimen and the necessity of continuing therapy for the appropriate time.

- Assess knowledge, learning ability and interest, developmental level, and obstacles to learning. *Assessment allows teaching tailored to the patient's needs and abilities.*
- Include significant others in teaching. *This allows clarification and reinforcement of teaching and learning.*
- Use teaching strategies and learning aids such as written and visual materials appropriate for age, level of education, and intellect. Provide clear, written instructions at the patient's level of literacy, knowledge, and understanding. *Teaching tailored to the patient is more effective and results in better learning. Written directions provide support and reinforcement.*

- Teach about TB and its treatment, including the following:
  - Nature of tuberculosis
  - Purpose of treatment and ordered follow-up
  - Importance of complying with the treatment regimen for its entire duration
  - Preventing TB spread to others
  - Importance of maintaining good general health by eating a well-balanced, nutritious diet, balancing rest and exercise, and avoiding exposure to infection
  - Names, doses, purposes, and side effects of prescribed drugs
  - Importance of avoiding alcohol and other liver toxins while taking antituberculosis drugs
  - Fluid intake needs of 2-1/2 to 3 quarts of fluid per day
  - Symptoms to report to the physician: chest pain, hemoptysis, or difficulty breathing; manifestations of drug toxicity (see Table 23-3). *This information is necessary for the patient to effectively manage TB and its treatment.*
- Document teaching and learning. Reinforce as needed. *Several teaching–learning sessions may be needed due to the amount and complexity of information.*

Ineffective Self-Health Management

Expected outcome: Will continue therapy as ordered for the recommended duration of treatment.

- Assess self-care abilities and support systems. *Assessment helps predict the ability to follow the ordered regimen.*
- Help identify barriers or obstacles to managing the ordered treatment. *Identifying potential barriers allows planning for solutions.*
- Assist to develop a plan for managing treatment. *A plan increases the sense of control and ownership and considers personal, cultural, and lifestyle factors.*
- Refer to smoking cessation programs, alcohol treatment and Alcoholics Anonymous, drug treatment and Narcotics Anonymous, and other support groups as appropriate. *Counseling, support groups, and other community resources provide additional assistance and support in managing TB and its treatment.*
- For homeless patients, arrange shelter placement or other housing and ongoing follow-up by easily accessed health care providers. *Active intervention for necessary services helps ensure compliance with treatment.*
- Refer to public health department for management and follow-up as indicated. *Public health follow-up often is required to prevent the spread of TB to other people.*

EVALUATING

To evaluate the effectiveness of nursing care for a patient with TB, collect data related to the patient's knowledge and understanding of TB and its treatment, ability and willingness to follow instructions for preventing the spread of TB to others, and compliance with the ordered treatment.

DOCUMENTING

Document continuing assessment data, including assessments related to potential adverse effects of prescribed drugs. Document teaching (including reinforcement of teaching) and the patient's understanding of information presented and willingness to comply with the prescribed treatment regimen.

CONTINUITY OF CARE

Continuing care for the patient with tuberculosis focuses on teaching to prevent spread of the disease to others and to ensure effective treatment to eradicate the organism.

Explain the effect, dose, and timing for all medications. Emphasize the importance of long-term therapy to cure TB. Discuss precautions and possible side effects of the drugs that should be reported to the health care provider as outlined in Table 23-3.

Teach the patient and family (and, as appropriate, caregivers) how to contain secretions. Stress the importance of having the patient personally dispose of tissues that contain sputum whenever possible. In long-term care and community-based settings, teach caregivers measures to prevent spread of the organism to other residents.

Refer to community services and agencies as appropriate. See the Clinical Reasoning Care Map at the end of this chapter for an opportunity to use the nursing process to plan care for a patient with tuberculosis.

Lung Abscess and Empyema

Lung abscess and empyema are potential complications of pneumonia and other respiratory infections. A *lung abscess* is local lung destruction or necrosis and pus formation. Aspiration pneumonia is the usual cause of lung abscess. **Empyema** is pus in the pleural cavity. Bacterial pneumonia, rupture of a lung abscess, and infection due to chest trauma are the major causes of empyema.

Manifestations typically develop about 2 weeks after the initiating event (aspiration, pneumonia, etc.). Signs of an acute infection with chills and fever, pleuritic chest pain, malaise, and anorexia develop. The cough may be productive of foul-smelling, purulent, and even blood-streaked sputum. Breath sounds are diminished, and crackles may be heard in the affected region. Rupture and drainage of an abscess into a bronchus is a frightening complication.

Intravenous antibiotic therapy is ordered. Postural drainage may be done to relieve obstruction and promote drainage. In some cases, bronchoscopy is used to drain an abscess. A chest tube may be used to drain an empyema.

See the section on pneumothorax for further discussion of chest tubes.

Most patients recover fully with appropriate treatment. Nursing care needs relate primarily to maintaining a patent airway and adequate gas exchange. When teaching, emphasize the importance of completing the prescribed antibiotic therapy. Antibiotic therapy may be continued for 1 month or more. Stress the need to contact the physician if symptoms do not improve or if they become worse. Infection from lung abscess can spread to lung and pleural tissue and also via the blood, causing systemic sepsis.

Emerging Respiratory Infections

Recent years have seen the emergence of respiratory infections caused by newly identified viruses or by viruses previously known to infect other species.

Severe pneumonia may complicate a new strain of influenza caused by the H1N1 virus (also called swine flu). Although rare, this complication occurs primarily in children, young adults, and pregnant women, and can quickly lead to acute respiratory distress syndrome and respiratory failure. While the manifestations of H1N1 influenza usually are mild, immediately report symptoms such as difficulty breathing, cyanosis, or a drop in oxygen saturation levels.

The H5N1 influenza virus (also called highly pathogenic avian [bird] influenza A) can cause severe respiratory illness in humans, although its incidence remains low. People contracting this virus are primarily those in close contact with infected poultry. At this time, human to human spread appears to be extremely rare.

Severe acute respiratory syndrome (SARS) is a lower respiratory illness caused by a newly identified virus called SARS-associated coronavirus (SARS-CoV). This virus spreads primarily by close human contact. Most people with SARS develop severe pneumonia, typically beginning with flulike symptoms, including high fever, headache and muscle aches, cough, and shortness of breath.

Inhalation anthrax has been identified as a potential biologic weapon. Inhalation anthrax causes initial flulike symptoms with malaise, dry cough, and fever. Severe dyspnea, stridor, and cyanosis develop abruptly, along with inflammation of lymph nodes in the mediastinum and thorax. Blood cultures and chest x-ray are used to diagnose inhalation anthrax. Fortunately, the antibiotic ciprofloxacin (Cipro) is effective for both prevention and treatment of inhalation anthrax.

People with these emerging infections require intensive and supportive nursing care. The nursing diagnoses and interventions identified for pneumonia and respiratory failure may be appropriate.

OBSTRUCTIVE LUNG DISORDERS

Key Concept Many diseases affect the airways and airflow. Decreased airflow increases the work of breathing and causes air trapping. Inhaled air mixes with trapped air, so less oxygen is available for gas exchange. Care focuses on promoting airway clearance and supporting gas exchange.

Airflow decreases when (1) secretions obstruct the airway; (2) airway walls are edematous or swollen; (3) smooth muscle of the airways constricts, reducing their size; (4) the lungs lose elasticity, making exhalation more difficult; and (5) supportive tissue is lost, allowing airways to collapse.

Asthma

Key Concept Asthma is characterized by chronic airway inflammation with recurrent acute episodes of respiratory distress. Treatment goals are to reduce the level of chronic inflammation and prevent acute exacerbations.

Asthma is a chronic inflammatory disorder of the airways characterized by recurrent episodes of wheezing, breathlessness, chest tightness, and coughing. Although it is more common in children than adults, about 5% of adults have asthma. It is becoming more common and is causing an increasing number of deaths.

PATHOPHYSIOLOGY

During symptom-free periods, there is little airway inflammation in patients with asthma. A variety of factors can trigger an acute inflammatory response, including allergens, environmental pollutants such as tobacco smoke and smog, and workplace pollutants. Respiratory infection is a common stimulus, as is exercise in cold, dry air for patients with exercise-induced asthma. Emotional stress can trigger an attack. Drugs such as aspirin and other NSAIDs, sulfites (used as preservatives), and beta-blockers can prompt an attack in some patients.

When a trigger occurs, an *acute* or *early response* develops. Inflammatory mediators such as histamine and prostaglandins constrict airways and increase capillary permeability. This, in turn, causes edema and increased mucus production, further narrowing airways. Airflow is reduced, and the work of breathing increases (Figure 23-7 ■).

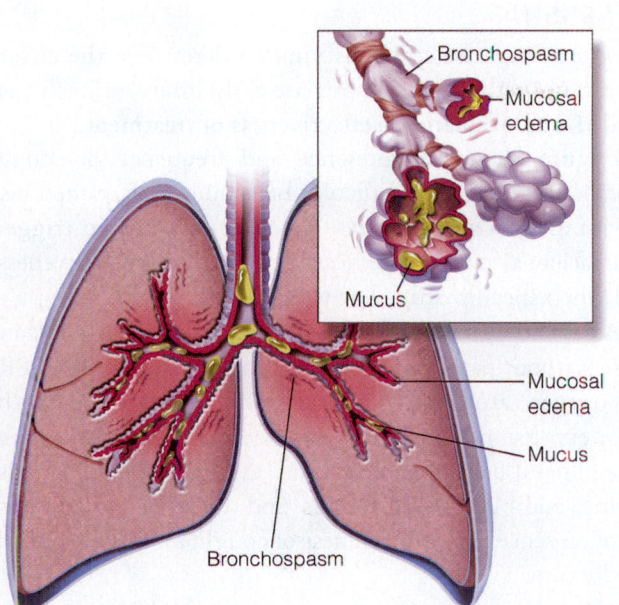

Figure 23-7. ■ In an acute asthma attack, the inflammatory response causes airway constriction and edema. Thick mucus is produced, further impairing airflow and increasing the work of breathing. (Source: Pearson Education.)

The *late phase response* develops 4 to 12 hours after exposure to the trigger, prolonging the attack. Inflammatory cells damage airway epithelium, produce mucosal edema, impair airway clearance, and prolong bronchoconstriction. Air is trapped beyond the narrowed airways, distending alveoli. Trapped air mixes with inspired air, reducing available oxygen for gas exchange. Blood flow is reduced to distended alveoli, further impairing gas exchange. Hypoxemia develops.

MANIFESTATIONS AND COMPLICATIONS

The frequency and severity of attacks vary. Some patients have infrequent, mild attacks, whereas others have nearly continuous symptoms.

An attack of asthma may develop abruptly or slowly. Early symptoms include a feeling of chest tightness and nonproductive cough. Tachypnea, tachycardia, wheezing, and prolonged expiration are common during an attack (Box 23-4■). The patient often has a sense of anxiety and apprehension. Patients with *cough-variant asthma* have persistent cough without accompanying wheezing or dyspnea, often delaying diagnosis.

During a severe attack, use of accessory muscles, intercostal retractions, and distant breath sounds may be noted. Severe dyspnea may allow the patient with asthma to speak only one or two words between breaths.

Respiratory failure can develop, marked by inaudible breath sounds, reduced wheezing, and an ineffective cough.

Respiratory failure is a medical emergency requiring prompt treatment to preserve life. Immediately report manifestations of impending respiratory failure.

Status asthmaticus is severe, prolonged asthma that does not respond to routine treatment. Without aggressive treatment, status asthmaticus can lead to respiratory failure. The patient may require intubation and mechanical ventilation.

COLLABORATIVE CARE

Asthma is diagnosed mainly by the patient's history and manifestations. Treatment focuses on controlling symptoms and preventing acute attacks. When an acute episode occurs, therapy focuses on restoring airflow and alveolar ventilation.

Diagnostic Tests

Diagnostic tests are used to identify possible triggers and to evaluate respiratory function during and between acute attacks. *Pulmonary function tests (PFTs)* are used to evaluate the degree of airway obstruction. *Peak expiratory flow rate (PEFR)* assesses airflow restriction and the effectiveness of treatment. Patients with asthma use inexpensive PEFR meters to monitor airflow and the need for treatment on a continuing basis. *Exhaled nitric oxide* is a noninvasive test to measure airway inflammation. *Pulse oximetry* and *arterial blood gases* evaluate oxygenation during an acute attack. *Skin testing* may be done to identify specific allergens that may trigger asthma attacks.

Preventive Measures

Asthma attacks often can be prevented by avoiding allergens and other triggers. Modifying the home environment (e.g., controlling dust, removing carpets, covering mattresses and pillows to reduce dust mites, and installing air filtering systems) may help. Pets may need to be removed from the household. Eliminating tobacco smoke in the house is also important. For exercise-induced asthma, wearing a mask that retains humidity and warm air when exercising in cold weather may prevent an attack. Early treatment of respiratory infections is vital.

BOX 23-4	MANIFESTATIONS OF ACUTE ASTHMA
■ Chest tightness	
■ Cough	
■ Dyspnea	
■ Wheezing	
■ Tachypnea and tachycardia	
■ Anxiety and apprehension	

Medications

Drugs are used to prevent and control asthma symptoms, reduce the frequency and severity of attacks, and reverse airway obstruction. Drugs used for long-term control are taken daily. These include anti-inflammatory agents, long-acting bronchodilators, and leukotriene modifiers. Quick-relief medications used to relieve bronchoconstriction and airflow obstruction include rapid-acting bronchodilators, anticholinergic drugs, and methylxanthines (Table 23-4■). Asthma medications often are administered locally, using a metered-dose inhaler (MDI), dry-powder inhaler (DPI), or nebulizer. These methods promote rapid action of the drug and limit their systemic effects. Products such as *Advair Diskus* (fluticasone/salmeterol) and *Symbicort* (budesonide/formoterol) provide both an anti-inflammatory corticosteroid and a bronchodilator for long-term asthma control. Box 23-5■ on page 570 provides teaching related to using an MDI or DPI.

Complementary Therapies

Herbal preparations such as atropa belladonna (the natural form of atropine, an anticholinergic drug that blocks bronchoconstriction), capsaicin, and grape seed extract may be helpful in managing and relieving symptoms of asthma. However, these preparations may interact with prescribed therapies. Stress the importance of discussing all herbal preparations with the physician and consulting with a qualified herbalist before taking any herbal preparation.

Biofeedback has been shown to have positive effects, reducing the frequency of asthma attacks and rescue inhaler use, as well as improving airflow (Barrows, 2013). Other complementary therapies such as yoga, breathing techniques, acupuncture, homeopathy, and massage also have been found to help control and relieve asthma symptoms.

NURSING CARE

PRIORITIZING NURSING CARE

Nursing care priorities for the patient experiencing a severe acute attack of asthma focus on maintaining effective ventilation and gas exchange. Once an acute attack subsides, the nursing focus is on teaching the patient how to monitor disease status and prevent acute episodes.

HEALTH PROMOTION

Discuss the link between parental smoking and childhood asthma with young adults and parents of young children. Encourage all patients not to start smoking or to quit. Provide information about smoking cessation classes and support groups. There is evidence that limiting antibiotic use in childhood may reduce the risk for asthma. Discuss appropriate and inappropriate antibiotic use with patients.

ASSESSING

Good nursing assessment is vital to determine the effects of an acute asthma attack, initiate early interventions when needed, and evaluate the effectiveness of treatment.

Inquire about the presence and frequency of cough, shortness of breath, or difficulty breathing. Ask about a history of asthma and allergies, exposure to a known trigger, the patient's current medications and their effectiveness, and when specific drugs last were used.

Assess LOC, mental status, skin color, and ability to converse without pausing for breath. Obtain vital signs, PEFR, and oxygen saturation. Note the respiratory rate and depth, chest expansion and use of accessory muscles, and the presence of nasal flaring or retractions. Auscultate lung sounds, noting audible breath sounds and presence of wheezes. Note presence and effectiveness of cough, as well as sputum production.

IDENTIFYING POTENTIAL COMPLICATIONS

Slow, shallow respirations; faint breath sounds; decreased wheezing; and an ineffective cough may indicate exhaustion and possible respiratory failure. Immediate intervention is vital.

DIAGNOSING, PLANNING, AND IMPLEMENTING

Ineffective Airway Clearance

Expected outcome: Airways will remain open and clear as evidenced by audible breath sounds throughout lung fields and no adventitious sounds (wheezes, crackles).

- Frequently assess respiratory status. Notify the charge nurse or physician of significant changes. *Respiratory status can change rapidly during an acute asthma attack.*
- Assess skin color and temperature and LOC every 1 to 2 hours or as indicated. *Cyanosis; cool, clammy skin; and changes in LOC (e.g., agitation, lethargy, or confusion) indicate worsening hypoxia.*
- Report abnormal or significant changes in oxygen saturation levels and ABG results. *Oxygen saturation and ABG values indicate the effectiveness of gas exchange and treatment.*
- Place in Fowler's or orthopneic (with head and arms supported on the over-bed table) position. *These positions reduce the work of breathing and increase lung expansion.*
- Administer oxygen as ordered. If a mask is used, monitor for feelings of claustrophobia or suffocation. *Supplemental oxygen reduces hypoxemia. Although the mask is very effective for delivering oxygen, it may increase anxiety.*
- Administer nebulizer treatments and provide humidification as ordered. *Bronchodilators and other drugs are given by nebulizer; humidity helps loosen secretions.*

TABLE 23-4	**Giving Medications Safely: Asthma Drugs**		
CLASS/DRUGS	**PURPOSE**	**NURSING IMPLICATIONS**	**PATIENT TEACHING**
Beta-agonists *Inhaled* ■ *Albuterol* (ProAir HFA, Proventil, Ventolin HFA) ■ Levalbuterol (Xopenex) ■ Metaproterenol (Alupent, Metaprel) ■ Pirbuterol (Maxair) ■ *Salmeterol* (Serevent) *Systemic* ■ Epinephrine ■ Terbutaline (Brethine)	These drugs stimulate sympathetic nervous system (SNS) receptors in the lungs, causing bronchodilation. Given orally, parenterally, or by metered-dose inhalers (MDIs), they are used to prevent and treat acute attacks. Their side effects include nervousness, irritability, tachycardia, and dysrhythmias, particularly when given systemically.	Use with caution in patients with hypertension, cardiovascular disease, hyperthyroidism, or diabetes. When given by MDI, wait 1–2 minutes between puffs to allow airways to dilate, permitting the second dose to reach distal airways. Chart response. Desired effect is reduced dyspnea and wheezing; anxiety, irritability, insomnia, and tremor are common side effects.	Use your inhaler or nebulizer as instructed. If you are taking this drug with another medication by inhalation, use this drug first to open airways. Rinse your mouth after using inhalers to reduce systemic effects. Keep a log of your use; if drug becomes less effective, or you need it more often, contact your doctor. Report irregular pulse and other side effects to your doctor.
Methylxanthines ■ Aminophylline (Somophyllin, Truphylline) ■ Theophylline (Bronkotabs, Theo-Dur, others)	Methylxanthines, which are related to caffeine, are primarily used to prevent nocturnal asthma in adult patients. Theophylline has a narrow margin of safety and a high risk for toxicity.	Monitor therapeutic blood levels (10–20 mcg/mL). Monitor for manifestations of toxicity: anorexia, nausea, vomiting, restlessness, insomnia, dysrhythmias, and seizures. Give with meals or a full glass of water or milk. Aminophylline is incompatible with many other intravenous drugs; administer in a separate line or flush the line with normal saline before and after giving any other drug.	Theophylline is ineffective to treat an acute asthma attack; do not delay other treatment by using these drugs. Check with your doctor before taking any over-the-counter drugs or other prescription drugs while taking theophylline. Do not smoke while you are taking this drug. Report adverse effects to your doctor.
Anticholinergics ■ Ipratropium bromide (Atrovent) ■ *Tiotropium* (Spiriva)	Anticholinergics dilate the bronchi. Ipratropium and tiotropium are available as inhalers, reducing anticholinergic side effects.	Assess for possible contraindications to the drug, including glaucoma, an enlarged prostate, or urinary retention. Provide ice chips, fluids, or hard candy to relieve dry mouth.	Take no more than the ordered number of doses per day. If the drug becomes less effective over time, notify your doctor. A dosage adjustment may be needed.
Corticosteroids ■ Beclomethasone (Vanceril, Beclovent, others) ■ Budesonide (Pulmicort Turbuhaler) ■ Flunisolide (AeroBid) ■ *Fluticasone* (Flonase, Flovent) ■ Triamcinolone acetonide (Azmacort)	These are potent anti-inflammatory drugs used to prevent and treat acute episodes. They reduce the frequency and severity of attacks and allow lower doses of other drugs. Giving these drugs by inhalation reduces systemic side effects.	Give inhaler doses after bronchodilators to improve transit of the drug to distal airways. Report common side effects: sore throat, hoarseness, and oropharyngeal *Candida albicans* infection.	Rinse your mouth after taking the drug; use good oral hygiene to reduce the risk of fungal infections. Do not use these drugs to treat an acute attack. The desired effect may not be noticed for several weeks. Call your doctor if you gain weight, retain fluid, or have muscle weakness, mood changes, or an appearance change.

TABLE 23-4	Giving Medications Safely: Asthma Drugs (continued)		
CLASS/DRUGS	**PURPOSE**	**NURSING IMPLICATIONS**	**PATIENT TEACHING**
Mast cell stabilizers ■ Cromolyn sodium (Intal, NasalCrom) ■ Nedocromil (Tilade)	These drugs reduce inflammatory airway responses and prevent airway constriction in response to cold air. They have a wide margin of safety.	Report potential adverse effects of wheezing and bronchoconstriction.	Use these drugs only to prevent asthma attacks; do not use to treat an acute attack.
Leukotriene modifiers ■ *Montelukast* (Singulair) ■ Zafirlukast (Accolate) ■ Zileuton (Zyflo)	Leukotriene modifiers interfere with airway inflammation, improving airflow and decreasing asthma symptoms. They are used to prevent asthma attacks; they are not used to treat an acute attack.	Give at least 1 hour before or 2 hours after meals. These drugs affect warfarin metabolism. Monitor for bleeding. Monitor liver enzymes, because these drugs may be toxic to the liver.	Several weeks may be required before a beneficial effect is noted. Take as ordered on an empty stomach. Call your doctor if you notice a change in color of stools or urine, or if jaundice develops.

Note: Medications identified in *italics* are among the 200 most frequently prescribed drugs in the United States.

BOX 23-5	PATIENT TEACHING

Using a Metered-Dose Inhaler or Dry-Powder Inhaler

Metered-Dose Inhaler
- Firmly insert the metered-dose inhaler canister into holder.
- Remove mouthpiece cap. Shake vigorously for 3 to 5 seconds.
- Exhale slowly and completely.
- Holding the canister upside down, close lips around mouthpiece, or hold mouthpiece directly in front of mouth.
- Press and hold canister down once while inhaling deeply and slowly for 3 to 5 seconds (see figure).
- Hold breath for 10 seconds. Release pressure on container and remove from mouth, and then exhale.
- Wait 20 to 30 seconds (or as directed) before repeating for a second puff.
- Rinse mouth after using inhaler.
- Rinse the inhaler mouthpiece after use; store in a clean location.

Dry-Powder Inhaler
- Remove the cap. Holding the inhaler upright, inspect to be sure the mechanism is clean and the mouthpiece is clear.
- If necessary, load the dose into the inhaler, following manufacturer's directions.
- Hold the inhaler level, with the mouthpiece end facing down.
- Breathe out slowly and completely. Tilt your head back slightly.

- Seal your lips around the mouthpiece. Breathe in rapidly and deeply through your mouth to activate the flow of medication.
- Remove the inhaler from your mouth, and hold your breath for 10 seconds. Then exhale slowly through pursed lips; do not exhale into the mouthpiece.
- Rinse your mouth or brush your teeth after using the inhaler.
- Store the inhaler in a clean, sealed plastic bag in a clean, dry location. Do not wash the inhaler unless directed by the manufacturer. Clean the mouthpiece weekly with a dry cloth.

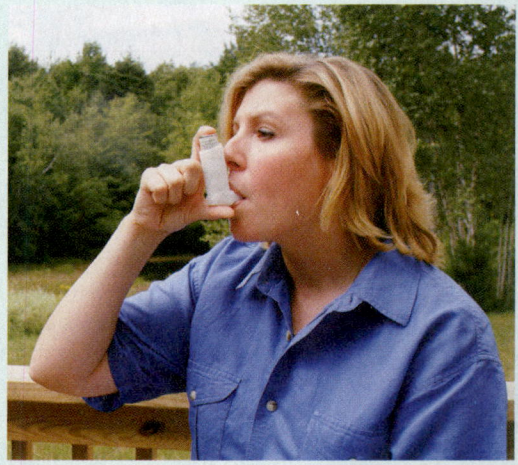

(Source: Michal Heron, Pearson Education.)

- Assist with chest physiotherapy, including percussion and postural drainage. *Percussion and postural drainage facilitate airway clearance.*
- Increase fluid intake. *Increasing fluids helps thin secretions.*
- Monitor effects of prescribed medications. *Medications used to improve airway status and facilitate breathing also may have significant adverse effects.*

Fatigue
Expected outcome: Will maintain effective respiratory rate, pattern, and oxygen saturation levels.

- Assist with ADLs as needed. *This allows energy conservation.*
- Provide rest periods between activities and treatments. *Rest helps prevent fatigue and reduce oxygen demands.*

■ Assist with breathing and relaxation techniques to control breathing pattern. *Pursed-lip breathing helps keep airways open; abdominal breathing improves lung expansion. Relaxation techniques reduce anxiety and help slow the respiratory rate.*

Anxiety

Expected outcome: Will demonstrate ability to manage anxiety within reasonable levels.

An acute asthma attack causes significant anxiety with a fear of suffocation. Hypoxia contributes to the sense of anxiety.

■ Provide physical and emotional support. Remain present during periods of acute anxiety. Schedule frequent time with the patient, and reassure about a prompt response to the call light. *The severely anxious patient may fear that he or she will die if someone is not on hand. Reassurance of readily available assistance and the presence of the nurse reduces anxiety.*

■ Listen actively to concerns; do not deny or negate the fear of dying or of being unable to breathe. *Active listening promotes trust and helps the patient express concerns.*

■ Help identify previously successful coping skills. *Coping skills can help the patient regain control.*

■ Provide clear, concise directions and explanations. Avoid presenting too much information. *Anxiety interferes with learning. Explanations may need to be repeated frequently.*

■ Reduce excessive stimuli and maintain a calm demeanor. *This promotes rest.*

■ Allow supportive family members to remain with the patient. *Significant others provide additional support and can help reduce anxiety.*

■ Assist with relaxation techniques such as guided imagery, muscle relaxation, and meditation. *These techniques help reduce anxiety and restore a sense of control.*

Ineffective Self-Health Management

Expected outcome: Will verbalize an understanding of the disease, measures to monitor its status, and prescribed therapeutic regimen.

■ Assess understanding of asthma and prescribed treatment. Reinforce teaching as indicated. *Assessment helps identify misperceptions about asthma and its management that may contribute to acute attacks.*

■ Help identify factors that contributed to the acute attack. *Awareness of contributing factors helps identify ways to prevent future attacks.*

■ Discuss the effect of asthma and its management on lifestyle and assist to identify ways to integrate daily treatment. *Asthma management can impact significant others as well as the patient, for example, eliminating smoking and pets in the household, removing carpets, and measures to reduce dust mites.*

■ Refer to counseling, support groups, or self-help organizations. *Services such as these can help with required lifestyle changes and the demands of treatment.*

MANAGING NURSING CARE

The patient experiencing an acute asthma attack may require assistance with ADLs such as hygiene, meals, and toileting. These activities are appropriate to assign to assistive nursing personnel.

EVALUATING

To evaluate the effectiveness of nursing care, collect data related to:

■ Respiratory status and breathing pattern.
■ Fatigue and activity tolerance.
■ Anxiety level.
■ Knowledge and understanding of measures to prevent future asthma attacks.

DOCUMENTING

Document initial and continuing assessment data, specifically noting response to treatment measures. Document all teaching provided, as well as the patient's and family's apparent understanding and acceptance of teaching.

CONTINUITY OF CARE

Teach about PEFR monitoring and using readings to manage use of short-acting inhalers. Provide information about all prescribed drugs verbally and in writing, including:

■ The drug name, its frequency, dose, and how to use it.
■ The desired effect and purpose of the drug.
■ Potential adverse effects and their management, including those that should be reported to the physician.
■ Potential interactions with other medications (including over-the-counter medications and herbal preparations) or with foods.
■ What to do if the medication becomes less effective or is needed with increasing frequency over time.

Provide teaching for caregiving staff in community-based settings as well as for patients, to ensure effective monitoring of asthma and correct use of MDI and DPIs. If specific triggers for asthma attacks have been identified, help identify ways to avoid these triggers. Because exercise, particularly in cold weather, often triggers an attack, instruct to warm up slowly before exercise and to wear a mask to retain air warmth and humidity while exercising. If necessary, help identify alternate indoor exercises. Discuss measures to prevent respiratory infections and support immune function, including adequate rest, good nutrition, and stress management. Recommend yearly influenza vaccine and immunization against pneumococcal pneumonia.

Help identify stress management techniques to incorporate into lifestyle. Refer to a local or regional agency for further teaching and support as needed or to Internet websites for local home care resources.

Chronic Obstructive Pulmonary Disease

> **Key Concept** Chronic obstructive pulmonary disease is a progressive disorder that gradually destroys lung tissue and obstructs airflow. Slowing disease progression and promoting the patient's functional status are both medical and nursing care goals for the patient with COPD.

Chronic obstructive pulmonary disease (COPD) is an inflammatory respiratory disease characterized by chronic and progressive obstruction of airflow in the lungs. It usually affects middle-aged and older adults. Smoking is the most common cause of COPD. Other risk factors are secondhand smoke exposure, air pollution, occupational pollutants, and family history of COPD.

COPD affects more than 15 million Americans. It affects Whites more often than Blacks, Hispanics, Native Americans, or Asian Americans. Not only is chronic lower respiratory disease (which includes COPD and asthma) the third leading cause of death, it is second only to heart disease as a cause of disability and lost work time.

PATHOPHYSIOLOGY

In COPD, the airways are narrowed and gradually obstructed by inflammation, excess mucus production, and loss of elastic tissue and alveoli. Two different processes, chronic bronchitis and emphysema, cause these airway and lung tissue changes. Alveolar ventilation is impaired, as is gas exchange between the alveoli and the blood.

Chronic bronchitis is a chronic inflammatory airway disorder that causes excessive secretion of thick, tenacious mucus and a productive cough lasting 3 or more months. Inhaled irritants, primarily cigarette smoke, lead to a chronic inflammatory process in the bronchial mucosa. Narrowed airways due to mucosal edema and excess secretions obstruct airflow (Figure 23-8 ■). Expiratory airflow is affected first. Ciliary function is impaired, so normal defense mechanisms cannot clear mucus and inhaled pathogens. Recurrent infection is common.

Emphysema is destruction of alveolar walls leading to large, abnormal air spaces in the lungs. As in chronic bronchitis, cigarette smoking is its major cause. Deficiency of $alpha_1$-antitrypsin, an enzyme that normally prevents lung tissue destruction, also causes emphysema.

When alveolar walls are destroyed, air spaces enlarge and the surface area for gas exchange decreases (Figure 23-9 ■).

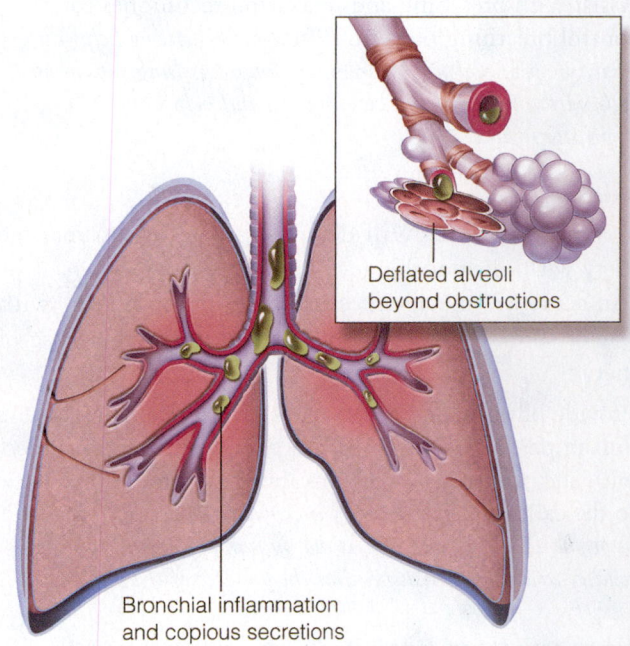

Bronchial inflammation and copious secretions

Deflated alveoli beyond obstructions

Figure 23-8. ■ In chronic bronchitis, airflow is obstructed by airway inflammation and excess mucous secretions. (Source: Pearson Education.)

The alveoli become less elastic and airways tend to collapse during exhalation. This causes air trapping in the lungs. Over time, the anterior–posterior chest diameter increases, and the patient develops a **barrel chest**. Expiration is prolonged.

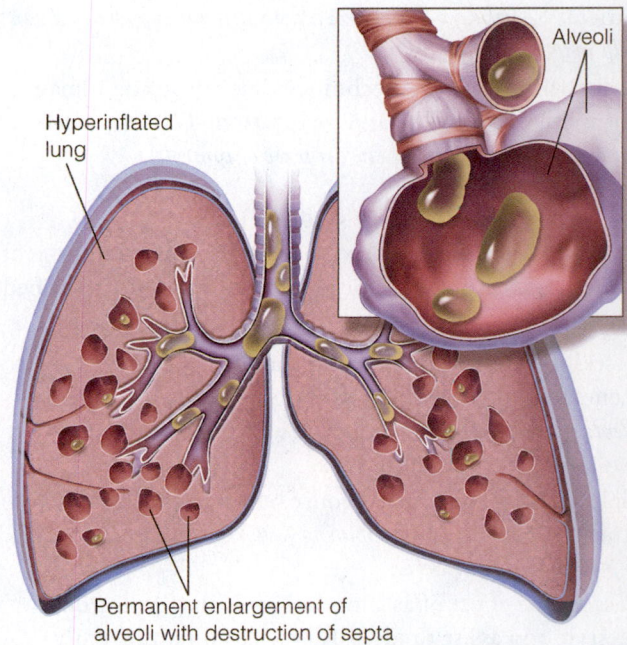

Hyperinflated lung

Alveoli

Permanent enlargement of alveoli with destruction of septa

Figure 23-9. ■ Emphysema is characterized by destruction of alveolar walls, enlarged air spaces, and loss of surface area for gas exchange. Loss of supportive tissue leads to airway collapse and air trapping in distal airways. (Source: Pearson Education.)

Manifestations

By the time COPD is diagnosed, the patient may have had a productive cough, dyspnea, and exercise intolerance for as long as 10 years. The cough usually occurs in the mornings ("smoker's cough"). Dyspnea becomes worse as the disease progresses; wheezing may be noted, particularly on expiration. Periodic episodes of increased sputum and difficulty breathing are common, often caused by respiratory infection. The patient often has a barrel chest, uses accessory muscles of respiration, and frequently assumes the *tripod position*, sitting and leaning forward (Figure 23-10■). The manifestations of COPD are summarized in Box 23-6■.

COLLABORATIVE CARE

Avoiding—never starting or stopping—smoking is the only way to prevent COPD and the only way to slow its progression. Early in the disease, airway obstruction can be reversed and disability minimized. As the disease progresses, airway obstruction becomes increasingly irreversible. Treatment focuses on reducing symptoms and maintaining optimal function.

Diagnostic Tests

The following tests are used to help diagnose COPD, assess the patient's status, and monitor the effectiveness of treatment:

- *Pulmonary function testing* is used to evaluate lung ventilation and function.
- *Serum alpha$_1$-antitrypsin* levels may be drawn to screen for a deficiency of this enzyme.

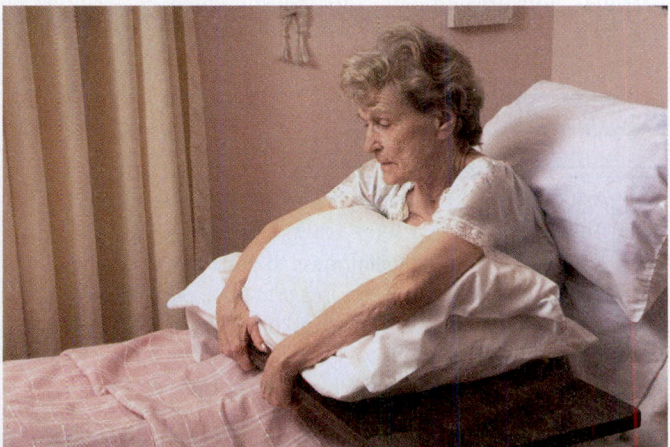

Figure 23-10. ■ Patients with emphysema often assume a position of sitting upright, leaning forward to ease breathing. (Source: Michal Heron, Pearson Education.)

BOX 23-6	MANIFESTATIONS OF COPD

- Chronic cough, often productive of thick sputum
- Dyspnea, exercise intolerance
- Exhalation phase of breathing is prolonged
- Barrel chest
- Distant breath sounds, possible wheezes and rhonchi
- Use of accessory muscles of respiration
- Possible cyanosis
- Weight loss, tissue wasting

- *ABGs* are drawn to evaluate the effect of COPD on gas exchange. During an acute episode, a low PO_2 (hypoxemia), high PCO_2 (hypercapnia), and low pH (respiratory acidosis) may be seen.
- *Pulse oximetry* is used to measure oxygen saturation of the blood. These levels may be used to continuously assess the need for supplemental oxygen.
- *Computed tomography (CT) scan* of the chest may be performed to determine the presence or absence of emphysema.

Medications

Smoking cessation is vital. Drug therapy in combination with traditional approaches to smoking cessation (referral to a clinic, support group, or counselor) improves the chances of success. Nicotine replacement therapy (gum, patches, inhaler, or nasal spray), bupropion (Wellbutrin, an antidepressant), or varenicline (Chantix, a smoking deterrent) may be prescribed.

Immunization against pneumococcal pneumonia and yearly influenza vaccine are recommended. A broad-spectrum antibiotic is ordered if infection is suspected.

Inhaled bronchodilators (administered by MDI, DPI, or nebulizer) are frequently ordered to manage COPD symptoms. A combination of bronchodilators with different mechanisms and duration of action may be prescribed. Theophylline, an oral bronchodilator, may be ordered because it also improves cardiac and respiratory muscle function. Review the nursing implications for bronchodilators as outlined in Table 23-4. Corticosteroids may be given to reduce inflammation and edema of the airways. Cough suppressants and sedatives are avoided. Alpha$_1$-antitrypsin may be given when this enzyme is deficient.

Oxygen Therapy

Patients with low resting oxygen saturation levels may need home oxygen therapy. Oxygen may be used intermittently, at night, or continuously. Home oxygen is available as liquid oxygen, compressed gas cylinders, or oxygen concentrators. During an acute episode, oxygen and ventilatory assistance using a continuous positive airway pressure

(CPAP) mask or mechanical ventilation may be required. Mechanical ventilation is discussed later in this chapter.

Other Therapies

In addition to smoking cessation, patients are advised to avoid other airway irritants and allergens. When air pollution is significant, the patient may need to remain indoors. Air filtering systems or air conditioning may be useful.

Increased fluid intake, effective cough, percussion, and postural drainage help clear secretions. A liberal fluid intake thins secretions. Forceful coughing is often less effective than leaning forward and repeatedly "huffing," with relaxed breathing between huffs. Percussion and postural drainage help clear secretions when they are thick or tenacious. Breathing exercises slow the respiratory rate and reduce fatigue. *Pursed-lip breathing* helps slow respirations and keeps airways open during exhalation by keeping positive pressure in the airways. *Abdominal breathing* helps reduce the work of accessory muscles of respiration (Box 23-7■).

A lung transplant or lung reduction surgery may be done in end-stage COPD. Lung reduction surgery reduces the volume of the lung, reshapes it, and improves elastic recoil. It improves pulmonary function and exercise tolerance and reduces dyspnea. (Nursing care of the patient undergoing lung surgery is discussed in Box 23-10, page 584.)

BOX 23-7	PATIENT TEACHING

Breathing and Coughing Techniques

Pursed-Lip Breathing

1. Inhale through nose with mouth closed.
2. Exhale slowly through pursed lips, as though whistling or blowing out a candle. Exhale twice as long as inhalation.

Diaphragmatic or Abdominal Breathing

1. Place one hand on abdomen, the other on the chest.
2. Inhale, concentrating on pushing abdominal hand outward while chest hand remains still.
3. Exhale slowly, while abdominal hand moves inward and chest hand remains still.

Controlled Cough Technique

1. After using bronchodilator, inhale deeply, and hold breath briefly.
2. Cough twice, first to loosen mucus, and then to expel secretions.
3. Inhale by sniffing to prevent mucus from moving back into deep airways.
4. Rest.

Huff Cough Technique

1. Inhale deeply while leaning forward.
2. Exhale sharply with a "huff" sound. This helps keep airways open while mobilizing secretions.

NURSING CARE

PRIORITIZING NURSING CARE

Because of the obstructive nature of COPD, maintaining clear airways is a high-priority nursing problem. Because this chronic disease affects all areas of life as it progresses, psychosocial issues also are a priority concern when planning nursing care.

HEALTH PROMOTION

Not smoking—quitting or never starting—is the best way to prevent COPD. Teach people of all ages about the risks of smoking. The Global Initiative for Chronic Obstructive Lung Disease (GOLD, 2011) recommends a five-step program that health care providers can use to help patients quit smoking (Box 23-8■).

ASSESSING

Patients with COPD need careful and frequent focused assessment. Inquire about shortness of breath or difficulty breathing; note its onset and duration and any known precipitating factors, such as a respiratory infection. Ask about cough and sputum production, including amount, color, and viscosity. Record the patient's smoking history, previous treatment for lung disease or asthma. Inquire about current medications, including oxygen, their effectiveness in managing symptoms, and when most recently used.

Note general appearance, apparent state of nutrition and health, anxiety, LOC, and mental status. Obtain height and weight. Observe for skin color, barrel chest and position. Observe respiratory rate and depth, chest expansion, use of accessory muscles, and ability to talk without pausing for breath. Obtain vital signs, including apical pulse and temperature. Auscultate breath sounds throughout, noting presence and any adventitious sounds such as crackles or wheezes.

BOX 23-8	STRATEGIES TO PROMOTE SMOKING CESSATION

1. **Ask** every patient at every office visit about tobacco use.
2. **Advise** all tobacco users to quit.
3. **Assess** the patient's willingness to quit.
4. **Assist** the patient to develop a quit plan; provide practical counseling, social support, supplementary materials, and recommend use of approved medications as appropriate.
5. **Arrange** follow-up, either in-person or by telephone.

Source: Global Initiative for Chronic Obstructive Lung Disease (GOLD). (2011). *Global strategy for the diagnosis, management, and prevention of chronic obstructive pulmonary disease.* Vancouver, WA: Global Initiative for Chronic Obstructive Lung Disease (GOLD).

IDENTIFYING POTENTIAL COMPLICATIONS

The patient with COPD is at risk for developing pneumonia, spontaneous pneumothorax, and respiratory failure (discussed in other sections of this chapter). Promptly report a change in skin color, elevated temperature, increased adventitious lung sounds or diminished breath sounds, decreasing oxygen saturation levels, or change in mental status or LOC (increasing apprehension and agitation, somnolence, or difficulty rousing the patient).

DIAGNOSING, PLANNING, AND IMPLEMENTING

Ineffective Airway Clearance

Expected outcome: Will maintain clear breath sounds throughout lung fields.

- Encourage fluid intake of at least 2,000 to 2,500 mL/day unless contraindicated. *Adequate fluid intake helps keep secretions thin.*
- Raise the head of the bed. Encourage activity to tolerance. *An upright position improves lung ventilation. Activity helps mobilize secretions and prevent them from pooling.*
- Assist to cough at least every 2 hours while awake. *Coughing helps mobilize secretions and maintain open airways.*
- Provide tissues and a paper bag to dispose of sputum. *This infection control measure reduces the spread of respiratory organisms to others.*
- Assist with percussion and postural drainage as needed. *Percussion helps loosen secretions in airways; postural drainage facilitates movement of these secretions out of the respiratory tract.*
- Provide rest periods between treatments and procedures. *Rest conserves energy and reduces fatigue.*
- Give expectorant and bronchodilator medications as ordered. *Using expectorants and bronchodilators before coughing, percussion, and postural drainage improves airway clearance.*
- Provide humidified oxygen as ordered. *Oxygen helps maintain blood and tissue oxygenation. Humidification decreases the drying effects of oxygen on respiratory tissues.*
- Prepare for transfer to intensive care if condition is deteriorating. *Respiratory failure is a possible complication of COPD that requires aggressive intervention to preserve life.*

Imbalanced Nutrition: Less Than Body Requirements

Expected outcome: Weight will remain stable.

- Obtain diet history. *The diet history is used to evaluate nutritional status.*
- Observe and document food intake, including types and amounts consumed. *This provides information about the possible need for supplements.*
- Monitor serum albumin and electrolyte levels. *These values provide information about nutritional status.*

- Consult with a dietitian to plan meals and supplements. *High-protein, high-calorie foods help maintain nutrition and reduce fatigue.*
- Provide frequent, small feedings with between-meal supplements. *Frequent, small meals help maintain intake and reduce fatigue associated with eating.*
- Assist to choose preferred foods from menu; encourage family members to bring food from home if allowed. *Providing food preferences encourages eating.*
- Keep snacks at bedside. *Snacks provide additional caloric intake.*
- Provide mouth care before meals. *This improves appetite.*

Compromised Family Coping

Expected outcome: Will express increased ability to cope with changes in family structure and responsibilities.

- Assess interactions and the effect of the illness on the family. *Assessment helps identify effective and disruptive behaviors.*
- Help identify strengths for coping with the situation. *Identifying strengths helps the patient and family regain a sense of control.*
- Encourage expression of feelings. Avoid judging the feelings as "good" or "bad," "right" or "wrong." *Active listening without judging promotes trust.*
- Help identify family members' behaviors and attitudes that may hinder effective treatment, such as continuing to smoke in the house. *Family members may be unaware of the effect of their behavior on the patient's ability to change habits and cope with a disabling disease.*
- Encourage participation in care. *This helps develop skills for use at home.*
- Refer to available support groups, pulmonary rehabilitation programs, and community agencies or services such as home health, homemaker services, or Meals-on-Wheels as appropriate. *Support groups, community services, and structured rehabilitation programs provide additional support and enhance coping abilities.*

Decisional Conflict (Smoking)

Expected outcome: Will use problem-solving and available resources to assist with smoking cessation.

- Encourage to express feelings; acknowledge concerns, values, and beliefs. *This demonstrates acceptance of the patient's right to make the decision. The nurse needs to avoid imposing personal values and beliefs about smoking on the patient.*
- Help plan a course of action for quitting smoking. *When the patient develops the plan, he or she has more ownership and interest in making it work.*
- Demonstrate respect for decisions and the right to choose. *Respect supports self-esteem and ability to cope.*

■ Refer to a counselor or other professional as needed. *Counselors or other people trained to assist with smoking cessation can help with the decision and plan.*

MANAGING NURSING CARE

The patient with COPD may require assistance with ADLs and the presence of a caring nurse during episodes of coughing or shortness of breath and anxiety. Such nursing care activities are appropriate to assign to assistive personnel.

EVALUATING

To evaluate the effectiveness of nursing care, collect assessment data related to airway clearance and respiratory status, nutritional status and diet intake, demonstrated coping behaviors by the patient and family, and a commitment to smoking cessation. Continuously monitor oxygen saturation to help evaluate the effectiveness of medical management.

DOCUMENTING

Document continuing assessment data and the patient's response to treatment and care measures. Note teaching provided and the patient's and family's understanding and acceptance of information. Document referrals made, including to a nutritionist, smoking cessation resources, and home care services.

CONTINUITY OF CARE

Teach the patient with COPD effective coughing and breathing techniques (see Box 23-7), how to prevent exacerbations, and management of the treatment regimen.

Advise patient to maintain a fluid intake of at least 2 to 2-1/2 quarts daily. Instruct to avoid respiratory irritants such as cigarette smoke (primary and secondary), other smoke sources, dust, aerosol sprays, air pollution, and very cold, dry air. Teach to avoid large crowds and people with known infections to prevent infection. Advise to obtain yearly influenza immunization. Discuss an exercise program, and encourage a balance of rest and activity as tolerated. Aerobic physical exercise (e.g., walking for 20 minutes at least three times weekly) improves exercise tolerance. Activities that strengthen the muscles used for breathing and ADLs, such as swimming and golf, also are helpful. Stress the importance of maintaining food intake, eating small frequent meals, and using nutritional supplements as needed. If a salt-restricted diet is ordered, teach about foods to avoid and suggest seasonings to improve taste without salt.

Instruct patients to report promptly early signs of infection or exacerbation of the disease to the physician: fever, increased sputum, purulent (green or yellow) sputum, URI, increased shortness of breath or difficulty breathing, decreased activity tolerance or appetite, increased need for oxygen.

Reinforce teaching about prescribed medications, including purpose, use, and expected effects. Instruct to avoid over-the-counter medications unless approved by the physician. Teach about other treatment measures, such as home oxygen, percussion, postural drainage, and nebulizer treatments. If special equipment is required, be sure to discuss its use, cleaning, and maintenance.

Finally, advise patients with COPD to wear an identification band and carry a list of their medications at all times.

NURSING CARE PLAN
Patient With COPD

Anna "Happy" Mercurio is an 83-year-old widow who lives with her two grown sons. During the past 15 years, she has become more short of breath and has developed a chronic cough. Ten years ago, emphysema was diagnosed. She is in the hospital with possible pneumonia and an acute exacerbation of COPD.

Assessment

Mrs. Mercurio denies smoking but says that her husband and two sons have been smokers "for practically their whole lives." She reports that she now must rest after just a few minutes of activity. Her cough is productive of moderate to large amounts of sputum, particularly in the mornings. Her dyspnea and sputum became worse 2 days ago; this morning, she was unable to get dressed without resting.

Mrs. Mercurio's skin is very warm and dry, her color dusky. She pauses frequently while talking to catch her breath. Respiratory rate 36, fairly shallow. Frequent cough productive of large amounts of thick, tenacious green sputum. Vital signs: P 115, irregular; BP 186/60; T 102.4°F (39°C). Weight 96 lb (43.6 kg), height 5'3" (160 cm). Appears barrel-chested with moderate kyphosis. Distant breath sounds with scattered wheezes and rhonchi throughout lung fields. Chest x-ray shows patchy infiltrates. Laboratory results include high RBC count, low serum albumin, and oxygen saturation of 86%.

Admitting orders include sputum for culture; intravenous penicillin G, 2 million units every 4 hours; ipratropium (Atrovent) inhaler, 2 puffs every 6 hours; beclomethasone (Vanceril) inhaler, 2 puffs every 6 hours; bed rest with bathroom privileges; oxygen per nasal cannula at 2 L continuously; regular diet.

Nursing Diagnosis

The following nursing diagnoses are identified for Mrs. Mercurio:

■ *Ineffective Airway Clearance* related to pneumonia and COPD

- *Impaired Gas Exchange* related to lung disease
- *Risk for Impaired Spontaneous Ventilation* related to respiratory muscle fatigue
- *Impaired Home Maintenance* related to activity intolerance

Expected Outcomes

The expected outcomes specify that Mrs. Mercurio will:
- Expectorate secretions effectively.
- Return to her previous level of respiratory function.
- Maintain oxygen saturation greater than 92%.
- Maintain spontaneous respirations without excess fatigue.
- Express willingness to allow help with household tasks.

Planning and Implementation

The following interventions are planned and implemented:
- Assess respiratory status and LOC every 1 to 2 hours until stable, and then at least every 4 hours.
- Monitor O_2 saturation continuously.
- Increase fluid intake to at least 2,500 mL/day.
- Provide bedside humidifier.
- Keep head of bed elevated to at least 30 degrees.
- Provide mouth care after inhaler treatments.
- Provide uninterrupted rest periods after respiratory therapy and other procedures.
- Refer to home health for nursing follow-up.
- Refer to social services for assistance with home maintenance.

Evaluation

Mrs. Mercurio's condition gradually improves. At discharge, she is able to provide self-care with less fatigue and dyspnea. She is using oxygen only at night, admitting that it is just for security. Although scattered wheezes are present, her sputum is thinner, white, and easily expectorated. She will continue oral penicillin V for an additional 10 days at home. She will continue to use Atrovent and Vanceril inhalers at home. Mrs. Mercurio's sons have agreed to smoke only in the garage or outside. A home health nurse will visit three times weekly. A housekeeper will clean and do laundry weekly. Mrs. Mercurio is glad to go home and grateful for the help she will receive.

Critical Thinking in the Nursing Process

1. Mrs. Mercurio had long-term exposure to secondhand smoke. How does secondhand smoke contribute to lung disease in adults and children?
2. The nursing care plan included the nursing diagnosis "Risk for Impaired Spontaneous Ventilation related to respiratory muscle fatigue." Review mechanics of respiration and how pH, carbon dioxide, and oxygen affect the respiratory drive.

3. The patient with COPD is at high risk for developing respiratory failure. What are the assessment findings of respiratory failure that you should report to the charge nurse or physician?

Note: Discussion of Critical Thinking questions appears on the companion website.

Cystic Fibrosis

Cystic fibrosis (CF) is an inherited disorder of childhood that causes excess mucus secretion. Its most damaging effects are to the lungs. Today, many people with CF live into adulthood.

PATHOPHYSIOLOGY AND MANIFESTATIONS

The genetic defect of CF causes excess mucus production in the lungs. Thick mucus plugs small airways and impairs normal airway clearing mechanisms. This leads to *atelectasis*, infection, *bronchiectasis*, and airway dilation. The lungs become scarred and stiff. Over time, COPD, *pulmonary hypertension* (increased pressures in the pulmonary vascular system), and right heart failure develop. The other primary features of CF are lack of pancreatic enzymes and impaired digestion and increased sodium and chloride in sweat.

The manifestations of CF include dyspnea, chest congestion, and a chronic cough productive of large amounts of thick, sticky sputum. A barrel chest and clubbing of the fingers and toes may be seen (Figure 23-11■). Digestive problems cause abdominal pain and *steatorrhea* (bulky, foul-smelling stool).

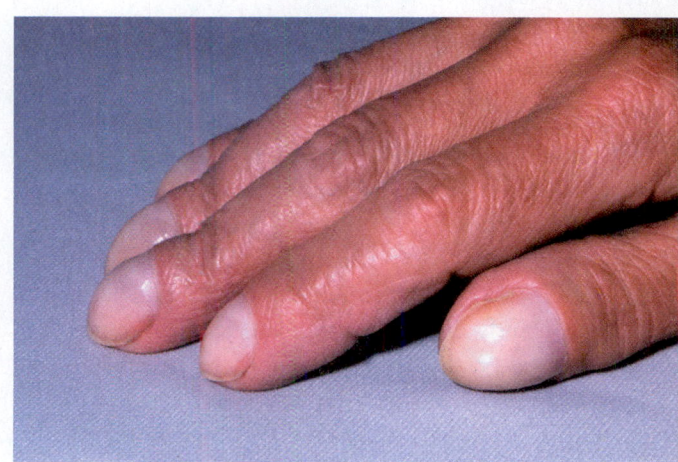

Figure 23-11. ■ Clubbing of the fingers caused by chronic hypoxia. (Source: © Medical-on-Line/Alamy.)

COLLABORATIVE CARE

Treatment goals for CF include preventing or treating respiratory complications and maintaining adequate nutrition.

A *pilocarpine iontophoresis sweat chloride test* is used to diagnose CF. Pilocarpine and a small electric current are used to increase sweating. The sweat is collected and analyzed.

Dornase alfa, an enzyme that helps liquefy mucus in CF, is given to improve airway clearance. This drug is given by aerosol. Prophylactic antibiotics often are given to prevent recurrent respiratory infections.

Chest physiotherapy with percussion, vibration, postural drainage, and coughing is essential for airway clearance. Oxygen therapy may be necessary. A liberal fluid intake helps to thin mucous secretions. Lung transplant currently is the only definitive treatment for CF. Single-lung, double-lung, and heart–lung transplants have been successful in CF patients.

NURSING CARE

Nursing care for the patient with CF is similar to that for patients with COPD. The genetic component of CF and the patient's age are important considerations. Patients with CF face a shortened life span and may have many questions about important decisions such as education, career, and starting a family.

Reinforce teaching for respiratory care techniques, including percussion, postural drainage, and controlled cough techniques. Stress the importance of avoiding respiratory irritants, such as cigarette smoke and air pollution. Discuss prevention of respiratory infection by maintaining immunizations, good general health, and avoiding large crowds and infected people.

Discuss the genetic transmission of CF. Refer for genetic testing if desired. Help sort through the impact of CF on future pregnancies and generations. Remember that the risk of CF may present an ethical dilemma about future pregnancies for patients and their families. Provide support as needed.

Atelectasis

Atelectasis is partial or total lung collapse and airlessness. It may be acute or chronic. The usual cause of atelectasis is obstruction of the airway to the affected area of lung. It may affect a small segment of a lung or an entire lobe. Atelectasis also may result from compression of the lung (e.g., a tumor) or an inability to keep alveoli open. The manifestations of atelectasis include absent or diminished breath sounds over the affected area, tachycardia, tachypnea, and dyspnea.

Prevention is the primary treatment for atelectasis. Patients with risk factors such as COPD, smokers undergoing surgery, and patients on prolonged bed rest need vigorous chest physiotherapy to keep airways open. Frequent respiratory assessment is important for early detection and treatment. Position the patient on the unaffected side, with the involved side up to promote drainage. Move the patient frequently, and encourage coughing and deep breathing. Encourage oral fluids to help thin secretions.

Bronchiectasis

Bronchiectasis is permanent dilation and destruction of large airways. It is usually due to repeated respiratory infections. Inflammation and airway obstruction weaken and dilate bronchial walls, causing secretions to pool. This pooling, in turn, promotes further infection and inflammation.

Bronchiectasis causes a chronic cough productive of large amounts of sputum. Other manifestations include hemoptysis, recurrent pneumonia, wheezing and shortness of breath, malnutrition, right-sided heart failure, and cor pulmonale (see the section of this chapter on pulmonary vascular disorders).

Treatment is similar to that for COPD. Antibiotics are ordered at the first sign of infection and may be used prophylactically. Inhaled bronchodilators also may be ordered. Chest physiotherapy is a vital part of care. Percussion and postural drainage help mobilize secretions. Oxygen may be ordered. If lung destruction is local, the affected segment may be surgically removed.

Nursing care of the patient with bronchiectasis is much the same as for COPD. Airway clearance is a primary problem, as is ineffective breathing pattern. Teaching is vital to help the patient and family manage the disease and prevent progression.

Occupational Lung Diseases

Occupational lung diseases damage the interstitial or connective tissue of the lung, restricting the ability of the lungs to expand and fill with air. These disorders frequently are called *restrictive lung disorders*.

Occupational lung diseases (Table 23-5 ■) are directly related to inhaling noxious substances in the work environment. There are two major classifications:

1. *Pneumoconioses*, caused by inhaling *inorganic* dusts and particulates.
2. *Hypersensitivity pneumonitis*, allergic responses to inhaled organic dusts.

PATHOPHYSIOLOGY AND MANIFESTATIONS

When a noxious substance is inhaled, the body's response depends on the size of the particles, whether it is organic or inorganic, where it lands in the respiratory tract, and the individual. Normal lung defenses attempt to remove

TABLE 23-5	**Occupational Lung Diseases**	
DISORDER	**CAUSE**	**HIGH-RISK POPULATION**
Pneumoconioses	Inorganic dusts	
■ Silicosis	■ Silica	■ Hard rock miners, foundry workers, sandblasters, pottery makers, granite cutters
■ Asbestosis	■ Asbestos	■ People involved in mining, milling, manufacturing, and application of asbestos products
■ Black lung disease	■ Coal	■ Coal miners
Hypersensitivity pneumonitis	Organic dusts	People exposed to cotton dust, moldy sugar cane fiber; farmers; people who raise birds

foreign matter; however, these defenses may be impaired by smoking, alcohol, or allergic reactions.

The inhaled substance and resulting inflammatory response damage the alveoli and interstitial tissue of the lung. The normally elastic fibers of the lung are replaced by scar tissue, leaving the lungs stiff and *noncompliant* (difficult to inflate). Lung volumes decrease, the work of breathing increases, and gas exchange is impaired, leading to hypoxemia.

The onset of occupational lung disease may be acute or gradual. A dry cough and dyspnea on exertion are common symptoms of interstitial lung diseases. Respirations are often rapid and shallow. Fine inspiratory crackles at the lung bases may be heard. Clubbing of the fingers and toes may develop.

COLLABORATIVE CARE

Prevention is important for all occupational lung diseases. Measures to contain dust and wearing personal protective devices that limit the amount of inhaled particles are essential for people who work in industries with known risks.

Diagnostic testing shows restricted ventilation, with reduced vital capacity and total lung capacity. Gas exchange is affected, leading to low oxygen saturation and hypoxemia, especially with exercise. The chest x-ray shows interstitial lung damage. A bronchoscopy may be done to obtain tissue for biopsy. Specialized lung scans can show the extent of scarring.

Management of occupational lung disease includes measures to identify and remove the cause, reduce inflammation, prevent progression, and support current lung function. Treatment is nonspecific. Anti-inflammatory drugs, such as corticosteroids, may reduce the inflammatory response and slow the progression of the disease. Generally, care is supportive, similar to that for patients with COPD.

NURSING CARE

Nursing care for patients with occupational lung diseases is similar to that for a patient with COPD.

Activity intolerance is a common problem. The patient's ability to perform ADLs may be significantly impaired. Nursing measures to reduce energy use and provide rest are essential. Caregiver role strain, either actual or potential, must be considered when the patient with severe disability is being cared for at home.

Ineffective coping may also be a priority nursing diagnosis. Many occupational lung diseases develop after 20 to 30 years of exposure to the hazardous material. Patients who began working after high school may develop signs of disease in their 40s and face the possibility of changing occupations or becoming disabled. The resulting role strain affects all family members.

CONTINUITY OF CARE

Teach patients at risk for occupational lung diseases how to reduce this risk. Nurses in industrial and public health settings should be alert to potential dangers. Teach workers about measures to reduce dust in their work area and the use of personal protective devices such as masks. Educate children of people with occupational lung disease about the risks associated with the occupation.

Teach how to avoid further lung damage; for example, avoid respiratory irritants such as cigarette smoke and heavy air pollution. Recommend influenza and pneumococcal pneumonia immunizations. Yearly tuberculin testing is recommended for patients with silicosis.

Teach pulmonary hygiene measures, such as maintaining fluid intake, coughing, and deep-breathing exercises. If oxygen therapy is ordered, teach about its use and care of the equipment. Always include teaching about the use and effects of any ordered medications.

If corticosteroid therapy is prescribed, stress the importance of taking the medication as prescribed and not stopping it abruptly. Include information about managing the side effects of corticosteroids by limiting sodium and increasing potassium in the diet, taking the medication with food or milk to minimize gastric irritation, and identifying early signs of infection.

Lung Cancer

Key Concept Lung cancer is the leading cause of cancer deaths in the United States. Nurses can impact this statistic through efforts to prevent smoking among teens and young adults and by assisting patients who smoke to quit.

Lung cancer is the leading cause of cancer deaths in the United States, causing an estimated 159,500 deaths in 2013. It has a grim prognosis: More than half of those with lung cancer die within 1 year of the diagnosis.

Cigarette smoking is the most important risk factor for lung cancer. About 85% of lung cancer is related to smoking. The disease is 10 to 30 times more common in smokers than nonsmokers. The more the person smokes and the longer the person smokes, the greater the risk. Other risk factors for lung cancer are exposure to secondhand smoke, radon gas, radiation, air pollution, and inhaled irritants, asbestos in particular.

PATHOPHYSIOLOGY

Most primary lung tumors arise in the cells lining the airways. Damaged bronchial cells mutate over time to become malignant. There are four major cell types that account for about 90% of lung cancers: small-cell carcinoma, adenocarcinoma, squamous cell carcinoma, and large cell carcinoma. These tumors differ by incidence, presentation, and manner of spread (Table 23-6■).

TABLE 23-6	Lung Cancer Cell Types		
	CELL TYPE	**LOCATION AND MANIFESTATIONS**	**SPREAD**
	Small-cell carcinoma Approximately 10%–15% of all lung cancers	Central mass; may cause endocrine symptoms (SIADH, Cushing syndrome) or thrombophlebitis	Aggressive; distant metastasis common at diagnosis
	Adenocarcinoma 40% of all lung cancers	Peripheral mass; few symptoms	Early metastasis to CNS, bone, adrenal glands
	Squamous cell carcinoma 25%–30% of all lung cancers	Central mass in large bronchi; cough, dyspnea, atelectasis, wheezing	Spreads by local invasion
	Large-cell carcinoma 10%–15% of all lung cancers	Large peripheral lesion; may cause gynecomastia or thrombophlebitis	Early metastasis

Lung cancer tends to be aggressive and locally invasive and metastasizes widely. Tumors begin as mucosal lesions that grow to obstruct the bronchi or invade adjacent tissue. Tumors frequently spread via the lymph system to nodes and other organs. Lung cancer usually is well advanced when diagnosed, with tumor cells in lymph nodes and distant metastasis.

MANIFESTATIONS AND COMPLICATIONS

Initial symptoms often are blamed on smoking or chronic bronchitis. In addition to manifestations of the tumor and cancer (Box 23-9■), lung cancers often produce hormone-like substances that cause indirect symptoms. These are known as *paraneoplastic syndromes* or manifestations.

Lung cancer metastasizes to the lymph nodes, brain, bones, liver, and other organs. Confusion, impaired balance, headache, and personality changes may be symptoms of brain metastasis. Tumor spread to the bone causes bone pain, pathologic fractures, and possible spinal cord compression. When the liver is affected, symptoms may include jaundice, anorexia, and upper right quadrant pain.

Superior vena cava syndrome, partial or complete obstruction of the superior vena cava, is a potential complication. Symptoms such as edema of the neck and face, headache, dizziness, vision changes, and syncope may develop abruptly or gradually. Veins of the upper chest and neck are dilated, and the skin is flushed or cyanotic. Laryngeal edema may cause dyspnea.

COLLABORATIVE CARE

Prevention of lung cancer should be a primary goal for all health care providers. Reducing tobacco use will have a greater positive effect on the death rate from lung cancer than treatment advances.

BOX 23-9	MANIFESTATIONS OF LUNG CANCER

Local
- Cough, hemoptysis
- Wheezing and dyspnea
- Chest pain, hoarseness, or dysphagia

General
- Anorexia, weight loss, anemia
- Weakness, fever

Paraneoplastic
- Fluid and electrolyte imbalances (hypercalcemia, hyponatremia, hypokalemia)
- Cushing syndrome
- Peripheral neuropathy, muscle weakness
- Thrombophlebitis, disseminated intravascular coagulation (DIC)

Because lung cancer is often advanced when diagnosed, the American Cancer Society and the United States Preventive Services Task Force (USPSTF) recommend lung cancer screening for people who are at high risk for lung cancer. Current smokers (or those who have quit within the past 15 years) age 55 to 79 years who have a 30-pack-year or greater smoking history should have (or be offered) yearly low-dose CT scan (ACS, 2013).

Diagnostic Tests

- *Chest x-ray* often shows the first evidence of lung cancer.
- Malignant cells may be identified by *sputum cytology*. This test requires collection of a sputum sample on arising.
- A *CT scan* is used to evaluate tumor size and location.
- *Bronchoscopy* may be done to visualize the tumor and obtain a specimen for biopsy. A cable-activated instrument is used to obtain a biopsy specimen.
- A *percutaneous needle biopsy* or aspiration of pleural fluid by *thoracentesis* may be done if the tumor is in the periphery of the lung.

Medications

Combination chemotherapy is the primary treatment for some types of lung cancer. It is used as an adjunct to surgery or radiation for other types. It may lengthen survival when metastases are present.

Other medications that may be ordered include bronchodilators to reduce airway obstruction and antibiotics to treat infection. Analgesics are ordered after surgery and for pain management in advanced cancers.

Surgery

Surgery is the only real chance for a cure in most lung cancers. At the time of diagnosis, however, most tumors are beyond the stage at which they can be completely removed. The goal of surgery is to remove all tumor cells, including involved lymph nodes.

The type of surgery depends on the location and size of the tumor, as well as the patient's health status (see Table 23-7■). As much functional lung as possible is preserved. Nursing care of the patient having lung surgery is outlined in Box 23-10■.

Radiation Therapy

Radiation therapy is used alone or in combination with surgery or chemotherapy. Before surgery, it is used to shrink tumors. When surgery is not an option, radiation therapy may be the treatment of choice. Complications such as superior vena cava syndrome may be treated with radiation.

Other Therapies

Pleural effusion is a frequent complication of lung cancer. As fluid collects in the pleural space, the lung cannot fully

TABLE 23-7	Types of Lung Surgery	
PROCEDURE	**DESCRIPTION**	**USED FOR**
Laser bronchoscopy	Bronchoscopy used to guide laser to resect tumor	Tumors localized in a main bronchus
Thoracotomy	Incision into the chest wall	Gain access to the lung for surgery
Wedge resection	Removal of a small section (wedge) of lung tissue	Small, peripheral lesions
Segmental resection	Removal of a single bronchovascular segment of a lobe	Localized peripheral lung tumors
Lobectomy	Removal of a single lung lobe	Tumors confined to a single lobe
Pneumonectomy	Removal of an entire lung	Tumors throughout a lung, in the main bronchus, or fixed to the hilum

expand and ventilation is impaired. A *thoracentesis* may be done to remove the excess pleural fluid. (Nursing care related to thoracentesis is discussed in Box 23-13 on page 589.)

NURSING CARE

PRIORITIZING NURSING CARE

Maintaining effective breathing, airway clearance, and gas exchange are the highest priorities for nursing care related to physiologic function. Because lung cancer frequently cannot be cured, its psychologic and emotional effects on the patient and family also are high priorities for caring.

HEALTH PROMOTION

Teaching people of all ages about the risks of cigarette smoking is the single most effective way of reducing the incidence of lung cancer. See Box 23-8 on page 576 for strategies to help patients stop smoking. In addition, work to reduce air pollution and to limit exposure of workers to materials such as asbestos.

ASSESSING

Obtain complete respiratory assessment data. Include smoking history and the duration of current symptoms. Obtain data related to both respiratory and cardiovascular status, especially if surgery is anticipated. Review laboratory and diagnostic test results, and report abnormal values to the charge nurse or physician.

Assess for concerns related to lung function, the cancer itself, and the planned treatment.

IDENTIFYING POTENTIAL COMPLICATIONS

Superior vena cava syndrome and metastasis to other body parts and organs are potential complications of lung cancer. Report development of facial or upper extremity edema, complaints of headache or dizziness, vision changes, or fainting. Immediately report stridor or increased difficulty breathing. Also report changes in skin color, complaints of back or bone pain, confusion, or personality changes, as these may be symptoms of metastasis.

BOX 23-10	NURSING CARE CHECKLIST

Lung Surgery

Before Surgery

☑ Provide routine preoperative care and teaching.
☑ Obtain baseline assessment data, particularly respiratory, cardiovascular, and nutritional status.
☑ Reinforce teaching, allowing time to practice breathing and coughing techniques.
☑ Establish a way to communicate if an endotracheal tube will be in place after surgery.
☑ Introduce to intensive care unit and policies if patient will return there after surgery.

After Surgery

☑ Assess and provide routine postoperative care.
☑ Frequently assess respiratory status (color, rate and depth, chest expansion, lung sounds, and oxygen saturation). Promptly report changes to the charge nurse or physician.
☑ Assist with coughing, postural drainage, and incentive spirometry. Suction as needed while intubated.
☑ Maintain intact chest tube drainage system. Initially measure output hourly, and then every 2 to 4 or 8 hours as indicated. Notify the physician if output exceeds 70 mL/hr and/or is bright red, warm, and free flowing.
☑ Assist to move in bed and ambulate as soon as possible.

DIAGNOSING, PLANNING, AND IMPLEMENTING

Ineffective Breathing Pattern

Expected outcome: Will maintain an effective respiratory rate and pattern.

- Assess and document respiratory status at least every 4 hours; more frequently as indicated. *Early identification of altered respiratory function is important to maintain tissue oxygenation.*
- Report abnormal oxygen saturation levels and blood gas results to the charge nurse or physician. *Changes in blood oxygen levels may indicate respiratory compromise.*
- Elevate the head of the bed to 60 degrees. *Elevating the head of the bed promotes lung expansion.*
- Assist to turn, cough, deep breathe, and use incentive spirometer. Help splint the chest with a pillow or blanket when coughing. *These measures promote airway clearance.*
- Administer oxygen as ordered. *Supplemental oxygen improves alveolar oxygenation and gas exchange.*
- Provide reassurance and emotional support. *Relief of anxiety promotes a more effective breathing pattern.*

Activity Intolerance

Expected outcome: Endurance will gradually increase, allowing completion of ADLs without shortness of breath or dyspnea.

Loss of functional lung tissue due to the tumor or surgery affects the ability to maintain normal activities.

- Document responses to activity, including pulse, respiratory rate, dyspnea, and fatigue. *Tachycardia, tachypnea, dyspnea, or fatigue with activities is a sign of activity intolerance.*
- Plan rest periods interspersed with activities and procedures. *Rest periods reduce oxygen demands and fatigue.*
- Assist to increase activities gradually. *Gradual increases in activity improve exercise tolerance.*
- Teach energy conservation measures, such as sitting while showering and dressing and wearing slip-on shoes. *These measures reduce oxygen demand and promote independence.*
- Encourage to remain as active as possible. *Maintaining activity levels improves physical and emotional well-being.*
- Allow family members to provide assistance as needed. *This helps the patient conserve energy and allows the family to feel useful.*

Pain

Expected outcome: Will report pain level of 2 or lower on a scale of 0 to 10.

- Assess and document pain. *Remember that pain is subjective; however, reluctance to cough or move may indicate unreported pain.*

- Provide analgesics as needed to maintain comfort. *Adequate pain relief promotes postoperative recovery and coping. Good pain management is vital to improve recovery from surgery and to allow a peaceful death for the terminal cancer patient.*
- For cancer pain, maintain a continuous medication schedule using opiates, NSAIDs, and other drugs as ordered. *Addiction is not a concern for the terminal cancer patient; adequate pain relief that does not allow "breakthrough" pain is vital.*
- Use adjunctive pain relief measures, such as massage, positioning, distraction, and relaxation techniques. *These techniques promote relaxation and enhance pain relief.*
- Allow significant others to remain with the patient. *Physical presence provides emotional support.*

Grieving

Expected outcome: Will express thoughts and feelings about the potential loss.

- Spend time with the patient and family. *Time is necessary to develop a trusting, therapeutic relationship.*
- Answer questions honestly; do not deny the probable outcome of the disease. *Honesty reinforces reality and promotes a sense of control over decisions to be made.*
- Encourage expression of feelings, fears, and concerns. *Open communication helps promote understanding and acceptance.*
- Assist to understand the grieving process and to accept responses as normal. *Explanation enhances understanding of the grieving process and the ability to cope.*
- Help identify strengths and effective coping measures. *Past successes in coping with crises can help with the present situation and help the patient develop a sense of control.*
- Encourage use of other support systems, such as spiritual and social groups. Refer to support groups, social services, and hospice care as indicated. *These support systems can help the patient and family cope with the diagnosis.*
- Discuss advance directives (the living will and durable power of attorney for health care). *These documents give more control over treatment when the patient is no longer able to express his or her own wishes.*

MANAGING NURSING CARE

The patient with lung cancer may require assistance with ADLs and the presence of a caring nurse during episodes of pain, coughing or shortness of breath, and anxiety. Such nursing care activities are appropriate to assign to assistive personnel.

EVALUATING

Collect data related to the patient's respiratory status, ability to complete ADLs and other activities, pain control, and acceptance of the probable outcome of the disease to evaluate the effectiveness of nursing care.

DOCUMENTING

Document continuing assessment data, particularly during the early postoperative period if surgery has been performed. Assess for and document any adverse responses to other cancer treatments such as chemotherapy and radiation therapy. Note the patient's and family's response to the diagnosis and treatment plan. Document any referrals provided, such as home health care or hospice.

CONTINUITY OF CARE

Provide honest information about lung cancer, the expected outcome, and planned treatment. Do not promote false hope.

Stress the importance of stopping smoking, especially if surgery has been done. The patient with lung cancer may have difficulty recognizing the need to stop smoking. Include information about the effects of nicotine and the tars in cigarette smoke on healing and already compromised lung tissue (Box 23-11 ■).

Provide information about planned treatments, explaining expected effects and usual side effects of each. Help identify ways to cope with noxious effects. If surgery has been done, discuss activities and exercises to improve strength and regain function. Stress the need to continue coughing and deep-breathing exercises at home. Provide information

about symptoms to report to the physician: fever, increasing dyspnea, cough, increased or purulent sputum, redness, pain, swelling, or incisional drainage.

Discuss medication use, including desired and adverse effects, and interactions with other drugs or foods. Teach how to use analgesics and other pain relief measures.

Provide information about hospice services, home health, cancer support groups, and American Cancer Society services.

BOX 23-11	PATIENT TEACHING

Effects of Cigarette Smoking

Tobacco was first used in religious ceremonies and to offer friendship. At one time, it was thought to help cure many common diseases. Tobacco is now known as the leading preventable cause of illness in the world.

Cigarette smoke contains about 4,000 chemicals, including more than 60 known carcinogens (cancer-causing agents). Nicotine is highly addictive, producing a feeling of well-being. Tar, the particulate matter in cigarette smoke, causes most of its ill effects in the lungs. Smoke paralyzes cilia, reducing clearance of tars from the bronchial tree.

Although most people recognize the harmful effects of smoking, quitting is difficult. The relapse rate after quitting is up to 80%, with most people resuming the habit within the first 3 months. See Box 23-8 for strategies to reduce tobacco use.

PULMONARY VASCULAR DISORDERS

Key Concept The cardiovascular and respiratory systems are closely linked. A good match of air movement and blood flow is essential to maintain gas exchange and oxygen delivery to all body tissues and organs.

Disorders previously discussed in this chapter affect airflow; this section discusses disorders that affect blood flow to the lungs.

Pulmonary Embolism

A **pulmonary embolism** is blockage of a pulmonary artery that disrupts blood flow to the lung. *Thromboemboli*, or blood clots, are the most common pulmonary emboli. Tumors, bone marrow fat, amniotic fluid, and foreign matter also can become emboli. Because a large pulmonary embolism can be fatal, prevention is the best treatment.

PATHOPHYSIOLOGY

Most pulmonary emboli begin as clots in the deep veins of the legs or pelvis. The risk factors are those for deep venous thrombosis (DVT): impaired venous blood flow, blood vessel damage, and altered coagulation. Prolonged immobility is the primary risk factor.

DVT may not be suspected until pulmonary embolism occurs. When the clot breaks loose from the vein wall, it travels through vessels that become gradually larger until it reaches the right side of the heart and enters the pulmonary artery. The pulmonary arteries and arterioles become smaller and smaller, and the clot is trapped, obstructing blood flow (Figure 23-12 ■). No blood flows through capillaries beyond the occlusion, so no gas exchange occurs in that portion of the lung. A large clot can obstruct blood flow to a major part of the lung, causing sudden death.

MANIFESTATIONS

The symptoms of a pulmonary embolism depend on its size and location (Box 23-12 ■). Small emboli may go unnoticed; larger emboli cause manifestations similar to a myocardial infarction (heart attack).

Fat emboli may occur after a long bone fracture (e.g., the femur) that releases bone marrow fat. Fat emboli cause a sudden onset of dyspnea, tachypnea, tachycardia, confusion, delirium, and decreased LOC. *Petechiae* may be seen on the chest and arms.

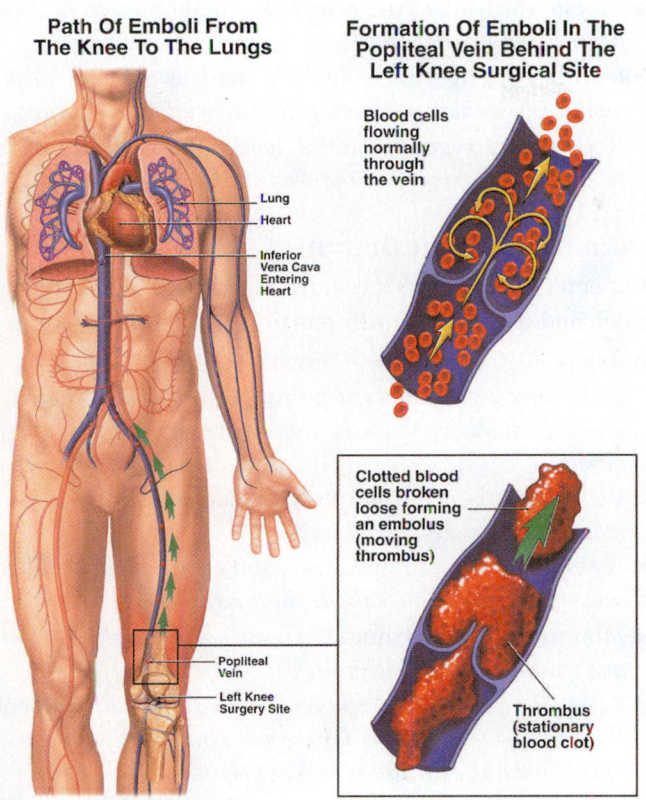

Path Of Emboli From The Knee To The Lungs

Lung
Heart
Inferior Vena Cava Entering Heart
Popliteal Vein
Left Knee Surgery Site

Anterior View

Formation Of Emboli In The Popliteal Vein Behind The Left Knee Surgical Site

Blood cells flowing normally through the vein

Clotted blood cells broken loose forming an embolus (moving thrombus)

Thrombus (stationary blood clot)

Figure 23-12. ■ Pulmonary emboli begin as clots that form in the deep veins of the legs or pelvis. These clots can break loose to become thromboemboli, travelling through the venous system to the right side of the heart. They are then carried into the pulmonary vascular system where they become lodged in a pulmonary artery or arteriole. (Source: © Nucleus Medical Art Inc./Alamy.)

COLLABORATIVE CARE

Preventive measures include elastic stockings (TED hose), pneumatic compression devices, anticoagulation therapy, and early ambulation to prevent venous stasis. Elevating the legs of immobilized patients and leg exercises also help prevent venous stasis and pulmonary emboli.

Treatment of a pulmonary embolism is supportive. Oxygen is given, and analgesics may be ordered to relieve pain and anxiety. The cardiac rhythm and hemodynamic pressures are monitored.

BOX 23-12	MANIFESTATIONS OF PULMONARY EMBOLISM

- Abrupt onset of dyspnea, chest pain
- Anxiety, apprehension
- Cough
- Tachycardia, tachypnea
- Diaphoresis
- Cyanosis

Diagnostic Tests

Plasma D-dimer levels are specific to the presence of a thrombus; elevated levels indicate formation of a blood clot. When a pulmonary embolism is suspected, *chest CT scan with contrast* is performed. A *ventilation–perfusion scan* may be ordered to evaluate blood flow in the pulmonary circulation. Other diagnostic tests may include chest x-ray, ECG to rule out myocardial infarction, and coagulation studies.

Medications

A fibrinolytic drug (e.g., t-PA) may be given to disintegrate a large pulmonary embolus and restore pulmonary blood flow. The primary risk of fibrinolytic therapy is bleeding, particularly intracranial bleeding.

Anticoagulants are ordered to prevent further clotting and embolization. Low-dose heparin is given to prevent DVT. When pulmonary embolus has occurred, an intravenous heparin infusion is ordered. The activated partial thromboplastin time (APTT) or PTT is monitored, and the patient is assessed for signs of abnormal bleeding. Heparin is continued until oral anticoagulant (warfarin) therapy is fully effective, 5 to 7 days after its initiation. Anticoagulants are continued for 2 to 3 months or longer. Bleeding is a risk for any patient taking anticoagulants.

Surgery

Pulmonary embolectomy may be performed using either an open or a percutaneous catheter approach to remove the thrombus. An umbrella-like filter may be inserted into the inferior vena cava of patients who have recurrent pulmonary emboli. This device traps large emboli while allowing blood to flow through the vena cava.

NURSING CARE

When a pulmonary embolus occurs, the patient has urgent nursing care needs and may be transferred to intensive care for close observation and monitoring.

PRIORITIZING NURSING CARE

Preventing DVT and pulmonary embolism is a priority of nursing care for all patients at risk. When pulmonary embolism does occur, maintaining effective gas exchange is the highest priority.

HEALTH PROMOTION

Teach patients to reduce the risk for DVT and pulmonary embolism:

- On automobile trips, stop every 1 to 2 hours for a brief stretch and walk to restore venous circulation.
- During long flights, get up every hour or so, and do leg exercises while seated.

- Do not cross legs.
- Exercise regularly (e.g., walking).
- Wear elastic hose when standing for prolonged periods. Avoid hose that bind around the knee or thigh.

ASSESSING

Because pulmonary embolism can be a medical emergency, assessment often is very focused. Inquire about chest pain, shortness of breath, and other manifestations. Ask about risk factors such as recent diagnosis of venous thrombosis, surgery, childbirth, or malignancy.

Objective assessment data include LOC; vital signs including heart and respiratory rate; skin color and temperature; heart and breath sounds; oxygen saturation; and neck vein distention.

IDENTIFYING POTENTIAL COMPLICATIONS

A pulmonary embolism that obstructs a major pulmonary artery can affect cardiac output and tissue perfusion. Frequently assess vital signs, urine output, and skin color and temperature. Immediately report manifestations of impaired cardiac output and shock.

clinicalALERT

A large pulmonary embolus may cause cardiac and respiratory arrest. Immediately initiate cardiopulmonary resuscitation (CPR) procedures if the patient is unresponsive and pulse and respirations are absent.

DIAGNOSING, PLANNING, AND IMPLEMENTING

Risk for Thromboembolism

Expected outcome: Will remain free of manifestations of venous thrombosis.

- Encourage early ambulation after surgery or illness.
- Apply elastic stockings or pneumatic compression devices as ordered.
- Assist with leg exercises.
- Discourage using pillows under the knees. *These measures promote venous return from the legs, reducing venous stasis and the risk for DVT and pulmonary emboli.*

Impaired Gas Exchange

Expected outcome: Will maintain SaO_2 levels within normal range for patient.

- Frequently assess respiratory status, including rate, depth, effort, and lung sounds. *Maintaining optimal ventilation facilitates gas exchange in well-perfused areas of the lung.*
- Report changes in LOC, mental status, and skin color to the charge nurse or physician. *A change in LOC or mental status and/or cyanosis may indicate hypoxemia.*

- Elevate the head of the bed. *This position promotes lung expansion and ventilation.*
- Start oxygen by nasal cannula or mask as ordered. *Supplemental oxygen increases alveolar and arterial oxygenation.*
- Report low oxygen saturation levels. *Pulse oximetry is used to assess gas exchange and the effect of interventions.*

Decreased Cardiac Output

Expected outcome: Vital signs, LOC, urinary output, skin color, and temperature will remain within normal ranges.

- Assess vital signs every 15 to 30 minutes initially, and then every 2 to 4 hours as indicated. *Frequent assessment is important during the early, unstable period after pulmonary embolus.*
- Record hourly urine output. *Decreased urine output may indicate impaired kidney perfusion.*
- Assess skin color, temperature, and capillary refill. *These assessments are used to evaluate tissue perfusion.*
- Monitor cardiac rhythm. *Monitoring allows early detection and treatment of dysrhythmias.*
- Assess for and report neck vein distention and peripheral edema. *Right-sided heart failure may result from pulmonary embolism due to increased pulmonary pressures.*
- Maintain intravenous and arterial lines. *The patient may be unstable and critically ill, requiring immediate interventions to maintain life.*
- Provide frequent skin care. *Impaired peripheral perfusion and tissue oxygenation increase the risk of skin breakdown.*
- Instruct to report chest pain or other symptoms. *Decreased cardiac output and an increased workload may cause angina.*

Anxiety

Expected outcome: Anxiety level will remain low to moderate, as evidenced by ability to follow directions and understand information.

- Reassure and provide emotional support. Accept fear of dying, and reassure that treatment usually restores respiratory function. *The fear of death is very real; reassurance helps relieve excess anxiety.*
- Remain with the patient as much as possible. *This helps reduce anxiety.*
- Explain procedures and treatments, using short, simple sentences. *Simple explanations reduce fear of the unknown.*
- Reduce environmental stimuli, and use a calm, reassuring manner. *These measures help reduce anxiety in both the nurse and the patient.*
- Allow family members to remain present as much as possible. *Calm, supportive family members provide further reassurance.*
- Administer morphine as ordered. *Morphine reduces both pain and anxiety.*

MANAGING NURSING CARE

Alert nursing assistive personnel to promptly report patient complaints of chest pain, shortness of breath, or changes in color or mental status, particularly in patients with known DVT or who are immobilized for an extended period.

EVALUATING

To evaluate the effectiveness of nursing care for the patient who is at risk for a pulmonary embolism, collect assessment data related to ambulation, manifestations of DVT, and respiratory status on a continuing basis. For the patient who experiences a pulmonary embolism, frequently evaluate mental status, respiratory status, and cardiovascular status, reporting significant changes to the physician or charge nurse. Assess the patient's return to previous health status after resolution of the acute event.

DOCUMENTING

Document measures instituted to prevent DVT and pulmonary embolism (e.g., leg exercises, ambulation, application of elastic hose or pneumatic compression devices) in all patients at risk. Document assessment data related to DVT, including complaints of calf or leg pain, swelling, or redness and warmth. Regularly document respiratory assessment data, noting any changes from previous findings. If a pulmonary embolism develops, document initial subjective and objective assessment data, emergency care measures instituted, and the patient's response to treatment. Document personnel notified, including the physician. Note diagnostic tests performed. If the patient is transferred to an acute care facility or critical care unit, document the transfer.

CONTINUITY OF CARE

Teach the patient and family or caregivers about prescribed anticoagulants, including symptoms of bleeding to report to the physician. Instruct to use a soft toothbrush and avoid taking aspirin (unless prescribed) and other over-the-counter drugs without the doctor's approval. Stress the importance of wearing an identification bracelet or tag to alert medical personnel about anticoagulant use. Provide information about preventing future episodes of venous thrombosis (see Health Promotion section).

Pulmonary Hypertension

Arterial pressure in the pulmonary system normally is low (25/8) compared with the systemic BP (120/80). **Pulmonary hypertension** is an abnormal elevation of the pulmonary arterial pressure. It can develop with no obvious cause, or it may occur as a result of chronic lung disease or another problem. Long-standing pulmonary hypertension can lead to *cor pulmonale*, with right ventricular hypertrophy and failure. COPD is the usual cause of cor pulmonale.

Manifestations of pulmonary hypertension include increasing dyspnea, fatigue, angina, and syncope (fainting or light-headedness) with exertion. Patients with cor pulmonale have a chronic productive cough, progressive dyspnea, wheezing, and signs of right heart failure (peripheral edema and distended neck veins). The skin is warm, moist, and dusky red.

Supplemental oxygen and drugs such as calcium channel blockers may be ordered for pulmonary hypertension. Rapid-acting direct vasodilators such as inhaled nitric oxide may be ordered. Salt and water intake may be restricted. Bilateral lung or heart–lung transplant may be done for primary pulmonary hypertension.

Nursing care is supportive, focusing on the underlying lung disease. *Impaired Gas Exchange* is a significant problem, as are problems such as *Activity Intolerance, Anxiety,* and *Fatigue*. See nursing assessment and interventions for COPD and for heart failure.

Provide information about pulmonary hypertension and cor pulmonale as appropriate. Include the disease process and manifestations to report to the physician, including change in activity tolerance, increased edema, and signs of respiratory infection or exacerbation. Discuss the importance of planned rest periods between activities and ways to conserve energy, such as using a shower chair. Stress the importance of not smoking due to its effects on the lungs and blood vessels. As always, teach about the purpose, use, and effects of medications.

PLEURAL DISORDERS AND TRAUMA

Key Concept   Trauma and disorders that affect the integrity or function of the chest wall, pleura, or lung itself can affect lung expansion and breathing. Initial and ongoing assessment of airway, breathing, and circulation (ABCs) is vital in these disorders.

A closed chest cavity with negative pressure in the pleural space (the potential space between the visceral and parietal pleura) is necessary for breathing. Excess fluid, air, or blood in the pleural space interferes with lung expansion and breathing. Chest and lung injury can result from penetrating or blunt trauma or inhalation injury.

Pleuritis

Pleuritis (*pleurisy*) is inflammation of the pleura that covers the lung surface and lines the inner chest wall. Pleuritis usually results from another process, such as a viral infection, pneumonia, or rib injury.

The onset of pleuritis is often abrupt, with characteristic localized sharp or stabbing pain (*pleuritic* pain). Deep breathing, coughing, and movement aggravate the pain. Breathing is rapid and shallow, and breath sounds are diminished. A *pleural friction rub* or harsh, grating sound may be heard over the affected area.

Treatment of pleuritis includes analgesics and NSAIDs to relieve the pain. Codeine may be ordered to relieve pain and suppress the cough.

Nursing care focuses on promoting comfort. Positioning and splinting the chest while coughing can be helpful. Wrapping the chest with 6-in.-wide elastic bandages may help relieve pain; care must be taken, however, to ensure that the lungs are still fully ventilated.

Advise that pleuritis usually lasts only a short time and resolves spontaneously. Instruct to report symptoms such as increased fever, productive cough, difficulty breathing, or shortness of breath to the physician. Discuss appropriate use of and precautions when taking NSAIDs and recommended analgesics.

Pleural Effusion

Pleural effusion is a collection of excess fluid in the pleural space (Figure 23-13■). Pleural effusions result from respiratory disorders (e.g., pneumonia, lung cancer, or trauma) or from systemic diseases such as heart failure or kidney disease.

A large pleural effusion presses on lung tissue, causing dyspnea and shortness of breath. Breath sounds are diminished or absent, and the affected area may sound dull when percussed. Chest wall movement may be limited.

When pleural effusion interferes with breathing, a *thoracentesis* may be done to remove the fluid. A large needle is inserted into the pleural space to remove the excess fluid (Figure 23-14■). Thoracentesis may be done at the bedside. Local anesthesia is used. The procedure requires less than 30 minutes to complete. Nursing care for the patient undergoing a thoracentesis is outlined in Box 23-13■.

Nursing care focuses on supporting respiratory function and assisting with procedures such as thoracentesis. With a large pleural effusion, diagnoses of *Impaired Gas Exchange* and *Activity Intolerance* are high-priority nursing problems. After thoracentesis, it is important to monitor for potential complications such as pneumothorax.

Teaching focuses on symptoms of recurrent effusion or complications after thoracentesis that should be reported

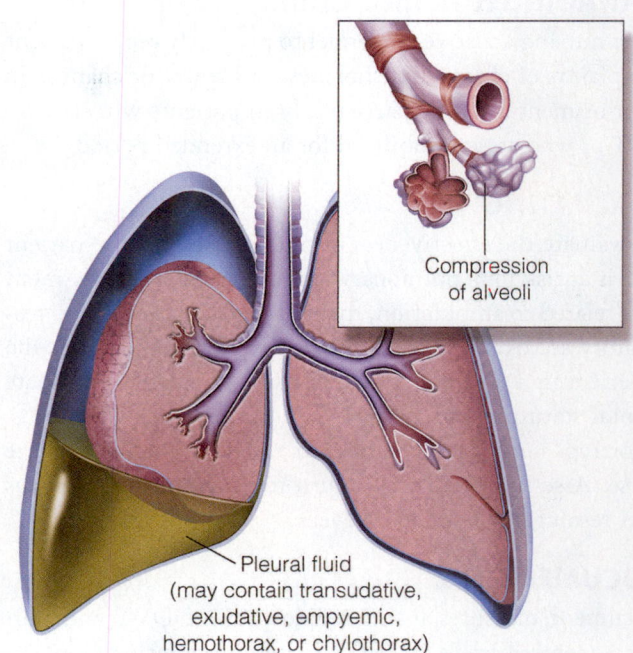

Compression of alveoli

Pleural fluid (may contain transudative, exudative, empyemic, hemothorax, or chylothorax)

Figure 23-13. ■ Pleural effusion. (Source: Pearson Education.)

to the physician. Instruct to report increasing dyspnea or shortness of breath, cough, hemoptysis, or pleuritic pain.

Pneumothorax

Accumulation of air in the pleural space is called **pneumothorax**. Pneumothorax can occur spontaneously, due to chronic lung disease, or as a result of trauma.

PATHOPHYSIOLOGY

When the pleura is breached, air enters the pleural space. Pressure in the pleural space is no longer negative, and the lung on the affected side collapses (Figure 23-15■). A small

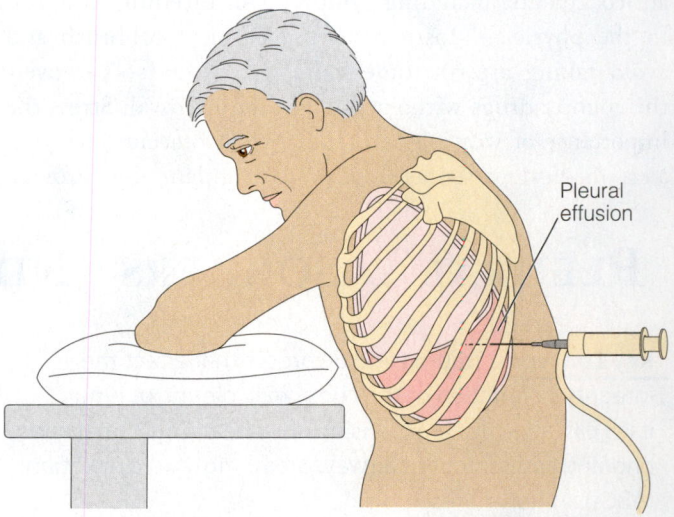

Pleural effusion

Figure 23-14. ■ Thoracentesis. A needle is inserted between the ribs into the pleural space to withdraw excess pleural fluid.

BOX 23-13 **NURSING CARE CHECKLIST**

Thoracentesis

Before the Procedure

- ☑ Verify a signed consent for this procedure has been obtained.
- ☑ Reinforce teaching.
- ☑ Administer cough suppressant if ordered.
- ☑ Bring supplies to the patient's room: thoracentesis tray, sterile gloves, local anesthetic, antiseptic solution, dressing, and an extra over-bed table or Mayo stand.
- ☑ Position patient sitting on side of bed, leaning forward with arms and head supported on an anchored over-bed table.
- ☑ Advise that pressure may be felt when the needle is inserted, but no pain should be experienced.

During the Procedure

- ☑ Support and assist patient to remain still and in position during the procedure.

- ☑ Provide emotional support as needed.
- ☑ Monitor respirations, pulse, and color, informing the physician of any changes.

After the Procedure

- ☑ Apply dressing to puncture site.
- ☑ Position patient as directed.
- ☑ Label any specimens (name, date, source, and diagnosis); send to laboratory for analysis.
- ☑ Record vital signs, breath sounds, and cough and assess for bleeding or crepitus at puncture site every 15 minutes × 4, every 30 minutes × 2, and then every 2 to 4 hours or as indicated.
- ☑ Obtain chest x-ray.
- ☑ Allow resumption of normal activities after 1 hour if no complications develop.

---

portion of the lung or the entire lung may be affected, depending on the amount and rate of air accumulation.

When a bleb (blister) on the lung surface ruptures (*spontaneous pneumothorax*), air moves freely into and out of the pleural space. As a result, the pneumothorax often is small. A gunshot wound or stab wound to the chest causes a *traumatic open pneumothorax (sucking chest wound)* that allows air to move freely through the chest wall. In a *tension pneumothorax*, injury to the chest wall or lungs allows air into the pleural space but prevents it from escaping. Air accumulates rapidly, and the lung on the affected side collapses. The heart, great vessels,

and trachea shift to the unaffected side of the chest, placing pressure on the opposite lung. Table 23-8 summarizes the major types of pneumothorax and their manifestations.

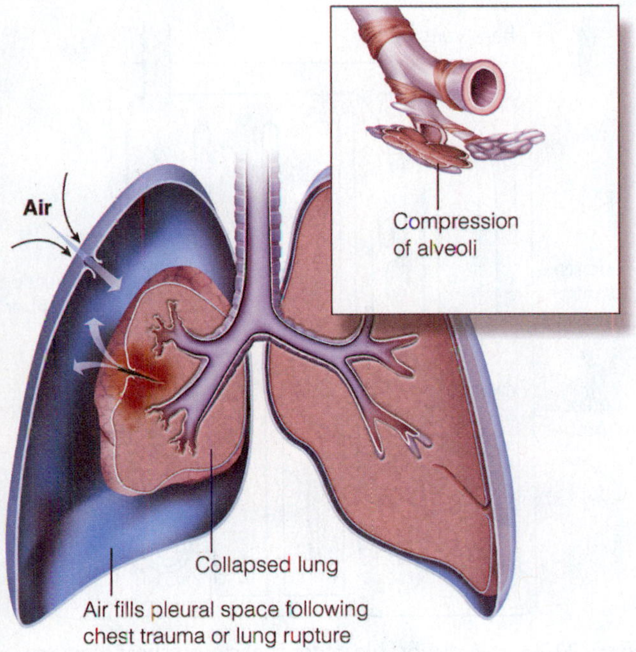

clinicalALERT

Tension pneumothorax is a medical emergency requiring immediate intervention to maintain the airway, breathing, and circulation.

MANIFESTATIONS

The manifestations of pneumothorax depend on its size, the extent of lung collapse, and any underlying lung disease. An abrupt onset of pleuritic chest pain and shortness of breath typically occurs with spontaneous pneumothorax. The heart and respiratory rates increase, and there is less chest wall movement on the affected side. Breath sounds are reduced on the affected side. Patients with secondary pneumothorax have a higher risk of developing complications due to their underlying lung disease.

Manifestations of traumatic pneumothorax may be unrecognized due to the presence of other injuries. If an open wound is present, air can be heard and felt moving into and out of the wound. In tension pneumothorax, the trachea shifts toward the unaffected side, and the patient becomes hypotensive and develops signs of shock.

COLLABORATIVE CARE

Diagnostic Tests

Often pneumothorax can be diagnosed simply by its manifestations. Oxygen saturation is measured to determine its effect on gas exchange. A chest x-ray is obtained to determine the size and extent of the pneumothorax.

Figure 23-15. ■ Pneumothorax. (Source: Pearson Education.)

TABLE 23-8	Types of Pneumothorax	
TYPE	**PATHOPHYSIOLOGY**	**MANIFESTATIONS**
Spontaneous Normal lung / Pleural space **A**	Rupture of a bleb (blister) on lung surface allows air from lungs into pleural space. ■ *Primary* occurs in previously healthy people, usually young men. Smoking is a risk factor. ■ *Secondary* affects people with COPD and other chronic lung diseases.	Abrupt onset Pleuritic chest pain Shortness of breath Tachypnea, tachycardia Unequal chest movement Decreased breath sounds on affected side Hyperresonant percussion tone
Traumatic Puncture wound through chest wall **B**	Result of chest trauma. ■ *Open* due to penetrating trauma that allows air from outside to enter pleural space. ■ *Closed* occurs when torn visceral pleura allows air from lung to enter pleural space; rib fracture a common cause. ■ *Health care related* due to lung trauma secondary to a procedure or mechanical ventilation.	Pain Dyspnea Tachypnea, tachycardia Decreased chest movement Absent breath sounds on affected side Air movement through an open wound
Tension Mediastinal shift to unaffected side / Wound in chest wall allows air to enter pleural space but not to escape **C**	Air enters pleural space through chest wall or from lungs but is unable to escape. Air accumulates rapidly, causing collapse of lung on affected side. Heart, great vessels, trachea, and esophagus shift toward unaffected side.	Hypotension, shock Severe dyspnea Tachypnea, tachycardia Decreased chest wall movement Absent breath sounds on affected side Trachea deviates toward unaffected side

Treatment

Treatment of pneumothorax depends on its severity. In a small simple pneumothorax, air is gradually reabsorbed, and the lung reexpands. With a larger pneumothorax, the air is removed from the pleural space to allow the collapsed lung to reexpand. A *thoracentesis* may be done by inserting a needle into the pleural space to withdraw air. Review Box 23-13 for nursing care of a patient having a thoracentesis or with a catheter with a one-way valve may be inserted into the pleural space. The one-way valve allows air to leave the pleural space but prevents it from entering.

Chest Tubes

The usual treatment for pneumothorax is *chest tubes* connected to a closed-drainage system. The drainage system has a one-way valve or a "water seal" that prevents air from entering the chest cavity during inspiration and allows air to escape during expiration. Applying low suction to the system helps reestablish negative pressure, allowing the lung to reexpand.

Several closed-drainage systems are available. Some use water to prevent air from entering the pleural space and to regulate suction (Figure 23-16■). Others are "dry" systems

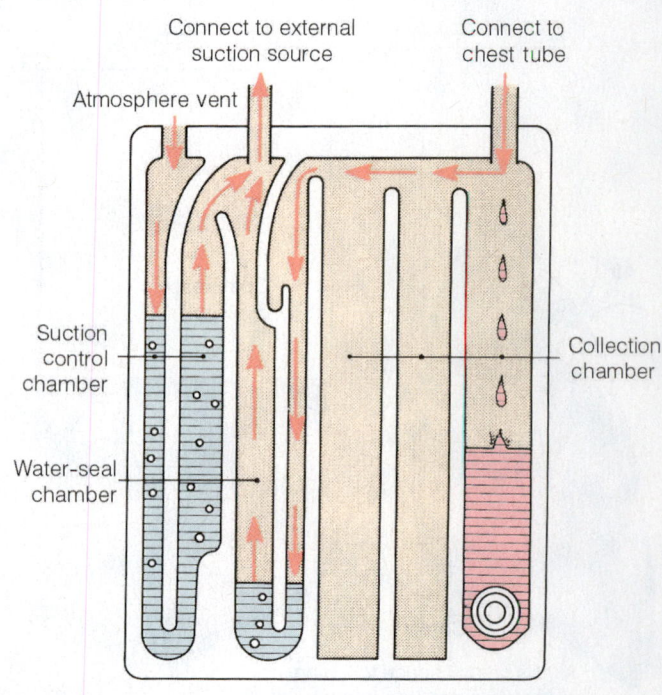

Figure 23-16. ■ A disposable water-seal closed chest drainage system.

that include a mechanical one-way valve to prevent air entry into the pleural space and a suction regulator. Chest tube drainage collects in a graduated chamber that allows easy measurement. To ensure system function, it is important to prevent damage and maintain the integrity of all tubes and connections. Box 23-14■ outlines nursing care for a patient with chest tubes.

NURSING CARE

PRIORITIZING NURSING CARE

Restoring ventilation and gas exchange is the highest priority of care for the patient with a pneumothorax.

HEALTH PROMOTION

Teach patients of all ages about the risks associated with smoking. Participate in programs to prevent smoking among children, adolescents, and young adults, and refer patients who smoke to smoking cessation programs. Advise all patients to wear a seat belt with shoulder harness when in an automobile. Discuss measures to prevent falls when working in high places.

ASSESSING

Collect assessment data from patients with risk factors for pneumothorax, such as chest or abdominal trauma (e.g., motor vehicle crash or fall from a height), COPD, or procedures such as central line insertion or thoracentesis. Assess patients with known pneumothorax for the effect of treatment measures. Ask about chest pain or difficulty breathing. Inquire about previous history of pneumothorax or chronic lung disease. Obtain smoking history.

Assess respiratory status, including dyspnea, rate and depth of respirations, chest wall movement, and lung sounds. Note LOC and skin color. Observe neck veins for distention and position of trachea.

IDENTIFYING POTENTIAL COMPLICATIONS

Immediately notify the physician if the trachea is displaced toward one side. This could indicate tension pneumothorax, a medical emergency that requires immediate treatment.

DIAGNOSING, PLANNING, AND IMPLEMENTING

Impaired Gas Exchange

Expected outcome: Will maintain an SaO_2 within normal or expected range.

When the lung collapses, gas exchange no longer occurs in the affected part of the lung.

- Document vital signs, oxygen saturation, and respiratory status at least every 4 hours. *Frequent assessment is necessary to monitor response to impaired lung function and treatment.*
- Raise the head of the bed. *This position facilitates lung expansion.*
- Administer oxygen as ordered. *Supplemental oxygen improves blood oxygen levels.*
- Provide emotional support. *Dyspnea and hypoxemia are frightening and produce anxiety.*
- Assist with frequent position changes and ambulation. *Movement promotes lung ventilation.*

BOX 23-14	NURSING CARE CHECKLIST

Chest Tubes

Before the Procedure

- ☑ Verify a signed consent for the procedure has been obtained.
- ☑ Reinforce teaching. Local anesthesia will be used; pressure may be felt during insertion. Breathing will improve when the chest tube is in place.
- ☑ Gather supplies as indicated: thoracostomy tray, local anesthetic, sterile gloves, drainage system, sterile water to fill water seal and suction chambers if needed.
- ☑ Position as ordered for the procedure.

During the Procedure

- ☑ Assist as needed. Provide physical and psychologic support.
- ☑ Notify the physician of changes in respiratory rate and effort, pulse, and color.

After the Procedure

- ☑ Document vital signs, breath sounds, oxygen saturation, color, and respiratory effort at least every 4 hours.

- ☑ Maintain closed system. Tape all connections; secure chest tube to chest wall.
- ☑ Keep collection device below chest level.
- ☑ Check tubes frequently for kinks or loops.
- ☑ If water-seal system is used:
  - ☑ Frequently check water-seal chamber. The water level should fluctuate with respiratory effort; if it does not, the system may not be patent or intact. Periodic air bubbles in the water-seal chamber are normal and indicate that trapped air is being removed from the chest.
  - ☑ Keep the device upright.
  - ☑ Add water to the suction control chamber as needed.
- ☑ Measure drainage every 8 hours, marking the level on the drainage chamber. Do not empty the chamber. Report drainage that is cloudy, in excess of 70 mL/hr, or red, warm, and free flowing.
- ☑ When chest tube is removed, immediately apply sterile occlusive dressing.

Risk for Injury

Expected outcome: Will remain free of complications associated with chest tube.

- Assess chest tube and drainage system at least every 2 hours. *The system must remain patent and intact to function effectively. Inadvertent removal of a chest tube or damage to the closed-drainage system allows air and pathogens to enter the chest cavity.*
- Secure chest tubes to chest wall and prevent tension on the tubes during care and ambulation. *Chest tubes are minimally secured with a suture and can be dislodged during activity.*
- Secure drainage tubing to sheet or gown. *Looping the drainage tubing prevents direct pressure on the chest tube itself.*
- Prevent kinking or occlusion of chest or drainage tube during repositioning. *This maintains the patency of the tubing.*
- Teach to keep drainage system below the level of the chest when sitting or ambulating. Suction usually can be disconnected during ambulation. *Ambulation promotes lung ventilation and reexpansion. Keeping the system lower than the chest promotes drainage.*
- Observe insertion site for redness, swelling, pain, or drainage. Report fever or signs of infection to the physician. *Disruption of skin integrity increases the risk for infection.*
- If the tube is inadvertently removed, promptly seal the wound with a sterile occlusive dressing. If a sterile dressing is not available, use other occlusive material such as foil or plastic wrap. Tape dressing on three sides only. *An occlusive dressing taped on three sides allows air to escape through the wound but prevents air from entering the wound on inhalation.*

MANAGING NURSING CARE

With instruction about maintaining the integrity of the chest tube drainage system, nursing care activities such as assisting with hygiene, ambulation, and ADLs may be assigned to assistive personnel.

EVALUATING

Frequently assess respiratory status and oxygenation to evaluate the effectiveness of nursing care. Observe for evidence of improved breathing and decreasing air leak.

DOCUMENTING

Document continuing respiratory assessment data, including the amount of drainage and functioning of the closed chest drainage system. Document all teaching provided. Note if referral has been made to a smoking cessation program and the patient's responsiveness to quitting smoking.

CONTINUITY OF CARE

Patients who have had a spontaneous pneumothorax have a 50% risk of recurrence. Stress the importance of quitting smoking to reduce the risk. Advise avoiding activities that can increase the risk, such as mountain climbing, flying in unpressurized aircraft, scuba diving, and possibly contact sports.

Instruct to gradually increase exercise and activity to previous levels. Stress the importance of follow-up care and monitoring. Advise to report the following to the physician: URI; fever, cough, or difficulty breathing; sudden, sharp chest pain; or redness, pain, swelling, tenderness, or drainage from the chest tube puncture wound.

Hemothorax

Hemothorax, blood in the pleural space, usually results from chest trauma or surgery. When blood collects in the pleural space, pressure on the affected lung impairs ventilation and gas exchange.

Hemothorax causes symptoms similar to those of a pneumothorax. Lung sounds are decreased. A dull percussion tone is heard over the collection of blood, usually at the lung base. Chest x-ray is used to confirm the diagnosis of hemothorax.

Thoracentesis or chest tubes are used to remove blood from the pleural space. With significant hemorrhage (e.g., after trauma or surgery), the blood may be collected for reinfusion.

Nursing care focuses on maintaining respirations, gas exchange, and cardiac output. In a large, slow-developing hemothorax, respiratory status is the primary concern. Nursing diagnoses and interventions are similar to those for pneumothorax. When hemothorax develops rapidly and hemorrhage is significant, shock is a risk.

Chest and Lung Trauma

Trauma, or injury due to an external source, can affect the chest wall as well as the lung itself. Chest wall injuries (including fractured ribs, flail chest, and underlying damage to lung tissue), smoke inhalation, and near-drowning are commonly seen.

RIB FRACTURE

Simple rib fracture, usually of a single rib, is the most common chest wall injury. This usually is a minor injury. In older adults or people with chronic lung disease, however, it can lead to problems such as pneumonia, atelectasis, and respiratory failure. If the fracture is displaced, bone can tear the pleura and cause pneumothorax.

A rib fracture causes pain on inspiration and coughing. Bruising may be seen over the fracture site. *Crepitus* (a

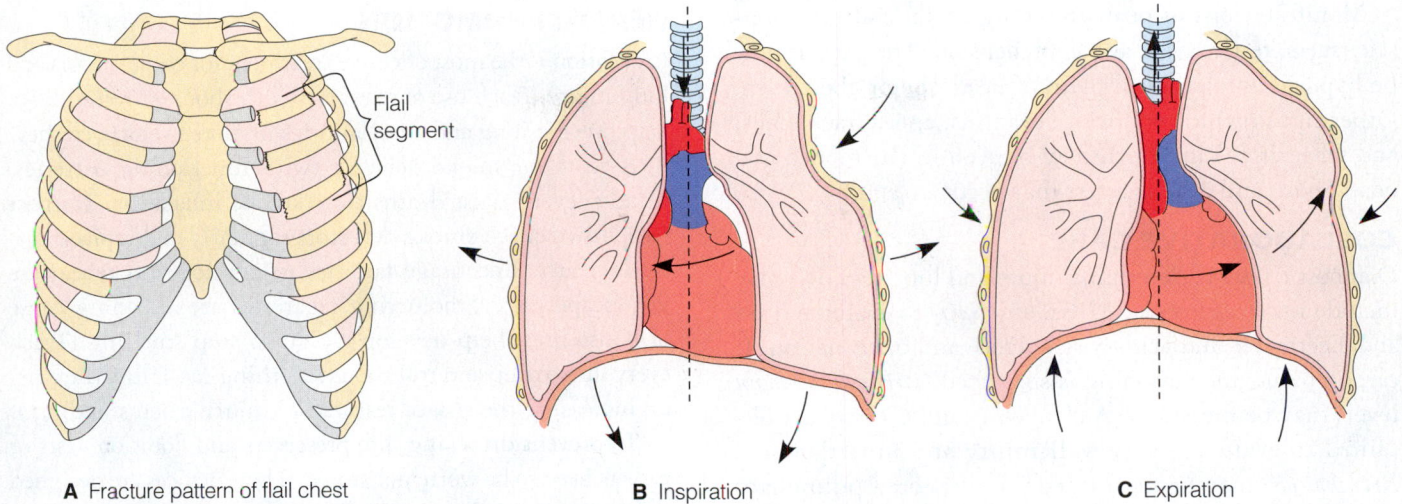

A Fracture pattern of flail chest   **B** Inspiration   **C** Expiration

Figure 23-17. ■ Flail chest with paradoxic chest wall movement.

grating sensation) may be felt with breathing. Breath sounds are diminished, especially in the bases, because of splinting.

Flail Chest

When two or more adjacent ribs are broken in several places, part of the chest wall becomes free-floating. This is a *flail chest.* The flail segment moves inward during inspiration and moves outward with expiration. This is called *paradoxic movement* (Figure 23-17■). Flail chest affects lung expansion and increases the work of breathing. The lung under the flail segment often is damaged.

In addition to paradoxic chest movement, flail chest causes pain and dyspnea. Chest expansion is unequal, and crepitus is present. Breath sounds are diminished, and crackles may be heard.

PULMONARY CONTUSION

Pulmonary contusion, or lung tissue injury, frequently occurs with chest trauma. When the chest is rapidly compressed and then decompressed (e.g., being thrown forward against the steering wheel then back in a motor vehicle crash), alveoli and pulmonary vessels rupture, causing tissue hemorrhage and edema. After the initial injury, inflammation further impairs breathing and gas exchange.

Manifestations of pulmonary contusion include shortness of breath, restlessness, apprehension, and chest pain. Copious sputum, possibly blood tinged, is present. Tachycardia, tachypnea, dyspnea, and cyanosis develop as well.

SMOKE INHALATION

Smoke inhalation is the leading cause of death in burn injury. Smoke inhalation is common when a burn occurs in a closed space and is suspected with burns on the face or upper torso or singed nasal hairs.

Smoke inhalation can lead to burns of airways, carbon monoxide or cyanide poisoning, and lung damage

from noxious gases. Manifestations of smoke inhalation include dyspnea, wheezes or crackles, and possibly ash-like material in sputum. Carbon monoxide is a colorless, odorless gas that binds readily with hemoglobin, reducing its ability to carry oxygen to cells of the body. The manifestations of carbon monoxide poisoning are listed in Box 23-15■. Survivors of severe carbon monoxide poisoning may have permanent neurologic damage. Cyanide inhalation can be fatal; other toxic chemicals can cause bronchospasm and edema of the airways and alveoli.

NEAR-DROWNING

Aspiration and oxygen deprivation are the primary problems in near-drowning. Significant hypoxemia and loss of consciousness can occur within 3 to 5 minutes of immersion; death can occur within 5 to 10 minutes. Immersion in very cold water may prolong survival.

The near-drowning victim who aspirates either fresh or salt water can develop pulmonary edema and respiratory failure. Freshwater drowning also causes blood cell hemolysis and electrolyte imbalances. In near-drowning, inhaled microorganisms and debris can lead to pneumonia.

BOX 23-15	**MANIFESTATIONS OF CARBON MONOXIDE POISONING**

Low Levels
- ■ Headache, dizziness
- ■ Dyspnea
- ■ Nausea
- ■ "Cherry-red" skin and mucous membranes

Higher Levels
- ■ Confusion, irritability, hallucinations
- ■ Visual disturbance
- ■ Hypotension
- ■ Seizures, coma

Manifestations of near-drowning include altered consciousness, restlessness, and apprehension. The patient may be hypothermic and complain of headache or chest pain. Other signs include vomiting, cyanosis, apnea, tachypnea, and wheezing. Pink froth may be seen in the mouth and nose. Shock and cardiac arrest may occur.

COLLABORATIVE CARE

Diagnostic tests to determine injury and lung function may include *serum electrolytes*, *ABGs*, and *SaO₂* to evaluate fluid and electrolyte and acid–base balance and oxygenation. If carbon monoxide poisoning is suspected, *carboxyhemoglobin* levels may be measured. A *chest x-ray* and *CT scan* are obtained to evaluate chest wall injury and lung damage. *Bronchoscopy* may be performed for suspected pulmonary contusion or smoke inhalation.

Simple rib fractures typically heal uneventfully. Analgesia is ordered to facilitate breathing, coughing, and movement. An intercostal nerve block may be done. Rib belts, binders, and taping of ribs are not recommended, because they can interfere with ventilation. With a flail chest, however, taping may be done to stabilize the chest wall. The ribs may be surgically stabilized when a large flail segment interferes with respiration.

Initial treatment of inhalation injury is removing the victim from the fire or water and providing effective cardiopulmonary resuscitation (CPR). Immediate restoration of effective breathing and circulation is key to preserving life. Oxygen is given as soon as available.

clinicalALERT

When the victim is hypothermic, resuscitation is continued until the body temperature is about 90°F (32°C). "Not dead until warm and dead" is a basic rule in hypothermia.

All patients with inhalation injury need supplemental oxygen. Coughing and suctioning are important to remove secretions and debris. Percussion and postural drainage may be done.

Intubation and mechanical ventilation may be ordered for flail chest, pulmonary contusion, and inhalation injuries because these patients often are critically ill. Intubation and mechanical ventilation are discussed in the next section of this chapter.

NURSING CARE

PRIORITIZING NURSING CARE

Promoting effective airway clearance and gas exchange are the nursing care priorities for patients with chest and lung trauma.

HEALTH PROMOTION

Prevention is the most effective treatment for chest trauma and lung injury. Teach use of seat belts with shoulder restraints to help prevent lung and chest injuries in motor vehicle crashes.

A working smoke detector (with functioning batteries) could prevent most deaths from smoke inhalation. Instruct patients to check smoke detectors regularly and replace batteries yearly. Encourage families to develop and rehearse a fire escape plan. Smoldering cigarettes are a leading cause of house fires; help develop a plan to stop smoking. Teach everyone to drop and roll should clothing catch fire. (Fire rises, increasing the risk of respiratory injury when standing.)

To prevent drowning, life preservers and flotation vests or jackets need to be worn, not stored. These devices are designed to keep the head above water. Encourage life vests when boating, water-skiing, or wind-surfing. Wet suits help prevent hypothermia in very cold water. Advise patients never to swim alone or when fatigued. Recommend covering or fencing swimming pools, hot tubs, and ponds to prevent entry and inadvertent drowning. Just as alcohol and driving do not mix, neither do alcohol and boating nor other water sports.

A population well trained in effective CPR provides the best second line of defense. Rapid restoration of breathing is essential to prevent brain damage. Encourage everyone to be trained and maintain current CPR certification. Work with local Red Cross and Heart Association chapters to increase the number of trained individuals.

ASSESSING

When chest trauma occurs, patient assessment may need to be very focused. Inquire about the circumstances surrounding the event; for example, in a motor vehicle crash, where was the victim in the vehicle? When smoke inhalation is suspected, did an explosion occur or were the victim's clothes on fire? Ask about the presence, location, severity, and type of pain. When possible, ask about current medications, any chronic conditions, and any known allergies.

Obtain vital signs including ease, rate, and depth of respirations. Assess LOC and mental status, skin color, and temperature. Note the presence of soot or burns around the nose or mouth and the quality of the voice. Observe equality of chest movement with breathing. If coughing is present, note the character of the sputum. Auscultate breath sounds, noting their presence or absence throughout all lung fields, as well as the presence of any adventitious sounds such as wheezes or crackles.

IDENTIFYING POTENTIAL COMPLICATIONS

Promptly report signs of respiratory distress, including anxiety, nasal flaring, or stridor. Look for midline position of the trachea and for equal chest wall movement. Report cherry-red skin or tongue color and other abnormal findings.

DIAGNOSING, PLANNING, AND IMPLEMENTING
Ineffective Airway Clearance

Expected outcome: Will maintain clear breath sounds throughout lung fields.

- Frequently assess respiratory status. Note the amount, color, and consistency of sputum. *The patient often is unstable; frequent assessment is necessary to rapidly detect changes.*
- Elevate head of bed. *This promotes alveolar ventilation.*
- Instruct to frequently cough, deep breathe, and change position. Encourage to use incentive spirometer. Assist with percussion and postural drainage as needed. *These measures help remove secretions and debris and prevent atelectasis or pneumonia after chest trauma.*
- Teach to splint affected area with a blanket or pillow when coughing. *Splinting improves ventilation and reduces pain.*
- Suction as needed. *Suctioning may be required when cough is ineffective or when intubated.*
- Stabilize endotracheal tube with tape and ties. *Stabilizing the tube prevents its displacement, which impairs effective ventilation.*
- Report decreased breath sounds, increased adventitious sounds; pink, frothy, or purulent sputum; chills or fever; or changes in vital signs or mental status. *Changes in respiratory status, vital signs, or mental status may indicate a complication such as pulmonary edema or pneumonia.*

Impaired Gas Exchange

Expected outcome: Will maintain SaO_2 within expected range.

- Report changes in skin color, oxygen saturation, and arterial blood gases. *Alveolar damage and pulmonary edema can significantly impair gas exchange.*
- Assess for anxiety or apprehension, restlessness, confusion or lethargy, or complaints of headache. *These may indicate hypoxia or hypercapnia.*
- Monitor intake and output; weigh daily. Maintain ordered fluid restriction. *Fluid volume excess can increase pulmonary edema and further impair gas exchange.*
- Maintain oxygen and mechanical ventilation as ordered. *These improve gas exchange.*
- Administer sedation as needed. *Sedation may be required to maintain effective mechanical ventilation.*
- Provide frequent mouth care. *Oxygen dries mucous membranes. Mouth care promotes comfort and reduces the risk for pneumonia in a ventilated patient.*
- Restrict activity and allow periods of uninterrupted rest. *These measures reduce oxygen consumption.*

Acute Pain

Expected outcome: Will report pain level at 2 or lower on a scale of 0 to 10.

- Frequently assess pain, using a standard pain scale. *Pain interferes with lung expansion and coughing.*

- Provide analgesics as ordered or on a schedule. *Regular analgesia controls pain more effectively than PRN doses.*
- Assess for respiratory depression related to narcotic analgesia. *Although pain control is important to maintain ventilation, narcotics can depress the respiratory center.*

Ineffective Cerebral Tissue Perfusion

Expected outcome: LOC and other neurologic signs will remain within expected parameters.

Inhalation injury can affect cerebral perfusion and oxygenation. Increased intracranial pressure (ICP) may develop after near-drowning.

- Frequently monitor neurologic status. Report changes promptly. *Change in LOC or behavior is the earliest sign of increased ICP.*
- Raise the head of the bed. Keep the head in a neutral position. *Elevating and keeping the head straight promotes blood and CSF circulation.*
- Maintain effective ventilation and oxygenation. *Hypercapnia and hypoxemia increase cerebral edema.*

EVALUATING

To evaluate the effectiveness of nursing care for the patient who has experienced pulmonary trauma, collect respiratory assessment data on a continuing basis. If the patient experienced smoke inhalation or near-drowning, frequently assess neurologic and cardiovascular status as well.

DOCUMENTING

Document continuing assessments, including neurologic, respiratory, cardiovascular, and pain status. Note the effectiveness of analgesia and other measures to relieve pain and the patient's ability to effectively ventilate all areas of the lungs. Document all teaching, including that related to identification and reporting of potential complications. Note teaching of the patient and family about safety measures to prevent pulmonary trauma.

CONTINUITY OF CARE

For a minor chest wall injury, discuss pain control and its importance in preventing complications. Teach to splint the rib cage during coughing. Stress the importance of coughing and deep breathing. Explain the reasons to avoid taping or wrapping the chest continuously. Describe complications to report to the physician: chills and fever, productive cough, purulent or bloody sputum, shortness of breath or difficulty breathing, and increasing chest pain. Emphasize the importance of avoiding respiratory irritants, such as cigarette smoke and pollutants.

A large pulmonary contusion can lead to long-term respiratory compromise. This can require changes in activities and possibly occupation.

CRITICAL RESPIRATORY CONDITIONS

Respiratory Failure

Key Concept Respiratory failure is the inability of the lungs to maintain effective respiration. Patients often require intensive care management with endotracheal intubation and mechanical ventilation.

Many of the conditions discussed in this chapter can lead to **respiratory failure**. In respiratory failure, the lungs are unable to oxygenate blood and remove carbon dioxide to meet the body's needs, even at rest. COPD is the usual cause of respiratory failure. Other lung diseases, trauma, neuromuscular disorders, and heart disease can also lead to respiratory failure.

PATHOPHYSIOLOGY AND MANIFESTATIONS

Respiratory failure is not a disease; it results from severe respiratory dysfunction. Blood oxygen levels are very low; the PO_2 may be less than 50 to 60 mm Hg (hypoxemia). Carbon dioxide levels rise as the lungs are unable to eliminate it. Tissue hypoxia and high PCO_2 levels (*hypercapnia*) lead to acidosis.

The manifestations of respiratory failure are caused by hypoxemia and hypercapnia (Box 23-16■). Hypercapnia causes vasodilation and depresses the central nervous system. As carbon dioxide levels increase, the respiratory center may be depressed. When this occurs, the usual stimulus to breathe is lost, and low blood oxygen levels provide the only stimulus to breathe. Providing oxygen without mechanical ventilation may remove any drive to breathe, with dire results.

The prognosis for acute respiratory failure depends on the underlying disease. Acute respiratory failure due to an uncomplicated drug overdose usually resolves quickly and completely. Respiratory failure due to chronic lung disease often has a prolonged course and less favorable outcome.

Acute Respiratory Distress Syndrome

Acute respiratory distress syndrome (ARDS) is a severe form of acute respiratory failure. ARDS is characterized by inflammatory pulmonary edema and progressive hypoxemia that does not respond to oxygen therapy. It can follow direct or indirect lung injury. Smoke inhalation and near-drowning are direct lung injuries that may lead to ARDS; shock and sepsis cause indirect lung damage and can precipitate ARDS. ARDS may also occur as a complication of diseases such as H1N1 influenza.

PATHOPHYSIOLOGY

A massive unregulated systemic inflammatory response damages the lungs. This damage occurs rapidly, often within 24 hours of the initial insult. Damage to the alveolar–capillary membrane allows plasma and blood cells to leak into the interstitial space and alveoli. Alveolar surfactant is inactivated, and the cells that produce it are damaged. Alveoli collapse, the work of breathing increases, and gas exchange is impaired. Hypoxemia develops and the PCO_2 rises.

MANIFESTATIONS

The manifestations of ARDS usually develop 24 to 48 hours after the initial insult. Dyspnea and tachypnea are initial symptoms. Breath sounds are initially clear. Increasing respiratory distress and *refractory hypoxemia* (low oxygen saturation and PO_2 levels that do not improve with supplemental oxygen) develop. As respiratory failure progresses, the patient may become agitated and confused or lethargic.

The prognosis for ARDS varies. Many patients recover fully. However, sepsis and multiple organ dysfunction syndrome (MODS) may develop. When this occurs, the prognosis is poor.

COLLABORATIVE CARE

Treatment of respiratory failure and ARDS focuses on the underlying cause or disease process, as well as supporting ventilation and correcting hypoxemia and hypercapnia.

Diagnostic Tests

Diagnostic tests include *arterial blood gases (ABGs)*. The arterial PO_2 may be less than 50 to 60 mm Hg, and the PCO_2 often is high, usually more than 50 mm Hg. The pH

BOX 23-16	MANIFESTATIONS OF RESPIRATORY FAILURE

Due to Hypoxemia
- Dyspnea, tachypnea
- Cyanosis
- Restlessness, anxiety, confusion
- Tachycardia, dysrhythmias
- Hypertension
- Metabolic acidosis

Due to Hypercapnia
- Dyspnea, respiratory depression
- Headache, drowsiness, coma
- Tachycardia, hypertension
- Heart failure
- Respiratory acidosis

is low, indicating acidosis. In ARDS, *chest x-ray* and *CT scan* show diffuse infiltrates and lung damage. *Ventilation-perfusion scans* and *exhaled carbon dioxide (capnography or ETCO₂)* are used to evaluate alveolar ventilation and gas exchange.

Medications

Bronchodilators may be given to reverse airway spasm and constriction. Infection is treated with antibiotics. Corticosteroids and NSAIDs may be ordered to reduce airway edema and inflammation. Surfactant therapy may be ordered for patients with ARDS.

Patients on mechanical ventilation often require sedation to reduce anxiety and analgesics to relieve pain. Benzodiazepines such as midazolam (Versed) provide sedation, and intravenous analgesics such as morphine relieve pain. These drugs also reduce the respiratory drive, facilitating mechanical ventilation. Occasionally, a neuromuscular blocking agent may be given to paralyze the respiratory muscles and allow the ventilator to control the patient's respirations. These patients require intensive care management.

Oxygen Therapy

Oxygen therapy is vital to treat the hypoxemia of acute respiratory failure. Patients with chronic COPD may need only 1 to 3 L by nasal cannula; higher flow rates often are necessary for other patients. High oxygen concentrations (40% to 60% or higher) are used only for short periods to avoid oxygen toxicity. Oxygen toxicity reduces lung compliance, increasing the work of breathing. A tight-fitting mask with continuous positive airway pressure CPAP) may be used to improve alveolar ventilation and allow lower oxygen concentrations.

Airway Management

Patients who need mechanical ventilation may be intubated with an endotracheal tube (ETT) extending from the mouth or nose into the trachea (Figure 23-18■). Most ETTs have an air-filled or foam cuff just above the end

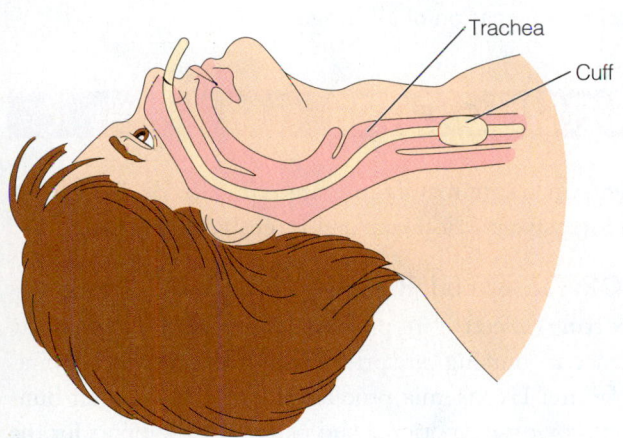

Figure 23-18. ■ Nasal endotracheal intubation.

| BOX 23-17 | NURSING CARE CHECKLIST |

Endotracheal Tube (ETT)

- ☑ Frequently assess respiratory status. Report changes to the charge nurse or physician.
- ☑ Monitor vital signs, skin color, LOC, and mental status at least every 4 hours.
- ☑ Secure ETT with an ETT holder (see figure). Mark tube placement in relation to the mouth or nose. Notify the charge nurse or physician if the tube becomes displaced.

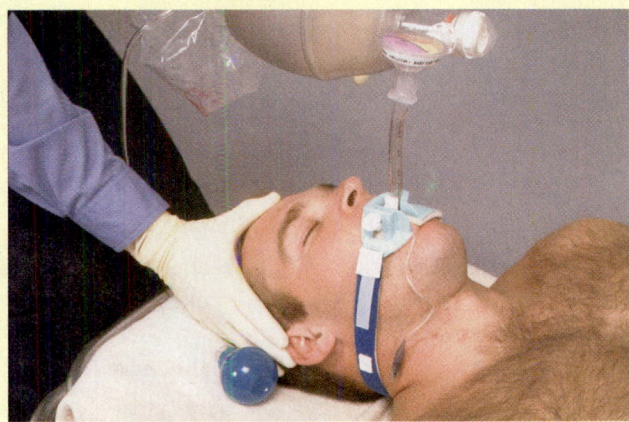

(Source: Pearson Education.)

- ☑ Provide oral and nasal care every 2 hours; assess oral and nasal mucosa for redness and irritation. Move oral ETT to opposite side of mouth every 8 hours.
- ☑ Using sterile technique, suction ETT as needed to remove secretions. Using clean technique, suction oropharynx as needed.
- ☑ Closely monitor ETT cuff pressure, maintaining recommended pressure.
- ☑ Provide humidified air or oxygen.
- ☑ Ensure that all ventilator alarms are in "on" position.
- ☑ Establish communication using hand signals, eye movement, a note pad, Magic Slate, or picture board.

of the tube that prevents air from escaping back into the upper airways during ventilation. A tracheostomy may be done if mechanical ventilation is needed for more than 3 or 4 weeks. Box 23-17■ outlines nursing care for the patient with an ETT.

Endotracheal intubation increases the risk for infection because the defenses of the upper airway are bypassed. ETTs pass through the larynx, so talking is not possible. Enteral or parenteral nutrition is required, because eating is not possible when an ETT is in place. A nasogastric feeding tube, gastrostomy, or jejunostomy may be used for enteral nutrition.

When the ETT is removed, the patient is placed on humidified oxygen and closely observed for respiratory distress (nasal flaring, dyspnea, wheezing, anxiety, decreased oxygen saturation levels). Reintubation may be necessary.

Sore throat and a hoarse voice are common after extubation. Oral intake is restarted slowly, with careful assessment of swallowing.

Mechanical Ventilation

Patients with respiratory failure may require mechanical ventilation to ensure alveolar ventilation and reduce the work of breathing.

VENTILATION TYPES, MODES, AND SETTINGS Mechanical ventilators can be set for a number of different modes or patterns of ventilation (Table 23-9 ■). In addition to the mode of operation, five other settings are used:

- The rate or number of breaths per minute, usually set at 10 to 15.
- The tidal volume or amount of air delivered with each breath. For adults, the tidal volume is usually set between 6 and 12 mL/kg (based on ideal body weight).
- The oxygen concentration of delivered air (FIO_2) is set at the lowest possible level to maintain oxygen saturation greater than 90%.
- The inspiratory–expiratory ratio, usually set at 1:2 to prevent air trapping.
- The pressure limit is set at 20% above peak airway pressures delivered (Smith et al., 2012).

COMPLICATIONS Although endotracheal intubation and mechanical ventilation can be life-saving, they also carry a risk for injury.

Table 23-9	Modes of Ventilator Operation
MODE	**DESCRIPTION**
Continuous mandatory ventilation (CVM or ACV, assist-control ventilation)	Ventilator controls volume or pressure and flow rate of all breaths. Patient can trigger ventilator with inspiratory effort; breaths will be delivered at a preset rate if patient fails to breathe.
Synchronized intermittent mandatory ventilation (SIMV)	Ventilator delivers a set number of mandatory breaths (synchronized with patient's breathing) per minute; patient can breathe on own between ventilator-assisted breaths.
Positive end-expiratory pressure (PEEP)	Used together with other ventilator modes; positive pressure is maintained in airways throughout respiratory cycle.
Continuous positive airway pressure (CPCP)	Airway pressures are maintained above atmospheric throughout the respiratory cycle.
Pressure support ventilation (PSV)	Pressurized inspiratory flow supports inspiratory effort, reducing work of breathing.

The intubated patient may develop pressure necrosis of the nose, lip, or trachea. Less saliva is produced, and mouth care can be difficult. Frequent mouth care, however, is an important intervention to reduce the risk for ventilator-associated pneumonia (VAD). If the tube is dislodged, ventilation of one or both lungs may be affected. Sterile technique must be used when suctioning to reduce the number of bacteria introduced into the respiratory tract. Secretions often become thick and tenacious, increasing the risk of atelectasis.

Mechanical ventilation can cause *barotrauma* (lung injury due to pressure). Pneumothorax and subcutaneous emphysema may result. Decreased cardiac output is a risk. GI bleeding is another potential complication. Many of these complications can be prevented by careful ventilator management and ETT care.

WEANING *Weaning* is the process of removing the ventilator. Patients who require mechanical ventilation for a brief period may be taken off the ventilator and extubated rapidly. A more gradual weaning process is used if mechanical ventilation has been prolonged. The patient is closely monitored during weaning. Vital signs, respiratory rate, dyspnea, oxygen saturation, and arterial blood gases are frequently assessed. If the oxygen saturation or PO_2 falls below specified limits, mechanical ventilation may be restarted.

Terminal weaning, gradual withdrawal of mechanical ventilation from a patient who is not expected to survive, may be done for a terminal illness or irreversible condition. The patient is moved to a quiet room or even home before removing the ventilator. Family members are encouraged to stay throughout the process. Ventilator support is gradually withdrawn, while analgesia and sedation are given to maintain comfort.

Other Therapies

A central catheter is inserted for hemodynamic monitoring. Fluid balance is carefully monitored. Enteral or parenteral feeding is provided to maintain nutritional status. The patient with ARDS may be placed in the prone position to improve oxygenation of all lung segments.

NURSING CARE

Patients in respiratory failure are critically ill. They need both intensive medical care and intensive nursing care.

PRIORITIZING NURSING CARE

Supporting effective respiration and maintaining airway clearance are nursing care priorities for the patient in respiratory failure. Hypoxemia produces intense fear and air hunger, so providing emotional and psychologic support for the patient and family is critical. When endotracheal intubation and mechanical ventilation interfere with the ability to communicate, the nurse must work to facilitate communication.

HEALTH PROMOTION

Education is the primary way to prevent respiratory failure. Teach all patients about the risks of smoking, water safety, the benefits of working smoke detectors, and ways to avoid inhalation injury. Teach patients with COPD and others at risk about ways to avoid respiratory infection, including the importance of immunization to prevent pneumococcal pneumonia and annual influenza vaccination.

ASSESSING

Frequent monitoring and assessment are critical. Initial assessment may be very focused, occurring concurrently with measures to support effective respiration. Obtain subjective data such as complaints of dyspnea and a history of COPD or acute pneumonia. Identify any recent episode of shock, sepsis, or other critical condition.

Carefully assess respiratory status, including rate, depth, and ease of breathing (retractions, use of accessory muscles, nasal flaring). Auscultate breath sounds for depth, equality, and adventitious sounds. Assess mental status, including LOC and level of anxiety. Obtain complete vital signs, including apical pulse and oxygen saturation. Document color of skin and mucous membranes, peripheral pulses, and capillary refill.

IDENTIFYING POTENTIAL COMPLICATIONS

Infection is a common complication of endotracheal intubation and mechanical ventilation. Document and report a change in the amount, color, viscosity, or odor of sputum. Frequently assess breath and lung sounds, reporting changes such as crackles or faint or absent breath sounds. Monitor fluid balance and bowel elimination. Gastrointestinal bleeding can develop; promptly report black, tarry, or obviously bloody stool. Monitor laboratory data; promptly report abnormal values and significant changes.

DIAGNOSING, PLANNING, AND IMPLEMENTING

Impaired Spontaneous Ventilation

Expected outcome: Effective respirations will be maintained.

■ Assess vital signs and respiratory status every 15 to 30 minutes. Report changes. *The patient in respiratory failure is critically ill; frequent assessment is vital to detect changes and evaluate interventions. Respiratory failure increases the work of breathing and can lead to fatigue and inadequate ventilation. This may occur before mechanical ventilation is established or during the weaning process.*

■ Promptly report changes in arterial blood gases and oxygen saturation. *These are important indicators of gas exchange and respiratory status.*

■ Administer oxygen as ordered. Observe closely for respiratory depression. *Supplemental oxygen may suppress the respiratory drive.*

■ Elevate the head of the bed. *Elevating the head of the bed to an angle of 30 to 45 degrees improves lung ventilation, decreases the work of breathing, and decreases the risk of ventilator-associated pneumonia.*

■ Promote rest. Assist with care, space procedures and activities, and allow uninterrupted rest periods. *Rest reduces oxygen and energy demands.*

■ Unless intubated and mechanically ventilated, avoid sedatives and respiratory depressant drugs. *These medications can further depress the respiratory drive, worsening respiratory failure.*

■ Prepare for endotracheal intubation and mechanical ventilation:
  ■ Obtain intubation tray with sterile endotracheal tubes and laryngoscope with a variety of adult blades.
  ■ Set up endotracheal suction and bring sterile catheter and glove kits and sterile normal saline to bedside.
  ■ Notify respiratory therapy department to set up ventilator.
  ■ Request portable chest x-ray to verify tube placement when procedure is completed.
  The patient with respiratory failure may require emergency intubation and mechanical ventilation to sustain respirations.

■ Explain procedure, reassuring patient that this is a temporary measure to reduce the work of breathing and allow rest. Instruct that endotracheal tubes interfere with talking, and establish a way to communicate. *Thorough explanations help reduce anxiety.*

Ineffective Airway Clearance

Expected outcome: Breath sounds will be clear throughout all lung fields.

■ Frequently assess respiratory status. *Increasing respiratory rate, crackles and rhonchi, frequent coughing, setting off of ventilator alarms, and increasing restlessness or anxiety may indicate ineffective airway clearance and a need for suctioning.*

■ Suction as needed to maintain patent airway. Box 23-18■ outlines the steps for endotracheal suctioning. *Suctioning removes secretions the patient is unable to clear.*

■ Obtain specimen for culture if sputum appears purulent or becomes odorous. *Sputum culture and sensitivity are done to identify pathogens and appropriate antibiotics to treat infection.*

■ Firmly secure endotracheal or tracheostomy tube. Prevent tension on tube during turning, positioning, or getting out of bed. *These measures help prevent displacement or inadvertent removal of the endotracheal tube or tracheostomy.*

■ Maintain fluid intake. Monitor intake and output. Weigh daily. *Adequate hydration helps liquefy secretions, but preventing fluid overload is important for lung function.*

BOX 23-18	PROCEDURE CHECKLIST

Endotracheal Suctioning

Before the Procedure

☑ Use Standard Precautions.

☑ Obtain all supplies.

☑ Identify patient; provide for privacy.

☑ Explain procedure. Suctioning is not painful, but is uncomfortable. Suctioning causes coughing, helping to clear the lungs.

☑ Elevate the head of the bed.

Procedure

☑ Regulate suction to no more than 80 to 120 mm Hg of suction.

☑ Open sterile saline, leaving cap loosely in place.

☑ Put on personal protective wear.

With an In-Line Catheter

☑ Attach catheter to suction tubing.

☑ Adjust the oxygen (FIO_2) to 100%; allow three breaths. Manipulating catheter through plastic shield (to maintain sterility), insert the catheter approximately 11 in. (28 cm, or 1 cm beyond end of ETT) with no suction; using a rotating motion, slowly withdraw catheter while intermittently applying suction.

☑ Apply suction for no more than 10 seconds (count seconds or watch clock—the time passes quickly), and then allow rest for three to five breaths. Repeat as needed for a total of no more than three times.

☑ Disconnect suction tubing from catheter, clear tubing, and turn off suction.

With a Separate Catheter-and-Glove Kit

☑ Open suction catheter/glove kit. Remove saline cup, and fill with sterile saline.

☑ Put on sterile gloves. Attach catheter to suction tubing, keeping dominant hand sterile; lubricate catheter with sterile saline.

☑ Use nondominant hand to adjust oxygen (FIO_2) to 100%; allow three breaths.

☑ Using nondominant hand, disconnect ventilator tubing from endotracheal tube.

☑ Holding suction catheter with dominant (sterile) hand and suction control valve with nondominant hand, insert the catheter approximately 11 in. (28 cm, or 1 cm beyond end of ETT) with no suction; using a rotating motion, slowly withdraw catheter while intermittently applying suction.

☑ Suction for no more than 10 seconds. Reconnect ventilator, and allow rest for three to five breaths; clear suction tubing with sterile saline.

☑ Repeat as needed for a total of no more than three times.

☑ Reconnect ventilator.

☑ Clear suction tubing; turn off and disconnect catheter, discarding it with the gloves.

☑ Provide three additional breaths at 100% oxygen, and then readjust to previous ordered level.

After the Procedure

☑ Assess lung sounds and tolerance of the procedure.

Sample Documentation

[date]
2100

Suctioned via endotracheal tube for moderate amount of thick, grayish sputum. Tolerated procedure well. Good breath sounds noted in all lung fields; scattered coarse crackles cleared with suctioning.

_____ S. Evans, LVN.

Note: Refer to a nursing fundamentals or skills text for more detailed instruction. Check state guidelines and facility policy before performing any procedure.

Risk for Injury

Expected outcome: Will experience no adverse effects of medical and nursing management.

The patient in respiratory failure is at risk for injury due to altered LOC, endotracheal intubation, and mechanical ventilation.

■ Assess frequently, including a head-to-toe assessment. *Frequent assessment allows early identification of potential problems.*

■ Maintain ETT cuff pressures as ordered. *Cuff pressures are maintained reduce the risk of damage to the trachea while preventing oropharyngeal secretions to enter the lungs.*

■ Do not bypass or turn off any ventilator alarms. *The intubated patient cannot call out for help. The patient who has received a neuromuscular blocker cannot breathe without ventilator support and cannot use the call bell.*

■ Report changes such as increasing air leak around ETT cuff and decreased breath sounds or chest movement. *These may indicate tracheal necrosis, displacement of the ETT, pneumothorax, or atelectasis.*

■ Turn and reposition frequently, stabilizing the ETT while moving. *Frequent position changes help prevent skin and tissue breakdown due to pressure.*

■ Keep skin and linens clean, dry, and wrinkle-free. Protect bony prominences with padding. *Because the patient may not perceive pain and pressure or move voluntarily, good skin care is mandatory.*

- Perform passive range-of-motion (ROM) exercises every 4 to 8 hours. *These exercises maintain joint flexibility and help prevent contractures associated with long-term immobility.*
- Administer H_2-blockers and antacids as ordered. *Stress gastritis and GI hemorrhage are common, preventable complications of mechanical ventilation.*

Decreased Cardiac Output

Expected outcome: Skin color, temperature, vital signs, urine output, and LOC will remain within expected range for patient.

- Monitor vital signs and hemodynamic pressures every 1 to 2 hours. Report changes to the charge nurse or physician. *Positive-pressure ventilation decreases cardiac output; applying PEEP further reduces cardiac output. Frequent assessment allows early detection of decreased cardiac output.*
- Measure urinary output hourly; report if less than 30 mL/hr. *A fall in urine output is an early sign of decreased cardiac output.*
- Assess LOC every 2 to 4 hours. *A change in LOC may indicate cerebral hypoxia.*
- Weigh daily. *Daily weight is the best indicator of fluid status; decreased cardiac output may cause fluid retention.*
- Maintain intravenous fluids as ordered. *Intravenous fluids are given to maintain vascular volume and prevent dehydration.*

Anxiety

Expected outcome: Anxiety level will remain within low to moderate range as demonstrated by stable vital signs, ability to understand and follow directions, and ability to rest when undisturbed by caregiving activities.

- Stay with the patient as much as possible. *The presence of a caregiver provides reassurance that help is readily available.*
- Explain all monitors, procedures, unusual sounds, and machinery. *Understanding the equipment and the meaning of beeps, buzzers, and alarms reduces anxiety.*
- Provide a simple means of communicating, such as a slate, picture board, or alphabet board. If a muscle-paralyzing drug has been given, use methods such as looking to the right for "yes" and left for "no." Reassure that the ability to speak will return once the ETT is removed. *The inability to speak and call out for help is frightening. Providing an alternate means of communication helps reduce anxiety.*
- Encourage family members to visit frequently and remain with the patient if possible. Assist family to provide as much care as possible. *Family visits help reduce anxiety and feelings of abandonment. Allowing family members to participate in care helps reduce their anxiety as well as the patient's.*
- Provide distraction with radio or television. *Distraction helps reduce the focus on machines and unusual sounds of monitors and alarms.*

- Reassure patients that intubation and mechanical ventilation are temporary measures and that they will be able to breathe independently again. *Patients may fear continued dependence on mechanical ventilation.*
- Provide sedation and antianxiety medications as needed, especially when a neuromuscular blocker has been used. *The patient whose voluntary muscles have been paralyzed remains mentally alert.*

MANAGING NURSING CARE

Nursing care activities such as assisting with hygiene and positioning are appropriate to assign to assistive personnel. The nurse retains responsibility for assessing and ensuring that care provided is safe and appropriate.

EVALUATING

To evaluate the effectiveness of nursing care for the patient with respiratory failure, collect assessment data related to breathing, respiratory status, and cardiac output; freedom from injury, tissue damage, and complications of immobility; and level of anxiety.

DOCUMENTING

Frequently document continuing assessment data, including respiratory rate, breath sounds, ease of respirations, equality of chest movement, and measures of cardiac output. Note ventilator settings and changes in laboratory data such as ABGs in response to changes in ventilator settings. When the patient is being weaned from a ventilator, note the heart and respiratory rate and ease as indicators of tolerance for lack of ventilator support. After extubation, document respiratory rate and ease. Promptly report any signs of respiratory distress such as nasal flaring, stridor, or intercostal retractions.

CONTINUITY OF CARE

Discuss factors that precipitated respiratory failure and measures to prevent it in the future. Discuss the importance of avoiding respiratory irritants. Encourage to remain indoors with an air filter or air conditioning when pollution levels are high, obtain influenza and pneumonia immunizations, and avoid exposure to cigarette smoke. Teach effective coughing and measures such as percussion, vibration, and postural drainage.

For the patient with ARDS, explain that ARDS did not result from their actions, but results from serious illness. Reassure that patients who survive the initial insult of ARDS generally recover without significant long-term adverse effects. Advise that recovery may be prolonged, however. Stress the importance of avoiding cigarette smoking.

Note: The references and resources for all chapters have been compiled at the back of the book.

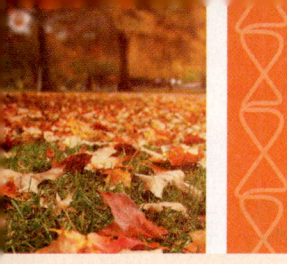

Chapter Review

KEY POINTS

- **Concept**: Effective lung ventilation and gas exchange can be affected by infectious diseases, airway restriction, structural changes of the lung tissue or chest wall, acute or chronic inflammatory disorders, and tumors.
- **Concept**: Inflammation of lung tissue can interfere with ventilation and gas exchange, affecting tissue oxygenation and carbon dioxide elimination. The nurse must assess for the potential effects of impairment and support and promote effective ventilation and gas exchange in patients with lung infections or inflammation.
- Pneumonia remains a leading cause of death, particularly in older adults. It interferes with gas exchange in the alveoli. It may be caused by bacteria, viruses, or other infectious organisms, or by aspiration of gastric contents. Nursing care for the patient with pneumonia focuses on maintaining airway clearance and gas exchange.
- Tuberculosis (TB) is a chronic infectious disease that can remain asymptomatic and undetected for years. A combination of antituberculosis drugs is given for 6 to 12 months to treat active TB. Controlling the spread of TB and promoting compliance with therapy are primary nursing responsibilities.
- **Concept**: Many diseases affect the airways and airflow. Decreased airflow increases the work of breathing and causes air trapping. Inhaled air mixes with trapped air, so less oxygen is available for gas exchange. Care focuses on promoting airway clearance and supporting gas exchange.
- **Concept**: Asthma is characterized by chronic airway inflammation with recurrent acute episodes of respiratory distress. Treatment goals are to reduce the level of chronic inflammation and prevent acute exacerbations.
- Asthma often can be controlled with medications and by avoiding triggers for acute attacks. Acute asthma can cause severe airway restriction, interfering with ventilation of alveoli and gas exchange. The nursing focus during an acute asthma attack is on promoting effective ventilation; once the episode resolves, teaching for self-care is the nursing focus.

- **Concept**: Chronic obstructive pulmonary disease (COPD) is a progressive disorder that gradually destroys lung tissue and obstructs airflow. Slowing disease progression and promoting the patient's functional status are both medical and nursing care goals for the patient with COPD.
- **Concept**: Lung cancer is the leading cause of cancer deaths in the United States. Nurses can impact this statistic through efforts to prevent smoking among teens and young adults and by assisting patients who smoke to quit.
- Cigarette smoking is the primary risk factor for lung cancer. Lung cancer often is advanced by the time it is diagnosed, so its prognosis is poor. Surgery offers the best hope for cure.
- **Concept**: The cardiovascular and respiratory systems are closely linked. A good match of air movement and blood flow is essential to maintain gas exchange and oxygen delivery to all body tissues and organs.
- Prevention of venous stasis and deep venous thrombosis (DVT) is the best treatment for pulmonary embolism. Elastic hose, early ambulation, and leg exercises are nursing care measures to prevent DVT.
- **Concept**: Trauma and disorders that affect the integrity or function of the chest wall, pleura, or lung itself can affect lung expansion and breathing. Initial and ongoing assessment of airway, breathing, and circulation (ABCs) is vital in these disorders.
- Pneumothorax (air in the pleural space) and hemothorax (blood in the pleural space) interfere with lung expansion and ventilation. Chest tubes are inserted to restore negative pressure in the pleural space. Nursing care focuses on maintaining safety and promoting comfort and lung reexpansion.
- **Concept**: Respiratory failure is the inability of the lungs to exchange oxygen and carbon dioxide to meet the needs of the body. Patients often require intensive care management with endotracheal intubation and mechanical ventilation.

PEARSON NURSING STUDENT RESOURCES

Find additional materials at **nursing.pearsonhighered.com**.

Clinical Reasoning Care Map

Caring for a Patient With Tuberculosis
NCLEX-PN® Focus Area: Physiologic Integrity, Reduction of Risk Potential

Case Study: Harry Facée, a 53-year-old man, arrives at a community clinic in a large metropolitan city. He complains of aching chest pain that has lasted for the past few days and says that now his sputum is bloody. He is afraid he might have lung cancer, so he feels he should see a doctor.

Nursing Diagnosis: Risk for Noncompliance

COLLECT DATA

Subjective

_____
_____
_____
_____
_____

Objective

_____
_____
_____
_____
_____

Does this present a threat to the patient's safety?
If yes, the priority intervention to address this threat would be:

_____

Nursing Care

_____
_____
_____
_____
_____
_____
_____
_____
_____

Interprofessional team members to include when planning care:

_____

How would you document this?_____

Compare your answers and documentation to those provided on the companion website.

Data Collected
(use only those that apply)

- Homeless for past 10 years; uses shelters only during very cold or wet weather
- Complains of chronic cough that now is productive of pink sputum
- Often wakes up drenched with sweat in the middle of the night
- Complains of increasing fatigue
- Vital signs: BP 152/86; P 92; R 20; and T 100.2°F (37.8°C)
- Clean; answers questions appropriately and intelligently
- Very thin, almost emaciated
- Sputum Gram stain positive for acid-fast bacillus

Nursing Interventions
(use only those that apply; list in priority order)

- Refer to local incentive shelter program for directly observed medical therapy and meals.
- Teach about prescribed medications, possible adverse effects, and importance of completing the entire prescribed regimen.
- Provide verbal and written information about tuberculosis.
- Emphasize importance of continued follow-up.
- Teach and demonstrate sputum and droplet control measures.

NCLEX-PN® Exam Preparation

TEST-TAKING TIP The concept of wellness is an important aspect of nursing care. Take care of your own health. Take a walk. Exercise increases mental sharpness. Do not stay up all night to study for your exam. Relax and get a good night's sleep.

1. The nurse collecting a history from a patient with chronic bronchitis would expect to find that the patient:
   1. worked in a cotton mill for 25 years.
   2. smoked cigarettes for 40 years.
   3. received a pacemaker at the age of 55.
   4. had a father who died of lung cancer.

2. Your patient had a tuberculin skin test with a positive result. The husband is concerned that he may also have TB. You explain that a positive skin test indicates that:
   1. the patient has active TB and the husband should immediately start prophylactic treatment.
   2. the patient has developed antibodies to TB; further testing is necessary to determine if the disease is active.
   3. tuberculosis is a bloodborne disease and the husband does not have to worry.
   4. the husband definitely has contracted the disease and should begin medications.

3. The nurse is caring for a patient with acute asthma. When reporting to the next shift, it is most important for the nurse to describe:
   1. medication effectiveness.
   2. intake and output results.
   3. lung assessment findings.
   4. level of consciousness.

4. When teaching use of a metered-dose inhaler (MDI), the nurse instructs the patient to:
   1. take quick shallow breaths in rapid succession while holding the canister down.
   2. use the inhaler containing the anti-inflammatory drug first, and then the bronchodilator.
   3. use the anti-inflammatory drug as needed to treat acute episodes of wheezing.
   4. rinse the mouth after using the inhaler to reduce systemic absorption of the drug.

5. Which of the following statements best represents a nurse's understanding of use of supplemental oxygen in patients with COPD?
   1. Because oxygen is flammable, the patient should not smoke.
   2. Oxygen is used only at night for patients with COPD.
   3. Oxygen is never used for patients with COPD because they may become dependent on it.
   4. The patient needs to be closely monitored for signs of respiratory depression.

6. Which of these statements by the patient would indicate that further instruction in preventing atelectasis is needed?
   1. "It is too painful to walk in the hallway today."
   2. "I need to drink extra water for lunch."
   3. "I don't need any pain medication right now."
   4. "I would like to have a laxative before I go to sleep."

7. When assisting with a thoracentesis, the nurse knows that the physician will insert the needle into the:
   1. thoracic cavity.
   2. pleural space.
   3. mediastinum.
   4. visceral space.

8. A patient with a chest tube trips while ambulating, accidentally pulling his chest tube out of the chest. The first thing the nurse should do is:
   1. call the physician.
   2. place an occlusive dressing over the wound.
   3. reinsert the tube.
   4. empty the collection device.

9. The nurse teaching a group of high school students about preventing lung damage or trauma evaluates teaching as effective when the students: **Select all that apply.**
   1. develop plans to form a cooperative exercise group.
   2. verbalize the importance of smoke detectors.
   3. organize a clinic for pneumococcal pneumonia vaccinations.
   4. start a smoking prevention campaign for their peers.
   5. develop a program to supply low-cost flotation devices to local boaters.

10. The nurse caring for a patient with COPD recognizes which of the following as an early sign of possible respiratory failure?
    1. Restlessness and tachypnea
    2. Deep coma
    3. Hypotension and tachycardia
    4. Decreased urine output

Answers and rationales for Review Questions appear in Appendix I.

Thinking Strategically About…

In this scenario, you will follow one patient, James Mueller, through the course of his illness. He will be seen in the doctor's office, in an acute care hospital, and in the home. Answer questions as they apply to the immediate events he is experiencing.

INITIAL OFFICE VISIT

After coughing up bloody sputum, James Mueller, 68 years old, comes to his physician's office to find out what is wrong. He has not been seen in the office for 2-1/2 years. Mr. Mueller describes himself as "pretty healthy," except for a smoker's cough. He has a 50 pack-year smoking history (one pack per day for 50 years, since age 18). He says he quit after a small heart attack 3 years ago but started again after 4 months. His cough has become productive and he admits to being more short of breath with activity than usual.

Mr. Mueller's vital signs are BP 162/86; T 98.4°F (36.9°C); P 78, regular; and R 20. His color is good; his skin is warm and dry. There are good breath sounds throughout all lobes, but wheezes are noted in the right chest.

CRITICAL THINKING

- Which diagnostic tests should the nurse anticipate the physician will order to diagnose Mr. Mueller?

PATIENT TEACHING

- What teaching is needed regarding collection of the sputum specimen?

After a complete physical examination, the doctor orders a chest x-ray and sputum specimen for culture and sensitivity and cytology. X-ray is available in the building, so it is completed right away. Mr. Mueller has the x-ray taken and then returns to the office for a report on the results. A sputum specimen will need to be sent to the lab for examination.

MANAGING CARE

- Are there any special procedures for handling the sputum specimen in order to send it to the lab?

HOSPITAL ADMISSION

The chest x-ray reveals a mass in Mr. Mueller's right lung. Mr. Mueller is admitted to the hospital for further diagnostic tests. The sputum specimen is positive for small-cell bronchogenic cancer. A CT scan shows a central mass with mediastinal and subclavicular lymph node involvement. A small mass is also seen on Mr. Mueller's lumbar spine. After talking with his physician and an oncologist, and discussing the information with his family, Mr. Mueller decides on a course of chemotherapy on an outpatient basis.

PRIORITIES IN NURSING CARE

- What are the priorities of care before Mr. Mueller is discharged?

PATIENT TEACHING

- What teaching should be provided to the patient and family regarding chemotherapy?

HOME CARE

After 3 months of chemotherapy, Mr. Mueller's tumor has not regressed, and a liver scan shows further metastasis. After discussion with his family, Mr. Mueller decides to stop treatment. The Muellers are referred to hospice for end-of-life care. With these services, Mr. Mueller is able to remain at home. His pain is managed with oral morphine sulfate (Roxanol). Mr. Mueller dies at home with family at his side 9 months after diagnosis.

COORDINATION OF CARE

- What kinds of services might be included with hospice end-of-life care?
- Identify members of the interprofessional team that may be involved in Mr. Muller's care at this time.

MANAGING CARE

- What care needs to be provided daily?
- What activities are important to include in end-of-life care?

DELEGATING

- Can administering pain medication be delegated to the home health aide who stays at the Mueller home?

CULTURAL CARE STRATEGIES

- If the Mueller family is Roman Catholic, are there any spiritual needs that must be considered in providing end-of-life care?

CRITICAL THINKING

- How can the nurse help if a patient decides to stop cancer treatment but the family disagrees with the decision?

DOCUMENTING

- Write a focus note about Mr. Mueller's death, including care and disposition of the body.

Note: Discussion of Unit questions appears on the companion website.

UNIT VI
Disrupted Gastrointestinal Function

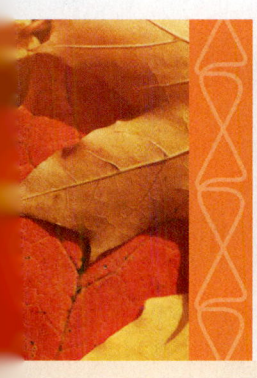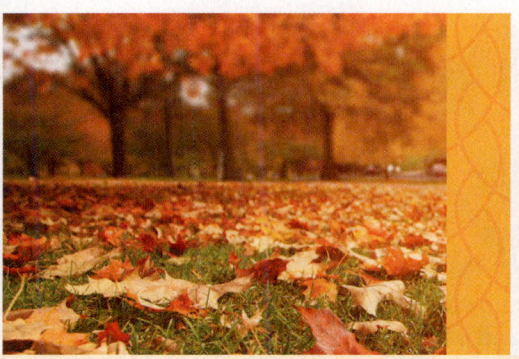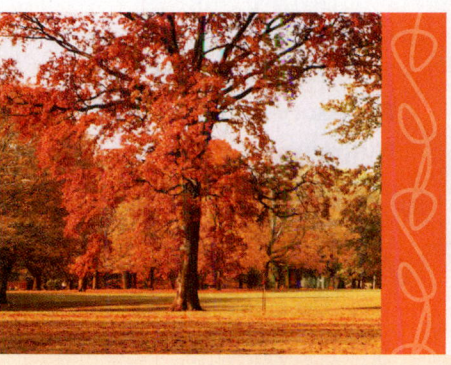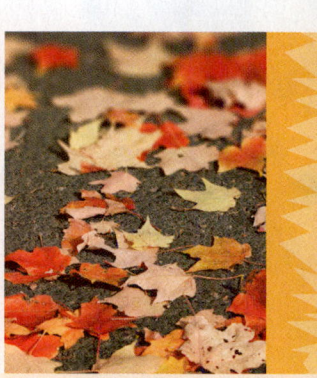

CHAPTER 24

The Gastrointestinal System and Assessment

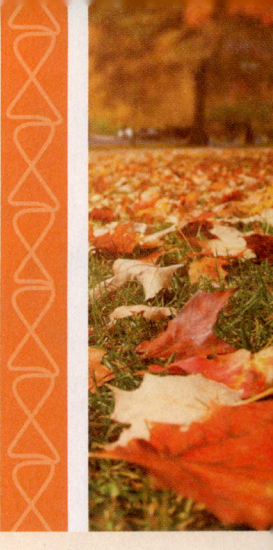

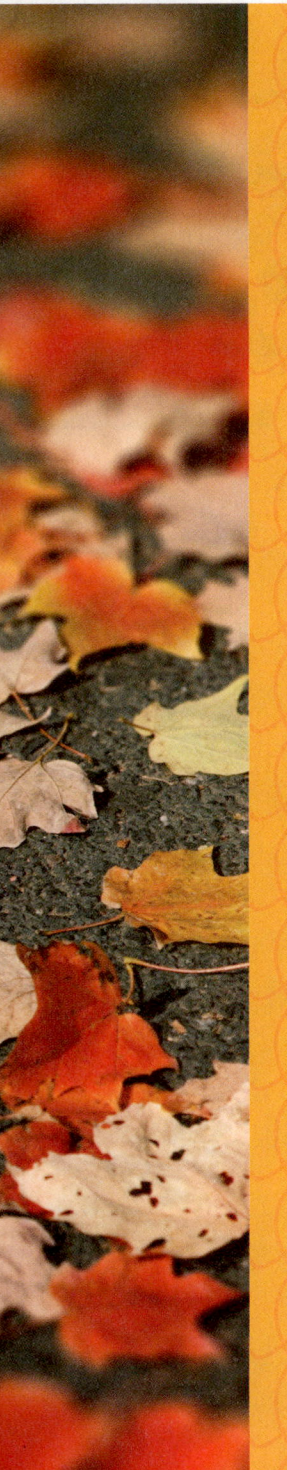

APPLIED LEARNING OUTCOMES

After completing this chapter, you will be able to:

1. Describe the structure and function of the gastrointestinal (GI) tract and accessory organs of digestion (liver, gallbladder, and pancreas).
2. Describe the physiologic processes involved in the ingestion, digestion, and elimination of foods and nutrients.
3. Identify sources and functions of various nutrients, including vitamins.
4. Collect, document, and communicate assessment data related to digestion, organ function, and nutritional status, identifying normal and abnormal data.
5. Provide patient-centered nursing care for patients undergoing diagnostic tests to identify disorders of nutrition or affecting the GI tract or accessory organs.

KEY TERMS

The key terms are defined on the pages listed below.

Nutrition is the process of ingesting, absorbing, using, and eliminating food in the body. The digestive organs involved in these processes are the gastrointestinal (GI) tract and the accessory digestive organs. The GI tract includes the mouth, pharynx, esophagus, stomach, small intestine, and large intestine (Figure 24-1 ■). The large intestine is primarily an organ of elimination. The accessory digestive organs include the liver, gallbladder, and pancreas.

The Gastrointestinal Tract

Key Concept   The purpose of the gastrointestinal system is to take in food, digest or break down the food into nutrients, absorb these nutrients into the blood, and eliminate what remains as solid waste.

The gastrointestinal tract is a continuous hollow tube. Once foods are ingested, they are broken down into products that can be absorbed as they move through the GI tract.

MOUTH, PHARYNX, AND ESOPHAGUS

The *mouth*, the upper opening of the GI tract, is lined with mucous membranes. In the mouth, the teeth chew and grind food into smaller parts. *Saliva* (produced by the salivary glands) moistens food for tasting, chewing, and swallowing. The digestive process starts in the mouth as enzymes in saliva (*amylase* and *lysozyme*) begin to break

down food. The tongue mixes food with saliva, forms the food into a mass (*bolus*), and initiates swallowing. Muscles in the pharynx move food to the esophagus. The esophagus carries food to the stomach through **peristalsis** (alternating waves of contraction and relaxation). The esophagus enters the stomach through the *cardiac* or *lower esophageal sphincter*. This sphincter, normally closed except during swallowing, keeps food in the stomach.

STOMACH

The *stomach*, connected to the esophagus at the upper end and to the small intestine at the lower end, can expand to hold up to 4 L of food and fluid (Figure 24-2 ■). The stomach continues the digestive process. Mechanical digestion in the stomach mixes partially digested food with gastric juices to produce **chyme**. Four to five liters of gastric juices are produced every day by specialized cells in the stomach lining:

- *Parietal cells* secrete hydrochloric acid and intrinsic factor. Hydrochloric acid is vital to protein digestion; intrinsic factor is necessary for vitamin B_{12} absorption.
- *Chief cells* produce pepsin, the primary enzyme in gastric juice, which digests protein.
- *Mucous cells* produce alkaline mucus that protects the lining of the stomach from gastric juices.
- *Enteroendocrine cells* secrete hormones that help regulate digestion.

The nervous system also controls gastric secretion. Seeing, smelling, or tasting food stimulates the parasympathetic nervous system to send signals via the vagus nerve that increase gastric secretion. Emotions such as anxiety or stress, on the other hand, inhibit gastric secretion and motility.

The *pyloric sphincter* controls emptying of the stomach into the duodenum. The stomach empties completely within 4 to 6 hours after a meal.

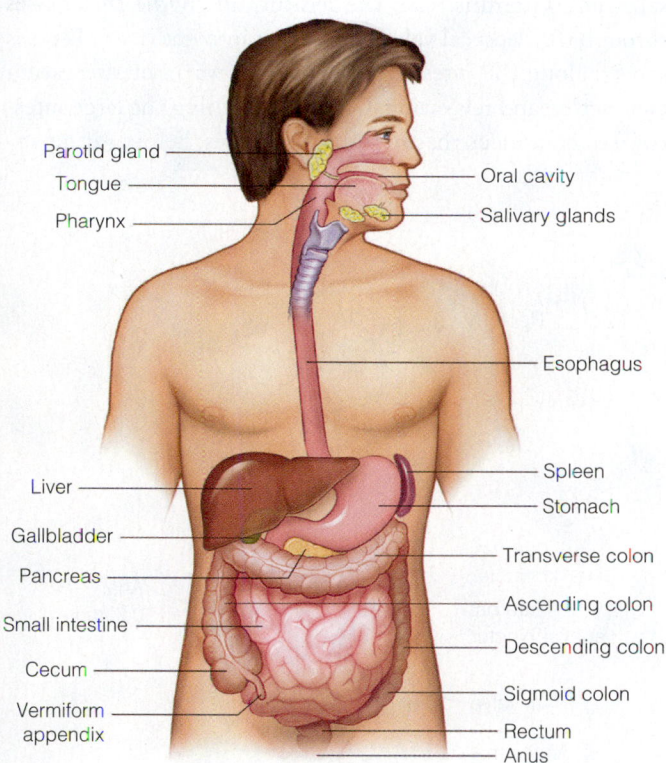

Parotid gland
Tongue
Pharynx
Oral cavity
Salivary glands
Esophagus
Liver
Spleen
Gallbladder
Stomach
Pancreas
Transverse colon
Small intestine
Ascending colon
Cecum
Descending colon
Vermiform appendix
Sigmoid colon
Rectum
Anus

Figure 24-1. ■ The gastrointestinal tract and accessory organs of digestion. (Source: Pearson Education.)

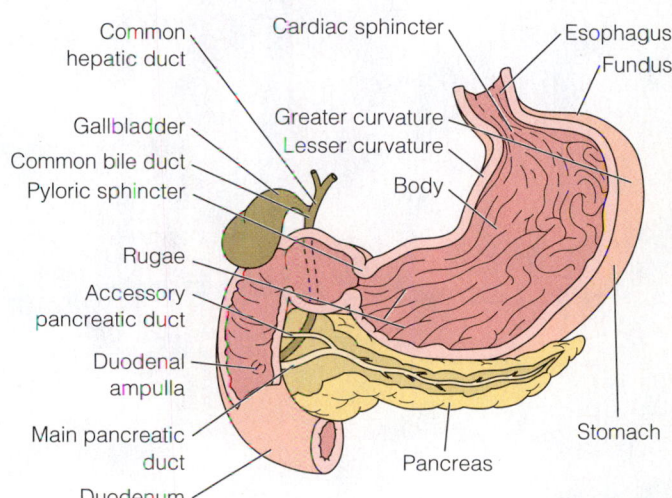

Common hepatic duct
Cardiac sphincter
Esophagus
Fundus
Gallbladder
Greater curvature
Lesser curvature
Common bile duct
Pyloric sphincter
Body
Rugae
Accessory pancreatic duct
Duodenal ampulla
Main pancreatic duct
Stomach
Pancreas
Duodenum

Figure 24-2. ■ Structures of the stomach and duodenum, including the common bile duct and pancreatic duct. The relationship of the pancreas and gallbladder to the stomach is also shown.

SMALL INTESTINE

The small intestine is about 6 m (20 ft) long but only about 2.5 cm (1 in.) in diameter. It hangs in coils in the abdomen, suspended by folds of peritoneal membrane and surrounded by the large intestine. The small intestine has three regions: the duodenum, the jejunum, and the ileum. The *duodenum* begins at the pyloric sphincter and extends for about 25 cm (10 in.). Pancreatic enzymes and bile from the liver enter the small intestine at the duodenum (see Figure 24-2). The *jejunum*, the middle region, is about 2.4 m (8 ft) long. It connects with the *ileum*, the distal 3.6 m (12 ft) of small bowel, which meets the large intestine at the ileocecal valve.

Food is chemically digested, and most of it is absorbed as it moves through the small intestine. Enzymes in the small intestine break down carbohydrates, proteins, and fats. Buffers produced by the pancreas neutralize the acid from the stomach. *Microvilli* (tiny cell projections), *villi* (finger-like projections of the mucosa), and deep folds of the mucosal layers increase the surface area of the small intestine to enhance absorption of food (Figure 24-3 ■).

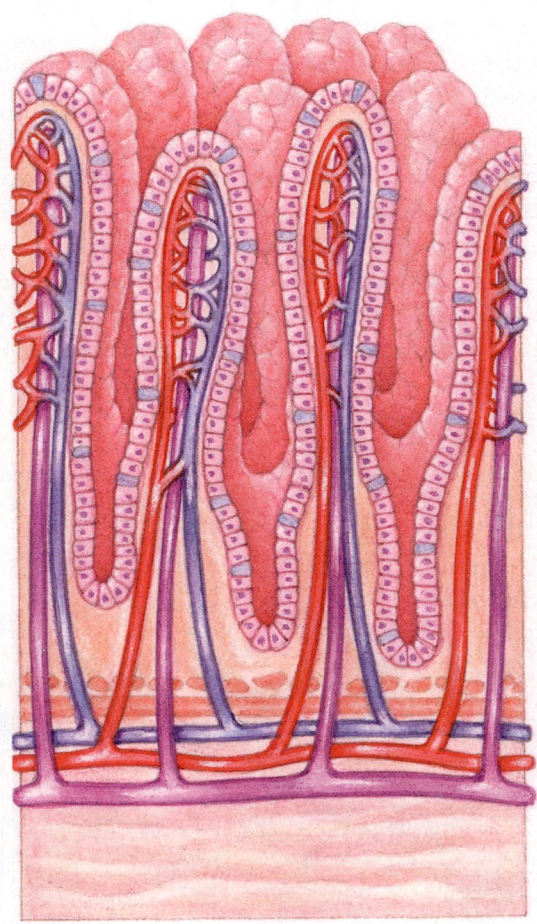

Figure 24-3. ■ A cross section of the small intestine, showing villi and deep mucosal folds that increase the surface area for absorbing nutrients. (Source: Dorling Kindersley Media Library.)

Almost all food products and water, as well as vitamins and minerals, are absorbed through the intestinal mucosa into the blood or lymph. Although up to 10 L of food, liquids, and secretions enter the GI tract each day, less than 1 L reaches the large intestine. Only indigestible fibers, some water, and bacteria enter the large intestine.

Bowel elimination is the end process in digestion. After foods are eaten and broken down into usable elements, nutrients are absorbed and indigestible materials are eliminated.

LARGE INTESTINE

The *large intestine*, or colon, begins at the *ileocecal valve* and terminates at the *anus*. It is about 1.5 m (5 ft) long. The first part of the large intestine, the *cecum*, includes the *appendix* (see Figure 24-1). The colon is divided into *ascending*, *transverse*, and *descending* segments. The descending colon ends at the S-shaped *sigmoid colon.* The sigmoid colon terminates at the rectum.

The *rectum* has transverse folds that help retain feces while allowing flatus to pass. The anorectal junction separates the rectum from the *anal canal*, which terminates at the anus. The *anus*, a hairless, dark-skinned area, is the end of the digestive tract. It has an internal involuntary sphincter and an external voluntary sphincter (Figure 24-4 ■). The sphincters are usually open only during defecation.

The major function of the large intestine is to eliminate indigestible food residue from the body. It absorbs water, salts, and vitamins from the semiliquid chyme that passes through the ileocecal valve, forming it into *feces* (*stool*). Feces is moved along the intestine by *peristalsis*, waves of alternating contraction and relaxation. Goblet cells lining the large intestine secrete mucus that lubricates the feces, helping it move.

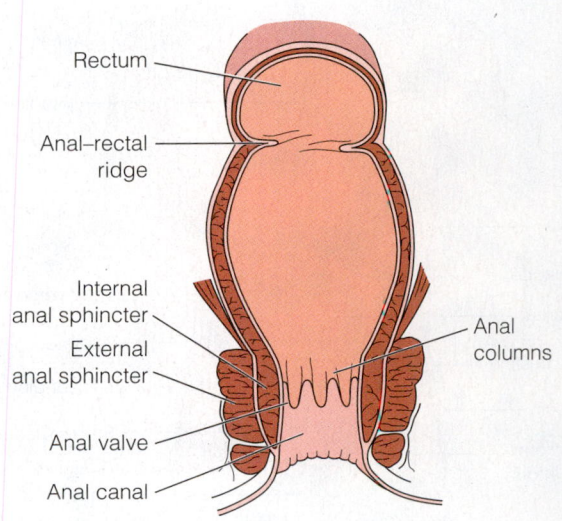

Rectum

Anal–rectal ridge

Internal anal sphincter

External anal sphincter

Anal valve

Anal canal

Anal columns

Figure 24-4. ■ Structure of the rectum and anus.

When feces enter the rectum and stretch the rectal wall, the *defecation reflex* causes the walls of the sigmoid colon to contract and the anal sphincters to relax. The reflex can be suppressed by voluntary control of the external sphincter. Defecation can be assisted by closing the glottis and contracting the diaphragm and abdominal muscles to increase intra-abdominal pressure (*Valsalva maneuver*).

COMMON CHANGES ASSOCIATED WITH AGING

Common changes in gastrointestinal function associated with aging can have a significant effect on nutrition,

general health, and well-being. Figure 24-5■ illustrates many of these changes. Some are normal consequences of the aging process; other changes, such as periodontal disease and tooth loss, do not result from the aging process itself, but are prevalent in older adults.

Periodontal disease, disease of the supporting structures of the teeth, is a common cause of tooth loss in older adults. It results from poor dental hygiene and environmental factors such as lack of access to fluoridated water supplies. In addition, genetics plays a role in periodontal disease, accounting for a significant portion of people affected. Loosening and

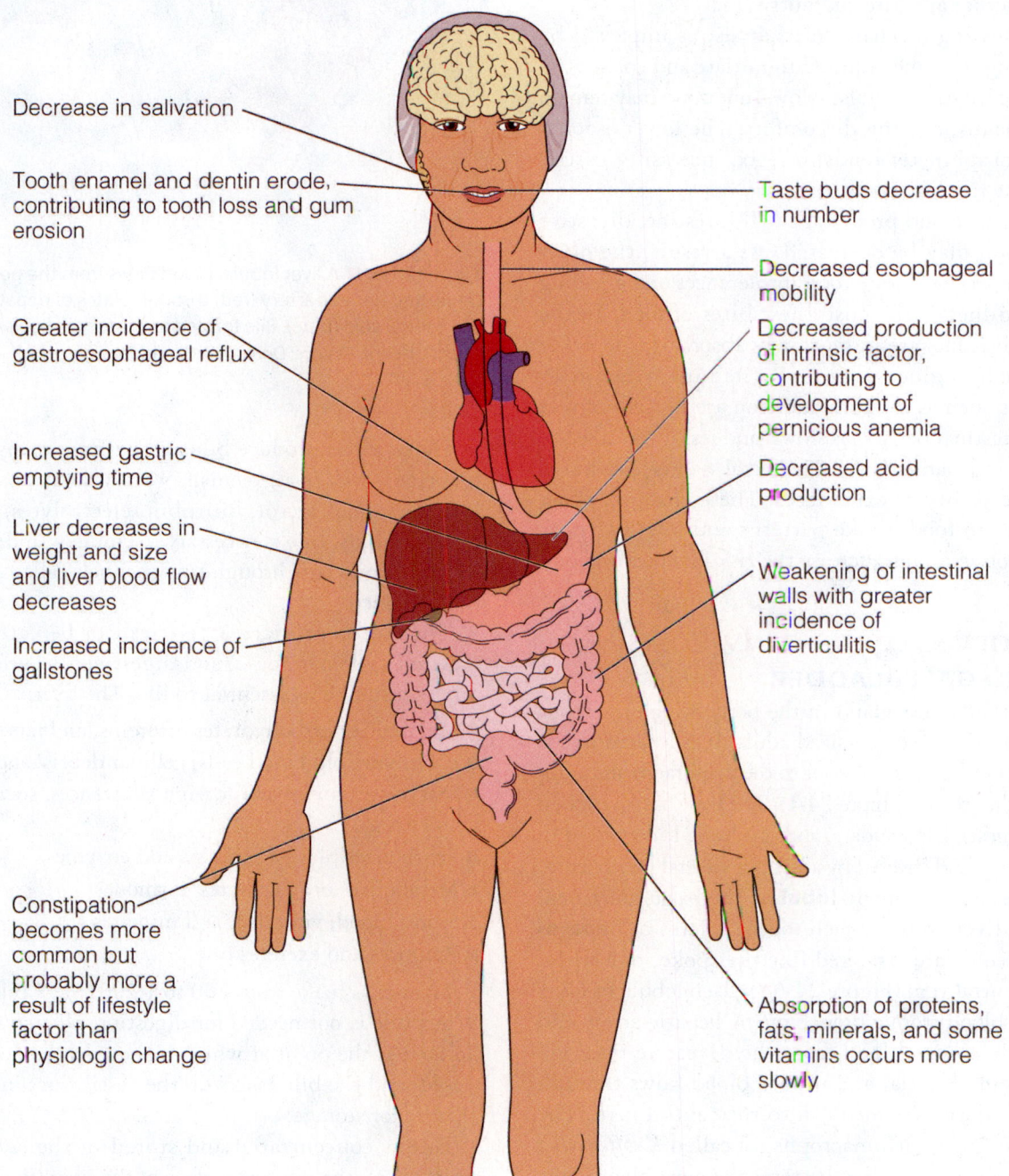

Decrease in salivation

Tooth enamel and dentin erode, contributing to tooth loss and gum erosion

Greater incidence of gastroesophageal reflux

Increased gastric emptying time

Liver decreases in weight and size and liver blood flow decreases

Increased incidence of gallstones

Constipation becomes more common but probably more a result of lifestyle factor than physiologic change

Taste buds decrease in number

Decreased esophageal mobility

Decreased production of intrinsic factor, contributing to development of pernicious anemia

Decreased acid production

Weakening of intestinal walls with greater incidence of diverticulitis

Absorption of proteins, fats, minerals, and some vitamins occurs more slowly

Figure 24-5. ■ Common changes in the gastrointestinal tract associated with aging. (Source: Pearson Education.)

loss of teeth affect the older adult's ability to chew food effectively. This, in turn, can lead to nutritional deficiencies as the person limits the intake of foods that are difficult to chew, for example, fresh fruits and vegetables or meat.

The tongue atrophies with aging, and the number of taste buds decreases. The resulting alterations in taste can lead to excessive use of salt to make food more flavorful and appealing. Saliva production decreases with aging. The mouth is dry, increasing the risk for irritation of the oral mucosa. The lack of saliva also interferes with the initial digestion of starches, which occurs in the mouth, and with swallowing. Sense of smell also tends to decline with aging, further impacting appetite and nutrition.

The swallowing mechanism itself also is impacted by age, increasing the time required to initiate and complete a swallow. Esophageal peristalsis slows, and food may remain in the esophagus, causing discomfort. The lower esophageal (cardiac) sphincter tends to relax, increasing gastric reflux and the risk for aspiration.

In the stomach and proximal small intestine, digestive juice secretion may be decreased. As a result, the older adult may experience more food intolerances and a feeling of satiety (fullness) after just a few bites of food. In the small intestine, fats are more slowly absorbed, and other nutrients such as glucose, some B vitamins, vitamin D, and minerals such as calcium and iron are less effectively absorbed. Intestinal peristalsis slows, and less mucous secretion occurs in the large bowel. The rectal wall is less elastic, affecting the ability to expel feces. These changes, along with changes in food intake patterns and lower activity levels common in aging, increase the risk for constipation.

Accessory Organs of Digestion
LIVER AND GALLBLADDER

The liver is the largest gland in the body, weighing about 1.4 kg (3 lb) in the average-sized adult. It is located in the right side of the abdomen, inferior to the diaphragm and anterior to the stomach (see Figure 24-1). The liver has four lobes: right (the largest), left, caudate, and quadrate. It is encased in a fibrous capsule and covered by a layer of visceral peritoneum.

Each lobe contains many **lobules**, the basic functional units of the liver. Within each lobule, plates of **hepatocytes** (liver cells) are arranged like the spokes of a wheel out from a central vein (Figure 24-6■). Each lobule receives oxygen-rich blood from a branch of the hepatic artery and nutrient-rich venous blood from the digestive tract via the portal vein. Arterial and venous blood flows through enlarged capillaries (*sinusoids*) into the central vein. The sinusoids are lined with macrophages called *Kupffer cells*, which remove debris, such as bacteria and aged blood cells, from the blood.

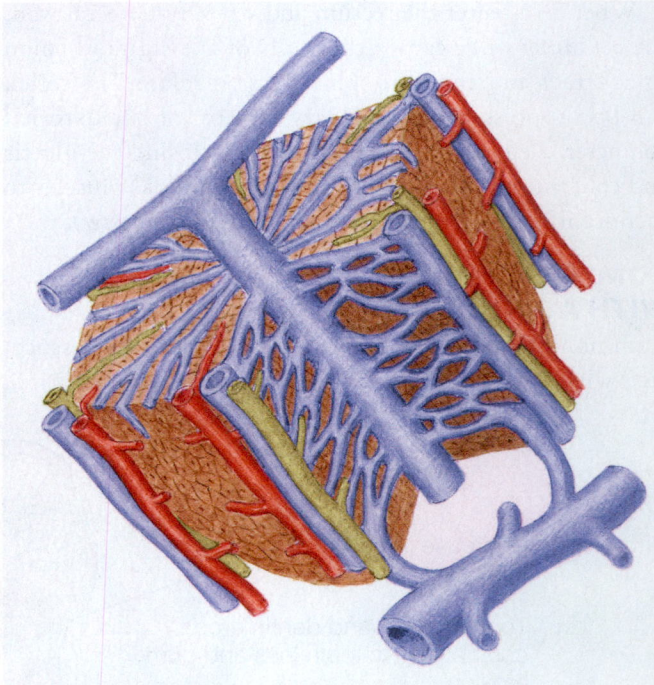

Figure 24-6. ■ A liver lobule. Blood flows from the portal vein (blue) and hepatic artery (red) through plates of hepatocytes to the central vein (blue). Bile formed in the lobule flows out to bile ducts (green). (Source: Dorling Kindersley Media Library.)

Hepatocytes produce bile and perform many metabolic functions. *Bile* is a greenish, watery solution containing bile salts, cholesterol, bilirubin, electrolytes, water, and phospholipids. Bile is necessary to emulsify and absorb fats. The bile flows out through tiny channels called *canaliculi* to the bile ducts.

The liver's primary activities can be categorized as metabolic, hematologic, and digestive. It performs many different functions essential to life. The liver:

- Metabolizes carbohydrates, proteins, and fats.
- Eliminates old blood cells, cellular debris, and bacteria.
- Inactivates toxins and foreign substances, such as alcohol and drugs.
- Synthesizes plasma proteins and enzymes.
- Metabolizes or inactivates hormones.
- Stores blood, vitamins, and minerals.
- Produces and excretes bile.

Liver cells make from 700 to 1,200 mL of bile every day. When bile is not needed for digestion, the *sphincter of Oddi* (located at the point at which bile enters the duodenum) is closed, and the bile backs up the cystic duct into the gallbladder for storage.

Bile is concentrated and stored in the *gallbladder*, a small sac on the inferior surface of the liver (Figure 24-7■). When food containing fats enters the duodenum, hormones

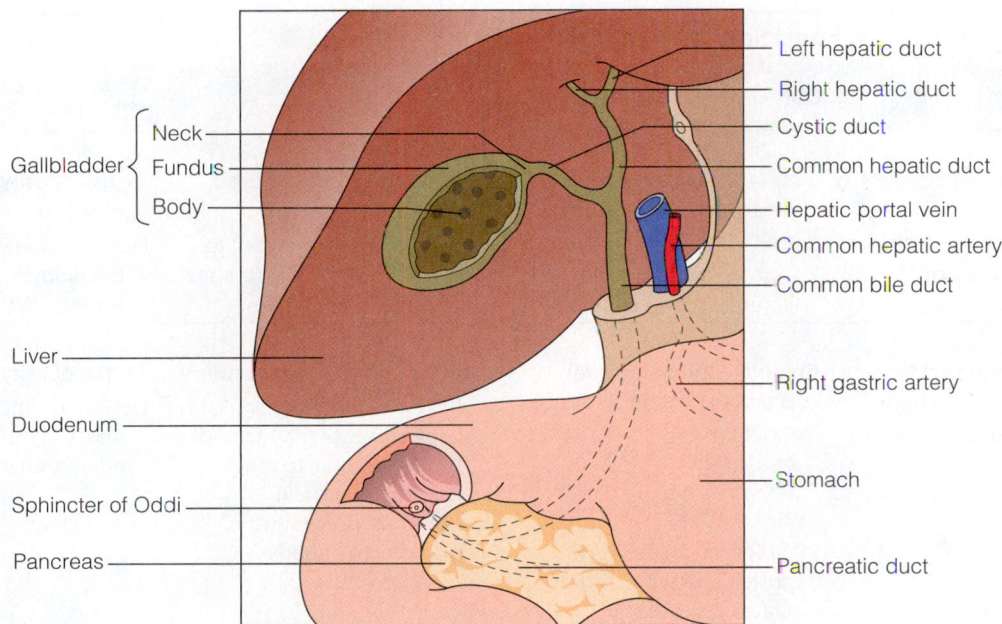

Figure 24-7. ■ The liver, gallbladder, common bile duct, and sphincter of Oddi.

stimulate the gallbladder to secrete bile into the cystic duct. The cystic duct joins the hepatic duct to form the common bile duct, from which bile enters the duodenum.

PANCREAS

The pancreas, a gland located between the stomach and the small intestine, produces enzymes necessary for digestion. It extends across the abdomen, with its tail next to the spleen and its head next to the duodenum (see Figure 24-1). The body and tail of the pancreas lie behind the stomach and the peritoneal membrane (**retroperitoneal**). The pancreas is actually two organs in one, having both exocrine and endocrine structures and functions. The exocrine portion secretes alkaline pancreatic juice into the pancreatic duct. The pancreatic duct joins with the common bile duct just before it enters the duodenum (see Figure 24-7). The pancreas also has endocrine functions (see the endocrine section for more information).

Every day, the pancreas produces 1 to 1.5 L of pancreatic juice containing bicarbonate to neutralize the acidic chyme as it enters the duodenum. The increased pH promotes digestion in the small intestine. Pancreatic secretion is controlled by the vagus nerve and the hormones secretin and cholecystokinin. Pancreatic juice contains enzymes that can digest all categories of foods: *Lipase* promotes fat breakdown and absorption; *amylase* completes starch digestion; and *trypsin*, *chymotrypsin*, and *carboxypeptidase* are responsible for half of all protein digestion. *Nucleases*, which digest nucleic acids, are also present in pancreatic juice.

CHANGES ASSOCIATED WITH AGING

The size of the liver decreases with age, and it becomes less able to regenerate. The incidence of gallstones increases with age due to changes in cholesterol metabolism and absorption. Ducts of the pancreas dilate and distend with aging. The effects of these changes on liver and pancreatic function are unclear.

Nutrients

Key Concept   Nutrition and diet influence overall health and an individual's risk for a number of diseases.

Nutrients are substances in foods that are used by the body for growth, maintenance, and repair. They include carbohydrates, proteins, fats, vitamins, minerals, and water (Table 24-1 ■).

Metabolism

After nutrients are ingested, digested, absorbed, and transported to the cells, they are metabolized to produce energy. **Metabolism** is the term for biochemical reactions that occur in the cells. Metabolism involves two basic processes. *Catabolism* breaks down complex structures into simpler forms, such as carbohydrates into adenosine triphosphate (ATP)—the fuel for cell processes. *Anabolism* combines simpler molecules to build more complex structures (e.g., amino acids into proteins). Water and carbon dioxide are waste products of metabolism. The energy produced by foods is measured in *kilocalories* (*kcal*), usually simply called *calories*.

TABLE 24-1	Nutrients, Food Sources, and Function		
NUTRIENT	**COMMON FOOD SOURCES**	**FUNCTION**	**EFFECT OF EXCESS OR DEFICIT**
Carbohydrates ■ Composed of simple or complex sugars ■ *Recommended intake:* 45% to 65% of total kcal/day or 130 g/day	Simple sugars: milk, sugar cane, sugar beets, honey, fruits Complex starches: grains, legumes, root vegetables	Converted to glucose, used by cells to make ATP Excess glucose converted to glycogen or fat for storage	Excess: obesity, dental caries, elevated serum triglycerides Deficit: tissue wasting (protein breakdown), metabolic acidosis (fat breakdown)
Proteins ■ Composed of amino acids ■ *Recommended intake:* 10% to 35% of total kcal/day or 46–56 g/day	Complete (or high-value) proteins contain all the essential amino acids: eggs; milk and milk products; and meat, fish, and poultry Plant (or *complementary*) proteins: legumes, nuts, grains, cereals, and vegetables	Vital for body structure and function *Nitrogen balance* maintained by intake equal to that needed for protein synthesis, preventing breakdown of body proteins	Excess: obesity Deficit: weight loss, tissue wasting, thin, sparse hair, edema, anemia
Fats (lipids) ■ Composed of triglycerides, phospholipids, sterols ■ *Recommended intake:* 20% to 35% of total kcal/day; saturated fat, 10% or less of total daily caloric intake; trans fats, 1% or less of total daily caloric intake	Saturated fats: animal fats, cocoa butter, palm and coconut oils Trans fats: hydrogenated (solid) vegetable fats (stick margarine, vegetable shortening) Unsaturated fats: liquid vegetable oils, soft margarines	Triglycerides: fuel supply, insulation; essential fatty acids help form cell membranes and hormones and carry fat-soluble vitamins A, D, E, and K Phospholipids: cell membranes Sterols: bile, sex hormones, adrenal hormones, vitamin D, and cholesterol	Excess: obesity, increased risk of heart disease Deficit: weight loss; skin lesions
Vitamins ■ Organic, essential nutrients; includes fat-soluble A, D, E, and K and water-soluble B complex (including niacin, biotin, folic acid) and C ■ *Recommended intake:* Varies by specific vitamin	Found in a variety of foods, including fruits, vegetables, grains, and animal products	Specific functions that promote growth, reproduction, and maintenance of health	Selected effects of deficits: Nails: iron—soft, spoon-shaped Hair: zinc—dry, dull, sparse Skin: vitamins A, B—flaky, dry; niacin—cracks; vitamin K—easy bruising; vitamin C—delayed healing Eyes: vitamin A—poor night vision; iron—pale conjunctiva
Minerals ■ Inorganic elements; includes sodium, potassium, calcium, magnesium, chloride, phosphorus ■ *Recommended intake:* Varies by mineral	Found in a variety of foods, including fruits, vegetables, grains, and animal products	Regulatory functions such as nerve conduction; muscle contraction; cardiac function; blood cell formation; fluid, electrolyte, and acid–base balance	Nervous system: thiamine—↓ deep tendon reflexes, peripheral neuropathies, confusion, apathy Musculoskeletal: thiamine—calf pain; vitamin C—joint pain GI: vitamin B complex—*cheilosis*, stomatitis, glossitis

TABLE 24-1	Nutrients, Food Sources, and Function *(continued)*		
NUTRIENT	**COMMON FOOD SOURCES**	**FUNCTION**	**EFFECT OF EXCESS OR DEFICIT**
Water ■ *Recommended intake:* 1,500–2,000 mL/day as fluid	Water Other liquids such as fruit juices, milk, coffee, tea, soft drinks Foods such as gelatin	Body structure and form Transport and exchange medium Medium for metabolic reactions within cells Insulation and temperature regulation Lubricant	Deficit: thirst, weakness, weight loss, ↓ BP, orthostatic hypotension, ↑ heart rate, poor skin turgor Excess: ↑ BP, ↑ heart and respiratory rates, shortness of breath, weight gain, edema

Assessment

Key Concept   Assessment of the GI system and its function includes gathering information about the patient's nutritional status, ability to ingest a variety of foods, and usual patterns of elimination.

In the focused assessment of the abdomen and gastrointestinal tract, the nurse collects data about the patient's nutritional status, as well as the GI system and its function.

HEALTH HISTORY

Ask the patient about current concerns related to food intake or tolerance, appetite, heartburn, nausea or vomiting, abdominal discomfort, diarrhea, or constipation. Inquire about recent weight changes and any associated factors (e.g., dieting). Question regarding food allergies or intolerances and their effects. Have the patient relate the usual pattern and amount of daily food intake. Ask specific questions about the teeth (including dentures or partial plates and their fit), mouth discomfort, and ability to chew and to swallow.

Have the patient describe any abdominal pain or discomfort, including its location, timing, and relationship to food intake. Ask about usual bowel habits and any recent changes that may have occurred, such as increased or decreased frequency of elimination, change in color or consistency of stool, or decreased caliber (size) of stools.

Ask about current medications, including use of over-the-counter drugs such as aspirin, ibuprofen, or other nonsteroidal anti-inflammatory drugs (NSAIDs); antacids; laxatives; and herbal or nutritional supplements. Inquire about chronic diseases such as diabetes, inflammatory bowel disease, or peptic ulcer disease. Question regarding any previous surgery of the GI tract or abdomen.

PHYSICAL EXAMINATION

Observe general health status, including skin color and condition, hair, and nails. Obtain height and weight.

Compare weight with ideal weight for height using height–weight charts (Box 24-1■). Determine *body mass index (BMI)* using the free BMI calculator available from the National Institutes of Health.

Using a light source, inspect the mouth, tongue, and teeth, noting the condition and moisture of the mucous membranes and gums and presence and condition of the teeth. Note any redness, irritation, color changes, or bleeding of mucous membranes or gums. Be sure to inspect under the tongue as well. Ask the patient to swallow, and observe the swallow reflex.

Inspect the abdomen, noting shape and contour, any visible vessels, striae, or other skin or color changes. Observe for visible peristalsis. Auscultate for bowel sounds, listening in all four quadrants (Figure 24-8■). Bowel sounds (clicks or gurgles) normally are heard every 5 to 15 seconds.

Percuss the abdomen in all four quadrants as indicated. Tympany normally is heard over the stomach and much of

BOX 24-1	HEALTHY WEIGHTS FOR ADULTS		
HEIGHT (CM/IN)	**WEIGHT (KG/LB)[a]**	**HEIGHT (CM/IN)**	**WEIGHT (KG/LB)[a]**
147/4'10"	41–54/91–119	175/5'9"	59–77/129–169
150/4'11"	43–56/94–124	178/5'10"	60–79/132–174
152/5'0"	44–58/97–128	180/5'11"	62–81/136–179
155/5'1"	46–60/101–132	183/6'0"	64–83/140–184
157/5'2"	47–62/104–137	185/6'1"	65–86/144–189
160/5'3"	49–64/107–141	188/6'2"	67–88/148–195
163/5'4"	50–66/111–146	191/6'3"	69–91/152–200
165/5'5"	52–68/114–150	193/6'4"	71–93/156–205
168/5'6"	54–70/118–155	196/6'5"	73–96/160–211
170/5'7"	55–73/121–160	198/6'6"	74–98/164–216
173/5'8"	57–74/125–164		

Note: The higher weights in the ranges generally apply to men; the lower weights more often apply to women.
[a]Without shoes or clothing.

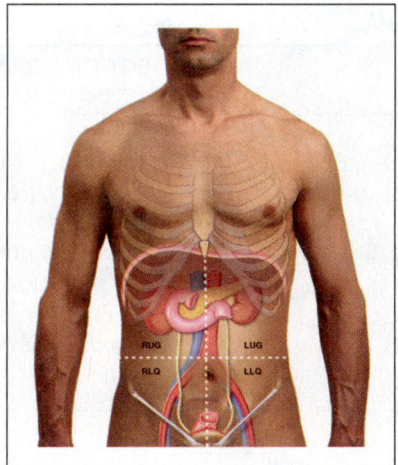

Right Upper Quadrant
Liver and gallbladder
Pylorus
Duodenum
Head of pancreas
Right adrenal gland
Portion of right kidney
Hepatic flexure of colon
Portions of ascending and
  transverse colon

Left Upper Quadrant
Left lobe of liver
Spleen
Stomach
Body of pancreas
Left adrenal gland
Portion of left kidney
Splenic flexure of colon
Portions of transverse and
  descending colon

Right Lower Quadrant
Lower pole of right kidney
Cecum and appendix
Portion of ascending colon
Bladder (if distended)
Right ovary and fallopian tube
Right spermatic cord
Right ureter

Left Lower Quadrant
Lower pole of left kidney
Sigmoid colon
Portion of descending colon
Bladder (if distended)
Left ovary and fallopian tube
Uterus (if enlarged)
Left spermatic cord
Left ureter

Midline
Aorta
Bladder
Uterus

○ = Umbilicus

Figure 24-8. ■ The four quadrants of the abdomen, with the organs located within each quadrant. (Source: Patrick Watson, Pearson Education.)

the bowel. A fecal mass, tumor, or full bladder may cause a dull percussion tone. The percussion tone also is dull over the liver.

Lightly palpate all abdominal quadrants, noting muscle tone or guarding and any areas of tenderness. If the patient has complained of abdominal pain, palpate the affected quadrant or area last. Document all assessment findings. Box 24-2 ■ presents a sample narrative documentation of the assessment of a patient with a gastrointestinal complaint.

NUTRITIONAL ASSESSMENT

Assessing the patient's nutritional status often is important, particularly for older adults and patients scheduled for surgery. A number of tools are available for nutritional screening, some developed specifically for older adults. One such tool, the Mini Nutritional Assessment (MNA) tool, can be used to determine whether an older adult is malnourished or at risk for malnutrition. The MNA uses questions related to food intake, history of weight loss, mobility, and psychologic stress, as well as objective data such as BMI and the presence or absence of acute disease, dementia, and psychologic conditions (DiMaria-Ghalili, 2012).

DIAGNOSTIC TESTS

A number of laboratory and diagnostic tests commonly are used to evaluate the structure and function of the gastrointestinal tract and the accessory organs of digestion. Some such as the hemoglobin and hematocrit and serum electrolyte levels are general indicators of health and illness;

| BOX 24-2 | DOCUMENTATION OF GASTROINTESTINAL AND NUTRITIONAL ASSESSMENT |

Patient: A 25-year-old woman presents at her primary care nurse practitioner's office with complaints of abdominal pain and frequent diarrhea for the past 3 to 4 weeks.

Assessment note: Current complaint of intermittent crampy abdominal pain and frequent diarrhea began gradually about 4 weeks ago. Denies other current or previous symptoms such as anorexia, nausea, vomiting, general malaise, or fever. No known exposure to contaminated food or water; has not traveled out of the region for over 6 months. Having 4–6 stools per day; has noticed some blood and mucus in stool. Crampy left lower quadrant abdominal pain is relieved after defecation. Denies previous problems with abdominal pain, diarrhea, or constipation. States she has been healthy all her life and able to maintain normal weight without dieting, but thinks she has lost several pounds since this problem began. Denies chronic diseases or known allergies to food or drugs. No previous surgery.

Appears somewhat anxious and uncomfortable. Color pink, skin warm and dry. Height 165 cm (65 in.), weight 50 kg (110 lb) (with clothing; without shoes) for a BMI of 18.3. BP 106/60; P 84; R 16; T 36.4°C (97.6°F) PO. Abdomen flat and symmetrical, no visible veins or striations noted. Active bowel sounds (10–12/min) noted in all quadrants. Tympanic percussion tone throughout. Tender to palpation in left lower quadrant, no guarding.

others provide specific information about GI function. The focus of this section is on those tests performed specifically to evaluate the structure and function of the gastrointestinal tract and its accessory organs.

Laboratory Tests

Several laboratory tests commonly are performed to evaluate the gastrointestinal system and the accessory organs of digestion. Table 24-2■ lists these tests, their normal values, what the test measures and its significance, and any nursing implications for the test.

Other Diagnostic Tests

Table 24-3■ lists special diagnostic procedures that may be used to evaluate the function of the GI tract or for specific disorders, such as gastroesophageal reflux or peptic ulcer disease. *(Text continues on p. 620.)*

TABLE 24-2	Common Laboratory Tests for Gastrointestinal Assessment		
TEST	**NORMAL ADULT VALUES**	**EXPLANATION**	**NURSING IMPLICATIONS**
Serum albumin and total protein	Total protein: 6.0–8.0 g/dL Albumin: 3.5–5.0 g/dL	Used to assess general nutritional status and liver function.	Requires no special precautions or fasting. Total protein levels lower during pregnancy or prolonged bed rest.
Serologic *H. pylori* testing	No detectable antibody	Positive result indicates the presence of antibodies to *H. pylori* bacteria; may or may not indicate current infection with *H. pylori*.	No special precautions or fasting required.
Stool specimen for ova and parasites	None present	Used to detect the presence of infective organisms.	Avoid contamination of the specimen with urine, use a clean bedpan or collection device; instruct the patient to avoid mixing stool with urine or toilet tissue.
Stool for occult blood	None	Used to assess for gastrointestinal (GI) bleeding.	Requires a single, random stool specimen. Patient may be advised to refrain from eating meats, poultry, and fish for 2–3 days before the test.
Fecal fat	Neutral fat: less than 50 globules/HPF Fatty acids: less than 100 globules/HPF	Used to confirm steatorrhea (impaired fat absorption).	Requires either random stool specimen or 24- to 72-hour stool specimen. Patient may be instructed to eat a high-fat diet for 3 days before testing.
Liver function tests Alanine aminotransferase (ALT or SGPT) Aspartate aminotransferase (AST or SGOT) Alkaline phosphatase (ALP) Gamma-glutamyl transferase (GGT) Serum bilirubin	All values are for adults. 10–35 units/L 8–35 units/L 42–136 units/L Women: 3–13 units/L Men: 4–23 units/L Total: 0.1–1.2 mg/dL Conjugated (direct): 0.1–0.3 mg/dL	Used to assess liver function, evaluate patients with jaundice, and detect liver disease such as hepatitis and alcoholic cirrhosis.	Fasting is required for the bilirubin level; samples for other liver function studies may be drawn without fasting. Water is permitted.
Urobilinogen (urine)	Random: negative 2-hour specimen: 0.3–1.0 Ehrlich units 24 hours: 0.5–4.0 mg (Ehrlich units/24 hours)	Used as a sensitive indicator of liver damage, hemolysis, or severe infections.	No food or fluid restrictions required. May require a 2-hour or 24-hour urine specimen.

(continued)

TABLE 24-2	Common Laboratory Tests for Gastrointestinal Assessment *(continued)*		
TEST	**NORMAL ADULT VALUES**	**EXPLANATION**	**NURSING IMPLICATIONS**
Pancreatic function tests			
Serum amylase	Adult: 60–160 units/L Older adult: slightly higher	Used to assess pancreatic and salivary gland function and to monitor treatment of pancreatitis.	
Serum lipase	Adult: 20–180 units/L		
Urine amylase	4–37 units/12 hours	Used to help diagnose pancreatitis.	Requires a 2- or 24-hour urine specimen. No food or fluid restrictions necessary.

TABLE 24-3	Diagnostic Tests for Gastrointestinal Assessment	
DIAGNOSTIC TESTS		
TEST	**EXPLANATION**	**NURSING IMPLICATIONS**
Gastric analysis	Used to assess hydrochloric acid secretion and for the presence of *H. pylori* in the stomach. The sample is collected via nasogastric tube or during endoscopy. A drug to stimulate gastric acid secretion may be given during the test.	Food, fluids, smoking, chewing gum, and some drugs are withheld for 8–12 hours before the test. Insert a nasogastric tube per institutional procedure and collect samples as ordered. Observe for and take precautions to prevent aspiration during tube insertion or during the test. Inform the patient about possible discomfort with tube insertion, the length of the test, and the procedure itself.
Urea breath test	Used to detect infection with *H. pylori* bacteria. Radio-tagged urea is administered orally. If *H. pylori* is present, exhaled ammonia and carbon dioxide can be measured.	Food and fluids are withheld for 4 hours before the test. Instruct to avoid using antacids, bismuth sulfate, antibiotics, and omeprazole (Prilosec) for 2 weeks before testing.
Ambulatory pH monitoring	Used to diagnose gastrointestinal reflux. A pH electrode inserted through the nose into the esophagus is connected to a data recorder worn on the belt. Recorded data are later analyzed by computer.	Teach per protocol about caring for the electrode and data recorder. The patient records symptoms and activities for a 24-hour period.
Acid perfusion (Bernstein test)	Used to reproduce heartburn manifestations, evaluate esophageal function, and identify gastric acid reflux.	Food and fluids are withheld for 8–12 hours before the test. Place the patient in high Fowler's position. A catheter is inserted through the nose into the esophagus. Dilute hydrochloric acid is instilled through the catheter until the patient develops pain; normal saline is then is instilled.
Esophageal manometry	Measures pressures of the esophageal sphincters and esophageal peristalsis.	Food and fluids are withheld for 8 hours before testing; some medications may be withheld as well. Gagging may occur during tube insertion; instruct the patient to breathe through the mouth to control. The test takes about an hour to complete.
Paracentesis	An invasive procedure used to detect bleeding, contamination, or infection in the peritoneal cavity.	Food and fluids are withheld as directed before the test. Explain that local anesthesia will be used, so it should not be painful; pressure will be felt, however, when the needle is inserted into the abdomen. Obtain baseline weight and vital signs. Instruct to void immediately before the test. Position seated with feet supported. Place a dressing over the puncture wound and monitor vital signs and wound drainage after the procedure. Label specimens and send with completed requisitions to the laboratory.

TABLE 24-3	Diagnostic Tests for Gastrointestinal Assessment *(continued)*	
IMAGING STUDIES		
TEST	**EXPLANATION**	**NURSING IMPLICATIONS**
Ultrasonography Abdominal ultrasound Gallbladder ultrasound Liver echogram	Echoes from high-frequency sound waves are used to detect and evaluate abdominal disorders, detect masses, and screen for abdominal aneurysms. Can detect gallstones and evaluate gallbladder emptying. Noninvasive.	Often performed at the patient's bedside. Food and fluids are withheld for 8 hours before the exam; cleansing enemas or other bowel preparation may be ordered. Advise the patient that this test is not painful and generally is completed in 30 minutes or less.
Radiologic studies	Used to identify the size and location of structures, and, when combined with use of an injected contrast medium, used to study blood flow through vessels and organs.	X-ray studies expose the patient to radiation; inquire about possible pregnancy before the exam. If contrast is used, inquire about allergies, particularly to iodine, seafood, or contrast media.
Abdominal x-ray (flat plate of the abdomen)	Used to evaluate abdominal pain, detect fluid collections, organ enlargement or rupture, masses, obstruction, or foreign bodies.	No fasting or contrast media is required for this x-ray.
Upper GI series (barium swallow, upper GI with small bowel follow-through)	Uses contrast media (barium), fluoroscopy, and still pictures to assess the structure and peristalsis of the esophagus, stomach, and upper small intestine.	Food, fluids, and smoking are restricted for 8 hours before the exam. Advise the patient that the test requires several hours to complete and to bring reading or other materials to pass time. Tell the patient that the barium is instilled through a weighted tube inserted into the small bowel; some discomfort may occur with insertion of the tube. Advise to increase fluid intake for 24–48 hours after the test to promote barium elimination. Advise the patient that stool will be chalky white for up to 3 days after the exam. When both an upper GI series and a barium enema are required, the barium enema is scheduled 1–2 days before the upper GI series to prevent interference with evaluation by retained barium. Monitor for barium excretion after the exam.
Barium enema (lower GI series)	Uses contrast media (barium) administered by enema to show the anatomy and movement of the colon.	Food and fluids are withheld as ordered; only liquids may be allowed the day before the test, but all food and fluid intake is prohibited for 8 hours before the test. Administer or instruct the patient to take laxatives, suppositories, or enemas as ordered the evening before and the morning of the exam. Inform that this procedure takes about 1 hour to complete and will require turning to several different positions. Advise the patient that a full sensation and urge to defecate are normally felt as the barium is instilled. The barium will be expelled in the toilet after the test is completed.
Oral cholecy-stogram	Uses orally ingested contrast media to detect stones or deformity of the gallbladder and to assess its ability to concentrate and excrete bile.	Assess for allergy to iodine, seafood, or other contrast media. Fat intake is restricted the evening before the test. Schedule before barium enema if ordered; may be scheduled on the same day as an upper GI series.
CT scans	Specialized radiographic procedures produce computer-generated images with significantly more detail than standard x-rays. May be done with or without contrast media.	If contrast is used, inquire about allergies (to iodine and seafood, in particular) and ensure that the patient is well hydrated to reduce the risk of kidney damage.

(continued)

TABLE 24-3	Diagnostic Tests for Gastrointestinal Assessment *(continued)*	
ENDOSCOPIC STUDIES		
TEST	**EXPLANATION**	**NURSING IMPLICATIONS**
Upper endoscopy (esophagoscopy, gastroscopy, esophagogastro-duodenoscopy, EGD)	Endoscopic examination of the esophagus, stomach, duodenum, and upper jejunum. Used to evaluate disorders such as difficulty swallowing, gastric reflux, and peptic ulcer disease. Also used to locate, diagnose, and control upper GI bleeding.	Requires fasting for 8 hours before the procedure. A local anesthetic and conscious sedation are used during the procedure. Remove dentures, check for loose teeth, and provide mouth care before the procedure. All food and fluids are withheld after the procedure until gag and cough reflexes have returned. Monitor for evidence of upper GI bleeding, abdominal or back pain, or difficulty swallowing or breathing. Inform the patient that sore throat, hoarseness, abdominal bloating, belching, and flatulence are common after the procedure. Warm saline gargles or throat lozenges may provide comfort. Instruct to notify the physician immediately if difficulty swallowing continues, or if the patient develops epigastric, chest, or shoulder pain, vomits blood, or has black, tarry stools or fever.
Colonoscopy, sigmoidoscopy	Visual examination of the large intestine from the anus to the ileocecal valve (or, in a sigmoidoscopy, the descending colon). Used as a screening examination to detect colorectal cancer and to evaluate chronic constipation, diarrhea, persistent bleeding, and abdominal pain. Polyps may be removed during the procedure, and tissue samples are taken.	Bowel preparation with cathartics and limited food intake occurs 24–48 hours before the exam. Conscious sedation is used during the procedure. Instruct the patient to report any abdominal pain, chills, fever, rectal bleeding, or purulent discharge after the procedure. If a polyp has been removed, advise the patient to avoid high-fiber foods for 1–2 days and heavy lifting for 7 days.
Capsule endoscopy	Uses a wireless camera inside a capsule that is swallowed. The camera takes multiple pictures as it travels through the digestive tract. These pictures are transmitted to a recorder on a belt worn around the waist. Capsule endoscopy allows visual inspection of the small intestine, which generally is inaccessible during other endoscopic procedures.	A laxative may be ordered for bowel preparation before the procedure. Instruct the patient to avoid eating and taking medications (except as ordered by the physician) for at least 12 hours before capsule endoscopy and to limit fluids to sips of clear water. Clear liquids may be resumed 2 hours after swallowing the capsule and solid foods 4 hours after swallowing the capsule. The procedure lasts approximately 8 hours or until the capsule is expelled during a bowel movement. The camera does not need to be retrieved and can safely be flushed away.
Endoscopic retrograde cholangiopan-creatography	Combines endoscopic and x-ray procedures to evaluate the pancreatic, hepatic, common bile ducts; ampulla of Vater; and gallbladder.	Food and fluids are withheld for at least 8 hours before the exam. A local anesthetic and conscious sedation are used. Care is similar to a patient undergoing upper endoscopy.

A variety of imaging techniques are used to diagnose gastrointestinal disorders. These procedures range from noninvasive to very invasive. The use of noninvasive ultrasonography has replaced many of the more invasive and uncomfortable procedures in recent years. Diagnostic imaging procedures with their nursing implications are summarized in Table 24-3.

Because the GI tract is a hollow tube accessible at each end (via the mouth and the anus), much of it can be visualized using a flexible endoscope or even a wireless camera inside a swallowed capsule. Endoscopes are fiberoptic instruments with a lighted lens that allow visual examination of organs and cavities of the body. Endoscopy is commonly used to evaluate the esophagus, stomach, colon, and peritoneal space. Endoscopy has significantly reduced the use of procedures such as x-rays using contrast media to evaluate the anatomy of the stomach and the colon. Common endoscopic procedures for evaluating the GI tract are outlined in Table 24-3.

clinicalALERT

Tests and procedures used to diagnose abdominal and gastrointestinal disorders often are invasive, requiring instrumentation or use of a contrast substance. Verify the presence of a signed informed consent before preparing patients for these procedures. Provide additional information as needed, and contact the physician if the patient does not understand the procedure and why it is being performed.

Note: The references and resources for all chapters have been compiled at the back of the book.

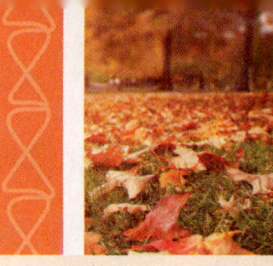

Chapter Review

KEY POINTS

- **Concept:** The purpose of the gastrointestinal system is to take in food, digest or break down the food into nutrients, absorb these nutrients into the blood, and eliminate what remains as solid waste.
- The gastrointestinal system, which includes the mouth, pharynx, esophagus, stomach, and small and large intestines, is a hollow tube that begins at the mouth and ends at the anus.
- Along with the accessory organs of digestion—the liver, gallbladder, and pancreas—the GI tract is vital to maintaining health and nutrition.

- **Concept:** Nutrition and diet influence overall health and an individual's risk for a number of diseases.
- **Concept:** Assessment of the GI system and its function includes gathering information about the patient's nutritional status, ability to ingest a variety of foods, and usual patterns of elimination.
- Diagnostic tests to evaluate GI system function include blood tests, such as the serum albumin and liver function tests; imaging studies, such as ultrasonography and x-rays; and direct examination of organs and tissue via endoscopy.

PEARSON NURSING STUDENT RESOURCES

Find additional materials at **nursing.pearsonhighered.com**.

NCLEX-PN® Exam Preparation

1 The nurse caring for a patient with dry mouth knows that this can affect the patient's nutrition because:

1. the patient needs to drink more water during a meal.
2. digestion begins in the mouth.
3. foods are likely to taste stronger.
4. the patient will eat more hard candy to stimulate saliva.

2 A patient is admitted with stenosis of the cardiac sphincter. The nurse knows that this will affect the patient's:

1. ability to swallow.
2. cardiac output.
3. blood pressure.
4. gastric emptying.

3 When assessing the abdomen of a patient, the nurse notes dullness to percussion in the lower left quadrant. One possible explanation for this finding is:

1. enlargement of the liver.
2. a full bladder.
3. air in the small intestine.
4. a fecal mass in the sigmoid colon.

4 A patient scheduled to undergo a colonoscopy asks the nurse just how the test is done. The nurse explains that this test involves:

1. instilling a contrast medium into the bowel and taking x-rays.
2. using ultrasonic waves to create and detect an echo off of abdominal structures.
3. inserting a flexible fiberoptic scope into the colon to visualize its mucous membranes.
4. taking multiple x-ray films that are then analyzed by computer to create a multidimensional image.

5 A patient loses a significant portion of the small intestine as a result of a gunshot wound. The nurse caring for the patient knows that this is likely to affect:

1. the absorption of most nutrients from food.
2. the ability to form a solid stool mass.
3. secretion of hydrochloric acid.
4. conjugation and elimination of bilirubin.

Answers and rationales for Review Questions appear in Appendix I.

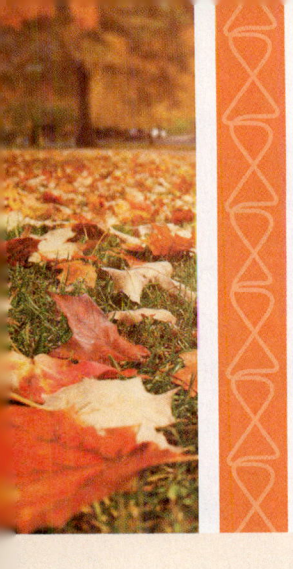

CHAPTER 25

Caring for Patients With Nutritional and Upper Gastrointestinal Disorders

BRIEF OUTLINE

DISORDERS AFFECTING EATING AND NUTRITION
Anorexia, Nausea, and Vomiting
Obesity
Malnutrition
Eating Disorders

DISORDERS OF THE MOUTH AND ESOPHAGUS
Stomatitis
Oral Cancer
Gastroesophageal Reflux Disease
Hiatal Hernia

Esophageal Cancer
DISORDERS OF THE STOMACH AND DUODENUM
Gastrointestinal Bleeding
Gastritis and Gastroenteritis
Peptic Ulcer Disease
Cancer of the Stomach

APPLIED LEARNING OUTCOMES

After completing this chapter, you will be able to:

1. Describe the causes, pathophysiology, and manifestations of common nutritional and upper GI disorders.
2. Conduct and document focused assessment of the patient with a nutritional or upper GI disorder, identifying and appropriately responding to unexpected or abnormal findings.
3. Use assessed data and current evidence and standards of practice for planning and evaluating care for patients with nutritional and upper GI disorders.
4. Demonstrate respect for patients' expressed needs, values, and preferences when implementing nursing care for patients with nutritional and upper GI disorders.
5. Safely administer medications and treatments for patients with nutritional and upper GI disorders.
6. Reinforce and document evidence-based teaching and learning for patients with nutritional and upper GI disorders and their families.

KEY TERMS

The key terms are defined on the pages listed below.

SPECIAL FEATURES

Key Concept Patients with nutritional and upper GI disorders require holistic nursing care that addresses nutritional needs, education, and psychosocial factors.

Nutritional disorders and diseases affecting the upper GI tract have the potential to affect multiple body systems and all aspects of the patient's health. These patients frequently receive care in community settings. However, when a complication develops, the patient may be acutely ill and have multiple nursing care needs.

DISORDERS AFFECTING EATING AND NUTRITION

Key Concept Nutritional disorders such as obesity and malnutrition are major causes of illness and disability. These disorders may be caused by lifestyle, diseases or their effects, problems of access to food and nutrients, or eating disorders.

Disorders affecting eating and nutrition range from simple to complex. Simple anorexia, nausea, and vomiting are common symptoms, frequently occurring with both major and minor illnesses. Nutritional disorders are major causes of illness and disability. The major nutritional disorders in the world today are obesity and malnutrition. Developmental, sociocultural, psychologic, and physiologic factors contribute to these disorders. Regardless of their cause, nutritional disorders affect many body systems and functions and often lead to serious health problems.

Anorexia, Nausea, and Vomiting

Anorexia is a loss of appetite. **Nausea** is a vague but unpleasant sensation of sickness or queasiness. It may or may not be accompanied by (and possibly relieved by) vomiting. **Vomiting** is the forceful expulsion of stomach contents. Anorexia, nausea, and vomiting commonly occur with food poisoning, gastroenteritis, or ingestion of toxins such as drugs or alcohol. When abdominal pain also is present, it may indicate a serious disorder. Chronic diseases such as chronic kidney disease and cancer and related treatments also frequently are accompanied by anorexia, nausea, and vomiting.

PATHOPHYSIOLOGY AND MANIFESTATIONS

The desire to eat is influenced by the contractions of an empty stomach as well as by appetite centers in the brain. Smell also contributes to appetite. *Anorexia*, loss of appetite, can result from many diverse diseases, as well as from drugs and psychologic factors such as fear, depression, or anxiety.

Nausea occurs when the vomiting center in the medulla of the brain is stimulated. The vomiting center can be stimulated by input from the GI tract; the inner ear; chemoreceptors that respond to drugs, toxins, diseases, or pregnancy; and by higher brain centers that respond to unpleasant sights, smells, or experiences.

Anorexia commonly precedes nausea, just as nausea frequently precedes vomiting. Vomiting is coordinated by the brainstem. *Emesis* (or *vomitus*) is produced when muscles of the rib cage, diaphragm, and abdomen contract, increasing pressures within the chest and abdomen. The gastroesophageal sphincter relaxes, and the larynx moves upward to expel gastric contents.

In addition to the subjective sensation of queasiness, nausea frequently is accompanied by manifestations such as pallor, sweating, tachycardia, and increased salivation. Vomiting may be accompanied by dizziness, lightheadedness, hypotension, and bradycardia.

Potential complications of vomiting include dehydration, hypokalemia, metabolic alkalosis (from loss of hydrochloric acid from the stomach), aspiration pneumonia, and esophageal tears.

COLLABORATIVE CARE

In most cases, anorexia, nausea, and vomiting are self-limited and require no treatment. If vomiting is severe or accompanied by other symptoms, acute care may be required to determine the underlying problem and prevent or treat complications.

Diagnostic tests may include serum electrolytes; pregnancy testing if indicated; liver, pancreatic, and renal function studies; and imaging studies (flat plate of the abdomen, abdominal CT scan) to detect GI obstruction. An upper endoscopy may be performed. CT scan or MRI of the head may be ordered if an intracranial problem is suspected as the cause.

Food is initially withheld, although clear liquids in small quantities are encouraged to prevent dehydration. Dry foods such as soda crackers also may reduce nausea and promote comfort.

Medications

Unless vomiting is related to pregnancy, antiemetic medications may be ordered to prevent or control nausea and vomiting. These drugs fall into several different classes and often are more effective when given in combination (Table 25-1 ■).

TABLE 25-1	**Giving Medications Safely: Nausea and Vomiting**		
CLASS/DRUGS	**PURPOSE**	**NURSING IMPLICATIONS**	**PATIENT TEACHING**
Serotonin receptor antagonists ■ Dolasetron (Anzemet) ■ Granisetron (Kytril) ■ Ondansetron (Zofran) ■ Palonosetron (Aloxi)	Drugs in this class suppress nausea and vomiting by blocking the effect of serotonin on nerves that stimulate the vomiting center. They are primarily used to prevent vomiting associated with chemotherapy, radiation therapy, and surgery.	Administer 30–60 minutes before chemotherapy or surgery as directed. May be given orally or intravenously (follow drug-specific directions). Monitor liver function and clotting studies; report abnormal levels to the physician.	Take this drug exactly as directed. It may be taken without regard to food intake. Headache is a common side effect of these drugs; use acetaminophen or another mild analgesic as directed by the physician.
Dopamine antagonists ■ Metoclopramide (Reglan) ■ Perphenazine (Phenazine, Trilafon) ■ Prochlorperazine (Compazine) ■ *Promethazine* (Phenergan) ■ Trimethobenzamide (Tigan)	These drugs block dopamine receptors in the chemoreceptor trigger zone (CTZ). They are used to suppress nausea and vomiting associated with surgery, cancer chemotherapy, and toxins. These drugs may cause sedation, hypotension, and *extrapyramidal symptoms* (muscle rigidity; slow, difficult movement). Older adults are more sensitive to their effects; a lower dose may be required.	Administer as ordered before surgery or before meals and procedures known to produce nausea and vomiting. These drugs may interact with other medications, increasing the risk for sedation and hypotension. Give with caution to older adults. Monitor closely for confusion, agitation, changes in vital signs. Promptly report extrapyramidal symptoms such as tremor, restlessness, hyperactivity, anxiety, or impaired coordination to the physician.	Use the drug as ordered; do not increase the dose unless recommended by the doctor. These drugs may cause drowsiness. Avoid using alcohol or other CNS depressants while taking these drugs. Change positions slowly because these drugs can cause light-headedness or dizziness. Promptly report changes in coordination, tremors, difficulty speaking or swallowing, or weakness to the physician.
Antihistamines ■ Cyclizine HCl (Marezine) ■ Dimenhydrinate (Dramamine) ■ Diphenhydramine (Benadryl) ■ Hydroxyzine (Vistaril, Atarax) ■ Meclizine (Antivert) ■ Scopolamine (Hyoscine, Transderm-Scop)	Antihistamines are primarily used to treat nausea and vomiting associated with motion sickness. They block histamine and acetylcholine receptors in the neural pathway from the inner ear to the vomiting center in the brainstem.	Do not give these drugs to patients with narrow-angle glaucoma, urinary retention, or bowel obstruction. May be given orally, parenterally, or rectally, depending on the preparation. Carefully monitor patients who are taking other CNS depressants or antihistamine preparations, tricyclic antidepressants, or monoamine oxidase inhibitors.	These drugs frequently cause drowsiness. Use caution when operating machinery or performing tasks requiring mental alertness. Avoid using alcohol or other substances that cause drowsiness or sedation while taking these drugs. The drug may cause dry mouth. Sips of water, ice chips, hard candies, and sugarless gum can be used for comfort. Use sunscreen and protective clothing to protect from sunburn while using these drugs.
Cannabinoids ■ Dronabinol (Marinol) ■ Nabilone (Cesamet)	Drugs in this class contain the same active ingredient as marijuana, thought to work by inhibiting the vomiting center in the medulla. They are used to relieve nausea and vomiting associated with cancer chemotherapy in patients who have not responded to treatment with other antiemetics.	Use with caution in older adults and people with a history of cardiovascular disease or substance abuse. These drugs are contraindicated for patients with a history of psychiatric disorders. Monitor for adverse effects such as dizziness, tachycardia, hypotension, impaired thinking and judgment, incoordination, irritability, and other mental symptoms.	Take the drug 1–3 hours before chemotherapy. Change positions slowly after taking this drug to prevent dizziness. You may experience distorted thinking, visual disturbances, confusion, and other mental symptoms while taking this drug. Keep this and all drugs out of the reach of children. Do not share this drug with anyone else.

Note: Medications identified in *italics* are among the 200 most frequently prescribed drugs in the United States.

Complementary Therapies

Mind–body interventions such as biofeedback, guided imagery, music therapy, and hypnosis may be effective for some patients with nausea. Ginger, an aromatic root frequently used in cooking, may also be helpful in relieving nausea and vomiting, particularly when due to motion sickness (Fontaine, 2011). It is safe for reducing nausea associated with pregnancy and may help relieve nausea associated with cancer chemotherapy. Ginger can inhibit platelet function and may increase the risk of bleeding in some patients.

NURSING CARE

Assessment of the patient is vital to help determine the cause of anorexia, nausea, and vomiting and to identify an underlying systemic disease or acute condition that requires immediate care (e.g., bowel obstruction). When the cause is known or no other acute symptoms are present, nursing interventions can promote comfort and prevent complications.

Nausea

Expected outcome: Nausea will be relieved as evidenced by subjective report and ability to eat.

The nursing diagnosis of nausea is defined as a subjective and unpleasant sensation in the throat or stomach that may lead to vomiting (Wilkinson, 2014).

- Monitor subjective complaints of nausea. *Nausea is a subjective sensation best described by the patient.*
- Monitor vital signs, skin turgor and condition, and weight. Maintain accurate intake and output records. Monitor the amount, color, and specific gravity of urine. *Nausea can cause aversion to food and fluids, leading to dehydration even when it is not accompanied by vomiting.*
- Administer antiemetic medication as ordered, before meals and before treatments or procedures known to stimulate nausea. *Preventing nausea is particularly important for patients receiving chemotherapy to avoid the association between the treatment and nausea.*
- Instruct to deep breathe to voluntarily suppress the vomiting reflex. *Controlling vomiting helps prevent dehydration and other complications associated with prolonged or severe vomiting.*
- Instruct the patient to consume small quantities of clear fluids and dry foods at separate times. *Separating the intake of dry foods and fluids helps reduce the nausea stimulus.*

Risk for Imbalanced Nutrition: Less Than Body Requirements

Expected outcome: Will tolerate the prescribed diet.

- Review medications and treatments for those that may contribute to anorexia. *Medications and unpleasant or painful treatments can affect the appetite. In some cases, changing the drug or treatment schedule (if possible) may improve the appetite.*

- Control unpleasant odors and sights in the area. *Noxious odors and sights (e.g., a commode or soiled dressing) inhibit the appetite and may stimulate nausea.*
- Monitor food intake. *A record of actual food intake provides information about the effects of anorexia and nausea and may suggest when intervention is necessary to prevent malnutrition.*
- Consult with a dietitian to develop a meal plan appropriate for the patient's culture and preferences. *A dietitian can determine the patient's calorie and protein requirements, providing a meal plan to meet these requirements. Familiar and preferred foods tend to stimulate the appetite.*
- Provide frequent small meals and snacks. *Large quantities of food can be overwhelming to a patient with anorexia, further suppressing the desire to eat.*

CONTINUITY OF CARE

Instruct the patient to initially limit intake to small quantities of clear liquids (tea, apple juice, broth, Jell-O) and dry foods such as soda crackers to help reduce nausea and prevent vomiting. Teach to avoid food-preparation odors if they produce nausea. Advise to restrict fluid intake for 1 hour before and after meals. Stress the need to maintain fluid intake to prevent dehydration and the importance of seeking additional medical help if unable to take in fluids or keep food down. Provide information about electrolyte replacement solutions such as sports drinks and commercially available electrolyte replacement solutions. Discuss the use of nutritional supplements such as Ensure for the patient with anorexia.

Obesity

> **Key Concept**   Obesity is associated with serious health problems such as hypertension, heart disease, cancers, disability, and death. Effective treatment of this prevalent disorder requires a multidisciplinary team approach.

Obesity is defined as excess adipose tissue or fat. *Overweight,* in contrast, is body weight greater than ideal for height; the excess weight may be from muscle, bone, or fat. Some people are overweight without being obese, such as body builders, for example. *Morbid obesity* is body weight of more than 100% over ideal weight.

Obesity occurs when excess calories are stored as fat. It is one of the most prevalent, preventable health problems in the United States (Box 25-1■). Nearly two-thirds of American adults are overweight; approximately one-third of adults are obese, making obesity the most prevalent health problem in the United States. **Bariatrics** is the medical specialty that focuses on preventing and treating obesity.

Obesity

Obesity is a prevalent health problem in the United States, where more than one-third (35.7%) of adults are obese. Its prevalence among adults varies by sex, race, and ethnicity. Although more men than women are overweight (70.7% of men to 61.4% of women), more women (34%) than men (30.2%) are obese. The prevalence of obesity varies among different ethnic groups (National Center for Health Statistics, 2013):

- Non-Hispanic Blacks—49.5%
- Mexican Americans—40.4%
- All Hispanics—39.1%
- Non-Hispanic Whites—34.3%

PATHOPHYSIOLOGY

Body weight is regulated by a complex set of factors. Overeating and physical inactivity do contribute to obesity, but they are not the entire cause of the problem. Factors such as appetite, hormones, heredity, and social and cultural influences also play a role in body weight.

Appetite is regulated by the central nervous system and by emotional factors. Appetite is stimulated by the hunger center in the hypothalamus in response to stimuli such as low blood sugar. *Satiety*, a feeling of fullness, counters appetite. The satiety center, also in the hypothalamus, is stimulated by gastric filling, a rise in nutrient levels, and hormones. Several hormones are involved in regulating obesity, including thyroid hormone, insulin, and leptin (a hormone that suppresses appetite and increases energy usage). There is a strong link between heredity and obesity. A person with one obese parent has a 40% chance of becoming obese; one with two obese parents has an 80% chance.

Physical inactivity is probably the most important factor contributing to obesity. Inactive people may consume fewer calories than active people and continue to gain weight due to lack of energy expenditure. Age-related loss of muscle mass combined with increased body fat, known as *sarcopenic obesity*, can lead to loss of strength and function, reduced quality of life, and early death for older adults.

Fat and calorie intake also contribute to obesity: People who eat more fat tend to have a higher body fat content than people who consume less fat and more complex carbohydrates and fiber. When more calories are consumed than are required to meet the body's energy needs, they are stored as fat.

Environmental and sociocultural influences—such as an abundant and readily accessible food supply, rewarding behavior with food, and spending significant amounts of time watching television—play a role in the prevalence of obesity in the United States.

Upper body obesity (or *central obesity*), identified by a waist/hip ratio greater than 1 in men and greater than 0.8 in women, is associated with a high risk of complications. **Lower body obesity** (or *peripheral obesity*), in which the waist/hip ratio is less than 0.8, is more common in women than men. Lower body obesity carries a lower risk for complications than does upper body obesity.

COMPLICATIONS

Obesity is associated with a higher risk for death and disease. Common complications associated with obesity include the following:

- Cardiovascular disease, such as high blood pressure, coronary heart disease, and heart failure
- Insulin resistance and type 2 diabetes
- Reduced male sex hormone levels in obese men and an increased risk for menstrual irregularities and polycystic ovarian syndrome (PCOS) in obese women

Box 25-2■ lists other complications associated with obesity.

COLLABORATIVE CARE

Because obesity is caused by many factors, its treatment is complex. Most experts recommend an individualized program combining exercise, diet, and behavior modification to meet the patient's specific needs.

Diagnostic Tests

- *Standard height–weight tables* can be used to determine a person's ideal weight.
- *Body mass index* (*BMI*) is used to determine obesity. A BMI of 19 to 24 kg/m^2 is considered healthy for adults. A BMI of 25 to 29.9 kg/m^2 is overweight; obesity is a BMI of 30 kg/m^2 or greater.
- *Fat-fold measures* (Figure 25-1■) provide an estimate of total body fat and its distribution.
- *Waist/hip ratio* is used to evaluate central obesity. It is calculated by dividing the waist measurement by the hip measurement.

- Cancers of the breast, uterus, prostate, and colon
- Cholecystitis and cholelithiasis
- Coronary heart disease
- Heart failure
- Hiatal hernia
- Hypertension
- Metabolic syndrome
- Muscle strains and sprains
- Osteoarthritis
- Peripheral vascular disease
- Postoperative complications
- Stress incontinence

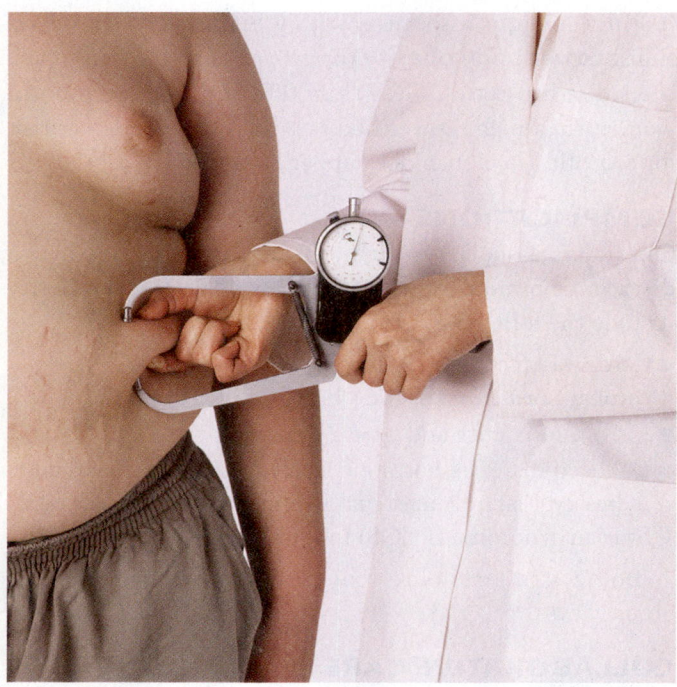

Figure 25-1. ■ A nurse measures skinfold thickness on the abdomen using calipers. (Source: Susanna Price / Dorling Kindersley Media Library.)

Other diagnostic tests may be done, such as a *thyroid profile*, *serum glucose* and *cholesterol*, and *lipid profile*. An *electrocardiogram* (*ECG*) may be ordered to evaluate effects of obesity on the heart.

Diet and Exercise

Treatment of obesity focuses on changing both eating and exercise habits. A pound of body fat is equivalent to 3,500 calories. To lose 1 lb, therefore, a person must increase activity to burn these calories or reduce daily caloric intake by 250 calories for 14 days.

Exercise is critical to weight loss and maintenance. After consulting with their health care providers, patients should engage in aerobic exercise of moderate intensity for 30 to 60 minutes a day, 5 or more days a week. This will reduce *adipose* (fatty) tissue, increase lean body mass (which burns more calories), and promote weight loss and long-term weight control.

The diet should be low in kilocalories and fat and contain adequate nutrients, minerals, and fiber. Selection of foods from all food groups helps ensure adequate nutrient consumption. The USDA food guide, MyPlate, and corresponding websites are a valuable guide (Figure 25-2■) to proper nutrition. Whole grains, foods with little or no added sugar, vegetables and fruits, lean protein sources, and use of unsaturated fats are emphasized. Regular meals with small servings are recommended. Weight loss should be gradual, no more than 1 to 2 lb/week. This usually means a diet of 1,000 to 1,500 calories/day. Fewer than 1,200 calories each day may lead to nutritional deficiencies and loss of lean tissue.

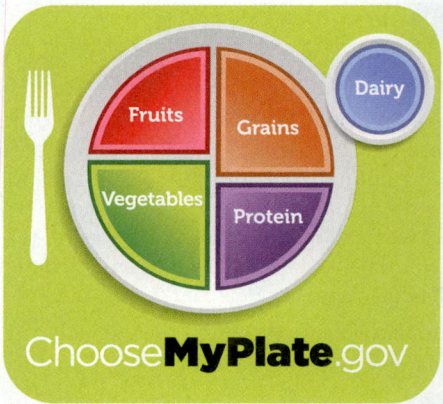

Figure 25-2. ■ MyPlate is designed to help Americans make healthy food choices and be active every day. (Source: U.S. Department of Agriculture and U.S. Department of Health and Human Services, 2010.)

Very-low-calorie diets (*VLCDs*) are generally only used in morbid obesity. These diets, which include only 400 to 800 calories/day, require medical supervision. A high protein intake allows dramatic weight loss while sparing muscle tissue. Exercise, nutrition, and behavior-modification counseling are important during the diet.

Behavior modification is a critical part of successful weight management. Keeping food records and identifying cues that create a desire to eat can help the dieter gain self-control. Weight loss and weight maintenance are separate but related issues. Most dieters regain lost weight within 2 years. Long-term weight management requires a lifelong commitment to changing food and eating habits, activity and exercise routines, and lifestyle. Physical activity is key to maintaining weight loss. People who exercise for 60 minutes a day most days of the week have a much greater likelihood of maintaining a healthy weight. Box 25-3■ outlines strategies for weight management.

Social support and group programs (Weight Watchers, Overeaters Anonymous, and Take Off Pounds Sensibly) provide weight loss strategies and peer support. Most programs charge a fee; paying for this kind of support may also encourage compliance.

Medications

Drugs may help people with obesity when used in combination with a comprehensive program that includes physical activity and a low-fat, low-calorie diet. An appetite suppressant such as phentermine (e.g., Adipex-P, Zantryl) inhibits the appetite center in the hypothalamus, producing gradual weight loss when combined with a reduced-calorie diet. Phentermine also is available in combination with topiramate, an antiepileptic drug, under the brand name Qsymia. Lorcaserin (Belviq), one of the newest appetite suppressants, activates serotonin receptors in the brain,

Behavioral Strategies for Weight Loss

Control the Environment

- Purchase low-calorie foods, shopping from a prepared list and on a full stomach.
- Keep all foods in the kitchen or pantry. Store them in opaque containers out of sight.
- Prepare exact portions of food to eliminate leftovers.
- Eat all foods in the same place, avoiding the kitchen.
- Do not eat while watching television or reading.
- Reduce frequency of eating out at restaurants, parties, and picnics.

Control Physical Responses to Food

- Eat a salad or drink a hot beverage before a meal.
- Eat slowly; take small bites and chew each bite thoroughly. Allow 20 minutes for a meal.
- Put eating utensils or food down between bites.
- Concentrate on the eating process; savor the food.
- Stop eating with the first feelings of fullness.

Control Psychosocial Responses to Food

- Make eating a pleasant experience, using attractive dinnerware and a formal setting.
- Use small plates and cups to make servings of food look larger.
- Concentrate on conversations and socialization during the meal.
- Use nonfood rewards for meeting a goal.
- Acknowledge small successes and improvements in all behavior.
- Substitute other pleasurable activities for eating (e.g., reading, exercise, hobbies).

Make Exercise a Daily Routine

- Make exercise a priority instead of trying to "fit it in" to a daily schedule.
- Try out different types of exercise to find one that is enjoyable.
- Form an exercise group or recruit an exercise "buddy."
- Plan strategies to maintain exercise during inclement weather.
- Wear comfortable and supportive clothing and shoes for exercising.

causing the person to feel full after eating smaller amounts and therefore to eat less.

Orlistat (Xenical) reduces the absorption of fat from the GI tract, leading to weight loss. It also lowers blood glucose and cholesterol levels, but is less effective in promoting weight loss than drugs that suppress the appetite.

Surgery

Surgery to treat obesity (called *bariatric surgery*) generally is reserved for morbidly obese individuals who have previous unsuccessful attempts at weight loss or who have serious comorbid conditions. Commonly used procedures restrict stomach capacity and absorption of nutrients from the stomach and duodenum (Figure 25-3■). In *gastric banding*

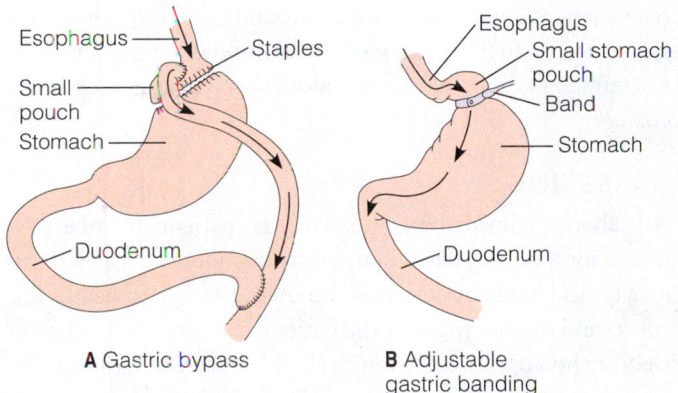

Figure 25-3. ■ Types of surgical procedures to treat obesity. (**A**) Gastric bypass surgery. (**B**) Adjustable gastric banding.

procedures, the capacity of the stomach is reduced using a band to create a small pouch just below the esophagus. *Adjustable banding* is the most common of these procedures. In adjustable gastric banding, a hollow band of silicone rubber is placed around the upper portion of the stomach. The band is inflated with saline solution to create a small stomach pouch with a narrow passage through to the rest of the stomach. The body feels full when the small pouch reaches capacity. The amount of band inflation can be adjusted using a port implanted under the skin.

Surgeries that affect nutrient absorption as well as capacity are more commonly used and, over time, are more effective in maintaining weight loss. In a *gastric bypass* procedure, a small stomach pouch is formed to restrict food intake, and a section of small intestine is attached to the pouch to bypass the lower stomach, duodenum, and upper jejunum. The risk of nutritional deficiencies, iron and calcium in particular, due to malabsorption is higher with these surgeries.

NURSING CARE

PRIORITIZING NURSING CARE

Overweight and obesity affect both the physical and emotional health of the patient. Helping the patient develop effective weight loss strategies is a priority of nursing care. In the obese patient undergoing surgery, assessing for and preventing complications are nursing care priorities.

HEALTH PROMOTION

Maintaining a healthy weight begins in childhood. Obese children and teenagers become obese adults. Promote healthy eating with a diet rich in whole grains, fruits, and vegetables and low in fat. Encourage all children and adults to be active, engaging in at least 30 minutes of aerobic activity daily. Encourage parents to limit time children spend watching television, using the computer, and playing electronic games. A gradual weight gain is common during adulthood. Encourage patients to reduce calories intake as energy needs change.

ASSESSING

Ask about eating habits, and have the patient describe food intake for a typical day. Identify activity and exercise patterns for a typical weekday and weekend. Ask about prior weight loss efforts and discuss whether the patient is satisfied with current weight and appearance. Inquire about recent changes in appetite or weight. Ask about any medical problems such as cardiovascular disease and diabetes. Assess height and weight, and compare actual weight to ideal body weight. Using a caliper, obtain fat-fold measurements (see Figure 25-1). Measure waist circumference at the level of the umbilicus.

IDENTIFYING POTENTIAL COMPLICATIONS

Carefully assess respiratory and cardiovascular status of obese patients, particularly those who have undergone surgery. Inquire about pain and comfort, carefully attending to new or increased complaints of pain. Frequently auscultate lung and heart sounds, peripheral pulses, and capillary refill. Maintain pulse oximetry, reporting low oxygen saturation levels. Monitor breathing pattern for signs of sleep apnea. Obtain capillary blood glucose measurements as ordered. Frequently assess the skin, particularly over pressure points and in folds.

DIAGNOSING, PLANNING, AND IMPLEMENTING
Imbalanced Nutrition: More Than Body Requirements

Expected outcome: Will acknowledge weight problem and verbalize components of an effective weight management program.

- Assist to identify factors that contribute to excess food intake. *Identifying cues to eating helps the patient eliminate or reduce these cues.*
- Establish realistic weight loss goals. *Success is more likely with small, reasonable goals (losing 1 to 2 lb/week) and a longer term goal of losing 5% to 10% of current body weight.*
- Assess knowledge and provide teaching about well-balanced eating plans. *Knowledge empowers the patient to make appropriate food choices.*
- Help develop an exercise plan that fits into the patient's lifestyle and includes enjoyable activities. Encourage 30 to 60 minutes of sustained activity daily. *A realistic, enjoyable exercise plan promotes participation and self-esteem.*
- Explore ability and willingness to make changes in daily patterns of eating, exercise, and lifestyle. *A commitment to losing weight and actively participating in weight loss strategies is necessary for long-term weight loss success.*

- Help identify behavior-modification strategies and support systems to promote weight loss and maintenance. *Lifestyle patterns that motivate the patient to continue exercising and eating sensibly promote success. Family and social support are critical to sticking with the plan.*
- Refer to a dietitian, nutritional counselor, or weight loss support program. *Professionals and support groups provide additional resources to help achieve and maintain weight loss.*
- Help plan strategies to deal with "stress eating" or relapses to previous eating patterns. *Overeating or not exercising can cause a sense of failure and lead to further overeating. Identifying strategies ahead of time helps the patient accept and deal with relapses.*

Risk for Impaired Tissue Integrity

Expected outcome: Skin and underlying tissues will remain intact.

The obese patient who has surgery (bariatric or other surgery) is at significant risk for pressure ulcers and impaired wound healing.

- Obtain a bed, chair, and mobility aids designed to accommodate an obese patient. If bed rest will be prolonged, obtain a pressure mattress. *Equipment specifically designed for obese patients promotes patient comfort and safety for the patient and caregivers.*
- Frequently assess the skin. Report changes such as bruising or redness promptly. *Early signs of pressure damage can be subtle.*
- Encourage use of incentive spirometer. Administer supplemental oxygen as ordered. Promote early ambulation. *The patient is at significant risk for respiratory complications due to immobility and sleep apnea. Ambulation promotes ventilation and airway clearance.*
- Maintain a diet high in protein and nutrients. *The obese patient is at risk for depletion of lean body mass and a negative nitrogen balance, which can affect healing.*

Chronic Low Self-Esteem

Expected outcome: Will acknowledge personal strengths.

Obese patients often experience "fat prejudice" in their family, workplace, or community. These experiences, coupled with the difficulty of finding attractive clothing or a chair large enough to sit on, can affect self-esteem. Hospitalized obese patients may be subject to frequent comments about their physical condition.

- Set small goals with the patient and offer positive feedback and encouragement. *Small goals provide more opportunities for success. Positive feedback and encouragement help develop self-esteem.*
- Explore the possibility of psychologic counseling with the patient. *Many patients benefit from counseling for issues related to self-esteem and depression.*

MANAGING NURSING CARE

Nursing care activities such as frequently repositioning the obese patient, using assistive devices during moving (e.g., overhead trapeze), and using protective padding to prevent tissue breakdown related to pressure or moisture in skin folds may be assigned to assistive personnel with appropriate training.

EVALUATING

To evaluate the effectiveness of nursing care, monitor weight, looking for a slow, progressive weight loss. Ask about eating and exercise patterns. Assess knowledge and willingness to consume a nutritionally sound diet. Discuss the patient's sense of success and self-image.

DOCUMENTING

Document progress in achieving weight loss goals, as well as any interventions or strategies to overcome barriers.

CONTINUITY OF CARE

The patient is ultimately responsible for managing and maintaining weight loss. Teaching and planning must therefore be individualized. Tailor teaching and weight loss strategies to address coexisting health problems. (For example, teach the overweight patient with diabetes about a diabetic, calorie-restricted diet. Develop an individualized exercise program for the overweight patient with heart disease.) Provide information about community or hospital-based programs and resources. Discuss strategies for incorporating exercise into the patient's daily schedule.

Malnutrition

Malnutrition is a condition that results from inadequate nutrient intake. It occurs when food and nutrient intake and absorption do not meet the needs for growth, development, or function. Malnutrition can result from lack of major nutrients (carbohydrates, proteins, and fats) or micronutrients (vitamins and minerals). It affects all body systems and increases the risk of disease and death. Malnutrition is common in hospitalized patients, often leading to poor wound healing and lower resistance to infection.

Other groups at risk for malnutrition include the young, the poor, older adults, the homeless, low-income women, and ethnic minorities. Malnutrition is particularly common among residents of long-term care settings. Patients may be undernourished because of poor food choices. Disorders such as *anorexia nervosa* (an eating disorder marked by a disturbed body image and fear of gaining weight) and *bulimia* (episodic binge eating and self-induced vomiting) are serious concerns, especially among teenagers and young adults (see the Eating Disorders section later in this chapter for more information about anorexia and bulimia). Fad diets

BOX 25-4	CONDITIONS ASSOCIATED WITH MALNUTRITION

- Aging
- AIDS
- Alcoholism
- Bariatric surgery
- Burns, trauma
- Cancer
- Chronic diseases (COPD, kidney disease)
- Eating disorders (anorexia, bulimia)
- Gastrointestinal disorders, short bowel syndrome
- Neurologic disorders
- Surgery

may also result in nutritional deficiencies. Gastrointestinal problems such as nausea or vomiting, altered digestion, or impaired absorption can lead to malnutrition, as can other illnesses (Box 25-4■).

PATHOPHYSIOLOGY

When food intake does not meet the body's energy needs, the body uses glycogen, body proteins, and fats to support metabolism. Glucose and glycogen stores, the energy sources in the body, are depleted within 12 to 24 hours of no food intake. When adequate calories are not available to meet energy needs, the body then turns to its proteins (in muscle and organs) and fats (in subcutaneous tissue). The size of all body compartments is reduced, and metabolically active tissues are lost, decreasing energy expenditure.

In hospitalized patients, the acute stress response to illness or trauma increases the metabolic rate and energy expenditure. This leads to **catabolism** (cell and tissue breakdown) and loss of lean body mass and protein stores. Inadequate protein and calorie intake can lead to *protein–calorie malnutrition* (*PCM*). Protein synthesis is impaired, delaying wound healing. Serum albumin levels fall, leading to edema. Immune function is impaired, increasing the risk of infection. The cardiovascular and GI systems also are impaired by malnutrition.

clinicalALERT

Approximately half of all hospitalized adults are malnourished or at risk for PCM. Carefully assess the patient's food and fluid intake, and alert the charge nurse or physician when poor appetite, dental problems, nausea, or NPO status interferes with intake.

MANIFESTATIONS AND COMPLICATIONS

Manifestations of malnutrition vary, depending on the nutrient deficit. Weight loss is the most apparent sign. Body mass and skin-fold thickness are reduced. Malnourished patients may have a wasted appearance;

dry and brittle hair; pale mucous membranes; peripheral edema; and a sore, smooth tongue.

In PCM, loss of subcutaneous fat and muscle proteins can impair mobility and increase the risk of skin and tissue breakdown (pressure ulcers). Wound healing is impaired. Serum albumin levels fall, with resulting abdominal edema, diarrhea, and impaired absorption of nutrients. The risk of infection increases. Cardiac output drops, increasing the risk for falls.

COLLABORATIVE CARE

Laboratory studies can provide additional assessment data to evaluate the effects of malnutrition on the patient. Patients with PCM have low *serum albumin* and *prealbumin* levels. On complete blood count (CBC), the *lymphocyte count*, *hemoglobin*, and *hematocrit* often are decreased due to iron deficiencies. *Serum electrolyte levels* also may be altered.

Medications

Malnourished patients generally need supplemental vitamins and minerals to restore adequate levels. A multivitamin and mineral supplement may be given, or therapy may be tailored to correct specific deficiencies.

Food and Fluid Management

The goal of treatment is to restore the malnourished patient to ideal body weight and replace necessary nutrients and minerals. In severe malnutrition, fluid and electrolyte imbalances are corrected first, and then food and nutrients are reintroduced gradually. Oral feedings and supplements are preferred. Small, around-the-clock feedings are generally tolerated best. Energy- and protein-rich foods or commercially available nutritional supplements (Carnation Instant Breakfast, Ensure, etc.) may be ordered. Intravenous solutions may be used to replace fluids and electrolytes.

ENTERAL FEEDINGS   **Enteral** or *tube feedings* may be used to meet all or part of the nutritional needs in patients who are unable to eat. Tube feedings are often administered through a soft, small-caliber nasogastric (NG) or nasoduodenal tube with a weighted tip. Box 25-5■ outlines the procedure for inserting an NG tube. Gastrostomy or jejunostomy tubes (discussed under Cancer of the Stomach later in this chapter), which are associated with a lower risk of aspiration, are increasingly used for enteral feedings.

A number of tube-feeding formulas are commercially available. All are nutritionally complete. Some formulas have added fiber to reduce the incidence of diarrhea, a common side effect of enteral feedings. Others have specific formulations for patients with chronic diseases such as chronic obstructive pulmonary disease (COPD) or kidney disease. Formulas may be diluted to half strength for the first day of therapy. If tolerated, they are given at three-fourths strength on the second day and at full strength thereafter.

Fluid and electrolyte status are monitored carefully, and additional water is given to meet the patient's specific needs. The volume of feedings is gradually increased, with a maximum feeding of 240 to 360 mL every 2 to 4 hours, or 2 L for a 24-hour period, based on the patient's caloric needs. Formulas may be administered as a bolus feeding, by continuous drip, or on a cyclic schedule (Box 25-6■). To prevent aspiration, elevate the head of the bed at least 30 degrees during feeding and for at least 1 hour after feeding.

PARENTERAL NUTRITION   **Parenteral nutrition** (*PN* or *hyperalimentation*) is intravenous administration of a solution that meets all the patient's nutritional needs (except for fiber). PN is used for both short- and long-term management of nutritional deficiencies when the patient is unable to eat. It may be used together with enteral feedings to meet the patient's nutritional needs. Patients who have undergone major surgery or trauma, or who are seriously undernourished, are often candidates for PN. Many patients are discharged to home with PN and are monitored by home health nurses.■

PN formulas have high concentrations of dextrose, protein (amino acids), electrolytes, vitamins, minerals, and fat emulsions. They are usually administered through a central vein, such as the subclavian vein. To initiate therapy, the physician often inserts a triple-lumen catheter that permits medications and other intravenous solutions to be given at the same time. Nursing responsibilities related to PN are outlined in Box 25-7■.

NURSING CARE

PRIORITIZING NURSING CARE

Nursing care priorities focus on the effects of malnutrition and its potential complications, such as increased risk for infection, deficient fluid volume, and skin breakdown.

HEALTH PROMOTION

Careful nursing assessment and interventions can help prevent malnutrition in the hospitalized or long-term care patient. Carefully monitor food intake. Assess patients' food likes and dislikes, and provide foods they are likely to eat. When the patient is placed on NPO status for surgery or tests, resume food intake as soon as possible. If allowed, encourage family members to provide favorite foods to promote intake. In long-term care settings, promote socialization during meals.

ASSESSING

Ask about eating habits and typical daily food intake. Ask about recent weight changes and contributing factors. Assess for anorexia, nausea, medications, or inability to buy and prepare food for meals. Ask about medical problems such as chronic lung or heart disease, thyroid problems,

BOX 25-5   PROCEDURE CHECKLIST

Inserting a Nasogastric Tube

☑ Gather all supplies.

☑ Verify the patient's identity and provide for privacy.

☑ Explain the procedure, using nonthreatening terms. Tube insertion is unpleasant, but once in place, little or no discomfort should be felt. Establish a means for the patient to indicate distress during the procedure, such as raising a finger. Emphasize the need to follow instructions to swallow during tube insertion.

☑ Follow Standard Precautions; wear clean gloves.

☑ Place in high Fowler's position with a towel or disposable pad on the chest.

☑ Occluding one naris at a time, ask the patient to breathe. Use the naris with the better airflow for insertion.

☑ Measure the tube: Hold the tip of the tube at the patient's nose and extend the tube to the earlobe and then to the distal sternum (see figure). If the tube is to be placed in the duodenum, add 8 to 10 in. (20 to 25 cm) to the measurement. Mark the tube.

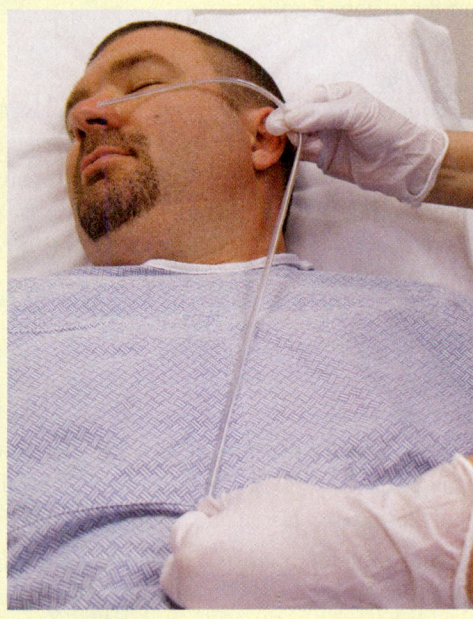

Measuring the appropriate length for nasogastric tube insertion. (Source: Patrick Watson, Pearson Education.)

☑ Provide a glass of water with a straw if allowed.

☑ For a small-bore tube, insert the guide wire or stylet into the tube.

☑ Using water-soluble lubricant, lubricate 3 to 4 in. of the tube tip.

☑ Gently insert the tube into the naris, directing it toward the ear. Use a smooth, continuous motion. Have the patient tip the head forward, chin to chest, and instruct to sip and swallow on command. Advance the tube 3 to 4 in. (7 to 10 cm) with each swallow until the point marked on the tube is at the opening of the naris.

☑ Pause briefly if the patient gags (do not withdraw the tube); instruct to take a few breaths through the mouth, and then resume advancing the tube. If gagging continues, check the mouth. If the tube is curled in the mouth, withdraw it until the tip is in the oropharynx before resuming.

☑ If the patient coughs and is unable to speak, withdraw the tube until the tip is visible. Have the patient tip the head further forward and swallow to prevent this from occurring.

☑ Verify tube placement. Withdraw a small amount of fluid from the tube and check the pH of the fluid. If the pH is 5 or lower, the tube is very likely in the stomach. If the pH is 6 or higher, confirm tube placement with an x-ray.

☑ Secure the tube with tape.

☑ Initiate feeding or gastric suction as ordered.

☑ Reposition and provide mouth and nose care.

Sample Documentation

[date] 1030   8 Fr. gastric feeding tube inserted via R naris. Small amount green drainage obtained, pH 4. Tolerated procedure well.

_____S. Williams, LPN.

Note: Refer to a nursing fundamentals or skills text for more detailed instruction. Check state guidelines and facility policy before performing any procedure.

---

or kidney disease. Look at psychosocial factors such as body image, loneliness, depression, and economic status. Determine food preferences.

Assess height, weight, and fat-fold measurements (see Figure 25-1). Wearing gloves, evaluate the mouth, looking for inflammation, gum disease, dental caries, or poorly fitting dentures. Assess ability to swallow liquids and semisolid and solid foods.

IDENTIFYING POTENTIAL COMPLICATIONS

Frequently assess for evidence of skin and tissue breakdown. Report abdominal or peripheral edema, diarrhea, or delayed wound healing. On admission and during treatment, monitor

serum albumin, serum electrolytes, and the hemoglobin and hematocrit. Report unanticipated changes and critical values.

DIAGNOSING, PLANNING, AND IMPLEMENTING

Imbalanced Nutrition: Less Than Body Requirements

Expected outcome: Will maintain weight within normal or expected range.

■ Monitor and record weight. Note the amount and type of foods eaten at meals and snacks. _These are important data to evaluate the effectiveness of nutritional therapy._

BOX 25-6	PROCEDURE CHECKLIST

Enteral Feedings

☑ Obtain ordered formula and all supplies. Verify the patient's identity. Use Standard Precautions.

☑ Elevate the head of the bed to at least 30 degrees during and for at least 1 hour after the feeding.

☑ Provide mouth care.

☑ Explain the procedure.

☑ Check residual stomach contents before intermittent feedings or every 4 hours if continuous. Check the pH of the aspirate to assess tube placement. Reinstill the aspirated contents.

☑ Withhold the feeding and notify the charge nurse or physician if more than 100 mL (gastrostomy tube) or 200 mL (NG tube) residual is obtained or if the pH is 6 or higher.

☑ Fill the feeding bag with the ordered amount of formula and water. Clear the tubing of air and/or attach it to a feeding pump.

☑ Attach the tubing to the feeding or gastrostomy tube. Set the flow rate by drip or on the pump and begin feeding.

Sample Documentation

[date] 1000   340 mL Sustacal with 100 mL water administered via gastric feeding tube. 75 mL residual obtained before feeding; reinstilled. Tolerated well with no evidence of aspiration.

_____S. Williams, LPN.

Note: Refer to a nursing fundamentals or skills text for more detailed instruction. Check state guidelines and facility policy before performing any procedure.

- Consult with the dietitian, patient, family, and caregivers to plan a nutritionally complete diet. _The best diet plan will not work if the patient does not eat it or if the caregivers do not prepare it._

- Provide mouth care before and after meals; eliminate foul odors; and offer frequent, small meals including foods the patient prefers. _Oral hygiene and a pleasant environment make food more appetizing. Small meals are generally more appealing and less overwhelming to a patient with anorexia._

- Provide a rest period before and after meals. _Eating requires energy, and the undernourished patient may have decreased physical strength._

Risk for Infection

Expected outcome: Remains free of infection as evidenced by temperature within normal range and absence of signs of inflammation.

- Monitor and record temperature; report any elevation to the charge nurse or physician. Note and report chills,

BOX 25-7	NURSING CARE CHECKLIST

Parenteral Nutrition

☑ Use aseptic technique at all times. Do not add any medication to the solution or administer medications or other IV solutions through the intravenous catheter into which PN is being administered.

☑ Use an infusion pump to ensure the correct rate of infusion.

☑ Keep accurate intake and output records. Monitor for and report manifestations of fluid and/or electrolyte imbalance.

☑ Check capillary blood glucose and administer insulin as ordered.

☑ Monitor and record vital signs, including temperature, reporting any changes to the charge nurse or physician.

☑ Carefully assess respiratory status. Report changes.

☑ Monitor for signs of infection, such as fever, malaise, redness, swelling, or drainage, at the catheter insertion site. Report these signs if noted.

---

malaise, confusion, local inflammation, or elevated WBC. _Early detection of infection may prevent complications._

- Maintain Standard Precautions and sterile technique for procedures as indicated. _Hand washing is the best strategy to prevent the spread of infection. Sterile technique is required for procedures such as changing dressings._

Risk for Deficient Fluid Volume

Expected outcome: Will remain free of signs of dehydration or fluid imbalance.

The malnourished patient is at risk for dehydration due to inadequate fluid intake, concentrated enteral feeding solutions, or parenteral nutrition.

- Monitor oral mucous membranes, skin turgor, urine output and specific gravity, level of consciousness, and laboratory results. _Dry mucous membranes, poor skin turgor, decreased urine output, and increased specific gravity may indicate dehydration. Dehydrated patients may have a decreased level of consciousness. Laboratory studies such as serum osmolality, electrolytes, and hematocrit also provide data about fluid balance._

- Weigh daily at the same time, on the same scale, and with the same clothing. Monitor intake and output. Document carefully. _Daily weights and intake and output records help monitor fluid balance._

- If fluids are allowed, offer them often in small amounts, considering the patient's preferences. _Small amounts are tolerated best; frequent drinking promotes adequate intake._

Risk for Impaired Skin Integrity

Expected outcome: Skin and underlying tissues will remain intact.

- Frequently assess the skin, noting areas of redness, abrasions, or other lesions. Record and report any abnormal findings or changes to the charge nurse or physician. *Early identification of pressure areas or lesions allows intervention to prevent further breakdown or complications.*
- Turn and reposition every 2 hours. Encourage passive and active range-of-motion exercises. *Pressure areas are at high risk for decreased circulation and breakdown. These measures reduce pressure and promote oxygenation of cells.*
- Keep skin dry and clean, and minimize shearing forces. Keep linens smooth, clean, and dry. Provide therapeutic beds, mattresses, or pads. *These measures promote comfort and reduce the risk of skin breakdown.*

MANAGING NURSING CARE

Nursing care activities such as obtaining daily weights, providing mouth care, assisting with meals and recording intake, and frequent repositioning for the patient with malnutrition are appropriate tasks to assign to assistive personnel.

EVALUATING

Collect the following data to evaluate the effectiveness of nursing interventions for the patient with malnutrition: consuming prescribed diet; evidence of weight gain; stable intake and output; laboratory values improving; remains free of infection or skin breakdown.

DOCUMENTING

Document weight, food and fluid intake, and responses to meals and snacks. Note skin condition, recording and reporting any areas of redness or early tissue breakdown.

CONTINUITY OF CARE

Diet therapy (including enteral feedings or parenteral nutrition) often is continued in the long-term care or home setting. Teach the patient and care providers about the importance of hand washing and proper food and supplement storage. If enteral feedings or PN will continue at home, instruct the patient, family, and caregivers how to (1) prepare and handle enteral or parenteral solutions, (2) add solutions to either the feeding tube or central line, (3) manage infusion pumps, (4) care for the feeding tube or central catheter, and (5) recognize and manage problems and complications. Teach the patient how and when to notify the home health agency or health care provider. Document all teaching and the learners' understanding of what has been taught. Assess compliance with the treatment plan on a continuing basis, especially when psychosocial factors contribute to malnutrition. Box 25-8 ■ describes strategies for older adults with malnutrition.

BOX 25-8	FOCUS ON OLDER ADULTS

Promoting Nutrition in the Older Adult

Changes that occur with aging can affect nutrition and the enjoyment of food in the older adult. The ability to taste salty and sweet flavors declines, and the sense of smell is reduced. Less saliva is produced, making it more difficult to swallow. Increased problems with teeth and gums or ill-fitting dentures affect eating. The lower esophageal sphincter relaxes, increasing the incidence of gastroesophageal reflux and heartburn. Less gastric acid is produced, impairing absorption of some nutrients. Peristalsis and digestion slow, often causing the older adult to feel full after eating small amounts. Medications taken for chronic diseases can lead to anorexia. Functional limitations may impair the ability to shop and cook. Psychosocial issues such as a fixed income, depression, social isolation, and loneliness contribute to the risk of nutritional problems. Older adults who eat alone often do not eat as well as those who share meals with companions.

To promote nutrition in older adults:

- Suggest congregate meals (usually offered through senior centers) and programs such as Meals-on-Wheels (for people who are homebound and physically unable to prepare meals).
- Discuss a well-balanced diet that includes whole grains, fresh fruit, and vegetables.
- Advise patients to avoid processed foods and foods high in fat, to drink adequate fluids, and to exercise regularly.
- Assist patients to shop wisely to get the most value for their money.

Eating Disorders

Eating disorders such as *anorexia nervosa* and *bulimia* affect eating and weight management. **Anorexia nervosa** is characterized by an intense fear of weight gain and weight less than 85% of expected for age and height. Patients with **bulimia nervosa**, in contrast, often have normal body weight. This disorder, which is more common than anorexia nervosa, is characterized by binge–purge behavior: Episodes of binge eating are followed by self-induced vomiting, laxative or diuretic use, or excessive exercise. Table 25-2 ■ compares the manifestations and complications of anorexia and bulimia.

Eating disorders often are difficult to treat. The intense fear of weight gain and disrupted body image cause patients with anorexia nervosa to resist increased food intake. A multidisciplinary team approach is necessary, involving nutritional, behavioral, and psychologic therapies. Refeeding of patients with anorexia nervosa must be approached slowly to avoid complications such as heart failure. Meals are supervised to prevent hiding of food. Antidepressant drugs may be prescribed.

TABLE 25-2	**Characteristics of Anorexia Nervosa and Bulimia**	
	ANOREXIA NERVOSA	**BULIMIA**
Onset and population	■ Adolescence ■ Women more than men	■ Late adolescence or early adulthood ■ Women more than men
Manifestations	■ Weight less than 85% of normal ■ Disturbed body image ■ Fear of weight gain ■ Refusal to eat, excessive exercise ■ Muscle wasting ■ Skin and hair changes ■ Amenorrhea ■ Low blood pressure, slow pulse ■ Low body temperature ■ Constipation ■ Insomnia	■ Weight normal or greater than normal ■ Binge–purge behavior ■ Scant menses or amenorrhea ■ Lacerations of palate (from induced vomiting) ■ Callous on fingers or back of hand
Complications	■ Electrolyte and acid–base imbalances ■ Low cardiac output, dysrhythmias ■ Anemia ■ Hypoglycemia ■ Osteoporosis ■ Delayed gastric emptying ■ Abnormal liver function	■ Enlarged salivary glands ■ Stomatitis ■ Loss of dental enamel ■ Fluid, electrolyte, and acid–base imbalances ■ Dysrhythmias ■ Esophageal tears, stomach rupture

NURSING CARE

Early identification and referral of patients with eating disorders are important to prevent adverse effects on growth and development. Be alert for patients who weigh less than ideal for height and yet complain of being overweight, relate a history of dieting, laxative or diuretic use, and significant amounts of exercise. *Imbalanced Nutrition: Less Than Body Requirements* is the priority nursing diagnosis. Other applicable nursing diagnoses include *Disturbed Body Image* and *Ineffective Family Coping*. Consider the following nursing care activities when caring for patients with an eating disorder:

■ Monitor weight, using standard conditions. *Weight provides a measurement of the effectiveness of interventions.*

■ Monitor food intake during meals and snacks, recording amount consumed. Continue close observation for at least 1 hour after meals; do not allow patient to use the bathroom alone. *Monitoring the patient during and after meals is important to prevent food hiding or disposal and purging after eating.*

■ Serve small, frequent, balanced meals, gradually increasing serving size. *Calorie intake is gradually increased to prevent complications of refeeding. "Normal" serving sizes may be overwhelming to the patient, reducing appetite and food intake.*

Ongoing treatment of eating disorders is vital. Patients and their families are referred to a multidisciplinary team for continuing care. Stress the importance of continuing treatment and involvement of the whole family for effective care.

DISORDERS OF THE MOUTH AND ESOPHAGUS

Key Concept Disorders of the mouth and esophagus can affect the ability to eat and maintain nutritional status. Although most disorders are appropriate for self-treatment, cancers of these organs require prompt diagnosis and treatment for successful resolution.

Any portion of the upper GI tract, from the mouth through the upper portion of the small intestine, can be affected by inflammation or cancer, affecting the ability to eat.

Stomatitis

Stomatitis (also called *oral mucositis*), inflammation of the oral mucosa, is a common problem. Patients with stomatitis may experience pain and difficulty eating. Stomatitis often develops secondarily to cancer, dental disease, or acquired immunodeficiency syndrome (AIDS). It may be caused by viral infection (herpes simplex) or fungal infection (*Candida albicans*). Chemotherapy or radiation therapy also can cause stomatitis. *Aphthous ulcers* (canker sores) are a type of stomatitis. These ulcers are usually less than 1 cm in diameter and can last weeks to months.

The manifestations of stomatitis vary, depending on the cause. Herpes lesions (cold sores) are clustered and painful, usually occurring on the lips and oral mucosa. Candidiasis (thrush) causes painful white patches with a red base (Figure 25-4 ■). Other manifestations of stomatitis include red and swollen oral mucosa, pain, and possible ulcerations.

COLLABORATIVE CARE

Treatment is directed at both the cause and symptoms of stomatitis. Lesions may be cultured or scrapings examined to determine the cause of stomatitis. Table 25-3 ■ lists nursing implications and patient teaching for selected drugs used to treat stomatitis.

NURSING CARE

Suspect stomatitis in a patient who refuses to eat or who complains about mouth pain. Wearing gloves, inspect the mouth and oropharynx. Document any visible lesions, as

well as the general condition of mucous membranes, teeth, and gums. Note the patient's breath. Foul breath odor may be noted in patients with stomatitis. Assess ability to chew and swallow, as well as food and fluid intake.

Assist with mouth care as needed after eating and at bedtime. If the patient is unable to tolerate a toothbrush,

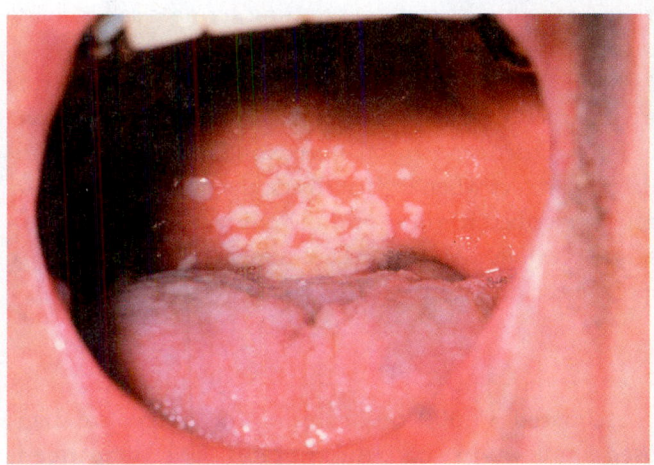

Figure 25-4. ■ Candidiasis of the mouth. (Source: © SPL/Custom Medical Stock Photo.)

TABLE 25-3	Giving Medications Safely: Stomatitis		
CLASS/DRUGS	**PURPOSE**	**NURSING IMPLICATIONS**	**PATIENT TEACHING**
Topical anesthetics/ anti-inflammatory agents			
■ Orajel ■ Viscous lidocaine ■ Anbesol ■ Triamcinolone acetonide	Provide temporary pain relief. Triamcinolone has an anti-inflammatory effect.	Assess for adverse or hypersensitivity reactions. Notify the primary care provider if they occur. Provide mouth care after eating and at bedtime.	Apply every 1–2 hours or as directed. Contact the primary care provider if symptoms worsen or do not improve within 1 week after starting treatment.
Topical antifungal agents			
■ Clotrimazole ■ Nystatin	Used to treat candidiasis. Effect is local rather than systemic.	These drugs are contraindicated in pregnancy. Instruct to dissolve troches or lozenges in mouth. For oral suspension, instruct to swish the solution throughout the mouth for at least 2 minutes and then either expectorate or swallow as directed.	Use the medication as prescribed. Do not eat or drink for 30 minutes after the medication. Contact the primary care provider if symptoms worsen or do not improve.
Antiviral agent			
■ Acyclovir (Zovirax)	Reduces the severity and duration of herpes lesions. May reduce frequency of outbreaks.	Administer with food or on an empty stomach.	Begin taking the medication at the first sign of an outbreak. Contact the primary care provider if symptoms worsen.

use sponge or gauze toothettes or a water pick with gentle pressure. Avoid alcohol-based mouthwashes. Encourage a high-calorie, high-protein diet tailored to the patient's likes and dislikes. Offer soft, lukewarm, or cool foods or liquids (eggnog, milkshakes, nutritional supplements, popsicles, and puddings) frequently in small amounts. Avoid spicy or irritating foods. Use straws or feeding syringes as needed to promote intake.

Provide clear and easily understood instructions for oral care. Instruct to avoid alcohol, tobacco, and spicy or irritating foods. Discuss nutritional needs and strategies to minimize discomfort when eating. Teach the patient and family about prescribed medications, including how and when to use and possible side effects. Discuss signs and symptoms to report to the physician.

Oral Cancer

An estimated 35,000 new cases of oral cancer are diagnosed annually in the United States. The incidence is more than twice as high in men as in women, particularly in men over 40. The major risk factor for oral cancer is tobacco use (both smoking and smokeless tobacco). Alcohol consumption and prolonged exposure to sunlight also are significant risk factors. Recent evidence links cancers of the oropharynx with the human papillomavirus (HPV) infection among White men and women (National Cancer Institute, 2014)

PATHOPHYSIOLOGY AND MANIFESTATIONS

Most oral cancers are squamous cell carcinomas. Tobacco and alcohol damage cells lining the mouth and oropharynx. These damaged cells grow more rapidly to repair the damage, increasing the risk for malignancy. Oral cancer may develop anywhere on the oral mucosa, including the lips, tongue, or pharynx (Figure 25-5 ■). Box 25-9■ lists manifestations of oral cancer.

COLLABORATIVE CARE

Biopsy is done to determine whether an oral lesion is benign or malignant. Treatment and the prognosis for cure of oral cancer depend on the stage of the tumor. Additional diagnostic studies such as CT scans or MRI may be done to stage the tumor. (See Chapter 12 for more information about staging and grading of cancer.)

Eliminating risk factors (tobacco and alcohol) is vital. Early lesions without cancerous cells may heal when exposure to these substances is eliminated. Early cancers may be treated with radiation therapy (external beam or implants), resection of the tumor, or both. Advanced oral cancers may require extensive surgery such as *radical neck dissection*, a potentially disfiguring procedure. Lymph nodes and some

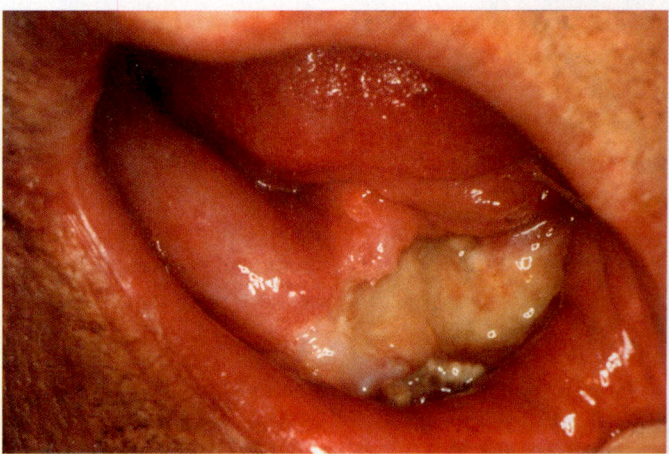

Figure 25-5. ■ Oral cancer. (Source: Biophoto Associates/Science Source.)

BOX 25-9	MANIFESTATIONS OF ORAL CANCER

- A sore or lesion in the mouth that does not heal
- *Leukoplakia:* irregular white patches on the lips, tongue, gums, tonsil, or oral mucosa
- *Erythroplakia:* slightly raised, irregular red patches that bleed easily when scraped
- Visible or palpable masses of the lips, cheek, or tongue
- Sore throat or a feeling of something caught in the throat
- Difficulty chewing, swallowing, or moving the jaw or tongue
- Asymmetry of the head, face, jaws, or neck
- Loosening of teeth, or dentures that no longer fit properly
- Swollen lymph nodes
- Blood-tinged sputum

muscles of the neck are removed, and a tracheostomy is performed during this procedure. The tracheostomy may be temporary or permanent. (See Chapter 22 for nursing care of the patient with a tracheostomy.) Chemotherapy is used as adjunctive treatment when the tumor has metastasized beyond the local area.

NURSING CARE

Teach all patients about the relationship between alcohol and tobacco use (especially smokeless tobacco) and oral cancer. Provide referrals to smoking cessation classes and Alcoholics Anonymous or alcohol treatment agencies as appropriate. Encourage parents to have young adolescent children vaccinated for HPV. Teach the early signs of oral cancer, demonstrating how to check tissues of the mouth.

Oral cancer and its treatment can affect airway clearance, food intake and nutrition, communication, and body image. Assess airway patency and respiratory status, particularly if the patient has undergone surgery to remove the tumor.

Place in Fowler's position and assist with turning, coughing, and using the incentive spirometer. Maintain adequate hydration to help loosen respiratory secretions and promote airway clearance.

Enteral feedings or parenteral nutrition may be necessary for patients with oral cancer. Monitor weight daily and food and nutrient intake. If the patient is able to eat, offer a soft, bland diet with enriched foods or dietary supplements. Offer small, frequent feedings, making mealtimes pleasant. Consider a dietary consultation to assess diet and plan appropriate supplements.

Provide a magic slate, flash cards, or picture or alphabet board as needed to facilitate communication. Allow ample time for communication and do not answer for the patient. Observe nonverbal communications to supplement verbal efforts. If the patient is unable to speak clearly, use yes/no questions and simple phrases. Keep the call light within easy reach and respond promptly. Alert all staff if the patient is unable to respond verbally over the intercom system. Consult with a speech therapist as needed.

Radical surgery of the head or neck can seriously affect body image. Assess coping, self-perception, and responses to surgery. Encourage the patient to express feelings regarding body image changes, and provide emotional support.

CONTINUITY OF CARE

For patients with oral cancer, teach about the cancer, its treatment, and any specialized care. As needed, teach caregivers how to change dressings and to provide tube or gastrostomy feedings, tracheostomy care, or central line care. Provide referrals to home health agencies as appropriate, and discuss support groups for cancer survivors or patients who have had head and neck surgery. If the patient and family have decided not to pursue treatment, support their decision and refer them to cancer support groups or hospice care.

Gastroesophageal Reflux Disease

The esophagus, essential for ingesting food and fluids, may be affected by inflammatory, mechanical, or cancerous disorders. The symptoms of these disorders often mimic other illnesses.

Gastroesophageal reflux is the backward movement of gastric contents into the esophagus. When the reflux of gastric contents causes inflammation and tissue damage to the esophagus, it is known as *gastroesophageal reflux disease* (*GERD*). GERD is common, affecting 15% to 20% of adults, many of whom experience daily symptoms.

PATHOPHYSIOLOGY AND MANIFESTATIONS

The lower esophageal sphincter normally prevents gastric contents from entering the esophagus. However, if the sphincter does not function effectively or gastric emptying is delayed, gastric contents may *reflux* (back up) into the lower esophagus. Factors contributing to reflux include increased volume of the stomach after meals, positioning, and increased gastric pressure due to obesity or restrictive clothing. Esophageal peristalsis and alkaline saliva normally clear and neutralize these corrosive gastric fluids, but this process may be impaired during sleep or by impaired esophageal peristalsis. Corrosive gastric fluids lead to tissue inflammation and may cause erosions, ulcers, or *strictures* (narrowing) of the esophagus. The risk of esophageal cancer is increased in patients with GERD.

Heartburn that increases after meals and is aggravated by bending over or lying down is the primary symptom of GERD. The patient may regurgitate sour material into the mouth or have difficulty or pain with swallowing. Sore throat, hoarseness, or chest pain also may be symptoms of GERD.

COLLABORATIVE CARE

Diagnostic tests used to establish the diagnosis of GERD include a barium swallow, upper endoscopy, and ambulatory pH monitoring.

GERD is managed with a combination of lifestyle changes and medications. Histamine-2 receptor blockers and proton-pump inhibitors are often ordered to suppress acid secretion in the stomach and promote esophageal healing. Table 25-5 later in the chapter discusses the nursing implications and patient teaching for these drugs.

Surgery may be used for patients who do not respond to more conservative GERD management. Surgeries such as laparoscopic fundoplication and Nissen fundoplication (Figure 25-6■) increase pressure in the lower esophagus, decreasing gastric reflux. In these procedures, the gastric fundus is wrapped around the distal esophagus.

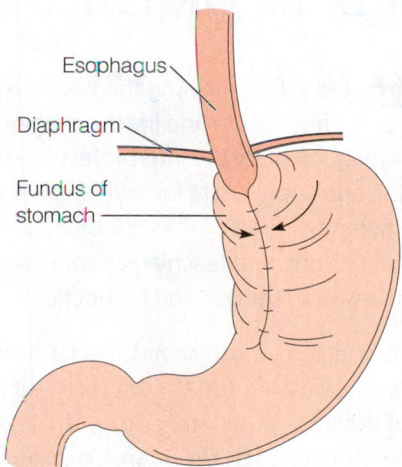

Esophagus

Diaphragm

Fundus of stomach

Figure 25-6. ■ Nissen fundoplication procedure. The fundus of the stomach is wrapped around the lower esophagus, and the edges are sutured together.

NURSING CARE

Nursing care for patients with GERD focuses on teaching. Instruct patients to avoid lying down within 3 hours after meals and to elevate the head of the bed on 6-in. blocks or use a foam wedge when sleeping. Discuss the need to avoid using alcohol and tobacco. Provide information about smoking cessation and support groups as needed. Weight loss, smaller meals, and avoiding bending may help to relieve symptoms. Discuss diet changes, such as avoiding acidic foods (e.g., orange juice) and foods that affect the lower esophageal sphincter or gastric emptying (fatty foods, peppermint, and chocolate).

Hiatal Hernia

A *hiatal hernia* occurs when part of the stomach protrudes through the opening of the diaphragm into the chest cavity. Hiatal hernias usually occur with aging or because of increased intra-abdominal pressure. Most people have no symptoms; however, upper GI bleeding or erosive esophagitis are potential complications of hiatal hernia.

With a *sliding hernia* (the more common type), part of the stomach slides through the opening of the diaphragm when the patient reclines and moves back into place when the patient stands. With a *paraesophageal hernia*, part of the stomach protrudes through the opening beside the esophagus.

The same medical, lifestyle, and pharmacologic interventions used for GERD are usually prescribed for patients with hiatal hernia. If the hernia becomes trapped, impairing blood flow to the hernia, surgery may be necessary. Nursing care for the patient undergoing hiatal hernia surgery is similar to that for a patient undergoing other abdominal or thoracic surgery.

Esophageal Cancer

Cancer of the esophagus is relatively uncommon in the United States, diagnosed in fewer than 17,000 people in 2013. Cigarette smoking and alcohol consumption, particularly in combination, are the major risk factors for esophageal cancer. Esophageal cancer is diagnosed four times more frequently in men than in women (American Cancer Society, 2013).

Most tumors affect the middle or lower third of the esophagus. The most common symptom, which often does not develop until late in the disease, is **dysphagia** (difficulty or pain in swallowing). Later symptoms include reflux, weight loss, regurgitation, and blood loss.

Treatment may involve surgery, radiation therapy, and/or chemotherapy. Controlling dysphagia is essential; many patients with esophageal cancer are undernourished because of dysphagia. Total parenteral nutrition (TPN) or enteral (tube) feedings may be needed to maintain weight and nutrition (see Boxes 25-6 and 25-7). A gastrostomy tube may be inserted.

After surgery, the patient is at high risk for aspiration and airway problems. Assess level of consciousness and respiratory status at least every hour after surgery. Encourage coughing and deep breathing every 1 to 2 hours and as needed.

Teach the patient, family members, and caregivers about the diagnosis and prescribed treatment, including wound care and follow-up care. If tube feedings or TPN will be continued at home, have the patient and caregivers demonstrate skills required to perform the procedure. Refer the patient to home health services or hospice as indicated.

DISORDERS OF THE STOMACH AND DUODENUM

Key Concept Disorders affecting the stomach and duodenum range from acute and life threatening, requiring emergent management by the interprofessional team, to self-limiting and appropriate for self-care. The nurse monitors patient responses to these disorders, providing support, interventions, and teaching as appropriate to maintain and restore nutrition and GI function.

The stomach and upper intestinal tract (duodenum and jejunum) are responsible for the majority of food digestion. Gastroenteritis, gastritis, peptic ulcer disease, and cancer of the stomach are the major disorders affecting food intake and digestion. These disorders also can lead to GI hemorrhage, one of the top 20 diagnoses leading to hospital admission. Nurses provide both acute care for the hospitalized patient and teaching for the patient who will manage these conditions at home.

Gastrointestinal Bleeding

Because the GI tract is constantly exposed to the environment, it can be affected by trauma, toxins, infection, inflammation, and insults such as ischemia. The rich blood supply of the GI tract can lead to significant bleeding when a vessel is affected.

safety**ALERT**

Gastrointestinal hemorrhage is a medical emergency requiring aggressive medical and nursing care.

Bleeding can occur in any portion of the GI tract. The upper GI tract (lower esophagus, stomach, and duodenum), however, is more commonly affected. Peptic ulcer disease, erosive gastritis, and esophageal varices are the three most common causes of upper GI hemorrhage. Gastritis and peptic ulcer disease are discussed later in this chapter; esophageal varices, usually seen as a complication of cirrhosis of the liver, are discussed in Chapter 27.

PATHOPHYSIOLOGY AND MANIFESTATIONS

Blood is irritating to the GI tract, typically causing nausea and vomiting (**hematemesis**, vomiting blood) when in the stomach. If bleeding has been slow and the blood is partially digested, it may look like "coffee grounds," not bright red blood. Blood in the GI tract stimulates peristalsis, leading to hyperactive bowel sounds and diarrhea. Stools may be black and tarry (**melena**) or frankly bloody (**hematochezia**); stool containing partially digested blood has a characteristic odor.

The effects of a GI bleed on other body systems depend on the speed and extent of the bleeding. Slow GI bleeding may not be identified until the patient develops symptoms of anemia. Although feces may not appear bloody, **occult** (hidden) bleeding may be detected by laboratory testing (e.g., guaiac or Hemoccult smears).

GI hemorrhage, with rapid loss of a significant amount of blood, depletes blood volume. Cardiac output falls, leading to tachycardia, hypotension, pallor, and decreased urine output. Peripheral blood vessels constrict to maintain blood flow to vital organs. Unless the blood volume is restored, hypovolemic shock progresses and may become irreversible. See Chapter 14 for more information about shock and its management.

COLLABORATIVE CARE

Diagnosis and treatment of an upper GI hemorrhage depends on the extent of the bleeding and the patient's condition. When GI hemorrhage is massive, stopping bleeding and restoring blood volume are the highest priorities; diagnostic testing is postponed until the patient's condition has been stabilized. When the bleeding is slow or chronic, diagnosis and treatment may be managed in a community-based setting.

Diagnostic Tests

- A *CBC with hemoglobin and hematocrit, serum electrolytes, osmolality,* and *blood urea nitrogen (BUN)* are obtained.
- *Blood type and crossmatch* may be done to prepare for transfusion.
- *Liver function studies* and a *coagulation profile* may be done to help identify the cause of bleeding.
- An *upper endoscopy* is performed as soon as possible to identify and, if possible, treat the source of bleeding.

Treatments

In acute hemorrhage, initial treatment focuses on stopping the bleeding and restoring cardiovascular stability. Intravenous fluids are administered through a large-bore intravenous catheter. Fresh whole blood or packed red cells may be given to restore blood volume and oxygen-carrying capacity.

Whenever possible, upper endoscopy is used to stop bleeding. The bleeding vessel is sealed using an injected sclerosing agent, heated probe, cautery, or laser. Rarely, emergency surgery is required to stop hemorrhage.

GASTRIC LAVAGE   Gastric lavage, washing out of stomach contents, may be done to remove blood from the GI tract, prevent vomiting, and prepare for upper endoscopy. See Box 25-10■ for nursing responsibilities related to gastric lavage.

NURSING CARE

PRIORITIZING NURSING CARE

Nursing care priorities for the patient with an acute GI bleed focus on restoring and maintaining the cardiac output and tissue perfusion, stopping the hemorrhage, and preventing further bleeding.

HEALTH PROMOTION

Preventing GI bleeding is critical to reduce risks associated with acute GI hemorrhage. Identifying patients at risk, monitoring gastric pH, and maintaining drug therapy to reduce gastric acidity are important preventive measures. All critically ill patients should be considered to be at risk for stress-related erosive gastritis.

ASSESSING

When hemorrhage is acute, assessment is very focused. If possible, ask about risk factors such as use of aspirin, platelet inhibitors, or anticoagulant medications, and any acute or chronic conditions that may contribute to bleeding (e.g., a clotting disorder, peptic ulcer disease, chronic hepatitis, or cirrhosis of the liver). If possible, note all current medications and any known allergies to medications or other substances.

Obtain vital signs and orthostatic vital signs (an early sign of hypovolemia). Place the acutely ill patient on a cardiac monitor and obtain a rhythm strip. Monitor oxygen saturation level. Note skin color and temperature, peripheral pulses, and capillary refill. Assess mental status, including level of consciousness and orientation. An indwelling catheter may be inserted to evaluate urine output.

IDENTIFYING POTENTIAL COMPLICATIONS

Report changes in skin color, temperature, and moisture, or slow capillary refill; agitation or a decline in mental status; or urine output less than 30 mL/hr. Development of cyanosis

BOX 25-10 PROCEDURE CHECKLIST

Gastric Lavage

☑ Obtain all supplies.

☑ Verify the patient's identity and provide for privacy.

☑ Use Standard Precautions.

☑ Explain the procedure. Instruct the patient to report any pain, difficulty breathing, or other problems during the procedure.

☑ Document baseline vital signs, abdominal girth, and bowel sounds.

☑ Place the patient in semi-Fowler's or Fowler's position. If hypotension is present, place in left side-lying position (see figure).

☑ Insert an NG tube (14 to 16 French, unless otherwise indicated) if one is not already in place, and verify placement. (See Box 25-5.)

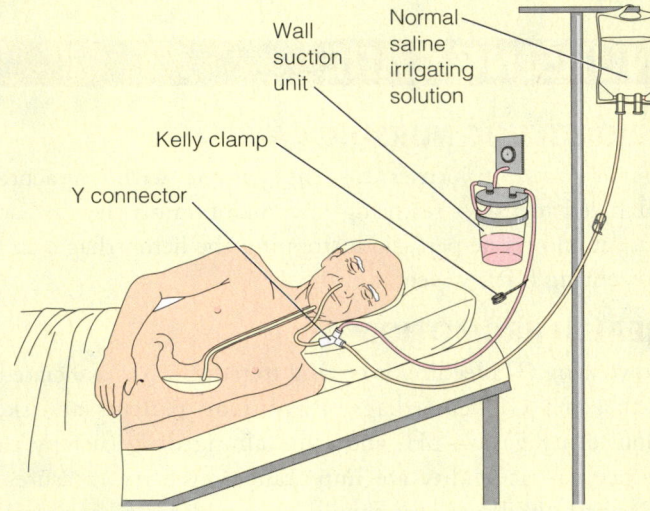

Wall suction unit

Normal saline irrigating solution

Kelly clamp

Y connector

A patient with a closed gastric lavage system.

Closed System Irrigation

Connect irrigating solution to NG tube with Y connector. Attach drainage or suction tube to other arm of connector. Empty the stomach, clamp drain tube or turn off suction, and allow 50 to 200 mL of solution to run into stomach by gravity. Stop solution and allow to drain or suction out. Repeat until ordered amount has been used or desired results are obtained. Measure the drainage, subtracting the amount of irrigant instilled, to obtain gastric output.

Intermittent Open System

Empty the stomach using suction or a 50-mL catheter-tip syringe. Measure and discard the aspirate. Using the syringe, draw up approximately 50 mL of irrigation solution, and instill it using gentle pressure. Withdraw and discard the solution into a measuring container. Continue until the desired amount of irrigant or desired results have been obtained.

☑ Monitor vital signs, respiratory status, and patient tolerance during the procedure.

☑ Notify the charge nurse or physician if the procedure is ineffective or the patient is unable to tolerate it.

Sample Documentation

[date] 1630   Gastric lavage with 750 mL normal saline. Irrigant returned clear; no bleeding noted. 50 mL gastric contents returned with irrigant. Tolerated procedure well with no abdominal or respiratory distress.

_____ S. Williams, LPN.

Note: Refer to a nursing fundamentals or skills text for more detailed instruction. Check state guidelines and facility policy before performing any procedure.

or mottling, impaired mentation, and inadequate urine output indicate ineffective tissue perfusion and oxygenation.

DIAGNOSING, PLANNING, AND IMPLEMENTING

Significant amounts of blood may be lost in a very short time with an acute GI hemorrhage, affecting cardiac output and tissue perfusion.

Bleeding

Expected outcomes: Demonstrates no further signs of GI bleeding. Vital signs, mental status, urine output, and skin color will remain stable and within expected range.

■ Frequently monitor and record vital signs and oxygen saturation until stable. Closely monitor urinary output.

clinicalALERT

Monitor urine output and report output of less than 30 mL/hr for 2 consecutive hours. Low urine output may indicate poor blood flow to the kidneys due to hypovolemia and decreased cardiac output, and an increased risk for acute kidney injury.

Weigh daily. _Careful monitoring is essential to identify possible shock and to intervene at an early stage._

■ Monitor stools and gastric drainage for visible and occult blood. Assess gastric drainage to estimate the amount and rate of hemorrhage. _Drainage is bright red with possible clots in acute hemorrhage and dark red or the color of coffee grounds when blood has been in the stomach for a period of time. Hematochezia is present in acute hemorrhage; melena indicates less acute bleeding._

■ Maintain intravenous infusions and assist with blood administration as needed. _Intravenous fluids and blood products are given to restore blood volume and oxygen-carrying capacity._

■ Frequently monitor hemoglobin and hematocrit. Monitor serum electrolytes and BUN. Report abnormal findings. _The hemoglobin and hematocrit provide data about the extent of blood loss and the blood's oxygen-carrying capacity. Electrolytes are lost through vomiting, gastric drainage, and diarrhea. Digestion and absorption of blood in the GI tract may cause elevated BUN levels._

- Insert an NG tube and maintain its position and patency. Initially, measure and record gastric output hourly, and then every 4 to 8 hours. *NG suction removes blood from the GI tract, preventing vomiting and possible aspiration. Gastric output is replaced with a balanced electrolyte solution to maintain homeostasis.*
- Assess abdomen, including bowel sounds, girth, and tenderness every 4 hours and record findings. *Borborygmi and abdominal tenderness are common in patients with acute GI bleeding. Increased abdominal girth, absent bowel sounds, or extreme tenderness with a rigid, boardlike abdomen may indicate perforation.*
- Prepare for possible endoscopy. *Endoscopy can identify bleeding sites and allow direct treatment of the erosion.*
- Maintain bed rest with the head of the bed elevated; ensure safety. *Loss of blood volume may cause orthostatic hypotension with syncope or dizziness upon standing.*

MANAGING NURSING CARE

Comfort and hygiene measures for the patient with acute GI bleeding and assisting with positioning and allowed activities may be appropriate to assign to assistive personnel.

EVALUATING

Monitor data related to cardiac output (vital signs, mental status, skin color and temperature, peripheral pulses, capillary refill, and urine output) to determine the effectiveness of medical and nursing interventions. Note the color of gastric and bowel output, and examine for occult blood to determine the effectiveness of interventions to stop and prevent further bleeding.

DOCUMENTING

Document assessments on a regular and continuing basis, reporting significant changes or abnormal data. Maintain accurate intake and output records. Note the patient's responses to interventions such as gastric lavage.

CONTINUITY OF CARE

After an acute GI hemorrhage, continuing care focuses on treating an underlying disease process and preventing future episodes of GI bleeding. The patient may be instructed to continue taking a gastric acid–reducing medication and avoid known gastric irritants such as aspirin and alcohol.

Patients with minor or slow GI bleeding often are managed in the community. Provide teaching about the cause of the bleeding and how to prevent future episodes. Provide verbal and written instructions for prescribed medications, such as acid reducers and oral iron supplements. Discuss diet recommendations; although a special diet to "soothe the stomach" rarely is indicated, foods rich in iron may be encouraged to treat anemia.

Discuss indicators of GI bleeding to be reported to the physician. If the source of bleeding has not been identified, provide instructions about prescribed follow-up diagnostic testing.

Gastritis and Gastroenteritis

Ingestion of irritating, toxic, or contaminated foods or substances can cause inflammation of the stomach and upper intestinal lining. **Gastritis**, inflammation of the stomach lining, is a common disorder, usually caused by ingesting irritants such as aspirin, alcohol, caffeine, or foods contaminated with certain bacteria. **Gastroenteritis** is inflammation of the stomach and intestines. It usually is caused by a bacterial, viral, or parasitic infection or by a toxin. Bacterial and viral infections are often termed *food poisoning*, because contaminated food is the usual route of entry. In recent years, *norovirus*, a highly contagious viral gastroenteritis transmitted by the fecal–oral route, has caused large outbreaks of illness of residents and health care workers in community-based and long-term care settings.

PATHOPHYSIOLOGY AND MANIFESTATIONS
Acute Gastritis

Normally, the stomach and duodenum are protected by the mucosal barrier (see Figure 25-7 in the section on peptic ulcers). In acute gastritis, a local irritant disrupts the mucosal barrier, allowing gastric juices to come into contact with the gastric tissue. This causes irritation, inflammation, and superficial erosions. The gastric mucosa rapidly regenerates, and healing occurs within several days.

Acute gastritis often is caused by drugs such as aspirin, nonsteroidal anti-inflammatory drugs (NSAIDs), corticosteroids, and chemotherapy. Bacterial toxins in contaminated food can cause an abrupt, severe gastritis. Ingestion of a strong alkali (e.g., ammonia) or acid severely damages the stomach and may lead to perforation, hemorrhage, and peritonitis.

Erosive or *stress-induced gastritis* (a severe form of acute gastritis) is a potential complication of conditions such as shock, severe trauma, or major surgery. Decreased blood flow to the gastric mucosa leads to superficial erosions and a significant risk for bleeding.

The patient with acute gastritis may have few symptoms. Possible manifestations are listed in Box 25-11■. Gastric bleeding may occur, causing hematemesis or melena.

clinicalALERT

Patients with stress gastritis often have no symptoms until signs of severe bleeding, shock, or an *acute abdomen* (severely painful, rigid, boardlike abdomen) develop.

MANIFESTATIONS OF GASTRITIS AND GASTROENTERITIS

Acute Gastritis
- Anorexia
- Nausea and vomiting
- Abdominal pain or discomfort
- Hematemesis (vomiting blood)
- Melena (black, tarry stool)

General
- Anemia
- Fatigue

Gastroenteritis
- Anorexia
- Nausea and vomiting
- Abdominal pain and cramping
- *Borborygmi* (loud, hyperactive bowel sounds)
- Diarrhea

General
- Malaise, weakness
- Dehydration
- Fever

Gastroenteritis

Acute bacterial or viral infection of the GI tract produces inflammation, tissue damage, and symptoms by two primary mechanisms:

1. *Production of enterotoxins.* Many bacteria produce and excrete a toxin that damages and inflames the GI tract. Enterotoxins impair intestinal absorption and can cause electrolytes and water to be secreted into the bowel, leading to diarrhea and fluid loss.

2. *Invasion and ulceration of the mucosa.* Other bacteria invade intestinal mucosa, causing ulceration, bleeding, fluid exudate, and water and electrolyte secretion.

Manifestations of bacterial and viral enteritis vary by organism but have several common features (see Box 25-11). Excess fluid in the bowel and increased bowel motility cause diarrhea with frequent, watery stools. Lost fluids and electrolytes can lead to dehydration, hypovolemia, and manifestations of fluid and electrolyte or acid–base imbalances.

Severe vomiting may lead to metabolic alkalosis. With diarrhea, metabolic acidosis is more likely. Potassium and sodium are lost, leading to possible hypokalemia and hyponatremia. The specific effects of certain GI infections are summarized in Table 25-4 ■.

COLLABORATIVE CARE

Identifying the cause, managing symptoms, and preventing complications are the primary goals of care. For patients at risk for erosive gastritis (e.g., critically ill patients), prevention is the primary focus. The patient's history and symptoms provide valuable clues about the cause. Gastritis and gastroenteritis usually are treated in community-based settings unless vomiting or diarrhea is severe or bleeding occurs.

Diagnostic Tests

The following diagnostic tests may be ordered:
- *Hemoglobin* and *hematocrit* are used to identify possible anemia due to bleeding.
- *Serum electrolytes* are obtained to evaluate the effect of vomiting and diarrhea on fluid and electrolyte balance.
- A *stool specimen* may be obtained for testing and examination for the suspected organism.
- *Gastric pH* and *gastric analysis* are used to assess the acidity of gastric fluid and hydrochloric acid secretion.
- *Endoscopy* may be done to inspect the gastric mucosa. Areas of bleeding may be treated directly.

Medications

Antiemetics and antacids may be ordered to relieve vomiting and gastric distress. An antidiarrheal drug may be prescribed to promote comfort and reduce fluid loss. Nursing measures related to the use of antidiarrheal agents are outlined in Table 26-2. Antibiotic therapy may be used to treat bacterial gastroenteritis.

Proton-pump inhibitors such as lansoprazole (Prevacid) or *omeprazole* (Prilosec) or histamine-2 (H$_2$)–receptor antagonists (e.g., cimetidine or *famotidine*) may be ordered to prevent or treat acute stress gastritis. Sucralfate (Carafate), a drug that works locally to protect gastric tissue, may also be used. Table 25-5 ■ outlines nursing implications and patient teaching for these drugs.

Food and Fluid Management

Maintaining fluid and electrolyte balance is a primary focus of care in gastritis and gastroenteritis. Initially, a short period of GI tract rest may be prescribed, but rehydration is critical for patients with severe vomiting and diarrhea. Oral rehydration is optimal. An oral glucose–electrolyte solution is often well tolerated in sips, even by the patient who is vomiting. Commercial or homemade preparations may be used. Intravenous fluids such as glucose in normal saline, Ringer, or lactated Ringer solution may be ordered when vomiting and diarrhea are severe. When tolerated, clear liquids (broth, tea, gelatin, carbonated beverages) are reintroduced, followed by heavier liquids (cream soups, puddings, milk), and finally solid foods.

Other Therapies

When acute gastritis results from ingesting a poisonous or corrosive substance (acid or strong alkali), the substance must immediately be diluted and removed. Vomiting is not induced because it might further damage the esophagus and trachea. Instead, gastric lavage is performed (see Box 25-10). Gastric lavage and catharsis also may be ordered if botulism is suspected and if the food has been recently ingested. Botulism antitoxin is administered as soon as

TABLE 25-4		Selected Causes and Characteristics of Gastroenteritis	
DISEASE AND ORGANISM	**INCUBATION**	**SOURCE**	**MANIFESTATIONS**
Norovirus	24–48 hours	Contaminated food or water; direct person-to-person spread	Abrupt onset of vomiting, watery nonbloody diarrhea, abdominal cramping, nausea; possible low-grade fever
Traveler's diarrhea *Escherichia coli*	24–72 hours	Contaminated food or water	Abrupt onset of diarrhea; vomiting rare
Staphylococcal food poisoning	2–8 hours	Contaminated food—meats and fish, dairy products	Severe nausea and vomiting; abdominal cramping and diarrhea; headache and fever
Botulism *Clostridium botulinum*	1.5–8 days	Improperly preserved foods such as home-canned vegetables, smoked meats, vacuum-packed fish	Diplopia, blurred vision; dry mouth, dysphagia; progressive muscle weakness and paralysis; possible nausea, vomiting, abdominal cramps
Clostridium difficile colitis	1–2 weeks	Opportunistic infection related to broad-spectrum antibiotic therapy Fecal–oral contamination; usually hospital acquired	Mild to moderate diarrhea; lower abdominal cramping May cause *pseudomembranous colitis* with acute symptoms of lethargy, fever, tachycardia, abdominal pain and distention, and dehydration
Hemorrhagic colitis *E. coli 0157:H7*	1–3 days	Undercooked beef; unpasteurized milk or apple juice	Severe cramping, watery to grossly bloody diarrhea; fever; complications of acute kidney injury and thrombotic thrombocytopenic purpura
Salmonellosis *Salmonella*	8–48 hours	Raw or improperly cooked meat, poultry, eggs, and dairy products	Diarrhea with cramping, nausea, and vomiting; low-grade fever, chills, weakness
Giardiasis *Giardia lamblia*	1–3 weeks	Fecal–oral spread through contaminated food or water; direct contact	Diarrhea, mild or severe; anorexia, nausea, vomiting; epigastric pain, cramping; flatulence and belching; may be asymptomatic
Amebiasis *Entamoeba histolytica*	2–4 weeks	Fecal–oral spread through contaminated food or water; direct contact	Usually asymptomatic; diarrhea with blood and mucus; abdominal cramping, tenderness, colic, tenesmus, and flatulence; nausea and vomiting; fever, fatigue, weight loss

possible when botulism is suspected. It can prevent paralysis from progressing but does not affect existing paralysis. Epinephrine is kept at the bedside because the antitoxin can cause anaphylaxis. The patient is observed closely for signs of respiratory distress. Respiratory support with endotracheal intubation and mechanical ventilation may be required.

clinicalAlert

Antidiarrheal agents are not used when botulism is suspected. To remove the toxin from the bowel, cathartics may be ordered for these patients.

Complementary Therapies

Complementary therapies such as herbal remedies or aromatherapy may be appropriate to recommend for patients with acute gastritis. Refer the patient to a health care provider trained in natural and herbal remedies or to an aromatherapist for an individualized treatment plan. Recommendations may include:

- Chamomile tea or the essential oil used in aromatherapy
- Garlic; one clove chopped fine and taken daily at bedtime
- Ginger; powdered, capsules, or made into a tea taken before or after meals
- Mint oil aromatherapy via a diffuser, in a bath, or diluted with a carrier oil and used for a soothing massage

NURSING CARE

PRIORITIZING NURSING CARE

The effects of acute gastritis or gastroenteritis and their manifestations on fluid balance and intravascular volume are the priority nursing care focus for the patient with these

TABLE 25-5	Giving Medications Safely: GERD, Gastritis, and Peptic Ulcer Disease		
CLASS/DRUGS	**PURPOSE**	**NURSING IMPLICATIONS**	**PATIENT TEACHING**
Proton-pump inhibitors ■ Esomeprazole (Nexium) ■ *Lansoprazole (Prevacid)* ■ Omeprazole (Prilosec) ■ *Pantoprazole (Protonix)* ■ Rabeprazole (AcipHex)	These drugs significantly reduce gastric acid secretion and the amount of acid in the stomach between and after meals. They are used to heal and prevent recurrence of peptic ulcers and for GERD.	Administer at bedtime or before breakfast. Do not open or crush capsules or tablets. Monitor liver function tests and report abnormal results. These drugs may slow the elimination of diazepam, warfarin, and phenytoin; monitor for adverse effects.	Take at bedtime or before breakfast. Take the drug for the full course of therapy, even if you feel better. Do not smoke, drink alcohol, or take aspirin or NSAIDs while taking this drug because they may interfere with healing. Adverse effects are rare with these drugs but should be reported to the physician.
H$_2$-receptor blockers ■ Cimetidine (Tagamet) ■ *Famotidine (Pepcid)* ■ Nizatidine (Axid) ■ *Ranitidine (Zantac)*	H$_2$-receptor blockers reduce stomach acid by blocking the acid-stimulating effects of histamine. This reduces the volume and concentration of hydrochloric acid in the stomach.	Should not be taken during pregnancy and lactation. Administer 30 minutes before meals and at bedtime or as ordered. Do not administer antacids within 1 hour before or after these drugs to ensure absorption. When given intravenously, do not mix with other drugs. Administer in 20–100 mL of solution over 15–30 minutes.	Take as directed, even after pain and gastric discomfort are relieved. Avoid taking antacids for 1 hour before and 1 hour after taking H$_2$ blockers. Report any of the following to the physician: diarrhea, confusion, rash, fatigue, malaise, or bruising.
Antacids ■ Aluminum hydroxide (Amphojel, ALternaGEL) ■ Magnesium hydroxide (Milk of Magnesia) ■ Calcium carbonate (Tums) ■ Magnesium hydroxide and aluminum hydroxide (Maalox, Mylanta, Gelusil)	Antacids buffer or neutralize gastric acid, generally by a local action. They help relieve pain and prevent further damage to the gastric mucosa.	Antacids interfere with absorption of many drugs; separate dosage times by at least 2 hours. Monitor for constipation or diarrhea. Notify the physician should either occur; a different antacid may be prescribed. Monitor for electrolyte imbalances in patients taking high doses of antacids.	Do not use sodium bicarbonate as an antacid because of its local and systemic effects. Take as prescribed; to work effectively, the antacid must be in the stomach. Avoid taking the antacid for approximately 2 hours before and after taking other medication. Report diarrhea or constipation to the physician. Continue taking the antacid for the duration prescribed; mucosal healing takes 6–8 weeks.
■ Sucralfate	Sucralfate creates a protective barrier against gastric juices. It does not neutralize gastric acid or affect its secretion.	Give on an empty stomach 1 hour before meals and at bedtime or as ordered. Sucralfate may interfere with absorption of other drugs; separate administration times by at least 2 hours.	This drug has few side effects. Constipation may rarely develop. If you have difficulty swallowing the tablets, an oral suspension is available.
Bismuth compounds ■ Bismuth subsalicylate (Pepto-Bismol) ■ Ranitidine bismuth citrate (Tritec)	Bismuth has a local antibiotic effect on *H. pylori*; it also may help prevent the bacteria from adhering to the gastric mucosa.	Do not give bismuth subsalicylate if fecal impaction is suspected. This drug is contraindicated for patients who are allergic to aspirin.	This drug may cause stools to turn dark or appear black. Do not take this drug if you are allergic to aspirin. Do not give this drug to children who have chickenpox or another viral illness.
■ Misoprostol (Cytotec)	Misoprostol is a synthetic prostaglandin used to prevent ulcers in patients who require long-term NSAID therapy.	Do not give during pregnancy because it may cause abortion of the fetus. Administer with meals and at bedtime.	Stress the importance of avoiding this drug during pregnancy. May cause diarrhea, abdominal pain, spotting, and uterine cramps. Report these effects to the doctor.

Note: Medications identified in *italics* are among the 200 most frequently prescribed drugs in the United States.

disorders. In an acute outbreak, preventing the spread of gastroenteritis is a major focus of nursing care.

HEALTH PROMOTION

Teach patients in all settings the following food and water safety measures:

- Maintain proper food temperatures. Promptly refrigerate cooked meats, dairy products, eggs, and egg products.
- Do not drink unpasteurized milk.
- Do not eat raw meat products. Cook hamburger until no redness remains.
- Follow directions precisely when home-canning foods; use a pressure canner when processing nonacidic foods, such as vegetables, mushrooms, meats, and fish.
- Boil home-canned foods for 10 to 15 minutes after opening to destroy any potential toxin.
- Destroy, without touching or tasting, any food that is discolored or comes from a container that has been punctured, is cracked or bulging, or does not have a tight seal.
- When using untreated water, boil, filter, or treat it with water purification tablets.
- Where water is untreated or sanitation is poor, avoid foods that cannot be peeled or cooked.
- When traveling out of the country, consume only bottled water unless local water supplies are clearly safe.

ASSESSING

Collect data regarding the onset, duration, and nature of the patient's symptoms. Ask specifically about foods, fluids, and other substances (e.g., aspirin or other drugs) that have been taken recently. Inquire about recent travel, changes in diet or water supply, or activities such as picnics or potluck meals. Ask about others in the family or household who also may be experiencing symptoms. Ask about the frequency and severity of vomiting and diarrhea and the nature of diarrheal stools. Ask about other manifestations such as abdominal pain or cramping. Inquire about measures taken to relieve the symptoms and the ability to take in and retain fluids. Inspect the abdomen and auscultate bowel sounds. Measure abdominal girth, and lightly palpate for tenderness. Measure and document the color and character of any emesis or stools.

IDENTIFYING POTENTIAL COMPLICATIONS

Inquire about evidence of bleeding in vomitus or stools. Note appearance and any visible distress. Assess vital signs, including orthostatic blood pressures. Obtain weight. Assess mucous membranes, skin turgor, and tongue. Monitor the results of laboratory and diagnostic testing, particularly the hemoglobin and hematocrit. Monitor serum electrolyte values and results of arterial blood gases for acid–base balance.

DIAGNOSING, PLANNING, AND IMPLEMENTING
Deficient Fluid Volume

Expected outcome: Vital signs, weight, urine output, skin, and mental status will remain within normal or expected ranges.

Nausea, vomiting, and abdominal distress are the primary manifestations of acute gastritis. Fluid and electrolyte imbalances may develop as a result.

- Frequently monitor vital signs, including orthostatic vital signs. *Tachycardia and orthostatic hypotension may indicate fluid volume deficit. Electrolyte imbalances may affect heart rate and rhythm, as well as blood pressure.*
- Monitor and record intake and output. Weigh daily. *Intake and output records and daily weights provide important data about fluid balance.*
- Provide meticulous skin and mouth care frequently. *Patients with fluid volume deficit are at high risk for impaired skin and mucous membrane integrity.*
- Report significant changes or deviations from normal laboratory values for electrolytes and acid–base balance. *Significant changes in electrolyte or acid–base balance may occur as a result of vomiting and poor food and fluid intake.*
- Provide fluids by mouth or parenterally as ordered. *Oral fluids are gradually reintroduced when the patient is no longer vomiting. Intravenous fluids restore or maintain hydration until adequate oral intake is resumed.*
- Administer antiemetic and other medications as ordered to relieve nausea and vomiting. *Medications can help prevent or relieve vomiting and can promote oral intake.*
- Provide for the safety of patients with orthostatic hypotension: Place the signal light within reach; put up the side rails; instruct the patient not to get up or walk without assistance. *Orthostatic hypotension may lead to fainting or falls.*

Risk for Infection

Expected outcome: Will remain free of infection.

- Maintain Standard Precautions with careful attention to appropriate use of gloves and hand washing. *When used in all health care facilities and with all patients, Standard Precautions limit the spread of disease-causing organisms present in blood, body fluids, and feces from one person to another.*
- Institute Contact Precautions for any patient who is incontinent and when an outbreak of gastroenteritis is suspected. Wear a mask when cleaning areas heavily contaminated with vomitus or feces. *Norovirus is highly contagious and can be transmitted via direct contact with contaminated clothing or surfaces.*

■ Place patients with symptoms of acute gastroenteritis in a private room. If several patients are affected, they may be confined to a specific area away from other patients/residents. *Isolating affected patients from others helps prevent the spread of the disease to other populations.*

■ Thoroughly clean contaminated surfaces, and then disinfect using an EPA-approved disinfectant or bleach. *Disinfectants work most effectively on clean surfaces.*

MANAGING NURSING CARE

Nursing care activities such as measuring intake and output and assisting with toileting and hygiene for the patient with gastritis or gastroenteritis are appropriate to assign to assistive personnel.

EVALUATING

Collect the following data to evaluate the effectiveness of nursing care: indicators of fluid and electrolyte balance, such as thirst, skin turgor, weight, intake and output, mental status, and laboratory values; appetite and food intake; skin condition, color, and other indicators of nutritional status.

DOCUMENTING

Document manifestations of the disorder and the response to treatment. Document continuing assessment data, particularly any episodes of vomiting, diarrhea, and the presence of blood in emesis or stool. Note the patient's ability to resume normal food and fluid intake.

CONTINUITY OF CARE

Teaching is a vital component of nursing care for patients who are managed at home or in a community-based care setting. Teach patients how to identify and avoid causative factors, manage acute symptoms, and reintroduce fluids and foods, and when to contact the physician (unrelieved vomiting, severe weight loss, changes in mental status, or lack of urine output). Emphasize that fluid replacement is more important than eating while diarrhea is severe. Advise use of a glucose–electrolyte solution such as Pedialyte or Gatorade. A solution of 1 quart (1 L) of clean water, 1 teaspoon (5 mL) each of table salt and baking soda, 4 teaspoons (20 mL) of granulated sugar, and desired flavoring (e.g., lemon juice or extract) can be made at home to replace water and electrolytes. Discuss manifestations of dehydration or hypovolemia that require a physician's care.

Teach the importance of good hand washing to prevent spread of infection to others. Instruct to wash hands thoroughly with soap and running water for at least 10 seconds after each defecation. Wash contaminated clothing and linens separately in hot water and detergent. Emphasize the need to keep toilet areas clean and to maintain good personal hygiene. Advise avoiding rectal contact during sexual activity.

Peptic Ulcer Disease

A **peptic ulcer** is a break in the mucous lining of the stomach or duodenum where it comes in contact with gastric juice. *Peptic ulcer disease* (PUD) is a chronic health problem that primarily affects adults (often duodenal ulcers in young and middle adults, and gastric ulcers in older adults). Chronic *H. pylori* infection and ingestion of aspirin and other NSAIDs are the major risk factors. Cigarette smoking doubles the risk of PUD.

PATHOPHYSIOLOGY

The mucosal barrier protects the gastric mucosa (Figure 25-7■). It is maintained by (1) bicarbonate secreted by epithelial cells, (2) mucous gel produced in response to prostaglandins, and (3) an adequate blood supply to the mucosa. Ulcers develop when the mucosal barrier is unable to prevent damage by gastric digestive juices.

The mucosal barrier can be damaged by poor circulation, decreased mucus, or reflux of bile or pancreatic enzymes into the stomach or duodenum. Aspirin and other NSAIDs inhibit prostaglandins and mucous gel production.

About three-fourths of the people with PUD have *H. pylori* infection. This bacterium secretes substances that break down mucous gel and also appears to stimulate acid production in the stomach. It also causes an inflammatory response in the lining of the stomach. Cigarette smoking contributes by inhibiting bicarbonate secretion.

Ulcers may develop in the esophagus, stomach, or duodenum. In the stomach, the lesser curvature and area closest to the pylorus are most often affected (Figure 25-8■). Ulcers may be superficial or deep, affecting all layers of the mucosa (Figure 25-9■).

MANIFESTATIONS

Epigastric pain is the classic symptom of PUD. The pain is often described as gnawing, burning, aching, or hunger-like. It occurs when the stomach is empty (2 to 3 hours after meals and during the night) and is relieved by eating. It may radiate to the back. The patient may complain of heartburn or regurgitation and vomiting. Older adults with PUD may have no symptoms or may complain of vague discomfort, chest pain, or dysphagia. Weight loss or anemia may be present. Manifestations of PUD are listed in Box 25-12■.

Complications

Potential complications of PUD include hemorrhage, obstruction, and perforation. *Hemorrhage* results from ulceration and erosion into blood vessels of the gastric mucosa. Erosion into small blood vessels may cause slow bleeding and black, tarry stools. Erosion into a larger vessel can lead to sudden, severe bleeding with hematemesis or

Normal gastric mucosa

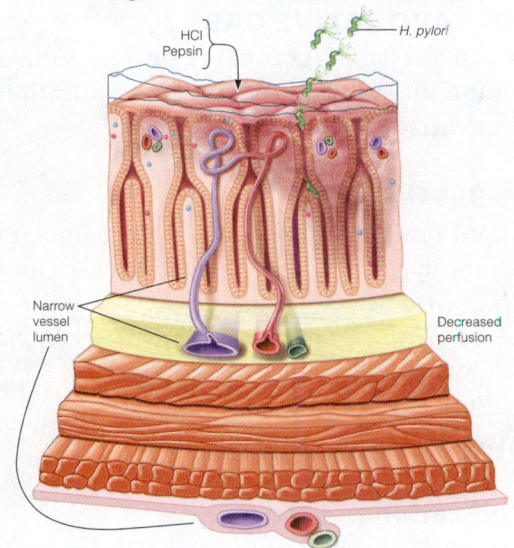

In the stomach and duodenum, the mucosal barrier constantly bathes surfaces, protecting the mucosa from damage.

Mucus serves as a barrier to hydrogen ion and pepsin in gastric juices. A thin layer of bicarbonate forms between the mucus and cell membranes.

Adequate blood flow to the gastric mucosa, prostaglandins, and nitric oxide are necessary to maintain the mucosal barrier.

Disruption of the mucosal barrier and inflammation

Ischemia, aspirin and other NSAIDs (which inhibit prostaglandins), alcohol, and bile acids can disrupt the mucosal barrier.

Helicobacter pylori, a common pathogen that infects the gastric mucosa, also disrupts the mucosal barrier.

When this critical barrier is disrupted, gastric acid and digestive juices reach the mucosa, damaging it. In the presence of *H. pylori* infection, excess gastric acid, impaired blood flow, or inhibited prostaglandin production, the inflammatory process causes further damage, leading to ulceration of the mucosa.

Erosion and ulcer formation

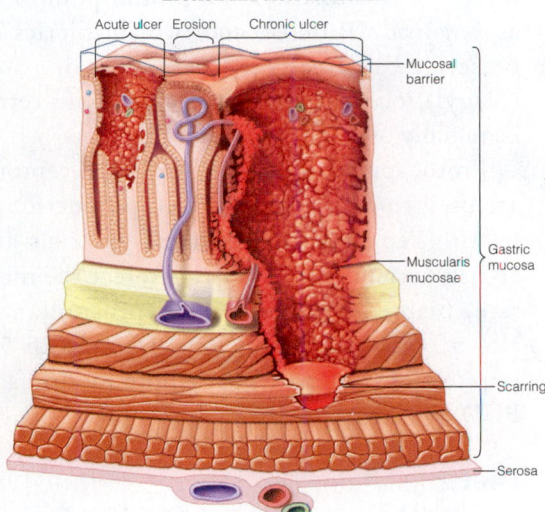

Superficial ulcers, called erosions, affect the mucosa.

True ulcers extend into deeper layers of the gastrointestinal wall, damaging blood vessels and potentially penetrating the entire wall.

Hemorrhage and peritonitis are potential acute complications of peptic ulcers.

Figure 25-7. ■ The gastric mucosa, mucosal barrier, and peptic ulcer formation. When the mucosal barrier is damaged, erosions and ulcers may form in the gastric mucosa and deeper layers of the GI wall.

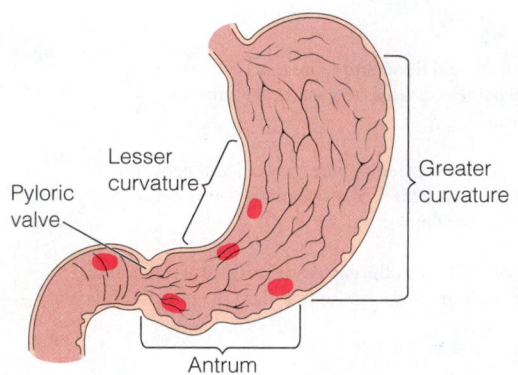

Figure 25-8. ■ Sites commonly affected by peptic ulcer disease.

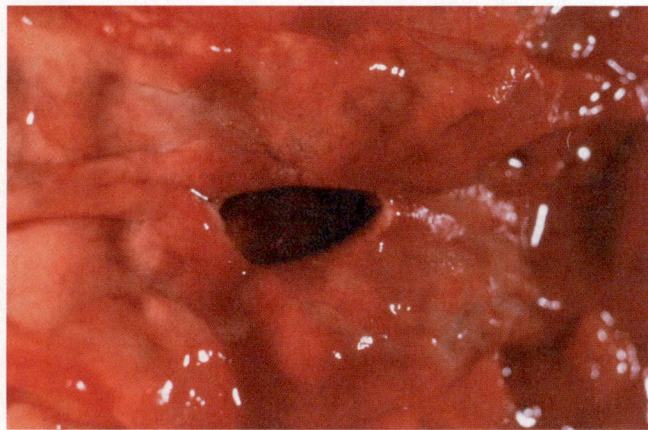

Figure 25-9. ■ A peptic ulcer as seen through an endoscope. (Source: CNRI/Science Source.)

BOX 25-12	MANIFESTATIONS OF PUD AND ITS COMPLICATIONS

- Epigastric pain: gnawing, burning, hunger-like; relieved by eating
- Heartburn, regurgitation

Hemorrhage

- Occult or obvious blood in the stool
- Hematemesis
- Fatigue, weakness, dizziness
- Orthostatic hypotension
- Shock

Obstruction

- Feeling of epigastric fullness
- Nausea and vomiting

Perforation

- Severe upper abdominal pain, radiating to the shoulder
- Rigid, boardlike (acute) abdomen
- Absent bowel sounds
- Signs of shock: diaphoresis, tachycardia, rapid and shallow respirations
- Fever

hematochezia and signs of shock. Box 25-12 lists manifestations of PUD complications.

PUD can cause *obstruction* of the upper GI tract. This usually occurs gradually. If the obstruction becomes complete, vomiting occurs.

Perforation of the ulcer through the mucosal wall is the most dangerous complication of PUD. When perforation occurs, gastric or duodenal contents enter the peritoneum, causing inflammation and *peritonitis*. Chemical peritonitis from GI secretions develops immediately; bacterial peritonitis from contamination of the normally sterile peritoneal cavity follows. When an ulcer perforates, the patient develops immediate manifestations of an acute abdomen, with pain, guarding, and absent bowel sounds. Signs of shock may be present. Older adults may have less specific manifestations of perforation; pain may be absent.

COLLABORATIVE CARE

Treatment of PUD focuses on relieving symptoms, healing ulcers, and preventing complications and ulcer recurrence.

Diagnostic Tests

- *Upper endoscopy* (*gastroscopy*) is done to inspect the mucosa of the upper GI tract and obtain samples for biopsy and *H. pylori* testing.
- A *urea breath test* may be done to detect *H. pylori* infection.
- *CBC* is performed to assess for anemia.
- *Stool* is tested for occult blood.

Medications

Drug therapy is used to eradicate *H. pylori* and heal existing ulcers. A combination of a proton-pump inhibitor such as *omeprazole* (Prilosec) and two antibiotics is commonly prescribed to treat *H. pylori* infection. Metronidazole (Flagyl), clarithromycin (Biaxin), and tetracycline are commonly used antibiotics for this therapy.

Proton-pump inhibitors and H_2-receptor antagonists are used to reduce gastric acid production, to promote healing, and to prevent stress gastritis and ulcers in at-risk patients. Agents that protect the mucosa (sucralfate, bismuth, antacids, and prostaglandin analogs) also may be prescribed. Review Table 25-5 for nursing implications and patient teaching for drugs used to treat PUD.

Diet

No special diet is prescribed for PUD. Encourage patients to eat a well-balanced diet with meals at regular intervals. Bland or restrictive diets are no longer recommended.

Mild alcohol intake is not harmful. Discourage smoking because it slows the rate of healing and increases the frequency of relapses.

Treatment of Complications

Patients with complications of PUD require additional treatment measures.

In *hemorrhage* associated with PUD, restoring and maintaining circulation is the priority of care, followed by measures to stop bleeding. See the preceding section on GI bleeding for interdisciplinary and nursing care related to hemorrhage.

If *obstruction* is suspected, an NG tube is inserted to relieve pressure and vomiting (gastric decompression). Endoscopy is performed to visualize and dilate the obstruction using balloon therapy. Surgery may be required to relieve the obstruction.

Perforation requires immediate treatment. The patient is kept NPO; intravenous fluids are given. To minimize peritoneal contamination, an NG tube is inserted and connected to suction to remove gastric contents. The patient is placed in Fowler's or semi-Fowler's position so that peritoneal contaminants will pool in the pelvis. Intravenous antibiotics are given to treat bacterial infection by intestinal flora. Many perforations seal spontaneously, but some require closure by laparoscopic surgery.

Surgery

When drug therapy and lifestyle management cannot control the symptoms or complications of PUD, surgery may be necessary. Acute perforation or massive hemorrhage may require emergency surgery. See the section on gastric cancer that follows for more information about surgical procedures, their complications, and nursing care of the patient undergoing gastric surgery.

NURSING CARE

PRIORITIZING NURSING CARE

In the patient with uncomplicated peptic ulcer disease, the discomfort associated with the disease and the effects of that discomfort on nutrition are the primary focus for nursing care. When the patient is admitted with an acute bleed related to PUD, restoring blood volume and cardiac output are the immediate priorities of care.

HEALTH PROMOTION

Although PUD can be unpredictable, advise patients to avoid risk factors such as cigarette smoking and excessive use of aspirin or NSAIDs. Encourage patients with manifestations of GERD (discussed earlier in this chapter) to seek treatment as it also is associated with *H. pylori* infection.

ASSESSING

Ask the patient about reported pain, documenting its location, character, timing and relationship to meals, and measures that relieve or aggravate the pain. Inquire about related symptoms such as nausea, heartburn, or indigestion. If vomiting is reported, ask about its color, consistency, and amount. Note reported color and consistency of feces, including any recent changes. Finally, ask about current and previous treatment measures and use of tobacco, aspirin or NSAIDs, and other medications.

Obtain vital signs, including orthostatic blood pressures. Observe the shape and contour of the abdomen; auscultate bowel sounds; and lightly palpate for tenderness or guarding. Test gastric contents and stool for occult blood.

IDENTIFYING POTENTIAL COMPLICATIONS

If the patient is being admitted with a possible complication such as bleeding, obstruction, or perforation, determine the onset and severity of symptoms. Carefully observe the patient's general appearance, watching for signs of acute distress. Focus interview questions and physical assessment to collect data quickly.

DIAGNOSING, PLANNING, AND IMPLEMENTING
Acute Pain

Expected outcome: Will report pain at a level of 3 or lower on a 0–10 scale.

- Assess pain, reporting any changes in intensity or character to the charge nurse or physician. *A change in the nature or severity of pain may indicate a complication of PUD or a separate problem.*

clinicalALERT

Pain may indicate a complication of PUD or may be related to another process (e.g., coronary heart disease, gallbladder disease).

- Administer medications as ordered. *Medications for PUD help prevent pain and promote healing. Administration at bedtime helps prevent nighttime ulcer pain that typically occurs between 1:00 and 3:00 a.m.*
- Limit food intake after the evening meal; eliminate bedtime snacks. *Eating before bed can stimulate gastric acid and pepsin production, increasing the chance of nighttime pain.*

Potential Complication: Bleeding

Expected outcome: Will demonstrate no further signs of GI bleeding.

- Irrigate the NG tube with room temperature saline as ordered. Calculate intake and output, subtracting the amount of irrigant from gastric output. *Irrigation helps remove irritating blood from the gut and may slow bleeding.*

- Prepare for upper endoscopy or surgery as planned. *Endoscopy or emergency surgery may be performed to repair the bleeding site or sclerose bleeding vessels.*
- After an acute bleed and in patients at risk for GI bleeding, monitor gastric pH as ordered and check emesis and feces for occult blood. Administer drugs to reduce gastric acidity as ordered. *The patient remains at risk for GI bleeding. Monitoring for occult blood helps identify slow bleeding or recurrent hemorrhage. Reducing the acidity of gastric secretions reduces the risk of bleeding.*

Imbalanced Nutrition: Less Than Body Requirements

Expected outcome: Will consume prescribed diet without nausea or vomiting.

- Assess diet, including pattern of food intake, eating schedule, and foods associated with pain. *This step increases patient awareness and identifies whether nutrient intake is adequate.*
- Arrange consultation with a dietitian. *A dietitian can help plan meals that meet the patient's nutritional needs and preferences. Foods that increase pain should be avoided. Providing six small meals per day generally helps increase food tolerance and decrease discomfort after meals.*
- Document and report complaints of anorexia, fullness, nausea, vomiting, or symptoms of dumping syndrome. *Problems with gastric emptying may be associated with PUD or surgery to treat PUD. It is important to monitor and report symptoms, because a change in therapy or food intake may be necessary.*

EVALUATING

To evaluate the effectiveness of nursing care for a patient with PUD, collect data regarding pain, weight, nutritional status (including food intake), fluid balance, and circulation (vital signs, peripheral pulses and capillary refill, mental status, and urinary output). Frequently monitor for and promptly report any manifestation of complications of the disease or gastric surgery.

DOCUMENTING

Document continuing assessment data and the effects of interventions (e.g., relief of pain after antacid administration). Document all teaching provided and the patient's understanding of information presented. As indicated, document compliance with prescribed regimen.

CONTINUITY OF CARE

Because PUD is a chronic disease, it is managed primarily by the patient at home. Teach patients about treatment measures and counter common misconceptions and myths (e.g., teach that drinking milk or cream every 2 hours "to coat the stomach" is not recommended and can increase

serum cholesterol levels and the risk for heart disease). Provide written and verbal instruction about medications, including the importance of continuing therapy even when symptoms are relieved. Teach patients taking metronidazole to eradicate *H. pylori* infection to avoid alcohol in any form while taking the drug and for a minimum of 48 hours after discontinuing the medication. Discuss the relationship between peptic ulcers and factors such as smoking. If indicated, refer the patient to a smoking cessation clinic. Stress the importance of avoiding aspirin and NSAIDs, as well as the need to read the labels of over-the-counter medications to identify the presence of aspirin.

Discuss symptoms of PUD complications, such as abdominal pain or distention, vomiting, black or tarry stools, light-headedness, or fainting. Emphasize the importance of contacting the physician if symptoms of a complication develop.

Reinforce stress and lifestyle management techniques that may help prevent flare-ups. Refer the patient to resources for stress management, such as classes, counseling, and formal or informal groups.

NURSING CARE PLAN
Patient With Peptic Ulcer Disease

Sean O'Donnell is a 47-year-old policeman who has had "heartburn" and epigastric pain for years. Last year, after becoming weak, light-headed, and short of breath, he was found to be anemic, and a duodenal ulcer was identified. He took famotidine (Pepcid) and ferrous sulfate for 3 months before stopping both, saying he had "never felt better in his life." Sean has now been admitted to the hospital with active upper GI bleeding.

Assessment

Mr. O'Donnell is alert and oriented, although apprehensive. Skin pale and cool; BP 136/78, P 98. Abdomen distended and tender with extremely active bowel sounds. NG tube inserted; 200 mL bright red blood obtained. Laboratory results include hemoglobin 8.2 g/dL and hematocrit 23%. An endoscopy is done to control Mr. O'Donnell's bleeding, and he receives two units of packed red blood cells as well as intravenous fluids to replace his lost blood volume.

Nursing Diagnosis

The following nursing diagnoses are identified for Mr. O'Donnell:

- *Deficient Fluid Volume* related to acute upper GI bleeding
- *Bleeding (Gastrointestinal)* related to active peptic ulcer disease
- *Ineffective Therapeutic Regimen Management* related to lack of understanding of the need for continued treatment

Expected Outcomes

The expected outcomes for the plan of care specify that Mr. O'Donnell will:

- Regain homeostasis, with stable vital signs and normal hemoglobin and hematocrit.
- Remain free of further bleeding and other complications of peptic ulcer disease.
- Demonstrate knowledge and understanding of prescribed treatment measures.
- Identify ways to promote ulcer healing and prevent recurrence.
- State manifestations to report to his primary care provider.

Planning and Implementation

The nurse plans and implements the following interventions for Mr. O'Donnell:

- Monitor and document vital signs, mental status, intake and output, and abdominal assessment every 4 hours until stable, and then every 8 hours.
- Maintain intravenous fluids and blood replacement as ordered.
- Monitor laboratory values (hemoglobin, hematocrit, serum electrolytes), reporting abnormal values to the charge nurse or physician as indicated.
- Explain PUD and ulcer healing, clarifying misconceptions.
- Discuss the importance of following the treatment plan to ensure healing and prevent further ulcers from developing.
- Discuss the effect of smoking, aspirin, and NSAIDs on PUD. Provide information about alternative analgesics.
- Provide written and verbal instructions about prescribed medications.
- With the patient, plan a medication schedule that fits his lifestyle.
- Discuss stress reduction strategies such as exercise, meditation, controlled breathing, and other relaxation exercises.

Evaluation

Mr. O'Donnell is discharged after 72 hours. He has had no further bleeding and is eating a normal diet. His hemoglobin and hematocrit levels have improved; other blood values are within normal limits. His physician has prescribed omeprazole (Prilosec), amoxicillin, and clarithromycin for 2 weeks to eradicate *H. pylori* infection confirmed during the endoscopy. He will continue to take the omeprazole daily at bedtime for another 6 weeks. He verbalizes an understanding of the need for these medications, when to take them, and what side effects he should report. He had used ibuprofen regularly for tension headaches, but says he is willing to try acetaminophen and relaxation techniques to "avoid

ending up in here again!" He states that the hardest part of going back to work will be reducing his coffee consumption.

Critical Thinking in the Nursing Process

1. What is the likely reason Mr. O'Donnell developed another peptic ulcer and hemorrhage after having been treated for a previous episode?
2. Discuss the relationship between aspirin and NSAIDs and peptic ulcer disease.
3. What additional lifestyle changes would you recommend for Mr. O'Donnell?

Note: Discussion of Critical Thinking questions appears on the companion website.

Cancer of the Stomach

Except for skin cancer, cancer of the stomach is the most common cancer in the world, but it is less common in the United States (see Box 25-13■). Chronic *H. pylori* gastritis is the major risk factor for gastric cancer. Older adults are more likely to develop gastric cancer than young and middle-aged adults.

PATHOPHYSIOLOGY AND MANIFESTATIONS

Gastric carcinomas usually develop in the distal portion of the stomach. Half of all gastric cancers occur in the antrum or pyloric region (Figure 25-10■). Lesions spread by direct extension to tissues surrounding the stomach, particularly the liver. Lymph node involvement and metastasis occur early due to the rich blood and lymphatic supply to the stomach. Metastatic lesions are often found in the liver, lungs, ovaries, and peritoneum.

Early symptoms of gastric cancer are vague (early satiety, anorexia, indigestion, and possibly vomiting). There may also be ulcer-like pain, typically occurring after meals and unrelieved by antacids. As the disease progresses, weight loss occurs, and the patient may be *cachectic* (very thin and malnourished).

BOX 25-13	**FOCUS ON DIVERSITY**

Stomach Cancer

The incidence of stomach cancer in the United States differs significantly by gender, ethnicity, and socioeconomic status:

- In all ethnic groups, the incidence is higher in men than it is in women; among Whites, men are twice as likely to be affected as women.
- The incidence of stomach cancer is highest among Asian Americans, followed closely by African Americans, Native Americans, and Hispanic/Latinos.
- Diets rich in smoked foods, salted meat or fish, and pickled vegetables and low in fresh vegetables are associated with a higher risk for stomach cancer. (American Cancer Society, 2014)

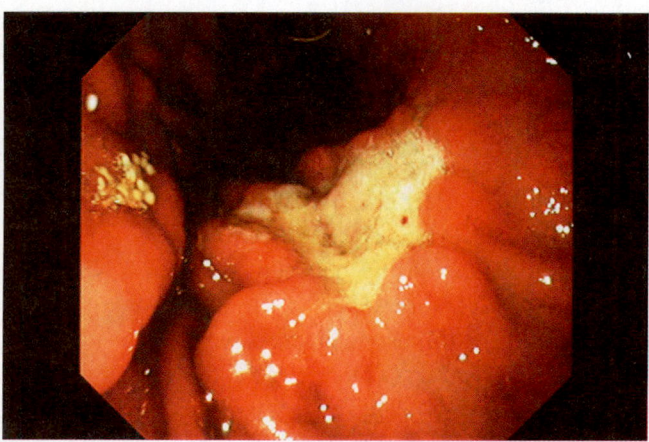

Figure 25-10. ■ Cancer of the stomach. (Source: Jean-François Rey/ Science Source.)

COLLABORATIVE CARE

An abdominal mass may be palpable in the patient with gastric cancer, and there may be occult blood in the stool. The diagnosis is confirmed with an endoscopy and biopsy of the lesion.

Surgery

When gastric cancer is diagnosed before metastases develop, a partial or total gastrectomy is done. In a *partial gastrectomy,* a portion of the stomach is removed, usually the distal half to two-thirds (Figures 25-11A and B ■). A *total* **gastrectomy** (removal of the entire stomach) is rarely done because of its impact on digestion and nutrition. Extensive gastric cancer, however, may require it. In a total gastrectomy, an **anastomosis** (surgical connection) connects the esophagus to the duodenum or jejunum (Figure 25-11C). A jejunostomy tube may be inserted during surgery to promote postoperative nutrition. Nursing care of the patient having gastric surgery is outlined in Box 25-14 ■.

BOX 25-14	NURSING CARE CHECKLIST

Gastric Surgery

Before Surgery

☑ Provide routine preoperative care and teaching.

After Surgery

☑ Provide routine postoperative care as outlined in Chapter 10.

☑ Assess position and patency of NG tube, connecting it to low suction. Unless contraindicated, gently irrigate with sterile normal saline if tube becomes clogged.

☑ Assess color, amount, and odor of gastric drainage, noting any changes, the presence of clots, or bright bleeding. Chart all assessments and notify the charge nurse or physician of clots or bright bleeding.

☑ Monitor bowel sounds and abdominal girth.

☑ Maintain intravenous fluids while nasogastric suction is in place.

☑ Resume oral food and fluids as ordered. Initial feedings are clear liquids, progressing to full liquids and then frequent small feedings of regular foods. Monitor bowel sounds and for abdominal distention frequently during this period.

☑ Begin discharge planning and teaching. Consult with a dietitian for diet instructions and menu planning; reinforce teaching. Teach the patient how to recognize and prevent potential postoperative complications, such as infection, dumping syndrome, postprandial hypoglycemia, or pernicious anemia.

COMPLICATIONS OF SURGERY   *Dumping syndrome* is the most common problem after a partial gastrectomy. After pyloric resection or bypass, concentrated *chyme* (partially digested food) may enter the small bowel rapidly. Water is pulled from the vascular system into the intestine, decreasing blood volume and dilating the intestine. Early symptoms of dumping syndrome occur within 5 to 30 minutes after eating; they include nausea and possible vomiting,

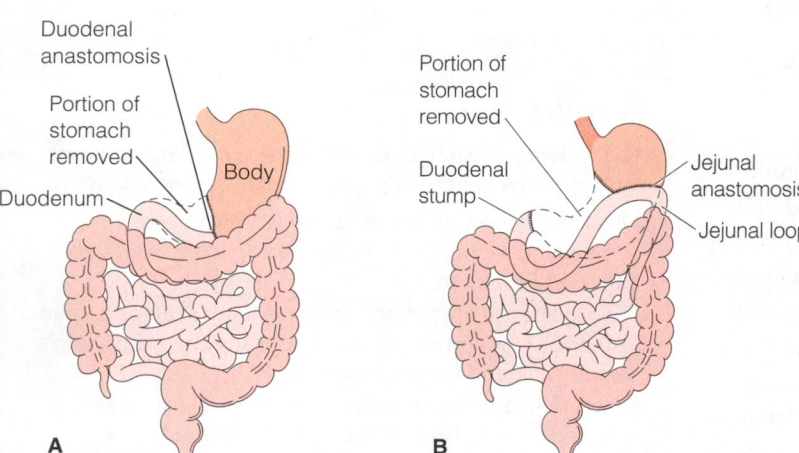

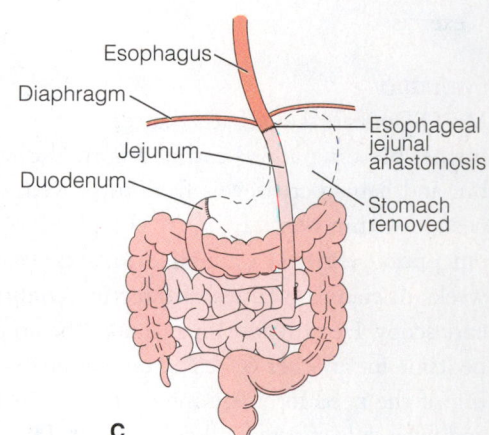

Figure 25-11. ■ Partial and total gastrectomy procedures. (**A**) Partial gastrectomy with anastomosis to the duodenum. (**B**) Partial gastrectomy with anastomosis to the jejunum. (**C**) Total gastrectomy with anastomosis of the esophagus to the jejunum.

epigastric pain, cramping, **borborygmi** (loud, hyperactive bowel sounds), and diarrhea. Systemic symptoms from decreased blood volume include tachycardia, orthostatic hypotension, dizziness, flushing, and diaphoresis. The rapid entry of undigested carbohydrates into the jejunum stimulates the pancreas to release excess insulin, and the patient develops symptoms of hypoglycemia 2 to 3 hours later.

Dumping syndrome is managed primarily by planning dietary intake to delay gastric emptying and allow smaller boluses of undigested food to enter the intestine. Meals are small and more frequent. Liquids and solids are taken at separate times instead of together. Proteins and fats in the diet are increased, because they exit the stomach more slowly than carbohydrates; carbohydrates, especially simple sugars, are reduced. The patient is taught to rest in a recumbent or semirecumbent position for 30 to 60 minutes after meals.

After gastric surgery, patients are at risk for nutritional deficiencies because of reduced absorption and inability to eat large meals. Nearly 50% of patients who undergo gastric surgery experience significant weight loss due to insufficient calorie intake.

Other Treatments

Radiation, chemotherapy, or both may be used to reduce the risk of spread of the cancer. For the patient with more advanced disease, treatment is palliative and may include surgery and chemotherapy. These patients may require a gastrostomy or jejunostomy feeding tube. Gastrostomy tubes are inserted into the stomach through a stoma in the epigastric region (Figure 25-12 ■). The tube may initially be plugged or connected to low suction. Tube feedings may be restarted shortly after the procedure. Box 25-15 ■ describes nursing care of the patient with a gastrostomy or jejunostomy tube.

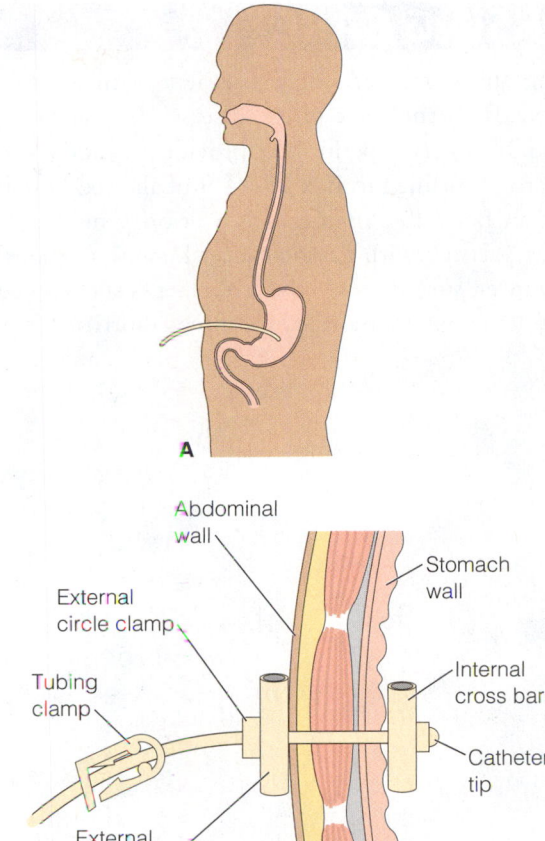

Figure 25-12. ■ (A) Gastrostomy tube placement. **(B)** The tube is held in place by cross bars.

Because gastric cancer is often advanced by the time of diagnosis, the prognosis is poor. The 5-year survival rate of all patients treated for gastric carcinoma is 10%.

| **BOX 25-15** | **NURSING CARE CHECKLIST** |

Gastrostomy or Jejunostomy Tube

Nursing Care

- ☑ Use Standard Precautions.
- ☑ Assess tube placement by aspirating stomach contents and checking the pH of the aspirate (see Box 25-5 for expected pH readings for the stomach and small intestine).
- ☑ Inspect the skin around the stoma for healing, redness, swelling, and any drainage. If drainage is present, note the color, amount, consistency, and odor. Document findings and report to the charge nurse or physician.
- ☑ Assess the abdomen for distention, bowel sounds, and tenderness; document.
- ☑ Until the stoma is well healed, use sterile technique for dressing changes and site care. Clean technique is appropriate for use once healing is complete.

- ☑ Cleanse the site with normal saline or soap and water. A well-healed stoma site may be cleansed in the shower with the tube clamped or plugged. Allow to air dry. Apply a protective barrier cream as needed.
- ☑ Redress the wound using a stoma dressing or folded 4 × 4 gauze pads.
- ☑ Irrigate the tube with 30 to 50 mL of water; clean the tube inside and out as indicated or ordered. A special brush may be used to clean the inside of soft gastric tubes.
- ☑ Provide mouth care or remind the patient to do so.
- ☑ If the patient is to be discharged with a gastrostomy or jejunostomy tube, teach the patient and family how to care for the tube and administer feedings. Refer to a home health agency or visiting nurse for support and reinforcement of learning.

NURSING CARE

Nursing and home care for the patient with gastric cancer depends on the stage of the disease and the treatment planned. If surgery is performed, provide pre- and postoperative care as outlined in Box 25-14. Imbalanced Nutrition: Less Than Body Requirements is a priority nursing diagnosis for patients with gastric cancer because of the effects of the cancer, surgery, and other treatments such as chemotherapy or radiation therapy. Parenteral nutrition may be necessary to maintain weight and nutrition. Refer to home health services as needed for assistance with dressing changes, tube feedings, or parenteral nutrition.

Because disease is usually advanced at the time of diagnosis, provide grief counseling and refer the patient and family to cancer support groups or hospice services as appropriate.

Note: The references and resources for all chapters have been compiled at the back of the book.

Chapter Review

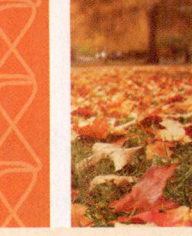

KEY POINTS

- **Concept:** Patients with nutritional and upper GI disorders require holistic nursing care that addresses nutritional needs, education, and psychosocial factors.
- **Concept:** Nutritional disorders such as obesity and malnutrition are major causes of illness and disability. These disorders may be caused by lifestyle, diseases or their effects, problems of access to food and nutrients, or eating disorders.
- **Concept:** Obesity is associated with serious health problems such as hypertension, heart disease, cancers, disability, and death. Effective treatment of this prevalent disorder requires a multidisciplinary team approach.
- **Concept:** Disorders of the mouth and esophagus can affect the ability to eat and maintain nutritional status. Although most disorders are appropriate for self-treatment, cancers of these organs require prompt diagnosis and treatment for successful resolution.
- **Concept:** Disorders affecting the stomach and duodenum range from acute and life threatening, requiring emergent management by the interprofessional team, to self-limiting and appropriate for self-care. The nurse monitors patient responses to these disorders, providing support, interventions, and teaching as appropriate to maintain and restore nutrition and GI function.
- Tobacco and alcohol use contribute to a number of upper GI disorders, including GERD, oral and esophageal cancers, and peptic ulcer disease. Encourage all patients to stop smoking or using smokeless tobacco and to consume alcohol in moderate amounts, if at all, to reduce their risk of these disorders.
- Both esophageal and gastric cancers often are diagnosed late in the disease because their symptoms may be vague. Encourage all patients with complaints of dysphagia, a sensation of gastric fullness, or heartburn to seek medical evaluation.
- Gastroenteritis is usually caused by a food- or water-borne pathogen. The symptoms, duration, and treatment of gastroenteritis depend on the organism; however, most cases of gastroenteritis are self-limiting and require no treatment other than supportive care.
- Upper GI hemorrhage usually occurs as complication of peptic ulcer disease and gastritis. The manifestations and immediate treatment of upper GI hemorrhage differ, depending on the rapidity of bleeding and the amount of blood lost. Preparing the patient for upper endoscopy is a major nursing responsibility, along with supporting cardiovascular function and tissue perfusion.
- *H. pylori* infection is the primary cause of peptic ulcer disease and a major risk factor for stomach cancer. Effectively treating the infection can reduce or eliminate the risk for future exacerbations of PUD.
- Promptly report a change in the nature of abdominal pain in a patient with PUD, especially if the pain is accompanied by vomiting, guarding of the abdomen, or a change in bowel sounds. These manifestations could indicate an obstruction or perforation into the peritoneal cavity.

PEARSON NURSING STUDENT RESOURCES

Find additional materials at **nursing.pearsonhighered.com**.

Clinical Reasoning Care Map

Caring for a Patient With Imbalanced Nutrition
NCLEX-PN® Focus Area: Prevention and Health Maintenance

Case Study: Sam Elliott has gained 30 lb since retiring 2 years ago, and now the most active thing he does each day is "walk to the end of the driveway to get the mail." He reports having juice, oatmeal, a muffin, and coffee with cream for breakfast and meeting friends midmorning for dough-nuts and coffee. Lunch is usually a bologna-and-cheese sandwich with chips and a root beer. He has cheese, crackers, and wine before a dinner of meat, potatoes, vegetables, and dessert. He tells the nurse, "I have never had to diet. I just don't know how to get this weight off."

Nursing Diagnosis: Imbalanced Nutrition: More Than Body Requirements

COLLECT DATA

Subjective	Objective
_____	_____
_____	_____
_____	_____
_____	_____
_____	_____

Does this present a threat to the patient's safety?

If yes, the priority intervention to address this threat would be:

_____

Nursing Care

_____
_____
_____
_____
_____
_____
_____
_____

Interprofessional team members to include when planning care:

_____

How would you document this? _____

_____

Compare your answers and documentation to those provided on the companion website.

Data Collected
(use only those that apply)

- Height 5'10" (178 cm)
- Easily fatigued
- Weight 201 lb (91.3 kg)
- "Needs to lose weight"
- Shortness of breath with activity
- LDL 180 mg/dL
- BP 138/90
- Fasting blood glucose 103 mg/dL
- Reports feeling hungry most of the time
- Cholesterol 240 mg/dL
- Stool negative for occult blood

Nursing Interventions
(use only those that apply; list in priority order)

- Suggest food substitutions that will reduce fat intake.
- Instruct the patient to lose 30 lb in 60 days.
- Instruct the patient to jog 45 minutes a day.
- Provide a list of local support groups and weight loss programs.
- Discuss Food Guide MyPlate.
- Instruct the patient to exercise at least three times a week, gradually increasing time.
- Discuss role of exercise in weight loss and control.

NCLEX-PN® Exam Preparation

1 Which of the following would be an expected finding when assessing a patient who has central or upper body obesity?

1. Weight 250 lb, height 5'10"
2. Serum cholesterol 180 mg/dL
3. Waist circumference 38", hip circumference 37"
4. Obesity in the patient's parents

2 When planning care for a patient who has a diagnosis of malnutrition, the nurse would include which of these goals?

1. Will gain 1 to 2 lb/week
2. Will consume a 1,500-calorie diet
3. Will state need to exercise 60 minutes five times per week
4. Will limit intake of unsaturated fats and whole-grain carbohydrates

3 When caring for a patient who has stomatitis, the nurse should give priority to which of these treatment measures?

1. Encourage consumption of raw fruits and vegetables.
2. Administer viscous lidocaine before each meal.
3. Assess the patient's gag reflex.
4. Encourage the patient to use a mouthwash after each meal.

4 During the initial assessment, the nurse notes a small, painless, dark-colored lesion on the patient's tongue. The patient states that the sore has been in his mouth for several months. Which of the following interventions should be the next priority?

1. Document findings and notify the health care provider.
2. Tell the patient to report any changes in the size or color of the lesion.
3. Prepare the patient for a biopsy of the lesion.
4. Immediately notify the charge nurse.

5 The nurse reinforcing teaching for a patient with gastroesophageal reflux disease includes which of the following in the instructions? **Select all that apply.**

1. Avoid lying down for several hours after eating.
2. Use of alcohol and tobacco in moderation is allowed.
3. Stop taking the prescribed proton-pump inhibitor once symptoms are relieved.
4. Raise the head of the bed on 6-in. blocks.
5. Peppermint and chocolate candies can help relieve symptoms.

6 A 58-year-old male is admitted with the diagnosis of esophageal cancer with erosion to the middle portion of the esophagus. Which of the following is most important to report immediately?

1. Aspiration pneumonia
2. Bright bleeding from the mouth
3. Weight loss
4. Difficulty swallowing

7 During the insertion of a nasogastric tube, the patient begins to gag. The nurse should:

1. withdraw the tube completely.
2. briefly halt the insertion.
3. have the patient sip water to assist the tube to advance.
4. check for placement.

8 The patient is receiving enteral feedings of Ensure (240 mL/can) at a rate of 60 mL/hr. The nurse anticipates that each can of the formula will run for _____ hours.

9 The health care provider has prescribed an antibiotic for a patient with peptic ulcer. The patient asks you why this type of medication is being given. The appropriate response is:

1. "This medication will help reduce the gastric acid in your stomach."
2. "The antibiotic will help to rid the stomach of the *H. pylori* bacteria."
3. "It will increase the production of mucus in the stomach."
4. "It is used only as a prophylactic to prevent colonization of bacteria in the stomach."

10 When developing a teaching plan for a patient who has undergone a partial gastrectomy, which of the following would the nurse include related to preventing dumping syndrome?

1. Diet low in protein and fats
2. Taking a walk before each meal
3. Eating three meals a day
4. Resting in a semirecumbent position after eating

Answers and rationales for Review Questions appear in Appendix I.

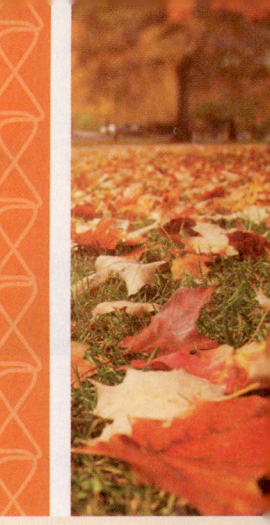

CHAPTER 26
Caring for Patients With Bowel Disorders

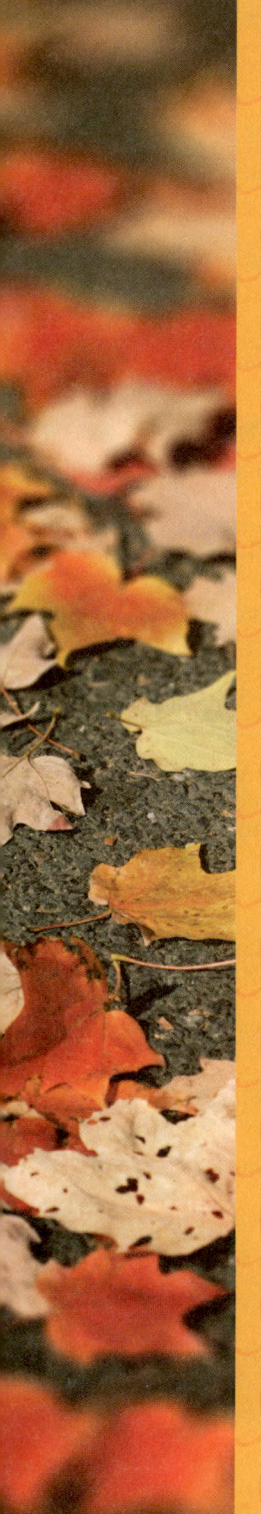

BRIEF OUTLINE

DISORDERS OF INTESTINAL MOTILITY AND ABSORPTION
Diarrhea
Constipation
Irritable Bowel Syndrome
INFLAMMATORY DISORDERS
Appendicitis
Peritonitis
Inflammatory Bowel Disease

STRUCTURAL AND OBSTRUCTIVE DISORDERS
Colorectal Cancer
Hernia
Bowel Obstruction
Diverticular Disease
ANORECTAL DISORDERS
Hemorrhoids
Anorectal Lesions

APPLIED LEARNING OUTCOMES

After completing this chapter, you will be able to:

1. Discuss the pathophysiology, manifestations, and management of bowel disorders.
2. Provide evidence-based nursing care and teaching related to measures used to manage bowel disorders.
3. Effectively care for the patient undergoing intestinal surgery, respecting the patient's culture, preferences, and expressed needs.
4. Provide individualized care for patients with a colostomy or ileostomy.
5. Conduct focused assessment of patients with bowel disorders, identifying, documenting, and reporting abnormal or unexpected data.
6. Contribute to nursing care planning and evaluation for patients with bowel disorders.

KEY TERMS

The key terms are defined on the pages listed below.

SPECIAL FEATURES

Key Concept Inflammation, obstructions, absorption disorders, and changes in structure can alter bowel elimination, affecting health, causing pain, or necessitating surgery. Nurses focus on providing physical care, emotional support, and teaching.

"Normal" patterns of defecation vary widely, from two to three stools per day to as few as three stools per week. Few body functions respond as readily to both internal and external factors as the process of defecation. Factors such as food and bacteria directly affect the gastrointestinal (GI) tract and the number and consistency of stools. Indirect factors (psychologic stress or voluntary postponement of defecation) also affect elimination patterns.

DISORDERS OF INTESTINAL MOTILITY AND ABSORPTION

Diarrhea

Diarrhea is an increase in the frequency, volume, and water content of stool. It is a symptom, not a primary disorder. Causes of diarrhea include bacterial toxins, infections, malabsorption syndromes, medications, systemic diseases, and psychogenic factors (e.g., pretest diarrhea).

PATHOPHYSIOLOGY

Diarrhea can result either from impaired water absorption or from increased water secretion into the bowel. Impaired water absorption occurs when the rate of peristalsis increases or when the absorptive surface of the bowel decreases. Increased water secretion into the bowel may occur as a result of infection (e.g., *Escherichia coli*, *Clostridium difficile*), unabsorbed fat, and some drugs. Inflammatory disorders cause plasma, blood, and mucus to accumulate in the bowel.

MANIFESTATIONS AND COMPLICATIONS

Patients with diarrhea may have several large, watery stools per day or very frequent small stools containing blood, mucus, or pus. The manifestations depend on the cause, duration, and severity of the diarrhea, as well as the area of bowel affected.

clinical**ALERT**

Immediately report bloody diarrhea to the charge nurse or physician because it may indicate bleeding or hemorrhage in the GI tract. GI bleeding can lead to significant blood loss and hypovolemic shock.

Diarrhea can have devastating results because water and electrolytes are lost in the stool. Patients, particularly very young or older, debilitated patients, can become dehydrated. Hypovolemic shock may occur with rapid fluid losses. Potassium, magnesium, and bicarbonate loss may lead to electrolyte and acid–base imbalances. (See Chapter 7 for further discussion of the effects of these imbalances.)

COLLABORATIVE CARE

Care of the patient with diarrhea focuses on identifying and treating the underlying cause. The diarrhea itself may need to be treated for comfort and to prevent complications.

Diagnostic Tests

- A *stool specimen* may be ordered for culture and to look for blood, pus, mucus, or excess fat (*steatorrhea*). Microscopic examination is done to identify blood cells and parasites. Because parasites may not be in the stool at all times, a series of three stool specimens, spaced 2 to 3 days apart, may be ordered.
- Blood is drawn to assess for fluid, electrolyte, and acid–base imbalances.
- A *sigmoidoscopy* may be done to allow direct examination of the bowel mucosa.

Dietary Management

Fluid replacement is a priority for patients with diarrhea. If the patient is able to take oral fluids, a glucose and balanced electrolyte solution is used (e.g., Pedialyte, Gatorade). Solid food is withheld during the first 24 hours of acute diarrhea to provide bowel rest. Then frequent, small meals can be added. The BRAT (bananas, rice, applesauce, and toast) diet is frequently recommended as a good way to reintroduce solid foods. Milk and milk products are added last. Raw fruits and vegetables, fried foods, bran, whole-grain cereals, condiments, spices, coffee, and alcoholic beverages are avoided during recovery. Patients with chronic diarrhea may need to eliminate certain foods and nonfood substances that can aggravate diarrhea (Table 26-1■). These patients need a diet that is high in calories and nutritional value. Vitamin supplements may be necessary, particularly the fat-soluble vitamins (A, D, E, and K). Parenteral nutrition may be required. A balanced electrolyte intravenous solution may be required to replace fluid losses.

Medications

Antidiarrheal medications may not be used until the cause of diarrhea has been identified, because they could worsen or prolong the disease. Opium derivatives and absorbents such as Pepto-Bismol are commonly used to treat acute diarrhea (Table 26-2■). Opium derivatives also may be used with caution for patients with chronic diarrhea. A potassium supplement may also be prescribed.

TABLE 26-1	Foods That May Aggravate Chronic Diarrhea	
FOODS	**REASON**
Milk, ice cream, yogurt, soft cheeses, cottage cheese	Contain lactose, which requires the enzyme lactase to digest; lactase deficiency common
Apple juice, pear juice, grapes, honey, dates, nuts, figs, fruit-flavored soft drinks	Contain fructose, which can draw fluid into the bowel when consumed in large quantities
Table sugar	Contains sucrose, which requires the enzyme sucrase to digest
Apple juice, pear juice, sugarless gums and mints	May contain sorbitol, a sugar that is not absorbed and can pull fluid into intestine
Breads, cereals, pasta, desserts and pastries; breaded meats; beverage mixes, beers and ales, root beer; gravy, white sauce, nondairy creamer	Contain gluten, a cereal protein found in wheat, rye, oats, or barley, that is not tolerated by people with celiac disease, a hereditary disorder
Antacids	Magnesium-containing antacids increase peristalsis and can draw fluid into the bowel
Coffee, tea, cola drinks, over-the-counter analgesics	Contain caffeine, which can increase peristalsis

Complementary Therapies

Complementary and alternative therapies may be appropriate to relieve discomfort associated with diarrhea. Gentle abdominal massage using oil containing chamomile, lavender, or peppermint may help relieve abdominal cramping and discomfort. Herbal tea made with black pepper, chamomile, rosemary, or sandalwood also may be used to promote comfort.

NURSING CARE

Nursing care of the patient with diarrhea is directed toward identifying the cause, relieving the symptoms, preventing complications, and, if the cause is infectious, preventing the spread of infection to others.

PRIORITIZING NURSING CARE

Although the diarrhea itself is a priority nursing care focus, the effects of the diarrhea on fluid balance and skin integrity are of importance in planning and implementing nursing care.

HEALTH PROMOTION

Teach all patients about the importance of hand washing, particularly after using the toilet and before handling food. Discuss safe food handling to prevent bacterial contamination (e.g., thorough cooking of meats, prompt refrigeration, maintaining safe food temperatures). Advise about ways to ensure safe drinking water, particularly with people planning overseas travel or wilderness camping.

ASSESSING

The patient's history and physical examination often provide enough information to identify the cause of diarrhea. Ask about the onset and duration of symptoms, including any related events such as travel, diet changes, or possible exposure to contaminated food and water. Have the patient describe the frequency, character, and timing (day or night, relationship to food intake) of stools. Inquire about associated symptoms such as abdominal or rectal pain or cramping, nausea, vomiting, or anorexia. Ask about any known chronic diseases such as inflammatory bowel disease or diabetes, and have the patient identify all current medications, including natural or herbal remedies.

Obtain vital signs, including orthostatic vitals. Note general appearance, including nutritional status and current distress. Inspect mucous membranes for color and moisture; assess skin color, temperature, moisture, and turgor; observe abdomen for shape and distention; auscultate bowel sounds; and palpate lightly for tenderness.

IDENTIFYING POTENTIAL COMPLICATIONS

Dry, shiny mucous membranes, poor skin turgor, and orthostatic hypotension are indicators of hypovolemia and should be reported to the charge nurse or primary care provider. Hyperactive bowel sounds may be expected in acute diarrhea. However, bowel sounds that are high pitched and "tinkling" or hypoactive or absent may indicate a complication and should be reported. Also report hemoglobin, hematocrit, serum electrolyte, and osmolality levels and urine specific gravity results that are outside the normal or expected range.

DIAGNOSING, PLANNING, AND IMPLEMENTING

Diarrhea

Expected outcome: Will report that stools are decreasing in number and are becoming increasingly solid.

■ Monitor and record the frequency and characteristics of bowel movements. *This provides a measure of the effectiveness of treatment.*

TABLE 26-2	Giving Medications Safely: Antidiarrheal Medications		
CLASS/DRUGS	**PURPOSE**	**NURSING IMPLICATIONS**	**PATIENT TEACHING**
Absorbants and protectants ■ Bismuth subsalicylate (Pepto-Bismol)	Bismuth salts act in the intestines to bind substances that can cause diarrhea. They are safe and available over the counter. Bismuth subsalicylate is used to prevent and treat traveler's diarrhea because it has an antimicrobial effect as well.	Assess for contraindications, such as chronic inflammatory bowel disease. If fever is present, check with the physician before administering. Give at least 1 hour before or 2 hours after other oral medications; bismuth may interfere with the absorption of other drugs. Observe for potential constipation.	Take at the onset of diarrhea and after each loose stool. If diarrhea persists for more than 48 hours, contact your doctor. Chew bismuth tablets for maximal effectiveness. This drug may cause the tongue and stool to darken. If you are allergic to aspirin, do not use bismuth subsalicylate. Avoid taking aspirin while taking bismuth subsalicylate.
Opium and opium derivatives ■ Camphorated tincture of opium (paregoric) ■ Difenoxin (Motofen) ■ Diphenoxylate (Lomotil, Logen, others) ■ Loperamide hydrochloride (Imodium)	Opium and related drugs act on the CNS to slow peristalsis and allow more water absorption. They also decrease the sensation of a full rectum and increase anal sphincter tone. Paregoric is a controlled prescription drug. Opium derivatives have few narcotic or abuse-promoting effects and are more commonly used.	Assess for contraindications and drug interactions before giving these drugs. Administer paregoric undiluted with water. Observe for increased effects of other CNS depressants, such as alcohol, narcotic analgesics, or barbiturate sedatives. Report abdominal distention to the charge nurse or physician.	Take as recommended at the onset of diarrhea and after each loose stool. These drugs may be habit forming; use for no more than 48 hours. Avoid using alcohol and over-the-counter cold preparations while taking these drugs. These drugs may cause drowsiness; avoid driving or operating machinery while taking them.
Synthetic hormone ■ Octreotide acetate (Sandostatin)	Octreotide stimulates fluid and electrolyte absorption from the GI tract and slows intestinal motility. It is primarily used to treat chronic diarrhea associated with certain tumors and HIV disease.	Do not use solution if it is discolored or has particulates. Administer room temperature solution slowly by subcutaneous injection. Refrigerate vials for long-term storage; use room temperature solution within 24 hours.	Rotate injection sites using the hips, thighs, or abdomen. Administer between meals and at bedtime to minimize nausea and diarrhea. Do not use this medication if you are pregnant.

■ Measure abdominal girth and auscultate bowel sounds every shift as indicated. *These indicate the effectiveness and possible complications of treatment, such as constipation or obstruction.*

■ Administer antidiarrheal medications as prescribed. *These medications promote comfort and prevent excess fluid loss.*

■ Limit food intake for acute diarrhea; slowly reintroduce solid foods in small amounts. *Limiting food allows the bowel to rest and lets the mucosa heal.*

Risk for Deficient Fluid Volume

Expected outcome: Will maintain stable weight, vital signs, urine output, and mental status.

■ Record intake and output; weigh daily; assess skin turgor, mucous membranes, and urine specific gravity every 8 hours. *These assessments help monitor fluid volume status.*

■ Monitor vital signs, including orthostatic vitals, every 4 to 8 hours. *A drop in blood pressure of more than 10 mm Hg on moving from lying to sitting or from sitting to standing indicates orthostatic hypotension and possible fluid volume deficit. The pulse rate typically increases as well.*

■ Remind the patient to ask for help when getting up. *The patient with orthostatic hypotension may become dizzy or light-headed on rising.*

■ Provide fluid and electrolyte replacement solutions as indicated. Ensure ready access to fluids. Assist the debilitated patient with fluid intake. *If tolerated, oral fluids are encouraged to prevent dehydration. Fluids may be replaced intravenously if necessary. A fluid intake of 3,000 mL or more per day may be necessary to replace losses.*

Risk for Impaired Skin Integrity

Expected outcome: Skin and underlying tissues will remain intact.

- Provide good skin care. Frequently reposition, and protect pressure areas. *Poorly hydrated skin is at increased risk for breakdown.*
- Assist with perianal cleaning as needed. Use warm water and soft cloths. Apply protective ointment or skin barrier cream. *These measures help prevent tissue irritation, trauma, and breakdown.*

EVALUATING

To evaluate the effectiveness of nursing interventions for patients with diarrhea, collect data related to stool frequency, nutritional status, weight, fluid volume status, and skin integrity. Monitor laboratory results, particularly serum electrolytes and serum osmolality, and acid–base balance, on a continuing basis.

DOCUMENTING

Document the number and characteristics of stools, complaints of abdominal pain or cramping, physical assessment data, and treatment measures initiated throughout the patient's care. Note compliance with fluid and dietary intake recommendations. Document teaching provided and reinforced, as well as the patient's (and, as appropriate, the family's) understanding of information presented.

CONTINUITY OF CARE

Teach about the causes of diarrhea and preventive measures such as food and water safety. Discuss measures to prevent the spread of bacteria, especially good hand washing after every bowel movement. Stress the importance of seeking medical intervention if diarrhea continues or is severe or prolonged.

Discuss the importance of maintaining fluid intake to replace lost water and electrolytes. Encourage use of Gatorade or a similar product rather than water for fluid replacement. A solution of 1 quart (1 L) of water, 1 teaspoon (5 mL) each of table salt and baking soda, 4 teaspoons (20 mL) of granulated sugar, and desired flavoring (e.g., lemon extract or juice) can be made at home to replace water and electrolytes. Another solution that can be made at home is a mixture of 1 teaspoon of salt and 8 teaspoons of sugar in 1 L of water, plus 4 ounces of orange juice.

Explain that food intake is not vital or recommended during episodes of acute diarrhea. When food is reintroduced, the BRAT diet may be recommended as a way to reintroduce solid food.

If an antidiarrheal drug is used, review its precautions and limitations. For the patient with chronic diarrhea, provide information on foods to avoid (see Table 26-1) and foods to include to maintain adequate nutritional status. Patients who are not lactose intolerant may benefit from consuming yogurt with active cultures, which contain the same nonpathogenic bacteria (probiotic cultures) as are normally found in the intestine.

Constipation

Constipation is defined as infrequent or difficult passage of stools. Patients may complain of constipation when they have less than one stool per day, even if feces are of normal consistency and are not difficult to expel. The term *constipation* is appropriate only when the patient has two or fewer bowel movements weekly or when defecation is excessively difficult or requires straining, and when these symptoms persist for an extended period of time.

Constipation affects older adults more often than younger people. Although intestinal transit slows somewhat with aging, more significant factors contributing to constipation include general health, diet, medications, and activity levels (Box 26-1). Use of narcotic analgesic medications is a significant risk factor for constipation.

PATHOPHYSIOLOGY AND MANIFESTATIONS

Acute constipation may be due to an organic cause, such as a tumor or partial bowel obstruction. Lifestyle and psychogenic factors (e.g., ignoring the urge to defecate or feeling the need to defecate on schedule) are the most frequent causes of chronic constipation. In older adults, habitual use of laxatives can lead to constipation when laxatives are withdrawn. Other common causes of constipation are listed in Table 26-3. The patient with significant constipation may develop a *fecal impaction* (hardened stool). Small amounts of watery mucus or liquid stool may pass around the impaction. The patient has a full sensation in the rectal area and abdominal cramping.

COLLABORATIVE CARE

On examination, the abdomen may appear distended, and bowel sounds may be reduced. Digital examination of the rectum in the patient with an impaction reveals a palpable hard or puttylike fecal mass. Simple or chronic constipation is best treated with education and modification of diet and exercise routines. Foods that have a high fiber content, such as fresh fruits and vegetables, whole-grain breads, and cereals, are recommended.

Diagnostic Tests

If constipation is acute or does not resolve, diagnostic studies such as *serum electrolytes* and *thyroid function tests* may be

Constipation

Slowed peristalsis, decreased activity levels, reduced food and fluid intake, and decreased sensation contribute to a higher incidence of constipation in older adults. Chronic diseases, mobility problems, and medications also increase their risk for constipation.

Because cultural influences and advertising lead many people to believe that a daily bowel movement is important for health, the older adult may come to rely on laxatives, suppositories, or enemas to facilitate movement of soft stool every 2 to 3 days.

When assessing the older adult, focus on bowel patterns and factors contributing to actual or perceived constipation. Ask about normal elimination (frequency, timing, size, and consistency). Assess dietary habits, including types and amounts of foods and fluids normally consumed. Assess the patient's mouth and teeth for possible barriers to consuming foods high in fiber. Evaluate medications (including over-the-counter) for their effects on elimination. Discuss daily activity and the ability to respond to the urge to defecate.

Teach about normal bowel elimination and expected changes that occur with aging. Discuss the following measures to promote regular elimination:

- Increase dietary fiber intake to provide bulk and keep stools soft and easy to expel. Fresh fruits and vegetables, whole grains, high-fiber breakfast cereals, and unprocessed bran added to other foods are good sources of dietary fiber.
- Drink six to eight glasses of water per day (unless contraindicated). Drinking a cup of warm water after breakfast may help stimulate the urge to defecate.
- Remain physically active to promote bowel function and maintain muscle tone. Good abdominal muscle tone helps expel feces.
- Respond to the urge to defecate when it is felt. Delaying defecation may contribute to constipation.
- Do not use laxatives, suppositories, or enemas on a regular basis unless advised by the physician. Bulk-forming agents (FiberCon, Citrucel, or Metamucil) are safe for long-term use. It is important to drink at least six to eight glasses of water daily when using any laxative.
- Report to your primary care provider any change in bowel habits such as constipation or diarrhea, abdominal pain, black or bloody stools, nausea or anorexia, weakness, or unexplained weight loss.

TABLE 26-3	Common Causes of Constipation
FACTOR	**RELATED CAUSE**
Activity	Lack of exercise; impaired mobility; bed rest
Dietary	Highly refined, low-fiber foods; inadequate fluid intake
Drugs	Antacids containing aluminum or calcium salts; narcotic analgesics; many antidepressants, tranquilizers, and sedatives; antihypertensives; iron salts
Large bowel	Diverticular disease, inflammatory disease, tumor, obstruction; changes in rectal or anal structure or function
Systemic	Advanced age; pregnancy; neurologic conditions (e.g., stroke); endocrine and metabolic disorders (e.g., hypothyroidism)
Psychogenic	Voluntary suppression of urge; perceived need to defecate on schedule; depression
Other	Chronic laxative or enema use

narcotic analgesics for chronic pain may need both a stool softener and a stimulant laxative on a regular basis to manage associated constipation. Cathartics and enemas interfere with normal bowel reflexes and should not be used to manage simple constipation. Commonly ordered laxatives are listed in Table 26-4■.

clinicalALERT

Laxatives should *never* be given if a bowel obstruction or impaction is suspected, nor be given to people with abdominal pain of unknown cause. Administering laxatives or cathartics when the bowel is obstructed may damage the bowel and lead to perforation.

Enemas

Significant or chronic constipation or a fecal impaction may require administration of an enema. Enemas may also be prescribed to prepare the bowel for diagnostic testing or examination. They are *never* used when there may be obstruction or risk of perforation. The following types of enemas may be prescribed:

- A *saline enema* using 500 to 2,000 mL of warmed normal saline solution is the least irritating to the bowel.
- *Tap-water enemas* use 500 to 1,000 mL of water to soften feces and irritate the bowel mucosa, stimulating peristalsis and evacuation.
- *Soap-suds enemas* consist of a tap-water solution to which soap is added as a further irritant.
- *Phosphate enemas* (e.g., Fleet) use a hypertonic saline solution to draw fluid into the bowel and irritate the mucosa, leading to evacuation.

ordered. A *barium enema, flexible colonoscopy,* or *virtual colonography* (CT scan of the colon) may be done to identify structural lesions of the colon.

Medications

Laxatives and cathartics were among the earliest drugs used by humans. Milder preparations are generally known as *laxatives; cathartics* have a stronger effect. Most laxatives are appropriate only for short-term use. Patients who require

TABLE 26-4	Giving Medications Safely: Cathartics and Laxatives		
CLASS/DRUGS	**PURPOSE**	**NURSING IMPLICATIONS**	**PATIENT TEACHING**
Bowel preparation cathartics **Magnesium citrate** ■ Citrate of magnesia ■ Citro-Nesia ■ Citroma **Polyethylene glycol and electrolytes** ■ Colyte ■ GoLYTELY ■ X-Prep	These cathartics are often used before colon x-ray studies or colonoscopy. They promote bowel evacuation by drawing fluid into the bowel, which distends the colon and stimulates peristalsis, causing diarrhea and bowel cleansing. Electrolytes may be added to the solution to minimize electrolyte imbalance.	Chill the solution to enhance palatability. Evacuation begins within 1 hour and continues until stool is clear and free of solid matter. *Magnesium citrate* Administer on an empty stomach followed by a full glass of water. *Polyethylene glycol* Administer 8 ounces of solution every 10 minutes.	Expect some degree of abdominal cramping. Do not eat solid food 3 to 4 hours prior to, nor within 2 hours of, ingesting polyethylene glycol solution. Do not use this medication for routine treatment of constipation.
Laxatives **Bulk-forming agents** ■ Bran ■ Calcium polycarbophil (FiberCon, Fiberall, others) ■ Methylcellulose (Citrucel) ■ Psyllium mucilloid (Metamucil, Naturacil, others)	Bulk-forming agents contain indigestible vegetable fiber. This natural fiber creates bulk and draws water into the intestine, softening the stool mass.	Mix the agent with a full glass of cool liquid just before administering. Do not administer to patients with possible impaction or bowel obstruction.	These agents may be mixed with water, milk, or fruit juice. Take in the morning or with meals. To reduce the risk of impaction, do not take at bedtime. With these and all laxatives, drink at least six to eight glasses of water daily.
Stool softeners ■ Docusate (Colace, Surfak, Doxidan, others)	Stool softeners draw water into the stool and form an emulsion of fat and water, softening the stool. They are used to prevent straining and reduce the discomfort of expelling hard stools.	Administer with ample fluids. Stool softeners may affect drug absorption. Do not give within 1 hour of other oral medications. Do not crush or open caplets; a liquid form is available for patients who have difficulty swallowing.	Do not use for longer than 1 week. Take in the morning or evening; avoid taking it at the same time as other medications.
Osmotic and saline laxatives/cathartics ■ Lactulose (Cholac, Heptalac, others) ■ Sorbitol ■ Magnesium hydroxide (Milk of Magnesia) ■ Magnesium citrate ■ Polyethylene glycol (Klean-Prep)	These laxatives contain poorly absorbed salts or carbohydrates that draw water into the intestine to increase stool volume, decrease its consistency, and stimulate peristalsis. These drugs also may stimulate peristalsis by irritating the bowel mucosa. Their use should be limited to acute, short-term use; chronic use may suppress normal bowel reflexes.	Assess for contraindications, such as bowel obstruction, fluid or electrolyte imbalances, heart failure, or renal failure. Administer with a full glass of liquid, preferably in the morning to avoid sleep disturbance. Monitor fluid and electrolyte status; skin turgor; mucous membranes; intake and output; daily weight; and serum electrolytes.	Do not use these drugs on a regular basis to treat or prevent constipation. Notify your doctor if you develop abdominal pain, bloody stool, excessive skin or mucous membrane dryness, rapid weight loss, dizziness, or other unusual symptoms. These agents work in 3 to 6 hours; take them in the morning to avoid sleep disturbance.
Irritant or stimulant laxatives ■ Bisacodyl (Dulcolax, Bisco-Lax, Carter's Little Pills, Theralax, others) ■ Phenolphthalein (Evac-U-Gen, Evac-U-Lax, Feen-A-Mint, Phenolax, others) ■ Cascara sagrada ■ Senna (Senna laxative, Fletcher's Castoria) ■ Castor oil	These laxatives stimulate intestinal motility and secretions. They cause watery stool, often accompanied by abdominal cramping and pain. They are used as a secondary measure to relieve constipation and for bowel preparation before diagnostic testing.	Assess for contraindications such as abdominal pain and cramping, nausea and vomiting, and anal or rectal fissures. Food may affect absorption; give on an empty stomach. Do not crush enteric-coated bisacodyl tablets. This may hasten their dissolution in the stomach, leading to gastric distress.	Do not use for more than 1 week because these drugs can be habit forming. Do not use if you are pregnant or lactating. Laxatives that contain phenolphthalein may turn urine pink or red. Stop taking the drug and contact your doctor if you develop difficulty breathing, dizziness or light-headedness, or a rash.

TABLE 26-4	Giving Medications Safely: Cathartics and Laxatives *(continued)*		
CLASS/DRUGS	**PURPOSE**	**NURSING IMPLICATIONS**	**PATIENT TEACHING**
Lubricants			
■ Mineral oil	Mineral oil forms an oily coating on feces, preventing water reabsorption and softening stool. It reduces absorption of the fat-soluble vitamins A, D, E, and K and may damage the liver and spleen; pneumonia may develop from aspiration of oil droplets into the lungs.	Do not give with stool softeners, which may increase systemic absorption and the effects of the mineral oil. Administer in the evening before bedtime to reduce the effect on vitamin absorption and minimize the risk of aspiration. Assess for manifestations of vitamin deficiency.	Long-term use of mineral oil is not recommended. Do not use mineral oil if you have hemorrhoids or rectal lesions; oil leakage may cause itching and interfere with healing. Suck on a lemon or orange slice after taking mineral oil to reduce the oily aftertaste.

■ *Oil-retention enemas* instill mineral or vegetable oil into the bowel to soften the fecal mass. The instilled oil is retained overnight or for several hours before evacuation.

Excess use of enemas, especially tap-water or phosphate, can impair bowel function and cause fluid and electrolyte imbalances.

Complementary Therapies

Unless it is associated with bowel obstruction or another serious disorder, complementary and alternative therapies may be helpful to relieve constipation. Exercise, particularly activities such as swimming, walking, or sit-ups, strengthens abdominal muscles and makes defecation easier. Exercise often also stimulates the urge to defecate. Abdominal massage with a massage oil containing orange, black pepper, ginger, or marjoram may reduce discomfort and stimulate an urge to defecate. Certain herbal preparations, such as dandelion root, chicory root, cascara sagrada, and senna, have a laxative effect and may be used for brief periods to relieve constipation.

NURSING CARE

In many cases, nursing care measures can relieve constipation and help prevent it from recurring.

PRIORITIZING NURSING CARE

Educating patients about "normal" bowel habits and health promotion measures to prevent constipation are the nursing care priorities for patients in the community. In settings such as long-term care, residential, or rehabilitation facilities, nursing care priorities are also on prevention. Patients in these settings are at high risk for becoming constipated, increasing the importance of monitoring and assessing bowel function on a continuing basis.

HEALTH PROMOTION

For many people, education can prevent constipation. Discuss normal bowel habits, explaining that a daily bowel movement is not the norm for everyone. Stress the importance of responding to the urge to defecate when felt. Teach the importance of maintaining a diet high in natural fiber. Encourage to reduce intake of meat and refined foods that are low in fiber. Emphasize the importance of maintaining a generous daily fluid intake. Discuss the relationship between regular exercise and bowel regularity. Encourage the patient to engage in some form of exercise, such as walking, daily.

Constipation

Expected outcome: Will resume normal or usual pattern of bowel elimination.

■ Assess and document pattern of defecation, including time of day, amount, and stool consistency. *Information about bowel habits helps identify physiologic versus perceived constipation. Whether real or perceived, constipation disrupts daily activities and life satisfaction.*

■ Assess diet, fluid intake, and activity. Evaluate for other contributing factors, such as use of narcotic analgesics, prescribed bed rest, painful hemorrhoids, and perianal surgery. *These provide clues about possible causes of constipation. The patient may require a bulk laxative or stool softener while contributing factors are present.*

■ Assess abdominal shape and girth, bowel sounds, and tenderness. If impaction is suspected, examine the rectum digitally, using a lubricated, gloved finger. *Constipation may cause abdominal distention, reduced bowel sounds, and some abdominal tenderness. Digital removal of stool impacted in the rectum may be required.*

■ Provide additional fluids to maintain an intake of at least 2,500 mL per day. *Adequate hydration facilitates normal bowel elimination.*

■ Encourage drinking of a glass of warm water before and after breakfast. Provide time and privacy after breakfast for bowel elimination. *Warm water provides mild stimulation of bowel peristalsis. Privacy helps encourage a pattern of natural elimination.*

■ Consult with the dietitian to increase dietary fiber (unless contraindicated). Provide foods such as natural bran, prunes, or prune juice. *Natural fiber adds bulk to the stool and has a mild stimulant effect.*

- Encourage activity. *Activity stimulates peristalsis and strengthens abdominal muscles, facilitating elimination.*
- Obtain an order for a stool softener, laxative, or enema if indicated. *Pharmacologic agents may be necessary to relieve acute constipation. Patients with restricted mobility or diet restrictions may need a bulk-forming laxative to prevent constipation.*

MANAGING NURSING CARE

Enema administration may be delegated to assistive personnel who have appropriate training and demonstrated competence.

CONTINUITY OF CARE

Discuss restricting the use of laxatives and enemas, and stress that bulk-forming laxatives are the only safe preparations for long-term use. Teach the patient that straining to have a bowel movement can lead to hemorrhoids and tissue damage. Suggest abdominal massage to reduce discomfort and promote elimination.

Irritable Bowel Syndrome

Irritable bowel syndrome (IBS) is a motility disorder characterized by alternating periods of constipation and diarrhea. It affects up to 20% of people in Western civilization.

PATHOPHYSIOLOGY AND MANIFESTATIONS

Central nervous system (CNS) regulation of the motor and sensory functions of the bowel is altered in IBS. Intestinal motility can be affected by eating, stress, hormones, and drugs. Motility of both the small and large intestine increases in response to stimulation by food intake, hormones, and physiologic and psychologic stress in patients with IBS. In addition, sensory responses to the movement of chyme through the bowel are exaggerated. Excess mucus may be secreted in the colon as well.

Stress may increase the manifestations of IBS but does not cause them. The patient with IBS may experience a change in the frequency or consistency of stools, straining, urgency, or a sensation of incomplete evacuation. Other manifestations of the disorder are listed in Box 26-2■.

COLLABORATIVE CARE

The diagnosis of IBS is based on the patient's history, the pattern of symptoms and elimination, and physical examination.

Diagnostic Tests

A *stool specimen* is examined for occult blood, WBCs, and ova and parasites (to rule out infectious causes). *Sigmoidoscopy* or *colonoscopy* may be done to visually examine the bowel mucosa and measure pressures within the large bowel.

BOX 26-2	MANIFESTATIONS OF IRRITABLE BOWEL SYNDROME

- Abdominal pain and tenderness:
  - Often in right lower quadrant
  - Intermittent and colicky or dull and continuous
  - May be relieved by defecation
- Alternating constipation and diarrhea; stool may contain mucus
- Abdominal bloating and flatulence
- Possible nausea, vomiting

A *small-bowel series* (also known as an upper GI series with small-bowel follow-through) and barium enema may be ordered. For the small-bowel series, the patient is given an oral barium preparation, and the small intestine is examined under fluoroscopy. The entire GI tract may demonstrate increased motility.

Treatment

Management is directed toward relieving the symptoms and reducing or eliminating precipitating factors. Stress reduction, exercises, or counseling may benefit the patient. Regular use of bulk-forming laxatives can help reduce bowel spasm and reestablish a normal pattern of elimination. Antidepressant medications, particularly selective serotonin reuptake inhibitors such as sertraline (Zoloft) and fluoxetine (Prozac), may help relieve abdominal pain and spasm. Tegaserod (Zelnorm) is a serotonin agonist drug approved for treating women with constipation related to IBS.

Although no specific diet is recommended, reduced milk intake may help some patients. In contrast, patients who are not lactose intolerant may benefit from consuming yogurt with active cultures, which contain the same nonpathogenic bacteria as are normally found in the intestine (probiotic cultures). Restricting gas-forming foods, fruits and berries, or caffeinated drinks may also be helpful. Some patients benefit from limiting their intake of sugars such as lactose (milk sugar), fructose (fruit sugar), or sorbitol (see Table 26-1). Patients in whom diarrhea predominates may benefit from a gluten-free diet (Di Sabatino & Corazza, 2012). Adding fiber to the diet reduces the incidence of both loose diarrheal and hard constipated stools. Complementary therapies such as use of herbs (peppermint oil, ginger, chamomile, valerian, or rosemary), biofeedback training, or hypnotherapy may provide relief for symptoms of IBS.

NURSING CARE

When patients with IBS are seen in the acute care setting, the disorder usually is a secondary condition. The previous sections on diarrhea and constipation provide selected nursing interventions for patients experiencing these manifestations.

When teaching, emphasize that the symptoms are real, believed, and not "all in the mind." Discuss related factors, such as stress, anxiety, and depression. Assist the patient to explore any relationship between mental stress and bowel manifestations. Teach stress- and anxiety-reduction techniques, such as exercise and progressive relaxation. Refer to a counselor for assistance in dealing with psychologic factors.

Help identify possible dietary influences on elimination patterns, and suggest changes such as increased water and fiber intake that may help relieve symptoms. Encourage changes in exercise and dietary patterns and use of stress-reduction techniques to gradually eliminate the need for prescribed medications.

Stress the importance of notifying the primary care provider if symptoms change, because the manifestations of IBS may mask symptoms of an organic problem, such as a tumor.

INFLAMMATORY DISORDERS

> **Key Concept**   Inflammatory bowel disorders may be either acute or chronic. Supporting physiologic function is the priority for acute inflammatory disorders, whereas teaching and supporting psychosocial function are vital for patients with chronic inflammatory bowel disorders.

The GI tract is constantly exposed to the external environment, making it particularly vulnerable to inflammation and infection. Most pathogens that affect it are ingested in food or water. *Gastroenteritis*, a general term for infection of the GI tract, is discussed in Chapter 25. Acute disorders such as appendicitis and peritonitis occur when bacteria normally residing in the GI tract infect damaged or normally sterile tissue.

Appendicitis

Appendicitis (inflammation of the appendix) is the most common reason for emergency abdominal surgery in the United States. The appendix is in the right lower quadrant region at *McBurney's point* (Figure 26-1 ■). Its function is not fully understood, but it regularly fills with and empties digested food. Appendicitis is most common in adolescents and young adults and is slightly more common in males than females.

PATHOPHYSIOLOGY

The appendix can become obstructed by a *fecalith* (hard mass of feces), stone, inflammation, or parasites (e.g., pinworms). As a result of the obstruction, the appendix becomes distended with fluid. This increases pressure within the appendix and impairs its blood supply. The lack of blood supply leads to inflammation, edema, ulceration, and infection of the tissue. Within 24 to 36 hours, the appendix becomes necrotic and perforates if treatment is not initiated.

Appendicitis is classified by the stage of the process. In *simple appendicitis,* the appendix is inflamed but intact. In *gangrenous appendicitis,* the appendix has areas of tissue necrosis and microscopic perforations. With a *perforated appendix,* the appendix has ruptured, contaminating the peritoneal cavity with its contents.

MANIFESTATIONS AND COMPLICATIONS

Generalized or upper abdominal pain is often the initial symptom of acute appendicitis. The pain gradually intensifies and localizes in the right lower quadrant of the abdomen. It is aggravated by moving, walking, or coughing. Localized and rebound tenderness are noted at McBurney's point. *Rebound tenderness* is demonstrated by relief of pain during palpation followed by pain on release of pressure. Extension of the right hip increases the pain. Less acute pain and local tenderness may delay diagnosis in pregnant women and older adults. The patient may have a low-grade

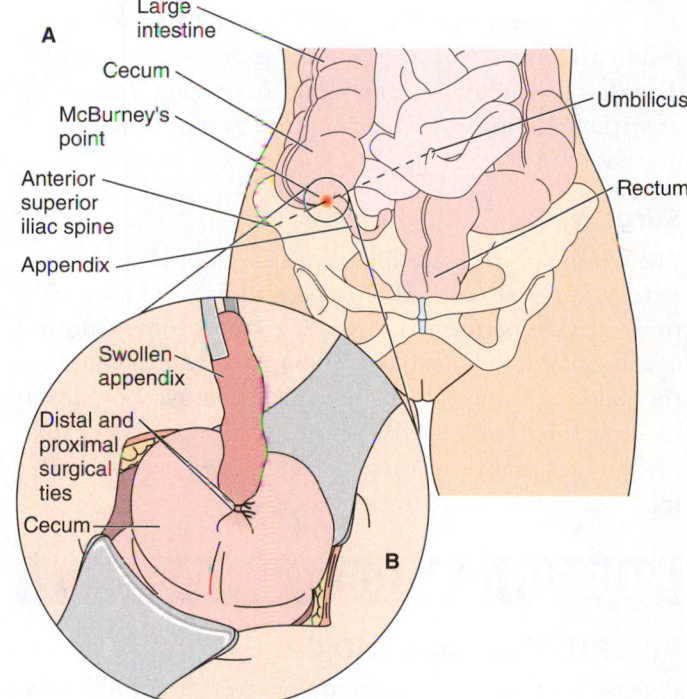

Figure 26-1. ■ **(A)** McBurney's point, located midway between the umbilicus and the anterior iliac crest in the right lower quadrant, is the usual site for localized pain and rebound tenderness due to appendicitis. **(B)** In an appendectomy, the appendix and cecum are identified. The base of the appendix is clamped and tied off; the appendix is then removed.

BOX 26-3	MANIFESTATIONS OF ACUTE APPENDICITIS

- Generalized abdominal pain becoming localized, usually in right lower quadrant
  - Aggravated by movement, right hip extension
- Rebound tenderness (pain on release of pressure of palpation)
- Anorexia, nausea, vomiting
- Low-grade fever

fever, anorexia, nausea, and vomiting. Manifestations of appendicitis are summarized in Box 26-3■.

Perforation is the major complication of acute appendicitis. It is manifested by increased pain, a rigid, boardlike abdomen, and a high fever. It can result in a small, localized abscess, local peritonitis, or significant generalized peritonitis.

COLLABORATIVE CARE

Because the acutely inflamed appendix can perforate within 24 hours, prompt diagnosis and treatment are important. The patient is admitted to the hospital, and intravenous fluids are initiated. Oral food and fluids are withheld until a diagnosis is confirmed.

Diagnostic Tests

Diagnostic testing and preoperative treatment are limited. The *white blood cell (WBC) count* is usually elevated in appendicitis. An *abdominal ultrasound* is done to confirm the diagnosis if symptoms are atypical. *Abdominal CT scan* with or without contrast media can often provide a definitive diagnosis of appendicitis.

Surgery

The treatment of choice for acute appendicitis is an *appendectomy,* surgical removal of the appendix. The appendectomy may be performed through a **laparotomy** (surgical opening of the abdomen) or by **laparoscopy** (exploration of the abdomen using an endoscope). *Laparoscopic appendectomy* requires three very small incisions, and recovery is rapid. Antibiotic therapy is initiated before surgery and continues for at least 48 hours postoperatively.

NURSING CARE

PRIORITIZING NURSING CARE

Because appendicitis can rapidly progress from inflammation to perforation, prompt assessment is vital.

ASSESSING

Assessment of the patient with suspected appendicitis focuses on describing the pain, as well as its onset, severity, and duration. Ask about recent food or fluid intake,

allergies, and current medications. Ensure that informed consent has been obtained before surgery. If time allows, teach postoperative turning, coughing, deep breathing, and pain management. Report WBC results as soon as available.

DIAGNOSING, PLANNING, AND IMPLEMENTING

safetyALERT

Withhold all food and fluids from the patient with suspected appendicitis, because surgery is the treatment of choice. Do not administer laxatives or enemas, apply heat, or palpate the abdomen because these measures may cause perforation of the appendix.

Risk for Infection

Expected outcome: Will remain free of signs of inflammation or infection.

Inflammation and edema of the appendix interfere with its blood supply, increasing the risk for tissue necrosis and rupture.

- Monitor for signs of perforation and peritonitis preoperatively. *A primary goal of care is to prevent complications. Perforation may be signaled by a sudden relief of pain as the appendix ruptures, followed by increased generalized pain, abdominal distention, and a rigid, boardlike abdomen.*
- Monitor vital signs. *An elevated pulse and rapid, shallow breathing may indicate perforation of the appendix with infection and peritonitis. The temperature may be elevated. If sepsis develops, the blood pressure may fall.*
- Maintain intravenous fluids until the patient is able to drink adequate amounts postoperatively. *Intravenous fluids help maintain fluid and electrolyte balance and vascular volume.*
- Postoperatively, monitor wound, abdominal girth, and pain. *Swelling of the wound, increased abdominal girth, or increased pain may indicate internal bleeding, infection, or peritonitis.*

Acute Pain

Expected outcome: Will report pain at a level of 2 or less on a scale of 0 to 10.

- Assess pain, including its character, location, severity, and duration. Report any unexpected changes in description of pain. *Careful pain assessment can provide important clues about diagnosis and possible complications. For example, generalized abdominal pain with guarding of abdominal muscles may indicate peritonitis.*
- Administer prescribed analgesics. *Preoperatively, pain medication can be given after a diagnosis is established. Postoperatively, provide analgesics to promote comfort and enhance mobility.*

- Assess effectiveness of medication after administration. If pain is not relieved, contact the charge nurse or physician. *Pain unrelieved by analgesics may indicate a complication.*
- Provide alternative methods of pain relief, including distraction, therapeutic touch, massage, meditation, or visualization. *These techniques can enhance comfort and the effectiveness of analgesics.*

CONTINUITY OF CARE

After an uncomplicated appendectomy, the patient is usually dismissed from the acute care setting either the day of surgery or the day after surgery. Teach wound or incision care. Instruct to report swelling, redness, drainage, bleeding, or warmth at the operative site to the surgeon. If a dressing is present, teach proper hand washing and dressing change procedures. Instruct the patient to report any fever or increased abdominal pain.

Discuss activity restrictions. Heavy lifting may be restricted for up to 6 weeks. Depending on the surgery, driving and return to work may be allowed within 1 to 2 weeks. Community health or home health care nurses may be required if the patient has a preexisting illness or has trouble performing activities of daily living (ADLs) and self-care.

Peritonitis

Peritonitis is inflammation of the peritoneum, a double-layered membrane that lines the walls and organs of the abdominal cavity. It is a serious complication of many acute abdominal disorders. Peritonitis results when the normally sterile space between the layers of the peritoneum is contaminated. A perforated appendix or gastric ulcer, traumatic injury such as a gunshot wound, or contamination during abdominal surgery can lead to peritonitis.

PATHOPHYSIOLOGY

Perforation of a peptic ulcer, rupture of the appendix, or contamination of the abdominal cavity by bowel contents during surgery allows chemicals and bacteria from the GI tract to enter the normally sterile peritoneal cavity. *Chemical peritonitis* develops immediately after perforation of a peptic ulcer, as gastric juices (hydrochloric acid and pepsin) enter the peritoneal cavity. *Bacterial peritonitis* results when bacteria that are normally confined within the bowel enter the peritoneal cavity. Normal inflammatory and immune defense mechanisms may effectively eliminate small numbers of bacteria or localize the infection. Massive or continued contamination, however, leads to generalized inflammation of the peritoneal cavity. The inflammatory process causes a fluid shift into the peritoneal space (*third-spacing*). Peristalsis slows or stops (**paralytic ileus**) due to the inflammation.

MANIFESTATIONS AND COMPLICATIONS

The signs and symptoms of peritonitis depend on the severity and extent of the infection, as well as the age and general health of the patient. Both abdominal and systemic manifestations are present (Box 26-4■). The patient often presents with an *acute abdomen.* An acute abdomen is characterized by an abrupt onset of severe pain, often accompanied by boardlike abdominal muscle rigidity.

clinical**ALERT**

The older, chronically debilitated, or immunosuppressed patient may have few of the classic signs of peritonitis. Increased confusion and restlessness, decreased urinary output, and vague abdominal complaints may be the only manifestations.

Complications of peritonitis may be life threatening and either localized or systemic. Formation of an *abscess* is the most common complication. *Septicemia,* the presence of pathogens in the blood, may develop. Without prompt treatment, shock may result from hypovolemia or sepsis. Shock (see Chapter 14) requires immediate, aggressive treatment to prevent multiple organ failure and death. *Adhesions* or bands of scar tissue may develop after peritonitis and subsequently cause a bowel obstruction.

COLLABORATIVE CARE

Care of the patient with peritonitis focuses on identifying and treating both the peritonitis and its cause.

Diagnostic Tests

The WBC is significantly elevated in peritonitis. *Blood cultures* are obtained to identify possible *bacteremia* (bacterial invasion of the blood), which often precedes septicemia. *CT scan* or *ultrasound* may show free fluid or an abscess in the abdomen. A *paracentesis* may be done to obtain peritoneal fluid for analysis.

BOX 26-4	MANIFESTATIONS OF PERITONITIS

Abdominal
- Diffuse or localized pain, usually severe
- Tenderness with rebound
- Boardlike rigidity or guarding of abdominal muscles
- Diminished or absent bowel sounds
- Progressive abdominal distention
- Anorexia, nausea, and vomiting

Systemic
- Fever, malaise
- Tachycardia, tachypnea
- Restlessness, confusion
- Oliguria

Management

Intestinal decompression is initiated to relieve abdominal distention. A nasogastric or long intestinal tube (Figure 26-2■) is inserted and connected to continuous drainage. Suction is maintained, and the patient is NPO until peristalsis returns (bowel sounds are heard and flatus is being passed). Intravenous fluids and electrolyte replacements are provided. Parenteral nutrition is given until oral intake resumes. The patient is placed on bed rest in Fowler's position to help localize the infection and to make breathing easier. Oxygen is often ordered.

A broad-spectrum antibiotic is prescribed until the infecting organism has been identified. Then antibiotic therapy is modified to the specific organism(s). The patient may receive narcotic analgesics and sedatives to promote comfort and rest.

Surgery

Laparoscopic surgery may be performed to identify and treat the source of infection. A laparotomy may be done to close a perforation, remove damaged and inflamed tissue, or remove an abscess. *Peritoneal lavage* (washing of the peritoneal cavity with warm, isotonic fluid) may be done during surgery and continued for up to 3 days after surgery. The solution is infused into the upper portion of the peritoneal cavity and removed via drains in the pelvis. Careful attention to fluid and electrolyte status and strict aseptic technique are necessary.

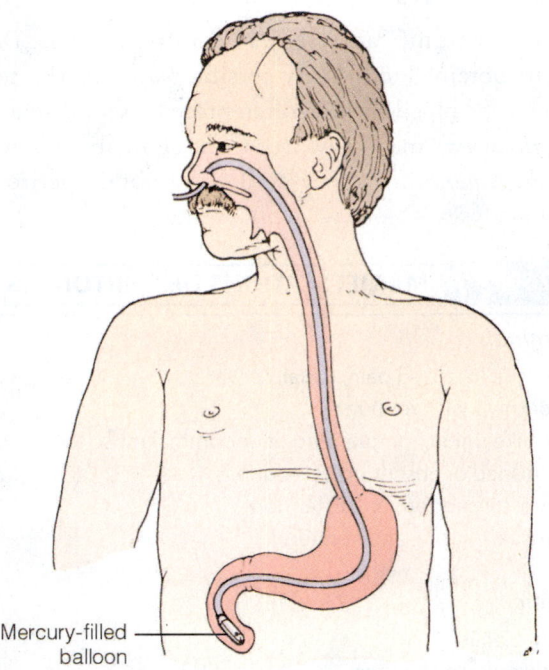

Mercury-filled balloon

Figure 26-2. ■ The weighted tip or inflated balloon at the end of an intestinal tube is drawn into the intestine by gravity and peristalsis.

Patients who have had laparotomy for peritonitis often return from surgery with drains such as a Jackson-Pratt. In some cases, the incision may be left unsutured. The abdomen may be closed temporarily with mesh containing a nylon zipper or Velcro to allow repeated exploration of the abdomen and drainage of infectious sites.

NURSING CARE

Peritonitis is a serious illness. Patients require intensive nursing and medical interventions to recover fully.

PRIORITIZING NURSING CARE

Supporting the patient and managing responses to the acute inflammatory process are the priorities for nursing care of the patient with peritonitis.

ASSESSING

Frequent, focused nursing assessment of patients with peritonitis is vital. Assessment focuses on monitoring the patient's current status, progress of recovery, and identifying possible complications.

Frequently assess the patient's pain, including location, intensity, and character. Ask about feelings of fear or anxiety and the patient's ability to cope.

Assess mental status and level of consciousness at least every 4 to 8 hours. Obtain vital signs, including temperature, hourly or as indicated. If ordered, note hemodynamic measurements such as venous or arterial pressures. Check urine output hourly.

Assess drainage from GI tube and surgical drains every 4 hours or as ordered. Record amount, color, odor, and type of drainage; report changes. Using the same measuring tape and a marked location on the abdomen (usually at the umbilicus), measure abdominal girth every 8 hours.

IDENTIFYING POTENTIAL COMPLICATIONS

Increasing abdominal pain, pain that is not relieved by prescribed analgesics, or pain that differs in nature from previously reported pain may indicate a complication and should be reported to the charge nurse or physician. Report changes in mental status, level of consciousness, or vital signs, as these may indicate systemic infection or another complication. Report urine output of less than 30 mL/hr for 2 consecutive hours. Notify the charge nurse or physician of increasing abdominal girth.

DIAGNOSING, PLANNING, AND IMPLEMENTING

Acute Pain

Expected outcome: Will report pain at a 2 or lower on a scale of 0 to 10.

- Place in Fowler's or semi-Fowler's position with the knees and feet elevated. *This position helps minimize stress on abdominal structures and facilitate respirations, promoting comfort.*
- Administer analgesics as ordered on a routine basis or using patient-controlled analgesia (PCA). Frequently evaluate response to analgesics. *Routine administration of analgesics helps maintain pain control, facilitating healing and movement.*
- Promptly report a change in the location, severity, or character of pain. *A significant change in the location or nature of the pain or pain that is unrelieved by narcotic analgesics may indicate a new problem or a complication.*
- Teach and assist to use alternative pain management techniques along with analgesics. *Meditation, visualization, massage, and progressive relaxation augment analgesics and increase comfort.*

Deficient Fluid Volume

Expected outcome: Will maintain adequate hydration as evidenced by stable vital signs, clear mental status, urine output greater than 30 mL/hr, and warm, pink, moist skin with good turgor.

- Record vital signs, intake and output, weight, and moisture of skin and mucous membranes as indicated. Measure or estimate fluid losses through abdominal drains and on dressings. *Fluid losses occur through third-spacing, GI suction, and drainage from surgical wounds and drains. This can lead to hypovolemia.*
- Monitor laboratory values, such as hemoglobin and hematocrit, urine specific gravity, and serum electrolytes. Report changes to the physician. *These values provide information about the patient's fluid and electrolyte status.*
- Maintain intravenous fluids and electrolytes as ordered. *GI drainage may be replaced milliliter for milliliter with a balanced electrolyte solution. In addition, fluid intake must be maintained intravenously while the patient is NPO.*
- Provide good skin care and frequent oral hygiene. *Fluid loss increases the risk of skin breakdown and ulceration of mucous membranes.*

Risk for Infection

Expected outcome: Will remain free of infection.

- Monitor for signs of infection, including fever, tachycardia, redness and swelling around incisions and drain sites, increased or purulent drainage, and cloudy, malodorous, or scant urine. *Surgical interventions and stress on immune defenses increase the risk for further infection.*
- Obtain cultures of purulent drainage from any site. *Early identification allows appropriate intervention to be instituted.*
- Practice meticulous hand washing before and after providing care. Use strict aseptic technique for dressing changes and wound or peritoneal irrigations. *Hand washing reduces transient bacteria on the skin and remains the most important method of controlling infection. Interruption of the skin barrier increases the risk for infection.*
- Maintain fluid balance and adequate nutrition through either enteral or parenteral feedings, as indicated. *Adequate nutrition and fluid balance are necessary for optimal immune system function.*

Anxiety

Expected outcome: Will be able to rest when undisturbed and follow directions when necessary.

- Assess the patient's and family's anxiety level and coping skills. *This provides a basis on which to plan interventions.*
- Present a calm, reassuring manner. Encourage the patient and family to express their concerns; listen carefully, and acknowledge their validity. *This helps establish trust.*
- Minimize changes in caregiver assignments. *Consistency of nursing care and care providers helps reduce anxiety. Complex wound care and irrigation procedures are best performed by people who are very familiar with prescribed techniques.*
- Explain all treatments, procedures, tests, and examinations. Reinforce and clarify information provided by physicians. *Understanding what is being done helps reduce anxiety and promote acceptance.*
- Teach and assist with relaxation techniques such as meditation, visualization, and progressive relaxation. *These measures promote positive coping skills and reduce physical manifestations of anxiety.*

MANAGING NURSING CARE

Nursing care activities such as obtaining vital signs, measuring intake and output, and assisting with positioning and hygiene for the patient with acute peritonitis may be appropriate to assign to assistive personnel who have appropriate training and demonstrated competence.

EVALUATING

Collect the following data to evaluate the effectiveness of nursing care for the patient with peritonitis: level of pain and effectiveness of analgesics; weight, urine output, and other indicators of fluid volume status; temperature, wound healing and drainage, and other indicators of infection; and indicators of anxiety and effective coping.

DOCUMENTING

Document continuing assessment data, including subjective complaints of pain and the effect of analgesia in relieving pain. Also document the type and amount of drainage from nasogastric or intestinal tubes and wound drains. Note wound healing (as appropriate), drainage from the incision, and any foul odor on dressings or of drainage.

CONTINUITY OF CARE

Teaching is vital throughout hospitalization and before discharge. The patient's and family's ability to manage wound care, nutrition, and ADLs helps to drive the decision for discharge home, to rehabilitation, or to a transitional care setting. Provide complete information to caregivers in community-based care settings regarding the disease, surgery, or other procedures performed, current medications, wound care needs, and nutritional status, as well as the patient's expressed preferences.

Begin teaching for home care before discharge. Provide verbal and written instructions for wound care, dressing changes, and irrigation procedures. Allow the patient and family members to practice and demonstrate procedures before discharge. Include information on where to obtain necessary supplies. Discuss medications, including the name and purpose of the drug and potential adverse effects and their management.

Describe the signs and symptoms of further infection (redness, heat, swelling, purulent drainage, chills, and fever) and other potential complications. Emphasize the need to report adverse responses promptly to the primary care provider. Reinforce instructions about activity restrictions. Discuss the importance of consuming a diet with adequate calories and protein to promote healing and optimal immune function. Provide a referral to home health services for assessment, wound care, and further teaching, as needed.

Inflammatory Bowel Disease

Chronic **inflammatory bowel disease** (IBD) includes two closely related disorders, ulcerative colitis and Crohn's disease. IBD is more common in the United States and northern Europe than it is in countries of the southern hemisphere. Its incidence also varies among cultural groups (Box 26-5■). These conditions are similar in many ways:

BOX 26-5 FOCUS ON DIVERSITY

Inflammatory Bowel Disease
- American Jews of European descent have a higher incidence of IBD than persons in other cultural/ethnic groups.
- The incidence of IBD is increasing among African Americans and Hispanics, who previously had a lower incidence than Whites.
- Asians have a lower incidence of IBD than do Whites, African Americans, and Hispanics.

Source: Crohn's & Colitis Foundation of America, 2013.

- Their cause is unknown, although factors such as infection, altered immune responses, genetic makeup, and lifestyle are thought to play a role.
- Both affect primarily young adults and may also affect older adults.
- Both are chronic and recurrent.
- Diarrhea is the predominant symptom of each.
- Both may have associated manifestations, such as arthritis.

Ulcerative colitis and Crohn's disease also differ from one another in several ways: Ulcerative colitis tends to affect the large bowel in a continuous pattern, whereas Crohn's disease affects any part of the GI tract in a patchy pattern. Table 26-5■ compares the manifestations and complications of ulcerative colitis and Crohn's disease. Figure 26-3■ illustrates the multisystem effects of chronic inflammatory bowel disease.

PATHOPHYSIOLOGY
Ulcerative Colitis

Ulcerative colitis is a chronic inflammatory disorder involving the mucosal layers of the colon and rectum. It affects primarily the young, although it is also seen in people between ages 60 and 80. Factors such as infection, diet, and environment may contribute to the development of ulcerative colitis.

TABLE 26-5	Manifestations and Complications of Inflammatory Bowel Disease	
	ULCERATIVE COLITIS	**CROHN'S DISEASE**
Manifestations	■ 5 to 30 stools per day ■ Blood and mucus in stool ■ Left lower quadrant crampy abdominal pain; relieved by defecation ■ Weight loss ■ Anemia, low serum protein levels ■ May have systemic symptoms	■ Diarrhea common but less severe ■ No obvious blood or mucus in stool ■ Right lower quadrant or central abdominal pain, cramping or steady ■ Significant weight loss ■ Anemia, multiple nutrient deficits ■ Fever, general malaise, fatigue
Complications	■ Toxic megacolon, perforation, massive hemorrhage ■ Colon cancer	■ Obstruction, fistula or abscess formation, malabsorption ■ Colon cancer

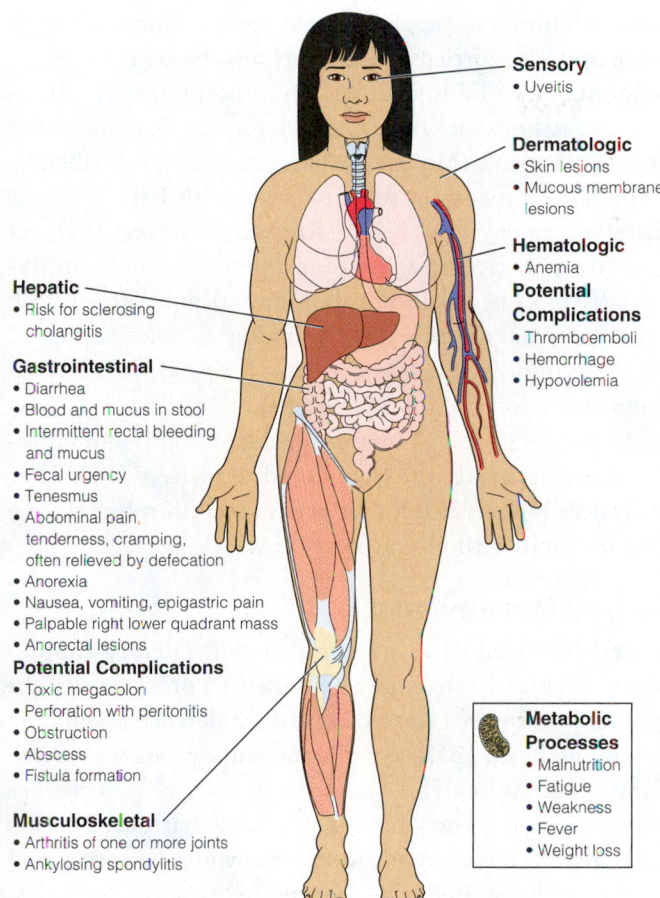

Sensory
• Uveitis

Dermatologic
• Skin lesions
• Mucous membrane lesions

Hematologic
• Anemia

Potential Complications
• Thromboemboli
• Hemorrhage
• Hypovolemia

Hepatic
• Risk for sclerosing cholangitis

Gastrointestinal
• Diarrhea
• Blood and mucus in stool
• Intermittent rectal bleeding and mucus
• Fecal urgency
• Tenesmus
• Abdominal pain, tenderness, cramping, often relieved by defecation
• Anorexia
• Nausea, vomiting, epigastric pain
• Palpable right lower quadrant mass
• Anorectal lesions

Potential Complications
• Toxic megacolon
• Perforation with peritonitis
• Obstruction
• Abscess
• Fistula formation

Musculoskeletal
• Arthritis of one or more joints
• Ankylosing spondylitis

Metabolic Processes
• Malnutrition
• Fatigue
• Weakness
• Fever
• Weight loss

Figure 26-3. ■ The multisystem effects of inflammatory bowel disease.

The inflammation of ulcerative colitis usually begins in the rectum. It may progress proximally along the colon, involving the bowel in a continuous pattern. The mucosa becomes inflamed and edematous and bleeds easily. The mucosa ulcerates, sloughs, and is lost in the feces. As scar tissue forms, the bowel wall thickens and shortens. In most people, only the rectum and sigmoid colon are affected. Less commonly, the entire colon may be involved.

MANIFESTATIONS   A gradual onset of diarrhea with intermittent rectal bleeding and mucus is common. In the most common form, acute attacks of colitis last 1 to 3 months and occur at intervals of months to years. Diarrhea is the chief symptom. In mild cases, the patient may have fewer than four stools per day with intermittent rectal bleeding and mucus and few systemic manifestations. In patients with severe ulcerative colitis, most of the large intestine may be involved. These patients may have more than 6 to 10 bloody stools per day and are at risk for dehydration and malnutrition. Rectal inflammation causes fecal urgency and *tenesmus* (straining). Left lower quadrant cramping relieved by defecation is common. Systemic manifestations include fatigue, anorexia, and weakness. Patients with severe disease may develop a related arthritis.

COMPLICATIONS   Complications of ulcerative colitis include *colon perforation,* the leading cause of death in these patients. *Toxic megacolon* is characterized by paralysis of the colon with significant distention, usually in the transverse segment of the large bowel. Manifestations of toxic megacolon include fever, tachycardia, hypotension, dehydration, abdominal tenderness, and cramping. An acute decrease in diarrhea stools may signal toxic megacolon. Patients with ulcerative colitis have a high risk for developing colon cancer.

Crohn's Disease

Crohn's disease (*regional enteritis*) is a chronic, relapsing inflammatory disorder that can affect any part of the GI tract from the mouth to the anus. The distal portion of the small intestine and the ascending colon are most commonly affected.

Crohn's disease causes inflammatory lesions of the bowel mucosa that may affect all layers of the bowel wall. These inflammatory lesions are localized, surrounded by normal tissue. Ulcers and deep fissures develop, and fistulas may form between loops of bowel or between the bowel and other organs (Figure 26-4■). Inflammation and scarring cause the bowel to narrow and become partially or fully obstructed. Over time, the bowel wall thickens and loses flexibility and looks somewhat like a rubber hose. Malabsorption and malnutrition may develop because inflammation and ulcers prevent absorption of nutrients, especially vitamin B_{12} and bile salts.

MANIFESTATIONS   Most people with Crohn's disease experience continuous or episodic diarrhea. Stools are liquid or semiformed and typically do not contain blood. Patients have abdominal pain and tenderness, and a mass may be

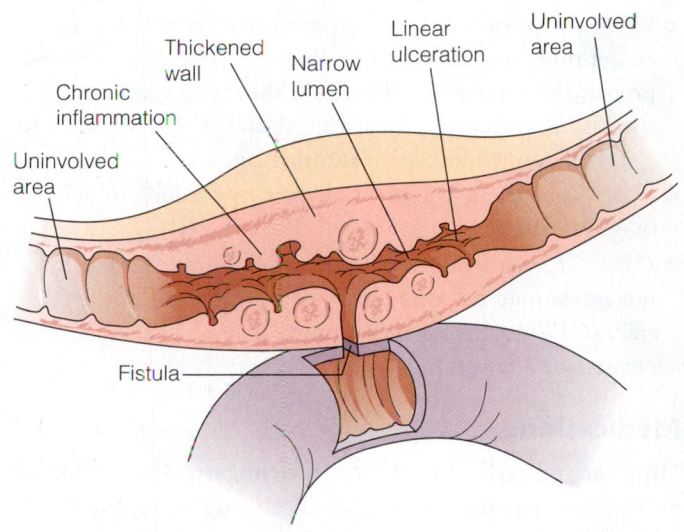

Chronic inflammation   Thickened wall   Narrow lumen   Linear ulceration   Uninvolved area

Uninvolved area

Fistula

Figure 26-4. ■ An illustration of the major characteristics of Crohn's disease in the small intestine.

palpable in the right lower quadrant. Many patients with Crohn's disease develop lesions of the rectum and anus, such as fissures, ulcers, fistulas, and abscesses. Systemic manifestations such as fever, malaise, and fatigue are common.

COMPLICATIONS Intestinal obstruction, abscess, and fistula are so common that they are considered part of the disease process. Intestinal obstruction causes abdominal distention, cramping pain, borborygmi, and sometimes nausea and vomiting. When an abscess forms, the patient develops chills and fever, a tender abdominal mass, and leukocytosis. Fistulas may be asymptomatic, particularly if they occur between loops of small bowel. A fistula between the small bowel and colon may increase diarrhea, weight loss, and malnutrition. When a fistula involves the bladder, recurrent urinary tract infections occur. Long-standing Crohn's disease increases the risk of cancer of the small intestine or colon by five to six times.

COLLABORATIVE CARE

Treatment of IBD is supportive, directed toward managing symptoms and controlling the disease process. Supportive care measures include rest, stress reduction, drugs, and nutritional support. When the disease does not respond to treatment or complications develop, surgery may be required.

Diagnostic Tests

Diagnostic testing is used to establish the diagnosis of IBD.

- A *stool specimen* is examined for blood and mucus and is sent for culture to rule out infectious causes.
- *Complete blood count (CBC), serum albumin level,* and serum levels of multiple vitamins are drawn to evaluate nutritional status. *ESR* (erythrocyte sedimentation rate) and *C-reactive protein* (CRP) provide evidence of inflammation.
- *Sigmoidoscopy* or *colonoscopy* is performed to visualize the bowel mucosa and collect tissue for biopsy. Harsh bowel preparations are avoided because they may exacerbate the disease. Instead, a clear liquid diet is ordered for 2 to 3 days before endoscopic examination.
- *Upper endoscopy* or *capsule endoscopy* may be done to help diagnose IBD.
- *Upper GI series with small-bowel follow-through* and a *barium enema* may be done for x-ray examination of the GI tract. *CT enterography* increasingly is used to evaluate the entire small bowel.

Medications

Drugs are prescribed to terminate acute attacks of IBD and reduce the frequency of relapse. Locally acting and systemic anti-inflammatory drugs are used to manage IBD.

Sulfasalazine (Azulfidine) and related drugs are poorly absorbed from the GI tract and act as local anti-inflammatory agents on the bowel mucosa. For an acute episode, corticosteroids may also be used to reduce inflammation (Table 26-6 ■). Immunosuppressive drugs such as azathioprine (Imuran), cyclosporine (Sandimmune), or methotrexate (Mexate, others) may be prescribed to maintain remission for some patients with IBD. Biologic therapies, the newest class of drugs used to treat IBD, act selectively, targeting specific immune responses. Infliximab (Remicade), adalimumab (Humira), and certolizumab pegol (Cimzia) are examples of biologics. See Chapter 11 for more information about caring for patients receiving drugs that affect the immune response.

Antibiotics such as metronidazole (Flagyl) and ciprofloxacin (Cipro) are commonly used to manage IBD. They are generally more helpful for patients with Crohn's disease than for those with ulcerative colitis.

Dietary Management

A well-balanced diet is recommended. Dietary supplements such as Ensure may be added to promote weight gain and nutritional status. Lactose intolerance is common in patients with IBD, so milk and milk products may be eliminated. When the disease primarily affects the colon, increasing dietary fiber may reduce diarrhea. Patients with obstruction or small-bowel narrowing, however, need a low-roughage diet (e.g., no raw fruits and vegetables, popcorn, nuts).

During an acute exacerbation, the patient is usually kept NPO. Total parenteral nutrition (TPN) is administered to maintain nutritional status. As the episode resolves, an elemental diet that contains all essential nutrients in a residue-free formula (e.g., Ensure) may be ordered. These measures reduce intestinal motility and allow the bowel to rest.

Surgery

Surgical removal of the colon cures ulcerative colitis. Most patients, however, choose surgery only when other treatments are ineffective or manifestations of the disease interfere with ADLs. Surgery may also be indicated for complications of Crohn's disease, such as bowel obstruction, fistulas, or abscesses.

Patients with ulcerative colitis may undergo a total **colectomy**, surgical removal of the colon. When the colon is removed, the terminal ileum may be brought to the surface of the abdomen to form an **ostomy**, an opening that allows elimination of fecal material. The surface opening of the ostomy is called a *stoma* (Figure 26-5 ■). The precise name of the ostomy depends on the location of the stoma (e.g., an **ileostomy**, as illustrated in Figure 26-6 ■, is an ostomy made in the ileum of the small intestine). A permanent ileostomy allows feces to drain directly (and constantly)

TABLE 26-6	Giving Medications Safely: Inflammatory Bowel Disease		
CLASS/DRUGS	**PURPOSE**	**NURSING IMPLICATIONS**	**PATIENT TEACHING**
Local anti-inflammatory agents ■ Sulfasalazine (Azulfidine) ■ Mesalamine (Asacol, Pentasa, others) ■ Olsalazine (Dipentum) ■ Balsalazide (Colazal)	These drugs have a local anti-inflammatory effect on intestinal mucosa. The drug inhibits prostaglandin production in the bowel. Prostaglandin is an important mediator of the inflammatory process; blocking its production reduces inflammation. These drugs may be administered by rectal suppository, enema, or mouth.	Do not give to patients who are pregnant or allergic to sulfonamides or salicylates. Give oral forms with a full glass of water. Monitor for adverse effects: a. Rash, dermatitis, hives, or pruritus b. Bleeding, easy bruising, fever c. Low blood cell counts d. Changes in urine output or renal function studies e. Evidence of hepatitis or myocarditis Teach patients how to administer the drug by enema or suppository as appropriate.	Take oral preparations after meals to decrease GI effects. Drink at least 2 quarts of fluid per day. Use sunscreen to prevent sunburns. Do not take aspirin, vitamin C, or any other over-the-counter medications containing aspirin or vitamin C without consulting with your doctor. Oral contraceptives may be less effective; use alternative methods of contraception. Notify your doctor if you develop a rash or hives, sore throat or mouth, bleeding gums, joint pain, easy bruising, or fever.
Corticosteroids ■ *Methylprednisolone (Medrol, Solu-Medrol)* ■ *Prednisone*	Glucocorticoids have potent anti-inflammatory effects and are used to treat acute episodes of IBD. They can be given by enema, mouth, or IV infusion. Because of their multiple and significant side effects, they are used for short periods only.	Notify the physician if the patient has peptic ulcer disease, glaucoma or cataracts, diabetes, or a psychiatric disorder. Monitor vital signs, weight, and intake and output during therapy. Assess for edema. Administer in the morning as ordered. Give oral forms with meals. Monitor for adverse effects: a. Infection b. Hyperglycemia c. Hypokalemia d. Fluid retention e. Peptic ulcers or gastritis f. Mental status changes	Take as prescribed; do not take additional doses. Do not stop the drug abruptly. Notify your doctor if you develop adverse effects. Take with food or meals. Monitor weight. Contact your doctor if you gain more than 5 lb. Moderate salt intake and avoid high-sodium foods and snacks. Increase intake of foods high in potassium, such as fruits, vegetables, and lean meats. Carry a card or wear a tag identifying corticosteroid use.

Note: Medications identified in *italics* are among the 200 most frequently prescribed drugs in the United States.

through the stoma. The surgeon may create an internal pouch from the terminal ileum to collect feces until the patient drains it with a catheter. A nipple valve prevents leakage of the stool between catheterizations.

A pouch formed from the terminal ileum may also be sutured to the anal canal (Figure 26-7■). This procedure allows more normal bowel elimination and helps preserve body image. The patient may return from surgery with a temporary ileostomy, which is later closed.

Nursing care of the patient having bowel surgery is outlined in Box 26-6■. Nursing care of the patient with an ostomy is described in Box 26-9.

NURSING CARE

PRIORITIZING NURSING CARE

Measures to manage diarrhea and its effects on the patient's health and well-being are the highest priority for nursing care of the patient with IBD. Among nursing care priorities are the psychosocial effects of frequent diarrhea as well.

HEALTH PROMOTION

Although IBD cannot, at this time, be prevented, effective management may help prevent complications of the disease. Stress the importance of effectively managing this

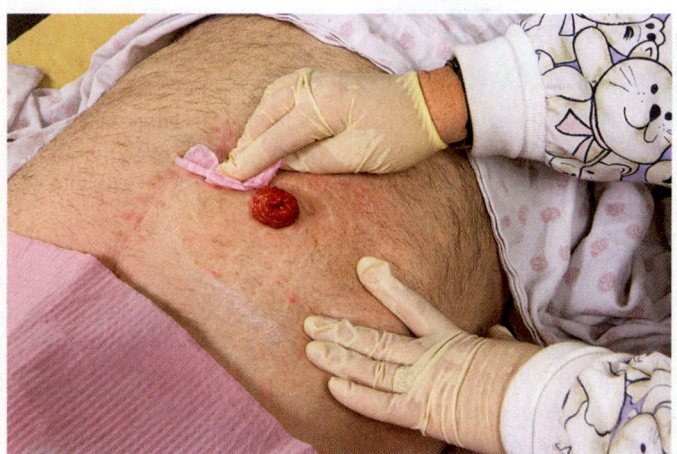

Figure 26-5. ■ A healthy appearing stoma. (Source: Ronald May, Pearson Education.)

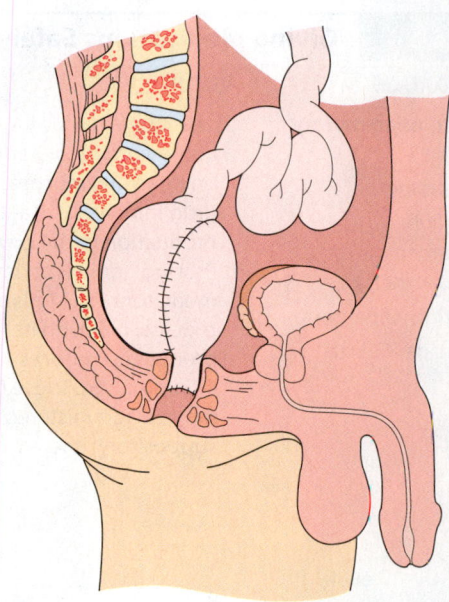

Figure 26-7. ■ An ileoanal anastomosis with reservoir.

Ask about other manifestations, such as anorexia, nausea or vomiting, general malaise, fatigue, and recent weight changes. Ask about current management, including medications, and previous treatments such as surgery.

Note the patient's general appearance and apparent overall health. Obtain vital signs, including orthostatic vitals, height, and weight. Inspect the abdomen, noting its shape and the presence of surgical scars or stomas; auscultate bowel sounds, and gently palpate for tenderness, guarding, or masses.

DIAGNOSING, PLANNING, AND IMPLEMENTING

Diarrhea

Expected outcome: Will report decreasing number of daily stools; perianal skin will remain intact.

■ Monitor the appearance (including presence of mucus and occult or bright bleeding) and frequency of bowel movements using a stool chart. *The severity of diarrhea often correlates well with the severity of the disease and the need for fluid replacement. Large amounts of bright or dark blood may indicate a complication of the disease.*

■ Administer anti-inflammatory and antidiarrheal medications as ordered. *Anti-inflammatory medications can reduce the severity and manifestations of the disease. Unless contraindicated, antidiarrheals reduce fluid loss and increase comfort.*

■ Assess perianal area for irritated or denuded skin from the diarrhea. Use or provide gentle cleansing agents (Peri-Wash, Tucks, or cotton balls saturated with witch hazel) and zinc oxide–based cream to use after bowel movements. *Digestive enzymes in the stool are very corrosive to the skin.*

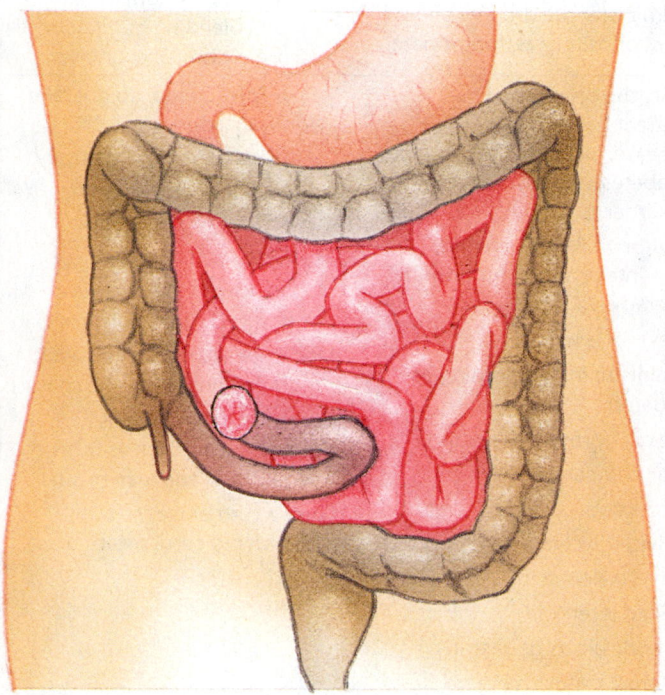

Figure 26-6. ■ An ileostomy formed when the terminal ileum and entire colon are removed. (Source: Pearson Education.)

chronic disease and promptly reporting a recurrence or increased symptoms.

ASSESSING

Assessment for patients with IBD focuses on their current health status, presence of complications, and psychosocial factors related to the disease.

Inquire about the onset, severity, and timing of current symptoms, including the number of stools per day and the presence of blood or mucus in feces. Have the patient describe symptoms such as abdominal pain, cramping, or distention, its timing, and factors that aggravate or relieve discomfort.

BOX 26-6	NURSING CARE CHECKLIST

Bowel Surgery

Before Surgery

☑ Provide routine preoperative care and teaching as outlined in Chapter 10.

☑ Assess understanding and clarify information as indicated.

☑ Reinforce preoperative teaching: pain management, expected tubes, turning, coughing, and deep breathing after surgery.

☑ Insert a nasogastric tube if ordered preoperatively.

☑ Perform bowel preparation procedures as ordered.

After Surgery

☑ Provide routine care for the surgical patient (see Chapter 10).

☑ Monitor bowel sounds and abdominal distention.

☑ Assess nasogastric tube position and patency; connect to low suction. If the tube becomes clogged, gently irrigate with sterile normal saline.

☑ Assess color, amount, and odor of drainage from surgical drains and the ostomy (if present), noting any changes or the presence of clots or bright bleeding. Initial ostomy drainage may be bright red and then become dark and finally clear or greenish yellow during the first 2 to 3 days. Report significant changes in color, amount, or odor.

☑ Frequently assess respiratory status, including rate, depth, and lung sounds.

☑ Encourage frequent turning, coughing, and deep breathing. Provide a pillow or blanket to splint the abdominal incision or assist the patient to splint the incision.

☑ If an abdominoperineal resection has been performed, alert all personnel to avoid rectal temperatures, suppositories, or other rectal procedures.

☑ Maintain intravenous fluids as ordered.

☑ Provide antacids, H_2-receptor blockers, and antibiotic therapy as ordered.

☑ Reintroduce oral intake with clear liquids, gradually progressing to frequent small feedings of regular foods. Monitor bowel sounds and abdominal distention frequently during this period.

☑ Encourage ambulation to stimulate peristalsis.

☑ Begin discharge planning and teaching. Consult with a dietitian for diet instructions and menu planning; reinforce teaching. Teach about potential complications, such as abdominal abscess or bowel obstruction, their manifestations, and prevention.

Risk for Deficient Fluid Volume

Expected outcome: Weight, urinary output, and vital signs will remain stable and within established range.

- Maintain accurate intake and output records, including emesis and diarrheal stools. *The patient with IBD can experience significant fluid losses during an acute exacerbation of the disease. Accurate records help determine fluid replacement needs.*

- Document vital signs every 4 hours. *Elevated pulse and respiratory rates may indicate fluid volume deficit.*

- Weigh daily. Assess for other indications of fluid deficit. *Weight loss may indicate dehydration from persistent diarrhea. Warm, dry skin; poor skin turgor; dry, shiny mucous membranes; weakness; lethargy; and complaints of thirst are manifestations of dehydration.*

- Maintain fluid intake by mouth or intravenously as indicated. *Adequate fluid replacement is vital. If enteral supplements or TPN is ordered, additional fluids may be necessary to meet the patient's needs.*

- Provide good skin care. *A fluid deficit increases the risk for skin breakdown.*

Imbalanced Nutrition: Less Than Body Requirements

Expected outcome: Will consume 100% of prescribed diet.

- Carefully monitor food intake. *Accurate assessment of food intake provides a way to estimate the patient's calorie intake in relation to nutritional needs.*

- Provide a high-calorie, high-protein diet with nutritional supplements as ordered. Consider food preferences as allowed. Arrange for dietary consultation. *Calories and protein are important to replace lost nutrients and meet metabolic needs. Nutritional supplements help restore losses and promote intake. A dietary consultant can design a diet to meet the patient's specific needs and food preferences.*

- Provide parenteral nutrition as necessary. *Parenteral nutrition can help reverse nutritional deficits and promote weight gain when the patient is unable to consume adequate amounts of food.*

- Engage family members, especially the primary food preparer, in dietary teaching. *Families can reinforce teaching, encourage intake, and help the patient follow the recommended diet.*

- Monitor hemoglobin and hematocrit, serum electrolytes, and serum albumin levels. *Laboratory values provide information about specific nutrient losses as well as the patient's overall nutritional status.*

Disturbed Body Image

Expected outcome: Will acknowledge impact of IBD on personal roles, relationships, and responsibilities.

The inability to control, or even predict, fecal elimination can interfere with the patient's body image and self-concept.

- Encourage discussion about the effect of the disease or treatment on the patient's feelings, self-perception, and relationships (including intimate). Accept the patient's feelings and perceptions; do not discount them. *This demonstrates understanding and acceptance and gives the patient an opportunity to express his or her thoughts and feelings.*

- Discuss possible effects of treatment options openly and honestly. Encourage the patient to make choices and decisions about care. *Open discussion allows the patient to make more informed decisions and increases the patient's sense of control.*
- Involve the patient in care. Teach coping strategies (e.g., odor control, dietary modifications), and support their use. *This encourages and facilitates independence and healthy adaptation to the disease.*
- Provide care in an accepting, nonjudgmental manner. *Acceptance of the patient despite potential embarrassment about odors or diarrhea enhances self-esteem.*
- Arrange for interaction with others who have IBD or ostomies. *People who have experienced a similar problem can understand the patient's feelings better.*

MANAGING NURSING CARE

When caring for the patient with inflammatory bowel disease, nursing care activities such as obtaining vital signs, measuring intake and output, documenting food intake and stool count, emptying an ostomy bag, and skin care and hygiene measures may be assigned to assistive personnel who have appropriate training and documented competency.

EVALUATING

Collect data related to the following to evaluate the effectiveness of nursing interventions for the patient with IBD: number of diarrheal stools per day, maintenance of skin integrity, hydration status, weight, ability to consume an adequate diet, and apparent coping with current situation.

DOCUMENTING

Document continuing assessment data and response to treatment, as well as food and fluid intake and output. Note teaching provided and the patient's and family's understanding and acceptance of information.

CONTINUITY OF CARE

Teaching is a vital component of care for the patient with IBD, because it is the patient who manages the disease on a day-to-day basis. Teach about the disease process, short- and long-term effects, and the relationship of stress to exacerbations of the illness. Talk about risks and benefits of various treatment options. Present information on stress management. Provide information about prescribed medications (names, desired effects, adverse reactions and their management, and schedules for tapering doses if ordered). Discuss manifestations of potential complications and their management. Discuss the increased risk for colorectal cancer and the need for regular medical follow-up.

Give verbal and written instructions about the recommended diet, and refer to a dietitian as necessary. Emphasize the need to consume a diet of good nutritional value, and note any specific restrictions (e.g., milk and milk products with lactose intolerance). Discuss use of nutritional supplements as needed. Emphasize the need to maintain a fluid intake of at least 2 to 3 quarts per day to replace fluids lost through the stool. Instruct to drink more fluid in hot weather, during exercise or strenuous work, or when feverish. Explain possible indications of malabsorption and impaired nutrition, self-care measures, and when to seek medical intervention. If home parenteral nutrition is planned, teach catheter care and troubleshooting, as well as TPN administration. Have the patient and a family member demonstrate catheter care techniques and initiation of feedings before discharge.

If surgery is planned, instruct about the surgery and follow-up care. Contact an enterostomal therapy (ET) nurse to meet with the patient and family. Teach ostomy care as indicated. Provide resources for obtaining ostomy supplies. Discuss the use of enteric-coated and timed-release drugs that may not be absorbed adequately before elimination through an ileostomy. Provide a list of local ostomy support groups, such as the Foundation for Colitis and Ileitis and the United Ostomy Association. Refer for home care as needed after discharge.

NURSING CARE PLAN
Patient With Ulcerative Colitis

Cortez Lewis is 42 years old and has had ulcerative colitis for 18 years. She has been treated with prednisone and sulfasalazine. During her most recent exacerbation, she had abdominal pain, cramping, frequent bloody diarrhea stools, and a 26-lb (12-kg) weight loss. A recent colonoscopy showed that her colon is extensively involved. On admission, Mrs. Lewis states, "I'm tired of fighting this disease. I am a prisoner in my home because of the diarrhea." She is admitted for a total colectomy and ileostomy.

Assessment

The nursing assessment on admission reveals that Mrs. Lewis weighs 115 lb (52.2 kg). Her vital signs are BP 104/72; T 98°F (36.6°C); P 72; R 26. Her skin is cool and pale. Her hemoglobin and hematocrit are low, as is her serum albumin at 2.4 g/dL (normal: 3.5 to 5 g/dL).

Nursing Diagnosis

The following nursing diagnoses are established for Mrs. Lewis:

- *Imbalanced Nutrition: Less Than Body Requirements* related to impaired absorption

- *Risk for Deficient Fluid Volume* related to abnormal fluid losses
- *Risk for Impaired Tissue Integrity* related to drainage from ileostomy
- *Acute Pain* related to surgery
- *Risk for Sexual Dysfunction* related to presence of ileostomy
- *Risk for Situational Low Self-Esteem* related to presence of ileostomy

Expected Outcomes

The expected outcomes are that Mrs. Lewis will:

- Tolerate prescribed diet.
- Maintain adequate fluid balance, as demonstrated by assessment data, vital signs, and laboratory results.
- Demonstrate appropriate ostomy care.
- Report pain at 2 or less on a scale of 1 to 10.
- Verbalize feelings about sexuality and discuss issues with her husband.
- Return to work and social activity 6 weeks after surgery.

Planning and Implementation

The nurses plan and implement the following nursing interventions for Mrs. Lewis:

- Discuss dietary modifications related to ileostomy, including foods to avoid and the need to limit high-fiber foods and to chew them well.
- Teach the importance of maintaining a high fluid intake and how to assess its adequacy. Review manifestations of dehydration.

- Teach to empty and change either a one- or two-piece ostomy pouch.
- Teach to assess her stoma and peristomal skin with each pouch change.
- Refer to the local United Ostomy Association.
- Provide names of local medical supply companies that sell ostomy appliances.

Evaluation

On discharge, Mrs. Lewis is independently caring for her ileostomy appliance. The ET nurse has given her written and verbal instructions on ileostomy care. Mrs. Lewis verbalizes her understanding of the recommended diet and medications that should be avoided (timed-release forms). The ET nurse has also discussed sexual aspects of having an ileostomy and has given Mrs. Lewis information about resources available online.

Critical Thinking in the Nursing Process

1. Why is the patient with an ileostomy at risk for dehydration? What assessments can Mrs. Lewis use at home to monitor her fluid volume status?
2. Why would Mrs. Lewis's hemoglobin and hematocrit be low on admission?
3. What suggestions would you provide to the patient with an ileostomy who is concerned about the bag being visible under her clothing or leaking?

Note: Discussion of Critical Thinking questions appears on the companion website.

STRUCTURAL AND OBSTRUCTIVE DISORDERS

Key Concept   The movement of intestinal contents through the bowel can be partially or completely obstructed by a mass, structural abnormality, or loss of peristalsis. It is important that the nurse recognize and respond appropriately to manifestations of bowel obstruction.

PATHOPHYSIOLOGY

Nearly all colon cancers begin as *polyps,* benign precancerous lesions of the large intestine. The tumor typically

Colorectal Cancer

Colorectal cancer, malignancy of the colon or rectum, is the third most commonly occurring cancer and the second leading cause of cancer deaths in the United States (see Box 26-7■). About 143,000 new cases of colorectal cancer were diagnosed in 2013, and nearly 51,000 people died from this disease. The specific cause of colorectal cancer is unknown. A number of risk factors have been identified (Box 26-8■), but only about one-fourth of patients diagnosed with colorectal cancer fall into a high-risk group. Therefore, screening for the disease is important.

BOX 26-7	FOCUS ON DIVERSITY

Colorectal Cancer

- Colorectal cancer is common among all peoples of the United States.
- African Americans have the highest rates of colorectal cancer of all cultural and ethnic groups in the United States.
- The incidence of colorectal cancer is also high among Jews of Eastern European descent.
- Hispanics in the United States have a lower rate of colorectal cancer than non-Hispanic Whites but a higher rate than is seen in Spanish-speaking countries of Central and South America.
- Asian Americans have the lowest incidence of colorectal cancer.

grows undetected in the rectum or sigmoid colon (the regions of the bowel most frequently affected, as illustrated in Figure 26-8■). By the time symptoms occur, the disease has often spread into deeper layers of the bowel tissue and adjacent organs. Colorectal cancer spreads by direct extension to involve the entire bowel wall. It may extend into neighboring structures (liver or genitourinary tract). It may "seed" other areas of the peritoneal cavity through the bowel wall or during surgery. Metastasis to regional lymph nodes is common, although sometimes distal nodes contain cancer cells while regional nodes remain normal. Cancerous cells may also spread through the lymphatic or circulatory system to the liver, lungs, brain, bones, and kidneys.

MANIFESTATIONS AND COMPLICATIONS

Bowel tumors usually grow slowly. There may be 5 to 15 years of growth from the first malignant cells until symptoms occur. Manifestations depend on the location and type of tumor, its size, and complications. Bleeding with defecation is often what leads patients to seek care. A change in bowel habits, for example, constipation or frequent small

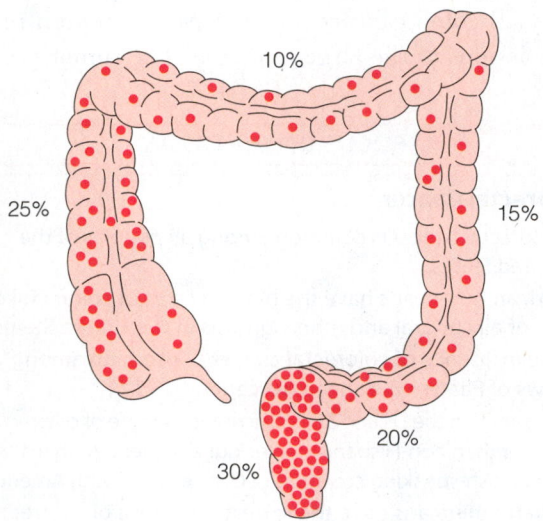

Figure 26-8. ■ The distribution and frequency of cancers of the colon and rectum.

stools, is another early symptom. In advanced disease, pain, anorexia, and weight loss occur, and a palpable abdominal or rectal mass may be present. Occasionally, anemia from occult bleeding is found before other symptoms are noted.

The prognosis for colon cancer depends most on the stage of the disease at diagnosis and initial treatment. More than half of all people diagnosed with colorectal cancer survive 10 years.

Bowel obstruction due to tumor growth is the primary complication associated with colorectal cancer. Bowel wall perforation and tumor spread to adjacent organs may also occur.

COLLABORATIVE CARE

Because colorectal cancer is often a silent disease and treatment at an early stage has a high cure rate, the American Cancer Society recommends routine screening of all people beginning at age 50:

- Annual *fecal occult blood test (FOBT)* or *fecal immunochemical test (FIT)* or *stool DNA (sDNA) test*
- Flexible *sigmoidoscopy* or *CT colonography (virtual colonoscopy)* or double-contrast *barium enema* every 5 years
- Flexible *colonoscopy* every 10 years

Screening exams are initiated earlier and performed more frequently for patients with IBD, a history of polyps, or a strong family history of colorectal cancer.

Diagnostic Tests

The patient with suspected colorectal cancer may undergo extensive diagnostic procedures:

- *Sigmoidoscopy* or *colonoscopy* is done to detect and visualize tumors and to collect tissue for *biopsy*. Tumors typically appear as raised, red, centrally ulcerated, bleeding lesions.
- *CBC* is done to evaluate for anemia.
- *Carcinoembryonic antigen (CEA,* a protein found in colorectal cancers) levels are measured. They are used primarily to predict prognosis and to detect tumor recurrence after surgery.
- *Chest x-ray* is obtained to detect tumor metastasis to the lung. *CT scans, magnetic resonance imaging (MRI),* or *ultrasound examinations* may identify involvement of other organs.

Surgery

The treatment of choice for colorectal cancer is surgical removal of the tumor, adjacent colon, and regional lymph nodes. Small, localized tumors may be removed by laser endoscopy, eliminating the need for abdominal surgery. Most patients with colorectal cancer undergo a *colectomy* (removal of the affected part of the colon with anastomosis of remaining bowel). Most tumors of the

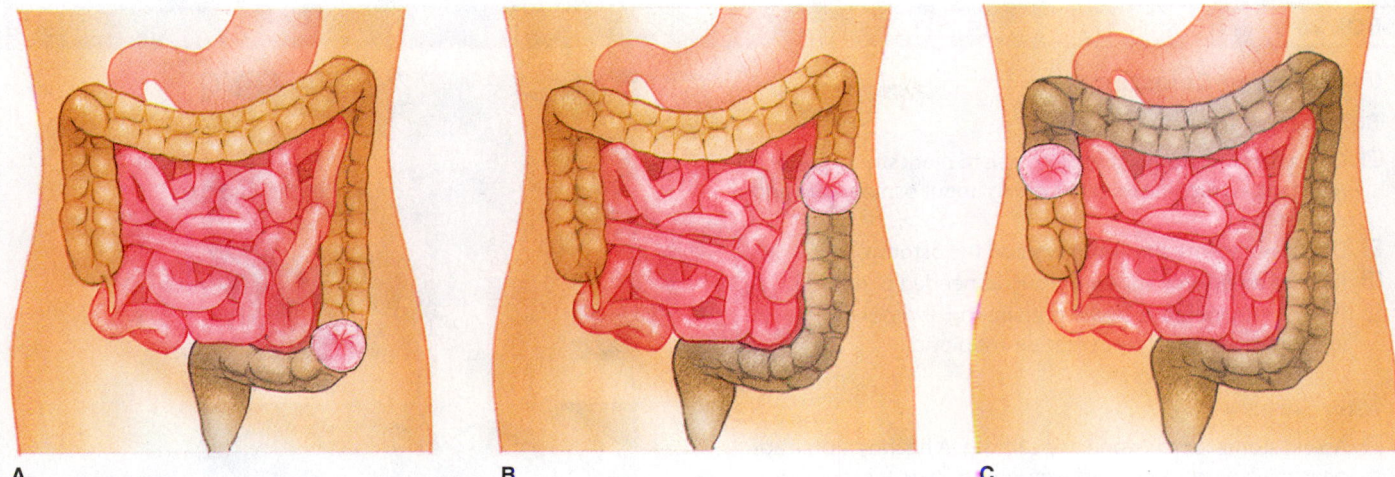

Figure 26-9. ■ Locations and types of colostomies. (**A**) Sigmoid colostomy. (**B**) Descending colostomy. (**C**) Ascending colostomy. (Source: Pearson Education.)

ascending, transverse, descending, and sigmoid colon can be removed by colectomy. Whenever possible, the anal sphincter is preserved, and **colostomy** (ostomy made in the colon) is avoided. Tumors of the rectum, however, usually require an *abdominoperineal resection,* in which the sigmoid colon, rectum, and anus are removed through both abdominal and perineal incisions. A permanent colostomy is created for elimination of feces. Nursing care of the patient having bowel surgery was described in Box 26-6.

A colostomy may be created if the bowel is obstructed by the tumor or as a temporary measure to promote healing of anastomoses. Colostomies take the name of the portion of the colon from which they are formed (Figure 26-9■). The color, consistency, and frequency of fecal output vary, depending on the type of colostomy. With a sigmoid colostomy, fecal output closely resembles normal stool. Elimination often occurs in a predictable pattern (e.g., in the morning after breakfast), allowing some patients to simply cover or cap the stoma at other times. As the location of the ostomy becomes more proximal, for example, with an ascending or transverse colostomy, feces is lighter in color, more liquid (less formed), and expelled more frequently and less predictably. Patients may need to wear an ostomy pouch at all times. Fecal output from an ileostomy is unformed, liquid, and continuous, necessitating continuous wearing of an ostomy appliance.

In a *double-barrel colostomy,* created to allow bowel healing, two separate stomas are created (Figure 26-10■). The distal colon is not removed, but feces are diverted through the proximal stoma. Small amounts of mucus may be expelled from the distal stoma. A double-barrel colostomy is usually temporary. Nursing care of the patient with a colostomy is outlined in Box 26-9■.

Adjunctive Therapy

Radiation and chemotherapy are often used in conjunction with surgery to treat colorectal cancers. Pre- or postoperative radiation therapy is used to reduce the recurrence of rectal tumors in the pelvic area. Chemotherapeutic agents are also used postoperatively as adjunctive therapy for colorectal cancer. (Further discussion about radiation and chemotherapy and their nursing implications is included in Chapter 12.)

NURSING CARE

PRIORITIZING NURSING CARE

Nursing care for the patient with colorectal cancer is aimed at providing emotional support, teaching, and addressing the surgical patient's needs.

HEALTH PROMOTION

To reduce the risk for and incidence of colorectal cancer, teach all patients about American Cancer Society dietary recommendations, including decreasing intake of fat, refined sugar, and red meats and increasing intake of dietary fiber, fresh fruits, and vegetables.

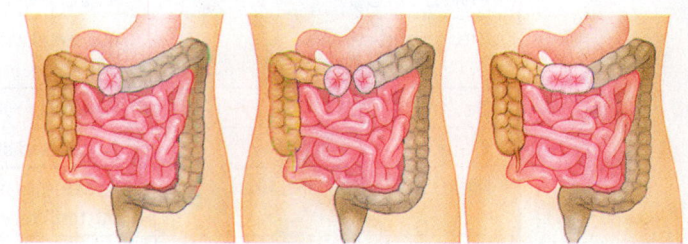

Figure 26-10. ■ A transverse colostomy is illustrated in the figure to the left. The center figure shows a double-barrel colostomy. A transverse loop colostomy is shown on the right. (Source: Pearson Education.)

BOX 26-9	NURSING CARE CHECKLIST

Ileostomy or Colostomy

Before Surgery

☑ Contact enterostomal therapy nurse to mark stoma placement and to provide initial teaching about ostomy care and appliances.

☑ Discuss concerns about surgery and the ostomy.

☑ Refer to an ostomy support group as needed or desired.

☑ Provide preoperative bowel preparation as ordered (cathartics, enemas, preoperative antibiotics).

After Surgery

☑ Assess stoma location and appearance. A healthy stoma appears pink or red and moist (see Figure 26-5). It should protrude approximately 2 cm from the abdominal wall. Report dark or pale color, *prolapse* (protrusion of bowel through the skin opening, making the stoma longer in length), or *retraction* (indentation of the stoma below skin level) of the stoma to the charge nurse or physician.

☑ Position a collection bag or drainable pouch over the stoma (see Figure A). Monitor and record color and consistency of ostomy output.

☑ Empty a drainable pouch or replace the colostomy bag when it is no more than one-third full (Figure B). Measure the drainage, and record as output.

☑ Assess and cleanse skin surrounding the stoma, and protect with caulking agents, such as Stomahesive or Karaya paste, and a skin barrier wafer as needed (Figure C). Change the bag or pouch if leakage occurs or the patient complains of burning or itching skin.

☑ A small needle hole high on the colostomy pouch will allow flatus to escape. For odor control, this hole may be closed with a Band-Aid and opened only while the patient is in the bathroom.

☑ Report abnormal assessment findings, such as a rash, purulent drainage, ulcerated skin, or bulging around the stoma, to the charge nurse or physician.

☑ Before discharge, teach ostomy care, pouch management, skin care, and irrigation (as indicated). Allow time for practice.

☑ Emphasize the importance of adequate fluid intake, particularly for patients with an ileostomy or proximal colostomy.

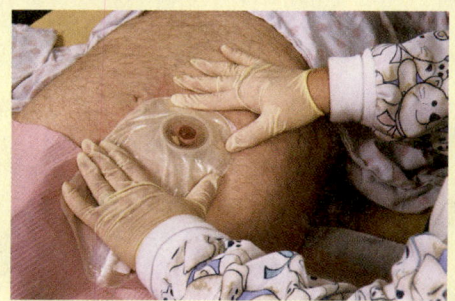

A

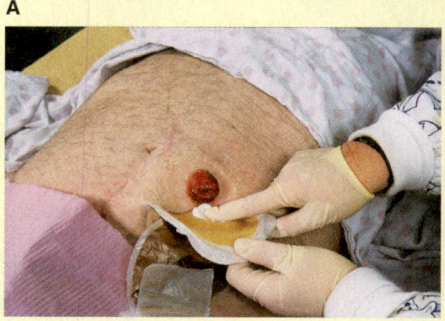

B

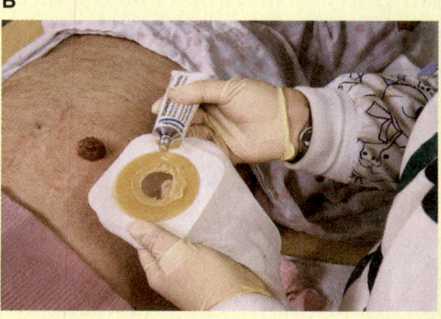

C

(Source: Ronald May, Pearson Education.)

☑ Discuss dietary concerns. A low-residue diet (Table 26-7 ■) may initially be recommended. Foods that may cause excessive odor or gas (e.g., vegetables such as asparagus or cabbage, dried beans, beer and carbonated drinks, or dairy products) are typically avoided, as are foods that can cause a blockage (e.g., popcorn, corn, nuts, caraway seeds, cucumbers, celery, fresh tomatoes, and berries).

TABLE 26-7	Low-Residue Diet
FOOD GROUP	**ALLOWED**
Breads and cereals	Products made from refined flours (e.g., white bread) or finely milled grains
Desserts	Gelatins, puddings; ice cream without fruit or nuts
Fruits	Juices and strained fruits; cooked or canned fruits; bananas
Meats and other proteins	Roasted, baked, or broiled meat, poultry, or fish; smooth peanut butter; cream and mild cheeses; milk
Potatoes, rice, and pasta	Peeled potatoes; white rice; most pasta products
Vegetables	Juices and strained vegetables; cooked or canned vegetables
Other	Coffee, tea, carbonated beverages; cream sauce and plain gravy

Stress the importance of regular health examinations, including recommended screening procedures after age 50. Also stress that people of any age should seek medical treatment if blood is noted in or on the stool. Teach patients that a change in bowel habits may be a warning sign for bowel cancer.

ASSESSING

Nursing assessment of the patient with colorectal cancer focuses on the effects of the disease and its treatment on the patient's ability to function and maintain ADLs.

- Subjective: onset of symptoms and current manifestations (including pain); treatment (current and previous); effect of disease and its treatment on ADLs and ability to maintain usual life roles.
- Objective: general appearance; vital signs; abdominal assessment and appearance of any incisions or ostomies; type of fecal output from ostomy.
- Laboratory data: CBC; hemoglobin and hematocrit; serum electrolytes and albumin; CEA level if done.

DIAGNOSING, PLANNING, AND IMPLEMENTING

Acute Pain

Expected outcome: Will report pain as a 2 or lower on a scale of 0 to 10.

The patient with colorectal cancer may experience pain from surgical incisions, "phantom" rectal pain, and tumors pressing on nerves and other organs. Postoperatively, patient-controlled analgesia (PCA) and regularly administered analgesics are used to manage pain. If the tumor is inoperable, continuous analgesia delivery (CAD) systems may also be used.

- Assess frequently for pain, using a standard pain scale. Document intensity, location, and character of the pain. *Pain is a subjective experience; careful assessment improves pain management. Controlling pain facilitates healing and recovery.*
- Assess the effectiveness of pain medications and monitor for adverse effects. *The prescribed dose may need to be increased or decreased based on the patient's response.*
- Assess abdomen for distention, tenderness, and bowel sounds; incision for inflammation or swelling; and drainage catheters and tubes for patency. *Poorly controlled pain may indicate an infection, impaired tube drainage, or a complication such as bleeding, peritonitis, or paralytic ileus.*
- Administer analgesics before an activity or procedure. *The analgesic can help prevent discomfort with movement or ambulation.*
- Provide nonpharmacologic relief measures, such as positioning, diversion, guided imagery, and relaxation techniques. *These techniques can enhance the effects of analgesia.*

- Splint incision with a pillow, and teach how to self-splint when coughing and deep breathing. *Splinting the incision reduces discomfort associated with muscle contraction and allows more effective coughing and deep breathing.*

Grieving

Expected outcome: Will express fears, thoughts, and feelings about potential loss.

- Work to develop a trusting relationship with the patient and family. Demonstrate respect for cultural, spiritual, and religious values and beliefs. *Providing support during the initial stages of grieving can improve physical recovery, psychologic coping, and eventual adaptation. This increases your effectiveness in helping patients work through the grieving process.*
- Encourage expression of fears and concerns and discussion about the potential impact of loss on individual family members, as well as family structure and function. *Sharing concerns with one another provides support and helps family members develop coping strategies.*
- Help the patient and family identify strengths, support systems, and successful coping mechanisms used in past experiences. *These resources can help in dealing with the current situation.*
- Refer to cancer support groups, social services, or counseling as appropriate. *These provide additional resources for support in the grieving process.*

Risk for Sexual Dysfunction

Expected outcome: Will adapt modes of sexual expression to accommodate illness-related physical changes.

Sexual function may be impaired by surgery, radiation therapy, chemotherapy, or medications prescribed after surgery. In addition, patients with an ostomy may feel undesirable and fear rejection. They may be concerned about odors or pouch leakage during sexual activity.

- Provide opportunities for patient and family to express their feelings about the ostomy. *By doing this, the nurse acknowledges that feelings of anger and depression are normal responses to this change in body function.*
- Provide consistent, secure colostomy care. *An accepting attitude and consistent care that controls odor and leakage instill confidence in the patient.*
- Encourage expression of sexual concerns within the patient's comfort zone. Provide reassurance that sexual function often improves with healing. *Sexuality is a very private concern, and most people will discuss it with only someone they trust. Many people think an initial decrease in libido means that sexual activity will never be possible again.*
- Refer to social services or a family counselor for further interventions. *Patients are often discharged from acute care settings before concerns about sexual activity begin to surface. Ongoing counseling provides a continuing resource.*

■ Arrange for a visit by a member of the United Ostomy Association. *A person who is living successfully with an ostomy is a valuable source of information and support and can often address questions the patient hesitates to ask.*

MANAGING NURSING CARE

Nursing care activities such as assisting with daily living activities, measuring intake and output, and emptying ostomy drainage bags may be assigned to assistive personnel who have appropriate training and documented competence.

EVALUATING

To evaluate the effectiveness of care for the patient with colorectal cancer, monitor pain levels and the effectiveness of analgesia and other measures to promote comfort. Assess emotional and psychologic responses to the disease and treatment measures (e.g., colostomy, chemotherapy). Also assess learning and understanding of the disorder, planned treatment, and care of incisions and ostomies.

DOCUMENTING

Document the patient's and family's responses to teaching and treatment measures, as well as continuing assessment data. If an ostomy is created, document stoma appearance, fecal output, and teaching related to ostomy care.

CONTINUITY OF CARE

Teach the patient and, as appropriate, caregivers about care of the ostomy and possible complications to report. Provide a list of resources for ostomy supplies. Refer to the local ostomy association or group. Discuss management of adverse effects if radiation and chemotherapy are planned.

If the cancer is advanced, provide information about pain and symptom management. Discuss the hospice philosophy and available services. Provide referrals as needed.

See the Clinical Reasoning Care Map at the end of this chapter for an opportunity to apply the nursing process for a patient with colorectal cancer.

Hernia

A *hernia* is protrusion of an organ or structure through a defect in the muscular wall of the abdomen. Hernias may contain loops of bowel or other internal organs. They may be congenital or acquired. Acquired hernias are associated with weakening of the normal musculature. They may be related to surgery, trauma such as heavy lifting, or gradual increases in intra-abdominal pressure caused by pregnancy, obesity, or ascites.

PATHOPHYSIOLOGY AND MANIFESTATIONS

Hernias are classified by their location (Figure 26-11■). Most hernias occur in the groin and are known as *ingui-*

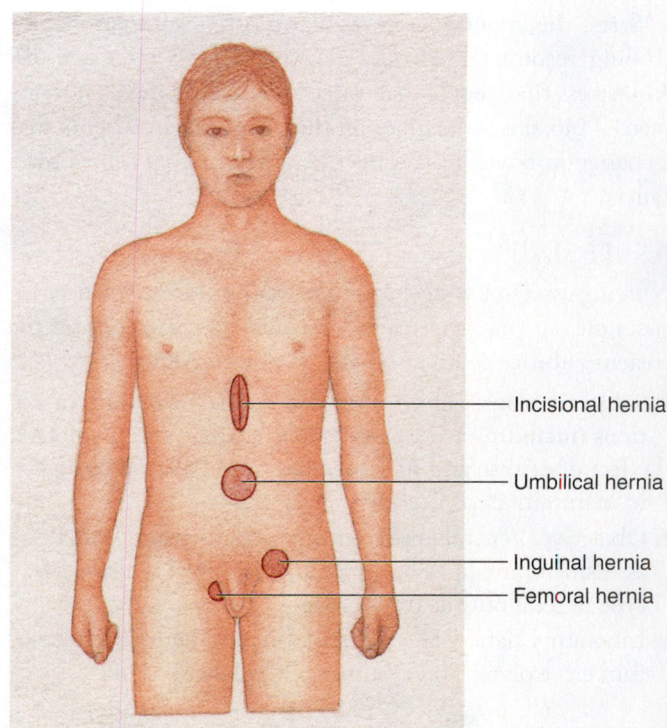

Figure 26-11. ■ Locations of different types of hernia. (Source: Dorling Kindersley Media Library.)

nal hernias. Inguinal hernias are usually caused by incomplete closure of the tract that develops as the testes descend into the scrotum before birth (Figure 26-12■). They often do not become apparent until increased intra-abdominal pressure causes abdominal contents to enter the channel in adulthood. In older adults, weakness of the posterior inguinal wall can also lead to an inguinal hernia. Inguinal hernias often produce no symptoms and are discovered during routine physical examination. A lump, swelling, or bulge in the groin may be noted with lifting or straining. The patient may complain of pain that radiates into the scrotum.

Umbilical and ventral (*incisional*) hernias occur in the abdominal wall. *Umbilical hernias* may be congenital or

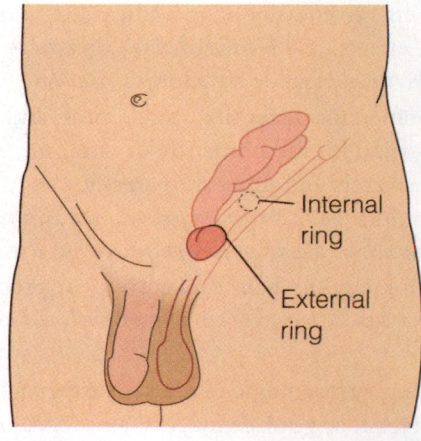

Figure 26-12. ■ An inguinal hernia. (Source: Pearson Education.)

acquired; pregnancy, obesity, and ascites are common risk factors. *Ventral hernias* result from inadequate healing of a surgical incision.

If a hernia is *reducible,* contents of the sac return to the abdominal cavity when intra-abdominal pressure is reduced (as with lying down) or with manual pressure. When the contents of a hernia cannot be returned to the abdominal cavity, it is said to be *irreducible* or *incarcerated.* Contents of an incarcerated hernia are trapped, usually by a narrow opening to the hernia. *Obstruction* occurs when the lumen of the bowel contained within the hernia becomes occluded, much like the crimping of a hose.

A *strangulated hernia* occurs when the blood supply to tissue within the hernia is compromised. This can lead to infarction (necrosis) of affected bowel with severe pain and perforation. Manifestations of a strangulated hernia include abdominal pain and distention, nausea, vomiting, tachycardia, and fever.

COLLABORATIVE CARE

The diagnosis of a hernia is made by examining the patient in a supine and sitting or standing position. A bulge may be seen or felt when the patient coughs or bears down. No laboratory or diagnostic testing is usually required, unless bowel obstruction or strangulation is suspected.

All types of hernia are surgically repaired (*herniorrhaphy*) unless specific contraindications to surgery exist. Heavy lifting and heavy manual labor are restricted for approximately 3 weeks after surgery. When surgery is not an option, the patient may be taught to reduce the hernia by lying down and gently pushing down against the mass. A binder or truss may be worn to prevent or control the protrusion.

NURSING CARE

The patient undergoing a herniorrhaphy has few acute nursing care needs apart from preoperative assessment and immediate postoperative care. Operative nursing care is similar to care of a patient with an appendectomy.

Risk for Ineffective Tissue Perfusion (Gastrointestinal)

Expected outcome: Will remain free of manifestations of bowel obstruction or strangulation.

■ Assess comfort. Notify the primary care provider if the hernia becomes painful or tender. Promptly report an acute increase in abdominal, groin, perineal, or scrotal pain. *Pain or tenderness of the hernia may indicate incarceration. An abrupt increase in pain may indicate bowel ischemia due to strangulation. Rapid identification of the problem is vital to prevent major complications such as peritonitis.*

■ Assess bowel sounds and abdominal distention at least every 8 hours. *A change in bowel sounds—either cessation of*

sounds or hyperactive, high-pitched sounds—and increasing abdominal girth may indicate obstruction.

■ If signs of possible obstruction or strangulation occur, place the patient in the supine position with the hips elevated and knees slightly bent. Keep NPO, and begin preparations for surgery. *This position helps relax abdominal muscles and may facilitate reduction of the hernia. Strangulation or obstruction require immediate surgical intervention.*

CONTINUITY OF CARE

Most teaching related to hernias is done during routine health examinations. Teach patients what hernias are and the risk factors for their development. Reassure patients that surgical intervention is generally without complications, even in older adults, and carries a lower risk than not repairing the hernia. Teach patients how to reduce hernias if necessary, and stress the importance of seeking immediate medical intervention if signs of strangulation or obstruction occur. When surgery is planned, instruct the patient to notify the physician should he or she develop an upper respiratory infection and cough, because forceful coughing is not recommended postoperatively. Reinforce postoperative teaching about pain management and activity restrictions after surgery.

Bowel Obstruction

A *bowel obstruction* occurs when intestinal contents are unable to move through the bowel. An obstruction can occur in any portion of the intestinal tract. The small intestine (especially the ileum) is the most common site.

PATHOPHYSIOLOGY

A bowel obstruction may be either mechanical or functional. With a *mechanical obstruction,* the bowel is obstructed by a physical barrier like scar tissue or a tumor. *Adhesions* (bands of scar tissue) are the most common cause of mechanical bowel obstruction. They usually result from previous abdominal surgery or inflammation. They may cause partial or complete obstruction. Tumors, a twisted bowel, or loops of bowel trapped within a hernia may also cause mechanical bowel obstruction (Figure 26-13■). With *functional obstruction (paralytic ileus),* the bowel lumen remains patent, but peristalsis stops. Paralytic ileus is common in acutely ill patients. It is associated with GI surgery, peritoneal inflammation, and certain drugs such as narcotic analgesics.

When obstruction occurs, gas and fluid collect in the bowel behind (proximal to) the obstruction, stretching its lumen. Extracellular fluid and electrolytes are drawn into the bowel, further distending it. This increases pressure within the bowel, which may affect blood flow and lead to ischemia and necrosis of the bowel wall. Hypovolemia and shock may result from fluid trapping within the intestine.

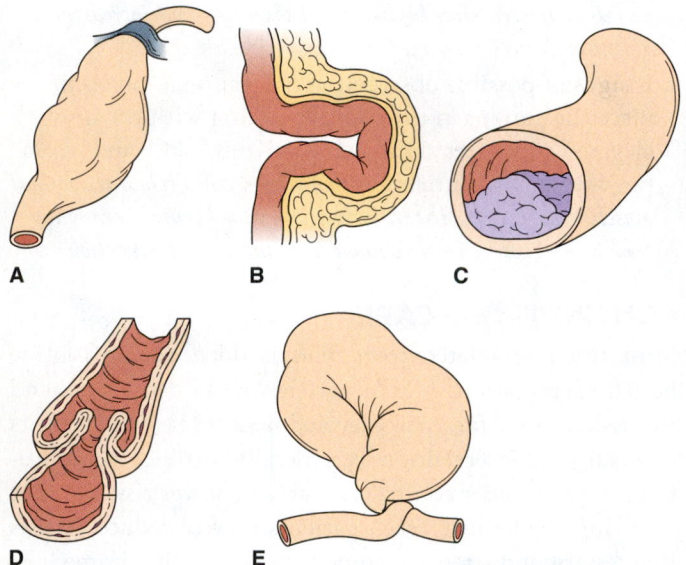

Figure 26-13. ■ Selected causes of mechanical bowel obstruction. (**A**) Adhesions, (**B**) incarcerated (irreducible) hernia, (**C**) tumor, (**D**) intussusception (telescoping of the bowel), (**E**) volvulus (twisting of the bowel).

MANIFESTATIONS AND COMPLICATIONS

The manifestations of a small-bowel obstruction depend on how fast the obstruction develops and where it occurs (Box 26-10■). Cramping or colicky abdominal pain that becomes progressively more severe is common. Vomiting is also common, particularly with obstructions of the small intestine. The vomitus may smell like feces. Early in the obstructive process, bowel sounds are hyperactive and loud (borborygmi); they may be high pitched. As the obstructive process continues and with functional obstruction, few or no bowel sounds are heard. The abdomen becomes distended and tender.

Hypovolemic shock with multiple organ failure and death can result from bowel obstruction. The mortality rate for small-bowel obstruction is approximately 10% (mostly in older adults). Strangulation of the bowel significantly increases the risk of death.

BOX 26-10	MANIFESTATIONS OF BOWEL OBSTRUCTION

- Abdominal pain: cramping or colicky; may be intermittent; increasing intensity; tenderness to palpation; severe, continuous pain may indicate bowel ischemia and possible perforation
- Vomiting; may smell like feces
- Borborygmi and high-pitched, tinkling bowel sounds; diminished or absent bowel sounds
- Abdominal distention; visible peristaltic waves
- Signs of hypovolemia and shock: orthostatic hypotension, tachycardia, tachypnea; decreased urine output

COLLABORATIVE CARE

Management of the patient with a bowel obstruction focuses on relieving the obstruction and providing supportive care. Restoration and maintenance of fluid and electrolyte balance is vital to prevent complications.

Diagnostic Tests

Abdominal x-rays or *CT scan* are used to confirm the diagnosis of a bowel obstruction. In addition to plain films, contrast media may be used. Evaluation for iodine or seafood allergies before the exam is important, because the contrast medium used may contain iodine.

Gastrointestinal Decompression

Most partial and functional small-bowel obstructions are successfully treated with GI decompression using a nasogastric tube or long intestinal tube. An intestinal tube (see Figure 26-2) may be inserted through the nose or via gastrostomy. A balloon or weighted tip draws the tube from the stomach into the intestine by peristalsis. Low suction removes fluid and gas until peristalsis resumes or the obstruction is relieved.

Surgery

Surgery may be required to relieve mechanical bowel obstruction. Before surgery, a nasogastric tube is inserted to relieve vomiting and distention and to prevent aspiration. Intravenous fluids and electrolytes are given to restore fluid and electrolyte balance. Intravenous antibiotics are administered prophylactically. Nursing care of the patient having bowel surgery was described in Box 26-6.

NURSING CARE

PRIORITIZING NURSING CARE

Nurses provide care for patients undergoing nonsurgical treatment for bowel obstruction as well as those who require surgery to relieve the obstruction. Preventing complications of obstruction and surgery are the priority areas of focus for nursing care.

HEALTH PROMOTION

Health promotion activities such as increasing dietary fiber intake, maintaining generous fluid intake, and staying physically active help prevent bowel obstruction, particularly in older adults. Stress the importance of complying with dietary restrictions for patients who have experienced previous or repeated small bowel obstructions.

ASSESSING

Nurses can help identify bowel obstructions early in older adults, homebound patients, or long-term care residents, thus significantly reducing morbidity. Assess all patients who complain of abdominal pain or who stop eating. Inspect the abdomen for distention, listen for bowel sounds, and notify the charge nurse or physician of abnormal findings.

IDENTIFYING POTENTIAL COMPLICATIONS

In patients with a suspected or confirmed bowel obstruction, frequent assessment for complications such as fluid and electrolyte imbalance, acid–base imbalances, hypovolemic shock, perforation, and peritonitis is necessary. Monitor laboratory data and report abnormal or unexpected values. Promptly report the patient whose abdomen becomes quiet, rigid or boardlike to the touch, and extremely painful and/or tender.

DIAGNOSING, PLANNING, AND IMPLEMENTING

Deficient Fluid Volume

Expected outcome: Vital signs, mental status, urine output, and weight will remain stable.

The obstructive process draws body fluids into the bowel and often causes vomiting. As a result, the patient is at risk for a fluid volume deficit.

- Monitor vital signs and hemodynamic pressures hourly. *Tachycardia, a drop in blood pressure, and tachypnea may indicate hypovolemia. Hemodynamic pressures provide measures of fluid volume status.*
- Measure urine output hourly and nasogastric output every 2 to 4 hours. Maintain intravenous fluids and blood replacement as ordered. *Urine output of less than 30 mL/hr indicates decreased cardiac output and hypovolemia. Nasogastric output is measured as a guideline for fluid replacement. Intravenous fluids are given to meet current needs and replace losses.*
- Measure abdominal girth every 4 to 8 hours. Mark the area to be measured on the abdomen. *A reference mark allows consistent, accurate measurements. Increased abdominal girth indicates increasing intestinal distention.*
- Notify the charge nurse or physician of changes in status. *Changes can indicate the need for immediate surgery.*

Ineffective Breathing Pattern

Expected outcome: Will maintain clear, audible breath sounds throughout lung fields.

Abdominal distention from a bowel obstruction can place pressure on the diaphragm. Pain from abdominal surgery may lead to shallow breathing. Aspiration of GI contents during vomiting is also a risk in the patient with bowel obstruction.

- Assess respiratory rate, pattern, and lung sounds every 2 to 4 hours. Monitor oxygen saturation levels. *Diminished breath sounds or crackles in the lung bases indicate poor ventilation. Tachypnea, shortness of breath, dyspnea, or fall in oxygen saturation (lower than 90% to 92%) may indicate respiratory compromise. Notify the charge nurse or physician.*
- Elevate the head of the bed. *This reduces pressure on the diaphragm.*

- Provide a pillow or folded bath blanket to use in splinting the abdomen while coughing postoperatively. *The ease and effectiveness of coughing are improved when abdominal muscles and incisions are splinted.*
- Maintain the patency of nasogastric or intestinal suction. *Suction prevents further abdominal distention or aspiration of intestinal contents during vomiting.*
- Encourage use of incentive spirometry or other assistive devices. *Assistive devices help the patient open distal airways and prevent atelectasis.*
- Contact respiratory therapy as indicated. *Additional measures to maintain pulmonary status may be available.*
- Provide oral hygiene at least every 4 hours. *Dehydration and nasogastric suction lead to dry mouth and throat, increasing the risk of bacterial growth. Many respiratory infections are the result of aspirated organisms.*

EVALUATING

To evaluate the effectiveness of nursing care, collect continuing assessment data related to the obstruction itself (abdominal girth, bowel sounds, pain and tenderness), fluid volume status (vital signs, weight, intake and output, skin and mucous membrane temperature and moisture, skin turgor), and potential complications such as atelectasis (respiratory assessment including breath sounds over all lung fields).

DOCUMENTING

Document continuing assessment data; intake and output; amount, color, and odor of nasogastric drainage; vomitus; or stool. If surgery has been performed, document appearance of the wound, and the type, color, and amount of any drainage noted on the dressing or from wound drains. Monitor bowel sounds on a continuing basis, and document when they return and when the patient begins to pass flatus.

CONTINUITY OF CARE

Instruct the patient and family about wound care, activity level after discharge, return to work, and any other recommended restrictions or procedures. If a temporary colostomy has been created, teach the patient and family about its care. For the patient with recurrent obstructions, discuss cause, early identification of symptoms, and preventive measures.

Diverticular Disease

Diverticula are acquired saclike projections of bowel mucosa through the muscular layer of the colon (Figure 26-14 ■). They occur most often in the sigmoid colon. Diverticular disease affects millions, but few people have symptoms. A diet of highly refined and fiber-deficient foods is a major risk factor for diverticula. Other risk factors include aging, a sedentary lifestyle, and postponing bowel movements.

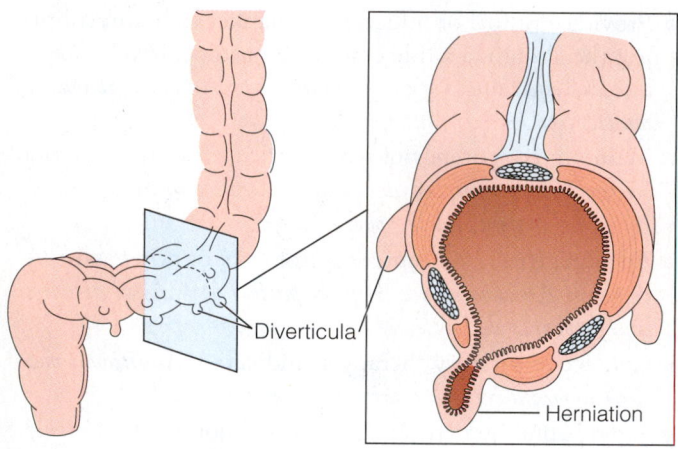

Figure 26-14. ▪ Diverticula of the colon.

PATHOPHYSIOLOGY AND MANIFESTATIONS

Diverticula form when increased pressure within the bowel causes the mucosa to herniate through defects in the wall. *Diverticulosis* is the presence of diverticula. It is usually asymptomatic. Patients may experience episodic left lower quadrant pain, constipation, and diarrhea.

Diverticulitis is inflammation and perforation of a diverticulum, usually in the sigmoid colon. The process is similar to that which occurs when appendicitis develops. Infection occurs when undigested food becomes trapped in a diverticulum, and its blood supply is impaired, allowing bacterial invasion. Perforation results from ischemia and necrosis of the mucosa.

Pain is a common manifestation of diverticulitis. It is usually left sided and may be mild to severe and either steady or cramping. Constipation or diarrhea, nausea, vomiting, and low-grade fever may occur. Complications include hemorrhage, peritonitis, abscess or fistula formation, and bowel obstruction.

COLLABORATIVE CARE

Management of diverticular disease ranges from no prescribed treatment to surgical resection of affected colon. In addition to the history and physical exam, a *flexible sigmoidoscopy* or *colonoscopy* or a *CT scan* may be performed to establish the diagnosis.

A diet high in fiber is prescribed for patients with diverticulosis (Table 26-8 ▪). The patient is generally advised to avoid foods with small seeds (e.g., popcorn, caraway seeds, figs, or berries), which could obstruct diverticula.

TABLE 26-8	High-Fiber, High-Residue Foods
FOOD GROUP	**RECOMMENDED FOODS**
Cereals and grains	Wheat or oat bran; cooked whole-grain cereals; dry cereals such as bran flakes, corn flakes, shredded wheat; whole-grain breads or crackers; brown rice
Fruits	Unpeeled raw apples, peaches, and pears; oranges
Vegetables	Dried beans (black, red, pinto, or kidney), lima beans; broccoli; peas; corn; squash; raw vegetables such as carrots, celery, and tomatoes; potatoes with skins

Bowel rest and antibiotic therapy are prescribed during an acute episode of diverticulitis. The patient initially may be NPO with intravenous fluids and parenteral nutrition. Feeding is resumed gradually, progressing from clear liquids to a soft, low-roughage diet with added psyllium seed to soften stool and increase its bulk. The high-fiber diet is resumed after full recovery. Surgery may be required if the patient develops an abscess or peritonitis. Review Box 26-6 for nursing care of the patient having bowel surgery.

NURSING CARE

The nurse's role for diverticulosis is mainly educational. Teach patients in all settings about the benefits of a high-fiber diet in preventing diverticular disease, bowel cancer, and other disorders. In residential or foster care settings, work with dietary staff and care providers to increase the amount of fiber in residents' diets, unless contraindicated.

Emphasize the importance of maintaining a high-fiber diet to reduce the incidence of complications of diverticulosis. Discuss how to increase dietary fiber, and refer to a dietitian as needed. Provide instruction about complications of the disease and their manifestations.

For the patient with acute diverticulitis, explain prescribed treatment and food and fluid limitations. Also explain why dietary fiber is limited during acute inflammation but increased for chronic management. Provide discharge instruction for patients undergoing surgery. Refer to community health care agencies as needed.

ANORECTAL DISORDERS

Key Concept   Anorectal disorders can cause significant pain and interfere with normal bowel elimination patterns. Patients are generally treated in the community and the nursing role is primarily educational.

Anorectal conditions include hemorrhoids, as well as lesions such as fissures, abscess, fistulas, and pilonidal disease.

Hemorrhoids

When pressure on the veins of the anus and anal canal is increased or venous return is impaired, the veins weaken and distend, forming **hemorrhoids** (or *piles*). Virtually all adults have hemorrhoids, usually asymptomatic.

Straining to defecate is the most common cause of hemorrhoids. Pregnancy increases intra-abdominal pressure and is an important cause of hemorrhoids. Contributing factors include prolonged sitting, obesity, chronic constipation, and a low-fiber diet.

Internal hemorrhoids develop above the mucocutaneous border or junction of the anus (Figure 26-15■). They rarely cause pain and usually present with bright red bleeding that is unmixed with stool. It can vary from streaks on toilet tissue to enough to color the water in the toilet. The patient may experience a feeling of incomplete stool evacuation. As they enlarge, hemorrhoids may *prolapse* or protrude through the anus.

External hemorrhoids develop below the mucocutaneous junction. Bleeding is rare with external hemorrhoids. Anal irritation, a feeling of pressure, and difficulty cleaning the anal region may be manifestations of external hemorrhoids.

"Normal" hemorrhoids are not painful. Prolapsed hemorrhoids may become strangulated, leading to thrombosis (clotting). Thrombosed hemorrhoids cause extreme pain. Internal hemorrhoids that are associated with liver disease may rupture and bleed profusely.

COLLABORATIVE CARE

Management of hemorrhoids is conservative unless complications occur. Internal hemorrhoids are diagnosed by *anoscopic* exam. A sigmoidoscopy or colonoscopy may be done to rule out colorectal cancer, which can produce similar symptoms.

A high-fiber diet and increased water intake to increase stool bulk, improve its softness, and reduce straining is effective for most patients with hemorrhoids. Bulk-forming laxatives (e.g., Metamucil, Citrucel) or stool softeners such as docusate sodium (DSS, Colase, Surfak, others) may be prescribed. Suppositories and local ointments (e.g., Preparation H, Nupercaine) have an anesthetic and astringent effect that reduces discomfort and irritation of surrounding tissues. They have little or no effect on the hemorrhoid itself. Warm sitz baths, bed rest, and local astringent compresses may be recommended to shrink edematous prolapsed hemorrhoids after digital reduction.

Prolapsed or thrombosed hemorrhoids may require additional treatment. *Sclerotherapy* involves injecting a chemical irritant into tissues surrounding the hemorrhoid to cause inflammation and scarring. *Rubber band ligation* involves placing a rubber band snugly around the hemorrhoid and surrounding mucosa, causing the tissue to necrose and slough within 7 to 10 days. Repeat treatments may be necessary. In *hemorrhoidectomy*, hemorrhoids are surgically excised.

NURSING CARE

Most patients with hemorrhoids are treated in outpatient settings. Nurses have frequent opportunities to teach preventive measures for hemorrhoids. Stress the importance of dietary fiber, liberal fluid intake, and regular exercise to maintain stool bulk, softness, and regularity. Discuss the need to respond to the urge to defecate rather than postpone it. Also discuss constipation management, including use of bulk-forming laxatives. Stress that stool softeners should be used for only short-term relief. Discuss appropriate use of over-the-counter preparations for hemorrhoid symptom relief.

Discuss signs of possible complications, such as chronic bleeding, prolapse, and thrombosis. Also discuss the link between manifestations of hemorrhoids and colorectal cancer. Urge the patient to seek medical care for persistent, unresolved, or progressive symptoms.

When a hemorrhoidectomy is performed, the patient requires more direct nursing care. Postoperative care of the patient with perianal surgery is outlined in Box 26-11■. Anal packing may be left in place for 24 hours after surgery. Closely observe for bleeding when it is removed. Postoperative pain can be significant because of rich innervation of the anal region and possible muscle spasms.

Anorectal Lesions

ANAL FISSURE

An *anal fissure* is an ulcer on the anal margin. Irritating diarrheal stools, childbirth trauma, habitual cathartic use, and anal intercourse may cause anal fissures. Tissues surrounding the fissure become chronically inflamed. Pain

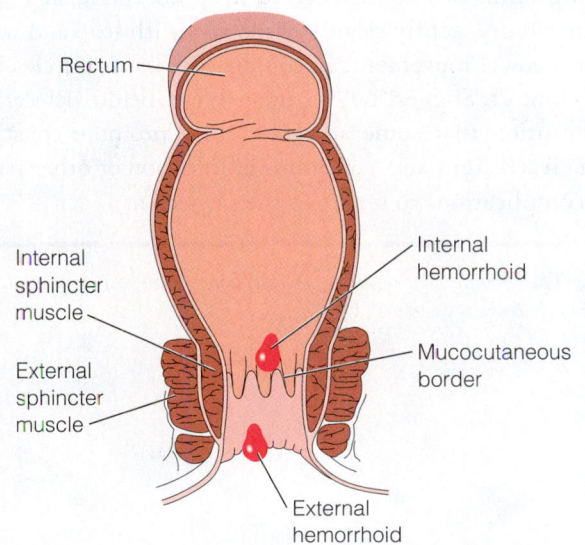

Figure 26-15. ■ Internal hemorrhoids are located above the mucocutaneous border, whereas external hemorrhoids develop below this junction.

Perianal Surgery (Postoperative)

☑ Monitor vital signs and urinary output every 4 hours.

☑ Inspect rectal dressing every 2 to 3 hours; observe closely for bleeding.

☑ Assist to position of comfort, usually side-lying.

☑ Provide analgesics as ordered and before first bowel movement.

☑ Apply ice packs over rectal dressing as ordered.

☑ Assist with sitz bath three to four times per day, providing a rubber ring or donut device for comfort.

☑ Provide a flotation pad for sitting.

☑ Give stool softeners as ordered.

☑ Encourage fluid intake of at least 2,000 mL per day.

Patient and Family Teaching

☑ Take sitz bath after each bowel movement for 1 to 2 weeks after surgery.

☑ Drink at least 2 quarts of fluid per day.

☑ Eat adequate dietary fiber, and exercise moderately.

☑ Take stool softeners as prescribed.

☑ Report to the physician the following symptoms: rectal bleeding, continued pain on defecation, a temperature greater than 101°F (38.3°C), purulent rectal drainage.

and small amounts of bright red bleeding occur with defecation. Anticipated pain may lead to constipation, which further aggravates symptoms. Treatment involves increased fluid and dietary fiber intake, as well as bulk-forming laxatives. A topical agent such as hydrocortisone cream may be prescribed.

ANORECTAL ABSCESS

Bacterial invasion of tissue around the anus can lead to *anorectal abscess*. Pain, which may be aggravated by sitting or walking, is the primary manifestation of an anorectal abscess. External swelling, redness, heat, and tenderness are apparent on examination. If the abscess does not drain spontaneously, an incision and drainage (I&D) is performed. Anorectal abscesses rarely resolve with antibiotic therapy alone.

ANORECTAL FISTULA

A *fistula* is a tunnel or tubelike tract with openings at each end. Anorectal fistulas have one opening in the anal canal and the other usually in skin around the anus. A fistula may develop spontaneously or result from an anorectal abscess or Crohn's disease. Drainage is intermittent or constant and may be purulent. It may be accompanied by local itching, tenderness, and pain with defecation. The fistula may heal spontaneously, or a *fistulotomy* may be performed. The primary opening of the fistula is closed, and the tract is opened to allow healing by secondary intention, from the inside out.

PILONIDAL DISEASE

Pilonidal disease is an acute abscess or chronic draining sinus in the sacrococcygeal area. Beneath the abscess or sinus is a cyst that often contains hair tufts. Pilonidal disease usually affects young hirsute (hairy) males; it is probably caused by trapping of hair in deep tissues. It may be congenital. The cyst is generally asymptomatic unless it becomes infected. Infection causes pain, tenderness, redness, heat, and swelling of the affected area. Purulent discharge may be noted. Pilonidal disease is treated with incision and drainage. The sinus tract and underlying cyst are excised and closed.

NURSING CARE

Teach the patient with a perianal lesion to maintain a high-fiber diet and liberal fluid intake to decrease discomfort with defecation. Stress the importance of responding to the urge to defecate to prevent constipation.

After surgical treatment of any of these disorders, teach the patient to avoid soiling the dressing with urine or feces during elimination. Instruct to keep the perianal region clean and dry, gently cleansing the area with soap and water after a bowel movement. Encourage sitz baths for cleaning and comfort. Suggest taking an analgesic before defecation, but caution that some analgesics may promote constipation. Teach signs and symptoms of infection or other possible complications to report to the physician.

Note: The references and resources for all chapters have been compiled at the back of the book.

Chapter Review

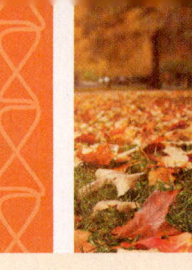

KEY POINTS

- **Concept:** Inflammation, obstructions, absorption disorders, and changes in structure can alter bowel elimination, affecting health, causing pain, or necessitating surgery. Nurses focus on providing physical care, emotional support, and teaching.
- Diarrhea and constipation are common bowel symptoms that, while often functional (no identified pathology), may indicate a serious disorder such as infection, inflammation, or obstruction. It is important to collect and document complete assessment data about patients' complaints of changes in patterns of bowel elimination.
- When prolonged or severe, diarrhea can lead to serious fluid and electrolyte imbalances, as well as excoriation of perianal tissues. Nursing care for the patient with diarrhea focuses on preventing complications such as dehydration and promoting comfort.
- Constipation is often a functional disorder caused by inadequate fluid intake, lack of dietary fiber, or voluntary retention of stool. Encourage all patients (unless specifically contraindicated) to consume generous amounts of water and a diet high in fiber.
- Most laxatives are appropriate for short-term use (1 week or less) only. Bulk-forming laxatives may be used for longer periods if necessary.
- **Concept:** Inflammatory bowel disorders may be either acute or chronic. Supporting physiologic function is a priority for acute inflammatory disorders, whereas teaching and supporting psychosocial function are vital for patients with chronic inflammatory bowel disorders.
- A rigid, boardlike abdomen and severe abdominal pain usually indicate acute inflammation of the peritoneum and a need for immediate medical intervention. Patients with peritonitis require intensive nursing care and continuing assessment.

- IBD, which includes ulcerative colitis and Crohn's disease, is a chronic condition that can have significant effects on nutritional status and body image. The nursing care focus is educational, helping the patient learn to manage the disorder and maintain optimal health.
- **Concept:** The movement of intestinal contents through the bowel can be partially or completely obstructed by a mass, structural abnormality, or loss of peristalsis. It is important that the nurse recognize and respond appropriately to manifestations of bowel obstruction.
- Rectal bleeding may indicate hemorrhoids (a common, benign condition) or colorectal cancer. Patients with rectal bleeding should undergo testing (e.g., colonoscopy) for colorectal cancer.
- Advise all patients over the age of 50 to undergo regular screening for colorectal cancer as recommended by the American Cancer Society. Patients with IBD have a significantly increased risk for colorectal cancer and should begin screening exams at an earlier age.
- Early manifestations of a bowel obstruction include high-pitched, tinkling bowel sounds. Later manifestations include absent bowel sounds, abdominal distention, and possible vomiting. Intestinal decompression relieves obstruction for some patients; others require surgery to correct or remove the obstruction if mechanical.
- **Concept:** Anorectal disorders can cause significant pain and interfere with normal bowel elimination patterns. Patients are generally treated in the community, and the nursing role is primarily educational.
- A warm sitz bath is an appropriate nursing measure for patients with an anorectal disorder (unless contraindicated by specific procedures performed).

PEARSON NURSING STUDENT RESOURCES

Find additional materials at **nursing.pearsonhighered.com**.

Clinical Reasoning Care Map

Caring for a Patient With Colorectal Cancer

NCLEX-PN® Focus Area: Reduction of Risk Potential

Case Study: William Cunningham is a 65-year-old man who has noticed small amounts of blood in his stools for the past 3 months. His physician finds a palpable mass on digital rectal exam and orders a colonoscopy. A large rectal lesion is found; biopsy shows it to be adenocarcinoma. Mr. Cunningham is scheduled for an abdominoperineal resection and sigmoid colostomy.

Nursing Diagnosis: Risk for Impaired Skin Integrity

COLLECT DATA

Subjective	Objective
_____	_____
_____	_____
_____	_____
_____	_____
_____	_____

Does this present a threat to the patient's safety?

If yes, the priority intervention to address this threat would be:

_____

Nursing Care

_____
_____
_____
_____
_____
_____
_____

Interprofessional team members to include when planning care:

_____

How would you document this? _____

_____

Compare your answers and documentation to those provided on the companion website.

Data Collected
(use only those that apply)

- Sense of pressure in rectum
- Intermittent constipation
- BP 118/78; T 98.4°F (36.9°C); P 82; R 18
- Height 5'10" (178 cm), weight 185 lb (84 kg)
- States, "I really don't want a colostomy, but if that is what it takes to keep me well, I'm ready to get it over with."

Nursing Interventions
(use only those that apply; list in priority order)

- Provide analgesia as ordered, evaluating its effectiveness.
- Frequently assess stoma and peristomal skin condition.
- Discuss foods that cause odor and gas.
- Teach colostomy care.
- Maintain consistent nursing personnel assignment to facilitate trust.
- Refer to the local United Ostomy Association.
- Provide a list of local resources for ostomy supplies.
- Provide for privacy when teaching and discussing concerns about ostomy.

NCLEX-PN® Exam Preparation

> **TEST-TAKING TIP** Although assessment is the first step in the nursing process, in emergent situations it may be done concurrently with interventions. When an exam question is addressing the nursing process, obtain assessment data before implementing nursing interventions unless the patient's safety and physiologic function are at risk.

1 The first priority for a nurse admitting a patient with severe diarrhea to an acute medical unit would be to:
1. prevent skin breakdown.
2. assess the patient's fluid volume status.
3. administer an antidiarrheal medication.
4. obtain a thorough patient history.

2 An older adult patient complains that her bowels move only two or three times a week. The most appropriate response by the nurse would be:
1. "You should start using a laxative to ensure a daily movement. I'll write down some safe laxatives for you."
2. "Reducing the amount of fiber in your diet may help. I'll give you a low-residue diet plan."
3. "Let's talk to the doctor about getting you scheduled for a colonoscopy to evaluate your large intestine."
4. "That pattern may be normal for you. Tell me about your stool—is it hard or difficult to expel?"

3 A patient comes to the walk-in clinic complaining of abdominal pain that started about 2 hours previously. In his assessment, the nurse notes tenderness in the right lower quadrant, and checks for rebound. Rebound tenderness is characterized by:
1. relief of pain with palpation followed by pain when pressure is released.
2. intensification of pain when the area is palpated.
3. a rigid, boardlike abdomen that is extremely tender.
4. pain in the affected quadrant when the opposite quadrant is palpated.

4 A patient with a newly created sigmoid colostomy asks if the bag will need to be worn constantly. Your best response would be:
1. "I think you should discuss this with an enterostomal therapist."
2. "Usually, patients learn to live with a colostomy bag. I'll get an educational video for you to watch."
3. "Your colostomy is at the level of the lower bowel, so you may be able to have regular daily bowel movements."
4. "I will ask the physician for an antidiarrheal medication."

5 A patient has been admitted with severe diarrhea. The nurse bases his decision on whether to administer the prescribed antidiarrheal medication on the understanding that antidiarrheal medication:
1. should not be used until the cause of diarrhea has been determined.
2. should be administered upon manifestation of diarrhea to prevent losses of fluids and electrolytes.
3. should be withheld until stool cultures and samples have been obtained.
4. should not be administered until fluid and electrolyte status have been established.

6 The nurse is teaching a patient with newly diagnosed ulcerative colitis about her prescription for sulfasalazine (Azulfidine). Which of the following does the nurse include in teaching? **Select all that apply**.
1. "Take this pill with a small sip of water at least an hour before meals."
2. "Use sunscreen while you are taking this drug to prevent sunburns."
3. "If you use oral contraceptives, use additional protection while taking this drug."
4. "A skin rash is a common side effect of this drug; it will abate with time."
5. "While you are using this drug, use aspirin, not acetaminophen, for pain relief."

7 When a patient is prescribed a low-residue diet, which of the following menu choices indicates an understanding of the diet?
1. Steak, baked potato, carrot sticks, lemon meringue pie
2. Steamed fish, baked potato, green beans, fresh fruit cup
3. Broiled chicken breast, mashed potatoes, whipped squash, angel food cake
4. Fried chicken, mashed potatoes, corn, angel food cake

8 The nurse caring for a patient with a possible bowel obstruction would immediately report which of the following?
1. Hypoactive bowel sounds
2. A flat, soft abdomen
3. Fecal-smelling nasogastric tube drainage
4. Increased pain with a rigid, boardlike abdomen

9 A patient recovering from bowel surgery is asking for regular food. The nurse's most appropriate response would be:
1. "When you start passing gas and your bowel is working again, it will be safe to start eating again."
2. "When you no longer require narcotic pain medication, it will be safe to reintroduce food."
3. "The IV fluids you are receiving are adequate nourishment."
4. "When you are able to ambulate, introducing food will be considered."

10 The nurse talking to a community group includes which of the following in her discussion of colorectal cancer?
1. "When you have reached the age of 50, you should have an annual digital rectal exam and a flexible sigmoidoscopy or colonoscopy every 10 years."
2. "People with inflammatory bowel disease need a flexible sigmoidoscopy or colonoscopy every 5 years after age 50 for early detection of polyps."
3. "When you have reached the age of 50, you need to have a lab test called carcinoembryonic antigen to determine the need for colonoscopy."
4. "When you have reached the age of 50, you need to have annual checks due to the rapid growth of bowel tumors."

Answers and rationales for Review Questions appear in Appendix I.

CHAPTER 27
Caring for Patients With Gallbladder, Liver, and Pancreatic Disorders

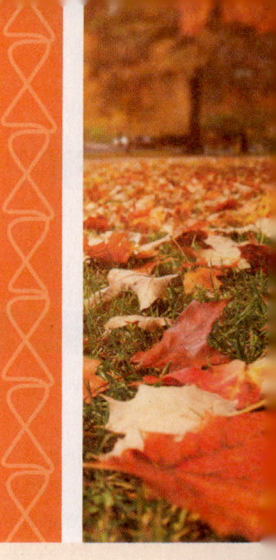

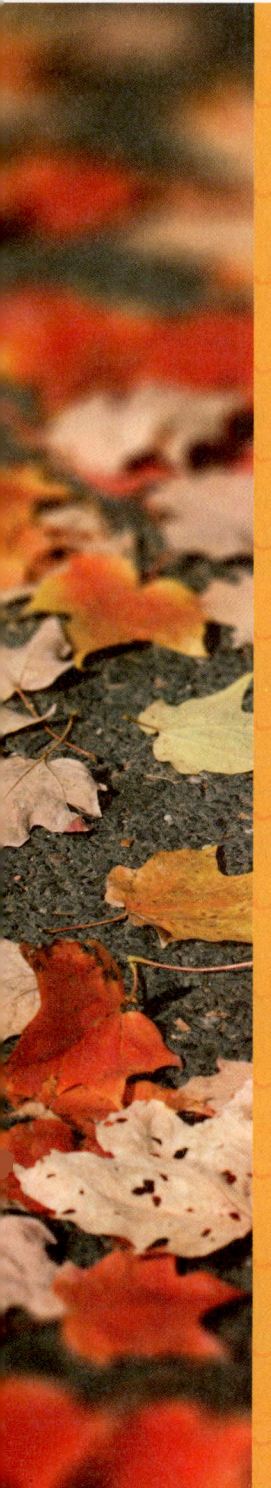

BRIEF OUTLINE

GALLBLADDER DISORDERS
Gallstones
LIVER DISORDERS
Common Features of Liver Disorders
Hepatitis

Cirrhosis
Cancer of the Liver
EXOCRINE PANCREAS DISORDERS
Pancreatitis
Cancer of the Pancreas

APPLIED LEARNING OUTCOMES

After completing this chapter, you will be able to:

1. Describe the pathophysiology, manifestations and effects, and complications of common disorders of the gallbladder, liver, and exocrine pancreas.

2. Collaborate with the interprofessional team to provide safe and effective care for patients with disorders of the gallbladder, liver, and exocrine pancreas.

3. Safely administer medications to patients with disorders of the gallbladder, liver, or exocrine pancreas.

4. Provide culturally appropriate and evidence-based nursing care for the patient who has surgery of the gallbladder, liver, or pancreas.

5. Use the nursing process and expressed values, needs, and preferences of the individual to assess, plan, provide, and evaluate care for patients with disorders of the gallbladder, liver, or exocrine pancreas.

KEY TERMS

The key terms are defined on the pages listed below.

SPECIAL FEATURES

Key Concept The gallbladder, liver, and exocrine pancreas are important in the digestion, absorption, and metabolism of food. Disorders of these organs have multiple effects on food intake and nutrient usage.

Because the gallbladder, liver, and exocrine pancreas—collectively known as the accessory organs of digestion—work together, one organ's functioning frequently affects that of another. Inflammation, obstruction, scarring, and tumors are the primary disease processes that affect these organs.

Patients who have a disorder of the gallbladder, liver, or pancreas may experience severe pain and a host of metabolic and nutritional disturbances. Nursing care priorities focus on helping the patient maintain good nutritional status, reducing the risk for complications, promoting comfort, and addressing psychosocial needs of the patient and family.

GALLBLADDER DISORDERS

Key Concept Gallstones can obstruct the flow of bile from the liver into the gut, causing inflammation and pain. Accurate diagnosis and appropriate treatment are necessary to preserve physiologic function and promote comfort.

Gallstones

Gallstones (*calculi*) are common, affecting an estimated 20 million people in the United States. **Cholelithiasis**, the formation of stones within the gallbladder or duct system that transports bile, is the most common gallbladder disorder. Gallstones are also the most common cause of obstructed bile flow. Risk factors for cholelithiasis include older age, female gender, obesity, family history, and use of oral contraceptives or estrogen therapy (Box 27-1■).

PATHOPHYSIOLOGY

Most gallstones are formed in the gallbladder, prompted by the interaction of abnormal bile composition, ineffective bile flow, and inflammation of the gallbladder. Gallstones usually contain cholesterol, bile pigments, and small amounts of other materials, such as calcium salts (Figure 27-1■). Several factors raise the level of cholesterol in bile: obesity, a high-calorie, high-fat diet, and drugs that lower blood cholesterol levels. Ironically, very low-calorie diets and fasting also increase the concentration of cholesterol in bile and slow its flow in the biliary system.

Gallstones usually form in the gallbladder. When the stones are small and remain in the gallbladder, they are frequently asymptomatic and the patient is unaware of their presence. Stones may, however, migrate into bile ducts, causing ductal inflammation (*cholangitis*). It is often this migration and resulting inflammation that cause the symptoms of cholelithiasis.

Cholecystitis is inflammation of the gallbladder. It usually results from stones obstructing the cystic or common bile duct (Figure 27-2■). The obstruction causes increased pressure and ischemia of the gallbladder. In addition, retained bile causes chemical irritation. The gallbladder becomes acutely inflamed as a result. The inflammation

BOX 27-1	RISK FACTORS FOR GALLSTONES

- Age over 60
- Family history
- Race or ethnicity: Native American or Mexican heritage
- Obesity, high blood triglyceride levels, glucose intolerance
- Rapid weight loss; very low calorie diets or bariatric surgery
- Female gender, oral contraceptive use, or hormone replacement therapy
- Biliary stasis: pregnancy, fasting, prolonged total parenteral nutrition
- Disorders: diabetes mellitus, cirrhosis, small intestinal disorders, sickle cell disease

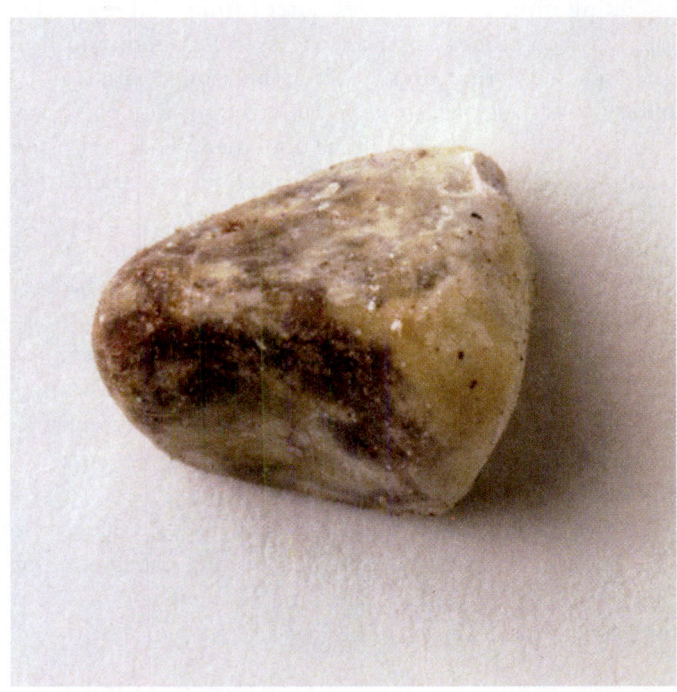

Figure 27-1. ■ Gallstone made up of cholesterol, bile pigments, and calcium salts. (Source: Susanna Price / Dorling Kindersley Media Library.)

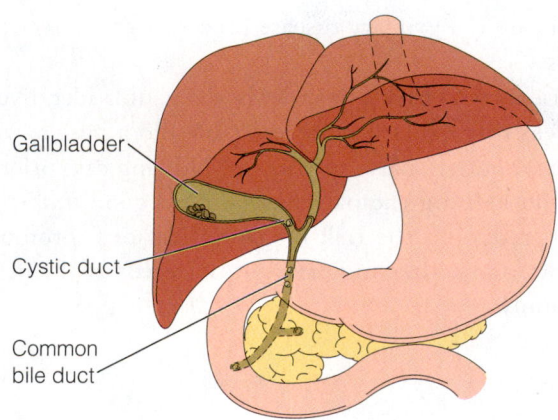

Figure 27-2. ■ Common locations of gallstones.

causes edema and further obstruction of bile flow. Ischemia can lead to necrosis and perforation of the gallbladder. Chronic cholecystitis is caused by repeated attacks of acute cholecystitis.

If the common bile duct is obstructed, bile backs up into the liver and possibly the pancreas, producing jaundice, pain, possible hepatic damage, pancreatitis (discussed later in this chapter), or sepsis.

MANIFESTATIONS AND COMPLICATIONS

Cholelithiasis is often asymptomatic. When symptoms do develop, they often relate to movement of a stone through the bile ducts or inflammation of the gallbladder and bile ducts.

Early manifestations of cholelithiasis are often vague, including mild gastric distress after eating a large or fatty meal. When stones obstruct the cystic or common bile duct, pressure increases behind the stone. This causes **biliary colic**, a severe, steady pain in the right upper quadrant or epigastric region of the abdomen. The pain often begins within a few hours after a meal and may radiate to the back or right shoulder.

Acute cholecystitis is characterized by severe epigastric or upper right quadrant pain that radiates toward the back or right shoulder blade. This steady pain results from contraction of the ducts and may be initiated by a large, high-fat meal. The pain lasts longer than biliary colic, continuing for 12 to 18 hours. Anorexia, nausea, and vomiting frequently occur along with the pain. *Chronic cholecystitis,* a complication of repeated episodes of acute cholecystitis or untreated gallstones, is often asymptomatic or may cause mild, nonspecific symptoms such as vague gastric upset or mild right upper quadrant pain after eating. See Box 27-2■ for the manifestations of cholelithiasis and cholecystitis.

Bile duct obstruction can lead to reflux (backflow) of bile into the liver, with resulting jaundice, pain, and possible liver damage. Pancreatitis can result from obstruction of the common bile duct.

BOX 27-2	MANIFESTATIONS OF CHOLELITHIASIS AND CHOLECYSTITIS

Cholelithiasis
- Often asymptomatic
- Epigastric fullness, gastric distress after a meal
- Biliary colic: severe, steady right upper quadrant or epigastric pain; often follows a meal

Acute Cholecystitis
- Severe epigastric or right upper abdominal pain; may radiate to back
- Pain precipitated by large, high-fat meal
- Right upper quadrant guarding and tenderness
- Nausea and vomiting
- Fever
- Possible jaundice

Perforation of the gallbladder and peritonitis are possible complications of cholecystitis. Other complications include infection, fistula formation, and cancer.

COLLABORATIVE CARE
Diagnostic Tests

Gallstones are often diagnosed through a right upper quadrant *abdominal ultrasound*. This test is noninvasive and requires no special preparation. An *oral cholecystogram* may be performed in nonacute situations. *Gallbladder scans,* also called liver-biliary scans or HIDA scans, use nuclear medicine techniques to assess acute cholecystitis. Laboratory tests may show elevated white blood cell (WBC) count, serum bilirubin, alkaline phosphatase, alanine transaminase (ALT), and aspartate transaminase (AST) levels.

Medications

Patients who refuse surgery or for whom surgery would pose a high risk (e.g., a frail older adult) may be treated with oral bile acids to dissolve stones. Ursodiol (Actigall) or chenodiol (Chenix) may be used to treat small cholesterol stones. These drugs work by reducing the cholesterol content of gallstones, gradually dissolving the stone. Nurses need to monitor blood levels of liver enzymes and watch for possible diarrhea in patients taking these drugs. Several years of therapy may be required, and stones frequently recur after treatment is stopped. If infection is suspected, antibiotics may be prescribed. Parenteral narcotic analgesics may be necessary to relieve the pain of acute cholecystitis.

Dietary Management

Because dietary fat stimulates gallbladder contraction, patients are usually placed on a low-fat diet. Examples of foods to avoid are listed in Box 27-3■. A high-fiber diet with ample fresh fruits and vegetables is protective against

BOX 27-3	**HIGH-FAT FOODS TO AVOID IN CHOLECYSTITIS**

- Whole-milk products (e.g., cheese, cream, ice cream)
- Deep-fried foods and pastries (e.g., donuts, french fries, batter-fried fish)
- Avocados
- Sausage, bacon, hot dogs
- Gravies made with fat or cream
- Most nuts
- Snack foods (e.g., potato chips, tortilla chips)
- Peanut butter
- Chocolate

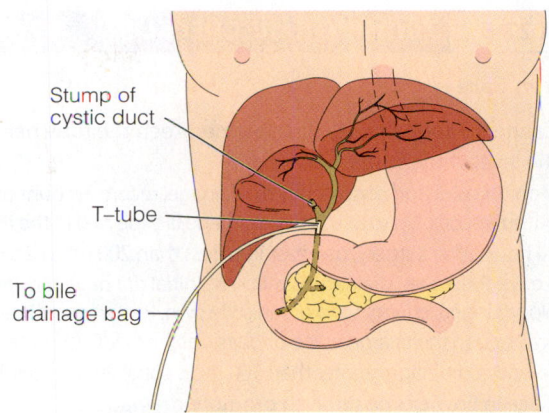

Figure 27-3. ■ A T-tube placed in the common bile duct. Bile flows by gravity into a collection device placed below the level of the abdomen.

gallstones and cholecystitis. Patients who are obese are encouraged to lose weight to reduce surgical risks. All food and fluids may be withheld during an attack of acute cholecystitis; total parenteral nutrition (TPN) may be used to maintain the patient's nutritional status.

clinicalALERT

Certain very low-calorie diets increase the risk for gallstones. Ask patients with symptoms of gallbladder disease about their current diet and any recent changes.

Surgery

Most patients with symptomatic gallbladder disease are treated with *laparoscopic cholecystectomy*. This minimally invasive surgery allows a hospital stay of 24 hours or less, and the patient is often able to return to work within a week. See Box 27-4■ for nursing care of the patient having laparoscopic cholecystectomy.

clinicalALERT

During laparoscopic cholecystectomy, the abdomen is inflated with carbon dioxide. This can cause shoulder pain after surgery. Carefully assess the patient's pain and provide adequate analgesia. Inform the patient that the pain will be relieved when the gas is absorbed.

Nursing care for patients who require a traditional cholecystectomy is similar to that required by any patient having abdominal surgery. (See Chapter 10 for more information about care of the surgical patient.) This surgery requires an upper abdominal incision. Coughing, deep breathing, and early ambulation are vital to prevent respiratory complications postoperatively.

Patients may return from surgery with a T-tube (Figure 27-3■). Inserted after common bile duct exploration, a T-tube keeps the duct open and promotes bile flow until edema decreases. Excess bile is collected in a drainage bag secured below the surgical site. Nursing care of a patient with a T-tube is outlined in Box 27-5■.

Complementary Therapies

Goldenseal, an herb, has been used to treat cholecystitis. It stimulates bile and bilirubin secretion and inhibits the growth of many of the bacteria known to infect the gallbladder. Studies have shown goldenseal to be effective in relieving all manifestations of cholecystitis. It should not be used during pregnancy and lactation, however, because it can stimulate the uterus.

BOX 27-4	**NURSING CARE CHECKLIST**

Laparoscopic Cholecystectomy

Before Surgery

- ☑ Reinforce preoperative teaching, including the procedure, postoperative care, and pain management.
- ☑ Provide routine preoperative care as outlined in Chapter 10.

After Surgery

- ☑ Monitor vital signs every 15 minutes for 2 hours or until stable and then every 4 hours until discharge.
- ☑ Provide routine postoperative care.
- ☑ Assess location and severity of pain; provide analgesia as needed.
- ☑ Assist out of bed and with ambulation as ordered.
- ☑ Reinforce and provide postoperative and discharge teaching:
  - ☑ Wound care
  - ☑ Pain management
  - ☑ Diet and activity
  - ☑ Medications
  - ☑ Follow-up appointments and care

BOX 27-5 | **NURSING CARE CHECKLIST**

T-Tube Care

☑ Connect T-tube to a sterile container; keep the tube below the level of the surgical wound.

☑ Monitor color and consistency of drainage; record amount on output record. Up to 500 mL of drainage is expected in the first 24 hours after surgery, decreasing to less than 200 mL in 2 to 3 days; thereafter, drainage is minimal. Initial drainage may be blood tinged, changing to greenish brown. Report excessive drainage to the charge nurse or physician immediately (after 48 hours, drainage greater than 500 mL is considered excessive).

☑ Place in Fowler's position to promote drainage.

☑ Assess skin for bile leakage during dressing changes; apply a protective skin barrier if necessary.

☑ Teach patient how to manage tube when turning, ambulating, and performing activities of daily living.

☑ Clamp the T-tube only as ordered by the physician.

☑ If indicated, teach the patient care of the T-tube, how to clamp it, and signs of infection.

NURSING CARE

PRIORITIZING NURSING CARE

For most patients with gallbladder disease, the priority of nursing care is managing symptoms of the disorder and promoting comfort.

HEALTH PROMOTION

Although many risk factors for gallstones cannot be controlled, several can. Encourage patients who are overweight or obese to reduce dietary fat and caloric intake and increase their intake of fresh fruits, vegetables, and whole grains. Discuss the health benefits of daily exercise. Encourage patients to avoid very-low-calorie diets and "yo-yo" dieting. For patients with high blood cholesterol levels, discuss the potential benefits of cholesterol-lowering drugs such as the statins.

ASSESSING

Focused assessment of patients with gallstones includes both subjective and objective data. Ask about the patient's pain, including its location, character, timing, and frequency. Inquire specifically about any relationship between food intake and pain. Note complaints of other symptoms such as nausea, vomiting, epigastric upset or heartburn, and their relationship to eating. Have the patient describe the color of any emesis and the color and consistency of feces. Observe the patient's general appearance and apparent comfort. Note skin color and any evidence of jaundice of the skin or sclera. Inspect the abdomen for distention; auscultate bowel sounds, and lightly palpate for tenderness and guarding, particularly over the right upper quadrant.

IDENTIFYING POTENTIAL COMPLICATIONS

Promptly report an abrupt relief of pain in a patient experiencing acute biliary colic or cholecystitis. Abrupt pain relief may signal perforation of the distended gallbladder. Monitor temperature because continued fever may indicate infection or abscess formation.

DIAGNOSING, PLANNING, AND IMPLEMENTING
Acute Pain

Expected outcomes: Will verbalize understanding of relationship between consuming foods high in fat and pain. Will report pain at a level of 2 or lower on a scale of 0 to 10.

- Teach patients to avoid fat in their diets. (See Box 27-3 for foods to avoid.) *Fat initiates gallbladder contractions and is a stimulus for pain.*
- Administer narcotic analgesics as ordered for severe pain. *Severe pain can cause muscle spasm and increased gastrointestinal symptoms. Parenteral analgesia may be required.*
- Place in Fowler's position. *Fowler's position decreases pressure on the inflamed area and may help relieve pain.*

Nausea

Expected outcome: Will report relief of nausea and ability to tolerate small amounts of food and fluids.

- Monitor complaints of nausea. Document amount, color, and consistency of any emesis. Monitor food and fluid intake. *Nausea may result from cholecystitis or be caused by pain. It increases the risk of a nutritional deficit; vomiting can lead to fluid volume deficit.*
- Administer prescribed antiemetics. *Giving antiemetic medication before meals and procedures helps promote food intake and prevent vomiting.*
- Promptly remove noxious items and odor-producing substances (e.g., food, commodes). *The sight or smell of food and noxious substances can stimulate or aggravate nausea.*
- Provide oral care and clean bedding (as needed) after each emesis. *This reduces nausea stimuli.*
- Withhold food and fluids during episodes of nausea and vomiting. Offer cold, low-fat, or fat-free foods and foods with little odor in small quantities when the patient is able to eat. *Attempting to eat when nauseous may precipitate vomiting. Cold, low-fat foods are better tolerated, as are small quantities rather than large meals.*

MANAGING NURSING CARE

Nursing care activities for the patient with gallbladder disease such as monitoring vital signs, recording intake and output, emptying, measuring and recording T-tube drainage, and assisting with ambulation are appropriate to assign to assistive personnel with documented training and competence.

EVALUATING

To evaluate the effectiveness of nursing interventions, collect data related to level of comfort, ability to consume the ordered diet and fluids, respiratory status, and freedom from infection.

DOCUMENTING

Document the patient's manifestations and responses to treatment measures. Note diagnostic tests, procedures, or surgery if performed, and continuing assessment data after the procedure. Document teaching provided and reinforced to the patient and family and their apparent understanding of instructions.

CONTINUITY OF CARE

Patients with cholelithiasis may manage their disease at home with medical interventions, or they may require prompt surgical intervention. Reinforce teaching about the disease, prescribed medications, diagnostic procedures, and treatment options. Discuss the relationship of food intake to episodes of acute cholecystitis, and the importance of maintaining a low-fat, low-calorie diet if indicated. Explain the role of bile and the function of the gallbladder in terms that the patient and family can understand.

Provide preoperative teaching, discussing what to expect before and after surgery. Discuss measures to reduce discomfort, promote healing, and prevent complications.

After surgery, prepare the patient for discharge and home care. Discuss pain control, monitoring for and preventing infection, and T-tube care. Include instructions about activities, diet, and returning to work. Inform about signs or symptoms to report to the physician.

Refer the patient to a dietitian to review low-fat foods; include the person preparing foods. Most patients start with a low-fat diet and gradually add fatty foods as tolerated. Refer the patient to home care services as indicated.

NURSING CARE PLAN
Patient With Cholelithiasis

Joyce Red Wing is a 44-year-old member of the Chickasaw tribe. Recently, she has noticed a dull pain in her upper abdomen that gets worse after eating fatty foods; the pain is accompanied by nausea. She remembers having similar pain after the birth of her last child. The diagnosis of cholelithiasis is made, and Ms. Red Wing is admitted for a laparoscopic cholecystectomy.

Assessment

Ms. Red Wing's admission history reveals that her usual diet consists of fatty foods, particularly tacos or fried bread and biscuits with gravy for breakfast. She reports not wanting to eat much of anything lately. She states that she has never had surgery before and hopes "everything goes well." She has a good understanding of the procedure to be done. Physical assessment findings: T 100°F (37.7°C); BP 130/84; P 88; R 20. Weight 130 lb (59 kg), a 5-lb weight loss from her usual; 5'3" (160 cm) tall. Abdomen tender to palpation in the upper right quadrant. No jaundice, chills, or other evidence of complications noted.

Nursing Diagnosis

The following nursing diagnoses are identified for Ms. Red Wing:

- *Anxiety* related to concerns about surgery
- *Acute Pain* related to surgery
- *Deficient Knowledge (Low-Fat Diet)* related to lack of nutritional information

Expected Outcomes

The expected outcomes specify that Ms. Red Wing will:

- Verbalize reduced anxiety related to undergoing surgery.
- Maintain adequate pain control postoperatively.
- Follow prescribed diet postoperatively.

Planning and Implementation

The following interventions are planned and implemented:

- Teach about the gallbladder and the function of bile.
- Discuss pre- and postoperative care, including plans for discharge, pain management, wound care, activities, and follow-up.
- Provide analgesia as needed.
- Review specific high-fat foods to avoid and ways to maintain weight.

Evaluation

Ms. Red Wing is discharged the morning after surgery. She has no signs of infection and is able to care for her incisions. She identifies the importance of eating a low-fat diet and keeping her weight stable, as well as gradually resuming activities. Ms. Red Wing states that she "is glad it is over, but it wasn't as bad as I thought it would be at first." She has an appointment to see her surgeon in 1 week.

Critical Thinking in the Nursing Process

1. What is the rationale for a low-fat diet with cholelithiasis? Discuss nutritional practices as they relate to cholelithiasis and Ms. Red Wing's culture.
2. Why would it be important to place Ms. Red Wing in Fowler's position after surgery?
3. List five areas to cover in predischarge teaching for Ms. Red Wing.

Note: Discussion of Critical Thinking questions appears on the companion website.

LIVER DISORDERS

Key Concept   The liver is constantly exposed to blood that may contain pathogens, toxins, and malignant cells, making it vulnerable to inflammation, damage, and tumors. Because the liver has many essential functions, liver disorders affect all other body systems.

With the exception of the skin, the liver is the largest organ in the body and one of the most complex. It is responsible for metabolizing food and nutrients, detoxifying drugs and alcohol, and synthesizing blood proteins and clotting factors. The liver is also a storehouse for glycogen, vitamins and minerals, and blood. It is vulnerable to inflammation, damage, and tumors because it is constantly exposed to a large amount of blood. More than 600 drugs, chemicals, herbal preparations, and other substances have been identified as damaging to the liver (*hepatotoxic*). Some of the more common substances are listed in Box 27-6■.

Common Features of Liver Disorders

Although many different disorders can affect liver function, the effects and manifestations of these disorders can be very similar. These common features relate to impaired liver cell function, impaired bilirubin excretion, and altered blood flow through the liver.

IMPAIRED LIVER CELL FUNCTION

When liver cells are damaged or their function is impaired, effects such as the following are seen:

- The production of albumin and clotting factors is impaired. Low albumin levels can lead to edema. Plasma proteins normally draw fluid from the tissues into the bloodstream (called an *oncotic draw*); this draw is reduced when protein levels are low. Lack of clotting factors increases the risk for bleeding.
- The metabolism and storage of glucose is affected, affecting energy and blood glucose levels (either hyperglycemia or hypoglycemia).
- Less bile is produced, impairing absorption of fats and fat-soluble vitamins. Vitamin K, a fat-soluble vitamin, may be deficient, affecting clotting and increasing the risk for bleeding.
- Impaired hormone metabolism (including estrogen and testosterone) leads to feminization in men and irregular menses in women.

JAUNDICE

Liver disorders impair the metabolism and excretion of bilirubin. Bilirubin is a pigment released from hemoglobin when aging red cells are removed from the circulation and destroyed. In the liver, bilirubin is converted to a water-soluble form and excreted in the bile. When bilirubin is not metabolized and excreted, it accumulates in tissues, leading to **jaundice** (yellow staining of tissues). Jaundice (also called *icterus*) is often first seen in the sclera of the eyes and then in the skin. It can develop for several different reasons:

- *Hemolytic jaundice* develops when excess RBCs are destroyed (hemolysis) and the liver is unable to process all the released bilirubin.
- *Hepatic jaundice* occurs when damaged liver cells (*hepatocytes*) are not able to metabolize and excrete bilirubin. Feces may appear clay colored because of the lack of bilirubin in bile. The urine is dark because the kidneys excrete bilirubin in the urine.
- Obstruction of bile flow within the biliary system (the gallbladder and bile ducts) impairs bilirubin excretion, leading to *obstructive jaundice.* Stools are light or clay colored due to lack of bile pigment, and urine is dark.

BOX 27-6	COMMON KNOWN HEPATOTOXINS

Alcohol
Nonprescription medications (e.g., acetaminophen)
Prescription medications
- Amoxicillin/clavulanic acid, erythromycin, and nafcillin, antibiotics
- Atorvastatin, lovastatin, and other statins to lower blood cholesterol levels
- Azathioprine and methotrexate, immunosuppressants
- Chlorpromazine, an antipsychotic drug
- Isoniazid, pyrazinamide, and rifampin, antituberculosis drugs
- Phenytoin, carbamazepine, and valproic acid, anticonvulsants

Complementary therapies
- Comfrey tea
- Jin bu huan, a Chinese remedy
- Pennyroyal oil, margosa oil, and clove oil in large doses

Environmental toxins
- Arsenic
- Carbon tetrachloride
- Copper
- Fluorine
- Toluene
- Vinyl chloride

PORTAL HYPERTENSION

The portal venous system is the major source of blood to the liver. It drains the gastrointestinal tract, the spleen, and surface veins of the abdomen. Inflammation, swelling, and scarring of the liver restricts blood flow through its lobules (its functional units; see Figure 24-6). Restricting blood flow through the liver increases pressure in the portal venous system (think about the pressure that builds up when a hose is crimped). This is known as **portal hypertension**. Over time, portal hypertension can lead to:

- Congestion and dilation of veins in the gastrointestinal tract and the abdominal wall. As a result:
  a. The appetite is suppressed (anorexia).
  b. Collateral vessels develop in the distal esophagus (known as **esophageal varices**), stomach, and rectum.
  c. The spleen enlarges (splenomegaly).
- **Ascites**, fluid in the peritoneal cavity, develops. Increased pressure forces fluid out of abdominal vessels and into the peritoneal cavity. Low blood protein levels contribute to ascites.
- Blood is shunted around the congested liver, allowing toxic waste products to accumulate. This can lead to **hepatic encephalopathy** (also called *portal systemic encephalopathy*), with confusion, agitation, and impaired consciousness.
- Blood flow to the kidneys is affected, leading to a type of acute kidney failure known as **hepatorenal syndrome**.

See the section of this chapter on cirrhosis for more information about the effects and complications associated with portal hypertension.

Hepatitis

Key Concept Hepatitis is usually an acute viral disease that primarily affects the liver. Preventing the spread of hepatitis is an important nursing and public health responsibility.

Hepatitis is inflammation of the liver. It is usually caused by a virus but may also be caused by alcohol, toxins (e.g., drugs), or gallbladder disease. Acute and chronic forms of hepatitis exist. Damage to liver cells resulting from hepatitis can lead to cirrhosis, discussed in the next section of this chapter.

Hepatitis is common. An estimated 33% of adults in the United States have been infected with hepatitis A at some time during their lives, and an estimated 4.4 million people have chronic hepatitis B or C (Centers for Disease Control and Prevention [CDC], 2013).

PATHOPHYSIOLOGY

Inflammation of liver tissues disrupts its metabolic functions and the elimination of bilirubin. Although the underlying pathology of hepatitis varies, its effects and manifestations are similar. Much depends on the extent of liver damage and the patient's health status at the time.

Viral Hepatitis

Nearly all cases of acute viral hepatitis are caused by one of five viruses, designated by letters of the alphabet. Hepatitis A virus (HAV) and hepatitis B virus (HBV) are the most common, although the incidence of hepatitis C virus (HCV) is increasing. Viral infection causes liver cell injury and necrosis. The liver cell damage may be directly caused by the virus or may result from the body's immune response to the virus. The manifestations of viral hepatitis are similar for all types, but other characteristics of the disease vary. Table 27-1■ compares the onset, incubation, mode of transmission, and other characteristics of the more common types of viral hepatitis.

Hepatitis A causes epidemics and sporadic cases of hepatitis. It is transmitted by the fecal–oral route, either by direct contact with an infected individual or via contaminated food, water, or shellfish. The source of infection is often not identified. Hepatitis A is usually a mild, self-limited illness that does not become chronic.

Hepatitis B is usually transmitted by intimate sexual contact or from an infected mother to her fetus. It is also usually a self-limited disease in adults, although a small percentage of patients develop chronic infection. *Carriers* can transmit HBV while having no symptoms of the disease. Patients with chronic hepatitis B have an increased risk for liver cancer. Health care workers are at risk for hepatitis B. Following Standard Precautions and obtaining hepatitis B immunization are important preventive strategies.

Hepatitis C is nearly always transmitted by blood and contaminated needles. This type of viral hepatitis affects African Americans and Mexican Americans more frequently than Whites. Although the initial illness is often asymptomatic, hepatitis C often leads to chronic liver disease and is the most common indication for liver transplant. A vaccine has been developed but is not commonly administered.

TABLE 27-1	**Common Types of Viral Hepatitis**		
	HEPATITIS A (HAV)	**HEPATITIS B (HBV)**	**HEPATITIS C (HCV)**
Incubation (in weeks)	2–6	8–24	5–12
Onset	Abrupt	Slow	Slow
Transmission	Fecal–oral	Blood and body fluids; perinatal	Blood and body fluids; perinatal
Communicable	2 weeks before to 1 week after onset of symptoms	1–2 months before symptoms; when hepatitis B surface antigen (HBsAg) present in blood	When HCV present in blood
Carrier state	No	Yes	Yes
Possible complications	Rare	Chronic hepatitis, cirrhosis, liver cancer	Chronic hepatitis, cirrhosis, liver cancer
Laboratory findings	Anti-HAV antibodies	Positive HBsAg; anti-HBV antibodies	Anti-HCV antibodies
Prevention	Hepatitis A vaccine (primary dose + booster in 6–12 months)	Hepatitis B vaccine (primary dose + second 1–2 months later + third 2–5 months after second)	None
Prophylaxis	Hepatitis A vaccine and/or standard immune globulin before or within 2 weeks of exposure	Hepatitis B immune globulin (HBIG) within 1–2 days of exposure; second dose 28–30 days after exposure	None

The *hepatitis delta virus (HDV)* causes infection only in people who have active hepatitis B. It causes more severe infection than hepatitis B alone. *Hepatitis E* is rare in the United States, occurring more commonly in underdeveloped areas of southeast Asia, parts of Africa, and Central America. It is transmitted by water contaminated by feces.

Chronic Hepatitis

Chronic hepatitis, a chronic infection of the liver, may lead to cirrhosis, liver cancer, or liver failure. It may develop with HBV and HCV infections. The manifestations of chronic hepatitis are often mild and nonspecific, such as general malaise, fatigue, and an enlarged liver.

Noninfectious Hepatitis

Alcoholic hepatitis is acute or chronic inflammation of the liver caused by alcohol. Although it is often reversible, alcoholic hepatitis can lead to necrosis of liver cells. It is the most common risk factor for cirrhosis (discussed in the next section of this chapter) in the United States. Many drugs (e.g., acetaminophen and tetracyclines) and other toxins (e.g., poisonous mushrooms, heavy metals, and carbon tetrachloride) can damage the liver, causing inflammation and necrosis (*toxic hepatitis*). Gallstones that block normal bile flow can also lead to inflammation of the liver, a condition known as *hepatobiliary hepatitis.*

MANIFESTATIONS

The manifestations of hepatitis may be mild or very severe. The course of acute viral hepatitis generally follows three phases.

The *preicteric* (before jaundice) *phase* may develop abruptly or insidiously. The **icteric** (jaundice) *phase* of the disease develops after 5 to 10 days. Early symptoms may worsen when jaundice develops and then begin to improve. During this phase, the skin, mucous membranes, and sclera of the eyes appear yellow. During the *posticteric* or *convalescent phase,* the patient begins to feel better, with an improving appetite, and jaundice disappears. Box 27-7■ summarizes the manifestations of each phase of hepatitis.

BOX 27-7	**MANIFESTATIONS OF ACUTE VIRAL HEPATITIS**

Preicteric or Prodromal Phase

- "Flulike" symptoms: malaise, fatigue, headache, muscle aches, nasal discharge, sore throat
- Gastrointestinal: anorexia, nausea, vomiting, diarrhea, or constipation
- Joint pain
- Mild and constant right upper abdominal pain

Icteric Phase

- Jaundice
- Pruritus
- Clay-colored stools, dark urine
- Mild weight loss

Posticteric or Convalescent Phase

- Well-being improves, energy increases
- Jaundice resolves

COLLABORATIVE CARE

Usually no specific treatment is required for acute viral hepatitis. Prevention, early identification of the disease, and teaching are vital.

Diagnostic Tests

- Blood is drawn to assess for *viral antigens* (e.g., hepatitis B surface antigen) or *antibodies* to the viral agents that cause hepatitis (see Table 27-1).
- *Liver function tests* are measured. Serum levels of these enzymes increase when the liver is inflamed or damaged.
- *Serum bilirubin* levels are also measured. Total bilirubin usually is elevated, as are both direct (conjugated) and indirect (unconjugated) bilirubin levels.
- *Prothrombin time* may be prolonged if the liver is not able to manufacture the protein needed for blood coagulation.

Prevention

Vaccines and immune globulin injections are available to prevent hepatitis A and B. Vaccines are recommended for people who are at increased risk for exposure to the disease. Immune globulin is used to prevent the disease after known or suspected contact with the virus. Table 27-1 lists recommended immunizations.

Hepatitis A vaccine is recommended for adults traveling internationally, homosexual men, drug users, and people with chronic liver disease. It is also recommended for all infants between 12 and 24 months of age.

When exposure to HAV has occurred, illness can often be prevented by a single dose of immune globulin given within 2 weeks of exposure. Immune globulin is recommended for people in close contact with someone who has hepatitis A, for child care workers where a case of hepatitis A has been identified, and for restaurant patrons where a food handler has developed hepatitis A.

Hepatitis B vaccine is recommended for all infants, adolescents who have not been immunized, and adults at risk for exposure to hepatitis B. All health care workers including nurses should be vaccinated. Box 27-8■ summarizes who should receive hepatitis B vaccine.

After exposure to hepatitis B, both hepatitis B vaccine and hepatitis B immune globulin (HBIG) are given to prevent infection. With perinatal exposure, infants are given both the vaccine and HBIG within 24 hours of birth.

Medications

Patients with a mild or moderate case of hepatitis B generally require no medications. However, an antiretroviral drug such as lamivudine (Epivir, Heptovir) or adefovir dipivoxil (Hepsera) may be given to treat severe cases. Patients with chronic hepatitis B may be treated with interferon alpha or pegylated interferon (long-acting interferon).

BOX 27-8	POPULATION FOCUS

People Who Should Be Vaccinated for Hepatitis B

- People at risk for sexual transmission: homosexual or bisexual men, prostitutes, people with multiple partners or recently diagnosed sexually transmitted disease
- Injection drug users
- Male prison inmates
- People on hemodialysis
- Health care workers
- Patients and staff of institutions for the developmentally disabled
- High-risk populations: Alaska Natives, Pacific Islanders, and immigrants from HBV-endemic areas
- Household members and partners of HBV carriers
- International travelers to HBV-endemic areas
- Recipients of certain blood products, such as clotting factors

---

Acute hepatitis C is usually treated with interferon alpha, an antiviral agent, to reduce the risk of chronic hepatitis C. Patients with chronic hepatitis C undergo combination therapy with long-acting pegylated interferon and the antiviral drug ribavirin (Rebetol, Virazole).

Other Therapies

Supportive care for patients with acute viral hepatitis includes adequate rest and a high-calorie diet. Alcohol and drugs that are toxic to the liver are avoided. Intravenous fluids may be given if nausea and vomiting interfere with intake. In most cases, clinical recovery takes 3 to 16 weeks.

Complementary Therapies

Herbalists in Europe have used milk thistle to treat liver disease for more than 2,000 years. Silymarin is believed to be the active ingredient in milk thistle. It helps prevent complications and promote more rapid recovery. It also benefits patients who have liver damage due to toxins, cirrhosis, and alcoholic liver disease. It appears that silymarin:

- Promotes liver cell growth.
- Is a powerful antioxidant.
- Blocks toxins from entering and damaging liver cells.
- Reduces inflammation in the liver.

Licorice root may also be used by herbalists to treat hepatitis. It has both antiviral and anti-inflammatory effects, but long-term use may lead to hypertension and affect fluid and electrolyte balance.

Other herbal remedies may help relieve the adverse effects of interferon (flulike symptoms, fatigue, dizziness, anorexia, nausea, diarrhea, and cough). These include ginger for nausea and St. John's wort for depression. Refer patients interested in complementary therapies for hepatitis to a certified herbalist.

NURSING CARE

PRIORITIZING NURSING CARE

For most patients, hepatitis is a self-limiting disease that requires little treatment beyond supportive care (rest and a balanced diet). The primary focus for nursing care is preventing transmission of the disease to others. Standard Precautions, which treat all body fluids as potentially contaminated, are adequate to prevent spread of the disease to others. Because hepatitis A is spread via the fecal–oral route, careful handling of feces and meticulous hand washing are vital.

HEALTH PROMOTION

Teaching is the primary measure to prevent hepatitis. Stress the importance of hand washing after toileting and before handling food. Inform patients about recommended immunizations and, as appropriate, about measures to prevent hepatitis when exposure is known or suspected. Discuss safer-sex practices such as abstinence, mutual monogamy, and using condoms. Talk about the dangers of injection drug use and of sharing equipment or needles.

ASSESSING

Patients with acute hepatitis often present with classic manifestations of hepatitis. However, patients who have chronic hepatitis may have more vague manifestations. Ask about known or possible exposure to hepatitis, including opportunities such as recent travel, close contact with someone known to have hepatitis, occupational exposure, or high-risk behaviors such as injection drug use. Inquire about recent flulike symptoms, appetite, and discomfort or pain. Ask to describe any changes in skin or eye color and the color of feces and urine.

Note the patient's general appearance and color of skin and sclera. Inspect the abdomen for distention, auscultate bowel sounds, and palpate lightly for tenderness.

DIAGNOSING, PLANNING, AND IMPLEMENTING

Risk for Infection (Transmission)

Expected outcome: Other patients and close contacts of the patient will remain infection-free.

- Use Standard Precautions and meticulous hand washing. *One of the most important goals when caring for patients with acute viral hepatitis is preventing the spread of infection. Proper aseptic technique can prevent transmission of the viruses.*
- For patients with hepatitis A, use Standard Precautions and contact isolation if fecal incontinence is present. *The fecal–oral route is the primary mode of transmission of hepatitis A.*
- Encourage at-risk patients to obtain hepatitis A or hepatitis B immunizations, or both. *Prevention is a key strategy for reducing the incidence and long-term consequences of viral hepatitis.*

Activity Intolerance

Expected outcome: Will maintain activities of daily living without excessive fatigue.

- Encourage rest as needed to relieve fatigue. *Fatigue and possible weakness are common in patients with hepatitis. Adequate rest promotes optimal immune function and recovery.*
- Plan nursing care activities that promote rest, allowing gradual resumption of activities. *As the patient recovers, fatigue and activity tolerance improve.*

Imbalanced Nutrition: Less Than Body Requirements

Expected outcome: Will consume 100% of prescribed or recommended diet.

- Encourage smaller, more frequent meals. *Patients with hepatitis often experience significant anorexia and possible nausea. Smaller meals are frequently better tolerated.*
- Help the patient select a palatable diet with adequate calories. Suggest supplements such as Ensure as needed to maintain intake. Low-fat diets are sometimes better tolerated. *Sufficient energy is required for healing.*
- Encourage eating more food at times when nausea and anorexia are minimal. *Many patients with acute hepatitis are nauseated in the afternoon and evening hours.*
- If nausea and vomiting persist, give intravenous fluids as ordered. Monitor fluid and electrolytes, and assess for signs of dehydration. *Prompt assessment of fluid and electrolyte imbalance allows early treatment to maintain homeostasis.*

EVALUATING

To evaluate the effectiveness of nursing care, collect data such as the following:

- Household members remain free of infection.
- Patient can verbalize appropriate measures to prevent spreading the disease.
- Patient gets adequate rest.
- Weight remains stable.

DOCUMENTING

Document continuing assessment data, including trends in serum bilirubin and liver function tests. Also document teaching provided to the patient and family and their understanding and apparent willingness to comply with precautions. If prophylactic measures are provided or immunizations administered, note the date and time administered. Report to the local health department cases of hepatitis A among food handlers, child care workers, and others at high risk for spreading the disease to the public.

CONTINUITY OF CARE

Most patients with acute viral hepatitis are cared for at home and in community-based settings. Teach the patient, family members, and members of the household how to prevent spread of the disease. Recommend prophylactic treatment and immunization for household contacts and others at risk for contracting the disease. Instruct the patient with hepatitis A not to prepare food for other members of the family until he or she is no longer infectious. Include instructions for cleaning eating utensils and soiled linens. Emphasize the importance of not sharing toothbrushes, razors, or dirty needles and the need to abstain from sexual activity until the patient is no longer infectious. Stress the importance of avoiding hepatotoxins, such as alcohol and acetaminophen, until the liver is fully healed. Discuss the need to undergo follow-up evaluations and the importance of following diet and activity recommendations for the full period of recovery.

Cirrhosis

> **Key Concept** Cirrhosis is a chronic liver disease that affects its metabolic, detoxification, and other functions. Blood flow through the liver is impaired, leading to portal hypertension. Patient care focuses on preserving function and preventing complications.

Cirrhosis is a chronic liver disease that destroys the structure and function of liver lobules. It has devastating effects and often leads to death.

Alcoholic liver disease (*Laënnec* or *alcoholic cirrhosis*) is the most common type of cirrhosis. The risk for alcoholic cirrhosis is directly related to the amount of alcohol consumed, the number of years of alcohol consumption,

and blood alcohol levels. Cirrhosis may also result from chronic hepatitis B or C, toxic liver damage due to drugs or chemicals (*postnecrotic cirrhosis*), heart failure, or obstructed bile flow (*biliary cirrhosis*).

PATHOPHYSIOLOGY

In cirrhosis, functional liver tissue is gradually destroyed and replaced with fibrous scar tissue. As hepatocytes and liver lobules are destroyed, the metabolic functions of the liver are lost. Scar tissue forms constrictive bands within liver lobules and disrupts blood and bile flow within the liver. Impaired blood flow through the liver increases pressure in the portal venous system, leading to portal hypertension (Figure 27-4■). Obstructed bile outflow damages liver cells. Loss of functioning liver lobules ultimately leads to liver failure.

In alcoholic cirrhosis, metabolic changes in the liver lead to fatty infiltration of hepatocytes. At this stage, the disease can be reversed with abstinence from alcohol; the liver will heal. With continued alcohol abuse, inflammatory cells infiltrate the liver, causing loss of functional liver tissue and formation of scar tissue. The liver becomes nodular and shrunken.

MANIFESTATIONS AND COMPLICATIONS

The manifestations and complications of cirrhosis result from both impaired liver function and altered blood flow through the portal venous system. Early in the course of the disease, the liver is enlarged and tender. The patient may complain of right upper quadrant pain. Other early

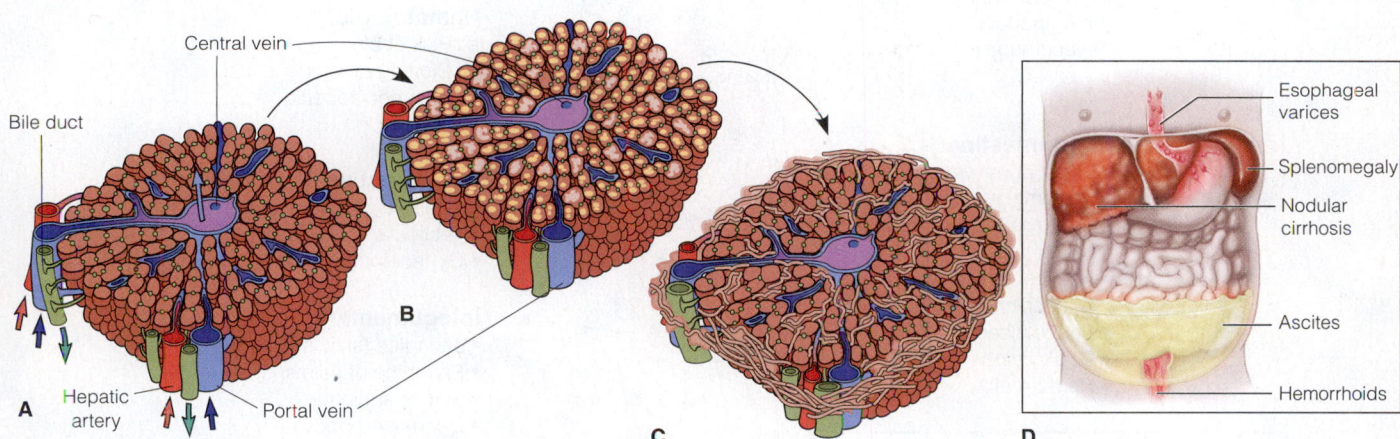

Figure 27-4. ■ Alcoholic cirrhosis and portal hypertension. (**A**) The liver contains multiple lobules made up of plates of hepatocytes surrounded by small capillaries called sinusoids. Blood from the portal vein (which drains the gut) and hepatic artery mixes and flows through these sinusoids to the central vein of the lobule. Hepatocytes produce bile, which drains outward to bile ducts. (**B**) Alcohol metabolism produces toxins that inflame and damage the liver and hepatocytes. This damage causes fat to accumulate in liver cells and lobules. With continued alcohol intake, inflammation produces additional damage. (**C**) Scar tissue forms within the damaged lobule. Small islands of liver cells continue to regenerate, forming nodules. Gradually, scarring outpaces regeneration, and the liver becomes shrunken, hard, and nodular. (**D**) Bands of scar tissue restrict blood flow through the sinusoids. Pressure in the portal venous system increases. Collateral vessels become dilated and congested, forming *varices* (fragile, distended veins) in the esophagus, stomach, and rectum. The spleen enlarges, and *ascites* (fluid in the abdomen) develops. Confusion, agitation, and altered levels of consciousness develop as the liver fails.

signs include weight loss, weakness, and anorexia. Bowel function may be disrupted. As the disease progresses, symptoms of liver failure and portal hypertension develop (Figure 27-5■).

Portal hypertension is elevated blood pressure in the portal venous system of the gut. Blood is *shunted* (rerouted) from vessels of the portal system into lower pressure vessels, causing congestion of veins in the esophagus, rectum, and abdomen.

Ascites is an accumulation of serous fluid in the peritoneal cavity. Portal hypertension is the primary cause of ascites, because fluid is forced out of capillaries by high pressure within the vessels. Impaired liver function affects the production of plasma proteins (e.g., albumin), reducing plasma osmotic pressure. This allows fluid to escape from blood vessels, leading to ascites and peripheral edema. Fluid and electrolyte imbalances also contribute to edema and ascites.

Splenomegaly (enlargement of the spleen) develops as blood is shunted from the portal system into the splenic vein. It can lead to anemia and low platelet and WBC counts. Low platelets (*thrombocytopenia*) and decreased

clotting factor production by the liver lead to increased risk for bleeding. Infection is a risk due to low WBC counts (*leukopenia*).

Esophageal varices are enlarged, fragile, and overdistended veins in the distal esophagus that result from portal venous congestion. Patients with esophageal varices are at high risk for bleeding. Even high-roughage foods (e.g., bacon) can lead to hemorrhage of these fragile vessels. *Upper gastrointestinal bleeding* is a frequent complication of cirrhosis. Bleeding, which can be massive, may result from varices, gastritis, or peptic ulcer.

As the liver is progressively destroyed, its ability to metabolize proteins is impaired. Ammonia and toxic wastes accumulate in the blood. These substances affect the central nervous system (CNS). *Hepatic encephalopathy* is characterized by altered levels of consciousness, cognition, and motor function. *Asterixis* (liver flap) is an early sign of hepatic encephalopathy. It is a muscle tremor that causes involuntary jerking movements that make it difficult to keep the extremities still (Figure 27-6■). *Hepatorenal syndrome* (renal failure associated with end-stage liver disease) may also

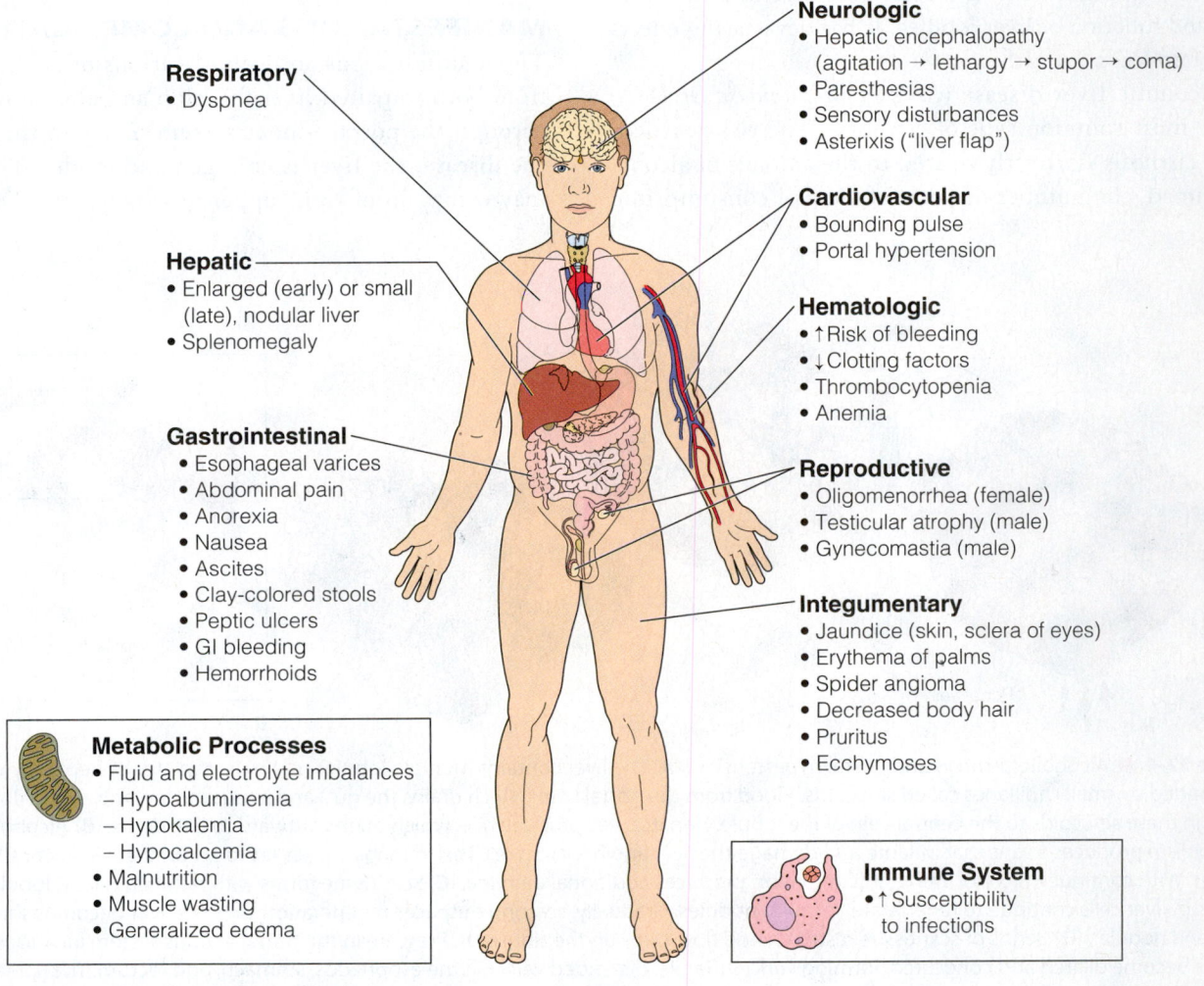

Figure 27-5. ■ The multisystem effects of cirrhosis.

Respiratory
• Dyspnea

Hepatic
• Enlarged (early) or small (late), nodular liver
• Splenomegaly

Gastrointestinal
• Esophageal varices
• Abdominal pain
• Anorexia
• Nausea
• Ascites
• Clay-colored stools
• Peptic ulcers
• GI bleeding
• Hemorrhoids

Metabolic Processes
• Fluid and electrolyte imbalances
  – Hypoalbuminemia
  – Hypokalemia
  – Hypocalcemia
• Malnutrition
• Muscle wasting
• Generalized edema

Neurologic
• Hepatic encephalopathy
  (agitation → lethargy → stupor → coma)
• Paresthesias
• Sensory disturbances
• Asterixis ("liver flap")

Cardiovascular
• Bounding pulse
• Portal hypertension

Hematologic
• ↑Risk of bleeding
• ↓Clotting factors
• Thrombocytopenia
• Anemia

Reproductive
• Oligomenorrhea (female)
• Testicular atrophy (male)
• Gynecomastia (male)

Integumentary
• Jaundice (skin, sclera of eyes)
• Erythema of palms
• Spider angioma
• Decreased body hair
• Pruritus
• Ecchymoses

Immune System
• ↑ Susceptibility to infections

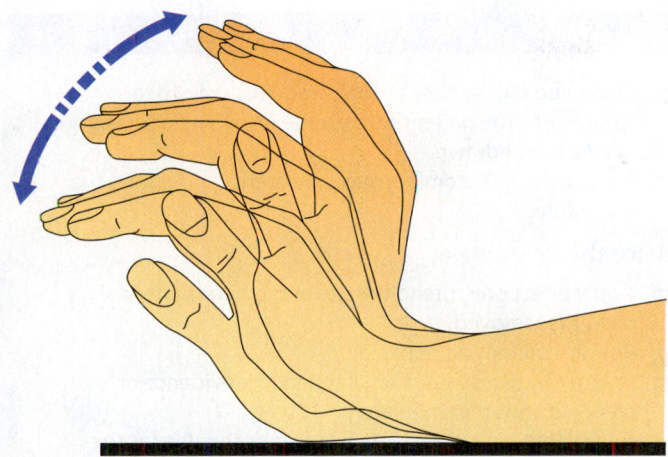

Figure 27-6. ■ Asterixis.

develop. Its cause is unknown, and treatment is generally ineffective.

COLLABORATIVE CARE

The goal of cirrhosis treatment is to prevent further liver damage and manage the effects and complications of cirrhosis. Holistic care that addresses physiologic, psychosocial, and spiritual needs is important. It is vital to include the family in the plan of care, particularly if alcohol abuse is the cause.

Diagnostic Tests

A number of laboratory and diagnostic tests may be ordered:

■ *Liver function tests* are elevated in cirrhosis, although not to the extent seen in hepatitis.

■ A *complete blood count (CBC)* is done to evaluate for possible anemia, leukopenia, and thrombocytopenia.

■ *Blood chemistries,* including serum electrolytes and glucose, protein, albumin, and ammonia levels, are done to evaluate liver function and its effects.

■ *Coagulation studies* are ordered to evaluate the patient's risk for bleeding.

■ An *abdominal ultrasound* is performed to evaluate liver size, identify nodules, and detect ascites.

■ *Liver biopsy* (Figure 27-7■) may be ordered to determine the type and severity of cirrhosis. Nursing care for the patient having a liver biopsy is outlined in Box 27-9■.

■ An *upper endoscopy* may be done to assess for esophageal varices.

Medications

Substances that are toxic to the liver, such as alcohol and acetaminophen, are avoided. Drugs metabolized by the liver, including barbiturates and sedatives cand hypnotics, are also avoided. Doses of other drugs may need to be

adjusted, because impaired liver function may alter their metabolism and subsequent excretion.

Several groups or classes of drugs commonly are prescribed for patients with cirrhosis. Diuretics are ordered to reduce edema and ascites. Spironolactone (Aldactone), a potassium-sparing diuretic, or the potent loop diuretic *furosemide* (Lasix) may be used. Medications to reduce ammonia absorption from the bowel frequently are used, particularly when blood ammonia levels are high. Two drugs used for this purpose are lactulose and rifaximin (Xifaxan) (see Table 27-2■).

Beta-adrenergic blockers such as propranolol or nadolol (Corgard) may be given to reduce portal hypertension. Vitamin K is given to promote clotting. Platelets and other blood products such as fresh-frozen plasma or salt-poor albumin may be administered to restore blood cells and replenish plasma proteins. Histamine-2 antagonists or antacids are ordered to manage associated gastritis and upper gastrointestinal bleeding. Oxazepam (Serax) is an antianxiety/sedative drug that is not metabolized by the liver and may be used to treat acute agitation.

Dietary and Fluid Management

Abstinence from alcohol is vital for patients with cirrhosis. Dietary support is also essential. The diet should be palatable and include adequate protein and calories. If serum

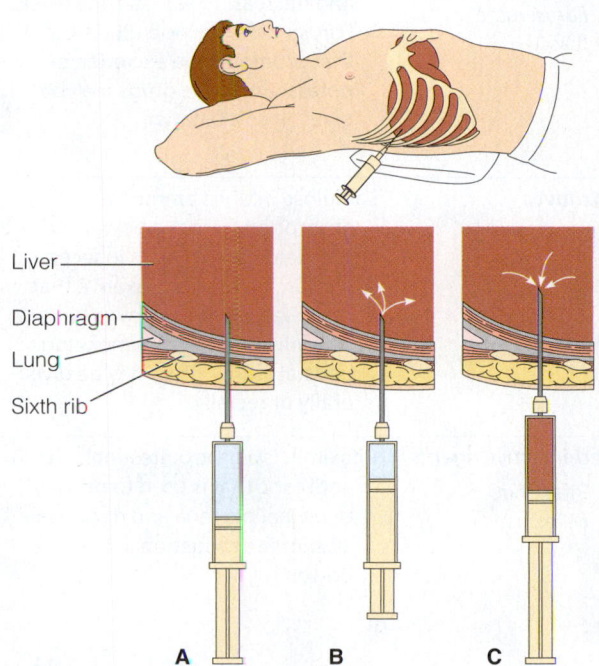

Liver
Diaphragm
Lung
Sixth rib

A B C

Figure 27-7. ■ Liver biopsy. (**A**) The patient exhales completely and holds breath, bringing the liver and diaphragm to their highest position. The needle is inserted between the sixth and seventh ribs. (**B**) A small amount of saline is injected to clear the needle of blood and tissue. (**C**) A tissue sample is aspirated into the needle. The needle is then withdrawn and the patient can resume breathing. Pressure is applied to the site.

BOX 27-9   NURSING CARE CHECKLIST

Liver Biopsy

Before the Procedure

☑ Verify that informed consent for the procedure has been obtained.

☑ Reinforce teaching about the procedure and its purpose.

☑ Keep NPO as ordered, usually 4 to 6 hours before the procedure.

☑ Assess and record baseline vital signs.

☑ Review prothrombin time and platelet count; administer vitamin K as ordered.

☑ Have the patient empty bladder immediately before the test.

☑ Place patient in supine position on far right side of bed; turn head to left and extend right arm above head for better visualization of the biopsy site.

During the Procedure

☑ Help patient hold breath after expiration to keep diaphragm and liver high in the abdominal cavity during needle insertion (see Figure 27-7).

☑ Obtaining biopsy tissue usually requires only 10 to 15 seconds. The patient can resume breathing after the needle is withdrawn.

☑ Some pain or discomfort may be experienced during the procedure.

After the Procedure

☑ Apply direct pressure to the site immediately after the needle is removed.

☑ Position patient on right side.

☑ Frequently assess site and vital signs for evidence of bleeding; report immediately.

☑ Advise that pain may occur in the right shoulder as the anesthetic loses effect.

☑ Keep NPO for 2 hours (or as ordered) and then resume usual diet.

☑ Instruct to avoid coughing, lifting, or straining for 1 to 2 weeks.

TABLE 27-2   Giving Medications Safely: Cirrhosis

CLASS/DRUGS	PURPOSE	NURSING IMPLICATIONS	PATIENT TEACHING
Diuretics ■ Spironolactone (Aldactone) ■ *Furosemide* (Lasix)	Spironolactone is a potassium-sparing diuretic that reduces ascites by increasing urine output and decreasing aldosterone levels. Furosemide is a loop diuretic that promotes the excretion of potassium. These drugs may be given in combination.	Monitor vital signs and serum electrolytes and osmolality. Report changes to the charge nurse or physician. Weigh daily. Monitor and record intake and output.	Take diuretics in the morning and early afternoon to avoid sleep disruption caused by increased urine output. Report increases in weight or edema to your physician. Keep scheduled appointments for laboratory testing and with your physician.
Laxatives ■ Lactulose (Cephulac, Chronulac)	Lactulose inhibits ammonia absorption from the bowel and promotes its excretion in feces. It is also an osmotic laxative that pulls water into the bowel lumen, softening stool and stimulating peristalsis. The drug may be given orally or rectally.	Assess bowel sounds and abdominal girth. Maintain accurate stool chart. Adjust dose to achieve two to three soft stools per day as ordered. Monitor electrolytes and hydration status.	Mix with fruit juice, water, or milk to make more palatable. Drink adequate fluids. Report diarrhea to your physician. If this drug causes nausea, take it with a soda or crackers. Do not stop the medication.
Anti-infective agents ■ Rifaximin (Xifaxan)	Rifaximin is a gastrointestinal antibiotic that is used to destroy intestinal bacteria and decrease ammonia production in the bowel.	Ask about known allergy to rifaximin, rifampin, or related drugs. Do not administer and notify the physician if the patient has bloody diarrhea. Monitor CBC and report abnormal results.	May be taken with or without food. This medicine may cause dizziness. Notify your doctor if you develop any of the following: itching, skin rash, or hives; difficulty breathing; fever; swelling of the hands, feet, or lower legs; or bloody diarrhea.

Note: Medications identified in *italics* are among the 200 most frequently prescribed drugs in the United States.

ammonia levels are high or the patient has signs of hepatic encephalopathy, animal proteins in the diet may be restricted. Sodium intake is restricted to less than 2 g/day to reduce edema. Fluids may be limited as needed to control ascites, edema, and heart failure. Patients who are NPO may require TPN. Vitamin and mineral supplements are ordered as indicated, particularly thiamine, folate, and B_{12}. The fat-soluble vitamins, A, D, and E, may need to be given in a

BOX 27-10   NURSING CARE CHECKLIST

Liver Transplant

Before Surgery

☑ Reinforce preoperative teaching provided by the transplant team.

☑ Provide psychologic support.

☑ Provide routine preoperative care and teaching as outlined in Chapter 10.

☑ Prepare the patient for returning from surgery to the intensive care unit.

After Surgery

☑ Provide routine postoperative care as indicated by postoperative day.

☑ Manage pain and promote respiratory function through coughing, deep breathing, incentive spirometry, and early ambulation.

☑ Administer drugs to prevent rejection (e.g., cyclosporine A, corticosteroids, and azathioprine) as ordered.

☑ Carefully monitor for infection because these drugs suppress the immune response.

☑ Monitor renal function and blood glucose levels.

☑ Monitor for signs of rejection: increasing temperature (an early sign), discomfort over transplant site, anorexia, decreased bile drainage from drain, arthralgia (joint pain), abnormal liver function tests.

☑ Promptly report abnormal assessment data to the charge nurse or physician.

☑ Provide discharge teaching:

  ☑ Avoid infections, recognizing signs of infection and the importance of reporting all fevers.

  ☑ Recognize signs of rejection.

  ☑ Follow verbal and written instructions and a schedule for all prescribed medications. Stress importance of reporting adverse effects and maintaining regular follow-up appointments.

  ☑ Prepare for potential body image changes associated with steroid use and for the psychologic effects of receiving a transplanted organ.

---

water-soluble form. Patients with alcohol-induced cirrhosis may also need a magnesium supplement.

Surgical Procedures

Various surgical procedures may be used to manage the effects and complications of cirrhosis. *Liver transplant* is the only definitive treatment and is not appropriate for all patients with cirrhosis (e.g., patients who continue to abuse alcohol). Nursing care of the patient having a liver transplant is outlined in Box 27-10■.

Paracentesis (removal of fluid from the peritoneal cavity) may be done if ascites is severe. Excess fluid in the peritoneal cavity puts pressure on the diaphragm, increasing the work of breathing. Removing this fluid improves breathing, but fluid will reaccumulate unless the underlying cause of ascites is corrected. Albumin may be given after paracentesis; it increases the intravascular oncotic pressure and slows the development of ascites.

A *transjugular intrahepatic portosystemic shunt (TIPS)* may be used to relieve portal hypertension for some patients. The shunt directs venous blood from the portal vein to the hepatic vein, allowing it to bypass the liver (Figure 27-8■). It can be inserted in a vascular catheterization lab, avoiding the need for surgery. After the procedure, observe the patient closely for evidence of bleeding, either at the insertion site (the jugular vein) or internally. Monitor vital signs, color, and level of consciousness frequently and report changes to the charge nurse or physician.

Bleeding esophageal varices are a potentially life-threatening complication of cirrhosis. Blood and fluids are given to stabilize vital signs. Once the patient's condition is stable, upper endoscopy is performed to identify and treat the varices. A sclerosing agent may be injected into the enlarged vessel, causing inflammation and clotting. In band ligation, bleeding vessels are occluded using small rubber bands. In an acute situation, a multiple-lumen gastrointestinal tube such as a Sengstaken–Blakemore tube may be inserted to *tamponade* (place pressure on) the bleeding varices (Figure 27-9■).

safetyALERT

When caring for a patient with a multiple-lumen NG tube, *always* keep an appropriate syringe at the bedside to deflate the esophageal balloon in case the patient develops respiratory distress.

NURSING CARE

Nursing care of the patient with cirrhosis presents many challenges, because liver dysfunction affects many body systems. Psychosocial and spiritual aspects of care are as vital as the physical care needs of the patient.

PRIORITIZING NURSING CARE

The priority nursing care focus for patients with cirrhosis may vary, depending on the stage of the disease, its effects on other body systems, and the presence of complications.

HEALTH PROMOTION

Talk with all patients about the relationship between alcohol and drug abuse and liver disorders. Excess alcohol

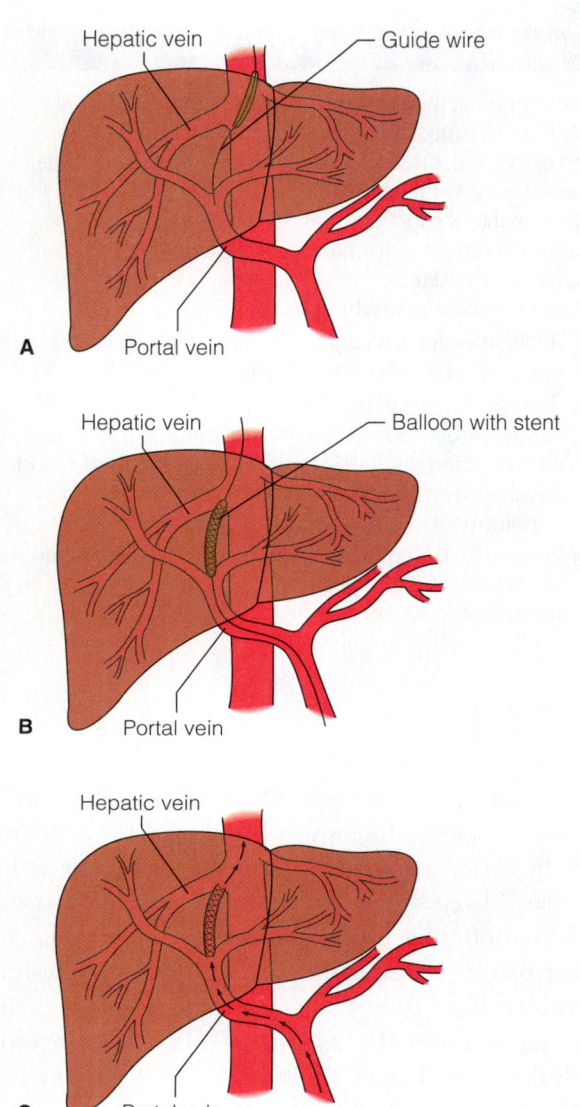

Figure 27-8. ■ Transjugular intrahepatic portosystemic shunt (TIPS). (**A**) A catheter inserted via the internal jugular vein is guided into the hepatic vein. From there, a new route connecting the hepatic and portal veins is created through liver tissue. (**B**) An expandable metal stent is positioned between the portal and hepatic veins. (**C**) The catheter and guide wire are removed, leaving the stent in place.

use is the leading cause of cirrhosis. Injection drug use, which increases the risk for hepatitis B and C, is also a behavior to avoid.

ASSESSING

Patients with cirrhosis may have vague symptoms or be acutely ill with bleeding, respiratory distress, or neurologic manifestations of hepatic encephalopathy. The extent of assessment data collected depends on the situation. Ask about current symptoms, including upper abdominal pain; anorexia, nausea, or vomiting; and itching or a change in the color of skin or the sclera. Obtain information about

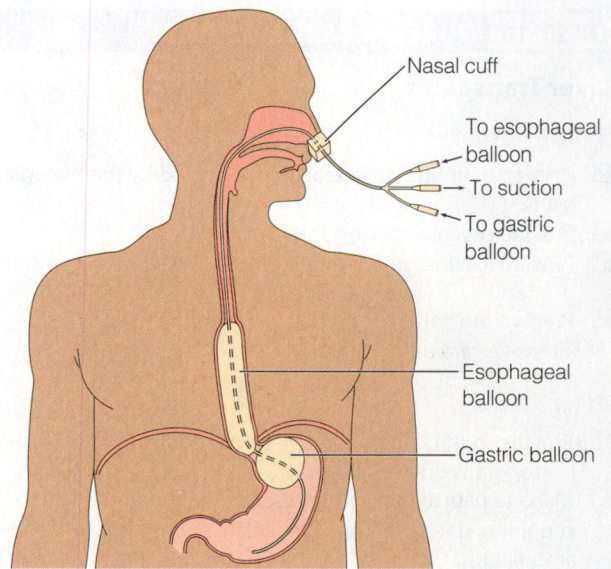

Figure 27-9. ■ A triple-lumen nasogastric (Sengstaken–Blakemore) tube used to control bleeding esophageal varices.

risk factors for cirrhosis such as alcohol use (amount per day or per week), exposure to drugs or toxins, or a history of chronic hepatitis or gallbladder disease.

Note the patient's general appearance, apparent nutritional status, mental status, and level of consciousness. Observe skin and sclera for color, bruising, dryness, or excoriations. Inspect the abdomen for shape and distention. Auscultate bowel sounds and lightly palpate for tenderness. Observe and test any emesis or feces for evidence of blood.

DIAGNOSING, PLANNING, AND IMPLEMENTING
Excess Fluid Volume

Expected outcome: Weight, neck vein distention, and abdominal girth will decrease.

- Weigh daily. Monitor intake and output. *Impaired salt and water regulation caused by cirrhosis can lead to problems such as peripheral edema, ascites, and heart failure. Changes in daily weight are an accurate indicator of fluid balance, as is monitoring intake and output.*
- Assess for neck vein distention and peripheral edema. *Neck vein distention and peripheral edema are indicators of excess fluid.*
- Measure abdominal girth daily. With the patient supine, position the measuring tape around the abdomen at the level of the umbilicus. Mark the skin with indelible marker. *This ensures consistent, accurate measurements about the presence and amount of ascites.*
- Provide a low-sodium diet and restrict fluids as ordered. *Sodium causes water retention, which patients with cirrhosis need to avoid.*

Risk for Acute Confusion

Expected outcome: Will demonstrate logical, organized thought processes.

The priority of care for the patient who is experiencing manifestations of high serum ammonia levels and hepatic encephalopathy is preserving safety and implementing measures to reduce its effects.

- Avoid unnecessary medications that can affect the CNS. *Careful use of medications can help avoid worsening manifestations of encephalopathy.*
- Assess level of consciousness and mental status. Monitor for changes in behavior, handwriting, speech, and development of *asterixis* (a flapping tremor of the hands). Notify the charge nurse or physician of changes. *Accumulated nitrogenous waste products affect the CNS and thinking processes. Early identification of problems allows prompt intervention—subtle changes in neurologic functioning are important.*
- If possible, have the same nurses care for patient. *Consistent care may allow early recognition of neurologic changes.*
- Provide diet as prescribed; teach the family the importance of maintaining diet restrictions. *Nitrogenous by-products from dietary protein increase serum ammonia levels; dietary protein may be limited during acute episodes of hepatic encephalopathy.*
- Administer medications as ordered to prevent gastrointestinal bleeding and reduce gastrointestinal production of nitrogenous waste products. Give laxatives and stool softeners as needed to avoid constipation. *These measures help decrease ammonia production in the bowel and serum ammonia levels.*
- Orient to time, place, and person; provide simple explanations for care at the patient's level of understanding. Maintain a calm environment; minimize external stimuli. *These measures help prevent agitation and anxiety when thinking is impaired.*

Risk for Bleeding

Expected outcome: Vital signs, level of consciousness, urine output, and skin color and temperature will remain within normal ranges.

The patient with esophageal varices is at significant risk for massive hemorrhage and hypovolemic shock.

- Monitor vital signs. *Increased pulse and decreasing blood pressure may indicate hemorrhage.*
- Institute bleeding precautions. (See Box 27-11■ for specific interventions.) *Preventive measures can decrease the incidence of active bleeding.*
- Monitor coagulation studies and platelet count. *The results determine the need to continue bleeding precautions and administer vitamin K as ordered.*

BOX 27-11	BLEEDING PRECAUTIONS

- Prevent constipation.
- Avoid rectal temperatures or enemas.
- Avoid injections; if needed, use small-gauge needle and apply pressure.
- Assess for bruises or purpura (hemorrhage into the skin).
- Apply pressure to bleeding sites.
- Apply direct pressure to venipuncture sites for at least 5 minutes.
- Use only a soft toothbrush.
- Avoid blowing nose.
- Assess oral cavity for bleeding gums.
- Administer H_2-blockers or antacids as ordered to prevent gastrointestinal bleeding.

Risk for Suffocation

Expected outcome: Will maintain effective ventilation as evidenced by respiratory ease and clear breath sounds throughout lung fields.

Patients with a Sengstaken–Blakemore or other multiple-lumen nasogastric tubes (see Figure 27-9) to control bleeding esophageal varices have special care needs. These patients are usually in intensive care units for close monitoring.

- Secure and maintain the original position of the tube. Use soft wrist restraints as needed to prevent the patient from pulling on the tube. Keep a large syringe at the bedside to deflate the balloons should the tube become displaced. *If the tube is dislodged while the esophageal balloon is inflated, the airway can be obstructed.*
- Place in Fowler's position. Suction the oropharynx as needed. *The esophageal balloon impairs the ability to swallow oral secretions. Elevating the head of the bed reduces the risk of aspiration and promotes gas exchange.*
- Monitor and release balloon pressures as ordered. *The gastric balloon helps keep the distal end of the tube in the stomach, preventing the esophageal balloon from obstructing the airway. The inflated balloons place pressure on gastric and esophageal tissues; they may be periodically deflated to reduce the risk of tissue necrosis.*

safetyALERT

Always deflate the esophageal balloon before deflating the gastric balloon.

- Frequently check the nares for tissue damage. Keep the nasal cuff (a small piece of foam) in place. *Pressure sores can develop on the nares through which the tube is inserted.*

Ineffective Breathing Pattern

Expected outcome: Will maintain oxygen saturation levels within expected range without dyspnea.

- Place in high-Fowler's position with feet elevated; assist to chair as tolerated. Avoid supine position when possible. *The sitting position permits full expansion of the lungs and allows gravity to pull fluid and abdominal organs away from the diaphragm.*
- Monitor respirations, lung sounds, and oxygen saturation levels. Report abnormal findings or changes in status. *Continuing respiratory assessments are important to prevent problems from impaired ventilation and oxygenation.*
- Administer oxygen as ordered. *Oxygen therapy may be necessary to prevent hypoxia.*

Impaired Skin Integrity

Expected outcome: Skin and underlying tissues will remain intact.

- Use warm water rather than hot water when bathing. *Hot water can dry the skin further and increase itching.*
- Avoid soap for bathing, apply an emollient or lotion without alcohol to moisten skin, and do not rub the skin. *These measures help prevent dry skin and pruritus.*
- Apply mittens or mitts to hands as needed to prevent scratching. *Patients with encephalopathy may not understand why they should not scratch.*
- Turn at least every 2 hours, use an alternating pressure mattress, and assess skin for breakdown. *Position changes relieve pressure and promote tissue oxygenation.*

MANAGING NURSING CARE

Nursing care activities such as obtaining daily weights and vital signs, measuring and recording intake and output, and assisting the patient with cirrhosis with hygiene and daily living activities are appropriate to assign to assistive personnel.

EVALUATING

To evaluate the effectiveness of nursing care, collect data related to outcomes for the identified nursing diagnoses. For example:

- Are the weight and abdominal girth stable?
- Is behavior and mental status normal for the patient?
- Has the patient remained free of bleeding?
- Is the patient's respiratory status improved?
- Has the skin remained intact?

DOCUMENTING

Document continuing assessment data, including mental status, respiratory effort, abdominal girth, daily weight, and intake and output. Note any diagnostic or therapeutic procedures performed and the patient's response to and recovery from these procedures. Document teaching provided to the patient and family and their apparent understanding and acceptance of information and prescribed care measures (e.g., alcohol avoidance, dietary restrictions).

BOX 27-12	ASSESSMENT

Assessing for Discharge: Cirrhosis

Patient

- Self-care: ability to perform activities of daily living; to prepare and eat the prescribed diet
- Knowledge: understanding of disease and its progression; preventing complications; diet and fluid restrictions; toxins to avoid; when to contact the physician
- Psychosocial: support network and significant others; willingness to abstain from alcohol and other drugs; ability to cope with long-term effects or with liver transplant; evidence of grieving
- Home environment: factors affecting the patient's ability to abstain from alcohol (e.g., roommates, type and location of housing)

Family and Caregivers

- Members of household: ability and willingness to help with food preparation, family responsibilities, and care
- Availability of and referral to home health and social services
- Support groups and Alcoholics Anonymous meetings or other alcohol treatment options

CONTINUITY OF CARE

Community-based and home care for the patient with cirrhosis requires a coordinated team effort that includes the patient, family, the physician, nurses, and social services. Box 27-12■ outlines assessment data to consider in planning for discharge.

Include family members in all teaching, particularly when alcohol abuse and hepatic encephalopathy are considerations. Consistently reinforce teaching; repeat explanations as needed. Reinforce teaching about the prescribed diet and any fluid restrictions. If necessary, refer to a dietitian for diet planning. Provide written and verbal instructions about all medications and when to contact the physician. Teach follow-up care and any home care considerations after procedures such as liver biopsy or TIPS placement. Stress the importance of avoiding all substances toxic to the liver, including alcohol and over-the-counter medications containing acetaminophen. If the patient is in end-stage liver disease, refer for hospice care as appropriate.

NURSING CARE PLAN
Patient With Alcoholic Cirrhosis

Richard Wright is a 48-year-old man who has alcoholic cirrhosis. He is admitted to the hospital with ascites and malnutrition. He has had three previous admissions for cirrhosis, the most recent being 6 months ago.

Assessment

Mr. Wright is lethargic but responds appropriately to verbal stimuli. He complains of "spitting up blood the past week or so" and says, "I just don't feel hungry." He has lost 20 lb (9 kg) since his previous admission. He is jaundiced and has petechiae and ecchymoses on his arms and legs. His admitting nurse notes 3+ pitting edema of his ankles and feet. His abdomen is distended and tight, with distended superficial veins. Vital signs are the following: T 100°F (37.7°C); BP 110/70; P 110; R 24.

Laboratory test results include RBC 4.0 million/mm^3, WBC 3,700/mm^3, platelets 75,000/mm^3; elevated serum ammonia, total bilirubin, and serum sodium levels; low serum potassium, total protein, and albumin levels.

The diagnosis of alcohol-induced cirrhosis with gastritis is made. Mr. Wright is started on spironolactone (Aldactone), magaldrate (Riopan), lactulose, an 800-mg sodium, low-protein diet, and fluid restriction of 1,500 mL/day.

Nursing Diagnosis

The following nursing diagnoses are identified for Mr. Wright:

- *Excess Fluid Volume* related to electrolyte imbalance and low serum albumin
- *Imbalanced Nutrition: Less Than Body Requirements* related to anorexia and possible alcohol abuse
- *Acute Confusion* related to high ammonia levels
- *Risk for Bleeding* related to low platelets and malnutrition

Expected Outcomes

The expected outcomes for the plan of care specify that:

- Abdominal girth will decrease by 1 to 2 cm per day; peripheral edema will decrease to no more than 1+.
- Weight will increase by 1 lb (0.45 kg) per week while losing excess fluid.
- Will be alert and oriented to time, place, and person.
- No further active bleeding will occur.

Planning and Implementation

The following nursing interventions are implemented:

- Weigh daily before breakfast.
- Consult dietitian to plan a low-salt, low-protein, high-calorie diet.
- Frequently assess mental status; promptly report changes.
- Measure abdominal girth every shift.
- Institute bleeding precautions.
- Keep head of bed elevated; assist to chair with legs elevated as tolerated.
- Refer to home health and community agencies for discharge follow-up.

Evaluation

Mr. Wright is discharged after 7 days. His weight has decreased by 4 lb (1.8 kg), but decreased peripheral edema (now 1+) and abdominal girth indicate that this is due to loss of excess fluid. He does not experience any further bleeding. His serum ammonia levels return to normal. Lactulose will be continued on discharge.

Mr. Wright and his teenage children have made contact with Alcoholics Anonymous and Al Anon; they also have appointments to meet with a psychiatric social worker and primary caregiver.

Critical Thinking in the Nursing Process

1. Why was Mr. Wright lethargic on admission? Why does bleeding into the gastrointestinal tract increase serum ammonia levels?
2. Discuss the relationship between portal hypertension, low serum protein levels, and ascites.
3. Outline a 1-day meal plan for Mr. Wright that is low in protein, high in calories, and low in salt.

Note: Discussion of Critical Thinking questions appears on the companion website.

Cancer of the Liver

Primary liver cancer is the eighth leading cause of cancer deaths in the United States (American Cancer Society [ACS], 2013). It affects men three times more often than women. Alcohol-induced cirrhosis and chronic hepatitis B or hepatitis C are the primary risk factors for primary liver cancer in the United States.

Most primary liver cancers arise from the hepatocytes; about 10% develop in the bile duct. Regardless of where the cancer develops, the progress for primary hepatic cancer is poor, in part because the disease is often not diagnosed before it reaches an advanced stage. Metastases to the lungs are common.

Manifestations of liver cancer include malaise, painful mass in the right upper quadrant, epigastric fullness, weight loss, anorexia, and fever. Patients may present with ascites, jaundice, or signs of liver failure. Liver biopsy establishes the diagnosis. Magnetic resonance imaging (MRI), ultrasound, and CT scans can aid in diagnosis, as can tests for serum markers such as alpha-fetoprotein (AFP).

Partial *hepatectomy* (resection and removal of a portion of the liver) is possible when the cancer is limited and has not spread beyond the liver. Liver transplant is a potential option. Radiation therapy is used to shrink the tumor, decreasing pressure on surrounding organs and reducing pain. Chemotherapy may be used as adjunctive treatment for liver cancer.

Preventive nursing care focuses on teaching about the causes of liver cancer and their prevention. Avoiding alcohol, particularly in excess, is also a preventive measure. For the patient with liver cancer, pain control is a priority. Refer patients with inoperable liver cancer to hospice services and cancer support groups.

EXOCRINE PANCREAS DISORDERS

Key Concept Disorders of the exocrine pancreas affect the secretion of digestive enzymes and may affect its endocrine functions as well. Manifestations may be acute and severe, or vague, slowing diagnosis and treatment.

The pancreas is both an exocrine and an endocrine gland. As an exocrine gland, it produces enzymes that empty through ducts into the small intestine. As an endocrine gland, it produces hormones that enter the bloodstream directly.

Pancreatitis

Pancreatitis (inflammation of the pancreas) can be either acute or chronic. *Acute pancreatitis* usually develops in middle life; gallstones and alcoholism are the primary risk factors for acute pancreatitis. Alcoholism is also the primary risk factor for *chronic pancreatitis,* a disease that eventually destroys the pancreas and leads to pancreatic insufficiency. Patients with pancreatitis are often acutely ill, and they may require lifelong treatment.

PATHOPHYSIOLOGY
Acute Pancreatitis

Acute pancreatitis occurs when the pancreas is damaged or its duct to the duodenum is blocked, allowing pancreatic enzymes to accumulate within the pancreas itself (Figure 27-10■). Pancreatic duct obstruction by a gallstone or spasm of the sphincter of Oddi (associated with alcohol use) can obstruct the outflow of pancreatic enzymes. When this happens, a self-destructive process known as *autodigestion* begins.

In the milder form of acute pancreatitis, *interstitial edematous pancreatitis,* the pancreas becomes inflamed and edematous. This process is often self-limiting and patients recover completely.

The more severe form, *necrotizing pancreatitis,* is an acute inflammatory process. Pancreatic tissue bleeds and becomes necrotic, and secondary bacterial infection can lead to abscess formation. Patients with necrotizing pancreatitis may recover completely, have recurrent attacks, or develop chronic pancreatitis.

MANIFESTATIONS AND COMPLICATIONS The onset of acute pancreatitis is often sudden. The patient develops continuous severe epigastric and abdominal pain. This pain commonly radiates to the back and is relieved somewhat by sitting up and leaning forward. The onset of

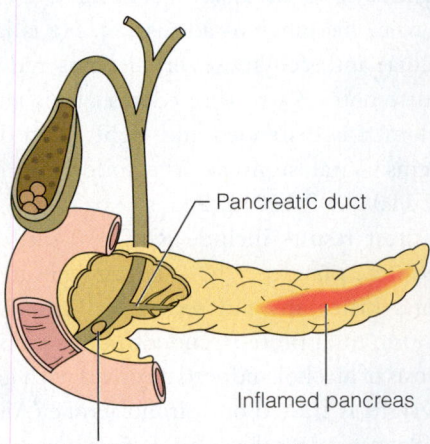

Acute Pancreatitis

- Pancreatic duct
- Inflamed pancreas
- Gallstone blocks pancreatic duct

Figure 27-10. ■ Acute pancreatitis occurs when the pancreatic duct is blocked by a gallstone, preventing pancreatic enzymes from entering the gut.

pain often occurs after a fatty meal or excessive alcohol consumption. Other manifestations are listed in Box 27-13■.

Patients with acute pancreatitis may develop hypovolemic shock due to vasodilation and a fluid shift into the small bowel. Bleeding into the retroperitoneal space may occur, as evidenced by bruising in the flanks (*Turner sign*) or around the umbilicus (*Cullen sign*). A *pancreatic pseudocyst*

BOX 27-13   **MANIFESTATIONS OF PANCREATITIS**

Acute Pancreatitis
- Acute severe epigastric pain; may radiate to back
- Nausea, vomiting
- Abdominal distention, decreased bowel sounds
- Low-grade fever
- Tachycardia, hypotension
- Cool, clammy skin
- Elevated WBC, serum amylase, and lipase
- Low serum calcium and magnesium

Chronic Pancreatitis
- Persistent or recurring episodes of upper abdominal pain radiating to the back
- Anorexia, nausea, vomiting, weight loss
- Flatulence and constipation
- Steatorrhea (fatty, frothy, foul-smelling stools)
- Elevated serum amylase and lipase
- Elevated glucose levels

(a collection of blood, fluid, and pancreatic secretions in the abdominal cavity) may develop. If the pseudocyst ruptures, peritonitis results. *Pancreatic abscess* (a collection of secretions and necrotic products within the pancreas) may be fatal. These complications usually occur 2 to 3 weeks after the onset of pancreatitis.

Chronic Pancreatitis

Chronic pancreatitis, which gradually destroys the pancreas, may follow acute pancreatitis or may have no identified cause. Alcoholism is the primary risk factor for chronic pancreatitis in the United States; worldwide, malnutrition is the major risk factor. In chronic pancreatitis, small ducts of the pancreas are blocked by calcified (stonelike) proteins. This causes an inflammatory process in which normal pancreatic tissue is destroyed and replaced by scar tissue. Chronic pancreatitis is progressive and irreversible. It ultimately leads to pancreatic insufficiency. Without normal pancreatic enzymes, malabsorption of nutrients occurs. If endocrine function of the pancreas is affected, diabetes mellitus develops. The manifestations of chronic pancreatitis are listed in Box 27-13.

Malabsorption, malnutrition, and peptic ulcer disease are the primary complications of chronic pancreatitis. In addition, chronic pancreatitis increases the risk for pancreatic cancer and narcotic addiction (due to frequent episodes of severe pain).

TABLE 27-3	Laboratory Values in Pancreatic Disorders
TEST	**SIGNIFICANCE**

Serum amylase
  Critical value greater than 500 IU/L
Serum lipase
  Critical value greater than 600 IU/L
	Elevated in acute pancreatitis and acute episodes of chronic pancreatitis; may be elevated in pancreatic cancer

Urine amylase	Elevated in acute pancreatitis

Serum calcium
  Critical value less than 6 mg/dL
Serum magnesium
  Critical value less than 1 mg/dL
	Decreased in acute pancreatitis

White blood cells (WBCs)	Elevated in acute pancreatitis
Carcinoembryonic antigen (CEA) Normal value less than 5 ng/mL	Elevated in pancreatic cancer

COLLABORATIVE CARE
Diagnostic Tests

- Laboratory tests may be ordered to confirm the diagnosis of pancreatitis. See Table 27-3■ for changes in laboratory results related to pancreatic dysfunction.
- *Abdominal x-ray* or *abdominal ultrasound* may show inflammatory changes or the presence of gallstones in acute pancreatitis.
- *CT scans* help differentiate acute and chronic pancreatitis.
- *Endoscopic retrograde cholangiopancreatography (ERCP)* is used to diagnose chronic pancreatitis.
- *Percutaneous fine-needle aspiration biopsy* may be done to distinguish between chronic pancreatitis and pancreatic cancer.

Treatment

Treatment of acute pancreatitis focuses on eliminating its causes (e.g., gallstones or alcohol abuse), minimizing additional damage to the pancreas by reducing pancreatic secretions, relieving pain, and preventing complications. The patient is initially given nothing by mouth. A nasogastric tube may be inserted and connected to suction, and intravenous fluid therapy or TPN is initiated. Enteral nutrition with a nasogastric or nasojejunal feeding tube may be instituted to reduce the risk of TPN-associated complications. These measures decrease pancreatic enzyme production while maintaining hydration and nutrition. Oral food and fluids are resumed when serum amylase levels return to normal, bowel sounds are present, and pain has disappeared. Intake begins with clear liquids and progresses to a low-fat diet as tolerated.

Parenteral narcotic analgesics may be required for pain relief. Endoscopic exploration of the pancreatic and common bile duct to remove obstruction may be performed when pancreatitis is severe and the patient is critically ill. Once the acute episode resolves, a laparoscopic cholecystectomy is done to reduce the risk of future episodes.

Treatment for chronic pancreatitis includes pain management, nutritional support, and replacement of deficient enzymes and hormones. Narcotic analgesics are avoided if possible, because the risk of addiction is high. Octreotide (Sandostatin) is a synthetic hormone that suppresses pancreatic enzyme secretion. It may be used to relieve the pain of chronic pancreatitis. Alcohol is forbidden; it may precipitate an attack. Pancreatic enzyme supplements (Table 27-4■) are given to manage *steatorrhea* (fat in stools).

Omeprazole (Prilosec), ranitidine (Zantac), or a similar drug is prescribed to reduce gastric acidity (which stimulates pancreatic enzyme production). Diabetes resulting from chronic pancreatitis is treated (see Chapter 36). Surgery may be performed to drain pseudocysts or dilate an obstructed duct.

TABLE 27-4	Giving Medications Safely: Chronic Pancreatitis		
CLASS/DRUGS	**PURPOSE**	**NURSING IMPLICATIONS**	**PATIENT TEACHING**
Pancreatic enzyme replacement			
■ Pancrelipase (Ku-Zyme, Pancrease, Ultrase, Viokase)	Pancrelipase promotes starch and fat digestion by replacing the pancreatic enzymes protease, amylase, and lipase. It improves nutrition and decreases the number of bowel movements.	Monitor frequency and consistency of stools. Weigh every other day. Record weights. Administer with meals. Monitor for side effects: rash, hives, respiratory difficulty, hematuria, gout, or joint pain.	Take the drug with meals or snacks. If medicine is enteric coated, do not crush, chew, or mix with foods such as milk or ice cream. Be sure to follow prescribed diet.

NURSING CARE

PRIORITIZING NURSING CARE

Relieving the acute, severe pain often associated with acute or chronic pancreatitis is the priority for nursing care.

HEALTH PROMOTION

Treating or eliminating risk factors for pancreatitis are the primary preventive measures for this disorder. Advise alcohol abstinence, and refer patients who abuse alcohol to a treatment program or Alcoholics Anonymous. Encourage patients with a known history of gallstones to seek treatment promptly should symptoms of acute pancreatitis develop.

ASSESSING

Assessment data focus on identifying the onset of symptoms and risk factors for pancreatitis. Ask the patient to describe the pain: its onset, intensity using a standardized pain scale, character (steady, boring, stabbing, radiating), duration, relieving and aggravating factors, and any associated symptoms, such as sweating, nausea, or vomiting. Also ask about any history of previous attacks or a history of gallbladder disease. Inquire about alcohol use (number of drinks per day or per week, most recent alcohol consumption). Ask about food intake for the day before the onset of the pain.

Observe for nonverbal cues of pain: restlessness or rigid stillness; tense facial features; clenched fists; rapid, shallow breathing; tachycardia; diaphoresis. Listen for bowel sounds and gently palpate the abdomen for tenderness. Report assessment data to the charge nurse or physician.

DIAGNOSING, PLANNING, AND IMPLEMENTING
Acute Pain

Expected outcome: Will report pain at a level of 2 or lower on a scale of 0 to 10.

■ Administer ordered narcotic analgesics on a regular schedule or teach the patient to use patient-controlled analgesia (PCA). Assess the effectiveness of analgesia. *Severe, established pain is difficult to control. Unrelieved pain may increase secretion of pancreatic enzymes.*

■ Maintain nothing by mouth (NPO) status and nasogastric tube patency as ordered. *Gastric secretions stimulate pancreatic secretion, aggravating pain. Withholding food and maintaining nasogastric suction reduce gastric secretions and help relieve nausea and vomiting.*

■ Maintain patient on bed rest in a calm, quiet environment. *Reducing physical movement and mental stimulation decreases metabolic rate, gastrointestinal secretion, and resulting pain.*

■ Provide comfort measures:
  ■ Provide oral and nasal care every 1 to 2 hours.
  ■ Assist to a comfortable position, such as side-lying with knees flexed and head elevated 45 degrees.
  ■ Encourage relaxation techniques and guided imagery to decrease pain.
  ■ Explain all procedures and care; listen carefully to concerns and evaluation of pain relief.

The patient who is NPO needs frequent mouth care for comfort. Inflammation and stretching of the peritoneum cause pain. Sitting up, leaning forward, or lying in a fetal position tends to decrease the pain. Alternative pain relief measures help reduce anxiety and help the patient gain a sense of control.

■ Ask the family and visitors to avoid bringing food into the patient's room. *The sight of food may stimulate pancreatic secretions.*

Risk for Imbalanced Nutrition: Less Than Body Requirements

Expected outcome: Weight will remain stable within expected parameters.

■ Weigh daily at the same time. *Decreasing weight may indicate poor nutritional status.*

■ Maintain stool chart; include frequency, color, odor, and consistency of stools. *Pancreatitis affects fat absorption, so undigested fats are excreted in the stool. Steatorrhea may indicate an increase in the severity of pancreatitis.*

- Regularly assess bowel sounds. *Nasogastric suction usually is discontinued within 24 to 48 hours after the return of bowel sounds, which indicates that the patient is regaining bowel motility.*
- Administer intravenous fluids and TPN or enteral nutrition as prescribed. *Inflammation increases metabolism and nutritional needs. TPN may be ordered to maintain nutritional status while the patient is NPO.*
- When eating resumes, provide small, frequent feedings and a high-carbohydrate, low-protein, low-fat diet. Avoid caffeine (coffee, tea, colas), spicy foods, or gas-producing foods. *Small, frequent feedings are better tolerated. A low-protein, low-fat diet minimizes pancreatic enzyme secretion, reducing inflammation and pain. Caffeine and spicy or gas-producing foods may increase pancreatic secretion and pain.*

Risk for Injury

Expected outcome: Vital signs, oxygen saturation, urine output, and mental status will be stable.

- Assess vital signs (including orthostatic blood pressures), peripheral pulses, skin color, temperature, and turgor every 1 to 2 hours until stable and then every 4 hours. Record data and report abnormal findings to the charge nurse or physician. *Frequent assessment of cardiovascular and fluid volume status is important because fluid losses associated with vomiting, diaphoresis, third-space shifts, and nasogastric suction can affect cardiac output and tissue perfusion.*
- Monitor respiratory status including breath sounds. Encourage to cough and deep breathe hourly. *Abdominal pain causes shallow respirations and impaired ventilation, increasing the risk of atelectasis or pneumonia. Coughing and deep breathing improve ventilation and mobilize secretions.*
- Measure urine output hourly; maintain accurate intake and output. Report output of less than 30 mL/hr to the charge nurse or physician. *A drop in urine output may be an early indication of decreased cardiac output, which increases the risk of acute kidney injury.*
- Frequently assess mental status, level of consciousness, and behavior. *Impaired mental status may indicate poor cerebral oxygenation, alcohol withdrawal, or other complications of acute pancreatitis.*

MANAGING NURSING CARE

Nursing care activities such as obtaining vital signs and daily weights, measuring and recording I&O and fecal output, and providing assistance with mouth care, hygiene, and positioning for the patient with pancreatitis are appropriate to assign to assistive personnel.

EVALUATING

When evaluating the effectiveness of nursing care for a patient with acute pancreatitis, collect data such as pain level, weight, ability to resume eating, and stability of cardiovascular and respiratory status.

DOCUMENTING

Document continuing assessment data and measures employed to relieve pain and their effects. Also document patient and family teaching about the disorder and their apparent understanding of teaching.

CONTINUITY OF CARE

When appropriate, teach the patient and family members about the disease and how to prevent further attacks. Discuss specific risk factors and needs, such as the following:

- Alcohol abstinence is vital to prevent future attacks of acute or chronic pancreatitis. (Refer as needed to community agencies, support groups such as Alcoholics Anonymous, or individual counseling.)
- Smoking and stress stimulate the pancreas and should be avoided.
- Possible treatment for gallstones if appropriate, including options such as laparoscopic cholecystectomy.
- Instruct to take pancreatic enzymes and insulin as ordered. Refer to a diabetes educator as appropriate.
- Advise to maintain a low-fat diet and avoid crash dieting or binge eating, which can bring on attacks. Discuss foods to avoid, such as spicy foods, caffeinated beverages, and gas-forming foods. Refer to a dietitian or nutritionist as needed for diet planning and teaching.
- Instruct to report signs of infection promptly (a fever of 102°F [38.8°C] or higher, pain, rapid pulse, malaise) to the physician. An abscess may form months after the initial attack, necessitating further intervention.
- Refer to a community or home health agency as needed for home care.

Cancer of the Pancreas

Although cancer of the pancreas is not common, its incidence is increasing in the United States and is now among the 10 most frequently diagnosed cancers. Pancreatic cancer is the fourth leading cause of cancer deaths in the United States (ACS, 2013). Older adults, African Americans, and men have a greater risk of developing pancreatic cancer. Smoking is a major risk factor for pancreatic cancer. Its incidence is twice as high in smokers as in nonsmokers. The prognosis for pancreatic cancer is poor: Less than 6% of people diagnosed with pancreatic cancer survive five years. Even when the disease is diagnosed at an early stage, median survival is 24 months.

Early manifestations of pancreatic cancer include anorexia, nausea, weight loss, flatulence, and dull epigastric pain. The pain increases in severity as the tumor grows. Cancer of the head of the pancreas, the most common site, often obstructs bile flow through the common bile duct, causing jaundice, clay-colored stools, dark urine, and pruritus (itching). Late manifestations include a palpable abdominal mass and ascites.

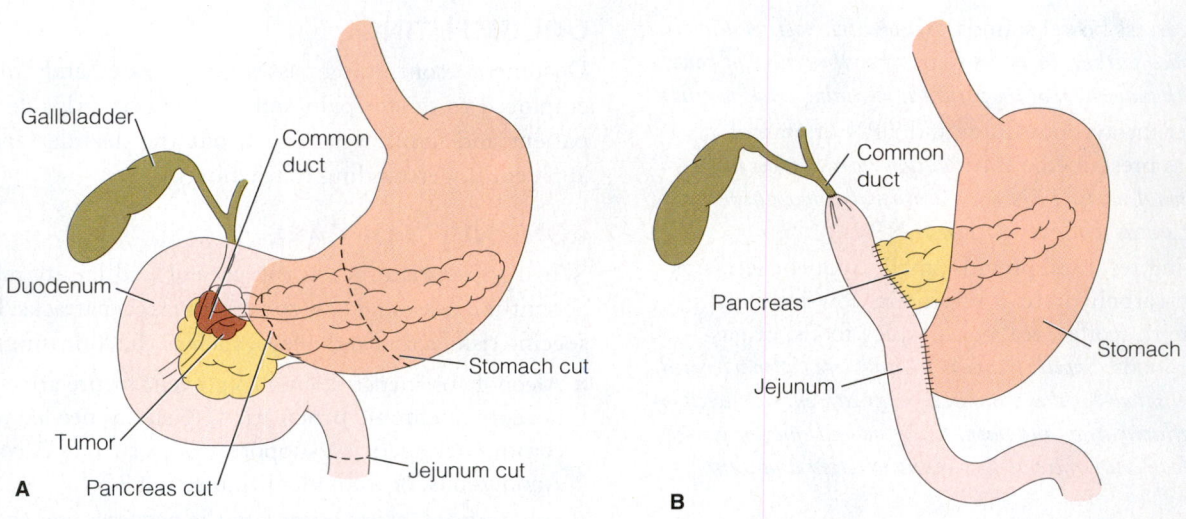

Figure 27-11. ■ Whipple procedure. (**A**) Areas that are removed. (**B**) Anastomosis of the stomach and pancreas to the jejunum.

With early diagnosis, surgery provides the best chance of cure. If the head of the pancreas is affected, a pancreatoduodenectomy (*Whipple procedure*) is done to remove the head of the pancreas, the duodenum, the distal third of the stomach, a portion of the jejunum, and part of the common bile duct. The common bile duct is then sutured to the end of the jejunum, and the remaining pancreas and stomach are sutured to the side of the jejunum (Figure 27-11 ■). Alternately, a distal pancreatectomy (removal of the body and tail of the pancreas and the spleen) or a total pancreatectomy (removal of the pancreas, part of the stomach and small intestine, the gall bladder and bile duct, the spleen and nearby lymph nodes) may be performed. Radiation and chemotherapy are often used in addition to surgery.

Postoperative nursing care of the patient undergoing Whipple procedure is similar to that of the patient undergoing intestinal surgery (see Chapter 26). The patient with pancreatic cancer has multiple problems that require nursing care. (Chapter 12 discusses nursing care for patients with cancer.) The nursing diagnoses and interventions discussed for the patient with pancreatitis are also appropriate for the patient with pancreatic cancer.

Note: The references and resources for all chapters have been compiled at the back of the book.

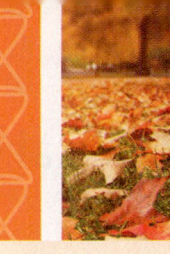

Chapter Review

KEY POINTS

- **Concept:** The gallbladder, liver, and exocrine pancreas are important for the digestion, absorption, and metabolism of food. Disorders of these organs have multiple effects on food intake and nutrient usage.
- **Concept:** Gallstones can obstruct the flow of bile from the liver into the gut, causing inflammation and pain. Accurate diagnosis and appropriate treatment are necessary to preserve physiologic function and promote comfort.
- The nursing role in caring for patients with gallstones usually involves providing pre- and postoperative care for patients undergoing cholecystectomy. Most patients recover uneventfully.
- **Concept:** The liver is constantly exposed to blood that may contain pathogens, toxins, and malignant cells, making it vulnerable to inflammation, damage, and tumors. Because the liver has many essential functions, liver disorders affect all other body systems.
- Alcohol abuse is a significant risk factor for liver and pancreatic disorders. Prevention, early identification, and treatment of alcohol abuse reduce the risk of these disorders.
- **Concept:** Hepatitis is usually an acute viral disease that primarily affects the liver. Preventing the spread of hepatitis is an important nursing and public health responsibility.
- Hepatitis B and C can lead to a carrier state in which the infected patient has no symptoms of the disease but can spread it to others.
- Hepatitis B and C can also become chronic and ultimately lead to cirrhosis and liver failure.

- **Concept:** Cirrhosis is a chronic liver disease that affects its metabolic, detoxification, and other functions. Blood flow through the liver is impaired, leading to portal hypertension. Patient care focuses on preserving function and preventing complications.
- Cirrhosis destroys the structure and function of liver lobules. Its complications, including portal hypertension, ascites, esophageal varices, and hepatic encephalopathy, affect multiple body systems.
- Bleeding from esophageal varices may be massive and requires prompt control to maintain cardiac output.
- Liver transplant is the only definitive treatment for cirrhosis.
- **Concept:** Disorders of the exocrine pancreas affect the secretion of digestive enzymes and may affect its endocrine functions as well. Manifestations may be acute and severe, or vague, slowing diagnosis and treatment.
- Acute pancreatitis often develops as a complication of gallstones, whereas chronic pancreatitis is more frequently related to alcohol abuse. Although acute pancreatitis often resolves without long-term effects, patients with chronic pancreatitis may require nutritional support and supplemental pancreatic enzymes and hormones to manage its effects.
- The gallbladder, liver, and pancreas can be primary or secondary cancer sites. Pancreatic cancer frequently is fatal because symptoms are often absent or vague until the tumor is advanced. When tumors are identified early, surgery is the treatment of choice for these cancers.

PEARSON NURSING STUDENT RESOURCES

Find additional materials at **nursing.pearsonhighered.com**.

Clinical Reasoning Care Map

Caring for a Patient With Pancreatitis
NCLEX-PN® Focus Area: Physiologic Adaptation

Case Study: Rose Schliefer, 59 years old, is home after a 2-month hospitalization for acute pancreatitis. The pancreatitis was caused by gallstones. Mrs. Schliefer spent 3 weeks in intensive care and underwent surgery for the gallstones and to drain a pseudocyst. At discharge she was on a soft, low-protein, low-fat diet and was able to walk in the hall. She has been referred for home health services.

Nursing Diagnosis: Imbalanced Nutrition: Less Than Body Requirements

COLLECT DATA

Subjective	Objective
_____	_____
_____	_____
_____	_____
_____	_____
_____	_____
_____	_____
_____	_____

Does this present a threat to the patient's safety?

If yes, the priority intervention to address this threat would be:

_____

Nursing Care

_____
_____
_____
_____
_____
_____
_____

Interprofessional team members to include when planning care:

_____

How would you document this? _____

_____

Compare your answers and documentation to those provided on the companion website.

Data Collected
(use only those that apply)

- Thin; appears anxious and tired
- States she lost 30 lb (13.6 kg) in the hospital
- Weight 102 lb (46 kg), height 66 in. (168 cm)
- Vital signs within normal limits
- Well-healed upper abdominal scar and two stab wounds on sides of abdomen noted; scabs present on stab wounds
- Skin cool and dry, poor turgor
- Alert and oriented, responds appropriately
- Blood glucose 80 mg/dL
- States main problems are lack of energy and lack of appetite
- Family expresses concern about ability to provide care

Nursing Interventions
(use only those that apply; list in priority order)

- Explain causes of fatigue.
- Help Mrs. Schliefer develop activity goals and identify steps to achieve goals.
- Plan daily rest periods, especially before meals.
- Discuss dietary restrictions and how to adapt to usual diet.
- Assist family to plan six small meals a day.
- Obtain a shower chair.
- Assist family to identify and divide responsibilities for care.
- Encourage patient to identify strengths and concerns.

NCLEX-PN® Exam Preparation

1 A patient diagnosed with cholelithiasis requests medication for pain relief. Which of the following medications is the physician most likely to prescribe?
1. Acetaminophen (Tylenol)
2. Morphine sulfate
3. Codeine
4. Ibuprofen (Motrin)

2 A patient returns to his room after an open cholecystectomy. He has a T-tube in place attached to a drainage bag. The nurse would report which of the following assessments to the charge nurse or physician?
1. There is less than 50 mL output from the T-tube each 8-hour shift.
2. Patient experiences nausea and vomiting 30 minutes after eating.
3. T-tube drainage decreases after 24 hours.
4. Patient requires pain medication every 4 to 6 hours.

3 A patient will manage her cholelithiasis at home using medical interventions. The nurse reinforces which of the following in discharge teaching?
1. Sleep in prone position to decrease pain.
2. Report episodes of pain that occur before meals.
3. Use a heating pad for pain relief.
4. Adhere to a low-fat, low-calorie diet.

4 A patient who was diagnosed with hepatitis A states he was told by the nursing assistant that his disease could be transmitted only through blood contact. The appropriate action by the nurse would be to:
1. provide the correct information to the patient and nursing assistant.
2. take no further action because the information is correct.
3. remove all precautions because hepatitis A cannot be transmitted.
4. place a sign on the patient's door stating "Blood Precautions."

5 A patient is diagnosed with hepatitis B. Which of the following information, if obtained during the admission assessment, would indicate a risk factor?
1. She ate in a restaurant 2 weeks ago.
2. She uses barrier protection during sexual intercourse.
3. She is an intravenous drug user.
4. She has never received a blood transfusion.

6 A patient with cirrhosis is scheduled for discharge. The LPN/LVN recognizes the need for further teaching if the patient states:
1. "I will use a soft toothbrush for oral hygiene."
2. "I will follow the prescribed diet."
3. "I will report increased difficulty breathing to my physician."
4. "I will limit alcohol intake to two servings per day."

7 The nurse evaluates a 54-year-old patient with cirrhosis for improvement in her ascites. Which of the following assessment findings may indicate improvement? **Select all that apply.**
1. Weight loss of 3 lb in the past 72 hours
2. Abdominal girth 2 cm less than previous measurement
3. Urinary output 30 mL/hr
4. Tea-colored urine
5. Complaints of increasing shortness of breath

8 A 45-year-old patient with liver disease is prescribed lactulose (Chronulac) 30 mL every 6 hours. Recognizing the action of this medication in the treatment of liver disease, the nurse would expect to assess which positive response to the medication?
1. Increased urine output
2. Reduced serum ammonia levels
3. Reduced steatorrhea
4. Increased serum potassium levels

9 A patient is admitted to the nursing unit with a diagnosis of acute pancreatitis. The patient complains of severe pain. Place the following nursing activities to promote patient comfort in the order in which the nurse would do them.
1. Insert the ordered nasogastric tube and connect to low intermittent suction.
2. Administer prescribed parenteral narcotic analgesic.
3. Place an NPO sign over the patient's bed and notify dietary services.
4. Place in a side-lying position with knees flexed and elevate the head of the bed 45 degrees.
5. Promote rest by darkening the room and placing a sign on the door to limit visitors.

10 The nurse is caring for a patient with acute pancreatitis. Which nursing assessment should receive the highest priority?
1. Assess intake and output.
2. Assess cardiovascular status and fluid volume status.
3. Assess bowel sounds and fecal output.
4. Assess mental status.

Answers and rationales for Review Questions appear in Appendix I.

Thinking Strategically About . . .

You are an LPN/LVN working in a medium-sized hospital emergency room. You work closely with an RN to provide care for several patients at a time.

Jamie, a 19-year-old college student, presents at the emergency department complaining of general lower abdominal pain that started the previous evening. The pain has localized to the right lower quadrant and became severe about 6 hours ago. She reports anorexia for the past 2 days. She complains of nausea and has vomited twice today. Jamie's vital signs are T 102.6°F (39.2°C); P 96; R 24; BP 110/70. Her abdomen is flat, with marked tenderness in the right lower quadrant. Guarding is present throughout her abdomen. Her WBC is 15,400/mm3. A diagnosis of acute appendicitis with possible perforation is made.

Nguyen, a 29-year-old, comes to the emergency department complaining of mild right upper quadrant abdominal pain, nausea, and muscle and joint pain. Although her natural skin tones are indicative of her Asian heritage, her sclera have become icteric over the past 24 hours. Nguyen was born and raised in the United States but returned from visiting her extended family in rural Laos 3 weeks ago. The doctor suspects hepatitis A. Her vital signs are T 98.6°F (37°C); P 88; R 22; BP 118/78. Her abdomen is flat, soft, with marked tenderness in the right upper quadrant.

Robert, a 55-year-old auto mechanic, comes to the emergency department with rectal bleeding. He has been experiencing constipation off and on for the past 3 months. Occasionally the stool has been very dark brown to black. This morning he had several drops of bright red blood in the toilet and on the toilet paper. He states he feels some pressure in the rectum. Robert's vital signs are stable with a slightly elevated pulse of 94 and a blood pressure of 132/62. He is overweight. His abdomen is rotund, soft without pain or tenderness.

CRITICAL THINKING

- How does Jamie's WBC compare with a normal WBC? What is the reason for blood value?

- If Nguyen has hepatitis A, what are possible sources of the infection?

- The nurse should anticipate the patient's diagnosis to prepare for medical and nursing care. What are some possible causes of Robert's rectal bleeding?

PRIORITIES IN NURSING CARE

- If these three patients come to the emergency department at the same time, in what order should they be seen? Why?

MANAGEMENT OF CARE

- What nursing care is indicated when a patient presents with an acute abdomen?

- What are the similarities in care of these three patients?

- What are the differences in care of these three patients?

DELEGATING

- What aspects of the care of these patients could be delegated to you as the LPN/LVN?

PATIENT TEACHING

- What preoperative teaching should be included in Jamie's care?

- If Nguyen has hepatitis A, what teaching must be done before she is discharged?

- Write the instructions you would give Robert regarding collecting a stool specimen for occult blood at home.

CULTURAL CARE STRATEGIES

- Do you anticipate cultural issues in caring for Nguyen?

DOCUMENTING AND REPORTING

- For each patient, what data would the LPN/LVN report to the RN?

- Write a focus note describing Robert's rectal bleeding.

Note: Discussion of Unit questions appears on the companion website.

UNIT VII
Disrupted Urinary Function

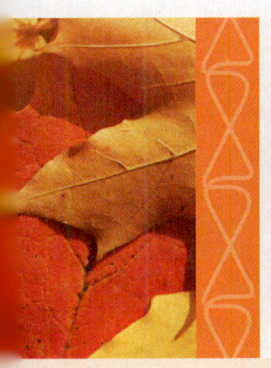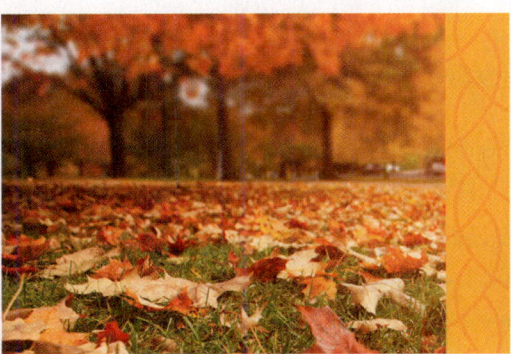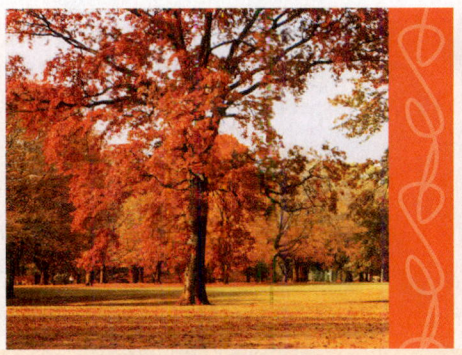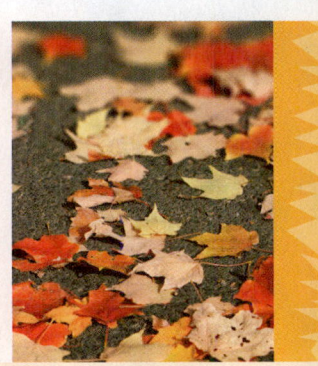

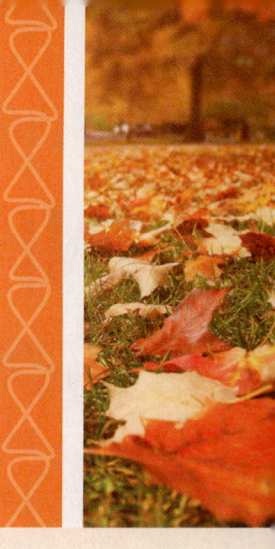

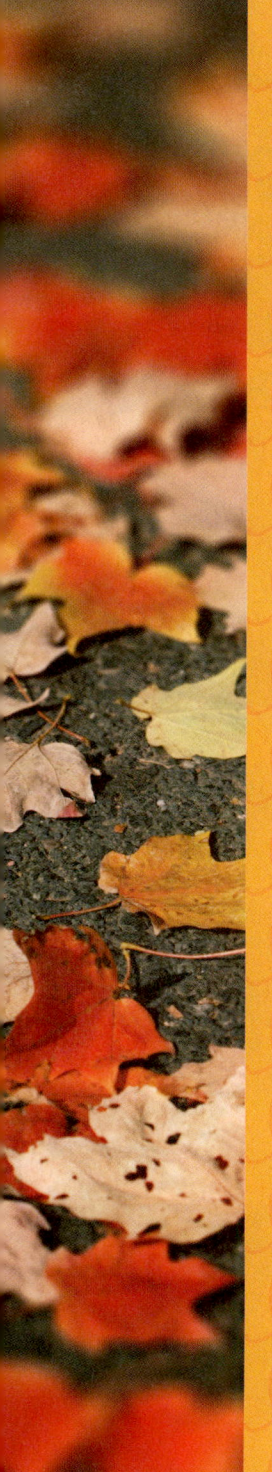

CHAPTER 28

The Urinary System and Assessment

BRIEF OUTLINE

Structure and Function of the Urinary System
Assessment

APPLIED LEARNING OUTCOMES

After completing this chapter, you will be able to:

1. Identify and describe the structures and functions of the renal and urinary system.
2. Collect subjective information and physical assessment data related to the urinary system and kidney function.
3. Provide appropriate nursing care for patients undergoing diagnostic tests to identify disorders of the urinary system or kidneys.

KEY TERMS

The key terms are defined on the pages listed below.

The urinary system plays a vital role in eliminating wastes and regulating fluid and electrolyte balance in the body. Changes in its structure or function can affect the entire body; likewise, it is affected by other body systems, particularly the cardiovascular and endocrine systems.

Structure and Function of the Urinary System

Key Concept The urinary system, including the kidneys, ureters, urinary bladder, and urethra, eliminates waste and plays a critical role in maintaining homeostasis (balance) of the body.

The urinary system includes the paired kidneys and ureters, the urinary bladder, and the urethra (Figure 28-1 ■). The urinary system is important in maintaining and regulating the body's internal environment. It excretes metabolic wastes and excretes or conserves water and solutes, as needed. The kidneys help regulate acid–base balance and blood pressure, and they secrete a hormone important for red blood cell production. Because these are vital functions, any disorder of the urinary system can affect the entire body.

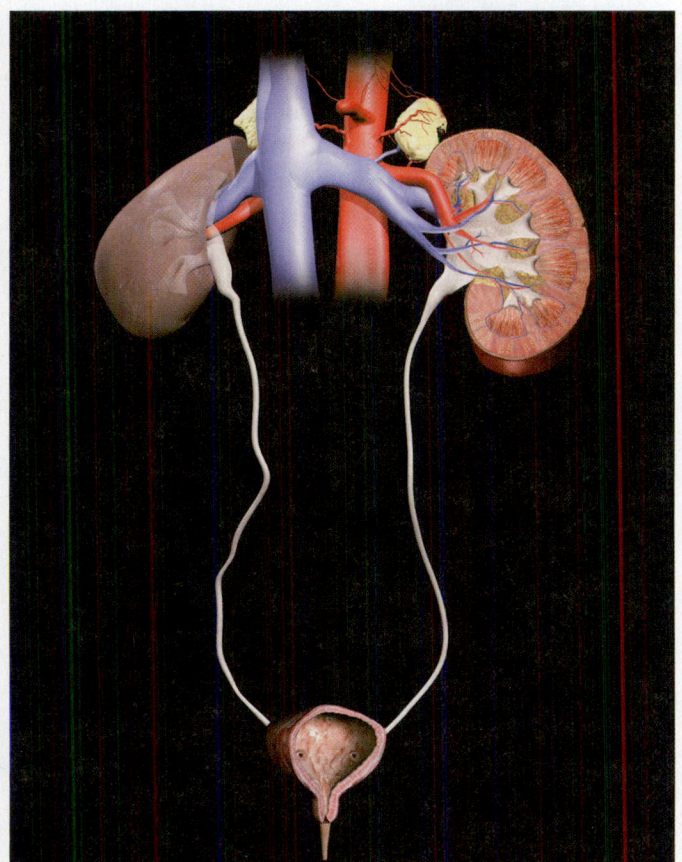

Figure 28-1. ■ The kidneys, ureters, and bladder. (Source: Dorling Kindersley Media Library.)

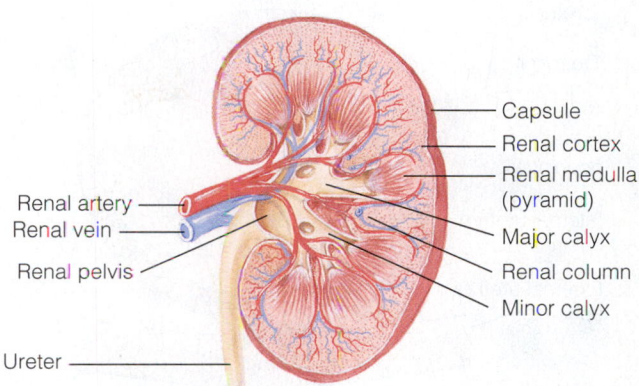

Figure 28-2. ■ An illustration of the internal structures of the kidney.

KIDNEYS

The two kidneys sit behind the peritoneum (in the *retroperitoneal* space) on either side of the spine. They are partially protected by the rib cage. These highly vascular, bean-shaped organs are about the size of a closed fist. On the inner (*concave*) surface of each kidney is a notch known as the *hilum,* where the ureter, renal artery, renal vein, lymphatic vessels, and nerves enter or exit. The *renal fascia,* a layer of dense connective tissue, protects and anchors the kidney.

Each kidney has three distinct regions: the cortex, medulla, and pelvis (Figure 28-2 ■). The outer region, or *renal cortex,* contains the **glomeruli**, small clusters of capillaries. The glomeruli are part of the **nephrons**, the functional units of the kidney (see Figure 28-4). Each kidney contains approximately 1 million nephrons, which process the blood to make urine.

In the *renal medulla,* or inner portion of the kidney, nephrons form the *renal pyramids.* These pyramids channel urine into branches of the innermost region, the *renal pelvis.* These branches are known as *calyces* (singular, *calyx*). Urine is channeled from the pelvis through the ureter and into the bladder for storage.

URETERS

The *ureters* are bilateral tubes about 10 to 12 in. (25 to 30 cm) long. They move urine from the kidney to the bladder by peristaltic waves. The ureters contain smooth muscle and are innervated by the autonomic nervous system.

URINARY BLADDER

The urinary bladder is a hollow, muscular organ that lies behind the symphysis pubis. The ureters enter the bladder at its base, an area known as the *trigone* (Figure 28-3 ■). The urethral opening is at the third point of this triangular region. Bladder muscle tone in this area prevents a backflow of urine from the bladder into the ureters.

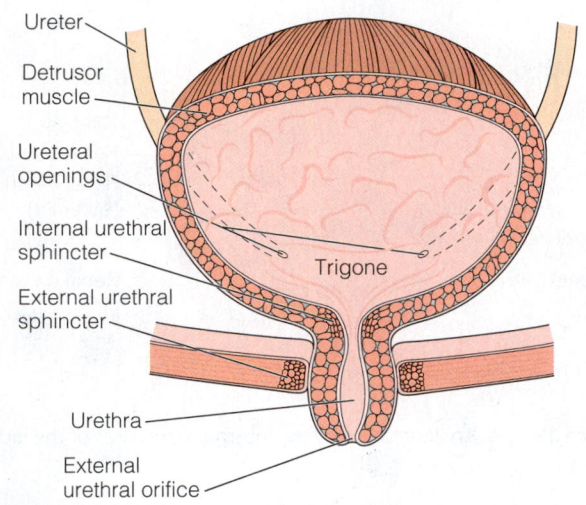

Ureter
Detrusor muscle
Ureteral openings
Internal urethral sphincter
Trigone
External urethral sphincter
Urethra
External urethral orifice

Figure 28-3. ■ Anatomy of the urinary bladder.

The bladder is lined with epithelial mucosa. The muscle (*detrusor muscle*) is arranged in layers that allow the bladder to expand or contract. Healthy adults usually feel the urge to void when the bladder contains 300 to 500 mL of urine. However, the bladder can hold more than twice that amount if necessary. The *internal urethral sphincter* relaxes in response to a full bladder, signaling the need to urinate. A second *external urethral sphincter* formed by skeletal muscle is under voluntary control.

URETHRA

The *urethra* is a thin-walled muscular tube that channels urine out of the body. It extends from the base of the bladder to the *urinary meatus (opening)*. In females, the urethra is approximately 1.5 in. (4 cm) long; the urinary meatus is anterior to the vagina. In males, the urethra is about 8 in. (20 cm) long; it serves as a channel for semen as well as urine. The prostate gland encircles the urethra at the base of the bladder in males. The male urinary meatus is at the end of the glans penis.

URINE FORMATION

The kidneys process about 180 L (47 gallons) of filtrate each day. Of this, only 1% is excreted as urine; the rest is returned to the circulation. Urine is formed by the processes of glomerular filtration, tubular reabsorption, and tubular secretion (Figure 28-4■).

Glomerular Filtration

Glomerular filtration is a passive process in which fluid and solutes move from the blood in the glomerulus into the glomerular capsule (Bowman's capsule). The amount of fluid filtered from the blood into the capsule per minute is called the **glomerular filtration rate** (GFR). Normal GFR in adults is 120 to 125 mL/min. Blood pressure and

volume are the primary factors controlling GFR. A drop in blood pressure or blood volume causes the GFR and urine output to fall.

The GFR is regulated by a number of mechanisms. Afferent (incoming) arterioles constrict or dilate in response to blood pressure changes. Specialized cells in the afferent arteriole and distal convoluted tubule (the *juxtaglomerular apparatus*) respond to changes in blood flow by releasing renin, an enzyme that affects systemic blood pressure. Glomerular filtration is also affected by the sympathetic nervous system.

Tubular Reabsorption

Tubular reabsorption begins as the filtrate enters the proximal tubules. In healthy kidneys, virtually all organic nutrients such as glucose and amino acids are reabsorbed. Water and electrolyte reabsorption is continuously regulated and adjusted to maintain homeostasis. Reabsorption occurs by both active and passive mechanisms.

Tubular Secretion

Through the process of *tubular secretion,* excess potassium and waste products such as hydrogen ion (H^+), creatinine, and ammonia are eliminated from the body. Both passive and active mechanisms work to eliminate waste products and regulate acid–base balance.

Urine Concentration

In the loop of Henle, urine is concentrated, and further wastes are excreted through reabsorption and secretion. In the distal tubule, antidiuretic hormone (ADH) determines the final dilution or concentration of urine. When ADH is secreted, water is reabsorbed in the distal convoluted tubule and collecting duct, and urine is more concentrated. When ADH is not secreted, water cannot be reabsorbed, and urine is more dilute.

Urine is about 95% water and 5% solutes. Solutes normally excreted in the urine include urea, sodium, potassium, phosphate, sulfate, creatinine, uric acid, calcium, magnesium, and bicarbonate. The characteristics of normal urine are listed in Table 28-1■.

ENDOCRINE FUNCTION OF THE KIDNEYS

Besides producing urine, the kidneys produce renin and erythropoietin, and they activate vitamin D. The enzyme *renin,* produced by the juxtaglomerular apparatus, converts the plasma protein angiotensinogen to angiotensin I. Angiotensin I is converted in the lungs to angiotensin II. Angiotensin II is a potent vasoconstrictor that raises blood pressure. It also stimulates the adrenal glands to release aldosterone, which promotes sodium and water retention. The net effect of the *renin–angiotensin–aldosterone* system is to raise the blood pressure and blood volume.

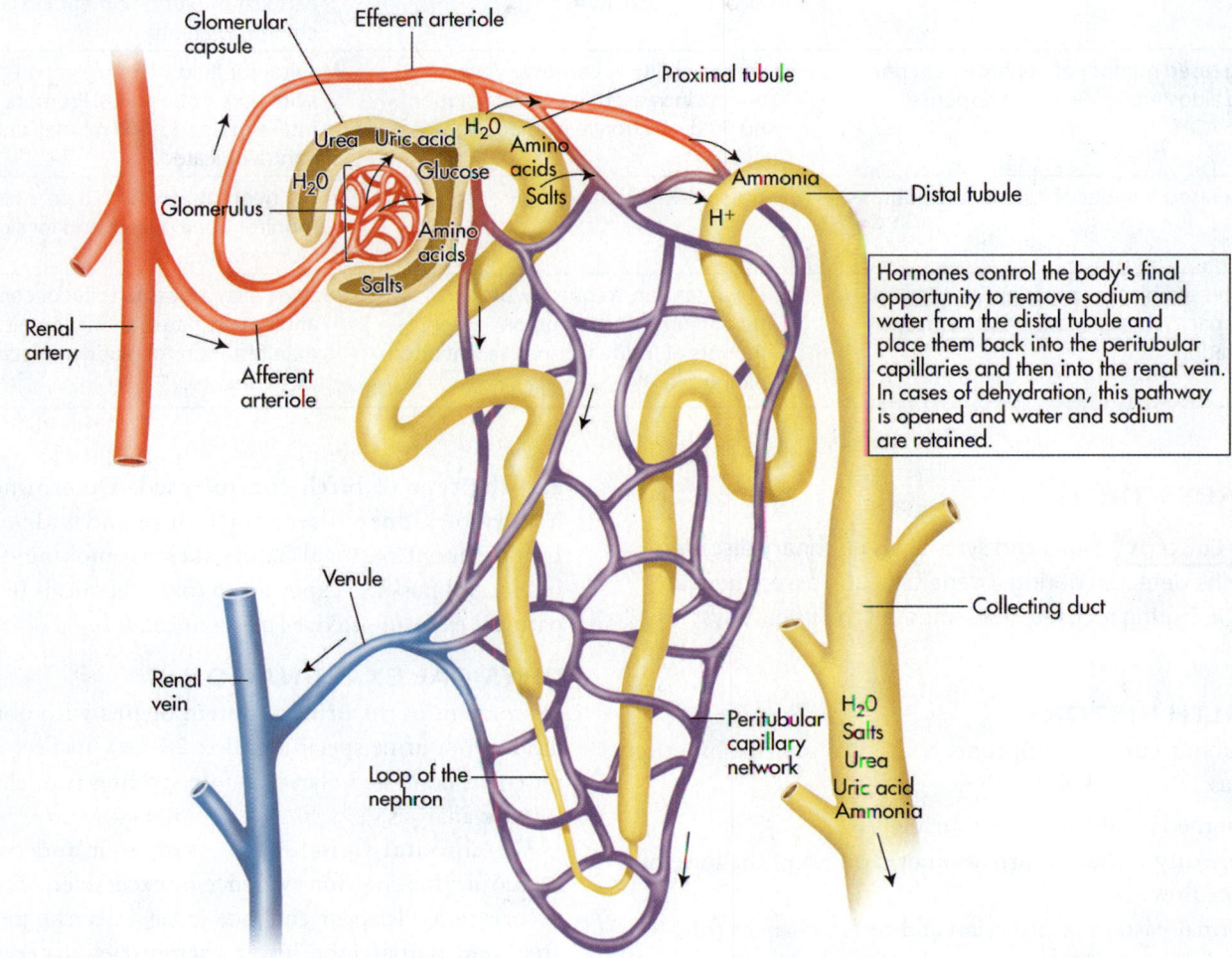

Glomerular Filtration

Blood from the renal artery is filtered in the glomerulus. The filtered product which contains water, salts, nutrients, and waste products is called the glomerular filtrate.

Tubular Reabsorption

Nutrients and salts are actively reabsorbed and transported to the peritubular capillary network and some water is passively reabsorbed into the peritubular capillaries.

Tubular Secretion

Some substances are actively secreted from the peritubular capillaries into the distal tubule for removal from the body.

Hormones control the body's final opportunity to remove sodium and water from the distal tubule and place them back into the peritubular capillaries and then into the renal vein. In cases of dehydration, this pathway is opened and water and sodium are retained.

Figure 28-4. ■ The structure of the nephron and the processes of urine formation. (Source: Pearson Education.)

TABLE 28-1	Characteristics of Normal Urine on Urinalysis
Color	Light straw to amber yellow; clear
Odor	Aromatic
Specific gravity	1.005–1.030
pH	4.5–8.0
Protein	Negative to trace (0–5 mg/dL)
Glucose	Negative
Ketones	Negative
RBC	1–2/low-power field (LPF)
WBC	3–4/LPF
Casts	Negative to occasional
Bacteria	Negative

Erythropoietin is produced by the kidneys in response to cellular hypoxia. It stimulates the bone marrow to produce red blood cells.

Vitamin D is important for calcium regulation in the body. It is inactive when it enters the body either through the diet or by exposure to ultraviolet light (sunlight). It is activated in two steps by the liver and then the kidneys.

AGE-RELATED CHANGES IN KIDNEY FUNCTION

Nephrons are lost with aging, reducing kidney mass and the GFR. By age 80, the GFR may be less than half of what it was at age 20. The kidneys are less able to concentrate urine in the older adult. This fact, combined with diminished thirst in older adults, increases the risk for dehydration (see Table 28-2 ■).

TABLE 28-2	Nursing Implications of Age-Related Changes in Urinary Function	
CHANGE	**EFFECT**	**NURSING IMPLICATIONS**
Decreased GFR	Decreased excretion of drugs primarily eliminated by the kidneys; increased risk of drug toxicity	Monitor patients carefully for signs of toxicity, especially when giving digoxin, certain antibiotics, cimetidine, and chlorpropamide.
Decreased number of nephrons; changes in aldosterone levels and response to ADH	Decreased ability to conserve water and sodium; increased risk of dehydration and fluid, electrolyte, and acid–base imbalances	Monitor for fluid, electrolyte, and acid–base imbalances. Promote fluid intake of up to 2,500 mL/day unless contraindicated.
Decreased number of functional nephrons	Increased risk of kidney failure	Avoid nephrotoxic drugs if possible; monitor urine output and for signs of kidney failure.
Decreased bladder muscle strength and capacity; increased difficulty emptying bladder	Urinary retention, frequency, urgency, and nocturia more common; larger amounts of residual urine present after voiding	Provide easy access to toilet or commode and appropriate lighting; monitor for manifestations of bladder infection or incontinence.

Assessment

Key Concept Signs and symptoms of urinary disorders may be detected during a general health assessment as well as during focused assessment of the urinary system.

HEALTH HISTORY

Ask about current symptoms related to urinary function such as:

- Color, odor, and amount of urine
- Difficulty initiating urination or changes in the force of urine flow
- Normal pattern of urination and recent changes from usual pattern
- Involuntary urine loss (leak), timing, and circumstances
- Usual type and amount of fluid intake
- Painful urination (**dysuria**)
- **Nocturia**, urinating more than one time at night
- Blood in the urine (**hematuria**) or cloudy, foul-smelling urine (**pyuria**)
- Discharge from the penis or urinary meatus
- Abdominal, suprapubic, or flank pain

Inquire about the onset, duration, and severity of symptoms, as well as associated symptoms such as nausea, general malaise, or fever. If pain is present, ask about the specific location and nature of the pain (sharp, burning, dull, constant, stabbing, intermittent), as well as its intensity.

Ask about previous urinary tract infections or surgeries. Determine what medications the patient is taking (if any). Ask about chronic diseases such as diabetes, heart failure, or kidney failure. Also ask women if pregnancy is a possibility

and the type of birth control used. Determine family history of kidney disease or failure and kidney stones. Inquire about personal habits such as smoking or alcohol intake and possible exposure to toxic chemicals (e.g., occupational exposure to dyes or chemicals).

PHYSICAL EXAMINATION

Assessment of the urinary system begins with obtaining a clean-catch urine specimen (Box 28-1■). Inspect the urine for color, odor, and clarity before sending it to the laboratory for analysis.

Obtain vital signs. Assess skin color and condition, including looking for evidence of excessively dry skin or excoriations. Inspect the face (especially the periorbital area) and palpate the lower extremities for evidence of edema. Expose the abdomen, and observe its contour and symmetry. Auscultate bowel sounds. Lightly palpate the abdomen for tenderness, including the suprapubic region. With the patient sitting and the back exposed, percuss the kidneys for tenderness (Figure 28-5■).

As indicated, inspect the genital area and urinary meatus for redness, swelling, discharge, or ulcerations. In the male, retract the foreskin if present with your gloved hands and gently compress the glans penis to expose the meatus (Figure 28-6■). Position the female patient recumbent with the knees raised and spread apart. Spread the labia using gloved hands to expose the meatus.

Box 28-2■ presents a sample documentation of the urinary system.

DIAGNOSTIC TESTS

Laboratory tests of blood and urine samples, ultrasound and x-ray studies, and direct visualization techniques are used to evaluate the urinary system.

BOX 28-1	NURSING CARE CHECKLIST

Collecting a Midstream Clean-Catch Urine Specimen

☑ Explain the purpose of the procedure and specimen.

☑ If alert and ambulatory, provide instructions and supplies for the patient to obtain the specimen:

   ☑ Clean the genital and perineal area with soap and water.

   ☑ Use each antiseptic towelette one time as follows:

      ☑ Female patients: Cleanse front to back.

      ☑ Male patients: Use a circular motion to clean the meatus. If uncircumcised, retract the foreskin before cleaning.

   ☑ Start urine flow and then place the container into urine stream to collect the specimen.

   ☑ Tightly cap the container, and if necessary, rinse and dry the outside.

☑ If the patient requires assistance:

   ☑ Obtain all supplies; use Standard Precautions.

   ☑ Provide perineal care.

   ☑ Position on clean bedpan, commode, or toilet.

   ☑ Cleanse perineal area with antiseptic towelettes as instructed earlier.

   ☑ Ask to begin voiding. Place the specimen container into the stream of urine, taking care to avoid touching perineal tissues or hair. Collect 30 to 60 mL of urine.

   ☑ Cap container, avoiding contamination of the inside of the cap.

☑ Label container and send with requisition to the laboratory.

☑ Document specimen collection and any pertinent information.

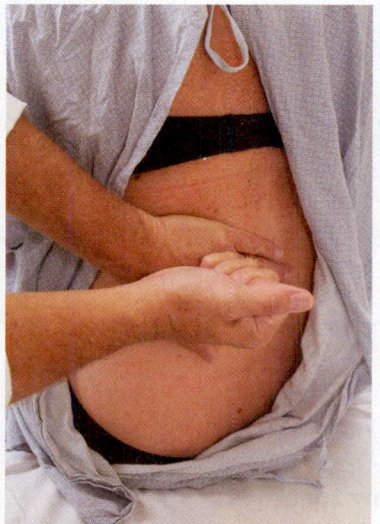

Figure 28-5. ■ Percussing the kidney. (Patrick Watson, Pearson Education.)

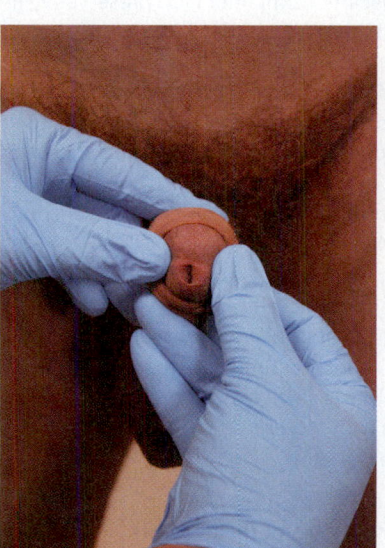

Figure 28-6. ■ Inspecting the urinary meatus of the male. (Patrick Watson, Pearson Education.)

BOX 28-2	DOCUMENTING URINARY SYSTEM ASSESSMENT

Patient: Nguyen Trong, 26 y.o., presents with complaints of urinary frequency, urgency, and burning on urination that began the evening previously.

Assessment note: States she had to urinate 3 times during the night and says her urine is dark, cloudy, and "smells bad." Denies previous history of UTI or kidney problems. Is not sexually active, denies possibility of pregnancy. Does not use birth control. Has little information about family history as her family remains in Vietnam. No known allergies or chronic diseases, not taking any medications currently.

BP 108/64, P 68, R 16, T 99.8°F PO. Skin pink, warm, and dry. Good turgor. No edema noted. Abdomen flat, slightly tender to palpation in suprapubic region. No tenderness on percussion of kidneys. Clean-catch urine specimen obtained; urine dark brown, cloudy, malodorous. Sent to lab for urinalysis.

Laboratory Tests

URINE STUDIES   The urinalysis (UA) is a key part of the diagnostic evaluation of the urinary system. Results of normal UA are listed in Table 28-1. When abnormal results are obtained or a disorder of the kidneys or urinary tract is suspected, urine may be subjected to further analysis. Tests commonly performed on urine are outlined with their nursing responsibilities in Table 28-3■.

RENAL CLEARANCE   Two substances found in the blood are routinely used to evaluate kidney function. *Urea* is formed in the metabolism of dietary and body proteins. *Creatinine* is produced in relatively constant quantities by muscle cell metabolism. Both of these substances are eliminated from the body by the kidneys by filtration and secretion; neither is reabsorbed. For this reason, *blood urea nitrogen (BUN)* and

TABLE 28-3	Laboratory Studies of Urine		
TEST	**EXPECTED RESULTS**	**EXPLANATION**	**NURSING IMPLICATIONS**
Urinalysis	See Table 28-1	Urinalysis includes both chemical and microscopic analysis of the urine. Chemical analysis is generally performed by dipstick. Microscopic analysis is used to identify cells (blood cells or bacteria), casts (protein structures that develop in the tubules of the kidneys), or crystals.	Use midstream clean-catch technique to collect specimen in a sterile container. Provide appropriate teaching for the patient to obtain the specimen. Use sterile technique to obtain a specimen from the drainage tubing if an indwelling catheter is in place.
Culture and sensitivity	No bacteria present	Urine is placed in or on an appropriate growth medium. If pathogens are present, they are microscopically identified. When combined with sensitivity testing, the specimen is grown in or on media containing disks of various antibiotics to identify those drugs that inhibit bacterial growth.	Obtain a specimen either by midstream clean-catch technique, by straight catheterization, or from an indwelling catheter using sterile technique. Promptly send the specimen to the laboratory.
24-Hour urine tests ■ Protein ■ Creatinine	 25–150 mg/24 hr 1–2 g/24 hr	Urine creatinine and protein are used to help identify kidney disease. Protein molecules are generally too large to be filtered through the glomerular membrane, thus little protein is normally present in urine. Increased levels indicate kidney disease, urinary tract infection, or other serious conditions.	Obtain specimen container with appropriate preservative (if indicated) from the laboratory. Determine whether specimen should be kept refrigerated or on ice during collection period. Follow procedures outlined in Box 28-3 for patient teaching and specimen collection.

serum creatinine levels in the blood are effective indicators of renal function.

The GFR can be estimated (the *eGFR*) using the patient's serum creatinine level, age, gender, and race (Black or another race). The GFR can also be calculated by determining the amount of blood plasma cleared of creatinine during a specific period of time. This is known as the *creatinine clearance test.* The creatinine clearance test generally requires collection of a 24-hour urine sample, although shorter collection periods may be used. A blood sample to measure the serum creatinine is obtained at some point during urine collection. Nursing responsibilities for collecting a 24-hour urine specimen are outlined in Box 28-3■. Normal values of the BUN, serum creatinine, eGFR, and creatinine clearance tests are in Table 28-4■. Serum albumin levels can be affected by kidney disease; Table 28-4 also includes normal values for the serum albumin.

Imaging Studies

X-rays, nuclear scans, and ultrasound examinations are used to assess the urinary system. Table 28-5■ outlines nursing responsibilities and patient teaching related to these exams.

BOX 28-3	NURSING CARE CHECKLIST

24-Hour Urine Specimen

☑ Note any diet or medication changes required during the collection period.

☑ Obtain specimen container with preservative (if indicated). Label with identifying data, the test, time started, and time of completion.

☑ Obtain a clean urine-collection device and place it in the room.

☑ Post notices—on chart, in Kardex, on the door, over the bed, and over the toilet—alerting all personnel that all urine is to be saved.

☑ At start time, have patient empty bladder completely and *discard* urine.

☑ Save all urine for next 24 hours in the container, placing container on ice or refrigerating as indicated. If any urine is missed, the collection must be restarted.

☑ At end of collection time, have patient empty the bladder completely and save this urine in the container. Take entire specimen with requisition to the lab.

☑ Chart appropriately.

Teaching

☑ Save all your urine for the 24 hours.

☑ Urinate (and save) before moving bowels. Do not put any toilet tissue in the urine container.

Table 28-4	Laboratory Tests Used to Evaluate Renal Function	
TEST	**SPECIMEN**	**NORMAL VALUE**
Blood urea nitrogen (BUN)	Blood	5–25 mg/dL; slightly higher in older adults
Serum creatinine	Blood	0.5–1.2 mg/dL Slightly lower in older adults
Estimated glomerular filtration rate (eGFR)	Blood	Greater than 60 mL/min/1.73 m^2 May be a less accurate indicator of renal function in older adults
Creatinine clearance	Blood 24-Hour urine	85–135 mL/min May be slightly lower in females Values lower in older adults
Cystatin C	Blood	Less than 0.70 mg/mL
Serum albumin	Blood	3.5–5 g/dL

- *Ultrasound* examination of the bladder or kidneys may be performed to evaluate their size, shape, and position. This is a noninvasive examination that requires no preparation of the patient other than explanation of the procedure. For this exam, the patient may be instructed either to empty the bladder before the exam or to consume several glasses of water and come to the exam with a full bladder. Nurses may perform ultrasonic bladder scans to evaluate for urinary retention and to determine postvoiding residual volume.
- An abdominal x-ray known as the *KUB (kidney, ureter, bladder)* may be done to evaluate the size, shape, and position of organs in the urinary tract. This is a plain x-ray that requires no special preparation, although the patient may be asked to either empty the bladder or allow it to fill before the x-ray.
- *Intravenous pyelography (IVP)* uses a contrast medium and x-rays to evaluate the urinary tract. The contrast medium is injected intravenously. It is filtered from the blood by the kidneys, allowing x-rays to show the contrast entering the kidney pelvis, flowing through the ureters, and into the bladder. This allows evaluation of renal function (by measuring the time required for filtration), and the position, size, shape, and structure of urinary tract organs. *Retrograde pyelography* may be done as an alternative to IVP. In this exam, contrast media is instilled into the collecting system of the urinary tract (renal pelvis, ureters, and bladder).
- *Renal arteriogram (angiogram)* is done to visualize and evaluate renal blood vessels and blood flow through the kidneys. It is used to identify vessel abnormalities or clots, as well as such problems as renal tumors or cysts.
- *CT scan* or *magnetic resonance imaging (MRI)* may also be done to visualize structures of the urinary tract. CT scan may be done with or without contrast media. If contrast is used, care of the patient is similar to that provided for IVP.
- *Renal scan (kidney scan)* is a nuclear medicine scan used to evaluate blood vessels and perfusion of the kidneys and the ureters. It can demonstrate blood flow obstructions to the kidneys as well as the functions of the nephron (filtration and tubular transport). It can also show obstructions of the ureters or backflow of urine from the bladder into the ureters (*reflux*).
- *Cystoscopy,* direct visualization of the urethra and bladder using an endoscope, is used to diagnose conditions such as urethral strictures, bladder stones, tumors, and congenital abnormalities. This invasive examination is performed in an endoscopy laboratory or cystoscopy room of the surgical suite.

TABLE 28-5	Diagnostic Studies of the Urinary System	
TEST	**NURSING RESPONSIBILITIES**	**PATIENT TEACHING**
Intravenous pyelography	Before the procedure: - Informed consent is required. - Assess and clarify understanding of the procedure. - Ask about and report allergies to seafood, iodine, or x-ray contrast media. - Teach or administer laxatives as ordered. Allow clear liquids only for 8 hours before the test. After the procedure: - Monitor vital signs and urinary output. - Report signs of reaction to contrast media such as dyspnea, tachycardia, itching, hives, or flushing. - Check injection site for redness, pain, and warmth. Apply warm packs to the site if indicated.	- IVP uses x-rays to show the structures of the kidney, ureters, and bladder by injecting a dye that is rapidly excreted in the urine. The test takes about 30 minutes. - As the dye is injected, you may experience flushing or burning, nausea, and a metallic taste. - Immediately notify the physician if you develop a rash, difficulty breathing, rapid heart rate, or hives. - Increase fluid intake after the test is completed.

(continued)

TABLE 28-5	Diagnostic Studies of the Urinary System *(continued)*	
TEST	**NURSING RESPONSIBILITIES**	**PATIENT TEACHING**
Renal arteriogram	Before the procedure: ■ Informed consent is required. ■ Assess and clarify understanding of the procedure. ■ Ask about and report allergies to seafood, iodine, or x-ray contrast media. ■ Teach or administer laxatives and/or cleansing enemas as ordered (usually preceding evening). ■ No food or fluids are allowed for 8–12 hours before the test. ■ Withhold anticoagulants as ordered. After the procedure: ■ Monitor vital signs, peripheral pulses, and urinary output. ■ Monitor for bleeding from the femoral artery. ■ Limit activities for 24 hours.	■ This test uses dye injected into the renal artery to show the blood vessels and structure of the kidneys on x-rays. ■ You may receive a light sedative before the procedure, as well as a local anesthetic where the arterial catheter is inserted. The test takes 1 to 2 hours to complete. ■ After the test is completed, you will be on limited activity for 24 hours. ■ Immediately report bleeding from the catheter site, rapid heart rate, difficulty breathing, rash, or itching to your nurse or care provider.
Renal scan	■ Informed consent is required. ■ Clarify and reinforce teaching. ■ Obtain weight. ■ Provide two to three glasses of water before the procedure and encourage fluids after. ■ Have patient void before the procedure.	■ Increase fluid intake before and after the renal scan. ■ No special diet or other preparation is required. ■ A dilute radioactive substance will be injected into a vein to allow visualization of the kidneys. ■ The test takes 1 to 4 hours.
Portable ultrasonic bladder scan	■ Perform the scan within 15 minutes of voiding if evaluating for residual urine. ■ Position supine; expose the lower abdomen. Using warmed ultrasound gel, place the probe just above the pubic bone to scan. ■ Obtain several readings to ensure accuracy; the largest reading is the most accurate. ■ Print the bladder outline, and document residual urine. Notify the charge nurse or physician of the results. ■ Remove ultrasound gel from the skin with a moist cloth. Clean the scanner, following unit protocol.	■ Explain the procedure and its purpose. This procedure is generally not done on pregnant patients. ■ The scanner shows an outline of the bladder and displays the volume of urine in milliliters (mL).
Cystoscopy	■ Informed consent is required. ■ Assess and clarify understanding of the procedure and its purpose. ■ Teach or assist with bowel preparation as ordered. ■ Withhold food and fluids for 8 hours before the procedure as ordered. ■ Administer sedation and other medications as ordered.	■ The procedure takes about 30 to 45 minutes. Local or general anesthesia is used. ■ You may feel pressure or an urge to urinate as the scope is inserted. ■ Do not attempt to stand up without assistance after the procedure because you may feel dizzy or faint. ■ Burning on urination for a day or two after the procedure is considered normal. ■ Contact your doctor immediately if you have bright red bleeding, low urine output, abdominal or flank pain, chills, or fever. ■ Warm sitz baths and medications help relieve discomfort. ■ Increase fluid intake to decrease pain, ease voiding, and reduce the risk of infection. ■ Laxatives may be ordered to prevent constipation and straining after the procedure.

Voiding Studies

Voiding studies are used to evaluate voiding and lower urinary tract function, urinary retention, and urinary incontinence. *Uroflowmetry* is a noninvasive test that measures the volume and rate of urine flow. For this test, the patient voids into a toilet equipped with a funnel and uroflowmeter. Before the test, the patient is instructed to drink fluids and avoid urination for several hours. The patient is placed in a specially equipped bathroom and advised to avoid discarding toilet tissue into the funnel or collection container. Privacy is provided, and the patient voids into the urometer funnel without straining. In a *cystometrogram* (*CMG,* or *voiding cystogram*), a measured amount of fluid is instilled into the bladder, and pressures during filling and voiding are measured. The patient is asked to identify when the urge to void is felt and when it is no longer possible to delay urination.

Note: The references and resources for this and all chapters have been compiled at the back of the book.

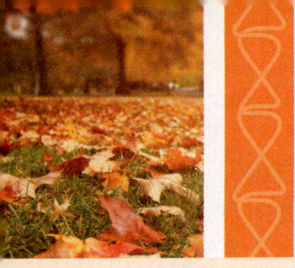

Chapter Review

KEY POINTS

- **Concept:** The urinary system, including the kidneys, ureters, urinary bladder, and urethra, eliminates waste and plays a critical role in maintaining homeostasis (balance) of the body.
- The urinary system eliminates waste and plays a critical role in maintaining homeostasis (balance) of the body.
- This system includes the paired kidneys, which produce urine, and the urinary drainage system, including the ureters, urinary bladder, and urethra. Unimpaired urine flow through the system is vital.
- The functional unit of the kidney is the nephron. The glomerulus of the nephron filters blood; this filtrate is then concentrated and refined in the tubule of the nephron to become urine. The urine flows from the collecting tubule into the renal pelvis and ureters to be stored in the bladder.
- **Concept:** Signs and symptoms of urinary disorders may be detected during a general health assessment as well as during focused assessment of the urinary system.
- Nursing assessment of urinary function generally is completed toward the end of the exam to allow the patient to develop trust and comfort with the nurse before discussing and examining potentially embarrassing topics or regions.
- Both blood tests and urine studies are used to evaluate the function of the urinary system. Imaging studies such as x-rays and ultrasound are important mechanisms for evaluating its structure.

PEARSON NURSING STUDENT RESOURCES

Find additional materials at **nursing.pearsonhighered.com**.

NCLEX-PN® Exam Preparation

1 A patient is complaining of pain in the right flank region. Which follow-up question would be most important for the nurse to ask?

1. Have you noticed any changes in your urine?
2. Do you have diabetes?
3. Has your appetite or weight changed recently?
4. Does the pain wake you from sleep?

2 The nurse caring for a patient with acute tubular necrosis knows that this is likely to affect:

1. blood flow to the kidney pelvis.
2. urine collection and voiding.
3. the formation of urine in the nephron.
4. the ability to maintain continence.

3 Digoxin 0.25 mg daily has been prescribed for an 80-year-old patient. The nurse observes closely for:

1. evidence of drug excretion without the desired effect.
2. excretion of the drug unchanged in the urine.
3. impaired urination due to effects of the drug.
4. manifestations of drug toxicity due to impaired excretion.

4 The nurse, preparing a patient who is scheduled for a creatinine clearance test, includes which of the following in the instructions? **Select all that apply.**

1. Note the time of the first saved urine sample as the start of the 24-hour collection.
2. Save a portion of each voiding for 24 hours.
3. Empty the bladder at the start time and discard this urine.
4. Avoid putting any toilet paper in the saved urine.
5. Prevent feces from contaminating the saved urine.

5 The nurse reviewing urinalysis (UA) results for a patient notes that there is 2+ protein in the urine. The most appropriate response by the nurse is to:

1. do nothing, as this is within normal limits for the UA.
2. limit the patient's protein intake.
3. report the result to the physician.
4. request a repeat urinalysis to verify the results.

Answers and rationales for Review Questions appear in Appendix I.

CHAPTER 29
Caring for Patients With Kidney and Urinary Tract Disorders

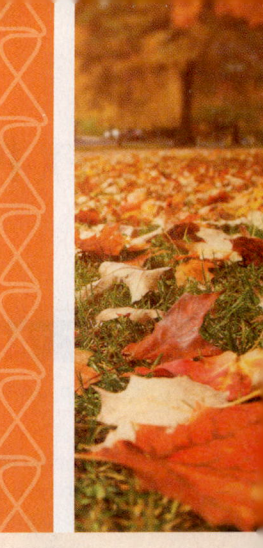

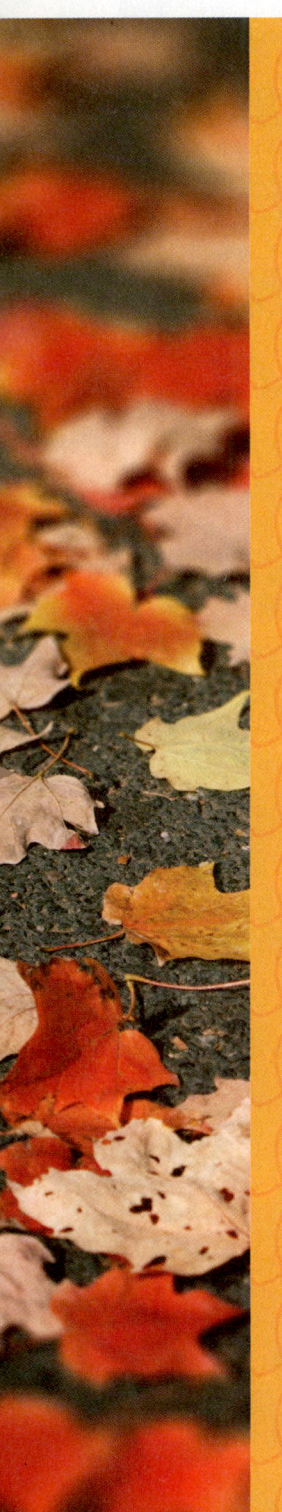

BRIEF OUTLINE

VOIDING DISORDERS
Urinary Incontinence
Urinary Retention
INFECTIOUS AND INFLAMMATORY DISORDERS
Urinary Tract Infections

Glomerulonephritis
OBSTRUCTIVE DISORDERS
Kidney Stones
Hydronephrosis
CONGENITAL KIDNEY DISORDERS

Polycystic Kidney Disease
CANCER OF THE URINARY TRACT
KIDNEY FAILURE
Acute Kidney Injury
End-Stage Renal Disease

APPLIED LEARNING OUTCOMES

After completing this chapter, you will be able to:

1. Describe the risk factors, pathophysiology, and potential complications of common disorders of the kidneys and urinary tract.
2. Compare and contrast the manifestations of common disorders of the kidneys and urinary tract.
3. Collaborate with the interprofessional team to provide safe and effective care for patients with these disorders.
4. Provide patient-centered, culturally appropriate, and evidence-based nursing care for the patient having surgery of the kidneys or urinary tract.
5. Use the nursing process and expressed values, needs, and preferences to assess, plan, implement, and evaluate individualized care for patients with disorders of the kidneys or urinary tract.
6. Use appropriate electronic resources in planning and documenting care for patients with kidney or urinary tract disorders.
7. Participate in studies directed at improving the outcomes for patients with disorders of the kidneys or urinary tract.

KEY TERMS

The key terms are defined on the pages listed below.

acute kidney injury, 766
azotemia, 749
cystectomy, 761
cystitis, 744
dialysate, 770
dialysis, 770
dysuria, 745

glomerulonephritis, 749
hematuria, 745
hydronephrosis, 758
kidney failure,766
nephrotoxins, 766
nocturia, 745
proteinuria, 749

pyelonephritis, 744
pyuria, 745
renal colic, 755
uremia, 768
urgency, 745
urinary incontinence, 739
urolithiasis, 755

SPECIAL FEATURES

PATHOPHYSIOLOGY ILLUSTRATED: Acute Glomerulonephritis, 750
NURSING CARE PLAN: Patient With Acute Glomerulonephritis, 754
NURSING CARE PLAN: Patient With Bladder Cancer, 765
PATHOPHYSIOLOGY ILLUSTRATED: Acute Kidney injury, 767
CLINICAL REASONING CARE MAP: Caring for a Patient With Urinary Incontinence, 778
UNIT VII WRAP-UP: Thinking Strategically About..., 780

In this chapter, disorders of the kidneys and the urinary system (ureters, urinary bladder, and urethra) are discussed. Review Chapter 28 for more information about structures of the urinary tract, their purpose, and urine formation.

When caring for patients with kidney and urinary tract disorders, it is important to consider the patient's modesty in voiding and possible reluctance to talk about the genitals. Patients often experience embarrassment about being exposed during examinations, tests, and procedures. Fear of potential changes in body function is also an important consideration when caring for patients with kidney and urinary tract disorders. These issues can interfere with the patient's willingness to seek help for problems.

VOIDING DISORDERS

Voiding disorders are common, although they are often unreported because of modesty, embarrassment, difficulty discussing elimination, and the perception that the disorder is a normal part of the aging process.

Urinary Incontinence

Key Concept   Urinary incontinence is a common and underreported problem, particularly among older adults. It is not a normal consequence of aging, and in most cases, it can be treated effectively.

Urinary incontinence (UI), or involuntary urination, is a common problem that can cause physical problems (e.g., skin breakdown, infection, and rashes), as well as embarrassment, isolation and withdrawal, feelings of worthlessness and helplessness, and depression.

PATHOPHYSIOLOGY AND MANIFESTATIONS

Urinary continence requires a bladder that is able to expand and contract and sphincters that can maintain a higher pressure in the urethra than that in the bladder. When pressure within the bladder is higher than urethral resistance, urine can escape. Any condition that increases bladder pressures or reduces resistance within the urethra can cause incontinence. Pelvic muscle relaxation, impaired neural control, and bladder problems are common contributing factors.

UI is commonly categorized as stress incontinence, urge incontinence, voiding difficulties, reflex incontinence, and functional incontinence (Table 29-1■). Mixed UI, usually defined as a combination of stress and urge UI, is common.

UI in Older Adults

Incontinence should *never* be considered a normal part of aging. However, age-related changes contribute to UI.

TABLE 29-1	Types of Urinary Incontinence		
TYPE	**DESCRIPTION**	**PATHOPHYSIOLOGY**	**CONTRIBUTING FACTORS**
Stress	Loss of small amounts of urine when intra-abdominal pressure increases (sneezing, laughing, lifting)	Pelvic muscle relaxation; weakness of urethra and surrounding tissues decreases urethral resistance.	■ Multiple pregnancies ■ Decreased estrogen levels (menopause) ■ Prostate surgery
Urge, overactive bladder	Involuntary urine loss associated with a strong need to void	Overactive detrusor muscle increases bladder pressure, causing inability to inhibit voiding.	■ Decreased bladder capacity ■ Bladder irritation ■ Central nervous system disorders
Voiding difficulties	Urinary retention with bladder overdistention and frequent loss of small amounts of urine (25–50 mL)	Outlet obstruction or impaired detrusor muscle activity leads to overfilling and increased pressure.	■ Neurologic disorders or trauma ■ Enlarged prostate ■ Fecal impaction ■ Anticholinergic drug effects
Reflex	Involuntary loss of moderate amount of urine occurring without warning	Altered spinal cord activity causes hyperreflexia of the detrusor muscle.	■ Neurologic disorders or trauma
Functional	Inability to get to toilet facilities to urinate	Self-care deficit interferes with ability to respond to urge to void.	■ Physical disability or impaired mobility, neurologic disorders ■ Diuretic therapy or sedation ■ Lack of facilities, privacy, or caregiver assistance

Bladder capacity usually declines with age, and involuntary bladder muscle contractions are more common. In women, decreased estrogen levels and pelvic muscle relaxation cause urethral resistance to decrease, so stress incontinence may occur. Decreased estrogen may also lead to dysuria and urgency. Other risk factors in older adults include constipation, low fluid intake, immobility, chronic degenerative diseases or dementia, medications, diabetes, and stroke. Incontinence increases the risk for falls, fractures, pressure ulcers, urinary tract infection, and depression. It contributes to caregiver stress and may be a major factor in institutionalizing the patient.

COLLABORATIVE CARE

The focus of collaborative care is to identify and correct the cause if possible. If the underlying problem cannot be corrected, techniques may be taught to manage urine output.

Evaluation begins with a complete history, including the duration, frequency, volume, and associated circumstances of UI. A voiding diary (Figure 29-1■) is often used to provide detailed information. The history includes any chronic or acute illnesses, previous surgeries, and current medications (prescription and over the counter).

Physical assessment includes abdominal, rectal, and pelvic exams, as well as evaluation of mental and neurologic status, mobility, and dexterity. Women with UI often have weak abdominal and pelvic muscle tone, protrusion of the bladder or urethral wall into the vagina (cystocele or urethrocele), and thin vaginal tissues. In men, an enlarged prostate gland is commonly identified.

Diagnostic Tests

Diagnostic tests to identify the cause of UI may include a *postvoid residual urine* measurement using ultrasonic bladder scan to determine how completely the bladder empties with voiding. Less than 50 mL of residual urine is expected; when 100 mL or more of residual urine is present, further tests are done. Additional studies may include *cystometrography* to evaluate bladder pressures and *uroflowmetry* to evaluate voiding patterns. See Chapter 28 for more information about uroflowmetry procedures.

Treatment

Drugs that contract the smooth muscles of the bladder neck may reduce episodes of mild stress incontinence. Duloxetine (Cymbalta) is the drug of choice for treating stress UI that is not fully controlled with nonpharmacologic measures (e.g., teaching, pelvic muscle exercise).

Urge incontinence may be treated with drugs to inhibit detrusor muscle contractions and increase bladder capacity. The drugs may include *oxybutynin* (Ditropan), *tolterodine* (Detrol), and solifenacin (VESIcare). The anticholinergic effects of these drugs may cause dry mouth and eyes, constipation, confusion, and urinary retention.

When UI is associated with postmenopausal atrophic vaginitis, estrogen therapy may be effective. Both systemic estrogens and local creams are used.

When incontinence is associated with a cystocele or urethrocele, or is due to an enlarged prostate gland, surgery may be performed. *Bladder neck suspension* is used to treat urethrocele. Nursing care of the patient having a bladder neck suspension is outlined in Box 29-1■.

Prostatectomy is indicated when an enlarged prostate gland obstructs urine outflow. (See care of the patient with a prostatectomy in Chapter 31.)

COMPLEMENTARY THERAPIES   Biofeedback and relaxation techniques may help reduce the frequency of UI. Biofeedback uses electronic monitors to teach conscious control over

---

DATE _____

Please complete this chart prior to your visit. Choose a 24-hour period when it is convenient for you to measure and record the following: The amount of fluid you void (urinate), the amount of fluid you drink and type of beverage, the time, when leakage episodes occur, whether or not you have an urge to void just prior to leaking, and the activity you are doing when you leak or need to void.

VOIDING DIARY

DIARY.URO

Void Amount (oz.)	Fluid Intake Amount (oz.)	Time	Leak?	Urge prior to leak?	Activity
14 oz.		6:23 am	yes	yes	Awakening
8 oz.	14 oz. coffee	6:35			
		8:05	yes	yes	reading
	16 oz. coffee	8:30			
10 oz.		9:10	yes	yes	watch TV
10 oz.		9:30	"	"	"

Figure 29-1. ■ A sample voiding diary.

Bladder Neck Suspension

Before Surgery

☑ Provide routine preoperative care and teaching.

☑ Instruct to avoid straining and the Valsalva maneuver post-operatively.

After Surgery

☑ Provide routine postoperative care.

☑ Frequently assess vaginal drainage or dressing. Notify the charge nurse or physician of bright red bleeding on dressing, from vagina, or in urine.

☑ Monitor and record quantity, color, and clarity of urine. Pink urine should gradually clear.

☑ Tape urinary catheters in position to prevent dislodging or pulling on incisions.

☑ Encourage activity and ambulation.

☑ Carefully monitor urine output after catheter removal.

☑ If a urethral or suprapubic catheter is in place at discharge, teach appropriate care.

☑ Stress importance of keeping scheduled appointments and contacting the physician if signs of a urinary tract infection or other complications develop.

physiologic responses to stimuli such as a partially full bladder. Developing awareness of stimuli allows the patient to gain voluntary control over urination. Biofeedback is widely used to manage UI.

NURSING CARE

PRIORITIZING NURSING CARE

Obtaining complete assessment data to help direct an accurate diagnosis and appropriate treatment is a nursing care priority, as is preventing complications of UI, such as skin irritation and falls.

HEALTH PROMOTION

Although UI rarely has serious physical effects, its psychosocial effects can be significant. UI can lead to lowered self-esteem, social isolation, and even institutionalization. Inform all patients that UI is not a normal part of aging and that treatments are available. To reduce the incidence of UI, teach all women to perform pelvic floor muscle (Kegel) exercises (Box 29-2■) to improve perineal muscle tone. Advise women to ask their care provider about hormone therapy (either topical or systemic) during menopause to maintain perineal tissue integrity. Also advise older men to have routine prostate examinations to prevent urethral obstruction and overflow incontinence. Pelvic floor muscle exercises may also benefit men who experience UI after prostatectomy.

Pelvic Floor (Kegel) Exercises

- Identify the pelvic muscles by:
  - Attempting to stop the flow of urine during voiding and holding for a few seconds.
  - Tightening the muscles of the vagina around a gloved finger or tampon.
  - Tightening the muscles around the anus as though trying to avoid passing flatus.
- Perform exercises: Tighten pelvic muscles, hold for 10 seconds, and relax for 10 to 15 seconds. Continue the sequence (tighten, hold, relax) for 10 repetitions.
- Keep abdominal muscles and breathing relaxed while performing exercises.
- Initially, exercises should be performed twice per day, working up to four times a day.
- Exercise at a specific time each day or in conjunction with another daily activity (e.g., bathing or watching the news). Establish a routine, because these exercises should be continued for life.

ASSESSING

Collect subjective assessment data by asking about problems with urine loss, its frequency, and any contributing factors. Inquire about frequency, urgency, and burning on urination. Identify current medications and their timing. Assess patterns of fluid intake and output. Also assess the abdomen for evidence of bladder distention or tenderness. Perform a mental status examination if indicated. Review any laboratory results, such as serum glucose and urinalysis for possible contributing factors such as diabetes or evidence of urinary tract infection.

DIAGNOSING, PLANNING, AND IMPLEMENTING

When planning care for patients with UI, consider mental and neurologic status, mobility, and motivation. Behavioral techniques require long-term commitment, as well as the physical and mental ability to implement them. Nursing interventions such as scheduled toileting, bladder training, and prompted voiding combined with praise can reduce the need for diapers, incontinence pads, and indwelling catheters in institutionalized patients.

Impaired Urinary Elimination

Expected outcome: Will experience fewer episodes of unintended urine loss.

- Monitor patterns of fluid intake and urination, including voluntary voiding and wetting accidents. *These data help identify the type and pattern of incontinence.*

- Teach pelvic floor muscle exercises, called Kegel exercises (see Box 29-2). Instruct to consciously tighten pelvic muscles and relax the abdomen when the need to void is perceived. *Improved pelvic muscle strength helps prevent stress incontinence and decrease urge incontinence.*
- Reduce toileting delays. Ensure that the call light is within reach. Place a bedside commode in the room or provide clear access to the bathroom. Dress in loose-fitting clothing with elastic waistbands or Velcro closures. *These actions reduce the risk of wetting accidents.*
- Ensure adequate fluid intake during daytime hours. After the evening meal, limit beverages, especially those that irritate the bladder, such as beverages containing caffeine or NutraSweet and citrus juices. *It is important to maintain fluid intake to prevent dehydration and bladder irritation by concentrated urine. Limiting evening fluid intake and bladder irritants reduces the risk of nighttime incontinence.*
- Administer diuretic drugs in the morning and midafternoon. *This timing allows the peak effect of the medication to occur while the patient is awake and more able to respond to the urge to void.*

Toileting Self-Care Deficit

Expected outcome: Will experience no incontinent episodes related to difficulty responding to urge to urinate.

In institutions, functional incontinence (see Table 29-1) can be a significant problem in previously continent people. With functional incontinence, the primary problem is an outside factor that interferes with the ability to respond to the urge to void.

- Assess physical and mental capabilities and limitations, usual pattern of voiding, and ability to assist with toileting. *A thorough assessment helps address specific needs.*
- Provide assistive devices such as raised toilet seats, grab bars, a bedside commode, or night-lights. *Assistive devices help maintain independence and prevent falls.*
- Plan a toileting schedule to achieve approximately 300 mL of urine output with each voiding. *Allowing the bladder to fill until the urge to void is felt helps maintain normal bladder capacity.*
- Position for ease of voiding—sitting for females and standing for males—and provide for privacy. *Normal positioning and privacy enhance the ability to void.*
- Provide the majority of fluids during times of day when the patient is most able to remain continent. *Unless restricted, maintain a fluid intake of at least 1.5 to 2 L per day.*

Social Isolation

Expected outcome: Will engage in social interactions and activities with others.

The patient with any form of UI is at risk for social isolation due to embarrassment, fear of not having ready access to a bathroom, body odor, or other factors.

- Refer for urologic examination and evaluation of incontinence. *Patients who assume that UI is a normal part of aging may not be aware of treatment options.*
- Explore alternative coping strategies with patient, significant others, staff, and other health team members. *Protective pads or shields, good perineal hygiene, scheduled voiding, and clothing that does not interfere with toileting can enhance continence.*

MANAGING NURSING CARE

Nursing care activities such as toileting assistance, using bladder ultrasound to measure residual volume, and providing assistance with hygiene for the patient with UI are appropriate tasks to assign to assistive personnel.

EVALUATING

To evaluate the effectiveness of nursing actions for the patient with UI, keep a diary of fluid intake, voidings, and wetting accidents. Look for a decrease in the number of wetting episodes. Identify factors that contribute to wetting episodes, such as delayed toileting or difficulty manipulating clothing. Assess the patient's willingness to participate in social activities.

DOCUMENTING

Document assessment data, teaching provided, and the patient's ability and apparent willingness to continue with prescribed treatment measures, lifestyle changes, and exercises.

CONTINUITY OF CARE

Appropriate home care and teaching can help keep the patient in the home, reduce caregiver stress, and reduce the risk of institutionalization. Assess the home environment (whether in the community or a residential living facility) for possible barriers to urinary elimination, such as:

- Inadequate lighting, particularly at night
- Narrow doorways that may interfere with access to the toilet
- Inadequate toilet facilities

Teach the patient to keep a voiding diary to help identify factors contributing to incontinent episodes. Instruct to maintain a generous fluid intake of 1.5 to 2 quarts of fluid per day. Advise restricting fluid intake after the evening meal. Discuss bladder irritants such as caffeine, citrus juices, and artificial sweeteners and advise limiting their use. Teach Kegel exercises. Discuss the potential risks and benefits of hormone replacement therapy, surgery, and physical therapy with women. Encourage overweight patients to lose weight.

Discuss scheduled voiding and bladder training techniques with caregivers. Suggest taking the patient to the toilet every 2 to 4 hours. To increase bladder capacity, the time between voidings may be gradually increased. Provide a list of resources for assistive devices such as a bedside commode, urinal, grab bars, or raised toilet seat.

Urinary Retention

Normal bladder emptying may be disrupted by an obstruction to urine flow or by a functional problem.

PATHOPHYSIOLOGY

When the bladder cannot empty, it becomes overstretched. This, in turn, affects detrusor muscle contraction and further impairs urination.

Benign prostatic hypertrophy (*BPH,* or enlargement of the prostate) is a common cause of urinary retention. Difficulty initiating and maintaining urine flow is often the presenting complaint in men with BPH. Acute inflammation associated with infection or trauma of the bladder, urethra, or perineal tissues may also interfere with the ability to urinate. Scarring caused by repeated urinary tract infections can narrow the urethra and obstruct output.

Surgery, particularly abdominal or pelvic surgery, can affect detrusor muscle function, leading to acute urinary retention. Medications may also affect bladder contraction. Drugs with anticholinergic effects may cause urinary retention. These include antianxiety drugs, antidepressant drugs, and many common over-the-counter cough, cold, allergy, and sleep-promoting drugs. Voluntary urinary retention (particularly common among nurses) may lead to overfilling of the bladder and a loss of detrusor muscle tone.

Neurologic diseases or trauma may interfere with normal mechanisms of bladder emptying (*neurogenic bladder*). The result may be either a *spastic bladder* that does not fill normally before emptying (reflex incontinence) or a *flaccid bladder* that overfills without reflexive emptying.

MANIFESTATIONS AND COMPLICATIONS

The patient with urinary retention is unable to empty the bladder completely. Overflow voiding or incontinence may occur (see Table 29-1). Assessment reveals a firm, distended bladder that may be displaced to one side of midline.

Acute or chronic urinary retention can lead to complications such as hydronephrosis (distention of the kidney with urine), acute kidney injury, and urinary tract infection. These conditions are discussed later in this chapter.

COLLABORATIVE CARE

A portable bladder scan or straight catheterization may be performed to assess retained urine and determine the extent of urinary retention.

For the patient with a mechanical obstruction to urine flow, retention is treated by removing or repairing the obstruction. Medications such as tamsulosin (Flomax) or terazosin (Hytrin) improve urinary flow in patients with BPH, whereas others such as finasteride (Propecia, Proscar) or dutasteride (Avodart) may be prescribed to reduce the size of an enlarged prostate gland. The prostate gland may be resected if necessary. Cholinergic medications such as bethanechol chloride (Urecholine) may be ordered to promote bladder emptying in patients with acute urinary retention or neurogenic bladder. Modification of the patient's medication regimen may be necessary.

Techniques to stimulate reflex voiding and promote complete bladder emptying are used for neurogenic bladder. These include using trigger points, for example, stroking or pinching the abdomen, inner thigh, or glans penis. Pulling pubic hairs or tapping the suprapubic region can also stimulate urination.

The *Credé method* (applying pressure over the symphysis pubis with the fingers of one or both hands) may promote complete bladder emptying. Applying manual pressure to the abdomen and using the *Valsalva maneuver* (bearing down while holding one's breath) also promotes bladder emptying.

Intermittent straight catheterization after surgery can prevent overdistention of the bladder (Box 29-3■). Intermittent catheterization is less likely to cause a urinary tract infection than an indwelling catheter and so is preferred. Patients with chronic urinary retention may perform intermittent self-catheterization every 3 to 4 hours.

BOX 29-3   PATIENT TEACHING

Patient Self-Catheterization Checklist

- Wash hands before and after the procedure, and clean the urinary meatus with soap and water.
- Attempt to void. If urine is not of sufficient quantity (at least 100 mL) or if you cannot void at all, do self-catheterization.

Female

- While sitting, locate the urethra by looking in a mirror or feeling it with a fingertip.
- Lubricate the meatus with a water-soluble lubricant.
- Take a deep breath and insert the catheter tip 2 to 3 in. or until urine flows.

Male

- While sitting, hold the penis with slight upward tension and extend it to its full length.
- Lubricate the catheter from the tip to about 6 in. downward.
- Take a deep breath and insert the catheter 6 to 7 in. or until urine flows.

Both

- Hold the catheter securely and allow urine to drain until the flow stops.
- Withdraw the catheter and wash it with soap and water. Store in a clean container.

NURSING CARE

Obtaining a timely focused assessment and relieving bladder distention are the priorities of nursing care for the patient with urinary retention. Not only is a full bladder uncomfortable, but urine can back up to the ureters and kidneys, leading to acute kidney injury.

Careful nursing assessment can identify patients with problems of urinary retention. Note intake and output, paying close attention to voiding patterns as well as total output. Notify the charge nurse or physician if it has been 8 or more hours since the patient has voided. Gently palpate the lower abdomen just above the symphysis pubis for tenderness and firm distention. Percussing the lower abdomen may be helpful; a full bladder has a dull percussion tone. If ordered or allowed by unit protocol, perform an ultrasonic bladder scan to measure the amount of urine present in the bladder.

Measures to promote urination can be helpful. Place the patient in normal voiding position (sitting for females and standing for males) and provide privacy. Run water in the sink or shower, place the patient's hands in warm water, pour warm water over the perineum, or provide a warm sitz bath as additional measures. Provide adequate time for voiding; allow up to 10 minutes.

When catheterization is necessary, use strict sterile technique. Nursing care related to catheterization is listed in Box 29-4■.

CONTINUITY OF CARE

Assess the patient's ability to provide self-care. Determine the patient's and family's or caregivers' understanding of the problem, ability to recognize manifestations of urinary retention, and ability to perform maneuvers to stimulate voiding. If intermittent catheterization is required, assess vision, ability to see the urinary meatus, and motor skills for inserting the catheter. Assess access to water and facilities for hand washing and for cleaning the catheter. Discuss the manifestations of acute urinary retention and urinary tract infection, and stress the importance of notifying a health care provider if these develop.

BOX 29-4	NURSING CARE CHECKLIST

Urinary Catheterization

- ☑ Use Standard Precautions.
- ☑ Use sterile technique for catheter insertion.
- ☑ If possible, use intermittent catheterization instead of an indwelling catheter to reduce the risk of infection.
- ☑ Use an appropriate size catheter. A small catheter may leak; a large catheter may traumatize tissues.
- ☑ Provide perineal care before catheterization and for patients with an indwelling catheter. Use soap and water, rinsing carefully. Avoid pulling on an indwelling catheter.
- ☑ Do not drain more than 750 to 1,000 mL from the bladder at one time.
- ☑ Assess amount, color, clarity, and odor of urine. Collect a urine specimen as needed.
- ☑ Monitor intake and output.
- ☑ Secure tubing of an indwelling catheter to prevent trauma.
- ☑ Maintain gravity drainage; prevent loops of tubing or elevation of the drainage container higher than the bladder.
- ☑ Document procedure, results, and patient responses.

INFECTIOUS AND INFLAMMATORY DISORDERS

Urinary Tract Infections

> **Key Concept** Urinary tract infections (UTIs) are common among adult women and patients in hospitals and long-term care facilities. UTIs can lead to sepsis or chronic kidney disease, making prevention through patient and caregiver teaching a major nursing responsibility.

Urinary tract infections (UTIs) are common, leading to more than 7 million office visits per year (AUA Foundation, 2011). Women are more likely to experience UTI than men. About 40% of women and 12% of men report having at least one UTI during their lifetime. The incidence of UTI increases with aging in both sexes. Unfortunately, hospital-acquired infections are among the most common UTIs.

UTIs can affect any portion of the urinary tract, although **cystitis** (inflammation of the bladder) is the most common site of infection. They are broadly classified according to the region and primary site affected. Lower UTIs include *urethritis* (inflammation of the urethra), *prostatitis* (inflammation of the prostate gland), and cystitis. The most common upper UTI is **pyelonephritis** (inflammation of the kidney and renal pelvis).

PATHOPHYSIOLOGY AND MANIFESTATIONS

The urinary tract is normally sterile above the urethra. The most important factors that keep it sterile are adequate urine volume, unimpeded urine flow, and complete bladder emptying. Other defenses include acid urine, ureteral peristalsis, bacteriostatic properties of the urinary tract, and a *vesicoureteral junction* (where the ureters enter the bladder) that prevents backflow of urine toward the kidneys (Figure 29-2■). In males, a long urethra and the antibacterial effect of zinc in prostatic fluid are also important.

Bacteria from the intestines (most commonly *Escherichia coli*) often infect the urinary tract by ascending from the perineal tissues into the lower urinary tract. Changes in the urinary tract associated with aging further increase the risk for UTIs in older adults. Box 29-5■ lists risk factors for UTI.

Cystitis

Cystitis (inflammation of the urinary bladder) is the most common UTI. The bladder mucosa becomes inflamed and congested with blood. Pus may form, and the mucosa

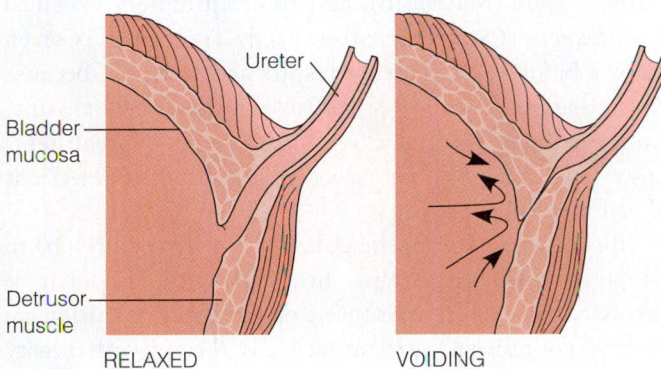

Figure 29-2. ■ Vesicoureteral junction. Note how the increased intravesical pressure during voiding occludes the distal portion of the ureter, preventing reflux.

BOX 29-5	RISK FACTORS FOR UTI

- Instrumentation of the urinary tract (e.g., catheterization, cystoscopy)
- Structural abnormalities, obstructions, or strictures
- Incomplete bladder emptying
- Chronic diseases such as diabetes

Females

- Short, straight urethra
- Proximity of urinary meatus to the vagina and anus
- Tissue trauma and possible contamination during sexual intercourse
- Use of a diaphragm for birth control
- Personal hygiene practices

Males

- An enlarged prostate gland

Older Adults

- More alkaline (less acid) urine
- Higher incidence of diabetes and glucosuria (glucose in the urine promotes bacterial growth)
- Incomplete bladder emptying, urinary retention
- Changes in vaginal pH in women; decreased prostatic secretions in men

may bleed. The inflammatory process causes the classic manifestations of cystitis (Box 29-6■). Older adults with UTI may be asymptomatic or may present with nocturia, incontinence, confusion, behavior change, lethargy, anorexia, or "just not feeling right."

Although cystitis is generally uncomplicated and often resolves spontaneously, the infection can ascend to involve the kidneys. In older adults or people with impaired immune responses, bacteremia, sepsis, and shock are possible serious complications.

Catheter-Associated UTI

Patients with indwelling urinary catheters are at significant risk for developing *bacteriuria*, bacteria in the urine. The longer the catheter remains in place, the greater the risk for infection. Bacteria reach the bladder by either migrating through urine within the catheter or moving up the urethra outside the catheter. Bacteria enter the catheter system at the connection between the catheter and drainage system or through the emptying tube of the drainage bag. Contamination of perineal skin by bacteria normally residing in the bowel is a common source of infection in catheterized women.

Catheter-associated UTIs are often asymptomatic and may not be recognized until the patient develops manifestations of systemic infection.

Pyelonephritis

Pyelonephritis is an inflammatory disorder affecting the renal pelvis and *parenchyma* (the functional portion of the kidney tissue). It may be acute, caused by a bacterial infection, or chronic, associated with other disorders.

Bacteria usually enter the kidney from the lower urinary tract. Risk factors include pregnancy (because of

BOX 29-6	MANIFESTATIONS OF UTI

Cystitis

- **Dysuria**—difficult or painful urination
- Frequency
- **Urgency**—a sudden, compelling need to urinate
- **Nocturia**—voiding two or more times at night
- **Pyuria**—presence of pus in the urine (cloudy appearance, foul odor)
- **Hematuria**—blood in the urine
- Lower abdominal (suprapubic) discomfort

Pyelonephritis

- Symptoms of cystitis
- Flank pain, costovertebral tenderness
- Vomiting, diarrhea
- Fever, shaking chills
- Malaise

slowed ureteral peristalsis), obstruction, and congenital malformation. *Vesicoureteral reflux* (a condition in which urine moves from the bladder back toward the kidney) is a common risk factor in children. It may occur in adults when bladder outflow is obstructed.

E. coli is responsible for most cases of acute pyelonephritis. The infection spreads from the renal pelvis to the cortex. The inflamed kidney becomes edematous. Localized abscesses may form, and the inflammatory process can destroy kidney tissue.

The onset of acute pyelonephritis is typically rapid, with chills and fever, malaise, and vomiting, as well as localized manifestations of flank pain and costovertebral tenderness (see Box 29-6). The patient may also have symptoms of cystitis. As with cystitis, older adults may present with a change in behavior, confusion, incontinence, or a general deterioration in condition.

Chronic pyelonephritis leads to fibrosis and scarring of the renal pelvis and calyces. The tubules are gradually destroyed. Chronic kidney disease is a possible consequence.

COLLABORATIVE CARE

Treatment of UTIs focuses on eliminating the cause, preventing relapse or reinfection, and identifying and correcting any contributing factors.

Diagnostic Tests

A *urinalysis* is ordered to identify blood cells and bacteria in the urine. A midstream, clean-catch urine specimen should be used. If necessary, urine may be obtained by a straight catheterization or "mini-cath," using aseptic technique. A urine *culture and sensitivity* may also be done to identify the causative organism. A *complete blood count (CBC) with differential* is done to assess for systemic responses to infection.

In men and in adult females with recurrent UTI, more extensive diagnostic testing may be done. An *intravenous pyelogram (IVP)* or CT scan is used to examine the kidneys, ureters, and bladder for abnormalities that may contribute to UTI. *Voiding cystourethrography* allows assessment of bladder and urethral abnormalities. *Cystoscopy* is used to diagnose conditions that may contribute to UTIs such as an enlarged prostate, urethral strictures, bladder stones, tumors, and congenital abnormalities.

Medications

An uncomplicated UTI is treated with a 3-day or a 7- to 10-day course of antibiotics. Drugs such as sulfonamides, *trimethoprim–sulfamethoxazole* (TMP–SMZ, Bactrim, Septra), *nitrofurantoin* (Macrobid), and fluoroquinolones such as *ciprofloxacin* (Cipro) are often used. Treatment is often started before urine culture results are obtained, because these drugs are effective against the usual organisms. Compliance is better with a 3-day course of treatment; however, it is not used for patients with recurrent infections or acute pyelonephritis.

In contrast, acute pyelonephritis usually requires 10 to 21 days of antibiotic therapy. Intravenous antibiotics may be necessary if the infection is severe or nausea and vomiting are present. For resistant or recurrent UTIs, therapy with urinary anti-infectives may last from 2 weeks to 6 or 12 months (Table 29-2■).

Other Therapies

Most catheter-associated UTIs are effectively treated by removing the catheter and administering a short course of antibiotic. Intermittent catheterization is a safer option than an indwelling catheter for patients who are unable to void or completely empty their bladder. Instilling anesthetic lubricating gel into the urethra before catheterization also reduces the risk of infection by reducing trauma to urethral tissues.

Complementary and alternative therapies to prevent and supplement treatment of UTI are presented in Box 29-7■.

NURSING CARE

PRIORITIZING NURSING CARE

Ensuring effective urinary elimination and treatment of the infection are nursing care priorities.

HEALTH PROMOTION

Teach measures to prevent UTI to all patients, particularly to young, sexually active women. Encourage a generous fluid intake of 2.0 to 2.5 quarts per day, increasing intake during hot weather or strenuous activity. Discuss the need to

TABLE 29-2	Giving Medications Safely: UTI		
CLASS/DRUGS	PURPOSE	NURSING RESPONSIBILITIES	PATIENT TEACHING
Sulfonamides ■ Sulfisoxazole (Gantrisin) ■ Sulfamethoxazole (Gantanol) ■ *Trimethoprim–sulfamethoxazole* (TMP–SMZ, Bactrim, Septra)	Sulfonamides are effective and inexpensive for treating UTIs. They are the drug of choice for most UTIs. They may be given alone or in combination with another antibiotic or with a urinary analgesic.	Assess for allergies to sulfa drugs. Stop the drug and notify the physician if a rash develops. Administer on an empty stomach, 1 hour before or 2 hours after meals, with a full glass of water. Assess for bruising, bleeding, fever, and signs of systemic infection. Assess for other drugs that may interact with sulfonamides. Closely monitor diabetic patients receiving oral hypoglycemic agents for hypoglycemic reactions.	Take all the medication as ordered. If you miss a dose, take it as soon as you can. Drink at least eight full glasses of water per day. Avoid cranberry juice. Notify your doctor if you are taking any other medications. If you are diabetic, monitor blood glucose closely. Do not take if you are pregnant or breastfeeding. Use sunscreen to reduce the risk of sunburn. Your urine may turn orange. This is harmless.
Urinary anti-infectives ■ Methenamine (Mandelamine, Hiprex) ■ Nalidixic acid (NegGram) ■ *Nitrofurantoin* (Furadantin, Macrodantin) ■ Trimethoprim (Proloprim, Trimpex)	Urinary anti-infectives are often used to prevent UTIs in patients with chronic infections. They may also be used if the patient is allergic or sensitive to commonly used antibiotics.	Ensure fluid intake of 1,500 to 2,000 mL/day. Give drug with meals to minimize GI side effects. Monitor liver and renal function studies. Monitor closely for adverse effects. Do not administer to pregnant patients. These drugs interact with many other medications. Monitor closely for adverse effects.	Continue taking these drugs even after symptoms have cleared. Drink six to eight glasses of water or fluid per day. Take with meals or food to minimize gastric upset. Do not take if you are pregnant or could become pregnant. Use sunscreen to prevent sunburn. Your urine may turn brown; this is not harmful.
Urinary analgesic ■ *Phenazopyridine* (*Pyridium*)	Phenazopyridine is a urinary analgesic that may be used to relieve pain, burning, frequency, and urgency associated with UTIs. It does not treat the infection and must be used along with antibiotic therapy.	Phenazopyridine stains the urine reddish orange. Yellow-tinged sclera or skin may indicate toxicity. Stop the drug and notify the physician. Do not give to patients with impaired renal function; monitor liver and kidney function tests.	Protect your clothing to prevent staining. Do not use for more than 24 to 48 hours. If symptoms continue, contact your doctor. If your skin or eyes appear yellow, stop taking the drug and notify the physician. Take the drug after meals to minimize gastric upset.

Note: Medications identified in *italics* are among the 200 most frequently prescribed drugs in the United States.

void when the urge is felt, emptying the bladder every 3 to 4 hours. Instruct women to cleanse the perineal area from front to back after voiding and defecating. Teach them to void before and after sexual intercourse to flush out bacteria introduced into the urethra and bladder. Advise women to avoid bubble baths, feminine hygiene sprays, and vaginal douches that may dry perineal tissues. Wearing cotton briefs and avoiding underwear made of synthetic materials is also helpful. Postmenopausal women may benefit from hormone replacement therapy or estrogen cream. Unless contraindicated, suggest consuming two or more glasses of low-sugar cranberry juice daily.

BOX 29-7 COMPLEMENTARY THERAPIES

Preventing UTIs

Cranberry products are effective in preventing UTI, especially in women with recurrent UTIs. Cranberry interferes with the ability of bacteria to attach to epithelial cells in the urinary tract. Juice appears to be more effective than cranberry capsules, particularly when consumed more than twice a day (Brown, 2012). Blueberries contain a compound that prevents bacteria from attaching to the bladder wall to cause cystitis as well. Bilberry (a relative of the blueberry) is also recommended and is available as an herbal extract in capsules. Saw palmetto is another herbal urinary anti-infective used primarily by men with prostate enlargement. Bromelain (an enzyme derived from pineapple) may increase the effectiveness of antibiotic therapy for treating UTIs. Vitamin C supplements can help treat and prevent UTIs. Dietary changes to prevent UTIs include reduced intake of sugar, alcohol, and fat.

ASSESSING

It is important to collect both subjective and objective assessment data from patients with a suspected or confirmed UTI. These data provide information that can be used to help the patient recover fully from the infection and prevent future UTIs.

- *Subjective data:* symptoms, including onset and duration; associated symptoms (abdominal or back pain, fever, nausea, or vomiting); previous UTIs, including frequency and treatment; current method of birth control, possibility of pregnancy; chronic diseases, medications, recent lifestyle changes (e.g., recent marriage or a new sexual relationship); hygiene practices (perineal cleansing after elimination, use of feminine hygiene sprays or bubble baths)
- *Objective data:* vital signs, including temperature; general appearance and apparent state of health; lower abdominal or costovertebral tenderness; obtain clean-catch midstream urine specimen
- *Laboratory studies:* WBC and differential; urinalysis and culture; serum glucose as indicated

IDENTIFYING POTENTIAL COMPLICATIONS

Significant systemic symptoms such as chills, fever, nausea, and vomiting may indicate sepsis from untreated or ineffectively treated UTI and should immediately be reported to the health care provider. Manifestations of early septic shock (tachycardia, low urine output, dizziness) may develop with overwhelming sepsis. Remember that the skin may be flushed and warm in early septic shock due to fever.

DIAGNOSING, PLANNING, AND IMPLEMENTING

UTI interferes with comfort and normal patterns of urination. If not effectively treated, the infection can ascend to the kidneys and lead to chronic kidney problems.

Impaired Urinary Elimination

Expected outcome: Will regain usual patterns of urinary elimination.

- Monitor urinary output and color, clarity, and character of urine, including odor. *The patient with a UTI often experiences dysuria, frequency, urgency, and nocturia. Urine may appear rusty or blood tinged, cloudy, and malodorous. Urine normally returns to clear yellow within 48 hours. If it does not, report to the charge nurse or physician.*
- Provide for easy access to a bedpan, urinal, commode, or bathroom. Make sure lighting is adequate and pathways are clear. *Frequency, urgency, and nocturia increase the risk of urinary incontinence and injury due to falls.*
- Encourage fluid intake unless contraindicated. Tell the patient to avoid caffeinated drinks. *Increased fluid dilutes urine, reducing irritation of the inflamed bladder and mucosa. Caffeine can increase bladder spasms and mucosal irritation.*

Readiness for Enhanced Self-Health Management

Expected outcome: Will complete prescribed treatment regimen within expected timeframe.

- Work with the patient to develop a plan for taking medications, such as taking them with meals (unless contraindicated) or setting out all doses for the day in the morning. *Missed doses of antibiotic can result in subtherapeutic blood levels and reduced effectiveness and development of drug-resistant bacteria. Taking medication in association with a regular daily activity such as meals helps patients to remember doses.*
- Instruct to complete the full course of antibiotic therapy even though symptoms resolve rapidly. Explain that noncompliance can lead to recurrent infection and potential long-term problems. *Although symptoms may be relieved within 1 to 2 days, this may not be adequate time to eliminate bacteria from the urinary tract.*
- Instruct to keep appointments for follow-up and urine culture. *Follow-up urine culture, scheduled 1 to 3 days after single-dose therapy and 7 to 14 days after conventional therapy, is vital to ensure complete eradication of bacteria and to prevent relapse or recurrence.*

CONTINUITY OF CARE

Because both upper and lower UTIs are usually managed in the community, teaching is the most important nursing intervention. Teach patients and their families about the risk factors that contribute to UTIs. Discuss measures to prevent future UTIs:

- Empty bladder at least every 2 to 4 hours while awake. Avoid voluntary urinary retention.
- Maintain intake of 2 to 2.5 quarts or 8 to 10 glasses of fluid per day.

- Complete the prescribed treatment and keep follow-up appointments. Failure to do so increases the risk of unresolved and recurrent infections.
- Unless contraindicated, drink two or more glasses of cranberry juice per day and consume blueberries regularly.

Like many infectious processes, UTI often occurs when immune defenses are low. Inform patient that lack of adequate rest, poor nutrition, and high levels of emotional stress are often associated with UTIs. Discuss possible lifestyle changes to reduce future risk for UTIs. Teach patients to identify the early manifestations of UTIs, and stress the importance of seeking medical intervention promptly.

The patient with an indwelling urinary catheter is at continued risk for UTIs. Provide information about alternatives such as scheduled toileting, incontinence pads or diapers, and external catheters. Teach the patient with urinary retention or a family member to perform straight catheterization every 3 to 4 hours using clean technique (see Box 29-3). If no alternative to an indwelling catheter is feasible, teach patients and their families how to care for the catheter. This includes perineal care, managing and emptying the collection bag, maintaining a closed system, and bladder irrigation or flushing if ordered. Stress the importance of maintaining a generous fluid intake and supporting immune function to prevent upper UTI.

Glomerulonephritis

> **Key Concept** Glomerular disorders cause loss of proteins and blood cells in the urine, decrease the glomerular filtration rate, and affect urine formation and waste elimination. Depending on the cause, the patient may recover fully or may eventually develop chronic kidney disease and end-stage renal failure.

Disorders and diseases involving the glomerulus and nephron are the leading cause of chronic kidney disease in the United States. The glomerulus is a tuft of capillaries surrounded by the glomerular capsule. Filtration, the first critical step in urine formation, occurs in this portion of the nephron. **Glomerulonephritis** is an inflammatory condition that primarily affects the glomerulus. It may be an acute or a chronic disorder. Glomerulonephritis may be a primary kidney disorder or may develop secondarily to a systemic disease such as lupus erythematosus.

PATHOPHYSIOLOGY AND MANIFESTATIONS

Glomerulonephritis affects both the structure and function of the glomerulus. It damages the capillary membrane, allowing blood cells and proteins to escape from the vascular compartment into the filtrate. *Hematuria* (blood in the urine) may be either gross or microscopic. **Proteinuria**

(protein in the urine) increases progressively with increased glomerular damage. Loss of plasma proteins in the urine causes *hypoalbuminemia* (low levels of albumin in the blood). Edema develops as a result, caused by reduced osmotic draw within blood vessels.

When glomerular filtration is disrupted, the glomerular filtration rate (GFR) falls and **azotemia** (increased blood levels of nitrogenous wastes, including urea and creatinine) occurs. The fall in GFR activates the renin–angiotensin–aldosterone system, leading to salt and water retention and hypertension (Figure 29-3■).

Acute Glomerulonephritis

Acute glomerulonephritis usually follows an infection with group A beta-hemolytic *Streptococcus,* such as strep throat. Immune complexes become trapped in the glomerular membrane, causing an inflammatory response and drawing WBCs to the area. Inflammation damages the glomerular capillary walls and makes them more porous. Plasma proteins and blood cells escape into the urine (Figure 29-4■). The inflammatory response also obstructs glomerular capillaries, impairing blood flow and reducing the GFR. Both kidneys are involved. This is primarily a disease of childhood, but it can affect adults.

Manifestations of acute glomerulonephritis typically develop abruptly, 10 to 14 days after the initial infection (Box 29-8■). Older adults may have fewer symptoms. Nausea, malaise, arthralgias, and proteinuria are common manifestations; hypertension and edema, commonly present in children and younger adults, are seen less often in older adults.

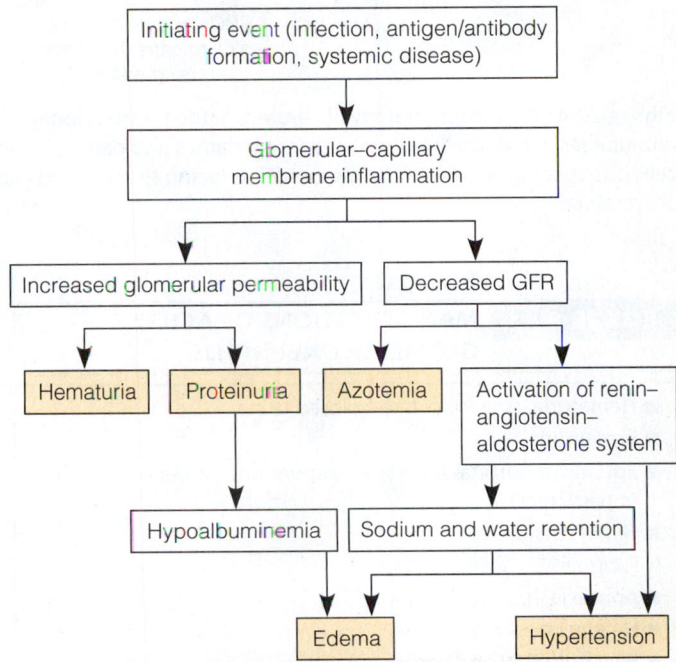

Figure 29-3. ■ The pathophysiology of glomerulonephritis.

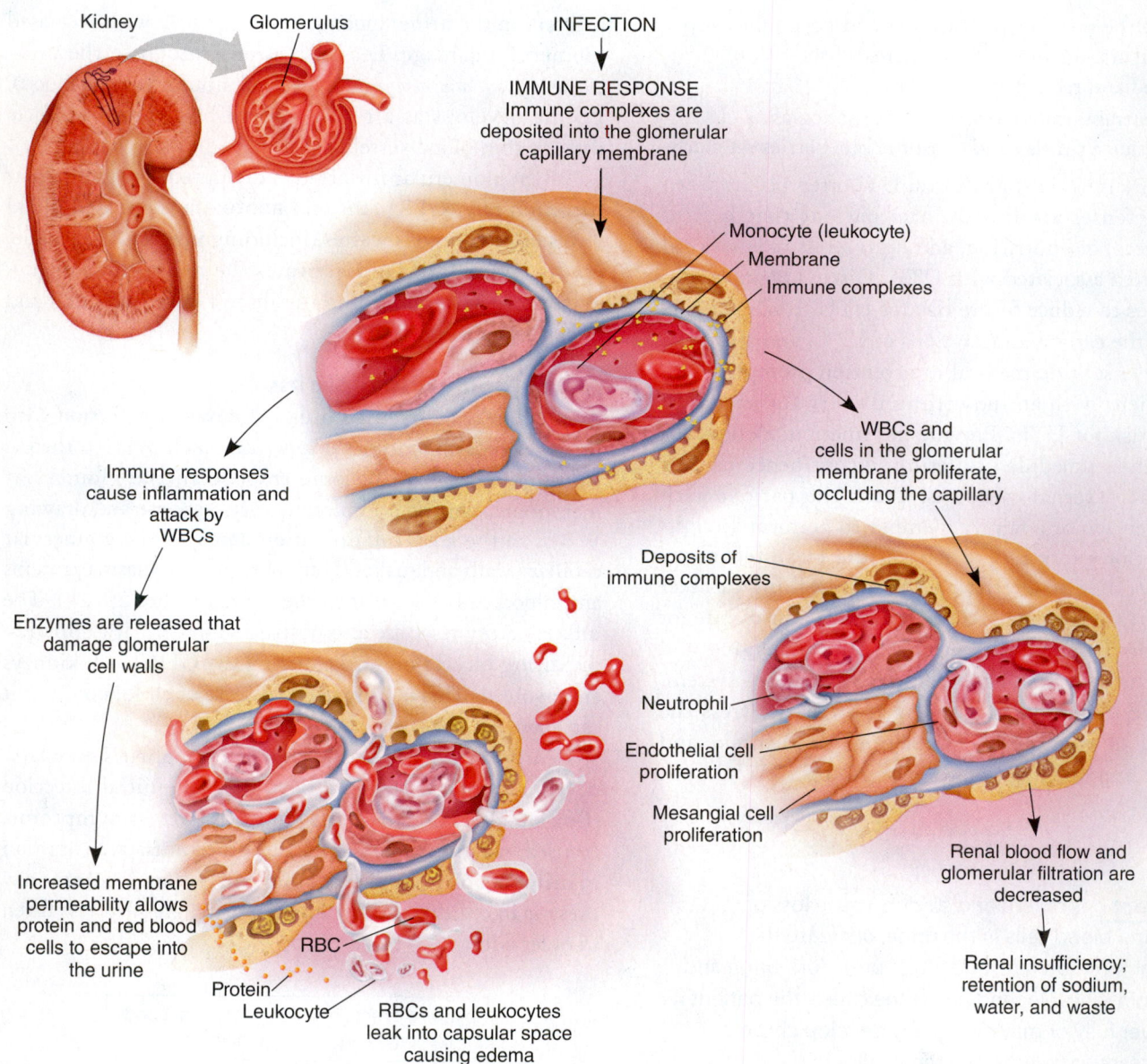

Kidney   Glomerulus

INFECTION

IMMUNE RESPONSE
Immune complexes are
deposited into the glomerular
capillary membrane

Monocyte (leukocyte)
Membrane
Immune complexes

WBCs and
cells in the glomerular
membrane proliferate,
occluding the capillary

Immune responses
cause inflammation and
attack by
WBCs

Enzymes are released that
damage glomerular
cell walls

Deposits of
immune complexes

Neutrophil

Endothelial cell
proliferation

Mesangial cell
proliferation

Increased membrane
permeability allows
protein and red blood
cells to escape into
the urine

RBC

Protein

Leukocyte

RBCs and leukocytes
leak into capsular space
causing edema

Renal blood flow and
glomerular filtration are
decreased

Renal insufficiency;
retention of sodium,
water, and waste

Figure 29-4. ■ Pathophysiology Illustrated: Acute Glomerulonephritis. Infection with group A beta-hemolytic *Streptococcus* causes an immune response. The immune response inflames and damages the glomeruli. Protein and RBCs escape through the glomeruli. Damaged cells obstruct blood flow to the glomeruli, reducing the GFR and causing renal insufficiency. As a result, sodium, water, and waste products are retained.

BOX 29-8	MANIFESTATIONS OF ACUTE GLOMERULONEPHRITIS

- Hematuria; cola- or coffee-colored urine
- Proteinuria
- Edema: periorbital and facial; dependent (upper extremities in particular)
- Hypertension
- Fatigue
- Anorexia, nausea, vomiting
- Headache
- Elevated BUN and serum creatinine

The symptoms may subside spontaneously within 10 to 14 days. Most people recover completely, but about 40% of adults develop chronic glomerulonephritis, never regaining full kidney function.

Nephrotic Syndrome

Nephrotic syndrome is not a disease but a group of symptoms. It results when glomerular tissues are damaged and there is significant protein lost in the urine. There is no one cause of nephrotic syndrome. In adults, it may result from a primary kidney disorder or a systemic disease such as diabetes or lupus.

Patients with nephrotic syndrome have proteinuria, low serum albumin levels, high blood lipids, and edema. Edema may be severe, affecting the face and periorbital area as well as dependent tissues (Figure 29-5■). *Thromboemboli* (mobilized blood clots) are a relatively common complication of nephrotic syndrome. Peripheral veins and arteries, pulmonary arteries, and renal veins may be occluded.

Nephrotic syndrome may resolve without long-term effects, although adults are less likely to recover completely than children. Many have persistent proteinuria and progressive renal impairment that may eventually lead to kidney failure.

Chronic Glomerulonephritis

Chronic glomerulonephritis is usually the result of kidney damage by a systemic disease such as diabetes. In many cases, however, no previous kidney disease or apparent cause can be identified. Chronic glomerulonephritis is characterized by slow, progressive destruction of glomeruli and nephrons. The kidneys decrease in size, and their surfaces become granular or rough as nephrons are destroyed.

Symptoms develop slowly, and the disease is often not recognized until signs of renal failure are evident. Kidney failure may develop years to decades after the disease is diagnosed.

DIABETIC NEPHROPATHY   *Diabetic nephropathy* is kidney disease that is common in the later stages of diabetes mellitus. It is the leading cause of chronic kidney disease in the United States. Initial evidence of kidney damage is typically seen 10 to 15 years after the onset of diabetes. Chronic kidney disease develops within 15 to 20 years of the initial diagnosis. In diabetic nephropathy, damage to the glomerulus impairs filtration and waste elimination.

COLLABORATIVE CARE

Care of the patient with acute or chronic glomerulonephritis focuses on identifying and treating the underlying disease process and preserving kidney function. In most cases, there is no specific treatment to achieve a cure.

Diagnostic Tests

Laboratory tests may help determine the cause of glomerulonephritis and evaluate its effects on kidney function. *Throat* or *skin cultures* are done to identify possible streptococcal infection. An *antistreptolysin-O (ASO) titer* identifies antibodies to group A beta-hemolytic streptococci.

The *BUN* and *serum creatinine* levels increase in kidney disease. The *eGFR* and *creatinine clearance,* very specific indicators of renal function and the GFR, fall. *Serum electrolytes* show the effect of impaired kidney function on fluid and electrolyte balance.

A *urinalysis* is done to identify blood cells and protein in the urine. A 24-hour urine specimen may be ordered to measure protein and creatinine in the urine.

In addition, a *renal ultrasound* may be done to evaluate kidney size. A *kidney scan* (see Table 28-5) or *biopsy* may also be ordered. Nursing care for a patient undergoing a kidney biopsy is outlined in Box 29-9■.

Medications

There is no specific drug treatment for glomerulonephritis. Penicillin or other antibiotics may be ordered for the patient with poststreptococcal glomerulonephritis to kill any remaining bacteria. Antihypertensives are prescribed to maintain the blood pressure within normal levels. Blood pressure management is important because hypertension is associated with a poorer prognosis in patients with glomerular disorders. Angiotensin-converting enzyme (ACE) inhibitors or angiotensin-receptor blockers (ARBs) have a protective effect on the kidney in patients with glomerular disorders and may be ordered. Glucocorticoids (e.g., prednisone) or other immunosuppressive drugs may be used with some types of acute glomerulonephritis or nephrotic syndrome to reduce the risk of kidney failure.

Drugs are avoided that are known to be nephrotoxic (damaging to the kidney), such as some antibiotics, x-ray contrast dyes, and nonsteroidal anti-inflammatory drugs (NSAIDs).

Plasma Exchange Therapy

Plasma exchange therapy (plasmapheresis) removes harmful antibodies in the plasma by passing the blood through a blood cell separator and reinfusing the red blood cells

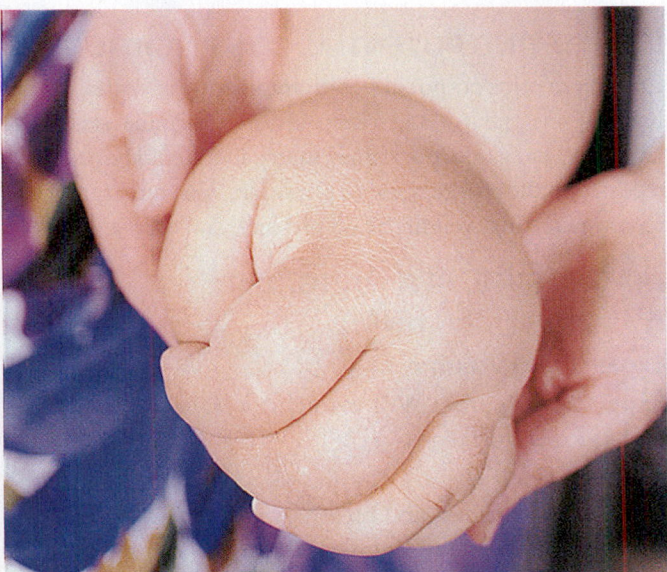

Figure 29-5. ■ Severe edema in a patient with nephrotic syndrome. (Source: Alain McLaughlin, Pearson Education.)

BOX 29-9 **NURSING CARE CHECKLIST**

Kidney Biopsy

Nursing Care

☑ Informed consent is required. Clarify and reinforce teaching.

☑ Withhold food and fluids for 8 hours before the procedure.

☑ After the procedure, apply pressure dressing and position supine to maintain pressure on the biopsy site.

☑ Monitor closely for bleeding during the first 24 hours after the procedure:

  ☑ Check vital signs frequently. Report tachycardia, hypotension, or other signs of shock.

  ☑ Monitor the biopsy site for bleeding.

  ☑ Check hemoglobin and hematocrit, comparing with preprocedure values.

  ☑ Report complaints of flank or back pain, shoulder pain, pallor, light-headedness.

  ☑ Monitor urine output. Initial hematuria should clear within 24 hours.

☑ Report manifestations of abdominal pain, guarding, and decreased bowel sounds.

☑ Encourage fluids.

Patient and Family Teaching

☑ Local anesthesia is used. The procedure may be uncomfortable but should not be painful.

☑ When the needle is inserted, you will be instructed to hold your breath.

☑ The entire procedure takes about 10 minutes.

☑ Avoid coughing for 24 hours after the procedure. Avoid strenuous activity such as heavy lifting for about 2 weeks after the procedure.

☑ Report symptoms such as flank, back, shoulder, or abdominal pain or light-headedness to your doctor because they may indicate a complication.

(RBCs) with an equal amount of albumin or plasma. It may be used to treat acute glomerulonephritis. This procedure is usually done in a series rather than a one-time-only treatment. Informed consent is required for this procedure.

Dietary Management

When edema is significant or the patient is hypertensive, sodium intake may be restricted. Dietary proteins may be increased when protein is being lost in the urine. However, if azotemia is present, dietary protein is restricted. Patients with nephrotic syndrome are placed on a low-sodium diet, often with a moderate protein restriction. When proteins are restricted, those included should be complete proteins such as meat, fish, eggs, soy, or poultry. These proteins supply all the essential amino acids required for growth and tissue maintenance.

NURSING CARE

PRIORITIZING NURSING CARE

Because there is no specific treatment for glomerulonephritis, nursing care focuses on the effects of the disorder on the patient's comfort and ability to maintain activities of daily living (ADLs).

HEALTH PROMOTION

Advise effective treatment of streptococcal infections in all age groups to help reduce the risk for acute glomerulonephritis. Stress the importance of completing the full course of antibiotic therapy to eradicate bacteria. Teach patients with diabetes about the risk for kidney damage. Discuss measures to reduce the risk, such as effectively managing blood glucose levels, treating hypertension, and avoiding drugs and substances that are potentially damaging to the kidneys.

ASSESSING

Assessment data provide valuable clues about the cause and effects of glomerulonephritis on the patient. Inquire about the onset and duration of manifestations such as changes in urine output or color, weight gain or edema, and other symptoms such as nausea and vomiting. Ask about recent sore throat or other infection and its treatment. Note any history of previous kidney disorders, UTIs, or chronic diseases such as diabetes or lupus. Have the patient identify all current medications.

Obtain the vital signs and weight. Note any edema, particularly of the face, around the eyes, or of the upper extremities. Inspect the throat and skin for evidence of infection. Obtain a urine specimen, and note the color, clarity, and character of the urine. Review laboratory data such as the serum creatinine, BUN, eGFR, and creatinine clearance.

IDENTIFYING POTENTIAL COMPLICATIONS

Changes in urine output (a significant increase or decrease, fixed low specific gravity) and rising serum creatinine and BUN levels may indicate acute kidney injury and should be promptly reported to the charge nurse or physician. Also monitor for and report increasing weight, blood pressure, and edema.

DIAGNOSING, PLANNING, AND IMPLEMENTING

Excess Fluid Volume

Expected outcome: Will maintain weight and vital signs within expected range.

■ Monitor vital signs, including blood pressure, apical pulse, respirations, and breath sounds, at least every 4 hours. Report any significant changes. *Excess fluid volume increases the workload of the heart and the blood pressure. Tachycardia or dysrhythmias may be present. Tachypnea, dyspnea, and crackles may be noted.*

- Record intake and output (I&O) every 4 to 8 hours or more frequently as indicated. *Accurate I&O records help determine fluid volume status.*
- Weigh daily under consistent conditions. *Daily weights are an accurate indicator of fluid volume status.*
- Assess location and degree of edema. *Edema associated with glomerulonephritis often affects low-pressure tissues such as the face, around the eyes, and the upper extremities.*
- Arrange dietary consultation to plan the diet when sodium is restricted and when proteins are either restricted or increased. *Providing appealing foods can help maintain adequate nutrition despite anorexia and nausea.*
- Provide frequent position changes and good skin care. *Tissue perfusion may be altered by edema, increasing the risk of skin breakdown.*

Fatigue

Expected outcome: Will balance activity and rest and use energy-conserving measures when performing ADLs.

- Provide for rest by scheduling procedures and activities. Assist with ADLs as needed. *Rest reduces fatigue and improves the patient's ability to tolerate and cope with treatments and activities. The goal is to conserve limited energy reserves.*
- Teach the patient and family about the relationship between fatigue and the disease process. Limit visitors and visit length. *Understanding the cause of fatigue helps the patient and family to cope with reduced energy and comply with prescribed rest.*

Risk for Infection

Expected outcome: Will remain free of signs and symptoms of infection.

- Monitor temperature, pulse, and mental status every 4 hours. *Fever, elevated pulse, increasing lethargy, or confusion may be early signs of infection.*
- Assess frequently for other signs of infection, such as purulent wound drainage, productive cough, abnormal breath sounds, and red or inflamed lesions. Monitor for indications of UTIs such as dysuria, frequency and urgency, and cloudy, foul-smelling urine. *Infection may be masked by the prescribed drugs. Frequent assessment allows early identification.*
- Practice good hand washing. Provide a private room and restrict ill visitors. *Drugs used to treat acute glomerulonephritis may reduce the ability to resist infection.*

Ineffective Role Performance

Expected outcome: Will identify strategies to meet role expectations within prescribed activity limits.

Activity may be limited to minimize proteinuria. Fatigue and muscle weakness may limit physical and social activities. In addition, facial edema affects self-concept and may lead to isolation.

- Encourage self-care and participation in decision making. *Increased autonomy helps to restore self-confidence and reduce powerlessness.*
- Support coping measures, helping identify personal strengths. Whenever possible, enlist the support of family, other patients, and friends. *This support helps the patient gain confidence and provide physical, psychologic, emotional, and social support.*
- Discuss the effect of the disease and treatments on roles and relationships. Help the patient and family develop a plan to deal with potential changes and maintain usual roles to the extent possible. *Planning ahead reduces stress and helps the patient and family maintain a sense of control.*
- Refer to social services and support groups as needed. *Groups can help the patient and family cope with and adapt to the disease.*

MANAGING NURSING CARE

As appropriate and allowed by the designated duties and responsibilities of assistive personnel, the nurse may assign nursing care activities such as measuring vital signs and intake and output, obtaining daily weights, and assisting with daily activities for the patient with glomerulonephritis.

EVALUATING

To evaluate the effectiveness of nursing care for the patient with glomerulonephritis, collect data such as:

- Weight, presence of edema, and skin integrity; freedom from infection.
- Ability to follow, prepare, and consume the prescribed diet.
- Planning for additional rest and modification of usual roles and relationships.

DOCUMENTING

Document continuing assessment data and trends in symptoms, objective data, and laboratory results. Also document all teaching and the patient's and family's apparent understanding and acceptance of the information and treatment plan.

CONTINUITY OF CARE

Glomerulonephritis may be self-limiting or progressive. Its course ranges from weeks to years. Self-management is essential, necessitating a good understanding of the disorder and treatment regimen.

Teach about the disease and prognosis. Discuss the prescribed treatment, including activity and diet restrictions. Provide information about the use and potential effects, both beneficial and adverse, of all prescribed medications. Discuss the importance of contacting the physician before taking any other medications. It is vital to avoid drugs that are potentially toxic to the kidneys. Discuss the risks, manifestations, prevention, and management of complications such as edema and infection. Because the patient and family may be monitoring kidney status to a certain extent themselves, teach the signs, symptoms, and implications of improving or declining renal function.

NURSING CARE PLAN
Patient With Acute Glomerulonephritis

Jung-Lin Chang is a 23-year-old graduate student who goes to the university health center when he notices that his urine is brown and foamy. The physician admits him to the infirmary and orders a throat culture, ASO titer, CBC, BUN, serum creatinine, and urinalysis.

Assessment

Connie King, the admitting nurse, notes that Mr. Chang's history is negative for past kidney or urinary problems. He states that he had a "pretty bad" sore throat a couple of weeks ago. He took a few antibiotics he had left from a previous bout of strep throat, increased his fluids, and did not see a doctor. The sore throat resolved, and he felt well until noticing the change in his urine. He thought the puffiness around his eyes was due to lack of sleep and fatigue. He has eaten little the past 2 days.

Assessment findings include BP 136/90, P 98, R 18, and T 98.8°F (37.1°C) PO; weight 165 lb (75 kg), up from his normal of 160 lb (72.5 kg); and moderate periorbital edema and edema of his hands and fingers.

Lab results show a negative throat culture but high ASO titer. His CBC is normal, BUN 42 mg/dL, and serum creatinine 2.1 mg/dL. Urinalysis shows the presence of protein, RBCs, and RBC casts. A subsequent 24-hour urine contains 1,025 mg of protein, compared with the normal of 30 to 150 mg/24 hr.

Mr. Chang is diagnosed with acute poststreptococcal glomerulonephritis. His orders include bed rest with bathroom privileges, fluid restriction (1,200 mL/day), and a low-sodium diet.

Nursing Diagnosis

- *Excess Fluid Volume* related to plasma protein loss and sodium and water retention
- *Risk for Imbalanced Nutrition: Less Than Body Requirements* related to anorexia
- *Anxiety* related to prescribed activity restriction
- *Deficient Knowledge: Glomerulonephritis* related to lack of information

Expected Outcomes

The expected outcomes for the plan of care are that Mr. Chang will:

- Maintain blood pressure within normal limits.

- Return to usual weight with no evidence of edema.
- Consume adequate calories, following prescribed dietary limitations.
- Verbalize less anxiety regarding ability to continue with his program of study.
- Demonstrate an understanding of acute glomerulonephritis and his prescribed management regimen.

Planning and Implementation

- Monitor vital signs every 4 hours. Notify the physician of significant changes.
- Record intake and output every 8 hours.
- Schedule fluids: 650 mL day shift, 450 mL evening shift, and 100 mL night shift.
- Weigh daily.
- Arrange for dietary consultation.
- Provide small meals with high-carbohydrate snacks.
- Encourage Mr. Chang to talk about his condition and its potential effects.
- Enlist friends and family to listen and provide support.
- Teach about acute glomerulonephritis and prescribed management regimen.
- Instruct in the appropriate use of antibiotics.

Evaluation

Mr. Chang is released from the infirmary after 4 days. He decides to return to his parents' home for the 6 to 12 weeks of convalescence prescribed by his doctor.

Mr. Chang's renal function gradually returns to normal with no further azotemia and minimal proteinuria after 4 months. He verbalizes an understanding of the relationship between the episode of strep throat, his inappropriate use of antibiotics, and the glomerulonephritis. He says, "I may not always remember to take every pill on time in the future, but I sure won't save them for the next time again!"

Critical Thinking in the Nursing Process

1. How did Mr. Chang's use of "a few" previously prescribed antibiotics to treat his sore throat affect his risk for developing poststreptococcal glomerulonephritis?
2. What additional risk factors did Mr. Chang have for developing glomerulonephritis?
3. What teaching should the nurse provide to reduce his risk for future episodes of acute glomerulonephritis?

Note: Discussion of Critical Thinking questions appears on the companion website.

OBSTRUCTIVE DISORDERS

Key Concept   The urinary tract can be affected by obstructive processes such as stones and tumors. Early recognition of obstructive processes and restoring unobstructed urinary output are critical to maintain kidney function.

Kidney Stones

Stones (or *calculi*) can affect any portion of the urinary tract, obstructing urine flow (Figure 29-6■). **Urolithiasis** (development of stones within the urinary tract) is the most common cause of obstructed urine flow. In the United States, stones most commonly form within the kidney (*nephrolithiasis*). Males are affected by kidney stones more often than females by a 4:1 ratio. Risk factors for kidney stones include personal or family history of urinary stones; dehydration; excess calcium, oxalate, or protein intake; gout; hyperparathyroidism; or urinary stasis. In other parts of the world, bladder stones are common. Here, bladder stones usually develop only in patients requiring an indwelling catheter for extended periods of time.

PATHOPHYSIOLOGY

Calculi (stones) are masses of crystals formed from materials normally excreted in the urine. Most are made of calcium. Stones form when a poorly soluble salt (e.g., calcium phosphate) crystallizes. When the concentration of the salt in the urine is very high, very little stimulus is needed to start crystallization. A meal high in the mineral or decreased fluid intake, as occurs during sleep, may prompt stone formation. When fluid intake is adequate, no stone growth occurs. Stone development is also affected by the pH of the urine and naturally occurring compounds that inhibit stone development.

Calcium stones are often associated with hypercalcemia. Risk factors for calcium stones include hyperparathyroidism and immobility (which causes calcium to move out of the bones into the bloodstream), as well as alkaline urine and dehydration.

MANIFESTATIONS AND COMPLICATIONS

Manifestations of urinary calculi are due to obstructed urine flow, distention, and tissue damage from the rough-edged stone. Symptoms vary by stone location (Box 29-10■). Stones at any level may cause manifestations of UTI, including chills and fever, frequency, urgency, and dysuria.

Urinary tract obstruction by a kidney stone may cause few symptoms if it develops slowly. Acute obstruction causes severe pain in the flank region, possibly radiating to the genitals. If the obstruction is not relieved, the kidney may be damaged. Urine production continues; however, the obstruction blocks its outflow from the kidney to the bladder or from the bladder out. This leads to increased pressure and distention of the urinary tract behind the obstruction. *Hydronephrosis* (discussed in the next section of this chapter) and *hydroureter* (distention of the ureter with urine) may result. Impaired urine excretion also increases the risk of infection.

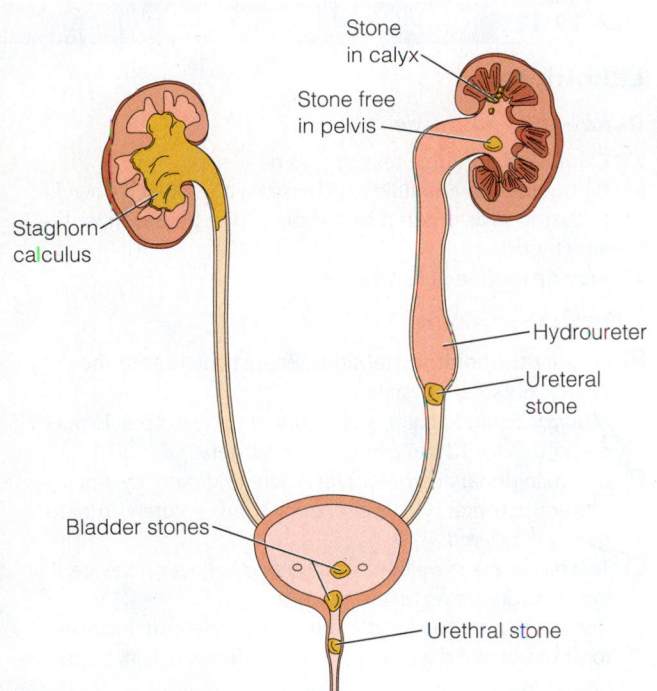

BOX 29-10	MANIFESTATIONS OF URINARY STONES

Kidney Pelvis
- May be asymptomatic
- Dull, aching flank pain

Ureter
- **Renal colic**: Acute, severe, intermittent flank pain on affected side
- Pain radiating to suprapubic region, groin, and scrotum or labia
- Nausea, vomiting
- Pallor; cool, clammy skin
- Microscopic hematuria

Bladder
- May be asymptomatic
- Dull suprapubic pain
- Microscopic or gross hematuria

Figure 29-6. ■ Potential locations of stones within the urinary tract.

COLLABORATIVE CARE
Diagnostic Tests

Diagnostic tests are used to confirm the diagnosis and determine the type of stone. A *urinalysis* is done to detect hematuria. Any stones passed are analyzed to identify their composition. The nurse is often responsible for retrieving stones. All urine is strained and may be saved. Any visible stones or sediment is sent for analysis.

A *KUB x-ray* is done to identify the presence of calculi in the kidneys, ureters, and bladder. *IVP, renal ultrasound, CT scan,* or *MRI* may be used to locate calculi and identify hydroureter or hydronephrosis. *Cystoscopy* is used to visualize and possibly remove calculi from the urinary bladder and distal ureters.

Medications

Pain relief is vital for acute renal colic. Narcotic analgesics are used to provide analgesia and relieve ureteral spasms. Analgesics are often administered intravenously for rapid pain relief. Indomethacin (an NSAID) in suppository form can reduce the amount of narcotic analgesia required. An oral alpha-adrenergic blocker such as tamsulosin (Flomax) is prescribed to relax ureteral muscle and promote passage of the stone.

After stone analysis, medications may be prescribed to prevent further stone formation. Thiazide diuretics are frequently ordered for calcium stones. They reduce urinary calcium excretion and can prevent future stones.

Food and Fluid Management

The diet may be modified to prevent further stone formation. Fluid intake is increased to 2.5 to 3 L per day to prevent concentration of stone-forming salts. Intake should be spaced throughout the day and evening. The patient may be advised to drink one to two glasses of water at night to maintain dilute urine during sleep.

Foods that contributed to stone formation may be limited in the diet. For calcium stones, however, restricting calcium intake may actually increase the risk of stone formation while also promoting bone loss. A low-sodium, restricted-protein diet is more effective in preventing recurrence of calcium stones. Oxalate, found in foods such as spinach, nuts, and chocolate, may be limited in patients found to have calcium oxalate stones. Organ meats, sardines, and other high-purine foods are eliminated from the diet of patients who form stones containing uric acid.

Surgery

Stones that are too large to be passed spontaneously (>5 mm in diameter) may require removal. *Lithotripsy* (crushing of calculi using sound or shock waves) is the preferred treatment. It may be done by laser or using an external lithotriptor device. In *extracorporeal shock-wave*

lithotripsy (ESWL), shock waves generated outside the body are directed at the stone (Figure 29-7■). These shock waves travel harmlessly through soft tissue but pulverize the stone into fragments that are small enough to be eliminated in the urine. Box 29-11■ outlines nursing care for patients having a lithotripsy.

Stones in the renal pelvis or calyces may require nephrostomy for removal. A small incision is made in the flank, and a nephroscope is inserted to visualize the renal pelvis. The stones may then be removed or crushed. With *percutaneous lithotripsy,* the stone is fragmented using a small ultrasonic transducer or a laser beam (Figure 29-8■). Fragments

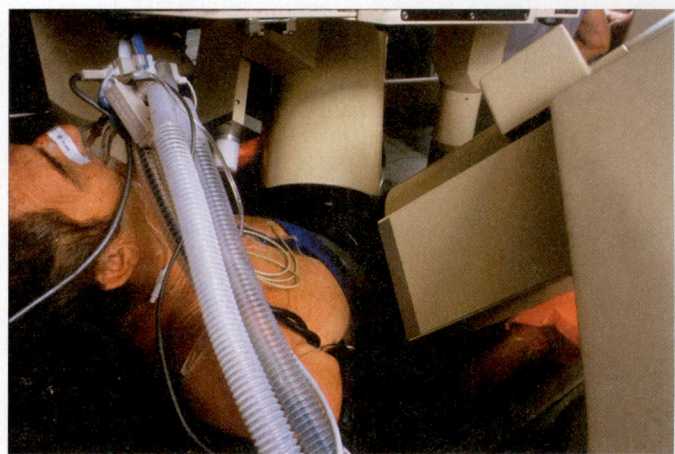

Figure 29-7. ■ Extracorporeal shock-wave lithotripsy. Energy pulses created by the generator travel through soft tissue to shatter the kidney stone into fragments, which are then eliminated in the urine. (Source: © SIU Biomed Com/Custom Medical Stock Photo.)

BOX 29-11	NURSING CARE CHECKLIST

Lithotripsy

Before the Procedure

- ☑ Clarify and reinforce teaching as needed.
- ☑ Withhold food and fluids and assist with or teach bowel preparation as ordered by radiology, the physician, or the anesthetist.
- ☑ Provide routine preoperative care.

After the Procedure

- ☑ Frequently monitor vital signs. Report changes to the charge nurse or physician.
- ☑ Monitor amount, color, and clarity of urine output. Expect hematuria for 12 to 72 hours after surgery.
- ☑ Maintain urinary catheter placement and patency. Anchor ureteral catheters or nephrostomy tubes securely. Irrigate gently if ordered.
- ☑ Teach care of indwelling catheter and collection device. If an incision was made, teach site care.
- ☑ Instruct patient to report drainage of urine from incision for more than 4 days, symptoms of infection, pain, bright hematuria.
- ☑ Teach measures to reduce the risk of further stone formation.

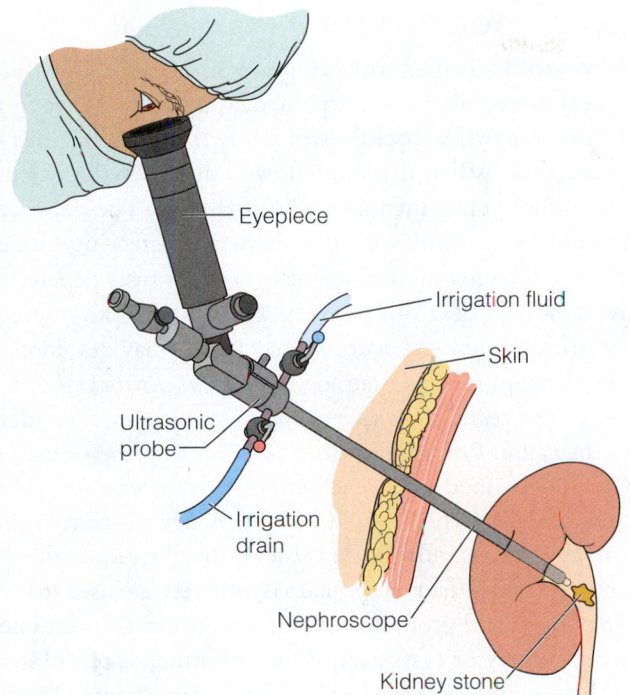

Figure 29-8. ■ Percutaneous lithotripsy. A nephroscope is inserted through the skin into the renal pelvis, and the stone is fragmented using ultrasonic waves or laser.

are removed by irrigation and suction or allowed to pass with urine flow.

Bladder stones may be crushed and removed by *cystoscopy*. Cystoscopy may also be used to advance a catheter or basket catheter into a ureter to remove a stone. A laser may be used to disintegrate a ureteral stone via a ureteroscope. Stone fragments are then flushed out with fluid.

Nephrolithotomy may be required to remove a staghorn calculus. A *staghorn calculus* is a stone that forms in the renal pelvis, growing to invade the calyces and renal parenchyma. If kidney damage has been severe, a partial or total *nephrectomy* (removal of the kidney) may be necessary. (See Box 29-16 later in this chapter for nursing care of patients having kidney surgery.)

NURSING CARE

PRIORITIZING NURSING CARE

Relieving the patient's pain and retrieving stone fragments for analysis are the priorities for nursing care of the patient with urinary stones.

HEALTH PROMOTION

Discuss the importance of maintaining an adequate fluid intake with all patients. Stress the need to increase fluid intake during warm weather and strenuous exercise or physical labor. Encourage all patients to remain as physically active as possible to prevent bone loss and possible hypercalciuria (excessive calcium in the urine).

ASSESSING

The patient with a urinary stone is often in acute distress when seeking care. The nursing assessment is brief and focused. Ask about the onset, character, intensity, location, and radiation of pain, as well as associated symptoms such as nausea and vomiting. Inquire about previous episodes of pain or a history of kidney stones. Ask about most recent food and fluid intake and any factors that may have contributed to dehydration (e.g., physical labor on a hot day). Be sure to ask about known allergies to medications or foods (seafood in particular).

IDENTIFYING POTENTIAL COMPLICATIONS

Dull, aching flank pain may indicate total obstruction of urine flow and hydronephrosis. Signs of acute kidney injury, including oliguria, edema, hypertension, nausea and vomiting, and elevated serum creatinine and BUN levels, may develop if urine flow from both kidneys is obstructed. Signs of obstructed urine flow should be promptly reported to the physician to prevent permanent kidney damage.

DIAGNOSING, PLANNING, AND IMPLEMENTING

Acute Pain

Expected outcome: Will report pain at a 3 or lower on a pain scale of 0 to 10.

- Administer analgesia as ordered. *Pain control is vital to reduce anxiety and stress and to facilitate healing.*
- Unless contraindicated, increase fluid intake and encourage ambulation. *Increased fluids and ambulation increase urinary output, help to move the stone through the ureter, and decrease pain.*

Impaired Urinary Elimination

Expected outcome: Will regain normal patterns of urinary elimination.

- Measure urine output; document hematuria, dysuria, frequency, urgency, and pyuria. *Low urine output is a possible indicator of obstruction. Hematuria is often associated with calculi and with procedures for stone removal. A change in the degree of hematuria may indicate stone passage or a complication. Dysuria, frequency, urgency, and cloudy urine are symptoms of UTI and may indicate the need for antibiotic treatment.*
- Strain all urine for stones, saving recovered stones for laboratory analysis. *Analysis of recovered stones helps direct treatment to prevent further stone formation.*

■ Maintain patency of all catheters if present. Secure catheters well and label as indicated. Use sterile technique for all irrigations or other procedures.
A kinked or plugged catheter obstructs urine flow, increasing the risk of further urinary system damage. Labeling catheters prevents mistakes, such as inappropriate irrigation or clamping. Aseptic technique minimizes the risk of infection.

MANAGING NURSING CARE

As appropriate and allowed with identified responsibilities of assistive personnel, the nurse may assign nursing care activities such as measuring intake and output, straining urine to retrieve stones, and assisting with activity for the patient with kidney stones.

EVALUATING

Collect data about pain level and urine output (amount, color, character) to evaluate the effectiveness of nursing care for the patient with urinary stones.

DOCUMENTING

Document continuing pain assessment, relief measures provided, and their efficacy. Also document urine output, including color and amount, and any fragments or stones retrieved and sent for analysis. Note all teaching provided and the patient's understanding of measures to prevent future episodes of urinary stones.

CONTINUITY OF CARE

Because a history of lithiasis increases the risk of future stone formation, teaching is essential. Assess level of understanding and previous learning. Clarify all diagnostic and therapeutic procedures. Patients whose pain can be managed with oral analgesics may be managed at home. Teach the patient to:

■ Collect and strain all urine, saving any stones.
■ Report stone passage to the physician and bring the stone in for analysis.
■ Observe the amount and character of urine, reporting any changes to physician.

Discuss factors that increase the risk of urinary stones and how to minimize this risk. Emphasize the importance of drinking 2.5 to 3 quarts of fluid per day, following dietary recommendations, and taking medication as prescribed. Discuss the relationship between urolithiasis and UTI. Teach prevention, recognition, and management of UTIs.

When the patient is discharged with dressings, a nephrostomy tube, or a catheter, teach dressing changes, tube care, and assessment of the wound and skin. Emphasize the need to keep tubes and catheters patent. Teach how to empty drainage bags, how to assess urine output, and when to contact the physician.

Hydronephrosis

Hydronephrosis (abnormal dilation of the renal pelvis and calyces) can result from urinary tract obstructions or from *vesicoureteral reflux* (backflow of urine from the bladder to the ureters). When urine outflow is obstructed, pressure in the renal pelvis increases, and it dilates. The nephrons and collecting tubules may be damaged, affecting kidney function. The manifestations of hydronephrosis depend on how rapidly it develops (Box 29-12■). If both kidneys are affected, symptoms of acute kidney injury may develop.

Hydronephrosis is diagnosed by *renal ultrasound* or *CT scan*. Other tests, such as *cystoscopy,* may be done to identify the cause. Prompt treatment is vital to preserve kidney function. Immediate treatment involves reestablishing urine flow from the affected kidney. A nephrostomy tube, ureteral stent, or indwelling catheter may be required.

Ureteral stents (small, specialized catheters) are used to keep ureters open and promote healing. Stents can be positioned during surgery or cystoscopy. One or both ends of the stent may be pigtail or J-shaped to keep it in place (Figure 29-9■).

BOX 29-12	MANIFESTATIONS OF HYDRONEPHROSIS

Acute
■ Colicky flank pain; may radiate into groin
■ Hematuria, pyuria
■ Fever
■ Nausea, vomiting, abdominal pain

Chronic
■ Intermittent, dull flank pain
■ Hematuria, pyuria
■ Fever
■ Palpable mass

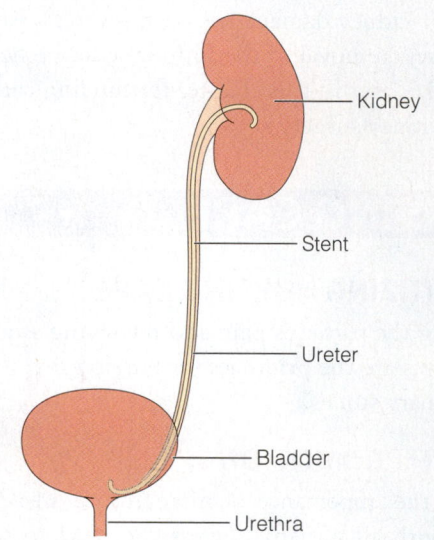

Figure 29-9. ■ A ureteral stent.

A stent may be temporary, or it may be used for longer periods when ureteral obstruction is due to tumors, strictures, or other causes. Box 29-13■ describes nursing care for a patient with a ureteral stent.

Nursing care focuses on preventing hydronephrosis and ensuring urinary drainage. Monitoring intake, urine output, and bladder emptying helps identify impaired urine outflow. Monitoring urine output is vital for patients with risk factors such as pelvic or abdominal tumors, urinary calculi, adhesions and scarring from previous surgeries, or neurologic deficits. Ensuring urinary drainage is also vital in the patient with a ureteral stent, nephrostomy, or surgical intervention for hydronephrosis. Label catheters and drainage tubes clearly, and measure outputs separately. Prevent kinking

or obstruction. Irrigate tubes only as ordered by the physician.

BOX 29-13	NURSING CARE CHECKLIST

Ureteral Stent

☑ Label all drainage tubes and stents for easy identification. Secure positions.

☑ Attach each catheter and stent to a separate closed drainage system.

☑ Monitor for infection or bleeding: fever, tachycardia, pain, hematuria, and cloudy or malodorous urine.

☑ Encourage fluids, especially those that acidify urine, such as apple and cranberry juice.

☑ For an indwelling stent, teach follow-up care and recognition and prevention of complications.

CONGENITAL KIDNEY DISORDERS

Polycystic Kidney Disease

Polycystic kidney disease is a hereditary disease in which cysts form on the kidneys, the kidneys enlarge, and their function is gradually destroyed. It is a relatively common disease that affects both children and adults.

PATHOPHYSIOLOGY AND MANIFESTATIONS

In polycystic kidney disease, cysts develop in the nephrons. These fluid-filled sacs can range in size from microscopic to several centimeters in diameter. Both kidneys are affected. As the cysts fill, enlarge, and multiply, the kidneys also enlarge (Figure 29-10■). The cysts gradually destroy functional kidney tissue. Cysts may also develop elsewhere (e.g., liver, spleen, pancreas). Cardiac valve disorders affect up to 25% of

people with polycystic kidney disease, although these often produce no symptoms. Patients are also at risk for developing cerebral aneurysms, which may rupture and bleed.

Adult polycystic kidney disease is slowly progressive, with symptoms usually noticed in the 30s or 40s. Common manifestations include flank pain, microscopic or gross hematuria, proteinuria, and polyuria and nocturia. UTIs and stones are common. Most patients develop hypertension. The kidneys become enlarged, palpable, and knobby. Eventually, signs of kidney failure develop.

COLLABORATIVE CARE

Management of adult polycystic kidney disease is supportive. A *renal ultrasound* is done to diagnose polycystic kidney disease.

Care is taken to avoid further kidney damage by nephrotoxins, UTI, obstruction, or hypertension. A fluid intake of 2,000 to 2,500 mL per day is encouraged to help prevent UTI and kidney stones. ACE inhibitors or other antihypertensive drugs are ordered to manage hypertension. Ultimately, patients with polycystic kidney disease develop kidney failure and require hemodialysis or kidney transplantation. The section on kidney failure later in this chapter gives more information about dialysis and kidney transplants.

NURSING CARE

Although each patient has individual nursing care needs, the following nursing diagnoses may be appropriate for the patient with polycystic kidney disease:

■ *Excess Fluid Volume* related to impaired renal function

■ *Grieving* related to potential loss of kidney function

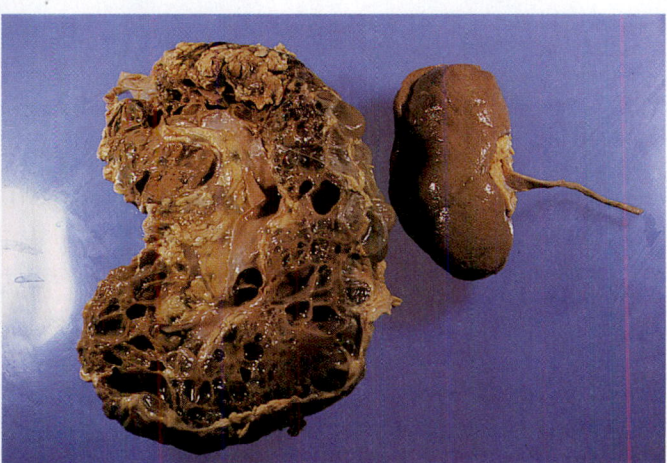

Figure 29-10. ■ A polycystic kidney and a normal kidney for comparison. (Source: Arthur Glauberman/Science Source.)

- *Ineffective Self-Health Management* related to lack of information about how to maintain kidney function
- *Ineffective Coping* related to the potential for transmitting an inherited disorder to offspring

CONTINUITY OF CARE

Teach about polycystic kidney disease and how to maintain good kidney function. Instruct to drink about 2,500 mL of fluid per day. Provide additional information about preventing UTIs, such as hygiene measures. Discuss early manifestations of UTI, and stress the importance of seeking prompt treatment to prevent further kidney damage. Advise avoiding medications that are potentially damaging to the kidneys and checking with the primary care provider before taking any new drug.

Offspring of patients with adult polycystic kidney disease have a 50% chance of inheriting the disorder. Discuss genetic counseling and screening of family members, especially if renal transplantation is likely and family members are potential donors.

CANCER OF THE URINARY TRACT

Key Concept Painless hematuria is a frequent initial manifestation of urinary tract cancer. Advise all patients with hematuria to see their physician for evaluation.

Any part of the urinary tract can be affected by a malignant tumor. The most common site is the bladder, accounting for 52% of urinary tract tumors, followed by the kidney (46%). Bladder cancer is the 10th leading cause of cancer deaths, followed closely by kidney cancer. Tumors of the urinary tract may lead to obstruction, kidney failure, hemorrhage, and invasion of surrounding tissues.

The major risk factors for urinary tract cancers are carcinogens in the urine and chronic inflammation (Box 29-14■). Cigarette smoking is the major risk factor. The risk in smokers is twice that of people who do not smoke.

Cancer of the urinary tract usually affects people over age 55. It is diagnosed in men two to four times more often than in women. The incidence of bladder cancer is higher in White males than in Black or Hispanic men. Many patients with bladder cancer have more than one tumor at the time of diagnosis.

PATHOPHYSIOLOGY

Bladder tumors begin as cells change and develop into superficial or invasive lesions (Figure 29-11■). Most are papillomas, with a polyplike structure attached by a stalk to the bladder mucosa. These lesions may be either superficial or invasive. The prognosis for a full recovery is good, although papillomas frequently recur. When metastasis occurs, the pelvic lymph nodes, lungs, bones, and liver are most commonly involved.

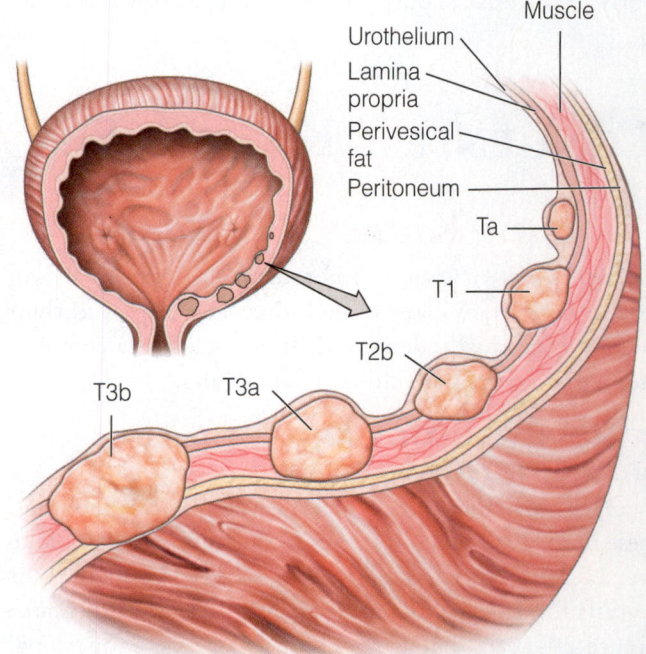

Figure 29-11. ■ Stages of bladder tumor development and invasiveness, beginning at the 3 o'clock position of the bladder and continuing in a clockwise manner. As the tumor grows, it invades progressively deeper tissues of the bladder, and, eventually, adjacent tissues. (Source: "Figure 27.07—Stages of Bladder Tumor Development and Invasiveness, Beginning at the 3 o'clock Position of the Bladder and Continuing in a Clockwise Manner" from Medical Surgical Nursing: Critical Thinking in Patient Care, 5e by Priscilla LeMone; Karen Burke; and Gerene Bauldoff. Published by Pearson Education, © 2011.

Kidney tumors can occur anywhere in the kidney and tend to invade the renal vein. They often have metastasized to other organs such as the lungs, bone, lymph nodes, liver, or brain at the time of diagnosis.

MANIFESTATIONS

Painless hematuria is the most common initial manifestation of bladder and kidney cancers. Hematuria may be either gross (visible) or microscopic and may be intermittent. Frequency, urgency, and dysuria are other manifestations of bladder cancer.

BOX 29-14	RISK FACTORS FOR CANCER OF THE URINARY TRACT

- Male gender, age over 55, urban residence
- Cigarette smoking
- Occupational exposure to dyes or chemicals
- Chronic UTI or urinary stones (bladder or kidney)

Other symptoms of kidney tumors include flank pain, a palpable mass, fever, fatigue, weight loss, and anemia or polycythemia (elevated RBCs). Kidney tumors may produce hormones or other substances that can cause such manifestations as hypercalcemia, hypertension, and hyperglycemia.

COLLABORATIVE CARE

When *urinalysis* shows hematuria, a *urine cytology* may be done to assess for cancer cells. *Bladder ultrasound* is a noninvasive test to detect bladder tumors; *renal ultrasound* is done when kidney cancer is suspected. A *cystoscopy* is done to visualize and biopsy a bladder lesion. *Kidney biopsy* (see Box 29-9) is performed to diagnose kidney cancer.

Medications

Chemotherapeutic drugs may be instilled into the bladder as the primary treatment for bladder cancer or to prevent recurrence of the tumor after surgery. Bacillus Calmette–Guérin (BCG Live, TheraCys) causes a local inflammatory reaction that eliminates or reduces superficial tumors. Other chemotherapeutic drugs may also be used. Bladder irritation, frequency, dysuria, and contact dermatitis are possible adverse reactions to *intravesical* (within-bladder) chemotherapy.

Surgery

Surgery for bladder tumors ranges from simple resection of noninvasive tumors to removal of the bladder and surrounding structures (Table 29-3■). In a total or radical **cystectomy**, the bladder and adjacent muscles and tissues are removed. In men, the prostate and seminal vessels are also removed, resulting in impotence. In women, the uterus, fallopian tubes, and ovaries are removed, resulting in sterility. When the bladder is removed, a *urinary diversion* is created to collect and drain urine. The most common urinary diversion is the *ileal conduit* (Figure 29-12■); alternatively, a *continent urinary diversion* may be created. Box 29-15■ describes nursing care of the patient undergoing a cystectomy and urinary diversion.

Radical nephrectomy (removal of the affected kidney and surrounding tissue) is done when cancer affects the kidney. The kidney may be removed using laparoscopic surgery. Frequently, however, an open technique is used to allow inspection of surrounding tissues. If the cancer has spread beyond the kidney, chemotherapy or radiation therapy may be prescribed. Box 29-16■ describes nursing care of the patient undergoing a partial or total nephrectomy.

Other Therapies

Radiation therapy may be used as an adjunct treatment, to shrink tumors before surgery. It may also be used together with chemotherapy to reduce the risk of tumor recurrence and for treating inoperable tumors.

TABLE 29-3	Bladder Cancer Surgeries	
PROCEDURE	**DESCRIPTION**	**NURSING CONSIDERATIONS**
Transurethral resection of bladder tumor (TURBT)	Tumor removal via cystoscope inserted through urethra	■ Maintain continuous bladder irrigation as ordered, ensure catheter patency. ■ Monitor for excessive bleeding. ■ Encourage fluids up to 2,500–3,000 mL/day. ■ Give stool softeners to prevent straining.
Partial cystectomy	Resection of the tumor and a portion of the bladder wall	■ Maintain urethral and/or suprapubic catheter patency to reduce pressure on suture lines. ■ Monitor for excessive bleeding.
Complete or radical cystectomy	Removal of the entire urinary bladder and surrounding tissues	■ Permanent urinary diversion required. ■ Maintain stent position and patency. ■ May have urethral catheter to drain pelvic cavity.
Ileal conduit	Portion of ileum formed into pouch; ureters inserted into pouch and open end is brought to surface to form stoma	■ Continuous urine drainage requires appliance. ■ Risk of infection is significant. ■ Good skin care is vital due to constant contact with urine.
Continent internal ileal reservoir or continent ileal bladder conduit	Pouch created from ileum; nipple valves formed by telescoping tissue where brought to skin and where ureters attach prevent urine leakage and reflux	■ Drainage-collection device is not necessary. ■ Patient must be willing and able to perform clean intermittent self-catheterization every 2 to 4 hours to drain pouch.

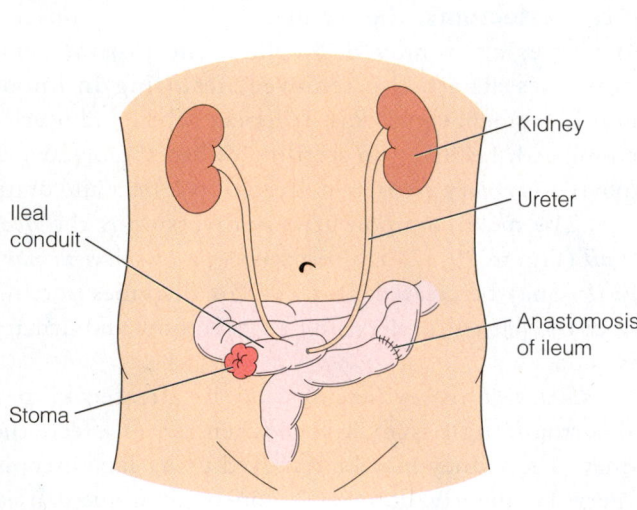

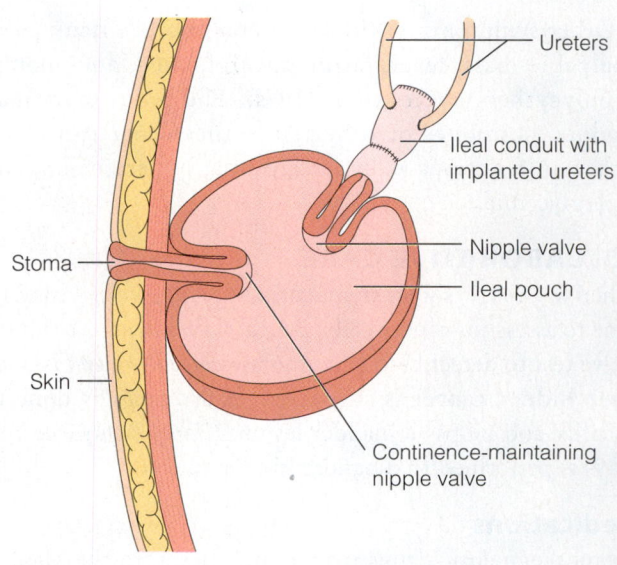

Figure 29-12. ■ Urinary diversion procedures. (**A**) An ileal conduit. A segment of ileum is separated from the small intestine and formed into a tubular pouch with the open end brought to the skin surface to form a stoma. (**B**) A continent urinary diversion. Formation of nipple valves where the ureters enter the pouch and where the stoma is formed allows the patient to periodically drain the pouch using clean catheterization.

BOX 29-15	NURSING CARE CHECKLIST

Cystectomy and Urinary Diversion

Before Surgery

☑ Assess knowledge of the surgery to be performed and expected outcomes of surgery. Clarify any misunderstandings.

☑ Begin teaching about postoperative tubes and drains, as well as stoma care.

☑ Contact the enterostomal therapist to determine the stoma site(s). Assist in identifying the site, avoiding skin folds, the belt line, and areas not easily seen by the patient.

☑ Provide routine preoperative care as ordered.

After Surgery

☑ Provide routine postoperative care as ordered.

☑ Monitor intake and output. Assess urine output hourly for the first 24 hours and then every 4 hours or as ordered. Notify the charge nurse or physician if less than 30 mL/hr.

☑ Assess urine color and consistency. Expect pink or bright red urine to clear by third postoperative day. Urine may be cloudy due to mucus produced by bowel mucosa, but excessive cloudiness or malodorous urine may indicate infection.

☑ Assess the stoma and surrounding skin every 2 hours for the first 24 hours and then every 4 hours for 48 to 72 hours. The stoma should appear bright and moist. Notify the charge nurse or physician if the stoma blanches when touched or is pale, gray, or cyanotic.

☑ Irrigate the ileal pouch catheter with 30 to 60 mL of sterile normal saline every 4 hours or as ordered. Stents placed in each ureter during surgery may be visible in the stoma opening. Note the visible length of each stent; do not irrigate stents unless specifically ordered by the physician. Notify the charge nurse or physician when the stent washes into the urinary drainage pouch.

☑ Change the urinary drainage pouch as ordered. Prevent urine flow during cleaning by placing a rolled gauze square or tampon over the stoma opening. Cleanse skin surrounding the stoma with soap and water, rinse, and pat or air dry.

☑ Trim the opening of the clean bag or seal to no more than 1 to 2 mm (1/16 to 1/8 in.) wider than the stoma. Apply over stoma, preventing wrinkles or creases in the seal to prevent leakage and protect the skin.

☑ Monitor for and report changes in serum electrolyte values, acid–base balance, and renal function tests such as BUN and serum creatinine.

☑ Teach stoma and urinary diversion care, including odor management, skin care, increased fluid intake, pouch application and leakage prevention, self-catheterization for patients with continent reservoirs, and signs of infection and other complications.

NURSING CARE

PRIORITIZING NURSING CARE

The patient with cancer of the urinary tract faces an uncertain future. The priority focus for nursing care is ensuring effective urinary elimination. When a cancerous kidney has been removed, managing postoperative pain, preventing respiratory complications, and preserving renal function of the remaining kidney are also nursing care priorities. Psychologically, the patient may experience grieving due to the cancer diagnosis.

BOX 29-16	NURSING CARE CHECKLIST

Nephrectomy

Before Surgery

☑ Assess understanding and reinforce teaching.

☑ Provide routine preoperative care and teaching as ordered.

After Surgery

☑ Provide routine postoperative care.

☑ Assess urine output hourly for the first 24 hours and then every 4 to 8 hours.

☑ Label and secure all catheters, stents, nephrostomy tubes, or drains. Irrigate only as ordered by the physician.

☑ Monitor for signs of hemorrhage or infection.

☑ Frequently monitor respiratory status and assist with respiratory care.

☑ Support grieving process and adjustment to the loss of a kidney.

☑ Teach home care:

☑ Maintain fluid intake of 2,000 to 2,500 mL/day.

☑ Gradually increase exercise to tolerance, avoiding heavy lifting for a year after surgery. Avoid contact sports to reduce the risk of injury to the remaining kidney.

☑ Care of the incision and any remaining drainage tubes, catheters, or stents.

☑ Prescribed medications, including their purpose, dose, scheduling, and potential side effects.

☑ Signs and symptoms of UTIs and other complications to report to the physician.

HEALTH PROMOTION

Encourage all patients not to smoke. Provide referral to smoking cessation programs or clinics for patients who wish to quit smoking. Encourage patients at high risk for developing urinary tract cancer to have periodic examinations, including urinalysis and possible urine cytology.

ASSESSING

Painless hematuria is the most common early manifestation of urinary tract cancer. Direct any patient with blood in the urine to seek medical evaluation and care.

IDENTIFYING POTENTIAL COMPLICATIONS

Be alert for possible signs that the tumor has invaded adjacent tissues or metastasized. Report such manifestations as cough, shortness of breath, signs of liver dysfunction (jaundice, nausea, fatigue, upper right quadrant pain), changes in bowel function (constipation, pain), and other symptoms such as weight loss, frequent infections, fatigue, and anemia.

DIAGNOSING, PLANNING, AND IMPLEMENTING

Impaired Urinary Elimination

Expected outcome: Will maintain urine output that is within expected range for amount, color, clarity, and odor.

■ Monitor amount, color, and clarity of urine output from all catheters, stents, and tubes hourly for the first 24 hours postoperatively and then every 4 to 8 hours. *Output of less than 30 mL per hour may indicate low blood volume, impaired kidney function, or impaired drainage. A change in urine color or clarity may indicate infection or other complication.*

■ Label all catheters, stents, and their drainage containers. Maintain separate closed gravity drainage systems for each. *Clear labeling of tubes can prevent errors in irrigating and calculating outputs. Separate closed systems minimize the risk of infection.*

■ Secure catheters and stents with tape; prevent kinking or occlusion; maintain gravity flow by keeping drainage bags lower than the kidneys. *Impaired urine flow can lead to kidney damage or place pressure on suture lines.*

clinicalALERT

Prevent kinking, twisting, or tension on drains and tubes. Do not clamp. Irrigate carefully and only with a physician's order. Notify the physician or charge nurse immediately if any tube becomes obstructed or dislodged.

■ Encourage fluid intake of 3,000 mL/day. *Increased fluid intake reduces the risk of infection and dilutes urine, which is less irritating to the skin around the stoma site.*

■ Use strict aseptic technique in caring for all urinary catheters, tubes, stents, drains, and incisions. *Asepsis is vital to prevent infection of the urinary tract.*

■ After removal of any stents or ureteral catheters, monitor urine output closely for 24 hours. *Edema or stricture of ureters may impede output.*

■ Encourage activity. *Ambulation promotes urine drainage and helps prevent calcium loss from bones, which could lead to urinary calculi.*

Risk for Impaired Skin Integrity

Expected outcome: Skin will remain intact without evidence of irritation or breakdown.

■ Assess skin surrounding the stoma for redness, excoriation, or signs of breakdown. Also assess for urine leakage from catheters, stents, or drains. Keep the skin clean and dry. *Urine irritates the skin, increasing the risk of breakdown. Meticulous skin care can prevent breakdown.*

■ Ensure gravity drainage of urine-collection device or empty bag every 2 hours. Change urine-collection appliance as needed, removing any mucus from stoma. *Overfilling may damage the seal, allowing leakage and urine contact with skin.*

Pain

Expected outcome: Will report pain at a level of 2 or lower on a standard 0 to 10 pain scale.

Pain management after open nephrectomy presents a challenge due to the type and location of the incision. Intercostal blocks, patient-controlled analgesia (PCA), or routine analgesic administration may be ordered.

- Assess frequently for adequate pain relief, using a pain scale and nonverbal signs such as grimacing, tense body position, increased pulse, blood pressure changes, or rapid, shallow respirations. Notify the physician of inadequate pain relief. *The patient may assume that pain is to be expected or may fear becoming addicted to analgesics. Responses to analgesics vary, and the prescribed dose may need to be adjusted.*
- Assess the incision for inflammation or swelling and drainage catheters and tubes for patency. *An obstructed catheter can lead to complications and increased pain.*
- Use adjunctive pain relief measures such as positioning, diversion, and relaxation techniques. *These can enhance the effects of analgesia.*

clinicalALERT

Assess for abdominal distention, tenderness, and bowel sounds. Intra-abdominal bleeding, infection, or paralytic ileus can cause pain that may be confused with incisional pain.

Ineffective Breathing Pattern

Expected outcome: Breath sounds will be audible and free of adventitious sounds throughout all lung fields.

- Place in semi-Fowler's position and side-lying positions as allowed and tolerated. *Lung expansion is improved in semi-Fowler's and Fowler's positions.*
- Assess respiratory status frequently, including rate and depth, cough, breath sounds, oxygen saturation, and temperature. *Pneumothorax or atelectasis on the operative side is common.*
- Change position frequently; ambulate as soon as possible. *These measures promote ventilation and airway clearance.*
- Encourage frequent (every 1 to 2 hours) deep breathing, spirometer use, and coughing. Assist to splint the incision. *These measures promote alveolar ventilation, gas exchange, and airway clearance.*

Disturbed Body Image

Expected outcome: Will demonstrate acceptance of appearance and gradually resume self-care.

- Use active listening and respond to concerns. *Surgical procedures and adjunctive cancer treatments can significantly affect the patient's body image. Grieving is a normal response.*

- Encourage the patient to look at, touch, and care for the stoma and appliance as soon as possible. Allow to proceed gradually, providing support and encouragement. *A willingness to provide self-care indicates adaptation to the changed body image.*
- Discuss concerns about resuming usual activities, perceived changes in relationships, and sexual relations. Refer to a support group or a person who has successfully adjusted to a urinary diversion. *If a radical cystectomy has been done, the patient will no longer be able to bear children and may experience erectile dysfunction. Patients and families may be reluctant to ask about sexual topics. Support groups allow open discussion of concerns and anxieties.*
- Demonstrate respect for cultural, spiritual, and religious values and beliefs; encourage use of these resources to cope with losses. *Value and belief systems can provide a structure and form for dealing with the grieving process.*
- Refer to cancer support groups, social services, or counseling as appropriate. *Support groups and counseling services provide additional resources for coping.*

MANAGING NURSING CARE

As appropriate and allowed within the designated duties and responsibilities of assistive personnel, the nurse may delegate nursing care activities such as measuring intake and output, obtaining daily weights, and assisting with ambulation and ADLs for the patient with cancer of the urinary tract. The nurse retains responsibility for managing stents and catheters and changing the urinary diversion appliance during the postoperative period.

EVALUATING

When evaluating the effectiveness of nursing care, collect data regarding urinary output, skin integrity, and the patient's and family's acceptance of and ability to care for any urinary diversion or catheters.

DOCUMENTING

Document continuing assessments, including the amount, color, clarity, and odor of urine output from all catheters or stomas. Note the presence of stents, including visible length. Document timing, location, and intensity of pain and effectiveness of analgesia. Note the patient's and family's response to the stoma and teaching about its care if one was created. Document all teaching provided and the understanding of the patient and family.

CONTINUITY OF CARE

For many patients, surgery for bladder cancer means a lifelong change in urinary elimination. Before discharge, assess the patient's and family's knowledge and understanding of the cancer diagnosis and recommended treatment plan.

When the tumor has been resected, stress the importance of regular follow-up care and monitoring for tumor recurrence.

Teach the patient who has had a urinary diversion to care for the stoma and surrounding skin. Discuss strategies to prevent urine reflux and infection. Teach signs and symptoms of UTI and renal calculi. If a continent urinary diversion has been created, teach self-catheterization using clean technique.

If renal cancer was detected at an early stage and cure is anticipated, teaching for home care focuses on protecting the remaining kidney. Emphasize the need to maintain a generous fluid intake of 2,000 to 2,500 mL/day, increasing fluid intake during hot weather and when exercising. Stress measures to prevent UTI, such as urinating when the urge is perceived, hygiene, and voiding before and after sexual intercourse. Discuss manifestations of UTI that should promptly be reported to the physician. With men, discuss the importance of regular screening for an enlarged prostate after ages 45 to 50. Encourage the patient to avoid contact sports such as football or hockey and use measures to prevent motor vehicle crashes and falls, which could damage the remaining kidney.

Stress the importance of follow-up care and of notifying the physician promptly if signs of a complication develop. Refer the patient and family to a cancer support group, and as appropriate, discuss hospice care.

NURSING CARE PLAN
Patient With Bladder Cancer

Ben Hussain is a 61-year-old man who became alarmed and called his doctor when his urine became bright red. Urinalysis and cytology showed gross hematuria and abnormal cells. A cystoscopy and biopsy confirmed an invasive bladder tumor. He is admitted to the hospital for a radical cystectomy and ileal diversion.

Assessment

Mr. Hussain's admission history indicates that he has lost 10 to 15 lb during the last few months. He had smoked two to three packs of cigarettes per day for 40 years, but he cut back to a pack a day about a year ago. Mr. Hussain says he is "a little nervous about surgery and what they're going to find." Ms. Mills, the admitting nurse, notes that he fidgets and talks rapidly throughout their interview. He is concerned about how he will handle the pain after surgery, because he has never been hospitalized before his cystoscopy. Physical assessment findings include BP 154/86; P 84; R 18; T 98.2°F (36.7°C) PO. He has scattered crackles throughout his lung fields. Mr. Hussain's urine is clear and bright pink. The remainder of his assessment is essentially normal.

Nursing Diagnosis

The following nursing diagnoses are identified for Mr. Hussain:

- *Anxiety* related to undetermined extent of disease and fear of pain
- *Readiness for Enhanced Knowledge* about ileal diversion
- *Impaired Urinary Elimination* related to cystectomy and ileal diversion
- *Risk for Impaired Gas Exchange* related to smoking history and effects of anesthesia

Expected Outcomes

The expected outcomes of the plan of care for Mr. Hussain are that he will:

- Verbalize a decrease in anxiety.
- Demonstrate ability to manage PCA for postoperative pain control.
- Report pain at an acceptable level (2 or less on a scale of 0 to 10) postoperatively.
- Demonstrate care for his ileostomy stoma, surrounding skin, and collection appliance before discharge.
- Maintain urine output with acceptable color and clarity and no signs of infection.
- Maintain adequate gas exchange as evidenced by good skin color, O_2 saturation greater than 95%, and clear lung sounds upon auscultation.

Planning and Implementation

The following nursing interventions are planned and implemented for Mr. Hussain:

- Allow time to answer questions and verbalize fears pre- and postoperatively.
- Provide written as well as verbal explanations as needed.
- Maintain PCA or epidural infusion postoperatively. Monitor effectiveness of pain relief.
- Explain all procedures related to stoma and appliance care as they are being performed.
- Encourage Mr. and Mrs. Hussain to look at the stoma and touch it when ready.
- Teach stoma, skin, and appliance care, emphasizing techniques to prevent skin irritation and UTI.
- Monitor urine output, color, clarity, and consistency hourly for 24 hours, then every 4 hours for 24 hours, and then every 8 hours. Report output less than 30 mL/hr, bright bleeding, and excessively cloudy or malodorous urine.
- Assist to use an incentive spirometer hourly while awake. Ambulate as soon as possible. Assess lung sounds every 4 hours, reporting increased crackles or diminished breath sounds.
- Refer to a local stoma group on discharge.

Evaluation

On discharge, Mr. Hussain has helped clean the stoma and surrounding skin several times. His wife is able to empty the drainage bag and change the appliance, cutting the opening to fit. His urine is pale yellow and slightly cloudy. Mr. Hussain is ambulating independently and using oxycodone (Percocet) twice a day for pain relief. His lungs are clear, and he is very proud of having "survived" 7 days without a cigarette. He says, "Now I'm going to shoot for 7 weeks, then 7 months, and then 7 years without a smoke!" A home health referral is made to continue teaching Mr. Hussain to care for his diversion and appliance.

Critical Thinking in the Nursing Process

1. How does cigarette smoking contribute to the increased risk of urinary tract tumors?
2. The first time Mr. Hussain changes his urostomy appliance, he experiences a leak. What hints can you give Mr. Hussain to prevent leaks from occurring?
3. How would you respond if Mr. Hussain said "I'm not only giving up on cigarettes, I'm also giving up on sex from here on"?

Note: Discussion of Critical Thinking questions appears on the companion website.

KIDNEY FAILURE

Key Concept   Kidney failure may occur in response to an acute insult or as the end-stage of chronic kidney disease. Nurses play a key role in preventing and recognizing acute kidney injury and in teaching patients with chronic kidney disease how to prevent or delay the onset of kidney failure.

Kidney failure is a condition in which the kidneys are unable to remove accumulated waste products from the blood. It may be acute or be the end stage of chronic kidney disease. It is characterized by azotemia (a buildup of nitrogenous waste products in the blood) and fluid, electrolyte, and acid–base imbalances.

Acute Kidney Injury

Acute kidney injury (AKI) is characterized by an abrupt and rapid decline in renal function. It is often reversible with prompt treatment. It is relatively common, affecting at least 10,000 people in the United States every year, most often those who are critically ill with another serious health condition. Major trauma or surgery, infection, hemorrhage, severe heart failure, and lower urinary tract obstruction are risk factors. *Iatrogenic* causes of AKI include drugs and contrast dye used in x-rays. Older adults are at particular risk.

PATHOPHYSIOLOGY

The most common causes of AKI are *ischemia* (poor perfusion) of the kidney and **nephrotoxins** (agents that damage the kidney tissue). Causes of AKI can be classified as prerenal, intrinsic (or intrarenal), and postrenal (Table 29-4■). Prerenal AKI is the most common, causing more than half of all cases of AKI. Prerenal AKI results from conditions that affect the blood supply to the kidney, for example, hemorrhage and shock or heart failure. It is readily reversed when blood flow is restored and the kidney tissue itself is undamaged. If blood flow is not restored, continued ischemia can lead to acute tubular necrosis and intrinsic AKI. *Intrinsic* AKI results from acute damage to the nephrons by inflammation (e.g., acute glomerulonephritis), by vascular disorders (e.g., severe hypertension), or by exposure to nephrotoxins (Figure 29-13■). The risk for *acute tubular necrosis (ATN)* is particularly high when ischemia and exposure to a nephrotoxin occur at the same time. Obstruction of urine outflow can lead to *postrenal* AKI.

TABLE 29-4	Causes of Acute Kidney Injury	
CATEGORY	**CAUSE**	**RISK FACTORS**
Prerenal	Impaired blood flow to kidney	Hemorrhage, dehydration, heart failure, shock
Intrinsic	*Acute tubular necrosis:* tubular cell damage due to prolonged ischemia (more than 2 hours) and/or exposure to nephrotoxins	Ischemia, nephrotoxic drugs or substances; red blood cell destruction (e.g., transfusion reaction); muscle tissue breakdown due to trauma, heatstroke
	Acute glomerular or vascular injury, acute nephritis	Acute glomerulonephritis; malignant hypertension; nephrotoxic drugs
Postrenal	Obstruction of urine outflow	Urethral obstruction by enlarged prostate or tumor; ureteral or kidney pelvis obstruction by calculi

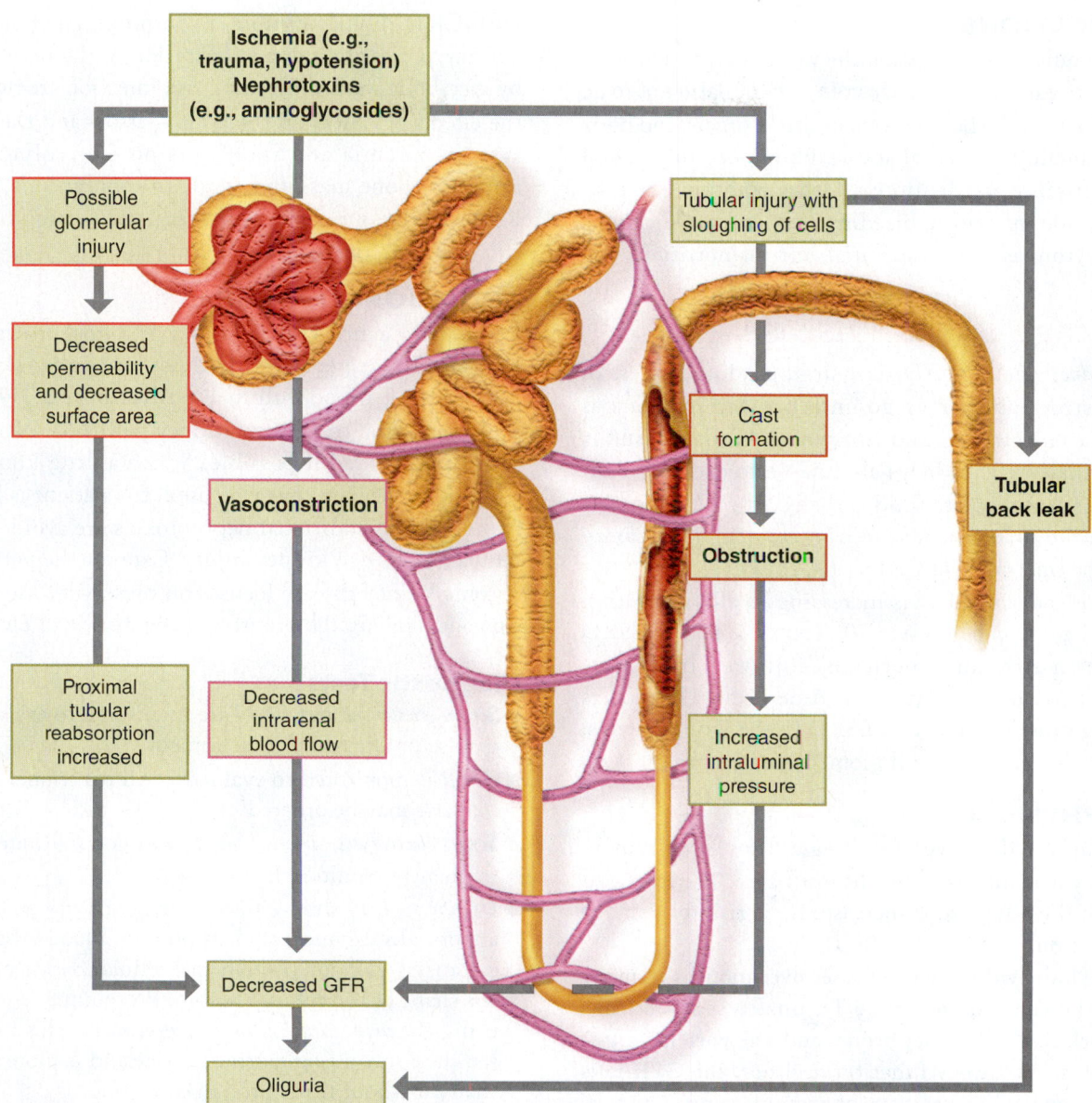

Figure 29-13. ■ Pathophysiology Illustrated: Acute kidney injury. The kidney is injured by ischemia (poor blood supply), a nephrotoxic drug or substance, or acute disease. The damage can affect the glomerulus, capillaries, or the tubules, leading to decreased glomerular filtration and urine output.

MANIFESTATIONS

Acute kidney injury is generally identified by rising BUN or serum creatinine levels. The GFR falls, tubular cells become necrotic and slough, and the nephron is unable to eliminate wastes effectively. *Oliguria,* urine output less than 400 mL/day, may be present. The course of AKI due to ATN includes three phases: initiation, maintenance, and recovery.

1. The *initiation phase* begins with the initiating event. This phase has few symptoms and is often recognized only after the patient has moved into the maintenance phase.
2. The *maintenance phase* of AKI is marked by a sharp drop in the GFR. Oliguria may develop, although many patients continue to produce urine. However,

the kidney is unable to eliminate metabolic wastes, water, electrolytes, and acids effectively. Azotemia can cause confusion and disorientation, as well as anorexia, nausea, and vomiting. Salt and water retention lead to edema. Hypertension and heart failure may develop. Hyperkalemia causes muscle weakness, nausea and diarrhea, and dysrhythmias. Metabolic acidosis results when the kidneys are unable to eliminate hydrogen ions. In this phase, anemia may develop and immune function is impaired, increasing the risk for infections.

3. The *recovery phase* of AKI is characterized by improving kidney function, urine output, and blood values. It lasts for up to 1 year.

COMPLICATIONS

AKI can significantly affect the kidneys' regulatory functions and ability to excrete wastes. **Uremia**, accumulation of toxic waste products in the body, affects multiple organs and body functions, including mental status. Fluid, electrolyte, and acid–base balance are disrupted. Other potential complications include infections, bleeding, cardiac complications (e.g., dysrhythmias and pericarditis), and malnutrition.

End-Stage Renal Disease

Chronic kidney disease (CKD) is a slow, gradual process of kidney destruction. It may go unrecognized for years as nephrons are destroyed and functional kidney tissue is lost. Eventually, the kidneys are unable to excrete metabolic wastes and regulate fluid and electrolyte balance. At this point, the patient is said to have *end-stage renal disease (ESRD),* the final stage of CKD.

The incidence of ESRD is increasing in all age groups, particularly in people over age 70. The incidence of ESRD is highest in African Americans, followed by Native Americans, Asians, and European Americans. Diabetes is the leading cause of CKD and ESRD in the United States, followed by hypertension and glomerulonephritis.

PATHOPHYSIOLOGY

As nephrons are destroyed by disease, those that remain hypertrophy to compensate for the lost tissue. The increased demand on these nephrons increases their risk for damage and destruction.

Chronic kidney disease progresses over months to many years. In the early stage (stage 1), unaffected nephrons do the work of the lost nephrons, and the patient is free of symptoms. As kidney function declines, the GFR falls slightly (stage 2), but the patient remains symptom-free. In stage 3, the GFR is moderately decreased. Any further insult to the kidneys at this stage (infection, exposure to nephrotoxins) can precipitate *end-stage renal failure.* By the time the patient reaches stage 4 of CKD, symptoms of *uremia* develop. In the final stage (ESRD), renal replacement therapies such as kidney transplant or dialysis are necessary.

MANIFESTATIONS

CKD may not be identified until uremia develops. Early symptoms of uremia include nausea, apathy, weakness, and fatigue. As it progresses, the patient may develop frequent vomiting, increasing weakness, lethargy, and confusion. The multisystem effects of ESRD and uremia are illustrated in Figure 29-14■ and listed in Box 29-17■.

COMPLICATIONS

A number of complications are associated with CKD. Cardiovascular disease is a leading cause of death in patients with CKD. Hypertension is common. The patient may develop pericarditis due to irritation of the pericardial sac by metabolic wastes. Bleeding and infection are risks due to the effects of ESRD on the bone marrow and the immune system. Uremia and its effects on electrolyte balance can affect bone mass and result in spontaneous fractures. Reproductive function is affected, and women have difficulty carrying pregnancy to term.

COLLABORATIVE CARE

Preventing acute kidney injury is a goal in the care of all patients, especially for those in high-risk groups. Maintaining blood volume, cardiac output, and blood pressure is vital to preserve kidney perfusion. Nephrotoxic drugs are avoided if possible. When a drug known to be toxic to the kidneys must be used, the patient is kept well hydrated, and additional nephrotoxins are avoided to help reduce the risk of kidney injury. Care for the patient with chronic kidney disease focuses on preserving kidney function and slowing the progress of the disease to ESRD.

Diagnostic Tests

- *Serum creatinine* and *BUN* are monitored to evaluate the disease progress and its treatment.
- *eGFR* is monitored to evaluate renal function. *Creatinine clearance* may be ordered.
- *Serum electrolytes, arterial blood gases,* and *CBC* are also frequently monitored.
- *Urinalysis* may show a fixed specific gravity at 1.010 and abnormal substances such as protein, blood cells, and cell casts. *Casts* are protein and cellular debris molded in the shape of the tubular lumen. Proteinuria is monitored using the *urine albumin to creatinine ratio.* This test requires only a single urine sample and is more accurate than a 24-hour urine protein collection.
- A *kidney biopsy* may be done to identify the underlying disease process (see Box 29-9).

Medications

Most medications are excreted by the kidneys. This fact is critical to remember when caring patients with AKI and CKD. All nephrotoxic drugs (e.g., NSAIDs) are avoided or used only with extreme caution. Drug dosages may be adjusted because excretion is slowed and half-life is prolonged.

Angiotensin-converting enzyme (ACE) inhibitors and angiotensin receptor blockers (ARBs) are used to reduce proteinuria and slow the progression of CKD. Antihypertensive drugs such as ACE inhibitors or ARBs may also be given to lower blood pressure when necessary. Diuretics such as furosemide (Lasix) may be ordered to reduce fluid volume, lower blood pressure, and lower serum potassium levels.

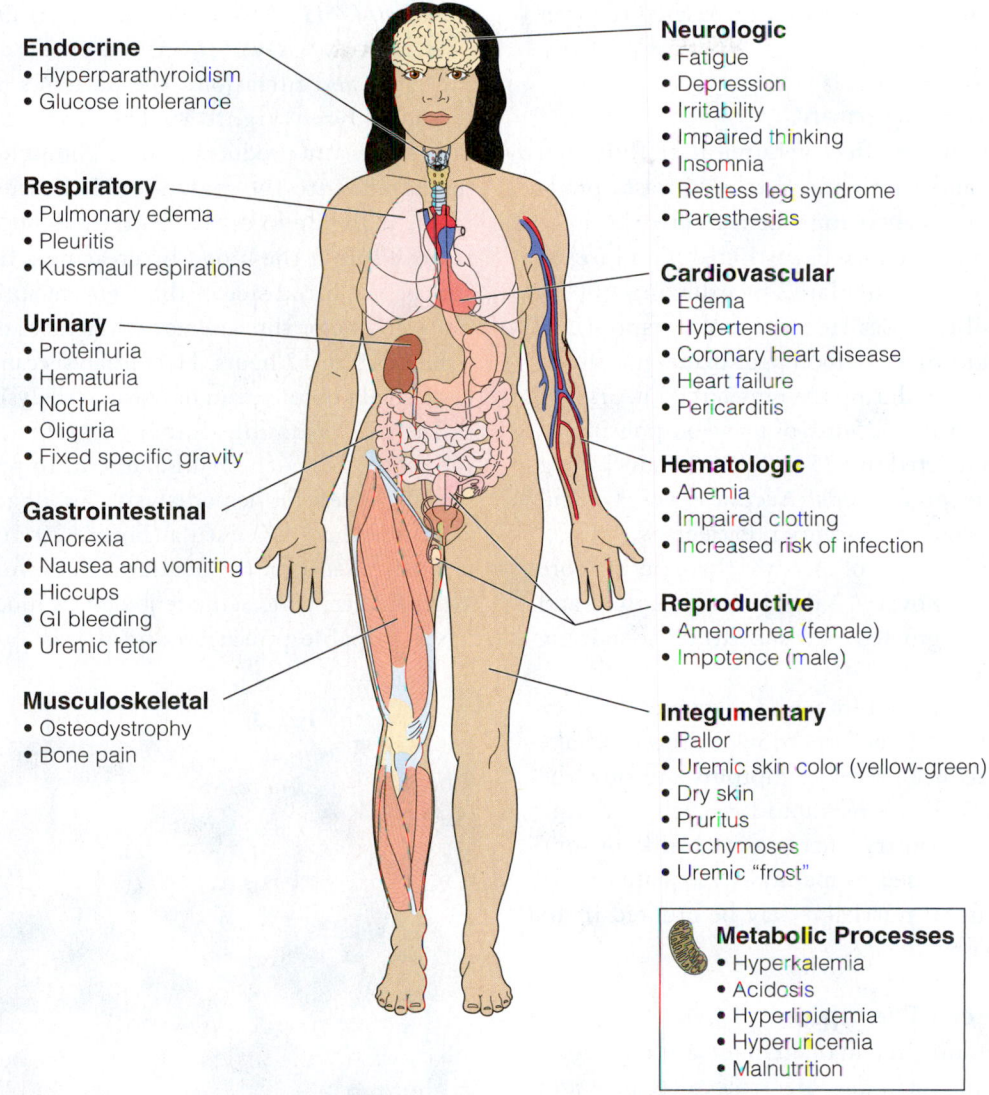

Endocrine
- Hyperparathyroidism
- Glucose intolerance

Respiratory
- Pulmonary edema
- Pleuritis
- Kussmaul respirations

Urinary
- Proteinuria
- Hematuria
- Nocturia
- Oliguria
- Fixed specific gravity

Gastrointestinal
- Anorexia
- Nausea and vomiting
- Hiccups
- GI bleeding
- Uremic fetor

Musculoskeletal
- Osteodystrophy
- Bone pain

Neurologic
- Fatigue
- Depression
- Irritability
- Impaired thinking
- Insomnia
- Restless leg syndrome
- Paresthesias

Cardiovascular
- Edema
- Hypertension
- Coronary heart disease
- Heart failure
- Pericarditis

Hematologic
- Anemia
- Impaired clotting
- Increased risk of infection

Reproductive
- Amenorrhea (female)
- Impotence (male)

Integumentary
- Pallor
- Uremic skin color (yellow-green)
- Dry skin
- Pruritus
- Ecchymoses
- Uremic "frost"

Metabolic Processes
- Hyperkalemia
- Acidosis
- Hyperlipidemia
- Hyperuricemia
- Malnutrition

Figure 29-14. ■ The multisystem effects of end-stage renal disease and uremia.

BOX 29-17	MANIFESTATIONS OF END-STAGE RENAL DISEASE AND UREMIA

- Anorexia, nausea, vomiting
- Difficulty thinking, concentrating, fatigue, insomnia
- Edema, high blood pressure
- Restless leg syndrome, numbness, tingling of hands and feet
- Dry, itchy skin; pallor and yellowish skin color
- Irregular menses, impotence
- Anemia with fatigue, weakness, depression
- Bone tenderness, pain, muscle weakness
- Electrolyte imbalances (high potassium, phosphate, and magnesium levels; low calcium levels)
- Metabolic acidosis leading to increased respiratory rate and depth, malaise, weakness, headache

Sodium bicarbonate or calcium carbonate may be used to manage the electrolyte imbalances and acidosis accompanying renal failure. When serum potassium levels are dangerously high, a potassium-binding exchange resin such as sodium polystyrene sulfonate (Kayexalate, SPS Suspension) may be given by oral or rectal route. Intravenous insulin and glucose may also be given to rapidly lower serum potassium levels.

Folic acid and iron supplements are used to combat anemia. Epoetin alfa may be used to stimulate RBC production in patients with CKD who are severely anemic. A multiple-vitamin preparation is also often prescribed, because anorexia, nausea, and dietary restrictions may limit nutrient intake. To reduce the risk of cardiovascular disease, the major cause of death in CKD, a statin drug such as atorvastatin (Lipitor) may be ordered to lower serum cholesterol levels.

Food and Fluid Management

When the kidneys cannot effectively regulate fluid and electrolyte balance and eliminate metabolic waste products, intake of these substances must be regulated.

Fluid and sodium intake may be restricted. Fluid intake for patients with AKI is calculated by allowing 500 to 800 mL for insensible losses (respiration, perspiration, bowel losses) and adding the amount of urine output (or lost in emesis or diarrhea) during the previous 24 hours. For example, if the patient has 325 mL of urine output, intake for the next day is restricted to 825 to 1,125 mL, including both oral and intravenous fluids. Accurate weights and intake and output records are essential. Patients with CKD should notify the physician of any weight gain of more than 5 lb (2 to 2.5 kg) over a 2-day period. Sodium and potassium intake are regulated. Salt substitutes containing potassium are avoided.

The patient with renal failure needs adequate nutrients and calories to prevent tissue breakdown. Protein intake may be limited to reduce uremic symptoms and slow the progression of CKD. Proteins should be rich in amino acids (i.e., meat, fish, poultry, cheese, eggs, milk, or soy). Carbohydrates are increased to maintain adequate calorie intake. Total parenteral nutrition may be ordered if the patient is unable to eat.

Renal Replacement Therapies

When medication and diet management are no longer effective to maintain fluid and electrolyte balance and prevent uremia, dialysis or kidney transplant is considered.

Dialysis is the diffusion of solutes across a membrane from an area of higher concentration to one of lower concentration. It is used to remove excess fluid and waste products in renal failure. In dialysis, blood is separated from a dialysis solution (**dialysate**) by a semipermeable membrane. Water and solutes such as urea and electrolytes diffuse across this membrane, but proteins do not. Dialysis compensates for the kidneys' inability to eliminate excess water and solutes.

The decision to start dialysis is not an easy one. Like insulin therapy for a diabetic, dialysis manages the effects of kidney failure but is not a cure, and it requires a daily commitment. Patients on dialysis may have difficulty maintaining a job because of the hours required for treatment. Many families fall apart with the day-to-day stress. Even with dialysis, patients may have constant flulike symptoms and feel controlled by their illness. In the end, patients may choose to discontinue treatment, preferring death over continued dialysis.

HEMODIALYSIS In *hemodialysis,* electrolytes, waste products, and excess water are removed from the body by diffusion and filtration. The patient's blood is pumped to the dialyzer (Figure 29-15■), where solutes (electrolytes and waste products) diffuse through a semipermeable membrane into the dialysate. Medications can be added to the dialysate to diffuse into the blood. Excess water is removed from the blood by creating a higher fluid pressure on the blood side of the membrane. Patients typically undergo two or three sessions of hemodialysis per week for a total of 9 to 12 hours. Hemodialysis can be done at home but usually occurs in an outpatient dialysis center.

In AKI, a double-lumen catheter may be inserted into the subclavian or jugular vein to provide temporary vascular access for hemodialysis. For longer-term access, an arteriovenous (AV) fistula (Figure 29-16■) is commonly created, usually on the nondominant arm. Often the radial artery and cephalic vein are joined. A functional AV fistula has a palpable pulsation and a *bruit* (audible murmur)

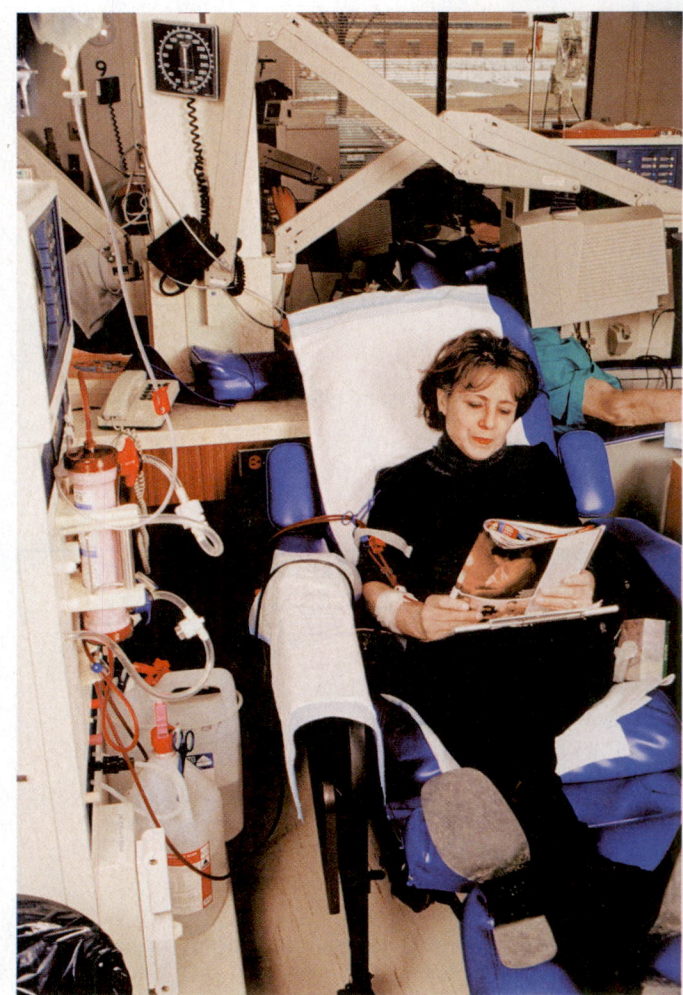

Figure 29-15. ■ A woman undergoing hemodialysis.
(Source: Carolyn A. McKeone/Science Source.)

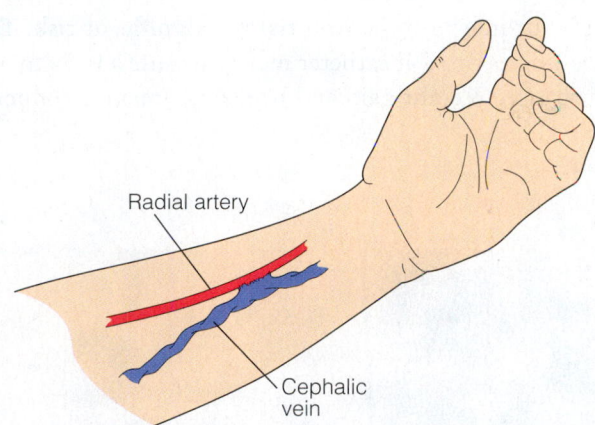

Radial artery

Cephalic
vein

Figure 29-16. ■ An arteriovenous fistula.

on auscultation. Patients with CKD may have an AV graft for vascular access. The graft, made of synthetic material, connects the artery and vein. Box 29-18■ outlines nursing care for the patient undergoing hemodialysis.

clinicalALERT

Do not take blood pressures or allow blood draws or IV starts on the nondominant arm of patients in renal failure, to avoid damaging blood vessels. If a fistula or graft is in place, avoid taking blood pressures or doing venipunctures on the affected arm.

Patients on hemodialysis may develop both systemic and fistula complications. Hypotension is the most frequent complication occurring during hemodialysis. Muscle cramps are also a common complication during hemodialysis. Bleeding may occur due to altered clotting and the use of heparin during dialysis. Infection is a significant risk.

AV fistula problems include infection and clotting or thrombosis. These complications may cause fistula failure and require development of a new site. AV fistula failure can have a psychologic impact, resulting in depression and an altered self-concept.

CONTINUOUS RENAL REPLACEMENT THERAPY Continuous renal replacement therapy (CRRT) allows more gradual fluid and solute removal than hemodialysis. It may be used for patients whose condition is unstable. Blood is continuously circulated (artery to vein or vein to vein) through a porous hemofilter, allowing excess water and solutes to drain into a collection device. Fluid may be replaced with a balanced electrolyte solution as needed during treatment. The slower process of CRRT reduces the adverse effects associated with hemodialysis but may require prolonged immobilization.

PERITONEAL DIALYSIS In *peritoneal dialysis,* the highly vascular peritoneum serves as the dialyzing surface. Warmed dialysate is instilled into the peritoneal cavity through a peritoneal catheter (Figure 29-17■A). Metabolic waste

BOX 29-18	NURSING CARE CHECKLIST

Hemodialysis

Before Dialysis

☑ Use Standard Precautions at all times.

☑ Document vital signs, including orthostatic blood pressures (lying and sitting), apical pulse, and respirations and also lung sounds and weight.

☑ Assess vascular access site for a palpable pulsation or vibration (*thrill*), an audible bruit, and signs of inflammation. Promptly report absence of pulsation, thrill, or bruit, as well as evidence of inflammation to the charge nurse or physician.

☑ Alert all personnel to avoid using the arm with the vascular access site (or the nondominant arm if a site has not yet been established) for blood pressure or venipuncture.

After Dialysis

☑ Document vital signs, weight, and vascular access site assessment. Monitor for orthostatic hypotension, tachycardia, and weight loss.

☑ Monitor BUN, serum creatinine, serum electrolytes, and hematocrit.

☑ Report possible adverse effects of dialysis such as muscle cramping, headache, nausea and vomiting, altered level of consciousness, seizures, or hypotension.

☑ Assess for bleeding at the access site or elsewhere.

☑ If a transfusion was given during dialysis, report symptoms of transfusion reaction, such as chills and fever; dyspnea; chest, back, or arm pain; and hives or itching.

☑ Provide psychologic support; listen actively for feelings of grief, hopelessness, or anger.

☑ Refer for social services and counseling as indicated.

products and electrolytes diffuse into the dialysate while it remains in the abdomen. Excess water is drawn into the dialysate by osmosis. The fluid is then drained by gravity out of the peritoneal cavity into a sterile bag. Peritoneal dialysis is significantly less costly than hemodialysis but is used by fewer people with renal failure in the United States.

Continuous ambulatory peritoneal dialysis (CAPD) is the most common form of peritoneal dialysis used today (Figure 29-17■B). Two liters of solution are instilled into the peritoneal cavity, and the catheter is sealed. The patient can then continue normal daily activities, emptying the peritoneal cavity and replacing the dialysate every 4 to 6 hours. No special equipment is needed. A variation of CAPD is *continuous cyclic peritoneal dialysis (CCPD)*. CCPD uses a delivery device during nighttime hours; the fluid remains in the peritoneal cavity during the day. CAPD can be performed anywhere, and CCPD allows for home treatment at night, leaving the patient free during the day. See Box 29-19■ for nursing care of the patient having peritoneal dialysis.

Peritoneal dialysis is less likely to cause rapid fluid and electrolyte shifts than hemodialysis, but it is less efficient in removing waste products. It does not require vascular access, but infection (peritonitis) is a significant risk. The indwelling peritoneal catheter may also cause a body image disturbance. Weight gain and hyperglycemia are common

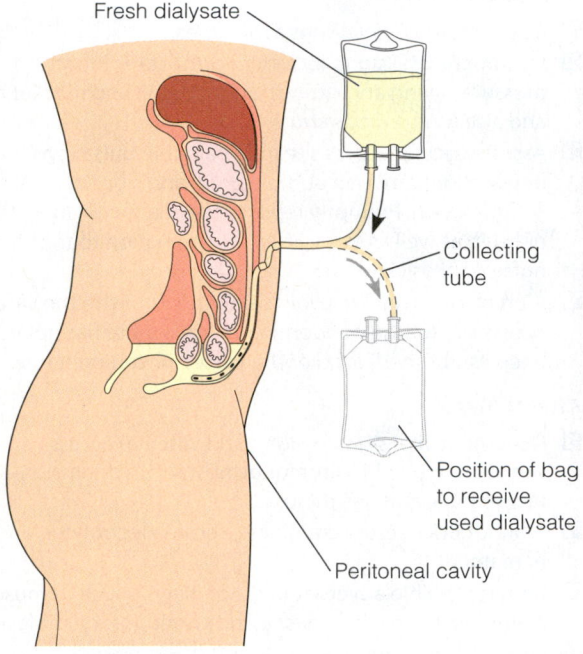
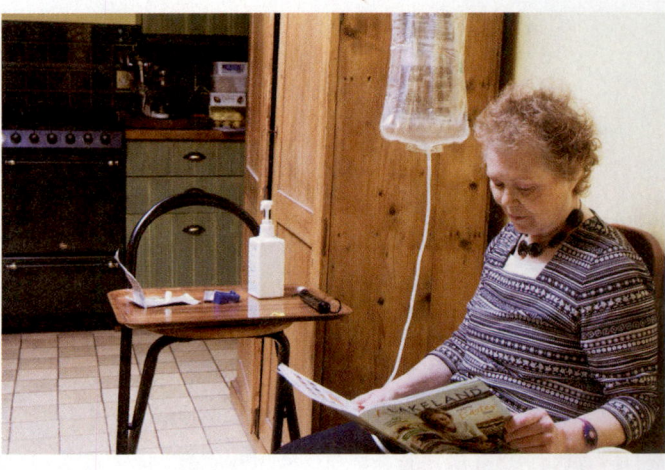

Figure 29-17. ■ (**A**) Peritoneal dialysis. (**B**) A woman undergoing continuous ambulatory peritoneal dialysis at home. (Source for B: Life-in-View/Science Source.)

BOX 29-19   NURSING CARE CHECKLIST

Peritoneal Dialysis

Before Dialysis

- ☑ Use Standard Precautions at all times.
- ☑ Document vital signs, including temperature, orthostatic blood pressures (lying and standing), apical pulse, and respirations and lung sounds.
- ☑ Weigh daily or between dialysis runs as indicated.
- ☑ Measure and record abdominal girth.
- ☑ Ask the patient to urinate before peritoneal catheter insertion.
- ☑ If manual peritoneal dialysis is used, warm prescribed dialysate solution to body temperature (98.6°F or 37°C) using a warmer. Dialysis cyclers automatically warm the solution.
- ☑ Explain all procedures and expected sensations.

During Dialysis

- ☑ Use aseptic technique during dialysis and when caring for the peritoneal catheter.
- ☑ Prime dialysis tubing with solution and connect it to the peritoneal catheter, avoiding kinks. Clamp drainage tubing.
- ☑ With the patient sitting or in Fowler's position, instill dialysate into peritoneal cavity over approximately 10 minutes. Clamp tubing and allow the solution to remain in the abdomen for the prescribed dwell period.

- ☑ During instillation and the dwell time, observe for dyspnea, tachypnea, or other signs of respiratory distress.
- ☑ After the prescribed dwell time, open drainage tubing clamps and allow dialysate to drain by gravity into a sterile container. Observe solution for clarity and any evidence of blood, feces, odor, or cloudiness. Promptly report abnormal findings to the charge nurse or physician.
- ☑ Accurately record amount and type of solution instilled, including any added medications, the dwell time, and amount and character of the drainage.
- ☑ Monitor laboratory values, including BUN, serum creatinine, and serum electrolytes.
- ☑ Troubleshoot for possible problems during dialysis:

  - ☑ Slow instillation of dialysate: Raise the container and reposition the patient. Check tubing and catheter for kinks. Check abdominal dressing for wetness, indicating leakage around the catheter.
  - ☑ Excess dwell time.
  - ☑ Poor dialysate drainage. Lower the bag; reposition the patient, and check tubing for kinks.

After Dialysis

- ☑ Record vital signs, including temperature. Report significant changes from baseline.
- ☑ Time meals to correspond with solution drainage.
- ☑ Maintain dietary restrictions as ordered.
- ☑ Teach peritoneal dialysis procedure as indicated.

problems for patients undergoing peritoneal dialysis, as calories and sugar are absorbed from the dialysate.

Kidney Transplant

Kidney transplant, implanting a functioning kidney, is the treatment of choice for many patients with end-stage renal disease. The patient is no longer tied to a dialysis catheter, machine, or center. Dietary and fluid restrictions are reduced, and the body image is one of increased "wholeness."

About 34% of transplanted kidneys in the United States are from living donors, many of whom are related to the recipient. The rest are from deceased donors. Individuals with normal kidneys who are in good physical health and have the same ABO blood group as the recipient may serve as donors. Predonation counseling is essential because of the risks involved. Deceased donor kidneys are obtained from people who meet the criteria for brain death, are younger than 60 years, and are free of systemic disease, malignancy, or infection, including HIV and hepatitis B or C. Kidneys are removed before or immediately after cardiac arrest and are preserved by hypothermia or continuous perfusion until they are implanted.

The donor kidney is usually placed in the lower abdominal cavity of the recipient (Figure 29-18■). It is connected to arterial and venous blood supplies, and its ureter is connected to one of the recipient's ureters or directly to the bladder, using a tunnel technique to prevent reflux. Review Box 29-16 for pre- and postoperative nursing care for a living kidney donor. Box 29-20■ provides nursing care for the kidney recipient.

Unless the donor and recipient are identical twins, the body mounts a normal immune response to reject the transplanted organ. Drugs are given to suppress the immune system and the inflammatory response. Even with immunosuppressive drugs, the transplanted kidney can be rejected at any time. *Acute rejection* develops within months of the transplant. The patient may have few symptoms of rejection other than a fall in urine output and increasing BUN and serum creatinine levels. Corticosteroid drugs and biologic therapies (monoclonal antibodies) are given to treat rejection. *Chronic rejection* is a major cause of transplant loss.

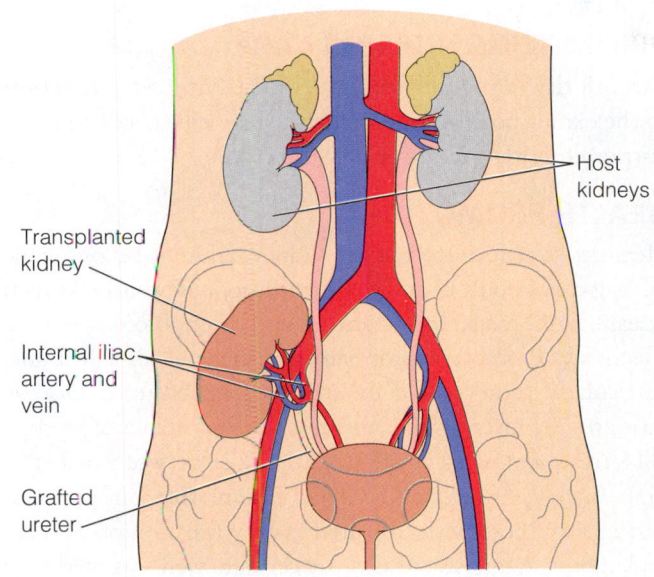

Host kidneys

Transplanted kidney

Internal iliac artery and vein

Grafted ureter

Figure 29-18. ■ Placement of a transplanted kidney.

BOX 29-20	NURSING CARE CHECKLIST

Kidney Transplant

Before Surgery

☑ Assess knowledge and reinforce teaching. Discuss concerns about surgery, the organ donor, and possible complications.

☑ Provide routine preoperative care.

After Surgery

☑ Provide routine postoperative care.

☑ Record urine output every 30 to 60 minutes initially. Maintain closed urinary drainage system.

☑ Closely monitor vital signs, arterial pressure, and hemodynamic pressures as ordered.

☑ Maintain intravenous fluids as ordered.

☑ Administer diuretics as ordered.

☑ Remove urinary catheter within 2 to 3 days or as ordered. Encourage voiding every 1 to 2 hours and assess frequently for urinary retention after catheter removal.

☑ Monitor serum electrolytes and renal function tests.

☑ Monitor for possible complications:

  ☑ Hemorrhage, as indicated by swelling at the operative site, increased abdominal girth, and changes in vital signs and level of consciousness.

  ☑ Urine leakage into the peritoneal cavity, as indicated by abdominal swelling and tenderness and decreased urine output.

  ☑ Renal artery thrombosis, indicated by the abrupt onset of hypertension and a fall in GFR.

  ☑ Infection, indicated by possible fever, change in level of consciousness, cloudy or malodorous urine, or purulent drainage from the incision.

  ☑ Rejection, as indicated by fever, swelling and tenderness over the graft site, decreased urine output, and declining renal function.

☑ Reinforce teaching, including medications and potential side effects, vital sign and weight monitoring, signs of organ rejection, and any prescribed diet changes.

☑ Provide psychologic support; address concerns and provide information as needed.

It can develop months to years after the transplant and does not respond to increased immunosuppression.

Patients receiving immunosuppressive drugs to prevent transplant loss have an increased risk of infections. Tumors may develop. Infants born to mothers undergoing immunosuppressive therapy have a higher risk of congenital defects. Corticosteroid use may lead to bone problems, peptic ulcer disease, and cataracts. Other potential complications of kidney transplant include hypertension and an increased risk of coronary heart disease and stroke.

NURSING CARE

PRIORITIZING NURSING CARE

The priority for nursing care is on preserving renal function to the extent possible and managing the effects of impaired output of fluids and waste products.

HEALTH PROMOTION

Measures to reduce the risk for kidney failure focus on maintaining cardiac output and tissue perfusion, preventing kidney disease, and managing diabetes and high blood pressure effectively. Promote appropriate treatment of all infections, particularly those caused by streptococcal bacteria. Discuss measures to prevent UTI, and stress the importance of prompt UTI treatment. Discuss the relationship between diabetes, high blood pressure, and CKD. Ensure that all patients, particularly those with impaired kidney function or who are undergoing diagnostic tests or surgery, are well hydrated.

ASSESSING

Nurses caring for patients at risk for developing renal failure collect data related to the cardiovascular system and kidney perfusion, as well as data related to urinary function.

Subjective Data

Collect information about current symptoms, including urine output (color, quantity, any difficulty initiating urine flow or emptying the bladder completely). Ask about recent weight changes and any noticeable swelling of the face or extremities, and other symptoms such as nausea or vomiting. Inquire about current or previous kidney problems, chronic diseases such as diabetes or blood pressure, recent surgery or diagnostic tests, and current or recent medications.

Objective Data

Document vital signs, current weight, and intake and output (if known); level of consciousness and mental status; skin color, temperature, and moisture, and presence of any edema; auscultate heart, lung, and bowel sounds. Obtain a urine specimen for analysis, noting the color, clarity, character of the urine, and its specific gravity.

IDENTIFYING POTENTIAL COMPLICATIONS

Be alert for and promptly report manifestations of uremia (see Box 29-17). Anorexia and nausea are early symptoms. Observe for increasing BUN and serum creatinine levels and decreasing eGFR. The patient with renal failure is at risk for GI bleeding; promptly report coffee-ground emesis or evidence of bleeding in feces. Cardiovascular disease is common in patients with CKD; immediately report complaints of chest pain, shortness of breath, or a sense of impending doom. Monitor the appearance of AV fistula or graft site, presence of pulsation or thrill, and for an audible bruit. Report the absence of palpable or audible pulsation of the graft. Assess for and promptly report signs of infection (fever, malaise, abdominal pain, cloudy dialysate) in the patient undergoing peritoneal dialysis. When caring for a patient who has had a kidney transplant, monitor for and promptly report signs of rejection, including decreasing urine output, manifestations of uremia, and changes in laboratory results.

DIAGNOSING, PLANNING, AND IMPLEMENTING

Excess Fluid Volume

Expected outcome: Will regain fluid balance as evidenced by weight and vital signs within expected range, decreased edema, and absence of manifestations such as shortness of breath.

- Maintain accurate I&O records. *Accurate I&O records help determine treatment, especially fluid restriction. Hourly urine output measurements may be required in acute kidney injury.*

- Weigh daily or as ordered. Use consistent technique and timing to ensure accuracy. *Weight often provides a more accurate assessment of fluid volume than I&O records, particularly in patients who are producing little or no urine.*

- Document vital signs at least every 4 hours. *Changes in vital signs may indicate either fluid volume excess or deficit. Hypertension can further damage the kidneys.*

- Frequently assess heart and breath sounds. Assess the degree of peripheral edema and neck vein distention. *Excess fluid volume increases the risk for heart failure and pulmonary edema. An S_3 or S_4 gallop rhythm or crackles in the lungs may indicate heart failure and should be reported to the charge nurse or physician.*

- Unless contraindicated, place in Fowler's position. *Fowler's position facilitates breathing and lung expansion and reduces the workload of the heart.*

- Restrict fluids as ordered. Provide frequent mouth care and encourage using hard candies to decrease the thirst response. If ice chips are used to relieve thirst, include as intake (generally calculated as half of an equivalent volume of fluid; an 8-oz or 240-mL container of ice chips yields 120 mL of water). *Fluid restriction helps minimize fluid retention and the complications of fluid volume excess, especially in the patient with AKI.*

- Administer medications with meals. *This reduces total liquid consumed.*
- Turn frequently and provide good skin care. *Edema can lead to skin breakdown, especially in the older or debilitated patient.*
- Administer diuretics as ordered and monitor response. *Diuretics may promote urination.*
- Monitor serum electrolytes and for manifestations of imbalances. Report abnormal results. *Electrolyte imbalances may develop because of water retention and impaired renal function.*

Imbalanced Nutrition: Less Than Body Requirements

Expected outcome: Will consume adequate calories to maintain weight within expected range.

The manifestations of uremia and dietary restrictions often affect food intake. The patient may not eat enough to meet metabolic needs. *Catabolism* (breakdown of body proteins to meet energy needs) worsens azotemia and uremia.

- Monitor and document food intake, including the amount and type of food consumed. *Food intake records help determine the adequacy of nutritional intake and identify the need for nutritional supplements.*
- Administer antiemetic drugs 30 to 60 minutes before eating. *Anorexia, nausea, and vomiting are common. Antiemetics reduce nausea and the risk of vomiting with food intake.*
- Provide mouth care just before meals. *The patient may have a metallic taste and bad breath. Mouth care improves taste and stimulates the appetite.*
- Provide frequent, small meals or between-meal snacks. *These measures promote food intake in the fatigued or anorectic patient.*
- Arrange for a dietary consultation. Provide preferred foods to the extent possible, and involve the patient in planning menus. Allow family to prepare meals within dietary restrictions and encourage family members to eat with the patient. *The patient is more likely to eat favorite foods. Involving the patient in planning promotes a sense of control and learning about dietary restrictions. Familiar foods and social interaction encourage eating and heighten the patient's enjoyment of meals.*
- Monitor serum electrolytes and albumin. *Changes in values may indicate either improving or declining nutritional status.*
- Administer and monitor enteral nutrition as ordered. *Enteral nutrition may be necessary to prevent catabolism and increasing azotemia in the patient with renal failure.*

Risk for Infection

Expected outcome: Will remain free of signs of infection.

Renal failure affects immune function, increasing the risk for infection. Invasive treatments and catheters further increase this risk.

- Use Standard Precautions and good hand washing at all times. *Hand washing and Standard Precautions help prevent spread of infection to and from the patient. Patients on hemodialysis have an increased risk of hepatitis B, hepatitis C, and HIV infection.*
- Use strict aseptic technique when handling ports, catheters, and incisions. *Aseptic technique is vital to reduce the risk of introducing an infectious organism.*
- Monitor temperature and vital signs at least every 4 hours. *An elevated temperature or increased pulse rate may indicate infection.*
- Monitor WBC count and differential. *High or low WBC counts may indicate an infection. Increasing numbers of immature WBCs in circulation may also indicate infection.*
- Culture urine, peritoneal dialysis fluid, and other drainage as indicated. *Culture is used to determine the presence of pathogens.*
- Turn or ambulate frequently; encourage coughing and deep breathing. *These measures decrease the risk of respiratory infection.*
- Restrict visits from obviously ill family members. Teach the patient and family how to reduce the spread of infection. *The patient and family need to know and understand how to reduce the risk of infection at home and in the community.*

Disturbed Body Image

Expected outcome: Will express willingness to use suggested resources after discharge.

- Involve the patient in decision making and encourage self-care. *Patient involvement increases autonomy, improves acceptance, and promotes independence.*
- Encourage expression of feelings and concerns. Accept perceptions and feelings without criticism. *Self-expression enhances the patient's self-worth and acceptance.*
- Work with the patient to develop and achieve realistic goals. Provide positive reinforcement and feedback. Support positive gains. *Adapting to a change in body image and self-concept requires time and often occurs in a series of small steps. Realistic goals allow the patient to see progress. Reinforcement helps develop positive coping strategies.*
- Encourage contact with a support group. Refer for counseling or social services as indicated. *Peer support and counseling can help the patient and family develop effective coping and adaptation strategies.*

MANAGING NURSING CARE

As appropriate and allowed by the designated duties and responsibilities of assistive personnel, the nurse may delegate nursing care activities such as providing oral and skin care and assisting with ADLs for the patient with kidney failure. Before assigning tasks such as obtaining vital signs, measuring intake and output, obtaining daily weights, and assisting with meals and fluid intake, ensure that assistive personnel have a clear understanding of restrictions (e.g., avoiding blood pressure measurement on the designated arm or fluid restrictions) and the importance of accurate measurements.

EVALUATING

When evaluating the effectiveness of nursing interventions for the patient with kidney failure, collect data related to fluid volume status, such as weight, intake and output, degree of edema, and cardiovascular status. Assess skin and mucous membrane integrity as well. Evaluate food and nutrient intake and compliance with prescribed diet. Assess for freedom from infection. Look at coping strategies employed by the patient, as well as active participation in care.

DOCUMENTING

Document assessment data on a regular and continuing basis. Note the relationship between any changes in assessment findings and treatments provided. Document status of the AV fistula if present or the clarity and amount of peritoneal dialysate returned. Also document all teaching provided to the patient and family and their apparent understanding and acceptance of information.

CONTINUITY OF CARE

Kidney failure may be an acute disorder or the final stage of CKD. Even when manifestations of AKI resolve before discharge, the healing process lasts for up to 1 year. Both AKI and CKD can require long-term, day-to-day management.

Early teaching focuses on the nature of the disorder and its projected course. Teach patients with AKI about the extended recovery period and the importance of avoiding exposure to nephrotoxins. Teach patients with CKD about ways to slow the progress of the disorder (e.g., managing diabetes and hypertension, following dietary recommendations) and the importance of avoiding further insults to the kidneys. Provide information about drugs that are potentially damaging to the kidneys (e.g., NSAIDs and some antibiotics) and the importance of checking with the physician before taking any new drug (prescribed or over the counter).

Educate all patients about prescribed dietary, sodium, and fluid restrictions. Involve the patient, a dietitian, and the family member usually responsible for cooking in teaching. Include strategies to improve flavor and to relieve thirst when fluid is restricted.

Teach the patient on hemodialysis how to assess and protect the fistula or shunt. Refer home dialysis helpers for formal training. Teach and demonstrate catheter care and the dialysis procedure to the patient who will perform CAPD and a family member or significant other. When a kidney transplant has been done, teach about the prescribed medications, their adverse effects and management, infection prevention, and signs and symptoms of organ rejection.

Refer patients to local or state chapters of the National Kidney Foundation or the American Association of Kidney Patients.

Note: The references and resources for all chapters have been compiled at the back of the book.

Chapter Review

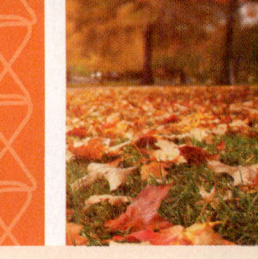

KEY POINTS

- **Concept:** Urinary incontinence is a common and underreported problem, particularly among older adults. It is not a normal consequence of aging and in most cases can be treated effectively.
- Urinary retention, a less common problem than UI, may be either acute (e.g., postoperative urinary retention) or chronic. Chronic urinary retention is the result of neurologic trauma or disease; nursing responsibilities focus on teaching self-care measures.
- **Concept:** Urinary tract infections are common among adult women and patients in hospitals and long-term care facilities. UTI can lead to sepsis or chronic kidney disease, making prevention through patient and caregiver teaching a major nursing responsibility.
- A 3-day course of antibiotic therapy is often effective for treating uncomplicated UTIs. Advantages of this shortened course are improved compliance and reduced adverse effects when compared with longer courses of treatment. Nursing care focuses on teaching health promotion to prevent future UTI.
- **Concept:** Glomerular disorders cause loss of proteins and blood cells in the urine, decrease the GFR, and affect urine formation and waste elimination. Depending on the cause, the patient may recover fully or eventually develop CKD and end-stage renal failure.
- Acute glomerulonephritis is usually due to an abnormal inflammatory response to beta-hemolytic streptococcal infection (strep throat). It generally resolves uneventfully in children and most adults.
- **Concept:** The urinary tract can be affected by obstructive processes such as stones and tumors. Early recognition of obstructive processes and maintaining unobstructed urinary output are critical to maintain kidney function.
- Patients with a history of kidney or other urinary stones have a high risk of developing stones in the future. Emphasize the importance of maintaining a generous fluid intake, avoiding dehydration, and, for calcium stones, staying physically active.
- **Concept:** Painless hematuria is a frequent initial manifestation of urinary tract cancer. Advise all patients with hematuria to see their physician for evaluation.
- Cancers of the urinary bladder and kidney are among the 10 most common cancers. When discovered early, treatment is often successful in eradicating the cancer. When advanced, radical surgery such as nephrectomy or cystectomy with urinary diversion may be needed.
- Nursing care for patients with cancer of the urinary system focuses on maintaining urinary output, preventing infection, and teaching and supporting the patient and family.
- **Concept:** Kidney failure may occur in response to an acute insult such as impaired blood flow or a nephrotoxic drug or as the end-stage of CKD. Nurses play a key role in preventing and recognizing acute kidney injury, as well as in teaching patients who are at risk for CKD how to prevent or delay the onset of kidney failure.
- AKI usually affects seriously ill older adults who experience hypovolemia or shock or who are exposed to a nephrotoxic drug or substance. It often resolves with treatment, and kidney function is restored.
- ESRD is the final stage of CKD and a long-term process of kidney destruction (due to diabetes, hypertension, or a primary kidney disease). Patients with ESRD often require treatment to replace lost kidney function, such as dialysis or a kidney transplant.

PEARSON NURSING STUDENT RESOURCES

Find additional materials at **nursing.pearsonhighered.com**.

Clinical Reasoning Care Map

Caring for a Patient With Urinary Incontinence
NCLEX-PN® Focus Area: Health Promotion and Maintenance

Case Study: Anna Giovanni, a 76-year-old widow, lives alone. Her eldest daughter is concerned that her mother seems increasingly reluctant to leave the apartment to visit friends and family. She reports a strong odor of urine throughout her mother's apartment and that her mother's bed is often wet.

Nursing Diagnosis: Urinary Incontinence

COLLECT DATA

Subjective	Objective
_____	_____
_____	_____
_____	_____
_____	_____
_____	_____
_____	_____

Does this present a threat to the patient's safety?

If yes, the priority intervention to address this threat would be:

_____

Nursing Care

_____
_____
_____
_____
_____
_____
_____

Interprofessional team members to include when planning care:

_____

How would you document this?_____
_____

Compare your answers and documentation to those provided on the companion website.

Data Collected
(use only those that apply)

- Relates urine leakage when laughing, coughing, and on hearing the sound of running water
- Often unable to reach bathroom in time at night
- Hysterectomy at age 52
- Estrogen-replacement therapy for approximately 10 years after hysterectomy
- Takes digoxin 0.125 mg qd, furosemide 40 mg bid, and KCl 20 mEq tid
- Moderate cystourethrocele
- Atrophy of vaginal tissues
- Pelvic floor strength weak
- Urinalysis within normal limits
- Postvoiding residual urine 5 mL
- Average of nine daytime voidings and four at night
- Urine leakage usually occurs in late afternoon and at night

Nursing Interventions
(use only those that apply; list in priority order)

- Suggest commercial products for protecting clothing and furniture.
- Change afternoon dose of furosemide from 9 p.m. to 4 p.m.
- Suggest decaffeinated tea and noncitrus fruit juices (grape, apple, and cranberry).
- Encourage voiding by the clock, gradually increasing intervals from every 45 to 60 minutes to every 2 to 2.5 hours. Advise shorter intervals for 2 to 3 hours after furosemide doses.
- Teach how to identify pelvic floor muscles and perform Kegel exercises.
- Provide bedside commode for nighttime use.
- Encourage minimizing fluid intake after evening meal.
- Schedule follow-up visits and evaluations to reinforce teaching.

NCLEX-PN® Exam Preparation

1 A 79-year-old patient with benign prostatic hypertrophy has not voided in the past 8 hours. The FIRST action by the LPN/LVN would be to:
1. provide 500 mL fluids orally.
2. perform a catheterization with a 14-Fr. straight catheter.
3. palpate the lower abdomen.
4. notify the physician.

2 A 50-year-old woman experiences stress incontinence. Which of the following assessment findings indicates a risk factor for this condition?
1. Total abdominal hysterectomy 9 years ago
2. Smoking one pack of cigarettes per day
3. Exercising four times a week
4. History of two pregnancies

3 An LPN/LVN evaluates for residual urine on a patient; 30 mL of clear yellow urine is returned. The appropriate action by the nurse would be to:
1. notify the physician.
2. document the finding in the medical record.
3. implement measures to assist the patient to void.
4. increase patient's fluid intake.

4 The nurse establishes a nursing diagnosis of *Urinary Incontinence* related to weak pelvic floor muscles for a 69-year-old patient. Which of the following would be an appropriate nursing intervention?
1. Encourage the patient to drink orange juice and tea at each meal.
2. Schedule furosemide (Lasix) 40 mg at 8 p.m. daily.
3. Teach the patient to perform Kegel exercises every 2 hours while awake.
4. Restrict fluid intake to 500 mL/day.

5 The nurse teaching a patient to help prevent urinary tract infections includes which of the following instructions? **Select all that apply**.
1. Drink at least one 8-ounce glass of orange juice daily.
2. Increase your water intake to six or more glasses per day.
3. After voiding or defecating, wipe from back to front.
4. Wear cotton briefs under clothing.
5. Void before and after sexual intercourse.

6 A 19-year-old is admitted with acute glomerulonephritis. The nurse expects to obtain which of the following assessment findings?
1. "Strep throat" 2 weeks ago
2. Pneumonia 1 week ago
3. Gastroenteritis
4. Influenza 3 weeks ago

7 For a patient with a ureteral stone, a priority nursing action is to:
1. wash hands.
2. restrict fluids.
3. strain all urine.
4. collect a sterile urine specimen.

8 A female patient is discharged after a right nephrotomy to remove a urinary calculus. Discharge teaching should include:
1. maintaining oral fluid intake of 1,500 mL daily.
2. avoiding all sources of calcium.
3. signs and symptoms of urinary tract infection.
4. maintaining alkaline urine.

9 A patient is diagnosed with chronic kidney disease. The nurse explains that dietary management of a patient with chronic kidney disease includes:
1. a high-protein, low-carbohydrate diet.
2. a low-protein, high-carbohydrate diet.
3. a high-fat, moderate-sodium diet.
4. a low-fat, high-sodium diet.

10 A patient has an arteriovenous fistula in his left arm for hemodialysis access. The nurse recognizes the need for further teaching if the patient states:
1. "My wife gets the best blood pressure in my left arm."
2. "I check my fistula for pulsations."
3. "I remind the lab personnel to take blood from my right arm."
4. "I sleep on my left side with my left arm extended."

Answers and rationales for Review Questions appear in Appendix I.

Thinking Strategically About . . .

You are an LPN/LVN working in a large urology clinic that provides diagnostic and outpatient treatment services, including hemodialysis and minor surgical procedures.

Walter, 45 years old, has been a type I diabetic since the age of 20. He was diagnosed with diabetic nephropathy 10 years ago and has now progressed to end-stage renal disease. He enters the nephrology unit for temporary hemodialysis to treat uremia and to prepare for peritoneal dialysis. During the nursing assessment, Walter states that he thought his lack of appetite, nausea, vomiting, and fatigue during the past month were caused by "a touch of the flu." His weight remained stable, so he did not worry about not eating much. His BP is 178/100; P 96; R 20. His skin is cool and dry, with minor excoriations on his forearms and lower legs. Walter has a fetid breath odor. A few fine crackles are noted in lung bases bilaterally. Both lower extremities have 3+ pitting edema to just below the knees; his hands also appear edematous. Bowel sounds are hypoactive. Urinalysis shows gross proteinuria.

Howard, a 62-year-old house painter, comes to the clinic for a follow-up appointment after TURBT 5 days ago. Preoperatively, Howard experienced urgency and painless hematuria. He assumed he had prostatic hypertrophy that he knew is common in his age group. The 3-cm tumor was located in the bladder neck, superior to the prostate gland. Howard was discharged with a Foley catheter in place to keep the bladder empty. Today he will learn that the pathology report confirmed bladder cancer. Chemotherapy will be discussed with Howard and his wife, Jane.

India, a 43-year-old registered nurse, is to be seen for repeat renal calculi. Over the past 6 months, she has passed four stones, which are mostly of calcium origin. India admits she does not drink enough water so she would not have to urinate so often at work. Today she is experiencing a dull ache in the right flank but states "it is not as sharp or as severe as the pain of passing a kidney stone."

CRITICAL THINKING

- What is a likely cause of the excoriations on Walter's extremities?
- What is the likely cause of Howard's preoperative symptom of urgency?
- What is a likely cause of the dull ache in India's right flank?

PRIORITY OF CARE

- Which of these patients should you attend to first? Why?
- What question will you ask Howard to determine whether he has been caring for the Foley catheter properly?

- What diagnostic exams would you anticipate the doctor ordering to determine the cause of India's repeated renal calculi?

MANAGEMENT OF CARE

- Which members of the interdisciplinary team should be included in planning for Walter's care?
- Because of Howard's diagnosis of cancer, what referrals may be needed for Howard and his wife?

DELEGATING

- The physician orders the following:
  - Walter: weight and height, clean-catch urine specimen, blood for serum creatinine, BUN, and CBC; schedule creatinine clearance test
  - Howard: remove Foley catheter after obtaining urine specimen for culture; provide printed educational materials about bladder cancer and its treatment to Howard and his wife
  - India: obtain clean-catch urine specimen; schedule for renal ultrasound

Which of these orders can you delegate to the medical assistant? Which should you retain responsibility for implementing? Include your rationale.

PATIENT TEACHING

- What teaching is important to provide for each of these patients?
- Identify credible online resources you can suggest for use by these patients and their families to learn more about their condition, prognosis, and treatment options.

REPORTING

- Often, large medical clinics such as this one employ a variety of nurses and technicians. To whom should the LPN/LVN report patient concerns or questions?

Note: Discussion of Unit questions appears on the companion website.

UNIT VIII
Disrupted Reproductive Function

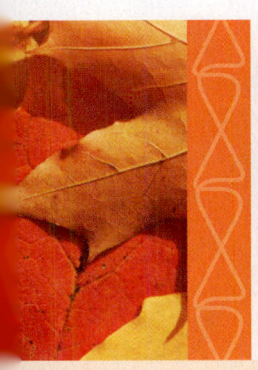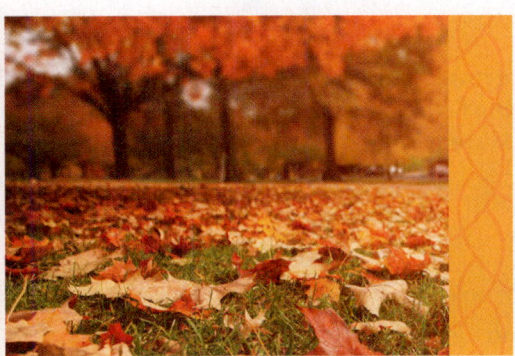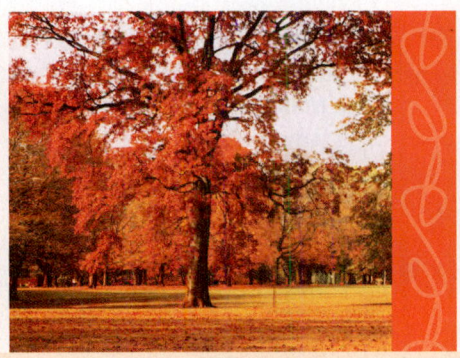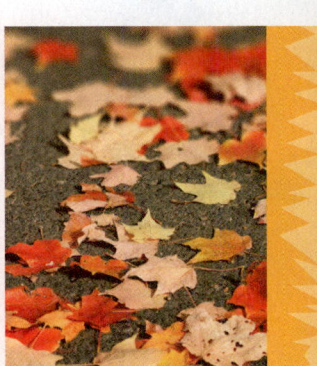

Cultural Care Strategies:

Assessing Communication Variables From a Cultural Perspective . . . 860

Unit VIII Wrap-Up

Thinking Strategically About . . . 878

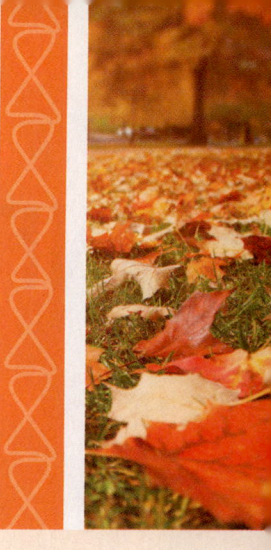

CHAPTER 30
The Reproductive System and Assessment

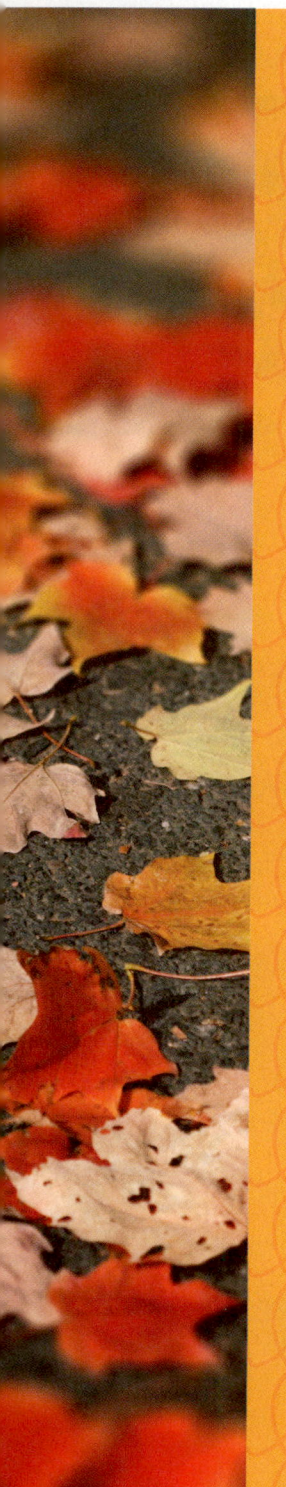

BRIEF OUTLINE

Structure and Function of the Male Reproductive System

Structure and Function of the Female Reproductive System

Age-Related Changes in the Reproductive System

Assessment

Contraception

APPLIED LEARNING OUTCOMES

After completing this chapter, you will be able to:

1. Describe the major structures and functions of the male reproductive system.
2. Describe the major structures and functions of the female reproductive system.
3. Anticipate the normal age-related changes in the male and female reproductive systems.
4. Collect subjective and objective assessment data related to the reproductive system.
5. Provide appropriate nursing care for patients undergoing diagnostic tests related to the reproductive system.

KEY TERMS

The key terms are defined on the pages listed below.

The reproductive organs, in conjunction with the endocrine system, also produce hormones that are important in biologic development and sexual function and behavior.

Structure and Function of the Male Reproductive System

The reproductive system in males includes the paired testes, ducts, accessory glands and organs, and the external genitalia, the penis and scrotum (Figure 30-1■).

TESTES AND SCROTUM

The *testes* produce sperm and testosterone. Sperm is produced in the *seminiferous tubules* of the testes. Leydig cells within the testes produce testosterone.

The testes are suspended in the scrotum by the spermatic cord. The *scrotum* is a sac or pouch that contains the testes and regulates their temperature. The best temperature for producing sperm is about 2 to 3 degrees below body temperature. When the temperature is too low, the scrotum contracts to bring the testes up against the body. When the testes are too warm, the scrotum relaxes to allow the testes to lie farther away from the body.

Spermatogenesis

Spermatogenesis is sperm production. This process begins with puberty and continues throughout a man's life, with approximately 500 million sperm produced daily (Martini, Nath, & Bartholomew, 2012). Spermatogenesis takes 64 to 72 days and includes the following processes:

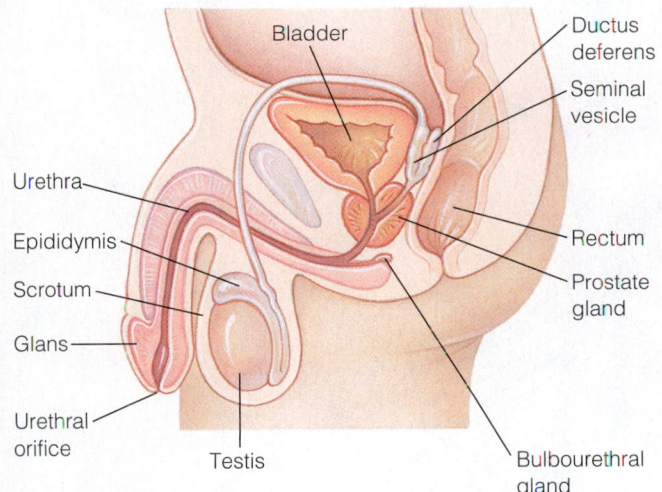

Figure 30-1. ■ The male reproductive system.

1. Sperm stem cells (*spermatogonia*) divide to produce daughter cells (*spermatocytes*) that have the same number of chromosomes (46) as the parent cell.
2. Spermatocytes further divide to produce *spermatids*, immature cells with half the number of chromosomes (23). Spermatids contain one of each chromosome of the 23 chromosome pairs of the human genome and are the father's genetic contribution to a new offspring.
3. Spermatids mature into sperm cells with a head and a tail. The head contains enzymes that allow the sperm to penetrate and fertilize the ovum. The tail allows the sperm to move. When the sperm and ovum fuse, the resulting cell has the normal 46 chromosomes in 23 pairs, including 23 chromosomes from the father via the sperm and 23 chromosomes from the mother via the ovum.

Male Sex Hormones

The male sex hormones are called **androgens**. Most are produced in the testes, although a small amount is produced by the adrenal glands. *Testosterone,* the primary male sex hormone, is essential to develop male secondary sex characteristics and to develop and maintain sexual function. It promotes metabolism, muscle and bone growth, and **libido** (sexual desire).

DUCTS AND SEMEN

Sperm mature and are stored in the *epididymis,* a long coiled tube that lies over the outer surface of each testis. When a man is sexually excited, the epididymis contracts to push the sperm through the *vas deferens* to mix with seminal fluid.

Seminal fluid is made of secretions from the seminal glands (also called seminal vesicles), the epididymis, the prostate gland, and Cowper glands. It nourishes the sperm, provides volume to the semen, and increases its alkalinity. An alkaline pH is essential to mobilize the sperm and ensure fertilization of the ovum. Sperm mixed with seminal fluid is called *semen.* During **ejaculation** (expulsion of seminal fluid), semen enters the urethra for expulsion.

The total amount of ejaculate is 1.5 to 5 mL. The normal sperm count is 60 to 150 million per mL (Kee, 2014).

PROSTATE GLAND

The *prostate gland* is about the size of a walnut. It encircles the urethra just below the urinary bladder (see Figure 30-1). Secretions of the prostate gland make up about one-third of the volume of the semen. These secretions enter the urethra through several ducts during ejaculation. Contraction of the muscular prostate causes the semen to be ejaculated.

PENIS

The penis is composed of a *shaft* and a tip called the *glans,* which is covered by the *foreskin* (or *prepuce*). The foreskin is removed according to cultural custom in a procedure called *circumcision* (see Box 30-1■).

Circumcision

Circumcision is removal of the foreskin of the penis. It is a culture-bound practice most prevalent in the Middle East, Africa, Southeast Asia, and the United States. It is relatively rare in Europe, Latin America, most of Asia, and Oceania. Circumcision is considered religious law in Judaism and an established tradition in Islam. It is usually performed in infancy, but in some cultures it is a rite of a boy's passage into manhood. Some consider it a hygienic practice. Evidence shows that circumcised men who have sex with women are less likely to contract HIV than those who are not circumcised.

The penile shaft contains three columns of erectile tissue: The two lateral columns are called the *corpora cavernosa,* and the central mass is called the *corpus spongiosum.*

Erection occurs when a reflex triggers the parasympathetic nervous system to stimulate arteriolar vasodilation, filling erectile tissue with blood. The erection reflex may be initiated by touch, pressure, sights, sounds, smells, or thoughts of a sexual encounter. After ejaculation, the arterioles constrict, and the penis becomes flaccid.

Structure and Function of the Female Reproductive System

The female reproductive system includes the paired ovaries and fallopian (or uterine) tubes, uterus, vagina, the external genitalia (including the mons pubis, labia, clitoris, and glands), and the breasts. In women, the urethra and urinary meatus are separated from the reproductive organs; however, they are in such close proximity that a health problem with one often affects the other.

INTERNAL STRUCTURES

The internal organs of the female reproductive system include the ovaries, fallopian (or uterine) tubes, uterus, and vagina (Figure 30-2 ■).

Ovaries and Ovulation

In adult women, the ovaries are flat, almond-shaped glands located below the ends of the fallopian tubes. The ovaries produce the female hormones estrogen and progesterone and store immature ova called *oocytes.*

The ovaries produce estrogens, progesterone, and androgens in a cyclic pattern. **Estrogens** are steroid hormones essential to the development and maintenance of female secondary sex characteristics. Along with other hormones, estrogens also help prepare the female reproductive organs for growth of a fetus. They help maintain skin, bone, and blood vessel structure; affect serum cholesterol and high-density lipoprotein (HDL) levels; enhance blood clotting; and affect sodium and water balance. Estrogen secretion varies with the menstrual cycle (see later discussion).

Progesterone primarily affects breast glandular tissue and the endometrium. During pregnancy, it relaxes smooth muscle to decrease uterine contractions. It also increases body temperature. Androgens (produced in small amounts by the adrenal glands as well as the ovaries) are responsible for normal hair growth patterns at puberty and also have metabolic effects.

memoryALERT

Remember progesterone as the hormone that is "pro," which means "promoting," and "gester," which means gestation or pregnancy. So the function of progesterone is to maintain pregnancy.

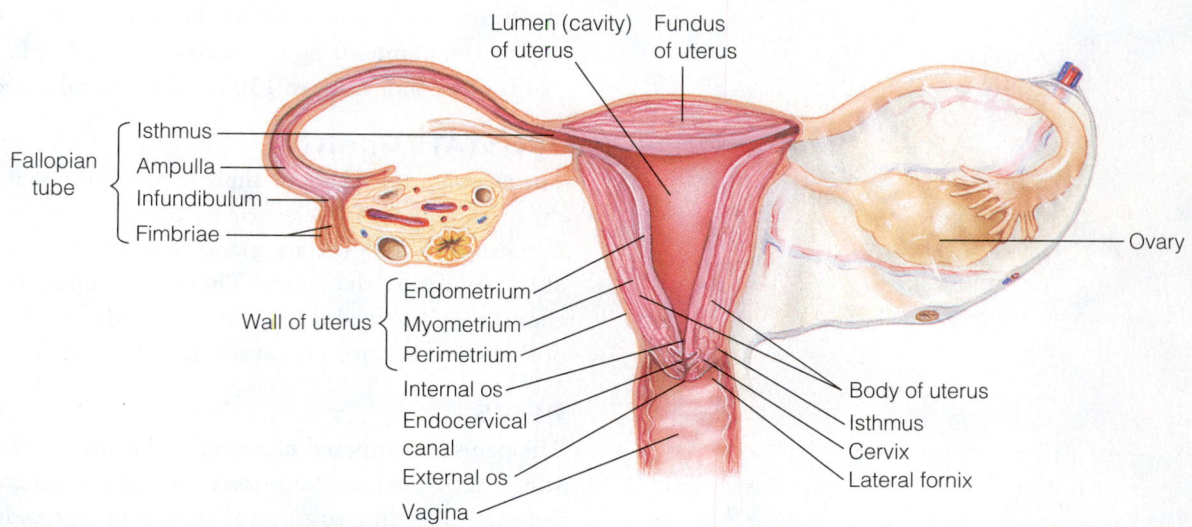

Figure 30-2. ■ The internal organs of the female reproductive system.

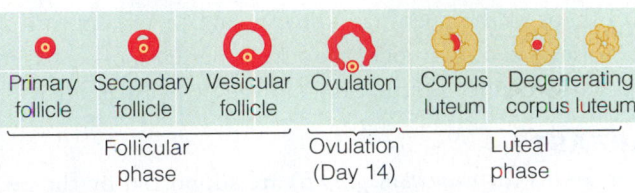

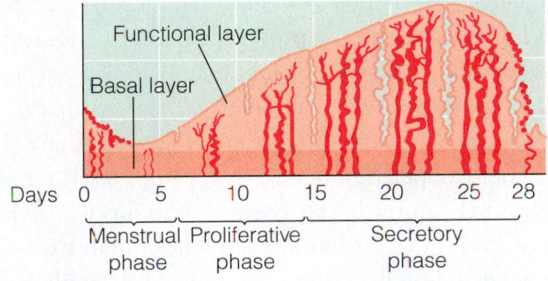

B Uterine cycle

Figure 30-3. ■ (A) Changes in ovarian follicles during the 28-day ovarian cycle. **(B)** Corresponding changes in the endometrium during the menstrual cycle.

The *ovarian cycle* has three phases lasting about 28 days. The *follicular phase* lasts from the 1st to the 10th day of the cycle. The *ovulatory phase* lasts from the 11th to the 14th day, ending with ovulation. The *luteal phase* lasts from the 14th to the 28th day (Figure 30-3 ■).

Each ovary contains many small structures called *ovarian follicles*. Each follicle contains an immature ovum, called an *oocyte*. Each month, several follicles mature, stimulated by *follicle-stimulating hormone (FSH)* and *luteinizing hormone (LH)*. The mature follicles (*graafian follicles*) produce estrogen, which stimulates development of *endometrium* (mucous membranes lining the uterus). When the estrogen level is high enough to stimulate the anterior pituitary gland, a surge of LH is produced. LH stimulates development of the oocyte into a mature ovum and causes the ovarian follicles to rupture, releasing the ova. This is the process of *ovulation*. Each ruptured follicle then becomes a *corpus luteum*, which produces estrogen and progesterone to support the endometrium until conception occurs or the cycle begins again. If pregnancy does not occur, the corpus luteum degenerates, and its hormone production ceases. Falling progesterone and estrogen levels allow LH and FSH levels to increase, and a new cycle begins.

Fallopian (Uterine) Tubes

The *fallopian tubes* are thin tubes about 4 in. (10 cm) long and 1 cm in diameter. They are attached to the uterus on one end. The distal ends of the fallopian tubes are open, with projections called *fimbriae* that drape over the ovary.

The ovum is released from the ovary and is moved into the fallopian tube when it contacts the fimbriae, which move it into the tube.

The fallopian tubes are made of smooth muscle and lined with cilia. Movement of the cilia and smooth muscle contractions move the ovum through the tubes toward the uterus. Fertilization of the ovum by sperm usually occurs in the outer portion of one of the fallopian tubes.

Uterus

The *uterus* is a thick-walled, pear-shaped muscular organ located between the bladder and rectum. Ligaments support it within the abdominal cavity. Its function is to receive the fertilized ovum and provide a site for growth and development of the fetus.

The uterine wall has three layers. The outer layer, the *perimetrium,* merges with the peritoneum. The middle layer, the *myometrium,* has muscle fibers that run in various directions, allowing expansion during pregnancy and contractions during the menses and childbirth. The *endometrium* lines the uterus. Its innermost layer is shed during menstruation.

The uterus is made up of three parts: the fundus, the body, and the cervix (see Figure 30-2). The cervix projects into the vagina. The uterine opening of the cervix is called the *internal os;* the vaginal opening is called the *external os.* The *endocervical canal* between the openings allows discharge of menstrual fluid and entrance of sperm. The cervix is a firm structure that softens in response to hormones during pregnancy.

The endometrium of the uterus responds to changes in estrogen and progesterone during the ovarian cycle to prepare for implantation of the fertilized embryo. It is receptive to embryo implantation for only about 7 days each month, during the time when the embryo would normally reach the uterus from the fallopian tube.

The menstrual cycle begins at the onset of menstruation (Figure 30-3B). During the *menstrual phase,* the inner endometrial layer detaches and is expelled as menstrual fluid. As the maturing follicle begins to produce estrogen, the *proliferative phase* begins. The inner endometrial layer is repaired and thickens, whereas spiral arteries proliferate and tubular glands form. Cervical mucus becomes thin, making it easier for sperm to move into the uterus. During the *secretory phase,* progesterone increases endometrial vascularity and prepares it to support the fertilized ovum. Cervical mucus thickens, blocking the internal os, which becomes the "mucus plug" and helps protect the inside of the uterus from bacteria if pregnancy occurs. If fertilization does not occur, hormone levels fall. Spasm of spiral arteries causes degeneration and sloughing of the inner endometrial layer, starting the process again.

Vagina

The vagina is a fibromuscular tubular structure about 3 to 4 in. (8 to 10 cm) long located between the bladder and urethra and the rectum. The upper end contains the cervix in an area called the *fornix*. The mucous membrane walls of the vagina form folds, called *rugae*. Vaginal mucus is relatively acidic and bacteriostatic. Estrogen and normal vaginal flora help maintain its acid pH. The vagina is the birth canal, allows excretion of menstrual fluid, and is an organ of sexual response.

EXTERNAL GENITALIA

The external genitalia include the mons pubis, the labia, the clitoris, the vaginal and urethral openings, and glands (Figure 30-4■).

The *mons pubis* is a pad of adipose tissue anterior to the symphysis pubis. After puberty, the mons is covered with hair.

The labia are divided into two structures. The *labia majora* are folds of skin and adipose tissue covered with hair that enclose the labia minora. The *labia minora* are hairless and contain some erectile tissue. The area between the labia is called the *vestibule.* It contains the openings of the vagina and urethra, as well as *Bartholin glands.* These glands secrete lubricating fluid during sexual stimulation. *Skene glands,* which open onto the vestibule on each side of the urethra, produce fluid to moisten the vestibule.

The *clitoris* is an erectile organ, similar to the penis in the male. Like the penis, it is highly sensitive and distends with blood during sexual arousal. The vaginal opening, called the *introitus,* is surrounded by a connective tissue membrane called the hymen, which determines the size and shape of the opening. The hymen is typically torn by the insertion of tampons, the first experience of sexual intercourse, pelvic examination, or even physical activity.

BREASTS

The *breasts* (or *mammary glands*) are supported by the pectoral muscles and are richly supplied with nerves, blood, and lymph (Figure 30-5■). The areola, a pigmented area near the center of the breast, contains sebaceous glands and a nipple. The *nipple* usually protrudes and becomes erect in response to cold and stimulation. The primary purpose of the breasts is to supply nourishment for the infant.

The breasts are made of adipose, connective, and glandular tissue. Cooper ligaments, which support the breast, extend from the outer breast tissue to the nipple, dividing the breast into 15 to 25 lobes. Each lobe contains *mammary glands* connected by milk ducts that open to the nipple.

Age-Related Changes in the Reproductive System

With aging, the secretion of androgens, estrogens, and gonadotropic hormones declines. Reduced hormone levels lead to changes in secondary sex characteristics of both men and women.

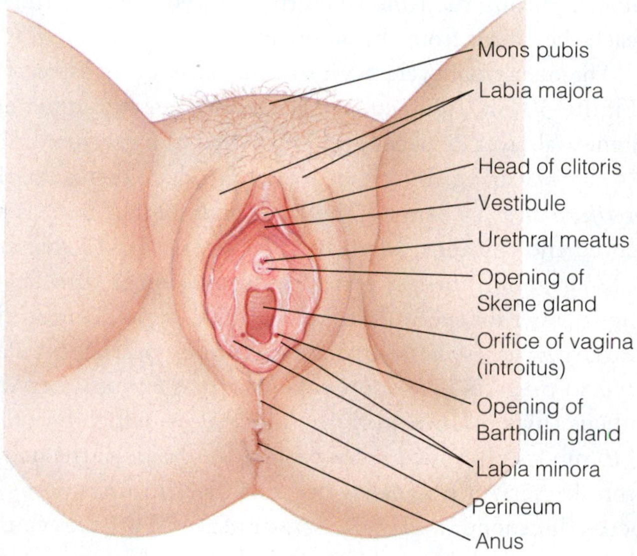

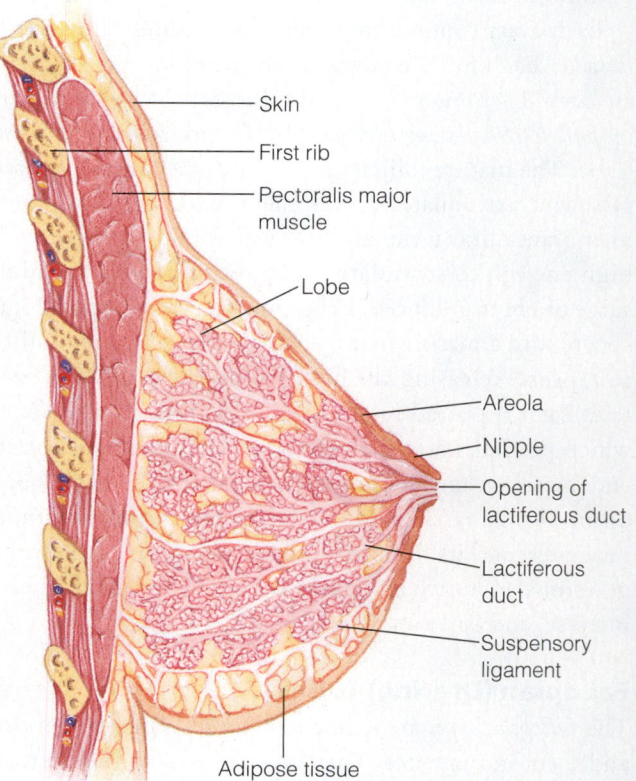

- Skin
- First rib
- Pectoralis major muscle
- Lobe
- Areola
- Nipple
- Opening of lactiferous duct
- Lactiferous duct
- Suspensory ligament
- Adipose tissue

Figure 30-5. ■ Structure of the female breast.

Mons pubis
Labia majora
Head of clitoris
Vestibule
Urethral meatus
Opening of Skene gland
Orifice of vagina (introitus)
Opening of Bartholin gland
Labia minora
Perineum
Anus

Figure 30-4. ■ The female external genitalia.

In women, lower estrogen levels lead to atrophy of the ovaries, uterus, and vaginal tissue. Subcutaneous fat is lost from perineal tissues, and pelvic floor muscles weaken, increasing the risk for stress incontinence. The vagina becomes smooth and shiny as its elasticity is lost. Vaginal secretions diminish and become more alkaline. With loss of hormonal support, the breasts and nipples decrease in size. Fibrosis and calcification may develop in the ducts of the breasts.

In men, the sperm count reduces with aging, although male fertility may extend into old age. The testes become firmer. Although the size of the penis diminishes, the ability to achieve erection is maintained. The prostate enlarges benignly in most older men. Prostate enlargement that interferes with urinary elimination is not normal and is covered in Chapter 31.

MENOPAUSE

Menopause is the cessation of menstruation for one year. *Perimenopausal* (approaching-menopause) symptoms occur usually when women are over 45 years of age. This time is also called "the change of life" and marks the end of a woman's childbearing years. In perimenopause when menstrual periods are irregular but still occurring, women may still be fertile. Menopause is a natural process due to a naturally decreasing estrogen level over years of time. However, it can also be induced immediately by surgery to remove the ovaries, where most estrogen is produced. Menopausal symptoms include the following:

- Menstrual periods that are lighter, irregular, and farther apart
- Sudden feelings of heat all over or in the upper body
- Hot flashes (or flushes) due to instability of vascular tone
- Nighttime sweating
- Vaginal dryness
- Changeable mood
- Difficulty concentrating mentally
- Less hair on head, more on face

Some women choose to take hormone replacement therapy (HRT) to decrease the symptoms of low estrogen. HRT is discussed in Chapter 32.

Assessment

Assessment of reproductive function is often left until the latter part of an interview and examination to allow development of trust and comfort between the patient and the nurse.

> **Key Concept**   Assessment of the reproductive system can include patient history, physical examination, surgical procedures (e.g., laparoscopy), and laboratory tests. Nurses have collaborative or independent roles in these procedures, depending on the demands of each assessment.

HEALTH HISTORY

It is important to use familiar terms, to ask questions in a nonthreatening manner, and to avoid judging the patient's responses. When interviewing, move from more general questions, for example, about previous pregnancies and a woman's menstrual cycle, to questions about problems such as sexually transmitted infections or difficulty maintaining an erection. For both male and female patients, first ask about the presenting problem. Identify its onset, manifestations, and effect on activities of daily living (e.g., difficulty urinating or dribbling, excessive menstrual flow). Inquire about possible contributing factors, such as a recent change in prescription medications or using a different brand of condom. Also ask about associated symptoms, such as fever or abdominal pain.

Because the urinary and reproductive systems are so closely linked in men, ask about problems such as difficulty urinating or dribbling when urinating. Also ask about urethral discharge or any rash or sores on the penis.

In women, ask about the color, amount, and character of vaginal bleeding and its relationship to the menstrual cycle. Inquire about any vaginal discharge, including its onset, color, character, and odor, and any itching or rashes.

Obtain a history of any chronic diseases such as diabetes, heart disease, multiple sclerosis, or spinal cord problems. Ask about a family history of cancer; the risk for endometrial and breast cancer is higher in women with a family history of these cancers. Also ask both men and women about possible intrauterine exposure to diethylstilbestrol. This drug was used to prevent miscarriage during the 1940s and 1950s and has been linked to an increased risk for urinary tract deformity and sterility in men and cervical and vaginal cancer in women. Determine what medications the patient is taking. Ask about physical or psychosocial stressors that may contribute to sexual problems.

Explore the patient's lifestyle, specifically asking about use of alcohol, cigarettes, or street drugs. Inquire about sexual history (number of sexual partners), history of specific sexual problems (e.g., impotence or dyspareunia, painful intercourse) or sexual trauma, use of erectile-enhancing drugs like sildenafil citrate (Viagra), use of contraceptives, and current sexual satisfaction.

PHYSICAL ASSESSMENT

The scope of practice of the LPN/LVN will not include all components of the thorough assessment of the reproductive system described here. However, knowing the process of reproductive system assessment and the meaning of findings will help the nurse explain the process and results to the patient.

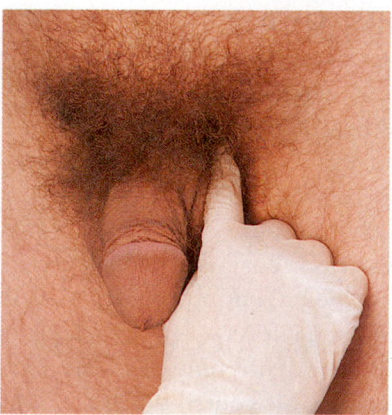

Figure 30-6. ■ Palpating the male inguinal area for bulges.

Men

Inspect and palpate the breasts, including the areola and nipple. Although breast problems are less common and easier to detect in men, it is important to not overlook this part of the examination.

Inspect and use a gloved hand to palpate the inguinal area and groin for bulges (Figure 30-6■). Inspect the penis; if the patient is uncircumcised, retract the foreskin (or ask the patient to do so). Also inspect the urinary meatus (see Chapter 28). Look specifically for skin irritation or sores and drainage from the meatus. Replace the foreskin. Inspect the skin around the base of the penis, and palpate the shaft of the penis. Inspect the scrotum; palpate each of the testes and epididymis.

Women

Inspect both breasts with the patient seated. Inspect first with the arms at the sides, then overhead, followed by the hands pressed on hips, and then leaning forward. Observe size, symmetry, contour, skin color, texture, venous patterns, and any lesions. Inspect the areolae and nipples. Position the patient supine, with a small pillow under the shoulder and the arm over the head. Palpate each breast, axilla, and supraclavicular area. Although various patterns of palpation can be used, it is important to palpate all areas of the breast including the axillary tail (see Chapter 32). Note any tenderness, and describe any identified masses by location, size, shape, consistency, mobility, and borders. Palpate the nipple and compress it between the thumb and index finger. Note any discharge and its color and consistency.

With the patient in **lithotomy position** (supine position with the knees flexed and separated) and using a gloved hand, inspect and palpate the labia majora for excoriation, rashes, lesions, or bulging. Separate the labia minora; inspect and palpate the labia minora. Inspect the clitoris, vaginal opening, and perineum. Ask the patient to strain

or "bear down," looking for bulging of the vaginal wall, protrusion of the cervix or uterus, or urinary incontinence.

Box 30-2■ presents two examples of documentation of assessment data collected related to the reproductive system.

DIAGNOSTIC TESTS

A variety of diagnostic tests may be used to identify disorders affecting the reproductive system, including diagnostic examinations, laboratory testing, imaging studies, and special procedures. Diagnostic examinations, such as digital prostate exam and clinical breast exam, are discussed in the chapters that follow. Diagnostic examinations and studies of the reproductive system often require use of invasive techniques and procedures, such as a pelvic exam using a vaginal speculum and bimanual palpation of pelvic organs for women and digital rectal exam in men. Box 30-3■ outlines nursing care of the woman undergoing a pelvic examination.

Laboratory Tests

Commonly used laboratory tests to evaluate the reproductive system are outlined, with normal values and their nursing implications, in Table 30-1■.

(Text continues on p. 791.)

BOX 30-2	DOCUMENTING ASSESSMENT OF THE REPRODUCTIVE SYSTEM

Male patient: George Jackson, a 68 y.o. African American male, presents at his physician's office. Assessment note: Complains of increasing difficulty starting to urinate and dribbling on completion of urination. States he thinks the problem began about 6 months ago but has recently become more noticeable. Also notes that it takes longer to fully empty his bladder, and he sometimes has to "bear down" to empty it completely. Denies other urinary symptoms, irritation of the urethra or penis, or difficulty maintaining an erection.

Appears healthy and younger than his stated age. Skin warm and dry; color has normal red undertones. BP 158/88, P 78, R 16, T 98.0°F. Pulses strong and equal ×4 extremities. Clean-catch urine specimen obtained. Urine clear, amber, and no visible sediment. External genitalia appear normal; no inflammation, lesions, or discharge noted. No tenderness or bulges noted on palpation of inguinal and groin regions.

Female patient: Michelle Wu, a 55 y.o. Asian American woman, presents at her gynecologist's office. Assessment note: Complains of perineal and vaginal itching, burning, and discharge. States symptoms began about 24 hours ago and have become so intense that she "can't stand it any longer." Denies previous history of vaginitis, recent antibiotic prescription, or other precipitating factors of which she is aware.

Appears healthy but acutely uncomfortable. Skin warm and dry. BP 128/76, P 84, R 18, T 97.6°F. Clean-catch urine specimen obtained. Urine clear yellow; no sediment noted. External genitalia red and inflamed. No clear line of demarcation between inflamed and normal-appearing tissue. Creamy discharge with a slight "fishy" odor noted at vaginal os; no mucous tissue bleeding noted.

BOX 30-3   NURSING CARE CHECKLIST

Pelvic Examination

Before the Procedure

☑ Obtain equipment: disposable exam gloves, light source, sterile cotton swabs, spatula, water-soluble lubricant, slides, fixative spray, vaginal specula of various sizes.

☑ Have the patient empty the bladder; obtain a clean-catch urine specimen if indicated.

☑ Explain the procedure, answering any questions.

☑ If the physician is male, reassure the woman that a female nurse will remain in the room.

☑ Ask the patient to remove all clothing and put on a gown. Provide a sheet for draping during the procedure.

During the Procedure

☑ Place the patient in lithotomy position with the knees flexed and separated.

☑ Position the light source to illuminate the perineal area.

☑ Assist the physician, nurse practitioner, or other care provider as needed during the examination.

☑ Provide continuing support for the patient.

After the Procedure

☑ Provide tissues and a towelette for cleansing lubricant from the perineal tissues.

☑ Provide a mini-pad to protect garments if any bleeding is expected (e.g., after a cervical biopsy). Allow privacy while the patient dresses.

☑ Prepare requisitions and slides for laboratory testing as indicated.

☑ Provide information about when to expect test results, follow-up appointments, and answer any further questions.

TABLE 30-1   Diagnostic Laboratory Tests

TEST	NORMAL ADULT VALUES	EXPLANATION	NURSING IMPLICATIONS
Blood tests used to evaluate testicular and ovarian function, infertility, and sexual dysfunction			
Progesterone	Female: 20–2,800 ng/dL, depending on menstrual phase Male and postmenopausal female: less than 100 ng/dL	Progesterone (produced by the ovaries, adrenal glands, and the placenta) levels are used to identify ovulation and assess corpus luteum function.	Note sex, age, and day of last menstrual period or trimester of pregnancy on the requisition or lab slip. Schedule these tests either before or at least 7 days after any nuclear medicine scans because radioisotopes can interfere with results.
Serum estradiol	Male: 15–50 pg/mL Female (menstruating): 20–500 pg/mL, depending on menstrual phase Female (postmenopausal): 60–260 pg/mL	Estradiol (an estrogen produced by the ovaries and the testes) decreases significantly after menopause. Levels are used to evaluate female infertility or amenorrhea.	
Follicle-stimulating hormone (FSH)	Male: 4–25 mU/mL Female (menstruating): 4–90 mU/mL, depending on menstrual phase Female (postmenopausal): 40–170 mU/mL	FSH (produced by the anterior pituitary gland) levels are measured to evaluate menstrual disorders, amenorrhea, or infertility in women and testicular dysfunction in men.	
Luteinizing hormone (LH)	Male: 5–25 mIU/mL Female (menstruating): 2–150 mIU/mL, depending on phase Female (postmenopausal): 40–100 mIU/mL	LH (produced by the anterior pituitary gland) levels are used to evaluate delayed sexual development, amenorrhea, menstrual irregularity, and infertility.	
Serum testosterone	Male: 300–1,000 ng/dL Female: 30–100 ng/dL	Testosterone (produced by the testes, ovaries, and adrenal glands) levels are measured to evaluate function of the testes and ovaries, male infertility, and sexual dysfunction.	

(continued)

TABLE 30-1	Diagnostic Laboratory Tests *(continued)*		
TEST	**NORMAL ADULT VALUES**	**EXPLANATION**	**NURSING IMPLICATIONS**
Laboratory tests used to detect and evaluate cancer of the reproductive organs			
Papanicolaou (Pap) smear	Within normal limits	The Pap smear is used to detect inflammation or infection and cell changes characteristic of premalignancy or malignancy of the vagina and cervix.	Schedule the test when the patient is not menstruating. Instruct to avoid sexual intercourse, douching, or vaginal medications for 48 hours before the exam. Have the patient void before the exam. Place the patient in lithotomy position. Support the patient during and after the exam. Note age, date of last menstrual period, and source of specimen on the requisition.
Tumor markers			
Human chorionic gonadotropin (HCG)	Male and nonpregnant female: less than 0.01 IU/mL Pregnant female: 0.01–0.04 IU/mL in week 1; as high as 100 IU/mL in weeks 5–12; decreases to 5–15 IU/mL last trimester	HCG is normally produced by the placenta; some malignant tumors (e.g., of the testes or ovaries) also produce HCG, causing serum levels to rise.	Schedule either before or at least 7 days after a nuclear scan because radioisotopes interfere with results. Note age, sex, and date of last menstrual period on requisition.
Alpha-fetoprotein (AFP)	Less than 15 ng/mL	AFP, normally present in maternal circulation during pregnancy, is used as a tumor marker for liver cancer, testicular cancer, and other malignancies.	
Prostate-specific antigen (PSA) Total PSA (tPSA) If PSA is elevated or previous result is doubled, the following tests are indicated: Free PSA % Free PSA	Male: 0–4 ng/mL Benign prostatic hyperplasia (BPH): 4.0–10 ng/mL Prostate cancer: 10–120 ng/mL 2.5–4 ng/mL >1.0 ng/mL >25%	PSA is produced exclusively by the prostate gland. Levels rise in benign prostatic hypertrophy and especially in malignancy of the prostate. The greater the percentage of free PSA, the lower the risk of cancer of the prostate. Free PSA <25% is an indication for a biopsy of the prostate gland.	Schedule test before or at least 2 weeks after any manipulation of the prostate (DRE, biopsy, etc.) No food or fluid restriction is required. This test may cause false positive results (elevated test result without a need for surgery).
Cancer antigen 125 (CA 125)	Less than 35 U/mL (less than 35 kU/L)	CA 125 is produced by malignant cells; it is used to detect ovarian cancer and monitor its progression after removal of the tumor.	Schedule before or at least 7 days after any nuclear scan because radioisotopes interfere with test results.
Tests to detect genital infections			
Syphilis serology: ■ RVDRL (Venereal Disease Research Laboratory) ■ Rapid plasma regain ■ Fluorescent treponemal antibody absorption	Negative or nonreactive	These tests are used to detect antibodies produced in response to infection with *Treponema pallidum*, the spirochete that causes syphilis.	Instruct the patient to avoid alcohol intake for 24 hours before the test and to avoid food intake for 8 hours before testing. Instruct to abstain from sexual contact until test results are known. Positive test results must be reported to the state health department. If positive, instruct patient to abstain from sexual contact until effectively treated and to notify all sexual partners of test results.

TABLE 30-1	Diagnostic Laboratory Tests *(continued)*		
TEST	**NORMAL ADULT VALUES**	**EXPLANATION**	**NURSING IMPLICATIONS**
Genital culture (cervix, vagina, prostate fluid, urethral secretions)	Negative	Cultures of genital secretions are done to diagnose the cause of vaginitis, vulvovaginitis, urethritis, and urethral discharge. The infection may be sexually transmitted or result from causes unrelated to sexual contact. A number of different organisms can cause genital infections.	Men: Instruct to avoid urinating for at least an hour before the test because this will reduce the number of organisms present. Women: Instruct to avoid douching for 24 hours before the exam because this will reduce the number of organisms present. Obtain the specimen before antibiotic therapy is started. Position men supine; advise that temporary nausea, sweating, light-headedness, or weakness may occur during specimen collection, but this is brief and temporary. Place women in lithotomy position; advise that discomfort may occur, but it should not be painful. Follow specific instructions for preparing slides such as a wet prep or saline prep.

Imaging Studies

Radiologic studies, including x-rays and CT scans, are often done as screening tests either to detect malignancy or to evaluate organs of the reproductive system.

Mammography is a radiological procedure used to screen for breast cancer in women who have no symptoms. It can detect tumors that are too small to be detected by clinical breast exam or self-breast exam. Tumors as small as 5 mm in diameter can be identified on mammography. Mammography, which involves x-rays of each breast taken from different angles, also helps differentiate between benign breast changes and malignancy. Suggest that women who have tender breasts avoid coffee, colas, chocolate, and other products containing caffeine or methylxanthines for 5 to 7 days before mammography. Instruct the patient to:

- Avoid using deodorants, creams, lotions, or powders on the day of the test.
- Remove all jewelry and clothing above the waist.
- Put on a hospital gown with the opening in front.

Plain x-ray films (abdominal x-ray) and abdominal CT scan may be ordered to evaluate for enlargement of reproductive organs or malignancy. Preparation and nursing care of the patient vary; in many cases, no special preparation is required. If contrast media is used, ask the patient about any allergies to drugs, iodine, seafood, or previous reactions to contrast media.

A number of ultrasonography examinations may be used to detect reproductive system problems. Although these exams generally do not expose the patient to radiation and many are noninvasive, some specialized ultrasound exams are more invasive. Table 30-2■ outlines commonly used ultrasound procedures for evaluating the reproductive system.

Endoscopy

Several endoscopy procedures are used to evaluate the reproductive system. These procedures allow direct visualization of the organs of the abdominal and pelvic cavities. In addition, tissue can be obtained during procedures for biopsy.

Abdominal laparoscopy is done using local anesthesia and intravenous (conscious) sedation. During this procedure, the peritoneal cavity is filled with gas to allow better visualization of its organs (Figure 30-7■). It may be combined with laparoscopic ultrasound. The instruments are inserted through small abdominal incisions. Nursing care of the patient undergoing abdominal laparoscopy is outlined in Box 30-4■.

In men, *cystoscopy* may be used to evaluate the size of the prostate gland and obtain tissue for biopsy. This procedure is discussed further in Chapter 28.

TABLE 30-2	Diagnostic Ultrasound Studies	
DIAGNOSTIC TEST	**PURPOSE**	**NURSING IMPLICATIONS**
Breast ultrasound	Primarily used to differentiate cystic from solid masses of the breast. May also be used to guide a needle biopsy of a breast mass.	These exams are noninvasive and require no special preparation of the patient. Provide support during the procedure. Assist the patient to clean off ultrasound gel residue after the procedure.
Abdominal ultrasound	Used to demonstrate structures of the abdomen and pelvis, including size, position, and shape.	
Pelvic ultrasound (females)	Used to identify malignancy, benign or malignant uterine tumors, and to monitor ovulation in women. Both abdominal and vaginal approaches are used. For the vaginal approach, the transducer is covered with a condom and coated with transducer gel.	Place the patient in lithotomy position when the transvaginal approach is used. Instruct to increase fluids and not void before the procedure to ensure a full bladder. Provide support during the procedure. Allow to empty the bladder as soon as possible.
Transrectal ultrasonography (TRUS) (males)	Used to assess the prostate gland, urethra, seminal vesicles, and vas deferens. May also be used to guide a needle biopsy of the prostate.	Instruct to use a disposable phosphate (Fleet) enema the evening or early morning before the procedure. Have the patient void before the procedure. Place the patient in lithotomy position. Administer sedation if ordered and provide support during the procedure.

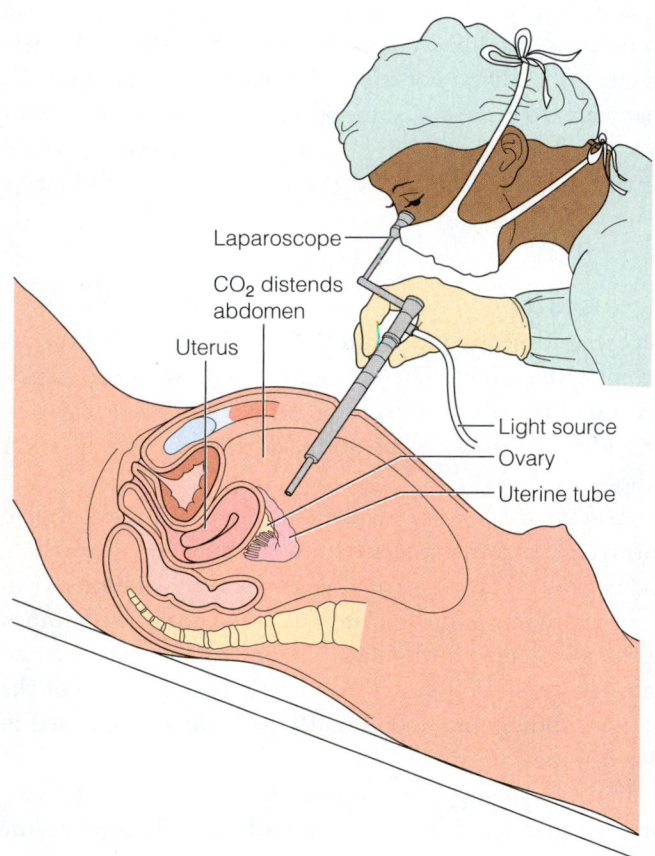

Laparoscope
CO2 distends abdomen
Uterus
Light source
Ovary
Uterine tube

Figure 30-7. ■ Laparoscopy. A flexible, lighted instrument (laparoscope) is inserted through a small incision to visualize the abdominal and pelvic cavities.

Colposcopy is used to examine tissues of the vagina and cervix using a brightly lighted microscope. It can identify early premalignant changes in cervical tissue and is performed when Pap test results are abnormal. This procedure is usually accompanied by *endocervical curettage* (scraping of cervical tissue) to obtain cell samples for examination and biopsy. Colposcopy should be scheduled early in the patient's menstrual cycle (between days 8 and 12). This invasive procedure requires informed consent. Instruct the patient to avoid using any vaginal creams or medications before the procedure. The patient is placed in lithotomy position during the procedure. Tell the patient that she will feel a pinch or momentary cramping sensation when the specimen is obtained. Provide psychologic support, because this procedure is often performed when an abnormal Pap smear result has been obtained. Instruct the patient to refrain from sexual intercourse or insertion of anything into the vagina (e.g., tampons) until the cervix has healed, approximately 7 to 10 days.

Contraception

Contraception is the avoidance of pregnancy while maintaining the ability to have heterosexual sexual intercourse. It is an important part of the discussion of reproductive issues. Table 30-3 ■ shows the variety of contraceptive (birth control) methods currently available and how they are used.

The role of the nurse is to provide information for women and their partners for the purpose of enabling patients to make an informed choice for themselves. Even when the nurse has strong personal feelings about this subject, the decision about whether to use contraception and what type to use belongs to the patient, without judgment by the nurse.

Note: The references and resources for all chapters have been compiled at the back of the book.

BOX 30-4 NURSING CARE CHECKLIST

Laparoscopy

Before the Procedure

- ☑ Obtain informed consent.
- ☑ Reinforce teaching; clarify any questions the patient or family members have.
- ☑ Instruct female patient to douche (vaginal cleansing) and both male and female patients to scrub around the umbilicus with povidone-iodine or other recommended antiseptic solution the night before the procedure.
- ☑ Ask to empty the bladder before the procedure.
- ☑ Obtain baseline vital signs and assessment data.

After the Procedure

- ☑ Monitor vital signs. Report data outside the established baseline or parameters. Report temperature greater than 101°F (38.3°C) PO.
- ☑ On female patients, apply a perineal pad. Instruct to change at least every 4 hours; keep a pad count.
- ☑ Observe dressings and surrounding tissue for drainage, bleeding, or hematoma formation.
- ☑ Monitor pain and provide analgesia as ordered. Instruct to report excessive pain at once.
- ☑ Explain that shoulder pain or release of gas through the vagina may occur.
- ☑ Maintain intravenous fluids until oral fluid intake is resumed.
- ☑ Provide discharge instructions, including potential problems about which the patient should notify the physician: bleeding, intense abdominal pain, fever, fluid leakage, malaise, or difficulty breathing. Explain that hiccups may occur; a drug can be prescribed if they are disruptive.

TABLE 30-3 Contraceptive Methods

BIRTH CONTROL		HOW TO USE	PRESCRIPTION NEEDED	PROTECTS AGAINST STIs
Monthly oral contraceptive		Take one pill every day as directed. A period occurs every 28 days.	Yes	No
Extended-regimen oral contraceptive		Take one pill every day for 3 months as directed. A period occurs every 3 months.	Yes	No
Patch		Apply to skin and change weekly. A period occurs every 28 days.	Yes	No
Vaginal ring (hormonal)		Insert monthly and leave in place for 21 days. A period occurs every 28 days.	Yes	No
Injection		Get injections every 3 months. A period occurs every 28 days.	Injections given in health care professional's office or clinic	No
Hormonal intrauterine contraceptive (IUC)		Inserted in the uterus by a health care provider and can remain for up to 10 years, depending on type.	IUC inserted in health professional's office or clinic	No

(continued)

TABLE 30-3	Contraceptive Methods *(continued)*			
BIRTH CONTROL		**HOW TO USE**	**PRESCRIPTION NEEDED**	**PROTECTS AGAINST STIs**
Nonhormonal intrauterine contraceptive (IUC)		Inserted in the uterus and can remain for up to 10 years.	As above	No
Plan B® emergency contraception levonorgestrel tablets 0.75 mg		Take the first tablet as soon as possible, ideally within 72 hours but up to 120 hours of unplanned intercourse or contraceptive failure. Take the second tablet 12 hours after the first one. This method prevents pregnancy.	No	No
Spermicide		Apply every time before sex.	No	No
Diaphragm		Insert every time up to 24 hours before sex. Keep in place for 6 hours after sex.	Yes, for fitting	No
Female condom		Insert every time before sex.	No	Yes
Male condom		New condom must be worn every time during sex.	No	Yes (latex only)
Female sterilization (tubal ligation or tubes tied)		No action required after surgery.	No; performed surgically	No
Male sterilization (vasectomy)		No patient action required after surgery, except surgeon may order sperm count afterward.	No, performed surgically as outpatient	No

Chapter Review

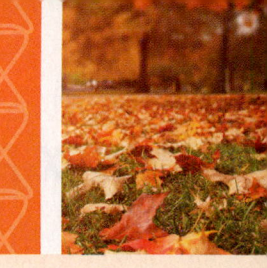

KEY POINTS

- **Concept:** The male and female reproductive systems include the structures and functions necessary for sexual intercourse and sexual reproduction.
- In men, the lower urinary and reproductive systems are closely related, with the urethra and penis serving as organs for both urine elimination and ejaculation of semen. In women, the urinary and reproductive systems, although anatomically close to one another, are totally separated in structure and function.
- **Concept:** Assessment of the reproductive system can include patient history, physical examination, surgical procedures (e.g., laparoscopy), and laboratory tests. Nurses have collaborative or independent roles in these procedures depending on the demands of each assessment.
- Modesty and fear may inhibit open discussion of reproductive system concerns and problems; establishing a trusting relationship with the patient is vital.
- Although blood tests can be used to identify some reproductive system disorders, diagnostic tests frequently require direct examination of structures. These procedures vary from minimally invasive to very invasive (laparoscopy, cystoscopy).

PEARSON NURSING STUDENT RESOURCES

Find additional materials at **nursing.pearsonhighered.com**.

NCLEX-PN® Exam Preparation

TEST-TAKING TIP The NCLEX-PN may ask you about the role of the practical nurse in various diagnostic procedures. You need to know how to prepare the patient, collect specimens, assist with setting up sterile fields for invasive procedures, and care for the patient after the procedure.

1. A patient asks the nurse how it is possible for the egg to make it all the way from the ovary to the uterus when it does not have a tail to propel it like the sperm. The nurse's response is based on the knowledge that movement of the egg to the uterus occurs:
   1. only when the egg has been fertilized by a sperm.
   2. by smooth muscle contraction and ciliary movement.
   3. by gravity.
   4. through chemical messengers that attract the ovum.

2. Place the following structures in the order in which a sperm travels from its production through ejaculation.
   1. Vas deferens
   2. Testes
   3. Urethra
   4. Epididymis
   5. Seminal vesicle

3. A 45-year-old woman sees her gynecologist because she has stopped menstruating and is concerned that it may be related to her exercise or signal a problem of the reproductive organs. Follow-up laboratory tests show the following: serum estradiol 12 pg/mL, FSH 60 mU/mL, LH 33 mU/mL. The nurse correctly interprets these results as:
   1. typical of a woman after menopause.
   2. indicative of pregnancy.
   3. significantly abnormal.
   4. within normal limits for women of all ages.

4. A patient had an abdominal laparoscopy this morning. What is the most important subjective assessment by the nurse?
   1. The amount of incisional bleeding
   2. The patient's blood pressure
   3. Presence of severe pain
   4. Drainage on the perineal pad

5. A male patient tells the nurse that his doctor's office called and told him that he needs to come in for a DRE and PSA now that he is over age 50. He says he was too embarrassed to admit that he did not know what that meant and wonders if there is anything he needs to know ahead of time. Which is the most appropriate response by the nurse?
   1. "No, no special preparation is required for a digital rectal exam and prostate-specific antigen test."
   2. "Yes. The day surgery unit will call you a week before because informed consent is required for these invasive procedures."
   3. "No. These tests are performed in the doctor's office. All required preparation will occur there under the doctor's direction."
   4. "Yes. You should have the PSA (a blood test) drawn before the doctor does the digital rectal exam."

Answers and rationales for Review Questions appear in Appendix I.

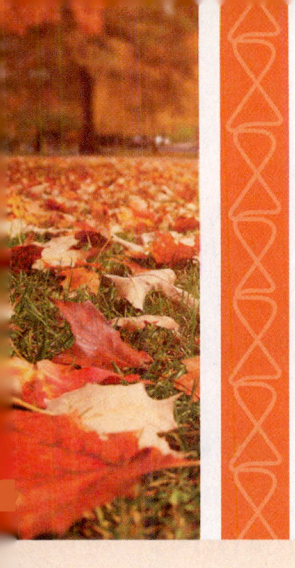

CHAPTER 31
Caring for Male Patients With Reproductive System Disorders

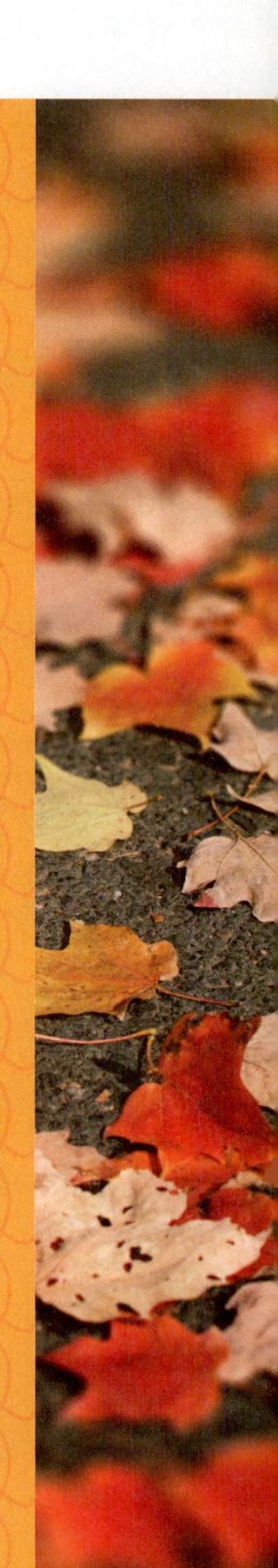

BRIEF OUTLINE

PROSTATE DISORDERS
Benign Prostatic Hyperplasia
Cancer of the Prostate
Prostatitis
DISORDERS OF THE TESTES AND SCROTUM
Structural and Inflammatory Disorders
Infertility
Scrotal Masses and Trauma
Testicular Cancer

DISORDERS OF THE PENIS
Phimosis
Peyronie Disease
Priapism
Cancer of the Penis
DISORDERS OF SEXUAL EXPRESSION
Erectile Dysfunction
Ejaculatory Dysfunction

APPLIED LEARNING OUTCOMES

After completing this chapter, you will be able to:

1. Describe the pathophysiology and manifestations of common disorders of the male reproductive system.
2. Administer and discuss nursing implications for medications used to treat disorders of the male reproductive system.
3. Apply the nursing process to provide care for patients with disorders of the male reproductive system.
4. Contribute to the plan of care for male patients undergoing surgery for reproductive system disorders.

KEY TERMS

The key terms are defined on the pages listed below.

SPECIAL FEATURES

The male reproductive system may be affected by structural and functional disorders, infectious and inflammatory disorders, and malignancies. Some disorders are life threatening.

> **Key Concept** Disorders of the male reproductive system and their treatments pose a risk to the patient's fertility, sexuality, and urinary function. The patient's body image and self-concept may also be affected by these changes.

Reproductive system disorders are associated with increased psychosocial risks when compared with disorders in other body systems.

PROSTATE DISORDERS

Benign Prostatic Hyperplasia

> **Key Concept** Enlargement of the prostate gland, **benign prostatic hyperplasia** (BPH), affects most men over the age of 50. The incidence of BPH increases with age.

More than 90% of men over 70 years old have BPH. Its cause is unknown, but risk factors have been identified. These include age, family history, race, ethnicity, and hormonal factors. BPH tends to develop earlier in African Americans than in European, Asian, or Native Americans. Its incidence is lowest in native Japanese men.

PATHOPHYSIOLOGY

BPH only develops in men who have testes; it does not affect men who had their testes removed before puberty. *Testosterone,* the primary androgen produced mainly in the testes, is converted to dihydrotestosterone (DHT) in the prostate gland. DHT stimulates growth of the prostate. Although testosterone levels decrease with aging, estrogen (produced in small amounts in men) levels increase. Estrogen appears to make the prostate more responsive to DHT, promoting its growth. Increases in estrogen levels in relation to testosterone levels may contribute to BPH.

BPH develops as small nodules that form and grow in the central and transition zones of the prostate, next to the urethra. The expanding prostate compresses surrounding tissue, narrowing the urethra (Figure 31-1■).

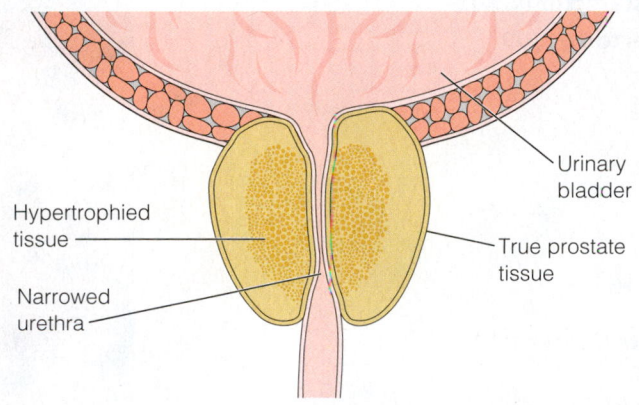

Figure 31-1. ■ Benign prostatic hyperplasia (BPH).

Hypertrophied tissue

Narrowed urethra

Urinary bladder

True prostate tissue

MANIFESTATIONS AND COMPLICATIONS

Narrowing of the urethra partially or completely obstructs the urethra, impairing urine flow and bladder emptying. Obstruction causes the symptoms of BPH, including weak urinary stream, difficulty initiating urine flow, dribbling, and urinary retention. *Nocturia* (voiding more than once at night) is an early symptom. The manifestations of BPH are summarized in Box 31-1■.

If BPH is not treated, increased pressure in the bladder causes urine *reflux* (backflow) into the ureters. This can eventually lead to *hydronephrosis,* which can affect kidney function (see Chapter 29). Fortunately, these complications are rare because the symptoms associated with BPH force most men to seek help before significant urinary retention and bladder distension develop.

COLLABORATIVE CARE

Some men are diagnosed with BPH during a routine physical examination before symptoms develop. Others wait until the discomfort from dysuria, urgency, and urinary retention becomes almost unbearable before seeking care.

Diagnostic Tests

■ A *digital rectal exam (DRE)* reveals an enlarged and asymmetrical prostate gland. To perform DRE, the primary care provider inserts a lubricated, gloved finger into the rectum to palpate the posterior surface of the prostate gland. This allows estimation of the size, shape, and consistency of the gland (firm but soft is normal; hard indicates BPH).

■ A routine *urinalysis* is done to detect signs of urinary tract infection.

BOX 31-1	MANIFESTATIONS OF BENIGN PROSTATIC HYPERPLASIA

- Nocturia (early symptom)
- Diminished force of urinary stream
- Hesitancy in starting voiding
- Dribbling after voiding
- Incomplete bladder emptying
- Frequency, urgency
- Urge incontinence
- Dysuria, hematuria

- *Prostate-specific antigen (PSA)* levels may be somewhat higher than normal in BPH (see Table 30-1). In contrast, PSA levels are significantly elevated with prostate cancer.
- *Uroflowmetry* may be done to determine the degree of urethral obstruction.

Medications

Several drugs may be used to shrink the enlarged prostate and reduce the manifestations of BPH. Finasteride (Proscar, an androgen inhibitor) inhibits the conversion of testosterone to DHT in the prostate, causing the gland to shrink. It is most effective in men with significantly enlarged prostate glands. This drug can decrease libido and can cause impotence.

Alpha$_1$ blockers such as terazosin (Hytrin), doxazosin (Cardura), and tamsulosin (Flomax) relax smooth muscles in the prostate, the urethra, and the bladder neck. Smooth muscle relaxation reduces urethral obstruction and improves urinary flow and symptoms of BPH.

Complementary Therapies

Saw palmetto is an herbal therapy that reduces the symptoms of BPH. Its effects are similar to those of finasteride, although its mechanism of action is unknown. The usual dose is 640 mg per day. The side effects of saw palmetto include constipation, diarrhea, headache, and urine retention. It should not be taken by pregnant women (Fontaine, 2011).

Surgery

Patients with BPH may need surgery to relieve urinary obstruction. Only the portion of the prostate gland surrounding the urethra is removed in BPH. *Transurethral incision of the prostate (TUIP)* and *transurethral resection of the prostate (TURP)* are the most common procedures used. In the TUIP procedure, small incisions are made in the prostate and the bladder neck to widen the urethra. No tissue is removed, and this procedure can be done on an outpatient basis.

In a TURP, obstructing prostate tissue is removed using the wire loop of a *resectoscope* inserted through the urethra (Figure 31-2■). Damage done by the procedure to the epithelial lining of the urethra heals, restoring the integrity of the urethral tube. Irrigating fluid carries resected tissue into the bladder to be flushed out on completion of the procedure. TURP is a relatively low-risk procedure with few complications. After surgery, *retrograde ejaculation* (discharge of seminal fluid into the bladder instead of through the urethra) is common. Fluid volume excess with hyponatremia, also known as *transurethral syndrome,* is a potential complication of TURP. Nursing care for the patient having a TURP is outlined in Box 31-2■.

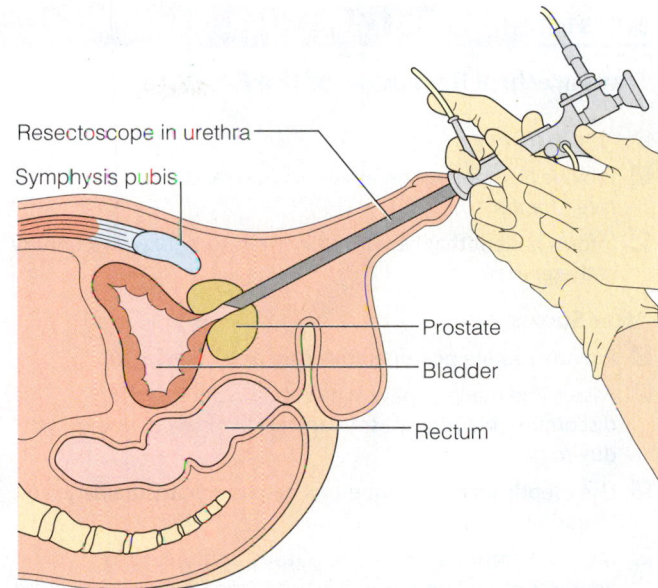

Figure 31-2. ■ Transurethral resection of the prostate (TURP). A resectoscope inserted through the urethra is used to remove excess prostate tissue.

Lasers or microwaves may also be used to destroy excess prostate tissue to treat BPH. One such procedure is the holmium laser enucleation of the prostate (HoLEP) (Mayo Clinic Staff, 2011). These minimally invasive procedures can be done on an outpatient basis.

NURSING CARE

PRIORITIZING NURSING CARE

Monitoring for adverse effects of the disorder and its treatment and educating the patient are priority nursing responsibilities.

ASSESSING

Ask older men about difficulty voiding, including difficulty starting and stopping the flow of urine, decrease in the size of the urinary stream, and any symptoms such as burning, frequency, urgency, or nocturia. Monitor urine output, including amount (total and per voiding), color, clarity, and odor.

DIAGNOSING, PLANNING, AND IMPLEMENTING

Although BPH itself is not a life-threatening condition, its consequences (urinary retention) can be.

Ineffective Self-Health Management

Expected outcome: Patient will explain the disease process of BPH and list two self-care strategies for affected men.

- Provide information about BPH and its treatment. Refer patient to a primary care provider or urologist.

BOX 31-2	NURSING CARE CHECKLIST

Transurethral Resection of the Prostate

Before Surgery

☑ Provide routine preoperative care and teaching (see Chapter 10).

☑ Inform patient that he will return from surgery with a urinary catheter in place.

After Surgery

☑ Provide routine postoperative care (see Chapter 10).

☑ Assess and manage pain, which may include urethral discomfort, bladder spasms, and abdominal cramping due to gas.

☑ Use aseptic technique when managing urinary drainage and irrigation.

☑ Maintain accurate intake and output, accounting for amounts of irrigating solution used. Irrigant may be counted as intake, or depending on hospital protocol, the amount of irrigant instilled may be subtracted from urinary output to accurately determine the amount of urine output.

☑ When allowed, encourage a liberal fluid intake.

☑ Frequently assess catheter patency; record color and character of urine. Light red to red urine with small clots is expected for up to 24 hours after surgery. The urine should gradually clear of clots and become light pink to yellow after 24 to 48 hours.

☑ For the first 24 to 48 hours, monitor for hemorrhage (frankly bloody urine, large blood clots, decreased urinary output, increasing bladder spasms, decreased hemoglobin and hematocrit, tachycardia, and hypotension). Notify physician if manifestations occur.

☑ Explain that the catheter may cause a sensation of needing to void. Instruct the patient to avoid straining to void or when having a bowel movement. A stool softener may be prescribed to prevent straining at stool.

☑ If a continuous bladder irrigation (CBI) is present, maintain irrigating fluid flow rate to keep the output light pink or colorless.

☑ Report changes in vital signs, mental status, and laboratory results.

☑ If CBI is not used, follow agency procedure and physician orders for irrigating the indwelling catheter (usually when the urine is frankly bloody or has numerous larger blood clots or when bladder spasms increase).

☑ After catheter removal, assess amount, color, and consistency of voided urine. Explain that burning, dribbling, and small clots in the urine are common after catheter removal.

☑ Teach Kegel exercises (see Chapter 29, Box 29-2) and to start and stop the urine stream several times during each voiding to increase strength of muscles used to stop urine flow and reduce incontinence.

☑ Maintain antiembolic stockings and pneumatic compression devices as ordered. Assist with leg exercises and ambulation as ordered.

Most men are aware that BPH is very common but are unsure of the function or exact location of the prostate gland. To make decisions, patients need to know about possible treatment options and their effects.

■ Advise patient to drink at least 3 L of fluids daily (Mayo Clinic Staff, 2011), unless contraindicated by heart or kidney disease. *Fluids help prevent urinary tract infections and reduce dysuria.*

■ Advise to restrict alcohol intake, especially late at night, to minimize problems with nocturia. *Nocturia can pose a safety risk (for falling) in older men who may have age-related changes in vision, muscle strength, and coordination.*

Excess Fluid Volume

Expected outcome: Will have normal fluid volume, as evidenced by a normal serum sodium level and urine volume.

■ Assess for manifestations of fluid volume excess and hyponatremia (see Chapter 7). *Irrigating fluid absorbed through disrupted tissues of the urethra and bladder can lead to water absorption, causing fluid volume excess and hyponatremia.*

clinicalALERT

Transurethral syndrome, resulting from the large amounts of irrigating fluid used during and after surgery, can affect cardiovascular or pulmonary status and lead to altered mental status.

■ Weigh daily. Monitor intake and output, including bladder irrigation fluid used during and after surgery. Subtract the amount of irrigating solution used after surgery from the amount of output in the urinary catheter drainage bag to determine the urine output. *Frequent assessments help identify fluid volume excess early. Weight is an accurate indicator of fluid volume status.*

■ Restrict fluids and administer diuretics as ordered. *Fluid restriction conserves sodium, and diuretics decrease total fluid load.*

Impaired Urinary Elimination

Expected outcome: Will experience no complications of urinary catheterization (e.g., infection or skin irritation) and will be continent of urine when catheter is removed.

■ Change from leg drainage bag to a larger night drainage bag at bedtime. *A bag suspended from the bed frame at night permits gravity drainage of urine and prevents reflux of urine back into the bladder.*

- Avoid strapping the leg bag on too tightly. *Tight straps can decrease venous return and increase risk for thrombophlebitis and complications such as pulmonary emboli.*
- Place a soft cloth between the leg bag and thigh *to decrease friction and absorb dampness under the bag, reducing the risk of skin irritation.*
- Empty the leg bag every 3 to 4 hours *to prevent overfilling.*

clinicalALERT

Promptly report any unexpected changes in urine color, consistency, or odor to the physician. Report continued hematuria, evidence of frank bleeding, or large blood clots, as well as a lack of or significant decrease in urine output, because these may be manifestations of a complication such as hemorrhage or infection.

- Obtain a bladder scan (see Table 28-5) as ordered or as indicated to assess urinary retention after catheter removal. *Bladder scan is a noninvasive method of assessing bladder emptying, which can be performed at the patient's bedside.*

MANAGING NURSING CARE

As appropriate and allowed by the designated duties and responsibilities of assistive personnel, the nurse may delegate nursing care activities such as measuring urine output and obtaining daily weights for the patient after urological surgery or procedures.

EVALUATING

Collect the following data to evaluate the effectiveness of nursing interventions for a patient with BPH or who has had surgery to treat BPH:

- Urine output, including amount, color, clarity, and odor
- Ability to control urine flow without incontinence or dribbling
- Knowledge and understanding of treatment options
- Ability to manage home care and understanding of when to contact the physician

DOCUMENTING

Document continuing assessment data for patients treated medically in the community and for patients who undergo surgery. Include ability to initiate urine flow, amount and appearance of urine output, and residual urine remaining in bladder. If surgery is performed, document presence and degree of hematuria. Note level of pain, its location and type, as well as analgesia provided and its effectiveness. Document all teaching and recommendations for follow-up appointments or care.

CONTINUITY OF CARE

Patients are often discharged within 2 days after a TURP. When TURP is done on an outpatient basis, the patient may be discharged with an indwelling urinary catheter. Provide home care instructions as noted under Impaired Urinary Elimination. Box 31-3■ outlines discharge instructions after prostate surgery. Address concerns about sexuality after prostate surgery, providing referral to counseling or support services as indicated.

BOX 31-3	PATIENT TEACHING

Prostate Surgery

Activity

Healing requires 4 to 8 weeks. Avoid strenuous activity and heavy lifting. Do not drive for 2 weeks. Take long walks but take stairs slowly and carefully. Continue leg exercises (dorsiflexing the foot) to prevent blood clots in the legs. You can take showers but avoid tub baths while the catheter is in place (National Institutes of Health, 2012).

Bleeding

Bleeding may occur after a bowel movement, coughing, or increased exercise. If you notice blood in the urine, increase fluids and rest until urine is clear. If you have clots or are unable to urinate, call your doctor immediately. Avoid aspirin and non-steroidal anti-inflammatory drugs (NSAIDs) for at least 2 weeks.

Bowel Movements

Keep bowel movements regular and soft to avoid pressure on the prostate area. Eat fruits and other high-fiber foods, and take stool softeners as ordered.

Diet

Resume your normal diet. Increase fluids to 3 L (13 cups) daily. Avoid alcohol unless otherwise advised by your physician.

Sexual Intercourse

Do not have sex for 6 weeks after surgery to avoid bleeding. You may still have erections even with the catheter in place. When you resume sex, ejaculate may flow back into the bladder; if this is so, you will express little or no semen.

Urination

After the catheter is removed, you may experience some burning, stinging, or leakage for several weeks, and you may pass small blood clots occasionally. These symptoms disappear as the area heals. Use pads to control leakage.

Work

If work is not strenuous, you may return in 4 weeks. Otherwise, wait 6 to 8 weeks.

Contact your doctor immediately if:

- You are unable to urinate.
- Bleeding is excessive or is not controlled by fluids and rest.
- You have chills and fever or severe abdominal pain.
- Your scrotum becomes swollen and tender.
- You have pain in one calf, chest pain, or difficulty breathing.

Cancer of the Prostate

Cancer of the prostate is the most common type of cancer in North American men and the second leading cause of cancer death, after lung cancer. It is primarily a disease of older men, increasing in incidence with age and rarely occurring before age 40 (Box 31-4■). Other risk factors include a family history of the disease. Occupational exposure to certain chemicals, a diet high in animal fat, and high serum testosterone levels may also contribute to the risk.

When diagnosed early, prostate cancer is curable. When the cancer is confined to the prostate at diagnosis, the 5-year survival rate is 100%. Prostate cancers may grow slowly or aggressively.

PATHOPHYSIOLOGY

Prostate cancer is usually an *adenocarcinoma,* arising from glandular epithelial cells. It usually begins in the peripheral, posterior tissue of the gland. As the tumor grows larger, it may compress the urethra, obstructing urine flow. The tumor may spread locally to involve the seminal vesicles or bladder. It rarely invades the bowel.

Tumor metastasis is common in the late stage of the disease. The pelvic lymph nodes are the most frequently involved. Distant metastases usually affect bony tissue, especially the pelvic bones and spinal column. Prostate cancer may also spread to the liver and lungs.

MANIFESTATIONS AND COMPLICATIONS

In the early stages, prostate cancer usually causes no symptoms. As the tumor grows and spreads, manifestations of urinary obstruction, metastasis, and general symptoms of the disease develop, as described in Box 31-5■.

BOX 31-4 | **FOCUS ON DIVERSITY**

Prostate Cancer

At all ages, African American men have a higher incidence of prostate cancer than European American men. African Americans are also more likely to die of prostate cancer, with a mortality rate more than double that of other racial and ethnic groups. Increasing awareness of the risk for prostate cancer and screening procedures is particularly important in populations of African American men. To improve care and reduce the risk for advanced prostate cancer, recommend that all African American men have a yearly DRE and serum PSA from age 45 on. Access to the health care providers who can diagnose prostate disorders is critical for people with low income or without health insurance. People with low income of all races are more likely to seek help for urinary disorders late in the disease. Accurate information about health care and insurance systems is important for people who have previously been uninsured.

BOX 31-5 | **MANIFESTATIONS OF PROSTATE CANCER**

Genitourinary
- Dysuria, hesitancy, reduced urinary stream
- Frequency, nocturia, hematuria
- Erectile dysfunction
- Hard, enlarged prostate on DRE

Musculoskeletal
- Bone or joint pain
- Back pain

Neurologic
- Lower extremity weakness
- Bowel or bladder dysfunction

Systemic
- Weight loss
- Anemia, fatigue

Compression fractures of the spine are common, potentially causing loss of mobility and bowel and bladder function. Tumors may eventually involve bone marrow, resulting in severe anemias and impaired immune function.

COLLABORATIVE CARE

Because prostate cancer is curable when diagnosed early, screening measures for early detection help reduce mortality. The American Cancer Society recommends offering an annual DRE and serum PSA check after age 50. Men at high risk, including African American males and men with a strong family history of prostate cancer, should receive annual screening exams including DRE and serum PSA beginning at age 45.

Many treatment options are available for prostate cancer. Watchful waiting may be the treatment of choice if the tumor is slow growing and the patient is older or has a limited expected life span (less than 10 years).

Diagnostic Tests

- *DRE* is done as a screening measure and when an enlarged prostate is suspected. In prostate cancer, the gland is enlarged and hard during palpation.
- *Serum PSA levels* increase significantly in prostate cancer.
- *Transrectal ultrasonography* is used to help differentiate prostate cancer from BPH (see Table 30-2).
- A *tissue biopsy* is done to establish the diagnosis of prostate cancer. Tissue is obtained by either needle biopsy or transrectal ultrasound-guided biopsy. See Box 31-6■ for nursing care of the patient undergoing a transrectal ultrasound-guided biopsy.
- *Bone scan, MRI,* or *CT scans* may be done to identify possible tumor metastasis.

Transrectal Ultrasound-Guided Biopsy of the Prostate

Before the Procedure

☑ Reinforce teaching. The patient will remain awake; a local anesthetic will be used. The patient will have a feeling of rectal fullness, which may be very uncomfortable. A sharp pain (a "pinch") may be felt as the biopsy is obtained.

☑ Instruct to avoid aspirin products and nonsteroidal anti-inflammatory agents for a week before the biopsy.

☑ Ensure that enema has been given before the examination if ordered.

☑ Obtain a signed consent.

After the Procedure

☑ Monitor vital signs and urine output for an hour after the procedure.

☑ Instruct to avoid strenuous activity for the rest of the day.

☑ Monitor for hematuria and some bloody streaks in the stool (these are expected for 24 to 48 hours after the procedure). Ejaculate may also contain blood for up to 2 weeks.

☑ Report unusual bleeding, such as blood clots in urine, bloody stools, or signs of infection, such as rectal pain, dysuria, and urgency.

Hormone Therapy

Hormone therapy is used to treat advanced prostate cancer. It can be accomplished by removing the testes (**orchiectomy**) or using drugs. Drugs that block the effects of testosterone and other androgens inhibit tumor growth but do not cure prostate cancer. In advanced prostate cancer, hormone therapy may improve length and quality of life. The disadvantages of hormone therapy are side effects such as loss of libido, erectile dysfunction (or *impotence*), hot flashes, and **gynecomastia** (breast enlargement). The patient who has had an orchiectomy may have body image problems due to loss of the testicles. Silicone testicle prostheses may be used to replace a patient's removed testes. These prostheses may help the patient with his body image after orchiectomy, because they provide the appearance that testicles are present and prevent shrinkage of the scrotum.

Radiation Therapy

Radiation therapy may be used to treat prostate cancer, avoiding many of the adverse effects of prostate surgery, such as impotence and urinary incontinence. Radiation may be delivered by either external beam or implants of radioactive seeds (*brachytherapy*). Radiation therapy may also be used to reduce the size of bone metastasis, control pain, and restore function in patients with advanced prostate cancer. (See Chapter 12 for nursing care of the patient receiving radiation therapy.)

Surgery

Prostatectomy, surgical removal of the prostate gland, may be done to treat prostate cancer. In a *simple prostatectomy*, only the prostate tissue is removed. A *radical prostatectomy* involves removal of the prostate, prostatic capsule, seminal vesicles, and a portion of the bladder neck. Prostatectomy may be done by several different approaches. Table 31-1■ outlines different types of prostatectomy procedures with their specific nursing implications.

Some patients have problems with urinary incontinence, erectile dysfunction, and bleeding after radical prostatectomy. The incidence of all these risks is lower with robotic-assisted laparoscopic prostatectomy (RALP) than with open radical prostatectomy (ORP). Approximately 80% of patients undergoing radical prostatectomy have the RALP procedure. In robotic prostatectomy, the surgeon sits at a computer console near the operating table and guides the instruments while viewing the surgical site on the monitor (Patel & Sivaraman, 2012). The patient may experience less tissue trauma and bleeding and thus may return to normal activity more quickly than with traditional procedures.

To prevent or treat urinary incontinence, an artificial urinary sphincter may be surgically implanted (Figure 31-3■). The patient with an artificial urinary sphincter must be able to manipulate the pump in the scrotum and recognize when a problem with the appliance occurs.

Cryosurgery is a possible treatment option. Guided by ultrasound, a cryoprobe is inserted into the tumor. Prostate tissue is destroyed by intermittent freezing and thawing. This surgical treatment is associated with a risk of bladder outlet injury, urinary incontinence, impotence, and rectal damage.

NURSING CARE

PRIORITIZING NURSING CARE

The effects of the enlarged prostate, the tumor, and treatment options on urinary elimination are the nursing care priority for patients undergoing treatment for prostate cancer. Because sexual dysfunction is a very real potential effect of treatment, it is also a nursing care priority.

ASSESSING

In most cases, nursing assessment of a patient with prostate cancer is done on admission to a facility for radiation therapy or surgery. Refer to Chapter 12 for assessment data to collect before radiation therapy. For the patient undergoing prostate surgery, see Chapter 10 for pre- and postoperative assessment data to collect. In addition, inquire about the patient's understanding of his disease and the planned treatment.

TABLE 31-1   Approaches to Prostatectomy

ILLUSTRATION	DESCRIPTION	NURSING IMPLICATIONS
Robotic-assisted laparoscopic prostatectomy (RALP) RALP is the most commonly used procedure. 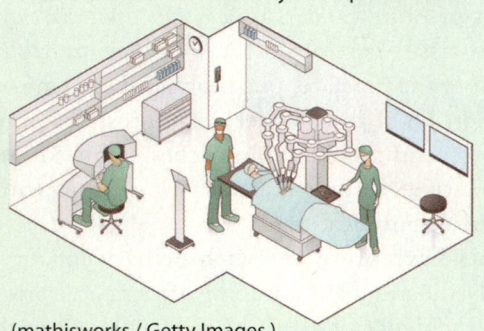 (mathisworks / Getty Images.)	The prostate is removed through a laparoscope as a less invasive procedure. The surgeon views the surgical area on a console with a magnified 3-D image. The robotic part has miniaturized hand-and-finger controlled instruments with more ease of manipulation.	Assess the small abdominal incisions from the laparoscopic instruments. Also assess urine output for amount and bleeding.
Open radical prostatectomy (ORP) Retropubic prostatectomy 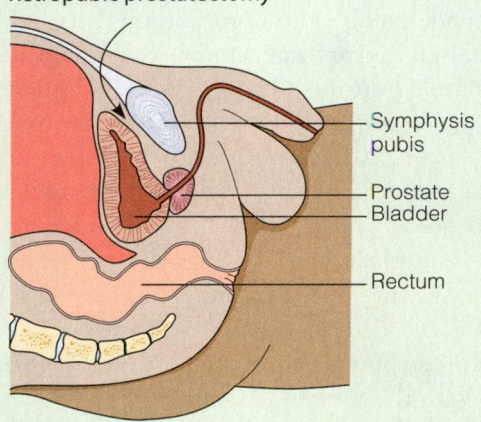 Symphysis pubis — Prostate — Bladder — Rectum	The prostate gland is removed through an abdominal incision; the bladder is left intact.	Assess abdominal incision for urine drainage (none should be present) and signs of infection, such as redness, increased or purulent drainage, or poor healing. Report to charge nurse or physician.
Suprapubic prostatectomy 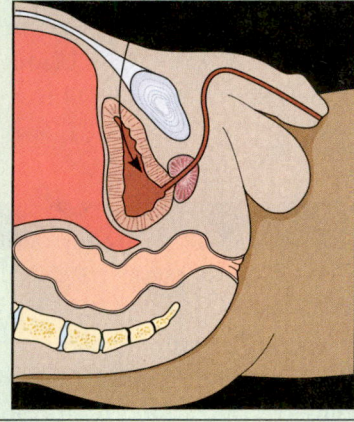	The prostate gland is removed through an abdominal incision into the bladder.	Assess urine output from suprapubic and urethral catheters. Also assess abdominal dressing for urine drainage; change saturated dressings frequently. Consult with a skin care specialist if necessary. After urethral catheter removal, clamp suprapubic catheter as ordered and encourage voiding. Assess residual urine by unclamping the catheter and measuring urine output after voiding.
Perineal prostatectomy 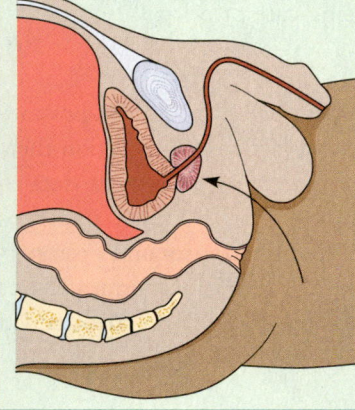	The prostate gland is removed through a perineal incision between the scrotum and anus.	Assess perineal incision for drainage and evidence of infection. Avoid rectal temperatures or enemas. Use a T-binder or padded scrotal support to hold dressing in place. After dressing removal, heat lamps or sitz baths may be used to promote comfort and healing. Teach perineal irrigation as ordered and after bowel movements.

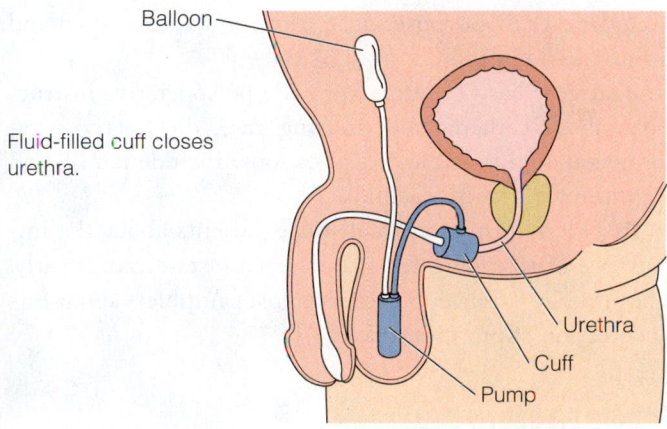

Balloon

Fluid-filled cuff closes urethra.

Urethra

Cuff

Pump

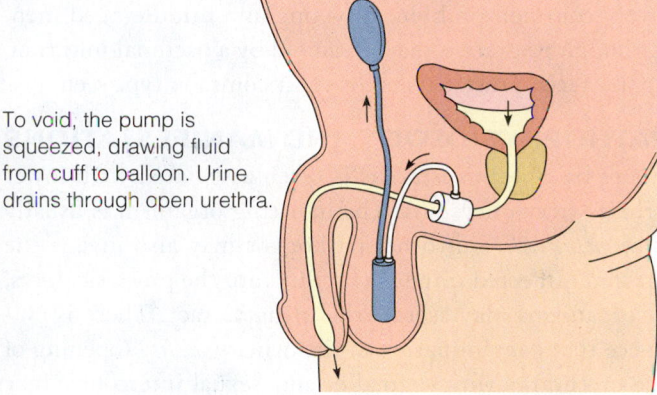

To void, the pump is squeezed, drawing fluid from cuff to balloon. Urine drains through open urethra.

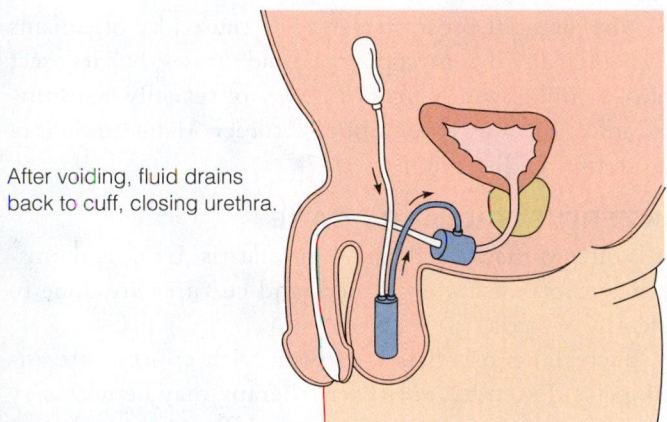

After voiding, fluid drains back to cuff, closing urethra.

Figure 31-3. ■ Operation of an artificial urinary sphincter.

Impaired Urinary Elimination (Risk for Incontinence)

Expected outcome: Will maintain urinary continence after treatment for prostate cancer.

■ Assess the degree of incontinence and its impact on lifestyle. *Knowledge of the amount and type of incontinence and its effect on the patient's life is used to plan appropriate nursing interventions.*

■ Teach pelvic muscle exercises (Kegel exercises), and help plan a regular schedule to perform the exercises. *Pelvic*

muscle exercises can improve urine retention in the patient with stress incontinence.

■ Refer to physical therapy or a continence specialist for additional measures. *Exercises, restricting some types of fluids, and other measures such as bladder training can often improve continence.*

■ Teach methods to control dampness and odor.
  a. Advise maintaining a liberal fluid intake, only limiting fluids after dinner. *Restricting fluids does not prevent incontinence, although it may prevent nighttime episodes. Fluid restriction causes more concentrated urine, increasing odor problems.*
  b. Suggest using absorbent pads worn inside the underwear and changed as needed. *Most pads help control odor and dampness, increasing comfort.*

■ Explore options such as an external collection device (external catheter or Texas catheter) for total incontinence. *This device, which collects urine as it leaves the urinary meatus, may improve self-esteem and allow resumption of social activities.*

■ Encourage expression of feelings about the impact of incontinence on quality of life. *Listening to these concerns with sensitivity can help the patient work through feelings and adapt to the inability to remain continent.*

Sexual Dysfunction

Expected outcome: Will discuss feelings about sexual function and options for treatment if indicated after prostate surgery.

■ Encourage discussion of sexual function between the patient, his partner, and his physician. *Most older men are active sexually and fully capable of sustaining an erection. Some men may refuse therapy because they fear the effect of treatment on sexuality. Open discussion of concerns assists with decision making about treatment options.*

■ Discuss various treatment options and their effects on sexual function. *The incidence of erectile dysfunction varies with different therapies for prostate cancer.*

■ Encourage the patient to discuss concerns about sexuality with a counselor or therapist. *A therapist or counselor may be able to suggest alternative ways for expressing sexuality.*

Acute Pain

Expected outcome: Will report pain at a level 3 or less on a 0 to 10 scale (after using pharmacological and nonpharmacological pain control methods) after prostate surgery.

■ Assess intensity, location, and quality of pain. Because most patients with prostate cancer are over age 65, many have pain from other conditions, such as osteoarthritis. Careful assessment helps identify its cause and direct treatment.

- Teach pain-control methods, including pharmacologic and nonpharmacologic measures. (See Chapters 8 and 12 for more information about pain control in the patient with cancer.) *Adequate pain management enhances quality of life and allows the patient to remain active.*

EVALUATING

To evaluate the effectiveness of nursing interventions for the patient with prostate cancer, collect data such as the following:

- Ability to control urination and remain continent
- If incontinent, ability to control odor and dampness and maintain social activities
- Willingness to discuss sexuality and consider the effects of treatment on sexuality
- Pain level on a standard pain scale

See the Clinical Reasoning Care Map at the end of this chapter on caring for a patient with prostate cancer.

DOCUMENTING

Document all instruction provided about prostate cancer and its treatment, as well as responses of the patient, spouse, and family to the information and treatment options. Also document continuing assessment data, including effects of the tumor on urinary output, cancer manifestations, and any symptoms of possible tumor metastasis.

CONTINUITY OF CARE

Patients with prostate cancer face both the diagnosis of cancer and a number of treatment options. The patient and family must deal with often conflicting advice from the urologist, medical and radiation oncologists, friends, the media, and advocate groups. Provide accurate information about available treatments and their effects. Encourage discussion of concerns. Provide information about prostate cancer support groups (if available). Men struggling with treatment choices may learn about the options from men who have experience.

Emphasize the importance of keeping appointments for treatment and follow-up. After treatment, yearly DRE and PSA levels are done. Discuss early warning signs of metastasis to the spinal column, such as intermittent back pain, which is aggravated by activity. Other symptoms include leg weakness. Provide verbal and written instructions about prescribed medications, including their purpose, dose, timing, and expected and unintended effects.

If surgery has been done, provide postoperative instructions about catheter and dressing care, diet, activity resumption, and possible complications. Include family and significant others in teaching.

Provide information to all male patients about the importance of screening tests to detect prostate cancer early. The American Cancer Society has free pamphlets about early detection of prostate cancer.

Prostatitis

Prostatitis (inflammation of the prostate gland) is a relatively common problem in young and middle-aged men. Although prostatitis may be caused by a bacterial infection, nonbacterial prostatitis is the most common type seen.

PATHOPHYSIOLOGY AND MANIFESTATIONS

Acute bacterial prostatitis is often associated with lower urinary tract infections. The infecting organism is usually *Escherichia coli,* but other pathogens may also invade the prostate. Infected urine may reflux into the prostatic ducts, or organisms may ascend the urinary tract. There is evidence that contamination of the urinary *meatus* (opening of the urethra) during vaginal or anal sexual intercourse may play a role in ascending infections.

Nonbacterial prostatitis may be caused by organisms such as chlamydia, mycoplasmas, and viruses, but its exact cause is unknown. It may be a type of sexually transmitted infection or an autoimmune disorder. Manifestations of prostatitis are listed in Box 31-7■.

INTERDISCIPLINARY CARE

It is often difficult to diagnose prostatitis. Urine and prostatic secretions are examined, and cultures are done to identify bacteria.

Bacterial prostatitis is treated with appropriate antibiotics. Extended antibiotic therapy may be necessary (up to 4 months) to eradicate the infection. Nonbacterial prostatitis is treated symptomatically. NSAIDs are useful for pain, and anticholinergics may reduce voiding symptoms.

BOX 31-7	MANIFESTATIONS OF PROSTATITIS

- Pain, burning on urination
- Frequency, urgency
- Chills, fever
- Low back, perineal, or genital pain
- Pain after ejaculation
- Obstructed urine flow

NURSING CARE

Instruct patients with prostatitis to increase fluid intake to about 3 L daily and to void often. Advise them to maintain regular bowel habits. These measures help decrease pain with voiding and defecation. Local heat, such as sitz baths, may help relieve pain and irritation. Stress the importance of finishing the course of antibiotic therapy to effectively treat the infection. In nonbacterial prostatitis, frequent ejaculation may help decrease congestion of the gland.

Honest, open discussion with the patient is important. It may help to explain nonbacterial prostatitis as a chronic inflammatory disorder, similar to arthritis. Address misconceptions about the disease with the patient and his partner. Sexual intercourse is actually helpful, and men cannot "infect" their partners.

DISORDERS OF THE TESTES AND SCROTUM

Structural and Inflammatory Disorders

TESTICULAR TORSION

Testicular torsion, or twisting of the testes and spermatic cord, is a potential medical emergency. Boys and young men up to age 20 are at greatest risk for testicular torsion. Its cause is unclear, although elevated hormone levels and abnormal attachment of the testicles to the scrotum may contribute. Trauma to the scrotum may precipitate the condition in patients who are already predisposed.

Testicular torsion causes acute scrotal pain with a sudden onset. Nausea and vomiting frequently occur. The *cremasteric reflex* (retraction of the testicles when the skin on the inside of the thigh is stroked) may be depressed or absent.

clinicalALERT

Advise men with symptoms of testicular torsion to seek immediate medical treatment because a delay in treatment can result in necrosis and loss of the affected testicle.

Diagnostic studies such as testicular scanning may be used to evaluate blood flow to the testicle. Emergency surgery is done to relieve testicular and spermatic cord twisting and to fix the testicle within the scrotum. Impaired blood flow to the testicle can lead to testicular ischemia and necrosis. If the testicle is necrotic or severely damaged, it will be removed.

An episode of torsion is frightening for the adolescent male. He is usually very embarrassed by the problem and may imagine that early sexual activity or even fantasies that result in erections are responsible. Because adolescents are not likely to volunteer these concerns, the nurse should relieve some of these anxieties by informing the patient that the disorder is not caused by patient behavior. Postoperative nursing care is similar to that for patients with scrotal surgeries, as discussed later in the section on testicular cancer. Discussion with patients concerning potentially embarrassing topics is a skill nurses must develop. A nurse's anxiety or shame can be contagious to the patient. Make your teaching and conversation with the patient clear, concrete (not abstract), and matter of fact. The nurse's ease and confidence will make the patient feel more relaxed.

CRYPTORCHIDISM

Cryptorchidism is failure of one or both testes to descend through the inguinal ring into the scrotum. In most males, the testes descend without intervention in the first year of life. Cryptorchidism is primarily a childhood problem, although on rare occasions, it is missed and discovered later in adolescent or adult life. When the problem continues into adolescence and adulthood, cryptorchidism increases the risk for testicular cancer and problems of fertility. Men who have a history of cryptorchidism should be especially vigilant about testicular self-examination (TSE). Teach the patient how to perform TSE (see Box 31-8 on page 809). Emphasize the importance of regular exams, and teach the patient that persistent undescended testicles should be reported to the physician.

EPIDIDYMITIS

Epididymitis is inflammation of the epididymis (see Figure 30-1). It is usually caused by an infection spread from the bladder, urethra, prostate gland, or seminal vesicles. In younger men, the cause is often a sexually transmitted organism such as *Chlamydia trachomatis* or *Neisseria gonorrhoeae.* In older men, epididymitis is usually associated with a urinary tract infection or prostatitis. Early manifestations include pain and local swelling; the scrotum may swell to the extent that it interferes with walking. Fever and general malaise may also develop. Sterility is a potential complication of epididymitis. Antibiotics are prescribed to treat epididymitis. Nursing care focuses on relieving symptoms of the disorder. Ice packs, if ordered, may be applied to the scrotum to relieve pain. A scrotal support is usually applied. The patient may wish to seek evaluation for the possibility of infertility at a later date.

ORCHITIS

Orchitis is inflammation of the testicle. It is commonly caused by an infection from other parts of the genitourinary tract. It can also occur as a complication of mumps; the mumps virus is excreted in the urine. Adult men with mumps are at highest risk for this complication. Trauma, including vasectomy and other scrotal surgeries, may cause inflammation of the testes. Manifestations of orchitis include severe testicular pain and swelling. Possible complications include hydrocele and abscess. These can lead to infertility or impotence. Bacterial orchitis is treated with antibiotics. Treatment for viral orchitis may be symptomatic. An abscess may require surgical drainage or orchiectomy. Nursing care is very similar to that of the patient with epididymitis and other scrotal disorders.

Infertility

Infertility is the inability to conceive a child during a year or more of unprotected intercourse. *Sterility* is the absolute inability to conceive. When the sperm count drops below 20 million/mL of semen, the patient is likely to be infertile. Male infertility usually results from a testicular disorder, such as cryptorchidism or orchitis. Less often, it may be caused by a systemic disease, hormonal disorder, or obstructed outflow of sperm from the testes. In many cases, no specific cause can be found for the infertility.

A sperm count is obtained to evaluate infertility in men. If an identifiable cause such as an endocrine disorder or varicocele (see next section) can be identified and treated, this may restore fertility. In many cases of male infertility, patients are counseled about options such as using a sperm donor or adopting a child.

Nursing care for the infertile male patient focuses on providing information and psychologic support for the man and his partner.

Scrotal Masses and Trauma

Scrotal masses such as hydroceles, spermatoceles, and varicoceles (Figure 31-4■) are usually benign and treatable.

SCROTAL MASSES

A *hydrocele* is a collection of fluid in the sac that encloses the testes. The cause is not always identifiable, but it may follow epididymitis, orchitis, injury, or a tumor. Scrotal enlargement may be the only manifestation of hydrocele, although it may cause pain or a tight sensation in the scrotum. Hydrocele is diagnosed by transillumination or ultrasound of the scrotum. Treatment is usually not necessary. If the hydrocele causes embarrassment or significant pain, a hydrocelectomy may be performed.

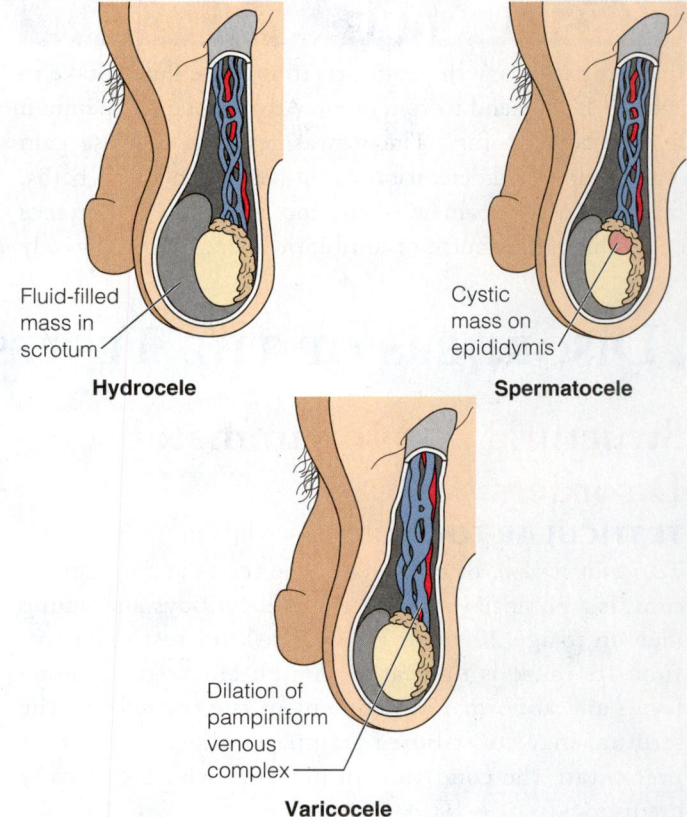

Fluid-filled mass in scrotum

Hydrocele

Cystic mass on epididymis

Spermatocele

Dilation of pampiniform venous complex

Varicocele

Figure 31-4. ■ Common scrotal masses.

A *spermatocele* is a mobile, usually painless mass in the epididymis that contains dead sperm cells. The cause is thought to be leakage of sperm due to trauma or infection. Treatment is usually not necessary.

A *varicocele* is abnormal dilation of the spermatic veins above the testis. It is caused by incompetent or absent valves in the veins and almost always occurs on the left side. The dilated veins form a soft mass (often described as a "bag of worms") that can cause dull pain in the scrotum. This condition can decrease the sperm count and cause atrophy of the testicle, resulting in infertility. Varicoceles are usually treated, especially in younger patients.

SCROTAL TRAUMA

Scrotal trauma is usually minor, resulting in temporary hematomas caused by minor crushing or straddle-type injuries. More severe crush injuries can rupture the testicles. Occasionally, the patient's clothing and scrotal skin can be trapped in moving machinery, resulting in avulsion injuries. Such an accident can tear the skin away from the penis and scrotum, sometimes releasing scrotal contents. Penetrating injuries of the scrotum due to knife or gunshot wounds can also occur. Treatment of scrotal trauma varies, depending on the extent and type of scrotal damage involved.

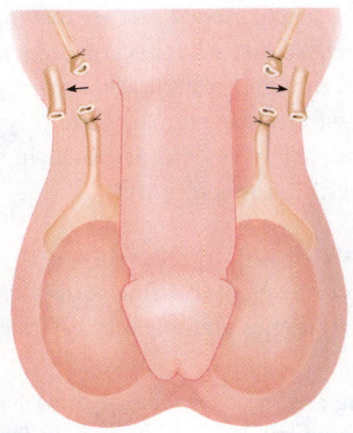

Figure 31-5. ■ Vasectomy.

VASECTOMY-RELATED PROBLEMS

The most common surgery of the scrotum is **vasectomy**, a sterilization procedure in which a portion of the spermatic cord is removed (Figure 31-5■). This surgery rarely causes long-term complications. However, some patients develop scar tissue, which causes chronic pain. Other complications include chronic testicular pain and epididymal obstruction.

NURSING CARE

Obtain assessment data such as the following from patients who have a history of scrotal trauma, surgery, or who complain about scrotal swelling or pain:

■ Ask about the onset, duration, and severity of symptoms.
■ Inspect the scrotum for swelling, redness, and bruising or discoloration. Using a gloved hand, gently palpate each testis and epididymis for tenderness, warmth, or masses.

Teach the patient with a scrotal disorder about the disorder and its treatment. If surgery is planned, discuss the patient's fears about the surgery, pain management, and measures to reduce bleeding (see next section). Postoperatively, observe for swelling and discoloration of the scrotum. Report excessive swelling or discoloration to the physician, because this could indicate excessive bleeding. Discuss the possible effects of surgery on fertility, and actively listen to the patient's concerns.

Testicular Cancer

Testicular cancer is the most common cancer in men between the ages of 15 and 35. Fortunately, it is one of the most treatable cancers, with a cure rate of greater than 90%.

Although its cause is unknown, risk factors for testicular cancer include the following:

■ Age: Testicular cancer usually develops between ages 15 and 40 but may occur at any age.
■ Cryptorchidism (undescended testicle)

■ Family history
■ Race and ethnicity: Men living in the United States, the United Kingdom, and Scandinavia have a higher risk of developing testicular cancer than African and Asian men.
■ Smoking
■ Exposure to endocrine disruptors (some pesticides, polychlorinated biphenyls, and dibutyl phthalate, a chemical used to manufacture cosmetics such as nail polish) may have a role in increasing the risk (National Health Service, 2012).

Unfortunately, most men who develop testicular cancer have no risk factors. Therefore, beginning at the age of 15, all men should perform monthly TSE (Box 31-8■).

PATHOPHYSIOLOGY AND MANIFESTATIONS

Testicular cancer grows within the testicle, eventually replacing most of the normal tissue. Usually only one testicle is affected. Local spread is limited, but it often spreads rapidly through lymph and blood vessels to other organs. Spread by lymph vessels usually causes disease in retroperitoneal lymph nodes. Dissemination of the disease through the vascular system can lead to metastasis in the lungs, bone, or liver. The classic presenting symptom of testicular cancer is a painless hard nodule. Occasionally, the patient may have a dull ache in the pelvis or scrotum. Acute pain related to the tumor is rare.

COLLABORATIVE CARE

Care focuses on diagnosing and eliminating the cancer and preventing or treating metastasis. Treatment depends on

BOX 31-8	TESTICULAR SELF-EXAMINATION

■ Examine your testicles during or just after a warm shower or bath. Soap on your hands and scrotum allows easy manipulation of tissue.
■ Gently roll each testicle between your thumb and fingers. The testicles normally feel smooth, rounded, walnut sized, and freely movable.

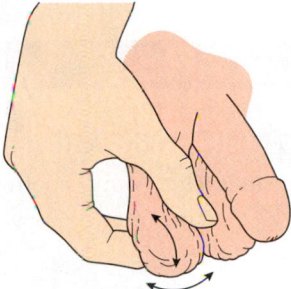

■ If one testicle is significantly larger than the other, or if you feel any hard lumps, contact your health care provider immediately.
■ Examine your testicles on the same day of each month (e.g., the first day of the month) to help you remember.

the stage of the cancer at diagnosis: Stage I is confined to the testicle; stage II includes regional lymph node involvement; in stage III, distant metastases are present.

When testicular cancer is suspected, blood is drawn to identify tumor markers such as *alpha-fetoprotein, human chorionic gonadotropin, alkaline phosphatase,* and *lactic dehydrogenase.* Elevated levels indicate probable testicular cancer. These markers are also measured after surgery to help monitor the effectiveness of treatment.

An *ultrasound of the testicle* is performed to rule out other causes of the mass. *CT scans* are done to detect possible metastasis to the lungs or abdominal organs. Biopsy is often done at the time of surgery.

Medications

Stage III testicular cancer is treated with a combination of surgery and chemotherapy. A combination of chemotherapy drugs is used. (See Chapter 12 for more information about chemotherapy for cancer and management of chemotherapy side effects.)

Surgery

Surgery to remove the affected testicle and spermatic cord (called a *radical orchiectomy*) is the primary treatment for early testicular cancer. This operation is performed through an incision in the inguinal area. Lymph nodes in the retroperitoneal area may also be removed, taking care to preserve the nerves necessary for ejaculation. After removal of the testis, a saline-filled prosthesis may be inserted into the scrotum.

Radiation Therapy

After surgery, radiation therapy is used to treat cancer in the retroperitoneal lymph nodes, the most frequent site of metastasis. The patient may experience temporary diarrhea, nausea, or decreased bone marrow function. These problems are usually mild. (See Chapter 12 for more information about nursing care related to radiation therapy.)

NURSING CARE

PRIORITIZING NURSING CARE

The patient with an orchiectomy is often discharged on the day of surgery. Nursing care focuses on teaching and psychologic support.

ASSESSING

Key Concept Nurses can be instrumental in identifying testicular cancer at an early, treatable stage. They should ask men if they have noticed any change in the size or texture of their testicles.

In some cases, the patient's partner may notice a change in the size or feel of one testicle compared with the other. Palpate the scrotum and testicles, noting any difference in size or changes from the normal. Promptly report to the physician a testicle that is hard, irregular in shape, or fixed (not movable within the scrotum).

Deficient Knowledge

Expected outcome: Will describe correct use of postoperative self-care strategies and when to call the physician for complications.

- Discuss using analgesics, ice bags, and a scrotal support to reduce postoperative pain. *Ice provides local analgesia and helps reduce scrotal swelling. A scrotal support is particularly helpful when the patient ambulates. See Chapter 10 for routine pre- and postoperative care and teaching.*
- Instruct to contact the physician if complications develop: the incision comes open, bleeding beyond slight oozing after 24 hours, or rapid scrotal swelling. *Because the patient is usually discharged early, complications may not develop until after discharge.*

Risk for Sexual Dysfunction

Expected outcome: Will discuss feelings about sexual function and possible altered sexual function after surgery for testicular cancer.

- Assess current sexual function. To do this, establish an atmosphere of openness and permission to discuss sexual concerns. *After the initial shock of the diagnosis, patients often have intense concerns about sexual and reproductive issues, which can be relieved only by information.*
- Help the patient express his concerns about altered sexual function and appearance. *The ability to express sexuality is a basic human need. The patient may fear the loss of this ability and will grieve its loss if treatment affects it.*
- Reinforce teaching about the expected effect of surgery on sexuality. Reassure that erectile function is rarely affected by testicular cancer and treatment. *If the treatment involves only an orchiectomy, there should be no lasting effects on sexual or reproductive function.*
- Discuss the option of preserving sperm in a bank before treatment. *This option may help relieve fears about the ability to father children in the future. Sperm banking must be done before treatment with surgery, chemotherapy, or radiation therapy.*

EVALUATING

To evaluate the effectiveness of nursing care for patients with testicular cancer, collect data such as the following:

- Ability to demonstrate and relate the importance of regular TSE
- Understanding of ways to reduce pain and swelling after surgery

- Knowledge of manifestations of complications and when to contact the physician
- Willingness to discuss or ask questions about effect of treatment on sexuality and reproduction

DOCUMENTING

Document education provided, the patient's and family's understanding of the information, and recommendations or appointments for follow-up care.

CONTINUITY OF CARE

clinicalALERT

Teach all young men how to perform TSE and stress the importance of establishing a routine.

Shower cards that demonstrate TSE on one side and breast self-exam on the other are available through the American Cancer Society. These cards serve as useful reminders.

Include families in teaching for the patient with testicular cancer. If the patient is sexually active, his partner needs information about the effects of treatment on sexuality and reproduction. If the patient is a teenager, his parents are often involved in postoperative care. The patient facing cancer needs the support of knowledgeable loved ones.

Teach postoperative care, including incision care, use of ice and a scrotal support, and signs and symptoms of complications to report to the physician.

Discuss the need for continuing follow-up after treatment for testicular cancer. Surveillance includes periodic physical examinations, chest x-rays, tumor markers, and CT scans of retroperitoneal nodes for 5 to 10 years after orchiectomy.

DISORDERS OF THE PENIS

Phimosis

Phimosis is constriction of the foreskin so that it cannot be pushed back over the glans penis. It may be present at birth or may follow infection or injury. Phimosis increases the risk of secondary infections, scarring, and perhaps cancer of the penis. Severe phimosis can interfere with urination. If the foreskin is forcibly retracted behind the glans, it may become trapped, impairing blood flow to the glans. Circumcision (removal of the foreskin) may be necessary to correct the condition. Teach patients and parents about the importance of hygiene measures to prevent infection and possible phimosis. Also teach patients with phimosis the importance of hygiene and how to perform self-examination for cancer of the penis.

Peyronie Disease

Peyronie (pa-ro-NEE) disease causes a hard fibrous layer of plaque (similar to scar tissue) to develop under the skin on one side of the penis. When the penis is erect, the scar tissue is less flexible than the rest of the penile tissue and causes the penis to curve. The plaque is caused by thickened layers of tissue and is benign. The condition can cause pain and can cause sexual intercourse to be difficult. Sometimes Peyronie disease resolves without treatment. Surgical treatment is usually postponed for 1 to 2 years after onset of symptoms to allow the disorder to resolve spontaneously if it can. Some affected patients have hardened connective tissues in other parts of their bodies. It usually occurs in men aged 45 to 60. Nurses may be able to help patients by talking with them about body image issues.

Priapism

Priapism is a sustained, painful erection that is not associated with sexual arousal. It is caused by impaired blood flow in the corpora cavernosa of the penis. Priapism may be idiopathic or be secondary to certain conditions or drugs (Box 31-9■). The sustained erection of priapism is often painful and harder than normal. If the condition continues, there is a risk of tissue damage and impotence.

Initial treatment of priapism includes analgesia, sedation, and fluids. In patients with sickle cell disease, transfusion and oxygen are provided. Ice packs to the perineum may provide relief. If other measures are ineffective, surgery may be done to temporarily drain blood out of the penis.

Inspect the penis for degree of erection and color; palpate its firmness and degree of rigidity. Monitor urine

BOX 31-9	RISK FACTORS FOR PRIAPISM

Illnesses/Conditions
- Sickle cell disease
- Leukemia
- Metastatic cancer
- Spinal cord trauma

Drugs
- Drugs to treat erectile dysfunction (see Table 31-2)
- Papaverine
- Psychotropic drugs
- Alcohol
- Marijuana

output. Report oliguria or signs of acute urinary retention. Provide analgesics as ordered to manage pain. Address the patient's anxiety about the condition, pain, treatment, and threat to sexual function. Reassure the patient that potency is usually maintained after surgical shunting of circulation. The patient may be acutely embarrassed by the erection; address his concerns and reassure him that the erection is not within his control.

Cancer of the Penis

Cancer of the penis is rare in North America. Older men are most often affected. Its cause is uncertain. Phimosis, tightening of the foreskin that prevents retraction over the glans, is a significant risk factor. Penile cancer is also linked to viral infections, human papillomavirus in particular. Other risk factors include exposure to ultraviolet (UV) light, unprotected sex with multiple partners, and cigarette smoking.

PATHOPHYSIOLOGY AND MANIFESTATIONS

Squamous cell carcinoma accounts for 95% of all penile cancers. The tumor usually develops as a nodular or wartlike growth or a red velvety lesion on the glans or foreskin. The tumors tend to grow slowly. Penile cancer spreads to regional lymph nodes and, very late in the disease, may spread to the bone, liver, or lungs. If the lesion is treated before nodes are involved, chances for a cure are good. Manifestations include a mass or persistent sore or ulcer at the distal end of the penis, involving the glans or foreskin. Most of these lesions are painless; however, they may ulcerate and bleed. Purulent, foul-smelling discharge may be noted under the foreskin.

COLLABORATIVE CARE

Cancer of the penis is diagnosed by biopsy of the lesion and any suspicious lymph nodes. Small, localized lesions may be treated with a topical chemotherapy drug, external-beam radiation, laser, or surgical excision. The penis may be partially or totally amputated if the cancer has spread into deeper structures. If a total *penectomy* is done, a perineal urethrostomy is created to preserve urinary drainage. Patients with distant metastases may be treated with chemotherapy.

NURSING CARE

When providing routine care, observe the penis for any visible lesions. If a lesion is noted, promptly report it to the physician. After surgery, monitor the surgical site for healing and any signs of infection. Carefully monitor intake and output, and provide routine postoperative care. Inform the patient that dribbling after voiding may occur for several weeks after surgery. Teach perineal care to reduce the risk of skin irritation and breakdown. Sitz baths may help relieve pain and promote healing. Carefully listen to concerns, being aware of the effect of a penectomy on body image, self-concept, and sexuality.

DOCUMENTING

Document assessment data, including any lesions. Note instructions provided, and the patient's and family's understanding of information.

CONTINUITY OF CARE

To help prevent cancer of the penis, teach patients about the risks of unprotected sex, and encourage condom use. Inform patients about the possible link between UV rays and penile cancer, and encourage men to shield their genitals when sunbathing or using tanning salons. Discuss the importance of seeking prompt treatment for any lesion or abnormal drainage noted on the penis.

DISORDERS OF SEXUAL EXPRESSION

Erectile Dysfunction

Erectile dysfunction (ED) or **impotence** is the inability to attain and maintain an erection that allows satisfactory sexual intercourse. An estimated 10 to 15 million men in the United States have ED. Most are older than age 65. This problem may involve total inability to achieve erection, an inconsistent ability to achieve erection, or the ability to sustain only brief erections.

There are many possible causes of ED, including many chronic diseases, such as diabetes and atherosclerosis, and many drugs. In most men, the cause of ED is primarily physiologic. Psychologic factors also contribute and are believed to cause 10% to 20% of cases of ED.

PATHOPHYSIOLOGY

A number of physiologic mechanisms work together to cause an erection. For an erection to occur, the blood supply to the penis must be adequate, normal nervous system and hormonal actions are necessary, and appropriate psychologic and social responses need to occur. Interruption of any of these factors and certain drugs can lead to impotence.

Atherosclerosis can interfere with the arterial blood supply to the penis. Surgeries such as radical prostatectomy or chronic diseases such as diabetes or multiple sclerosis can disrupt innervation. Decreased testosterone levels can also lead to ED. Many drugs, including antihypertensive medications, psychotropic drugs, hormones, and others, can disrupt the normal mechanisms to achieve erection, leading to impotence.

COLLABORATIVE CARE

ED can often be effectively managed using drugs, mechanical devices, or surgery.

Diagnostic Tests

Diagnostic tests are done to help identify the cause of the problem:

- *Blood tests,* such as a chemistry profile and testosterone, prolactin, thyroxine, and PSA levels, are done to identify systemic disorders that may be causing the dysfunction.
- *Nocturnal penile tumescence and rigidity (NPTR)* monitors erections that occur during rapid eye movement (REM) sleep. This test may be done in a sleep laboratory or at home with a portable device.
- *Cavernosometry* and *cavernosography* evaluate blood flow to and from the penis.

Medications

ED can be treated with drugs that work in a variety of ways. Sildenafil (Viagra, a phosphodiesterase type 5 inhibitor) for ED was approved for use in 1998. Sildenafil and related drugs do not directly cause an erection but enhance the natural response to sexual stimuli. At recommended doses, no effect occurs in the absence of sexual stimulation. Table 31-2■ discusses nursing implications for these drugs. The onset and duration of action of these drugs vary; review information specific to the prescribed drug before teaching.

clinicalALERT

Sildenafil and related drugs can cause a dangerous drop in blood pressure when used together with nitrates (including nitroglycerin to treat angina). Advise men who use nitrates to prevent or treat angina to talk to their cardiologist before taking ED drugs, and instruct all men using these drugs to avoid use of recreational nitrates, which can be used to prolong erection.

Testosterone replacement may also be ordered for men with ED. Alprostadil (prostaglandin E_1) can be administered by inserting a semisolid pellet into the urethra or by direct injection into the penis. This drug stimulates an erection, but many men discontinue treatment because of the mode of delivery or dissatisfaction with lack of spontaneity. Transdermal nitroglycerin paste applied directly to the penis is another option to promote blood flow and erection.

Mechanical Devices

Men who cannot take sildenafil may use a *vacuum constriction device* that draws blood into the penis with a vacuum, trapping it there with a constricting band at the base of the penis. This device, however, is cumbersome and may be an unacceptable option for many men.

Surgery

When ED does not respond to less invasive methods of treatment, a semirigid or inflatable prosthesis may be implanted (Figure 31-6■). Patients are generally satisfied with the results of a penile implant. Partners are also likely to report satisfaction, although the more firm erection can cause pain or prolong the duration of intercourse for an unacceptable period. Patient and partner teaching is mandatory. Counseling by a sex therapist may be needed to facilitate adaptation to the implant.

TABLE 31-2	Giving Medications Safely: Drugs for Erectile Dysfunction		
CLASS/DRUGS	**PURPOSE**	**NURSING IMPLICATIONS**	**PATIENT TEACHING**
Phosphodiesterase type 5 inhibitors ■ *Sildenafil* (Viagra), *tadalafil* (Cialis), *vardenafil* (Levitra)	These drugs are used to treat erectile dysfunction in men. They work together with nitric oxide and an enzyme released during sexual stimulation to increase the firmness and duration of an erection. The duration of effect varies among these drugs.	Contraindicated for men taking any form of nitrate drug (including recreational nitrates); combination can cause significant hypotension. Relatively contraindicated for men who have cardiovascular disease. May cause priapism, especially in men with other risk factors. Approved only for use in men.	Take the drug approximately 30 minutes to 1 hour before sexual activity. Drug effect may diminish after 2 to 36 hours; do not take more than once a day. If you have high blood pressure or cardiovascular disease, check with your doctor before taking. Promptly report erection that lasts more than 4 hours, chest pain, or shortness of breath.

Note: Medications identified in *italics* are among the 200 most frequently prescribed drugs in the United States.

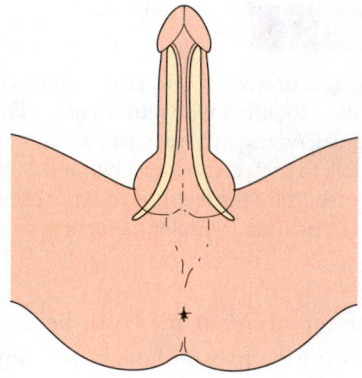

A Semirigid

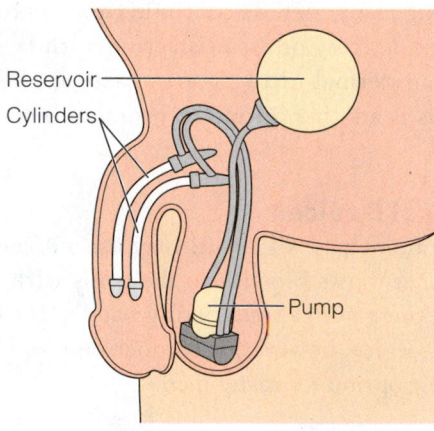

Reservoir

Cylinders

Pump

B Inflatable

Figure 31-6. ■ Types of penile implants. (**A**) Semirigid rods implanted in the corpora cavernosa keep the penis in a constant state of semierection. (**B**) With an inflatable penile implant, the patient compresses a pump in the scrotum to fill cylinders in the corpora cavernosa and achieve an erection. Pressing a release valve returns the fluid to a reservoir.

NURSING CARE

PRIORITIZING NURSING CARE

The focus for the nurse in caring for a patient with ED is straightforward, therapeutic communication and reinforcement of teaching.

ASSESSING

Problems with ED are often revealed in the course of a health assessment interview. Ask about chronic diseases such as diabetes and thyroid conditions, hypertension and other cardiovascular disease, kidney failure, and neurologic conditions. Inquire about medications such as antihypertensive drugs (which often cause ED), antidepressants, tranquilizers, and sedatives. Explore psychosocial stressors that may contribute to ED. Discuss lifestyle and use of alcohol or street drugs. Finally, ask specific questions about sexual function, including a history of premature ejaculation, impotence, or other sexual problems.

DIAGNOSING, PLANNING, AND IMPLEMENTING

Key Concept Sensitive, straightforward communication with patients experiencing sexual problems is most therapeutic. The nurse's communication is an important part of intervention with these patients.

Willingness of the nurse to discuss the patient's sexuality is often important to bring the subject of ED into the open and to inform the patient (and partner) that treatment is available.

Sexual Dysfunction

Expected outcome: Will discuss feelings about sexual dysfunction and consider possible treatments.

■ Assess for risk factors such as a new medication or recent surgery. *Although most older men have at least one risk factor for ED, identifying specific risk factors can help focus treatment strategies.*

■ Ask specific questions about sexual function and current sexual practices. *Men with ED and their partners often live in isolation with the problem for many years. The partner may be unaware of the problem or may believe the patient has lost his attraction to the partner. The patient may keep his problem secret because of an intense feeling of shame. Many patients greet the information about the high incidence of ED with a sense of relief that they are not alone.*

■ Discuss previous methods of coping with ED. *Current coping strategies provide insight into the problem and help guide teaching.*

■ Provide information about treatment options. *Information provides hope for successful resolution of the problem and helps the patient and his partner identify acceptable treatment options.*

■ Refer the patient and his partner for counseling. *Although ED is primarily a physiologic problem, many patients benefit from counseling to address psychologic issues of ED.*

EVALUATING

To evaluate the effectiveness of nursing care for a patient with ED, collect data such as the following:

■ Willingness to discuss sexual function with a health care professional

■ Willingness to share concerns with partner

■ Knowledge of medical and surgical treatment options, their risks, and benefits

DOCUMENTING

Document teaching provided, as well as the patient's and partner's apparent understanding and acceptance of information. Note any referrals provided.

CONTINUITY OF CARE

To reduce the risk of ED, advise patients to remain physically active, consume a low-fat diet, and avoid cigarette smoking and excess alcohol intake. Discuss the potential effects of high-risk medications on sexual function with patients during teaching. Provide information about various treatment options for ED, including their cost, intended benefit, and potential risks or drawbacks of each option. Stress the importance of contacting the primary care provider before taking any prescription or over-the-counter drug to treat ED. Encourage partners to be involved in the treatment plan.

NURSING CARE PLAN
Patient With Erectile Dysfunction

Donald Lawton, 68 years old, has been married for 40 years. At age 52, he was diagnosed with type 2 diabetes mellitus. He has had stable angina controlled with sublingual nitroglycerin for the past 5 years. Two years ago, he noticed that his erections were not as rigid as usual. Gradually, the problem has worsened until he can no longer attain an erection adequate for sexual intercourse. His libido remains unaffected. He relates shame and embarrassment and is unable to discuss this problem with anyone, including his wife.

Assessment

Mr. Lawton talks to his doctor after his wife threatens to leave him, claiming neglect. He is referred to a urologist. Mr. Lawton says he values his relationship with his wife and that sexual intimacy has been important to them. He says their sexual activity has always been limited to foreplay and sexual intercourse, expressing mild distaste about other forms of sexual intimacy. He reports feeling as if he is no longer a man and that he is ashamed that he can no longer satisfy his wife. This has affected their entire relationship and communications.

Mr. Lawton's serum testosterone levels are normal. Nocturnal penile tumescence and rigidity monitoring in the sleep laboratory reveal an absence of erections during REM sleep. The urologist prescribes *vardenafil* (*Levitra*) and suggests couples counseling.

Nursing Diagnosis

The following nursing diagnoses are identified for Mr. Lawton:

- *Sexual Dysfunction* related to diabetes
- *Ineffective Sexuality Patterns* related to lack of knowledge and poor communication patterns with wife
- *Disturbed Body Image* related to change in erectile function

Expected Outcomes

The expected outcomes for the plan of care are that Mr. Lawton will:

- Demonstrate the ability to discuss sexual concerns with his wife.
- State acceptance of the change in his erectile function.
- Verbalize understanding of the use and potential adverse effects of vardenafil.

Planning and Implementation

The following interventions are planned and implemented for Mr. Lawton:

- With permission, include his wife in discussions and teaching sessions.
- Encourage couples counseling.
- Listen to concerns about ED, and encourage communication.
- Teach about vardenafil, its use, precautions, and potential adverse effects.

Evaluation

Mr. Lawton begins to discuss his sexual and relationship problems more readily. He and his wife begin to attend counseling. Mrs. Lawton states that she had been afraid her husband no longer found her attractive and that he had found another woman. She greets the knowledge of the true nature of the problem with relief and concern. Privately, Mr. Lawton tells the nurse that he feels his marriage is improving and that even though "things will never be the same," he is beginning to look forward to some mutual exploration. Mr. Lawton is able to use *vardenafil* without adverse effects, and 4 months later reports that he and his wife are "90% satisfied with the result."

Critical Thinking in the Nursing Process

1. Mr. Lawton's ED was directly related to his diabetes. Describe the pathophysiology of diabetes-induced ED (see Chapter 36).
2. How does the NPTR test differentiate between physiologic and psychologic causes of ED?
3. Discuss the importance of Mr. and Mrs. Lawton's lack of communication on the development of their sexual problems. Include possible reasons for their difficulty in discussing sexual concerns.

Note: Discussion of Critical Thinking questions appears on the companion website.

Ejaculatory Dysfunction

There are many types of ejaculatory dysfunction. *Premature ejaculation* is often caused by psychologic factors; diabetes can also cause premature ejaculation. *Delayed ejaculation* may be related to aging changes, such as decreased penile sensation or decreased libido. Ejaculation can also be affected by drugs to treat hypertension, depression, anxiety, and narcotic medications. *Retrograde ejaculation* (semen discharged into the bladder rather than through the urethra) is usually related to treatment of prostate disorders or testicular cancer.

Medical and nursing care for patients with ejaculatory problems focuses on assessing the problem and patient teaching. Of these problems, premature ejaculation is most easily treated. Wearing a condom and techniques such as relaxation and guided imagery can delay sexual excitement and ejaculation. The patient's partner can be taught how to avoid excessive stimulation until ejaculation. If the problem persists, referral to a specialist is appropriate.

Note: The references and resources for all chapters have been compiled at the back of the book.

Chapter Review

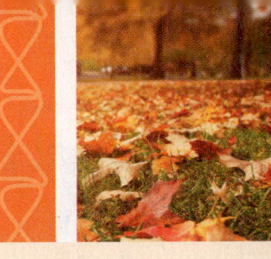

KEY POINTS

- BPH is the most common problem affecting the male reproductive system, followed by prostate cancer. Their risk is increased in older adults.
- **Concept:** Disorders of the male reproductive system and their treatments pose a risk to the patient's fertility, sexuality, and urinary function. The patient's body image and self-concept may also be affected by these changes.
- **Concept:** Enlargement of the prostate gland, BPH, affects most men over the age of 50. The incidence of BPH increases with age.
- The manifestations of BPH and prostate cancer are similar: urinary frequency, urgency, and hesitancy, a reduced urine stream, and nocturia. Physical examination and diagnostic testing are necessary to differentiate these disorders.
- Monitoring for adverse effects of reproductive system disorders and their treatment and educating the patient are priority nursing responsibilities.
- In both BPH and prostate cancer, medications or "watchful waiting" may be appropriate treatment; surgery, however, is often the treatment of choice. Minimally invasive procedures such as balloon dilation, laser prostatectomy, or TUIP may be used to treat BPH. Prostate cancer, on the other hand, is treated with a prostatectomy.
- After a prostatectomy, the patient is at risk for deep venous thrombosis and pulmonary embolism. Preventive measures such as leg exercises, elastic hose, pneumatic compression devices, and early ambulation are important to prevent these complications.
- Although testicular cancer is rare, its risk is highest in young men (15 to 35 years old). Teach all young men to perform TSE and stress the importance of doing it on a regular basis.
- **Concept:** Nurses can be instrumental in identifying testicular cancer at an early, treatable stage. They should ask men if they have noticed any change in the size or texture of their testicles.
- Most patients with ED can be effectively treated with medication or an implanted prosthetic device.
- **Concept:** Use the skill of sensitive, straightforward communication with patients experiencing sexual problems. The nurse's communication is an important part of intervention with these patients.

PEARSON NURSING STUDENT RESOURCES

Find additional materials at **nursing.pearsonhighered.com**.

Clinical Reasoning Care Map

Caring for a Patient With Prostate Cancer
NCLEX-PN® Focus Area: Safety and Infection Control

Case Study: William Turner is a 71-year-old African American. He lives at home with his wife, who had a stroke 2 years ago. Mr. Turner has been in good health except for a "touch" of osteoarthritis in his hips and hands. He reports a gradual onset of urinary urgency during the past 2 years. During a routine physical examination, a hard nodule is palpated on his prostate gland, and his PSA level is found to be elevated. A radical retropubic prostatectomy is performed. He is discharged home several days later with an indwelling catheter in place. The home health nurse visits Mr. Turner 2 days after his discharge.

Nursing Diagnosis: Ineffective Self-Health Maintenance

COLLECT DATA

Subjective

_____

_____

_____

_____

_____

_____

Objective

_____

_____

_____

_____

_____

_____

Does this present a threat to the patient's safety?

If yes, what is the priority intervention to address this threat?

_____

Nursing Care

_____

_____

_____

_____

_____

Interprofessional team members to include when planning care:

_____

How would you document this? _____

_____

Compare your answers and documentation to those provided on the companion website.

Data Collected
(use only those that apply)

- History of osteoarthritis in hands and hips
- Home clean and neat
- Fully dressed, carrying large night urinary drainage bag
- Relates difficulty getting out of house to buy groceries due to embarrassment of being seen with drainage bag
- Reports inability to change from large drainage bag to leg bag due to arthritis
- Vital signs within normal limits
- Pelvic incision healing well with no evidence of infection
- Lung sounds clear
- Urine pale yellow, not malodorous
- Uncertain about whether to continue pelvic muscle and dorsiflexion exercises at home
- Questions need for follow-up visits now that his cancer is cured

Nursing Interventions
(use only those that apply; list in priority order)

- Provide teaching for Mr. Turner and care assistants as appropriate.
- Discuss potential postoperative complications.
- Explore available support systems to identify people to assist with catheter care.
- Discuss the possibility of stress incontinence after the catheter is removed.
- Reinforce the need for perineal muscle exercises while the catheter is still in place.
- Reinforce the importance of follow-up care to monitor the disease and healing.

NCLEX-PN® Exam Preparation

1 After a transurethral prostatectomy (TURP), a patient confesses to the nurse that although he is able to maintain an erection, he "can't seem to produce anything" on orgasm. The nurse recognizes this as indicative of:

1. nocturia.
2. impotence.
3. decreased libido.
4. retrograde ejaculation.

2 After TURP surgery, the nurse irrigates the bladder:

1. on an every-4-hour schedule.
2. as needed to clear blood clots and reduce spasms.
3. to reduce the sensation to void.
4. to prevent hyponatremia.

3 A patient is about to be discharged after TURP. What statement indicates the need for additional instruction?

1. "I will continue taking one regular daily aspirin for my heart."
2. "I will not take a tub bath while the catheter is in place."
3. "I should not have sex for six weeks."
4. "I need to drink ten eight-ounce glasses of fluids a day."

4 A patient is one day postoperative from a TURP. In what order would the nurse address the patient's following complaints?

1. Pain and bladder spasms
2. Leakage around the irrigation catheter
3. Blood clots in urinary catheter
4. Dyspnea and chest pain
5. Poor appetite and an "off" taste

5 Which of the following instructions should the nurse include when teaching a patient with nonbacterial prostatitis?

1. Restrict fluids to avoid painful voiding.
2. Have frequent sex.
3. Wear a condom to avoid infecting their partner.
4. Finish the antibiotic therapy.

6 A 63-year-old patient with no prior history of prostate problems has an elevated PSA level. He asks the nurse if this means that he has prostate cancer. The most appropriate response is:

1. "Yes. Prostate cancer increases the PSA level."
2. "No. The PSA increases when there is a prostate infection."
3. "Although the PSA increases with prostate cancer, it also increases in benign prostatic hypertrophy. Further tests are necessary."
4. "PSA levels increase with aging, so this test is ineffective to detect or diagnose prostate cancer."

7 A patient with prostate cancer asks why the physician is planning to remove his testicles when the cancer is in his prostate gland, not his scrotum. The nurse responds based on the knowledge that:

1. removing the testes reduces testosterone needed to support tumor growth.
2. prostate cancer frequently metastasizes to the testes.
3. this measure is important to prevent the patient from engaging in sexual relations.
4. removing the testes is easier than administering hormones to treat prostate cancer.

8 Which of the following is an accurate statement regarding sildenafil (Viagra)?

1. Sildenafil is helpful in patients who have cardiovascular disease.
2. Sildenafil works better when combined with a nitrate drug.
3. Sildenafil may cause priapism.
4. Sildenafil is taken bid on an empty stomach.

9 A 19-year-old man presents at the walk-in clinic complaining of severe pain in his scrotum that began suddenly about an hour ago. The nurse should:

1. obtain a complete medical history from the patient.
2. advise the patient to call his personal physician for an appointment.
3. provide a narcotic analgesic to relieve the pain.
4. notify the physician immediately.

10 A young woman tells the nurse that she has noticed that one of her husband's testicles is much harder than the other. She wonders if this is normal because it is not painful. The nurse responds that:

1. this is a normal variation in many men.
2. if the testicle becomes painful, her husband should see his physician.
3. testicular cancer usually presents as a hard, painless nodule; he should see his physician.
4. this is a common manifestation of an infected testicle; her husband should see his physician for an antibiotic prescription.

Answers and rationales for Review Questions appear in Appendix I.

CHAPTER 32

Caring for Female Patients With Reproductive System Disorders

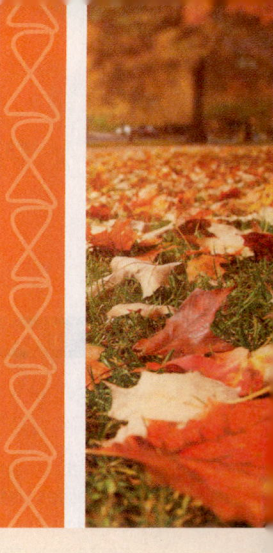

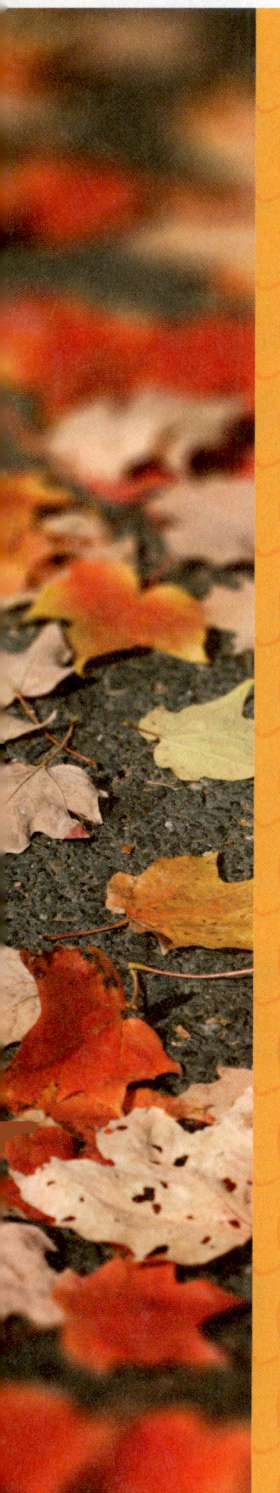

BRIEF OUTLINE

APPLIED LEARNING OUTCOMES

After completing this chapter, you will be able to:

1. Describe the pathophysiology of commonly occurring disorders and changes of the breast and female reproductive system.
2. Compare and contrast the manifestations of benign and malignant disorders of the breast and female reproductive system.
3. Provide appropriate preoperative and postoperative nursing care for the patient having gynecologic surgery.
4. Use the nursing process when providing nursing care for female patients with perimenopausal symptoms and disorders of the breast and reproductive system.
5. Teach current screening recommendations for breast cancer.

KEY TERMS

The key terms are defined on the pages listed below.

SPECIAL FEATURES

Disorders of the female reproductive system may affect a woman's ability to bear children, her sexuality, and her sense of well-being as a woman. For many women, the ability to reproduce affects self-concept and general health. Women experiencing reproductive system problems may be asked to disclose personal, intimate information, which may be embarrassing and uncomfortable. Sensitivity on the part of the nurse is vital to establishing a caring, therapeutic relationship with the patient.

DISORDERS RELATED TO THE MENSTRUAL CYCLE

Key Concept Menstruation is a normal event, occurring cyclically on a monthly basis. It is an almost universal experience for women, and yet it is often misunderstood. Some cultures have beliefs that women are unclean, have special powers, or are less able to function while menstruating. None of these superstitions is accurate.

Menstruation is a normal physiological process, which usually proceeds without major difficulty. It occurs in most women between the ages of approximately 12 and 50. Monthly menstruation often causes minor discomfort, such as breast tenderness, a feeling of heaviness and congestion in the pelvic area, uterine cramping, and backache. This section presents common disorders that are related to the menstrual cycle: premenstrual syndrome (which occurs before menstruation), dysmenorrhea (during menstruation), and abnormal uterine bleeding (during or between menstrual periods).

Premenstrual Syndrome

Premenstrual syndrome (PMS) is a common disorder characterized by emotional and physical symptoms that occur on a monthly cyclic basis during the luteal phase of the menstrual cycle (between ovulation and the start of menstruation). Women with more severe mood symptoms may be diagnosed with premenstrual dysphoric disorder (PMDD) (Youngkin, Davis, Schadewald, & Juve, 2013).

PATHOPHYSIOLOGY AND MANIFESTATIONS
The pathophysiology of PMS is not clearly understood. Hormonal changes such as altered estrogen–progesterone ratios, increased prolactin levels, and rising aldosterone levels during the luteal phase of the menstrual cycle (see Figure 30-3) are thought to contribute to the problem. Increased aldosterone levels cause salt and water retention and edema. Neurotransmitters such as monoamine oxidase and serotonin affect emotions and probably play a role in the depressed mood symptoms of PMS.

It is estimated that 20% to 40% of women of reproductive age experience PMS symptoms severe enough to meet the diagnostic criteria set by the American College of Obstetricians and Gynecologists (ACOG). The ACOG guideline for diagnosing PMS requires that one or more of the following symptoms must be present for at least 5 days in the 2 weeks prior to menses (the luteal phase). The symptoms in this group are abdominal bloating, breast tenderness, headaches, fluid retention, increased appetite, cravings, weight gain, acne, fatigue, heart palpitations, gastrointestinal disturbances, mood swings, irritability, anxiety, depression, crying easily, and poor mental concentration. To qualify as PMS symptoms, they must be present for at least three menstrual cycles in a row, must resolve within 4 days of the beginning of menstruation, and must cause significant impairment or distress in normal daily activities (Youngkin et al., 2013).

The multisystem effects of PMS are shown in Figure 32-1■. The manifestations of PMS and their intensity vary markedly among patients.

COLLABORATIVE CARE
The goals of care for PMS are to relieve manifestations and help the patient develop self-care strategies for episodes of PMS. The patient is advised to keep a daily diary of symptoms for several months to evaluate their timing and severity.

Management focuses on diet, exercise, relaxation, and stress management. A diet is recommended that is high in whole foods (e.g., whole grains, beans, nuts, fruits, and vegetables) and low in processed foods and refined sugars (e.g., high-fructose corn syrup, cane juice, fructose, dextrose, sucrose, malt syrup, fruit juice concentrate, and sugar). It is also recommended that use of alcohol be limited. Reduced salt intake helps to minimize fluid retention. Caffeine is restricted to reduce irritability. Increased intake of calcium, magnesium, and vitamin B_6 may be helpful. Exercise is beneficial, and adequate rest is also necessary. The patient needs to balance periods of activity and rest. Techniques for relaxation and stress management include deep abdominal breathing, meditation, muscle relaxation, and guided imagery.

Suppression of ovulation with hormone therapy has shown effectiveness for treating severe PMS symptoms. Oral contraceptives have been used for this purpose, especially in women who also desire contraception.

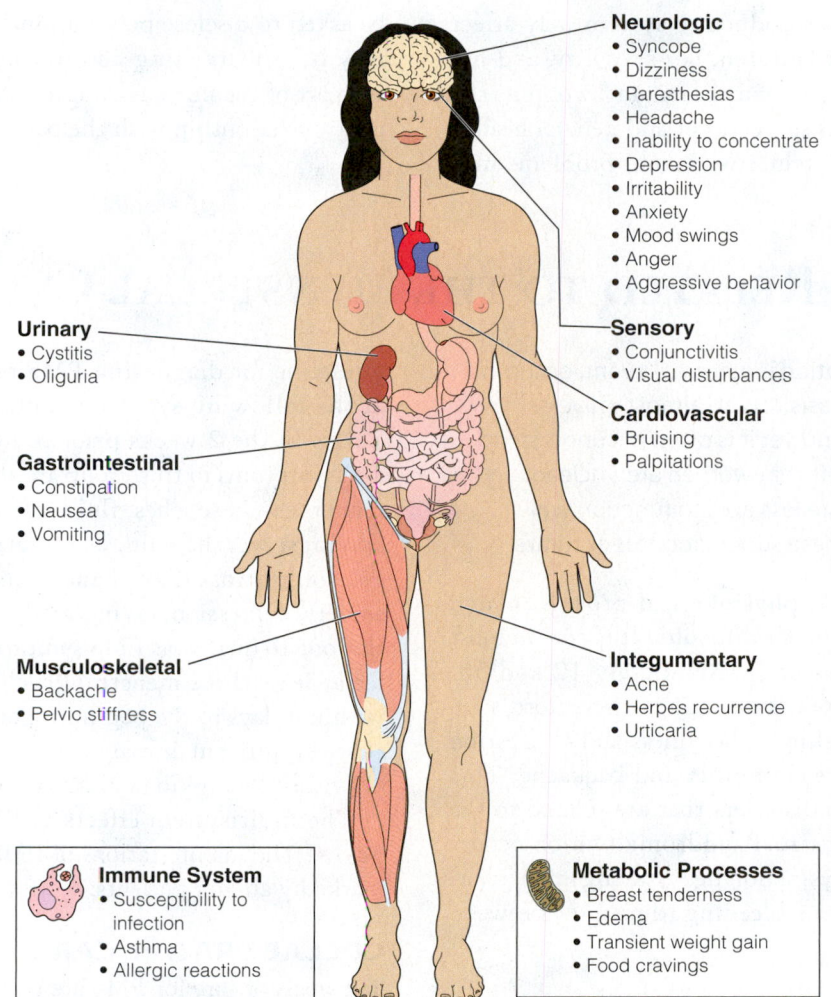

Neurologic
• Syncope
• Dizziness
• Paresthesias
• Headache
• Inability to concentrate
• Depression
• Irritability
• Anxiety
• Mood swings
• Anger
• Aggressive behavior

Sensory
• Conjunctivitis
• Visual disturbances

Cardiovascular
• Bruising
• Palpitations

Urinary
• Cystitis
• Oliguria

Gastrointestinal
• Constipation
• Nausea
• Vomiting

Musculoskeletal
• Backache
• Pelvic stiffness

Integumentary
• Acne
• Herpes recurrence
• Urticaria

Immune System
• Susceptibility to infection
• Asthma
• Allergic reactions

Metabolic Processes
• Breast tenderness
• Edema
• Transient weight gain
• Food cravings

Figure 32-1. ■ The multisystem effects of premenstrual syndrome.

Complementary therapies may also be used for PMS. Black cohosh is used for dysmenorrheal and other PMS symptoms, evening primrose oil is used for PMS, and valerian is effective for uterine cramping (Fontaine, 2011). Reflexology (manipulation of reflex zones on feet, hands, and more rarely on ears) has been found to ease PMS symptoms.

PREMENSTRUAL DYSPHORIC DISORDER

PMDD is similar to PMS, because it can present with all the PMS symptoms. To be diagnosed with PMDD, however, the patient must also have more consistent and debilitating premenstrual mood symptoms. PMDD occurs in 3% to 8% of the reproductive female population. The history of a depressive disorder increases a woman's vulnerability to premenstrual symptoms, especially the severity and duration of mood changes (Youngkin et al., 2013). Women with PMDD are more likely than those with PMS to respond well to antidepressant medications, but other therapies are similar (Osborn, Watson, & Wraa, 2010).

NURSING CARE

Nursing care for the patient with PMS focuses on teaching the patient to manage manifestations of the disorder.

Readiness for Enhanced Self-Health Management

Expected outcome: Will explore self-care and coping measures for PMS or PMDD.

■ Encourage keeping a journal of menstrual cycle, physical symptoms, and mood changes. *Recognizing the signs and timing of PMS is the first step in developing ways to cope with the problem.*

■ Review symptoms, relating them to diet, activity, and stress levels. *Identifying relationships helps develop strategies to reduce and manage the symptoms of PMS.*

■ Explore self-care measures that have helped the patient cope with mood alterations in the past. Encourage coping strategies such as relaxation techniques and exercise. *Using some drugs or alcohol to relieve PMS may actually make symptoms worse.*

- Review daily activities and suggest ways to balance rest periods and activity. *Rest decreases energy and oxygen consumption, increasing the amount available to muscles.*
- Explore ways to rearrange or reschedule activities to reduce stress during PMS symptoms. *Planning ahead provides more control and promotes effective coping.*
- Teach self-care measures to relieve pain: heat application, relaxation techniques (e.g., breathing exercises, imagery techniques, or meditation), and exercise. *Heat relieves muscle spasms and dilates blood vessels, increasing blood supply to the pelvis and uterus. Relaxation and exercise promote release of naturally produced pain relievers (endorphins).*

EVALUATING

Assess the patient's level of understanding about PMS and symptom management.

DOCUMENTING

Document information provided, as well as the patient's apparent willingness to employ suggested measures to relieve symptoms.

CONTINUITY OF CARE

Teach the patient that PMS is not a disease but a response to hormone changes of the menstrual cycle. Understanding the condition allows the patient to assume control, manage anxiety, and use appropriate strategies to reduce symptoms. Discuss dietary measures, relaxation techniques and exercise, stress reduction techniques, and support systems in teaching about PMS management.

Dysmenorrhea

Dysmenorrhea is pain associated with menstruation. It is the most common gynecologic disorder experienced by menstruating women. It is described as cramping pain in the lower abdomen, and although the associated symptoms vary, 45% to 95% of menstruating women suffer from dysmenorrhea (Youngkin et al., 2013).

memory**ALERT**

Dysmenorrhea comes from the Greek words *dys* (difficult, painful, or abnormal), *meno* (month), and *rrhea* (flow). A complex term like this is much simpler to remember if you know the Greek roots.

PATHOPHYSIOLOGY AND MANIFESTATIONS

In *primary dysmenorrhea,* no disease process is identified. Prostaglandins stimulate muscles in the uterus to contract. These contractions can cause mild cramping to severe muscle spasms. As the muscles contract, blood flow to the uterus is restricted, causing ischemia and pain. Abdominal pain begins with the onset of menses and lasts 12 to 48 hours. Pain may radiate to the lower back and thighs. Other manifestations may include headache, nausea, vomiting, diarrhea, fatigue, or breast tenderness. Psychologic factors, such as anxiety and tension, may contribute to dysmenorrhea. Childbirth tends to decrease the incidence and severity of symptoms.

Secondary dysmenorrhea is related to an underlying disorder that causes scarring or injury of reproductive organs. Endometriosis, fibroid tumors, pelvic inflammatory disease, or ovarian cancer may cause painful menses. These conditions are discussed later in this chapter.

Mittelschmerz, pain on ovulation, is a transitory pain that occurs 14 days before the start of menstruation. It is considered a normal variation, not a pathological symptom.

COLLABORATIVE CARE

Care of the patient with menstrual pain focuses on identifying its cause and managing pain. Drugs such as mild analgesics, prostaglandin inhibitors such as nonsteroidal anti-inflammatory drugs (NSAIDs), or oral contraceptives may be recommended to relieve pain. Nonpharmacologic measures include dietary changes, exercise, relaxation, and stress management. Dietary measures like those for PMS, such as increasing the intake of whole foods and decreasing processed foods, can be effective. Decreasing intake of sodium, caffeine, and alcohol and increasing intake of protein, calcium, magnesium, and vitamin B_6 may be helpful. A balance of rest and exercise is important. Techniques for relaxation and stress management include deep abdominal breathing, meditation, muscle relaxation, and guided imagery. Use of a heating pad also helps reduce pain. As with PMS, complementary therapies such as aromatherapy, herbal preparations, reflexology, acupressure, or massage may be helpful.

NURSING CARE

Nursing care focuses on helping the patient develop effective coping strategies. Discuss using an NSAID such as ibuprofen on a regular basis during periods of menstrual pain. Teach nonpharmacologic pain relief measures, and encourage use of these as well for pain relief. Stress the benign nature of primary dysmenorrhea, being sure to validate the reality of the pain and discomfort. Discuss healthy diet changes and exercise, as well as stress management techniques. Teach safe use of heat for pain relief. Provide information about engaging in sexual intercourse or masturbation, explaining that orgasm may help relieve the cramping pain.

Dysfunctional Uterine Bleeding

Key Concept Dysfunctional uterine bleeding has several causes but the one that the interprofessional team cannot afford to miss is bleeding due to malignancy.

Dysfunctional uterine bleeding (DUB) is vaginal bleeding that is abnormal in amount, duration, or time of occurrence. It is usually related to hormonal imbalances or pelvic tumors, either benign or malignant.

PATHOPHYSIOLOGY AND MANIFESTATIONS

Hormonal imbalance, especially progesterone deficiency with relative estrogen excess, causes endometrial tissue to proliferate. Unless this tissue is supported by adequate progesterone, sloughing occurs. Depending on ovarian function and the hormone imbalance, irregular, prolonged, or profuse vaginal bleeding may occur. *Anovulation,* absence of ovulation, is associated with both estrogen and progesterone deficiencies. Emotional upsets or physiological stress can also cause hormonal imbalances and thus affect menstruation. Pelvic tumors can also cause abnormal bleeding. They are discussed in later sections of this chapter.

Amenorrhea is the absence of menstruation. It is usually caused by hormone imbalance. Because a certain percentage of body fat is required for menstruation to occur, anorexia nervosa or excessive athletic activity or training can also cause amenorrhea. Amenorrhea is a normal consequence of pregnancy, breastfeeding, and menopause. It is an expected effect of removal of the uterus or ovaries.

Oligomenorrhea, scant menses, is usually related to hormonal imbalances. *Menorrhagia,* excessive or prolonged menstruation, may result from endocrine or reproductive system disorders. Clotting disorders and anticoagulant medications can also cause menorrhagia. Repetitive long or heavy cycles can lead to excessive blood loss, fatigue, anemia, hemorrhage, and sexual dysfunction.

Metrorrhagia, bleeding between menstrual periods, may be a sign of cervical or uterine cancer. For this reason, it is important to evaluate metrorrhagia promptly and thoroughly. Midcycle spotting associated with ovulation occurs in many women and is not considered metrorrhagia.

Postmenopausal bleeding may be caused by endometrial polyps, endometrial hyperplasia, uterine or cervical cancer, vaginal tissue atrophy, or hormone replacement therapy. The possibility of cancer makes early evaluation and treatment essential.

COLLABORATIVE CARE

The care of the patient with DUB focuses on identifying and treating the underlying disease. A careful history and physical examination are obtained. Abdominal and pelvic exams are done to rule out abdominal masses. Trauma from abuse should also be ruled out. The patient may need to keep a menstrual history and basal body temperature chart for several months to determine whether ovulation is related to bleeding.

Diagnostic Tests

- *Complete blood count (CBC)* to assess the severity of DUB.
- *Thyroid function tests* to rule out thyroid disorders such as hyper- or hypothyroidism as the cause of DUB.
- *Serum estradiol (estrogen)* and *progesterone* levels to evaluate ovarian function.
- *Serum HCG* and *LH* levels to evaluate pituitary function.
- *Pap smear* to rule out cervical cancer.
- *Pelvic ultrasound* to detect lesions such as fibroid or cancerous tumors. See Table 30-2 Diagnostic Ultrasound Studies for nursing care related to pelvic ultrasound.
- *Laparoscopy* to visualize pelvic structures or hysteroscopy to detect abnormalities of the uterine cavity. Nursing care for the patient undergoing a laparoscopy is outlined in Box 30-4 Nursing Care Checklist for Laparoscopy.
- *Endometrial biopsy* may be done to microscopically examine endometrial tissues.

Medications

For many patients, menstrual irregularities can be treated with hormones. Oral contraceptives or progesterone preparations may be ordered. Oral iron supplements may be prescribed to replace iron lost through menstrual bleeding.

Surgery

DUB is the leading cause of hysterectomy. However, the least invasive intervention that proves effective is preferred, beginning with a therapeutic dilation and curettage (D&C), then endometrial ablation, uterine balloon heart therapy, and, finally, hysterectomy.

In a *therapeutic D&C,* the cervical canal is dilated and the uterine wall is scraped. D&C is used to diagnose and treat DUB and certain other disorders. It is contraindicated for any woman who has been taking anticoagulant drugs. Nursing care of the patient undergoing D&C is outlined in Box 32-1■.

Endometrial ablation permanently destroys the endometrial layer of the uterus. It can be done by laser surgery or electrosurgical resection. Another endometrial ablation technique is *uterine balloon heat therapy,* in which a specialized balloon is inserted through the cervix into the uterus and then filled with heated liquid. The result is destruction of the lining of the uterus. This outpatient procedure can be done using local anesthesia. Endometrial ablation is done for women who do not respond to drug therapy or D&C. This procedure ends menstruation and reproduction.

BOX 32-1   NURSING CARE CHECKLIST

Dilation and Curettage (D&C)

Before Surgery
- ☑ If ordered, ask the patient to come in the day before surgery for insertion of a laminaria stent to absorb cervical secretions and slowly begin to dilate the cervix.
- ☑ Provide routine preoperative care (see Chapter 10).

After Surgery
- ☑ Provide routine postoperative care (see Chapter 10).
- ☑ Monitor circulation and sensation in the legs; avoid placing a pillow under the knees.
- ☑ Instruct to use perineal pads and avoid tampons for 2 weeks.
- ☑ Explain that the next menstrual period may be delayed.
- ☑ Instruct to avoid intercourse until after follow-up visit and cessation of vaginal discharge.
- ☑ Advise to rest, avoid heavy lifting for several days, and report bright red or excessive bleeding (more than a normal menstrual period).

Hysterectomy, or removal of the uterus, may be done if other treatments are unsuccessful or malignancy is found, particularly if childbearing is no longer desired. In premenopausal women, the ovaries are usually left in place. In postmenopausal women, a total hysterectomy, or panhysterectomy, may be done, removing the uterus, fallopian tubes, and ovaries.

Hysterectomy may be done using an abdominal approach, a vaginal approach, or a vaginal approach with laparoscopic visualization of the pelvic cavity. Recovery is faster after vaginal or laparoscopic hysterectomy than with an abdominal hysterectomy. The abdominal approach, however, may be used when better access to and visualization of the pelvic cavity is needed. Nursing care of the patient undergoing a hysterectomy is outlined in Box 32-2 ■.

A newer alternative to abdominal or vaginal hysterectomy is *supracervical laparoscopic hysterectomy*. In this outpatient procedure, a laparoscope is inserted through a small incision near the umbilicus. The uterus is removed with a laser, leaving the cervix intact. It is less invasive than a hysterectomy done with an abdominal or vaginal incision.

clinical**ALERT**

Pelvic surgery, including hysterectomy, increases the risk of deep venous thrombosis and pulmonary embolism. Encourage leg exercises and early ambulation to promote venous return. Advise women who smoke to stop. Promptly report symptoms such as leg or calf pain, swelling of one leg, chest pain, or difficulty breathing.

BOX 32-2   NURSING CARE CHECKLIST

Abdominal or Vaginal Hysterectomy

Before Surgery
- ☑ Assess understanding and reinforce teaching as needed. Provide emotional support.
- ☑ Instruct to cleanse abdominal and perineal areas as ordered.
- ☑ If ordered, administer a small cleansing enema and have patient empty bladder.
- ☑ Provide routine preoperative care as ordered (see Chapter 10).

After Surgery
- ☑ Provide routine postoperative care (see Chapter 10).
- ☑ Report excess bleeding, especially after a vaginal hysterectomy.
- ☑ Monitor for potential complications, such as infection, ileus, venous thrombosis, and pulmonary embolus.
- ☑ Assess vaginal drainage; teach perineal care.
- ☑ Advise to restrict physical activity, such as heavy lifting and stair climbing, as well as douching, tampons, and sexual intercourse for 4 to 6 weeks (3 to 4 weeks for the vaginal procedure).
- ☑ Instruct to shower, avoiding tub baths, until bleeding has stopped.
- ☑ Instruct to report the following to the physician:
  - ☑ Temperature greater than 100°F (37.7°C)
  - ☑ Vaginal bleeding greater than a typical menstrual period or that is bright red
  - ☑ Urinary incontinence, urgency, burning, or frequency
  - ☑ Severe pain
- ☑ Encourage expression of feelings and concerns.
- ☑ If appropriate, provide information about hormone replacement therapy.
- ☑ Reinforce the importance of regular gynecologic examinations even after hysterectomy.

NURSING CARE

PRIORITIZING NURSING CARE

DUB often causes anxiety and may threaten self-image, sexuality, or reproductive potential. In many cases, helping the patient deal with the psychologic and emotional effects of DUB and its treatment (e.g., therapeutic D&C or hysterectomy) is the highest nursing care priority.

ASSESSING

Nursing assessment focuses on subjective data related to the onset of symptoms, timing and amount of menstrual flow (in pads per day and duration of period), and associated symptoms such as pain or cramping, weakness, or excessive fatigue.

clinical**ALERT**

Advise women with complaints of bleeding between periods or after menopause to promptly seek medical attention because this can be a sign of endometrial or cervical cancer.

DIAGNOSING, PLANNING, AND IMPLEMENTING
Ineffective Coping

Expected outcome: Will describe her psychosocial support system and state how she will manage the stress of DUB and its treatment.

- Discuss results of diagnostic tests and examinations with the patient face to face. *This allows for open exchange of information.*
- Provide information about causes, treatment, risks, long-term effects, and prognosis for DUB. *Knowledge allows the patient to assume responsibility for her own health and become involved in her own treatment plan.*
- Evaluate coping strategies and psychosocial support systems. Teach appropriate coping strategies if indicated. *The possibility of surgery or cancer may be a crisis for the patient and her support system. Effective coping strategies help in dealing with this situational crisis.*

Sexual Dysfunction

Expected outcome: Will discuss her feelings about sexuality as they relate to DUB.

- Discuss sexual intercourse during menstruation. Explain that orgasm may help relieve symptoms. Emphasize that it is necessary to use contraception to prevent pregnancy even during menstruation. *Orgasm frequently provides at least temporary relief of the cramping pain. Some women mistakenly believe that birth control measures are unnecessary during menstruation.*
- Provide an opportunity to express concerns related to effect of DUB on lifestyle and sexual functioning. *Some women abstain from sexual activity due to symptoms of DUB. Encouraging verbalization of concerns can assist to develop strategies to minimize the impact of DUB on sexuality and lifestyle.*
- Encourage frequent rest periods. *Rest conserves energy and may allow sexual function to resume.*
- Provide information about alternative methods of sexual expression. *Methods of sexual expression other than vaginal intercourse may satisfy the needs of both partners.*

EVALUATING

Collect data related to the following to evaluate the effectiveness of nursing interventions:

- Verbalize strategies to cope with symptoms and treatment of disorder.
- Discuss her feelings about sexuality as they relate to DUB.
- Discuss acceptable and satisfying sexual practices with partner.

DOCUMENTING

Document assessment data on a continuing basis to show changes in the patient's condition. This is particularly important for the postoperative patient who has undergone a D&C or hysterectomy. Document the number of perineal pads saturated as an estimate of bleeding. Also document care and teaching, as well as the patient's emotional responses to information and treatment options.

CONTINUITY OF CARE

Provide support, reassurance, and information to help the patient and her family understand her disorder and its treatment. Teach self-care measures to help minimize the effects of DUB on activities of daily living (ADLs).

Discuss using ordered drugs, including oral contraceptives, iron supplements, or other agents, including dosage and side effects. Encourage the patient to take an iron supplement with orange juice (or other high vitamin C food) to improve absorption, and avoid taking it with foods high in calcium (e.g., milk), which interfere with its absorption. Provide information about maintaining a balanced diet, increasing iron-rich foods, such as eggs, beans, liver, beef, and shrimp. Encourage a fluid intake of 2,000 to 3,000 mL/day.

Emphasize the need to report recurring episodes of DUB (particularly in postmenopausal women) to the health care provider immediately.

Infertility

Ten to fifteen percent of couples are classified as infertile. **Infertility** means inability to get pregnant with unprotected intercourse for at least one year. For approximately 40% to 50% of infertile couples, the cause is female infertility. The man's sperm is the cause 30% to 40% of the time, and for the remaining 10% to 30%, the cause involves both partners or is unknown (Mayo Clinic Staff, 2011).

The main symptom for most women is an abnormal menstrual cycle, either too long or too short. There may be no other signs or symptoms. Abnormal ovulation is the most frequent cause of abnormal menstrual cycles and female infertility. Table 32-1 ■ (Mayo Clinic Staff, 2011) shows more details about infertility.

The nursing responsibility for patients with infertility is primarily health promotion. Nurses teach patients about risk factors for infertility and how they can change their behavior to prevent or decrease those factors. Nurses also assist with diagnostic and treatment procedures, including preparing and reinforcing teaching of patients for these procedures. The psychosocial side of infertility is also important in nursing treatment. Fertility has many meanings including femininity, fulfillment of life goals of the affected couple and their families, responsibility to family to carry on lines of inheritance, religious obligation, and many others depending on the culture and values of the patient. The nurse must be sensitive to these issues and allow patients to express their feelings about the meaning of this struggle for them.

TABLE 32-1 Female Infertility

RISK FACTORS	CAUSES	DIAGNOSTIC TESTS	MEDICAL TREATMENT AND MEDICATIONS	PREVENTION AND TEACHING: NURSING INTERVENTIONS
Age greater than 32. Follicle decline and loss increase. After 35 the risk of miscarriage and chromosomal abnormalities increases. **Smoking** increases risk for miscarriage and ectopic pregnancy. **Weight** Significant overweight or underweight reduces fertility. **Sexually transmitted infections** Chlamydia and gonorrhea can damage fallopian tubes. **Heavy alcohol intake** Increases incidence of abnormal ovulation and endometriosis. **High caffeine intake** Intake of greater than 900 mg (six cups) of coffee per day can decrease fertility.	**Ovulation disorders** Decreased or absent ovulation from abnormal regulation of ovulatory hormones or ovarian abnormalities: ■ Abnormal FSH and LH secretion ■ Polycystic ovary syndrome ■ Luteal phase defect ■ Early ovarian failure **Damage to fallopian tubes from:** ■ Sexually transmitted infections ■ Ectopic pregnancy ■ Damage from previous surgery **Endometriosis** Tissue that normally grows in the uterus implants and grows in other locations. **Cervical stenosis** Malformation or damage to the cervix affecting the opening for sperm or mucus production **Uterine causes** Benign tumors (fibroids) in uterus can prevent implantation although some people with fibroids can conceive. **Unexplained infertility** Sometimes the cause of infertility cannot be found. Couples in this position often eventually conceive.	**Ovulation testing** Blood test for levels of hormones produced after ovulation. **Laparoscopy** Physician views uterus, ovaries, fallopian tubes. Endometriosis and scarring can be removed or repaired. **Hysterosalpingography** X-ray to diagnose flow of fluid between uterus and fallopian tubes. **Ovarian reserve testing** Series of blood and imaging tests for women at risk for decreased supply of eggs. **Hormone testing** Tests specific hormones (e.g., FSH and prolactin) to determine whether medical condition affects fertility.	**Stimulating ovulation with fertility drugs (all increase the incidence of multiple pregnancies)** Fertility drugs, the main treatment for ovulation disorders, regulate or induce ovulation. ■ Clomiphene citrate stimulates pituitary gland to produce FSH and LH to induce ovulation in women with polycystic ovary syndrome or other ovulation disorders. ■ Gonadotropins increase production of FSH and LH from other sources. Human menopausal gonadotropin (HMG) injection contains FSH and LH, which directly stimulate ovaries to ovulate. FSH stimulates ovaries to produce mature egg follicles. HCG is combined with above drugs to stimulate the ovarian follicle to release eggs. ■ Metformin, an oral drug, is used when insulin resistance is the suspected cause of infertility. ■ Aromatase inhibitors (used for some breast cancers) may induce ovulation. **Surgery** ■ Tissue removal for endometriosis or pelvic adhesions ■ Tubal reversal surgery to reconnect fallopian tubes ■ Tubal surgeries to correct anomaly ***In-vitro fertilization*** retrieves mature eggs, fertilizes them with sperm in a dish, and returns them to the uterus 3 to 5 days after fertilization. Requires daily hormone injections. Highest risk of multiple births.	**Maintain normal weight.** (See Risk Factors.) Exercise moderately; strenuous intense exercise of more than 7 hr/week can decrease ovulation. **Quit smoking.** Tobacco has negative effects on fertility as well as on fetal health and the general health of the mother. **Reduce stress.** Couples experiencing the greatest stress have poorer results with infertility treatment. Nurses can encourage new methods for coping with stress and suggest healthy alternatives. **Limit caffeine.** Patients should be drinking significantly less than six cups of coffee per day.

PERIMENOPAUSE

Menopause

Menopause (or the *climacteric*) is the period during which menstruation permanently ceases. It marks the natural biologic end of reproduction. **Perimenopause** includes the 4 or 5 years surrounding menopause, during which estrogen production declines, and the menses permanently cease due to loss of ovarian function. It extends for 1 year after the final menstrual period. At this point, a woman is said to be postmenopausal.

Menopause is a normal physiologic process. However, the hormonal changes that occur can lead to unpleasant side effects. These side effects may vary from simply annoying to disruptive and difficult.

In the United States, menopause occurs usually between ages 45 and 55. *Surgical menopause* occurs when the ovaries are removed in premenopausal women, causing immediate loss of estrogen production and thus menopause. Certain health risks increase after menopause, including heart disease, osteoporosis, and breast cancer.

PHYSIOLOGY AND MANIFESTATIONS

During menopause, the number of ovarian follicles declines significantly, and the follicles that remain are less sensitive to FSH and LH. (Review the ovarian cycle in Chapter 30). As follicles cease to develop, ovarian estrogen production ceases. The ovaries continue to produce androgens, and small amounts of a less active form of estrogen are produced by the adrenal glands. This remaining estrogen is insufficient to maintain the female secondary sexual characteristics. This causes a loss of breast tissue, body hair, and subcutaneous fat. The ovaries and uterus shrink in size. The skin becomes less elastic, and vaginal and perineal tissues atrophy. Vaginal lubrication decreases.

An imbalance between estrogen and FSH from the pituitary gland causes *vasomotor instability*. This instability can lead to night sweats and hot flashes, palpitations, and headaches. The woman may have an increased incidence of vaginitis, as well as **dyspareunia** (pain during sexual intercourse). Menstrual cycles become irregular and eventually stop. Other common manifestations of menopause include possible irritability, anxiety, insomnia, difficulty concentrating, and depression.

COLLABORATIVE CARE

Care related to menopause focuses on managing symptoms, teaching about menopause, and discussing postmenopausal health risks.

Medications

Hormone replacement therapy (HRT) is often used to relieve unpleasant manifestations of menopause and reduce some of the risks associated with estrogen deficiency. It relieves hot flashes and night sweats. It also decreases vaginal dryness and perineal tissue atrophy, which can lead to painful intercourse and urinary incontinence. Long-term benefits of HRT include reduced bone loss, with a lower risk for osteoporosis and resulting fractures, as well as a lower risk for colon cancer.

HRT, however, is not without risk. Nausea, vomiting, weight gain, breast tenderness and engorgement, and vaginal bleeding are common side effects of HRT. Fluid retention may be a problem. Long-term estrogen replacement increases the risk of endometrial cancer and ovarian cancer. A combination of estrogen with progestin reduces the risk of these cancers but may contribute to bloating and irritability. HRT increases the risk of breast cancer and the formation of blood clots with resulting pulmonary emboli. Although initially thought to reduce the risk for coronary heart disease, HRT actually appears to increase this risk. Patients on HRT may also develop gallbladder disease. The decision to use HRT ultimately falls to the patient, in consultation with her care provider. Table 32-2■ provides nursing implications and patient teaching related to HRT.

Women for whom HRT is inappropriate or who choose not to use HRT may take drugs known as selective estrogen receptor modulators (SERMs), such as raloxifene (Evista), to prevent some of the long-term effects of menopause. SERMs act like estrogen in some tissues but not in others and appear to reduce the risk of breast cancer and osteoporosis significantly in menopausal women. They do not prevent the manifestations of menopause, and they do increase the risk of venous thromboembolism.

Complementary Therapies

Several complementary therapies may be used to help relieve perimenopausal symptoms. Black cohosh is used as an estrogen enhancer; chasteberry for hormone balancing; St. John's wort for mood changes; motherwort for palpitations and hot flashes; skullcap for anxiety; and dong quai for an estrogen enhancement. Hypnotherapy, meditation, and homeopathy are also used (Fontaine, 2011). Massage and aromatherapy massage have also been found effective for treatment of perimenopausal symptoms (Darsareh, Taavoni, Joolae, & Haghani, 2012).

NURSING CARE

PRIORITIZING NURSING CARE

Menopause is not a disorder but a normal part of the life and reproductive cycle. The nursing role during menopause focuses on education.

TABLE 32-2	Giving Medications Safely: Hormone Replacement Therapy		
CLASS/DRUGS	**ACTION PURPOSE**	**NURSING IMPLICATIONS**	**PATIENT TEACHING**
■ *Conjugated estrogens/ medroxyprogesterone acetate* (Premarin, Prempro, Premphase) ■ Estradiol/norethindrone acetate (CombiPatch)	These drugs replace lost estrogen to minimize the manifestations of menopause and potentially reduce some of the long-term risks of menopause. Progesterone is added to the estrogen to reduce the risk of endometrial cancer.	Notify physician of contraindications to HRT: pregnancy, breast cancer, undiagnosed vaginal bleeding, thrombophlebitis, or history of stroke. Women currently using any form of HRT should complete current cycle before changing products.	This replaces hormones lost during menopause. Do not use if you think you may be pregnant. You may have spotting or irregular menstrual bleeding while on HRT. Have yearly Pap smear and mammogram. Talk to your doctor every 6 months about continuing HRT; visit annually. Promptly report unusual bleeding, abdominal pain, or other adverse effects to your doctor.

Note: Medications identified in *italics* are among the 200 most frequently prescribed drugs in the United States.

HEALTH PROMOTION

Women who exercise regularly after menopause feel better and enjoy life more. Health behaviors that promote a sense of well-being in perimenopausal women include daily physical activity with a preference for weight-bearing exercise, a healthy diet, social contacts with women who are also perimenopausal, low alcohol intake, and nonsmoking.

ASSESSING

Collect subjective assessment data such as date of the last menstrual period, timing and regularity of the menstrual cycle, and duration and amount of menstrual flow. Ask the patient if there is any risk that she could be pregnant. Inquire about menopausal symptoms such as night sweats, hot flashes, vaginal irritation or discomfort with intercourse, and measures that she has taken to relieve symptoms.

DIAGNOSING, PLANNING, AND IMPLEMENTING
Deficient Knowledge (Menopause)

Expected outcome: Will express ways to cope with effects of menopause.

■ Discuss symptoms the patient is experiencing, and suggest strategies for coping (see Continuity of Care). *Appropriate information helps both understanding and decision making. Many effects of menopause can be managed with lifestyle and other nondrug strategies.*

■ Provide information about the benefits and risks of HRT. *Information helps the patient decide whether HRT is right for her.*

clinicalALERT

Advise women who choose HRT to stop smoking and to consider limiting the number of years of HRT to 5 or less to reduce the short- and long-term risks.

■ Recommend a daily calcium intake of 1,500 mg for patients not on HRT and 1,000 mg for patients on HRT. *Adequate calcium is important to help reduce the risk of osteoporosis associated with menopause.*

■ Emphasize the importance of aerobic and weight-bearing exercise. *Exercise reduces the rate of bone loss, helps maintain optimal weight, and reduces cardiovascular risk. It also enhances mood, possibly by increasing endorphin production.*

Sexual Dysfunction

Expected outcome: Will express concerns about sexual functioning after menopause.

■ Encourage the woman to express feelings and concerns about the effects of menopause on her sex life. *The patient may not be comfortable expressing her feelings until the nurse shows comfort with the topic and encourages her.*

■ Suggest spending more time in foreplay and using water-soluble gels (e.g., Replens) for vaginal lubrication. *These measures can prevent vaginal pain and irritation and improve the quality of the sexual experience for the patient and her partner.*

Risk for Situational Low Self-Esteem

Expected outcome: Will state concerns or fears about changes in lifestyle associated with menopause.

■ Encourage expression of fears and concerns related to changes in interpersonal and family roles. *Some women associate aging with "uselessness" and unattractiveness.*

■ Encourage volunteer activities or employment for the woman who has extra time. *This promotes a sense of usefulness and contribution to society. Activities involving young people can help reduce anxiety about the loss of reproductive ability.*

■ Discuss the importance of a healthy lifestyle in maintaining physical attractiveness. Identify risk factors and high-risk behaviors. *Lifestyle habits and behaviors (e.g., cigarette smoking and sun exposure) contribute to the aging process. Active women who exercise and eat a well-balanced diet look better and feel better.*

BOX 32-3 | **PATIENT TEACHING**

Coping With Symptoms of Menopause

Vaginal Dryness
- Use a water-soluble lubricant for comfort during intercourse.
- Avoid vaginal douches or perineal powders.

Hot Flashes
- Let people know when you are having a hot flash—it is nothing to be ashamed of!
- Use relaxation techniques such as meditation or guided imagery during hot flashes.
- Stay active—activity relieves hot flashes and stress and improves sleep.

- Avoid hot-flash triggers such as alcohol, caffeine, sugar, hot or spicy foods, and very large meals.
- Dress in layers of natural fabrics.
- Splash face and neck with cool water or put something cool on wrists and forehead.
- Lower the thermostat, especially at night.

Irritability or Depression
- Stay involved in work or meaningful volunteer activities.
- Maintain balance—work, exercise, do something you enjoy, and get enough rest every day.

EVALUATING

To evaluate the effectiveness of nursing care and teaching, assess the patient's level of understanding about the perimenopausal period and measures to reduce unpleasant effects. Openly discuss the effects of menopause on sexuality and self-esteem with the patient to evaluate coping.

DOCUMENTING

Document teaching provided and the patient's response to and apparent understanding of information. Note the patient's decision regarding HRT or herbal preparations to deal with the manifestations of perimenopause.

CONTINUITY OF CARE

Emphasize that menopause is a normal physiologic process, not a disease or an illness, and that symptoms are temporary and manageable. Discuss ways of coping with undesirable side effects (Box 32-3■). Explain that making healthy lifestyle changes and reducing risk behaviors may reduce the need for HRT. Health maintenance and self-care are increasingly important: Encourage yearly mammograms, clinical breast examinations, Pap tests, and monthly breast self-examination and self-monitoring for vaginitis. Although eating yogurt that contains cultures of acidophilus bacteria is a commonly used home remedy for preventing vaginitis, the research results are not conclusive. Therefore, the nurse should not recommend this treatment.

DISORDERS OF FEMALE REPRODUCTIVE TISSUE

Disorders of female reproductive tissue include endometriosis, cysts, polyps, and benign tumors known as uterine leiomyomas (fibroids). Malignant tumors of reproductive tissue are discussed in the next section of this chapter.

Endometriosis

Endometriosis is a common condition in which endometrial tissue is found outside the uterus. Endometrial tissue may be found on the ovary and other pelvic organs or tissues and, rarely, in other organs, such as the lungs. Risk factors may include a family history of endometriosis; early menarche; and short, regular menstrual cycles with heavy flow.

PATHOPHYSIOLOGY

The cause of endometriosis is unknown. It may be caused by backflow of menstrual blood carrying endometrial cells through the fallopian tubes into the abdomen. Cells that can develop into endometrium may be implanted during embryonic development, or endometrial cells may spread through the blood or lymph to other sites. Inflammation or immune responses may contribute to endometriosis.

The **ectopic** (abnormally located) endometrial tissue responds to the ovarian cycle, and bleeding occurs during menses. The implants regress during pregnancy and atrophy at menopause. Bleeding of the ectopic tissue may cause cysts, scarring, inflammation, and adhesions. Scarring can lead to infertility and problems such as bowel obstruction.

MANIFESTATIONS

The manifestations of endometriosis occur just before and during the menses. They include dysmenorrhea with backache and cramps, painful defecation, dysuria, dyspareunia, and infertility. These manifestations may vary, depending on the site of ectopic tissue.

COLLABORATIVE CARE

Endometriosis is often diagnosed by the history and physical exam. Firm, tender nodules are found in the pelvic cavity, and the uterus may be retroflexed. A *pelvic ultrasound* may be done, or a laparoscopy is performed to visualize the abnormal endometrial tissue.

Medications

Mild analgesics and NSAIDs are used to relieve pain associated with endometriosis. Hormones such as oral contraceptives, progesterone, or danazol (an androgen hormone) may be given to suppress ovarian function, at least temporarily. Suppressing ovarian function allows the ectopic tissue to shrink.

Surgery

Ectopic lesions may be treated by laser or electrocautery via laparoscopic surgery. When the disease is severe and childbearing is no longer desired, a bilateral **salpingo-oophorectomy** (BSO, removal of both fallopian tubes and ovaries) and hysterectomy may be performed. Nursing care for the patient undergoing a hysterectomy was outlined in Box 32-2.

NURSING CARE

PRIORITIZING NURSING CARE

Helping the patient to deal with the manifestations and potential complications of endometriosis is the nursing care priority.

ASSESSING

When assessing the patient with endometriosis, collect subjective data such as:

- Pain—timing in relation to menses; location, quality, and duration
- Other symptoms such as painful defecation, dysuria, painful intercourse, or other manifestations associated with menses
- Pregnancy history or desire for and attempts to conceive a child
- Effect of the condition on attitudes, roles, and relationships

DIAGNOSING, PLANNING, AND IMPLEMENTING

Pain is often the primary manifestation of endometriosis. Discomfort can be severe, impairing productivity and leading to lost work time.

Acute Pain

Expected outcome: Will rate pain a 3 or less on a 0 to 10 scale throughout hospitalization.

- Evaluate the severity and timing of the pain. *Although the severity of the pain may not directly relate to the severity of the disease, it will help guide the choice of treatment.*

- Discuss using drugs and nonpharmacologic measures for pain relief. *Heat to the abdomen or back, relaxation techniques (e.g., yoga and meditation), exercise, and biofeedback can help the patient manage pain, particularly when used together with analgesics.*
- Suggest trying alternative positions for sexual intercourse. *Different positions may reduce discomfort during intercourse for the patient with endometriosis.*

Anxiety

Expected outcome: Will discuss feelings about fertility.

- Encourage discussion of concerns about infertility. Answer questions honestly. *Knowledge helps the patient gain a sense of control and relieve anxiety and fear.*
- Discuss the advantages of having children soon and in rapid succession and using oral contraceptives between pregnancies to minimize bleeding. *Ectopic endometrial tissue regresses during pregnancy and with oral contraceptives, reducing scarring.*
- Provide information about measures to promote conception, including measuring basal body temperature and other techniques to identify ovulation. *Using measures such as these helps optimize the chance of conception.*

EVALUATING

To evaluate the effectiveness of nursing interventions for the patient with endometriosis, collect information about the patient's ability to manage associated discomfort and cope with the effects of the disorder.

DOCUMENTING

Document care and teaching, as well as the patient's understanding of the disorder and management options.

CONTINUITY OF CARE

Teach the patient and family about endometriosis and treatment options, including their side effects. Discuss the possible benefits of having children earlier in life, rather than delaying parenthood. If the patient has undergone surgery, provide instructions for home care, including managing incisions, preventing infection, and follow-up care.

Ovarian Cysts

A cyst is a fluid-filled sac. Cysts can develop in the vulva, endometrium, or ovaries. This section focuses on ovarian cysts.

PATHOPHYSIOLOGY AND MANIFESTATIONS

Ovarian cysts may be either follicular cysts or corpus luteum cysts. Follicular cysts develop when a mature follicle does not rupture or when the fluid in an immature follicle does not reabsorb after ovulation. Corpus luteum cysts occur when the follicle does rupture, but the resulting corpus luteum remains enlarged after ovulation. Most cysts regress spontaneously within two or three menstrual cycles. They are often asymptomatic, although the pain associated with cyst rupture may be severe enough to be confused with the pain of appendicitis.

Polycystic ovary syndrome (PCOS) is characterized by numerous follicular cysts. It is an endocrine disorder in which LH, estrogen, and androgen hormone levels are higher than normal and FSH levels are low. This hormone imbalance causes irregular menstrual periods, *hirsutism* (excessive hair growth), acne, obesity, and infertility. Women with PCOS often have insulin resistance and may develop type 2 diabetes early in adulthood. PCOS also increases the risk of endometrial cancer, hypertension, and abnormal cholesterol levels.

COLLABORATIVE CARE

Care focuses on identifying and correcting the disorder and preventing its recurrence.

Diagnostic Tests

Diagnostic tests may be used to diagnose and differentiate ovarian cysts from other disorders:

- *LH, FSH,* and *serum testosterone* levels are measured. The FSH–LH ratio is reversed in PCOS, and serum testosterone levels are higher than normal.
- *Glucose tolerance tests* may be done to identify possible type 2 diabetes.
- *Laparoscopy* is done to visualize ovarian cysts.

Medications

Oral contraceptives are often ordered to balance hormones and regulate the menses in women with PCOS. If the patient wishes to become pregnant, clomiphene (Clomid, Serophene) may be prescribed to stimulate ovulation. Other drugs such as progesterone or the corticosteroid dexamethasone can be given to control manifestations of hirsutism.

Surgery

Follicular cysts may be punctured through laser surgery, or a wedge resection of the ovary may be done to restore ovulation. Rarely, **oophorectomy** (removal of the ovary) is performed if the cysts are very large.

NURSING CARE

Unless surgery is performed, the focus of nursing care for patients with ovarian cysts is on education. Provide information about the disorder and prescribed treatment. Discuss the benign and temporary nature of most ovarian cysts other than PCOS. Reinforce teaching about the risks and benefits of treatment options with the patient. Encourage the patient with PCOS to share concerns about potential risks and the effect of the disorder on the ability to conceive. Teach measures to reduce the risk of heart disease (control hypertension, exercise and diet management to control cholesterol levels, avoid smoking, and manage stress) and type 2 diabetes (weight loss, exercise, and diet management). Stress the importance of regular follow-up with a health care provider knowledgeable about PCOS. Teach the manifestations of endometrial cancer, and stress the importance of promptly notifying the health care provider if symptoms develop.

Uterine Fibroid Tumor

Fibroid tumors, or *uterine leiomyomas,* are benign tumors of the uterus or cervix. They are common among all women of childbearing age (Box 32-4■) and are a leading reason for hysterectomy.

Fibroid tumors are classified by their location in the wall of the uterus (Figure 32-2■). *Intramural* tumors are within the uterine wall. *Subserous* fibroids are beneath the outer layer of the uterus, projecting into the peritoneal cavity. *Submucous* fibroid tumors are beneath the endometrial lining of the uterus.

BOX 32-4	FOCUS ON DIVERSITY

Uterine Fibroid Tumors in African American Women
Uterine fibroid tumors are three to nine times more common in African American women than in European American women: 40% to 50% of African American women between ages 30 and 60 develop fibroid tumors, whereas only 20% of European American women in this age group develop them.

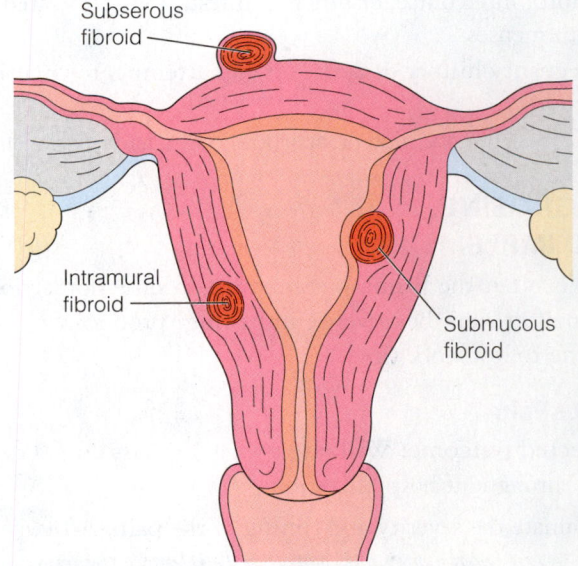

Figure 32-2. ■ Sites of uterine fibroid tumors.

The cause of fibroid tumors is not clear, but they are probably related to estrogen secretion. Small tumors may be asymptomatic. Large fibroids can crowd other organs, causing pelvic pressure, pain, dysmenorrhea, menorrhagia, and fatigue. Depending on tumor location, constipation and urinary urgency and frequency are common. The uterus is enlarged. Excessive bleeding often causes anemia.

In asymptomatic women who wish to bear children, fibroid tumors are monitored. Drugs may be given to reduce tumor size and slow their growth. *Laparoscopic myomectomy,* removal of the tumor without removing the entire uterus, may be performed in young women who wish to have a child. Hysterectomy is performed if tumors are large and in women who are menopausal.

If surgery is deferred, patient teaching emphasizes the importance of regular follow-up appointments to monitor tumor growth. If surgery is chosen, teaching emphasizes pain control techniques and appropriate preoperative and postoperative teaching (see the previous discussion of the patient undergoing a hysterectomy). Dietary modifications to increase iron intake, prevent constipation, and promote healing are important.

INFECTIONS OF THE FEMALE REPRODUCTIVE SYSTEM

Infections affecting the female reproductive tract may be local or systemic. Many are sexually transmitted infections (STIs), which are discussed in Chapter 33. The most common local infections are vaginal, including simple vaginitis, candidiasis, and trichomoniasis. Systemic infections include pelvic inflammatory disease, toxic shock syndrome, and HIV/AIDS.

Vaginitis

Vaginitis, inflammation or infection of the vagina, is common. Vaginal infections are classified by cause and may be fungal (candidiasis), protozoan (trichomoniasis), or bacterial (*Gardnerella*) infections.

Risk factors for vaginitis include unprotected sexual activity, multiple sexual partners, using a broad-spectrum antibiotic, obesity, diabetes, immunosuppression, pregnancy, vaginal changes associated with aging (dryness and tissue atrophy), and poor personal hygiene. Sexual activity and swimming in contaminated water are risk factors for trichomoniasis.

PATHOPHYSIOLOGY AND MANIFESTATIONS

The low pH of vaginal secretions, normal vaginal flora, and estrogen normally protect against vaginal infections. An infection is more likely to develop when any or all of these factors are disrupted. When conditions are favorable, microorganisms invade the vulva and vagina. Simple vaginitis is the most common vaginal infection in women of reproductive age. *Gardnerella vaginalis* is the causative organism in many cases. Candidiasis (moniliasis or yeast infection) is caused by the organism *Candida albicans*. Candida organisms are part of the normal vaginal environment, causing problems only when they multiply rapidly. When decreased estrogen levels, antibiotics, fecal contamination, or other factors alter the normal vaginal flora, *Candida* organisms multiply, causing a yeast infection.

Trichomoniasis, a protozoan infection, is an STI. This organism is frequently carried asymptomatically by the male partner.

Most vaginal infections cause vaginal discharge, itching or burning, and dysuria. The specific manifestations of various vaginal infections are outlined in Table 32-3 ■.

COLLABORATIVE CARE

Vaginitis is common, and self-care is often appropriate. Many topical agents are available over the counter. A woman's first vaginal infection should be diagnosed by a health care provider, who should also teach the patient about which symptoms may be treated with over-the-counter antifungal drugs and which symptoms require a provider's prescription.

clinicalALERT

Patients with persistent or recurrent episodes of vaginitis should be carefully evaluated. Repeated vaginal yeast infections may be a manifestation of decreased immune function, such as in diabetes or HIV infection.

Diagnostic Tests

- Vaginal secretions are cultured and examined microscopically for the presence of "clue cells," a sign of bacterial vaginitis.
- *Wet mount* or *wet prep* with potassium hydroxide reveals a fishy odor in bacterial vaginitis. The slide is examined microscopically to detect *hyphae* (filaments or threads) and *Candida* spores.
- *Normal saline wet prep* is used to detect the presence of protozoa if trichomoniasis is suspected.
- *Glucose tolerance tests* or *HIV screening* may be done at the time of the initial assessment.
- *Pregnancy tests* may be done because certain treatments are contraindicated during pregnancy.

TABLE 32-3	**Vaginal Infections**			
INFECTION	**TYPE OF DISCHARGE**	**OTHER MANIFESTATIONS**	**TREATMENT**	**NURSING CARE**
Candidiasis (*Monilia*, yeast infection)	Thick white patches adhering to cervix and vaginal wall, resembling cottage cheese; little odor	Itching of vulva and vaginal area, redness, painful intercourse	Butoconazole, miconazole, clotrimazole, or terconazole creams, vaginal tablets, or suppositories	Teach perineal hygiene and use of vaginal applicators. Instruct to complete entire treatment.
Simple vaginitis (bacterial vaginosis, *Gardnerella* vaginosis)	Thin, white, "milklike," or gray with fishy odor, especially when mixed with potassium hydroxide	None to mild itching or burning in vulvar area; clue cells on microscopic examination	Oral metronidazole or metronidazole gel; clindamycin cream or oral clindamycin	Teach perineal hygiene. Instruct to complete treatment. Discuss relationship to pelvic inflammatory disease.
Trichomoniasis	Frothy, yellow or white, foul odor	Burning and itching of vulva	Oral metronidazole for patient and sexual partner	Teach perineal hygiene; avoid unprotected intercourse until treatment is completed.
Atrophic vaginitis (senile vaginitis)	Thin, opaque discharge, may be blood tinged, odorless; pale, smooth, thin, dry vaginal walls	Painful intercourse, itching, vaginal dryness	Topical estrogen cream; water-soluble lubricant for intercourse	Discuss symptoms of menopause and sexual techniques to minimize trauma.

Medications

Drugs used to treat vaginitis vary with the organism, as shown in Table 32-3. In many cases, the patient's sexual partner must also be treated to prevent reinfection. Mild vinegar douches may be ordered but should not be used routinely. Frequent douching washes away normal flora, affecting the natural defense mechanism against bacterial invasion. Vaginal sprays are not advisable at any time.

NURSING CARE

PRIORITIZING NURSING CARE

Nursing care focuses on teaching the patient and, if necessary, her sexual partner to comply with the treatment regimen, use safer sex practices, and prevent future transmission of the infection.

HEALTH PROMOTION

To prevent vaginitis, teach all women about personal hygiene and safer sex practices. Teach women to avoid douching, wearing nylon underwear (should wear underwear made of natural materials such as cotton), and wearing tight pants that encourage a moist perineal environment. Unprotected sexual activity, particularly with multiple partners, greatly increases the risk of vaginal infections and STIs.

Many postmenopausal women experience atrophic vaginitis due to the thinning and drying of the vaginal mucosa that result from lack of estrogen. Teach these patients about using water-soluble lubricants for intercourse and topical estrogen creams (which require a prescription) to minimize the undesirable vaginal effects of menopause.

ASSESSING

Collect subjective assessment data from the patient with complaints of vaginal discharge or itching. Subjective data includes the onset, duration, and severity of the symptoms, as well as any associated manifestations (e.g., dysuria, frequency, and urgency, or abdominal pain) and circumstances (e.g., antibiotic therapy). Ask patient to describe the amount, color, odor, and consistency of vaginal discharge. Inquire about perineal care (use of bubble baths, perineal powders or sprays, and douching) and usual dressing habits (underwear of synthetic materials and tight jeans or pants). Ask if the patient could be pregnant and about menstrual history. Inquire about any chronic diseases such as diabetes or HIV infection and current medications. Finally, ask what self-care measures she has used to treat her symptoms.

DIAGNOSING, PLANNING, AND IMPLEMENTING
Deficient Knowledge (Prevention of Vaginitis)

Expected outcome: Will state appropriate methods for preventing vaginitis.

- Explain how the infection is transmitted. *The infection may be acquired through sexual activity, from inappropriate perineal hygiene measures, or overgrowth of certain organisms that normally reside on perineal and vaginal tissues. A clear understanding of how the infection developed allows the patient to use measures to prevent future infections.*

- If advised, emphasize the need for both the patient and her partner to complete the course of treatment. *Many infections are asymptomatic in one partner. Incomplete treatment allows the infection to recur and reinfect the partner.*
- Teach hygiene measures such as the following:
  - Avoid bubble baths, douches, feminine hygiene sprays, synthetic underwear, and tight pants.
  - Cleanse the perineum from front to back after voiding and defecating.
  - Cleanse genitals before and after sexual intercourse.

These measures help maintain the normal vaginal environment and prevent irritation and contamination of perineal tissues that can increase the risk of infection.

Acute Pain

Expected outcome: Will rate pain as 3 or less on a 0 to 10 pain scale throughout infection.

- Suggest using cool compresses and mild vinegar douches. *Cool compresses relieve itching. Vinegar has a fungicidal and bactericidal effect.*
- Recommend sitz baths to alleviate discomfort. *Sitz baths cleanse the perineal area and wash away irritating discharge.*

EVALUATING

To evaluate the effectiveness of nursing interventions, collect data related to the patient's and her partner's understanding of the treatment and prevention of vaginitis, as well as the patient's level of comfort.

DOCUMENTING

Document subjective and objective assessment data, including the duration and circumstances of the infection, appearance of perineal tissues, and character of any vaginal discharge, including its odor. Also document teaching provided, as well as the patient's understanding of the information and willingness to comply with recommended treatment measures.

Pelvic Inflammatory Disease

Pelvic inflammatory disease (PID) is an infection of the pelvic organs (fallopian tubes, ovaries, uterus, and cervix). It is usually caused by infection with *Neisseria gonorrhoeae* or *Chlamydia trachomatis.* Patients with PID are often infected with more than one organism. PID is a major cause of female infertility.

PID usually affects young, sexually active women who have multiple partners. Other risk factors include use of an intrauterine device (IUD) for birth control. Oral contraceptives and barrier contraceptives such as condoms reduce the risk of PID.

PATHOPHYSIOLOGY

Infectious organisms enter the vagina and travel to the uterus during intercourse or other sexual activity. They can also enter during childbirth, abortion, or reproductive tract surgery. The infection then spreads through the fallopian tubes, leading to inflammation and obstruction due to scar tissue. It settles on the ovary and also may enter the lymphatic system or bloodstream, leading to systemic infection.

MANIFESTATIONS

The manifestations of PID include high fever, vaginal discharge, severe lower abdominal pain, nausea, malaise, and dysuria. Scarring of the fallopian tubes can lead to infertility and an increased risk of ectopic pregnancy. The patient may also experience pain during intercourse and dysmenorrhea.

COLLABORATIVE CARE

The diagnosis of PID is often based on the history and physical examination.

Diagnostic Tests

Endocervical secretions are cultured to identify the infecting organism. The *WBC* is often markedly elevated, a sign of infection. *Ultrasonography* is performed to rule out ectopic pregnancy. *Laparoscopy* may show inflammation, edema, and possible abscess of pelvic structures.

Medications

Treatment is usually started with antibiotics that are effective to treat gonorrhea and chlamydia. If PID is not acute, outpatient antibiotic treatment is prescribed. In acute cases, however, the patient is hospitalized. Analgesics are given, and antibiotics and fluids are administered intravenously. In either case, the woman's sexual partner is treated at the same time.

Surgery

The surgeon may insert a drain into an abscess, if present, and remove any adhesions. If the infection is overwhelming or chronic, a hysterectomy with BSO may be necessary.

NURSING CARE

PRIORITIZING NURSING CARE

Promoting prompt and effective treatment of PID and compliance with the prescribed treatment is the priority for nursing care.

HEALTH PROMOTION

PID is often preventable through the use of safer sex practices. Sex education for adolescents should include personal hygiene when using tampons (not to leave them in too long) and safer sex practices. Early detection of PID can reduce complications, so teaching should include reporting to a health care provider abdominal pain associated with fever and nausea.

ASSESSING

Ask about abdominal pain, including its location, intensity, character, timing, and duration. Inquire about associated symptoms such as nausea, vomiting, and vaginal drainage. Ask if the patient could be pregnant. Inquire about risk factors such as multiple sexual partners, having one sexual partner who has multiple partners, unprotected sexual activity, and recent STIs.

Objective data include vital signs and temperature, shape and contour of the abdomen, bowel sounds, and abdominal tenderness. Note the color, odor, and amount of any vomitus or vaginal drainage.

DIAGNOSING, PLANNING, AND IMPLEMENTING

PID can have severe, even life-threatening complications. Scarring of the fallopian tubes can lead to infertility, ectopic pregnancy or pelvic abscess. Adhesions (bands of scar tissue) within the pelvis can obstruct the bowel.

Risk for Injury

Expected outcome: Will not experience complications of PID.

- Maintain bed rest in semi-Fowler's position. *This promotes drainage and helps localize the infection in the pelvic cavity.*
- Maintain Standard Precautions and meticulous hand washing. Wear gloves when handling perineal pads and linens. Disinfect bedpans and toilet seats. *These measures help prevent spread of the infection to others.*
- Administer antibiotics as ordered, monitoring closely for adverse effects. *Antibiotics used in acute PID are potent agents; some can have life-threatening side effects.*
- Teach to recognize and report potential complications such as ectopic pregnancy, abscess, or bowel obstruction. *Reporting early manifestations of these potential complications reduces the risk of delayed treatment.*

Deficient Knowledge (STI Prevention)

Expected outcome: Will state how to use safer sex practices.

- Explain how infection is spread and how to prevent future infections. *Knowledge of the spread of infections allows control in preventing exposure to future infections.*
- Stress the importance of completing the treatment regimen and of follow-up visits. *Incomplete treatment can lead to chronic infection and bacteria that are resistant to antibiotics. Noncompliance and recurrence are common.*

- Teach perineal care, especially wiping from front to back. *This reduces transmission of fecal organisms to reproductive tissues and reduces the incidence of urinary tract infections.*
- Instruct to avoid using tampons until the infection has completely cleared. Advise changing tampons or pads at least every 4 hours. *Menstrual flow provides a favorable environment for microorganisms to multiply.*
- Discuss safer sex practices and family planning. Instruct to remove diaphragms 6 to 8 hours after use. IUDs are contraindicated. Latex condoms offer the most effective protection against infection. *These measures help prevent recurrence of infection.*
- Teach to report any unusual vaginal discharge or odor to the health care provider. Emphasize the importance of seeking treatment if her partner develops an STI. *Treatment is most effective early in the disease process. STIs such as gonorrhea and chlamydia are often asymptomatic in women.*

EVALUATING

To evaluate the effectiveness of nursing care for the patient with PID, collect data related to manifestations of the disease and its complications, as well as the patient's and her partner's understanding of and willingness to use measures to prevent future infections.

DOCUMENTING

Document continuing assessment data and the patient's response to treatment measures (e.g., reduced fever and abdominal pain). Also document all teaching provided and the patient's and partner's apparent understanding and acceptance of measures to prevent future episodes of PID.

CONTINUITY OF CARE

Emphasize the importance of completing the prescribed treatment and keeping follow-up appointments as directed to ensure eradication of the infection. Discuss safer sex practices and measures to prevent recurrence of PID. Address the manifestations of potential complications of PID.

clinical**ALERT**

Stress the importance of seeking care promptly if manifestations of ectopic pregnancy (intermittent colicky abdominal pain), sharp abdominal or shoulder pain, symptoms of bowel obstruction (severe abdominal pain and distention, nausea and vomiting) develop.

Inform the patient that the patency of the fallopian tubes can be evaluated after several menstrual cycles to allow for complete resolution of the inflammatory process.

Toxic Shock Syndrome

Toxic shock syndrome (TSS) is a rare but acute illness caused by *Staphylococcus aureus* infection. Although it may be related to using tampons during menstruation, TSS has also been associated with the use of vaginal barrier contraceptives such as the sponge, the diaphragm, and the cervical cap. About half of all cases of TSS are related to other factors, such as childbirth, abdominal surgery, septic abortion, burns, and skin lesions.

PATHOPHYSIOLOGY

TSS is caused by virulent strains of *Staphylococcus aureus* that enter the bloodstream through open blood vessels during the menses, the placental site after childbirth, or other open wounds. Once inside the body, the organism produces toxins that cause vasodilation, hemodynamic instability, and shock. TSS can be fatal. The clinical manifestations of TSS are presented in Box 32-5■.

Collaborative Care

The goals of care for a patient with TSS are to identify the source of the infection, eradicate the infection, and restore stability of the cardiovascular and other body systems. The diagnosis is based on the history and physical examination as well as culture of the blood. Wounds and vaginal secretions are cultured for *Staphylococcus aureus*. Treatment includes administering intravenous fluids to restore blood volume and blood pressure. Antibiotics are given to eliminate the infection. Drugs to restore the blood pressure and perfusion of vital organs may also be given.

NURSING CARE

PRIORITIZING NURSING CARE

The focus in caring for patients with TSS in the acute phase is to restore stable vital signs and hemodynamic stability. As the patient recovers, the priority is to provide teaching, both about causes and potential consequences of the infection and about the importance of completing the course of treatment.

HEALTH PROMOTION

Prevention of TSS is the best form of health promotion. Women need to know that tampons should be changed at bedtime, in the morning, and every 4 hours during the day. Barrier contraceptives should always be used and removed according to prescribed instructions. Self-care measures for prevention are in Box 32-6■. Prevention of complications by early diagnosis includes reporting to the health care provider any purulent vaginal discharge.

ASSESSING

Ask about the onset and duration of symptoms. Inquire about use of tampons, diaphragm, or vaginal barrier contraceptive devices. Ask about other risk factors, such as recent surgery or abortion or disruption of the skin by an infection or wound.

Obtain complete head-to-toe physical assessment data, including vital signs.

DIAGNOSING, PLANNING, AND IMPLEMENTING

Patients with TSS may be critically ill, requiring intensive nursing care.

Ineffective Tissue Perfusion

Expected outcome: Will have stable vital signs, within normal limits.

- Administer intravenous fluids and blood expanders as ordered. *Vascular dilation causes blood pooling and impaired organ and tissue perfusion. Increasing intravascular volume improves venous return, cardiac output, and tissue perfusion.*
- Administer oxygen as ordered. Monitor oxygen saturation, reporting levels less than 95% to the charge nurse or physician. *Increasing the oxygen content of blood increases oxygen reaching peripheral tissues.*

BOX 32-5	MANIFESTATIONS OF TOXIC SHOCK SYNDROME

- High fever
- Nausea, vomiting, abdominal pain, diarrhea
- Muscle pain
- Sore throat
- Headache
- Dizziness, low blood pressure
- Diffuse red rash, conjunctivitis
- Peeling skin on palms and soles
- Altered mental status

BOX 32-6	PATIENT TEACHING

Preventing Toxic Shock Syndrome

- Use the lowest absorbency tampon possible to contain menstrual flow.
- Change tampons at least every 4 hours, and use sanitary pads at night.
- Wash hands with soap before inserting a tampon, diaphragm, or vaginal medication.
- Remove diaphragms when recommended after intercourse. Do not use during menses.
- Do not use tampons during the first 12 weeks after childbirth.
- If you have had TSS, avoid using tampons or a diaphragm.

Decreased Cardiac Output

Expected outcome: Will have stable fluid balance status, including normal blood pressure, pulse, and urine output.

In the patient with TSS, low circulating blood volume may decrease cardiac output.

- Monitor vital signs hourly or more often, as indicated. *An increase in pulse and respiratory rates is often the earliest sign of shock. The blood pressure may remain within normal limits, even though tissues are not receiving adequate blood flow.*
- Monitor urine output hourly; notify the physician if urinary output falls below 30 mL per hour. *Urine output falls when the kidneys do not receive adequate blood flow. This indicates compromised perfusion to other tissues as well and an increased risk for renal and other organ system failure.*
- Monitor respiratory status, including rate, depth, and breath sounds. *Rapid fluid administration increases the risk of pulmonary edema, which increases the work of breathing and interferes with gas exchange.*

EVALUATING

To evaluate the effectiveness of nursing care for the patient with TSS, collect data about the patient's vital signs and fluid volume status.

DOCUMENTING

Document continuing assessment data, especially vital signs and urine output, and the patient's response to treatment measures. Note all teaching provided, referrals made for continuing care, and follow-up appointments.

CONTINUITY OF CARE

Teach the patient and family about the causes of TSS and self-care measures to prevent future infection (see Box 32-6).

Emphasize the importance of completing the prescribed course of antibiotics, even after manifestations have subsided. Stress the need to keep follow-up appointments. Advise women who have had TSS to avoid using tampons and vaginal barrier contraceptives. Stress the importance of reporting manifestations of the disorder to primary care provider, because women who have had TSS have a high risk for recurrence.

MALIGNANT TUMORS

Cervical Cancer

Cervical cancer is common. Early detection and intervention have substantially reduced the incidence of invasive cervical cancer and deaths due to cervical cancer.

Most cervical cancers are related to infection of the cervix with human papillomavirus (HPV). See Chapter 33 for information about Gardasil, the vaccine given to prevent HPV infection. The other risk factors for cervical cancer include early sexual experience, multiple sex partners, HIV infection, unprotected sex, smoking, and a poor diet.

PATHOPHYSIOLOGY

Most cervical cancers begin as changes in squamous cells of the cervix. These changes are called *cervical intraepithelial neoplasia (CIN).* Over a number of years, these cells become more abnormal and the number of affected cells increases, developing into carcinoma *in situ.* Carcinoma *in situ* is localized, but if it is not treated, it becomes invasive, spreading into the underlying connective tissue. Cervical cancers spread by direct invasion of surrounding tissues such as the vagina, bladder, and rectum, as well as by metastasizing to the pelvis and other organs.

MANIFESTATIONS

Early cancer causes no symptoms. Invasive cancer produces bleeding and leukorrhea (whitish discharge from the vagina), which increase as the cancer progresses. Other manifestations include pain in the back or thighs, hematuria, bloody stools, anemia, and weight loss.

COLLABORATIVE CARE
Screening

A *Pap smear* is used to screen for cervical cancer. Cells and secretions from the cervix are collected and spread on a glass slide for examination. Infectious or abnormal cell changes can be identified. Abnormal cells may be described as atypical, mild dysplasia, or moderate to severe dysplasia (carcinoma *in situ*). See Box 30-3 and Table 30-1 for nursing responsibilities related to a Pap smear. Abnormal Pap smear results are reported by the type and severity of cellular changes (Table 32-4■).

Diagnostic Tests

- If the initial *Pap smear* shows abnormal cells, it is repeated.
- The *Digene Hybrid Capture II HPV test* may be done to identify the presence of high-risk strains of HPV.
- *Colposcopy* (endocervical curettage) and *biopsy* of the suspicious area may be done if the second Pap smear shows abnormal cells. Box 32-7■ describes nursing implications for cervical biopsy.
- *MRI* or *CT* of the pelvis, abdomen, or bones may be done to evaluate for tumor spread.

TABLE 32-4	Abnormal Pap Smear Result Classifications	
DYSPLASIA	**CERVICAL INTRAEPITHELIAL NEOPLASIA (CIN)**	**BETHESDA SYSTEM**
Benign	Benign	Normal
Benign with inflammation	Benign with inflammation	Normal, atypical squamous cells of undetermined significance (ASC-US)
Mild dysplasia	CIN I	Low-grade squamous intraepithelial lesion (SIL)
Moderate dysplasia	CIN II	High-grade SIL
Severe dysplasia	CIN III	
Carcinoma *in situ*		
Invasive cancer	Invasive cancer	Invasive cancer

BOX 32-7   NURSING CARE CHECKLIST

Cervical Biopsy

Before the Procedure

☑ Explain the procedure. Discomfort is minimal, although cramping may be felt during cervical dilation.

☑ Have patient empty her bladder.

After the Procedure

☑ Cleanse the area, apply a perineal pad, and assist to a comfortable position.

☑ Explain that minor bleeding and vaginal discharge are expected; use perineal pads and avoid tampons for at least 1 week.

☑ Caution to avoid sexual intercourse until discharge has stopped.

☑ Instruct to notify physician of heavy bleeding, pain, foul-smelling discharge, fever, or malaise.

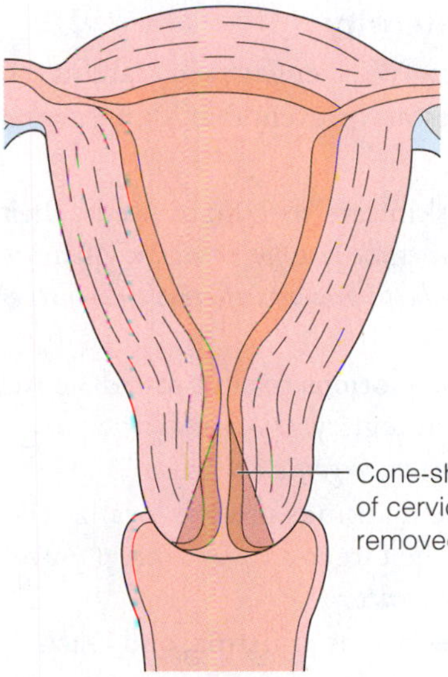

Cone-shaped area of cervical tissue removed and biopsied

Figure 32-3. ■ Conization, removal of a cone-shaped section of the cervix.

Treatment

When the tumor is limited to cervical tissue (not invasive), it may be excised by laser, heated or cooled probes, or cauterization. *Conization,* removal of a cone-shaped wedge of cervical tissue (Figure 32-3■), may be done if the lesion extends into the endocervical canal.

Radioactive implants of needles, tubes, or seeds into the uterine cavity (brachytherapy) are used to treat locally invasive tumors. For invasive lesions, hysterectomy or radical hysterectomy (removal of the uterus, fallopian tubes, lymph nodes, and ovaries) is performed. A *pelvic exenteration*—removal of all pelvic contents, including the bowel, vagina, and bladder—may be done for locally invasive cancer. A colostomy is created for bowel elimination and a urinary diversion for urine elimination. Radiation therapy is also used to treat invasive cervical cancer. External radiation beam therapy may be used before surgery to decrease the size of the tumor. Chemotherapy may be used when surgery or radiation therapy cannot be used or if the cancer has metastasized (see Chapter 12).

NURSING CARE

PRIORITIZING NURSING CARE

Nursing care priorities include helping the patient deal with the physical and psychologic effects of cervical cancer, reinforcing teaching needed to make informed decisions, and minimizing the adverse effects of treatment.

HEALTH PROMOTION

The vaccine Gardasil prevents infection with the four HPV types that cause 70% of all cervical cancers and 90% of genital warts (see Chapter 33 for more information about Gardasil). Safer sex practices, starting sexual intercourse at a later age, and having few sexual partners are also preventative of HPV infection. Regular pelvic exams with Pap smears can diagnose cervical cancer early and prevent further complications.

ASSESSING

Because the patient with cervical cancer rarely has symptoms until the cancer is advanced, nursing assessment focuses on collecting data related to risk factors for cervical cancer. Ask:

- The age at which the patient began having sexual intercourse
- Number of partners
- Use of barrier protection (male or female condoms)
- History of sexually transmitted diseases
- Smoking history

DIAGNOSING, PLANNING, AND IMPLEMENTING

Impaired Tissue Integrity

Expected outcome: Will engage in careful skin care and have no unnecessary/preventable skin breakdown or infection.

- Teach wound and skin care specific to needs. *Open and damaged tissue increases the risk for infection. Meticulous skin and wound care helps prevent infection and further tissue destruction.*
- Apply non–oil-based lotions to skin to reduce itching and help maintain integrity. *Oil-based lotions are not recommended for tissue undergoing radiation.*
- Instruct to preserve markings used to localize the radiation beam to the target area. *Markings are used in future radiation treatments.*
- Observe for manifestations of fistula, and teach the patient to do the same. *Fistulas may form as a complication of radiation to the pelvic or abdominal cavities.*

Fear

Expected outcome: Will express feelings and ask questions about the diagnosis of cervical cancer. She will also identify her psychosocial support group.

- Explain that most women with cervical cancer survive for 5 years or more and that the earlier the cancer is detected, the better the prognosis. *The cure rate for early cervical cancer is 90%. This fact can provide hope, an essential ingredient in recovery.*
- Allow time to express concerns and ask questions. *Unexpressed feelings and fears and lack of understanding may cause the patient to view the situation as worse than it is.*
- Refer to counselor or support group for additional information. *Cancer survivors provide proof that people can survive the diagnosis and treatment of cancer and lead normal, productive lives.*

Disturbed Body Image

Expected outcome: Will state her feelings about surgery for cervical cancer.

- Actively listen and acknowledge concerns about effect of the disease and its treatment on self-concept, attractiveness, and sexuality. *Hysterectomy represents loss of a significant body part, which can significantly change body image. If surgery is extensive, the patient may also need to adjust to the presence of a colostomy and urinary diversion.*
- Encourage the patient and family to share their feelings and concerns with one another. *Family members provide support for each other and can be instrumental in helping the patient adjust to the change in body image and function.*
- Allow the patient and family to grieve for not only lost body image and function but also the potential loss of life. *Cervical cancer presents a threat to overall life span, as well as a threat to reproductive function.*
- Assist the patient and family to identify and use coping mechanisms that have been successful in the past. *Coping mechanisms help the patient and family deal with stressors during diagnosis and treatment of the disease.*
- Help the patient select clothing, wigs, and cosmetics, as appropriate, to project a positive body image. *Appearance to the outside world is a significant contributor to body image.*

EVALUATING

To evaluate the effectiveness of nursing interventions, collect data related to skin integrity and absence of infection. Ask the patient and family members about coping with the diagnosis and treatment and provide additional information and support as needed.

DOCUMENTING

Document all information and teaching provided and the patient's and family's apparent understanding of treatment options. Also document continuing assessments, postoperative care, and the patient's response to other treatments such as radiation therapy.

CONTINUITY OF CARE

Teach all patients and the public how to control risk factors for cervical cancer. Stress the importance of regular pelvic exams and Pap smears throughout the life span. Teach young women about the relationship between early sexual activity, multiple partners, and risk for sexually transmitted diseases and cervical cancer. Discuss safer sex alternatives and using condoms for protection. Emphasize the importance of continued screening exams for the older patient who may not see a gynecologic specialist on a regular basis.

Patient and family teaching vary according to the stage of the cancer and the treatment selected. Provide information concerning radiation, chemotherapy, or surgery, as indicated. Refer the patient to home health services or a cancer support group.

NURSING CARE PLAN
Patient With Cervical Cancer

Anna Eliza Gillam is a 45-year-old divorced woman with four children ranging in age from 16 to 23. She was married at age 18 and had several sexual partners before marriage. She has had three sexual partners since her marriage ended. Her Pap smear 2 weeks ago showed atypical cells. A repeat Pap smear and biopsy of a cervical lesion is positive for squamous cell carcinoma of the cervix.

Assessment

The nursing assessment reveals: BP 130/80; P 72; R 18; T 99.2°F (37.3°C). Weight 142 lb (64.5 kg), approximately 15% over ideal for height. Smokes about one-half pack of cigarettes per day and does not drink alcohol.

Ms. Gillam is very fearful and has told no one about her abnormal Pap smear. She says that she has had back pain radiating down her thighs for several months and a foul vaginal discharge that increases after intercourse. Until 2 weeks ago, she had not had a Pap smear for 5 years.

Laparoscopy shows the disease to be widespread in the pelvic cavity. A CT scan is scheduled.

Nursing Diagnosis

The nursing diagnoses for Ms. Gillam include the following:

- *Decisional Conflict* related to treatment options
- *Acute Pain* related to metastasis and surgery
- *Risk for Impaired Skin Integrity* related to radiation
- *Grieving* related to cancer diagnosis and potential loss of life

Expected Outcomes

The expected outcomes for the plan of care specify that Ms. Gillam will:

- Gain knowledge to make informed decisions about treatment options.
- Develop strategies for pain control.
- Maintain skin and tissue integrity during radiation therapy.
- Develop effective coping strategies for dealing with life-threatening illness and pain.

Planning and Implementation

The following interventions are planned and implemented for Ms. Gillam:

- Explore treatment alternatives, including the prognosis with each option.
- Administer pain medications as ordered.
- Inspect skin surfaces daily before and after radiation therapy.
- Provide information about additional strategies for pain control.

- Refer to a local cancer support group.
- Refer to clinical social worker for discharge and home care planning.
- Assess response to treatment and understanding of her disease.
- Recommend a high-protein, high-carbohydrate diet.

Evaluation

Ms. Gillam has begun radiation therapy after pelvic exenteration. She controls her pain with relaxation and imagery techniques, requiring only occasional analgesics. Her skin is reddened but intact in the area of radiation. Ms. Gillam seems optimistic and has quit smoking. She and her family are continuing to attend the cancer support group meetings.

Critical Thinking in the Nursing Process

1. Develop a teaching outline to use with groups about reducing modifiable risks for cervical cancer.
2. After an abnormal Pap smear, a second smear reveals inflammatory changes consistent with HPV but no cell changes. What advice will you provide to the patient?
3. Explain the terms *noninvasive* and *invasive* in relation to cervical cancer and its methods of treatment.

Note: Discussion of Critical Thinking questions appears on the companion website.

Endometrial Cancer

Endometrial cancer is common. It usually affects women between ages 50 and 70. In addition to age, risk factors for endometrial cancer include early menarche, late menopause, history of infertility, extended use of tamoxifen or estrogen therapy (without progestins), obesity, and diabetes. Endometrial cancer is curable. With early diagnosis and treatment, the 5-year survival rate exceeds 90%.

PATHOPHYSIOLOGY

Most endometrial malignancies are slow to grow and metastasize. These tumors tend to be associated with estrogen excess and begin with endometrial hyperplasia. This type of endometrial cancer occurs more commonly in perimenopausal white women. Endometrial cancers seen in postmenopausal Asian and African American women may be more aggressive and are not associated with known risk factors.

The tumor usually begins in the fundus of the uterus, invades the muscle of the uterus, and spreads throughout the female reproductive tract. Metastasis occurs by the lymphatic system and bloodstream, as well as through the fallopian tubes to the peritoneal cavity. Target areas for metastasis include the lungs, liver, and bone.

MANIFESTATIONS

Abnormal uterine bleeding after menopause is the most common manifestation of endometrial cancer. This bleeding is usually painless but may be moderate to large in amount. Vaginal discharge is another sign of endometrial cancer. On pelvic examination, the uterus is often enlarged.

COLLABORATIVE CARE

The preliminary diagnosis of endometrial cancer is made based on the history and physical examination. An endometrial biopsy or D&C is performed to obtain cells for examination. (Review Box 32-1 for nursing responsibilities related to a D&C.)

Treatment

The treatment of choice for primary endometrial carcinoma is a total abdominal hysterectomy and BSO (removal of the uterus, fallopian tubes, and both ovaries). Pelvic lymph nodes may also be resected during surgery. Radiation therapy may be done before surgery to shrink the tumor or after surgery to eliminate cancer cells in lymph nodes. Progesterone is ordered to treat recurrent disease. Chemotherapy is less effective than other forms of therapy, although it may be used to treat disseminated disease.

NURSING CARE

Nursing care involves helping the patient deal with the physical and psychologic effects of endometrial cancer, make informed decisions, and minimize the adverse effects of therapy. The patient who has had a hysterectomy requires pre- and postoperative nursing care (review Box 32-2). Encourage the patient to perform self-care and resume normal ADLs.

Disturbed Body Image

Expected outcome: Will discuss feelings about having endometrial cancer and feelings about treatments that cause changes in appearance (e.g., hair loss).

- Review the side effects of treatment (hair loss, nausea, vomiting, fatigue, diarrhea, stomatitis, and surgical scarring) and help develop a plan to deal with these effects. *This promotes a sense of control.*
- Provide information about measures to alleviate adverse effects of chemotherapy, such as premedicating with antiemetic drugs, using viscous lidocaine for stomatitis, and obtaining a wig or using hats and scarves to cover the head. *Knowledge helps reduce the sense of helplessness patients often feel in dealing with these effects.*

CONTINUITY OF CARE

Provide information about the disease and proposed specific treatments. To patients receiving radiation therapy, emphasize the importance of keeping appointments. If necessary, help them arrange transportation to and from the facility. Teach appropriate skin care. Explain the expected side effects of radiation implant therapy. Pain control measures are also an essential part of the teaching plan. Emphasize the importance of follow-up care as recommended.

Ovarian Cancer

Ovarian cancer is the most lethal of the gynecologic cancers, because it is often asymptomatic until it becomes advanced, and there is no early diagnostic test. In most cases, the disease has spread beyond the ovaries at the time of diagnosis. Ovarian cancer is more common in European American women than in African American women. However, the mortality rate is higher in African American women.

Risk factors for ovarian cancer include older age, early menarche and late menopause, history of infertility, treatment for infertility with clomiphene (Clomid), and a personal or family history of breast or ovarian cancer.

PATHOPHYSIOLOGY

Because the ovaries contain several different tissue types, there are different types of ovarian cancers. These cancers grow and spread at different rates. The most common type of ovarian cancer is an epithelial tumor. Malignant tumors usually present as solid masses with areas of necrosis and hemorrhage.

Ovarian cancer spreads by shedding cancer cells into the peritoneal cavity and by direct invasion of the bowel and bladder. Tumor cells also spread through the lymph system and blood to lymph nodes and such organs as the liver and the lungs.

MANIFESTATIONS

Early ovarian cancer generally has no symptoms. When manifestations do develop, they are often vague and mild, such as indigestion, urinary frequency, abdominal bloating, and constipation. Pelvic pain sometimes occurs. An enlarged abdomen with ascites (a collection of fluid in the abdomen) is a late manifestation of ovarian cancer.

COLLABORATIVE CARE

Although an enlarged ovary may be palpated on physical examination, diagnostic tests usually are required to detect ovarian cancer. These tests may include:

- *CA125,* a tumor marker, may not be elevated in early ovarian cancer and is not specific for ovarian cancer.
- *Transvaginal ultrasonography* may be done to detect ovarian masses.
- *Laparoscopy* is performed to obtain tissue for biopsy and determine organ involvement.

Surgery is the treatment of choice for ovarian cancer. In most cases, a total hysterectomy with BSO is performed, and other organs and tissues in the abdomen are inspected for spread of the cancer. After surgery, chemotherapy may be used to eliminate cancer cells in other tissues. Paclitaxel (Taxol), a chemotherapy drug, may help achieve and maintain remission. See Chapter 12 for more information about nursing care of the patient receiving chemotherapy.

NURSING CARE

Nursing care for the patient with ovarian cancer is similar to the nursing care for patients with other gynecologic cancers. The side effects of treatment and generally poor prognosis affect the quality of life and have major psychosocial implications. Anticipatory grieving may begin at the time of diagnosis.

Educate women who have significant risk factors for ovarian cancer, such as a positive family history of the disease or previous breast cancer, about the importance of having regular pelvic examinations. Regular screening with transvaginal ultrasound and CA125 measurements may be suggested for this high-risk group. Teach patients not to ignore symptoms such as indigestion, nausea, or urinary frequency, because these may be early manifestations of ovarian tumors. Emphasize, however, that ovarian cancer usually has no symptoms in early stages. Instruct any woman with a palpable abdominal mass to see her primary care provider.

Discuss recommended treatment with women who have ovarian cancer. Suggest ways to minimize or manage side effects. Provide emotional and psychologic support throughout the course of the disease, and refer the patient to hospice services when appropriate.

Cancer of the Vulva

Cancer of the vulva usually affects women between the ages of 60 and 70. In younger women, it is strongly associated with STIs, particularly HPV. Herpes simplex virus type 2 (HSV-2) infection is also a risk factor for vulvar cancer.

The prognosis of vulvar carcinoma is generally good, with an 85% to 90% 5-year survival rate when there is no lymph node involvement.

PATHOPHYSIOLOGY AND MANIFESTATIONS

Cancer of the vulva usually arises in epithelial cells. The primary site is usually the labia majora, but it may also be found on the labia minora, clitoris, vestibule, and other perineal tissues. It spreads by direct extension into surrounding tissues, as well as through the lymph system to regional and pelvic lymph nodes.

Cancer of the vulva often causes no symptoms, and lesions are discovered on routine examination or self-examination. The lesion may appear as a white macular patch, a small raised lump, an ulceration, or a red painless sore.

Persistent pruritus (itching) and irritation of the vulva is the most common symptom. Perineal pain and bleeding occur with advanced disease.

COLLABORATIVE CARE

Visible lesions are carefully examined, excised, and biopsied. Early, noninvasive lesions are excised using laser surgery, cryosurgery, or electrocautery. For more advanced disease, vulvectomy may be performed (Figure 32-4■).

In a simple *vulvectomy*, the vulva, labia majora and minora, clitoris, and prepuce are removed. In a radical vulvectomy, subcutaneous tissue and regional lymph nodes are removed as well. If surgery is contraindicated, lesions may be treated with locally applied chemotherapy or by laser.

NURSING CARE

PRIORITIZING NURSING CARE

Disruption of perineal tissues is a priority nursing problem for patients being treated for cancer of the vulva. Sexuality is also significantly affected and must be considered as a nursing care problem. Body image is also affected; see also the nursing interventions for Disturbed Body Image under the section on cervical cancer.

Impaired Tissue Integrity

Expected outcome: Will not experience infection of perineal tissues.

- Teach the patient and her partner or other family member how to irrigate perineal tissues. *Irrigation helps prevent skin breakdown and infection.*
- After irrigation, apply dry heat using a heat lamp positioned about 18 in. from the area; emphasize safety precautions, including use of a low-wattage bulb (40 to 60 watts). *Dry heat helps promote healing and comfort.*

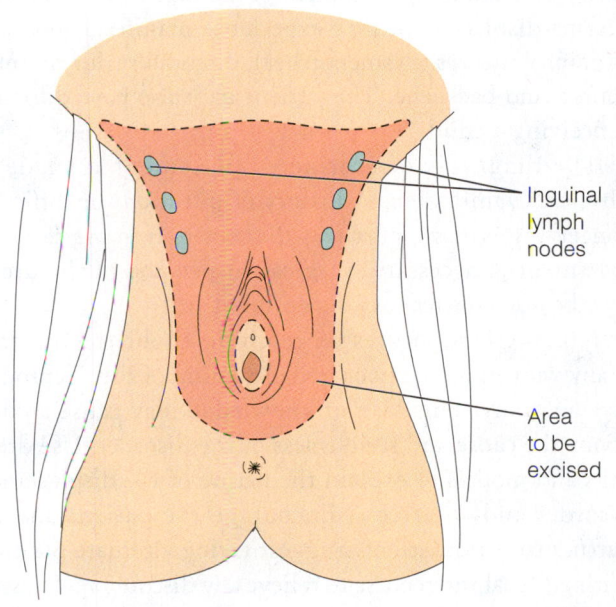

Figure 32-4. ■ Vulvectomy for cancer of the vulva.

- Discuss dietary measures (high protein, iron, and vitamin C) to promote healing. *These nutrients promote collagen formation and wound healing.*

CONTINUITY OF CARE

Because many patients who undergo treatment for cancer of the vulva are older, consider referral to home health services for wound management. Discuss early manifestations of infection or impaired healing, and stress the importance of contacting the physician if these develop. Instruct the patient to cleanse the perineum by pouring warm water over it after voiding and using a sitz bath after defecation. If lymph nodes have been removed, the patient may experience lower extremity edema. Teach the patient to elevate the feet and legs when sitting and wear antiembolic elastic hose or other devices for improving venous return when out of bed.

STRUCTURAL DISORDERS OF THE FEMALE REPRODUCTIVE SYSTEM

Structural disorders of the female reproductive system include displacement of the uterus from its normal position within the pelvis, prolapse of pelvic organs, and vaginal fistulas.

Uterine Displacement

The uterus is not fixed within the pelvis. It is normally positioned with the body and fundus facing anteriorly and the cervix more posterior, but its position may vary among women. An *anteverted* uterus is tilted toward the bladder, whereas a *retroverted* uterus is tilted toward the rectum (Figures 32-5A and B■). Changes in the upper portion of the uterus in relation to the cervix can also occur (Figures 32-5C and D). An *anteflexed* uterus is flexed forward on itself. Backward flexion of the uterus is called *retroflexion.*

Uterine displacement can be congenital or acquired. Childbirth or inflammation and scarring within the pelvic cavity can lead to displacement of the uterus. Patients with uterine displacement may experience manifestations such as painful menses (dysmenorrhea), discomfort during intercourse, and backache. The patient may also have difficulty conceiving a child.

The diagnosis of uterine displacement is made by physical examination. A history of infections or difficulty conceiving will support this diagnosis. In most cases, no treatment is necessary. Surgical suspension of the uterus may be done to treat associated infertility.

Nursing care focuses on teaching about the disorder. Many women have a poor understanding of their reproductive anatomy. This lack of knowledge may cause anxiety about the cause and seriousness of the disorder. Use drawings and models to explain the nature of the displacement disorder and its effects. Encourage the patient and her partner to ask questions. Suggest trying alternate positions during sexual intercourse to relieve any discomfort. Reassure the patient that the ability to have an orgasm is not affected.

Pelvic Organ Prolapse

Relaxation or damage of the pelvic floor muscles puts additional tension on the ligaments and structures that support the bladder, uterus, and rectum within the pelvis. When this occurs, these organs may prolapse or drop down.

PATHOPHYSIOLOGY AND MANIFESTATIONS
Cystocele

A **cystocele** is prolapse of the urinary bladder into the vagina. It develops as the ligaments that support the bladder are stretched. Thinning of the vaginal wall commonly occurs during menopause, increasing the risk of cystocele. Cystocele is often accompanied by a urethrocele or prolapse of the urethra into the vagina. The patient with a cystocele often develops stress incontinence. Other manifestations include urinary frequency and urgency and difficulty emptying the bladder. Frequent bladder infections may develop due to urinary retention.

Rectocele

Rectocele, protrusion of the anterior rectal wall into the vagina, may be caused by trauma during childbirth or chronic constipation with straining to defecate. The patient may have a sense of pelvic pressure and difficulty defecating.

Uterine Prolapse

Prolapse of the uterus into the vagina can vary from mild to complete prolapse outside the body (Figure 32-6■). **Uterine prolapse** is caused by stretching of the ligaments that normally support the uterus within the pelvis. Increased pressure within the abdomen can also lead to uterine prolapse. The patient experiences a heavy or dragging sensation in the groin and lower back that is relieved by lying flat. She may notice a mass protruding from the vagina, especially after bearing down or with heavy lifting. Constipation, urinary incontinence, and painful intercourse are common.

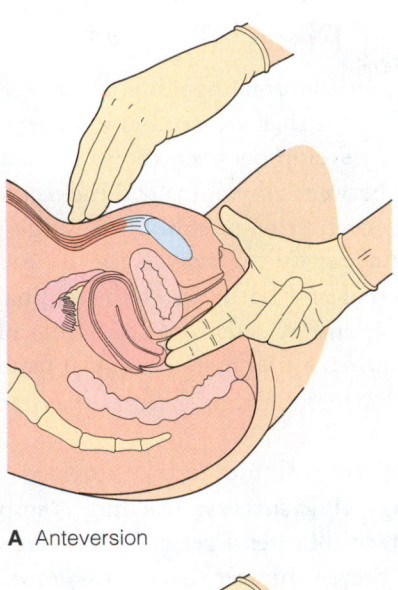

A Anteversion

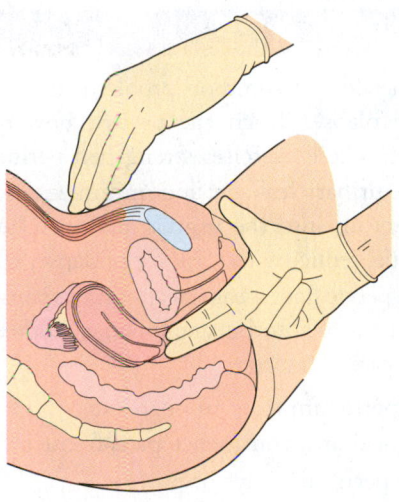

B Retroversion

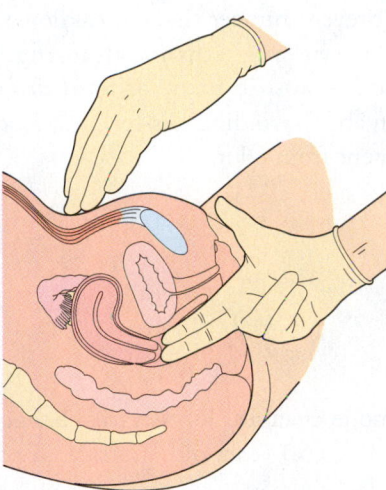

C Anteflexion

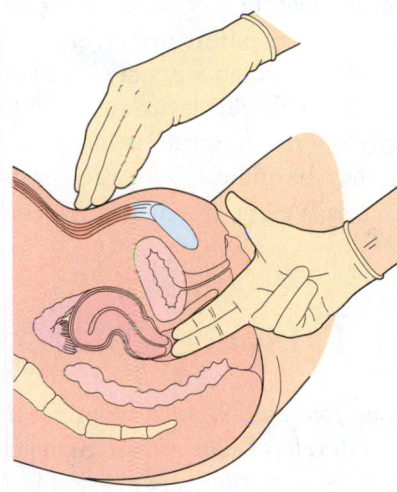

D Retroflexion

Figure 32-5. ■ Common uterine displacements.

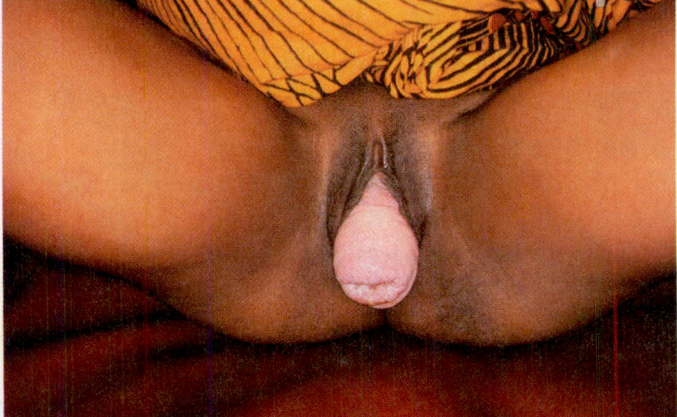

Figure 32-6. ■ Complete uterine prolapse with inversion of the vagina. (Source: Scott Camazine/Science Source.)

COLLABORATIVE CARE

If pelvic organ prolapse is suspected, the patient is asked to bear down or cough during pelvic examination to help identify the problem.

Kegel exercises or physical therapy may be ordered to strengthen weakened pelvic muscles. Pelvic organ prolapse is often treated surgically with procedures to repair the vaginal wall, shorten pelvic muscles, and resuspend pelvic organs. In postmenopausal patients, hysterectomy is the preferred treatment for significant uterine prolapse.

When surgery is contraindicated or refused by the patient, a pessary may be inserted into the vagina to provide temporary support for the uterus or bladder. At regular intervals, the pessary is removed, cleaned, and reinserted.

NURSING CARE

Stress incontinence is a common problem in patients with pelvic organ prolapse. Teach the patient how to perform Kegel exercises. These exercises strengthen perineal muscle tone, minimize urinary leakage, and minimize descent of the bladder and rectum into the vagina. Estrogen helps maintain pelvic tissue, reducing the risk for prolapse, which is the reason that the pelvic floor weakens after menopause. Suggest using perineal pads to absorb urine leakage, and teach appropriate perineal care measures:

- Cleanse the perineum from front to back.
- Change perineal or incontinence pads frequently.
- Avoid using perineal sprays or powders.

Suggest reducing or eliminating caffeine intake and minimizing consumption of diet sodas. Both caffeine and artificial sweeteners can aggravate urinary incontinence.

Teach the patient for whom a pessary is ordered how to insert, remove, and care for the device.

Because obesity is a risk factor for pelvic organ prolapse, diet counseling may be indicated. Suggest self-help diet organizations such as Weight Watchers or TOPS.

Vaginal Fistula

A *fistula* is an abnormal opening or passage between two organs or spaces that are normally separated. A vaginal fistula may develop between the vagina and the urinary bladder or between the vagina and the rectum. The fistula may be a complication of childbirth, surgery, or radiation therapy. Bladder cancer may also lead to vaginal fistula. Urine or stool and flatus enter the vagina through this abnormal opening, causing complaints of involuntary leakage of urine or gas. A small vaginal fistula may resolve without treatment. Larger fistulas may require surgical repair.

Nursing care is similar to that provided for any patient undergoing pelvic surgery. Teaching is important. Stress the importance of careful perineal cleansing to reduce irritation and prevent further tissue breakdown. Suggest perineal irrigation or sitz baths for cleansing. Perineal pads may be used to absorb urine or fecal drainage. Provide information about avoiding gas-forming foods to minimize embarrassment from odor.

BREAST DISORDERS

Breast disorders are common. Women are primarily affected, but men can also develop them. Breast tissue changes in response to hormones, nutrition, and physical and environmental factors. Most women notice increased tenderness and lumpiness before menses. More than half of all women who menstruate regularly find a lump in the breast; 80% of these lumps are not cancerous. When a woman discovers a breast lump, her first response is often fear: of breast cancer, of losing her breast, and perhaps of losing her life. Because American society views the breast as a significant part of feminine beauty, breast problems often threaten a woman's self-image.

Nurses play a critical role in teaching about normal breast tissue, common disorders, and screening and risk factors for breast cancer. It is also important for nurses to teach patients how to examine their breasts for the purpose of recognizing the usual "geography" of their own breast tissue. When women know the size, shape, and symmetry of their breasts, the consistency of the different areas, and the appearance of the skin, they will be empowered to recognize changes that should be brought to the attention of their health care providers.

Fibrocystic Breast Changes

Fibrocystic breast changes are noncancerous changes in breast tissue, causing swelling, pain, tenderness, and lumpiness. They are thought to be caused by an excessive response to cyclic hormone changes. Fibrocystic changes are common in women 30 to 50 years old and rare in postmenopausal women.

PATHOPHYSIOLOGY

Fibrocystic changes are classified as nonproliferative or proliferative changes. *Nonproliferative* fibrocystic changes involve fibrosis of connective tissue, cyst formation, and inflammation (Figure 32-7 ■). These changes do not increase the risk for breast cancer. *Proliferative* fibrocystic changes involve cell growth, with an increase in cell numbers, especially of epithelial gland cells. The risk for cancer is higher in patients with proliferative breast changes. Both forms of fibrocystic changes may be present in the same person.

MANIFESTATIONS

Fibrocystic breast changes cause bilateral or unilateral breast pain or tenderness and a sense of fullness that increases just before menstruation. Lumps may be felt in the breasts, and discharge from the nipple may be noted. Multiple, mobile cysts can form, usually in both breasts. Fluid may be aspirated from these cysts.

COLLABORATIVE CARE

Diagnosis of fibrocystic breast changes is based on the history, physical exam, and mammography. A needle biopsy may be done to rule out malignancy.

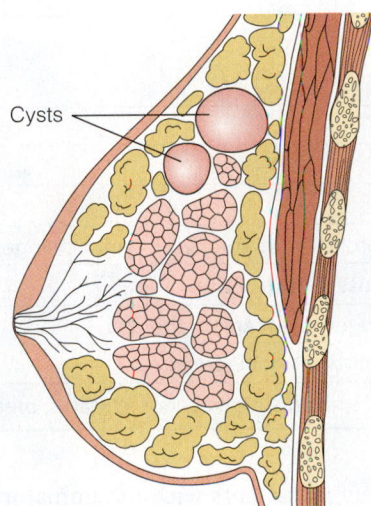
Cysts

Figure 32-7. ■ Fibrocystic breast changes.

Aspiration of a large cyst may relieve pain. A well-fitting supportive brassiere worn day and night helps relieve discomfort. Some women report that avoiding caffeine and chocolate relieves symptoms; both contain methylxanthines, believed to contribute to fibrocystic changes. Women who smoke report a reduction in breast lumps when they quit smoking. Mild analgesics and local heat or cold are also recommended. Vitamin E also may help relieve breast pain.

NURSING CARE

The nursing role for women with fibrocystic breast changes is primarily educational. Provide preoperative teaching and psychologic support before breast biopsy. After the procedure, discuss home care and possible complications that should be reported to the physician. Reinforce teaching about measures to promote comfort. Suggest that although research has not confirmed the role of abstaining from caffeine or taking vitamin E to relieve discomfort, many women find these measures beneficial.

Mastitis

Mastitis is inflammation that causes tenderness, swelling, and redness of the breast. It usually affects lactating women, caused by organisms from the infant's nose and throat.

Mastitis is treated with antibiotics. Increasing fluid intake, wearing a supportive bra, and taking mild analgesics, such as aspirin or ibuprofen, help relieve symptoms. If lactating, the woman should continue to breast-feed from the unaffected breast and express milk from the affected breast.

Nursing care of the woman with mastitis includes teaching about the importance of hand washing, breast and nipple care, and, in lactating women, regular, thorough emptying of the breasts to prevent engorgement.

Disorders Related to Breast Reconstruction

Since 2009, each year an estimated 4 million women undergo breast reconstruction surgery in the United States. Breast reconstruction is usually done after mastectomy or for breast augmentation. Several problems are associated with breast implants:

- Scarring may occur around the implant, causing excessive firmness and distortion of the breast.
- The implant may rupture or leak silicone gel through the capsule, causing local inflammation.
- Although implants do not appear to increase the risk of breast cancer, they make early detection more difficult.

Other disorders, such as connective tissue disease and chronic fatigue syndrome, have been linked with silicone breast implants, although a connection has not been proved. Most current implants are saline filled.

Removing the implant is not recommended unless it has ruptured or the patient has symptoms of an autoimmune disorder. Reinforce teaching for patients who have reconstructive breast surgery after mastectomy for cancer that local cancer recurrence is usually superficial and easily detected by palpation. Recurrent cancer is treated the same for patients with implants as for those without them.

Breast Cancer

Breast cancer is second only to lung cancer as a cause of cancer-related deaths among women. It also strikes men, although rarely. Although the incidence of breast cancer remains stable, mortality rates are decreasing (see Box 32-8 ■).

Breast cancer is not one disease, but many, depending on the affected breast tissue, the effect of estrogen on the tumor, and the age of the person at onset. The two most significant risk factors for breast cancer are female gender and age over 50. Other risk factors for breast cancer are listed in Table 32-5 ■.

BOX 32-8	FOCUS ON DIVERSITY

Breast Cancer in African American Women
The incidence of breast cancer is decreasing, with the largest declines occurring in younger women. Although the incidence of breast cancer is lower in African American women than in Caucasian women, the mortality rate is higher. It is often detected at a later stage, and survival rates for African American women are lower at all stages.

TABLE 32-5	Breast Cancer Risk Factors
Gender	Female
Race	White
Age	Over 50
Family history	Breast cancer in mother or sister
Medical history	Cancer of other breast; endometrial cancer; proliferative fibrocystic breast changes
Menstrual history	Early menarche (before age 12); late menopause (after age 50)
Reproductive history	First birth after age 30; prolonged use of estrogen replacement therapy
Radiation exposure	Multiple chest x-rays or fluoroscopic exams, particularly before age 30
Lifestyle	More than two alcoholic drinks daily; obesity; smoking; high economic status; breast trauma

PATHOPHYSIOLOGY

Breast cancer is unregulated growth of abnormal cells in breast tissue. It begins as a single transformed cell, which then multiplies. Breast cancer is hormone dependent: It does not develop in women without functioning ovaries who have never received estrogen replacement therapy. Most tumors occur in the ductal areas of the breast. Breast cancers are classified as noninvasive (*in situ*) or invasive. Invasiveness refers to penetration of the tumor into surrounding tissue. Two atypical types of breast cancer are inflammatory carcinoma and Paget disease.

Noninvasive (*in Situ*) Carcinoma

In *noninvasive* breast cancer, malignant cells proliferate within the ducts or lobules of the breast without invading surrounding tissue. The nipple and the subareolar region are usually involved. Noninvasive cancers are typically diagnosed when the mass is seen on mammography rather than by a palpable breast mass or nipple discharge. They appear to increase the risk for invasive breast cancer.

Invasive Carcinoma

Most breast cancers are *invasive*, arising from the intermediate ducts of the breast. These tumors can be differentiated by cell type. However, the prognosis and treatment of the disease depend on the stage of the disease (see later section on staging), rather than on cell type. Invasive breast cancers spread to involve surrounding breast tissue, lymph, and blood vessels. The cancer can metastasize to distant sites through the bloodstream or lymphatic system. The common sites of metastasis of breast cancer are regional lymph nodes, bone, brain, lung, liver, and skin.

Inflammatory Carcinoma

Although rare, inflammatory breast cancer is the most malignant form of breast cancer. The patient presents with a diffuse redness, warmth, and edema of the breast. A discrete mass may not be palpable. Metastases develop early and widely in patients with inflammatory carcinoma. The prognosis for this type of breast cancer is poor.

Paget Disease

Paget disease is a rare breast cancer that involves the nipple ducts. Initial symptoms are itching or burning of the nipple with superficial erosion, crusting, or ulceration.

MANIFESTATIONS

Most breast tumors are discovered by the patient as small, hard, and painless lumps or masses. The mass is usually found in the upper outer quadrant of the breast. Nipple discharge is common and is usually milky fluid that may come from more than one duct. The nipple discharge associated with cancer, however, is clear or bloody fluid that leaks spontaneously, without nipple pressure (American Cancer Society, 2012). Other symptoms are listed in Box 32-9■. Skin changes such as dimpling, *peau d'orange* (Figure 32-8■), and engorged vessels on the affected breast may occur.

Patients with bone metastasis may have pathologic fractures, chronic pain, and hypercalcemia. Patients with lung metastasis may have difficulty breathing, and brain metastasis can affect mental processes.

COLLABORATIVE CARE

Treatment of breast cancer begins with detection and diagnosis. The earlier breast cancer is detected, the more likely it is that treatment will be effective in curing the disease or extending survival.

BOX 32-9	MANIFESTATIONS OF BREAST CANCER

- Small, hard, painless lump in breast
- Change in size or shape of breast
- Nipple discharge, especially if fluid leaks spontaneously
- Breast pain
- Dimpling, pulling, or retraction in an area of the breast
- Persistent skin rash near the nipple area
- Flaking or eruption near the nipple
- Unusual lump in the underarm or above the collarbone

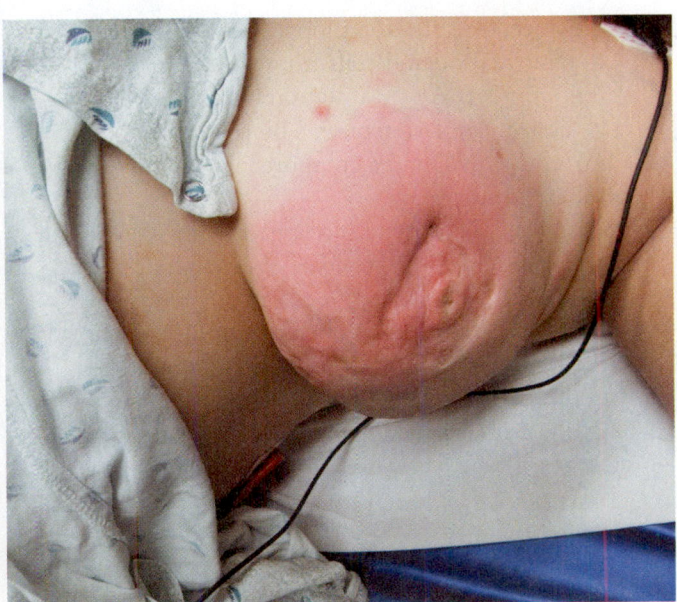

Figure 32-8. ■ This *peau d'orange* breast skin resembles the skin of an orange, for which it is named. (Source: © B. Slaven/Custom Medical Stock Photo.)

Breast Cancer Screening

Key Concept   Annual clinical breast examination and screening mammogram are now the recommended breast cancer screening protocol for women over age 40.

Breast cancer screening includes breast self-exam (BSE), clinical breast examination (CBE), and mammography. These are usually used in combination. BSE seemed very promising as a way to enable early diagnosis of breast cancer when it was introduced. However, research over the years has not shown that it offers benefit as a screening test. There is no difference in breast cancer survival 15 years after diagnosis between women who did routine BSE and those who did not. BSE groups had more false positive exams, leading to twice as many biopsies, many of which were unnecessary. BSE does not offer the accuracy and benefits of other screening tests for breast cancer (Kosters & Gotzsche, 2008).

The American Cancer Society's 2012 recommendations for breast cancer screening are:

- CBE every 3 years as part of a regular health exam by a health care provider.
- CBE every year, starting at age 40.
- Mammogram every year, starting at age 40.
- Women should know how their own breasts look and feel, and report changes to the health care provider.

BREAST SELF-EXAMINATION   All women should be familiar with their own breasts so they can identify changes if they develop. Although monthly BSE is no longer the preferred early detection strategy, nurses still teach women how to examine their own breasts so changes can be recognized and reported to the health care provider. A systematic format is the best approach to BSE (Figure 32-9 ■). Premenopausal women should perform BSE after their menstrual period, because hormonal changes increase breast tenderness and lumpiness before menses.

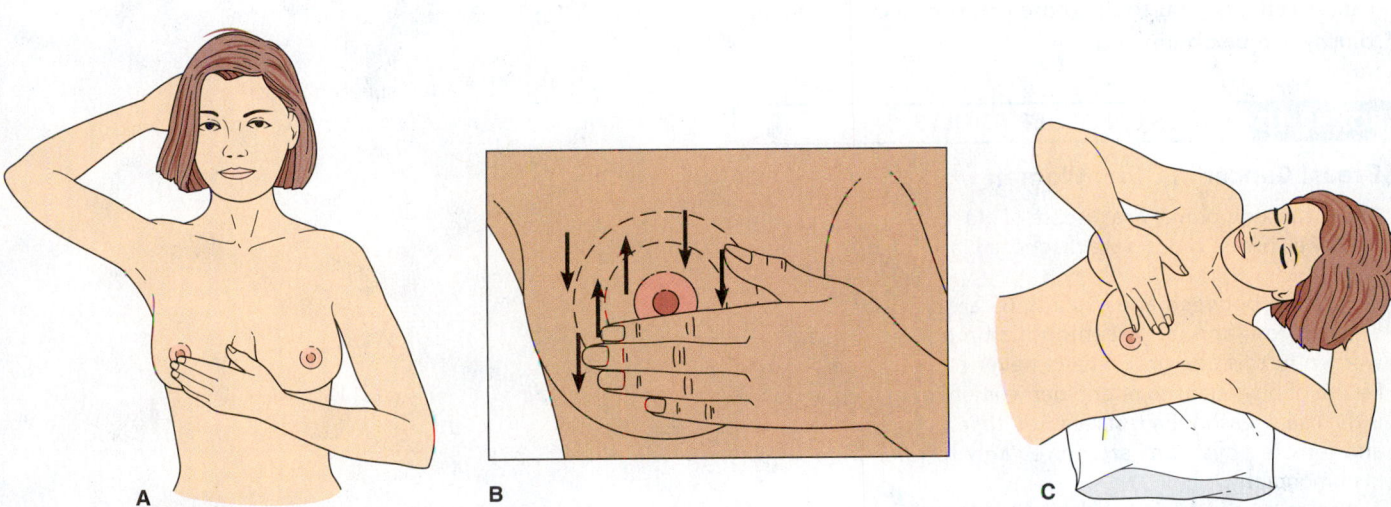

A   B   C

Figure 32-9. ■ Teaching breast self-examination, which is done so the woman has a baseline understanding of her own breast structure and appearance. First, look for dimpling, irregular shape, or discharge with hands relaxed by the sides, then observe again with hands clasped over the head, and then on the hips, with the body leaning forward. (**A**) Hold one hand behind the head and palpate the breast in dime-sized circles, working vertically up and down across the breast, examining the entire area from axilla to breastbone, and from below the breast to the collarbone. Squeeze the nipple between the thumb and forefinger, looking for clear or bloody discharge. (**B**) Pattern for examining the breast and surrounding tissue. (**C**) Palpate the breast again while lying down, with a pillow under the shoulder and back on the side being examined, to flatten the breast tissue.

CLINICAL BREAST EXAMINATION In CBE, a trained health professional inspects and palpates the breasts and axillae and checks for nipple discharge.

SCREENING MAMMOGRAPHY Mammography is a low-dose x-ray of the breast used to detect breast lesions before they can be felt. Although mammography can detect breast tumors 2 years before they are palpable, most of these tumors have been present for 8 to 10 years. Mammography compresses breast tissue. It is uncomfortable to painful, depending on breast size and tenderness and pain tolerance.

Box 32-10■ discusses concerns about screening and treatment for older women.

Diagnostic Tests

■ *Diagnostic mammography* is done to visualize a palpable breast mass or identify a possible tumor in a patient with other symptoms of breast cancer but no palpable mass.

■ *Ultrasonography* is done to localize and distinguish between solid and cystic masses.

■ *CT scans, MRI,* and *positron emission tomography* scans may be done to locate and evaluate possible metastasis of breast cancer.

■ *Cytologic examination* of fluid from nipple discharge may reveal the presence of cancer cells.

■ *Tissue biopsy,* or examination of tissue from the lesion for cancer cells, is vital to diagnose breast cancer. Tissue for biopsy can be obtained in several ways:

a. Fine-needle aspiration biopsy uses a fine needle to remove fluid and cells from the breast lesion (Figure 32-10A■). Aspiration biopsy may be done using a stereotactic biopsy device; mammography and a computer are used to guide the needle.

b. Core-needle biopsy uses a large, hollow-core needle to remove one or more cores of tissue from the breast lesion.

c. Excisional biopsy is an open technique, in which the lesion is surgically removed and the tissue is examined (Figure 32-10B).

Box 32-11■ outlines nursing care for a patient undergoing a breast biopsy.

■ In some centers, a *breast cancer risk profile* may be done to identify women who might benefit from aggressive therapy. This study subjects tumor cells to tests to determine their response to hormones, aggressiveness, and likelihood of recurring.

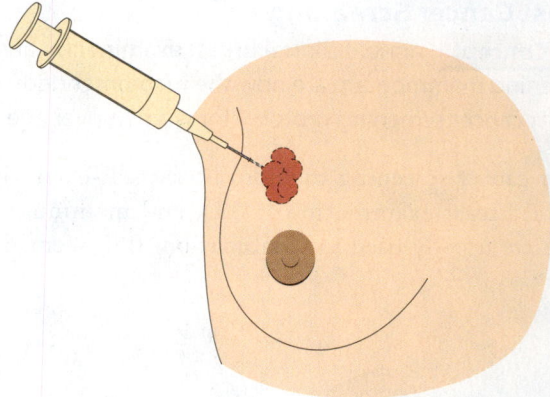

A Aspiration biopsy

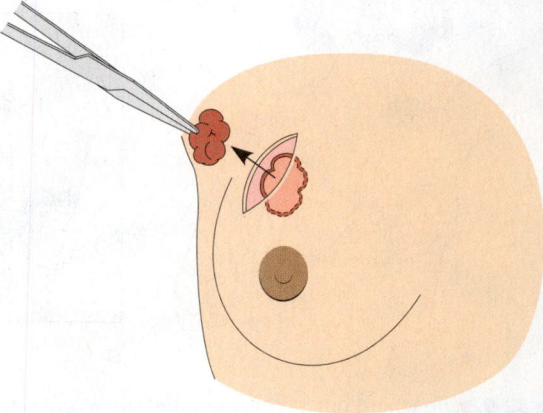

B Excisional biopsy

Figure 32-10. ■ Types of breast biopsy. (**A**) In an aspiration biopsy, a needle is used to aspirate fluid or tissue from the breast. (**B**) In an excisional biopsy, the breast lesion is removed surgically, and its tissue is examined.

BOX 32-10 FOCUS ON OLDER ADULTS

Breast Cancer in Older Women

Breast cancer is primarily a disease of older women: More than 60% of all breast cancers are diagnosed in women age 50 and older.

Women between ages 50 and 65 are the most likely to benefit from annual screening mammography, yet many women in this age group have never had a mammogram. Failure of physicians to refer older women for mammography is the usual reason the tests are not done. Nurse practitioners and female physicians are more likely to refer women for mammography.

Breast-conserving surgery is offered to older women less often than modified radical mastectomy. Yet the preference for type of surgical treatment, particularly for older women, is highly individual. Many older women wish to preserve their breasts. Nurses in their role as patient advocate can discuss the issue with providers and patients and influence whether patient preferences are considered before surgery.

BOX 32-11	NURSING CARE CHECKLIST

Breast Biopsy

Before the Procedure

☑ Provide routine preoperative care as ordered (see Chapter 10).

☑ Provide psychologic support.

Client and Family Teaching

☑ Teach the patient and family the following:
  ☑ The results will be available within a few days.
  ☑ A mild analgesic should be used to relieve discomfort.

Fine-Needle Aspiration Biopsy

☑ Tissue and fluid are withdrawn from the lesion using a fine needle. This procedure takes only a few minutes and may be done in the physician's office.

Core-Needle Biopsy

☑ The patient will lie on a special table with her breast protruding through a hole.

☑ Local anesthesia will be used.

During the Procedure

☑ Tissue from the lesion will be removed with a needle.

Excisional Biopsy

☑ The biopsy is done in ambulatory surgery with local anesthesia.

☑ The entire lesion and a small amount of surrounding tissue are removed.

☑ A nurse will explain what is happening, answer questions, and offer support during the biopsy.

☑ It is important to tell the doctor if pain occurs during the procedure.

☑ The incision is closed with sutures or tape and covered with a small dressing.

After the Procedure

☑ After the Procedure To relieve discomfort and bruising after the procedure, a well-fitting bra should be worn and ice packs may be applied.

Staging of Breast Cancer

Staging (classifying the tumor by size, lymph involvement, and metastasis) provides important information for deciding on treatment options. The choice of treatment also depends on age and the woman's preferences. Breast cancer tends to be more aggressive in premenopausal women (probably because of hormonal factors), requiring more aggressive treatment.

Medications

Systemic therapy (tamoxifen, chemotherapy, or biologic therapy) is used to prevent breast cancer or delay the recurrence of cancer in all patient groups.

Tamoxifen (Nolvadex) interferes with estrogen activity. It is used to treat existing breast cancer and reduce the risk for developing breast cancer in women who are at high risk (see Table 32-6■).

clinicalALERT

Although tamoxifen reduces the risk for developing breast cancer, it increases the risk of endometrial cancer, deep venous thrombosis, and pulmonary embolism. Teach women taking tamoxifen the early warning signs of endometrial cancer. Stress the importance of yearly pelvic examinations. Emphasize the need to stop smoking.

When tamoxifen is ineffective or poorly tolerated, other hormone therapies may be used. In premenopausal women, the ovaries may be removed to reduce estrogen levels. Drugs such as diethylstilbestrol (DES), megestrol acetate (Megace), or aminoglutethimide (Cytadren) may be prescribed. However, these drugs have more side effects than tamoxifen.

Chemotherapy is commonly used to treat breast cancer when lymph nodes in the axilla are involved. It is also used

TABLE 32-6	Giving Medications Safely: Tamoxifen		
CLASS/DRUGS	**PURPOSE**	**NURSING IMPLICATIONS**	**PATIENT TEACHING**
Estrogen blocker/antineoplastic agent			
■ Tamoxifen (Nolvadex)	Tamoxifen inhibits tumor growth by blocking estrogen receptor sites of cancer cells. It is used to reduce the risk of breast cancer in high-risk women, to prevent cancer recurrence after treatment, and as adjunctive therapy for advanced breast cancer. Tamoxifen increases the risk for endometrial cancer, deep venous thrombosis, and pulmonary embolism.	Assess for increased bone or tumor pain; provide analgesics as ordered. Monitor CBC, serum electrolytes, liver function tests, and thyroid hormone levels during treatment. Report abnormal results to the charge nurse or physician.	Use a diaphragm, condom, or other barrier contraception while taking this drug and for 1 month after. Promptly report bone pain, weight gain, swelling, shortness of breath, nausea or vomiting, changes in mental status, headache, blurred vision, menstrual irregularities, or vaginal bleeding. This drug may cause hot flashes. Do not smoke while you are taking this drug.

to prolong life in late metastatic disease. (See Chapter 12 for more information about chemotherapy and its nursing implications.)

Radiation Therapy

Radiation therapy is typically used after breast cancer surgery to destroy any remaining cancer cells that could cause recurrence or metastasis. It is usually used in combination with lumpectomy for early-stage breast cancer. If a tumor is unusually large, radiation can shrink the tumor before surgery. Palliative radiation therapy is also used to treat chest wall recurrences and help control pain and prevent fractures with bone metastases. Radiation is delivered by external beam or tissue implants.

Surgery

When breast cancer has not metastasized, the treatment of choice is surgery to remove the primary tumor combined with radiation therapy to reduce the risk of tumor recurrence or spread.

BREAST-CONSERVING SURGERY   Breast-conserving surgery involves removing the tumor and a disease-free margin surrounding the tumor (Figure 32-11A■). Lymph nodes under the arm (axillary nodes) are removed as well. Surgery is followed by whole-breast radiation to destroy remaining cancer cells. This treatment is as effective as total mastectomy in treating breast cancer.

MASTECTOMY   **Mastectomy** (removal of the breast) is often done to treat breast cancer. *Radical mastectomy* is removal of the entire affected breast, underlying chest muscles, and lymph nodes under the arms. *Modified radical mastectomy*

is removal of the breast tissue and lymph nodes under the arm, leaving the chest wall muscles intact (Figure 32-11B). Box 32-12■ outlines nursing care and teaching for the patient undergoing a mastectomy.

Axillary node dissection usually accompanies breast cancer surgeries. Dissection may be limited to a single node to check for cancer cells or may involve removal of all axillary lymph nodes. This surgery can lead to long-term complications, such as lymphedema, nerve damage, and adhesions. Exercises to promote optimal use of the affected arm are discussed in the Continuity of Care section that follows.

BREAST RECONSTRUCTION SURGERY   Breast reconstruction is common after mastectomy. It may be done at the time of surgery or at a later date, depending on factors such as physical condition, need for additional therapy, and preference. An implant may be used under the muscle if sufficient tissue to cover the implant is available (Figure 32-12A■). After radical surgery, muscle from the back or abdomen may be transplanted and used with or without an implant to reconstruct the breast (Figure 32-12B). A new nipple may be created by using tissue from the opposite nipple or other sites.

Metastatic Breast Cancer Treatment

If breast cancer has metastasized to other sites, the focus of treatment is palliation (symptom relief), extending life, and ensuring the comfort of the patient. Therapies such as radiation therapy, hormone therapy, chemotherapy, or surgery may be used for palliative treatment, depending on the sites of metastases. Quality of life may take precedence over quantity of life.

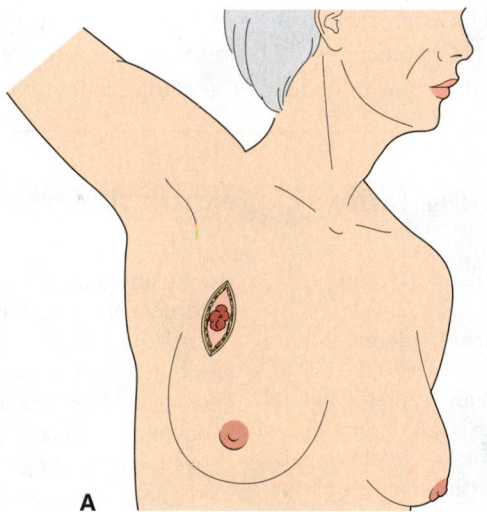
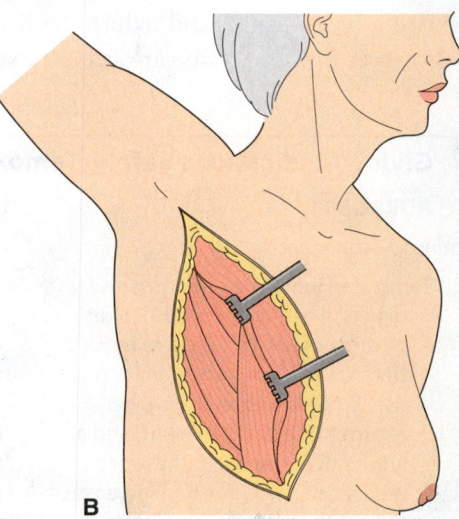

A   **B**

Figure 32-11. ■ Surgery for breast cancer. (**A**) In a lumpectomy, the tumor and a small margin of surrounding tissue are removed. (**B**) In a modified radical mastectomy, the entire breast and axillary lymph nodes are removed.

BOX 32-12   NURSING CARE CHECKLIST

Mastectomy

Before Surgery

- ☑ Provide routine preoperative care as outlined in Chapter 10.
- ☑ Reinforce teaching as needed.
- ☑ Allow access to support persons (significant others, religious or spiritual, or counselors).
- ☑ Offer emotional support.

After Surgery

- ☑ Provide routine postoperative care as outlined in Chapter 10.
- ☑ Reinforce teaching about postoperative care and exercises (discharge may occur within hours or the day after surgery).

Patient and Family Teaching

- ☑ Empty the drain and replace the dressing daily.
- ☑ Return for drain removal in 2 to 4 days or as ordered.

- ☑ Take the prescribed analgesic before pain becomes severe and before performing exercises.
- ☑ Report excessive bleeding to your doctor.
- ☑ Numbness and tingling in the axillary area are common.
- ☑ Begin arm and shoulder exercises to restore full mobility as recommended by your doctor.
- ☑ You may drive within 7 to 10 days and return to work within 4 to 6 weeks.
- ☑ Do not lift heavy objects with the arm on the operated side.
- ☑ Protect the affected arm from injury and infection: Wear rubber gloves when washing dishes, wear garden gloves when working outside, and avoid having blood pressures taken or blood drawn on the operative side.

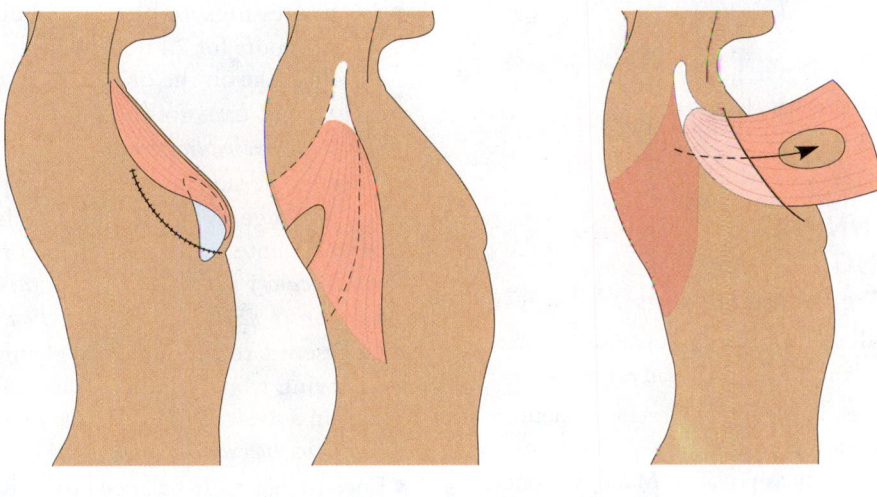

A Implant   **B** Latissimus dorsi myocutaneous flap

Figure 32-12. ■ Breast reconstruction surgeries. (**A**) An implant is inserted under the pectoris muscle. (**B**) A latissimus dorsi flap is used to reconstruct the breast.

NURSING CARE

PRIORITIZING NURSING CARE

Nursing care priorities for the patient with breast cancer focus on supporting the patient's decision making and grieving processes, as well as promoting rehabilitation after treatment.

ASSESSING

Obtain subjective information from all women about their risk factors for breast cancer, such as a history of the disease in a close female relative (mother, grandmother, sibling), early menarche or late menopause, and childbearing. Ask about their history and knowledge of recommendations for CBE and mammogram. Ask about breast pain, nipple discharge, change in breast size, or a change in the appearance or skin of the breast.

With the patient disrobed to the waist, inspect the breasts and nipples for size, symmetry, contour, skin color and texture, venous patterns, and lesions. With the patient supine and the arm behind the head, palpate each breast. Be sure to include the nipple and the axillary tail of breast tissue. Figure 32-9B shows one possible pattern for breast palpation. Note any palpable masses by location, size, shape, consistency, tenderness, mobility, and borders (sharp or poorly defined). Palpate each axilla for enlarged lymph nodes (Figure 32-13■).

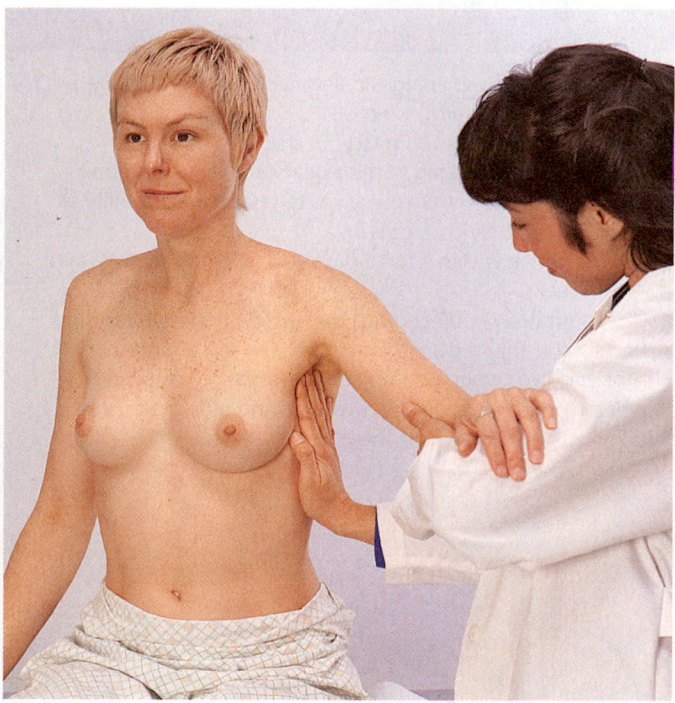

Figure 32-13. ■ Palpating the axillary lymph nodes.
(Source: Richard Tauber, Pearson Education.)

DIAGNOSING, PLANNING, AND IMPLEMENTING
Decisional Conflict (Treatment Options)

Expected outcome: Will state treatment options for breast cancer, including their advantages and disadvantages.

■ Discuss the disease process and reinforce teaching about treatment options. Provide an opportunity for questions. Answer as simply and directly as possible. Make eye contact with the patient and pay attention to body language. *Providing factual information and an opportunity to ask questions helps the patient make an informed decision during a highly stressful time. High stress inhibits the patient's ability to remember teaching, so reinforcement of teaching by the nurse is valuable.*

■ Focus on immediate concerns, and provide up-to-date written material for review. *Stress and anxiety interfere with the ability to process information. Written materials can be reviewed later.*

■ Listen in a nonjudgmental manner during the decision-making process. *Nonjudgmental, empathic listening helps the patient process information and make informed decisions.*

■ Provide opportunities to meet with other women who have had breast cancer surgery. *Breast cancer survivors can often answer questions the patient is unable or unwilling to ask of care providers. They can also be a resource after surgery.*

Grieving

Expected outcome: Will discuss feelings and concerns about having breast cancer.

■ Listen attentively to expressions of loss and observe for nonverbal cues (failure to make eye contact, crying, silence). *Breast surgery, even lumpectomy, alters the appearance of the breast and may also bring fears related to death. This loss is expressed through grief. Not all women grieve openly. Attending to nonverbal cues helps open discussion of feelings of loss and grieving.*

■ Spend time with the patient. Do not rush interactions. *Taking time to be with the patient communicates caring.*

■ Explain that periods of depression, anger, and denial after breast surgery are normal. *They are expected responses to loss and grieving.*

■ Enlist support from significant others to help the woman cope with her grief. *The patient's family and friends can provide support during the grieving process.*

Risk for Infection

Expected outcome: Will not experience infection in surgical area.

■ Assess dressings for bleeding, drainage, color, and odor every 4 hours for 24 hours. Circle any visible bleeding and drainage on the dressing as a baseline for subsequent assessment. *Excessive bleeding or drainage may indicate a postoperative complication that requires intervention.*

■ Observe incision and IV sites for pain, redness, swelling, and drainage. Assess the wound drainage system for patency; note the color and amount of drainage. *A local inflammatory response or wound drainage that is cloudy or malodorous may indicate an infection.*

■ Use aseptic technique when changing dressings, emptying wound drainage, and caring for intravenous tubing and sites. *Aseptic technique minimizes the risk of contamination with pathogens.*

■ Encourage a well-balanced diet. Refer to a dietitian as indicated. *Adequate nutrition promotes healing and immune function.*

■ Teach how to care for the incision and drainage system (cleansing, securing, and emptying). *The patient is often discharged before the drainage system is removed and needs teaching to provide self-care.*

■ Instruct to report fever, redness or hardness at the surgical site, or purulent drainage to the surgeon. *Early identification and treatment of infection can prevent more serious or long-term consequences.*

■ Instruct to avoid deodorants and talcum powder on the affected side until the incision is completely healed. *These substances may irritate the skin and impede healing.*

■ Discuss skin care during radiation therapy to reduce the risk of infection. *Radiation can cause dryness, itching, rash, or scaling of skin, increasing the risk of infection.*

Risk for Injury

Expected outcome: Will be free from lymphedema on the operative side.

Removing axillary lymph nodes increases the risk for problems such as lymphedema and infection.

- Use the arm on the nonsurgical side for taking blood pressures and blood samples. *Compression of the arm on the surgical side may cause lymphedema.*
- Elevate the affected arm on a pillow. *Elevating the arm permits drainage, prevents swelling, and promotes circulation.*
- Encourage range-of-motion (ROM) exercises of the affected arm. *Exercise helps develop new drainage channels.*
- Teach protective measures: Avoid constricting sleeves, avoid lifting heavy objects, use a heavy oven mitt or pot-holder when cooking, and promptly apply antibiotic ointment to any cut or burn. Wear gloves when working in the yard or garden to prevent skin injury. *These measures help prevent infection and lymphedema.*

Risk for Disturbed Body Image

Expected outcome: Will look at surgical site and discuss feelings about having mastectomy.

- Encourage verbalization of feelings. *Breast surgery can change body image. Talking about feelings of loss and change helps the patient cope with the changes her body is experiencing due to surgery and treatment.*
- Explain that redness and swelling will fade with time. *Surgical changes may be compounded by side effects of chemotherapy or hormone therapy. Knowing that the scar will fade may help develop a more realistic view of the changes.*
- Include the partner (as desired) in discussions about physical changes caused by surgery and treatment. *The patient may fear her partner's response to surgery. Open discussions facilitate adaptation of both partners to the changes.*
- Provide resources (pamphlets, books, referral to counselors or support groups) as appropriate. *Information and resources can assist with coping and adaptation to the changed body image.*
- Encourage the patient to look at the incision when she feels ready. *Often, the reality is not as frightening as was imagined.*
- Reassure her that the decision about a prosthesis or reconstruction can be made at a later time. *Physical and emotional healing help the patient make a better decision for long-term body image.*
- If the patient is interested, provide written material about breast reconstruction and encourage meeting with a plastic surgeon and with women who have had reconstruction. *These steps allow the patient to make a fully informed decision about available options.*

EVALUATING

To determine the effectiveness of nursing interventions, collect data such as the following:

- Make an informed choice of treatment options based on extent of disease and personal preferences.
- Express feelings of anger or sorrow related to potential consequences of breast cancer.
- Look at and touch incision; care for incision and drainage system.
- Remain free of infection or injury.

DOCUMENTING

Document teaching and discussions about treatment options. After surgery and during radiation or chemotherapy, document continuing assessment data, including healing, skin condition, adverse effects, and the patient's and family's emotional and psychologic responses to treatment. Note all teaching provided and the patient's understanding and acceptance of information presented.

CONTINUITY OF CARE

Limited postoperative exercises are started within 24 hours after surgery, beginning with ROM of the elbow, wrist, and hand. Encourage performance of ADLs, such as eating, combing her hair, and washing her face. If wound drains are present, tell to avoid abducting the arm or raising the elbow above shoulder height until drains are removed.

When wound healing is complete, abduction and external rotation of the upper arm may begin. Activities that require complete ROM include vacuuming and dusting. Forward and lateral elevation of the arms also increases function. Postmastectomy exercises such as "wall climbing," overhead pulley, rope turning, and arm swings (Figure 32-14■) should be discussed with the physical therapist.

Advise that adequate rest and emotional support are important to promote healing and recovery. Both radiation and chemotherapy can cause fatigue and other symptoms. Use measures (outlined in Chapter 12) to manage these symptoms.

Encourage participation in a breast cancer support group to share thoughts, feelings, experiences, and information about treatments, side effects, insurance problems, and other practical aspects of living with breast cancer. Discuss using online information services and discussion groups for additional information and support.

Discuss manifestations of breast cancer recurrence, either as a second primary tumor or as metastasis from the original site. Advise patient to report signs and symptoms promptly (new breast lumps, a persistent cough or shortness of breath, jaundice or pain in the upper right quadrant of the abdomen, bone pain, or lumps around the collarbone or under the arm).

Advise a wholesome, balanced diet for healing and to deal with the effects of treatment, particularly chemotherapy. Maintaining body weight during chemotherapy can be difficult because of nausea and vomiting. Discuss potential solutions such as eating cold foods, which may be better

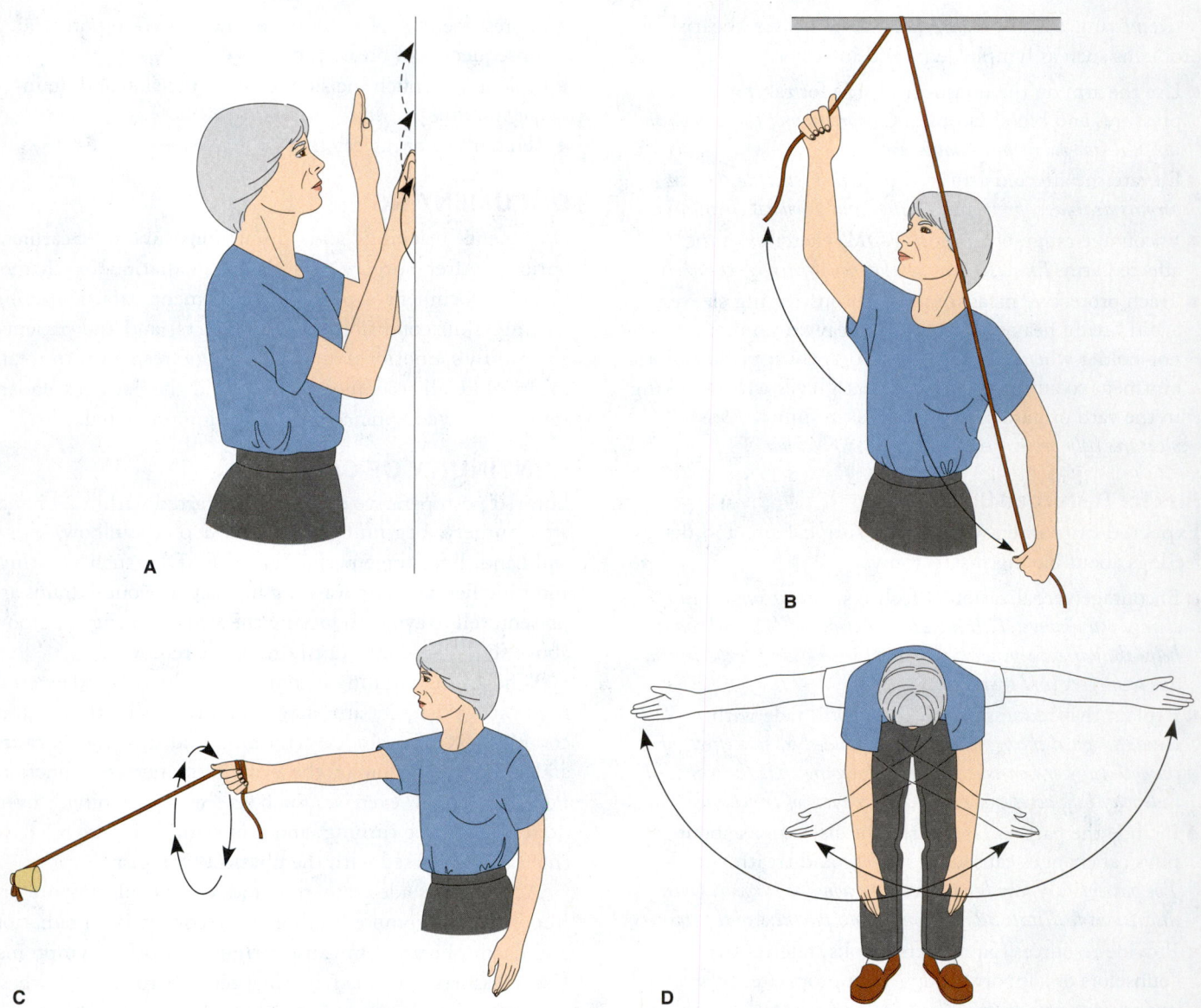

A

B

C

D

Figure 32-14. ■ Postmastectomy exercises. (**A**) Wall climbing: Stand facing wall with toes 6 to 12 in. from wall. Bend elbows and place palms against wall at shoulder level. Gradually move both hands up the wall parallel to each other until incisional pulling or pain occurs. (Mark that spot on wall to measure progress.) Work hands down to shoulder level. Move closer to wall as height of reach improves. (**B**) Overhead pulley: Using operated arm, toss 6-foot rope over shower curtain rod (or over top of a door that has a nail in the top to hold the rope in place for the exercise). Grasp one end of rope in each hand. Slowly raise operated arm as far as comfortable by pulling down on the rope on opposite side. Keep raised arm close to your head. Reverse to raise unoperated arm by lowering the operated arm. Repeat. (**C**) Rope turning: Tie rope to door handle. Hold rope in hand of operated side. Back away from door until arm is extended away from body, parallel to floor. Swing rope in as wide a circle as possible. Increase size of circle as mobility returns. (**D**) Arm swings: Stand with feet 8 in. apart. Bend forward from waist, allowing arms to hang toward floor. Swing both arms up to sides to reach shoulder level. Swing back to center and then cross arms at center. Do not bend elbows. If possible, do this and other exercises in front of mirror to ensure even posture and correct motion.

tolerated than hot foods. Suggest complementary therapies such as guided imagery and meditation to help cope with the adverse effects of treatment. Discuss the potential benefits of vitamin supplements (vitamins A, C, and E) to help promote healing and recovery.

Advise women who choose a prosthesis that a temporary lightweight prosthesis can be worn immediately after the drains and sutures have been removed. Because prostheses are expensive, advise not purchasing a permanent prosthesis until the wound has healed completely. Prostheses are available at medical suppliers and many larger department stores. Most private and government insurance policies pay for the first prosthesis.

Note: The references and resources for all chapters have been compiled at the back of the book.

Chapter Review

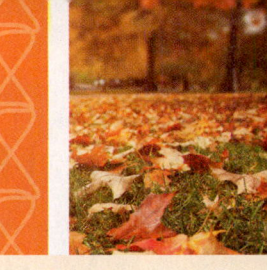

KEY POINTS

- Disorders affecting the female reproductive system often affect the patient's sexuality and body image in addition to their physical effects.
- **Concept:** Menstruation is a normal event, occurring cyclically on a monthly basis. It is an almost universal experience for women, and yet it is often misunderstood. Some cultures have beliefs that women are unclean, have special powers, or are less able to function while menstruating. None of these superstitions is accurate.
- **Concept:** Dysfunctional uterine bleeding has several causes but the one that the interprofessional team cannot afford to miss is bleeding due to malignancy.
- Menopause is the period during which menstruation permanently ceases. It marks the natural biologic end of reproduction.
- Many disorders of the female reproductive system, including structural disorders, endometriosis, ovarian cysts, uterine fibroid tumors, and PID, increase the risk of infertility.
- A number of tumors of the female reproductive system, including some breast, cervical, and endometrial cancers, are estrogen dependent. Women who have a history of early menarche, late menopause, few or no pregnancies or late childbearing, and estrogen replacement therapy have an increased risk for these cancers.
- Current technology has resulted in alternatives to hysterectomy as the primary treatment for many female reproductive disorders.
- Although specific genes have been identified that increase the risk of breast and ovarian cancer, the majority of these cancers occur in women who do not have the identified gene or genes.
- Screening measures such as clinical breast exam every 3 years by a health care provider until age 40, and annual CBE and mammogram after 40, significantly reduce the mortality rate of breast cancer.
- **Concept:** Annual CBE and screening mammogram are now the recommended breast cancer screening protocol for women over age 40.

PEARSON NURSING STUDENT RESOURCES

Find additional materials at **nursing.pearsonhighered.com**.

Clinical Reasoning Care Map

Caring for a Patient Experiencing Menopause

NCLEX-PN® Focus Area: Health Promotion and Maintenance: Growth and Development Through the Life Span

Case Study: Maria Villagrana, age 49, is having her annual checkup. She is concerned about recent symptoms, including palpitations, hot flashes, night sweats, and periods of anxiety and insomnia. During the past year, her menstrual periods have become short and erratic, and she has not menstruated for the past 3 months. Her most recent period lasted only 1 day.

Nursing Diagnosis: Grieving

COLLECT DATA

Subjective	Objective
_____	_____
_____	_____
_____	_____
_____	_____
_____	_____
_____	_____

Does this present a threat to the patient's safety?

If yes, the priority intervention to address this threat would be:

_____

Nursing Care

_____
_____
_____
_____
_____
_____
_____
_____
_____

Interprofessional team members to include when planning care:

_____

How would you document this? _____

_____

Data Collected
(use only those that apply)

- Often feels as though her "heart is running away with her"
- Hates thought of growing older
- Thinks her husband is losing interest in sex
- Wonders about decision not to have children
- Breaks down in tears for no reason
- Reports absentmindedness and difficulty concentrating
- BP 140/70; P 74; R 18; T 98.2°F (36.7°C)
- Smokes one pack of cigarettes daily
- Weighs 152 lb (69 kg) (approximately 25% over ideal body weight)
- No history of uterine or breast cancer
- High-fat, high-carbohydrate, low-protein, and low-fiber diet
- Calcium intake is less than 30% of recommended level
- Thyroid hormone levels normal
- FSH level elevated
- All other laboratory findings within normal ranges

Nursing Interventions
(use only those that apply; list in priority order)

- Teach coronary heart disease risk factors.
- Refer to smoking cessation program.
- Arrange sexual counseling for Mr. and Mrs. Villagrana regarding techniques, positions, and modifications to accommodate midlife changes.
- Arrange consultation with a registered dietitian.
- Refer to midlife women's support group at the local community center.
- Explain risks and benefits of HRT.

Compare your answers and documentation to those provided on the companion website.

NCLEX-PN® Exam Preparation

1 A woman experiencing frequent hot flashes and night sweats associated with perimenopause asks the nurse whether she should take hormones. The nurse's response is based on the knowledge that hormone replacement therapy: **Select all that apply.**

1. is recommended for all women during the 5 to 6 perimenopausal years.
2. is associated with a lower risk of breast cancer.
3. can reduce the risk of fractures associated with osteoporosis.
4. does little to relieve menopausal symptoms such as hot flashes and night sweats.
5. reduces the risk of developing coronary heart disease after menopause.

2 A patient with nonproliferative fibrocystic breast changes complains of monthly breast pain. She is likely to be advised to do all of the following. **Select all that apply.**

1. Consider prophylactic mastectomy to reduce her risk for breast cancer.
2. Use NSAIDs such as acetaminophen or ibuprofen for discomfort.
3. Try local heat or cold applications.
4. Eliminate caffeine and chocolate from her diet.
5. Wear a supportive brassiere to reduce discomfort.

3 A 23-year-old woman being seen for a pelvic exam and Pap smear confesses to the nurse that she is terrified of cervical cancer because her mother died of the disease at age 35. The nurse recommends measures to reduce her risk, including:

1. practicing monogamy and using barrier protection during sexual activity.
2. taking prophylactic tamoxifen until menopause.
3. having a pelvic examination and Pap smear every 6 months.
4. using oral contraceptives to regulate hormone secretion.

4 All of the following are good advice, but which is especially important for the woman taking tamoxifen?

1. Eat a low-fat, low-cholesterol diet.
2. Stop smoking.
3. Get regular aerobic exercise.
4. Get regular dental care.

5 A 52-year-old woman tells the clinic nurse that her husband felt a lump in the area between her breast and axilla. She wonders if this is anything to worry about, given that it really is not in her breast. The nurse's response is based on the knowledge that the most frequent location for breast cancer is:

1. upper outer quadrant.
2. periareolar area.
3. lower outer quadrant.
4. upper inner quadrant.

6 A patient has had a simple mastectomy with dissection of the lymph nodes. She has a Jackson–Pratt drain in place. The nurse's discharge instructions would include:

1. getting a permanent prosthesis as soon as possible.
2. how to empty the drain and clean around the insertion site.
3. keeping her arm elevated with the elbow above shoulder height as much as possible.
4. wrapping the chest and arm with elastic bandage to reduce scarring.

7 A patient, age 22, has primary dysmenorrhea. Which of the following statements indicates that she may need more instruction regarding self-care?

1. "It is okay to have sexual relations during my periods."
2. "A heating pad may help relieve symptoms."
3. "I should take an analgesic like ibuprofen right before and regularly during my period."
4. "I will need another form of birth control, since this means I can't continue taking the pill."

8 Your 65-year-old neighbor asks the nurse about some vaginal bleeding she has been having. She is postmenopausal and not on hormone replacement therapy. The nurse's best advice is:

1. that she still has some hormones present, stimulating a period.
2. to see her doctor immediately.
3. to increase her use of soy products.
4. that hormone replacement therapy would relieve this.

9 A patient relates a history of periods that last up to 2 weeks, with heavy bleeding for the first 5 days. The nurse appropriately charts this as:

1. amenorrhea.
2. metrorrhagia.
3. Mittelschmerz.
4. menorrhagia.

10 A patient has a history of PID. She is at increased risk for:

1. cervical cancer.
2. passing this tendency on to her daughter.
3. infertility and ectopic pregnancy.
4. toxic shock syndrome.

Answers and rationales for Review Questions appear in Appendix I.

CULTURAL CARE STRATEGIES

ASSESSING COMMUNICATION VARIABLES FROM A CULTURAL PERSPECTIVE

Mrs. Phuong Nguyen, a 25-year-old Vietnamese American woman, arrived in the emergency room in transition with very strong and closely spaced contractions. Despite her imminent delivery, she did not initiate conversation or communicate urgency about getting attention from the staff. She answered questions politely, nodding and smiling respectfully at the staff between occasional grimaces during the contractions. The only other sign of pain was her white knuckles as she grasped the armrests on the wheelchair in which she was placed. Many Vietnamese, as most Asians, believe that a woman must experience pain as part of childbirth and that expressing these feelings will bring on shame.

Communication

Verbal and nonverbal methods of communication vary among persons in different cultures. Communication presents the most significant challenge in working with patients from diverse cultural backgrounds, because the meaning of communication may vary by culture. The nurse who is aware of communication variables can be more attentive to nuances and different meanings of communication across cultures.

Communication embraces the entire world of human interaction and behavior. It provides the means by which people connect, and it is also the means by which culture is transmitted and preserved. Regardless of culture, individuals learn to think, feel, believe, and strive for what their culture considers proper. Both verbal and nonverbal communications are learned within one's culture (Giger, 2013). The nurse should be aware of these communication variables shown in the following table.

Nursing Implications

- Assess verbal and nonverbal communication for cultural variations in meaning. The nurse should be attentive to variations between and within cultures in relation to dialect, language style, volume of speech, touch, context of speech, and kinesics. A misinterpretation of communication due to cultural differences can create misunderstanding and deficits in meeting a patient's needs.

- Determine how respect can be communicated within a particular culture. In some cultures, a patient will not confide information until a relationship with the caregiver has developed. Thus use of "small talk" may be essential to develop a therapeutic relationship. In other cases, calling patients by their last names or greeting them by name is important. It may be helpful to greet an individual by title and first name, to approach and shake hands, or to smile with direct eye contact. In every case, it is important to assess the response of the individual, to determine the patient's comfort level, and to adapt communication strategies depending on the response of the individual.

Dialect	Dialect largely depends on geographic location. For example, patients from Appalachia, Australia, and England speak English quite differently from one another.
Language style	Words may have *different meanings* in different cultures. For example, the word *bad* may have a positive meaning to a teenager and have a more typical, negative meaning to an adult (Giger, 2013).
Volume of speech	Volume of speech may be culturally determined. Irish people, for example, frequently raise their voices. In contrast, others (e.g., the Japanese) tend to keep their voices low.
Touch	Use of touch varies widely among cultures. Because nurses use touch to reassure, provide affirmation, and decrease loneliness, we must be aware of how it is perceived. Depending on the situation and the culture of the person, touch can also be perceived as threatening, intrusive, or seductive.
Context of speech or emotional tone	Context of speech refers to the use of emotion when communicating. The African American, Jewish, or German patient is less likely to use an emotional tone than one who is Italian, Irish, or Mexican (Giger, 2013). Arabs may express their emotions openly through nonverbal cues and voice but may withhold some feelings from strangers. They may express agreement in front of strangers that does not reflect their true feelings. An Arab may tend to protect others from disagreements or indicate disagreement by simply raising an eyebrow rather than responding verbally.
Kinesics	Kinesics refers to the use of stances, gestures, and eye behavior when communicating with others. Vietnamese individuals typically nod and smile to indicate respect when interacting with a health care professional (Giger, 2013). However, they may or may not be agreeing with what is being said.

Self-Reflection Questions

1. What personal communication techniques do you use when approaching individuals for the first time?
2. What communication techniques do you observe among other cultures during your initial greeting?
3. What generally accepted communication techniques can you use to communicate respect to persons from another culture?

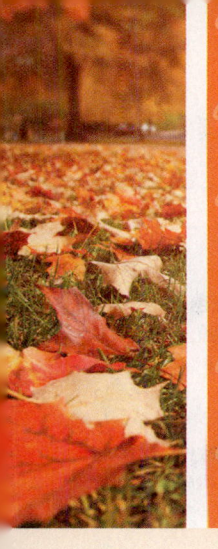

CHAPTER 33
Caring for Patients With Sexually Transmitted Infections

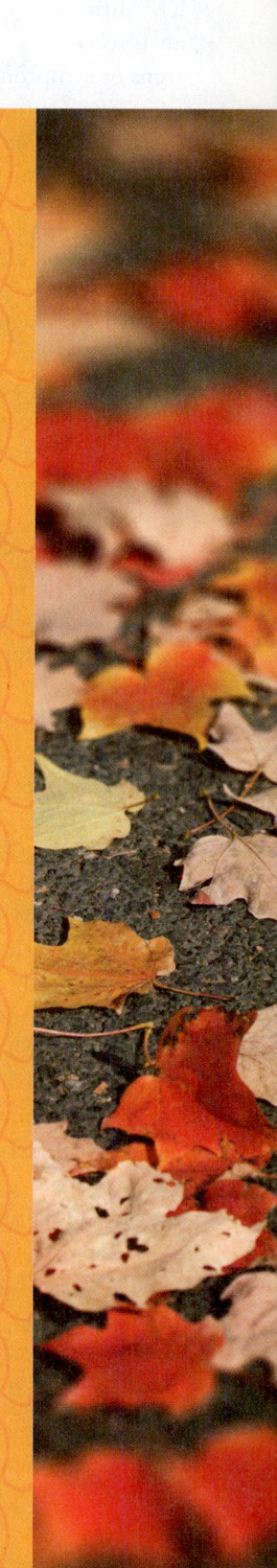

BRIEF OUTLINE

Sexually Transmitted Infections
Overview of STIs

Chlamydia
Genital Herpes
Genital Warts

Gonorrhea
Syphilis

APPLIED LEARNING OUTCOMES

After completing this chapter, you will be able to:

1. Describe sexually transmitted infection (STI).
2. Explain risk factors for STI.
3. Explain the pathophysiology of the most common STIs.
4. Explain laboratory and diagnostic tests used for STIs.
5. Discuss general measures to prevent and treat common STIs.
6. Explain the signs and symptoms of the most common STIs.
7. Plan safety measures to prevent patient–nurse transmission of communicable infections.
8. Discuss nursing implications for medications prescribed for patients with STIs.
9. Use the nursing process to provide individualized care for patients with STIs.

KEY TERMS

The key terms are defined on the pages listed below.

abstinence, 867
chancre, 872
female condom, 864
infertility, 862

mutual monogamy, 867
prodromal symptoms, 869
sexually transmitted
   infection (STI), 862

vesicles, 868
vulva, 863

SPECIAL FEATURES

NURSING CARE PLAN: Patient With Gonorrhea, 871
CLINICAL REASONING CARE MAP: Caring for a Patient With Syphilis, 876
UNIT VIII WRAP-UP: Thinking Strategically About..., 878

Sexually Transmitted Infections

Key Concept Any infection transmitted by sexual contact, including vaginal, oral, and anal intercourse, is referred to as a **sexually transmitted infection (STI)**, also known as a *sexually transmitted disease (STD)*.

The difference between an infection and a disease is that an infection is the presence of microorganisms without signs or symptoms and diseases (which are caused by infections) have symptoms (Planned Parenthood Federation of America, 2013). The terms are used interchangeably in the literature on this subject.

Key Concept Every sexually active person, and even some people who are not, are at risk for STIs.

Health care workers, including nurses, are at risk for contracting some STIs from their patients through unprotected contact with infected blood and body fluids.

Infants can be infected by their mothers *in utero* or during delivery. Children can be infected through incest or sexual abuse. Victims of sexual assault are also at risk.

People with multiple sexual partners have the highest risk of acquiring an STI. The incidence is also high in people of color in urban settings with lower socioeconomic status and less education (Box 33-1■). Drug abuse and unprotected sex are also risk factors for STIs (Box 33-2■). The incidence of STIs is highest among young people: Two-thirds of all STIs occur in people under age 25. However, people of all ages are at risk. Anyone who is sexually active can be infected with STIs.

STIs are very common. Every year, an estimated 15 million people in the United States acquire an STI. Half of all the people in the United States will get an STI at some time in their lives (Planned Parenthood Federation of America, 2013).

STIs affect the patient's general and reproductive health; some, such as HIV and hepatitis B, can be life threatening. Because of tissue trauma that occurs during sexual intercourse, many STIs are more easily transmitted from a man to a woman than from a woman to a man. Women often experience few early manifestations of the infection and have a greater risk for complications of STIs, such as pelvic inflammatory disease (PID), **infertility** (the inability to conceive or initiate pregnancy), and genital cancers.

clinicalALERT

Reporting STIs
All states require *reporting* of syphilis, gonorrhea, and HIV/AIDS to state and federal public health agencies. Chlamydia is reportable in most states; requirements for reporting other STIs vary by state. Due to the inconsistency of state requirements, the exact incidence of many STIs is unknown.

BOX 33-1	POPULATION FOCUS

Syphilis in Men Who Have Sex With Men

In 2000, the incidence of syphilis in the United States was the lowest since reporting began in 1941. The Healthy People 2010 goal was to have it nearly eradicated. However, since 2000, the incidence has risen in all racial and ethnic groups and in all areas of the country. Between 2006 and 2007, the rate increased 17.5%. The overall increase in primary and secondary syphilis cases during 2000–2007 was observed mostly in men. From 2006 to 2007, infections reported to the Centers for Disease Control and Prevention (CDC) increased among men from 8,293 to 9,769 cases (17.9%) and in women from 1,458 to 1,692 cases (10.0%). The increases in rates for males, and the ratios of males to females, suggest an increase in syphilis among men who have sex with men (CDC, 2009).

BOX 33-2	RISK FACTORS FOR STIs

- Personal or partner history of STI
- Adolescent sexual activity
- Use of oral contraceptives
- Unprotected sexual activity
- Multiple sexual partners
- Pregnancy

Overview of STIs

Although STIs are caused by many different organisms, including bacteria, viruses, and parasites, they have several characteristics in common:

1. Most can be prevented by the use of latex condoms (see following Health Promotion section).
2. They can be transmitted during both heterosexual and homosexual activities.
3. For treatment to be effective, sexual partners of the infected person must also be treated.
4. Two or more STIs frequently coexist in the same patient.

Some STIs can be cured with appropriate antibiotic treatment. Others, such as genital herpes and genital warts, are chronic conditions caused by viruses. These infections may be managed but not cured. Some, such as HIV and hepatitis B, are potentially fatal. (Note that the main discussion of HIV is in Chapter 11 and of hepatitis is in Chapter 27.) Common STIs, their manifestations, treatment, and possible complications are outlined in Table 33-1■. The five most common STIs in the United States are discussed next in greater detail.

HEALTH PROMOTION

Key Concept The most effective form of protection against STIs, as well as the recommendation of the CDC, is the latex condom. There are also good alternatives for people who are allergic to latex.

TABLE 33-1	Selected STIs, Manifestations, Treatment, and Complications		
DISEASE/ORGANISM	**MANIFESTATIONS**	**TREATMENT**	**COMPLICATIONS**
Chancroid* (rare in United States) *Haemophilus ducreyi*	**Females:** Frequently asymptomatic **Males:** Painful penile ulcers and *lymphadenopathy* (tender, enlarged lymph nodes)	Azithromycin PO once *or* ceftriaxone IM once *or* ciprofloxacin PO for 3 days *or* erythromycin PO for 7 days	Secondary infection of lesions, fistulas, chronic ulcers
Chlamydia *Chlamydia trachomatis*	**Females:** Asymptomatic; may have dysuria, vaginal or cervical discharge, vaginal bleeding, or pelvic pain **Males:** May be asymptomatic or have dysuria, white or clear urethral discharge, testicular pain (epididymitis)	Doxycycline PO for 7 days *or* azithromycin PO once Erythromycin PO is an alternative for pregnant patients.	**Females:** PID, infertility, pelvic abscesses, spontaneous abortion, stillbirth, postpartum endometritis **Neonates:** Ophthalmia neonatorum or pneumonia **Males:** Urethritis, epididymitis, prostatitis
Genital herpes Herpes simplex virus, usually type 2	Single or multiple small painful vesicles on an erythematous base on the genitals with associated pruritus, followed by painful ulcers	No cure; acyclovir PO *or* famciclovir PO *or* valacyclovir PO for 7–10 days or until symptoms resolve Docosanol 10% cream (Abreva) topically applied to the lesions can reduce outbreak duration (used with PO meds). Valacyclovir can be taken on a long-term daily basis to prevent transmission.	Herpes keratitis, a severe eye infection **Females:** Cervical cancer **Neonates:** Herpes affecting the eye, skin, mucous membranes, and central nervous system **Males:** Neuralgia, meningitis, urethral strictures, pus forming in lymph nodes
Genital warts (condylomata acuminata) caused by a type of human papillomavirus. The type that causes genital warts is not the type that causes cancer.	Single or multiple painless warts (small or large bumps or groups of bumps) on genitals or perianal area	No cure, usually recur. Cryotherapy, *or* podophyllin 10%–25% in tincture of benzoin compound applied to wart, *or* patient-applied podofilox topical solution or gel *or* imiquimod cream	Urinary obstruction and bleeding **Females:** Enlargement during pregnancy **Neonates:** Respiratory papillomatosis, a very rare chronic condition
Human papillomavirus (HPV): There are more than 40 types that can cause STIs.	Most people with HPV do not have symptoms. The virus infects the skin and mucous membranes of men and women, including the penis, vagina, **vulva** (perineal area outside the vagina), and anus.	Gardasil is an immunization given to young people to prevent HPV infection. There is no treatment for the virus itself, but any cancer it may cause has better outcomes if diagnosed early.	Some types cause cancer. They can cause cancer of the cervix, and less commonly the vulva, vagina, anus, and penis.
Gonorrhea* *Neisseria gonorrhoeae*	**Females:** Often asymptomatic; may have vaginal discharge, abnormal menses, dysuria **Males:** Dysuria, increased urinary frequency, purulent urethral discharge	Drug resistance is becoming a problem for gonorrhea. Currently, there is no evidence of resistance to the cephalosporins (Cefixime) PO *or* ceftriaxone IM in a single injection *plus* azithromycin PO in a single dose *or* doxycycline PO for 7 days to treat possible coexisting chlamydia.	**Females:** PID, infertility, ectopic pregnancy, abdominal adhesions **Males:** Prostatitis, urethritis, nephritis, epididymitis, infertility
Granuloma inguinale* (rare in United States) *Calymmatobacterium granulomatis*	Single or multiple subcutaneous nodules that erode to form painless, bleeding, enlarging ulcers	Trimethoprim–sulfamethoxazole PO for 21 days *or* doxycycline PO for 21 days	Secondary infection of lesions, *keloid* (excess scar tissue) on genitals, tissue necrosis, fever, malaise, secondary anemia, cachexia, and death

*Reporting to state and federal agencies required by law.

(continued)

TABLE 33-1	Selected STIs, Manifestations, Treatment, and Complications *(continued)*		
DISEASE/ORGANISM	**MANIFESTATIONS**	**TREATMENT**	**COMPLICATIONS**
Lymphogranuloma venereum* (rare in United States) *Chlamydia trachomatis*	Painless vesicle or ulcer, followed by regional lymphadenopathy, inguinal abscess	Doxycycline PO for 21 days *or* erythromycin PO for 21 days	Ruptured abscesses with draining sinuses or fistulas, nephropathy, hepatomegaly, or phlebitis
Pelvic inflammatory disease (PID) *Chlamydia trachomatis, Neisseria gonorrhoeae, Mycoplasma hominis,* and others	Pain and tenderness in lower abdomen, uterus and surrounding tissues; possible fever, chills, and elevated WBC and sedimentation rate	Combined drug therapy such as cefotetan IV *plus* doxycycline IV or PO *or* clindamycin IV *plus* gentamicin IV or IM; may require hospitalization	Ectopic pregnancy, pelvic abscess; infertility, recurrent or chronic PID, chronic abdominal pain, pelvic adhesions, depression
Syphilis* *Treponema pallidum*	**Primary:** Painless chancre at site of exposure; regional lymphadenopathy **Secondary:** Skin rash; oral mucous patches; generalized lymphadenopathy; mucous patch on vulva or anus; fever; malaise; patchy alopecia **Tertiary** (late): Tumors of skin, bone, liver; inflammation of aorta, aneurysms; central nervous system degeneration	Penicillin G IM in a single injection *or* doxycycline PO for 14 days. Syphilis of unclear or more than 1 year's duration: penicillin G IM weekly for 3 weeks *or* doxycycline PO for 28 days	**Primary and secondary:** Disease progression **Tertiary:** Heart failure, blindness, paralysis, skin ulcers, liver failure, mental illness
Trichomoniasis *Trichomonas vaginalis*	**Females:** Asymptomatic or may have frothy, excessive vaginal discharge, erythema, edema, and pruritus **Males:** Usually asymptomatic; may have urethritis, penile lesions, or inflammation	Metronidazole PO in a single dose or for 7 days	**Females:** Recurrent infections, salpingitis, low-birth-weight infants, prematurity*

*Reporting to state and federal agencies required by law.

Review Table 30-3 for the ability of various contraceptive methods to protect against STIs.

Some people have allergies to the lubricant or preservatives or chemicals used in condom manufacture, not to the latex rubber itself. The symptoms of this contact allergy are local irritation or itching and may be avoided by trying another brand of condom.

People who have systemic allergic reactions, such as skin reactions on the body in areas not in contact with the condom, respiratory distress, or anaphylaxis, must avoid latex altogether. Safer sex can still be practiced with nonlatex condoms. (Natural skin condoms protect from pregnancy, but *not* against STIs, so they are not safe enough.) The **female condom** is a lubricated polyurethane sheath inserted into the vagina and held in place by a flexible ring around the cervix (see Figure 33-1■ for instructions on its use). It can withstand oil-based lubricants or oils, which do not interfere with its function, and it leaves the woman in control of the safety side of intercourse. Males also have a good nonlatex choice in the polyurethane

(plastic) *male condom* (see Figure 33-2■ for instructions on its use). Polyurethane is not as flexible as latex, but in every other way it is as effective (Thomas, 2009).

Patients who are too embarrassed to purchase condoms at the store can go online and order them to be delivered through the mail. Latex allergy is becoming more common, so nurses must be aware of resources such as reputable websites or current printed information that can provide patient education about alternatives such as polyurethane condoms.

Chlamydia

Chlamydial infections are thought to be the most common STIs in the United States and the leading cause of PID (see Chapter 32). Because the infection is often asymptomatic, the incidence of the disease is thought to be nearly 10 times what is reported. Incidence is highest among sexually active teenagers. The risk factors for chlamydia are those for nearly all STIs (see Box 33-2).

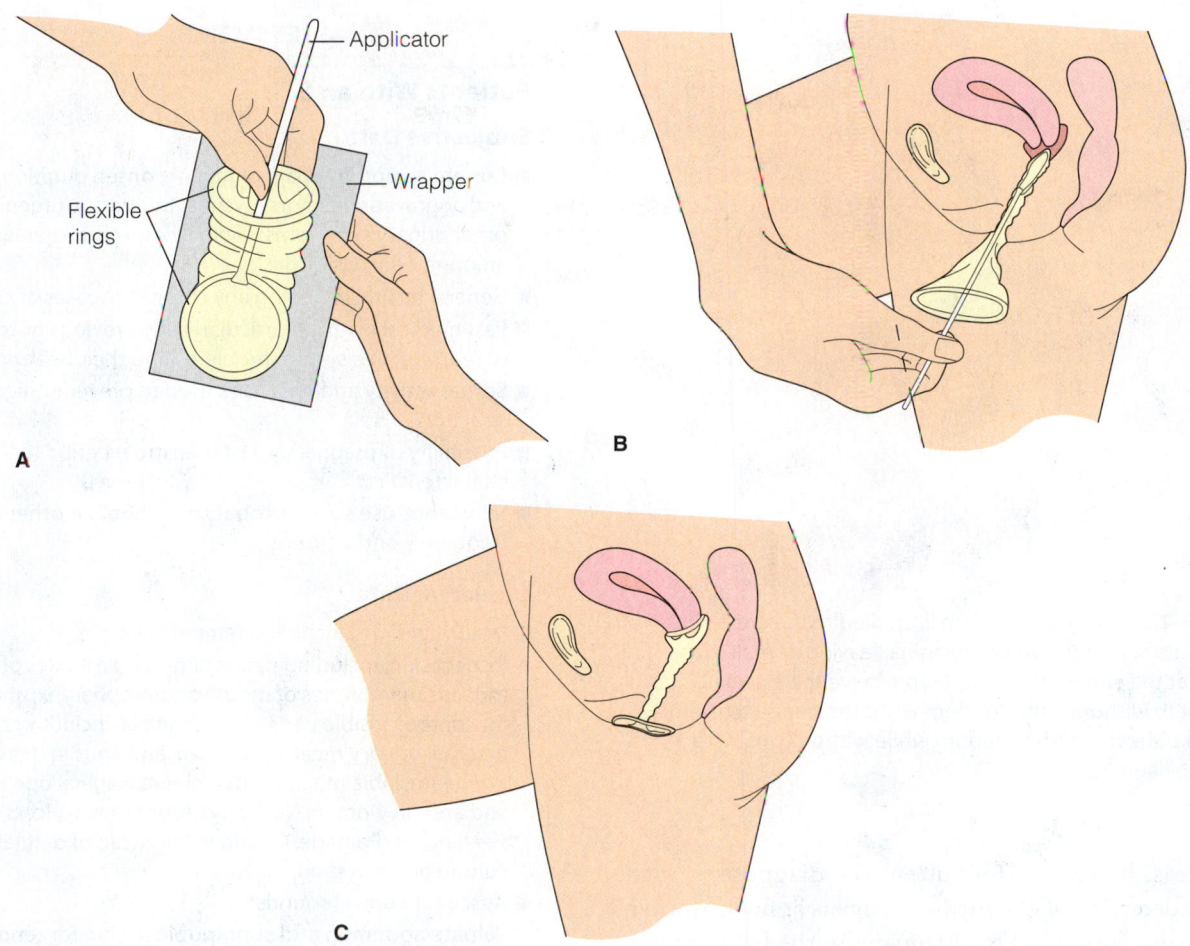

Figure 33-1. ■ Female condom. (**A**) Remove the condom and applicator from the wrapper by pulling up on the ring. (**B**) Insert the condom slowly by gently pushing the applicator toward the small of the back. (**C**) When properly inserted, the outer ring should rest on the folds of skin around the vaginal opening, and the inner ring (closed end) should fit loosely against the cervix.

PATHOPHYSIOLOGY

Chlamydia trachomatis is a bacterium that behaves like a virus, reproducing only within the host cell. It is spread by any sexual contact and to the neonate by passage through the birth canal of an infected mother. The incubation period is from 1 to 3 weeks. The bacteria typically invade the cervix in women and the urethra in men. In addition to causing genital infections, *C. trachomatis* causes *trachoma, a* chronic, contagious type of conjunctivitis prevalent in Asia and Africa, which can result in blindness.

MANIFESTATIONS AND COMPLICATIONS

Chlamydial infections are asymptomatic in most women until they have invaded the uterus and fallopian tubes. Early manifestations, when present, include dysuria, urinary frequency, and vaginal discharge. Nearly a third of men with chlamydia are also asymptomatic. Manifestations of the infection in men include dysuria, urethral discharge, and possible testicular pain. Although patients may be asymptomatic, they are still potentially infectious.

If untreated, chlamydial infection in women ascends into the upper reproductive tract, causing such complications as PID, which includes endometritis, salpingitis, and chronic pelvic pain. These infections are a major cause of infertility and ectopic pregnancy, a potentially life-threatening condition. Complications in men include epididymitis, prostatitis, sterility, and Reiter syndrome (an autoimmune disorder). In the newborn, chlamydia can lead to blindness or pneumonia.

COLLABORATIVE CARE

Because chlamydial infections are often asymptomatic, treatment is often begun on a presumptive basis. The CDC recommends screening asymptomatic women who are at high risk for chlamydia.

Diagnostic Tests

Chlamydial infection can be diagnosed in several ways. Infected tissue can be cultured to identify the presence of the bacteria. This test is expensive and not readily available

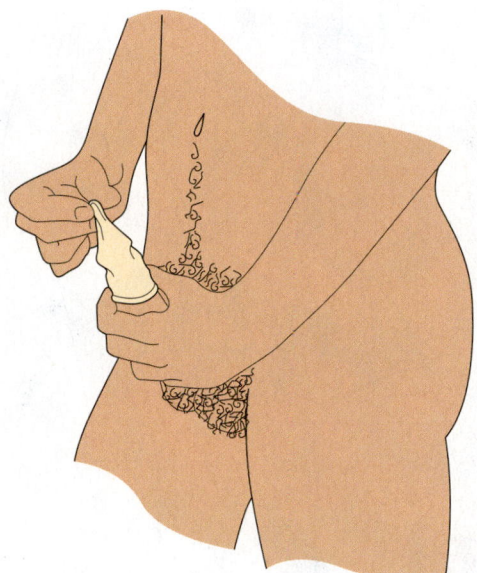

Figure 33-2. ■ The male condom is applied to the erect penis before contact with the vulva or vagina, leaving a small space available at the end of the condom to receive the ejaculate. It is important to withdraw the condom while the penis is still erect and to hold the rim of the condom while withdrawing it, to prevent spillage.

in all areas, however. More often, the diagnosis is made based on detection of chlamydial antigens or nucleic acid or by detecting antibodies to chlamydia in the blood or local secretions. These tests are particularly effective in diagnosing chlamydial infection in high-risk populations.

NURSING CARE

PRIORITIZING NURSING CARE

Teaching about the infection, its treatment, and potential effects on reproductive health for the patient and his or her partners is the priority for nursing care.

Nursing care of the patient with chlamydia focuses on identifying the infection, eradicating it, preventing future infections, and managing any complications.

ASSESSING

Box 33-3■ outlines nursing assessment as it relates to patients with an STI.

DIAGNOSING, PLANNING, AND IMPLEMENTING

Consider the following nursing diagnoses and interventions when planning and delivering care for a patient with an STI.

Ineffective Health Maintenance

Expected outcome: Will explain how to use safer sex practices.

| BOX 33-3 | ASSESSMENT |

Patients With an STI

Subjective Data

■ Current symptoms: pain or itching; onset, duration, relieving and aggravating factors; dysuria, frequency, urgency, or other urinary symptoms; vaginal or urethral drainage, color, amount, odor; visible lesions
■ General health, including any chronic diseases or conditions
■ Past medical history, particularly any previous history of STIs or reproductive system problems and their treatment
■ Sexual activity and measures used to prevent pregnancy or infection
■ Possibility of pregnancy; last menstrual period (date, characteristics)
■ Substance use such as tobacco, alcohol, or other drug use; frequency and amount

Objective Data

■ Note vital signs, including temperature.
■ Inspect skin, including palms of hands and soles of feet; mucous membranes of mouth and oropharynx; abdomen for contour, visible peristalsis; genitalia, including penis, external urinary meatus, scrotum, and anus in men; perineum, labia majora, labia minora, vaginal opening, and anus in women. Note any redness, rash, ulcers, lesions, swelling, or drainage. Obtain sterile swab of drainage for culture or Gram stain.
■ Auscultate bowel sounds.
■ Palpate abdomen and suprapubic region for tenderness; inguinal lymph nodes for swelling or tenderness (lymphadenopathy); perineal tissues for tenderness or swelling.

■ Teach about the disease, its transmission, treatment, and measures to prevent its spread or reinfection. *Understanding the disease and how it is spread helps the patient gain a sense of control and prevent future STIs.*
■ Discuss safer sex practices outlined in Box 33-4■. *Patients can prevent future STIs by making lifestyle changes and conscious decisions about safer sex practices.*
■ Emphasize the importance of referring all sex partners for testing and treatment as needed. *Unless both partners in a relationship are effectively treated, reinfection is likely.*
■ Stress the importance of completing the prescribed treatment plan and returning for follow-up visits as recommended. *Incomplete treatment may result in continued infection and organisms that are resistant to antibiotic therapy.*

Impaired Skin Integrity

Expected outcome: Will do own perineal hygiene to keep area clean and dry; will have intact skin.

Preventing STIs: A Checklist for Patients

- You can eliminate your risk entirely by not having sex with anyone (**abstinence**) or by having sex only with an uninfected partner who has sex only with you (**mutual monogamy**).
- The more sexual partners you have, the greater your risk of contracting an STI.
- Latex condoms, used consistently and correctly, can prevent many STIs, including HIV infection. Use a new condom each time, lubricating the condom with a water-based lubricant.
- The female condom reduces the risk of STIs, including HIV.
- Vaginal spermicides reduce the risk for gonorrhea and chlamydia but do not prevent HIV infection.
- If you suspect you have been exposed to an STI, see a doctor or clinic right away. Encourage your partner to seek treatment, too.
- Follow the doctor's instructions carefully and take all the medicine prescribed for you. Continue the medication even when the symptoms go away. (The infection sometimes remains active after symptoms go away.)
- Go back to your doctor for a follow-up exam according to his or her instructions.
- Do not have sex until you *and* your partner are completely cured.
- If you use drugs by injection, enroll in or continue a drug-treatment program. Do not use injection supplies that have been used by another person under any circumstances. Thoroughly and consistently clean injection equipment with bleach-water between uses.

- Teach the patient to keep perineal tissues clean and dry. Advise cleansing front to back after urinating and defecating, using soap and water as needed to clean the area, and a blow drier on cool setting to dry. *Keeping perineal tissues clean and dry promotes healing and reduces the risk of secondary infection of lesions.*
- Instruct to avoid perineal powders or sprays, as well as bubble baths. *Feminine hygiene sprays and bubble baths can excessively dry perineal tissues, increasing the risk of infection.*
- Advise patient to wear cotton underwear, avoiding tight-fitting jeans and pantyhose. *These measures allow moisture to evaporate rather than keeping it against the skin.*

Risk for Injury

Expected outcome: Will state the importance of taking all medications and adhering to therapeutic regimen, including ways to prevent future infection.

- Stress the importance of taking all prescribed medication. *Completing the prescribed course of antibiotic helps ensure elimination of the infecting organism and prevents development of drug-resistant organisms.*

- Instruct to abstain from sexual contact until patient and partners are cured and to use condoms to prevent future infections. *Abstinence prevents reinfection and spread of the STI. Condoms provide barrier protection, reducing the risk of infection during sexual activity.*
- Provide information about signs and symptoms of reinfection and other STIs. Stress the importance of prompt diagnosis and treatment of all STIs. *Successful treatment of the disease does not prevent future infections.*

Anxiety

Expected outcome: Will discuss feelings about having an STI.

- Emphasize that most STIs can be effectively treated, preventing serious complications and transmission to the fetus during pregnancy. *This information provides a sense of control and helps decrease anxiety.*
- Discuss with women of childbearing age that cesarean delivery can prevent transmission of an active infection to the neonate. *Understanding that infection of the neonate can be prevented helps relieve anxiety. The patient and her health care provider can discuss this further, but the nurse can initiate this conversation.*

Situational Low Self-Esteem

Expected outcome: Will discuss feelings about having an STI.

- Create an environment in which the patient feels respected and safe to discuss concerns about the disease and its effect on the patient's life. *Being treated with respect and privacy helps the patient realize that the disease does not change his or her worth as a person.*
- Provide privacy and confidentiality. *Patients are often embarrassed to discuss intimate details of their sex lives. STI carries a stigma, and nonjudgmental nurse–patient relationships help patients experience an STI as an infection and not a character flaw.*
- Communicate caring for the patient. *Unfortunately, many people affected by STIs lack family and other social support networks. The nurse's concern can enhance self-esteem.*

Sexual Dysfunction

Expected outcome: Will discuss feelings and ask questions about STI; will accept information about community resources for people with STIs.

- Provide a supportive, nonjudgmental environment to discuss feelings and questions about the effect of the STI on current and future sexual relationships. *Feelings of guilt, shame, and anger are natural responses to the diagnosis of an STI and can lead to a total avoidance of sexual intimacy.*

■ Offer information about support groups and other resources for people with specific STIs. *Information can offset feelings of shame and hopelessness. Many people have learned to live with and manage these disorders without infecting their partners or their children.*

Impaired Social Interaction

Expected outcome: Will state plans to resume social activities.

■ Help the patient understand that an STI is a consequence of sexual behavior, not a "punishment," and that it can be avoided in the future. *This knowledge enhances the patient's ability to relate to others.*

EVALUATING

To evaluate the effectiveness of nursing care, collect data such as the following:

■ Completed prescribed medication regimen as ordered?
■ Kept all recommended follow-up appointments?
■ Able to identify measures to prevent future STIs?
■ Engaging in safer sex practices with an uninfected partner?
■ Resumed social activities?
■ If pregnant, can state measures to prevent disease transmission to fetus?

DOCUMENTING

Document subjective and objective assessment data, including the circumstances under which the infection was obtained (if known) and the number of recent sexual partners. Also document all teaching provided and the patient's understanding and apparent willingness to comply with prescribed treatment. Note information provided about safer sex practices and the receptiveness of the patient and partner to safer sex practices.

CONTINUITY OF CARE

Nurses have a critical role in preventing STIs by teaching patients about these diseases, their prevention, treatment, and potential complications (see Box 33-4).

Stress the importance of complying with the prescribed treatment and referring partners for examination and treatment as needed. Discuss safer sex practices and using condoms to avoid reinfection. Teach about the complications of chlamydia, such as PID, and their manifestations. Instruct the patient to seek medical attention promptly if symptoms of PID develop. If the infection has progressed to PID, provide additional information about PID and its treatment (see Chapter 32).

Genital Herpes

Genital herpes (*Herpes genitalis*) is a chronic and sometimes asymptomatic STI. Currently, no cure is available for genital herpes. As many as 45 million people in the United

States are infected with the herpes simplex virus type 2 (HSV-2), the usual cause of genital herpes. Most of these people, however, have undiagnosed infections. Like other STIs, the incidence of genital herpes is highest among adolescents and young adults.

PATHOPHYSIOLOGY AND MANIFESTATIONS

HSV-2 is closely related to HSV-1, which commonly causes fever blisters or cold sores in the mouth. HSV-1 can also infect the genitalia; likewise, HSV-2 can infect other parts of the body. Genital herpes is spread by vaginal, anal, or oral–genital contact. Its incubation period is 3 to 7 days. Within a week after exposure, painful or itchy red papules appear in the exposed area. In men, the lesions usually occur on the glans or shaft of the penis. In women, the lesions often occur on the labia, vagina, and cervix. Anal intercourse may result in lesions in and around the anus. Oral infection will yield lesions (small painful vesicles on a red base) at the edges of the lips.

Soon after the papules appear, they form small painful **vesicles** (blisters) filled with clear fluid containing virus particles (Figure 33-3■). The skin around the vesicles is red and painful. The blisters break, shedding the virus and creating painful ulcers that last 6 weeks or longer.

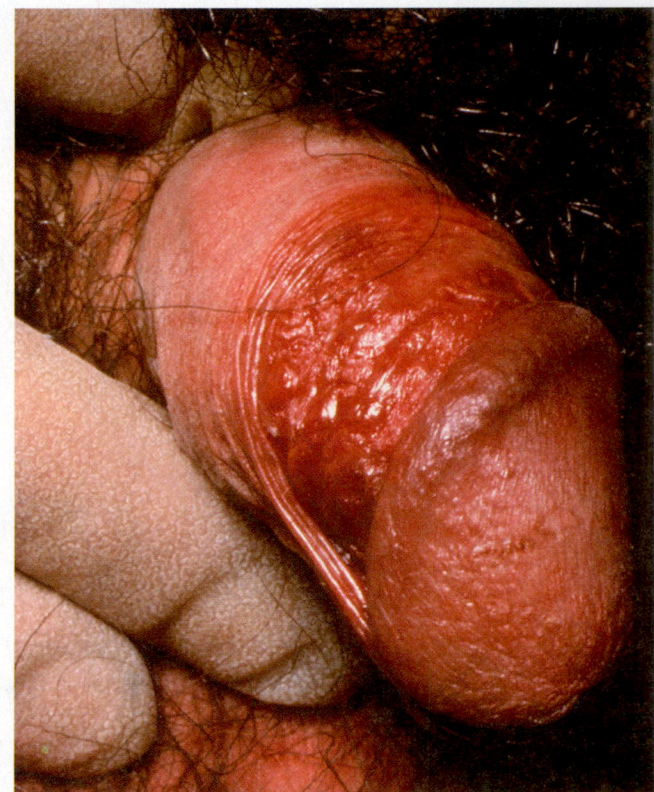

Figure 33-3. ■ Genital herpes blisters as they appear on the penis. (Source: Biophoto Associates/Science Source.)

Touching these blisters and then rubbing or scratching in another place can spread the infection to other areas of the body. The blister exudate forms a crust.

The first outbreak of herpes lesions is called the *first episode infection.* Subsequent episodes, or *recurrent infections,* are usually less severe and last for a briefer period. The period between episodes is called *latency.* During latency, the virus withdraws into the nerve fibers that lead from the infected site to the lower spine, remaining dormant until recurrence, at which time it retraces its path to the exposed area.

Prodromal symptoms (warning symptoms that occur before the outbreak of lesions) of herpes outbreaks include burning, itching, tingling, or throbbing at the sites where lesions commonly appear. There may be pain radiating to the legs, thighs, groin, or buttocks. The infection may be infectious during the prodromal period, so sexual contact should be avoided.

Recurrent infections have symptoms of herpetic lesions, general malaise or headache, fever, dysuria and urinary retention, and vaginal or urethral discharge.

Men are not likely to experience serious complications of genital herpes. Women, however, face more serious concerns. Neonatal infection from a mother with herpes can range from asymptomatic to widely disseminated, fatal disease. Transmission occurs during passage through the birth canal. The risk is highest during the first episode of infection. The baby may be delivered via cesarean section if the mother is having an active outbreak of genital herpes. Women also face an increased risk of cervical cancer. In rare cases, the herpes virus can spread to the brain, causing herpes encephalitis, a life-threatening complication.

> **Key Concept** Nurses may contract herpes infections of the skin (called *herpetic whitlow*) or of the eyes by contact with the herpes-shedding lesions of patients.

When herpes infection is in the blister stage, the blister fluid contains the herpes virus. Herpes virus is shed in relatively large amounts from leaking or bursting blisters. The crust that follows the broken blisters may also shed viruses. Health care workers can be exposed to these viruses on the skin of their hands and may develop *herpetic whitlow,* a herpetic skin infection that is contagious. Health care workers have also contracted herpes infections of the eyes and esophagus. Standard Precautions are adequate protection from these infections, thus gloves should always be worn when contact with the patient's herpes lesions is possible.

COLLABORATIVE CARE

Because there is no cure for herpes infection, treatment focuses on relieving symptoms and preventing spread of the infection. Teaching is an essential component of care.

Genital herpes is usually diagnosed by the history (including lesion characteristics and patterns of recurrence) and physical exam. Antiviral drugs such as acyclovir (Zovirax) or famciclovir (Famvir) help reduce the length and severity of the first episode and decrease the frequency of recurrent episodes. These drugs usually are given orally; for severe episodes, acyclovir can also be given intravenously.

Due to the stigma of having an STI, especially herpes, which is not curable, many people use the mental coping mechanism of denial to deal with their herpes infection. These people may be so stressed by the thought that they have herpes that they are not able to think about it or try to have it treated. They even deny to themselves that they are infected. They may think, "I don't have anything unless the doctor says I do." These denying patients put their partners at risk. They may say, "I didn't know I had herpes" or "My last outbreak was years ago, and I didn't know this was another herpes outbreak," when their partner is diagnosed with herpes. The nurse's best resource to treat denial is honest and nonjudgmental information. When the nurse teaches the patient in an accepting way and provides the most accurate information about treatment and prevention, patients are most likely to be able to listen and express their feelings.

NURSING CARE

In addition to the nursing care as outlined for chlamydia, the nursing diagnoses of Pain and Impaired Health Maintenance should be considered for the patient with genital herpes.

Acute Pain

Expected outcome: Will have pain 3 or less on a 0 to 10 scale during herpes outbreak.

- Teach the patient to keep herpes blisters clean and dry. A solution of warm water and soap can be used to cleanse the lesions two or three times daily. Lesions should be dried using a hair dryer on the cool setting. Instruct to wear loose cotton clothing that will not trap moisture; pantyhose and tight jeans should be avoided. *Keeping the lesions clean and dry reduces the risk of secondary infection and promotes healing.*

- For dysuria, suggest pouring water over the genitals while urinating. Encourage increased fluid intake. *These measures help relieve dysuria by diluting the urine that comes in contact with the painful lesions.*

clinical**ALERT**

Instruct the patient to use barrier protection for all sexual intercourse because the infection can be transmitted from the onset of prodromal symptoms until crusted lesions are healed and all symptoms are cleared.

CONTINUITY OF CARE

With teaching, patients with genital herpes can learn to manage this chronic disease with the least possible disruption in lifestyle and relationships. Teach the patient to recognize prodromal symptoms of recurrence, and discuss factors that seem to trigger recurrences (e.g., emotional stress, acidic food, sun exposure). Explain the need for abstinence from sexual contact from the time prodromal symptoms appear until 10 days after all lesions have healed.

Encourage the patient to use prescribed oral antiviral drugs to reduce the frequency and duration of outbreaks. Painful lesions can be protected with sterile Vaseline, docosanol cream (Abreva), or aloe vera gel. Because viral shedding can occur at any time during an outbreak, emphasize the importance of using latex condoms and careful hygiene practices (e.g., not sharing towels or other personal items).

Genital Warts

Genital and anal warts, also known as *condylomata acuminata* or *venereal warts,* are caused by human papillomavirus (HPV). HPV is a common virus with over 40 types that can cause STIs in humans, and it is one of the most common STIs in the United States. Most HPV infections are asymptomatic or unrecognized. Like most STIs, genital warts are usually found in young, sexually active adults and are associated with early onset of sexual activity and multiple sexual partners.

PATHOPHYSIOLOGY AND MANIFESTATIONS

HPV is transmitted by all types of sexual contact. The incubation period for genital warts is about 3 months. Many different types of HPV cause chronic genital infections.

Although most people who carry HPV have no symptoms, others develop single or multiple painless, cauliflower-like growths on the vulvovaginal area, perineum, penis, urethra, or anus (Figure 33-4■). Genital and anal warts are diagnosed primarily by their clinical appearance. In women, the growths may appear in the vagina or on the cervix and be apparent only during a pelvic examination. HPV may also be diagnosed by examination of cervical cells taken during a Pap smear or cervical biopsy.

Several subtypes of HPV are strongly associated with cervical dysplasia (abnormal cervical cells) and an increased risk of cervical cancer. HPV is also associated with a higher risk of vaginal, vulvar, penile, and anal cancers.

Potential complications of genital warts include destruction of normal tissue or obstruction of the urethra. Instruct the patient to report difficulty urinating or symptoms of urinary retention or infection. The virus can also rarely be transmitted to the fetus during pregnancy or delivery. The lesions enlarge during pregnancy and may obstruct the

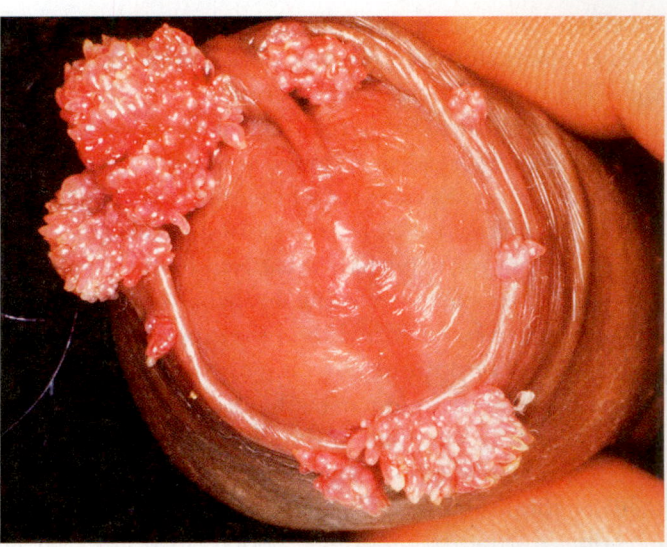

Figure 33-4. ■ Genital warts (condylomata acuminata) on the penis. (Source: Biophoto Associates/Science Source.)

birth canal, necessitating cesarean delivery. Infants infected with HPV can develop respiratory papillomatosis, a chronic respiratory condition. Stress the importance of telling the woman's regular health care provider about the infection.

COLLABORATIVE CARE
Vaccination

Gardasil is a vaccine that provides immunity against several types of HPV that cause genital warts and cervical cancer. The series of three injections over 6 months is recommended for girls and boys aged 11 and 12 years, before the age when they are more likely to be exposed to HPV. The vaccine is also recommended for previously unvaccinated people up to age 26 years, when the immune response is still optimal. However, people are sexually active into old age, so while early immunization is recommended, the vaccine is available to people of any age (CDC, 2013).

Treatment

Genital warts on the vulva, perineum, or penis can be treated with a topical agent (podophyllin resin) applied directly to the warts. This treatment is done in the physician's office, with the patient returning weekly until the warts are gone.

Genital warts may be removed by cryotherapy, electrocautery, or surgical excision. Carbon dioxide laser surgery is increasingly used to remove extensive warts.

NURSING CARE

In addition to the general nursing care for patients with an STI (see the section on chlamydia), the patient with genital warts needs pretreatment teaching if the warts are to be removed.

Emphasize the need for the patient and infected partners to return for regular treatment and abstain from sexual relations until lesions have resolved and to use condoms to prevent reinfection.

clinicalALERT

Stress the importance of annual Pap smears for female patients with HPV because of the increased risk for cervical cancer.

Gonorrhea

Gonorrhea, also known as *GC* or *clap,* is the most common reportable communicable disease in the United States. The rate of gonorrhea infection among African Americans is significantly higher than in non-Hispanic Whites. Among women, 15- to 19-year-olds have the highest rate of infection, whereas among men, 20- to 24-year-olds have the highest rate.

PATHOPHYSIOLOGY AND MANIFESTATIONS

Gonorrhea is caused by *Neisseria gonorrhoeae,* a gram-negative diplococcus. Its incubation period is 2 to 8 days. Gonorrhea is transmitted by direct sexual contact and during delivery as the neonate passes through the birth canal.

The organism initially targets the cervix and the male urethra. Without treatment, the disease spreads to other organs. In men, gonorrhea can cause acute, painful inflammation of the prostate, epididymis (Figure 33-5■), and periurethral glands and can lead to sterility. In women, it can cause PID, endometritis, salpingitis, and pelvic peritonitis. In the neonate, gonorrhea can infect the eyes, nose, or anorectal region.

Manifestations of gonorrhea in men include dysuria and serous, milky, or purulent urethral discharge. Some men also develop regional lymphadenopathy. Some men and most women have no symptoms until the disease is advanced. When manifestations of gonorrhea are present in women, they include dysuria, urinary frequency, or abnormal vaginal discharge.

COLLABORATIVE CARE

Drug resistance is becoming a problem with gonorrhea. Treatment of gonorrhea is directed toward eradicating the organism and any coexisting disease (see Table 33-1 for medications), preventing reinfection, and preventing spread of the disease.

Diagnostic Tests

In men, the diagnosis of gonorrhea can usually be confirmed by obtaining a smear of urethral discharge. Cultures are not necessary unless Gram stains of smears are negative despite

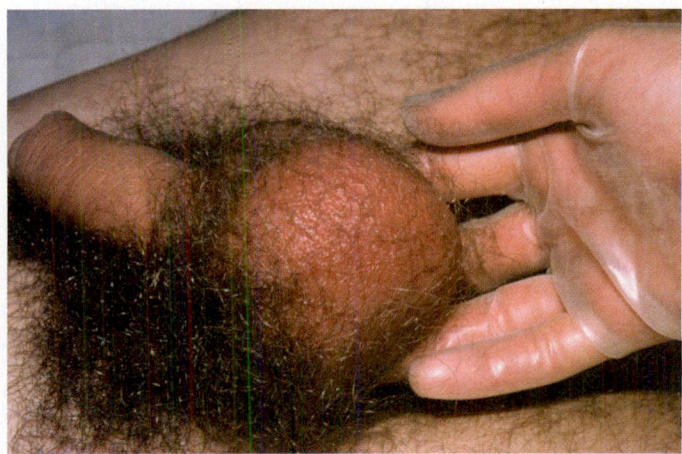

Figure 33-5. ■ Acute epididymo-orchitis caused by gonorrhea. (Source: © Wellcome Image Library/Custom Medical Stock Photo.—All rights reserved.)

typical clinical symptoms of gonorrhea. In women, cultures of cervical discharge are necessary to confirm the diagnosis of gonorrhea. Because cultures require 24 to 48 hours for confirmation, treatment is usually begun on a presumptive diagnosis.

People with gonorrhea are often infected with another STI. For this reason, the patient and his or her partners are tested for other STIs, such as syphilis, chlamydia, and possibly HIV.

NURSING CARE

Review Box 33-3 for areas to assess with patients who have STIs. Also review nursing care as described under chlamydia at the beginning of this chapter and the Nursing Care Plan provided here.

Emphasize the importance of taking the entire prescribed antibiotic dose as directed. Encourage referral of sexual partners for evaluation and treatment. Stress the need to abstain from all sexual contact until the patient and partners are cured of the disease, and instruct to use a condom to avoid transmitting or contracting infections in the future. Emphasize the need for a follow-up visit 4 to 7 days after treatment is completed to ensure that the infection has been cured.

NURSING CARE PLAN
Patient With Gonorrhea

Janet Cirit, a 33-year-old legal secretary, is unmarried and dating a man named Jim Adkins. Ms. Cirit visits her gynecologist because her periods have become irregular and she is having pelvic pain and abnormal vaginal discharge. Recently, she developed a sore throat, and the pelvic pain is keeping her awake at night.

Assessment

In the gynecologist's office, the nurse obtains a complete history, including questions about menstrual periods, pain associated with urination or sexual intercourse, urinary frequency, most recent Pap smear, birth control method, history of STI and drug use, and types of sexual activity. Ms. Cirit reports her symptoms and indicates that she is taking oral contraceptives for birth control so she and Mr. Adkins do not use a condom during sexual relations.

Physical examination reveals both pharyngeal and cervical inflammation and lower abdominal tenderness. Ms. Cirit's temperature is 98.5°F (37.0°C). She is not pregnant. Diagnostic tests are positive for gonorrhea and negative for chlamydia. WBC is slightly elevated, indicating possible salpingitis. Because Mr. Adkins has been Ms. Cirit's only sexual partner, it is clear that he needs to be treated as well.

Nursing Diagnosis

The following nursing diagnoses are identified for Ms. Cirit:

- *Acute Pain* related to the infectious process
- *Situational Low Self-Esteem* related to shame and guilt of having an STI
- *Ineffective Sexuality Patterns* related to impaired relationship and fear of reinfection

Expected Outcomes

The expected outcomes are that Ms. Cirit will:

- Report relief of pelvic pain.
- Verbalize an understanding of the cause and transmission of gonorrhea.
- Verbalize that she will insist her partner use condoms during future sexual activity.

Planning and Implementation

The following interventions are planned and implemented during care of Ms. Cirit:

- Administer ceftriaxone IM as ordered and document.
- Discuss feelings and concerns about the diagnosis of gonorrhea.
- Emphasize relationship of STI to behavior, not cleanliness or self-worth.
- Help identify ways to talk with a future sexual partner about condom use.

Evaluation

During her follow-up visit, Ms. Cirit states that she is feeling much better and sleeping well at night since the pain has ended. She has ended her relationship with Mr. Adkins and is considering joining a health club in the hope of increasing her level of fitness and perhaps meeting someone new.

Critical Thinking in the Nursing Process

1. What signs might have caused Ms. Cirit to suspect that Mr. Adkins had gonorrhea?
2. How are Ms. Cirit's signs and symptoms related to the infectious process of gonorrhea?
3. How might Ms. Cirit convince a future sexual partner to use condoms during sexual activity without spoiling the romantic aspect?

Note: Discussion of Critical Thinking questions appears on the companion website.

Syphilis

Syphilis is a complex systemic STI that, if not treated appropriately, can lead to blindness, paralysis, mental illness, cardiovascular damage, and death. Penicillin has significantly reduced the incidence of syphilis. The current rate of infection is increasing, especially among men who have sex with men. See Box 33-1 for more details. Incidence is higher among African Americans, American Indians, and Alaska Natives than among non-Hispanic Whites. Syphilis infection rates are highest in the South and in many urban centers, but the rate of infection is increasing in the western region of the United States.

Syphilis often occurs with one or more other STIs, such as HIV or chlamydia.

PATHOPHYSIOLOGY AND MANIFESTATIONS

Syphilis is caused by a spirochete, *Treponema pallidum*, which may infect almost any body tissue or organ. It is transmitted from open lesions during any sexual contact (genital, oral–genital, or anal–genital). The organism can survive for days in fluids. It may also be transmitted by infected blood or other body fluids such as saliva. The average incubation period is 20 to 30 days. Once it has entered the system, *T. pallidum* spreads through the blood and lymphatic system. Congenital syphilis is transferred to the fetus through the placental circulation.

Syphilis is characterized by three clinical stages: primary, secondary, and tertiary, with an extended period of latency between the last two stages. Each stage has characteristic clinical manifestations.

Primary Syphilis

The primary stage of syphilis is characterized by the appearance of a painless ulcer called a **chancre** (Figure 33-6■) at the site of inoculation (genitals, anus, mouth, breast, finger). Regional lymph nodes (e.g., inguinal nodes) may also be swollen. The chancre appears 3 to 4 weeks after the infectious contact. In women, a genital chancre may go unnoticed, disappearing within 4 to 6 weeks. In both primary and secondary stages, syphilis is highly infectious, even if no symptoms are evident.

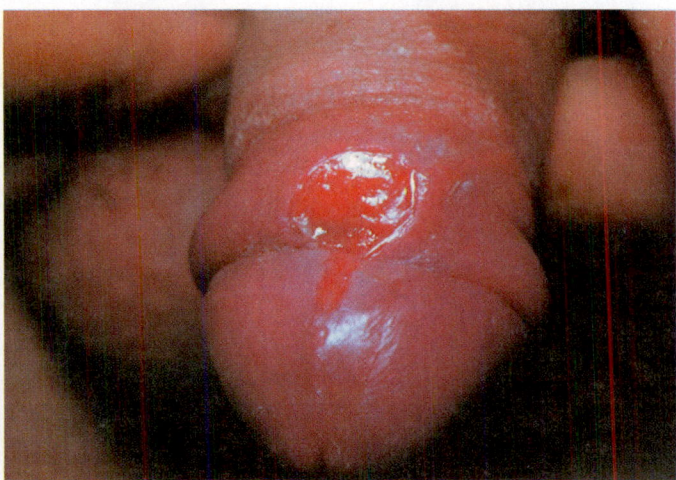

Figure 33-6. ■ Chancre of primary syphilis on the penis. (Source: © SPL / Custom Medical Stock Photo—All rights reserved.)

Secondary Syphilis

Manifestations of secondary syphilis may appear any time from 2 weeks to 6 months after the initial chancre disappears. These symptoms can include a skin rash, especially on the palms of the hands (Figure 33-7 ■) or soles of the feet; mucous patches in the oral cavity; sore throat; generalized lymphadenopathy; condyloma lata (flat, broad-based papules, unlike the pedunculated structure of genital warts) on the labia, anus, or corner of the mouth; flulike symptoms; and alopecia (absence of hair) in random spots on the scalp. These manifestations generally disappear within 2 to 6 weeks.

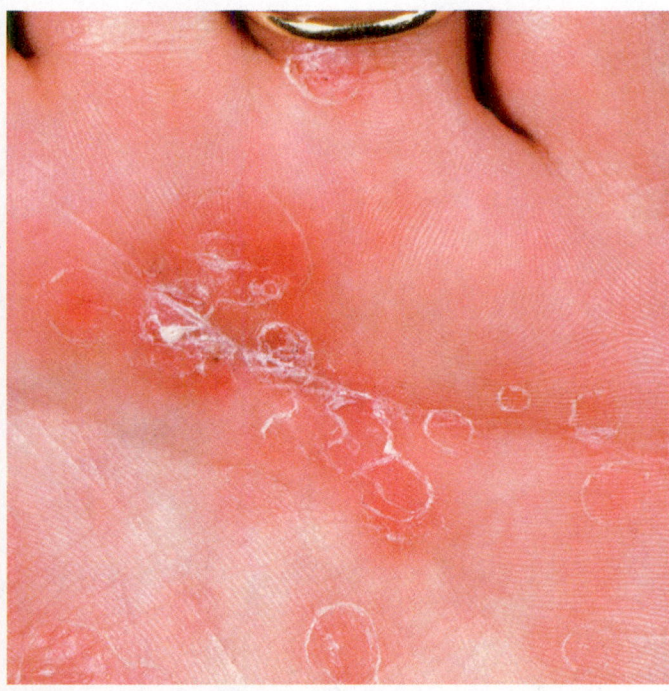

Figure 33-7. ■ Palmar rash of secondary syphilis. (Source: Biophoto Associates/Science Source.)

Latent-Stage Syphilis

The latent stage of syphilis can last up to 50 years. During this stage, no symptoms of syphilis are apparent, and the disease is not transmissible by sexual contact. It can be transmitted by infected blood, however. All prospective blood donors are screened for syphilis. In two-thirds of all cases, the latent stage persists without further complications. Unless treated, the remaining one-third of infected people progress to late-stage or tertiary syphilis. The latent stage is shortened in people with HIV disease.

Tertiary Syphilis

Tertiary syphilis can be manifested in two different ways. *Benign late syphilis* is characterized by localized infiltrating tumors (*gummas*) in skin, bones, and liver (Figure 33-8 ■). This form of tertiary syphilis generally responds promptly to treatment. A *diffuse inflammatory response* that involves the central nervous system and the cardiovascular system has a more insidious onset. Although the disease can still be treated at this stage, much of the cardiovascular and central nervous system damage is irreversible.

COLLABORATIVE CARE

As with other STIs, the goals of treatment for syphilis are to inactivate the spirochete and educate the patient about how to prevent reinfection or further transmission. In addition, patients should be screened for chlamydial infection and advised to have an HIV test.

Diagnostic Tests

The following tests are widely used to diagnose syphilis:

■ The *VDRL (Venereal Disease Research Laboratory)* and *RPR (rapid plasma reagin)* become positive about 4 to 6 weeks after infection. Because these tests are not specific, additional tests may be necessary.

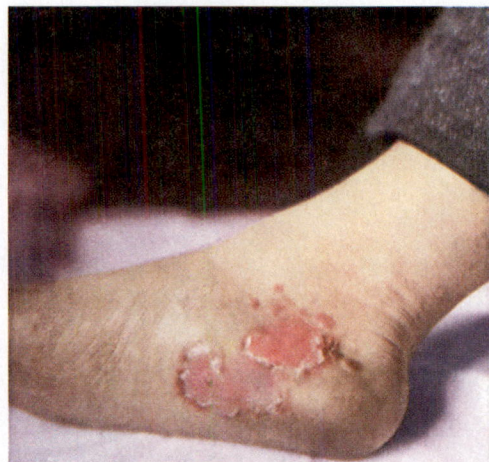

Figure 33-8. ■ Painful localized tumor of the skin (also occurs in liver and bone) called *gumma* of tertiary syphilis. (Source: Double Vision / Science Source.)

- The *FTA-ABS (fluorescent treponemal antibody absorption)* test is specific for *T. pallidum* and can be used to confirm VDRL and RPR findings.
- *Immunofluorescent staining* or *dark-field microscopy* can be used to identify the presence of *T. pallidum* in a specimen obtained from a chancre or by aspirating a lymph node.

NURSING CARE

The nursing assessment, diagnoses, interventions, and evaluation for a patient with syphilis are similar to that for a patient with chlamydia discussed earlier in this chapter. In addition, see the Clinical Reasoning Care Map at the end of the chapter for an opportunity to plan care for a patient with syphilis.

CONTINUITY OF CARE

Early symptoms of syphilis resolve with or without treatment. Teach patients that syphilis is a chronic disease that can be spread to others even when no symptoms are evident.

There is even a phase of the disease when the symptoms are expected to disappear. Stress the importance of (1) taking all prescribed medications, (2) referring all sexual partners for evaluation and treatment, (3) abstaining from all sexual contact for a minimum of 1 month after treatment, and (4) using a condom to avoid transmitting or contracting infections in the future. Emphasize the need for follow-up testing at 3 and 6 months for patients with primary or secondary syphilis and at 6 and 12 months for those with late-stage disease. Discuss integrating safer sex practices into the patient's lifestyle to prevent future episodes of STIs.

Note: The references and resources for all chapters have been compiled at the back of the book.

Chapter Review

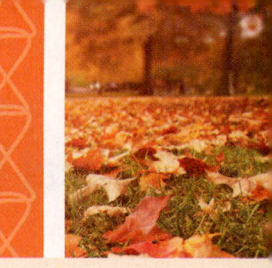

KEY POINTS

- **Concept:** Any infection transmitted by sexual contact, including vaginal, oral, and anal intercourse, is referred to as a sexually transmitted infection (STI), also known as a sexually transmitted disease (STD).
- **Concept:** Every sexually active person, and even some people who are not, are at risk for STIs.
- The risk for contracting an STI is directly related to lifestyle. Teach all patients to use safer sex practices such as abstinence, mutual monogamy with an uninfected partner, and barrier protection during sexual relations.
- **Concept:** The most effective form of protection against STIs, as well as the recommendation of the CDC, is the latex condom, and there are good alternatives (polyurethane condom) for people who are allergic to latex.
- Many STIs such as chlamydia, gonorrhea, and syphilis can be effectively treated with single-dose antibiotic therapy. Others, such as genital herpes and genital warts, are chronic viral infections that can be managed but not cured.
- HPV infection significantly increases a woman's risk for cervical cancer. Recommend that all women with HPV have annual Pap tests for early detection of cervical cancer.
- Gardasil is an immunization for several strains of HPV. The recommended schedule is that all girls and boys should be immunized at 11 or 12 years of age.
- Many STIs such as syphilis, gonorrhea, and other less common diseases must be reported to state and federal agencies.
- Screening and treatment of the patient's partner is necessary to prevent reinfection during or after treatment for an STI.
- Complications of STIs can include PID and problems of fertility, as well as systemic responses (e.g., cardiovascular and neurologic manifestations of tertiary syphilis).
- **Concept:** Nurses may contract herpes infections of the skin (called *herpetic whitlow*) or of the eyes by contact with the herpes-shedding lesions of patients. Some STIs are transmitted by blood-borne pathogens. Standard Precautions protect nurses from infection.

PEARSON NURSING STUDENT RESOURCES

Find additional materials at **nursing.pearsonhighered.com**.

Clinical Reasoning Care Map

Caring for a Patient With Syphilis
NCLEX-PN® Focus Area: Reduction of Risk Potential

Case Study: Eddie Kratz, a 22-year-old man, shares a small apartment with Marla Jones, who is 7 months pregnant with his child. Although he intends to marry Ms. Jones before the baby is born, he has continued a previous relationship with a woman named Justine Simpson. His sexual activities with Ms. Simpson have increased in frequency as Ms. Jones's pregnancy has advanced. Recently, Mr. Kratz has noticed a swelling in his groin and a sore on his penis.

Nursing Diagnosis: Risk for Injury, infection

COLLECT DATA

Subjective	Objective
_____	_____
_____	_____
_____	_____
_____	_____
_____	_____
_____	_____

Does this present a threat to the patient's safety?

If yes, the priority intervention to address this threat would be:

_____

Nursing Care

_____

_____

_____

_____

_____

_____

_____

_____

Interprofessional team members to include when planning care:

_____

How would you document this? _____

_____

Compare your answers and documentation to those provided on the companion website.

Data Collected
(use only those that apply)

- Regional lymphadenopathy
- Having unprotected sex with Ms. Jones and Ms. Simpson
- Syphilitic chancre on the shaft of the penis
- Believes that Ms. Jones is not having sex with anyone else but is not sure
- ELISA results negative for HIV
- Dark-field analysis of chancre exudate confirms syphilis

Nursing Interventions
(use only those that apply;
list in priority order)

- Teach the importance of treatment to the health of their infant.
- Explain the need for follow-up testing in 3 and 6 months.
- Refer Mr. Kratz and Ms. Jones for counseling about the impact of the disease on their relationship.
- Send reminders for follow-up at 3- and 6-month intervals.
- Administer and document IM injection of benzathine penicillin G as ordered.
- Discuss importance of abstaining from sexual activity until patient and partners are cured, and using condoms to prevent reinfection.
- Provide a copy of STI prevention checklist.
- Notify Ms. Jones and Ms. Simpson of need for testing.

NCLEX-PN® Exam Preparation

1 A woman has been diagnosed with a chlamydia infection. As the nurse explains her prescription to her, she states, "I don't need any medicine. I feel fine." The nurse's response is based on the knowledge that:
1. the body often clears chlamydia by itself.
2. fever and dysuria usually accompany chlamydia in women.
3. patients with STIs often deny symptoms.
4. if untreated, chlamydia can progress to PID.

2 Using azithromycin (Zithromax) instead of doxycycline (Vibramycin) can improve compliance primarily because Zithromax:
1. has fewer side effects.
2. is taken in a single oral dose.
3. costs less.
4. tastes better.

3 An 18-year-old college student has just been diagnosed with a first episode infection of herpes simplex type 2. She says, "I can't believe this. I'm so embarrassed. How could he? I trusted him." Your initial response is:
1. "You can't believe this has happened to you."
2. "You need to use barrier protection so you do not pass this on."
3. "You can't trust what these college guys tell you."
4. "We will provide you with prescriptions that will make you more comfortable."

4 Teaching the patient with genital warts (HPV) should include:
1. measures to relieve pain.
2. how to take acyclovir.
3. avoiding acidic foods.
4. importance of regular Pap testing.

5 A patient with newly diagnosed gonorrhea also undergoes testing for HIV infection. She asks why this is necessary. The nurse's response is based on the knowledge that:
1. it is likely the patient has been using injection drugs, increasing her risk for HIV.
2. gonorrhea is an opportunistic infection that usually does not occur in patients with intact immune systems.
3. other STIs including HIV often coexist in patients with gonorrhea.
4. both gonorrhea and HIV occur more frequently in women who have sex with other women.

6 A patient with syphilis is reluctant to take the prescribed antibiotic. The nurse stresses which of the following as the most important reason for treating this disease?
1. Treatment prevents transmission of the disease to others.
2. Treatment promotes healing of the initial chancre without secondary infection.
3. Treatment ensures that the disease will not progress to tertiary syphilis.
4. Treatment prevents reinfection of the patient.

7 A patient has been diagnosed with syphilis. Which allergy would necessitate a change in the usual treatment?
1. Penicillin
2. Eggs
3. Acyclovir
4. Sulfa

8 A male patient diagnosed with genital herpes says that he does not want to use condoms because they are uncomfortable. He asks if there is another way to prevent spreading this infection to his partners. The nurse responds that:
1. it is only necessary to use condoms when lesions are visible.
2. condoms should be used for all sexual relations, especially from the onset of prodromal symptoms until all lesions are healed.
3. it is not necessary to use condoms if sexual relations are limited to oral sex during outbreaks of the infection.
4. practicing mutual monogamy will prevent spreading this infection to others even if a condom is not used.

9 Which comment by a 20-year-old indicates the patient needs additional teaching about STIs?
1. "My boyfriend needs to see his doctor for treatment also."
2. "If we only engage in oral sex, we cannot transmit STIs."
3. "Use of latex condoms can prevent most STIs."
4. "Some STIs cannot be cured, but symptoms can be treated."

10 Important nursing responsibilities related to the sexually transmitted infections of syphilis and gonorrhea are: **Select all that apply.**
1. reporting cases of the infection to state agencies.
2. discussing the need for cesarean delivery with infected women.
3. emphasizing the need to identify and treat infected partners.
4. teaching safer sex practices to infected patients and their partners.
5. stressing the importance of abstinence until the infection is cleared.

Answers and rationales for Review Questions appear in Appendix I.

Thinking Strategically About . . .

You are an LPN/LVN working on a women's surgical unit of a large hospital. You are assigned to care for the following patients from 0700 to 1500.

- Rachel is a 44-year-old African American divorced mother of two teenage girls. She is moderately overweight, and smoked one pack of cigarettes daily until 4 years ago. Rachel's mother, two aunts, and one sister have had breast cancer. Her mother and one aunt died before age 45. Rachel has had annual mammograms and clinical breast examination and has done monthly BSE for the past 4 years. Two weeks ago, Rachel discovered a thickened area in her left breast. A biopsy revealed invasive lobular carcinoma.

  Rachel underwent a modified radical mastectomy and axillary node dissection yesterday without incident. She has a Shirley drain in place with a large dressing. IV fluids are being given by infusion pump.

  Rachel is debating whether to have reconstructive breast surgery. Her oncologist has recommended 6 months of chemotherapy, and she is concerned about side effects. She is afraid that treatment will limit her ability to keep her job and continue to meet her daughters' needs. She worries that breast cancer is the family legacy and that it will happen to her girls.

- Allison is a 33-year-old, European American, single, school teacher. She has a history of ovarian cysts since she was 16 years old. She was treated with contraceptive hormones by a variety of routes of administration. These treatments lasted a few months to a year and then became ineffective. She has undergone eight abdominal surgeries to drain ovarian cysts and cut adhesions. There are no further options for prevention of the ovarian cysts. Allison also has a history of three small strokes due to thromboemboli. She has been taking Plavix daily for 4 years.

  Even though Allison is single and has no children, she has decided to have an abdominal hysterectomy with bilateral salpingo-oophorectomy. She should be admitted to the surgical unit from the recovery room at approximately 1100.

- Evelyn, a 23-year-old European American secretary, has a history of PID as a result of chlamydia infection at age 17. Evelyn and her husband have been trying to have a baby. They were excited two weeks ago when Evelyn had a positive pregnancy test. She had an appointment to see her nurse practitioner next week. Yesterday morning she developed severe left lower quadrant pain and a small amount of vaginal bleeding. Evelyn's husband took her to the emergency room where a ruptured fallopian tube was diagnosed. Evelyn was bleeding into her pelvic cavity, resulting in a hemorrhage emergency. Laparoscopic surgery was performed and Evelyn is anticipating discharge today.

CRITICAL THINKING

- Explain the reason to monitor Rachel closely for breast cancer.
- Explain the significance of Allison's long-term use of Plavix and her surgical risk.

- Explain the relationship between Evelyn's PID caused by chlamydia and the ectopic pregnancy.

PRIORITIES IN NURSING CARE

- What care will you provide for Rachel and Evelyn before 1100 so you will have time to observe Allison closely after her abdominal surgery?

MANAGEMENT OF CARE

- Rachel requests a shower after breakfast. Explain your response to her request including any follow-up you will need to do.
- If Allison is admitted to the women's surgical unit at 1100, use the following table to identify what times you will provide routine assessments and care.

1100	1130	1200	1230	1300	1330	1400	1430	1500

- Identify criteria Evelyn must meet so she can be discharged.

PATIENT TEACHING

- What knowledge deficits does the nurse need to address with Rachel?
- What teaching needs to be provided to Evelyn before she is discharged?

CULTURAL CARE STRATEGIES

Many surgeons are reluctant to do a hysterectomy on a young woman who has not had children. Explain why Allison's doctor might have agreed to her surgical treatment.

DOCUMENTING AND REPORTING

At 1300, Allison's vital signs are 74/42, T 96.8, P 120, R 28. Her skin is cool. She rates her pain at 7–8 and she has been using the morphine PCA every 10 minutes. Oxygen saturation is 92% with O_2 at 2 L/min.

- What nursing interventions can you implement in this situation without the direction of the RN?
- What report will you give to the RN?

Document your findings at 1300.

Note: Discussion of Unit questions appears on the companion website.

UNIT IX
Disrupted Endocrine Function

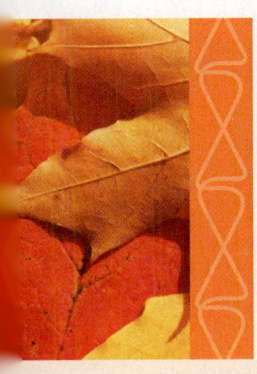 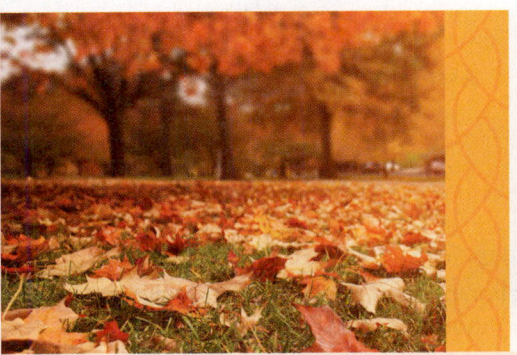 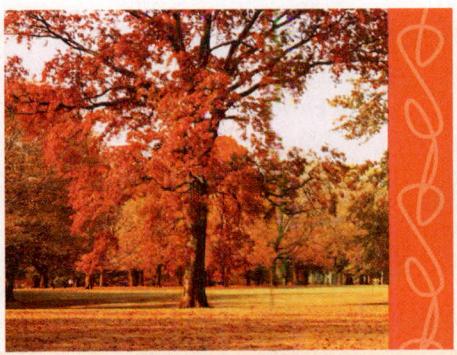 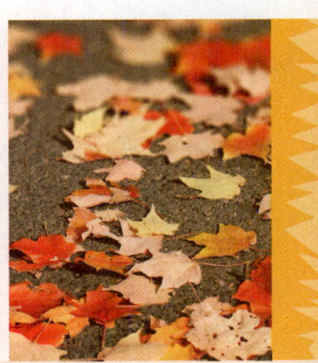

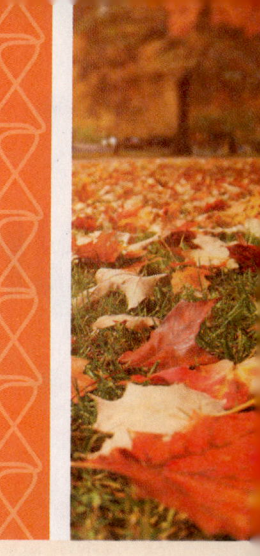

CHAPTER 34

The Endocrine System and Assessment

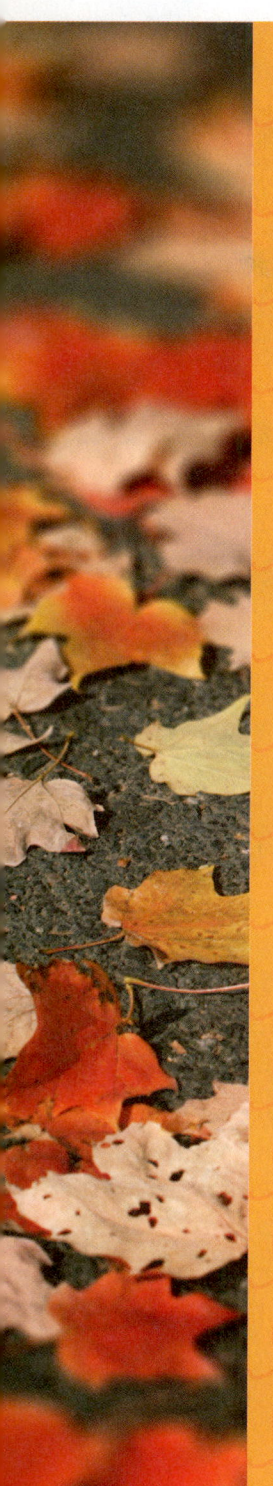

BRIEF OUTLINE

Structure and Function of
    the Endocrine System

Assessment

APPLIED LEARNING OUTCOMES

After completing this chapter, you will be able to:

1. Describe the structure and function of the organs of the endocrine system, including the pancreas, and the actions of hormones secreted by the endocrine glands.
2. Collect subjective and objective assessment data for patients with endocrine disorders.
3. Monitor the results of common tests used to diagnose endocrine disorders and report abnormal findings.
4. Implement nursing responsibilities for patients undergoing common diagnostic tests with endocrine disorders.

KEY TERMS

The key terms are defined on the pages listed below.

exophthalmos, 884	glycogenolysis, 883	hyperglycemia, 883
gluconeogenesis, 883	hormones, 882	hypoglycemia, 883

Key Concept The endocrine system plays a key role in regulating physiological processes such as growth, development, and metabolism through the release of hormones. Homeostasis is dependent on a balanced level of each type of hormone. Disorders of the endocrine system usually result from either too much or too little hormone production.

This chapter includes a discussion of the endocrine system and the pancreas. The primary function of the endocrine system is to regulate the body's internal environment. Hormones secreted by endocrine glands regulate growth, reproduction and sex differentiation, metabolism, and fluid and electrolyte balance. The endocrine system helps the body adapt to constant changes in the internal and external environment.

The pancreas produces hormones needed for the metabolism of carbohydrates, proteins, and fats. The pancreatic hormones insulin and glucagon are responsible for maintaining blood glucose levels.

Structure and Function of the Endocrine System

The major endocrine organs are the hypothalamus, pituitary gland, thyroid gland, parathyroid glands, thymus (see Chapter 11 for discussion on thymus gland), adrenal glands, pancreas, and gonads (reproductive glands) (Figure 34-1■). Table 34-1■ lists the endocrine organs with their hormones and the primary hormone action. This chapter focuses on the hypothalamus, pituitary gland, thyroid

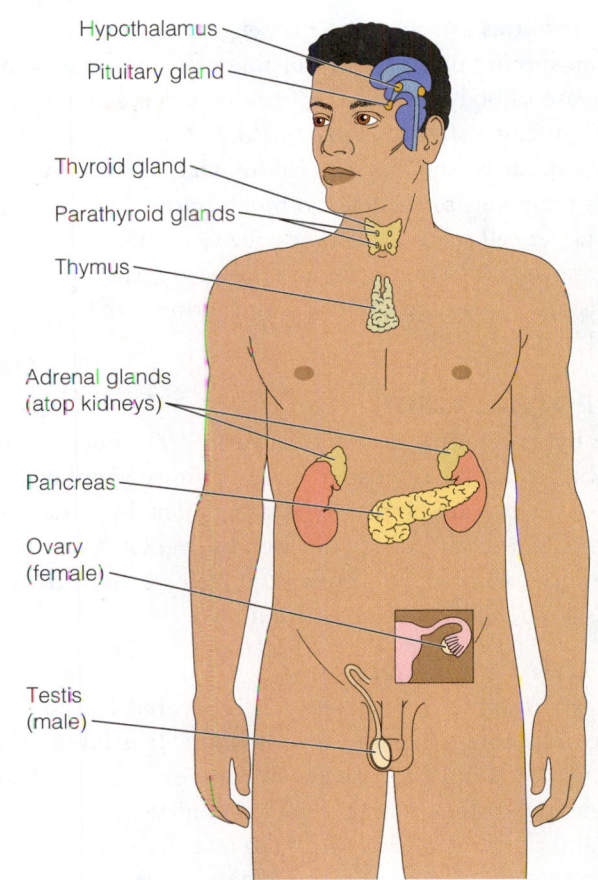

Figure 34-1. ■ Location of the major endocrine glands.

gland, parathyroid glands, and adrenal glands. The pancreas is discussed after the endocrine organs. Specific information about the gonads is presented in Chapters 31 and 32.

TABLE 34-1	Endocrine Organs, Hormones, and Functions	
ORGAN	**HORMONE**	**FUNCTION**
Anterior pituitary	Growth hormone (GH)	Promotes growth of body tissues
	Thyroid-stimulating hormone (TSH)	Stimulates secretion of thyroid hormone
	Adrenocorticotropic hormone (ACTH)	Stimulates adrenal cortex to secrete glucocorticoids
	Melanocyte-stimulating hormone	Controls pigmentation of the skin
	Follicle-stimulating hormone (FSH)	Stimulates ovary development and egg and sperm production
	Luteinizing hormone (LH)	Stimulates ovulation and secretion of sex hormones in males and females
	Prolactin	Stimulates breast milk production
Posterior pituitary	Antidiuretic hormone (ADH)	Promotes water retention by kidneys
	Oxytocin	Promotes uterine contraction and release of milk
Thyroid gland	Thyroid hormone (TH)	Increases metabolic rate
	Calcitonin	Lowers serum calcium levels
Parathyroid gland	Parathyroid hormone (PTH)	Increases serum calcium levels
Adrenal cortex	Glucocorticoids (cortisol)	Stimulates gluconeogenesis and increases blood glucose level; anti-inflammatory response
	Mineralocorticoids (aldosterone)	Regulates blood volume and electrolytes
Adrenal medulla	Epinephrine and norepinephrine	Increases sympathetic nervous system response to stress

Hormones are chemical messengers of the body. They act on specific target cells, causing either an increase or a decrease in body function. Hormone levels are regulated by a process called *negative feedback.* Negative feedback acts similar to the way the thermostat in a house regulates temperature. When too much hormone is released, the target cell sends back a message to reduce its hormone release. If too little hormone is released, the target cell sends back a message to increase the hormone to the normal level.

HYPOTHALAMUS

The hypothalamus is located in the brain between the cerebrum and the brainstem. The pituitary gland and the hypothalamus are physically attached. The hypothalamus controls anterior pituitary function by regulating temperature, fluid volume, and growth. It also responds to pain, pleasure, hunger, and thirst stimuli.

PITUITARY GLAND

The pituitary gland (*hypophysis*) is located in the skull beneath the hypothalamus of the brain. It is often called the *master gland* because its hormones regulate many different body functions. The pituitary gland has two parts: the anterior lobe (*adenohypophysis*) and the posterior lobe (*neurohypophysis*). The anterior lobe secretes six different hormones (Figure 34-2■). The posterior lobe releases antidiuretic hormone (ADH) and oxytocin.

THYROID GLAND

The thyroid gland is shaped like a butterfly and sits on either side of the trachea. This gland has two lobes connected by a structure called the *isthmus.* The thyroid gland needs an adequate supply of iodine to secrete thyroid hormone (thyroxine [T_4] and triiodothyronine [T_3]), which increases metabolism. The thyroid gland also secretes *calcitonin,* a hormone that decreases excess calcium levels in the blood.

PARATHYROID GLANDS

The parathyroid glands (usually four to six) are embedded on the posterior lobes of the thyroid gland. They secrete parathyroid hormone (*PTH,* or *parathormone*). PTH secretion increases when calcium levels in the plasma fall, and it decreases phosphorous levels. Normal levels of vitamin D are necessary for PTH to apply this effect on bone and kidneys.

ADRENAL GLANDS

The two adrenal glands are pyramid-shaped organs that sit on top of the kidneys. Each gland consists of two parts: an outer cortex and an inner medulla.

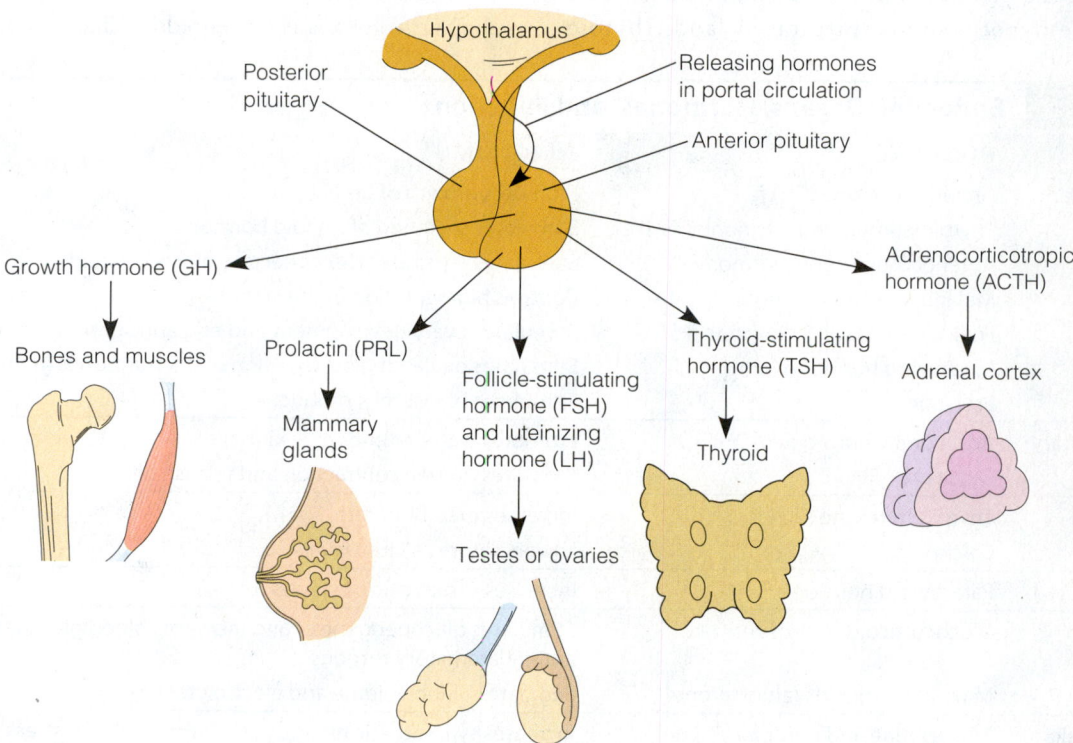

Figure 34-2. ■ Actions of the major hormones of the anterior pituitary.

Adrenal Cortex

The adrenal cortex secretes several different hormones called *corticosteroids.* They are classified into two groups, *glucocorticoids* and *mineralocorticoids,* and are essential to life. *Cortisol,* a glucocorticoid, affects carbohydrate metabolism. Its primary effect is to raise blood glucose levels by increasing gluconeogenesis, increasing lipolysis from fatty acids, and breaking down protein in times of stress. Glucocorticoids also have an anti-inflammatory response and affect emotions. The primary mineralocorticoid, *aldosterone,* maintains normal salt and water balance through its action on the kidneys. It is released when blood volume or blood pressure falls below normal levels and acts to save sodium and water, which in turn raises blood volume and pressure. Small amounts of *androgens* (sex hormones) are also released by the adrenal cortex.

Adrenal Medulla

The adrenal medulla produces two hormones (*catecholamines*): epinephrine (also called adrenaline) and norepinephrine (or noradrenaline). Both catecholamines constrict blood vessels and increase the heart rate and the force of heart contractions. Epinephrine and norepinephrine are released during times of stress and initiate the *fight-or-flight response.*

PANCREAS

The primary organ involved in diabetes mellitus is the pancreas. It is located behind the stomach between the spleen and the duodenum. The pancreas serves two major functions: (1) Acini cells secrete digestive enzymes into the duodenum, and (2) the *islets of Langerhans* release insulin and glucagon into the bloodstream. To prevent **hyperglycemia** (high blood glucose level) or **hypoglycemia** (low blood glucose level), these hormones must be in balance.

Insulin

Beta cells in the islets of Langerhans produce insulin. Insulin's primary function is to regulate blood glucose levels. This is accomplished through several mechanisms. Insulin eases the active transport of glucose into muscle and fat cells, where it is used as an energy source and for cell functions. It facilitates fat formation, inhibits the breakdown and movement of stored fat, and helps move amino acids into cells for protein synthesis. Glucose unused by the cells is stored in the liver and muscle cells as glycogen. If there is excess glucose at this point, it is converted into fat and stored as adipose tissue. Insulin release increases when blood glucose levels rise and decreases when blood glucose levels fall. When a person eats food, insulin levels rise in minutes, peak in 30 to 60 minutes, and return to baseline in 2 to 3 hours.

Glucagon

Alpha cells in the islets of Langerhans produce glucagon. Glucagon prevents blood glucose from decreasing below a certain level when the body is fasting or is between meals. It

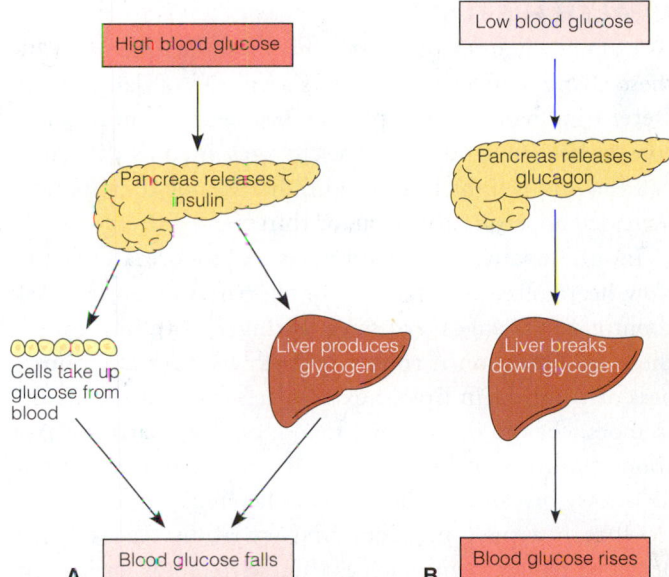

Figure 34-3. ■ Action of insulin and glucagon on blood glucose levels. (**A**) High blood glucose is lowered by insulin release. (**B**) Low blood glucose is raised by glucagon release.

makes new glucose (**gluconeogenesis**), converts glycogen into glucose in the liver and muscles (**glycogenolysis**), and prevents excess glucose breakdown. Usually, glucagon is released when blood glucose falls below about 70 mg/dL. The primary function of glucagon is to decrease glucose oxidation and increase blood glucose.

Blood Glucose Homeostasis

Normal blood glucose is maintained in healthy people primarily through the balancing actions of insulin and glucagon (Figure 34-3■). However, other hormones (known as counterregulatory hormones) can help increase blood glucose levels during periods of hypoglycemia, stress, growth, or increased metabolic demand. Counterregulatory hormones include cortisol, epinephrine, and growth hormone.

Definitions of normal blood glucose levels vary in clinical practice, depending on the laboratory that performs the assay. In this text, normal blood glucose is defined as 70 to 110 mg/dL.

Assessment

Key Concept   Because hormones affect all body tissues and organs, manifestations of endocrine dysfunction are often nonspecific. This makes assessment of endocrine function more difficult.

A health assessment interview to identify problems with the endocrine system may be part of a general health screening or may be focused on a specific complaint. The nurse collects data about the patient's medical, family, social, and personal history and also conducts a physical examination.

HEALTH HISTORY

Ask about changes in energy level and fatigue and how these changes affect the patient's activities of daily living. Determine whether the patient has become more sensitive to heat or cold. Explore changes such as difficulty swallowing; weight loss or gain; diarrhea or constipation; increased appetite, urination, or thirst; and salt cravings.

Inquire about high blood pressure, abnormally fast or slow heart rate, palpitations, or shortness of breath. Ask about vision changes, excessive tearing, or swelling around the eyes. Question if the patient experiences any numbness or tingling in lips or extremities, nervousness, hand tremors, change in memory, mood, or sleep patterns. Ask about thinning or loss of hair, dry or moist skin, brittle nails, easy bruising, or slow wound healing.

Obtain a past medical history about taking any hormone replacements such as thyroid, steroids, or insulin. Determine whether the patient has had previous surgery, chemotherapy, or radiation, especially of the neck area, as well as brain surgery or a head injury. It is important to consider genetic influences on the health of the adult. Inquire about endocrine disorders in immediate family members, including the family members' age of onset and gender. Ask the patient about a family history of diabetes mellitus, diabetes insipidus, goiter, growth problems, hypertension, and obesity. Obtain a sexual history regarding changes in sexual function or secondary sex characteristics. Ask women about problems with infertility, pregnancy, menstruation, or menopause.

PHYSICAL EXAMINATION

Begin by assessing the patient's general appearance and documenting vital signs, height, and weight. Note extremely short height. Assess skin color, temperature, texture, and moisture. Observe for rough, dry or smooth, flushed skin. Note bronze color over knuckles, purple striae over the abdomen, and bruising. Inspect the lower extremities for lesions and any signs of healing. Assess the texture and condition of hair and nails. Observe for thinning and loss of hair, as well as thick or thin, brittle nails. Look for excessive hair growth on face, chest, or abdomen.

Inspect the face for shape and symmetry. Inspect the eyes for the presence of **exophthalmos** (forward protrusion of the eyeballs). Determine visual acuity. Inspect the neck for visible signs of masses. Gently palpate the thyroid gland from behind the patient. Palpate only one side of the neck at a time (Figure 34-4 ■).

Assess for increased size of hands and feet, trunk obesity, and thin extremities. Inspect men for *gynecomastia*, enlargement of the breasts. Evaluate muscle strength and deep tendon reflexes. Assess for Chvostek sign and Trousseau sign

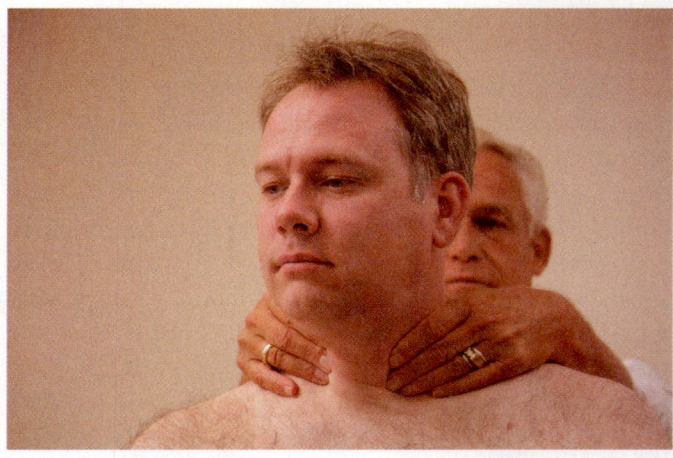

Figure 34-4. ■ Palpating the thyroid gland from behind the patient. (Patrick Watson, Pearson Education.)

(see Chapter 7, Figure 7-17). Assess the patient's ability to sense touch, hot/cold, and vibration in the extremities.

Auscultate lungs for adventitious sounds and heart for extra heart sounds. Palpate hands and feet for edema.

THE OLDER ADULT

There is an unclear relationship between aging and endocrine function. Aging causes fibrosis of the thyroid gland and decreases production of T_3 (triiodothyronine), reducing the older adult's metabolic rate and contributing to weight gain. The adrenal cortex decreases in weight, but the overall level of cortisol remains the same. The most common endocrine disorders in older adults include thyroid abnormalities and an increased risk for diabetes mellitus.

clinicalALERT

Fatigue, constipation, and mental impairment may be misdiagnosed as normal aging changes rather than being related to endocrine dysfunction.

DIAGNOSTIC TESTS
Laboratory Tests

To diagnose an endocrine disorder, several laboratory tests are used. Table 34-2 ■ lists these tests, their normal values, what the test measures and its significance, and any nursing implications for the test. Other nonspecific laboratory tests are done to give cues about endocrine disorders. A chemistry panel, which includes serum electrolytes such as sodium, potassium, calcium, and phosphate, and blood glucose levels monitor disease progression. For instance, serum sodium and blood glucose levels increase in Cushing syndrome but decrease in Addison disease. In diabetics,

TABLE 34-2	Common Laboratory Tests for Endocrine Disorders		
TEST	**NORMAL ADULT VALUES**	**EXPLANATION**	**NURSING IMPLICATIONS**
Pituitary			
Growth hormone (GH)	Less than 5 ng/mL for men Less than 10 ng/mL for women	Used to evaluate growth hormone excess or deficiency. Increased values indicate acromegaly.	The patient must be fasting, well rested, and not physically or emotionally stressed.
Water deprivation test	1–5 pg/mL	Increased level indicates SIADH, decreased level means diabetes insipidus.	Tell patient to withhold food, fluids, and smoking from midnight until the test.
Thyroid			
Thyroid-stimulating hormone (TSH)	0.35–5.5 mcg/mL	This is the most sensitive test to evaluate thyroid function by measuring pituitary TSH secretion.	No fluid restriction is required. Avoid shellfish several days before test.
T_3 T_4	80–200 ng/dL 4.5–11.5 mcg/dL	Measures triiodothyronine (T_3) and thyroxine (T_4) to evaluate thyroid function. Increased level indicates hyperthyroidism and decreased reflects hypothyroidism.	
Parathyroid			
Serum calcium	9–11 mg/dL	This test evaluates parathyroid function and calcium metabolism.	Fasting not required; however, the test is part of a chemistry panel in which fasting is required.
Serum phosphate	2.5–4.5 mg/dL	It measures serum phosphate. Increased levels in both tests indicate hyperparathyroidism; decreased levels indicate hypoparathyroidism.	
Adrenal			
Cortisol	8 to 10 a.m.: 5–23 mcg/dL 4 to 6 p.m.: 3–13 mcg/dL	This test measures total serum cortisol, which evaluates adrenal cortex function. Levels are increased in Cushing syndrome and decreased in Addison disease.	Tell patient not to eat or drink and to rest 2 hours before blood is drawn. Explain that two blood samples are drawn—one at 8 to 10 a.m., the other at 4 to 6 p.m.
Aldosterone	4–30 ng/dL sitting position Less than 16 ng/dL supine position	Levels are drawn to diagnose hyperaldosteronism.	Ask patient to be in supine position for 1 hour before test is drawn.
Urinary 17-ketosteroids (17-KS)	5–15 mg/24 hr for men 5–25 mg/24 hr for women	17-KS are metabolites of testosterone, which are released from adrenal cortex. Levels increase with Cushing syndrome and decrease in Addison disease.	Teach patient about 24-hour urine collection, which must be iced or refrigerated during collection.
Pancreas			
Fasting blood glucose	70–110 mg/dL	This test measures circulating blood glucose level. Increases are seen in diabetes mellitus, acute pancreatitis; decreased level is seen in Addison disease.	This test is done while fasting.
Glycosylated hemoglobin (HbA1c)	5.5%–7%	Test used to measure glucose control during the previous 3 months. Levels are increased in newly diagnosed or poorly controlled diabetic. It is not used to diagnose diabetes mellitus.	No fasting is required.
Two-hour oral glucose tolerance test (OGTT)	Less than 125 mg/dL	Determines the level of glucose 2 hours after drinking 75 g of glucose. Glucose level should return to premeal levels, but in diabetics, the level is higher than 200 mg/dL.	Patient is NPO for 12 hours before test. Then patient must drink entire 100 g of glucose and not eat anything else until blood is drawn.

(continued)

TABLE 34-2	Common Laboratory Tests for Endocrine Disorders *(continued)*		
TEST	**NORMAL ADULT VALUES**	**EXPLANATION**	**NURSING IMPLICATIONS**
Urine glucose	Negative	Estimates the amount of glucose in urine, which should be negative.	Collect a fresh urine sample; stagnant urine may alter test results.
Urine ketones	Negative	Measures ketones excreted in urine from incomplete fat metabolism. Positive result means lack of insulin or diabetic ketoacidosis.	Some drugs may interfere with both test results.
Urine test for microalbumin	0.2–2.0 mg/dL	Microalbumin is the earliest indicator for development of diabetic nephropathy. Elevated microalbumin levels increase the risk for end-stage renal disease.	Collect a fresh urine sample and send to laboratory for analysis.

TABLE 34-3	Imaging Studies	
TEST	**EXPLANATION AND PURPOSE**	**NURSING IMPLICATIONS**
Magnetic resonance imaging (MRI)	MRI uses a super magnet and radiofrequency signals to elicit a response from hydrogen nuclei. As a result, tumors of the pituitary gland and hypothalamus can be identified.	Assess for any metallic implants such as pacemakers or body piercings. If present, notify the imaging physician. Inform patient of the need to lie still during the test. Remove transdermal medication patches unless otherwise ordered; replace the patch after the MRI. Ask if the patient is pregnant; if so the test *must* not be performed. Ask about claustrophobia; if a problem, the patient may need to take a relaxing medication prior to the MRI.
Computed tomography (CT) scan	Specialized radiographic procedures that produce computer-generated images with significantly more detail than standard x-rays allow. May be done with or without contrast media. Abdominal CT is used to detect tumors of the adrenal gland and pancreas.	If contrast dye is used, ask about allergies to iodine and seafood. Patient must lie still during the procedure.
Thyroid scan	Iodine-125 is injected IV. A scanner passes over the thyroid making a graph of the radiation emitted. "Cold spots," which do not take up the I-125, indicate malignancy.	Ask about allergies to iodine and seafood. Patient may need to withhold thyroid drugs or medications containing iodine for weeks before the study. No fasting is needed.
Radioactive iodine (RAI) uptake test	Iodine-131 or I-125 (capsule or liquid form) is given and then the thyroid is scanned three times. Increased uptake indicates Graves disease; decreased uptake means hypothyroidism.	Patient fasts for 8 hours before the test but can eat 1 hour after radioiodine capsule or liquid has been taken. Thyroid drugs or medications containing iodine are held for weeks before the study.

BOX 34-1	DOCUMENTATION OF ENDOCRINE ASSESSMENT

Patient: A 48-year-old female has an appointment with her family physician to rule out a diagnosis of hyperthyroidism. She states she eats all the time but has lost 10 lb in the past 2 months. She has a family history of Graves disease.

Assessment Note: BP 168/90, P 110, R 26. Alert and oriented but cannot sit still and keeps fidgeting with purse. Hands visibly shake. Has difficulty focusing on interview questions. Appears exhausted. Eyeballs protrude and cannot close eyelids completely. Denies blurry vision. Patchy hair loss with thin, brittle nails noted. Skin warm, smooth, and moist. C/O heart palpitations, denies chest pain. Bowel tones hyperactive.

serum cholesterol and triglyceride levels are drawn to evaluate the risk of developing atherosclerosis.

For additional information about assessment techniques, see Chapter 5. See Box 34-1 ■ for an example of an endocrine assessment.

Imaging Techniques

The imaging techniques used to diagnose endocrine disorders are noninvasive. Table 34-3 ■ summarizes these diagnostic procedures and their nursing implications.

Note: The references and resources for all chapters have been compiled at the back of the book.

Chapter Review

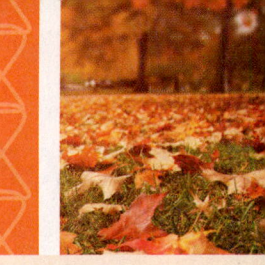

KEY POINTS

- **Concept:** The endocrine system plays a key role in regulating physiological processes such as growth, development, and metabolism through the release of hormones. Homeostasis is dependent on a balanced level of each type of hormone. Disorders of the endocrine system usually result from either too much or too little hormone production.
- The endocrine system consists of six major organs, anterior and posterior pituitary, thyroid, parathyroids, adrenal medulla and cortex, pancreas, and gonads. The pituitary gland is considered the "master gland" because its hormones regulate numerous body functions.
- Hormone regulation throughout the body is done through a process called negative feedback.
- Blood glucose homeostasis is maintained by the actions of insulin and glucagon. The counterregulatory hormones of cortisol, epinephrine, and growth hormone increase blood glucose during times of stress.

- **Concept:** Because hormones affect all body tissues and organs, manifestations of endocrine dysfunction are often nonspecific. This makes assessment of endocrine function more difficult.
- It is important to ask about endocrine disorders in immediate family members, including the family members' age of onset and gender. Common genetic endocrine disorders include diabetes mellitus, hypothyroidism, Graves disease, and Addison disease.
- Older adults are more prone to developing thyroid disorders and diabetes mellitus type 2.

PEARSON NURSING STUDENT RESOURCES

Find additional materials at **nursing.pearsonhighered.com**.

NCLEX-PN® Exam Preparation

1 Which one of the following hormones is responsible for promoting water retention by the kidneys?
1. Antidiuretic hormone (ADH)
2. Adrenocorticotropic hormone (ACTH)
3. Epinephrine
4. Aldosterone

2 The nurse is teaching the patient about a scheduled thyroid scan. Which of the following points should be emphasized to the patient?
1. "You should fast for 8 hours before this test is done."
2. "It is important to lie very still while the contrast dye is being injected."
3. "The radioactive dye is harmless to you."
4. "Two blood samples will be drawn, one in the morning and the other in the evening."

3 A patient is admitted to the medical unit with hyperparathyroidism. What laboratory test finding should the nurse expect to find?
1. Increased T_3 and T_4
2. Decreased protein
3. Decreased aldosterone
4. Increased serum calcium

4 What diagnostic test should the nurse anticipate being ordered to diagnose a patient with possible diabetes mellitus?
1. Water deprivation test
2. Glycosylated hemoglobin (Hb A1c)
3. 17-Ketosteroids
4. Serum cortisol

5 To assess the presence of the Chvostek sign in a patient, the nurse should:
1. palpate the thyroid gland.
2. inflate a blood pressure cuff above the antecubital space.
3. have the patient extend the leg when the hip is flexed.
4. tap the finger on the patient's cheek.

Answers and rationales for Review Questions appear in Appendix I.

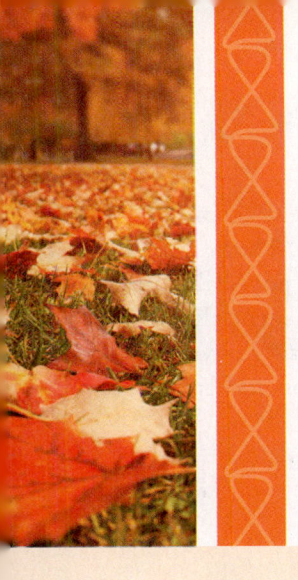

CHAPTER 35

Caring for Patients With Endocrine Disorders

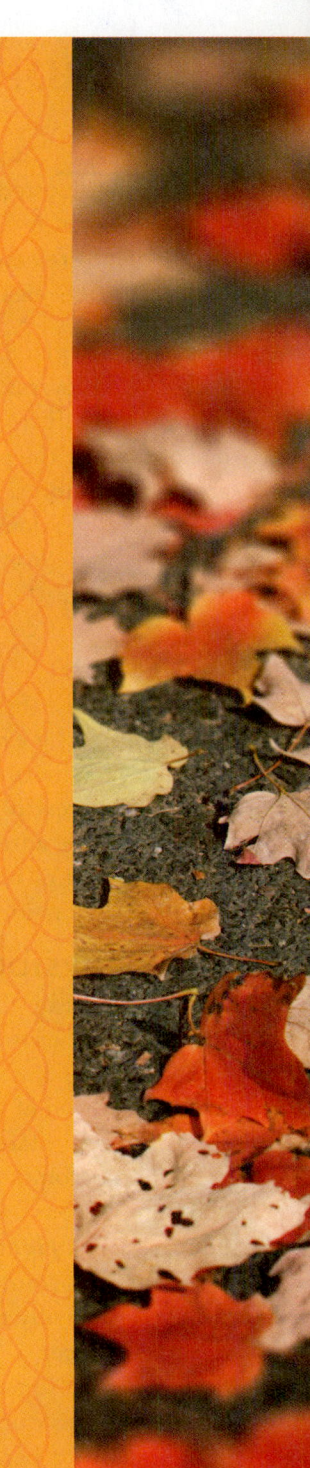

BRIEF OUTLINE

DISORDERS OF THE PITUITARY GLAND
Disorders of the Anterior Pituitary Gland
Disorders of the Posterior Pituitary Gland
DISORDERS OF THE THYROID GLAND

Hyperthyroidism
Hypothyroidism
Cancer of the Thyroid
DISORDERS OF THE PARATHYROID GLANDS
Hyperparathyroidism
Hypoparathyroidism

DISORDERS OF THE ADRENAL GLANDS
Cushing Syndrome
Addison Disease
Disorder of the Adrenal Medulla

APPLIED LEARNING OUTCOMES

After completing this chapter, you will be able to:

1. Describe the pathophysiology of the common disorders of the pituitary, thyroid, parathyroid, and adrenal glands.

2. Contrast the manifestations resulting from hypersecretion and hyposecretion of hormones from the pituitary, thyroid, parathyroid, and adrenal glands.

3. Identify laboratory and diagnostic tests used to diagnose endocrine disorders and report abnormal findings.

4. Administer medications and treatments knowledgeably and safely as ordered for patients with endocrine disorders.

5. Implement preoperative and postoperative nursing care for a patient undergoing either a subtotal thyroidectomy or an adrenalectomy.

6. Use the nursing process to care for patients with disorders of the pituitary, thyroid, parathyroid, and adrenal glands.

7. Reinforce teaching guidelines for patients receiving long-term hormonal replacement therapy.

KEY TERMS

The key terms are defined on the pages listed below.

SPECIAL FEATURES

The primary function of the endocrine system is to regulate the body's internal environment. Hormones secreted by endocrine glands regulate growth, reproduction and sex differentiation, metabolism, and fluid and electrolyte balance. The endocrine system helps the body adapt to constant changes in the internal and external environment.

When *hypersecretion* (increase) or *hyposecretion* (decrease) in hormone production occurs, individuals develop an endocrine disorder. Patients with endocrine disorders require care for multiple problems. They often face exhausting diagnostic tests, changes in physical appearance and emotional responses, and permanent alterations in lifestyle. Nursing care focuses on meeting physical and emotional needs and providing education and emotional support for the patient and family.

DISORDERS OF THE PITUITARY GLAND

Key Concept The pituitary gland, consisting of the anterior and posterior lobes, in conjunction with the hypothalamus, is the master gland of the body. The anterior lobe releases seven hormones, whereas the posterior lobe releases two hormones.

The pituitary gland's hormones affect the thyroid, adrenal cortex, ovary, uterus, mammary glands, testes, and kidneys. Disorders result from an excess or deficient production of one or more of the pituitary hormones. Pituitary disorders are less common than other endocrine disorders but can cause diverse, serious problems.

Disorders of the Anterior Pituitary Gland

Hyperpituitarism (hyperfunction of the pituitary gland) is characterized by excess production and secretion of one or more of its hormones. It most commonly causes oversecretion of growth hormone (GH). *Hypopituitarism* (hypofunction of the anterior pituitary gland) results in a lack of production of one or more of the gland's hormones. Pituitary tumors usually cause both conditions.

PATHOPHYSIOLOGY

GH, produced by the anterior lobe of the pituitary gland, stimulates the growth of the epiphyseal plates of the long bones and is necessary for skeletal and muscle growth. Excess secretion of GH before puberty and the closure of the epiphyseal plates results in *gigantism*. A person with gigantism becomes abnormally tall, often over 7 feet, but body proportions are normal. This condition is rare today due to early diagnosis and treatment. *Dwarfism* (short stature) occurs from inadequate production of GH during childhood. Usually the dwarf has normal body proportions and intelligence.

Acromegaly (enlargement of bones and connective tissue) develops during adulthood from hypersecretion of GH. Usually, a benign, slow-growing tumor (pituitary adenoma) stimulates the hypersecretion. Because epiphyseal plates close by adulthood, long bones cannot increase in length. However, other bones and connective tissue continue to grow at a very slow rate, causing an enlarged forehead and protruding jaw. With overgrowth of tissue in the hands and feet, patients require larger shoes, gloves, and rings. Manifestations can take as long as 10 to 15 years to develop. If untreated, complications such as hypertension, diabetes mellitus, cardiac enlargement, and cardiac failure can develop.

COLLABORATIVE CARE

Diagnosis is confirmed by MRI and CT scans, which show pituitary gland enlargement along with elevated serum GH levels. Acromegaly, caused by a pituitary adenoma, is treated by *transsphenoidal hypophysectomy* (surgical removal of the pituitary gland through an incision in the roof of the mouth) or irradiation of the pituitary tumor. Drug therapy with octreotide (Sandostatin) decreases GH production but does not reduce tumor size.

NURSING CARE

Nursing care of patients with anterior pituitary disorders focuses on helping them cope with body image changes and with anxiety about an unknown future after surgery. (See Chapter 38 for nursing care after cranial surgery.) Patients should be taught about the need for lifelong hormone replacement therapy.

Disorders of the Posterior Pituitary Gland

Disorders of the posterior pituitary are caused by too much or too little antidiuretic hormone (ADH). ADH regulates total body water by acting on the kidney to retain or release water. Receptors in the hypothalamus control the release of ADH in response to serum *osmolarity* (concentration of particles in the blood). When serum osmolarity increases (*hyperosmolarity*), ADH secretion increases, and renal water is reabsorbed, which decreases urine output. *Hyposmolarity* suppresses the release of ADH, so urine output increases.

DIABETES INSIPIDUS

Diabetes insipidus (DI) is a condition that results from ADH insufficiency. There are two types: neurogenic and nephrogenic. *Neurogenic DI* can result from damage to the pituitary gland after head injury or cranial surgery. *Nephrogenic DI* occurs when the kidneys fail to respond to ADH secretion. This condition may be due to renal failure.

Deficient supply of ADH causes a urinary output of 5 to 15 L per day. The patient develops *polydipsia* (excessive thirst). If unable to replace the water loss, the patient becomes dehydrated. Patients who cannot maintain an adequate fluid intake are at risk for hypernatremia. Additional manifestations are listed in Box 35-1■.

COLLABORATIVE CARE

Diagnosis of syndrome of inappropriate ADH secretion or DI is based on presence of manifestations, risk factors, and results of the water deprivation test (see Chapter 34, Table 34-2). Neurogenic DI is treated by giving additional fluids by mouth or 0.45% normal saline intravenous infusions to replace the lost water. In addition, patients are given ADH replacement therapy with desmopressin (DDAVP) or vasopressin (Pitressin). Sodium restriction and thiazide diuretics may be ordered for patients with nephrogenic DI.

NURSING CARE

PRIORITIZING NURSING CARE

Nursing care for the patient with DI focuses on managing fluid and electrolyte problems and replacing ADH.

Deficient Fluid Volume Related to Deficiency of ADH

Expected outcome: Will have balanced intake and output.

BOX 35-1	**MANIFESTATIONS OF DIABETES INSIPIDUS**

- Extreme thirst
- Polyuria (5 to 15 L/day)
- Urine specific gravity less than 1.005
- Very pale urine
- Weakness
- Dehydration:
  - Tachycardia
  - Poor skin turgor
  - Dry mucous membranes

- Monitor intake and output, urine specific gravity, vital signs, skin turgor, and neurologic function every 1 to 2 hours during the acute phase. Monitor daily weight. *Frequent monitoring alerts the nurse to potential complications.*
- Provide adequate fluids. Be sure patient is alert and can reach them. *Patient needs to drink extra fluids to reduce or prevent dehydration.*
- Give DDAVP or vasopressin as ordered. *DDAVP is given as oral tablets or via a metered-dose inhaler, and vasopressin is given as an injection to replace low ADH levels in neurogenic DI. Monitor for side effects of pounding headache and abdominal cramps, which indicate water intoxication.*
- Give thiazide diuretics and low-sodium diet as ordered. *Thiazide diuretics may increase the kidneys' responsiveness to vasopressin. A low-sodium diet is given to reduce hypernatremia.*

CONTINUITY OF CARE

Teach the patient with DI about the disease process, medications, and the need for follow-up care. Instruct patients who need long-term ADH replacement therapy in how to self-administer DDAVP intranasally. Teach them the manifestations of water excess from an overdosage of DDAVP.

SYNDROME OF INAPPROPRIATE ADH SECRETION

Syndrome of inappropriate ADH secretion (SIADH) is a condition that results from excess production of ADH. This disorder may be caused by lung tumors, pancreatic cancer, head injury, pituitary surgery, or the use of barbiturates, anesthetics, or diuretics.

Excess production of ADH leads to water retention, hyponatremia (low serum sodium levels), and serum hyposmolarity (excess dilution of the blood). The common manifestations of SIADH are decreased urine output and concentrated urine. Neurologic symptoms appear as brain cells swell. No edema is present because water is distributed between the intracellular and extracellular spaces. Manifestations are found in Box 35-2■.

clinicalALERT

Older adults are at an increased risk for developing hyponatremia. Because geriatric patients take many medications and have decreased kidney function, they should be monitored carefully for signs of SIADH.

COLLABORATIVE CARE

SIADH is treated by correcting the underlying cause and limiting fluid intake. Diuretics such as furosemide (Lasix) are given along with fluid restriction. Demeclocycline (Declomycin), a tetracycline antibiotic, is used to promote urine production in patients with SIADH. Patients with severe hyponatremia may receive intravenous hypertonic saline.

BOX 35-2	MANIFESTATIONS OF SIADH

- Headache
- Anorexia
- Muscle weakness
- Decreased urine output
- Dark yellow, concentrated urine
- Urine specific gravity greater than 1.030
- Weight gain without edema

- Monitor daily weight and auscultate lungs. *These measures detect the presence of excess fluid buildup.*
- Restrict fluids as ordered, usually less than 1,000 mL/day. *Fluid restriction prevents further dilution of the plasma and sodium levels.*
- Provide frequent mouth care. *Oral rinses or sucking on hard candy keeps mucous membranes moist.*
- Give diuretics as ordered. *Diuretics will help to decrease fluid volume excess.*
- Institute seizure precautions. *Dangerously low serum sodium levels can lead to seizures.*

NURSING CARE

Excess Fluid Volume Related to Excess Production of ADH

Expected outcome: Will have balanced intake and output.

- Monitor intake and output, vital signs, and level of consciousness frequently. *Frequent monitoring alerts the nurse to potential complications.*

CONTINUITY OF CARE

Teach patients with SIADH about the disease process and the importance of maintaining water restriction at home. They must know how to weigh themselves daily, and they should learn the number of milliliters of fluid in common beverage containers and how to measure urine output. Discuss medication action and side effects as needed, and stress the need for follow-up care.

DISORDERS OF THE THYROID GLAND

Key Concept Thyroid disorders occur most often in women. These disorders change body image and alter energy levels, creating fatigue or exhaustion.

Increased or decreased production of thyroid hormone (TH) affects the cardiovascular, gastrointestinal (GI), and neuromuscular systems, as well as the metabolic rate. Hyperthyroidism and hypothyroidism are among the most common endocrine disorders.

memoryALERT

Elevated TH levels *increase* metabolism; reduced TH levels *decrease* metabolic rate.

Hyperthyroidism

Hyperthyroidism (*thyrotoxicosis*) is caused by an excess production of TH. It develops more often in women and older adults. The main disorders are Graves disease and thyroid crisis.

PATHOPHYSIOLOGY AND MANIFESTATIONS

Hyperthyroidism is caused by an autoimmune response, by excessive doses of thyroid medication, or by excess secretion of TSH from the pituitary gland. Whatever the underlying cause, increased levels of TH increase the metabolic rate. As individuals age, the increased metabolic rate places a strain on the cardiovascular system. If left untreated, this condition can result in cardiac dysrhythmias and eventual heart failure. With increased metabolism of carbohydrates, proteins, and lipids, the person has an increased appetite, yet loses weight. If the condition is prolonged, nutritional deficiencies occur. The multisystem manifestations of hyperthyroidism are shown in Figure 35-1■.

Graves Disease

Graves disease, the most common cause of hyperthyroidism, is an autoimmune disorder. It develops eight times more often in women under the age of 40 than in the general population.

Increased production of TH results in a characteristic enlargement of the thyroid gland (*goiter*) (Figure 35-2■) and a forward protrusion of the eyeball known as *exophthalmos* (Figure 35-3■). Often, the sclera is visible above the iris. The upper lids may be retracted, and the person has a characteristic unblinking stare. Exophthalmos is usually bilateral, but it may involve only one eye. Inability to close the eyelids completely over the protruding eyeballs increases the risk of corneal dryness, infection, and ulceration. The treatment of Graves disease does not reverse these eye changes.

Thyroid Crisis

Thyroid crisis (thyroid storm) is an extreme state of hyperthyroidism but is rare today. This disorder may result from untreated hyperthyroidism or from hyperthyroidism along

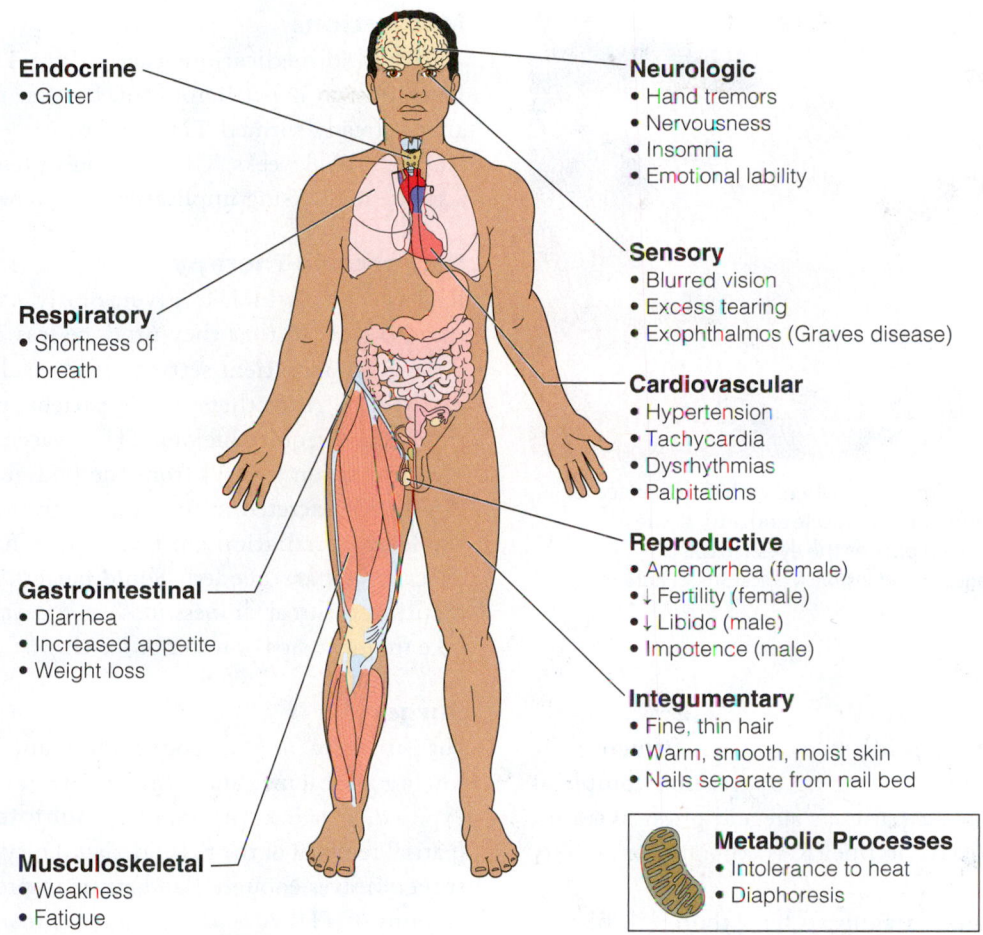

Endocrine
• Goiter

Respiratory
• Shortness of breath

Gastrointestinal
• Diarrhea
• Increased appetite
• Weight loss

Musculoskeletal
• Weakness
• Fatigue

Neurologic
• Hand tremors
• Nervousness
• Insomnia
• Emotional lability

Sensory
• Blurred vision
• Excess tearing
• Exophthalmos (Graves disease)

Cardiovascular
• Hypertension
• Tachycardia
• Dysrhythmias
• Palpitations

Reproductive
• Amenorrhea (female)
• ↓ Fertility (female)
• ↓ Libido (male)
• Impotence (male)

Integumentary
• Fine, thin hair
• Warm, smooth, moist skin
• Nails separate from nail bed

Metabolic Processes
• Intolerance to heat
• Diaphoresis

Figure 35-1. ■ Multisystem effects of hyperthyroidism.

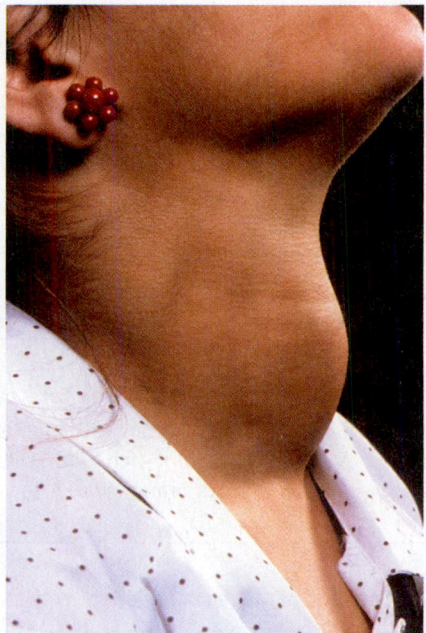

Figure 35-2. ■ Individual with enlargement of the thyroid gland (goiter). (Source: © Wellcome Image Library/Custom Medical Stock Photo.)

with a stressor, such as an infection, untreated diabetic ketoacidosis, physical or emotional trauma, or thyroid surgery. Thyroid crisis is a life-threatening condition and requires immediate medical attention.

Oversecretion of TH results in a sudden, rapid rise in metabolic rate. Manifestations include high fever (over 102°F), tachycardia, and hypertension. Restlessness and tremors are common, progressing to confusion, delirium, coma, and seizures.

Rapid treatment of thyroid crisis is essential to preserve life. The patient is admitted to the intensive care unit for close monitoring and treatment. Antithyroid medications such as propylthiouracil (Propyl-Thyracil) are given to reduce TH production. An external cooling blanket and acetaminophen are used to lower the severe hyperthermia. Cardiovascular and respiratory status is monitored closely throughout treatment.

clinicalALERT

Do not give aspirin during severe hyperthermia caused by thyroid crisis because it can increase TH levels.

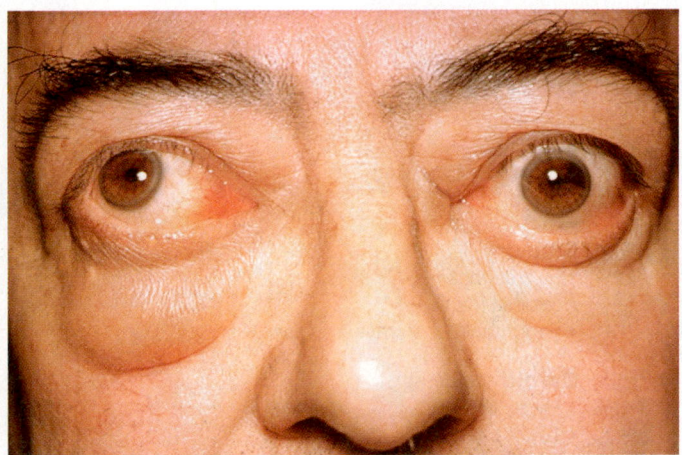

Figure 35-3. ■ Exophthalmos in a patient with Graves disease. This is caused by enlargement of muscle and fatty tissue surrounding the eye, which pushes the eyes outward. (Source: © Wellcome Image Library/Custom Medical Stock Photo.)

COLLABORATIVE CARE

Treatment of hyperthyroidism focuses on reducing the production of TH and preventing or treating complications. Depending on the patient's age and physical status, medications, radioactive iodine (RAI) therapy, or surgery may be used.

Hyperthyroidism is diagnosed by a thorough history and physical examination. In addition, the following laboratory tests can confirm a diagnosis: elevated serum T_3 and T_4 levels, decreased TSH levels, and increased RAI uptake.

Medications

Antithyroid medications that reduce TH production are given to treat hyperthyroidism. Because these drugs do not affect already-formed TH, therapeutic effects may not be seen for several weeks. The commonly prescribed drugs, their actions, and nursing implications are shown in Table 35-1■.

Radioactive Therapy

RAI (I-131), which is given orally, is used to destroy thyroid cells so that they produce less TH. Treatment is done in an outpatient setting, with results seen in about 6 to 8 weeks. After therapy, the patient may become hypothyroid and require lifelong TH replacement.

Elimination of RAI from the body takes about 2 to 3 days and is excreted in the urine, saliva, and feces. Because the level of radiation emitted is low, no radiation safety precautions are needed. Some patients may experience mouth and throat dryness for 2 to 3 days. Instruct them to take frequent sips of water or ice chips.

Surgery

For patients with large goiters that cause breathing or swallowing problems, and pregnant women who cannot be exposed to radiation therapy, a **subtotal thyroidectomy** (partial removal of the thyroid gland) may be indicated. This surgery leaves enough gland tissue to produce an adequate amount of TH. A *total thyroidectomy* (complete removal of the thyroid gland) is done to treat cancer of the thyroid, but the patient requires lifelong hormone replacement. Before surgery, the patient should be in as nearly a *euthyroid*

TABLE 35-1	Giving Medications Safely: Hyperthyroidism		
CLASS/DRUGS	**PURPOSE**	**NURSING IMPLICATIONS**	**PATIENT TEACHING**
Antithyroid drugs ■ Methimazole (Tapazole) ■ Propylthiouracil (Propyl-Thyracil)	Antithyroid drugs inhibit TH production.	Give at the same time each day to maintain stable blood levels. Monitor for itching, rash, fever, nausea, loss of taste, and agranulocytosis. Monitor for hypothyroidism: bradycardia, fatigue, weight gain.	Take at the same time each day. Do not discontinue abruptly. If taking warfarin, report any signs of bleeding. Report signs and symptoms of hypothyroidism to the physician.
Iodine sources ■ Potassium iodide, saturated solution (SSKI) ■ Strong iodine solution (Lugol's solution)	Inhibits TH release. Decreases vascularity of thyroid gland to make surgery safer.	Ask about allergies to shellfish. Dilute in water or orange juice to disguise bitter taste. Monitor for bleeding if patient takes anticoagulants.	Take at the same time each day. Avoid drugs with iodine and limit iodine-rich foods. Dilute in water or orange juice.
Beta-adrenergic blockers ■ *Propranolol* (Inderal)	Relieves thyrotoxicosis (e.g., heat intolerance, palpitations, nervousness, and tremors).	Do not give to patients with asthma or heart disease. Monitor for side effects of bradycardia, fatigue, and weakness.	Teach patient how to check pulse. Notify the physician of side effects: bradycardia, fatigue, and weakness.

Note: Medications identified in *italics* are among the 200 most frequently prescribed drugs in the United States.

Care of the Patient Having a Subtotal Thyroidectomy

Preoperative Care

☑ Review standard preoperative care in Chapter 10.
☑ Give ordered antithyroid medications and iodine preparations.

Postoperative Care

☑ Review standard postoperative care in Chapter 10.
☑ Place the patient in a semi-Fowler's position; support head and neck with pillows.
☑ Monitor and report the following complications to the physician:

  ☑ *Hemorrhage.* Assess dressing and the back of the neck for bleeding. Assess tightness of dressing. Monitor blood pressure and pulse for symptoms of hypovolemic shock.
  ☑ *Respiratory distress.* Assess respiratory rate, rhythm, depth, and effort. Provide humidification. Have suction equipment, oxygen, and a tracheostomy set available for immediate use.
  ☑ *Laryngeal nerve damage.* Assess for the ability to speak aloud and hoarseness.
  ☑ *Tetany.* Assess for tingling of toes, fingers, and lips; positive Chvostek and Trousseau signs. Keep IV calcium gluconate or calcium chloride at the bedside.
  ☑ *Thyroid storm.* Assess for high fever, hypertension, and tachycardia.

(balanced thyroid) state as possible. This is done by giving antithyroid drugs to reduce hormone levels and iodine preparations to decrease the vascularity and size of the gland.

After surgery, the patient is monitored for five common complications: hemorrhage, respiratory distress, laryngeal nerve damage, tetany, and thyroid storm. The vascularity of the thyroid gland and neck tissues increases the risk of hemorrhage. Respiratory distress can develop from hemorrhage and edema, which compresses the trachea. The laryngeal nerve is located near the thyroid gland and can be damaged during surgery. The parathyroid glands are found in and near the thyroid gland. During surgery they may be damaged or removed accidentally, causing hypocalcemia and tetany. Handling of the thyroid gland during surgery may trigger thyroid storm.

Additional nursing care of the patient having a subtotal thyroidectomy is discussed in Box 35-3■.

NURSING CARE

PRIORITIZING NURSING CARE

The nurse must consider the multisystem effects of hyperthyroidism when planning nursing care for the patient with this disorder. Although each patient has different needs, the priority problems include altered cardiovascular function, imbalanced nutrition, fatigue, visual deficits, and body image disturbance.

HEALTH PROMOTION

Although hyperthyroidism is unpreventable, it is important to teach patients the importance of regular health care visits to monitor TH levels. Patients are taught the special measures they must follow when taking antithyroid medications.

ASSESSING

Assessment data collected by the nurse can help determine how much hyperthyroidism is interfering with the patient's life and can identify risk factors for complications (Box 35-4■). The following nursing diagnoses address the most common problems: Risk for Decreased Cardiac Output, Risk for Imbalanced Nutrition: Less Than Body Requirements, Fatigue, Risk for Injury: Corneal Abrasion, and Disturbed Body Image.

IDENTIFYING POTENTIAL COMPLICATIONS

Two primary complications may occur: thyroid storm and heart disease. Older patients with a prolonged history of thyrotoxicosis have an increased risk for developing heart failure.

DIAGNOSING, PLANNING, AND IMPLEMENTING
Risk for Decreased Cardiac Output

Expected outcome: Blood pressure returns to patient's baseline, pulse rate between 60 and 100, respiratory rate 16 to 20 with clear breath sounds.

Patients With Hyperthyroidism

Subjective Data

- Changes in appetite, diet, or weight
- Palpitations, chest pain, or shortness of breath
- Complaints of nervousness, fatigue, or insomnia
- Vision changes
- Changes in emotional status
- Past medical history of taking THs

Objective Data

- Measure blood pressure, pulse, respirations, and temperature.
- Check height and weight.
- Observe patient during interview for nervousness.
- Assess condition of nails and hair.
- Inspect neck for visible signs of masses.
- Inspect eyes for signs of exophthalmos.
- Palpate the skin for moisture.
- Monitor and report elevated TSH, T_3, and T_4 levels.

- Monitor blood pressure, pulse rate and rhythm, respiratory rate, and breath sounds. Assess for peripheral edema. *Increased heart rate and cardiac output increase the body's oxygen needs. Stress on the heart may result in hypertension, dysrhythmias, angina, and heart failure. Patients with a preexisting cardiovascular disorder are at a special risk.*
- Teach relaxation procedures. *Stress increases circulating catecholamines, which further increase cardiac workload.*

Risk for Imbalanced Nutrition: Less Than Body Requirements

Expected outcome: Weight remains stable at baseline.

- Assess patient's daily food intake. Weigh at the same time each day and report losses. *Assessing food intake determines whether food intake is adequate to meet patient's needs. The body's inability to meet metabolic demands results in weight loss. Regular monitoring detects continued weight loss.*
- Encourage patient to eat a high-calorie, high-protein diet in six small meals a day. *Increased metabolism causes the body to use protein for energy. Smaller, more frequent meals are easier for patients to increase their daily food intake. This diet can prevent weight loss and muscle breakdown.*
- Teach patient to avoid high-fiber foods and highly seasoned foods that increase peristalsis or cause diarrhea such as apple or prune juice. *Increased GI action or diarrhea decreases nutrient absorption.*

Fatigue

The increased metabolic rate robs the patient of energy. The patient may be unable to perform normal activities of daily living (ADLs) and may have difficulty concentrating.

Expected outcome: Can perform ADLs without excessive fatigue or shortness of breath.

- Take pulse and blood pressure before and after an activity. Note any shortness of breath. *This determines how much the patient's activity is affecting the cardiovascular and respiratory systems.*
- Provide rest periods between activities. *Rest is needed to prevent total energy depletion.*
- Provide back rubs or cool showers as well as a cool, quiet environment. *This promotes relaxation while decreasing nervous energy. A cool, quiet environment reduces stimuli and stressors.*

Risk for Injury: Corneal Abrasion

If the patient is unable to close the eyelids because of exophthalmos, corneal dryness may develop. Without intervention, this could lead to blurred vision or corneal ulceration.

Expected outcome: Remains free of corneal abrasion.

- Ask the patient about feelings of grittiness or eye pain. Assess for incomplete lid closure. *These are signs of corneal abrasion. Prompt intervention is needed to prevent corneal ulceration and loss of visual acuity.*

- Teach the patient measures to prevent eye injury and maintain visual acuity: using tinted glasses or shields as protection; using artificial tears to moisten the eyes; using cool, moist compresses to relieve irritation; and promptly reporting any pain or changes in vision. *These measures decrease the risk of injury, provide comfort, and decrease periorbital edema.*

clinicalALERT

Teach the patient to cover or tape the eyelids shut at night if they do not close and to sleep with the head of the bed elevated.

Disturbed Body Image

Patients with hyperthyroidism often experience an altered body image due to the physical changes found with this disorder. These changes frighten both the patient and family members.

Expected outcome: Will state willingness to accept physical changes.

- Encourage the patient to discuss feelings and ask questions about the illness and treatment. Provide reliable information, and clarify misconceptions. *Body image is very important to patients. They need to understand what is causing the physical changes and whether they will last forever.*
- Explain the effects of the illness on the patient's physical and emotional status. *Family members can be sources of support as the patient adapts to the illness. They must understand that changes in appearance and behavior may be disease related and can be controlled with treatment.*

MANAGING NURSING CARE

As appropriate and allowed by the designated duties and responsibilities of assistive personnel, the nurse may delegate nursing care activities such as obtaining daily weights and assisting with meals and ADLs for the patient with hyperthyroidism. Before assigning tasks such as taking vital signs in the immediate postoperative period after a thyroidectomy, ensure that the assistive personnel have a clear understanding of the importance of accuracy in measurement and of reporting decreased blood pressure as well as increased heart and respiratory rate and temperature.

EVALUATING

Evaluate the care for the patient with hyperthyroidism by collecting data about the patient's blood pressure, resting pulse, breath sounds, weight, and energy level. Identify whether the patient has any visual problems related to exophthalmos. If the patient had a thyroidectomy, determine that the patient can state an understanding of all potential complications.

DOCUMENTING

Documentation includes assessment of vital signs, weight, and relief of manifestations such as hand tremors, nervousness, weakness, and diarrhea. Identify and record the patient's understanding of teaching related to medications, diet, and need for rest and sleep.

CONTINUITY OF CARE

Patients with hyperthyroidism primarily require self-care at home. Individualized planning and teaching for home care are important nursing responsibilities. Teach patients who are taking oral medications that the condition requires lifelong treatment. After a thyroidectomy, provide information about postoperative wound care. Teach patients the importance of regular follow-up with their health care provider. When teaching, focus on the signs and symptoms of hypothyroidism and hyperthyroidism, and tell patients when to seek medical care.

NURSING CARE PLAN
Patient With Graves Disease

Juanita Manuel is a 33-year-old mother of four small children. For the past 3 months, she has been hungry all the time and eating more than usual, but she has lost 15 lb. Her hands shake, she can feel her heart beating rapidly, and she finds herself laughing or crying for no apparent reason.

Assessment
T 101°F (38.3°C); BP 162/86; P 110; R 24. Her skin is moist and warm; her hair is thin and fine. Her eyeballs protrude, and she cannot close her eyelids completely. Her thyroid is enlarged, and she has increased T_3 and T_4 levels. Mrs. Manuel is diagnosed with Graves disease and is started on the antithyroid medication propylthiouracil, 150 mg orally every 8 hours.

Nursing Diagnosis
The following priority nursing diagnoses (among others) are established for this patient:

- *Risk for Imbalanced Nutrition: Less Than Body Requirements* related to weight loss of 15 lb
- *Risk for Injury: Corneal Abrasion* related to incomplete eyelid closure
- *Deficient Knowledge* related to a lack of knowledge about the disease process

Expected Outcomes
The expected outcomes for the plan of care are that Mrs. Manuel will:

- Gain at least 1 lb per week.

- Maintain normal vision and state ways to protect her eyes.
- State medical treatment and self-care needs.

Planning and Implementation
The following nursing interventions are done for Mrs. Manuel:

- Ask her to record her weight before breakfast daily.
- Encourage her to eat a high-calorie diet.
- Teach Mrs. Manuel how to apply artificial tears.
- Tell her to elevate the head of her bed to 45 degrees at night and tape eye shields over her eyes before sleep.
- Teach her about Graves disease, her medications, side effects, and the need for continued medical care.

Evaluation
By her next office visit, Mrs. Manuel had gained 1 lb (0.45 kg). She uses her eyedrops, wears the eye shields, and elevates the head of her bed at night. Mrs. Manuel states, "I'll always take my medicine. I never want to feel like that again!" She also says that she feels less anxious now.

Critical Thinking in the Nursing Process
1. Why were Mrs. Manuel's vital signs abnormal?
2. Why should Mrs. Manuel wear eye shields at night?
3. If Mrs. Manuel tells you that she plans to stop taking her medications, how would you respond to her? How would this put Mrs. Manuel at risk for complications?

Note: Discussion of Critical Thinking questions appears on the companion website.

Hypothyroidism

Hypothyroidism occurs when the thyroid gland produces an insufficient amount of TH. It is most common in women between the ages of 30 and 60, but the incidence increases after age 60.

> **clinicalALERT**
> Careful evaluation of symptoms is important in the older adult because manifestations of hypothyroidism may be misdiagnosed as normal manifestations of aging.

Thyroid deficiency may be caused by congenital defects in the gland, antithyroid medications, surgical removal of the gland, or iodine deficiency. The main disorders are goiter, Hashimoto thyroiditis, and myxedema coma.

PATHOPHYSIOLOGY AND MANIFESTATIONS
The underlying problem in hypothyroidism is failure of the thyroid gland. However, certain drugs (lithium carbonate, which blocks TH synthesis, and amiodarone [Cordarone],

which has high iodine content) lead to hypothyroidism. Hypothyroidism has a slow onset, with manifestations occurring over months or even years. With treatment, the mental and physical symptoms rapidly reverse in patients of all ages. Unfortunately, TH replacement may result in hyperthyroidism.

Because reduced TH levels decrease metabolic rate and heat production, the rest of the body systems slow. Many of the manifestations are opposite of those in hyperthyroidism (Figure 35-4■).

Goiter

When TH production decreases, the thyroid gland enlarges in an attempt to produce more hormone. This enlargement is called a **goiter** (see Figure 35-2). Because iodine is necessary for TH synthesis and secretion, iodine deficiency can result in hypothyroidism. The use of iodized salt has reduced this risk in the United States.

Hashimoto Thyroiditis

The most common cause of primary hypothyroidism is Hashimoto thyroiditis. It is classified as an autoimmune disorder because antibodies destroy thyroid tissue. The primary manifestation is the presence of a goiter. It is most common in women between 30 and 50 years of age and those with a family history of thyroid disease.

Myxedema Coma

Myxedema coma is a life-threatening form of hypothyroidism requiring immediate medical attention. It may be brought on by failure to take thyroid replacement medications, trauma, infection, exposure to cold temperatures, or use of central nervous system depressants (especially narcotics and tranquilizers). This crisis occurs most often in the winter months. Myxedema coma develops frequently in older women with chronic hypothyroidism.

The patient presents with seizures, lethargy quickly progressing to coma, and hypothermia. Without adequate TH, the respiratory and cardiovascular systems shut down, causing bradycardia and decreased respiratory rate. The precipitating cause must be identified immediately to prevent the high mortality rate. Treatment focuses on maintaining a patent airway, stabilizing cardiac function,

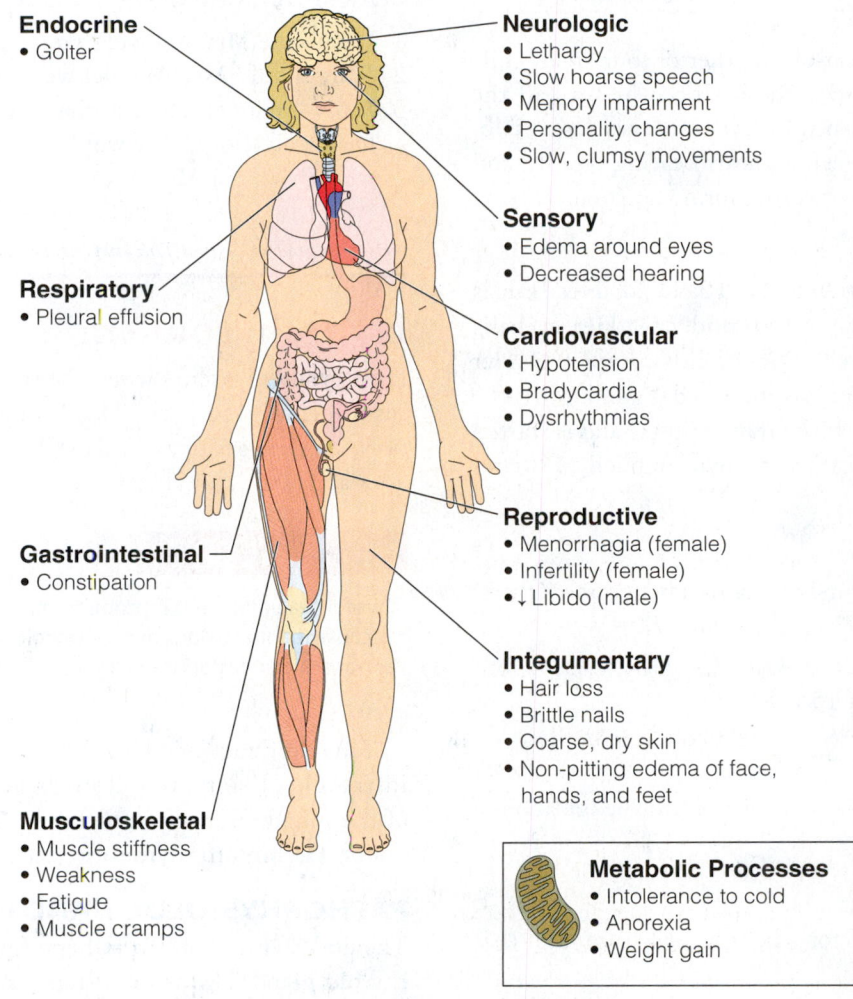

Figure 35-4. ■ Multisystem effects of hypothyroidism.

TABLE 35-2	Giving Medications Safely: Hypothyroidism		
CLASS/DRUGS	**PURPOSE**	**NURSING IMPLICATIONS**	**PATIENT TEACHING**
Thyroid preparations ■ Levothyroxine sodium (Synthroid, Levothroid) ■ Liothyronine sodium (Cytomel)	Increases blood levels of TH. Older adults usually require lower doses when treatment is first started.	Give 1 hour before breakfast. Check pulse before giving; call the physician when resting pulse is greater than 100. Monitor for side effects of nervousness and weight loss. Monitor for bleeding if taking anticoagulants. Check blood glucose levels closely in diabetics. Thyroid drugs alter insulin action. Report C/O chest pain immediately.	Take each morning before breakfast. Take pulse daily; call the physician when resting pulse greater than 100. Do not take with antacids or iron preparations. Take the medication for the rest of your life. Report unusual weight loss, nervousness, bleeding, or chest pain. If you have diabetes and use insulin, monitor blood glucose levels closely.

improving ventilation, and increasing temperature and TH levels by giving intravenous TH (levothyroxine).

COLLABORATIVE CARE

The medical treatment of the patient with hypothyroidism focuses on diagnosis, prevention or treatment of complications, and replacement of the deficient TH.

Hypothyroidism is diagnosed by a thorough history and physical examination. The presence of hypothyroidism manifestations and a decrease in TH, especially T_4, confirms the diagnosis.

Hypothyroidism is treated with TH. Drug therapy is started with small doses, which are gradually increased (Table 35-2■). When a goiter is large enough to cause respiratory difficulties or dysphagia, a subtotal thyroidectomy may be performed (see Box 35-3).

NURSING CARE

PRIORITIZING NURSING CARE

When planning care for the patient with hypothyroidism, the nurse takes into account that the disorder has a multisystem effect. The highest priority patient problems include cardiovascular function, nutrition, constipation, and activity level.

HEALTH PROMOTION

Individuals at a high risk for hypothyroidism should be screened regularly. High-risk people include those with a family history of thyroid disease, women over age 50, and those who have received neck radiation.

ASSESSING

Assessment data collected by the nurse can help determine the extent to which hypothyroidism is interfering with the patient's life and can identify risk factors for complications (Box 35-5■).

BOX 35-5	ASSESSMENT

Patients With Hypothyroidism

Subjective Data
■ Weight gain or constant constipation
■ Complaints of muscle or joint pain, intolerance to cold, or headaches
■ Change in memory, attention span, and personality
■ Preexisting goiter or use of THs

Objective Data
■ Measure blood pressure, pulse, respirations, and temperature.
■ Check height and weight.
■ Observe patient during interview for sluggishness, memory lapses, decreased attention span, and hoarse voice.
■ Inspect neck for visible signs of masses.
■ Palpate the skin for dryness and presence of edema.
■ Auscultate heart for irregularities and bradycardia.
■ Auscultate bowel sounds; decreased bowel sounds indicate decreased peristalsis.
■ Monitor and report decreased TSH, T_3, and T_4 levels.

IDENTIFYING POTENTIAL COMPLICATIONS

The primary complication of hypothyroidism is myxedema coma. Also, excessive TH replacement may worsen heart failure.

DIAGNOSING, PLANNING, AND IMPLEMENTING
Decreased Cardiac Output

Expected outcome: Blood pressure returns to patient's baseline, pulse rate between 60 and 100 with strong peripheral pulses.

■ Monitor blood pressure, apical pulse, and peripheral pulses. *Hypothyroidism causes hypotension and slow pulse rate. Hypotension and bradycardia reduce peripheral blood flow.*
■ Provide blankets to the patient and increase room temperature to avoid chilling. *Chilling increases metabolic rate and places increased stress on the heart.*

- Monitor respiratory rate and depth and for crackles. *Increased respiratory rate and crackles may indicate fluid overload secondary to decreased cardiac output.*

Imbalanced Nutrition: More Than Body Requirements

Expected outcome: Will attain weight appropriate to height.

- Weigh patient on first encounter and monitor weekly. *First weight establishes a baseline to evaluate success of interventions.*
- Consult with a dietitian regarding a reduced calorie diet. *Patients with hypothyroidism often gain weight due to decreased metabolic rate. Dietitian can develop a diet for weight loss.*
- Encourage patient to engage in exercise activities within patient's limits. *Fatigue may accompany decreased metabolism, leading to a sedentary lifestyle. Patient will need to understand the importance of exercise and weight reduction.*

Constipation

Expected outcome: Will have regular, soft formed stools.

- Increase fluid intake to 2,000 mL per day and provide low-calorie liquids. *Reduced appetite, food intake, activity level, and peristalsis contribute to the development of constipation. Adequate fluids are necessary to maintain soft stool.*
- Provide a high-fiber diet, including foods such as dried beans and peas, fruits with skin, whole-grain cereals and breads, popcorn, and brown rice. *Diets high in fiber increase fecal mass and assist moving feces through the intestines.*
- Encourage activity as tolerated. *Activity stimulates peristalsis.*
- Give stool softeners or laxatives as ordered. *These stimulate bowel elimination, but their use should be limited.*

Activity Intolerance

Expected outcome: Carries out ADLs with minimal fatigue or discomfort.

- Monitor blood pressure, pulse rate and rhythm, and respiratory rate before, during, and after activity level. *TH deficit reduces cardiac and respiratory function. Symptoms of cardiac stress include dyspnea, chest pain, palpitations, and dizziness.*
- Alternate activity with rest periods. Ask the patient to report any breathing difficulties, chest pain, heart palpitations, or dizziness. *Activity increases demands on the heart and should be balanced with rest, which decreases oxygen demands.*
- Assist patient with ADLs. *Meeting the needs of the patient promotes comfort and well-being.*

MANAGING NURSING CARE

As appropriate and allowed by the designated duties and responsibilities of assistive personnel, the nurse may delegate nursing care activities such as obtaining daily weights and assisting with meals and ADLs for the patient with hypothyroidism.

EVALUATING

Evaluate the care for the patient with hypothyroidism by collecting data about the patient's vital signs, nutrition intake, elimination patterns, and ability to perform ADLs. Determine the patient's understanding of medications, diet, and need for balancing activity with rest periods.

DOCUMENTING

Documentation includes assessment of vital signs, weight, and relief of manifestations such as lethargy, impaired memory, dry skin, fatigue, and constipation. Record effectiveness of patient teaching related to medications, diet, and importance of balancing rest and activity.

CONTINUITY OF CARE

The lifelong care required for patients with hypothyroidism can be accomplished at home. Teach the patient and family about self-care, compliance with lifelong prescribed medications, and the need for regular follow-up with a health care provider. The older adult may need referrals to social services or community health services, especially if home support is not available.

If the patient is lethargic or has memory problems, include the family in any teaching sessions and provide written instructions. Instruct them about the signs and symptoms of hypothyroidism, hyperthyroidism, and myxedema coma. Teach the importance of a high-fiber, low-calorie diet with adequate fluid intake. Emphasize the need to balance rest and physical activity and to avoid extreme cold temperatures and people with infections. Provide instruction about thyroid preparations as presented in Table 35-2. Additional resources for patient and families include American Thyroid Association and Endocrine Society.

Cancer of the Thyroid

Although thyroid cancer is relatively rare, with an estimated rate of 56,000 new cases annually, the rate is increasing. The most consistent risk factor is exposure to external radiation to the head and neck during childhood for treatment of sinus infections. Thyroid cancer affects women most often between the ages of 40 and 65.

Thyroid cancer appears as a small nodule in the thyroid. If undetected, it may grow and press on the esophagus or trachea, causing difficulty in swallowing or breathing. Diagnosis is made by measuring TH levels, by performing a radioisotope thyroid scan, and by needle biopsy of the nodule.

The usual treatment is subtotal or total thyroidectomy. A radical neck dissection is performed when lymph nodes are involved. TSH suppression therapy with levothyroxine may be given after surgery. RAI therapy, external radiation, and chemotherapy are additional therapeutic options. If the tumor has not metastasized, the 5-year survival rate is 97%. (See nursing care for the patient with cancer in Chapter 12.)

DISORDERS OF THE PARATHYROID GLANDS

Key Concept The parathyroid glands synthesize parathormone, and the thyroid gland produces calcitonin. Together these two hormones provide the proper level of serum calcium, which is essential for cardiac function, bone stability, nerve conduction, and muscle contraction.

Disorders of the parathyroid glands, hyperparathyroidism and hypoparathyroidism, are not as common as those of the thyroid gland. The main alterations in parathyroid function result in hypercalcemia and hypocalcemia. (See the Hypercalcemia and Hypocalcemia sections in Chapter 7.)

Hyperparathyroidism

Hyperparathyroidism results from increased secretion of *parathyroid hormone* (PTH), which regulates normal serum levels of calcium. This disorder occurs frequently in older adults and is three times more common in women. It is classified as either primary or secondary. Primary hyperparathyroidism is the most common and usually results from an adenoma (tumor) in one of the parathyroid glands. Secondary hyperparathyroidism may result from chronic renal failure.

PATHOPHYSIOLOGY AND MANIFESTATIONS

The increase in PTH causes calcium to leave the bones and enter the blood, resulting in *hypercalcemia*. Excess PTH also causes excretion of phosphate leading to *hypophosphatemia*. Many patients with hyperparathyroidism are asymptomatic. When symptoms occur, they affect the musculoskeletal, renal, and GI systems. The release of calcium and phosphorus from the bones results in bone decalcification and possible pathologic fractures. Elevated calcium levels alter neural and muscular activity, causing muscle weakness and atrophy. Kidney function is altered, leading to polyuria and renal *calculi* (stones) formation from calcium deposited in the kidney. The manifestations of hyperparathyroidism are summarized in Box 35-6■.

COLLABORATIVE CARE

Elevated levels of serum calcium, PTH, and alkaline phosphatase confirm a diagnosis of hyperparathyroidism. Once the diagnosis is confirmed, bone density studies are conducted to determine whether bone loss has occurred.

Treatment of hyperparathyroidism focuses on decreasing the serum calcium levels. Patients are urged to drink more than 2,000 mL per day and to increase activity. Those with acute hyperparathyroidism are hospitalized and given intravenous saline infusions and bisphosphonates such as

BOX 35-6	MANIFESTATIONS OF HYPERPARATHYROIDISM

- *Musculoskeletal*: chronic low back pain; pathologic fractures; muscle weakness; decreased muscle tone
- *Renal*: polyuria; renal calculi
- *Gastrointestinal*: abdominal pain; anorexia; nausea; constipation; peptic ulcers
- *Cardiovascular*: dysrhythmias; hypertension
- *Central nervous system*: malaise; fatigue; depression; impaired memory; psychosis; stupor

alendronate (Fosamax) or pamidronate (Aredia) to inhibit bone resorption. Calcitonin, a hormone produced by the thyroid gland, can reduce calcium release by the bones.

The main treatment for primary hyperparathyroidism is surgical removal of the parathyroid glands caused by an adenoma. Nursing care of the patient after removal of the parathyroid gland affected by the adenoma is essentially the same as that for the patient having a thyroidectomy (see Box 35-3).

NURSING CARE

PRIORITIZING NURSING CARE

Care focuses on interventions related to impaired physical mobility and risk for injury due to the patient's muscle weakness and altered mentation. It is important to monitor for manifestations of urinary tract infection. The patient may need additional interventions to decrease chronic pain and promote sound nutrition intake. (Nursing care of the patient with hypercalcemia is discussed in Chapter 7.)

CONTINUITY OF CARE

Once the patient's condition is stabilized, teach the patient and family how to adapt lifestyle at home. Consult a dietitian to discuss a calcium-restricted diet, as well as increased dietary fiber and fluid intake to prevent constipation. Teach the patient to contact the health care provider before taking any over-the-counter medications containing calcium.

Stress the importance of developing an exercise plan because immobility increases calcium excretion and the risk for kidney stones. Exercise is also important to maintain bone density, even with medications. Discuss safety hazards and injury prevention guidelines. Review the manifestations of hypercalcemia and hypocalcemia, and stress the importance of keeping annual appointments.

BOX 35-7	MANIFESTATIONS OF HYPOPARATHYROIDISM

- *Musculoskeletal:* muscle spasms and tremors; positive Chvostek and Trousseau signs
- *Integumentary:* hair loss; brittle nails; dry, scaly skin
- *Gastrointestinal:* abdominal cramps
- *Cardiovascular:* dysrhythmias
- *Central nervous system:* numbness and tingling in lips, hands, feet; irritability, depression, psychosis

Hypoparathyroidism

Hypoparathyroidism results from inadequate secretion of PTH. The usual cause is accidental damage to or removal of the parathyroid glands during a thyroidectomy. The lack of circulating PTH causes hypocalcemia and an elevated blood phosphate level.

PATHOPHYSIOLOGY AND MANIFESTATIONS

Reduced PTH levels impair kidney regulation of calcium and phosphate. Decreased activation of vitamin D leads to lower calcium absorption by the intestines. The low calcium levels increase neuromuscular activity, especially the peripheral motor and sensory nerves.

Patients with mild hypoparathyroidism may be asymptomatic. With more acute disease, neuromuscular manifestations result. **Tetany** (a continuous spasm of muscles) is the primary symptom of hypocalcemia. In severe cases, bronchospasm, laryngeal spasms, convulsions, and even death may occur. Nursing assessments for tetany include Chvostek sign and Trousseau sign (see Chapter 7). The manifestations of hypoparathyroidism are summarized in Box 35-7.

COLLABORATIVE CARE

Hypoparathyroidism is diagnosed by low serum calcium levels and high phosphorus levels in the absence of renal failure, an absorption disorder, or a nutritional disorder. Tetany usually occurs when serum calcium levels drop below 6 mg/dL.

The first priority for treating hypoparathyroidism is to increase calcium levels. Intravenous calcium gluconate is given immediately to reduce or prevent tetany. Because the patient can develop respiratory distress, the nurse must ensure a patent airway. Conscious patients are instructed to breathe in and out of a paper bag. This rebreathing technique increases acid levels in the blood, which temporarily stabilizes calcium levels.

clinicalALERT

Keep oxygen, suctioning equipment, and a tracheostomy set at the bedside.

The patient needs a calm environment to prevent excessive neuromuscular irritability. Dim lights, reduced noise, and few visitors are recommended. If the patient is at risk for seizures, pad the side rails. Placing the patient near the nurses' station decreases the patient's anxiety and enables the nurse to provide closer observation.

Long-term therapy includes supplemental calcium with oral calcium salts. The patient needs a diet high in calcium but low in phosphorus. Vitamin D therapy is given to increase GI absorption of calcium.

NURSING CARE

Nursing care of the patient with hypoparathyroidism must consider the patient's risk for injury due to tetany. There may be personality changes and impaired memory. The patient's need for a diet high in calcium must be included. (Nursing care for the patient with hypocalcemia is discussed in Chapter 7.)

CONTINUITY OF CARE

Patients with hypoparathyroidism need instruction for taking calcium and phosphate binders. Teach them the necessity of lifelong medication and follow-up care. Consult a dietitian to identify foods high in calcium and vitamin D and low in phosphorus. Milk and milk products are restricted because they contain high levels of phosphorus. More appropriate foods include spinach, soybeans, and tofu. Review the signs and symptoms of hypocalcemia and hypercalcemia with the patient and family. Teach patients to wear a MedicAlert bracelet identifying condition and medication therapy.

DISORDERS OF THE ADRENAL GLAND

Key Concept The adrenal glands regulate energy and fluid balance through glucocorticoids and mineralocorticoids. Cushing syndrome and Addison disease are polar opposites. Treatment eliminates manifestations of one disorder but creates manifestations of the other disorder.

Disorders of the adrenal gland involve either the adrenal cortex, which secretes cortisol and aldosterone, or the adrenal medulla, which releases epinephrine and norepinephrine. Hormones of the adrenal cortex are essential to life because they maintain homeostasis in response to stress. Disorders of the adrenal cortex cause physical, psychologic, and metabolic alterations that are potentially life threatening. The most common disorders are Cushing syndrome, Addison disease, and pheochromocytoma.

Cushing Syndrome

Cushing syndrome is a chronic disorder in which the adrenal cortex produces excessive amounts of the hormone cortisol. It is more common in women between the ages of 30 and 50. Several factors may lead to Cushing syndrome: (1) adrenal tumors causing an increased production of cortisol; (2) a tumor of the pituitary gland increases adrenocorticotropic hormone (ACTH) release, which stimulates the adrenal cortex to produce cortisol; (3) chronic glucocorticoid therapy; and (4) increased release of ACTH from lung or pancreatic tumors.

PATHOPHYSIOLOGY AND MANIFESTATIONS

With excess production of glucocorticoids, there are changes in carbohydrate, protein, and fat metabolism. There are fat deposits in the abdomen, fat pads under the clavicle, a "buffalo hump" over the upper back, and a round "moon" face (Figure 35-5■). Altered protein metabolism leads to muscle weakness and wasting in the extremities. Excess cortisol causes loss of collagen and connective tissue, leading to poor wound healing. As thinned skin stretches over the abdomen and buttocks, purple *striae* (stretch marks) appear (Figure 35-6■). Glucose metabolism is often altered, and diabetes mellitus may occur.

Decreased calcium absorption results in osteoporosis and compression fractures of the vertebrae. Mineralocorticoid

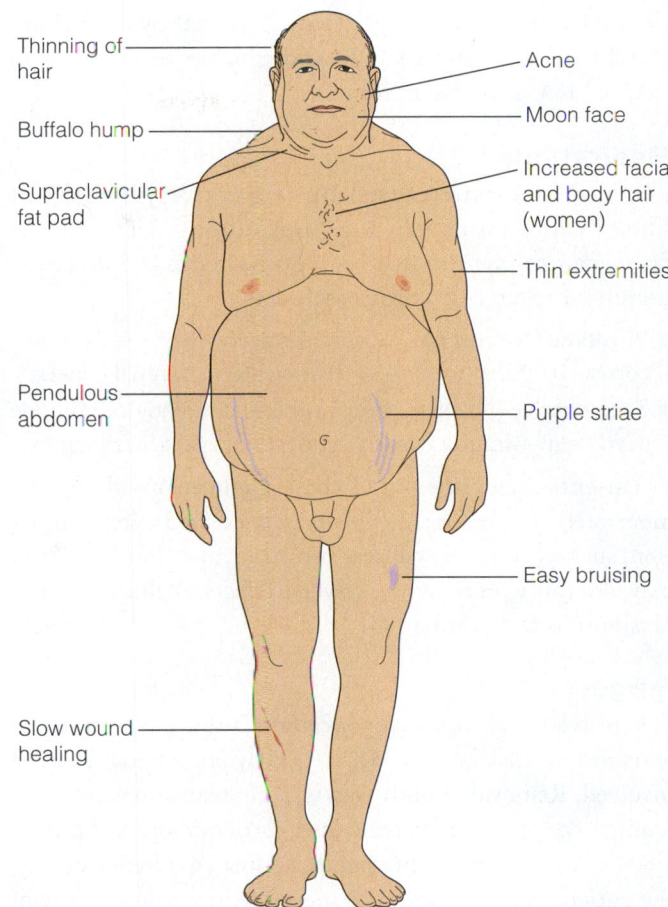

Figure 35-6. ■ Major clinical manifestations of Cushing syndrome.

release promotes sodium and water retention and potassium loss, leading to hypertension.

The inflammatory and immune responses are suppressed, so there is a greater risk for infection that can become life threatening. Increased gastric acid secretion may lead to peptic ulcers. Emotional changes range from euphoria to depression. In women, increased androgen levels cause **hirsutism** (excessive facial hair), acne, and menstrual irregularities. Emotional instability may range from depression to psychosis. Untreated Cushing syndrome can lead to multiple complications.

COLLABORATIVE CARE

The treatment of Cushing syndrome includes surgery, radiotherapy, or medication. For patients with a pituitary adenoma, the preferred treatment is surgery. Radiation therapy might be considered for inoperable pituitary gland tumor. Drug therapy is used when surgery is contraindicated.

Diagnostic Tests

Diagnosis of Cushing syndrome is confirmed by an increased plasma cortisol level and an elevated 24-hour urine test for 17-ketosteroids. Plasma ACTH levels are

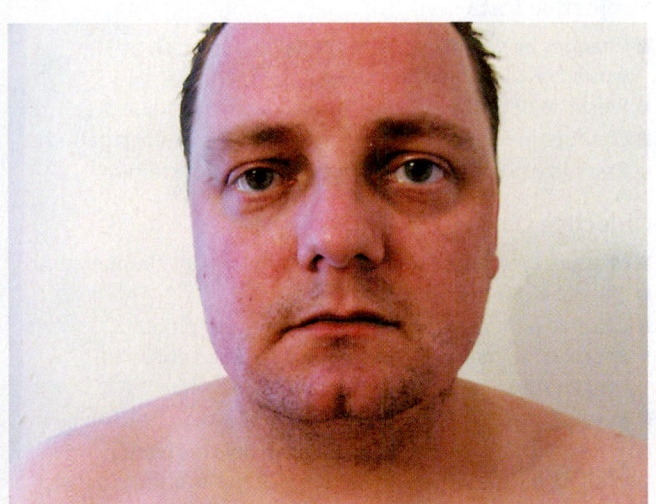

Figure 35-5. ■ A man with Cushing syndrome; this image shows the typical swollen facial features. (Source: © Mirrorpix/Splash News/Corbis.)

elevated when Cushing syndrome is caused by a pituitary gland tumor. Serum sodium and glucose levels are also elevated in Cushing syndrome.

Medications

Cushing syndrome caused by inoperable pituitary or adrenal tumors is treated with medications. Although the drugs control symptoms, they do not cure the disorder. Commonly prescribed drugs include:

- Mitotane (Lysodren)—suppresses activity of the adrenal cortex. It is also used to treat metastatic adrenal cancer.
- Ketoconazole (Nizoral), metyrapone, and aminoglutethimide (Cytadren)—inhibit cortisol synthesis by the adrenal cortex.

Patients receiving any of these medications should be monitored closely for side effects of decreased adrenal function, such as anorexia, nausea, vomiting, and diarrhea. They may also cause more serious adverse effects, including hypotension and tachycardia.

Surgery

When an adrenal cortex tumor causes Cushing syndrome, an *adrenalectomy* may be done. Usually, only one adrenal gland is involved. Removal of both glands, a bilateral adrenalectomy, requires the patient to take lifelong corticosteroid and mineralocorticoid replacement therapy. After an adrenalectomy, the patient is cared for in the intensive care unit because of the risk for Addisonian crisis, also known as adrenal crisis.

Surgical removal of the pituitary gland (*hypophysectomy*) is indicated when Cushing syndrome is the result of a pituitary tumor. (Nursing care for the patient having cranial surgery is discussed further in Chapter 38.)

Radiation Therapy

Radiation therapy is used in patients with an inoperable pituitary tumor causing Cushing syndrome. Radioactive isotopes may be implanted into the pituitary gland. If the pituitary gland is destroyed, lifelong replacement of pituitary hormones is necessary.

NURSING CARE

The nurse caring for the patient with Cushing syndrome must consider a wide variety of problems. The most common problems are related to fluid and electrolyte balance, injury, infection, and body image. (For additional information about patients with alterations in fluid and electrolyte balance, see Chapter 7.)

PRIORITIZING NURSING CARE

Patients with Cushing syndrome may need both acute and chronic interventions. When the patient is acutely ill, hospitalization may be needed. The priority problems during acute illness include excess fluid volume, risk for injury or infection, and altered body image. During the chronic phase, the nurse focuses on patient teaching for self-management at home.

HEALTH PROMOTION

Health promotion focuses on identifying individuals at risk for Cushing syndrome, such as patients who take long-term steroid therapy. Discontinuing steroids abruptly can lead to acute adrenal insufficiency. It is essential to include teaching about medication therapy.

ASSESSING

The nurse must collect assessment data to determine the extent to which Cushing syndrome is interfering with the patient's life. Assessment also identifies risk factors for complications (Box 35-8■).

IDENTIFYING POTENTIAL COMPLICATIONS

Electrolyte complications include hypernatremia, hypokalemia, and hyperglycemia. Patients are at risk for hypertension and heart failure. Compression fractures from osteoporosis may result in serious disability. Depression may predispose the patient to thoughts of suicide.

DIAGNOSING, PLANNING, AND IMPLEMENTING
Excess Fluid Volume

Expected outcome: Will lose excess fluid as demonstrated by weight loss and absence of edema.

BOX 35-8	ASSESSMENT

Patients With Cushing Syndrome

Subjective Data
- Changes in weight, increased facial or body hair, poor wound healing, or bruising
- Presence of back pain, muscle weakness, or fatigue
- Changes in memory, ability to concentrate, or sleep patterns
- Past history of frequent infections or use of steroids

Objective Data
- Measure blood pressure, pulse, respirations, and temperature.
- Check height and weight.
- Observe patient during interview for general body appearance, memory lapses, and decreased ability to concentrate.
- Assess for excess body hair and acne; thinning head hair.
- Inspect for thin, fragile skin; bruising; delayed wound healing; purple striae and fat deposits in the abdominal region; and edema.
- Monitor and report increased serum cortisol, glucose, and sodium levels and urine 17-ketosteroids.

- Monitor daily weight and intake and output every 8 hours. *Excess cortisol secretion causes sodium and water retention, which leads to fluid volume excess and weight gain. Body weight and intake and output are accurate indicators of fluid status.*
- Monitor blood pressure, rate and rhythm of pulse, respiratory rate, and breath sounds. Assess for peripheral edema. *Sodium and water retention is manifested by hypertension and a bounding, rapid pulse. Also, there may be crackles, wheezes, and dependent edema.*

clinicalALERT

Limit fluid intake to prevent the risk of fluid overload.

Risk for Injury

Expected outcome: Remains free from injury.

The patient with Cushing syndrome has muscle weakness and fatigue, increasing the potential for accidental falls. Excess cortisol increases the likelihood of osteoporosis and risk of pathologic fractures.

- Maintain a safe environment. Keep unnecessary clutter and equipment out of the way and off the floor. Ensure adequate lighting, especially at night. *A well-lit, clutter-free environment reduces the risk of injury.*
- Encourage the patient to use assistive devices for ambulation or ask for help if needed. Be sure corrective lenses are available and clean. Encourage the use of nonskid slippers or shoes. *Encouraging the patient to use assistive devices, corrective lenses, and nonslip footwear can decrease injury risk.*
- Provide rest between physical activities. *Rest conserves energy so that the patient is less likely to fall from fatigue.*
- Change patient's position frequently. *Patients with Cushing syndrome have thin, fragile skin, which increases the risk for tissue injury. Position changes and massage minimize pressure and improve circulation to keep skin intact.*
- Provide protection by using pillows, pads, foam mattress, and so forth. *These measures increase circulation and reduce tissue pressure.*

Risk for Infection

Expected outcome: Remains free of signs of infection.

- Place the patient in a private room and limit visitors. *The patient with impaired immunity must avoid exposure to infection.*
- Monitor temperature, pulse, and patient's feeling of well-being. *Increased temperature and pulse are systemic indicators of infection. Because Cushing syndrome decreases the inflammatory response, the patient may not show the usual manifestations of infection.*
- Use sterile technique for invasive procedures. *Aseptic technique reduces the risk of infection in the patient with an impaired immune system.*

- Assess wounds for pain, color, odor, and drainage. *Excess cortisol decreases protein synthesis, causing delayed wound healing and closure.*

clinicalALERT

A feeling of malaise may be the first indicator of infection, especially in the older adult.

- Use mild soap, dry gently and thoroughly, and apply lotion as needed. *Good hygiene promotes healthy skin to prevent bacteria from entering the body.*

Disturbed Body Image

Expected outcome: Verbalizes acceptance of body appearance.

The abnormal fat distribution, moon face, buffalo hump, striae, acne, and facial hair (in women) disrupt the way patients view themselves. They may be unable to perform usual activities because of their negative feelings about their appearance.

- Encourage the patient to express feelings about the physical changes. *Understanding the disease and adapting to changes are the first steps in regaining control of one's own body.*
- Spend time with the patient and listen carefully. *Each situation affects individuals differently, depending on their coping skills.*

MANAGING NURSING CARE

As appropriate and allowed by the designated duties and responsibilities of assistive personnel, the nurse may delegate nursing care activities such as providing skin care and assisting with meals and ADLs for the patient with Cushing syndrome. Before assigning tasks such as obtaining vital signs, measuring intake and output, obtaining daily weights, and assisting with ambulation, ensure that the assistive personnel clearly understands the importance of accurately measuring vital signs, limiting fluid intake, preventing falls or injury, and preventing infection.

EVALUATING

Collect the following data to evaluate the effectiveness of care for the patient with Cushing syndrome: (1) improved memory, (2) no falls or injuries, (3) normal temperature without signs of infection, (4) normal blood pressure, (5) no skin breakdown or edema, and (6) coping with physical changes. Serum sodium and potassium levels should return to normal.

DOCUMENTING

Documentation includes assessing the patient for a decrease in clinical manifestations and the response to interventions. Record patient teaching about medications, safety measures at home, fluid restriction, and diet modifications.

CONTINUITY OF CARE

The patient with Cushing syndrome requires education about self-care at home. Teach about safety measures if fatigue, weakness, and osteoporosis are present. Caution the patient to avoid extremes of temperature, infections, and emotional stress. Stress can lead to acute adrenal insufficiency, so it is important to teach the patient signs and symptoms of urinary tract, upper respiratory, and wound infections. Also, stress the importance of contacting the physician if cuts do not heal.

Instruct the patient about prescribed medications, including side effects and adverse reactions. Recommend wearing a MedicAlert bracelet, indicating the patient has Cushing syndrome and listing the medication therapy.

Provide instruction on a diet high in potassium and low in calories, sodium, and carbohydrates. Teach the patient and family why fluid intake is restricted. Be sure the patient and family understand and are able to perform protective skin measures. Stress the importance of regular visits to the physician. Provide the patient and family with additional resources such as National Adrenal Diseases Foundation and National Institute of Diabetes, Digestive, & Kidney Diseases.

Addison Disease

Adrenal cortex hypofunction may be *primary* (Addison disease) or *secondary,* from lack of pituitary ACTH. **Addison disease** is the most common form of adrenal cortex insufficiency. It occurs most frequently in women under the age of 60.

PATHOPHYSIOLOGY AND MANIFESTATIONS

In primary Addison disease, an autoimmune response destroys the patient's own adrenal cortex. This leads to reduced levels of glucocorticoids, mineralocorticoids, and androgens. The onset of Addison disease is slow, and manifestations develop when more than 90% of the gland is destroyed. Manifestations result from elevated ACTH levels and decreased aldosterone and cortisol (Box 35-9■). The primary complication of Addison disease is Addisonian crisis.

memory**ALERT**

Cortisol is essential to life. Severe cortisol deficiency can lead to circulatory collapse, shock, and death.

Addisonian Crisis

Addisonian crisis, or adrenal crisis, is a serious, life-threatening response to acute adrenal insufficiency. Major stressors such as surgery, trauma, or severe infections usually precipitate this condition. Addisonian crisis may also occur in patients who are abruptly withdrawn from corticosteroid medications.

BOX 35-9	MANIFESTATIONS OF ADDISON DISEASE

- *Integumentary*: bronze color over knuckles, knees, and elbows
- *Musculoskeletal*: weakness, muscle and joint pain
- *Cardiovascular*: postural hypotension; weak, irregular pulse
- *Central nervous system*: dizziness, lethargy, depression
- *Gastrointestinal*: anorexia, nausea, vomiting, diarrhea

The patient is monitored for hypotension; rapid, weak pulse; extreme weakness; and confusion resulting from circulatory collapse and shock. Potassium levels can reach dangerously high levels, leading to cardiac dysrhythmias. Other manifestations include high fever; severe pain in abdomen, back, and legs; and severe vomiting. The patient is managed in the intensive care unit for intravenous administration of fluids, glucose, sodium, and glucocorticoids. During the crisis stage, the patient is kept quiet to prevent increasing the stress response. Once the crisis has resolved, the patient requires teaching and follow-up.

COLLABORATIVE CARE

The patient with Addison disease requires early diagnosis and treatment. Medical treatment involves corticosteroid and mineralocorticoid replacement therapy. Corticosteroid therapy causes immunosuppression and can induce Cushing syndrome.

Diagnostic Tests

Addison disease is diagnosed through findings of decreased serum levels of cortisol and aldosterone and urinary 17-ketosteroids. Potassium is increased, and blood glucose and sodium levels are decreased. CT scan and MRI may identify atrophy of the adrenal glands.

Medications

Addison disease is treated by replacing corticosteroids and mineralocorticoids and by giving a diet high in sodium. Hydrocortisone is given orally to replace cortisol; fludrocortisone (Florinef) is given orally to replace mineralocorticoids. During a crisis such as surgery, serious illness, or trauma, increased doses of corticosteroids and mineralocorticoids are required to prevent Addisonian crisis. Nursing implications and patient teaching guidelines for these drugs are presented in Table 35-3■.

NURSING CARE

PRIORITIZING NURSING CARE

Patients with Addison disease may require acute and chronic interventions. Acutely ill patients need immediate hospitalization. Nursing care focuses on restoring fluid

TABLE 35-3	Giving Medications Safely: Addison Disease		
CLASS/DRUGS	**PURPOSE**	**NURSING IMPLICATIONS**	**PATIENT TEACHING**
Corticosteroids ■ Cortisone (Cortone) ■ Hydrocortisone (Cortef, Solu-Cortef) ■ Prednisone (Deltasone) ■ Dexamethasone (Decadron) ■ Prednisolone (Delta-Cortef) ■ Methylprednisolone (Solu-Medrol)	Used to replace glucocorticoids in acute and chronic adrenal insufficiency.	Give oral forms of the drug with food to reduce ulcers. Check stools for occult blood; urine for glycosuria. Report increased blood pressure, edema or weight gain, bruising, or weakness (Cushing syndrome). Assess for impaired wound healing.	Take medications with food; report any gastric distress or dark stools. Never abruptly stop the medication. Take medications for the rest of your life. Eat a diet high in potassium, low in sodium. Weigh yourself daily; report weight gain or edema (adrenal excess). Use safety measures to avoid accidents. Wear a MedicAlert bracelet. Report adrenal insufficiency: dizziness on sitting or standing, nausea and vomiting, pain, thirst, feelings of anxiety, malaise, infections.

and electrolyte balance and increasing nutritional intake. During the chronic phase, the patient needs support and teaching to manage the disease.

HEALTH PROMOTION

Health promotion interventions for the patient with Addison disease focus on careful assessments during birth, major trauma, or open-heart surgery. If the disease is present, it is essential to teach the patient about preventing or treating Addisonian crisis.

ASSESSING

Assessment data (Box 35-10■) can help determine the extent to which Addison disease is affecting the patient's life and can identify risk factors.

DIAGNOSING, PLANNING, AND IMPLEMENTING
Deficient Fluid Volume

Expected outcome: Patient intake and output will be balanced.

Addison disease leads to fluid volume deficit from loss of water and sodium often caused by vomiting and diarrhea. During the crisis phase, acute volume deficit may lead to hypotension and hypovolemic shock.

■ Monitor intake and output, and assess for signs of dehydration (dry mucous membranes; thirst; poor skin turgor; sunken eyeballs; scanty, dark urine; and weight loss). *Glucocorticoid and mineralocorticoid depletion causes fluid volume deficit.*

■ Monitor blood pressure (lying, sitting, and standing) and strength of peripheral pulses; monitor potassium level and ECG. *Fluid volume deficit may lead to hypotension and a rapid, weak, or thready pulse. As aldosterone levels fall, serum potassium levels increase, causing ECG changes.*

BOX 35-10	ASSESSMENT

Patients With Addison Disease

Subjective Data
■ Skin color changes
■ Presence of anorexia, nausea and vomiting, abdominal pain, and diarrhea
■ Complaints of weakness, muscle and joint pain, and dizziness
■ Feelings of lethargy or depression
■ Past history of steroid use, adrenal surgery, and recent infection

Objective Data
■ Measure blood pressure (standing and sitting), pulse, respirations, and temperature.
■ Check height and weight.
■ Observe patient during interview for lethargy or depression.
■ Test muscle strength.
■ Inspect exposed skin for bronze color.
■ Auscultate pulse for irregularities.
■ Monitor and report decreased serum cortisol, glucose, and sodium levels and increased potassium levels.

■ Weigh patient daily at the same time and in the same clothing. *Dehydration is characterized by weight loss.*

■ Increase oral fluids to 3,000 mL per day and increase salt intake. *Fluids and sodium are given to manage the fluid volume deficit and hyponatremia characteristic of adrenal insufficiency.*

clinicalALERT

Teach the patient to stand up slowly because dehydration causes orthostatic hypotension, increasing the risk for falls.

Activity Intolerance

Expected outcome: Will participate in ADLs as tolerated.

- Keep patient on bed rest and perform ADLs for patient. *This prevents stimulation of an overly stressed adrenal cortex.*
- Slowly increase physical activity. *Once adrenal cortex hormones are replaced, the patient will be able to regain normal physical activity.*

Imbalanced Nutrition: Less Than Body Requirements

Expected outcome: Will gain 1 lb per month until normal weight is reached.

- Provide a high-calorie diet in six small meals each day. Encourage patient to avoid potassium-rich foods. *A high-calorie diet is used to replace lost weight. Addison disease increases potassium levels that can affect cardiac muscle function.*
- Auscultate bowel tones and note presence of diarrhea. *Hyperactive bowel sounds and diarrhea indicate an inability to absorb nutrients.*

MANAGING NURSING CARE

As appropriate and allowed by the designated duties and responsibilities of assistive personnel, the nurse may delegate nursing care activities such as obtaining daily weights and assisting with meals and ADLs for the patient with Addison disease. Before assigning tasks such as obtaining vital signs, measuring intake and output, obtaining daily weights, and assisting with ambulation, ensure that the assistive personnel clearly understands the importance of accurately measuring vital signs, increasing fluid and sodium intake, and preventing falls.

EVALUATING

Collect the following data to evaluate the effectiveness of care for the patient with Addison disease: (1) no signs of dehydration or postural hypotension, (2) activity level increases, and (3) increased fluid and dietary intake. Determine whether the patient understood teaching about the lifelong management of Addison disease.

DOCUMENTING

Documentation includes vital signs, especially orthostatic blood pressures, skin status, mental status, and intake and output. Record patient teaching about medications, stress reduction measures, increased fluid intake, diet modifications, and manifestations of adrenal hormone excess.

CONTINUITY OF CARE

Educate the patient and family about the need for lifelong treatment and self-care. Explain the possible complications that can result from not following the treatment plan.

Teach patients that regular follow-up with the health care provider is important and how to recognize the signs and symptoms that require medical attention.

Discuss the relationship between hormone levels and stress. Teach patients and families how to adjust medication doses during times of physical and emotional stress. Instruct them about the manifestations of adrenal hormone excess and insufficiency.

Teach the patient and family how and when to administer corticosteroids and mineralocorticoids. Stress the importance of carrying at all times an emergency kit containing parenteral cortisone and a syringe/needle. Advise the patient to wear a MedicAlert bracelet that identifies both the disease and the medication therapy.

Remind the patient to increase oral fluid intake. Because corticosteroid medications can lower potassium and increase sodium levels, teach the patient to consume a diet high in potassium and low in sodium. Stress the importance of not skipping meals.

Disorder of the Adrenal Medulla

Pheochromocytoma is a benign tumor of the adrenal medulla. It commonly occurs in middle-aged adults. The tumor erratically produces excessive amounts of catecholamines (epinephrine or norepinephrine), which stimulate the sympathetic nervous system. This leads to a dramatic rise in the systolic blood pressure of 200 to 300 mmHg and a diastolic greater than 150 mmHg. Additional symptoms include pounding headache, tachycardia, profuse sweating, flushing, and palpitations. If untreated, this can lead to such life-threatening conditions as myocardial infarction and stroke.

A pheochromocytoma is diagnosed by increased catecholamine levels in the blood or urine, CT scan, and MRI. Surgical removal of the tumor(s) by laparoscopic adrenalectomy is the treatment of choice.

Nursing care during the acute attack and before surgery focuses on stabilizing the patient's blood pressure. The patient is admitted to the intensive care unit, where constant hemodynamic monitoring and intravenous antihypertensive medications are instituted. After surgery, the patient may require adrenal hormone replacement therapy. Sometimes patients remain hypertensive and require continual follow-up.

Note: The references and resources for all chapters have been compiled at the back of the book.

Chapter Review

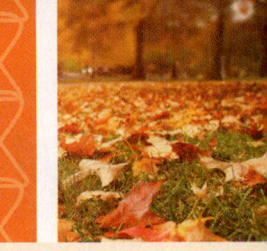

KEY POINTS

- **Concept:** The pituitary gland, consisting of the anterior and posterior lobes, in conjunction with the hypothalamus, is the master gland of the body. The anterior lobe releases seven hormones, whereas the posterior lobe releases two hormones.
- Deficient or excess production of GH (somatotropin) can result in dwarfism or acromegaly, respectively. Cranial surgery may be used to remove pituitary adenomas, causing acromegaly.
- Deficient secretion of ADH from the posterior pituitary gland can result in DI; excess secretion of ADH can lead to SIADH.
- **Concept:** Thyroid disorders occur most often in women. These disorders change body image and alter energy levels, creating fatigue or exhaustion.
- Hyperthyroidism is frequently caused by Graves disease, which increases metabolic rate. Surgery, radiation therapy, and medications are used to manage hyperthyroidism. Thyroid crisis, a life-threatening form of hyperthyroidism, requires immediate medical treatment.
- Hypothyroidism develops when the thyroid gland fails to secrete an adequate amount of THs. This causes metabolic processes to slow, as seen by the manifestations of lethargy, constipation, weight gain, and hypothermia. Lifelong thyroid medication therapy is needed to manage hypothyroidism.
- Although thyroid cancer is rare, patients may require surgery, radiation therapy, or chemotherapy to treat it.
- **Concept:** The parathyroid glands synthesize parathormone, and the thyroid gland produces calcitonin.

Together these two hormones provide the proper level of serum calcium, which is essential for cardiac function, bone stability, nerve conduction, and muscle contraction.
- Hypoparathyroidism usually results from accidental removal of the parathyroid glands during a thyroidectomy. Tetany, as manifested by positive Chvostek and Trousseau signs, is the primary complication of acute disease.
- Hyperparathyroidism results from excess PTH levels, causing hypocalcemia. The patient is at increased risk for pathologic fractures and renal calculi.
- **Concept:** The adrenal glands regulate energy and fluid balance through glucocorticoids and mineralocorticoids. Cushing syndrome and Addison disease are polar opposites. Treatment eliminates manifestations of one disorder but creates manifestations of the other disorder.
- Excess production of glucocorticoid hormones by the adrenal cortex results in Cushing syndrome, causing multisystem problems. Nursing care focuses on monitoring fluid status and preventing injury and infection.
- An adrenalectomy (removal of adrenal tumor) or hypophysectomy (removal of pituitary tumor) may be needed to treat Cushing syndrome.
- Addison disease is an acute deficiency of glucocorticoid (cortisol), mineralocorticoid (aldosterone), and androgen hormones. Cortisol and aldosterone are vital to sustain life. Addisonian or adrenal crisis is a life-threatening complication. Patients must understand the importance of lifelong treatment.

PEARSON NURSING STUDENT RESOURCES

Find additional materials at **nursing.pearsonhighered.com**.

Clinical Reasoning Care Map

Caring for a Patient With Hypothyroidism
NCLEX-PN® Focus Area: Psychosocial Adaptation

Case Study: Jane Lee is a 60-year-old retiree. She has gained 10 lb (4.5 kg) in the past 6 months, even though she is rarely hungry and eats much less than normal. Diagnostic tests reveal decreased serum T_4 level and increased TSH. The medical diagnosis of hypothyroidism is made, and Mrs. Lee is started on levothyroxine 0.05 mg daily.

Nursing Diagnosis: Disturbed Body Image

COLLECT DATA

Subjective	Objective
_____	_____
_____	_____
_____	_____
_____	_____
_____	_____
_____	_____
_____	_____

Does this present a threat to the patient's safety?

If yes, the priority intervention to address this threat would be:

_____

_____

Nursing Care

_____

_____

_____

_____

_____

_____

_____

_____

_____

Interprofessional team members to include when planning care:

_____

_____

How would you document this?_____

_____

Compare your answers and documentation to those provided on the companion website.

Data Collected
(use only those that apply)

- Rarely hungry, eats less than normal
- Dry skin and hair loss
- Eyelids will not close
- Weight gain of 10 lb in past 6 months
- Hoarse voice
- Puffy face and ankles
- Always cold
- Slurred speech
- No energy to do housework
- Hypertension
- Bradycardia

Nursing Interventions
(use only those that apply; list in priority order)

- Teach Mrs. Lee how to increase fluids and fiber in her diet.
- Recommend that Mrs. Lee join a weight reduction class.
- Teach Mrs. Lee about reversible body changes.
- Encourage her to allow her husband and daughter to help with housecleaning and cooking.
- Provide information that helps Mrs. Lee understand why the body changes occurred from hypothyroidism.
- Refer Mrs. Lee for a visual screening.

NCLEX-PN® Exam Preparation

TEST-TAKING TIP   Review the basic dietary requirements for specific diseases and illnesses (e.g., high-potassium, low-calorie, low-sodium diet for the patient with Cushing syndrome). Be familiar with the types of foods that contain sodium, calcium, iodine, and other elements.

1 A patient is admitted with Cushing syndrome. Which of the following laboratory tests results should the nurse expect to find?

1. Elevated serum potassium
2. Decreased serum sodium level
3. Decreased growth hormone level
4. Elevated serum glucose level

2 In caring for a patient who has had a subtotal thyroidectomy, what priority life-threatening complication should the nurse monitor for?

1. Hemorrhage
2. Tetany
3. Dehydration
4. Laryngeal nerve damage

3 A patient is diagnosed as having a goiter. What is the underlying cause of this condition?

1. Iodine deficiency
2. Excess thyroid-stimulating hormone
3. Deficient calcium levels
4. Excess cortisol

4 The nurse has taught a patient about taking prednisone (Deltasone). What statement by the patient indicates that the patient understands the instructions?

1. "I will consume higher calorie and sodium foods in my diet."
2. "I will not stop my medication unless I talk to my health care provider."
3. "I plan to take my pulse each morning before breakfast."
4. "If I experience nervousness or chest pain, I will call my health care provider."

5 For a patient diagnosed with Cushing syndrome, which of these nursing diagnoses should be addressed on the care plan?

1. Deficient Fluid Volume
2. Activity Intolerance
3. Body Image, Disturbed
4. Constipation, Acute

6 Which one of these nursing actions is the highest priority for a patient admitted with acute hypoparathyroidism?

1. Provide a quiet, dimly lighted room.
2. Assess for abdominal cramps.
3. Provide a diet high in calcium.
4. Assess for a patent airway.

7 Which of the following nursing interventions should be used when administering potassium iodide (SSKI) to a patient with hyperthyroidism? **Select all that apply.**

1. Do not give with an antacid.
2. Ask about allergies to shellfish.
3. Do not give to patients with asthma.
4. Monitor for itching and rash.
5. Dilute in milk or orange juice.
6. Monitor for bradycardia.

8 A patient newly diagnosed with SIADH is preparing for discharge. Which of the following teaching points should be included in the discharge instructions?

1. Teach the patient how to measure urine output.
2. Encourage the patient to eat a high-protein diet.
3. Instruct the patient on how to take the pulse every day.
4. Teach the patient to avoid crowds.

9 A patient is taking Synthroid (levothyroxine sodium) for 3 months. Which evaluation criteria would indicate a therapeutic response to this drug?

1. Decreased appetite
2. Decreased diarrhea
3. Normal heart rate
4. Weight loss of 5 lb

10 What clinical manifestation should the nurse expect to observe in a patient diagnosed with Addison disease?

1. Multiple bruises
2. Postural hypotension
3. Peripheral edema
4. Shortness of breath

Answers and rationales for Review Questions appear in Appendix I.

CHAPTER 36
Caring for Patients With Diabetes Mellitus

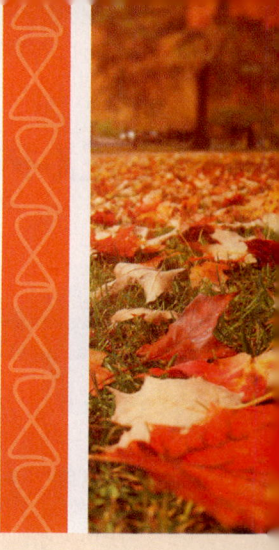

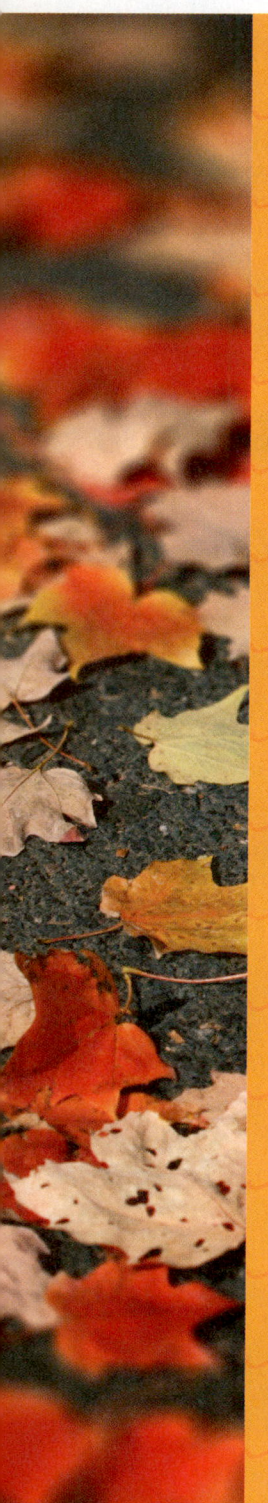

BRIEF OUTLINE

Overview of Diabetes Mellitus
Types of Diabetes Mellitus
Diabetes in the Older Adult
Pathophysiology
Collaborative Care

Complications of Diabetes Mellitus
Acute Complications
Chronic Complications
Complementary Therapies

APPLIED LEARNING OUTCOMES

After completing this chapter, you will be able to:

1. Differentiate risk factors, pathophysiology, and clinical manifestations between type 1 and type 2 diabetes mellitus.
2. Identify the diagnostic tests used to diagnose and monitor self-management of diabetes mellitus and report abnormal findings.
3. Administer insulin and oral antidiabetic agents ordered for patients with diabetes mellitus knowledgeably and safely.
4. Compare and contrast the causes, manifestations, and interdisciplinary care for diabetic ketoacidosis, hyperosmolar hyperglycemic state, and hypoglycemia.
5. Implement collaborative care of chronic complications for patients with type 1 and type 2 diabetes mellitus.
6. Reinforce teaching guidelines to patients with diabetes mellitus regarding self-management of medications, diet, exercise, and foot care.
7. Use the nursing process to collect data, establish outcomes, provide individualized care, and evaluate responses for the patient with diabetes mellitus.

KEY TERMS

The key terms are defined on the pages listed below.

dawn phenomenon, 927
diabetes mellitus, 913
diabetic ketoacidosis (DKA), 922
gangrene, 928
glycosuria, 914

hyperglycemia, 914
hyperosmolar hyperglycemic state (HHS), 924
hypoglycemia, 925
ketonuria, 923
ketosis, 914

microalbuminuria, 928
polydipsia, 914
polyphagia, 914
polyuria, 914
Somogyi effect, 927

SPECIAL FEATURES

Key Concept All body tissues and organs require a constant supply of glucose. Normal blood glucose levels are maintained through the actions of insulin and glucagon. Diabetes mellitus results from defects in the secretion of insulin, the action of insulin, or both.

Diabetes mellitus is a common chronic disease of adults. It is not a single disorder but a group of metabolic disorders characterized by hyperglycemia (too much glucose in the blood). This condition is due to an absolute deficiency of insulin, or insufficient supply of insulin and ineffective insulin action.

Patients with diabetes mellitus face lifelong changes in lifestyle and health status. Depending on the type of diabetes and the patient's age, patient needs and nursing care may vary greatly. Nursing care is provided in many settings for the diagnosis and care of the disease and treatment of complications.

Overview of Diabetes Mellitus

The American Diabetes Association (ADA) estimates that approximately 25.8 million people in the United States have diabetes. Unfortunately, 7 million people are undiagnosed. Approximately 1.8 million new cases are diagnosed each year. It is the sixth leading cause of death in the United States and more than $218 billion is spent annually on health care. Type 2 diabetes is increasing among older adults, African American women, Hispanic women, Native Americans, Asians, and Pacific Islanders. Even more alarming is the rapid increase in type 2 diabetes among children and adolescents, especially those who are obese.

Diabetes mellitus cannot be cured. However, control of blood glucose is essential to reduce complications that most often affect the cardiovascular system, kidneys, eyes,

and nerves. People with diabetes have a significantly higher risk for heart disease and stroke than people without diabetes. Diabetes is the leading cause of end-stage renal disease and the main cause of newly diagnosed blindness in people ages 20 to 74. Nontraumatic amputations occur more frequently in people with diabetes.

The term *diabetes*, or *DM*, when used throughout the chapter, refers to diabetes mellitus.

TYPES OF DIABETES MELLITUS

There are two broad categories of diabetes, type 1 DM and type 2 DM. *Type 1 DM* was formerly known as juvenile-onset diabetes mellitus, or insulin-dependent diabetes mellitus (IDDM). *Type 2 DM* was previously known as type II non-insulin-dependent diabetes mellitus (NIDDM) or adult-onset diabetes. The characteristics of type 1, type 2, gestational, and the other types of diabetes are shown in Table 36-1■.

DIABETES IN THE OLDER ADULT

Older adults may have either type 1 or type 2 DM, but most have type 2. Improved management strategies have increased the survival rates for people with type 1 DM. As older adults are living longer and the incidence of diabetes increases with age, more people over age 65 will develop DM. In addition, those older adults with diabetes tend to develop more severe chronic complications.

Complicating the problem is that over the age of 50, blood glucose levels rise. This makes it more difficult to diagnose older adults with DM. Sometimes people are mistakenly diagnosed with diabetes because they show normal aging changes. The usual physiologic changes of aging may mask manifestations of a diabetes onset and may also increase the potential for complications. For instance, urinary incontinence may be confused with polyuria. Other symptoms of diabetes, such as blurred vision and fatigue,

TABLE 36-1	Classification and Characteristics of Diabetes
CLASSIFICATION	**CHARACTERISTICS**
Type 1 diabetes	Autoimmune destruction of beta cells leads to a state of absolute insulin deficiency
	Usually occurs in childhood and adolescence, but may occur at any age
	Patient prone to developing ketoacidosis
	Insulin dependent (*If the patient does not receive insulin, he or she will die.*)
Type 2 diabetes	State of sufficient insulin to prevent ketoacidosis, but insufficient to lower blood glucose levels
	Usually occurs after age 30
	Most patients are obese or have an increased amount of abdominal fat.
	May become *insulin requiring*, but not insulin dependent (*If the patient does not receive insulin, he or she will become ill, but will not die.*)
Other types	Occur from genetic defects or associated with pancreatitis, Cushing syndrome, infection, or drugs such as glucocorticoids
Gestational	Any degree of glucose intolerance with the onset or first recognition of diabetes mellitus during pregnancy

Source: Data from American Diabetes Association. (2012a). Diagnosis and classification of diabetes mellitus. *Diabetes Care, 35* (Suppl.), S64–S71.

may be blamed on age. Peripheral vascular disease related to diabetes or cardiovascular disease may be undetected until serious wound healing problems occur. Older adults often have hypertension, requiring treatment with diuretics, which alters glucose tolerance test results.

The older adult with diabetes has multiple and complex health care problems and needs. Consider the following concerns when working with the older patient:

- Physical limitations due to arthritis and Parkinson disease as well as confusion can interfere with food preparation, activities of daily living, insulin administration and blood glucose testing, foot care, and hygiene.
- Lower fixed incomes and rising costs of medications, blood glucose–monitoring equipment, visits to the physician, and hospitalization may be a problem. Even though Medicare pays part of the medical expenses, the patient is still responsible for part of the cost.
- Cultural background and ethnic origin may encourage a fatalistic acceptance of illness and its complications. Chronic illness often interferes with family communication and relationships.
- Vision or hearing deficits may require the nurse to adapt teaching materials and methods.

PATHOPHYSIOLOGY

DM is a collection of metabolic diseases characterized by hyperglycemia. The two major types of diabetes mellitus are type 1 diabetes and type 2 diabetes, which are discussed next.

Type 1 Diabetes Mellitus

Type 1 diabetes usually occurs in children and adolescents, but it may occur at any age. Type 1 DM results from an autoimmune response that destroys the beta cells of the islets of Langerhans in the pancreas. The end result is that insulin is no longer produced. Insulin deficiency causes **hyperglycemia** (excess glucose in the blood) and a breakdown of body fats and proteins. Without insulin to move glucose into the cells, the cells begin starving so they burn fats and proteins for their energy source. During the burning of fats, **ketosis** develops, a toxic accumulation of *ketone bodies* (by-products from the burning of fatty acids).

When blood glucose exceeds the level the kidneys can process, glucose spills into the urine, and **glycosuria** (excess glucose in the urine) occurs. The body's state of hyperglycemia and glycosuria cause the three primary manifestations of type 1 DM: polyuria, polydipsia, and polyphagia. Hyperglycemia acts as an *osmotic diuretic*, meaning it draws fluid from the intracellular spaces into the general circulation. This causes **polyuria** (increased urine output). The increased urinary output leads to dehydration. The mouth becomes dry, and thirst sensors are

---

BOX 36-1	MANIFESTATIONS OF TYPE 1 AND TYPE 2 DIABETES MELLITUS

Type 1	Type 2
Polyuria	Polyuria
Polydipsia	Polydipsia
Polyphagia	Recurrent infections
Weight loss	Obesity
Fatigue	Fatigue
Malaise	Blurred vision
Blurred vision	Paresthesias

---

activated, causing the person to drink increased amounts of fluid (**polydipsia**).

Because glucose cannot enter the cell without insulin, energy production decreases. This decrease in energy stimulates hunger, and the person eats more food (**polyphagia**). Despite increased food intake, the person loses weight. Malaise and fatigue accompany the decrease in energy. Manifestations are listed in Box 36-1■.

Heredity plays a key role in the development of diabetes mellitus. The child of a diabetic has a 1 in 20 to 1 in 50 risk. Environmental factors may also trigger DM. Viral infections including mumps, rubella, cytomegalovirus, or Coxsackie 4 have been linked to type 1 DM.

Type 2 Diabetes Mellitus

Type 2 DM is characterized by hyperglycemia due to insufficient insulin production and insulin resistance. The inadequate insulin supply cannot lower blood glucose levels through the usual uptake of glucose by muscle and fat cells. However, sufficient insulin is produced to prevent the breakdown of fats; therefore, ketosis does not develop. Heredity plays an important role in its transmission. Other risk factors include obesity, physical inactivity, illnesses, increasing age, and belonging to a high-risk ethnic group.

The majority of people with type 2 DM are overweight. Obesity, especially of the upper body, reduces available insulin receptor sites in the cells of skeletal muscles and adipose tissues and leads to insulin resistance. About three-fourths of older adults with type 2 DM are overweight. All older adults with type 2 DM develop insulin resistance. Diabetics who lose weight through diet and exercise can lessen insulin resistance and improve insulin release. Sometimes insulin efficiency can improve enough so that the type 2 diabetic may no longer require oral antidiabetic agents.

Unfortunately, type 2 diabetes is often undiagnosed for years. People are unaware of its presence until health care is sought for another problem. The hyperglycemia found in type 2 DM is less severe than that of type 1 DM, so only polyuria and polydipsia are seen. Other manifestations include recurrent infections, blurred vision, fatigue, and paresthesias (see Box 36-1). Accumulated glucose in the tissues provides a breeding ground for bacterial infections. High glucose levels cause a cloudiness of the lens of the eye, leading to blurred vision, as well as destruction of peripheral nerves, resulting in paresthesias. Fatigue results from an inadequate amount of glucose being available to feed the cells.

memory**ALERT**

The relationship between glucose and insulin is like a lock and key. Insulin acts as the key to unlock the cell membrane so that glucose can enter the cell. Without insulin, glucose cannot leave the bloodstream, resulting in hyperglycemia.

COLLABORATIVE CARE

Treatment of the patient with diabetes focuses on maintaining blood glucose at levels as nearly normal as possible through medications, diet, and exercise.

Diagnostic Tests

Three laboratory tests are used to screen for the presence of diabetes mellitus: plasma glucose (PG) level, fasting blood glucose (FBG), and an oral glucose tolerance test (OGTT). Although any of the three tests may be used, in the clinical setting the FBG is preferred because it is easier to administer, more convenient, and more economical than the other two.

Diagnostic criteria recommended by the ADA include:

1. Classic diabetic symptoms plus *casual* PG concentration greater than 200 mg/dL (*casual* is defined as any time of day without regard to when last meal was eaten).
2. Eight-hour *fasting* plasma glucose (FPG, also known as FBS) greater than 126 mg/dL (*fasting* is defined as no calorie intake for 8 hours).
3. Two-hour PG greater than 200 mg/dL during an OGTT.

It is usually recommended that the diagnostic test be repeated on a subsequent day to confirm the diagnosis of diabetes mellitus. In addition, the ADA recommends measuring glycosylated hemoglobin (Hgb A1c) level. An Hgb A1c level greater than 6.5% is considered positive for a diagnosis of DM. Levels of 5.7%–6.4% indicate an increased risk for diabetes and cardiovascular disease.

Because of the risk for developing multisystem complications, routine screening should be done for any person who meets one or more of the following seven risk criteria:

1. Is obese (greater than 120% of standard body weight)
2. Has a first-degree relative with diabetes
3. Is a member of a high-risk ethnic population (e.g., African American, Hispanic American, Native American, Asian American, Pacific Islander)
4. Has delivered a baby weighing more than 9 lb or has been diagnosed with gestational diabetes mellitus

5. Is hypertensive (greater than 140/90)
6. Has a high-density lipoprotein (HDL) cholesterol level less than 35 mg/dL and/or a triglyceride level greater than 250 mg/dL
7. On previous testing, had impaired glucose tolerance or impaired fasting glucose

Delayed insulin release from the pancreas, decreased tissue sensitivity to insulin, or both lead to decreasing glucose tolerance in older adults. Because of these physiologic changes in persons over age 60, their FBG levels may be slightly increased.

Prediabetes is a term used to describe people who are at an increased risk for diabetes. It is characterized by increased Hgb A1c levels, FPG between 100 and 126 mg/dL, and a glucose tolerance between 140 and 200 mg/dL after fasting overnight. These test results indicate there is a risk for progression to diabetes. Approximately 79 million adults ages 40 to 74 have prediabetes. Studies suggest that weight loss and increased physical activity can prevent or delay diabetes.

Diagnostic Tests to Monitor Diabetes Management

The most common diagnostic tests to monitor diabetes management are FBG, Hgb A1c, urine glucose and ketone levels, and serum cholesterol and triglyceride levels. The ADA recommends that Hgb A1c levels should be measured twice per year and kept at 7% or less. Serum cholesterol and triglyceride levels are indicators of atherosclerosis and an increased risk of cardiovascular complications. The ADA recommends raising HDL cholesterol level to greater than 50 mg/dL, lowering LDL cholesterol level to less than 100 mg/dL, and lowering triglyceride level to less than 150 mg/dL (ADA, 2012b). FBS and Hgb A1c tests and normal results are summarized in Chapter 34, Table 34-2.

MONITORING BLOOD GLUCOSE   People with diabetes must monitor their condition daily by testing glucose levels. Two types of tests are available. The first type, direct measurement of blood glucose, is widely used in all types of health care settings and in the home. The second type is urine testing for glucose and ketones. Urine testing is less common today because not all patients who are hyperglycemic will spill glucose into their urine.

SELF-MONITORING OF BLOOD GLUCOSE   Self-monitoring of blood glucose (SMBG) allows the person with diabetes to monitor and achieve metabolic control. It is also useful when the person is ill or pregnant or has symptoms of hypoglycemia or hyperglycemia. The ADA recommends that all diabetics be taught some method of monitoring their blood glucose. SMBG should be done three or more times per day for patients with type 1 diabetes. For patients with type 2 diabetes, testing should be sufficient to help them reach glucose goals.

Equipment needed for SMBG includes:

- Some type of lancet device to perform a finger stick for obtaining a drop of blood (e.g., an Autolet, Penlet, or Soft Touch).
- A blood glucose–measuring machine (e.g., Glucometer, Accu-Chek, or OneTouch) if the most accurate measurement is desired or recommended.
- Test strips that change color when they come into contact with glucose or that can be read by machine (e.g., Glucostix and Chemstrip bG). If a meter is not being used, the strip is read by comparing its color with a color chart on the side of the container or on an insert.

Blood glucose–monitoring machines can provide a single reading or (if computerized) can provide a memory of previous glucose readings to show a pattern of control. Each machine has specific operating instructions that must be followed closely. If the timing of the blood on the strip is not exact, the test will be inaccurate. The machine must be cleaned according to the manufacturer's directions to ensure accuracy. Monitors that use no-wipe technology improve the accuracy of glucose measurement.

A new insulin pump receives information from a continuous glucose monitor (CGM) worn on the skin. The CGM has a sensor that is inserted under the skin, just like the insulin pump. This sensor sends data to the insulin pump screen, warning of high or low glucose levels. (Insulin pumps are discussed under equipment later in the chapter.)

URINE TESTING FOR KETONES AND GLUCOSE At one time, urine testing for glucose and ketones was the only available method for evaluating diabetic management. Although inexpensive and noninvasive, it has unpredictable results and cannot be used to detect or measure hypoglycemia.

Urine testing should be done in people with type 1 DM who have unexplained hyperglycemia during illness or pregnancy to monitor for hyperglycemia and ketoacidosis. Ketones may be detected through urine testing, and positive testing reflects the presence of the life-threatening complication diabetic ketoacidosis (discussed in Complications).

To test the urine for ketones:

1. Ask the patient to void, discard the urine, and drink a full glass of water.
2. Thirty minutes later, collect a urine sample.
3. For Acidtest tablets: Place the tablet on a white paper towel, place one drop of urine on the tablet, and wait for 30 seconds. If the tablet turns any shade from lavender to deep purple, the test is positive for ketones.
4. For Ketostix: Dip the reagent stick into the urine sample. Wait for 15 seconds and compare the color of the pad at the end of the stick to an accompanying color chart. Purple indicates ketonuria.

To test the urine for glucose:

1. Follow the same procedure to collect a urine sample.
2. Dip the reagent stick into the urine sample, and wait for the specified time. Compare the color of the pad at the end of the reagent stick with an accompanying color chart.

clinicalALERT

Normally, no glucose is found in the urine, so the presence of glucose indicates hyperglycemia.

Medications

Key Concept Administration of insulin is the primary management strategy along with diet and exercise for patients with type 1 DM. Type 2 DM is usually managed with antidiabetic drugs from multiple classes in addition to diet and exercise.

The pharmacologic treatment for diabetes mellitus depends on the type of diabetes. People with type 1 DM must have insulin; those with type 2 are usually able to control glucose levels with an antidiabetic medication, but they may require insulin when control is inadequate.

INSULIN Insulin is derived from pork pancreas or made in the laboratory. Synthetically produced insulin comes either from altered pork insulin or through genetic engineering using strains of *Escherichia coli* to form biosynthetic human insulin. Insulins are available in rapid-acting, short-acting, intermediate-acting, and long-acting preparations. (The common insulins, times of onset, peak, and duration of action are listed in Table 36-2■.)

clinicalALERT

Rapid-acting (e.g., lispro), regular, and Lantus insulins appear clear. All other insulins appear cloudy.

Insulin is dispensed in two concentrations, either as 100 units/mL (U-100 insulin) or as 500 units/mL (U-500 insulin). The standard concentration is 100 units/mL. U-500 insulin is used only in rare cases of insulin resistance when very large doses are needed.

Insulin is given in sterile, single-use, disposable insulin syringes, marked in units per milliliter. This means that in U-100 insulin, there are 100 units of insulin in 1 mL. Common syringe size is either 0.5 mL (50 units) or 1.0 mL (100 units). The advantage of the 0.5-mL size is that the distance between unit markings is greater so that it is easier to measure the dose accurately. Most insulin syringes are manufactured with the needle permanently attached

TABLE 36-2	Action of Insulin Preparations		
TYPE OF INSULIN	**ONSET (HR)**	**PEAK (HR)**	**DURATION (HR)**
Rapid-acting			
■ Lispro (Humalog)	0.25	0.5–1.5	3–4
■ Aspart (NovoLog)	0.25	1–3	3–5
■ Glulisine (Apidra)	0.25	0.5–1.5	3–5
Short-acting			
■ Regular (Novolin R, Humulin R)	0.5–1	2–3	4–6
Intermediate-acting			
■ NPH (Novolin N, Humulin N)	1–2	6–8	12–16
■ Novolin NPH 70/ regular 30	0.5	4–8	24
Long-acting			
■ Glargine (Lantus)	2	Peak not defined	24
■ Detemir (Levemir)	2	Peak not defined	24

in a 25- to 26-gauge, 0.5-in. size. Regular insulin may be given by either subcutaneous or intravenous (IV) routes; all others are given only subcutaneously.

Special Injection Products   Special injection products such as insulin pens are available. Insulin pens use a prefilled, multidose insulin cartridge with a disposable needle (Figure 36-1■). Patients who use the insulin pen dial the appropriate dose before injection. Prefilled pens should be stored at room temperature and must be discarded after 28 days. Pens not in current use should be stored in the refrigerator. Insulin pens are useful for people who are visually impaired or traveling.

Regular or rapid-acting insulins can be delivered through a continuous subcutaneous insulin infusion (CSII) device, also called an insulin pump. The CSII device has a small external pump, about the size of a pager that holds a syringe connected to a subcutaneous needle by tubing. The needle is placed into the subcutaneous tissue, usually the abdomen, and is changed every 3 days. This device delivers a constant amount of programmed insulin throughout each 24-hour period. It also delivers a bolus of insulin when programmed manually (e.g., before meals). Frequent blood glucose monitoring is necessary to program the amount of insulin to be delivered. The advantages of CSII include more normal glucose control and greater lifestyle flexibility. Disadvantages are an increased risk of ketoacidosis from a malfunctioning pump and infection at the needle insertion site.

Insulin Injection Sites   Recommended injection sites are the upper arm, the abdomen except for a 2-in. circle around the navel (the umbilicus), the anterior lateral part of the thigh, and the buttocks (Figure 36-2■). Absorption and peak action of insulin differ according to the site. The most rapid absorption site is the abdomen, followed by the arms, thighs, and buttocks.

To administer insulin, gently pinch a fold of skin and inject the needle at a 90-degree angle. If the person is very thin, a 45-degree angle may be required to avoid injecting into muscle. Do not massage the site after giving the injection because this may interfere with absorption. Rotation within injection sites is recommended to

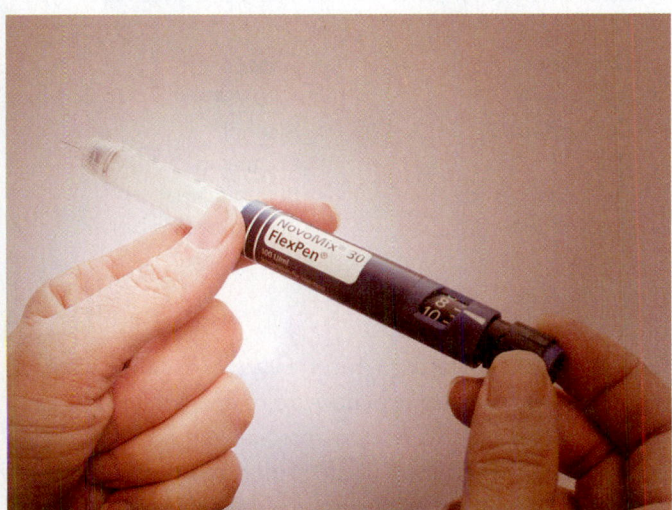

Figure 36-1 ■ Air shot clears cartridge and needle of air and primes needle for injection. (Source: Eddie Lawrence/Science Source.)

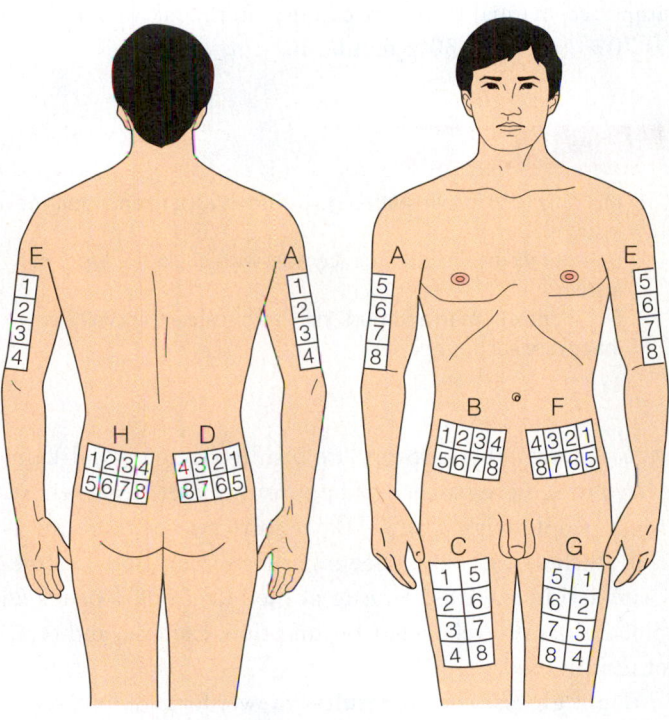

Figure 36-2 ■ Sites of insulin injection.

give more consistent blood glucose levels and to prevent lipodystrophy. The distance between injections should be about 1 in. There are several techniques to minimize painful injections that the nurse can use or can teach (if the patient is self-administering insulin). First, bring insulin to room temperature and remove all air from the syringe before administering the injection. If topical alcohol is used, be sure it has evaporated completely before giving the injection. Insert the needle quickly. Insert and remove the needle without changing needle direction. Instruct the patient to relax the muscles in the area before the injection and not to reuse needles (ADA, 2004).

Lipodystrophy (hypertrophy of subcutaneous tissue) or *lipoatrophy* (atrophy of subcutaneous tissue) may occur if the same injection sites are used repeatedly. The use of refrigerated synthetic or pork insulin may trigger the development of tissue hypertrophy or atrophy. These problems rarely occur with the use of human insulins. Lipodystrophy and lipoatrophy alter insulin absorption by delaying its onset. Lipodystrophy usually resolves if the area is unused for a minimum of 6 months.

Mixing Insulins People who require more than one type of insulin must mix their insulins to avoid multiple injections per dose. In addition, patients often need different doses of insulin throughout the day to provide adequate blood glucose control. The *procedure* for mixing insulins is described in Box 36-2■. Additional nursing implications and guidelines for teaching patients insulin administration techniques are listed in Table 36-3■. Patients who have difficulty mixing insulin because of poor eyesight or impaired manual dexterity can use premixed insulins such as 70% NPH and 30% regular insulin.

clinicalALERT

1. Mix only NPH insulin with regular, lispro, aspart, and glulisine insulins.
2. Do not mix insulin glargine (Lantus) with *any* other types of insulin.
3. Do not mix human and pork insulins because they will inactivate each other.

Insulin Regimens The appropriate insulin dosage is individualized to achieve balance among insulin, diet, and exercise. Most people with type 1 DM require two or more injections each day. Usually, they mix short-acting and intermediate-acting insulins. Timing of the injections depends on blood glucose levels, food consumption, exercise, and types of insulin used.

Tight glucose control results in fewer long-term complications. This can be achieved through an intensive insulin

regimen (three or four injections per day) (Table 36-4■). Whether the patient needs one or multiple daily injections, the goal is to avoid daytime hypoglycemia while achieving adequate blood glucose control overnight.

Sliding Scale Insulin. Hospitalized patients with type 1 and type 2 diabetes can experience drastic changes in serum glucose levels due to infection, surgery, acute illness, altered caloric intake, or physical and/or emotional stress. Sliding scale insulin provides subcutaneous regular insulin injections that are adjusted according to capillary blood glucose levels. When this regimen is used, blood glucose levels are measured every 6 hours or at specified times such as before meals and at bedtime. Maintaining tighter control of blood glucose levels during hospitalization decreases the risk of postoperative infections and shortens hospital stay.

ANTIDIABETIC AGENTS Oral antidiabetic agents are used to treat people with type 2 DM (Table 36-5■). All patients taking oral antidiabetics must be taught to monitor their blood glucose levels at least two to three times per week. Testing may be more frequent when patients have difficulty reaching their glucose goals.

Two injectable drugs, exenatide (Byetta) and pramlintide (Symlin), are being used to manage glucose levels better. Byetta mimics incretin, a naturally occurring hormone secreted by the gastrointestinal tract to slow gastric emptying and stimulate insulin release. It works best with type 2 diabetics who take oral antidiabetic drugs. Symlin, a synthetic form of amylin, decreases blood glucose levels after meals. It is used to supplement mealtime insulin in type 1 or type 2 diabetes. Both medications carry an increased risk of hypoglycemia.

clinicalALERT

Patients taking sulfonylureas can develop hyperglycemia or hypoglycemia when taken with the following drugs:

Monitor for Hyperglycemia	Monitor for Hypoglycemia
■ Corticosteroids	■ Alcohol
■ Estrogen	■ Coumadin
■ Thiazide diuretics	■ Beta-blockers
■ Epinephrine	■ Ranitidine (Zantac)

Nutrition Therapy

Diabetes management requires a careful balance between nutrient intake, daily expenditure of energy, and the dose and timing of insulin or oral antidiabetic agents. Persons with diabetes must eat a more structured diet in order to prevent hyperglycemia. The American Diabetes Association (ADA, 2008) established the following medical nutrition therapy (MNT) goals for adults with diabetes:

| BOX 36-2 | PROCEDURE CHECKLIST |

Mixing Insulins: 10 Units of Regular and 20 Units of NPH

☑ Wash hands.
☑ Inspect regular insulin for clarity. *Regular insulin is contaminated if cloudy.*
☑ Gently rotate NPH insulin to mix well. *Shaking insulin creates bubbles and prevents an accurate dose from being withdrawn.*
☑ Wipe off the top of both vials with an alcohol pad. *Prevents contamination of insulin.*
☑ Draw 20 units of air into the syringe, and inject air into the NPH vial (Figure A). Withdraw the needle. *Prepares vial by creating pressure.*

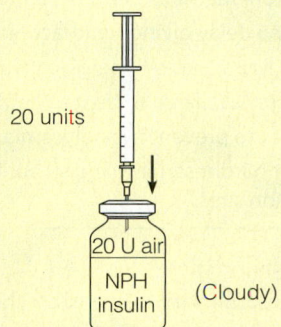

20 units

A Injecting air into the NPH vial.

☑ Draw 10 units of air into the syringe, and inject air into the regular vial (Figure B). *Prepares vial by creating pressure.*

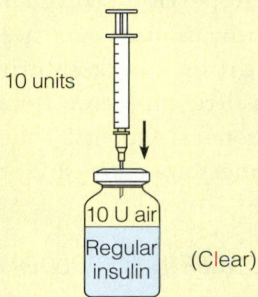

10 units

B Injecting air into the regular insulin vial.

☑ Invert the regular insulin vial, and withdraw 10 units of regular insulin (Figure C). Withdraw the needle. *Withdrawing regular insulin first prevents contaminating regular insulin with NPH insulin.*

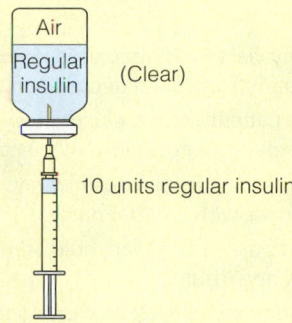

10 units regular insulin

C Withdrawing regular insulin.

☑ Insert the needle into the NPH vial, and carefully withdraw 20 units of NPH insulin (Figure D) for a total of 30 units of insulin in the syringe. *Accurate dosage is important for effectiveness.*

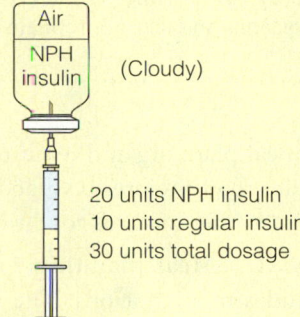

20 units NPH insulin
10 units regular insulin
30 units total dosage

D Withdrawing NPH insulin.

☑ Administer insulin.
☑ Dispose of the syringe properly and wash hands.

Sample Documentation

[date]   07:30 a.m. regular insulin 10 units and NPH insulin 20 units given subcutaneously in right upper arm.

_____R. Perry, LPN.

Note: Refer to a nursing fundamentals or skills text for more detailed instruction. Check state guidelines and facility policy before performing any procedure.

1. Achieve and maintain as near-normal blood glucose levels as safely possible by balancing food intake with insulin or oral antidiabetics.
2. Achieve and maintain optimal serum lipid levels to reduce the risk of vascular disease.
3. Achieve and maintain blood pressure levels in the normal range.
4. Prevent, or at least slow, the rate of development of chronic complications of DM by modifying nutrient intake and lifestyle.
5. Prevent and treat the acute complications of insulin-treated DM, short-term illnesses, and exercise-related problems.
6. Address individual nutrition needs, taking into account personal and cultural preferences and willingness to change.
7. Maintain pleasure of eating and only limit food choices as indicated.

Early in the diagnosis of diabetes, patients should be referred to a certified diabetic educator and registered

TABLE 36-3	Giving Medications Safely: Insulin and Patient Teaching
NURSING IMPLICATIONS	**PATIENT/FAMILY TEACHING**
■ Discard vials of insulin whose expiration date has passed.	■ Know the manifestations of diabetes mellitus.
■ Discard any vial that is discolored or contains clumps, granules, or solid deposits on the sides.	■ Store opened insulin vials in a cool place for up to 4 weeks; avoid exposure to extreme temperatures (36° to 46°F) or sunlight.
■ Check the patient's blood glucose level 30 minutes before giving an insulin injection.	■ Refrigerate unopened extra insulin vials; do not freeze them.
■ When drawing up insulin dose, always check the type and dose with another nurse.	■ Refrigerated insulin should be brought to room temperature before using it.
■ If a patient's meal is delayed, hold administration of rapid-acting insulin.	■ Demonstrate self-administration of insulin (review procedure checklist in Box 36-2).
■ Monitor and maintain a record of blood glucose readings before each meal and at bedtime or as ordered.	■ Know how to mix two types of insulin.
	■ Discard outdated or discolored insulin.
	■ Keep a regular insulin vial available for emergencies.
■ Monitor food intake; notify the physician when the patient eats an inadequate diet.	■ Check blood glucose before meals, at bedtime, and as prescribed.
■ Inspect injection sites for signs of lipodystrophy.	■ If breakfast is delayed, also delay giving rapid-acting insulin.
■ Monitor for signs and symptoms of hypoglycemia or hyperglycemia and take appropriate action.	■ Know the signs of hypoglycemia and hyperglycemia.
	■ Keep candy or sugar source available to treat hypoglycemia.
	■ Avoid alcoholic beverages to prevent hypoglycemia.
	■ Observe injection site for hardness, dimpling, or sunken areas; develop a plan for rotating injection sites.

dietitian for meal planning and teaching. The dietary plan should consider food preferences, food habits and values, culture, age, and other medical conditions (Table 36-6 ■).

MEAL PLANNING Meal planning for the person with diabetes includes many options. The standard ADA diet is no longer recommended by the American Diabetes Association. Instead, MNT focuses on developing a well-balanced diet that meets the patient's daily needs. Meal planning may be based on food groups, carbohydrate counting, the consistent-carbohydrate diabetes meal plan, or exchange lists. The ADA recommends daily dietary intake of carbohydrates, proteins, and fats (see Table 36-6). Altering foods and meal patterns is one of the most difficult parts of diabetes management. Careful consideration of individual preferences promotes dietary compliance.

Carbohydrate Counting Carbohydrates have the greatest effect on *postprandial* (after-meal) blood glucose levels. In this plan, patients are taught to count carbohydrates so they can administer a prescribed amount of regular insulin or lispro insulin for every 10 to 15 g of carbohydrate eaten in a meal. This method provides better glucose control than the traditional exchange list plan and is, therefore, replacing it.

Consistent-Carbohydrate Diabetes Meal Plan This diabetes meal plan focuses on creating meals with consistent-carbohydrate content. For example, breakfast each day contains the same amount of carbohydrates as the previous day. The same method is used for lunch and dinner.

Exchange Lists The exchange list diet is based on the person's ideal (or reasonable) weight, activity level, age, and occupation. These factors determine the total kilocalories that the person may consume each day. The distribution of foods throughout the day is based on six exchange lists. Foods in each list contain similar amounts of carbohydrate, protein, fat, and calories. Standard household measurements determine portion sizes. The number of servings is based on the calorie count needed by the patient. A food item on the list can be substituted ("exchanged") for another with little difference in calories or amount of carbohydrates, proteins, and fats. The meal plan prescribes how many exchanges are allowed for each food group per meal and snacks.

NUTRITIONAL CONCERNS FOR OLDER ADULTS An obese older adult with type 2 DM may need a diet, exercise, and weight-reduction program. To improve compliance with the diet plan, the nurse should consider the following factors: dietary likes and dislikes, eating habits, the person preparing the meals, age-related changes in taste and smell, and dental health. Other factors to consider include the age-related decline in calorie needs and reduced physical activity. The older adult who is overweight should reduce calorie intake in order to lose weight. Portion control is one strategy for reducing intake and therefore weight. The ChooseMyPlate website from the USDA shows the recommended food portion sizes (see Figure 25-2). Other dietary concerns include the fact that many older adults live on a fixed income, limiting their diet to canned meat, fruits, and vegetables. Coexisting illnesses and the use of multiple medications decrease appetite and reduce their energy to

TABLE 36-4	Insulin Regimens
REGIMEN	**INSULIN TYPE***

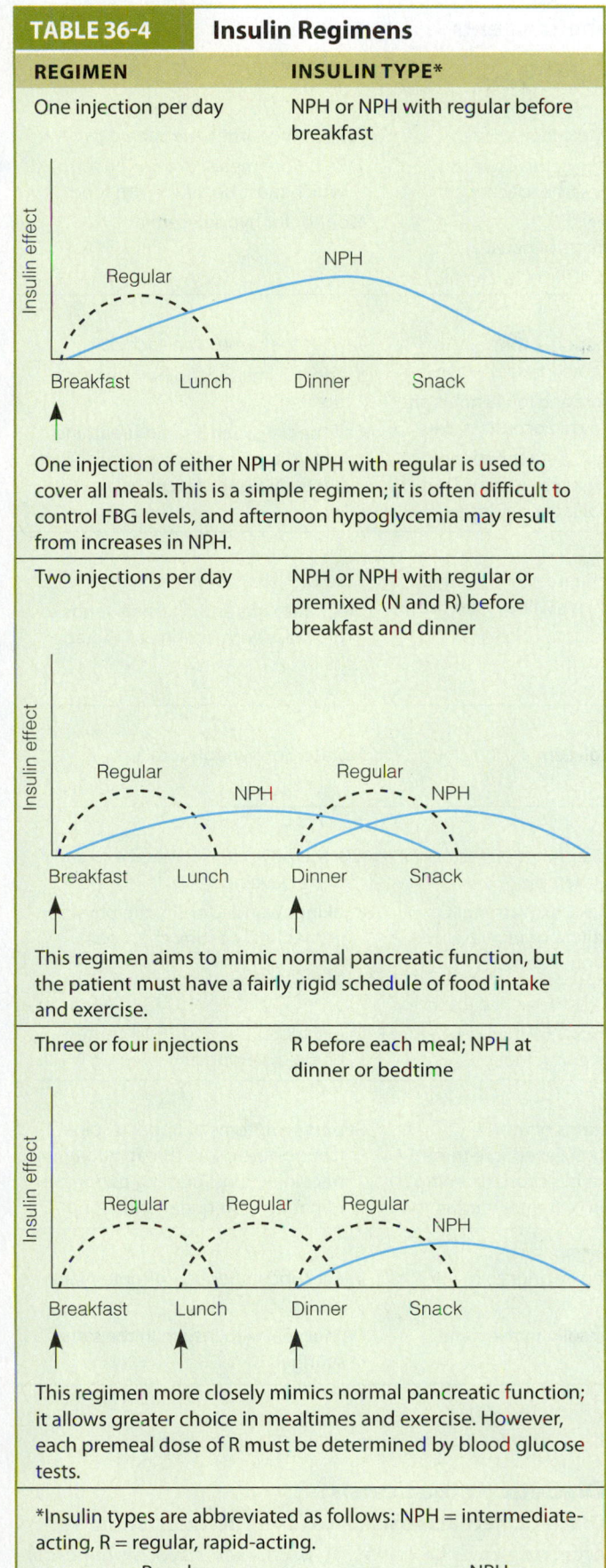

One injection per day — NPH or NPH with regular before breakfast

One injection of either NPH or NPH with regular is used to cover all meals. This is a simple regimen; it is often difficult to control FBG levels, and afternoon hypoglycemia may result from increases in NPH.

Two injections per day — NPH or NPH with regular or premixed (N and R) before breakfast and dinner

This regimen aims to mimic normal pancreatic function, but the patient must have a fairly rigid schedule of food intake and exercise.

Three or four injections — R before each meal; NPH at dinner or bedtime

This regimen more closely mimics normal pancreatic function; it allows greater choice in mealtimes and exercise. However, each premeal dose of R must be determined by blood glucose tests.

*Insulin types are abbreviated as follows: NPH = intermediate-acting, R = regular, rapid-acting.

_____ = Regular   _____ = NPH

plan, cook, or eat. Dietary restrictions may cause the older adult to avoid social gatherings. If possible, encourage older adults to eat their meals with others, which may increase their appetite.

Exercise

Exercise is extremely important for diabetic patients. It reduces blood glucose levels by increasing glucose use by the muscles. This potentially decreases the need for insulin. Exercise also decreases cholesterol and triglycerides, reducing the risk of cardiovascular disorders. People with diabetes should consult their primary health care provider before beginning or changing an exercise program. The ability to maintain an exercise program may be affected by fatigue and glucose levels.

The nurse should assess the patient's lifestyle before determining the type of exercise program. Lifestyle factors to consider are the patient's usual exercise habits, living environment, and community programs. The type of exercise the person usually enjoys is probably the one that he or she will continue throughout life. Whatever exercise the patient chooses, it must be done on a regular basis for at least 150 minutes per week.

Patients with diabetes should follow the recommendations of the ADA when exercising: Use proper footwear, inspect the feet daily and after exercise, avoid exercise in extreme heat or cold, and avoid exercise during periods of poor glucose control. The patient over age 35 should have an exercise-stress electrocardiogram before beginning an exercise program (see Chapter 16). General exercise guidelines for patients with type 1 and type 2 diabetes are listed in Box 36-3■.

Complications of Diabetes Mellitus

The person with diabetes mellitus, regardless of type, is at increased risk for acute and chronic complications involving multiple body systems. Altered blood glucose levels affect the vascular and nervous systems and cause an increased susceptibility to infection. Figure 36-3■ shows the progression from early manifestations to acute complications to chronic multisystem complications. A discussion of each of these complications with related interdisciplinary and nursing care follows.

ACUTE COMPLICATIONS

Key Concept   Uncontrolled or poorly managed DM can cause acute alterations in blood glucose levels, resulting in the complications of diabetic ketoacidosis, hyperosmolar hyperglycemic state, and hypoglycemia. It is essential that these complications be recognized and treated immediately.

TABLE 36-5	Giving Medications Safely: Oral Antidiabetic Agents		
CLASS/DRUGS	PURPOSE	NURSING IMPLICATIONS	PATIENT TEACHING
Sulfonylureas ■ *Glimepiride* (Amaryl) ■ *Glipizide* (Glucotrol, Glucotrol XL) ■ *Glyburide* (DiaBeta)	Increases release of insulin from pancreas and increases tissue response to insulin.	Assess for allergy to sulfonamides. Observe for hypoglycemia (sweating, hunger, shakiness, headache, tachycardia, anxiety). Assess for side effects of nausea, heartburn, or diarrhea.	Take at the same time each day. Take before meals, except Glucotrol XL, which must be taken with food. Monitor for hypoglycemia.
Biguanides ■ *Metformin* (Glucophage)	Reduces liver glucose production and improves glucose use in skeletal muscle.	Monitor renal function, especially in patients at risk for kidney disease. Hold 48 hours before and for 48 hours after injection with any radiocontrast dye. Call the physician if rapid breathing, drowsiness, or malaise occurs. These are early signs of lactic acidosis.	Take at the same time each day. If a dose is missed, do not double dose. Call the physician if rapid breathing, drowsiness, or malaise occurs. These are early signs of lactic acidosis.
Alpha-glucosidase inhibitors ■ Acarbose (Precose) ■ Miglitol (Glyset)	Slows digestion and absorption of carbohydrates to decrease rise in blood glucose after meals.	Do not give to patients with intestinal disorders; acarbose will worsen these conditions.	Take with the first bite of a meal. May cause gas and diarrhea; tends to decrease with continued therapy.
Meglitinides ■ Repaglinide (Prandin) ■ Nateglinide (Starlix)	Stimulates pancreas to secrete insulin.	Monitor for hypoglycemia.	Monitor for hypoglycemia.
Thiazolidinediones ■ Rosiglitazone (Avandia) ■ Pioglitazone (Actos)	Increases insulin sensitivity at receptor sites on liver, muscle, and fat cells.	Obtain baseline liver function tests before starting therapy. Avandia has a Black Box Warning: Can worsen heart failure or increase risk for myocardial infarction.	Call the physician if jaundice or dark urine develops. If taking Avandia, notify the physician immediately of any chest pain.
Incretin mimetics ■ Exenatide (Byetta)	Increases release of insulin from pancreas.	Inject subcutaneously 60 minutes before morning and evening meal.	Inject subcutaneously 60 minutes before morning and evening meal.
DPP-4 inhibitors ■ Sitagliptin (Januvia)	Decreases the release of glucose from liver and increases insulin secretion.	Monitor for symptoms of upper respiratory (cough, fever, sore throat) and urinary tract infections (burning during urination or frequent urination).	Report symptoms of upper respiratory (cough, fever, sore throat) and urinary tract infections (burning during urination or frequent urination).
Amylin hormone ■ Pramlintide (Symlin)	Delays gastric emptying and suppresses glucagon secretion after meals.	Inject subcutaneously prior to major meals. Do not mix with insulin in the same syringe.	Inject subcutaneously prior to major meals. Do not mix with insulin in the same syringe.

Note: Medications identified in *italics* are among the 200 most frequently prescribed drugs in the United States.

Diabetic ketoacidosis, hyperosmolar hyperglycemic state, and hypoglycemia are the primary acute complications of diabetes mellitus. These can be life threatening and require immediate medical treatment.

Diabetic Ketoacidosis

Diabetic ketoacidosis (DKA) is a life-threatening illness occurring in type 1 DM. It is characterized by hyperglycemia, dehydration, and coma. DKA often develops in a

TABLE 36-6	Nutrient Recommendations for Adults With Diabetes
NUTRIENT	**RECOMMENDED DAILY INTAKE**
Calories (kcal)	Amount needed to attain and maintain as close as possible the desired body weight.
Carbohydrates	Individualized to the patient's needs, glucose and lipid goals, with recommended allowances of 45%–60% of the daily diet.
Sweeteners	Saccharin (Sweet'N Low), aspartame or neotame (NutraSweet, Equal), sucralose (Splenda), and acesulfame potassium (Sunette) are safe when consumed within acceptable daily levels by FDA.
Protein	Approximately 15%–20% of the daily caloric intake; should be from both animal and vegetable sources. Patients with nephropathy need lower protein intake.
Saturated fat and cholesterol	Less than 7% of the daily calories should be from saturated fats, with dietary cholesterol limited to 300 mg or less per day.
Fiber	20–35 g of dietary fiber each day from legumes, fruits, vegetables, whole grain products, and fiber-rich cereals (5 g or more fiber/serving).
Sodium	The same as for the general population; no more than 3,000 mg/day.
Vitamins and minerals	Sufficient to meet daily requirements.
Alcohol	Limit alcohol intake to one drink or less per day for women and two drinks or less per day for men. Ingest with a meal to decrease the risk of hypoglycemia.

Source: Data from American Diabetes Association. (2008). Nutrition recommendations and interventions for diabetes. *Diabetes Care, 31* (Suppl. 1), S61–S74.

BOX 36-3   POPULATION FOCUS

Exercise Guidelines for Patients With Type 1 and Type 2 DM

1. Include a warm-up and cool-down period in your exercise program.
2. Check feet for blisters or other damage before and after exercise.
3. Consume adequate fluids, especially water, before, during, and after exercise.
4. Monitor SMBG before and after exercise.
5. Always carry quick-acting carbohydrate (Life-Savers or 5-g glucose tablets).
6. Always carry diabetic ID card and wear ID bracelet.

Type 1
- Exercise within 30–60 minutes of eating.
- Avoid exercise if ketones are present in the urine.

Type 2
- If taking sulfonylureas, eat a snack before exercising.
- Include resistance-exercise (muscle strengthening) in the program.

Source: American Diabetes Association. (2012b). Standards of medical care in diabetes: 2012. *Diabetes Care, 35* (Suppl. 1), S11–S63.

patient with undiagnosed and untreated diabetes. An individual who is sick, has an infection (the most frequent cause of DKA), who decreases or omits insulin, or has excessive physical or emotional stress is at a greater risk for developing DKA.

Without insulin, glucose cannot enter the cell, which stimulates the liver to increase glucose production, leading to hyperglycemia. This excess glucose acts as an osmotic diuretic (pulls fluid from extracellular space), causing polyuria and eventually leading to dehydration and sodium and potassium loss.

Because glucose cannot be used for energy, the fat stores break down, resulting in continued hyperglycemia and burning of fatty acids. This causes the formation of ketones. When more ketones are produced than the cell can use and the kidneys can excrete, *ketoacidosis* develops. Ketoacidosis alters acid–base balance, causing metabolic acidosis. The increased buildup of ketones depresses the central nervous system (CNS), leading to coma and death if left untreated (Figure 36-4■). The manifestations of DKA are listed in Box 36-4■.

memory**ALERT**

To compensate for the acidic state produced by DKA, the respiratory center increases the rate and depth of breathing. This is known as Kussmaul respirations.

TREATMENT OF DIABETIC KETOACIDOSIS   DKA is the most serious metabolic disturbance of people with type 1 diabetes. Hospital admission may be required when the person has a blood glucose of greater than 250 mg/dL and ketones in the urine (**ketonuria**).

DKA is treated with fluids (for dehydration), insulin (to reduce hyperglycemia and acidosis), and correction of electrolyte imbalances. If the patient is alert and conscious, fluids may be given orally. Unconscious patients require IV fluids. The nurse should be prepared to administer a 0.9% normal saline solution to replace the sodium losses at a rate of 500 to 1,000 mL/hr. After 2 to 3 hours, the

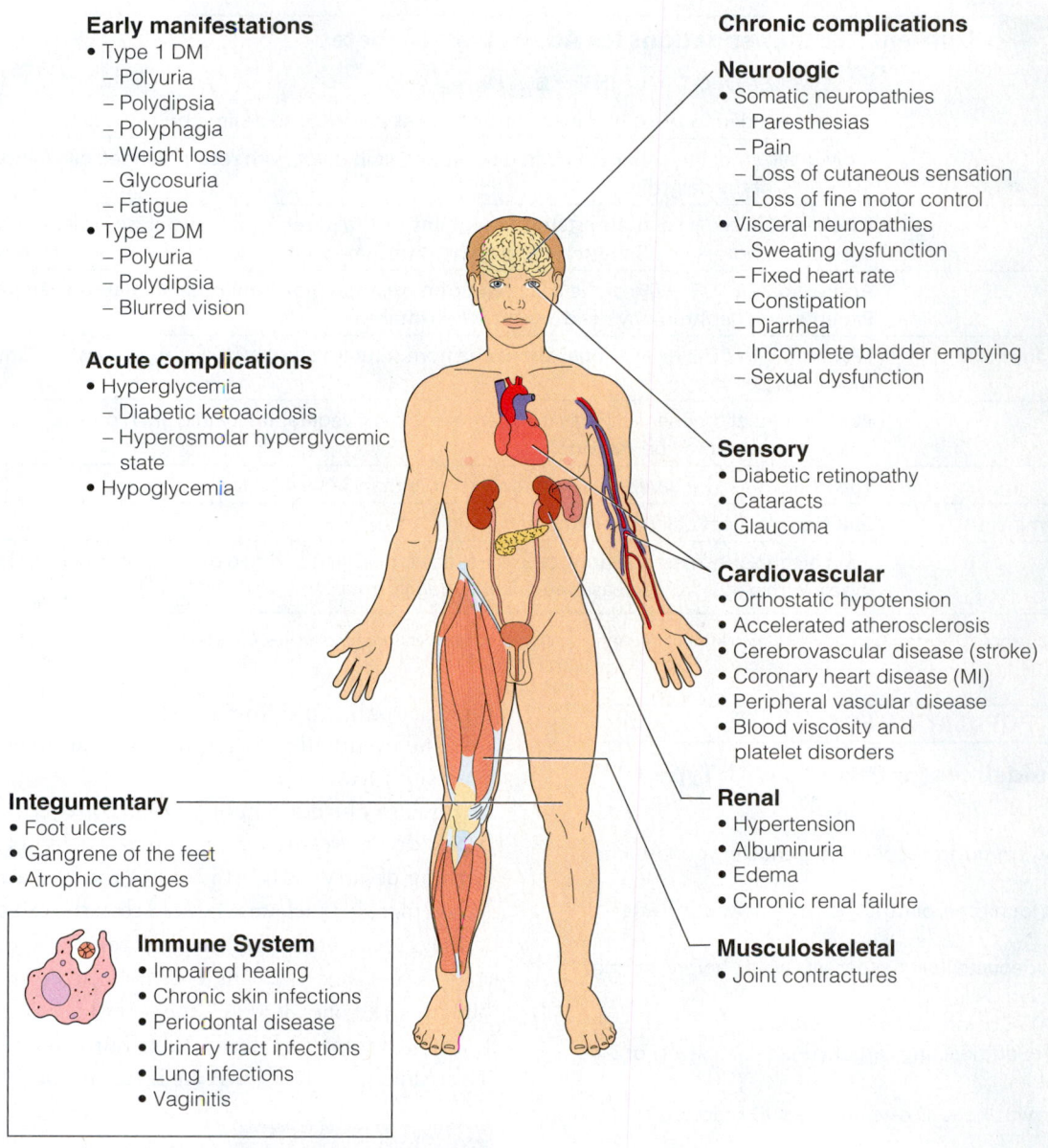

Early manifestations
- Type 1 DM
  - Polyuria
  - Polydipsia
  - Polyphagia
  - Weight loss
  - Glycosuria
  - Fatigue
- Type 2 DM
  - Polyuria
  - Polydipsia
  - Blurred vision

Acute complications
- Hyperglycemia
  - Diabetic ketoacidosis
  - Hyperosmolar hyperglycemic state
- Hypoglycemia

Integumentary
- Foot ulcers
- Gangrene of the feet
- Atrophic changes

Immune System
- Impaired healing
- Chronic skin infections
- Periodontal disease
- Urinary tract infections
- Lung infections
- Vaginitis

Chronic complications

Neurologic
- Somatic neuropathies
  - Paresthesias
  - Pain
  - Loss of cutaneous sensation
  - Loss of fine motor control
- Visceral neuropathies
  - Sweating dysfunction
  - Fixed heart rate
  - Constipation
  - Diarrhea
  - Incomplete bladder emptying
  - Sexual dysfunction

Sensory
- Diabetic retinopathy
- Cataracts
- Glaucoma

Cardiovascular
- Orthostatic hypotension
- Accelerated atherosclerosis
- Cerebrovascular disease (stroke)
- Coronary heart disease (MI)
- Peripheral vascular disease
- Blood viscosity and platelet disorders

Renal
- Hypertension
- Albuminuria
- Edema
- Chronic renal failure

Musculoskeletal
- Joint contractures

Figure 36-3 ■ Multisystem effects of diabetes mellitus.

IV solution is changed to 0.45% normal saline to prevent hypernatremia. When the blood glucose levels reach 250 mg/dL, dextrose is added to prevent rapid decreases in glucose, causing hypoglycemia. Potassium may be added to an IV solution if the patient's laboratory values show a deficit. Regular insulin is used to treat the patient's hyperglycemia. The degree of hyperglycemia and ketosis determines whether insulin is given by the subcutaneous or IV route. Typically, a continuous insulin infusion is started and maintained until the ketoacidosis is resolved.

clinicalALERT

Only regular insulin may be given by the IV route.

Hyperosmolar Hyperglycemic State

Hyperosmolar hyperglycemic state (HHS) occurs in people with type 2 DM. It is characterized by severely elevated blood glucose levels, extreme dehydration, and an altered level of consciousness. This condition usually develops slowly over several hours to days. It is a serious, life-threatening medical emergency that has a higher mortality rate than DKA because usually the patients are older and have other medical problems. Infection, surgery, renal and cardiac disease, and dialysis are a few factors that can trigger HHS.

The state of extreme hyperglycemia leads to osmotic diuresis and results in severe dehydration, especially of the brain. The manifestations result from the effects of

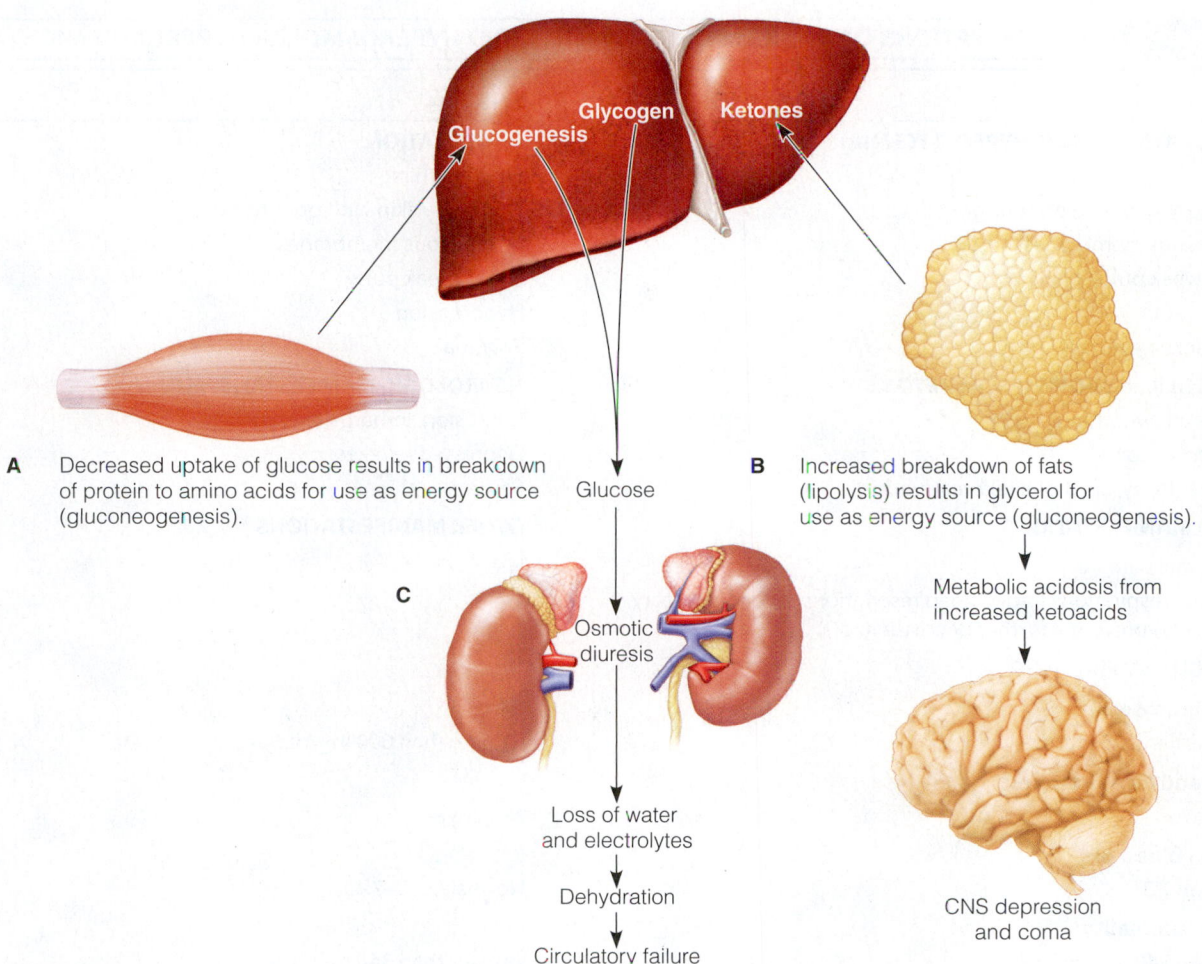

Figure 36-4. ■ In type 1 diabetes mellitus, without adequate insulin, muscle (**A**) and fat (**B**) cells are used as sources of energy. Amino acids from skeletal muscle are converted to glucose in the liver. Glycerol from fat cells is converted to glucose and fatty acids to form ketoacids, causing CNS depression and coma. Increased glucose (**C**) causes osmotic diuresis, leading to dehydration and decreased circulatory volume. The end result of these processes is diabetic ketoacidosis (DKA), which can be reversed with intravenous insulin to lower blood glucose. Intravenous fluids are given to reduce dehydration and raise blood pressure. Electrolytes are monitored and corrected.

hyperglycemia and dehydration (see Box 36-4). Ketosis does not occur like it does in DKA, because the type 2 diabetic has sufficient insulin.

TREATMENT OF HYPEROSMOLAR HYPERGLYCEMIC STATE   Treatment is similar to that of DKA, namely, correcting fluid and electrolyte imbalances and providing insulin to lower hyperglycemia. IV fluids of 0.9% normal saline are given, followed by 0.45% normal saline to correct the fluid and sodium losses. Insulin is administered to reduce the severe hyperglycemia. When blood glucose levels reach 250 mg/dL, insulin is discontinued because, in contrast to DKA, ketosis is not present.

Whether caring for the patient with DKA or HHS, the nurse is responsible for measuring the patient's vital signs, monitoring the level of consciousness, monitoring IV infusions, monitoring fluid status through intake and output,

and notifying the physician of the patient's response to treatment.

Hypoglycemia

Hypoglycemia can occur in people with type 1 DM and people with type 2 DM who are treated with antidiabetic agents. It may be caused by too much insulin intake, overdose of antidiabetic agents, too little food, or excess physical activity. The onset is sudden, and blood glucose is usually less than 50 mg/dL.

The brain requires a constant supply of glucose, so a hypoglycemic episode alters brain function. The manifestations of hypoglycemia (Box 36-5■) result from activation of the autonomic nervous system (ANS) and from impaired cerebral function. People who experience frequent hypoglycemic episodes during which the blood glucose level drops

BOX 36-4   MANIFESTATIONS OF DIABETIC KETOACIDOSIS AND HYPEROSMOLAR HYPERGLYCEMIC STATE

DKA	HHS
DEHYDRATION (FROM HYPERGLYCEMIA)	**DEHYDRATION**
Thirst	Extreme thirst
Warm, dry skin with poor turgor	Warm, dry skin with poor turgor
Dry mucous membranes	Dry mucous membranes
Rapid, weak pulse	Rapid, weak pulse
Hypotension	Hypotension
Soft, sunken eyeballs	Polyuria
METABOLIC ACIDOSIS (FROM KETOSIS)	**NEUROLOGIC MANIFESTATIONS**
Nausea and vomiting	Confusion, lethargy to coma
Lethargy to coma	Depressed reflexes
Acetone (fruity, alcohol-like) breath odor	Seizures
OTHER MANIFESTATIONS	**OTHER MANIFESTATIONS**
Abdominal pain	Nausea
Kussmaul respirations (rapid, deep respirations; a compensatory response to prevent a further decrease in pH)	
LABORATORY FINDINGS	
Blood glucose:	
Greater than 250 mg/dL	Greater than 600 mg/dL
Blood and urine ketones:	
Positive	Negative
Arterial blood pH:	
Less than 7.3	Normal (7.35–7.45)
Serum osmolality:	
Less than 340 mOsm/L	Greater than 340 mOsm/L

below 20 mg/dL may develop decreased cerebral function. Severe untreated hypoglycemia may lead to death.

clinicalALERT

As the body ages, the autonomic nervous system becomes less responsive. The older adult may not experience the manifestations caused by the autonomic nervous system.

Some people with long-standing type 1 diabetes may develop hypoglycemia unawareness. The normal compensatory mechanisms, which should raise blood glucose levels, fail. The person does not show any symptoms of hypoglycemia, even though they exist. Because treatment is delayed, the patient may experience more frequent and severe episodes of hypoglycemia.

TREATMENT OF HYPOGLYCEMIA   Hypoglycemia may occur at any time, but it most often develops before meals or in the middle of the night. Mild hypoglycemia is usually recognized and self-managed, but severe hypoglycemia requires treatment by health care providers.

Mild Hypoglycemia   When mild hypoglycemia (blood glucose between 60 and 70 mg/dL) occurs, immediate treatment is necessary. People experiencing hypoglycemia should take about 15 to 20 g of a rapid-acting sugar. Examples of fast-acting glucose are as follows:

- Three to four glucose tablets
- Half cup of fruit juice or regular soda
- Eight ounces of milk
- Five to six pieces of hard candy
- One tablespoon of sugar or honey

clinicalALERT

Do not add sugar to fruit juice, because it causes a rapid rise in blood glucose, which would require additional treatment.

BOX 36-5	MANIFESTATIONS OF HYPOGLYCEMIA

CAUSED BY RESPONSES OF THE AUTONOMIC NERVOUS SYSTEM

Hunger	Shakiness
Nausea	Irritability
Anxiety	Rapid pulse
Pale, cool skin	Hypotension
Sweating	

CAUSED BY IMPAIRED CEREBRAL FUNCTION

Strange or unusual feelings	Blurred vision
Headache	Decreasing levels of consciousness
Difficulty in thinking	Seizures
Inability to concentrate	Coma
Change in emotional behavior	
Slurred speech	

LABORATORY FINDINGS

Blood glucose	Less than 70 mg/dL
Blood and urine ketones	Negative
Plasma pH	Normal
Serum osmolality	Normal

If the manifestations continue, the 15/15 rule should be followed: Wait for 15 minutes, and then monitor blood glucose; if it remains below 70 mg/dL, eat another 15 to 20 g of carbohydrate. This procedure can be repeated until blood glucose levels return to normal. Once hypoglycemia is resolved, the patient should be encouraged to eat a complex carbohydrate and protein snack such as half a sandwich or cheese and crackers. People with diabetes should always carry a rapid-acting carbohydrate source. Patients experiencing frequent hypoglycemic episodes should consult their health care provider.

Severe Hypoglycemia Diabetic patients with severe hypoglycemia (blood glucose less than 50 mg/dL) are often hospitalized. If the patient is conscious and alert, 15 to 20 g of an oral carbohydrate may be given. When the patient is unconscious, 25 to 50 mL of 50% dextrose is given intravenously, followed by IV infusion of 5% dextrose in water (D_5W). IV glucose acts the fastest to raise blood glucose levels. When it is unavailable, glucagon 1 mg may be given by the intramuscular route to stimulate the release of glycogen. Because glucagon has a short action period, a carbohydrate snack is given to prevent a recurrence of hypoglycemia. Glucagon should be included in the patient's emergency kit, and family members should be taught how and when to administer it.

Other Alterations in Blood Glucose Levels

SOMOGYI EFFECT **Somogyi effect** is a rise in blood glucose to hyperglycemic levels in the morning after an episode of nighttime hypoglycemia. The morning hyperglycemia stimulates the release of counterregulatory hormones, which stimulate gluconeogenesis and glycogenolysis.

Patients with Somogyi effect are taught to monitor their blood glucose levels and assess for manifestations of nocturnal hypoglycemia: tremors, night sweats, and restlessness. Treatment focuses on increasing the bedtime snack or decreasing the evening dose of intermediate-acting insulin.

DAWN PHENOMENON **Dawn phenomenon** is a rise in blood glucose between 4 a.m. and 8 a.m. The exact cause is unknown but may be related to nighttime release of growth hormone. Treatment may include increasing the insulin dose or changing the injection time of the intermediate-acting insulin from dinnertime to bedtime.

CHRONIC COMPLICATIONS

Key Concept Long-term diabetes mellitus increases the risk for the development of microvascular and macrovascular disease. Retinopathy, nephropathy, and neuropathy result from microvascular changes, whereas cardiac and peripheral arterial disease occurs with macrovascular disease.

Chronic complications of diabetes mellitus result from consistently high glucose levels in the body. The longer the patient has been diagnosed with diabetes, the greater the chance of developing one or more of these complications. To reduce the potential for the chronic complications of diabetes, it is recommended that patients keep their blood glucose levels within the normal or near-normal range. The complications are categorized according to their effect on large blood vessels (macrovascular disease) or small blood vessels (microvascular disease).

Macrovascular Complications

The macrocirculation (the large blood vessels) in people with diabetes undergoes changes due to atherosclerosis; abnormalities in platelets, red blood cells, and clotting factors; and changes in arterial walls. (See Chapter 16 for more information about atherosclerosis.) Atherosclerosis has an increased incidence and earlier age of onset in people with diabetes. Macrovascular complications include coronary artery disease, hypertension, stroke, and peripheral vascular disease.

Coronary heart disease coupled with high lipid levels are major risk factors in the development of myocardial infarction in people with diabetes, especially in the middle to older adult with type 2 DM. Coronary heart disease is the most common cause of death in people with diabetes. Persons who have a myocardial infarction are more prone to develop heart failure as a complication of the infarction. They are also less likely to survive in the period immediately after the infarction than people without diabetes. (Myocardial infarction is fully discussed in Chapter 16.)

Hypertension often develops in those with DM. It affects more than 70% of all people with DM and is a major risk factor for cardiovascular disease and the microvascular complications of retinopathy and nephropathy. Weight loss, exercise, and decreased sodium and alcohol intake can reduce hypertension. When these methods are ineffective, antihypertensive medications are prescribed.

Stroke is two to six times more likely to occur in the type 2 diabetic. Although the exact cause is unknown, hypertension plays a major role in its development. The manifestations of impaired cerebral circulation are often similar to hypoglycemia or HHS and warrant immediate medical attention.

Peripheral vascular disease (PVD) of the lower extremities accompanies both types of DM, but the incidence is greater in type 2 DM. Atherosclerosis of the lower legs is usually bilateral, develops at an earlier age, progresses more rapidly, and develops equally in men and women. Occlusions can form in the large vessels below the knee, causing impaired peripheral circulation. Decreased arterial circulation can lead to lower leg ulcers and **gangrene** (necrosis or tissue death). Gangrene from diabetes is the most common cause of nontraumatic amputations of the lower leg. Manifestations of PVD are summarized in Box 36-6■. (PVD is discussed in Chapter 18.)

Microvascular Complications

Microvascular complications involve alterations in the microcirculation (the smaller blood vessels and capillaries), especially the eyes, kidneys, and nerves. Microvascular disease is also called microangiopathy.

Diabetic retinopathy is the collective name for the destructive retinal changes that occur in the person with diabetes. Changes in the retinal capillaries cause decreased blood flow to the retina, leading to retinal ischemia and possible retinal hemorrhage or detachment. Retinopathy has two stages: nonproliferative and proliferative. Varying degrees of visual impairment can occur at any stage. Retinopathy is the leading cause of blindness in people between ages 20 and 74. After 20 years of diabetes, most type 1 diabetics and 70% of type 2 diabetics have some degree of retinopathy. All diabetics have a greater risk for developing cataracts (opacity of the lens) as a result of increased glucose levels within the lens. Yearly eye exams by an ophthalmologist are recommended, as laser photocoagulation surgery can help to prevent the loss of vision.

Diabetic nephropathy is a disease of the kidneys characterized by the presence of albumin in the urine, hypertension, edema, and progressive renal insufficiency. This disorder is the most common cause of renal failure requiring dialysis or transplantation in the United States. Nephropathy occurs in 30% to 40% of type 1 diabetics in contrast to 15% to 20% in type 2 diabetics.

Changes in the glomerular capillaries in the kidney result in *glomerulosclerosis* (fibrosis of the glomerular tissue). This condition severely impairs the filtering function of the glomerulus so that albumin is lost in the urine.

The first indication of nephropathy is **microalbuminuria** (small amounts of albumin in the urine). With the presence of microalbuminuria, usually the patient progresses to end-stage renal disease or renal failure. (Renal failure is discussed in Chapter 29.) Because hypertension increases the progression of nephropathy, patients are treated with angiotensin-converting enzyme (ACE)–inhibiting drugs such as captopril (Capoten).

Diabetic neuropathy involves disorders of the peripheral nerves and the ANS. Diabetic neuropathies cause one or more of the following problems: sensory and motor impairment, postural hypotension, delayed gastric emptying, diarrhea, and impaired genitourinary function. Neuropathies result from thickening of the capillary membrane and destruction of myelin sheath, which impair nerve conduction.

Peripheral neuropathies are bilateral sensory disorders. Manifestations appear first in the toes and feet and progress upward to involve the fingers and hands. Initial manifestations include *distal paresthesia* (a feeling of numbness or tingling); pain described as aching, burning, or shooting; and a feeling of cold feet. People experience reduced feeling, touch, and position sense, increasing their risk for falls. Foot injuries are common due to impaired temperature and pain sensation. There is no specific treatment for peripheral neuropathy. Collaborative management focuses on controlling the neuropathic pain with tricyclic antidepressants, anticonvulsants such as gabapentin (Neurontin), or topicals like capsaicin (Zostrix) or a lidocaine patch.

BOX 36-6	MANIFESTATIONS OF PERIPHERAL VASCULAR DISEASE

- Loss of hair on lower leg, feet, and toes
- Atrophic skin changes: shininess and thinning
- Cool to cold feet
- Legs become red when dependent; legs become white when elevated
- Thick toenails
- Diminished or absent peripheral pulses
- Intermittent claudication—pain with walking
- Pain at rest, usually at night

Autonomic neuropathies involve numerous organ systems, including the following:

- *Cardiovascular:* fixed, slightly rapid heart rate and postural hypotension
- *Gastrointestinal:* delayed gastric emptying, resulting in irregular blood glucose control, constipation, and diarrhea
- *Genitourinary:* neurogenic bladder (inability to empty the bladder completely), leading to urinary retention and an increased risk of urinary tract infections; sexual dysfunction in men and women

THE DIABETIC FOOT   People with diabetes mellitus experience more problems with their feet and subsequent amputations because of macrovascular disease, neuropathy, and infection. Often, they experience some type of foot trauma without knowing it. Because they have lost their perception of pain, an injury may go unattended for days or weeks. Common sources of foot trauma are cracks and fissures caused by dry skin or infections such as athlete's foot, blisters from ill-fitting socks and shoes, ingrown toenails, and direct trauma (cuts, bruises, or burns). Foot care guidelines are discussed in Box 36-7■

Foot lesions usually begin as a superficial injury and then progress into an ulceration (Figure 36-5■). In time,

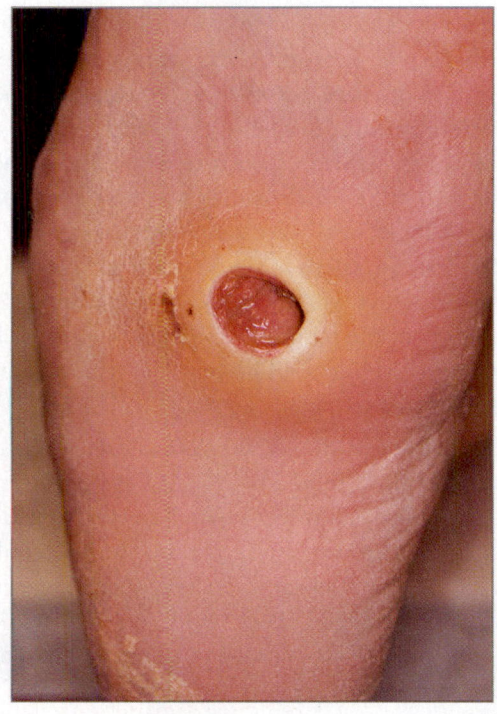

Figure 36-5. ■ Ulceration after trauma to the foot of a person with diabetes. (Source: Roberto A. Penne-Casanova/Science Source.)

BOX 36-7	PATIENT TEACHING

Sample Foot Care Teaching Session

Buying and Wearing Shoes and Stockings

- Shoes that allow 1/2 to 3/4 in. of toe room are best; there should be room for toes to spread out and wiggle. The lining and inside stitching should be smooth, and the insole should be soft. The sole should be flexible and cushion the foot. The heel should fit snugly, and the arch support should give good support.
- Do not wear open-toed shoes, sandals, high heels, or thongs; they increase the risk of trauma.
- Buy shoes late in the afternoon, when feet are at their largest; always buy shoes that feel comfortable and do not need to be "broken in."
- Shoes made of natural fibers (leather, canvas) allow perspiration to escape.
- Check the shoes before each wearing for foreign objects, wrinkled insoles, and cracks that might cause lesions.
- Stockings made of wool or cotton allow perspiration to dry.
- Do not wear garters, knee stockings, or pantyhose; they may interfere with circulation.
- Wear insulated boots in the winter.

Inspecting the Feet

- Check the feet daily for red areas, cuts, blisters, corns, calluses, or cracks in the skin. Check between the toes for cracks or reddened areas.
- Check the skin of the feet for dry or damp areas.
- Use a mirror to check each sole and the back of each heel.
- If you are unable to inspect the feet daily, be sure that someone else does so.

Care of Toenails

- Cut the toenails after washing, when they are softer and easier to trim.
- Cut the nails straight across with a clipper, and smooth edges and corners with an emery board.
- Do not use razor blades to trim the toenails.
- If you are unable to see well or to reach the feet easily, have someone else trim the nails. If the nails are very thick or ingrown, if the toes overlap, or if circulation is poor, get professional care.

General Information

- Take your shoes off at every visit to your health care provider.
- Never go barefoot. Wear slippers when leaving the bed during the night.
- Do not use commercial corn medicines or pads, chemicals (e.g., boric acid, iodine, or hydrogen peroxide), or over-the-counter cortisone medications on the feet.
- Do not put heating pads, hot water bottles, or ice packs on the feet. If the feet become cold at night, wear socks or use extra blankets.
- Do not apply lotion between toes because it promotes bacterial and fungal growth.
- Do not allow the feet to become sunburned.
- Do not put tape on the feet.
- Do not sit with the legs crossed at the knees or ankles or wear constrictive clothing.

the ulcer extends deeper into muscles and bone and can lead to abscess or osteomyelitis. Infections commonly occur in the traumatized or ulcerated tissue. Dry gangrene is manifested by cold, dry, shriveled, and black tissues of the toes and feet. If untreated, the whole foot eventually becomes gangrenous and requires amputation. Treatment consists of bed rest, antibiotics, and debridement.

Another foot problem is the Charcot foot, which often develops in patients with diabetic neuropathy. In Charcot foot, the joints of the foot and ankle are destroyed, leading to deformity of the foot. The foot deformity limits the patient's ability to walk.

INCREASED SUSCEPTIBILITY TO INFECTION   The person with diabetes has an increased risk of developing frequent bacterial and fungal infections. Normally, glucose is used efficiently throughout the body, but in people with diabetes, glucose accumulates in the epidermal layer of the skin. Moisture tends to collect under the armpits, breasts, groin, or genitalia. The higher-than-normal concentration of glucose in the skin coupled with the moisture creates a perfect breeding area for microorganisms. When the skin appears beefy red to violet red, an infection should be suspected. Fungal infections can develop under the nails, giving them a thick, yellow, crumbly appearance. Treatment focuses on prevention of infection.

memory**ALERT**

Any minor cut or injury in the patient with diabetes mellitus poses a significant risk for infection.

Special Concerns

SICK-DAY MANAGEMENT   When the person with diabetes is sick, blood glucose levels increase, even though food intake decreases. The person mistakenly alters or omits the insulin dose or oral antidiabetic agent, causing further problems. Dietary guidelines during illness focus on preventing dehydration and providing nutrition for promoting recovery. The nurse teaches the following sick-day management:

- Monitor blood glucose at least four times a day throughout the illness.
- Test the urine for ketones if the blood glucose level is greater than 250 mg/dL.
- Continue to take the usual insulin dose or oral antidiabetic agent.
- Drink 8 to 12 oz of fluid each waking hour.
- Eat 10 to 15 g of carbohydrate every 1 to 2 hours, such as:
  - Half cup regular Jell-O.
  - Half cup regular soft drink or fruit juice.
  - One whole Popsicle.
- Call the health care provider if you are unable to eat for more than 24 hours or if vomiting and diarrhea last for more than 6 hours.

SURGERY MANAGEMENT   Surgery is a stressor that releases excess counterregulatory hormones, causing hyperglycemia and insulin resistance. Protein stores are decreased. In addition, diet and activity patterns change, and medication types and dosages vary. As a result, surgical patients with diabetes are at a greater risk for postoperative infection, delayed wound healing, fluid and electrolyte imbalances, hypoglycemia, and DKA.

For patients with type 2 DM, oral antidiabetic agents are usually withheld 1 to 2 days before surgery, and patients are given regular insulin. Patients with type 1 DM follow a carefully prescribed insulin regimen to meet their specific needs.

The surgical procedure should be scheduled for early in the morning to decrease the fasting time. If there is no food intake after surgery, IV dextrose is given along with subcutaneous regular insulin every 6 hours. Although intake is decreased postoperatively, stress increases insulin requirements. Glucose control is also affected postoperatively by nausea and vomiting, anorexia, and gastrointestinal suction.

During the postoperative period, the patient with type 2 DM may continue to require insulin or may resume oral medications, depending on glucose levels. The patient with type 1 DM may require reduced insulin as healing progresses and stress-induced hyperglycemia diminishes. Regular blood glucose monitoring is essential, as are assessments for hypoglycemia.

Sometimes postsurgical patients require enteral tube feedings or total parenteral nutrition to meet their dietary needs. Both nutritional supplements contain glucose. Diabetic patients receiving these supplements must be monitored closely for hyperglycemia. Often, they need additional insulin to prevent acute hyperglycemia complications.

PANCREAS TRANSPLANTATION   Surgical management of diabetes involves replacing or transplanting the pancreas, pancreatic cells, or beta cells. Islet cell transplant has had moderate success. Greater success is seen when the kidneys and pancreas are transplanted at the same time. Before patients can be considered transplant candidates, an extensive physical and emotional evaluation is done. After the transplantation procedure, patients require lifelong immunosuppressant drugs.

COMPLEMENTARY THERAPIES

Acupuncture, biofeedback, exercise, and yoga may be used to relieve the chronic pain from peripheral neuropathy. No scientific evidence supports these techniques, and they are not harmful as long as patients continue with their diabetic medications, diet, and exercise plan.

Before diabetics take any herbal supplements, they should talk with their health care provider. The following supplements may increase blood glucose levels: ginkgo biloba, glucosamine, and green tea. In contrast, black cohosh, chromium, garlic, and ginseng are herbal supplements that may reduce blood glucose levels.

NURSING CARE

Nursing care differs for the person with newly diagnosed diabetes, the person with long-term diabetes, and the person with acute complications. Patients with diabetes require lifelong collaborative care.

PRIORITIZING NURSING CARE

Nursing care focuses on maintaining blood glucose levels within values that are as normal as possible to prevent acute and chronic complications. Emphasis is placed on teaching the patient self-management strategies related to nutrition, medications, exercise, hygiene, and safety precautions.

HEALTH PROMOTION

Health promotion focuses on preventing the complications of diabetes. Recommendations include reducing excess weight, following a well-balanced diet, and participating in a regular physical exercise program. People in the high-risk group should have a blood glucose test at 3-year intervals starting at age 45. These same activities, along with medication and self-monitoring, can decrease the potential for complications.

ASSESSING

Assessment data collected by the nurse can determine the extent to which DM is affecting the patient's life, identify risk factors for complications, and suggest guidelines for medical treatment or self-care (Box 36-8■).

IDENTIFYING POTENTIAL COMPLICATIONS

Acute complications include hypoglycemia, DKA, and HHS. Chronic complications involving the microcirculation include retinopathy, nephropathy, and neuropathy. Cardiac disorders such as coronary artery disease, stroke, and peripheral vascular disease are common macrocirculation complications. There is a significant increased risk for infection.

DIAGNOSING, PLANNING, AND IMPLEMENTING
Risk for Unstable Blood Glucose Level

Expected outcome: Maintains balance of nutrition, exercise, and blood glucose levels.

- Monitor blood glucose levels regularly and report values below 70 mg/dL or above 200 mg/dL. *Patients with diabetes are at risk for hypoglycemia or hyperglycemia.*
- Monitor the percentage of meals and snacks that the patient eats. *Anorexia, gastric fullness, and abdominal pain can reduce oral intake. To prevent hypoglycemia, the patient must consume the amount of food indicated in the diet plan.*

BOX 36-8	ASSESSMENT

Diabetes Mellitus

Subjective Data

- Presence of hyperglycemia manifestations: polyuria, polydipsia, polyphagia.
- History of any change in vision or speech, numbness or tingling in feet or hands, pain when walking, change in weight and appetite, slow-healing wounds, frequent infections, pain or burning with urination, or vaginal discharge.
- Family history of diabetes mellitus or hypertension.
- Use of insulin or oral antidiabetic medications.

Objective Data

- Monitor vital signs (blood pressure—standing and lying, pulse, respirations, temperature).
- Assess visual acuity and sensations of touch, position, pain, and temperature.
- Observe gait patterns, use of assistive devices for walking, and abnormal wear patterns on shoes.
- Inspect lower extremities for hair loss and lesions, redness over pressure points, cellulitis, or gangrene.
- Palpate peripheral pulses; assess color and temperature of lower extremities and edema.
- Monitor and report blood glucose levels above or below expected range.

- Identify food preferences, including ethnic/cultural needs. *Patients are more likely to eat food they like and that meets their ethnic/cultural requirements.*
- Provide meals and snacks on time. *Glucose and insulin control is more effective when meals are eaten on time.*
- Give insulin and/or antidiabetic agents as ordered. *To prevent hyperglycemia, insulin and/or antidiabetic agents must be given on time. Altered times might be necessary when food is delayed or diagnostic procedures are being done.*
- Encourage the patient to include physical exercise into daily routine. *Exercise increases the uptake of glucose by the muscles, which can promote better diabetes control.*

Risk for Impaired Skin Integrity

Expected outcome: Remains free from areas of skin breakdown.

- Teach foot care. Wash feet daily with lukewarm water and mild hand soap; pat dry, especially between the toes. Apply a thin film of lubricating lotion except between the toes. *Proper hygiene decreases the chance of infection.*

clinicalALERT

Teach the diabetic patient to always check the water temperature in the shower or bath with a bath thermometer before stepping in to prevent burns.

- Use alternating pressure mattresses, elbow and heel protectors, and foot cradle as ordered. *These devices reduce pressure on the skin to prevent skin breakdown.*
- Encourage fluid intake of at least 2,500 mL/day unless cardiac complications exist. *Adequate fluid intake prevents dry skin and the risk for skin breakdown. However, patients with cardiac disease may develop fluid overload with an excess intake.*
- Discuss the importance of not smoking. *Nicotine in tobacco causes vasoconstriction and decreases blood supply to the feet.*
- If boils, pimples, or skin breakdown occurs, notify the physician immediately. *Immediate intervention is needed to prevent the development of deep wounds and infection.*
- Rotate insulin injection sites. *Site rotation prevents lipodystrophy.*
- Conduct foot care teaching sessions as often as necessary (see Box 36-7). *Foot care is a priority in diabetes management to prevent serious problems.*
- Discuss the importance of maintaining blood glucose levels as near normal as possible. *Hyperglycemia increases the growth of microorganisms.*

clinicalALERT

Suggest the use of a hand mirror to check the bottom of the feet and the back of the heel.

Risk for Infection

Expected outcome: Remains free of signs of infection.

- Use and teach meticulous hand washing. *Hand washing is the best method for preventing the spread of infection.*
- Assess for manifestations of infection: fever; chills; tachycardia; cough; vaginal discharge; cloudy, foul-smelling urine; or redness, pain, swelling, or discharge at the injury site. *Common infections include urinary tract and nail infections, osteomyelitis, vaginal yeast infections, chronic gingivitis, and pyorrhea. Early diagnosis and treatment can control their severity and decrease complications.*
- Obtain specimens and send for culture and sensitivity test as ordered. *Before antibiotic therapy is begun, specimens must be sent for culture and sensitivity to identify the causative organism and appropriate antibiotic.*
- Keep the skin clean and dry, using mild soap and lukewarm water. *Clean, intact mucous membranes are the first line of defense against infection.*
- Provide catheter and perineal care. *Patients with diabetes are prone to developing urinary tract infections.*
- Use meticulous sterile technique when performing wound care or any invasive procedure. *These measures prevent infection in existing wounds or introduction of bacteria into the body.*

- Encourage adequate nutrition and fluid intake. *Maintaining satisfactory food and fluid intake reduces susceptibility to infection.*
- Assist patient with oral hygiene. Brush teeth with a soft toothbrush and fluoridated toothpaste at least twice a day and floss. *Proper oral hygiene reduces the risk of periodontal disease.*
- Teach female diabetics the symptoms and preventive measures of vaginitis caused by *Candida albicans:*
  - Symptoms are an odorless, white or yellow, cheese-like vaginal discharge and itching.
  - Sexual transmission is unlikely, but discomfort may cause the patient to avoid sexual activity. *Diabetes is a predisposing factor for* C. albicans *vaginitis. Poor personal hygiene and use of clothing that keeps the vaginal area warm and moist increase the risk of vaginitis.*

clinicalALERT

Teach women with DM to take preventive measures such as not douching, wiping from front to back after voiding, wearing cotton underwear, and avoiding tight jeans and nylon pantyhose.

Risk for Injury

Expected outcome: Remains free from injury.

- Reduce environmental hazards in the health care facility.
  - Orient the patient to new surroundings on admission.
  - Keep the bed at the lowest level with side rails raised if needed.
  - Keep the floors free of objects and wipe up spills immediately.
  - Use a night-light.
  - Teach the patient to wear shoes or slippers when getting out of bed.
  - Monitor for side effects of prescribed medications, such as dizziness or drowsiness. *Strange environments increase the risk of falls.*
- Teach about safety in the home and community.
  - Use a night-light, preferably one with a soft, nonglare bulb. (Note: Red light is better, because the eyes adjust more quickly.)
  - Turn the head away when switching on a bright light.
  - Avoid looking directly into headlights when driving at night.
  - Conduct a daily foot inspection.
  - Wear shoes and slippers with nonskid soles.
  - Do not use throw rugs.
  - Install hand grips in the tub and shower and next to the toilet. *Environmental hazards increase the risk of falls or other accidents. Glare is often responsible for falls when visual deficits exist.*

- Assist the patient with tasks requiring finger and hand dexterity. *Patients with neuropathies may lose their ability to grip handles of cups or sharp objects.*
- Assist the patient during ambulation; provide ambulatory aids as needed. Do not rush the patient. *These interventions decrease the potential for falls.*
- Advise the patient to get out of bed slowly. *Autonomic neuropathy can cause postural hypotension. When a patient rises too quickly, there is a risk for dizziness and falls.*
- Monitor for DKA in the patient with type 1 diabetes and for HHS in the patient with type 2 DM. Teach the patient and family to recognize and seek care for the manifestations of DKA or HHS. *DKA and HHS can be life threatening and require immediate medical treatment.*

clinicalALERT

Monitor frequently the older adult for symptoms of HHS, especially after major surgery.

- Monitor for and teach the patient and family to recognize and treat the manifestations of hypoglycemia. The person should carry some form of a rapid-acting sugar source at all times. *Severe hypoglycemia causes a decreased level of consciousness.*
- Recommend that patients wear a MedicAlert bracelet or necklace identifying themselves as having diabetes. *In case of sudden illness or accident, a MedicAlert tag alerts health professionals about the patient's diagnosis so that appropriate medical attention can be begun.*

Ineffective Coping

Expected outcome: Verbalizes effective coping strategies.

- Assess the patient's perception of the current situation. *This establishes how the patient feels about his or her diagnosis.*
- Assess the patient's emotional resources and support sources. *Chronic illness affects all dimensions of a person's life as well as the lives of family members.*
- Provide an atmosphere of trust and support. *A positive emotional environment helps patients feel comfortable about discussing their concerns.*
- Explore with the patient and family the effects of the diagnosis and treatment on finances, occupation, energy levels, and relationships. *Failure to cope successfully can lead to noncompliance and poor blood glucose control. Common frustrations associated with diabetes are the disease itself, the treatment modalities, and the health care system.*
- Provide information about support groups and community resources. *Support groups offer opportunities for mutual support and problem solving. Community resources may help the patient and family with other methods for coping with diabetes.*

MANAGING NURSING CARE

As appropriate and allowed by designated duties and responsibilities of assistive personnel, the nurse may delegate nursing care activities such as providing oral and skin care, assisting with ambulation, and daily living activities for the patient with diabetes mellitus. Before assigning tasks such as obtaining vital signs and blood glucose levels, measuring intake and output, and assisting with meals and fluid intake, ensure assistive personnel understand the importance of accuracy of measurement and reporting abnormal vital signs, CBG less than 70 mg/dL or greater than 110 mg/dL, increased or decreased output, and decreased fluid or food intake.

EVALUATING

To evaluate the effectiveness of care for a patient with DM, collect data related to the presence of chronic complications, such as frequent infections, unhealed wounds, decreased vision, altered kidney function, peripheral neuropathy, and hypertension. Evaluate the patient's ability to cope with a chronic disease and adherence to diet and medication regimes. It is important to identify the frequency with which the patient has experienced episodes of DKA or HHS and hypoglycemia.

DOCUMENTING

Document the patient's vital signs, CBG levels, the level of consciousness, skin integrity, and the presence of any acute or chronic complications. Notify the physician of the patient's response to treatment. Reinforcement of patient teaching related to medications, diet, and self-care must be documented, along with the patient's response to teaching. Note any referrals to diabetic educators and dietitians.

CONTINUITY OF CARE

Teaching the patient and family involves all aspects of diabetes management. The nurse's role is to reinforce teaching completed by other health care providers, such as registered nurses, certified diabetic educators, or dietitians. Because diabetes mellitus is a chronic disease, patients must be able to self-manage their disease at home.

During hospitalization, teaching should begin on admission. Before the actual teaching session starts, the nurse assesses the patient's and family's knowledge and learning needs, educational level, preferred learning methods and style, life experiences, and support systems. In addition, the nurse determines past diabetes management practices and identifies physical, emotional, and sociocultural needs.

It is important for the nurse and patient to establish mutual goals based on the assessment data. Responsibility for daily management lies with the patient. Family members must understand that their primary role is support. However, they must know how to provide physical care for the patient if necessary.

If the patient is newly diagnosed, the teaching first focuses on basic skills and then progresses to lifelong management strategies. Patients with a long-standing history of DM should not be overlooked. Often, they need a review of basic management strategies.

The following are some general guidelines for the nurse on teaching patients with diabetes mellitus:

- Listen to questions and provide information about common myths regarding diabetes.
- Present information in small segments.
- Explain medical terms so that the patient understands the meaning.
- Be specific about what the patient needs to know.
- Repeat and reinforce information as many times as necessary.
- Validate the person's knowledge and skills.
- Adapt teaching to the special needs of the older adult:
  - Diet changes may be difficult to implement. Favorite foods are hard to give up. Balanced meals at regular times may not have been part of the patient's lifestyle. Purchasing, storing, and preparing foods may be a problem. Dentures may not fit well. Changes in taste sensation may cause the patient to use more salt and sugar. A decreased thirst mechanism may lead to dehydration.
  - Exercise of any type may not have been part of the activities of daily living. Exercise is individualized to accommodate physical limitations caused by arthritis, Parkinson disease, chronic respiratory diseases, and/or cardiovascular diseases.
  - A chronic illness diagnosis threatens independence and self-worth. After years of taking care of themselves, older adults who have to depend on others may withdraw from social situations. Distance from family or death of a spouse may cause depression.
  - Money to purchase medications and supplies or visit health care providers must be taken out of a fixed income.
  - Visual and fine motor skill deficits can make insulin administration, blood glucose monitoring, food preparation, exercises, and foot care difficult or impossible.

Box 36-9■ summarizes the knowledge and skills needed for self-management of DM.

The ADA and American Dietetic Association provide information on all aspects of self-management. Most hospitals or outpatient settings offer diabetes educational programs and support groups. Blood glucose screenings are often provided at little or no cost as part of community health promotion activities. Restaurants provide diabetic meals on request. Encourage patients to explore resources in their own communities.

BOX 36-9 | **PATIENT TEACHING**

Teaching for Patient Self-Management of Diabetes

The nurse reinforces teaching and skills for patients with DM. The content of a teaching plan includes the following points:

- Information about how diabetes changes body metabolism.
- *Dietary plan:* How diet helps keep blood glucose in the normal range; why patients should eat complex carbohydrates and foods high in fiber but limit the intake of sugar, fat, sodium, and alcohol; how to read food labels for sugar and fat; integrating personal food preferences; eating meals away from home; relationship between diet, exercise, and medication.
- *Exercise:* How it helps lower blood glucose; the importance of a regular exercise program; types of exercise; and integrating personal exercise choices.
- *Glucose levels:* Self-monitoring of blood glucose; how to perform the tests accurately; how to care for equipment; what to do for high or low blood glucose; importance of monitoring Hgb A1c levels.
- *Medications:*
  - Insulin type, dosage, mixing instructions (if necessary); times of onset and peak actions; how to get and care for equipment; how to give injections; where to give injections; timing of insulin injections and mealtimes.
  - *Oral and/or injectable antidiabetic agents:* Type, dosage, side effects, interaction with other drugs.
- *Complications:*
  - Factors that cause DKA or HHS; manifestations of each; what to do when they occur.
  - Factors that cause hypoglycemia; manifestations; what to do when they occur.
- *Safety precautions:* Identify person to contact in an emergency; carry ID card and rapid-acting glucose; carry insulin and glucagon kit.
- *Hygiene:* Skin, dental, foot care.
- *Vision:* Yearly exam; supply sources for vision aids such as magnifying sleeve for insulin syringe or large-print instructions.
- *Sick days:* What to do about food, fluids, and medications.
- *Communication and follow-up:*
  - What signs and symptoms to report; whom to contact; when to report.
  - Importance of keeping follow-up appointments.
  - Resources such as American Diabetes Association, diabetic education classes, diabetic support groups, weight loss programs, and publications such as *Diabetes Forecast*.

NURSING CARE PLAN
Patient With Type 1 Diabetes

James Meligrito, 24 years old, is a first-year nursing student at a local community college. He attends school full time and works 20 hours a week as a campus student security guard. He works from 8 p.m. to 12 midnight, 5 nights a week.

Mr. Meligrito dislikes cooking and usually eats "whatever is handy." He was diagnosed with type 1 diabetes mellitus when he was 12. Currently, he takes a total of 32 units of insulin each day, 10 units of NPH, and 6 units of regular insulin each morning and evening. He monitors his blood glucose about three times a week. He feels that he is too busy for a regular exercise program and that he gets enough exercise in clinical and in weekend sports activities. He has not seen a health care provider for over a year.

One day during a 6-hour clinical, Mr. Meligrito notices that he is urinating frequently, is thirsty, and has blurred vision. He is very tired but blames all his symptoms on working too much and studying for school. He forgot to take his morning insulin and realizes he must have hyperglycemia but decides that he will be all right until he gets home in the afternoon. Around noon, he complains of abdominal pain, weakness, and a rapid pulse. When he reports his physical symptoms to his clinical instructor, she takes him immediately to the hospital emergency department (ED).

Assessment

In the ED, his blood glucose level is 300 mg/dL; Hgb A1c is 8.5%; urine shows the presence of ketones; and electrolytes are normal, with a pH of 7.1. Vital signs: T 99°F (37.2°C); P 140; R 28; BP 102/52. An IV of 1,000 mL 0.9% normal saline is started at a rate of 400 mL/hr. He receives 10 units of regular insulin IV. Three hours later, his blood glucose level is 160, with normal vital signs. He is sent home with an appointment the next morning with the hospital's diabetes clinical specialist, Carole Traci.

Nursing Diagnosis

The following priority nursing diagnoses are established for this patient:

- *Powerlessness* related to a perceived lack of control of diabetes due to demands on his time
- *Deficient Knowledge* regarding self-management of diabetes
- *Ineffective Therapeutic Regimen Management* related to difficulty in modifying his personal habits

Expected Outcomes

The expected outcomes for the plan of care are that Mr. Meligrito will:

- Identify those aspects of DM that can be controlled and participate in making decisions about self-managing care.
- Demonstrate an understanding of DM self-management through planned medication, diet, exercise, and blood glucose self-monitoring activities.

- Verbalize ways to modify his personal habits.

Planning and Implementation

Ms. Traci plans and implements the following nursing interventions with Mr. Meligrito during the diabetes education program:

- Mutually develop short-term and long-term goals for self-management of blood glucose control.
- Discuss Mr. Meligrito's personal habits and ways to modify them.
- Provide positive reinforcement for increasing his involvement in self-care activities.
- Review insulin administration, dietary management, exercise, self-monitoring of blood glucose, and healthy lifestyle.

Evaluation

After participating in weekly diabetes classes for 2 months, Mr. Meligrito has increased his understanding of and compliance with managing his diabetes. He states that he finally understands how insulin, food, and exercise affect his body, having previously thought they were "just things I should do when I wanted to." Mr. Meligrito developed a workable meal schedule and weekly grocery list. Mr. Meligrito and a friend have arranged to walk 2 to 3 miles three times a week on a community hiking trail. To gain a sense of control over his illness, Mr. Meligrito has also worked out a schedule that allows time for school, health care, and himself.

Critical Thinking in the Nursing Process

1. What factors caused Mr. Meligrito's diabetic ketoacidosis?
2. What evidence-based practice guidelines would the nurse implement when Mr. Meligrito arrives in the emergency department?
3. Consider that you are teaching Mr. Meligrito and another patient, Mr. McDaniel (age 75, newly diagnosed with type 2 DM). What components of your teaching plan would be the same, and what components would be different?

Note: Discussion of Critical Thinking questions appears on the companion website.

Note: The references and resources for all chapters have been compiled at the back of the book.

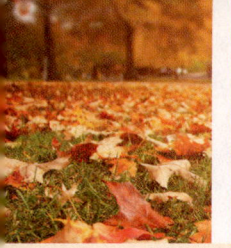
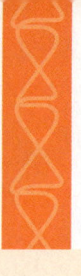

Chapter Review

KEY POINTS

- **Concept:** All body tissues and organs require a constant supply of glucose. Normal blood glucose levels are maintained through the actions of insulin and glucagon. Diabetes mellitus results from defects in the secretion of insulin, the action of insulin, or both.

- Type 1 DM is a metabolic disorder of the pancreas that results from beta cell destruction, leading to absolute insulin deficiency. Type 2 DM occurs from a progressive decrease in insulin secretion and an increase in insulin resistance.

- The incidence of type 2 DM is increasing among children and adolescents. Type 1 DM is the sixth leading cause of death by disease in the United States, usually due to cardiac problems.

- Risk factors for type 1 DM include heredity, viral infections, and chemical toxins found in smoked and cured meats. Heredity, obesity, sedentary lifestyle, older adult, race/ethnicity, hypertension, HDL cholesterol greater than 35 mg/dL, and triglyceride greater than 250 mg/dL increase the risk for type 2 DM.

- Classic manifestations of type 1 diabetes include the three "polys" (polydipsia, polyuria, polyphagia) plus weight loss and fatigue. In contrast, type 2 DM is characterized by polyuria, polydipsia, recurrent infections, and fatigue.

- Diabetes is diagnosed by plasma glucose level, oral glucose tolerance test, and fasting blood glucose. Tests used to monitor DM management include fasting blood glucose, glycosylated hemoglobin (Hgb A1c), serum cholesterol and triglyceride, and microalbumin.

- **Concept:** Administration of insulin is the primary management strategy along with diet and exercise for patients with type 1 DM. Type 2 DM is usually managed with antidiabetic drugs from multiple classes in addition to diet and exercise.

- Insulin is available in rapid-, short-, intermediate-, and long-acting preparations. Regular and NPH insulin can be mixed in the same syringe; Lantus insulin must be given alone. It is essential to monitor for hypoglycemia during the peak action of each insulin preparation.

- There are eight primary classes of antidiabetic drugs used to treat patients with type 2 DM. These drugs are ineffective for persons with type 1 DM.

- Patients must be taught guidelines for taking antidiabetic drugs, including side effects, adverse reactions, and when to notify their health care provider.

- Medical nutrition therapy (MNT) and a regular exercise program are essential components of diabetes prevention, management, and self-management education.

- **Concept:** Uncontrolled or poorly managed DM can cause acute alterations in blood glucose levels, resulting in the complications of diabetic ketoacidosis, hyperosmolar hyperglycemic state, and hypoglycemia. It is essential that these complications be recognized and treated immediately.

- Diabetic ketoacidosis (DKA) can occur in type 1 DM, whereas hyperosmolar hyperglycemic state develops mainly in type 2 DM; both are life-threatening complications. DKA is treated with a combination of intravenous fluid and electrolyte solutions and with insulin.

- Hypoglycemia is a sudden onset of blood glucose level less than 70 mg/dL. In conscious patients immediately give 15 to 20 g of a rapid-acting glucose to prevent prolonged neurologic damage. Unconscious patients with CBG less than 50 mg/dL should be given either 50 mL of 50% glucose intravenously or glucagon 1 mg IM.

- **Concept:** Long-term diabetes mellitus increases the risk for the development of microvascular and macrovascular disease. Retinopathy, nephropathy, and neuropathy result from microvascular changes, whereas cardiac and peripheral arterial disease occurs with macrovascular disease.

- Diabetic nephropathy is the leading cause of end-stage renal disease, and diabetes is the primary cause of all new cases of blindness.

- Because macrovascular changes predispose diabetic patients to cardiac disorders, they must understand ways to prevent atherosclerosis, hypertension, myocardial infarction, and stroke.

- Patients with poorly managed DM have a greater risk for peripheral vascular disease (PVD). PVD and peripheral neuropathy often lead to foot trauma, diabetic ulcers, gangrene, and amputation.

- Using the nursing process, nursing management focuses on a thorough assessment and implementing interventions that maintain normal blood glucose levels, prevent acute and chronic complications, maintain skin integrity, teach self-management, and increase coping skills.

PEARSON NURSING STUDENT RESOURCES

Find additional materials at **nursing.pearsonhighered.com**.

Clinical Reasoning Care Map

Caring for a Patient With Diabetes Mellitus
NCLEX-PN® Focus Area: Health Promotion and Maintenance

Case Study: Mrs. Vaughn, age 64, has type 2 diabetes mellitus and is visiting her physician for a 6-month checkup. As she walks to the exam, the nurse notices that she walks with a slight limp. She is helped to remove her shoes, and the nurse notices several red spots over the top of the toes on her right foot and a blister on her left heel. Mrs. Vaughn tells you that she does not know how this happened. "I never saw these red spots on my toes or the blister on my heel." She also says that she bought a new pair of shoes last week and has been wearing them every day.

Nursing Diagnosis: Impaired Skin Integrity

COLLECT DATA

Subjective	Objective
_____	_____
_____	_____
_____	_____
_____	_____
_____	_____

Does this present a threat to the patient's safety?

If yes, the priority intervention to address this threat would be:

_____

Nursing Care

_____
_____
_____
_____
_____
_____
_____
_____

Interprofessional team members to include when planning care:

_____

How would you document this?_____

_____

Compare your answers and documentation to those provided on the companion website.

Data Collected
(use only those that apply)

- Weight 160 lb
- Red spots on top of the toes on her right foot
- Fasting blood glucose 160 mg/dL
- Blister on the left heel
- Does not complain of any discomfort in her feet
- Says she uses a hot water bottle on her feet at night
- Complains of tingling in both feet

Nursing Interventions (use only those that apply; list in priority order)

- Teach her to wear new shoes for a short period of time each day.
- Discuss changes in her diet.
- Cleanse feet with normal saline.
- Teach her to monitor red areas for signs of skin breakdown.
- Apply lubricating lotion to her feet and between the toes.
- Discuss the importance of not smoking.
- Instruct the patient on proper foot care.

NCLEX-PN® Exam Preparation

1 A patient is taught self-monitoring of blood glucose (SMBG) in order to check his blood glucose before meals and administer insulin according to a sliding scale. The nurse will teach the patient to use which type of insulin?

1. Humulin N
2. Humulin R
3. Lantus
4. Humulin 70/30

2 A patient with diabetes mellitus experiences hypoglycemia during the night followed by episodes of hyperglycemia when the blood glucose is assessed in the morning. What disorder might these symptoms indicate?

1. Somogyi effect
2. Diabetic ketoacidosis
3. Dawn phenomenon
4. Hyperosmolar hyperglycemic state

3 A female patient with a history of diabetes mellitus visits her physician because of flulike symptoms. Which of the following indicates a need for further teaching when she discusses her sick-day care?

1. "I will check my blood glucose every four hours."
2. "I will check my urine ketones if my blood glucose is above 250 mg/dL."
3. "I will hold my daily insulin dose until I stop vomiting."
4. "I will consume 10 to 15 g of carbohydrates every 1 to 2 hours."

4 Which one of the following patients has the highest risk factors for developing type 2 diabetes mellitus?

1. 16-year-old Native American who plays basketball in high school
2. 30-year-old Caucasian with a family history of diabetes mellitus
3. 52-year-African American with a history of thyroid disease
4. 68-year-old Hispanic female who is overweight

5 A 16-year-old girl is diagnosed with type 1 diabetes mellitus. Which of the following statements made by the patient indicates a need for further instruction?

1. "When my blood sugar is stable, I will use pills for my diabetes."
2. "I will rotate my insulin injection sites."
3. "My blood glucose should be maintained between 70 and 110 mg/dL."
4. "I will perform foot care and inspect my feet daily."

6 A patient with diabetes mellitus received lispro (Humalog) 20 units at 7:30 a.m. What are the most likely times that the nurse would expect the patient to experience hypoglycemia?

1. Between 8:30 a.m. and 9:30 a.m.
2. Between 10:30 a.m. and 2:00 p.m.
3. Between 12:30 p.m. and 2:30 p.m.
4. Between 1:30 p.m. and 3:30 p.m.

7 A patient is admitted to the medical unit with a diagnosis of diabetic ketoacidosis. Which of the following clinical manifestations should the nurse expect to find?

1. Cool, clammy skin
2. Acetone breath odor
3. Slurred speech
4. Radial pulse 70, bounding

8 The nurse instructs a patient to mix Humulin N and Humulin R insulin. List the actions in the sequence in which the patient should perform them.

1. Inject air into the Humulin N vial first.
2. Gently rotate the Humulin N vial.
3. Withdraw Humulin R insulin first.
4. Wipe off the top of both vials with an alcohol pad.
5. Inspect Humulin R for clarity.

9 A conscious patient arrives in the emergency department with a blood glucose level of 50 mg/dL. What nursing intervention should the nurse anticipate doing for this patient?

1. Give lispro (Humalog) injection.
2. Give crackers and cheese.
3. Give glucagon injection.
4. Give a half cup regular soda.

10 The nurse instructs a diabetic patient on foot care. Appropriate instruction should include which of the following points? **Select all that apply.**

1. Cut the toenails straight across with a clipper.
2. Have a family member check a heating pad before applying to the feet.
3. Apply lotion or oil generously between the toes.
4. Wear closed-toe shoes made of soft leather.
5. If buying a new pair of shoes, shop in early morning.
6. Use a mirror to check the soles of the feet every day.

Answers and rationales for Review Questions appear in Appendix I.

You are an LPN/LVN working on a medical–surgical unit of a medium-sized hospital. You are assigned to care of the following patients from 0700 to 1900.

Jake Priestley, a 54-year-old male, was admitted with a diagnosis of type 2 diabetes mellitus, end-stage renal disease, and a small gangrenous infection of the left foot. He receives hemodialysis three times per week, and dialysis is scheduled for tomorrow. Physician's orders on admission are for bed rest, a dressing change b.i.d., and lab in the a.m.:

- Chemistry panel (Chem 16)
- Glycohemoglobin (glycosylated hemoglobin, Hgb A1c) level
- CBC

The patient will receive a 1,500-calorie, carbohydrate-consistent diet. He is on fluid restriction of 1,200 mL/24 hr. The physician ordered capillary blood glucose (Glucoscan) a.c. and h.s., with sliding scale insulin coverage.

A.M. LAB RESULTS	NORMAL VALUES	PATIENT VALUES
Potassium	3.5–5.3	5.6
Chloride	95–105	94
Creatinine	0.5–1.5	10
Blood urea nitrogen	5–25	50
Glucose	70–110	328

Grace, a 52-year-old female, has a history of difficulty swallowing and a "swelling" in her throat. She was diagnosed with hypothyroidism and a large goiter. Grace underwent a subtotal thyroidectomy this morning. You will assist the RN in admitting Grace to the surgical unit from the recovery room around 1000. Once she has stabilized, you will assume responsibility for her care.

Sky, a 38-year-old Native American woman, was admitted last evening with hypertension, electrolyte imbalance, elevated blood glucose, and recurrent respiratory infections. She reports irregular menstrual cycles for the past year and increased roundness of her face. The doctor suspects Sky has Cushing syndrome and has ordered a 24-hour urine specimen for 17-ketosteroids, serum electrolytes, and glucose levels. The 24-hour urine collection was started at 2030.

CRITICAL THINKING

- Which of Jake's lab values are of most concern to you? Why?
- Parathyroid glands can be traumatized or inadvertently removed during thyroidectomy. What effect can this have on the patient postoperatively?
- Because Cushing syndrome increases the production of cortisol, what effect would you expect on Sky's blood glucose level?

PRIORITIES IN NURSING CARE

- After you hear report on your patients, which of these patients should you see first? What are your top priorities for the next 30 minutes? What is your rationale for these choices?

MANAGEMENT OF CARE

- In what order will you provide Jake's care? Why?
- In planning care for Grace, what preparation should you do in her room before her arrival from the recovery room?
- What diversional activities can you plan for Sky while she is in the hospital?

DELEGATING

- You asked the CNA to take Jake's vital signs and CBG while you go to lunch. What follow-up must you do when you return?
- When you assume care for Grace, vital signs are stable, she is sitting in bed, and there is an ice pack on her neck. What part of her care can you delegate to the CNA?
- Once Sky has been instructed in collecting a 24-hour urine specimen, can this procedure be delegated to the CNA?

TEAMWORK AND COLLABORATION

- Jake expresses concerns about his self-care when he is discharged and about losing time at work with his foot wound. What interprofessional team members should be included in Jake's discharge planning?
- What teaching points and ways to evaluate his learning and self-care ability would the nurse emphasize to Jake?

CULTURAL CARE STRATEGIES

- If you are not familiar with Native American cultures, what questions should you ask Sky in order to provide culturally sensitive care?

DOCUMENTING AND REPORTING

- What part of Jake's care that has been delegated to you will you need to report to the RN?
- Who is responsible to document the care provided by the CNA?
- Write a focus note documenting your assessment of Grace at the point you assumed her care.

Note: Discussion of Unit questions appears on the companion website.

UNIT X
Disrupted Neurologic Function

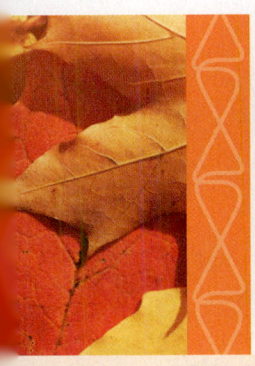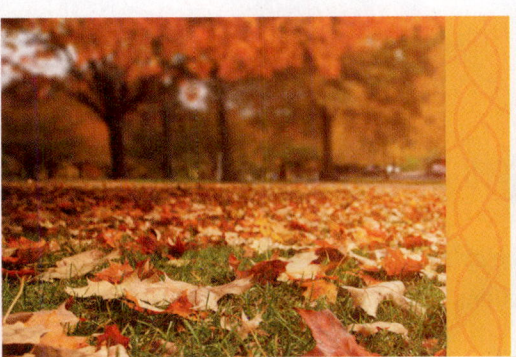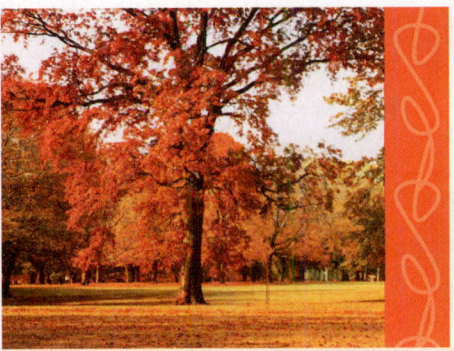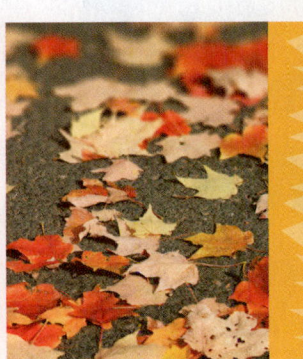

Unit X Wrap-Up

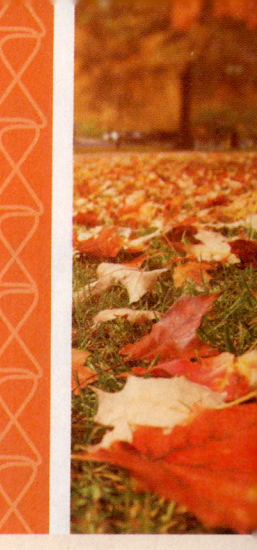

CHAPTER 37
The Nervous System and Assessment

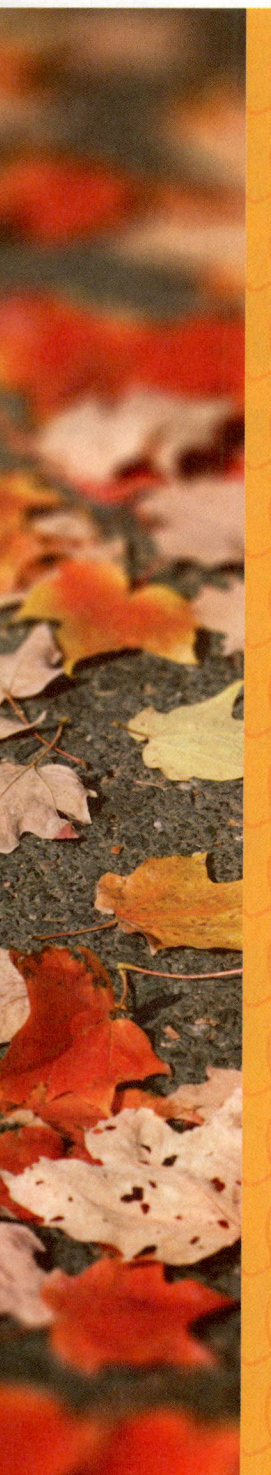

BRIEF OUTLINE

The Nervous System
Structure and Function of the Eye

Structure and Function of the Ear
Assessment

APPLIED LEARNING OUTCOMES

After completing this chapter, you will be able to:

1. Describe the structure and functions of the central and peripheral nervous systems, the eye, and the ear.
2. Identify subjective and objective assessment data to collect for patients with neurologic or sensory disorders.
3. Explain changes in neurologic function, vision, and hearing that occur with aging.
4. Identify nursing responsibilities for common diagnostic tests and monitor the results for patients with neurologic or sensory disorders.

KEY TERMS

The key terms are defined on the pages listed below.

ataxia, 951	myelin sheath, 943	ptosis, 951
cerumen, 949	neuron, 943	reflex, 945
dermatome, 945	neurotransmitter, 943	refraction, 949
dysphagia, 951	nystagmus, 951	spasticity, 951
flaccidity, 951	presbyopia, 952	synapse, 943

The nervous system consists of the brain, spinal cord, and peripheral nerves. It is a very complex system that controls all motor, sensory, and autonomic activities of the body. It responds to changes within the body and to environmental stimuli. When the nervous system malfunctions, the person may experience acute or chronic disorders.

The visual system includes internal and external structures, which are important for visual function. The auditory system functions to receive and perceive sounds as well as maintain position sense and balance. The major sensory organs, including the eyes and ears, are vital in providing input to the nervous system.

The Nervous System

The nervous system is divided into the central nervous system (CNS) and the peripheral nervous system (PNS). The brain and spinal cord make up the CNS. The PNS consists of 12 cranial nerves, 31 pairs of spinal nerves, and the autonomic nervous system.

A **neuron** (basic cell of the nervous system) is made up of a dendrite, a cell body, and an axon (Figure 37-1■).

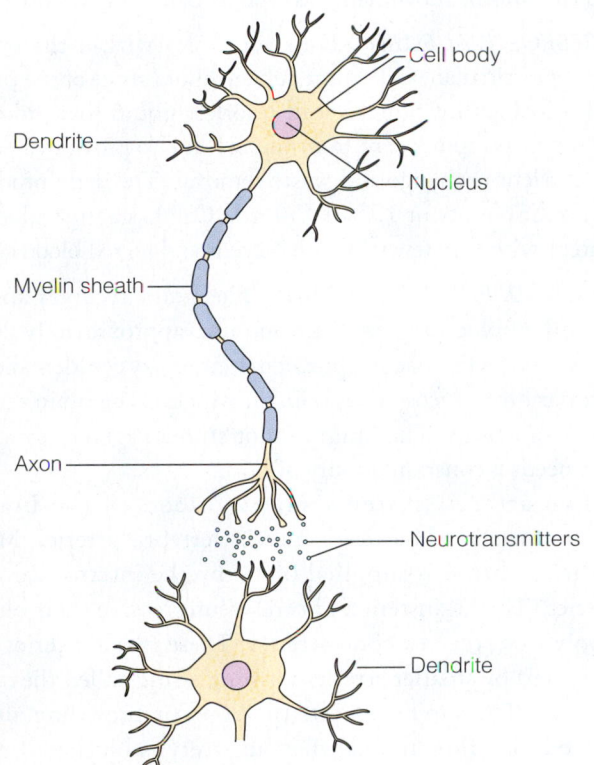

Dendrite

Cell body

Nucleus

Myelin sheath

Axon

Neurotransmitters

Dendrite

Figure 37-1. ■ A neuron.

Dendrites are short, branch-like extensions on the cell body. They carry impulses to the cell body from other cells. The cell body controls the function of the neuron. At the other end of the neuron is a single, long projection known as the axon. It carries impulses away from the cell body. Many axons are protected and insulated by a white fatty substance called **myelin sheath**. Nerves covered with a myelin sheath are known as *myelinated* or white nerve fibers. Axons without myelin are unmyelinated or gray nerve fibers.

Neurons are responsible for neurotransmission. Nerve impulses move from one neuron to another neuron across a **synapse**. A chemical **neurotransmitter** (see Figure 37-1) such as acetylcholine either helps the impulse cross the synapse or stops it. *Sensory* (or afferent) neurons carry impulses from the skin and muscles to the CNS. *Motor* (or efferent) neurons carry impulses from the CNS to the muscles for contraction and to glands in order to release secretions.

THE CENTRAL NERVOUS SYSTEM
The Brain
The brain is the control center of the nervous system. A rigid, bony skull protects the brain from external injury. Beneath the skull are three protective membranes or *meninges*: (1) dura mater, the outer layer; (2) arachnoid, the middle layer; and (3) pia mater, the inner layer directly attached to the brain (Figure 37-2■ *inset*). Arterial blood vessels are located in the *epidural space* between the skull and dura mater. Cerebrospinal fluid (CSF) is found in the *subarachnoid space* between the arachnoid and the pia mater.

There are four major regions of the brain: cerebrum, diencephalon, brainstem, and cerebellum (see Figure 37-2).

CEREBRUM   The cerebrum is the largest area of the brain and is divided into a right and left hemisphere. Deep grooves called *fissures* separate the hemispheres and separate the cerebrum from the cerebellum. The cerebral hemispheres are connected by a thick band of nerve fibers called *corpus callosum*, which lies deep in the brain. It allows communication between the two hemispheres. Each hemisphere receives sensory and motor impulses from the opposite side of the body. The right hemisphere controls sensation and movement of the left side of the body, whereas the left hemisphere controls sensation and movement of the right side of the body. In every individual, one hemisphere is more dominant than the other. The left hemisphere is responsible for speech, problem solving, reasoning, and calculations. The right hemisphere controls visual–spatial information such as art, music, and the surrounding physical environment.

The cerebrum consists of gray matter and white matter. The outer layer or *cerebral cortex* contains the gray matter, which is made up of neurons. The rest of the cerebrum is made up of myelinated nerve fibers called white matter.

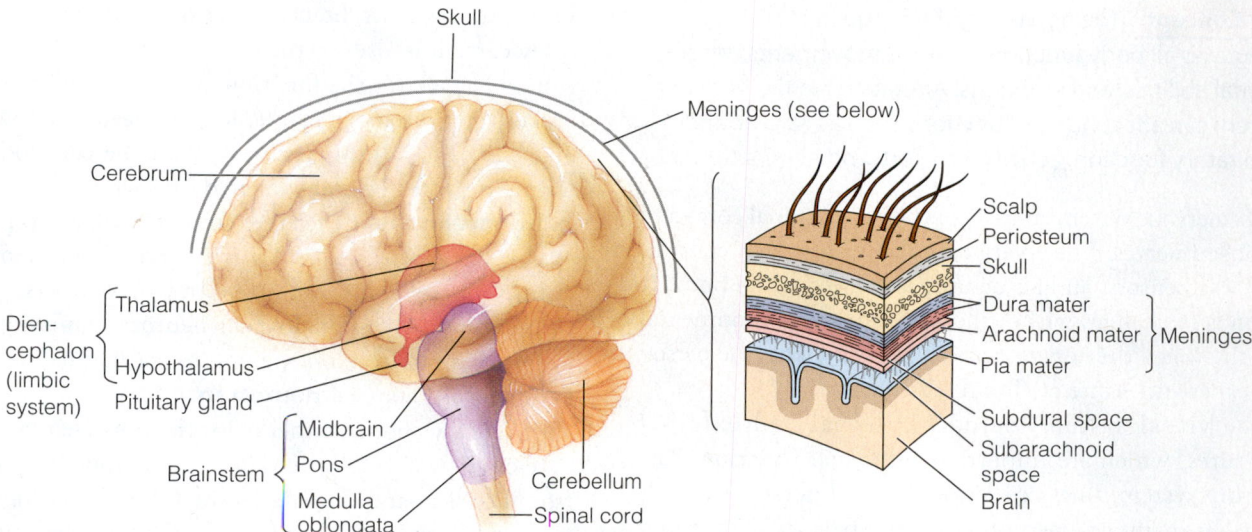

Figure 37-2. ■ The four major regions of the brain with an illustration of the meninges.

Each cerebral hemisphere is divided into four lobes: frontal, parietal, temporal, and occipital (Figure 37-3 ■). They are separated by fissures.

DIENCEPHALON The diencephalon contains the thalamus and hypothalamus. The thalamus relays all sensory information to the cortex. The hypothalamus regulates temperature, fluid balance, thirst, appetite, emotions, and the sleep–wake cycle.

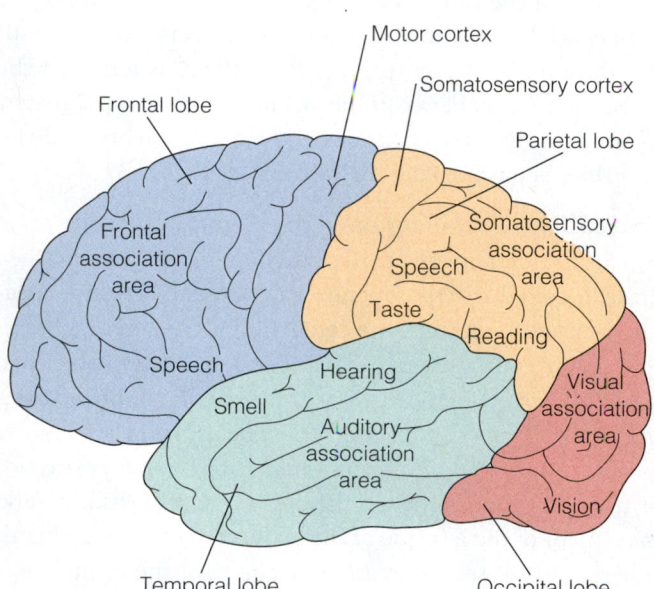

Figure 37-3. ■ Cerebral lobes with their functions. The *frontal lobe* controls voluntary motor activity on the opposite side of the body and determines emotions, motivation, complex thinking, judgment, and personality. Broca area promotes speaking ability. The *parietal lobe* interprets sensations and determines right from left and where the body is in relation to the environment. The *temporal lobe* processes taste, smell, and hearing stimuli; it is also important in long-term memory. Wernicke area promotes understanding of the spoken and written word. The *occipital lobe* processes visual stimuli.

BRAINSTEM The brainstem consists of the midbrain, pons, and medulla oblongata. The midbrain is the center for auditory and visual reflexes. It serves as a nerve pathway between the cerebral hemispheres and lower brain. The pons controls respiration. The medulla oblongata is located at the base of the brainstem. It controls heart rate, blood pressure, respirations, coughing, swallowing, and vomiting.

CEREBELLUM The cerebellum is connected to the midbrain, pons, and medulla. Like the cerebrum, it has two hemispheres. It coordinates involuntary muscle activity and fine motor movements as well as balance and posture.

CEREBROSPINAL FLUID Four ventricles within the brain make and circulate CSF in the subarachnoid space of the brain and spinal cord. CSF is a clear, colorless liquid that protects the brain and spinal cord from trauma. It also provides a place for nutrient exchange and waste removal. The daily production of CSF is about 125 to 150 mL. CSF has a high glucose content with very few white blood cells and no red blood cells.

BLOOD SUPPLY TO THE BRAIN The brain receives about 750 mL of blood each minute and uses approximately 20% of the body's cardiac output. This large oxygen demand is necessary for glucose metabolism, which is the brain's only source of energy. The brain cannot store oxygen or glucose so it needs a constant supply of both.

Two arterial systems supply blood to the brain: (1) internal carotid arteries and (2) vertebral arteries. Most of the cerebrum is supplied blood by the internal carotid arteries. The brainstem and cerebellum receive their blood supply from the vertebral arteries. These major arteries are connected by smaller arteries forming a ring called the *circle of Willis*. This circle protects the brain by providing alternative blood flow routes when an artery is blocked. Cerebral veins drain venous blood into the jugular veins.

BLOOD–BRAIN BARRIER   The *blood–brain barrier* is composed of astrocytes that are joined by tight junctions. This decreases permeability so that harmful substances in the blood cannot enter the brain. It allows only the passage of lipids, glucose, some amino acids, carbon dioxide, oxygen, and water. Substances such as urea, creatinine, some toxins, and most antibiotics cannot pass this barrier. However, brain injury or infection may cause a local breakdown of the barrier.

The Spinal Cord

The spinal cord exits the skull through the foramen magnum and extends to the first or second lumbar vertebra, where it ends in the cauda equina. It is about 17 in. long and 3/4 in. thick. The spinal cord is surrounded and protected by the vertebral column. The column consists of 7 cervical, 12 thoracic, 5 lumbar, 5 sacral, and 4 fused vertebrae, which form the coccyx.

The inside of the spinal cord is H shaped and consists of gray matter surrounded by white matter. The gray matter contains three specialized areas called horns: (1) the ventral horn (motor neurons), (2) dorsal horn (sensory neurons), and (3) lateral horn (sympathetic neurons). The white matter forms ascending and descending pathways known as *spinal tracts*. These tracts carry messages to and from the brain: ascending sensory pathways and descending motor pathways. On exiting the brain, motor and sensory nerve fibers cross to the opposite side of the spinal cord. This is why a stroke in the left hemisphere affects motor and sensory function on the right side of the body.

THE PERIPHERAL NERVOUS SYSTEM

The PNS links the CNS with the rest of the body. It receives and conducts information from the external environment and transmits signals to muscles and organs of the body. Spinal nerves, cranial nerves, and ganglia make up the PNS. The PNS is divided into the sensory and autonomic nervous systems. The sensory system connects the skin and muscles to the CNS. The autonomic nervous system controls visceral organs and some glands.

Spinal Nerves

There are 31 pairs of spinal nerves (Figure 37-4■). These nerves are named in reference to the corresponding vertebrae of the spine:

- Cervical: 8 pairs (C_1 to C_8)
- Thoracic: 12 pairs (T_1 to T_{12})
- Lumbar: 5 pairs (L_1 to L_5)
- Sacral: 5 pairs (S_1 to S_5)

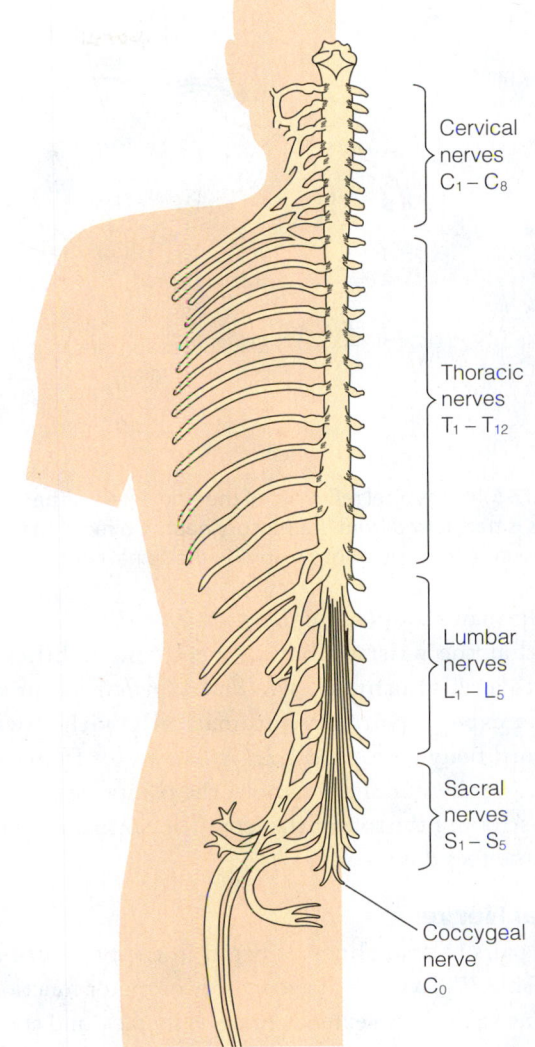

Cervical nerves $C_1 – C_8$

Thoracic nerves $T_1 – T_{12}$

Lumbar nerves $L_1 – L_5$

Sacral nerves $S_1 – S_5$

Coccygeal nerve C_0

Figure 37-4. ■ Distribution of spinal nerves.

Each spinal nerve contains sensory and motor fibers. The dorsal and ventral root of each spinal nerve attaches it to the spinal cord. Sensory fibers are in the dorsal root, with motor fibers in the ventral root. Damage to the dorsal root causes loss of sensation, whereas damage to the ventral root results in flaccid paralysis.

An area of the skin supplied by a single spinal nerve is called a **dermatome**. The dorsal roots of the spinal nerves carry sensations from specific dermatomes. Dermatomes are useful for locating pain sites and neurologic lesions.

Spinal nerves are also involved in reflexes. A **reflex** is an involuntary motor response to a stimulus. Reflexes follow a pathway known as a *reflex arc*. The reflex arc consists of a receptor, an afferent sensory neuron, the response center in the spinal cord or brain, an efferent motor neuron, and an effector muscle or gland (Figure 37-5■).

Common reflexes include stretch, deep tendon, withdrawal, and superficial. *Stretch reflexes* control muscle tone

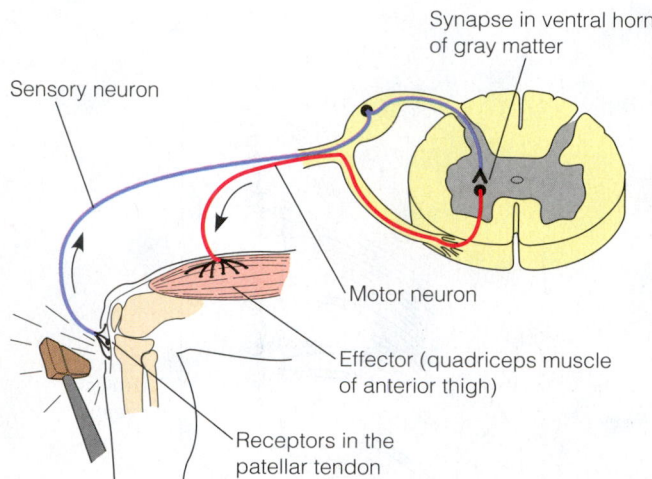

Figure 37-5. ■ A typical reflex arc of the spinal nerve. The stimulus is transferred from the sensory neuron directly to the motor neuron at the point of synapse in the spinal cord.

and help maintain posture. *Deep tendon reflexes (DTRs)* are assessed at the wrists, elbows, knees, and Achilles tendon with a reflex hammer. *Withdrawal reflexes* occur when a person expects pain and automatically withdraws the threatened body part. *Superficial reflexes* result from gently stimulating the skin. For example, the plantar reflex is elicited by stroking the sole of the foot. The normal response is to curl the toes downward.

Cranial Nerves

Twelve pairs of cranial nerves begin in the brain or brainstem (Table 37-1 ■). They have sensory or motor functions or both. The vagus nerve extends into the thoracic and abdominal areas, but the other 11 cranial nerves innervate only head and neck regions. Cranial nerves I (olfactory), II (optic), and VIII (vestibulocochlear) control sensory function only.

THE AUTONOMIC NERVOUS SYSTEM

The autonomic nervous system (ANS) is part of the PNS. It is responsible for maintaining the body's internal homeostasis. The ANS regulates respiration, heart rate, digestion, urinary excretion, body temperature, and sexual function.

There are two divisions: (1) the sympathetic nervous system (SNS) and (2) the parasympathetic nervous system. Fibers from both systems can affect the same structures. Generally when one system increases an action, the other system decreases the action. This process keeps the body in balance so that one action does not dominate.

The SNS prepares the body to handle stress. It plays a key role in the body's "fight-or-flight" response. The parasympathetic nervous system operates during nonstressful situations. It conserves the body's energy by regulating digestion, elimination, and other activities. The actions of the parasympathetic nervous system and SNS are shown in Figure 37-6 ■.

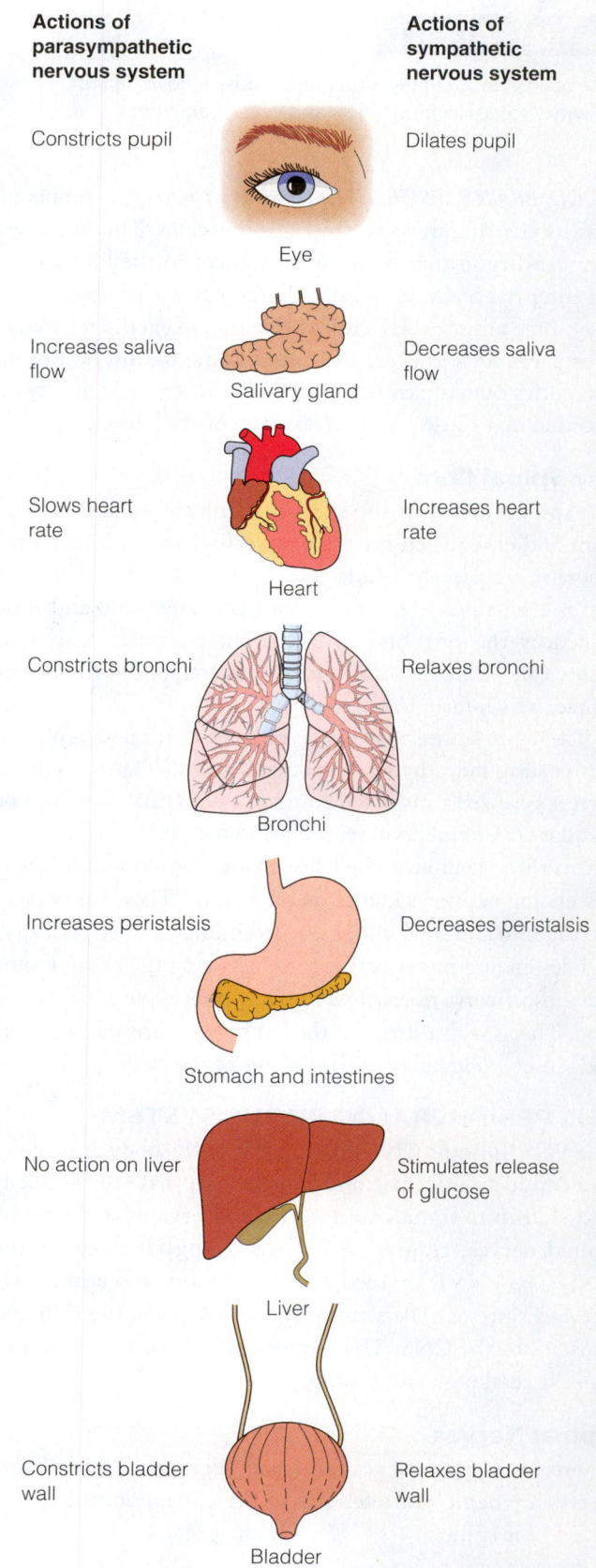

Figure 37-6. ■ Autonomic nervous system and the organs it affects. The left side shows the actions of the parasympathetic nervous system. The right side shows the actions of the sympathetic nervous system.

TABLE 37-1	The Cranial Nerves
CRANIAL NERVE	**FUNCTION**
I Olfactory	Smell
II Optic	Vision
III Oculomotor	Pupil constriction Eyeball movement Raising of upper eyelid
IV Trochlear	Eyeball movement
V Trigeminal	Sensation of the scalp, nose, mouth, and cornea Chewing
VI Abducens	Lateral movement of the eyeball
VII Facial	Movement of facial muscles Secretions from lacrimal and salivary glands Taste in anterior two-thirds of tongue
VIII Vestibulocochlear	Sense of hearing and equilibrium
IX Glossopharyngeal	Swallowing Gag reflex Sensation of pharynx and tongue Taste in posterior one-third of tongue Secretions of parotid gland
X Vagus	Swallowing Control of parasympathetic nervous system activities (e.g., heart rate, respiration, digestion) Sensation in pharynx and larynx
XI Accessory	Neck and shoulder movement
XII Hypoglossal	Tongue movement

Structure and Function of the Eye

Key Concept   The eyes and ears provide the major proportion of the body's sensory functions. Deficits in vision or hearing may limit self-care, safety, independence, communication, and relationships with others.

The eyes are complex structures. The primary function of the eye is to convert patterns of light from the environment into a message that is transmitted via the optic nerve to the brain. The brain gives meaning to the message, allowing us to make sense of what we see.

The eye is protected and supported by the *accessory structures*. They include (Figure 37-7■):

■ The *eyelids* and *eyelashes*, which protect the eye, trap dirt and debris, regulate the amount of light entering the eye, and spread tears.

■ The *conjunctiva*, a thin mucous membrane that covers the anterior surface of the eye, also lines the inner surfaces of the eyelids.

■ The *lacrimal apparatus* secretes and drains tears to cleanse and moisten the eye's surface. Tears are produced by the *lacrimal gland*. They contain an antibacterial enzyme that protects the eye from infections. Tears drain into the *lacrimal ducts* and from there into the nose.

■ The *eye muscles* control eye movement and help maintain the shape of the eyeball.

Each eye is a hollow sphere about 1 in. (2.5 cm) in diameter, surrounded and protected by bone and cushions of fat. The wall of the eyeball has three layers. The outermost layer consists of the white, fibrous *sclera* and the transparent *cornea* (Figure 37-8■). The sclera protects and gives shape to the eyeball. The border between the sclera and the cornea is called the *limbus* (see Figure 37-7). The cornea is a transparent window that allows light to enter the eye. It contains no blood vessels and is very sensitive to touch. When the cornea is touched, the eyelids blink (the *corneal reflex*) and tears are secreted.

The middle layer of the eyeball, the *uvea*, is very vascular. It includes the iris, the ciliary body, and the choroid. The *iris*, the colored part of the eye, regulates light entering the eye by controlling the size of the pupil. The *pupil* is the dark center of the eye through which light enters. The pupil constricts in bright light and dilates in dim light or darkness. The *ciliary body* encircles the lens. It controls the shape of the lens to focus light onto the retina. The *lens* is a transparent structure behind the pupil that can change shape to focus light onto the retina. Like the cornea, the lens contains no blood vessels. The vascular *choroid* nourishes the other layers of the eyeball and absorbs light, preventing it from scattering within the eyeball.

The *retina* is the innermost lining of the eyeball. It contains millions of light receptors called rods and cones. *Rods* are very light sensitive and allow us to see in dim light. *Cones* allow us to see in color and provide a sharper image than rods. Most cones are located in the *macula*, the area where light passing through the pupil and lens focuses on the retina. The macula provides our central vision. In the center of the macula, the *fovea centralis* allows detailed color vision. The optic nerve enters the eye at the *optic disk*.

The hollow eyeball is divided into two interior cavities. The larger *posterior cavity* behind the lens contains the clear gelatinous *vitreous body*. The vitreous body shapes and supports the eye.

The *anterior cavity* is further divided into the *anterior chamber* (the space between the cornea and the iris) and the *posterior chamber* (the space between the iris and

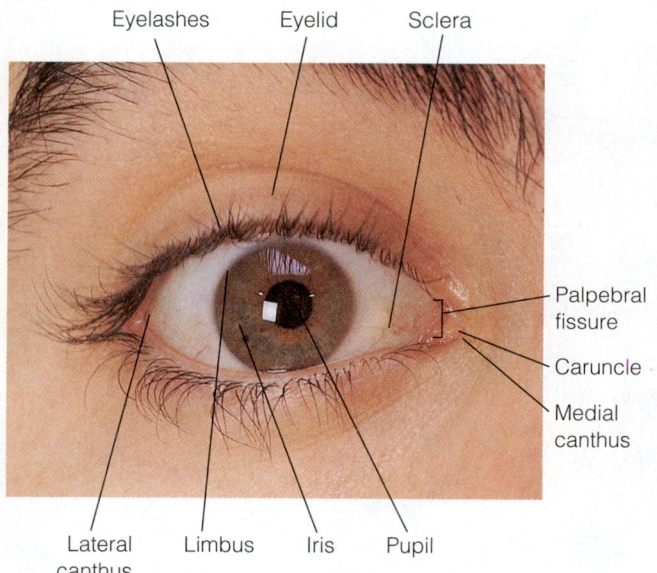

Figure 37-7. ■ The external and accessory structures of the eye. (Pearson Education.)

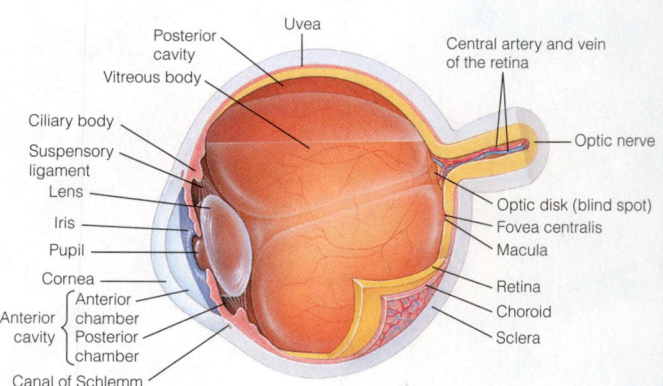

Figure 37-8. ■ The internal structures of the eye.

the lens). Aqueous humor, a clear fluid, circulates through the anterior cavity, nourishing the lens and cornea. Aqueous humor is constantly formed and drained to maintain a relatively constant pressure within the eye. The *canal of Schlemm* at the junction of the sclera and the cornea allows aqueous humor to flow between the anterior and posterior chambers.

As light enters the eye, it is bent (**refraction**) to focus on the retina. The cornea, aqueous humor, lens, and vitreous body bend light rays to focus the image. To change the point of focus from far to near, the lens changes shape, the pupil constricts, and the eyes converge. This is called *accommodation*.

The *optic nerves* are cranial nerves that meet at the *optic chiasma*. Here nerve fibers from the medial half of each retina cross to the opposite side to join nerve fibers from the lateral half of the other eye (Figure 37-9■). The impulses generated in the retina travel to the *visual cortex* in the occipital lobe of the brain. The brain translates the impulses into the image we see, our vision.

The visual fields of each eye overlap considerably, and each eye sees a slightly different view. This allows *depth perception*, the ability to identify differences in the distance between objects.

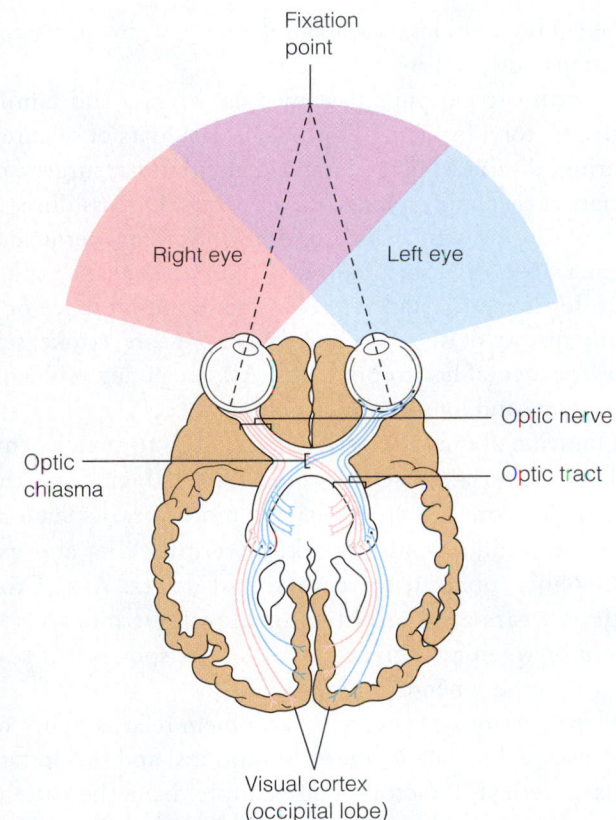

Figure 37-9. ■ The visual fields of the eyes and the optic pathways.

Structure and Function of the Ear

The ear has two primary functions: hearing and maintaining balance. The ear is divided into three areas: the external ear, the middle ear, and the inner ear (Figure 37-10■). All three areas are needed for hearing. The inner ear also helps maintain balance.

The *external ear* includes the auricle (or pinna), the auditory canal, and the tympanic membrane (eardrum). The *auricles* direct sound waves into the ear. The *auditory canal* is about 1 in. (2.5 cm) long. It focuses sound waves on the eardrum. Glands in the canal secrete **cerumen** (earwax), a yellow to brown waxy substance. Cerumen traps dirt and debris, protecting the tympanic membrane and middle ear from infection. The *tympanic membrane* (eardrum) separates the external ear and the middle ear.

The *middle ear* contains the auditory ossicles (bones): the malleus, the incus, and the stapes. These bones transmit vibrations from the tympanic membrane to the oval window of the inner ear. The middle ear is filled with air. It opens into the *eustachian tube*, which connects it with the nasopharynx. This proximity to the nasopharynx increases the likelihood for middle ear infections associated with upper respiratory infections. The eustachian tube helps equalize the pressure in the middle ear with atmospheric pressure.

The *inner ear* (*labyrinth*) is a maze of bony, fluid-filled chambers. The labyrinth has three regions: the vestibule, the semicircular canals, and the cochlea. The *vestibule* contains the oval window and joins the cochlea and the semicircular canals. Receptors in the vestibule respond to changes in gravity and head position, helping to maintain balance. The three *semicircular canals* also contain receptors that respond to head movements. The *cochlea* contains the *organ of Corti*, the receptor for hearing. The organ of Corti is the set of sensory hair cells innervated by cranial nerve (CN) VIII, the vestibulocochlear nerve.

Hearing is the perception and interpretation of sound. Sound waves entering the external auditory canal cause the eardrum to vibrate. The ossicles transmit this vibration to the oval window, setting fluid within the vestibule into motion. The fluid movement stimulates receptors in the organ of Corti, which then send signals to the brain via CN VIII. Nerve fibers from each ear cross, so the auditory centers on each side of the brain receive impulses from both ears. The brain can receive and interpret a wide variety of sounds, as well as localize the source of the sound.

The inner ear also provides information to the brain about head position. This information is used to coordinate body movements so that *equilibrium* and *balance* are maintained. Changing head position sends different patterns of nerve

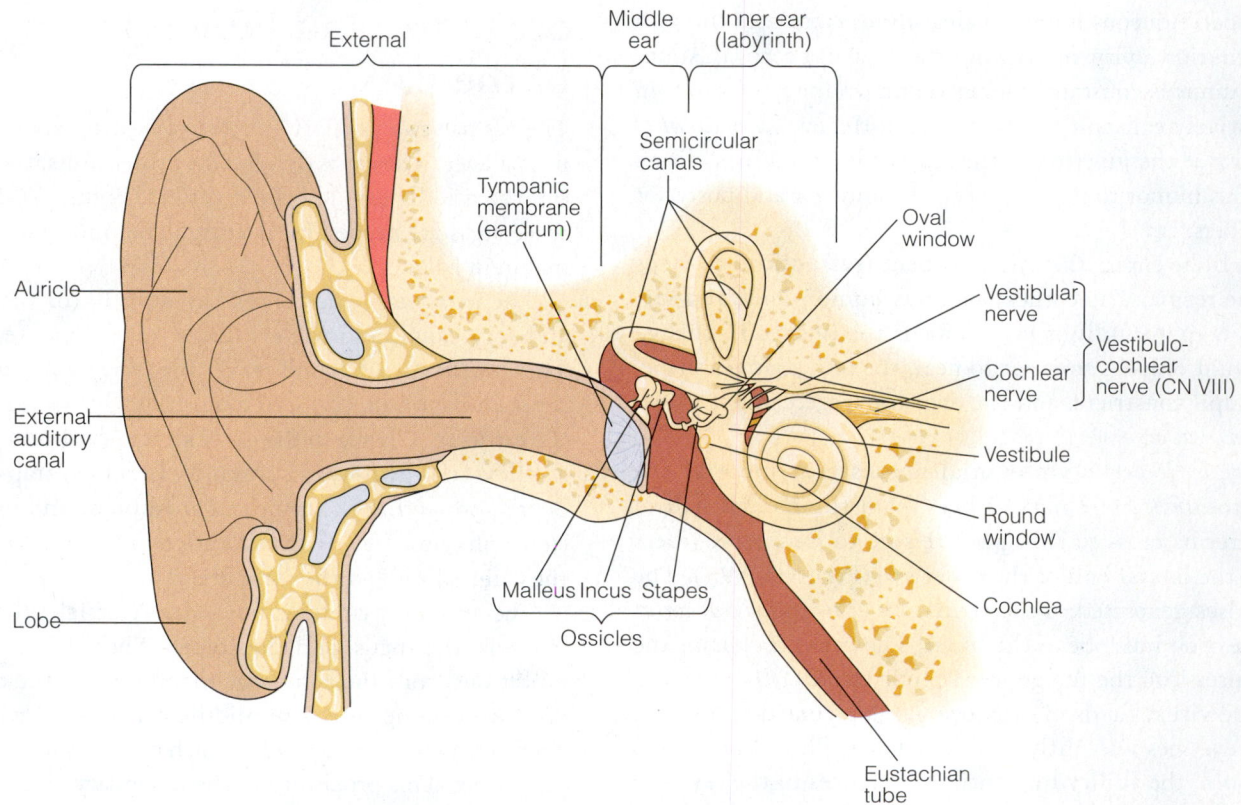

Figure 37-10. ■ Structures of the external, middle, and inner ear.

impulses to the brain from the inner ear. The brain interprets these messages, stimulating motor centers to coordinate body movements.

Assessment

HEALTH HISTORY

Focused assessment of the patient with a neurologic disorder begins with identifying the patient's level of consciousness (LOC). Start by asking the patient's name in a normal conversational volume. When the patient's LOC is altered, the nurse may need to ask the family for information. Assess the patient's respiratory status, including rate and depth of breathing. Depressed respiratory rate and depth can lead to hypoxia and decreased LOC.

Ask about numbness, tingling, sensations, tremors, problems with coordination or balance, loss of movement in any part of the body, or difficulty walking or using the hands. Determine when symptoms first began and whether they are constant or intermittent. If the patient is experiencing pain, ask if coughing, sneezing, or walking increases the pain.

Determine whether the patient has difficulty with speaking, seeing, hearing, tasting, or detecting odors. Inquire about memory, feelings of anxiety or depression, recent changes in sleep patterns, ability to perform activities of daily living, sexual activity, and weight changes. If the patient is taking any medications (prescription, over-the-counter, and natural or herbal preparations), ask about the purpose, frequency and duration of use, and any side effects.

Obtain the patient's past medical history and family health history, focusing on previous incidents of seizures; fainting; dizziness; headaches; and any trauma, surgery, or tumors of the brain, spinal cord, or nerves. Discuss illnesses such as cardiovascular disease, sinus infections, pernicious anemia, liver disease, and/or renal failure that may cause neurologic manifestations. Ask about the presence or a family history of diabetes, high blood pressure, stroke, seizures, or mental health problems. Ask about any problems with short- and long-term memory.

Question about occupational exposure to toxic chemicals or materials, use of protective headgear, and the amount of time doing repetitive motion tasks such as data entry and assembly work. Determine diet and use of alcohol, tobacco, or recreational drugs. Ask if the patient wears a helmet during bicycle or motorcycle riding or when participating in contact sports or if seat belts are used when driving.

If the patient presents with a problem related to one or both eyes, ask about its onset, symptoms, and precipitating and relieving factors. For example, have the patient describe the type of eye pain, when it began, and how long it lasts. Determine whether the patient notices rings of color around streetlights at night or has difficulty reading the paper.

Observe the patient for squinting or abnormal eye movements that indicate problems with eye function. Ask about watery, irritated eyes or changes in vision. Inquire about the use of eye medications, corrective eyewear, and care of eyeglasses or contact lenses. Identify any history of eye trauma, surgery, or infections, as well as the date and results of the last eye examination. Ask about a personal or family history of glaucoma, cataracts, diabetes, hypertension, thyroid disorders, and eye infections. Question whether there is a history of nearsightedness or farsightedness, cancer of the retina, or color blindness. Collect information about environmental or work exposure to chemicals or participation in sports or hobbies that increase the risk of eye injury.

Explore changes in hearing such as difficulty hearing high-pitched or low-pitched sounds, ringing in the ears (*tinnitus*), ear pain, drainage from the ears, or use of hearing aids. Ask about trauma, surgery, or ear infections, as well as infectious diseases such as meningitis or mumps. Determine the use of medications that may affect hearing such as aminoglycoside antibiotics. Obtain the patient's family history of hearing loss or ear problems and the date of the last ear examination.

PHYSICAL EXAMINATION

The focused physical examination for the patient with a neurologic problem begins by assessing the patient's posture, movement, and appearance and identifying orientation, mental state, and emotional state. Identify whether the patient can see, hear, and feel your touch.

Assess dress, hygiene, and grooming, as well as gait and posture. Observe the patient's actions and affect. Note the LOC; content and quality of speech; mood swings; personality changes; and orientation to time, place, and person. Assess for memory or perceptual deficits.

Obtain blood pressure in both arms (unless contraindicated), pulse, respiratory rate, and temperature. Note any abnormal breathing patterns such as increased or decreased rate and depth of breathing. Check pupil response to light by using a penlight. Normal response should be PERRLA (pupils equally round and reactive to light and accommodation). Observe for **ptosis** (drooping eyelids) and **nystagmus** (involuntary eye movement). Assess the ability to swallow a small drink of water, noting the presence of **dysphagia** (difficulty swallowing).

Determine the patient's ability to shrug the shoulders and stick out the tongue. Note that the tongue should be midline. Assess for facial droop. Have the patient turn head side to side against resistance. Perform the Romberg test.

Assess upper and lower extremities for weakness, atrophy, and tremors, as well as identifying decreased muscle tone (**flaccidity**) or increased muscle tone (**spasticity**). Ask the patient to squeeze your hands, push feet against the resistance of your hands, and raise both legs off the bed. Note if there

is any difference between left and right side. Assess gait and ability to stand on one foot and walk heel to toe. **Ataxia** is a lack of coordination and an unbalanced gait. Assess DTRs. Abnormal DTRs require further medical evaluation.

Assess distant vision by using the Snellen chart (see Figure 5-4) and asking the patient to cover one eye at a time to read the chart and then repeat the test for the other eye. Assess near vision in the same manner, using a Rosenbaum chart (Figure 37-11■). To test extraocular movements, ask the patient to follow a pen or your finger while keeping the head stationary. Inspect the eyelids for unusual redness or discharge. Note abnormal wideness of the lids, which may be due to *exophthalmos*. Inspect the cornea and iris for cloudiness or irregularities and the sclera for redness or yellow discoloration.

Assess for hearing loss by performing the whisper test and the Rinne and Weber tests (see Box 40-9). Inspect the auricle for redness, drainage, scales, or skin lesions. Palpate the auricles and over the mastoid process for tenderness, swelling, or nodules.

For more information about assessment techniques, see Chapter 5. See Box 37-1■ for an example of a neurologic assessment.

The Older Adult

In the older adult the brain atrophies, causing slower movement and reflexes, as well as a degree of forgetfulness. However, significant short- and long-term memory loss, mental status changes, altered coordination, loss of motor skills, and altered speech signal a need for further assessment. The patient may have difficulty changing position or standing up without assistance. This may be accompanied by dizziness, which is the result of anemia, ear infection, eye problems, stroke, or drug toxicity. These changes are often related to common chronic diseases that develop in older adults.

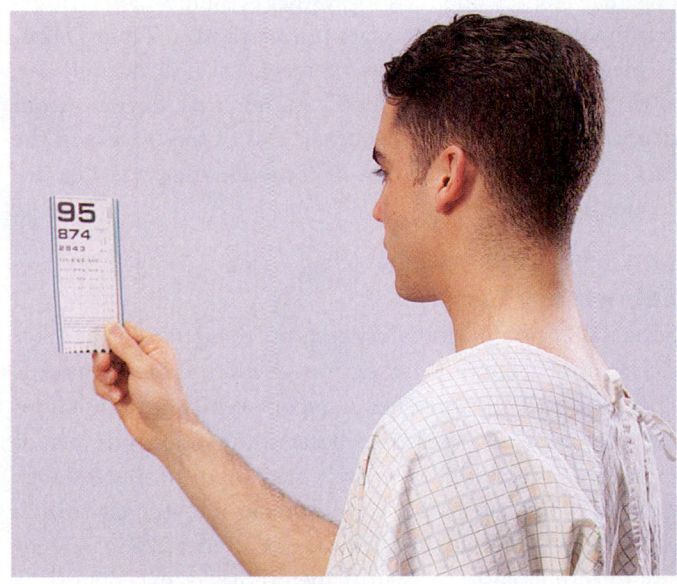

Figure 37-11. ■ Testing vision using a Rosenbaum eye chart.
(Richard Tauber, Pearson Education.)

<table>
<tr><td>

| BOX 37-1 | DOCUMENTATION OF NEUROLOGIC ASSESSMENT |
</td></tr>
</table>

BOX 37-1	**DOCUMENTATION OF NEUROLOGIC ASSESSMENT**

Patient: A 50-year-old male arrives on the neurologic unit at 5:00 p.m. after a motor vehicle crash. He is diagnosed with a concussion. He has no significant other medical problems.

Assessment note: Alert and oriented × 3. PERRLA. Able to move all extremities and resist pressure equally. Denies numbness or tingling in all extremities. Hand grasps strong and equal.

At 8:00 p.m. difficult to arouse. Oriented to person only. Pupils unequal with right greater than left, sluggish reaction. Speech slightly slurred. Left hand grasp weak. States numbness in left hand. Has difficulty raising left leg and has decreased ability to push against resistance. Charge nurse notified and physician paged.

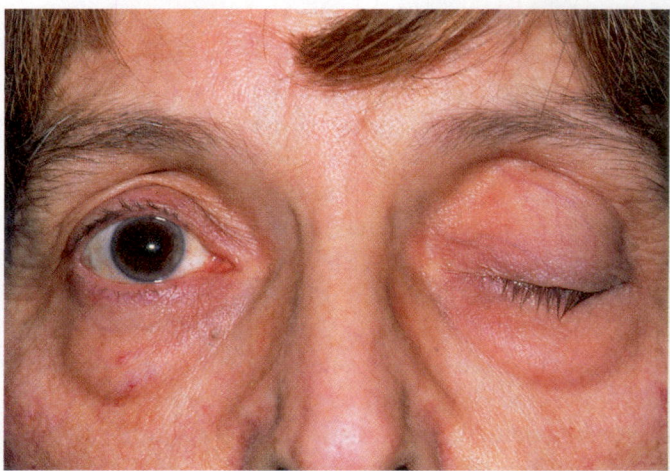

Figure 37-12. ■ Ptosis. (Source: Dr. P. Marazzi/Science Source.)

Often older adults experience sleep disorders and reduced pain perception. This may result from other chronic diseases and medication use or more serious neurologic dysfunction. Depression, delirium, and dementia develop in many older adults, signaling underlying disease. Confusion, memory loss, and depression are not associated with normal aging. Further information on assessing psychologic status may be found in Chapter 47.

A number of changes in the eye and vision occur with aging. The lens becomes less elastic, affecting near vision. This is known as **presbyopia**. Patients with presbyopia may feel that their arms have become too short to read the newspaper comfortably.

Eyelid muscles may lose tone, causing the lower lid to turn out (*ectropion*) or the upper lid to droop (ptosis, Figure 37-12■). The lid margin may turn inward (*entropion*), causing the lashes to irritate the eye. Tears are decreased, so the eyes may feel dry and scratchy. Other eye and vision changes commonly seen with aging are summarized in Table 37-2■.

Hearing difficulties may be mechanical or natural. Inability to hear high-frequency sounds may develop from degeneration in the cochlea or the loss of small hairs in the ears. Increased accumulation of cerumen or earwax can also reduce hearing ability.

DIAGNOSTIC TESTS
Laboratory Tests

Several nonspecific laboratory tests are done to rule out other causes of neurologic dysfunction. A blood glucose level is done to identify the presence of hypoglycemia. Serum sodium and osmolarity are measured because low sodium levels, or increased or decreased osmolarity, may cause an altered LOC. Arterial blood gases are used to rule out low oxygen or high carbon dioxide levels, another cause of altered LOC. To identify infectious diseases such as meningitis or encephalitis, a complete blood count (CBC) with differential and cultures from blood, urine, throat, and nose are done.

Elevated serum creatinine and BUN, which reflect decreased kidney function, can decrease LOC. Liver studies such as ALT, AST, and serum ammonia are elevated in liver failure, which also affect LOC. Blood and urine toxicology screenings are useful in identifying drug or alcohol toxicity.

Normal CSF is clear, is colorless, and contains no RBCs, a few WBCs, very little protein, and glucose of 50 to 70 mg/dL. A lumbar puncture is done to obtain CSF, which is sent for a culture and sensitivity and Gram stain, in order to identify intracranial infections. The nursing care before and after a lumbar puncture as well as patient teaching are summarized in Chapter 38 (see Box 38-2).

TABLE 37-2	Age-Related Changes in the Eye and Vision
CHANGE	**EFFECT ON VISION**
Decreased corneal sensation and tear secretion	Increased risk of damage due to foreign body or trauma; increased risk of infection
Constriction of the pupil	Reduced light entering the eye; difficulty with night vision
Decreased elasticity and increased density of the lens	Difficulty focusing, especially for near vision Increased problems with glare Decreased color perception (especially blues, greens, and violet)
Loss of rods at the periphery of the retina	Decreased peripheral vision
Loss of fat and subcutaneous tissue around the eyes	Eyes appear sunken; decreased peripheral vision

TABLE 37-3	Imaging Techniques	
DIAGNOSTIC STUDY	**EXPLANATION AND PURPOSE**	**NURSING IMPLICATIONS**
Radiography	Used to identify neurologic abnormalities such as lesions and tumors; when combined with use of an injected contrast medium, used to study blood flow through vessels.	If contrast medium is used, ask about allergies to iodine and seafood before the exam; ensure good hydration before and after the exam to reduce the risk of kidney damage. Although noninvasive, radiography exposes the patient to potentially damaging radiation. Ask women of childbearing age about possible pregnancy before the exam.
Skull and spine x-rays	Used to identify fractures, bone erosion, and calcifications.	Noninvasive test. Explain if different positions are needed.
Computed tomography (CT) scans	Specialized radiographic procedures that produce computer-generated images with significantly more detail than standard x-rays allow. May be done with or without contrast medium. Detects problems such as hemorrhage, edema, hematoma, infarction, tumor, brain abscess, aneurysm, as well as size and location of cerebrovascular accident (CVA).	See Box 38-8 for the nursing care checklist of a patient undergoing a CT scan of the head.
Magnetic resonance imaging (MRI)	MRI uses a super magnet and radiofrequency signals to elicit a response from hydrogen nuclei. Used to identify stroke, tumor, trauma, multiple sclerosis, and seizures.	The patient is not exposed to radiation during an MRI. Assess for metal implants such as pacemaker, shrapnel, or body piercing. Provide teaching, as the experience can be frightening.
Cerebral angiogram	Invasive procedure that combines x-ray and fluoroscopy (a radiographic image displayed on a screen) with injection of contrast medium into the vessel to illuminate blood flow through the vessel and evaluate its patency. Used to detect an aneurysm, brain tumor, and stroke.	Withhold fluids and food for 8 hours before test. Explain that the patient will have hot flush of head and neck when contrast medium is injected. **clinicalALERT** Closely monitor neurologic and vital signs; maintain pressure dressing and ice to the injection site. Immediately report bleeding or swelling to the charge nurse and physician.
Myelogram	X-ray of spinal cord and canal after injection of contrast medium. Identifies spinal cord tumors, herniated intervertebral disks, and arthritic bone spurs.	See Box 39-8 for nursing care of a patient undergoing myelogram. **clinicalALERT** Closely monitor neurologic and vital signs. Immediately report leakage or bleeding from lumbar puncture site to the charge nurse and physician.
Positive emission tomography (PET)	A radioactive agent is injected, and computed tomography measures metabolic activity of the brain. Used to detect brain cancer, Alzheimer disease, epilepsy, and Parkinson disease.	Withhold food and fluids 4 hours before the exam. Explain that an IV line will be inserted. Post-test, encourage oral fluids to aid removal of radioisotope.
Ultrasound	Echoes from high-frequency sound waves are used to study blood flow within a vessel.	
Carotid duplex study	Sound waves identify blood flow velocity to determine the presence of occlusive vascular disease.	Explain study to the patient.

Imaging Techniques

Imaging techniques used to identify neurologic function may be invasive and noninvasive. Table 37-3■ summarizes these diagnostic procedures and their nursing implications.

Electrographic Studies

Electrographic studies are used to evaluate electrical activity of the brain, nerve and skeletal muscles, and sensory pathways. These diagnostic procedures with their nursing implications are presented in Table 37-4■.

Diagnostic Tests for Visual and Auditory Systems

Specific studies are used for evaluating the visual and auditory systems. These tests and appropriate nursing implications are summarized in Table 37-5■.

Note: The references and resources for all chapters have been compiled at the back of the book.

TABLE 37-4	Electrographic Studies	
ELECTROGRAPHIC STUDY	**EXPLANATION AND PURPOSE**	**NURSING IMPLICATIONS**
Electroencephalogram (EEG)	Electrodes are placed on the scalp to record brain electrical activity. Done to diagnose epilepsy, brain tumor, abscess, or hematoma, and brain death.	Noninvasive procedure that does not cause electric shock. Assist the patient to wash electrode paste out of hair.
Electromyogram (EMG)	Needles are inserted into skeletal muscles (as on the legs) to record electrical activity. Used to diagnose such disorders as multiple sclerosis, myasthenia gravis, and spinal cord injury or disease.	Explain that there is slight discomfort when the needles are inserted. Tell the patient to avoid caffeine or nicotine for 3 hours before the test.
Evoked potentials	Visual or auditory stimulus evokes electrical activity related to nerve conduction along sensory pathways. Electrodes on the scalp and skin record the activity level. Done to diagnose multiple sclerosis, acoustic neuroma, Parkinson disease, spinal cord disease, or blindness.	Instruct the patient to wash hair before the exam.

TABLE 37-5	Diagnostic Tests for Visual and Auditory Systems	
DIAGNOSTIC TEST	**EXPLANATION AND PURPOSE**	**NURSING IMPLICATIONS**
Fluorescein stain	Fluorescein dye is injected onto the cornea, and the cornea is viewed with a slit lamp. The green staining allows identification of corneal ulceration or abrasion.	Explain that the dye may sting slightly when inserted, and the staining will wash away with tears.
Visual field testing	A semicircular bowl-like instrument shows light in different parts of the bowl to map field of vision. Used to evaluate the progression of glaucoma.	Procedure does not cause pain but can tire the patient.
Facial x-rays and CT scan	X-rays and CT scan are used to identify orbital fractures or the presence of foreign bodies in the eye.	Explain procedure to the patient.
Ultrasonography	A probe is placed against the cornea to measure for lens implant after cataract removal and to diagnose retinal detachment.	Explain to the patient that cornea is anesthetized before the procedure is done.
Audiometry	The patient wears earphones through which sounds are presented to determine the hearing range. Used to diagnose conductive hearing loss.	Explain that the test is done by an audiologist.
X-ray and CT scan	X-rays and CT scan are used to evaluate the auditory canal for diagnosing Ménière disease.	Explain procedure to the patient.
Caloric testing	In caloric testing, cold or warm water is injected into the semicircular canals. The patient is observed for nystagmus, nausea, vomiting, falling, or vertigo, indicating labyrinth disease.	Ensure patient safety by observing for vomiting and assisting as necessary to prevent aspiration.

Chapter Review

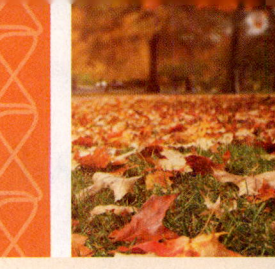

KEY POINTS

- **Concept:** The nervous system regulates and integrates all body functions, muscle movements, senses, mental abilities, and emotions. Alterations in the nervous system can affect human functions such as cardiac and respiratory function, activity, comfort, and elimination.
- The brain and spinal cord comprise the central nervous system (CNS). The peripheral nervous system (PNS) includes the cranial and spinal nerves along with the autonomic nervous system (ANS).
- The ANS consists of two divisions: sympathetic and parasympathetic. Both regulate visceral functions such as respiration, heart rate, digestion, urinary excretion, body temperature, and sexual function.
- Meninges and cerebrospinal fluid provide protective and metabolic functions in the CNS. The blood–brain barrier prevents harmful substances from entering the brain.
- The brain is divided into four lobes (frontal, parietal, occipital, temporal) and two hemispheres (right and left), each responsible for specialized functions.
- Numerous diagnostic tests such as computed tomography (CAT) scan, magnetic resonance imaging (MRI), and cerebral angiogram are used to detect stroke, brain tumors, or aneurysm.

- **Concept:** The eyes and ears provide the major proportion of the body's sensory functions. Deficits in vision or hearing may limit self-care, safety, independence, communication, and relationships with others.
- Vision results from light entering through the pupil that stimulates receptors in the retina and sends a message via the optic nerve to the occipital lobe. The brain interprets the image of what the eye sees.
- As adults age they often experience problems with night vision, glare, and near vision known as presbyopia. Common visual disorders include cataracts, glaucoma, and macular degeneration.
- Hearing occurs when sound waves vibrate the eardrum, travel to the ossicles and oval window, and stimulate the organ of Corti, which sends signals to the brain via cranial nerve VIII. Balance and equilibrium are maintained by the semicircular canals in the inner ear.
- More than 10% of adults, especially those over age 75, experience hearing deficits. Two diagnostic hearing tests, Rinne and Weber, are useful to identify the extent of hearing loss.

PEARSON NURSING STUDENT RESOURCES

Find additional materials at **nursing.pearsonhighered.com**.

NCLEX-PN® Exam Preparation

1 Which of the following visual changes should the nurse expect the older adult patient to report?
   1. Increased tear secretion
   2. Reduced ability to differentiate blue and green colors
   3. Reduced vision during daylight hours
   4. Difficulty focusing on objects in the distance

2 After electroencephalography (EEG), what nursing action should the nurse implement?
   1. Monitor for signs of bleeding at the insertion site.
   2. Encourage the patient to increase fluid intake.
   3. Monitor for nausea and vomiting.
   4. Assist the patient to shampoo the hair.

3 Which of these physiologic results would occur from the stimulation of the sympathetic nervous system? **Select all that apply.**
   1. Decreased peristalsis
   2. Slower heart rate
   3. Dilation of skin blood vessels
   4. Increased blood glucose levels
   5. Dilation of the pupils
   6. Constriction of the bronchi

4 When the patient has difficulty maintaining balance, what cranial nerve is involved?
   1. Cranial nerve III
   2. Cranial nerve V
   3. Cranial nerve VIII
   4. Cranial nerve XI

5 A patient arrives in the emergency department after a bicycle crash. Which of the following assessment questions is most important for the nurse to ask?
   1. "Were you wearing a helmet?"
   2. "Have you had difficulty sleeping at night?"
   3. "Do you have a family history of diabetes?"
   4. "Do you take any herbal preparations?"

Answers and rationales for Review Questions appear in Appendix I.

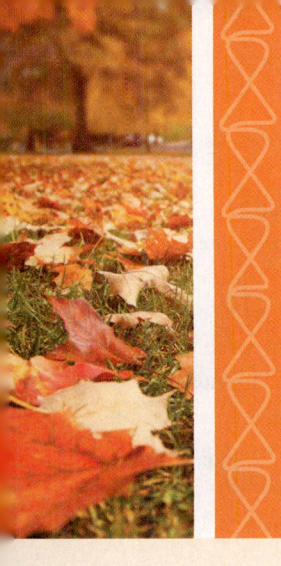

CHAPTER 38
Caring for Patients With Intracranial Disorders

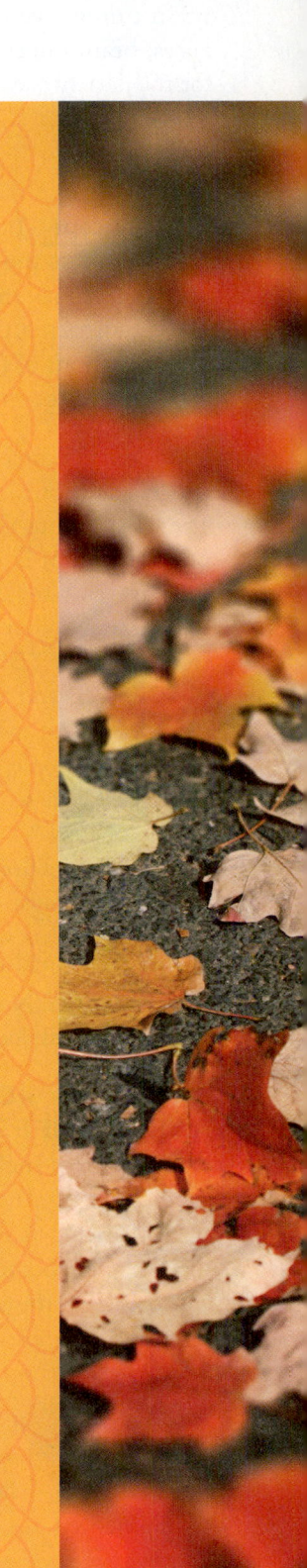

BRIEF OUTLINE

Head Injuries
Brain Tumor
Cerebrovascular Accident/Stroke
Cerebral Aneurysm

Seizure Disorder
Intracranial Infections
Headaches

APPLIED LEARNING OUTCOMES

After completing this chapter, you will be able to:

1. Identify common manifestations and neurologic effects of head injuries, increased intracranial pressure, tumors, cerebrovascular accident, seizures, brain infections, and headaches.
2. Identify laboratory and diagnostic tests used to diagnose intracranial disorders and report abnormal findings.
3. Implement collaborative care required for managing patients with increased intracranial pressure.
4. Apply the nursing implications for medications ordered for patients with intracranial disorders.
5. Provide appropriate preoperative and postoperative care for patients undergoing neurosurgery.
6. Use the nursing process to collect data, establish outcomes, provide individualized care, and evaluate nursing responses for the patient with an intracranial disorder.
7. Reinforce home care teaching guidelines for patients with altered neurologic function.

KEY TERMS

The key terms are defined on the pages listed below.

SPECIAL FEATURES

Intracranial disorders can be acute and life threatening or occur over a long period of time. These disorders often result in long-term problems that affect the patient's and family's quality of life.

This chapter presents common head injuries, followed by a discussion on increased intracranial pressure and altered level of consciousness. Additional topics include brain tumors, cerebrovascular accidents, aneurysms, seizures, brain infections, and headaches. Basic nursing care for the patient having neurosurgery is described.

Head Injuries

> **Key Concept**   Traumatic brain injury occurs when a blow or jolt to the head disrupts normal brain function. Its effects range from a brief change in consciousness to long-term coma, permanent disability, or death. Major complications of TBI are increased intracranial pressure and cerebral edema.

Head injuries can cause minor damage, such as that seen in scalp lacerations, or major damage to the skull or brain. The most serious form of head injury is traumatic brain injury (TBI). TBI is a leading cause of death and disability in the United States. Males ages 15 to 24, children ages 4 and younger, and older patients (75 years or older) are at an increased risk for TBI injuries (National Institute of Neurological Disorders and Stroke [NINDS], 2013d). The Centers for Disease Control and Prevention (CDC) estimate that at least 1.7 million people in the United States sustain head injuries each year. Of these, 275,000 are hospitalized, and 52,000 die. Approximately 3.2 to 5.3 million Americans live with long-term disabilities from an injury to the brain (CDC, 2011). Falls are the major cause of head injuries followed by motor vehicle accidents (MVAs), workplace or sports-related injuries, and violent assaults. Elevated blood alcohol levels often increase the risk of an MVA. Not wearing seatbelts or motorcycle helmets increases the risk for head injury when crashes occur.

PATHOPHYSIOLOGY AND MANIFESTATIONS

Head injuries include scalp lacerations, skull fractures, concussion, contusion, and hematomas. Scalp lacerations are classified as a minor head injury and often look worse than they are because they bleed profusely. A *skull fracture* is a break in the skull. It is usually caused by extreme force and can possibly result in brain damage. Skull fractures are either *open* (from a tear in the dura) or *closed* (the dura is not torn). There are four types of skull fractures:

1. *Linear*—a simple, clean break in the skull.
2. *Comminuted*—the skull is crushed into small, fragmented pieces.

3. *Depressed*—bone fragments may be pushed into the brain; usually caused by a powerful blow to the skull.
4. *Basilar*—occurs at the base of the skull and may extend to the paranasal sinus of the frontal bone or the middle ear found in the temporal bone. This can cause blood or cerebrospinal fluid (CSF) to leak from the nose (**rhinorrhea**) or the ears (**otorrhea**). Other manifestations include *Battle sign* (bruising over the mastoid process) and *periorbital ecchymosis*, sometimes called *raccoon eyes*. If CSF leakage is present, the risk of infection is high.

In any head injury, it is important to determine whether the brain has sustained damage. Brain damage may result from open or closed head injuries. *Open head injuries* occur in two ways. Severe blunt trauma can create an opening through the scalp, skull, and dura to expose the brain, as seen in a depressed skull fracture. An object such as a bullet or knife can penetrate the skull and damage the brain. Patients with open injuries have a higher risk for meningitis.

Closed head injuries usually result from an acceleration–deceleration injury, also called the coup–contrecoup phenomenon (Figure 38-1 ■). For instance, when the head hits an object (e.g., dashboard), the brain bounces forward (acceleration) and then rapidly rebounds and hits the back of the skull (deceleration). Thus the brain sustains bruising at two points, resulting in extensive brain damage. Other types of closed head injuries are **concussion** (brain injury resulting from violent shaking or impact) and **contusion** (bleeding into soft tissue resulting from a blunt force). The amount of damage from a head injury relates to how the injury occurred, the type of injury, and its location. Brain damage develops either from direct trauma to the tissue or from cerebral edema and increased **intracranial pressure** (pressure exerted within the cranium by the brain, blood, and CSF). *Diffuse axonal injury (DAI)* causes widespread

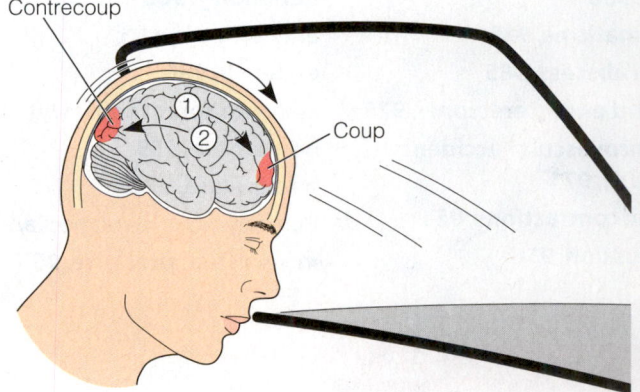

Figure 38-1. ■ Coup–contrecoup head injury. After the initial injury (coup), the brain rebounds within the skull and sustains additional injury (contrecoup) in the opposite part of the brain.

TABLE 38-1	Common Brain Injuries With Pathophysiology and Manifestations	
BRAIN INJURY	**PATHOPHYSIOLOGY**	**MANIFESTATIONS**
Concussion	Brain injury is caused by violent shaking of the brain.	Immediate loss of consciousness for less than 5 minutes Drowsiness, confusion, dizziness Headache, blurred or double vision
Contusion	Bruising of the brain tissue occurs when the brain strikes the inner skull, such as in coup–contrecoup injury. Can cause cerebral edema and increased intracranial pressure.	Varies with the size and location of the injury. Initial loss of consciousness; if LOC remains altered, the patient may become combative. Full consciousness is regained very slowly, and some residual deficits may persist.
Epidural hematoma	Severe blow to the brain causes arterial bleeding that collects between the skull and dura mater. May be caused by skull fractures or contusion. Common site is the temporal area.	Brief loss of consciousness followed by a short period of alertness and then rapid deterioration to a coma; *contralateral* (opposite side) hemiparesis; *ipsilateral* (same side) fixed pupil dilation, and seizures.
Subdural hematoma	Closed head injury causes venous blood to collect between dura mater and the subarachnoid layer.	There are three types of subdural hematomas: *Acute:* Symptoms appear 24–48 hours after injury; headache, drowsiness, slowed thinking, and confusion, with possible ipsilateral pupil dilation.
	Subacute occurs from less severe head injury.	*Subacute:* Symptoms appear 48 hours to 2 weeks later; headache, drowsiness, slowed thinking, and confusion.
	Chronic occurs most often in older adults, alcoholics, and those taking anticoagulants.	*Chronic:* Symptoms of slowed thinking, confusion, and drowsiness develop weeks to months after initial injury.
Intracerebral hematoma	Bleeding into the brain tissue; caused by gunshot wound or a depressed skull fracture.	Headache, decreasing LOC to coma; ipsilateral pupil changes and contralateral hemiparesis.

damage to cerebrum and brainstem. DAI is the leading cause of persistent vegetative state in which there is total loss of cognitive function. Table 38-1 ■ lists common brain injuries.

Intracranial hemorrhage is defined as bleeding within the skull and is the most serious type of brain injury. Intracranial hemorrhage may result from the tearing of cerebral arteries or veins or from direct trauma. This bleeding leads to the formation of a **hematoma** (an accumulation of blood). Blood accumulates in the epidural, subdural, or subarachnoid spaces, or within the cerebral lobes. Pressure on surrounding tissues leads to increased intracranial pressure. If the pressure is unrelieved, neurologic changes occur. Hematomas are classified by their location: epidural, subdural, or intracerebral (Figure 38-2 ■ and Table 38-1).

COMPLICATIONS
Increased Intracranial Pressure
The cranium has three compartments: (1) the brain (80%), (2) blood (10%), and (3) CSF (10%). Intracranial pressure is the pressure exerted within the cranium by these contents.

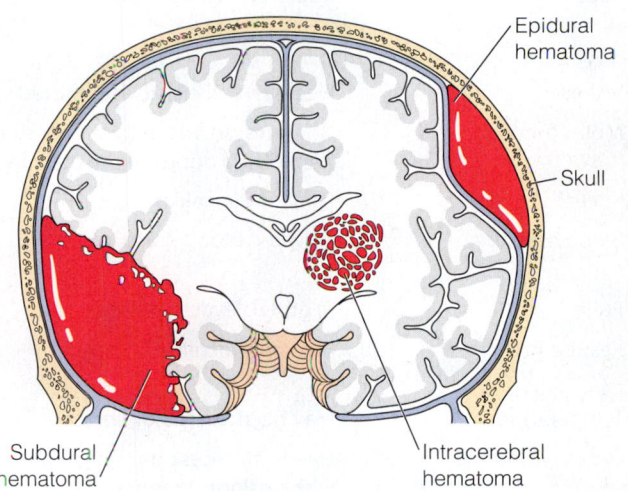

Figure 38-2. ■ Three types of hematomas: epidural, subdural, and intracerebral.

memoryALERT

The skull is a rigid bony structure that restricts the potential area of expansion. Increased pressure within the brain can damage neurons, causing cell death.

This pressure normally ranges from 5 to 15 mm Hg. If the volume of one component increases, the volume of the other components must decrease to keep the pressure within its normal range. This is known as the Monro–Kellie hypothesis. When this does not occur, increased intracranial pressure (IICP) develops. Normal activities such as coughing, sneezing, straining, or bending forward can briefly increase ICP. Brief pressure increases are not harmful; however, prolonged increases can damage delicate brain tissue. IICP can develop with a head injury, brain surgery, or meningitis.

Cerebral blood flow is vital to deliver the required oxygen and glucose. For the brain to function properly, an adequate amount of blood must travel to the brain. When ICP increases, cerebral vasoconstriction occurs, which reduces cerebral blood flow and causes ischemia. If ischemia lasts longer than 5 minutes, the result is irreversible brain damage. Cerebral blood flow is also affected by the amount of carbon dioxide and oxygen in the blood. Increased carbon dioxide levels ($PaCO_2$) and/or decreased oxygen levels (PaO_2) cause vasodilation of the cerebral arteries. Either one of these conditions will increase intracranial pressure.

Any increase in ICP causes changes in the patient's level of consciousness (LOC), pupil response, speech, motor function, and vital signs. The changes become more dramatic as ICP increases. Manifestations may be labeled as early or late (Table 38-2■) and develop slowly or rapidly. Not all manifestations occur in all patients. The location and cause of IICP will determine the symptoms. Because the symptoms may be subtle, the nurse must closely observe the patient for any changes. Two later symptoms, decorticate (flexion) and decerebrate (extension) posturing, indicate IICP in the patient and must be treated immediately. Cushing response occurs late in the development of IICP. This is an ominous sign of impending death.

clinicalALERT

The earliest sign of IICP is a change in the level of consciousness because the neurons of the cerebral cortex are most sensitive to glucose and oxygen deficit.

Cerebral Edema

Cerebral edema, an abnormal accumulation of fluid, increases the amount of extracellular or intracellular brain tissue volume. As the brain swells within the rigid skull, intracranial pressure increases. Brain injury, intracranial surgery, tumors, hemorrhage, and infections can cause cerebral edema. Edema rises to its highest level within 48 to 72 hours after an insult to the brain and then gradually subsides. Without early recognition and treatment, the patient's condition can deteriorate rapidly.

Head injuries severe enough to cause IICP can lead to altered LOC, brain herniation, and brain death. The following information shows how these additional complications affect the patient.

TABLE 38-2	Manifestations of Increased Intracranial Pressure	
MANIFESTATION	**EARLY IICP**	**LATE IICP**
Level of consciousness	Irritability; restlessness; personality changes; short-term memory changes; disorientation to time and then to place and person	Decreasing LOC that progresses to coma and no response to painful stimuli
Pupils	Pupils equal, round, and reactive to light (PERRL)	Sluggish response to light progressing to fixed (no response to light). Pupils may dilate on one side (ipsilateral), progressing to bilateral dilation.
Vision	Decreased visual acuity, blurred vision, diplopia	Cannot assess due to decreasing LOC or coma
Motor function	Weakness in one extremity or side progressing to hemiplegia opposite the brain injury side	Decorticate or decerebrate posturing
Speech	Difficulty speaking	Cannot assess due to decreasing LOC or coma
Blood pressure	Elevated blood pressure	*Cushing response:* increased systolic blood pressure, widening pulse pressure, bradycardia
Pulse	Slightly elevated pulse	
Respiration	Rate may increase	Decreased respiratory rate with altered respiratory patterns (e.g., Cheyne–Stokes)
Temperature	May be increased or decreased	Significantly elevated
Other symptoms	Headache worse on rising in the morning and with position changes	Continual headache Projectile vomiting Loss of pupil, corneal, gag, and swallowing reflexes

ALTERED LEVEL OF CONSCIOUSNESS   *Consciousness* means that the patient is oriented to time, place, and person, and responds appropriately to external stimuli. To maintain normal consciousness, the brain must receive its constant supply of oxygen and glucose. It also requires an intact reticular activating system (RAS), located in the brainstem. The RAS keeps a person alert and responsive to the environment.

Many neurologic conditions can affect the patient's LOC. Usually LOC is altered by IICP and cerebral edema because the increased pressure in the cranium reduces the blood supply to the brain. The following disorders will likely increase ICP and affect the person's ability to remain alert and oriented:

- Head injury
- Hematoma
- Cerebrovascular accident or stroke
- Tumors
- Infections

Any condition that reduces oxygen and glucose levels in the brain may decrease LOC. Patients at an increased risk include those with poorly controlled diabetes and those with long-term cardiac or respiratory disease. Drugs such as alcohol, narcotics, sedatives, and anesthetics depress the CNS, which in turn alters consciousness. Seizures and toxins produced by liver or kidney failure may also alter LOC.

The patient's altered LOC may be described using the terms in Box 38-1■. However, it is best for the nurse to describe the patient's actual behavior and response to stimuli instead of relying on a specific term. Altered LOC and behavior are early changes associated with IICP (see Table 38-2). As brain function deteriorates, more stimuli are needed to elicit a response from the patient. Eventually, no response is obtained.

The Glasgow Coma Scale (Table 38-3■) provides a quick guide for assessing LOC. It measures how well the patient responds with eye opening and verbal and motor responses. The lower the score, the worse the patient's condition. A Glasgow Coma score of 15 means the patient is fully alert,

TABLE 38-3	Glasgow Coma Scale	
BEHAVIOR	**RESPONSE**	**SCORE**
Eye opening response	Spontaneously	4
	To speech	3
	To pain	2
	No response	1
Best verbal response	Oriented to time, place, and person	5
	Confused	4
	Inappropriate words	3
	Incomprehensible sounds	2
	No response	1
Best motor response	Obeys commands	6
	Moves to localized pain	5
	Flexion withdrawal from pain	4
	Abnormal flexion (decorticate)	3
	Abnormal extension (decerebrate)	2
	No response	1
Total score:	*Best response*	15
	Comatose patient	8 or less
	Totally unresponsive	3

whereas a score of eight or less means the patient is in a coma. To prevent permanent brain damage, the nurse must act quickly. The physician must be notified, and measures must be started to lower IICP.

BRAIN HERNIATION   Brain herniation occurs late in the course of IICP. In an attempt to save the brain tissue, the brain shifts from an area of high pressure to low pressure. One common site of herniation is the foramen magnum (the hole at the base of the brain where the spinal cord exits). As pressure rises, the brain is pushed through the foramen magnum. This compresses the brainstem so that vital functions such as respiration cease. Without prompt recognition, the patient eventually dies.

BRAIN DEATH   Brain death occurs when cerebral blood flow stops, resulting in irreversible loss of brain function. (The criteria for determining brain death can be found in Chapter 14, Box 14-10.) If organ donation is planned, the appropriate agencies are contacted.

COLLABORATIVE CARE

It is most important to identify and prevent IICP in any patient with a neurologic problem. Medications are given immediately to lower ICP. Patients with severe brain injuries need their ICP monitored. Uncontrolled intracranial bleeding requires immediate surgery.

Diagnostic Tests

The type and extent of neurologic deficits are often discovered during the history and physical examination. The

BOX 38-1	TERMS FOR LEVELS OF CONSCIOUSNESS

Full Consciousness: alert; oriented to time, place, and person; fully understands written and spoken words

Confusion: unable to think rapidly and clearly; easily bewildered with short attention span and poor memory

Disorientation: disoriented to time, place, or person

Obtundation: appears drowsy and lethargic; responds to verbal and tactile stimuli but quickly drifts back to sleep

Stupor: generally unresponsive; may withdraw purposefully with vigorous or painful stimuli

Coma: unarousable; does not stir or moan in response to stimuli

following laboratory tests are ordered to determine the cause of the patient's altered LOC:

- *Blood glucose* is measured when hypoglycemia is suspected.
- *Arterial blood gases* monitor pH and levels of oxygen and carbon dioxide. They can identify hypoxia and increased carbon dioxide levels. See Chapter 7 for more information about arterial blood gases.
- *Toxicology screening* of blood and urine is done to identify alcohol or drug toxicity.
- *Serum creatinine and BUN* are measured when renal failure is suspected (see Chapter 28 for normal levels).
- *Liver function tests* (alanine transaminase {ALT}, aspartate transaminase {AST}) can evaluate liver function (Chapter 24).
- *Complete blood count with differential* is used to assess for anemia or infectious disease.

The following diagnostic tests are ordered to determine the cause of IICP:

- *Computed tomography (CT) scan* or *magnetic resonance imaging (MRI)* detects hemorrhage, edema, hematoma, or tumor.
- *Cerebral angiography* provides x-ray views of cerebral blood flow and is used when a stroke is suspected.
- *Lumbar puncture* provides a sample of CSF to analyze for possible meningitis. It is performed only when there is danger of IICP. Removal of CSF during IICP greatly increases the risk of brain herniation. Nursing interventions for the patient having a lumbar puncture are described in Box 38-2■.

Medications

Medications play an important role in managing patients with IICP. The most frequently ordered drugs include (1) osmotic diuretics, (2) loop diuretics, (3) anticonvulsants, (4) antipyretics, and (5) histamine antagonists or proton-pump inhibitors.

Intravenous (IV) fluids are used to maintain the patient's fluid and electrolyte balance and to prevent hypotension. Only 0.9% normal saline and lactated Ringer solution are given because they do not cross the blood–brain barrier and increase cerebral edema. They are infused at low rates such as 50 to 75 mL/hr. All IV solutions must be given using an IV pump to prevent volume overload.

Osmotic diuretics (e.g., mannitol {Osmitrol}) draw water out of the edematous brain tissue to be excreted by the kidneys. Large or frequent doses of mannitol cause dehydration and electrolyte losses. Loop diuretics decrease cerebral edema but cause less fluid and electrolyte losses.

clinicalALERT

Closely monitor the patient who is receiving diuretics for dehydration and electrolyte losses, especially sodium and potassium.

BOX 38-2	**NURSING CARE CHECKLIST**

Lumbar Puncture

Before the Procedure

☑ Obtain a signed consent form.

☑ Obtain lumbar puncture tray and additional equipment requested by the physician.

☑ Have the patient empty the bowel and bladder before the procedure begins.

☑ Position the patient in a lateral recumbent position on the side of the bed with the back toward the physician (see figure).

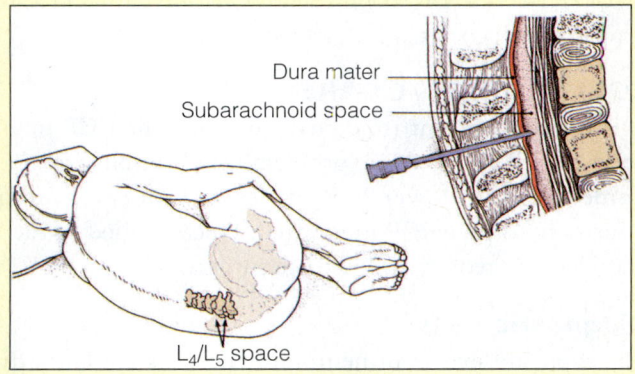

Dura mater
Subarachnoid space
L_4/L_5 space

☑ Assist the patient to take slow, deep breaths and maintain position during the procedure.

After the Procedure

☑ Monitor vital signs and neurologic signs, following facility policy.

☑ Monitor the puncture site for leakage of CSF or hematoma formation.

☑ Encourage fluid intake to replace fluids lost (up to 3,000 mL in 24 hours) if cardiac disease is not present.

☑ Give analgesics as prescribed for pain.

Patient and Family Teaching

☑ Reinforce and clarify information about the procedure.

☑ Explain the importance of not moving during the procedure.

☑ A Band-Aid will cover the place where the needle was inserted.

☑ After the procedure, remain flat in bed for 4 to 8 hours as ordered by the physician.

☑ If you have a headache or backache, take medications for pain.

A histamine H_2-receptor antagonist like ranitidine (Zantac) or a proton-pump inhibitor such as pantoprazole (Protonix) is given to prevent gastric irritation and ulcers. Antiemetics are used to prevent vomiting and the risk for aspiration.

Anticonvulsants are ordered to treat seizure activity associated with a head injury. The most commonly ordered anticonvulsant is phenytoin (Dilantin). Acetaminophen, an antipyretic, is used alone or in combination with a hypothermia blanket to treat hyperthermia. Hyperthermia raises cerebral metabolism and increases ICP.

Patients with severe TBI and continually elevated ICP or uncontrolled seizures may be given high-dose barbiturate therapy. Barbiturate therapy places the patient in a coma, reducing metabolism of the injured brain. Lowering metabolism allows the brain time to heal without permanent damage. During this therapy, the patient is closely monitored in the critical care unit.

ICP Monitoring

An ICP monitoring device is inserted into the skull to assess for IICP. This device is used only for patients in the critical care unit. Intracranial pressures are constantly monitored so that immediate treatment can be started before brain damage occurs. Because bacteria could enter the brain via the monitoring device, the patient is assessed for symptoms of meningitis.

Surgery

Different cranial surgical procedures are done to reduce the patient's ICP. A bone flap may be removed from the skull to allow room for the brain to expand (Figure 38-3 ■).

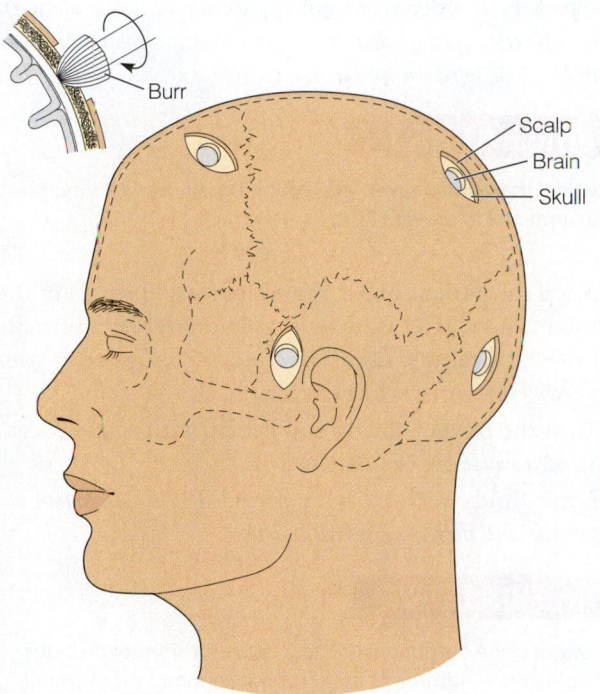

Figure 38-3. ■ Possible locations of burr holes.

Burr holes are holes drilled into the skull to remove a blood clot or evacuate a hematoma. A craniotomy can relieve the pressure of a brain tumor. Care of the patient after a craniotomy is presented under the section on brain tumor.

NURSING CARE

PRIORITIZING NURSING CARE

The patient with a head injury has multiple nursing needs. Besides preventing IICP, it is important to avoid its potential complications. If the patient is unconscious, care is directed at maintaining the airway, nutrition, and skin integrity, as well as preventing problems that can arise due to immobility and the risk of infection. Unconscious patients are usually cared for in the critical care unit. Persons with mild head injuries may be treated in the emergency department and then monitored at home.

HEALTH PROMOTION

Prevention is the key to avoiding head injuries. Public education continues to stress the importance of driving safely, the dangers of driving under the influence of alcohol or drugs, and the reasons for wearing seatbelts and cycle helmets. Most states have passed legislation requiring seat belts, child safety seats, air bags, use of headsets with cell phones, and prohibition of texting while driving. Other recommendations for reducing TBI include following gun safety rules; promoting farm safety; wearing of protective helmets by construction workers, miners, horseback riders, and snowboarders; and teaching older adults about preventing falls in the home.

ASSESSING

Patients with TBI need frequent nursing assessments to prevent IICP. The nurse observes and reports immediately to the physician any sudden change in neurologic function. Subjective and objective findings help to identify the type of nursing interventions the patient will need (Box 38-3 ■).

IDENTIFYING POTENTIAL COMPLICATIONS

The most common complications after a serious TBI include ineffective breathing patterns, cerebral edema, IICP, coma, and brain herniation. Comatose patients have an increased risk for developing seizures, meningitis, and complications of impaired mobility, such as pneumonia, pressure ulcers, DVT, contractures, and malnutrition.

BOX 38-3   **ASSESSMENT**

Patients With Increased Intracranial Pressure

Subjective Data

- When did change in LOC or memory occur first; onset slow or rapid.
- Presence of headache, nausea, or vomiting.
- Visual changes such as double vision or blurring.
- Ringing in the ears; dizziness or feeling faint.
- Any numbness or tingling in extremities.
- History of trauma, infection, cranial surgery, seizures, or loss of consciousness.
- Medication and alcohol use.

Objective Data

- Measure blood pressure, pulse, respirations, and temperature.
- Observe for memory lapses or altered thought processes.
- Assess LOC and orientation to time, place, and person. If the patient is unconscious or condition is unstable, use the Glasgow Coma Scale (see Table 38-3).
- Check pupil's response to light (PERRL).
- Assess strength of hand grip and movement of extremities.
- Note nausea or vomiting.
- Note the color and amount of drainage from ears and nose. Assess for halo sign: Collect fluid on gauze, noting the presence of a yellowish ring, which indicates CSF.
- Note the presence of raccoon eyes or Battle sign.

Additional Data for Unconscious Patients

- Note any change in breathing pattern.

- Assess for the Babinski reflex by stroking the bottom of the foot. An abnormal or positive response in adults is found when the big toe flexes upward and the other toes fan out. This indicates upper motor neuron disease.
- Assess the corneal reflex by touching the corneal surface with a wisp of cotton. Normally, the patient blinks.
- Assess the gag reflex by touching the back of the patient's throat gently with a tongue blade. Normally, the patient will show a gag reflex.
- Assess for abnormal posturing—decorticate (flexion) or decerebrate (extension) posturing; (see figure).
- Monitor and report diagnostic test results beyond expected range.

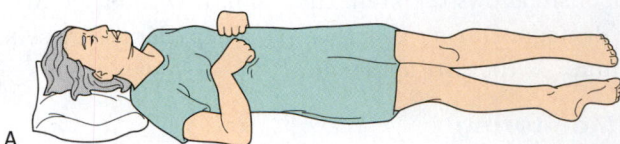

A

Decorticate (flexion) posturing

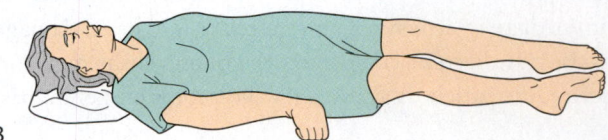

B

Decerebrate (extension) posturing

DIAGNOSING, PLANNING, AND IMPLEMENTING

Risk for Ineffective Tissue Perfusion: Cerebral

Expected outcome: Maintains adequate tissue perfusion.

- Assess for manifestations of IICP, including vital signs every 15 minutes to 1 hour and as necessary. Monitor temperature every 2 hours for hyperthermia. *Sudden changes in neurologic signs often indicate deterioration and the need for immediate treatment. Increased blood pressure and decreased pulse could indicate Cushing response, requiring immediate treatment. Increased temperature increases metabolic rate and further increases intracranial pressure.*
- Elevate the head of the bed 30 degrees and keep the head in a midline position. *These measures promote venous drainage from the head so that pressure does not build up.*
- Give oxygen as ordered. Use pulse oximetry to measure oxygen levels. Keep PaO₂ levels above 94% and PaCO₂ levels between 35 and 45. *The brain needs a constant supply of oxygen to prevent brain damage. Increased carbon dioxide levels can cause cerebral vasodilation, leading to cerebral edema.*

- Avoid hip flexion and abdominal distention. Give stool softeners as ordered. Monitor patency of nasogastric tube. *Hip flexion, gastric distention, and constipation can increase ICP. Stool softeners and a nasogastric tube may prevent IICP.*

clinical**ALERT**

Avoid Valsalva maneuver (e.g., coughing, straining during bowel movements) to prevent IICP.

- Keep the patient quiet, reduce noise and lights in the room, and cluster nursing activities over the shift. Speak softly and calmly. *Loud noises and bright lights plus constant nursing care activities can increase ICP.*
- Turn the patient slowly and gently with a turn sheet. *Sudden movement can increase ICP.*
- Limit fluid over a 24-hour period. *Fluid restrictions may prevent and decrease cerebral edema.*

clinical**ALERT**

Monitor urine output every 1 to 2 hours for signs of diabetes insipidus or syndrome of inappropriate antidiuretic hormone (SIADH).

- If the patient is combative, avoid using restraints. Have nursing staff or family sit quietly with the patient. *Restraining the patient increases ICP. Family may provide a soothing atmosphere.*
- Monitor for seizure activity and maintain seizure precautions:
  - Keep oral airway and suction equipment at bedside.
  - Pad side rails with blankets or seizure pads.
  - Keep the bed in low position with side rails up.

Patients with neurologic injuries are prone to developing seizures and are at risk for injury.

Ineffective Breathing Pattern

Expected outcome: Maintains an effective breathing pattern.

- Monitor respiratory rate, depth, and rhythm for changes. *As ICP increases, the risk of respiratory distress rises. IICP is known to cause respiratory arrest. Unconscious patients may lose their cough reflex. Head injuries will decrease respiratory function.*
- Assess the patient's ability to clear secretions. If the patient is unconscious or has a poor cough, suction the airway for less than 10 seconds with a physician order only. *Suctioning longer reduces oxygen levels and increases carbon dioxide levels, which can increase ICP.*

clinicalALERT

Never suction nasally the patient with a basilar skull fracture who is draining CSF from the nose or ears.

- Insert an oral airway as needed. *This prevents the tongue from obstructing the airway.*
- Turn the patient from side to side every 2 hours; keep in a side-lying position with the head of the bed elevated. *Turning prevents pooling of secretions in one area of the lungs. Side positioning prevents the tongue from obstructing the airway.*
- If the patient is unconscious, keep NPO and provide oral hygiene. *Oral hygiene removes secretions that could dry and be aspirated.*

clinicalALERT

To prevent aspiration, never give oral food or fluids to the unconscious patient.

Risk for Imbalanced Nutrition: Less Than Body Requirements

Expected outcome: Maintains weight within range for height and age.

- Give tube feeding through a nasogastric or gastrostomy tube or administer total parenteral nutrition (TPN) as ordered. *Head injuries increase the patient's metabolic rate and risk for malnutrition. Tube feedings or TPN are ordered to prevent malnutrition.*

- Before each tube feeding, check gastric residual. *Excess gastric residual means that the tube feeding is not being absorbed. This places the patient at risk for malnutrition and aspiration.*
- Monitor daily weights and serum albumin. *Daily weights help determine the patient's nutritional and fluid status. A decrease in serum albumin often indicates nutritional deficits.*

Risk for Impaired Skin Integrity

Expected outcome: Maintains intact skin integrity.

- Turn the patient every 2 hours. Use a special mattress or bed as available. Lift rather than drag the patient across the sheet. *Turning relieves pressure over bony prominences. Special mattresses (e.g., egg crate cushion or beds) distribute the patient's weight more evenly. Dragging can cause skin tears.*
- Prevent skin breakdown by:
  - Keeping bed linens clean, dry, and wrinkle free.
  - Bathing the patient daily with mild soap.
  - Cleansing the skin after urine and fecal soiling with a mild cleansing agent.
  - Providing adequate hydration.

Keeping linens clean, dry, and wrinkle free decreases the risk of skin injuries. Daily hygiene keeps the skin soft and supple. Adequate hydration prevents the skin from drying out and cracking.

- Provide oral care and lubricate the lips every 2 to 4 hours. *This removes dried crusts and prevents drying and cracking of oral mucous membranes.*
- Keep the cornea moist by instilling methyl cellulose solution (0.5% to 1%). Apply protective eye shields if the corneal reflex is absent. *Proper eye care prevents corneal abrasion and irritation.*

Impaired Physical Mobility

Expected outcome: Remains free of immobility complications.

- Maintain extremities in position of function with support devices. Remove support devices every 4 hours for skin care. Place a pillow in the axilla area; use hand splints; use foam boots on the feet. *Pillows in the axilla area prevent abduction of the shoulder. Hand splints may prevent flexion contractures of the hands. Foam boots are used to prevent footdrop.*
- Perform passive range-of-motion (ROM) exercises at least four times per day. *Passive ROM exercises done routinely maintain muscle tone and function, prevent contractures, and restore impaired motor function in unconscious patients.*
- Consult with physical therapy as ordered. *Physical therapists can provide expertise to prevent immobility complications and promote patient mobility as much as possible.*

clinicalALERT

Do not perform passive ROM on the patient with IICP.

Risk for Infection

Expected outcome: Remains free of signs of infection.

- Assess for a CSF leak and monitor for signs of infection. *Open head wounds such as a depressed skull fracture increase the risk for infection. They can be contaminated with dirt, hair, or other debris.*
- Test clear drainage from the ear and nose for glucose by using a glucose reagent strip. *Clear drainage that tests positive for glucose indicates the presence of CSF.*
- Keep the nasopharynx and external ear clean. Place a sterile piece of cotton in the ear and loosely tape a 4 × 4 gauze under the nose to collect any drainage. Change the dressings when they become wet. *Bacteria can enter through these openings when wet dressings are present.*
- Remind the patient not to blow the nose, cough, or stop a sneeze. *Blowing the nose or coughing increases ICP. Stopping a sneeze can force bacteria up into the brain.*
- Use strict aseptic technique when changing head dressings or handling the ICP monitoring device. *Aseptic technique decreases the risk of introducing bacteria.*

MANAGING NURSING CARE

As appropriate and allowed by the designated duties and responsibilities of assistive personnel, the nurse may delegate nursing care activities such as providing oral and skin care and assisting with activities of daily living (ADLs) for the patient with TBI. Before assigning tasks such as obtaining vital signs, daily weights and pulse oximetry readings, assisting with meals and fluid intake, and measuring intake and output, ensure assistive personnel have a clear understanding of the importance of accuracy in measurement.

EVALUATING

To evaluate the effectiveness of nursing care for a patient with IICP, monitor vital signs and assess the level of alertness and orientation; strong hand grip, extremity movement, and steady gait; and absence of diplopia, tinnitus, dizziness, nausea, vomiting, or abnormal pupil response. In the unconscious patient, collect data about breathing pattern, reflex response, posturing, and skin integrity.

DOCUMENTING

Documentation includes the results of a neurologic examination, including specific assessments for IICP and Glasgow Coma Scale rating. Document all teaching provided and the patient's and family's understanding for home care. Note specific instructions about skin care, ROM exercises, medication administration and side effects, and symptoms to report.

CONTINUITY OF CARE

The nurse assesses patients to determine whether they can manage their care at home or if they need to be transferred to a long-term care facility. Patients with a mild head injury should be observed for at least 24 hours. If they are not hospitalized, they must be closely monitored at home. For example, with a linear skull fracture, the family is taught to wake and observe the patient every 2 hours during the first 8 hours after the accident. The patient and family should return to the emergency department if the patient develops any of the following manifestations:

- Increasing drowsiness, confusion, or slurred speech
- Difficulty waking the patient
- Vomiting
- Blurred vision; one or both pupils dilated
- Prolonged headache
- Blood or clear fluid leaking from the nose or ears
- Weakness in the arm or leg
- Seizures

Patients and their families should receive a copy of the home care instructions that were reviewed in the emergency department. The nurse must document all teaching done for observation after a head injury.

Patients with a concussion may develop postconcussion syndrome. They may experience headache, poor concentration, dizziness, personality changes, and fatigue for weeks to months. Family support is important during this phase of recovery.

Patients with severe head injuries usually require extensive rehabilitation either as inpatients or outpatients. Rehabilitation may include physical, speech, and occupational therapy. The patient and family need teaching about medications, exercises and positioning, skin care, diet, use of assistive devices, and potential complications. Families providing long-term home care may need respite care and referrals to community resources and support groups. Helpful resources include National Head Injury Foundation and the Brain Injury Association of America.

Unconscious patients need placement in a long-term care facility. A social services department can help the family find a suitable facility and also assist with financial concerns. Because the prognosis of the patient is uncertain, the family may need support services from counselors and the clergy.

NURSING CARE PLAN
Patient With Increased Intracranial Pressure and Altered Level of Consciousness

---

Martin Straton, 52 years old, fell during his daily run in the park. He hit his head on the right side and was knocked unconscious. A bystander called an ambulance, which arrived in 10 minutes to transport Straton to the local hospital.

Assessment

BP 150/90, P 60, R 14. He responds to verbal and tactile stimuli but quickly falls back asleep. His right pupil is dilated and does not react to light. He is unable to move his extremities on the left side. Oxygen is given by a face mask. CT scan shows an epidural hematoma on the right side with edema. The neurologist discusses the need for immediate surgery with Mr. Straton's wife. He was taken to surgery in the evening for burr holes to evacuate the hematoma. His surgery is successful, and he is transferred to the critical care unit.

Nursing Diagnosis

After surgery, the following priority nursing diagnoses are established for this patient:

- *Risk for Ineffective Tissue Perfusion: Cerebral* related to increased intracranial pressure and edema
- *Risk for Aspiration* related to altered LOC
- *Risk for Impaired Skin Integrity* related to immobility
- *Risk for Imbalanced Nutrition: Less Than Body Requirements* related to inability to eat

Expected Outcomes

The expected outcomes for the plan of care are that Mr. Straton will:

- Maintain adequate cerebral tissue perfusion as evidenced by stable vital signs and neurologic status and no decrease in LOC.
- Have no aspiration as evidenced by clear lung sounds.
- Maintain intact skin.
- Maintain normal body weight.

Planning and Implementation

The following interventions are planned and implemented for Mr. Straton:

- Perform neurologic and respiratory assessment with vital signs every 2 hours or as needed. Monitor pulse oximetry.
- Use measures to reduce cerebral edema such as:
  - Elevate the head of the bed 30 degrees; keep the head in neutral alignment; avoid flexion of the head and hips.
  - Provide calm environment and allow for rest periods.
- Assess the ability to clear secretions; check the gag reflex every shift; and suction posterior pharynx as needed.
- Turn side to side every 2 hours, and maintain side-lying position. Turn slowly with a turn sheet.
- Maintain NPO status and provide frequent oral hygiene.
- Assess the skin over bony prominences every shift.
- Assess fluid status and document intake and output.

Evaluation

Twenty-four hours after surgery, Mr. Straton slowly starts to regain consciousness. His right pupil slowly reacts to light, and he moves his left extremities slightly. Mr. Straton continues to improve and is discharged to his home a week later.

Critical Thinking in the Nursing Process

1. Mr. Straton was found unconscious. What assessments would you make, and how could you maintain an open airway at the scene?
2. During the immediate postoperative period, Mr. Straton becomes confused and tries to pull out his ICP monitoring device. You know you cannot restrain him. What evidence-based practice interventions could you try?
3. Describe skin care measures for patients who are unconscious.

Note: Discussion of Critical Thinking questions appears on the companion website.

Brain Tumor

Brain tumors are abnormal growths within the cranium. Their cause is unknown, but prolonged exposure to certain chemicals and radiation increases the incidence. Brain tumors can occur at any age; the highest incidence is in adult men between the ages of 45 and 75.

Intracranial tumors are classified as either benign or malignant, based on tissue type and cell characteristics. The term *benign* can be misleading, because the tumor may be inaccessible by surgery, and as it grows, it presses on vital centers. If the compression increases, it leads to disability and death. Malignant tumors invade other areas of the brain and eventually cause death unless effectively treated.

Brain tumors are also categorized as primary or secondary. Primary tumors develop from cells and structures within the brain. Secondary brain tumors develop in areas outside of the brain and metastasize to the brain. The most common brain tumors are listed in Table 38-4■.

PATHOPHYSIOLOGY AND MANIFESTATIONS

Brain tumors invade, displace, and destroy brain tissue. As the tumor grows, it disrupts the normal balance of brain tissue, blood, and CSF within the skull. When the brain fails to compensate for the increase in volume, IICP develops. This will lead to the typical manifestations of IICP discussed earlier in the chapter. If untreated, the final result is brain herniation and death.

Manifestations are either local or generalized. Local manifestations relate to the location and function of that specific site, for example, frontal lobe or temporal lobe (Box 38-4■). Knowing the tumor site helps the nurse plan

TABLE 38-4	Classification of Brain Tumors
TUMOR	**CHARACTERISTICS**
Glioma	
■ Astrocytoma	Most common glioma
	Graded I to IV according to the degree of cell differentiation
■ Glioblastoma multiforme	Highly malignant
	Fast growing and highly invasive of other tissues
Meningioma	Slow-growing tumor developing in the meninges
Acoustic neuroma	Benign, slow-growing tumor of the acoustic nerve
Metastatic brain tumor	Slow growing and malignant
	Spreads from primary tumor sites in the lung and breast

BOX 38-4	MANIFESTATIONS OF BRAIN TUMORS

Frontal Lobe Tumors
- Personality changes, inappropriate behavior, impaired judgment, inability to concentrate, recent memory loss
- Headache
- Motor deficits
- Expressive aphasia

Parietal Lobe Tumors
- Sensory–perceptual deficits
- Visual field deficits

Temporal Lobe Tumors
- Psychomotor seizures

Occipital Lobe Tumors
- Visual field deficits

the patient's care. Tumors can press on cerebral blood vessels, decreasing their blood supply and causing dizziness. The more common generalized manifestations include headache; seizures; vomiting; and changes in memory, communication, and concentration. Headache, a prominent early symptom, is usually intermittent, worse in the morning, and associated with nausea and vomiting. Other manifestations may be seen, such as motor weakness, visual–spatial disorders, and sensory deficits.

COLLABORATIVE CARE

A brain tumor is treated with chemotherapy, radiation therapy, surgery, or any combination of these. The choice of treatment is based on the size and location of the tumor, the type of tumor, and the patient's overall health. The following tests aid in diagnosing a brain tumor:

- A *CT scan* or *MRI* is ordered to locate and define the size of the tumor for examination and grading.
- An *electroencephalogram* (*EEG*) is ordered if seizures are present.
- A *cerebral angiogram* is used to measure blood flow through the cerebral blood vessels.
- A *stereotactic needle biopsy* may be performed for some tumors.

Medications

A limited number of chemotherapy drugs are available to treat a brain tumor because the drugs cannot cross the blood–brain barrier. Mannitol, an osmotic diuretic, is used to open the blood–brain barrier, enabling chemotherapy to reach the tumor. Tumors in the meninges may be treated with chemotherapy through an Ommaya reservoir. This device is surgically implanted into the lateral ventricle of the brain (Figure 38-4 ■). It allows the chemotherapy to be absorbed along with CSF. Timed-release, biodegradable chemotherapy wafers can be placed directly into the tumor cavity after the tumor is removed by surgery. Patients with gliomas may receive the new oral chemotherapy drug temozolomide (Temodar).

Intracranial Surgery

Surgery can remove a tumor, reduce its size (also known as **debulking**), or relieve symptoms. Some of the common intracranial surgeries are the following:

- *Burr hole:* A hole is drilled into the skull to remove a clot or to relieve pressure.

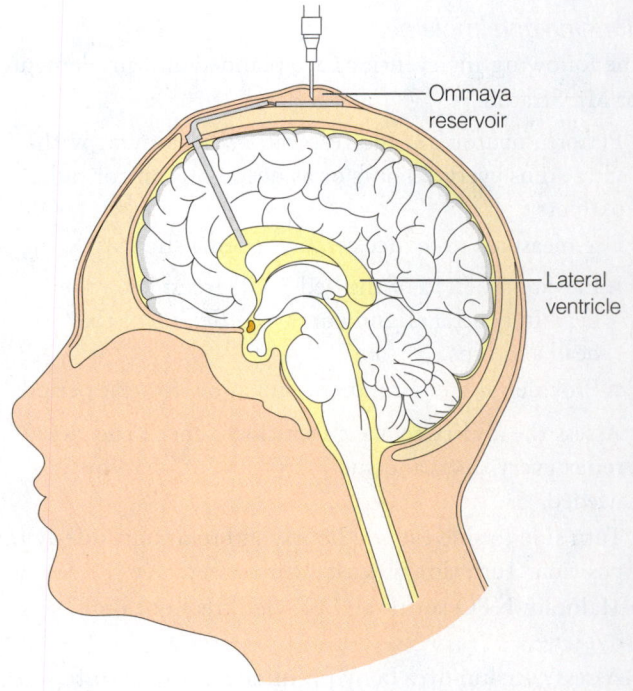

Figure 38-4. ■ Ommaya reservoir for medication administration.

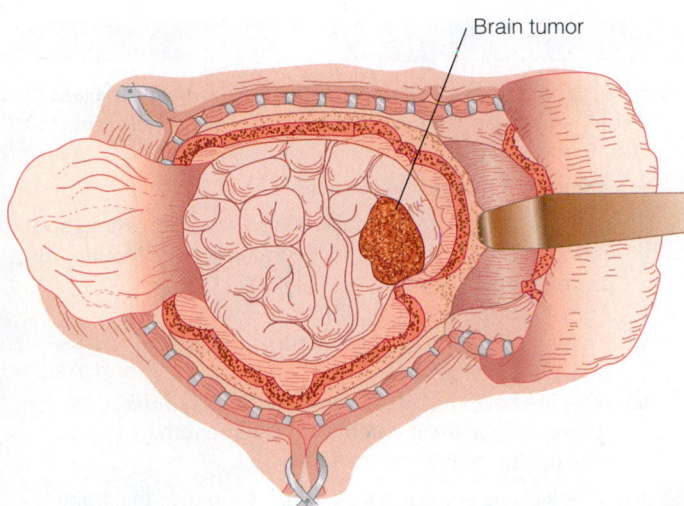

Figure 38-5. ■ In a craniotomy, a portion of the skull is opened surgically to allow access to the brain in order to remove the brain tumor shown in this diagram.

- *Craniotomy:* A surgical opening is made into the cranial cavity (Figure 38-5■). A craniotomy is done by making a series of burr holes. The bone between the holes (bone flap) is cut with a saw and then turned down. After the tumor is removed, the bone flap is sutured in place. A craniotomy is also used to repair defects after a TBI.
- *Craniectomy:* Complete removal of a bone flap decreases cerebral edema.
- *Cranioplasty:* Synthetic material, a metal plate, or wire mesh is inserted where the skull was removed.

Radiation Therapy

Radiation therapy may be given to slow tumor growth or after surgery. The purpose is to destroy abnormal tumor cells that are sensitive to radiation. Conventional external radiation may be given daily, five times per week for 6 weeks. A procedure called *stereotaxic radiation* or "gamma knife" is used for deep tumors. A stereotaxic frame is attached to the patient's head, allowing a large, single dose of radiation to be directed at a small specific site so that normal cells are not harmed.

NURSING CARE

The nursing care of a patient with a brain tumor requires support during diagnosis and specific interventions as determined by the treatment used. The diagnosis of a brain tumor is frightening. Both the patient and family need ongoing emotional support throughout all phases of care.

PRIORITIZING NURSING CARE

The patient with a brain tumor has many nursing care needs. Both patients and their families face an uncertain future. The patient may experience side effects from chemotherapy,

radiation, or surgery. After surgery, the patient may develop altered LOC, IICP, and seizures. The patient will require intensive care in the immediate postoperative period. Nursing care after a craniotomy is found in Box 38-5■. The patient may also experience anxiety and an altered body image.

HEALTH PROMOTION

Health promotion is limited to early recognition and the reporting of clinical manifestations that could indicate the presence of a brain tumor to a health care provider.

ASSESSING

Before delivering care, the nurse gathers information about the patient's history and performs a basic neurologic examination. If the patient is confused or has difficulty answering questions, the family should be included in the interview. Assessment data can identify how the brain tumor is interfering with the patient's life (Box 38-6■).

IDENTIFYING POTENTIAL COMPLICATIONS

The most common complications of a brain tumor include cerebral edema and IICP. Tumors located in the temporal and occipital lobes have a higher risk of causing seizures. After a craniotomy, there is a potential for airway obstruction.

DIAGNOSING, PLANNING, AND IMPLEMENTING
Anxiety

Expected outcome: Verbalizes that anxiety has decreased.

- Explain diagnostic procedures and treatment methods to the patient and family. Repeat information as needed. *The patient and family need time to adjust to the diagnosis and its implications. If urgent treatment is necessary, they will not have time to adjust. Explaining the procedures and treatments may decrease anxiety.*
- Encourage the patient and family to express their feelings. *Talking about their feelings and fears can reduce anxiety.*
- Provide emotional support by listening and staying with the patient. If the patient prefers, arrange for a member of the clergy to visit. *Provide a calm environment. Listening and the nurse's physical presence may make the patient feel calmer.*

Disturbed Body Image

Expected outcome: Verbalizes positive and negative feelings.

- Assess for signs and symptoms of a negative body image (e.g., refusal to look in the mirror, denial, and withdrawal from family and friends). *Physical changes; dependence on others for basic needs; and long-term speech, vision, and motor deficits can cause low self-esteem.*

BOX 38-5   NURSING CARE CHECKLIST

Patients Having a Craniotomy

Before Surgery

☑ Provide routine preoperative care (see Chapter 10).

☑ Assess understanding and the level of anxiety of the planned surgery.

☑ Prepare the family for how the patient will appear after surgery: a large dressing covering the head; possible swollen, bruised eyelids; and an endotracheal tube.

After Surgery

☑ Provide routine postoperative care (see Chapter 10).

☑ Review nursing care intervention for IICP.

☑ Monitor respiratory status every 1 to 2 hours and assess airway patency.

☑ Monitor oxygen saturation levels as needed.

☑ Position on the nonoperative side if a bone flap or large mass was removed to decrease venous collection and pressure on the surgical incision.

☑ Apply cool cloth over the patient's eyes. Reduce noise and bright lights in the room.

☑ For pain, use acetaminophen with codeine cautiously. Opioids such as codeine increase the risk for constipation and straining, which increase ICP.

☑ Assess and report CSF leak from ears, nose, or wound; a leak might indicate an opening in the dura that could allow bacteria into the brain.

☑ Provide interventions to prevent infection:

  ☑ Use strict aseptic technique when changing dressings and caring for wound drains and ICP monitor lines. Monitor for any purulent drainage.

  ☑ Administer prescribed antibiotics.

  ☑ Assess for manifestations of meningitis (see later discussion in this chapter).

  ☑ After the head dressing is removed (usually 3 days post surgery), clean the incision with half-strength hydrogen peroxide to remove dried blood.

☑ If CSF leak is present, place a sterile dressing over the drainage area and change when damp.

  ☑ If CSF leaks from the nose, elevate the head of the bed 20 degrees unless contraindicated. Do not suction nasally; do not clean the nose; tell the patient not to put fingers in the nose.

  ☑ If CSF leaks from the ear, position the patient on the side of leakage unless contraindicated. Do not clean the ear; tell the patient not to put fingers in the ear.

☑ Monitor for seizures and maintain seizure precautions.

■ Provide or arrange for a patient to have surgical cap, scarf, or turban. Assist the patient to obtain a wig or hairpiece. Reinforce the fact that the hair will grow back. *These interventions can decrease the patient's embarrassment about hair loss.*

BOX 38-6   ASSESSMENT

Patients With Brain Tumors

Subjective Data

■ Change in memory, ability to concentrate, personality, or behavior

■ Frequency and location of headache

■ Difficulty speaking; double or blurred vision; ringing in the ears

■ Dizziness or changes in coordination or balance

■ Any numbness, tingling, or weakness in extremities

■ History of seizures or brain tumors

Objective Data

■ Measure blood pressure, pulse, respirations, and temperature.

■ Observe for orientation to time, place, and person, and memory lapses.

■ Assess strength of hand grip and movement of extremities.

■ Assess gait by asking the patient to walk normally and then in a heel-to-toe fashion.

■ Assess coordination.

MANAGING NURSING CARE

As appropriate and allowed by the designated duties and responsibilities of assistive personnel, the nurse may delegate nursing care activities such as providing oral and skin care and assisting with ADLs for the patient with a brain tumor. Before assigning tasks such as obtaining vital signs and measuring intake and output, ensure assistive personnel have a clear understanding of the importance of accuracy in measurement.

EVALUATING

The nurse collects the following data to evaluate the effectiveness of nursing interventions for the patient after a craniotomy: absence of neurologic deficits, IICP, bleeding, signs of infection, level of anxiety, pain, and knowledge of follow-up care at home. Evaluate the patient's ability to accept the long-term consequences of a brain tumor and side effects of the treatments.

DOCUMENTING

Documentation includes neurologic assessment findings and any signs of infection, anxiety, or altered body image. Document the patient and family teaching about wound care, medications, symptoms of complications, and safety precautions.

CONTINUITY OF CARE

Patients diagnosed with a brain tumor have short- and long-term needs. They may require chemotherapy or radiation treatments. If surgery is planned, the patient and family need to discuss their fears about the potential side effects. Assess the patient's and family's capabilities and resources to provide care after discharge. Helpful resources are the American Cancer Society, American Brain Tumor Association, and Brain Tumor Society.

If chemotherapy or radiation therapy is ordered, the following information should be given to the patient and family:

■ Importance of keeping appointments for chemotherapy or radiation therapy
■ Adverse effects of chemotherapy or radiation
■ Skin care with radiation therapy
■ How to manage nausea or vomiting; nutritional support

After a craniotomy, the patient and family require emotional support. The recovery process is lengthy. It involves adapting to body image changes and managing motor and sensory deficits. Encourage the family to be involved in the patient's care. For example, they can assist the patient with personal hygiene and meals. As patients are able, they should be encouraged to take an active role in their own care.

The patient and family may need information about support groups and community resources. Patients with neurologic deficits are referred for physical, occupational, and speech therapy, and those with inoperable brain tumors are referred to hospice. Before the patient is discharged home, the nurse should provide verbal and written information on the following topics:

■ The use and side effects of anticonvulsant and anti-inflammatory medications
■ Wound care:
  ■ Do not shampoo hair until the incision is healed and then pat the incision dry after shampooing. Avoid a curling iron or hair dryer on hot setting until the hair has grown back.
  ■ When outside, wear a hat to prevent sunburn.
  ■ Protect the head until the wound is healed.
■ Signs and symptoms to report:
  ■ Swelling at the incision site; bloody, yellow, or clear drainage from ears, nose, or incision site
  ■ Increased drowsiness
  ■ Changes in behavior
  ■ Stiff neck, severe headache, and elevated temperature
  ■ New sensory or motor deficits, vision changes, or seizures
■ Safety precautions for motor deficits, sensory deficits, lack of coordination, seizures, and cognitive deficits
■ Importance of follow-up appointments

Cerebrovascular Accident (Stroke)

> **Key Concept**   An ischemic stroke results from a sudden decrease in blood flow to the brain, causing brain cell death. Early assessment and rapid medical intervention can save brain tissue and reduce the risk of permanent brain damage or death.

Cerebrovascular accident (CVA), also called **stroke** or *brain attack*, is an emergency condition that causes neurologic deficits from a decreased blood supply to a local area of the brain. Approximately 795,000 people suffer a CVA each year in the United States. CVAs are the fourth leading cause of death in the United States and frequently leave patients with some type of physical disability, such as hemiparesis, dysphagia, and aphasia. Strokes can occur at any age; the highest incidence is in people over 65 years of age. Males have an increased incidence, as do those with a family history of CVA. However, as women age, the risk for and death from CVA increases. African Americans have twice the risk of Caucasians. Hispanics have a higher rate of strokes at a younger age, often due to the presence of diabetes, hypertension, and obesity.

Other risk factors include hypertension, diabetes mellitus, obesity, atrial fibrillation, sleep apnea, physical inactivity, and atherosclerosis. Lifestyle habits such as smoking, high cholesterol diet, excessive use of alcohol, and cocaine and heroin use increase the risk. Newer oral contraceptives have lower risks for stroke, except in those who smoke or have hypertension. People living in the southeastern United States have the highest stroke mortality rate.

PATHOPHYSIOLOGY AND MANIFESTATIONS

A **transient ischemic attack (TIA)**, a brief episode of reversible neurologic deficits, lasts from a few minutes to less than 24 hours. It results from a temporary reduction of blood flow to a specific area of the brain. Usually TIA is caused by atherosclerosis or a small embolus, which obstructs a small cerebral blood vessel. TIA is often a warning signal of a future CVA. The patient may experience several TIAs before a CVA. The time between the TIA and a CVA ranges from hours to months. Manifestations include dizziness; visual loss in one eye; contralateral numbness or weakness of the fingers, arms, or legs; or **aphasia** (inability to express or receive and understand speech, as a result of brain damage).

A CVA is the sudden loss of neurologic function. CVAs are classified under two broad categories: ischemic and hemorrhagic. Ischemic CVAs may occur from a thrombus or an embolus. There are two types of hemorrhagic CVAs: intracerebral hemorrhage and subarachnoid hemorrhage (Table 38-5 ■). CVAs caused by thrombus occur most often in older adults who are resting or sleeping. Any one of

Table 38-5	Comparison of the Types of CVA (Stroke)		
TYPE	**CAUSE**	**ONSET**	**PATHOPHYSIOLOGY**
Ischemic stroke			
Thrombotic CVA	Atherosclerosis of large cerebral arteries	During or after sleep	Atherosclerosis causes plaque to build up in cerebral arteries. If plaque is not removed or treated, a thrombus or clot develops. This leads to ischemia in the brain tissue supplied by the vessel.
Embolic CVA	Atrial fibrillation, congestive heart failure (CHF), rheumatic heart disease Mitral valve disease Endocarditis	Sudden onset with immediate deficits	Embolus travels to a cerebral artery from a distant site, especially the heart. It usually lodges in a narrow portion of the cerebral artery, causing necrosis.
Hemorrhagic stroke			
Intracerebral hemorrhage	Hypertension	Occurs suddenly, often during some activity	Hypertension weakens a cerebral blood vessel, causing it to rupture. This leads to bleeding into the brain tissue or subarachnoid space.

these causes can partially or completely reduce blood flow to cerebral tissues. This decreases oxygen to the area of the brain supplied by the involved blood vessels. Initially, the brain cells are ischemic but quickly die, resulting in a cerebral infarction. If the brain experiences *anoxia* (lack of oxygen to the brain) for more than 10 minutes, irreversible brain damage occurs. Surrounding the damaged brain tissue, there is an area of minimally perfused cells called the *penumbra*. Maintaining survival of these cells depends on a timely return of adequate circulation. Thrombolytic agents are used early in the treatment of ischemic stroke to preserve the penumbra. Adequate collateral blood supply can decrease the amount of damage. Collateral circulation occurs when areas of the brain have decreased blood flow over a long period of time. Smaller blood vessels develop to supply blood to areas with reduced blood flow. Large areas of infarction usually result in severe disability or death.

When cerebral blood supply is altered, there is temporary or permanent loss of neurologic function. The signs and symptoms of a CVA vary, depending on the area of the brain involved, the size of the area, and collateral blood flow. Typical manifestations alter movement, sensation, thought, memory, behavior, or speech (Table 38-6■). However, the effects of a CVA are not limited to the nervous system. Complications of a CVA can affect respiration, elimination, and muscle function.

Right- and Left-Hemisphere Problems

Strokes usually occur in one hemisphere. Recent studies have shown that people who are left-hemisphere dominant (right-handed) show certain symptoms. A comparison of right- and left-hemisphere strokes is given in Box 38-7■.

Table 38-6	Manifestations and Complications of CVA (Stroke)
MANIFESTATIONS	**POTENTIAL COMPLICATIONS**
Motor deficits ■ Hemiplegia ■ Hemiparesis ■ Facial droop	*Respiratory problems* ■ Decreased ability to cough ■ Airway obstruction ■ Pneumonia
Speech deficits ■ Expressive aphasia, receptive aphasia, global aphasia ■ Dysarthria	*Gastrointestinal problems* ■ Dysphagia ■ Constipation
Visual deficits ■ Diplopia ■ Homonymous hemianopia	*Genitourinary problems* ■ Incontinence ■ Frequency ■ Urinary retention
Sensory–perceptual deficits ■ Agnosia ■ Apraxia ■ Neglect syndrome	*Musculoskeletal problems* ■ Contractures ■ Muscle atrophy ■ Footdrop ■ Shoulder adduction
Cognitive and behavior changes ■ Memory loss ■ Short attention span ■ Poor judgment ■ Poor problem-solving ability ■ Emotional lability ■ Depression	*Integumentary problems* ■ Decubitus ulcers

BOX 38-7	RIGHT-HEMISPHERE VERSUS LEFT-HEMISPHERE CEREBROVASCULAR ACCIDENT (STROKE)

Right-Hemisphere CVA	Left-Hemisphere CVA
Left hemiplegia	Right hemiplegia
Left visual field deficits	Right visual field deficits
Spatial–perceptual deficits	Aphasia
Denies or unaware of deficits	Aware of deficits
Easily distracted	Impaired intellectual ability
Poor judgment	Slow, cautious behavior
Impulsive	High level of frustration over losses

Motor Deficits

Motor deficits commonly follow a CVA. Depending on the area of the brain involved, CVAs may cause weakness, paralysis, or spasticity. Because the sensory and motor nerves cross at the neck, sensory and motor deficits develop on the opposite side of the damage. For example, a CVA in the right hemisphere causes deficits in the left side of the body and vice versa. This is known as *contralateral* (opposite side) deficit. The deficits include:

- *Hemiparesis:* weakness of the left or right half of the body.
- **Hemiplegia**: paralysis of the left or right half of the body (Figure 38-6■). Initially, the affected arm and leg are flaccid; they become spastic within 6 to 8 weeks. Spasticity can lead to adduction of the shoulder; flexion of the fingers, wrist, elbow, and knee; and external rotation of the hip. These problems limit the patient's mobility and increase risk for immobility complications, including thrombophlebitis, orthostatic hypotension, aspiration and pneumonia, contractures, and decubitus ulcers.

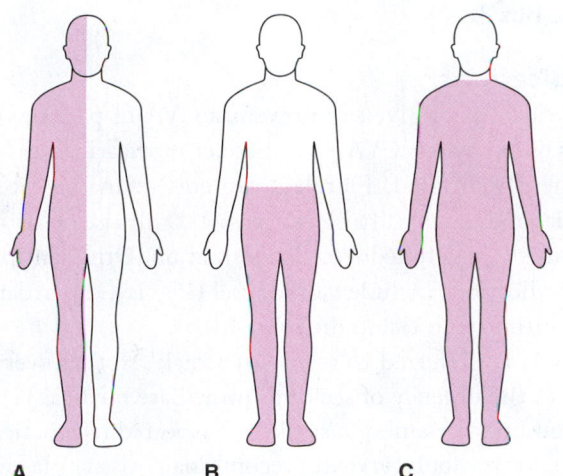

Figure 38-6. ■ Types of paralysis. (**A**) Hemiplegia is paralysis of one-half of the body. (**B**) Paraplegia is paralysis of the lower part of the body. (**C**) Tetraplegia is paralysis affecting all four limbs.

Speech Deficits

Speech deficits usually result from a CVA affecting the dominant hemisphere. The left hemisphere is dominant in all right-handed people and most left-handed people. Strokes cause many speech and language problems. Among these problems are:

- *Expressive aphasia:* an inability to speak or write due to damage of Broca area. The patient usually can understand what is being said.
- *Receptive aphasia:* an inability to understand the spoken word due to damage of Wernicke area. The patient can speak, but the words do not make sense.
- *Global aphasia:* a combination of expressive and receptive aphasia.
- *Dysarthria:* difficulty in speech caused by paralysis of the muscles that control speech.

Visual Deficits

When a CVA damages the parietal and temporal lobes, vision is impaired. The patient may experience diplopia or **homonymous hemianopia** (the loss of vision in half of the eye). The visual loss is opposite to the side affected by the stroke. The patient sees only one-half of the normal vision and must turn the head to see the environment (Figure 38-7■).

Sensory–Perceptual Deficits

A CVA may alter sensation and perception of temperature, vibration, pain, pressure, and *proprioception* (awareness of the body's position). The loss of these sensory abilities increases the patient's potential for injury. Common sensory–perceptual deficits include the following:

- *Agnosia:* the inability to recognize a familiar object such as a toothbrush.
- *Apraxia:* the inability to carry out a familiar routine (e.g., brushing teeth or combing hair), even when paralysis is not present.
- *Neglect syndrome* (or unilateral neglect): The patient ignores the affected side of the body; tends to bump into walls, walk to one side, or fail to dress the affected side.

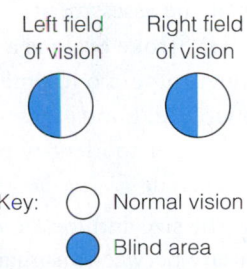

Figure 38-7. ■ Homonymous hemianopia. Loss of vision in the nasal field of the right eye and temporal field of the left eye.

Cognitive and Behavioral Changes

Patients who have had a CVA may have cognitive changes. For example, damage to the right-hemisphere frontal lobe can cause memory loss, decreased attention span, poor judgment, and an inability to solve problems. Behavioral changes include *emotional lability* (extreme emotion and mood swings, from crying to laughing) or loss of self-control, such as swearing or refusing to wear clothes. Depression is common, especially when there are functional and speech losses. Stress is poorly tolerated and is seen as uncontrolled anger.

Urinary and Gastrointestinal Problems

When the stroke damages only one hemisphere, bladder and bowel problems are usually short term. Initially, the patient may experience urinary frequency, urgency, or incontinence. These problems last longer when there are cognitive deficits. Constipation develops as a complication of immobility. A stroke can impair the ability to swallow. Factors such as attention deficits and weakness or lack of coordination of the tongue often contribute to this problem. *Dysphagia* may result in choking, drooling, aspiration, or regurgitation. Nursing care focuses on preventing aspiration and promoting adequate nutrition.

COLLABORATIVE CARE

The patient with a TIA receives medications or has surgery to prevent a stroke. Once a CVA has occurred, immediate medical attention is needed. At first, the medical team concentrates on diagnosing the type of CVA and preserving life. Drugs are ordered to reduce IICP and prevent neurologic deficits. After the acute phase, care focuses on the patient's rehabilitation.

memory**ALERT**

Patients with suspected stroke must receive immediate treatment (within 3 hours) to preserve as much brain function as possible.

Diagnostic Tests

Diagnosis begins with a complete history and physical examination. The time of the onset of stroke manifestations is an essential part of the assessment. The National Institutes of Health (NIH) Stroke Scale is a clinical evaluation tool used to assess neurologic outcome and the degree of recovery. The following diagnostic tests are used to detect the potential for a stroke or to identify physiologic changes once the CVA has occurred:

- *CT scan* identifies the size and location of the CVA. It is useful to differentiate between an infarction and hemorrhage. Nursing interventions for the patient having a CT scan of the head are described in Box 38-8.

BOX 38-8 NURSING CARE CHECKLIST

Patients Having CT Scan of the Head
Preparation of Patient
- ☑ Obtain a signed consent form.
- ☑ Check facility policy on withholding food and fluids. For a.m. test: NPO 8 hours before test. For p.m. test: May have a liquid breakfast.
- ☑ Give medications up to 2 hours before test.
- ☑ Identify for allergy to iodine dye (by asking about allergy to seafood).
- ☑ Remove hairpins, clips, and earrings.

Patient and Family Teaching
- ☑ Follow the guidelines for not drinking or eating before the test.
- ☑ If contrast dye is injected, a warm sensation may be felt in the face or body.
- ☑ The exam lasts from 30 to 90 minutes.
- ☑ The CT scanner is a narrow circular enclosure with a round opening. You are strapped to a special table while the scanner revolves around your head. This test is painless, but the scanner makes a loud clicking noise.
- ☑ Someone is always immediately available during the test.

- *MRI* detects areas of infarction earlier than a CT scan.
- *Cerebral arteriogram* identifies vessel abnormalities such as an aneurysm.
- *Doppler ultrasound* studies evaluate the flow of blood through the carotid arteries and identify if a vessel is partially or completely occluded.
- *Positron emission tomography* (PET) identifies the amount of tissue damage after a CVA.
- *Lumbar puncture* is used to obtain CSF for examination. Blood in the CSF indicates a hemorrhagic CVA (see Box 38-2).

Medications

Medications are given to prevent a CVA in patients with TIAs or a previous CVA. Antiplatelet medications are most frequently ordered. Platelets can collect in the cerebral arteries and potentially block a vessel. Daily use of low-dose aspirin effectively reduces clot formation. Other antiplatelet medications include clopidogrel (Plavix), dipyridamole (Persantine), and ticlopidine (Ticlid).

CVAs are referred to as "brain attack" so that everyone realizes the urgency of seeking immediate medical help. If a thrombotic or embolic stroke is suspected, the patient is given a thrombolytic drug, recombinant tissue plasminogen alteplase (Activase rt-PA). This drug dissolves blood clots, increases blood flow, and prevents damage to the brain cells. To be effective, it must be given intravenously between 3 and 4.5 hours after symptoms appear. It is not given when intracerebral bleeding is present.

Thrombotic strokes are treated with anticoagulant therapy. They do not dissolve an existing clot but prevent new clots from forming. Anticoagulants are never given to a patient who is bleeding within the brain. The most common anticoagulants are heparin; warfarin (Coumadin); and low-molecular-weight heparin, such as Lovenox. Antiplatelet medications or heparin is started 24 hours after thrombolytic therapy. See Chapter 18 for more information about anticoagulant therapy.

Initially, CVA can increase the patient's blood pressure to perfuse the penumbra. Lowering blood pressure within the first 48 hours could decrease perfusion to the brain's ischemic areas. Antihypertensive drugs are given only when the systolic blood pressure remains higher than 220 mm Hg. An anticonvulsant such as phenytoin may be given to control seizures.

Surgery

Surgery may be performed to prevent a stroke. Persons with a history of TIAs or in danger of having another CVA may undergo a **carotid endarterectomy**. Surgery removes atherosclerotic plaque or a thrombus (Figure 38-8■). Nursing care for the patient after a carotid endarterectomy is described in Box 38-9■. For the first 24 hours after surgery, the patient is cared for in the critical care unit. Transluminal angioplasty, a nonsurgical procedure, compresses plaque against the arterial wall, increasing blood flow to the cerebrum. Once the vessel is opened, a stent may be placed to maintain arterial patency.

Complementary Therapies

Patients taking antihypertensive medications should not take black cohosh because it increases the antihypertensive drugs' hypotensive effects. Feverfew, garlic, ginger root, and ginkgo can suppress platelet aggregation and increase

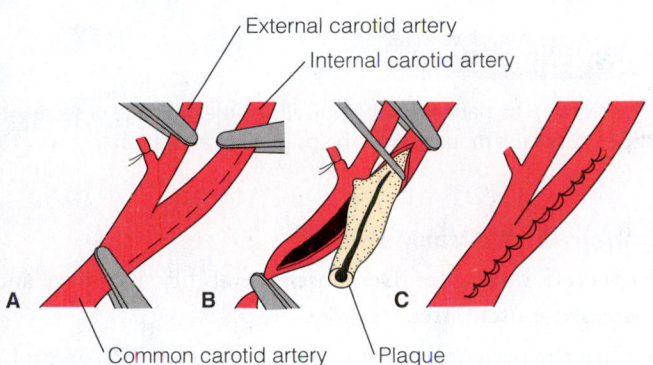

External carotid artery
Internal carotid artery

A   B   C

Common carotid artery   Plaque

Figure 38-8. ■ Carotid endarterectomy. (**A**) The occluded area is clamped off, and an incision is made in the artery. (**B**) Plaque is removed from the inner layer of the artery. (**C**) To restore blood flow through the artery, the artery is sutured or a graft is inserted.

BOX 38-9	NURSING CARE CHECKLIST

Post–Carotid Endarterectomy

☑ Position on the unoperated side with the head and neck in midline alignment and either maintain a flat position or elevate the head of the bed 30 degrees as ordered.

☑ Teach the patient to support the head with the hands when changing position.

☑ Maintain patency of wound drains.

☑ Monitor for *hemorrhage:* Assess the dressing and the area under the neck and shoulders for drainage.

☑ Monitor for *respiratory distress:* Assess respiratory rate, rhythm, depth, and effort. Assess for difficulty swallowing, tracheal deviation from the midline, and restlessness. Keep a tracheostomy set at the bedside.

☑ Monitor for *cranial nerve impairment:* Assess for facial drooping, hoarseness, dysphagia, tongue deviation, speech difficulty, or shoulder sag on one side.

☑ Monitor for *hypertension* or *hypotension:* Monitor blood pressure at least hourly. Report hypertension immediately because of the risk of CVA, artery rupture, or hypotension that could lead to myocardial ischemia.

the risk of bleeding for those patients taking aspirin and anticoagulants such as heparin and warfarin (Coumadin).

NURSING CARE

Patients with a CVA may fully recover or have some residual effects from the stroke. They may experience problems with mobility, speech, and swallowing and an inability to perform ADLs. As patients progress from the acute to the recovery phase, they are cared for in a long-term care facility, rehabilitation center, and the home.

PRIORITIZING NURSING CARE

Many nursing diagnoses are appropriate for the patient with a CVA. Each person is affected differently, depending on the amount of brain damage and the area involved. The priority of care during the initial period is preserving functional brain cells and preventing acute complications. Once the patient's condition is stable, problems of physical mobility, communication, sensory–perceptual deficits, bowel and urine elimination, and swallowing present the major nursing challenges.

HEALTH PROMOTION

Health promotion focuses on activities to prevent a stroke, especially in those with increased risk factors. Stress the importance of stopping smoking and drug use in all age groups. Regular cholesterol screening should be done to monitor for hyperlipidemia. To reduce obesity, which increases the risk for hypertension and type 2 diabetes mellitus, promote weight control through diet and exercise. The National Stroke Association (2013a) launched two campaigns: "Give me 5 for stroke" and "Act FAST" to provide stroke indicators for a person's walk, talk, reach, vision, and feel. Act FAST focuses on face, arm, and speech changes similar to those symptoms listed below. Both campaigns strive to increase public awareness about the signs of a stroke or TIA and the need to call 911 or seek immediate care when the following symptoms occur:

- Sudden weakness or numbness of face, arm, or leg, especially on one side of the body
- Sudden confusion, trouble speaking or understanding speech
- Sudden trouble walking, dizziness, loss of balance or coordination
- Sudden change in vision in one or both eyes
- Sudden severe headache without a cause

Women may experience different symptoms of a stroke than men. According to the National Stroke Association (2013b), women should report immediately any sudden face and limb pain, nausea, hiccups, general weakness, chest pain, shortness of breath, or palpitations.

ASSESSING

Subjective and objective information is obtained from the patient with a suspected TIA or CVA. On admission to the hospital, the patient is assessed for any neurologic deficits. If the patient's condition is unstable, respiratory and cardiac status is closely monitored. Box 38-10■ suggests additional data to collect.

IDENTIFYING POTENTIAL COMPLICATIONS

Serious complications after a CVA include IICP, aspiration pneumonia, and atelectasis. Other potential complications include dysphagia, constipation, incontinence, urinary retention, footdrop, and shoulder abduction. Impaired mobility can lead to pressure ulcers, contractures, muscle atrophy, DVT, and an increased risk for falls. Impaired swallowing can result in malnutrition. Aphasia alters communication ability, increasing the patient's level of anxiety and coping.

DIAGNOSING, PLANNING, AND IMPLEMENTING
Risk for Ineffective Tissue Perfusion: Cerebral

Expected outcome: Demonstrates stable or improved cerebral perfusion.

The acute phase of a CVA is 24 to 72 hours after admission. If the CVA is extensive, the patient is cared for in the critical care unit. ICP is monitored closely. See the section on IICP earlier in this chapter.

| BOX 38-10 | ASSESSMENT |

Patients With Cerebrovascular Accident (Stroke)
Subjective Data
- Change in memory or confusion
- Any sudden severe headache
- Difficulty speaking or understanding speech
- Visual changes such as double vision or blurring
- Any dizziness, loss of coordination or balance
- Any numbness, tingling, or weakness of the face, arm, or leg
- History of hypertension, previous TIA or CVA, diabetes, dysrhythmias, or cardiac disease
- History of alcohol abuse, smoking
- Use of antihypertensive, anticoagulant, or oral contraceptive medication

Objective Data
- Measure blood pressure, pulse, respirations, and temperature.
- Monitor for manifestations of IICP (see Table 38-2).
- Assess orientation; observe for memory lapses.
- Assess for slurred speech, expressive or receptive aphasia.
- Test facial sensation by stroking face with cotton ball.
- Assess strength of hand grip, movement of extremities, gait, and bilateral foot strength.
- Assess the ability to swallow.
- Note the presence of bowel and/or bladder incontinence; palpate bladder for distention.

Risk for Ineffective Airway Clearance

Expected outcome: Maintains patent airway.

- Monitor respiratory status and airway patency. Suction the airway as necessary. Place the patient in a side-lying position to prevent aspiration. Monitor respiratory status and give oxygen as ordered. *Breathing may be affected by the CVA. If the patient is unconscious, suctioning is important to prevent airway obstruction. The patient is at risk for developing atelectasis and pneumonia. Giving oxygen reduces the risk of hypoxia and hypercapnia that increases cerebral ischemia.*

clinicalALERT

Positioning the patient on the side allows the drainage of secretions out of the mouth, which helps prevent aspiration.

Impaired Physical Mobility

Expected outcome: Demonstrates ability to move and increased muscle strength.

- Turn the patient from side to side every 2 hours around the clock. Keep the body aligned and place extremities in proper position with pillows (Figure 38-9■). *Mobility can be impaired by weak extremities, muscle wasting, or hemiplegia. Proper positioning and turning maintain joint function*

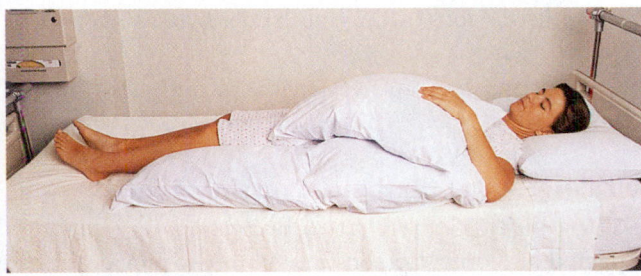

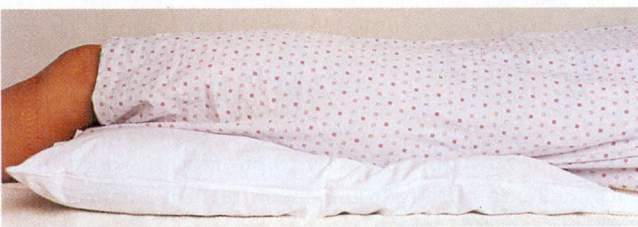

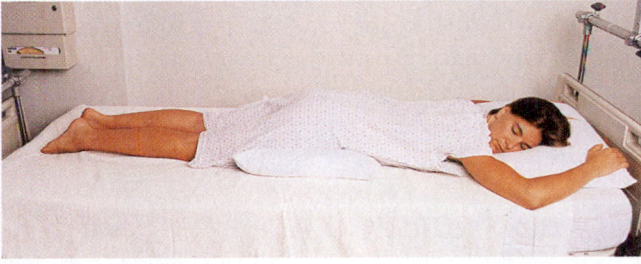

Figure 38-9. ■ Positioning the patient with hemiplegia is important to prevent deformity of the affected extremities. (**A**) With the patient in a supine position, place a pillow in the axilla (to prevent adduction) and under the hand and arm, with the hand higher than the elbow (to prevent flexion and edema). (**B**) When the patient is lying supine, use a pillow from the iliac crest to the middle of the thigh to prevent external rotation of the hip. (**C**) When the patient is in the prone position, place a pillow under the pelvis to promote hip hyperextension. (Pearson Education.)

and decrease skin breakdown and dependent edema in the hands and feet. These actions also reduce the risk of other complications resulting from immobility.

■ Monitor calves each shift for symptoms of thrombophlebitis: redness, warmth, and tenderness. *Patients on bed rest can develop thrombophlebitis.*

■ Do not use a footboard. Use hand splints as directed by the physical therapist. *Footboards are no longer recommended. Hand splints may prevent contractures of the fingers and wrist.*

■ Perform active ROM exercises on unaffected extremities and passive ROM exercises on affected extremities every 4 hours. *Active ROM exercises can improve muscle strength. Passive ROM exercises improve joint mobility.*

clinicalALERT

Active and passive ROM exercises increase venous return and decrease the risk of thrombophlebitis.

■ Collaborate with the physical therapist to teach the patient transfer and ambulation. *The physical therapist knows the correct transfer and ambulation techniques for the CVA patient.*

Impaired Verbal Communication

Expected outcome: Uses oral and other communication techniques as able.

Use the following guidelines when communicating with the patient:

■ Speak to the patient as an adult. Do not raise your voice when speaking to the patient.

■ Allow adequate time for the patient to answer.

■ Face the patient and speak slowly.

■ When you do not understand the patient's speech, be honest and say so.

■ Use short, simple statements and yes/no questions.

■ If patients cannot speak, ask them to nod the head or blink their eyes.
Communication may be altered by expressive or receptive aphasia. All of these techniques can decrease the patient's frustration and may motivate the patient to communicate.

■ Provide pad and pencil, magic slate, flash cards, computerized talking board, and/or picture board. *Other techniques may help the patient communicate.*

Risk for Injury

Expected outcome: Remains free from falls.

■ Keep the environment free of clutter and well lit. Keep the bed in the low position with side rails elevated. *Patients with a CVA are at risk for injury.*

■ Place items on the unaffected side. *Patients with a visual field deficit may ignore items on the affected side of the body.*

■ Teach the patient to turn the head and move the eyes toward the affected side of the body. *Patients with homonymous hemianopia cannot see half of their environment; turning the head and moving the eyes in one direction increases mobility and decreases the risk of injury.*

■ Approach the patient from the unaffected side and speak before touching. *These actions prevent startling the patient.*

■ If unilateral neglect is present, encourage the patient to handle affected extremities. *This increases the patient's awareness of the affected side.*

Impaired Urinary Elimination and Constipation

Expected outcome: Maintains normal bladder and bowel function.

■ Offer the bedpan or urinal, or assist the patient to bedside commode every 2 to 4 hours. *This reduces the risk of urinary incontinence and helps establish a regular voiding pattern.*

Frequent voiding of small amounts may indicate bladder dysfunction. Assess for bladder distention.

■ Promote daily intake of 2,000 mL, but limit oral intake at night. *Adequate fluid intake may prevent urinary tract infection (UTI). Limiting intake may prevent incontinence at night.*
■ Keep the skin dry and monitor for signs of redness. *Patients who are incontinent are at risk for skin breakdown.*
■ Reinforce the patient's pre-CVA bowel habits:
  ■ Drink 2,000 mL/day and eat a high-fiber diet.
  ■ Increase physical activity as tolerated.
  ■ Offer the bedpan or bedside commode at the same time each day, ensure privacy, and have the patient sit in an upright position.
  ■ Give stool softeners as ordered.

Increased fluids, fiber, and activity stimulate bowel activity. A regular daily time for bowel movements in the upright position and privacy promotes normal bowel elimination. Stool softeners help prevent hard stool that is more difficult to expel.

Impaired Swallowing

Expected outcome: Demonstrates effective swallowing without choking or aspiration.

■ Place the patient in an upright position for meals and 30 minutes afterward. Tilt the head slightly forward. *The patient's swallowing reflex or ability to concentrate may be affected by a CVA. Upright position and tilting head forward prevent aspiration.*

clinical**ALERT**

Do not feed a patient who does not have a functioning gag reflex. Ensure that dysphagia screening has been passed successfully.

■ Provide oral care before meals. *Oral care stimulates saliva and eases swallowing.*
■ Serve thickened liquids and pureed or soft food such as custard and canned fruits and vegetables. *Thickened liquids and pureed and soft foods are easier to swallow and may prevent aspiration.*
■ Encourage the patient to eat small bites of food and place food on the unaffected side of the mouth. *Small bites and using the unaffected side prevents food from collecting in the mouth and makes swallowing safer.*

clinical**ALERT**

After eating, check the patient's mouth for "pocketing" of food, especially on the affected side.

■ Limit distractions during mealtime. *Distractions increase the risk of aspiration.*
■ Have suction equipment available during mealtime. *Suction will be needed if the patient starts to choke or aspirate.*

Self-Care Deficit (Bathing, Dressing, Feeding, and/or Toileting)

Expected outcome: Demonstrates ability to provide self-care.

■ Encourage the patient to use the unaffected arm to bathe, brush teeth, comb hair, dress, and eat. *Self-care to the extent the patient is able reduces his or her frustration, increases independence, and improves self-esteem. Using the unaffected arm will promote the patient's feeling of independence.*
■ Teach the patient and family to put clothing on the affected extremity first and then dress the unaffected extremities. *This technique increases awareness of the affected extremity and promotes independence.*
■ Consult with an occupational therapist to teach the patient how to use assistive devices for eating, hygiene, and dressing. *An occupational therapist's role is to teach patients how to use their upper extremities and appropriate assistive devices.*

MANAGING NURSING CARE

As appropriate and allowed by the designated duties and responsibilities of assistive personnel, the nurse may delegate nursing care activities such as obtaining vital signs, measuring intake and output, providing oral and skin care, and positioning the patient with CVA. Before assigning tasks such as feeding or ambulation, ensure assistive personnel have a clear understanding of the importance of preventing aspiration and falls.

EVALUATING

Evaluate the effectiveness of nursing care of the patient with a CVA by assessing airway patency; the ability to swallow, communicate, move extremities, and self-care or need for assistance; and urinary and bowel patterns. Collect data on the patient's coping ability, willingness to participate in rehabilitation, and knowledge of medications and home care.

DOCUMENTING

Documentation includes vital signs, assessment of speech, ability to move extremities, strength of hand grip, swallowing, bowel and breath sounds, intake and output, and nutritional intake. Record the patient and family teaching about self-care, complications, medications, diet, assistive devices, ROM exercises, and safety measures. Note specific instructions about skin care, ROM exercises, medication administration and side effects, and symptoms to report.

CONTINUITY OF CARE

After a CVA, the patient and family face many changes. The middle-aged adult family member may become the caretaker for an older parent. An older adult may be unable to care for a spouse who has had a stroke. They may have to accept placement of the spouse in a long-term care facility.

Discharge planning includes assessing the patient's and family's ability to care for the patient. The patient and family need teaching before the patient can be sent home. The following topics should be included:

- Prevention of CVA; symptoms of TIA and CVA
- When to seek medical care (provide physician's name and emergency numbers)
- Complications such as aspiration, pneumonia, UTI, blood clots, and skin breakdown
- Medications: use, dose, and side effects
- Equipment modifications in the home; for example, a raised toilet seat, grab bars in the bathroom, a bath chair, a vise lid opener, a long-handled shoehorn
- Safety measures to prevent falls
- Demonstration of feeding techniques and use of assistive devices
- Demonstration of ROM exercises and the use of any splints
- Physical care (ADLs, transfer techniques, skin care)
- Psychologic support for the patient and family; respite care for the caregiver
- Community resources such as home health agency, Meals-on-Wheels, elder care (day care for adults); sources for special equipment (e.g., walker); support groups and stroke clubs
- Other helpful resources: American Heart Association, National Stroke Association

Rehabilitation is a lengthy process. The family will need to be patient as the patient relearns ADLs. Emphasize that physical function may continue to improve for up to 3 months, and speech may continue to improve even longer.

Cerebral Aneurysm

A cerebral **aneurysm** is an abnormal outpouching or dilation of a cerebral artery. It occurs at the point where the arterial wall is the weakest. The weakness is related to atherosclerosis, hypertension, or a congenital defect. Cerebral aneurysms usually develop in the circle of Willis. There are several types of aneurysms: (1) berry, (2) saccular, (3) fusiform, and (4) dissecting (Figure 38-10■). A ruptured cerebral aneurysm is the most common cause of a hemorrhagic CVA.

PATHOPHYSIOLOGY AND MANIFESTATIONS

At first, the weakened portion of the artery enlarges and presses on nearby cranial nerves. Unless it affects cranial nerve function, the person is asymptomatic. As the aneurysm enlarges, it may periodically leak blood into the brain. The person complains of headache, nausea, vomiting, and pain in the neck and back. If the leak can spontaneously seal itself with a clot, the patient again becomes asymptomatic. If the aneurysm keeps expanding, it is likely to rupture, forcing blood into the subarachnoid space at the base of the brain. This is known as a **subarachnoid hemorrhage**. Bleeding into the subarachnoid space causes meningeal irritation.

Manifestations of a subarachnoid hemorrhage include (1) sudden, explosive headache; (2) stiff neck (*nuchal rigidity*); (3) change in consciousness; (4) photophobia; (5) nausea and vomiting; and (6) cranial nerve deficits. The major complications are rebleeding and vasospasm. Rebleeding can occur within the first 48 hours and later in 7 to 10 days. The later rebleeding occurs when the initial clot breaks down as part of the body's normal process. A *cerebral vasospasm* occurs when one or more cerebral arteries narrow,

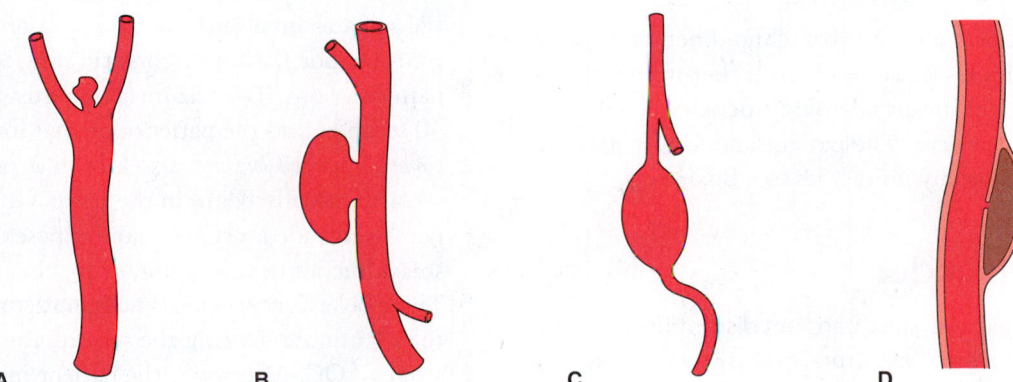

Figure 38-10. ■ Types of aneurysms. (**A**) A berry aneurysm is a small sac on a stem or stalk. (**B**) A saccular aneurysm is formed from a distended small portion of the vessel wall. (**C**) A fusiform aneurysm is an enlarged area of the entire blood vessel. (**D**) A dissecting aneurysm is formed when blood fills the area between the tunica media and the tunica intima.

leading to ischemia and infarction. Both complications have a high mortality rate.

COLLABORATIVE CARE

Diagnosis is made by a CT scan, angiography, and lumbar puncture. A *CT scan* of the brain shows the location and size of the aneurysm. *Cerebral angiography* is done to view the cerebral arteries, locate the aneurysm, and identify a vasospasm. The presence of blood in the CSF during a *lumbar puncture* confirms a subarachnoid hemorrhage.

Several medications are given to avoid rebleeding and vasospasm until surgery is possible. Calcium channel blockers, such as nimodipine (Nimotop), decrease vasospasm. The patient may be given anticonvulsants for seizure activity. Stool softeners prevent unnecessary straining that can increase intracranial pressure. Acetaminophen or codeine is used for pain control.

Surgery is the treatment of choice to prevent additional bleeding. It is preferred as soon as the patient's condition is stable. The skull is opened and either a metal clip is placed at the neck of the aneurysm or the involved artery may be clipped before and after the aneurysm to isolate the affected area. New coil or mesh stents may be placed around the neck of the aneurysm.

If the size or location of the aneurysm prohibits surgery, the patient is managed conservatively. The nurse monitors the patient for signs of deterioration by doing neurologic checks and taking blood pressure, pulse, and respirations hourly (more frequently if the patient's condition worsens). The following aneurysm precautions are instituted to prevent an increase in ICP and the risk of rebleeding:

- Place the patient in a private, quiet, darkened room.
- Limit visitors to two family members at any one time.
- Avoid activities that increase ICP, such as coughing, sneezing, straining, blowing the nose, moving self up in bed, or smoking.

Discharge teaching after a subarachnoid hemorrhage is similar to that for a CVA, as discussed earlier in this chapter. Patients with significant neurologic deficits are referred for rehabilitation services. The patient and family need to follow postop craniotomy guidelines (see Box 38-5).

Seizure Disorder

Key Concept   Seizures are a transient disruption in brain function caused by abnormal excessive electrical discharges from the cortical neurons in one or more areas of the brain. They can alter motor, sensory, and autonomic function, consciousness, or behavior. Epilepsy is classified as a chronic seizure disorder.

A **seizure** is a brief disruption of brain function caused by abnormal electrical activity in the nerve cells of the brain. This electrical activity may involve all or part of the brain and may cause sensory, motor, or autonomic manifestations. A **convulsion** is involuntary muscle contraction and relaxation, which involves the entire body.

Seizures can occur as an isolated event. For example, it is not uncommon for a patient to have a few seizures after a severe head injury. When seizures occur in a chronic pattern, the disorder is called **epilepsy** or *seizure disorder*. The cause of most seizure disorders is unknown. However, seizures beginning in adulthood usually result from other conditions such as a brain infection, CVA, or brain tumor. Approximately 2 million people in the United States are affected by epilepsy and seizures.

PATHOPHYSIOLOGY AND MANIFESTATIONS

Neurons carry messages by electrical impulses from the body to the cerebral cortex. If a few unstable neurons continue sending electrical impulses, a seizure occurs. A group of abnormally firing neurons that start a seizure is called an **epileptogenic focus**. The part of the body controlled by these neurons performs abnormally. Certain conditions such as hypoglycemia, high fever, and hypoxia can trigger seizure activity. When seizures occur, they greatly increase metabolism and therefore consumption of oxygen and glucose to the brain. Seizures are classified as partial or generalized.

Partial Seizures

Partial (or focal) seizures start in one area of the cerebral cortex. There are two types of partial seizures:

1. *Simple partial seizures* cause uncontrolled jerking movements of a finger, hand, foot, leg, or the face. This motor activity may spread to other body areas and is known as the *Jacksonian march*. Sometimes simple partial seizures involve the sensory part of the brain. Symptoms include flashing lights, tingling sensations, or hallucinations. The seizure activity usually lasts 20 to 30 seconds, and the patient does not lose consciousness.

2. *Complex partial seizures*, also known as psychomotor seizures, usually begin in the temporal lobe. Manifestations include repetitive, nonpurposeful actions: lip smacking, aimless walking, or picking at clothing. These behaviors are called **automatisms** and last less than 1 minute. During the seizure, the person has an altered LOC. Afterward, the patient may be confused or not remember the seizure. The seizure can be preceded by an **aura** (a warning sign that something is going to happen), such as an unusual smell, a sense of déjà vu, or a sudden intense emotion.

Generalized Seizures

Generalized seizures involve both hemispheres of the brain and result in loss of consciousness. There are two common forms of generalized seizures:

1. *Absence seizures* occur more frequently in children. They are characterized by a brief change in consciousness such as a blank stare, blinking of the eyes, eyelid fluttering, and lip smacking. All motor activity is stopped during the seizure. Because the seizure lasts only 5 to 10 seconds, the patient may be unaware of it. Some patients can experience many seizures per day.

2. *Tonic–clonic seizures* are the most common seizure disorder in adults and children. Because these seizures can develop suddenly, the patient risks potential injury such as head trauma, fractures, burns, or MVAs. Tonic–clonic seizures follow a typical pattern: (1) aura, (2) tonic phase, (3) clonic phase, and (4) postictal phase.

The patient experiences an aura such as a bright light, an odd taste in the mouth, or an unusual sound. A loud cry may be heard when air is forced out of the lungs. The patient falls to the ground, loses consciousness, and has tonic contractions followed by clonic contractions (Figure 38-11 ■). In **tonic contractions**, muscles are rigid with the arms and legs extended and jaws clenched. Pupils become fixed and dilated. Breathing stops briefly and cyanosis develops. During **clonic contractions**, movements are jerky as the muscles alternately contract and relax. The eyes roll back; tongue and cheek biting, as well as frothing from the mouth, may occur. Urinary and bowel incontinence are common. The entire seizure generally lasts about 1 to 2 minutes.

In the postictal phase, the patient is unconscious for up to 30 minutes. The patient regains consciousness slowly and may be confused and disoriented on waking. Individuals often experience headache, muscle aches, and fatigue after the seizure. Many people sleep for several hours afterward. Amnesia of the events before the seizure is normal.

Status Epilepticus

Status epilepticus is a continuous period of tonic–clonic seizures usually lasting 5 minutes or more in which the patient does not regain consciousness. Constant seizure activity can harm the brain's nerve cells due to depletion of oxygen and glucose and impaired ventilation. It also causes physical exhaustion and respiratory distress. Status epilepticus is considered a life-threatening medical emergency to prevent permanent brain damage. It can be triggered by abrupt discontinuation of anticonvulsant medication, acute head injury, or hypoxia.

COLLABORATIVE CARE

Initial treatment focuses on controlling the seizure. Long-term management involves identifying the cause and preventing future seizures. Collaborative care includes diagnostic testing, medications, and, in some cases, surgery.

Diagnostic Tests

A complete neurologic exam is done to identify the site of the seizures. The following diagnostic tests may be ordered:

- *EEG* can determine the type of seizure and locate the seizure focus. See Box 38-11 ■ for nursing implications with an EEG.
- *Skull x-rays* may identify possible skull fractures.
- *CT scan* or *MRI* may detect a tumor, CVA, or hemorrhage.
- *Blood studies* assess CBC, electrolytes, blood urea nitrogen (BUN), and blood glucose levels.

Medications

Most seizure activity can be decreased or controlled with anticonvulsant medication. The goal is to use the lowest

---

BOX 38-11   NURSING CARE CHECKLIST

Electroencephalogram

Preparation of the Patient

☑ Explain the procedure to the patient.

☑ Withhold tranquilizer and depressant medications 24 to 48 hours before and caffeine-containing foods (e.g., coffee, tea, cola, and chocolate).

☑ Shampoo hair the night before.

Patient and Family Teaching

☑ The test lasts from 1 to 2 hours.

☑ The test is painless. It is done while you lie on a stretcher or sit in a reclining chair.

☑ Electrodes are applied to the scalp with a thick paste.

☑ After the test, the nurse will help you remove the paste from your hair.

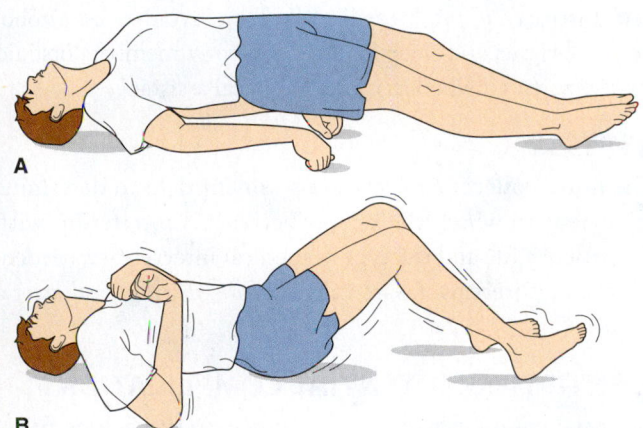

Figure 38-11. ■ Tonic–clonic contractions in generalized seizures. (**A**) Tonic phase. (**B**) Clonic phase.

TABLE 38-7	Giving Medications Safely: Antiepileptic Drugs		
CLASS/DRUGS	**PURPOSE**	**NURSING IMPLICATIONS**	**PATIENT TEACHING**
■ Clonazepam (Klonopin) ■ Carbamazepine (Tegretol) ■ Ethosuximide (Zarontin) ■ *Gabapentin* (Neurontin) ■ Lamotrigine (Lamictal) ■ Phenobarbital ■ Phenytoin (Dilantin) ■ Primidone (Mysoline) ■ Tiagabine (Gabitril) ■ Valproic acid (Depakene)	Antiepileptic drugs act in the motor cortex of the brain to prevent abnormal electrical discharges from the epileptic foci in this area. They control chronic seizures but do not cure seizure disorders. Also, they raise the seizure threshold so that a seizure cannot begin.	Give at the same time each day. Monitor for side effects (e.g., drowsiness, confusion, blurred vision, rash, or nystagmus). Check patients taking phenytoin for gingival hyperplasia. Monitor CBC, platelet count, and kidney and liver function tests for adverse reactions. Monitor serum drug levels for therapeutic range.	Take at the same time each day. Do not drive a car or operate machinery when drowsy. If taking Dilantin, brush and floss daily. Report rash, bleeding, or yellow eyes. Keep follow-up appointments with physician and lab for drug levels. Carry ID card identifying the type of seizures and the medications you are taking.

Note: Medications identified in *italics* are among the 200 most frequently prescribed drugs in the United States.

possible dose of medication with the fewest side effects. It takes several weeks to adjust the dose. Routine serum drug levels are drawn to determine effective doses and the potential for toxicity, as well as to identify patients who are not taking their medications. Each medication has a therapeutic and toxic level. Consult a drug handbook for the appropriate levels. If the patient's seizures are not well controlled, a second medication is added. Many patients often need these drugs for their entire life. Antiepileptic drugs may interact adversely with other drugs. Nursing implications are discussed in Table 38-7 ■.

Status epilepticus must be treated immediately. The first priority is to establish and maintain an airway. Then diazepam (Valium) or lorazepam (Ativan) are given intravenously to stop seizure activity. Because these drugs are short acting, the dose may need to be repeated. For longer control of seizure activity, phenytoin and phenobarbital are given.

Surgery

When medications do not control a patient's seizures, surgery may be an option. New techniques allow the patient to be awake during the surgery. While the patient is awake, the surgeon can map the area of abnormal electrical discharges and remove it. It is important to identify the abnormal area of epileptogenic tissue clearly, so that normal brain tissue is not removed. This procedure is most effective for partial complex seizures of the temporal lobe.

Complementary Therapies

Ginkgo decreases the effectiveness of phenytoin (Dilantin). Patients taking anticonvulsants should avoid drinking grapefruit juice because it reduces metabolism of these drugs, raising plasma levels.

NURSING CARE

Nursing assessments and interventions focus on care during and immediately after a seizure. Once the patient's condition is stable, patient and family teaching are emphasized for care at home. Preventing recurrent seizures is a major treatment goal.

PRIORITIZING NURSING CARE

Nursing care for patients with a seizure disorder focuses on providing care during and immediately after a seizure. Priorities of care for these patients include maintaining a patent airway, preventing injury, and decreasing anxiety.

HEALTH PROMOTION

Health promotion includes teaching the patient ways to reduce the incidence of seizure activity and to promote safety. Emphasize the importance of follow-up care, keeping appointments with physician and laboratory, and taking prescribed antiepileptic medications even when no seizure activity occurs. Review any state laws that apply to people with seizure disorders. Instruct the patient to limit caffeine, avoid excess alcohol intake, fatigue, and sleep loss. Teach family members first aid for a seizure and when to call for medical assistance.

ASSESSING

The nurse collects subjective assessment data to determine the extent to which the seizure activity is interfering with the patient's life and the type of medical intervention needed. Objective observations are made before, during, and after a seizure (Box 38-12 ■).

IDENTIFYING POTENTIAL COMPLICATIONS

Potential complications after seizure activity include physical injury and altered airway, breathing, and circulation. A life-threatening complication is status epilepticus.

Patients With Seizure Disorders

Subjective Data

- Describe where seizures begin in your body. What are you told happens during a seizure? How do you feel after the seizure? Do you have a warning sign (aura)?
- History of birth or head injuries, brain tumor or infections, CVA, liver or renal disease, alcohol or drug addiction
- Antiepileptic medications

Objective Data

- Observe before, during, and after a seizure:
  - Precipitating factors; sudden onset or warning aura; length of seizure; urine or bowel incontinence; clenched teeth; foaming or bleeding from the mouth
  - Where did the seizure begin; did it involve both sides? Were there tonic to clonic movements?
  - Loss of consciousness during and after seizure? How long?
  - Presence of automatisms (e.g., lip smacking, eyelid fluttering)
  - Rate, quality, or absence of respirations; presence of cyanosis
  - Amnesia about the seizure and events before it

DIAGNOSING, PLANNING, AND IMPLEMENTING

Risk for Ineffective Airway Clearance

Expected outcome: Maintains patent airway.

- Loosen clothing around the neck. *Loosening clothing can maintain a patent airway.*
- Turn the patient on the side. *During a seizure, the tongue may fall back and obstruct the airway. Secretions may pool at the back of the mouth. Turning the patient on the side allows secretions to drain from the mouth.*

clinicalALERT

Do not force anything into the patient's mouth because it could obstruct the airway.

- Give oxygen by mask as needed. *Seizures can cause hypoxia, so the patient may need supplemental oxygen.*
- Provide suction at the bedside. *Suction is used to prevent aspiration.*

Risk for Injury

Expected outcome: Remains free from injury during seizure activity.

- Maintain the bed in a low position and keep side rails up. *A low bed position helps the patient avoid falls and injuries. Side rails prevent the patient from falling out of bed during a seizure.*

- Place blankets or protective pads over the side rails. *Padding decreases the risk of injury.*
- If the patient is sitting or standing when the seizure begins, gently lower the patient to the floor. *Loss of consciousness during a seizure would cause the patient to fall.*
- If on the floor, place a folded towel or pillow under the patient's head. *The head is protected to prevent injury.*
- Never restrain the patient during a seizure. *Physically restraining the patient could cause fractures of the arms or legs.*
- Clear the area of objects that could cause harm. *This provides an environment free of potential harm.*

Anxiety

Expected outcome: Verbalizes that anxiety is reduced.

- Patients with a seizure disorder worry about having a seizure in public and fear rejection by others. Encourage the patient to identify potential concerns and misconceptions. *The patient needs time to accept the diagnosis and its effect on family, work, and future lifestyle. Misconceptions cause unnecessary worry and anxiety.*
- Provide information about community support groups. *Sharing information with other people with similar health problems may decrease the patient's anxiety.*
- Refer the patient to any local and state agencies for information about driving or operating dangerous machinery. *Accurate information decreases anxiety. The patient needs to know there are legal limitations on driving until a person is proven free of seizures. A driver's license may be reinstated after a seizure-free period and a letter from a physician.*

MANAGING NURSING CARE

As appropriate and allowed by the designated duties and responsibilities of assistive personnel, the nurse may delegate nursing care activities such as providing oral care and assisting with ADLs for the patient with seizure disorder. Ensure assistive personnel have a clear understanding of the importance of promoting patient safety during any seizure activity.

EVALUATING

To evaluate the effectiveness of nursing care for the patient with a seizure disorder, collect data regarding the type and number of seizures, any occurrence of injury during a seizure, and knowledge of medications. Evaluate the patient's level of anxiety to manage a potential chronic disorder.

DOCUMENTING

Describe any seizure activity, including precipitating factors, length and number of seizures, involvement of one or both sides of the body, tonic–clonic movements, automatisms, urine or bowel incontinence, apnea or cyanosis, and foaming from mouth. Record patient teaching about safety measures, medications and side effects, and importance of wearing an ID bracelet.

CONTINUITY OF CARE

Seizure disorders require lifelong management. Teach the patient and family to understand the disorder, medications, and injury prevention.

Discuss the care and observations necessary before, during, and after a seizure. Stress the importance of safety and keeping the airway patent. Teach the patient and family ways to prevent injury at home by (1) not smoking in bed or alone, (2) installing grab bars in the shower and tub area, (3) taking a shower rather than a tub bath to prevent drowning, and (4) keeping the bedroom and bathroom doors unlocked in case of an emergency.

The following points should be emphasized:

- Teach about medication use, side effects, and the need to take at prescribed intervals.
- Record any seizure activity and medications taken daily.
- Avoid activities that require alertness and coordination until medication levels are stable.
- Instruct to wear ID bracelet identifying seizure condition and medications.
- Avoid factors that may trigger a seizure: fasting, excessive stress, flashing or blinking lights.
- Provide information on the Epilepsy Foundation.

Intracranial Infections

Key Concept   Intracranial infections caused by bacteria, viruses, or fungi invade the CNS, resulting in inflammation of the brain and spinal cord. Meningococcemia, a severe and often fatal illness, occurs primarily in adolescents and young adults.

The most common inflammatory conditions of the brain are meningitis, encephalitis, and brain abscesses. They are caused by bacteria and viruses (Table 38-8■). If untreated, these conditions may lead to long-term neurologic deficits or death.

MENINGITIS

Meningitis is an inflammation of the meninges of the brain and spinal cord. Bacterial meningitis may result from *Neisseria meningitidis* (meningococcal meningitis), *Streptococcus pneumoniae*, or *Haemophilus influenzae.* Organisms enter the brain by way of (1) the bloodstream, (2) the respiratory tract, or (3) penetrating wounds of the skull or cranial surgery. Most often, meningitis is secondary to another infection, such as otitis media, an upper respiratory infection, or pneumonia. Viral meningitis, also called aseptic meningitis, is a less severe disease than bacterial meningitis. It is caused by several common viruses (see Table 38-8).

Once the bacteria or virus enters the central nervous system, it begins an inflammatory response in the meninges, CSF, and ventricles. The inflammatory process increases production of CSF. This can lead to cerebral edema and increased ICP. Although viral infection also triggers the inflammatory response, the course of the disease is shorter. Recovery is usually uneventful.

Manifestations show an irritation of the meninges, as outlined in Box 38-13■. Two positive signs of meningeal irritation are Brudzinski sign and Kernig sign. In Brudzinski sign, when the patient's neck is flexed, the knees and hips flex. Kernig sign is an inability to extend the leg when the hip is flexed at a 90-degree angle. The patient may also show signs of IICP, including decreased LOC, seizures, and changes in vital signs and respiratory pattern.

Complications of meningitis may include seizures, hydrocephalus, cerebral infarction, coma, and death.

TABLE 38-8	Comparison of Patient Susceptibility to Intracranial Infections	
INFECTION	**CAUSATIVE ORGANISM**	**SUSCEPTIBLE PATIENTS**
Bacterial meningitis ■ Pneumococcal meningitis	*Streptococcus pneumoniae*	Children under age 2; adults over age 65
■ *Haemophilus influenzae* meningitis	*Haemophilus influenzae*	Children under age 5
■ Meningococcal meningitis	*Neisseria meningitidis*	College students living in dormitories or military personnel in barracks
Viral (aseptic) meningitis	Herpes simplex and zoster; mumps; Epstein–Barr virus; cytomegalovirus (CMV); West Nile virus	All ages
Encephalitis	St. Louis, Eastern and Western equine, and West Nile virus transmitted by ticks and mosquitoes; herpes simplex; virus that causes mumps or chickenpox	All ages
Brain abscess	Streptococci, staphylococci, and pneumococci that cause secondary infection	30 to 40 years old; higher incidence in men

BOX 38-13	MANIFESTATIONS OF MENINGITIS

- Severe headache
- High fever
- Photophobia, diplopia
- Signs of meningeal irritation: nuchal rigidity (stiff neck), positive Brudzinski sign, and positive Kernig sign (see figure)
- Restlessness, irritability, confusion, altered LOC
- Signs of IICP (elevated blood pressure, bradycardia, change in respiratory pattern, decreased LOC, vomiting)
- Seizures
- Petechial rash (in meningococcal meningitis)

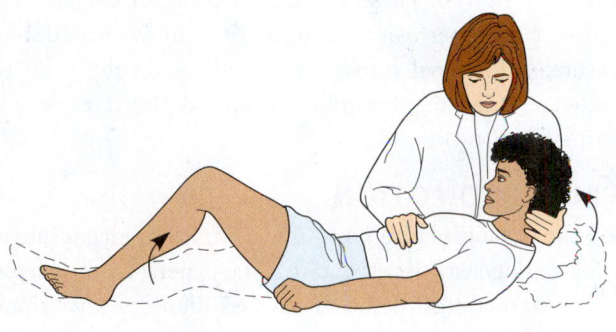

A

Positive Brudzinski sign

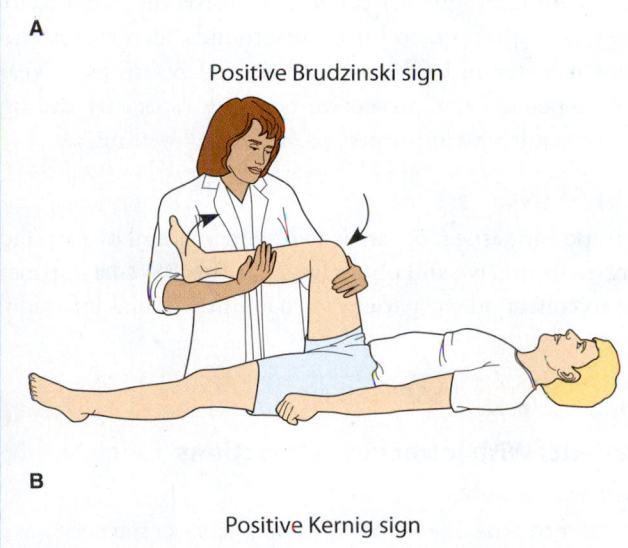

B

Positive Kernig sign

Meningitis may leave residual effects such as visual deficits, deafness, cranial nerve palsies, or hemiplegia.

Meningococcal meningitis can progress to the devastating complication of meningococcemia. This form of meningitis is spread by airborne droplets and is highly contagious. It can cause death within 10 to 12 hours after the patient develops a high fever and petechial rash. Death results from an overwhelming septicemia, vascular collapse, and adrenal hemorrhage.

ENCEPHALITIS
Encephalitis is an acute inflammation of the white and gray matter of the brain and spinal cord. It is almost always caused by a virus, but it may also be caused by bacteria or fungi (see Table 38-8). Many of the viruses are associated with certain seasons of the year or particular geographic regions. The virus may be transmitted by ticks or mosquitoes.

Encephalitis ranges from a mild infection to a serious disease that could be fatal. There is widespread inflammation of the white and gray matter of the brain and spinal cord. Nerve cells may be extensively damaged. Edema and areas of necrosis may lead to localized hemorrhage. IICP develops, progressing to brain herniation, unless treated. Certain viruses tend to affect specific areas of the brain. For example, herpes simplex virus involves the frontal and temporal lobes. Manifestations are similar to those of meningitis, including high fever, headache, stiff neck, seizures, confusion, and disorientation. As the disease progresses, the LOC deteriorates, and the patient becomes comatose.

BRAIN ABSCESS
A **brain abscess** is a collection of purulent material within the brain. Many brain abscesses occur from an infection in the middle ear or nasal sinuses. They may develop after a head injury or intracranial surgery. Other sources include bacterial endocarditis; osteomyelitis; and lung, pelvic, or skin infections. Streptococci and staphylococci are often the underlying causes.

The microorganisms in the brain tissue cause local inflammation. As the white blood cells destroy the organisms, pus forms. The body tries to protect the rest of the brain by forming a capsule around the pus. Unless the abscess is treated, the capsule enlarges and compresses nerves and brain tissue. Chronic inflammation can lead to edema and IICP.

Initially, the patient complains of a headache, fever, chills, and malaise. As the abscess expands, nausea, vomiting, drowsiness, confusion, weakness on one side, and seizures develop.

COLLABORATIVE CARE
Bacterial meningitis is a medical emergency that could be fatal within days. Treatment focuses on a rapid diagnosis and starting antibiotic therapy immediately. Depending on hospital policy, the patient may be placed in Airborne Precautions isolation. Management of viral meningitis focuses on relieving patient symptoms with antipyretics and analgesics. Antibiotic therapy and specific isolation precautions are not indicated for viral meningitis.

The treatment for encephalitis is similar to that for meningitis, with the exception that antiviral medications are used. Isolation is not necessary, because encephalitis is not transmitted from person to person.

Treatment of the patient with a brain abscess focuses on prompt beginning of antibiotic therapy. Other manifestations are treated symptomatically. When antibiotics are unsuccessful, the abscess may be surgically drained or, if encapsulated, removed during a craniotomy.

Diagnostic Tests

The diagnosis of bacterial or viral meningitis or encephalitis is based on clinical manifestations. Diagnosis of a brain abscess is more difficult because there are unclear symptoms. The following diagnostic tests may be ordered:

- *Lumbar puncture* is done to collect samples of CSF. The following findings indicate a positive diagnosis of bacterial meningitis: (1) CSF appears cloudy, (2) an elevated protein level and white blood cell count, (3) a decreased glucose level, and (4) elevated CSF pressure.
- *Culture and sensitivity* and *Gram stain* of the CSF can identify the bacteria or virus causing meningitis or encephalitis.
- *Cultures from the blood, urine, throat, and nose* are performed to identify the bacterial source of infection.
- *CT scan*, *MRI*, or *skull x-rays* may identify the infection source causing a brain abscess.

Medications

In cases of bacterial meningitis, high doses of IV ampicillin, third-generation cephalosporins, or vancomycin (Vancocin) are started immediately. The specific antibiotic is chosen after the culture and sensitivity report identifies the causative organism. Antibiotic therapy is given in high doses so that it will cross the blood–brain barrier and reach the CSF. (For an in-depth discussion of antibiotic therapy, see Chapter 9.) Drug therapy is continued from 7 to 21 days. The CDC recommends that isolation be continued for 24 hours after antibiotic therapy started. Antibiotics are also used to treat brain abscesses.

Anyone exposed to meningococcal meningitis is started on prophylactic antibiotic therapy immediately. The drugs of choice are rifampin (Rifadin) and vancomycin (Vancocin). All cases of meningitis must be reported to the local public health department.

Treatment for encephalitis consists of antiviral drugs such as acyclovir (Zovirax) and vidarabine (Vira-A). If started early in the disease course, they may decrease mortality. They are most effective if used before the patient becomes comatose.

Additional medications are given to relieve symptoms and to prevent complications from any one of the intracranial infections. Anticonvulsant medications prevent or control seizures. Antipyretics are used to reduce fever. Analgesics such as acetaminophen are given to relieve headache and neck pain. Osmotic diuretics and corticosteroids may decrease cerebral edema. The patient initially may require antiemetics to control nausea and vomiting. IV fluids may be necessary to prevent dehydration until the patient is able to take oral fluids.

NURSING CARE

Patients with intracranial infections are acutely ill. Depending on the extent of their illness, they may be cared for in the critical care unit or on a medical unit. If neurologic deficits are present, long-term nursing may be needed. The combination of fever, dehydration, and cerebral edema predisposes the patient to seizures.

PRIORITIZING NURSING CARE

When caring for patients with intracranial infections, it is essential to prevent patient injury, to monitor for decreased cerebral tissue perfusion, and to prevent increased temperature. Additional nursing care focuses on reducing the patient's headache, photophobia, and diplopia caused by meningeal irritation.

HEALTH PROMOTION

Vaccinations for meningococcal meningitis are recommended for college students and military personnel. Anyone exposed to meningococcal meningitis should receive rifampin (Rifadin) prophylactically. Emphasize the importance of destroying mosquito breeding grounds such as pools of stagnant water in bird baths, pools, and pet dishes. Wear insect repellant and protective clothing especially during peak mosquito-biting times, such as early evening.

ASSESSING

An important aspect of care is to obtain a careful history and identify subjective and objective data. Box 38-14■ outlines data to collect on the patient with an intracranial infection.

BOX 38-14	ASSESSMENT

Patients With Intracranial Infections

Subjective Data
- Presence of nausea, vomiting, photophobia, or stiff neck
- Confusion or headache
- Exposure to mosquitoes or ticks
- History of head injury, brain surgery, otitis media, or bacterial endocarditis

Objective Data
- Measure blood pressure, pulse, and temperature.
- Assess orientation, LOC, memory, and response to stimuli.
- Assess for dizziness, diplopia, drooping eyelids, pupil changes, and hearing difficulty due to cranial nerve damage.
- Assess for Brudzinski or Kernig signs (see Box 38-13, Figures A and B)
- Observe for any seizure activity, restlessness, and/or agitation.
- Inspect the skin for presence of petechial rash over the body.

IDENTIFYING POTENTIAL COMPLICATIONS

Intracranial infections can result in complications of IICP and hyperthermia. Seizure activity and confusion may accompany intracranial infections, increasing the risk of physical injury.

DIAGNOSING, PLANNING, AND IMPLEMENTING

Risk for Ineffective Tissue Perfusion: Cerebral

Expected outcome: Maintains adequate cerebral perfusion.

- Monitor for altered neurologic function. See interventions for IICP discussed earlier in this chapter. *Inflammation from intracranial infections increases the patient's risk for developing altered levels of consciousness, seizures, increased IICP, and cranial nerve dysfunction.*

Hyperthermia

Expected outcome: The patient's temperature returns to normal parameters.

- Monitor body temperature at least every 2 to 4 hours. *Patients with intracranial infections can spike high fevers, which could lead to seizures.*
- Remove unnecessary clothing and bed linen. Give antipyretic medications, tepid sponge baths, or use a cooling blanket as ordered. *Antipyretic drugs, tepid sponge baths, and a cooling blanket can reduce a fever. Removing unnecessary clothing and bed linen promotes cooling. The temperature is decreased slowly to prevent shivering, which can raise the temperature higher.*
- Monitor for signs and symptoms of dehydration, noting skin turgor, mucous membranes, and daily body weight. Measure and compare intake and output every 2 to 4 hours. Note urine concentration. *Fluids are restricted in patients with intracranial disorders to prevent cerebral edema. When a high fever exists, fluids are quickly lost, increasing risk for dehydration.*

Acute Pain

Expected outcome: Patient pain is absent or decreases to tolerable levels.

- Keep the room quiet and dim bright lights. Place a cool cloth over the patient's eyes. *Quiet, low lighting and cool cloth may decrease headache and photophobia.*
- Place the patient in position of comfort and provide gentle ROM exercises. *Positioning and ROM exercises may decrease muscle and joint aches, reduce joint stiffness, and promote circulation.*
- Give a mild analgesic such as acetaminophen or codeine. *Morphine sulfate is avoided because it can alter the size and reaction of the patient's pupils.*

MANAGING NURSING CARE

As appropriate and allowed by the designated duties and responsibilities of assistive personnel, the nurse may delegate nursing care activities such as assisting with ADLs and fluid and food intake for the patient with intracranial infections. Before assigning tasks such as obtaining vital signs and measuring intake and output, ensure assistive personnel have a clear understanding of the importance of accuracy in measurement.

EVALUATING

Evaluate the effectiveness of the nursing care for a patient with an intracranial infection by collecting the following data related to the absence of headache, neurologic irritation, and IICP; normal vital signs including temperature; and fluid volume status.

DOCUMENTING

Documentation focuses on vital signs; LOC; intake and output; neurologic deficits such as dizziness, diplopia, hearing loss, and seizures; and presence of headache, photophobia, and petechial rash. Record the patient and family teaching related to medications, symptoms to report, diet, and rest.

CONTINUITY OF CARE

After the acute phase of an intracranial infection, the patient requires several weeks of convalescence. The patient and family need to understand home management. The nurse assesses the patient's and family's abilities and resources to provide care after discharge.

Include the following topics in the teaching session:

- Medications: use, dose, and side effects. Emphasize the importance of taking all antibiotic or antiviral medication until completely gone to prevent new organisms from growing.
- Emphasize the importance of reporting fever, headache, or neck stiffness in people who had close contact with the patient with meningitis.
- Encourage adequate rest and sleep as well as a well-balanced diet.
- Advise to increase physical activity gradually.
- Stress the importance of reporting any signs or symptoms of ear infection, sore throat, or upper respiratory infection.

The patient with permanent neurologic deficits resulting from encephalitis is usually discharged to a rehabilitation setting or a long-term care facility. For infections transmitted by mosquitoes, the patient and family need to know how to destroy breeding sites of insect larvae. They are also taught to avoid mosquito and tick bites by wearing protective clothing and insect repellents.

Headaches

Headache is one of the most common symptoms people experience at all ages. They may result from brain tumors, meningitis, head injuries, stress, muscle tension, or a combination of these factors. Most headaches are mild and are relieved by a mild analgesic. Other headaches are chronic, intense, and recurring. Clinical manifestations vary according to the cause and type of the headache.

The cranium has many pain-sensitive structures. These include the skin, muscles, and periosteum of the skull; the nasal cavities and sinuses; parts of the meninges; cerebral blood vessels; and cranial nerves with sensory function. Stretching, inflammation, pressure, and dilation of the pain-sensitive structures can produce a headache. The most common types of headaches are migraine, cluster, and tension headaches (Table 38-9■).

MIGRAINE HEADACHE

Migraine headaches are the most common type of vascular headache. The exact causes are uncertain. It is believed that migraine headaches result from abnormal cerebral blood flow, increased release of serotonin, or abnormal genes that control the activities of certain brain cells. Migraines differ in intensity, duration, and frequency from patient to patient, and episodes may be different in the same person (see Table 38-9).

CLUSTER HEADACHE

The cluster headache is a form of vascular headache. It typically begins 2 to 3 hours after the person falls asleep. The attacks usually occur in clusters of one to eight daily for weeks or a few months and then they disappear for an extended period. Usually, the same side of the head is involved in each cluster of attacks. Cluster headaches can be triggered by alcohol consumption.

TENSION HEADACHE

Tension headaches often result from prolonged muscle contraction of the head and neck. They are poorly localized with a gradual onset. Occupations that require a prolonged period of abnormal posture such as bending over a desk often precipitate tension headache. Slouching while reading or watching television can lead to muscle contraction. Most headaches are tension headaches.

COLLABORATIVE CARE

The first priority of care is to identify the underlying cause of the headache. If the cause is treatable, the headache symptoms should decrease or disappear. Migraine headaches are managed by drug therapy, patient teaching, and controlling of triggers. Eliminating alcohol may reduce the incidence of cluster headaches. Improving poor posture and initiating comfort measures such as gentle massage or heat may help reduce tension headaches.

A thorough history and physical examination are part of the diagnosis and treatment. A brain scan, MRI, x-ray studies of the skull and cervical spine, EEG, and lumbar puncture for CSF are used to rule out other neurologic problems. Serum metabolic screens and hypersensitivity testing also may be performed if systemic problems are suspected.

Medications

The choice of medications for managing headaches depends on the specific type of headache. The goals are to reduce the frequency and severity of headaches and to limit or stop a headache when it occurs.

To reduce the frequency and severity of migraines, several prophylactic medications are ordered. Propranolol (Inderal) prevents dilation of cerebral blood vessels, and verapamil (Calan) controls cerebral vasospasms. Amitriptyline (Elavil) blocks the uptake of serotonin and catecholamines. Methysergide (Sansert) decreases serotonin action; however, it can produce severe side effects and must be used cautiously. Topiramate (Topamax), an anticonvulsant, may be effective in preventing migraines, but abrupt discontinuation can cause seizures.

Before a migraine becomes severe, ergotamine with caffeine (Cafergot) is given by oral, sublingual, rectal, or intranasal route. When given at the first sign of an attack,

TABLE 38-9	**Types of Headaches**		
TYPE	**RISK FACTORS**	**DESCRIPTION**	**MANIFESTATIONS**
Migraine	More common in women Family history of migraine headaches	May be triggered by stress; rapid changes in blood glucose levels; foods such as aged cheese, nuts, chocolate, caffeine, or alcohol. Often correlates with menstrual cycle. May last hours to days. Migraine with aura usually lasts less than an hour.	*No aura:* pulsating or throbbing headache on one side of the head. Accompanied by nausea, vomiting, and sensitivity to light and sound. *Aura:* Preceded by aura and then the same symptoms as above.
Cluster	More common in men between ages 20 and 40	Series of headaches over a 2- to 3-month period and then disappear for a long period of time.	Unilateral pain located around or behind the eye that can wake the patient; also nasal congestion, tearing, facial flushing.
Tension	More common in women	May be triggered by stress, eyestrain, or poor posture. These triggers can cause muscle contraction in neck, face, and scalp.	Bilateral pain, tightness, pressure, or viselike feeling; pain is most common on awakening.

ergotamine is effective in controlling up to 70% of acute attacks. Two serotonin agonists, sumatriptan (Imitrex) and zolmitriptan (Zomig), act rapidly to stop migraines. Sumatriptan (Imitrex) is available for oral, subcutaneous, or intranasal use.

Once a migraine attack is in progress, acetaminophen, ibuprofen, and ketorolac (Toradol) may be used for mild migraines. Opioids such as codeine or meperidine (Demerol) may be required for severe migraines. Antiemetics such as promethazine (Phenergan) or metoclopramide (Reglan) are given to control nausea and vomiting.

Many of the same medications used for migraines may treat cluster headaches. Some patients gain relief from a cluster headache by inhaling 100% oxygen at 12 to 15 L/min for 15 minutes or giving sumatriptan (Imitrex). Ergotamine tartrate may be given in suppository form at bedtime to prevent cluster headaches. Nonnarcotic analgesics such as aspirin or acetaminophen may be effective in relieving tension headaches.

Complementary Therapies

Biofeedback and meditation are used to reduce stress and possible tension headaches. Kava relaxes skeletal muscles, relieving tension that may lead to a tension headache. Some patients with migraines have received relief from acupuncture, massage, exercise, hot baths, biofeedback, and the herbal supplement feverfew. Other complementary therapies for headaches include riboflavin, vitamin D, and magnesium.

NURSING CARE

Nursing care begins by obtaining a history and description of the headache. It is important to identify the effects of recurring headaches on the patient's daily life. Box 38-15 ■ lists assessment data to collect. Nursing interventions focus on controlling the pain and discomfort of the headache.

Acute Pain

Expected outcome: Patient pain is absent or decreases to tolerable levels.

■ Ask the patient to rate the pain on a 0–10 scale (10 = the worst pain) or provide a visual analog of faces that show different levels of discomfort. *Rating scales provide objective data about the patient's subjective pain or discomfort. They can also evaluate the effectiveness of pain relief measures.*
■ Minimize light, noise, and activity. Provide rest in a quiet, nonstimulating environment when the headache is present. *Reducing environmental stimuli may decrease pain.*
■ Encourage the patient to use deep breathing or relaxation techniques. *These strategies reduce tension and may help the patient gain a sense of control over the pain.*

BOX 38-15 ASSESSMENT

Patients With Headaches
Subjective Data
■ Type of pain, frequency, duration, location, radiation, precipitating factors, time of day it occurs, relieving factors
■ Any light flashes or bright spots before the headache begins?
■ Does nausea, vomiting, or numbness accompany headache?
■ Interference with daily activities or associated with stress
■ Exposure to toxic chemicals at work
■ Family history of migraines
■ Medication and alcohol use

Objective Data
■ Observe for facial flushing and tearing (present with cluster headaches).
■ Observe for pallor, diaphoresis, and one-sided weakness (present with migraines).
■ Note presence of nausea, vomiting, or diarrhea.
■ Palpate neck and shoulder muscles for tightness (present with tension headaches).

■ Apply cold or warm cloth to the head and neck as ordered. *Cold causes vasoconstriction, which may reduce pain in vascular headaches. Heat reduces muscle tension and improves circulation.*
■ Offer a back massage. *Massage promotes muscle relaxation, which is especially useful for tension headaches.*

Collect the following information to evaluate the effectiveness of providing care to the patient with headaches: decreased or absence of pain; knowledge about medications; and lifestyle modifications to reduce headaches.

CONTINUITY OF CARE

Because headaches are managed at home, patient education is the main focus. Teach the patient how to limit attacks and to reduce the effects of headaches. Patients with long-term or migraine headaches may be referred for stress reduction or biofeedback classes. The teaching session should include the following points:

■ Teach about medication use, dosage, and side effects.
■ Report ergotamine side effects (e.g., numbness and tingling in fingers and toes, leg weakness, and aching muscles).
■ Avoid caffeine, cured meats, monosodium glutamate (MSG), and foods containing tyramine (chocolate, red wine, aged cheese); smoking.
■ Participate in regular moderate exercise.
■ Avoid fasting, fatigue, and irregular sleep patterns.
■ Keep a headache diary.
■ Identify comfort measures during a headache: darkened, quiet room and applying a cool cloth to the forehead.

Note: The references and resources for all chapters have been compiled at the back of the book.

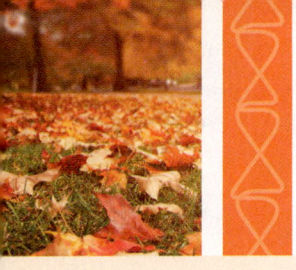

Chapter Review

KEY POINTS

- **Concept:** Traumatic brain injury (TBI) occurs when a blow or jolt to the head disrupts normal brain function. Its effects range from a brief change in consciousness to long-term coma, permanent disability, or death. Major complications of TBI are increased intracranial pressure and cerebral edema.

- The highest incidence for traumatic brain injuries (TBI) is for people between the ages of 1 and 35 and the older adult. In the older adult, falls are a frequent cause of brain trauma. TBIs include concussion, contusion, skull fractures, and intracranial hemorrhage.

- Subtle changes such as restlessness, drowsiness, altered LOC indicate an early change in neurologic function and must be reported and treated promptly.

- Increasing ICP is characterized by altered LOC, abnormal motor weakness, altered pupil size and reaction to light, increased blood pressure, and decreased pulse and respiratory rate. IICP is a medical emergency and must be treated immediately to prevent permanent brain damage or death. Patients with severe brain injuries have an increased risk for brain death.

- Brain tumors are abnormal growths within the cranium that can be benign or malignant. They can cause IICP as they grow within the confined space of the skull. Medical treatment may include debulking of the tumor, radiation, and chemotherapy.

- Intracranial surgery increases the risk of meningitis. It is extremely important to use aseptic technique when changing any wound dressing and to monitor for any purulent drainage.

- **Concept:** An ischemic stroke results from a sudden decrease in blood flow to the brain, causing brain cell death. Early assessment and rapid medical intervention can save brain tissue and reduce the risk of permanent brain damage or death.

- Strokes are caused by a thrombus, embolus, or hemorrhage. Primary risk factors for a stroke are hypertension, atherosclerosis, atrial fibrillation, smoking, and age.

- Older adults often ignore the symptoms of a TIA, mistakenly thinking it is part of the normal aging process because the symptoms disappear after a short time.

- Patients must be taught the warning signs of an impending CVA and lifestyle modifications to prevent a CVA. People with a higher risk for further CVAs from a thrombus are usually started on low-dose aspirin or anticoagulant therapy.

- **Concept:** Seizures are a transient disruption in brain function caused by abnormal excessive electrical discharges from the cortical neurons in one or more areas of the brain. They can alter motor, sensory, and autonomic function, consciousness, or behavior. Epilepsy is classified as a chronic seizure disorder.

- Seizures are categorized into those that affect only one part of the brain known as partial seizures. They are further subdivided into simple or complex partial seizures. Generalized seizures affect all of the brain and include tonic–clonic or absence seizures.

- Seizure disorders are managed with antiepileptic drugs. These medications must be taken on a regular schedule and not discontinued without medical supervision.

- During a generalized tonic–clonic seizure it is critical for the nurse to maintain a patent airway in the patient and to protect the patient from injury.

- **Concept:** Intracranial infections caused by bacteria, viruses, or fungi invade the CNS, resulting in inflammation of the brain and spinal cord. Meningococcemia, a severe and often fatal illness, occurs primarily in adolescents and young adults.

- Common manifestations of intracranial infections include fever, headache, nuchal rigidity, photophobia (light sensitivity) and positive Brudzinski and Kernig signs. Possible complications include seizures, altered LOC, and coma. CNS infections such as meningitis or encephalitis are usually treated with broad-spectrum antibiotics.

- Meningococcemia, a complication of meningococcal meningitis, can cause death in 10 to 12 hours. Any patient with a high fever and petechial rash must be seen by a physician immediately.

- Common types of headaches are migraine, cluster, and tension. Classic migraine headaches are preceded by an aura. Migraine attacks may be prevented with drugs such as propranolol (Inderal) and verapamil (Calan) and avoiding caffeine, smoking, and foods high in tyramine (aged cheese, chocolate, and nuts).

PEARSON NURSING STUDENT RESOURCES

Find additional materials at **nursing.pearsonhighered.com**.

Clinical Reasoning Care Map

Caring for a Patient After a Cerebrovascular Accident/Stroke
NCLEX-PN® Focus Area: Physiologic Integrity; Reduction of Risk Potential

Case Study: Mr. Boren, a 68-year-old African American male, had a CVA this morning. He is drowsy but responds to verbal stimuli by nodding his head to indicate "yes" when asked questions. He has flaccid paralysis in his left arm and left leg (he is left-handed). He shows visual field deficits that indicate homonymous hemianopia. A CT scan confirms the diagnosis of a right-brain CVA due to a thrombus of the middle cerebral artery. Mr. Boren is started on a continuous IV heparin infusion.

Nursing Diagnosis: Impaired Verbal Communication

COLLECT DATA

Subjective	Objective
_____	_____
_____	_____
_____	_____
_____	_____
_____	_____

Does this present a threat to the patient's safety?

If yes, the priority intervention to address this threat would be:

_____

Nursing Care

_____
_____
_____
_____
_____
_____

Interprofessional team members to include when planning care:

_____

How would you document this? _____

_____

Compare your answers and documentation to those provided on the companion website.

Data Collected
(use only those that apply)

- Lack of eye contact
- Left arm and leg flaccid
- Nods off while people speak to him
- Nods head to answer questions
- Makes a clenched fist of right hand when trying to speak
- Eyes look pleading

Nursing Interventions
(use only those that apply; list in priority order)

- Provide a large marker and tablet.
- Place objects, call bell, and tissues on Mr. Boren's unaffected side.
- Use short, simple sentences when talking to Mr. Boren.
- Provide adaptive devices (silverware with thick handles and nonslip plates) for Mr. Boren to use.
- Contact speech therapy for consultation.
- Encourage Mrs. Boren to visit at mealtimes.
- Explain all health care procedures.
- Maintain a calm, unhurried manner.

NCLEX-PN® Exam Preparation

TEST-TAKING TIP Focus on reviewing safety issues in the care of patients. Many issues are important, but there is usually one that will stand out as being the most relevant. Think critically about the situation, and eliminate safety issues that are common to all patient illnesses or diseases.

1 A patient was accidentally struck in the head by a baseball bat. Which clinical finding should the nurse anticipate as a serious complication?

1. Clear fluid draining from the ears
2. Large hematoma at the impact site
3. Headache
4. Complaints of dizziness

2 Which of the following risk factors in the patient's history is most likely to increase the potential in developing a CVA? **Select all that apply.**

1. Age 50 or older
2. Use of oral contraceptives for the past 10 years
3. Presence of atherosclerosis
4. Consumption of one beer per day
5. Overweight by 50 lb
6. Caucasian race

3 After a lumbar puncture, which nursing action should the nurse implement?

1. Remind the patient not to move the legs after the procedure.
2. Monitor the puncture site for CSF leakage.
3. Have the patient empty his or her bladder.
4. Limit the patient's fluid intake.

4 What teaching point should the nurse emphasize to a patient taking phenytoin (Dilantin) on a daily basis?

1. Check urine for brownish color.
2. Report fatigue and weakness.
3. Do not take with food.
4. Brush and floss daily.

5 A patient experienced a blow to the right frontal region of the head. If the patient begins to develop increased intracranial pressure, which manifestation should the nurse see first?

1. Decreased heart rate
2. Sluggish response by pupils to light
3. Irritability
4. Projectile vomiting

6 After a craniotomy for removal of a brain tumor located in the occipital lobe, what nursing intervention should the nurse implement?

1. Place the patient in a side-lying position.
2. Monitor for signs of cranial nerve impairment.
3. Give morphine for headache.
4. Monitor vital signs every 4 hours.

7 Which nursing diagnosis has the highest priority for a patient with status epilepticus?

1. Anxiety
2. Risk for Injury
3. Risk for Ineffective Airway Clearance
4. Risk for Ineffective Cerebral Tissue Perfusion

8 A patient is being discharged from the emergency department with a diagnosis of migraine headaches. It is most important to include which of the following teaching points?

1. Keep a headache diary.
2. Identify comfort measures during a headache.
3. Refer the patient to stress reduction classes.
4. Teach the patient how to reduce frequency of attacks.

9 The physician notes the following findings: positive Brudzinski and Kernig signs, IICP, sputum cultures positive for *Streptococcus pneumoniae*. Based on this information, what medical diagnosis should the nurse anticipate that the physician will make for this patient?

1. Encephalitis
2. Brain abscess
3. Bacterial meningitis
4. Subdural hematoma

10 A patient begins to seize while the nurse is conducting an assessment. Place these actions in the sequence that the nurse should do them.

1. Clear the area of objects that could cause injury.
2. Loosen the gown.
3. Turn the patient on his or her side.
4. Pad the side rails as soon as possible.
5. Provide supplemental oxygen.
6. Place a pillow under the patient's head.

Answers and rationales for Review Questions appear in Appendix I.

992 Unit X   Disrupted Neurologic Function

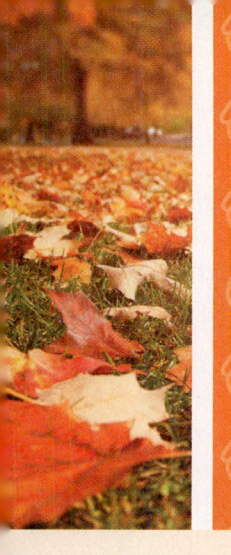

CHAPTER 39

Caring for Patients With Degenerative Neurologic and Spinal Cord Disorders

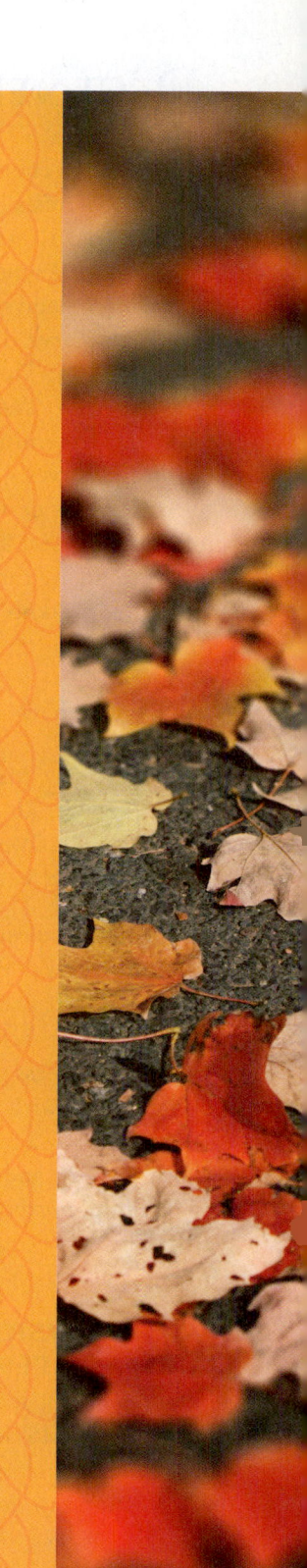

BRIEF OUTLINE

DEGENERATIVE NEUROLOGIC DISORDERS
Multiple Sclerosis
Parkinson Disease
Myasthenia Gravis

OTHER NEUROLOGIC DISORDERS
Huntington Disease
Amyotrophic Lateral Sclerosis
Guillain–Barré Syndrome
Trigeminal Neuralgia
Bell Palsy

Rabies
Tetanus
Creutzfeldt–Jakob Disease
SPINAL CORD DISORDERS
Spinal Cord Injury
Herniated Intervertebral Disk
Spinal Cord Tumor

APPLIED LEARNING OUTCOMES

After completing this chapter, you will be able to:

1. Describe the causes, pathophysiology, and manifestations of common degenerative neurologic disorders and spinal cord injuries.
2. Apply the nursing implications for medications and treatments ordered for patients experiencing degenerative neurologic disorders.
3. Describe the patient's functional ability according to the level of damage to the spinal cord.
4. Implement the collaborative care required for patients with quadriplegia and other spinal cord disorders.
5. Reinforce teaching to patients with a degenerative neurologic disorder.
6. Use the nursing process to assess, plan, and implement individualized care for the patient with degenerative neurologic and spinal cord disorders.

KEY TERMS

The key terms are defined on the pages listed below.

SPECIAL FEATURES

Degenerative neurologic disorders disrupt the central nervous system (CNS) and the peripheral nerves. They can cause devastating physical and emotional changes. The patient and family often face lifestyle and role changes and may even experience financial difficulties. The exact cause of these disorders is uncertain. Some may have a genetic or autoimmune cause.

Spinal cord injuries and herniated disk problems are also discussed in this chapter. Permanent damage to the spinal cord can also present physical and psychologic challenges to the patient and caregiver.

DEGENERATIVE NEUROLOGIC DISORDERS

Common degenerative disorders of the CNS include multiple sclerosis, Parkinson disease, myasthenia gravis, Huntington disease, and amyotrophic lateral sclerosis. Guillain–Barré syndrome is an example of a disorder affecting the peripheral nerves.

Cranial nerve disorders may be caused by trauma or inflammation. The pairs of cranial nerves are described in Chapter 38. The most common cranial nerve disorders affect the trigeminal (cranial nerve V) and facial (cranial nerve VII) nerves.

A variety of nervous system disorders may have toxic or infectious causes. These disorders are rare but require significant nursing care when they occur. Rabies, tetanus, and Creutzfeldt–Jakob disease are presented in the last part of this section.

Multiple Sclerosis

> **Key Concept**   Multiple sclerosis is the most frequent cause of nontraumatic chronic neurologic disability in young adults. Over time it progressively destroys the brain, optic nerves, and spinal cord.

Multiple sclerosis (MS) is a chronic, degenerative disease that damages the myelin sheath surrounding the axons of the CNS. Most patients experience periods of exacerbation (symptoms appear) followed by periods of remission, when symptoms are less obvious. In the end there is a progression of the disease with increasing loss of function.

MS affects Caucasian females more frequently between the ages of 20 and 40. A family history and living in the cold, damp, northern part of the United States increase the risk. The exact cause is unknown, but viral infections are thought to trigger an autoimmune response.

PATHOPHYSIOLOGY AND MANIFESTATIONS

Myelin sheaths make up what is known as white matter in the CNS. MS destroys the myelin sheath of the spinal cord, brain, and optic nerve and replaces it with *plaque*. The plaque can develop throughout the white matter of the CNS. This process is called **demyelination**. When the myelin is destroyed, nerve impulse conduction slows. The destroyed myelin is similar to a frayed electrical cord.

Manifestations vary according to the area of the nervous system affected (Figure 39-1■). They may appear suddenly and last for days to months. As the disease progresses, exacerbations last longer and occur more often. When the nerve cells are finally destroyed, the manifestations become permanent. Fatigue is a common but often ignored symptom that affects almost all patients. Medical care is sought when the patient develops diplopia, weakness, and tingling and numbness in the extremities. An unusual characteristic of MS is the worsening of motor symptoms after a hot shower or exercise.

As the disease progresses, the patient is prone to urinary tract infections (UTIs), pressure ulcers, joint contractures, injuries from falls, pneumonia, and depression. Death often results from pneumonia and a debilitated condition.

COLLABORATIVE CARE

The severity of the patient's symptoms guides the management plan. The treatment goal is to retain the patient's optimal level of functioning for as long as possible. As the patient becomes more disabled, speech, physical, and occupational therapists are consulted. Meeting the patient's and family's psychosocial needs is also an essential part of the care.

Diagnostic Tests

Initial manifestations may be vague or mild, making an early diagnosis difficult. A positive diagnosis is based on the patient's history, physical examination, and symptoms. Periodic diagnostic testing is done to follow the course of the disease. The following laboratory and diagnostic tests may be ordered:

■ *Cerebrospinal fluid (CSF) analysis* reveals increased T lymphocytes, protein, and immunoglobulin G (IgG). IgG indicates increased immune system activity.

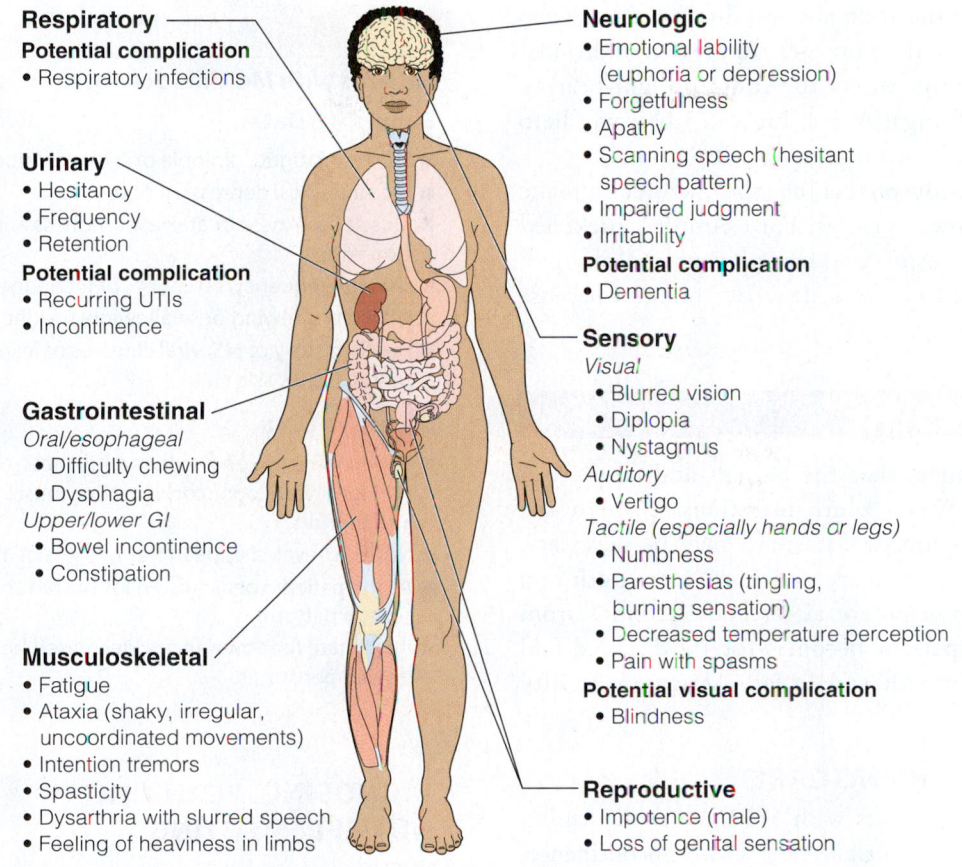

Respiratory
Potential complication
- Respiratory infections

Urinary
- Hesitancy
- Frequency
- Retention
Potential complication
- Recurring UTIs
- Incontinence

Gastrointestinal
Oral/esophageal
- Difficulty chewing
- Dysphagia
Upper/lower GI
- Bowel incontinence
- Constipation

Musculoskeletal
- Fatigue
- Ataxia (shaky, irregular, uncoordinated movements)
- Intention tremors
- Spasticity
- Dysarthria with slurred speech
- Feeling of heaviness in limbs

Neurologic
- Emotional lability (euphoria or depression)
- Forgetfulness
- Apathy
- Scanning speech (hesitant speech pattern)
- Impaired judgment
- Irritability
Potential complication
- Dementia

Sensory
Visual
- Blurred vision
- Diplopia
- Nystagmus
Auditory
- Vertigo
Tactile (especially hands or legs)
- Numbness
- Paresthesias (tingling, burning sensation)
- Decreased temperature perception
- Pain with spasms
Potential visual complication
- Blindness

Reproductive
- Impotence (male)
- Loss of genital sensation

Figure 39-1. ■ Multisystem effects of multiple sclerosis.

- *MRI* studies detect the plaque lesions in the white matter.
- *CT scan* of the brain shows atrophy and white matter lesions.

Medications

During an exacerbation, medications are used to decrease inflammation, which in turn limit manifestations and increase periods of remission. Corticosteroids and adrenocorticotropic hormone (ACTH) are most often used for this purpose. Another class of drugs, immunomodulators, seems to slow MS progression and reduce the number of attacks. These drugs include interferon beta-1a (Avonex), interferon beta-1b (Betaseron), glatiramer (Copaxone), and natalizumab (Tysabri). Natalizumab (Tysabri) may delay physical disability and reduce the frequency of attacks in people with relapsing MS. Patients with advanced MS are being treated with mitoxantrone (Novantrone), but use is limited because of its cardiotoxicity.

Muscle spasms along with pain develop in the patient's extremities, which may be reduced with baclofen (Lioresal) and dantrolene (Dantrium). Patients with severe spasticity may receive baclofen (Lioresal) by intrathecal route. Fatigue is managed with amantadine (Symmetrel) and modafinil (Provigil). Patients with urinary retention and frequency are given bethanechol (Urecholine) and propantheline (Pro-Banthine). Depression is managed with antidepressants.

Other Therapies

Physical therapists teach the patient ways to maintain balance. For example, the patient should stand with the feet slightly apart to give a wider base of support. The patient with ataxia is taught to use a walker or cane. Spasticity is managed with stretching exercises, gait training, and the use of braces or splints. Occupational therapy can assist the patient to maintain strength in the upper extremities. Surgery is used as a last resort to treat severe spasticity and uncontrolled pain.

Plasmapheresis (plasma exchange) is a procedure that removes plasma from whole blood. Its purpose is to remove T lymphocytes that cause inflammation. Patients unresponsive to corticosteroid therapy may receive plasmapheresis, but success is quite limited.

Nutrition

Diet therapy does not treat MS, but a well-balanced diet provides energy and strengthens the immune system. Reduced physical activity tends to cause weight gain and bone loss. Consult a dietitian about a diet low in calories but high in calcium and vitamin D. To prevent additional bone loss, encourage the patient to perform weight-bearing activities (e.g., walking). A diet high in fiber may help reduce the problem of constipation.

If the patient has dysphagia, change the diet to make chewing and swallowing easier. For example, thickened drinks and small bites of food can prevent choking and fatigue. Avoid serving crackers, dry toast, or chips because they may cause choking.

NURSING CARE

MS is a lifelong illness that the patient and family can manage at home. When acute infections threaten the patient's life, admission to a hospital may be necessary. As the disease advances, weakened muscle strength and spasticity increase the potential for complications from immobility. If the patient becomes totally disabled and the family cannot provide care, a long-term care facility will be necessary.

PRIORITIZING NURSING CARE

Priorities of care for patients with MS focus on managing fatigue, altered mobility, urinary and bowel incontinence, constipation, and altered respiratory status. In addition, the patient may be unable to perform activities of daily living (ADLs). Coping with changes in lifestyle may cause depression.

HEALTH PROMOTION

It is important for the patient to understand how to prevent fatigue and exacerbation of MS. The patient should be taught to avoid stress, extremes of cold and heat, high humidity, and physical overexertion. Discuss preventive measures to avoid urinary and respiratory infections. Women considering pregnancy should consult with their health care provider, as pregnancy can increase manifestations.

ASSESSING

Assessment data collected by the nurse can help identify the diagnosis, determine the extent to which the disease is interfering with the patient's life, and indicate the type of treatment required at this stage of the disease (Box 39-1 ■).

IDENTIFYING POTENTIAL COMPLICATIONS

The most common complications of MS include dysphagia, spasticity, respiratory and urinary infections, seizures, dementia, and blindness. As the disease progresses, the patient becomes immobile and cannot perform any self-care activities.

BOX 39-1	ASSESSMENT

Patients With Multiple Sclerosis

Subjective Data

- Extreme fatigue; diplopia or blurred vision
- Mood swings: depression to euphoria
- Muscle weakness or ataxia; numbness and tingling in extremities
- Urinary frequency, retention, or incontinence; constipation
- Difficulty chewing or swallowing; weight loss
- Family history of MS; viral illnesses or living in northern United States as a child

Objective Data

- Observe the patient for inattentiveness, difficulty finding the right word, poor coordination, muscle weakness, ataxia, and tremors.
- Note disheveled appearance or signs of incontinence.
- As the patient speaks, listen for slurred speech or hesitating speech pattern.
- Auscultate for bowel tones; decreased bowel tones indicate slowed peristalsis.

DIAGNOSING, PLANNING, AND IMPLEMENTING
Fatigue

Expected outcome: Will verbalize ways to conserve energy.

- Observe how fatigue affects the patient's ability to perform ADLs. *Knowing how fatigue affects the patient will assist in planning care.*
- Plan daily activities to include naps and rest periods. *Rest is essential to manage feelings of fatigue; relaxation periods can restore energy reserves.*
- Encourage the patient to perform tasks in the morning hours. *Fatigue usually worsens in the afternoon.*
- Advise to avoid extremes of temperature, such as hot showers or exposure to cold. *Constant body temperature may reduce exacerbations of this disorder.*

clinicalALERT

Fatigue in patients with MS is different from being "tired," so rest and sleep may not cause an improvement.

Self-Care Deficits

Expected outcome: Will perform ADLs to the extent possible.

- Encourage the patient to perform as much self-care as possible. *This promotes independence and decreases feelings of helplessness.*
- Allow adequate time to perform tasks. *Weak muscles and spasticity slow the patient's ability to perform all tasks.*

- Provide adaptive devices such as arm or wrist braces, long-handled combs, or modified clothing. Provide shower chair or raised toilet seat. *Adaptive devices encourage the patient to perform ADLs and may reduce fatigue.*

Ineffective Coping

Expected outcome: Will use effective coping strategies.

- Encourage the patient to verbalize his or her feelings. Consult with a counselor or psychiatrist as needed. *Patients with MS feel helpless and isolated. They often believe they cannot effectively manage the symptoms of MS.*
- Refer to a support group and provide information about the National MS Society. *Support groups and the National MS Society can offer suggestions for coping with MS.*
- Refer to state vocational rehabilitation agency as needed. *Vocational rehabilitation agencies can assist the patient with job retraining.*

MANAGING NURSING CARE

As appropriate and allowed by the designated duties and responsibilities of assistive personnel, the nurse may delegate nursing care activities such as providing oral and skin care and assisting with ADLs for the patient with MS. Before assigning tasks such as assisting with meals and fluid intake and ambulation, ensure that assistive personnel have a clear understanding of the importance of monitoring for difficulty swallowing and preventing falls.

EVALUATING

The nurse collects data to evaluate the effectiveness of care by assessing the degree of fatigue, neuromuscular and visual deficits, and mobility activities. Evaluate the patient's ability to perform ADLs, ability to cope with a chronic illness, and knowledge of medications, diet, and ways to prevent complications. For the immobile patient, evaluate for skin breakdown and pneumonia.

DOCUMENTING

Documentation includes presence of fatigue, neuromuscular deficits, self-care deficits, and coping strategies. Document teaching content related to medications, diet, potential complications, and stressors. Include interventions to assist with daily living, such as special devices for eating or ambulating.

CONTINUITY OF CARE

The newly diagnosed patient needs a realistic explanation of MS. Early in the course of the disease, refer patients to a support group. Encourage patients to keep a diary about symptoms and activities in order to identify stressors. Teaching is best done when the patient is in a period of remission. Discuss the following topics with the patient and family:

- Medications, side effects, and interactions with prescription or other drugs

- Adequate fluid intake, regular bowel and bladder elimination schedule, well-balanced meals, daily physical exercise, and weight control
- Ways to prevent complications such as pressure ulcers and respiratory and UTIs
- Ways to cope with pain, dysphagia, spasticity, and vision changes
- Importance of follow-up care with the physician, nurses, and rehabilitation team

If the patient is employed, discuss the availability of sick leave during periods of exacerbation. As the disease progresses, the patient will require assistance from many community agencies, including home health nursing. A helpful resource is the National MS Society.

NURSING CARE PLAN
Patient With Multiple Sclerosis

David Wilson, a 30-year-old from northern Michigan, is married with a 3-month-old baby. Over the past 2 months he has experienced increased urinary frequency and urgency. He also has had two episodes of visual "fuzziness" associated with double vision and dizziness when he stands up suddenly. He says, "I feel exhausted all of the time, even when I sleep 8 hours at night." His wife urges Mr. Wilson to make an appointment with a neurologist.

Assessment
Mr. Wilson sees a neurologist, who finds weakness in Mr. Wilson's legs and right arm when he tries to hold any object, as well as blurred vision, diplopia, hesitant speech, and forgetfulness. David states, "At times, my arms and legs feel so heavy. When my arm feels weak, I'm afraid of dropping my new infant son when I hold him." His wife says that she has tried to ignore how often David forgets to do routine household chores. An MRI confirms the diagnosis of MS. Mr. Wilson and his wife are fearful and unsure what this means for their future.

Nursing Diagnosis
The following priority nursing diagnoses are established for this patient.

- *Impaired Physical Mobility* related to leg weakness and muscle fatigue
- *Risk for Injury* related to extremity weakness, visual changes, and forgetfulness
- *Fatigue* related to neuromuscular destruction from the disease process

Expected Outcomes
Mr. Wilson is referred to physical and occupational therapy for evaluation. In addition, the Wilsons are referred to Ms. Jane Baldwin, a home health nurse. The expected outcomes of care are that Mr. Wilson will:

- Remain physically mobile, either by himself or through the use of assistive devices.
- Remain free of injury.
- Perform ADLs.

Planning and Implementation

- Implement weight-bearing activities such as daily walking to help conserve bone mass.
- Encourage Mr. Wilson to stand with his feet slightly apart to maintain balance.
- Implement exercises prescribed by the occupational therapist to maintain strength in the upper extremities and to carry out ADLs.
- Have the home health nurse assess the Wilsons' home for any potential hazards and ease of mobility.
- Suggest safety measures such as installing handrails in the stairwell and shower, removing throw rugs from the bathroom, adding a night-light in the bathroom, and wearing shoes with nonskid soles.
- Have Mrs. Wilson make lists of the household chores and encourage Mr. Wilson to help with the chores but to balance all activities with rest periods.
- Suggest guidelines to Mr. Wilson so that he can safely hold his infant son.
- Assist the Wilsons to set realistic goals and review possible coping strategies.
- Encourage the Wilsons to attend monthly support group meetings for MS patients and their families for 6 months.

Evaluation

Six months later, the physical therapist finds that Mr. Wilson requires the use of a cane to maintain his balance and is taught how to use it. Ms. Baldwin's follow-up visit notes that Mr. Wilson needs more assistance with mobility but is able to complete other ADL needs. She explores how Mr. and Mrs. Wilson are coping and suggests meeting with a family counselor. The family understands that Mr. Wilson will have periods of remission but that his physical condition will deteriorate over time. They are concerned about their future but are trying to remain positive.

Critical Thinking in the Nursing Process

1. Outline a plan for teaching Mr. and Mrs. Wilson about situations or factors that can cause an exacerbation of symptoms.
2. Describe evidence-based nursing approaches to use if Mr. Wilson develops problems with swallowing.
3. Explain how the effect of a chronic degenerative neurologic disease might differ in a young adult versus an older adult.

Note: Discussion of Critical Thinking questions appears on the companion website.

Parkinson Disease

Key Concept Parkinson disease (PD) is a slow progressive neurodegenerative movement disorder, resulting from a loss of dopamine. Levodopa is the most common drug used to increase dopamine levels in patients with PD.

Parkinson disease (PD) is a chronic, progressive, degenerative neurologic disease that alters motor coordination. It is one of the most common neurologic disorders, affecting approximately 1 million people in the United States. Most people are diagnosed after the age of 60 but the disease can develop in those younger than 40. PD seems to affect Caucasian men more often than women.

The cause of primary PD is unknown. *Secondary parkinsonism* may be caused by repeated head trauma, encephalitis, or exposure to carbon monoxide or cyanide poisoning. Drugs such phenothiazines, haloperidol (Haldol), and methyldopa (Aldomet) may induce parkinsonism. The symptoms disappear when the drug is stopped.

PATHOPHYSIOLOGY AND MANIFESTATIONS

PD results from a deficiency of **dopamine**, which is a chemical produced in the substantia nigra of the midbrain that controls complex movements, cognition, motivation, and pleasure. In PD, neurons in the cerebral cortex atrophy, and the number of dopamine receptors decreases. This results in a decrease in dopamine (a neurotransmitter responsible for voluntary motor function). The balance of dopamine (an inhibitory neurotransmitter) and acetylcholine (an excitatory neurotransmitter) is upset. When dopamine levels drop, acetylcholine is no longer inhibited. This means that acetylcholine causes constant excitement of the motor neurons, which is the basis for the manifestations of PD.

Manifestations are subtle and may be mistaken as signs of normal aging (Figure 39-2■). The onset is gradual, and the disease progresses slowly. There are three cardinal signs: (1) tremor, (2) rigidity, and (3) **bradykinesia** (slowed voluntary movements and speech). The classic "pill-rolling" tremor occurs when the thumb and fingers move like they are rolling a pill. Tremors disappear during sleep and movement. Muscle rigidity makes active and passive movement difficult. The extremity may move, but does so in a jerky movement called *cogwheel rigidity*. Other manifestations are noted in Box 39-2■.

COLLABORATIVE CARE

There are no specific tests to diagnose PD. Diagnosis is based on the patient's history and the presence of two of the three cardinal symptoms. A PET scan may show decreased levels of levodopa (a precursor of dopamine).

Interventions vary with the extent of the patient's manifestations and disability. The patient may be treated with

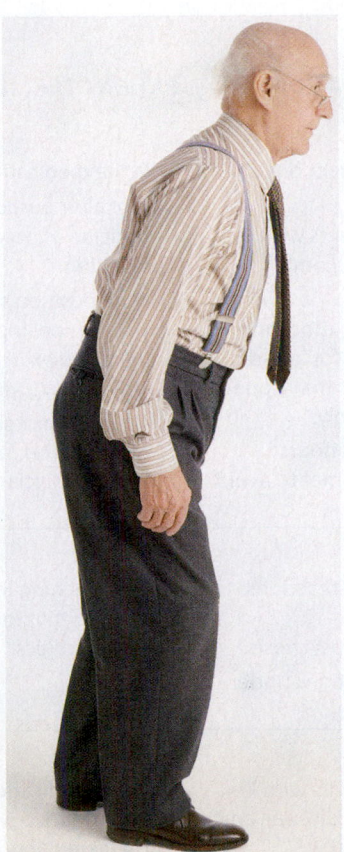

Figure 39-2. ■ In Parkinson disease, subtle changes in facial expression and movement occur. (Source: Susanna Price / Dorling Kindersley Media Library.)

BOX 39-2	MANIFESTATIONS OF PARKINSON DISEASE

- Tremor that moves from one arm to both arms and may involve lips, jaw, head, and lower extremities
- Muscle rigidity
- Stooped posture and shuffling gait
- Bradykinesia:
  - Inability to initiate voluntary movements
  - Slurred speech, low amplitude
  - Decreased blinking
  - Masklike, expressionless face
- Difficulty swallowing, drooling
- Postural hypotension
- Skin problems: excess sweating on the face and neck; excessively oily skin
- Depression, memory loss

medication, surgery, and rehabilitation. The goal is to retain the highest level of function for as long as possible.

Medications

Drug therapy does not cure PD, but rather is used to control symptoms. Four different classes of drugs are used:

dopaminergics, *dopamine agonists*, *anticholinergics*, and *monoamine oxidase inhibitors* (*MAOIs*) (Table 39-1 ■). Drugs are chosen based on the patient's symptoms, individual response, and the length of effectiveness. Initially, patients receive dopaminergics such as amantadine (Symmetrel) or anticholinergics. As the disease progresses, carbidopa–levodopa (Sinemet) is added. Over time, levodopa, a dopaminergic, loses its effectiveness, and side effects increase. Dopamine agonists are added to increase the effectiveness of levodopa. Eventually, drugs no longer control the symptoms, and the patient's condition declines. Catechol-*O*-methyltransferase (COMT) inhibitors, such as tolcapone (Tasmar), are a newer class of drugs that reduce symptoms caused by the "wearing-off" of carbidopa–levodopa. It is essential for patients with PD to receive their medications at the scheduled times to reduce "off-times."

Surgery

The most common procedure is deep brain stimulation (DBS). It involves surgically implanting a battery-operated neurostimulator device. An insulated wire is placed in the thalamus and connected to a pulse generator, which is placed under the skin near the clavicle. Once in place, the device sends mild electrical impulses into the brain. The impulses block the signals that cause PD tremors.

Two surgeries, thalamotomy or pallidotomy, may be used to relieve symptoms. Both procedures are done under local anesthesia. *Thalamotomy* destroys part of the thalamus to reduce tremors; it is reserved for younger people with extreme unilateral tremor. In the *pallidotomy*, part of the globus pallidus (basal ganglia located in cerebral cortex that is responsible for skilled movement) is destroyed to control rigidity and tremors.

Complementary Therapies

Yoga and t'ai chi are well-established therapies to improve strength, balance, and flexibility in patients with PD, along with traditional medicines. Massage therapy and acupuncture seem to decrease the muscle stiffness and aching that accompanies PD. No specific herbal supplements are recommended and should be used only with the guidance of a physician.

NURSING CARE

Patients with PD have complex needs. In the early stages, most patients remain at home with limited family assistance. As the patient's health deteriorates and care increases, the family may want to consider placement in a long-term care facility. Throughout this illness, the patient and family need continued support and counseling.

TABLE 39-1	**Giving Medications Safely: Parkinson Disease**		
CLASS/DRUGS	**PURPOSE**	**NURSING IMPLICATIONS**	**PATIENT TEACHING**
Dopaminergics ■ Levodopa (Larodopa) ■ *Carbidopa–levodopa (Sinemet)* ■ *Amantadine (Symmetrel)*	Levodopa is converted to dopamine in the brain, and carbidopa prevents levodopa from being destroyed. Levodopa is the most effective drug for PD. Amantadine, an antiviral drug, raises dopamine levels.	Check for drug interactions before giving. Do not give to patients with angle-closure glaucoma. Monitor for nausea, hypotension, confusion, and dyskinesia. Assess for "on–off" effect—symptoms may appear or improve suddenly. Hold levodopa for 8 hours before giving Sinemet to avoid toxicity.	Take the medication as directed. Do not alter dosages. Inform the physician of other drugs you are taking. Change position slowly to avoid hypotension. Increase fluid intake and exercise regularly. Report the "on–off" effect, decreased motor movements, insomnia, and rapid heartbeat to your physician.
Dopamine agonists ■ Apomorphine (Apokyn) ■ Bromocriptine (Parlodel) ■ Pramipexole (Mirapex) ■ Ropinirole (Requip)	They are given to decrease tremor, rigidity, and bradykinesia.	Monitor for adverse reactions: nausea, orthostatic hypotension, and psychosis. See nursing implications under the dopaminergics.	Patient teaching information is similar to that found under the dopaminergics.
Anticholinergics ■ Trihexyphenidyl (Artane) ■ Benztropine (Cogentin)	They decrease the activity of acetylcholine and are given during the early stages of the disease or when the patient can no longer take levodopa. These medications ease drooling, tremors, and rigidity.	Do not give to patients with glaucoma, cardiac disease, and prostatic hypertrophy. Check for drug interactions. Monitor for side effects of dry mouth, blurred vision, constipation, and urinary retention. Taper off slowly to avoid parkinsonism.	Take the medication as prescribed. Do not suddenly stop taking anticholinergics. Check with physician before taking with other medications. Report blurred vision, constipation, difficulty urinating, or increased temperature. Drink adequate amounts of fluid to prevent dehydration.
Monoamine oxidase inhibitors (MAOIs) ■ Rasagiline (Azilect) ■ Selegiline (Eldepryl)	It reduces tremor, rigidity, and bradykinesia.	Monitor for ataxia, insomnia, dizziness, or postural hypotension.	Take the medication as directed. Report signs of insomnia, difficulty moving, or dizziness.

Note: Medications identified in *italics* are among the 200 most frequently prescribed drugs in the United States.

PRIORITIZING NURSING CARE

Patients with PD develop problems similar to those of other degenerative neurologic disorders. Refer to the previous nursing care section in this chapter for discussion of fatigue, self-care deficits, and ineffective coping. This section focuses on mobility, communication, and nutrition. In later stages, the patient may develop airway management problems.

HEALTH PROMOTION

It is important to teach preventive measures when caring for patients with PD. They are at risk for developing malnutrition, falls, constipation, skin breakdown from incontinence, and joint contractures. Teach patients ways to prevent postural hypotension when changing positions. Also, address safety issues when taking their medications.

ASSESSING

Assessment should identify the patient's symptoms and the extent to which the disease is affecting the patient's daily life (Box 39-3 ■). It is important to note the patient's ability to function safely.

IDENTIFYING POTENTIAL COMPLICATIONS

Common complications associated with PD are malnutrition from dysphagia and an inability to prepare meals, falls from altered balance and posture, and impaired communication.

Patients With Parkinson Disease

Subjective Data

- Difficulty making decisions
- Mood swings; depression; insomnia
- Drooling or difficulty swallowing; weight loss
- Arm or leg stiffness; frequent falls
- Loss of dexterity or ability to write
- Urinary incontinence; constipation
- Past medical history of head trauma, exposure to metals, or carbon monoxide
- Use of major tranquilizers

Objective Data

- Measure height and weight.
- Observe the patient for infrequent blinking, expressionless face, slow slurred speech, stooped posture, shuffling gait, or depression.
- Assess for muscles that move in small jerky movements.
- Assess for tremors at rest that disappear with movement, or "pill-rolling" tremor.
- Palpate the skin for excessive sweating or oiliness; inspect for injury from falls.

Immobility predisposes the patient with PD to pneumonia, UTIs, and skin breakdown. Sleep disturbances are common, affecting quality of life. Dementia also occurs frequently.

DIAGNOSING, PLANNING, AND IMPLEMENTING

Impaired Physical Mobility

Expected outcome: Will maintain mobility without injury.

- Perform range-of-motion (ROM) exercises at least twice a day, emphasizing the trunk, neck, arms, hips, and legs. *ROM exercises promote joint function, strengthen muscles, and prevent contractures.*
- Assist with ambulation at least four times a day. *Exercise fosters independence and self-esteem.*
- Use assistive devices such as canes, splints, braces, or lift chairs as needed. *Assistive devices improve balance, protect joints, and help the patient maintain correct positioning.*
- Consult with a physical therapist. *Physical therapy can help to improve coordination, balance, gait, and transfers. Exercise is also important in preventing contractures.*

Impaired Verbal Communication

Expected outcome: Will communicate orally or with assistive devices.

- Teach the patient to face the listener and speak in short sentences. Allow extra time for self-expression. *These strategies reduce the patient's frustration in communicating.*

- Provide a write-on, wipe-off slate or flash cards with common phrases; or ask the patient to point to objects. *Individualizing communication decreases anxiety and isolation.*
- Suggest referral to a speech therapist to develop oral exercises and interventions to facilitate speaking. *The muscles of speech and swallowing are affected by PD. Speech therapists can teach breathing patterns to improve voice tone and pitch.*
- Try to anticipate the patient's needs. *This reduces the patient's frustration.*

Imbalanced Nutrition: Less Than Body Requirements

Expected outcome: Will maintain normal weight without difficulty swallowing.

- Place in upright position for all meals and for an hour afterward, cut food into small pieces, and keep suction equipment at the bedside *to decrease the risk for aspiration.* Massage the throat as the patient swallows *to help swallowing.*
- Reduce distractions during mealtime. *This allows the patient to focus on eating, chewing, and swallowing.*
- Obtain utensils that are easier for the patient to grasp. *Modified utensils help the patient eat and maintain a sense of self-esteem.*
- Increase daily fluid intake and fiber. *Fluids and fiber prevent constipation caused by several of the anti-Parkinson medications.*
- Weigh weekly. *Early recognition of weight loss allows for quicker intervention.*

clinicalALERT

Serve semisolid or thickened liquid foods to prevent aspiration.

MANAGING NURSING CARE

As appropriate and allowed by the designated duties and responsibilities of assistive personnel, the nurse may delegate nursing care activities such as assisting with ADLs for the patient with PD. Before assigning tasks such as assisting with meals and fluid intake and ambulation, ensure assistive personnel have a clear understanding of the importance of monitoring for difficulty swallowing and preventing falls.

EVALUATING

Evaluate the effectiveness of nursing care by collecting data related to the presence of common manifestations of PD and any complications. Determine the patient's ability to ambulate, chew, swallow, and communicate. Evaluate for safety risks; impaired body image; and knowledge of disease process, diet, safety, and medications.

DOCUMENTING

Documentation includes noting the patient's tremors, gait, motor function and muscle strength, speech pattern, skin integrity, and swallowing. Record referrals to speech and occupational therapy and dietitian. Patient and family teaching about safety measures, diet, medications, and exercise is documented.

CONTINUITY OF CARE

Persons with PD face such complications as skin breakdown from incontinence or immobility, falls, and joint contractures. As their condition progresses, they may develop malnutrition, constipation, or infection. Provide information about the disease; its management; and strategies for coping with tremors, dysphagia, and speech problems. Explain the purpose, side effects, and directions for taking each medication. Reinforce gait training, ROM exercises, and proper posture. Explain the importance of follow-up meetings with speech, physical, and occupational therapy.

Refer the patient to home health services so that the nurse can assess the home for potential hazards. Poor vision, stooped posture, and confusion increase the patient's risk for injury. Discuss safety measures such as removing loose rugs and excess furniture, installing a raised toilet seat and handrails in the bathroom, and providing adequate lighting throughout the home and in outside areas. Refer to local support groups and the American Parkinson's Disease Association.

Myasthenia Gravis

Myasthenia gravis is a chronic, autoimmune disorder affecting women under 40 and men older than 60 years of age. Patients experience periods of exacerbations and remissions. Stress, pregnancy, and secondary infections may trigger an acute onset.

PATHOPHYSIOLOGY AND MANIFESTATIONS

For an unknown reason, the thymus gland produces antibodies that block or reduce the number acetylcholine receptors at each neuromuscular junction. Nerve impulses cannot be sent to the cranial nerves that control muscles of the face, lips, tongue, neck, and throat. This causes weakness of the facial, speech, and chewing muscles. Characteristic manifestations first develop in the eye muscles causing diplopia and eyelid ptosis. Next the facial, speech, and chewing muscles are involved, causing slurred speech, nasal voice, difficulty chewing and swallowing, and fatigue. A smile appears as a snarl or grimace. There is progressive difficulty in performing fine motor tasks such as writing and progressive weakness of the respiratory muscles. Onset is gradual, and manifestations may vary each day.

Complications relate to the muscles involved and degree of muscle weakness. When pharyngeal and respiratory muscles are affected, swallowing and breathing become difficult. The patient faces the risk of aspiration and respiratory insufficiency. Two life-threatening emergencies are possible:

1. *Myasthenic crisis* is due to missed doses of medication or an infection. Patients suddenly develop increased muscle weakness, resulting in dysphagia, impaired speech, severe respiratory distress, and anxiety.
2. *Cholinergic crisis* is caused by overmedication with anticholinesterase (cholinergic) medications. The symptoms are similar to myasthenic crisis: severe muscle weakness plus nausea, vomiting, abdominal cramps, increased salivation, sweating, and bradycardia.

Either crisis requires immediate treatment and the possible need for mechanical ventilation.

COLLABORATIVE CARE

A physical examination of the facial, oculomotor, laryngeal, and respiratory muscles is done. Diagnosis is confirmed by injecting edrophonium chloride (Tensilon), a short-acting anticholinesterase. Patients with myasthenia gravis show dramatic improvement in muscle strength, but the improvement lasts only about 5 minutes. *Electromyographic (EMG) studies* show increased muscle fatigue. *CT scan* of the chest may show a tumor of the thymus gland.

Pyridostigmine (Mestinon) and neostigmine (Prostigmin), anticholinesterase medications, are the treatment of choice for myasthenia gravis. Dosage is adjusted until the patient's symptoms decrease. It is difficult to balance the correct dose without causing myasthenic or cholinergic crisis. The patient is taught to record all signs and symptoms carefully so that medication doses can be adjusted (Table 39-2 ■). Prednisone and cytotoxic agents, such as cyclosporine or azathioprine (Imuran), are added to block antibody production or decrease circulating antibodies.

Along with drug therapy, a **thymectomy** (surgical removal of the thymus gland) may be performed to remove the source of the antibodies. A short-term treatment option involves plasmapheresis. This procedure removes the antiacetylcholine receptor antibodies so that muscle weakness and fatigue decrease.

clinicalALERT

Administer anticholinesterase drugs on a strict time schedule. Patients with dysphagia may not be able to swallow the medication unless it is taken exactly on time. Doses taken too late may cause myasthenic crisis. Taking doses early may result in cholinergic crisis.

TABLE 39-2	Giving Medications Safely: Myasthenia Gravis		
CLASS/DRUGS	**PURPOSE**	**NURSING IMPLICATIONS**	**PATIENT TEACHING**
Anticholinesterase drugs ■ Neostigmine (Prostigmin) ■ Ambenonium (Mytelase) ■ Pyridostigmine (Mestinon, Regoncl) ■ *For diagnosis:* Edrophonium (Tensilon)	Anticholinesterase drugs prolong the action of acetylcholine to improve muscle contraction. Dose is adjusted to obtain maximum benefit with the fewest side effects. They are contraindicated in patients with urinary or GI tract obstruction, asthma, or hyperthyroidism.	Identify the patient's ability to swallow. Give the medication on a regular schedule at the exact time. Monitor for *myasthenic crisis:* severe muscle weakness and difficulty breathing, swallowing, or speaking. Notify the physician immediately. Monitor for cholinergic crisis: excess salivation and sweating, bradycardia, nausea, and vomiting. Notify the physician immediately.	Take the drug as directed on a regular schedule at the exact time. Report symptoms of *myasthenic crisis* immediately: severe muscle weakness; fast heartbeat; and difficulty breathing, swallowing, or speaking. Report symptoms of cholinergic crisis immediately: slow heartbeat, increased salivation or sweating, decreased blood pressure. Wear MedicAlert ID.

NURSING CARE

The nurse collects data about the patient's muscle weakness; speech, chewing, or swallowing difficulties; and changes in vision. Nursing care focuses on decreasing or preventing respiratory and swallowing problems, as well as reducing fatigue. The nursing diagnoses and interventions are similar to those presented earlier in caring for the patient with MS or PD.

Once the patient and family understand the disease and ways to cope with the physical and psychosocial problems, the patient can be managed at home. Review home care assessment and strategies found in the MS and PD sections.

Teaching should emphasize medication actions, side effects, scheduling, and symptoms of myasthenic and cholinergic crisis. Stress the importance of taking medications on an exact schedule. Advise the patient to wear a MedicAlert bracelet.

Refer the patient and family to local support groups, and provide information about the Myasthenia Gravis Foundation. Pregnancy should be discussed with the physician because it may cause manifestations to worsen. Also, medications such as neostigmine (Prostigmin) cross the placenta.

OTHER NEUROLOGIC DISORDERS

Huntington Disease

Huntington disease (HD) is a progressive, inherited neurologic disease. Men and women are affected equally between the ages of 30 and 50. HD is transmitted as an autosomal-dominant genetic trait. Each child of a parent with HD has a 50% chance of inheriting the disease. There is no cure for this disease.

HD involves a lack of a neurotransmitter, gamma-aminobutyric acid (GABA). This causes acetylcholine levels to drop and dopamine levels to rise. Unlike PD, in which a dopamine deficit slows movement, in HD, the excess dopamine causes uncontrolled movement. Without GABA, there is premature death of basal ganglia and cerebral cortex cells. All of these changes develop slowly, affecting (1) personality, (2) intellectual function, and (3) movement.

Emotional lability ranges from irritability and anger to depression. Delusions and hallucinations are not unusual. Memory and intellectual function decline to the point of dementia.

Chorea (constant, jerky, uncontrolled movements of the body) is a characteristic manifestation. The patient exhibits mild fidgeting or writhing and twisting of the entire body. Motor symptoms are worse with emotional stress, but decrease during sleep. Facial grimaces and tics affect speech, chewing, and swallowing, leading to choking and malnutrition. Bowel and bladder control are lost. As the chorea increases, the patient is confined to bed. Prognosis is poor, with inevitable total dependence. Death is usually from aspiration pneumonia.

There is no specific test for this disease. Diagnosis is based on symptoms and family history. A PET scan shows changes in the brain. Offspring concerned about their chances of developing HD should have genetic testing.

Medications are given to control the symptoms of HD. The chorea movements may be modified by tetrabenazine (Xenazine) or haloperidol (Haldol). Antidepressants and antipsychotics are prescribed in the early stage of the disease.

At first, the patient and family can manage care at home. Many families are overwhelmed with the future physical and psychologic debilitation that the disease brings. Refer them to local support groups, the Huntington's Disease Foundation, or a psychologist. As the patient's health declines, care is given similar to care for other deteriorating neurologic disorders. Eventually, skilled long-term care is needed.

Amyotrophic Lateral Sclerosis

Amyotrophic lateral sclerosis (ALS), also called *Lou Gehrig disease* after the famous baseball player who suffered from it, is a rapidly progressive, fatal neurologic disease. The exact cause is unknown. More men are affected between the ages of 40 and 60.

ALS involves loss of motor neurons in the spinal cord and brainstem. When electrical impulses cannot be sent from the brain to the voluntary muscles, the muscles lose strength and atrophy. Although body function decreases, the person remains mentally alert.

This disorder is characterized by muscle weakness; **fasciculations** (involuntary contractions of the voluntary muscles, or twitching); and muscle wasting of the arms, legs, and trunk. Brainstem involvement causes speech and swallowing difficulties. Toward the end, patients develop breathing problems, and death is from aspiration pneumonia or respiratory failure. About 50% of patients die within 2 to 5 years of diagnosis.

Diagnosis is based on the patient's symptoms. A series of different tests are done to rule out other conditions that mimic ALS. An EMG confirms muscle weakness. Muscle biopsies show loss of muscle fiber.

There is no cure for ALS. Only one medication, riluzole (Rilutek), seems to slow the destruction of motor neurons. Other medications include baclofen and diazepam to relieve muscle spasms. Psychologic support is important for the patient and family as the disease progresses. The patient and family should be referred to an ALS support group, social worker, or psychologist as needed.

For as long as possible, promote the patient's independence in performing daily ADLs. Nursing care is similar to that for the patient with MS, discussed earlier in this chapter. Before speech is lost, develop communication signals, such as blinking for yes/no answers. When swallowing or breathing problems develop, anticipate enteral feedings and mechanical ventilation. To manage the patient at home, the family is taught the following: (1) suctioning techniques and the Heimlich maneuver, (2) bowel and urinary catheter care, (3) enteral feedings, (4) skin care, and (5) turning and positioning the patient.

Guillain–Barré Syndrome

Guillain–Barré syndrome (GBS) is an acute, progressive inflammation of the peripheral nervous system (PNS). The cause is unknown, but GBS most often follows a recent respiratory or gastrointestinal (GI) viral or bacterial infection, viral vaccination, or surgery. Infection with *Campylobacter jejuni* causes about 60% of Guillain–Barré cases.

PATHOPHYSIOLOGY AND MANIFESTATIONS

A cell-mediated immune system reaction destroys the myelin sheath covering the peripheral nerves. Without myelin, impulses are poorly conducted to the sensory and motor nerves. This causes rapid, muscle weakness, loss of reflexes, and paralysis.

Manifestations of GBS start in the lower extremities and move upward. The first symptoms are bilateral weakness and numbness and tingling in the legs. Then weakness and sensory loss extend to the arms, torso, and cranial nerves. Paralysis of the respiratory muscles can alter respiratory function. Cranial nerve involvement causes chewing, swallowing, and talking problems. If the autonomic nervous system is affected, blood pressure and pulse changes develop. Throughout this process, the person remains alert and oriented.

The most serious complication is respiratory failure. If this develops, the patient will need endotracheal intubation and mechanical ventilation to prevent respiratory arrest. (See nursing care for the patient with mechanical ventilation in Chapter 23.) Other complications, such as skin breakdown and deep venous thrombosis (DVT), relate to the length of time the patient is paralyzed.

COLLABORATIVE CARE

Most patients with GBS recover with few or no residual effects. Recovery time depends on how fast the myelin sheath can rebuild itself. Average rehabilitation is about 6 months, but may take as long as 1 year. As the nerves recover, the patient's symptoms improve in reverse order.

Diagnosis of GBS is based on clinical symptoms and a recent viral infection. A lumbar puncture shows elevated CSF protein levels. The results of EMG studies show a definite slowing of nerve conduction.

Medical management consists of plasmapheresis and intravenous immune globulin. Plasmapheresis removes the antibodies that caused GBS. It is beneficial when used within the first 2 weeks. Patients typically have five exchanges over 8 to 10 days. The action of intravenous immune globulin is unclear, but the effects are similar to those of plasmapheresis. Antibiotics are prescribed for urinary tract or respiratory infections. Anticoagulants are given to prevent DVT and pulmonary embolism. Morphine is given to control muscle pain.

NURSING CARE

Patients are acutely ill and are managed in a critical care unit. Nursing assessments are done every 1 to 2 hours. Nursing interventions focus on preventing immobility problems; promoting adequate hydration, nutrition, and respiratory function; and providing psychosocial support. It is important to anticipate the needs of the patient and family. They are stunned by the rapid deterioration of function and fear permanent paralysis.

After the acute phase, the patient is transferred to a skilled nursing facility or home. Those with extensive paralysis need inpatient or outpatient physical, occupational, and speech therapy. The caregiver may need help from a homemaker or home health aide. When recovery is long, the caregiver will need respite care.

Trigeminal Neuralgia

Trigeminal neuralgia (*tic douloureux*) involves two sensory branches of the trigeminal nerve: the maxillary and mandibular (Figure 39-3■). The disease causes pain along one or both of these branches. It usually affects middle-aged and older adult women more often than men. The actual cause is unknown but may be from dental or surgical

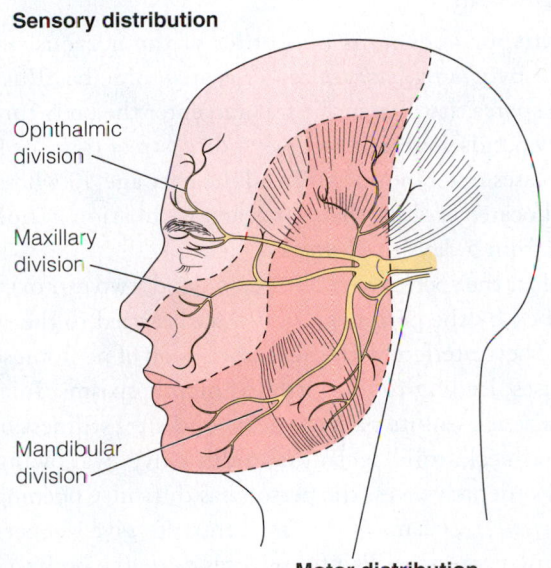

Sensory distribution

Ophthalmic division

Maxillary division

Mandibular division

Motor distribution

Figure 39-3. ■ Sensory and motor branches of the trigeminal nerve. There are three sensory branches: ophthalmic, maxillary, and mandibular.

procedures, facial trauma, infection, or pressure on the nerve by a tumor.

Trigeminal neuralgia is characterized by periodic, severe, one-sided facial pain lasting a few seconds to a few minutes. The pain is described as stabbing or burning in the forehead, along the nose, lips, or cheek. Attacks occur for several weeks and then suddenly disappear. The patient may remain pain free for days to years. With age, remissions become shorter.

Trigger zones on the face initiate an attack when they are stimulated. Simple actions such as shaving, chewing, brushing the teeth, or washing the face or wind or a change in temperature can set off an attack. An attack may cause wincing, grimacing, or tearing of the eye. To control pain, patients may refuse to wash, shave, eat, or talk.

Diagnosis is based on the characteristic location and type of pain. The drug most useful in controlling the pain is the anticonvulsant carbamazepine (Tegretol). When ineffective, other medications such as phenytoin (Dilantin), gabapentin (Neurontin), and baclofen (Lioresal) are added. If drug therapy fails, biofeedback and nerve blocks with local anesthetics are tried. Another option is a **rhizotomy** (the surgical severing of a nerve root to control pain). Only the sensory nerve root is destroyed. Motor function is preserved so that eating is unaffected. If the ophthalmic branch is damaged, the corneal reflex is lost.

Nursing care focuses on teaching self-care strategies, including medications and potential side effects. Because this is a chronic condition, long-term use of narcotics is avoided. Discuss ways to avoid trigger points, such as using room temperature water and soft cotton pads to wash the face. If the patient refuses to eat during periods of pain attacks, encourage a soft high-protein and high-calorie diet.

After surgery, the patient may lose sensation and corneal reflex on the involved side. Teach the patient to chew on the unaffected side, to avoid hot foods or liquids, and to brush the teeth and check for food pockets between gums and cheek after every meal. Men should use an electric razor to shave. Patients should also protect the face from very cold or windy conditions, and, if necessary, wear a protective eye shield.

Bell Palsy

Bell palsy (facial paralysis) is associated with the herpes simplex virus. Inflammation causes edema and pressure on the facial nerve, resulting in necrosis. This leads to sudden weakness and paralysis on one side of the face. Paralysis distorts the affected side, causing ptosis of the eyelid, tearing, mouth drooping, drooling, an inability to smile, and difficulty chewing (Figure 39-4■). There is also pain around or

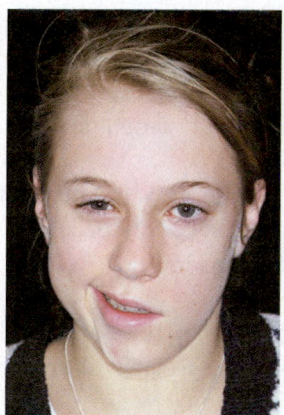

Figure 39-4. ■ The patient with Bell palsy shows the typical drooping of one side of the face. (Source: Dr. P. Marazzi/Science Source.)

behind the ear. Most patients improve within a few weeks to months, although some are left with residual paralysis.

Diagnosis is based on the patient's facial appearance. Treatment is a short-term course of steroids. Because it is linked to the herpes virus, patients are given antiviral drugs. Mild analgesics may reduce the facial pain. Nursing and home care is similar to that for the patient with trigeminal neuralgia. (Review the strategies listed after surgery.) In addition, teach the patient to apply warm, moist heat, such as gel packs, which increases circulation and relieves pain. A soft diet that does not require chewing and six small meals per day are helpful. Teach the patient to chew slowly on the unaffected side and to avoid hot foods.

The loss of blinking increases the risk for corneal drying. Demonstrate how to instill artificial tears four times a day and how to apply an eye patch at night. Be sure the patient understands how to inspect the eye each day and to report eye pain, redness, swelling, or discharge. Recommend wearing dark glasses or goggles when outside or working in dusty conditions.

Rabies

Rabies is a viral infection of the CNS caused by an animal bite. The rabies virus is carried by wild and domestic animals, including bats, skunks, foxes, raccoons, cats, and dogs. The virus spreads from the wound to the peripheral nerves and eventually travels to the CNS. Incubation period varies from 14 days to 3 months. Any animal that has bitten someone is observed for 1 to 2 weeks to detect rabies symptoms. Sick animals are euthanized, and their brains are examined for the rabies virus.

Clinical manifestations occur in stages. In the *prodromal stage*, the wound is painful, with a tingling sensation. The patient develops flulike symptoms such as malaise, fever, headache, and lethargy. This stage is followed by the *excitement stage*, during which the person experiences delirium, painful spasms of the larynx when attempting to drink (*hydrophobia*), and large amounts of thick mucus. Without treatment, death occurs in about 7 days from respiratory failure.

To prevent rabies, it is recommended that all household dogs and cats be immunized. Any animal bite or scratch is thoroughly cleaned with soap and water to remove the saliva and dilute the virus. The person is taken immediately to the emergency department to receive rabies immune globulin (RIG) as soon as possible after the bite if the bite is from a wild animal or a domestic animal that has not been immunized. This is followed by five doses of inactivated human diploid cell rabies vaccine (HDCV) intramuscularly on the day of exposure and on days 3, 7, 14, and 28 after exposure.

clinicalALERT

Never give RIG and HDCV in the same syringe or at the same site because they inactivate each other.

Patients who show signs of rabies are cared for in the critical care unit, with the room dark and quiet to decrease stimulation. Nursing care focuses on airway maintenance and seizure control. Standard Precautions are essential, because the rabies virus is present in the saliva of the patient. If an open wound of a health care provider is contaminated with infected saliva, the provider must receive postexposure immunizations.

Tetanus

Tetanus, or *lockjaw*, is a disorder of the nervous system caused by *Clostridium tetani*. This anaerobic bacillus produces spores that live in the soil and enter the body through open wounds contaminated with dirt, street dust, or feces. Most cases of tetanus occur in adults over age 50 whose tetanus booster is older than 10 years. Incubation period can range from 5 days to 15 weeks.

When the spores enter an open wound, two exotoxins are absorbed by the peripheral nerves and carried to the spinal cord. They interfere with the transmission of neuromuscular impulses, leading to uncontrolled muscle spasms. Initially, the patient exhibits pain at the wound site, stiffness of the jaw and neck, mild spasms, and difficulty swallowing. As the disorder advances, the person has difficulty opening the jaw (*trismus*). Spasms of the facial muscles give the person a grinning expression. Painful seizures cause the back to arch. Despite these physical effects, the patient remains alert and oriented. The mortality rate is high and usually due to asphyxia from spasms of the glottis and respiratory muscles.

There are no specific laboratory tests for tetanus. The diagnosis is based on the clinical manifestations. Active immunization can prevent tetanus. Children should receive tetanus toxoid as part of the diphtheria–tetanus–pertussis (DPT) immunization series. Adults should be given two doses of tetanus toxoid 4 to 6 weeks apart, with a third dose in 6 to 12 months. The Centers for Disease Control and Prevention (CDC) recommends a booster dose every 10 years.

If a wound is extensive or heavily contaminated or if the person's immunization status is unknown, give tetanus immune globulin (TIG) to destroy the tetanus toxins. This is followed by injections of tetanus toxoid according to the schedule mentioned before. All wounds, no matter how small, are thoroughly cleaned with soap and water. Foreign material is carefully flushed out or removed from a wound. Only hydrogen peroxide and iodine kill the tetanus organism.

Patients who develop tetanus are cared for in a critical care unit, with minimal stimulation. They are given penicillin to destroy the organism and anticonvulsants to stop any seizures. When muscle spasms and seizures are severe, paralytic agents are used. Airway obstruction is managed by mechanical ventilation. The recovery period varies from 2 to 5 weeks.

Creutzfeldt–Jakob Disease

Creutzfeldt–Jakob disease (CJD) is a rare, progressive neurologic disease causing brain degeneration. The disease is transmissible and fatal within 6 to 12 months after diagnosis. It primarily affects adults over age 60, with more cases in England, Chile, and Italy.

CJD destroys the brain's gray matter. On autopsy, the brain has numerous tiny holes resembling a sponge (called *spongiform encephalopathy*). The underlying cause seems to be an infective protein pathogen called a *prion*. It is resistant to normal chemical and physical sterilization methods. A few cases have been transmitted through corneal transplants and brain surgery.

Early manifestations include memory loss and personality and visual changes. Then the person rapidly develops dementia, muscle contractions, speech problems, and ataxia. Patients in the terminal stage are comatose until death.

Diagnosis is difficult because CJD mimics other degenerative neurologic diseases, such as Alzheimer disease. A thorough neurologic examination, EEG changes, and CT scan help confirm the diagnosis. However, the final diagnosis of CJD is made only by an autopsy.

No specific treatment exists for CJD. Medical and nursing care focus on providing support and comfort. Standard Precautions are followed when handling all blood and body fluids. A 5% bleach solution seems to be most effective in disinfecting contaminated surfaces and equipment. It is not necessary to place the patient in isolation.

A new disease, *new variant CJD*, seems to be linked to eating meat from animals infected with bovine spongiform encephalopathy (BSE), or "mad cow disease." It is a rare, degenerative, fatal brain disease that appears in younger patients. Because the disease is fatal and associated with infected cattle, the import of cattle is severely restricted from countries where BSE exists.

SPINAL CORD DISORDERS

The spinal cord, vertebrae, intervertebral disks, and spinal nerves are anatomically close to each other. Because of this, damage to the vertebrae or an intervertebral disk can affect the spinal cord and nerve impulse transmission through it. For example, if the patient suffers a thoracic vertebrae injury, pressure is applied to the spinal cord. Unless the pressure is relieved, the patient could be paralyzed.

Spinal Cord Injury

Key Concept Spinal cord injuries involve damage to the neurons of the spinal cord. They not only cause loss of independence but also pose numerous long-term physical and psychologic challenges for the patient and family.

A spinal cord injury (SCI) is usually caused by trauma. Adolescent and adult males experience most SCIs. Motor vehicle crashes cause most of the injuries, followed by falls, violent acts, and sports injuries. Approximately 12,000 new cases of SCI occur each year. Life expectancy for people with SCI continues to increase. The leading causes of death are pneumonia and septicemia, often during the first year after injury.

The spinal cord provides a two-way path to conduct impulses between the brain and body. Nerves in the spinal cord connect to the body through nerve roots that exit the spinal column. These nerves provide motor and sensory information to the entire body below the head. Just like the spinal column, the spinal cord is divided into cervical, thoracic, and lumbar regions. The cervical region carries sensations from the head, neck, diaphragm, shoulders, and arms. The thoracic region supplies nerves to the chest that help in breathing and nerves of the sympathetic nervous system. The lumbar region supplies nerves to the legs, pelvis, and bowel and bladder.

PATHOPHYSIOLOGY AND MANIFESTATIONS

A number of factors cause SCIs. The neck can be forcibly bent forward or backward, compressing the vertebrae. Diving into shallow water also compresses the vertebrae and spinal cord (Figure 39-5 ■). A bullet may penetrate the cord, or a fall may cause a fracture of the neck or back. Most injuries occur in the lumbar and cervical regions, where the vertebrae are not protected by other parts of the skeleton such as the rib cage or pelvis.

SCIs are classified according to the level of injury and the amount of cord damage. For example, an injury at the sixth cervical vertebra is called a C_6 SCI. Cord damage is described as complete or incomplete. A *complete SCI* results in total loss of motor and sensory function below the level of injury. *Incomplete injury* affects degrees of function below the level of injury. The level of injury determines whether the patient develops paraplegia or tetraplegia (see Figure 38-6). Damage at the thoracic level causes **paraplegia** (paralysis of the lower part of the body). High cervical injuries result in **tetraplegia**, formerly called quadriplegia, which is paralysis of the arms, trunk, legs, and pelvic organs.

As soon as bruising or compression occurs to the spinal cord, there is bleeding into the gray matter. At this point the damage may be reversible. However, the body's inflammatory response causes edema, hypoxia, and ischemia of the spinal cord. This process actually expands the injury area and may cause more damage than the original injury. If the cord has not suffered irreversible damage, corticosteroids given within the first 8 hours after injury may stop the inflammation. Tissue repair occurs over a period of 3 to 4 weeks, but the spinal cord does not regenerate.

The patient may have deficits in movement, sensation, and reflex activity. The level of injury determines the patient's deficits and potential for rehabilitation (Table 39-3 ■). Complications occur either immediately after an injury or later (Box 39-4 ■). Patients with tetraplegia are prone to more complications than those with paraplegia.

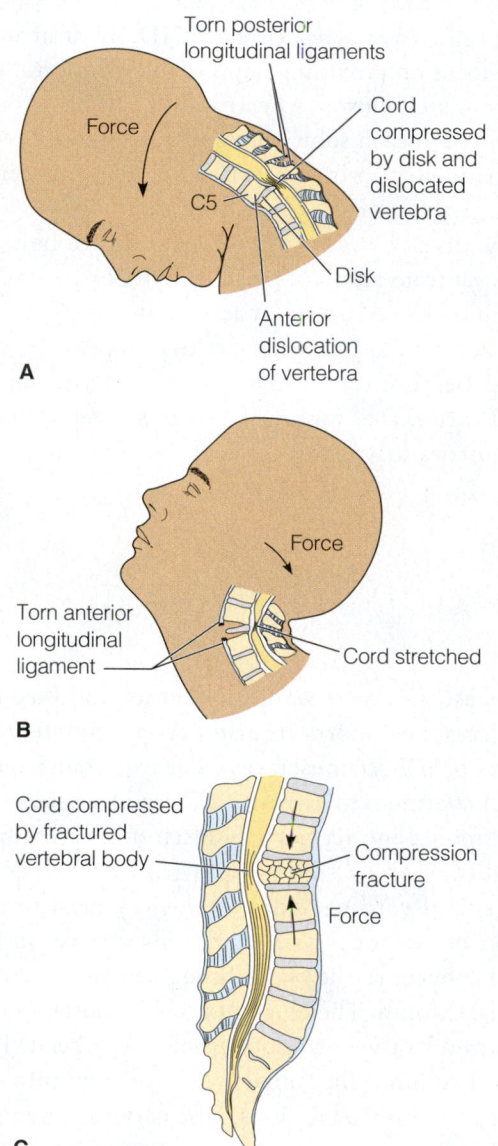

Figure 39-5. ■ Spinal cord injury mechanisms. (**A**) Hyperflexion. (**B**) Hyperextension. (**C**) Cord compression.

Labels in figure:
Torn posterior longitudinal ligaments
Force
C5
Cord compressed by disk and dislocated vertebra
Disk
Anterior dislocation of vertebra
A

Torn anterior longitudinal ligament
Force
Cord stretched
B

Cord compressed by fractured vertebral body
Compression fracture
Force
C

SPINAL SHOCK

Spinal shock is a temporary loss of reflex activity below the level of SCI. It typically occurs immediately or within a few hours after a complete SCI. There is loss of motor function, sensation, spinal reflexes, and autonomic function. Other manifestations include the following: (1) bradycardia, (2) hypotension, (3) loss of sweating and temperature control below the level of injury, (4) bowel and bladder dysfunction, (5) flaccid paralysis, and (6) loss of ability to perspire. Spinal shock usually lasts from days to weeks, and then reflex activity returns. Until it resolves, the patient needs medical support, such as intravenous (IV) fluids.

Autonomic Dysreflexia

Autonomic dysreflexia is an exaggerated sympathetic response in patients with SCIs at or above the T_6 level. This occurs because impulses from the autonomic nervous system are blocked by the SCI. Stimuli such as a full bladder, fecal impaction, or pressure ulcers trigger a hypertensive crisis. The patient develops pounding headache; bradycardia; blurred vision; flushed, diaphoretic skin above the lesion and pale, cold, and dry skin below it; goose bumps; and anxiety. If untreated, autonomic dysreflexia can cause seizures, stroke, or death.

TABLE 39-3	Functional Abilities by Level of Spinal Cord Injury				
LEVEL	FUNCTION	ADL	ELIMINATION	MOBILITY	
C_1–C_3	No movement or sensation below the neck; ventilator-dependent	D	D	Voice or sip-n-puff controlled electric WC	
C_4	Movement and sensation of the head and neck; some partial function of the diaphragm	D	D	Chin-operated electric WC	
C_5	Controls head, neck, and shoulders; flexes elbows	WA	D	Electric WC	
C_6	Uses shoulder; extends wrist	I or WA	WA	WC, self-transfer	
C_7 and C_8	Extends elbow; flexes wrist; some use of fingers	I	I	Manual WC	
T_1–T_5	Has full hand and finger control; full use of thoracic muscles	I	I	Manual WC	
T_6–T_{10}	Controls abdominal muscles; has good balance	I	I	Manual WC	
T_{11}–L_5	Flexes and abducts the hips; flexes and extends the knees	I	I	Ambulates with leg braces, short braces, or canes	
S_1–S_5	Full control of legs; progressive bowel, bladder, and sexual function	I	I	Ambulates with leg braces, short braces, or canes	

Abbreviations: D = dependent; I = independent; WA = with assistance; WC = wheelchair.

BOX 39-4	COMPLICATIONS OF SPINAL CORD INJURY

- *Integument:* decubitus (pressure) ulcers
- *Neurologic:* pain, hypotonia, autonomic dysreflexia
- *Cardiovascular and peripheral vascular:* spinal shock, orthostatic hypotension, bradycardia, DVT
- *Respiratory:* limited chest expansion, pneumonia
- *Gastrointestinal:* stress ulcers, paralytic ileus, stool impaction, stool incontinence
- *Genitourinary:* urinary retention, urinary incontinence, neurogenic bladder, UTIs, impotence, decreased vaginal lubrication
- *Musculoskeletal:* joint contractures, muscle spasms, muscle atrophy, pathologic fractures, hypercalcemia

clinicalALERT

Blood pressure readings in autonomic dysreflexia may be as high as 240/120 mm Hg.

Autonomic dysreflexia is a medical emergency. Elevate the head of the bed 45 degrees to lower the blood pressure. If this does not lower it, give antihypertensive medications as ordered. Monitor blood pressure every 2 to 3 minutes while assessing for the cause. If the patient has a Foley catheter, check the tubing for kinks or irrigate the catheter to check for patency. When the patient does not have a catheter, insert a straight catheter. Instill lidocaine jelly into the urethra before catheterization. If a fecal impaction is present, apply anesthetic ointment such as Nupercaine into the anus, wait 10 minutes, and manually remove the impaction.

COLLABORATIVE CARE
Immediate Care

Care of the patient with an SCI begins at the accident scene. Moving a patient at the scene can further damage the spinal cord. If the patient is moved incorrectly, pieces from a fractured vertebra could penetrate the cord and cause permanent damage. Patients are not moved unless there is a life-threatening danger, such as being burned, crushed, or drowned.

clinicalALERT

Manage all accident victims as if they have an SCI.

At the accident scene, assess the patient's airway, breathing, and circulation immediately. Next, assess the patient for complaints of neck pain or changes in movement or sensation. Then immobilize the neck with rolled towels or blankets and keep the patient in the supine position until emergency personnel arrive. They will apply a rigid cervical collar and place the patient on a spinal backboard in a neutral position.

In the emergency department, the patient is assessed for other injuries, respiratory distress, and neurologic deficits. The neck and spine remain immobilized throughout assessment and diagnostic testing. Oxygen is given to patients with cervical or thoracic injuries. An intravenous line and fluids are started to prevent shock. Until the patient's condition is stable, closely monitor for respiratory, cardiac, urinary, and GI complications. High-dose methylprednisolone (Solu-Medrol), a corticosteroid, may be given to prevent secondary spinal cord damage from edema and ischemia.

TABLE 39-4	Giving Medications Safely: Antispasmodics in Spinal Cord Injury		
CLASS/DRUGS	**PURPOSE**	**NURSING IMPLICATIONS**	**PATIENT TEACHING**
■ Baclofen (Lioresal) ■ Diazepam (Valium) ■ Dantrolene (Dantrium) ■ Tizanidine (Zanaflex)	They are used to control muscle spasm and pain associated with acute or chronic musculoskeletal conditions. They are not always effective in controlling spasticity resulting from cerebral or spinal cord conditions.	Assess the patient's spasticity and involuntary movements. Give with food to decrease gastric irritation. Monitor for drowsiness and dizziness. Monitor for therapeutic effect.	Take with meals to decrease gastric irritation. These drugs may cause drowsiness or dizziness. Change positions slowly and do not drive until drug response is known. Do not stop the drug abruptly without discussing with the physician.

Diagnostic Tests

The following diagnostic studies are used to diagnose SCIs:

- *Cervical spine x-rays* show fracture or displacement of the vertebrae.
- *CT scan* or *MRI* shows damage to the vertebrae, spinal cord, and tissues around the cord.
- *ABGs* determine baseline or identify any respiratory insufficiency.

Medications

Corticosteroids may be given to decrease or control edema of the cord. Muscle spasms are treated with antispasmodics such as baclofen (Lioresal) (Table 39-4■). *Proton-pump inhibitors* (e.g., pantoprazole [Protonix]) are used to prevent stress-related gastric ulcers. Thrombophlebitis is prevented with *anticoagulants.* Stool softeners may be given as part of a bowel-training program. During spinal shock, fluids and vasopressors are used to increase blood pressure, and atropine may be given to treat bradycardia.

Stabilization and Immobilization

Early management includes stabilizing and immobilizing the spinal cord. Thoracic and lumbar injuries are immobilized with braces or body casts. Cervical injuries are treated with cervical tongs (see Gardner–Wells tongs, Figure 39-6■) or a halo vest. The tongs are inserted into

the skull and attached to weights to keep the spine in correct alignment. The disadvantage is that the patient must be monitored closely for displacement of the tongs. If traction is interrupted, the patient faces additional spinal cord damage. Tongs are less frequently used today.

The halo vest (Figure 39-7■) is used for stable cervical or thoracic fractures without cord damage. It allows greater mobility, self-care, and participation in a rehabilitation program. This device is secured through four pins inserted into the skull, two in the frontal bone and two in the occipital bone. The halo ring is then attached to a rigid plastic vest lined with sheepskin. Nursing care is described in Box 39-5■.

Patients with cervical tongs and traction may be placed on a kinetic bed, which provides a continuous side-to-side slow rotation. The kinetic bed helps to prevent immobility

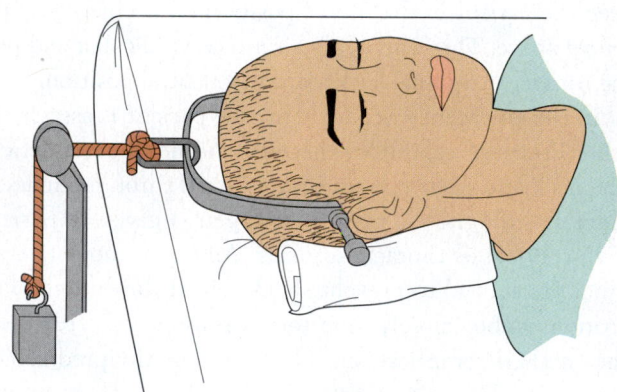

Figure 39-6. ■ Cervical traction with Gardner–Wells tongs.

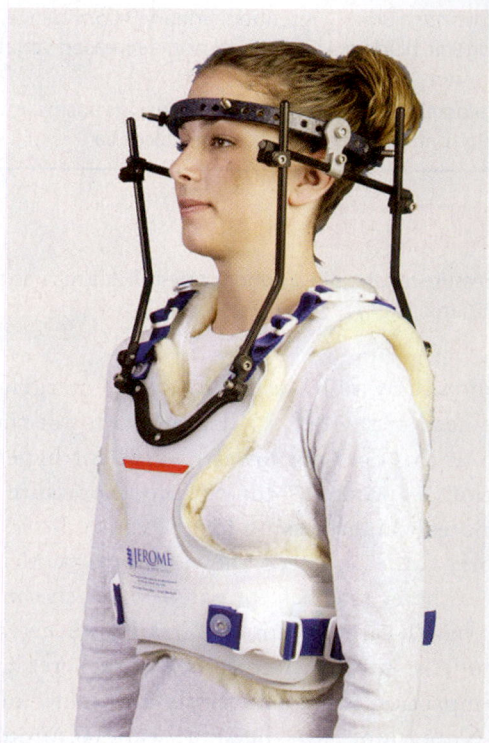

Figure 39-7. ■ Halo vest. (Pearson Education.)

BOX 39-5	NURSING CARE CHECKLIST

Patients in Halo Vests

☑ Inspect pins and traction bars for tightness; report loose pins to the physician.

☑ Check for access to the front of the vest for emergency intervention. Tape the appropriate wrench to the head of the bed.

☑ Never use the halo ring to lift or reposition the patient.

☑ Assess the pin sites for redness, edema, and drainage.

☑ Clean pin sites daily.

☑ Inspect the skin under the vest for pressure areas.

☑ To provide skin care, loosen the sides of the vest. Wash and thoroughly dry the skin. Prevent the lining from becoming wet.

☑ Change the sheepskin lining when it is soiled or weekly.

☑ Turn the patient every 2 hours.

☑ Provide mild analgesic for headache.

problems yet keep the spine aligned. Those with the halo vest can be placed in a regular bed.

Surgery

Surgery is necessary when bone fragments or a hematoma compresses the spine. It is also done to stabilize and support the spine. Different spinal surgeries may be performed, such as a spinal fusion, decompression laminectomy, or insertion of metal rods. These surgeries are discussed later in the chapter.

NURSING CARE

Patients with an SCI need acute care in the hospital followed by rehabilitation that involves all members of the health care team. The care plan focuses on preventing complications of immobility, promoting self-care, and teaching the patient and family.

PRIORITIZING NURSING CARE

SCIs can affect all body systems. The nurse monitors for and plans interventions to prevent problems with breathing, physical immobility, bowel and bladder elimination, skin integrity, nutrition, and self-esteem. Nursing care focuses on preventing complications of immobility, such as UTI, paralytic ileus, and pressure ulcers; promoting self-care; and educating the patient and family.

HEALTH PROMOTION

Injury prevention is the primary focus of health promotion. Programs that emphasize wearing seatbelts and using approved car infant seats and child booster chairs can significantly help to reduce the number of SCIs each year. Stress the need to use headsets with cell phones and

to avoid alcohol and drug use and texting when driving. Provide information to prevent falls and injury from heavy equipment in workplace and farm settings.

ASSESSING

On arrival at the hospital, the patient is assessed from head to toe. Box 39-6■ presents subjective and objective data to collect. During the acute phase, perform assessments at frequent intervals.

IDENTIFYING POTENTIAL COMPLICATIONS

Patients with complete cervical SCIs have the highest risk for complications. Life-threatening complications in these patients include autonomic dysreflexia, pneumonia, respiratory failure, pulmonary emboli, and sepsis. Other complications that can occur in all patients with SCI were summarized in Box 39-4.

DIAGNOSING, PLANNING, AND IMPLEMENTING
Ineffective Breathing Pattern

Expected outcome: Will maintain normal breathing patterns and respiratory rate.

- Monitor pulse oximetry levels. *It is important to measure oxygen levels in order to prevent respiratory problems.*

- Turn, cough, and deep breathe at least every 2 hours. Suction PRN. *These measures decrease the risk for pneumonia and atelectasis.*

- Administer supplemental oxygen as ordered. *Supplemental oxygen helps prevent hypoxemia.*

BOX 39-6	ASSESSMENT

Patients With Spinal Cord Injury

Subjective Data

- Breathing difficulty
- Loss of strength, movement, or sensation below the level of injury
- Numbness or tingling in extremities
- Presence of fear, anger, or depression
- Past history of traumatic injury (circumstances of the accident/injury)

Objective Data

- Measure blood pressure, pulse, and temperature.
- Measure respiratory rate, depth, and breath sounds; ability to cough; use of accessory muscles.
- Test motor strength.
- Assess sensation, noting areas where the patient cannot feel the touch.
- Palpate the bladder for fullness.
- Auscultate bowel sounds.
- Monitor and report diagnostic test results.

■ Increase fluids to 2,000 mL/day. *Increased fluids thin secretions, making them easier to expel and expectorate.*

Monitor for difficulty swallowing or coughing, respiratory stridor, and increased motor and sensory loss. Injuries above the C_4 level alter respiratory function from edema of the cord or paralysis of the respiratory, chest, and abdominal muscles.

Impaired Physical Mobility

Expected outcome: Will remain free from immobility complications, such as skin breakdown, DVT, and contractures.

■ Perform passive ROM exercises to all extremities at least twice a day. *ROM exercises help prevent contractures and improve circulation.*
■ Use splints, trochanter rolls, and foam boots *to prevent wrist drop, footdrop, and external rotation of the hips.*
■ Inspect the skin at least once per shift for pressure ulcers. Turn the patient every 2 hours. Use a special bed such as a kinetic bed if necessary. *The lack of sensation along with immobility increases the risk for pressure ulcers. Kinetic beds allow turning while keeping the spine in alignment.*
■ Provide diet high in protein, carbohydrate, and calories. *Stress from an SCI increases metabolism and the risk for malnutrition.*
■ Assess the lower extremities each shift for DVT. Apply antiembolic stockings (TEDs) or sequential compression devices (SCDs) and remove for 30 to 60 minutes each shift. *Immobile patients are at risk for DVT. TED hose and SCDs prevent blood from pooling in the lower extremities and reduce the risk for DVT.*

Removing TED hose or SCDs each shift promotes healthy skin and allows the nurse to assess skin integrity.

Impaired Urinary Elimination and Constipation

Expected outcome: Will remain free from UTIs and constipation.

■ During spinal shock, insert a Foley catheter or perform intermittent catheterization. After spinal shock, reinforce the bladder training program. *A catheter prevents urinary retention and possible bladder rupture. Patients have a high risk for UTIs; the use of catheters is limited.*
■ Teach the patient to use trigger voiding techniques, such as stroking inner thigh, pulling the pubic hair, or tapping on the suprapubic area or abdomen. *These trigger voiding techniques cause reflex activity that may initiate voiding.*

Palpate the bladder for fullness, because patients with cervical injuries cannot feel a full bladder.

■ Place the patient on a bedside commode if possible. *Upright position facilitates complete bladder and bowel emptying.*
■ Monitor for cloudy, foul-smelling urine and increase fluid intake. *These patients have a high potential for UTIs.*
■ Begin a bowel retraining program using stool softeners, rectal suppositories, and digital stimulation as needed. *These measures stimulate peristalsis and initiate bowel movements.*

Monitor for decreased or absent bowel tones that could indicate paralytic ileus.

Situational Low Self-Esteem

Expected outcome: Will demonstrate positive self-perception given physical abilities.

■ Allow the patient time to grieve or to express denial, depression, and anger over the changes in social, financial, and personal roles. *The patient needs time to adjust to the lifestyle changes.*
■ Provide accurate information based on the physician's prognosis. *Accurate information helps the patient understand his or her present and future needs.*
■ Include family and significant others to treat the patient as normally as possible. *These strategies can make the patient feel worthy and of value.*
■ Refer the patient and family to support groups. *Support groups can help the patient and family adjust to the changes.*

MANAGING NURSING CARE

As appropriate and allowed by the designated duties and responsibilities of assistive personnel, the nurse may delegate nursing care activities such as providing skin care, measuring vital signs and intake and output, and assisting with meals and fluid intake and ADLs for the patient with SCI.

EVALUATING

To evaluate the effectiveness of care for a patient with an SCI, collect data on respiratory and cardiac function, bowel and bladder elimination, and ability to manage ADLs. Determine absence of complications such as pressure ulcers, contractures, DVT, pneumonia, UTI, and stress ulcers.

DOCUMENTING

Documentation includes vital signs, motor and sensory deficits, respiratory depth, presence of crackles and wheezes, skin integrity, contractures, spasms, and bowel and bladder function. Patient and family teaching about skin care, bowel and bladder training, exercises, nutrition, medications, and potential complications is recorded.

CONTINUITY OF CARE

The nurse assesses the patient's ability to live independently and, if necessary, the family's ability to provide care. This assessment provides information about whether the patient can live at home or will need care in a rehabilitation center.

The patient's physical and emotional needs determine the type of rehabilitation program. Rehabilitation centers can offer specialized assistance but may not be near the patient's home. These centers teach the patient to function at the highest level possible.

Discharge responsibilities include teaching the patient and family how to provide medications, ADLs, exercises, bowel and bladder programs such as urinary catheterization, and skin care. Discuss ways to prevent potential complications such as constipation, urinary retention, pressure ulcers, contractures, DVT, autonomic dysreflexia, and infections. Emphasize indications for notifying the physician. A physical therapist will demonstrate the use of any assistive devices, such as wheelchair or crutches, and the need for position changes. Social services can arrange referral to a home health agency, transfer to a rehabilitation center, or a job retraining program. A home health nurse can evaluate the suitability of the living area in the home. Other helpful resources include National Spinal Cord Injury Association and American Paralysis Association.

Herniated Intervertebral Disk

A **herniated intervertebral disk**, also called *ruptured* or *slipped disk*, usually is more common in middle age when age-related changes occur. Disk injury can develop from trauma, lifting incorrectly, sudden twisting of the spine, or degenerative changes due to arthritis. The majority of herniated disks occur in the lumbar (L_4 or L_5 to S_1) or cervical regions. Herniated disks are a common cause of chronic back pain and reduced mobility.

PATHOPHYSIOLOGY AND MANIFESTATIONS

The intervertebral disks are located between the vertebrae of the spinal column. They are made of an inner *nucleus pulposus* and an outer fibrous ring, the *annulus fibrosus*. The disks allow the spine to absorb compression by acting as shock absorbers. A herniated intervertebral disk occurs when the nucleus pulposus protrudes through a weakened or torn annulus fibrosus (Figure 39-8■). When the disk herniates or "slips," it compresses the nearby spinal nerve root and causes motor and sensory changes, pain, and altered reflexes (Box 39-7■).

The herniation may be abrupt or gradual. Sudden straining of the back may cause immediate intense pain and muscle spasms. Gradual herniation resulting from degenerative changes and osteoarthritis has a slow onset of pain. The classic manifestation of a ruptured lumbar disk is recurrent low-back pain. **Sciatica** describes pain that follows along the sciatic nerve. The pain radiates down the posterior leg to the ankle and ranges from mild to excruciating. It is increased by sitting, straining, coughing, sneezing, and walking. Sciatica is usually elicited when the patient performs straight-leg raises.

COLLABORATIVE CARE

Medical care focuses on identifying the location of herniation and determining the type of treatment. Nursing care

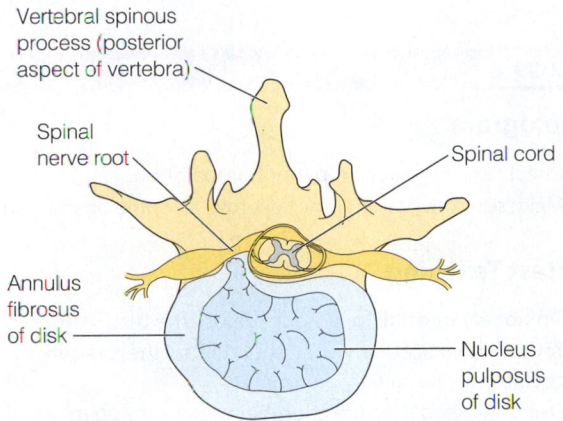

Figure 39-8. ■ A herniated intervertebral disk. The herniated nucleus pulposus is applying pressure against the nerve root.

BOX 39-7	MANIFESTATIONS OF HERNIATED INTERVERTEBRAL DISK

Lumbar–Sacral Area (L_4 to L_5 and S_1)
- Pain that radiates from hip down the leg, usually unilateral
- Muscle spasms
- Numbness and tingling of the leg and foot
- Decreased or absent knee and/or ankle reflexes

Cervical Area (C_5 to C_7)
- Neck stiffness
- Pain radiating from the shoulder down the arm to the hand
- Numbness and tingling of the neck, shoulder, arm, and possibly hand
- Decreased arm strength
- Decreased triceps reflex

is directed toward preparing patients for diagnostic tests. The nurse also cares for the patient after surgery and provides teaching for discharge.

Diagnostic Tests

A complete neurologic examination is part of diagnosing a herniated disk. Spinal *x-rays* can identify skeletal deformities and narrowing of the disk spaces. *CT scan* and *MRI* show the site of the herniation. *Myelogram* is used to both rule out tumors and locate the herniation. Nursing implications for myelogram are found in Box 39-8■. *EMG* identifies specific spinal nerves that are affected by the pressure.

Medications

Pain is managed with *nonsteroidal anti-inflammatory drugs (NSAIDs)*, such as aspirin, ibuprofen (Motrin), and naproxen (Naprosyn). Short-term opioids are used for acute pain but are discontinued with chronic pain because of the risk of dependency. Muscle spasms are treated with *muscle relaxants. Transcutaneous electrical stimulation (TENS)* may relieve uncontrolled pain. Oral corticosteroids such as prednisone or injected corticosteroids may be effective in relieving acute pain and decreasing inflammation.

Medical Management

Besides medication, the patient with disk herniation is managed conservatively for 2 to 6 weeks. Physical therapy, such as proper body mechanics and positioning, and exercises are prescribed to strengthen the back. Patients should sleep on a firm mattress. Those with cervical injuries may need to wear a cervical collar or brace. Warm, moist compresses to the neck are useful to relieve muscle spasms. Most patients respond well to these conservative treatments.

Surgery

Surgery is necessary when conservative measures fail or there are serious neurologic deficits. The following surgical procedures may be used:

- *Diskectomy:* removal of the herniated disk or disk fragments
- *Laminectomy:* removal of the vertebral lamina to relieve pressure on the nerves. This is the most common surgical procedure (Nursing care is discussed in Box 39-9■.)
- *Spinal fusion:* insertion of bone graft (from iliac crest) between the vertebrae, which fuses the vertebrae so they are more stable
- *Microdiskectomy:* microsurgery performed through a very small incision to remove the nucleus pulposus of the herniated disk

The surgical approach depends on the location and size of the ruptured disk. The posterior approach is used for lumbar surgery. An anterior or posterior approach is used for cervical disks.

After a successful surgery, the majority of patients are able to return to their jobs in about 6 weeks. They may experience a few small areas of permanent numbness in the involved leg.

NURSING CARE

Patients with a herniated disk experience pain and possibly reduced mobility. These problems can affect everyday life. Nursing care focuses on managing pain and preventing any further injury.

PRIORITIZING NURSING CARE

Nursing care for the patient with a herniated intervertebral disk focuses on pain management and education. Pain management is essential during conservative therapy and after surgery. Teaching focuses emphasizing the importance of doing the prescribed physical therapy exercises.

BOX 39-8	NURSING CARE CHECKLIST

Myelogram

- ☑ Check facility policy for patient preparation.
- ☑ Make sure the patient is not allergic to iodine or shellfish.

Pretest Teaching

- ☑ Do not eat or drink for 4 hours before the test.
- ☑ You will be placed on a table that tilts so the dye can circulate in the spinal column.
- ☑ Dye is injected through a lumbar puncture. You may feel warmth or a burning sensation. Tell the physician if you feel pain.
- ☑ Stay in bed and follow the doctor's orders for position.
- ☑ Immediately report fever, stiff neck, or seizures.

Post-Test Nursing Care

- ☑ Monitor vital signs and assess neurologic status every 1 to 4 hours for 24 hours.
- ☑ Monitor lumbar puncture site for leakage of CSF or bleeding every 4 hours. Notify the physician of leakage or bleeding.
- ☑ Increase fluids to 2,400 to 3,000 mL in 24 hours. (This may reduce the headache.)
- ☑ Make sure that the patient voids within 8 hours after the examination.
- ☑ Give analgesics and antiemetics as needed for pain, headache, or nausea.
- ☑ If oil-based dye is used, keep the patient flat for 6 to 8 hours, according to facility policy. If water-based dye is used, elevate the patient's head at least 60 degrees for 8 hours, or as ordered.

BOX 39-9   NURSING CARE CHECKLIST

Laminectomy

Before the Procedure

☑ Provide routine preoperative care (see Chapter 10).

☑ Teach patient logrolling technique.

After the Procedure

☑ Provide routine postoperative care (see Chapter 10).

☑ After a cervical laminectomy:
  ☑ Place a small pillow under the neck.
  ☑ Keep cervical collar in place.

☑ After a lumbar laminectomy:
  ☑ Keep the bed flat or elevate the head of the bed slightly.
  ☑ Place a small pillow under the head and a pillow under the knees.

☑ Logroll the patient every 2 hours.

☑ Assess sensation and movement of arms and hands (cervical) and lower extremities and feet (lumbar). Report motor or sensory impairment immediately.

☑ Inspect dressing for drainage with halo sign; test for glucose.

☑ Palpate the operative site for a hematoma. Maintain wound suction and patency of drains.

☑ Assess for urinary retention. Patient should void within 8 hours after surgery.

☑ For cervical laminectomy, assess for difficulty swallowing, hoarseness, increased swelling at the neck, or labored breathing.

HEALTH PROMOTION

A key preventive strategy is using proper body mechanics. Provide this information to all workers, including nurses, who use lifting in their jobs. Important points to emphasize include the following:

- Begin any lifting with feet apart to give a broad base of support.
- Use large arm muscles to lift and legs to push when lifting.
- Slide, roll, push, or pull an object rather than lift it.
- When lifting, bend the knees and lift up over your center of gravity.
- Work as close as possible to the object that is to be lifted.

ASSESSING

The patient is assessed for the degree to which a herniated intervertebral disk affects the patient's daily life. Data can determine possible treatment options (Box 39-10■).

IDENTIFYING POTENTIAL COMPLICATIONS

Patients with a herniated intervertebral disk are at risk for developing chronic, permanent neurologic deficits. Extensive deficits may cause prolonged disability and an inability to work.

BOX 39-10   ASSESSMENT

Patients With Herniated Intervertebral Disk

Subjective Data

- Pain radiating from hip to foot or neck to hand
- Muscle weakness or spasms
- Numbness and tingling of the leg, foot, or neck, shoulder, arm, or hand
- Neck stiffness
- Difficulty sleeping at night
- Medical history of falls, sudden straining of back, heavy lifting, osteoarthritis, or having a myelogram

Objective Data

- Observe for abnormalities of the posture when standing.
- Assess ROM of affected extremity and level of muscle weakness in arm or leg.
- Assess the location and type of pain and aggravating and relieving factors.
- Test patellar, Achilles, or triceps reflexes.
- Note changes in gait, for example, walking with a limp.
- Monitor and report diagnostic test results.

DIAGNOSING, PLANNING, AND IMPLEMENTING

Acute Pain

Expected outcome: Will report that pain has decreased to an acceptable level.

- Teach the patient to avoid turning or twisting the spinal column when changing positions. Elevate the patient's head and place a small pillow under the knees (for herniated lumbar disk) or under the neck (for herniated cervical disk). *Proper positioning can decrease intervertebral disk pressure and prevent muscle spasms.*
- Use a firm mattress or place a board under the mattress. *A firm bed supports the spinal column and muscles.*
- Give muscle relaxant and analgesic medications on a regular basis around the clock. *Giving the medications around the clock lessens periods of severe pain.*
- Apply moist heat as ordered. *Moist heat increases blood flow and relaxes muscles.*
- Do not refer to the patient as an addict. *Patients with chronic pain develop a tolerance to pain medications and may require higher dosages.*
- When chronic pain is unrelieved, refer the patient to a pain management clinic. *These clinics offer specialists in pain management techniques.*

clinicalALERT

Patients with chronic pain often develop tolerance to their pain medications, which does not mean addiction.

MANAGING NURSING CARE

As appropriate and allowed by the designated duties and responsibilities of assistive personnel, the nurse may delegate nursing care activities such as measuring vital signs, assisting with positioning and ambulation, and ADLs for the patient with herniated intervertebral disk.

EVALUATING

To evaluate the effectiveness of nursing care for a patient with a herniated disk, collect and record data related to absence of pain, muscle spasms, numbness, tingling, and neurologic deficits. Evaluate the patient's understanding of home care after surgery.

DOCUMENTING

Document the presence of pain, muscle spasms, numbness and tingling, and any neurologic deficits. Record patient teaching about proper body mechanics; pain control; and, if applicable, follow-up after surgery.

CONTINUITY OF CARE

Preparing the patient for care at home may involve teaching about pain control or follow-up after surgery. Review medications and potential side effects. Teach the patient and family about relaxation techniques. Listening to the patient is important to determine the best methods for pain management. If needed, discuss referral to a pain management center with the physician. Patients may be referred to physical therapy for back-strengthening exercises.

The patient is taught to maintain proper body positioning and body mechanics. The following are some of the guidelines to reinforce:

- Sleep on a firm mattress or use a bedboard. Use a small pillow under the neck and sleep on the side with the knees flexed.
- Sit in straight-backed chairs.
- Avoid activities that flex the spine, such as bending or lifting, and do not twist the back.
- Wear flat-heeled shoes that provide good support.

After surgery, discuss incision site care and the symptoms of wound infection and healing. The patient and family also need to understand the patient's limitations. For example, driving is prohibited for the first 6 weeks. All activities that involve bending, twisting, and lifting are avoided. Patients should not lift more than 10 lb. Review the use of a cervical collar, back brace, or corset. Reinforce indications for when to seek medical care. Those with chronic pain may need psychologic counseling to help accept limitations and lifestyle changes.

Spinal Cord Tumor

Spinal cord tumors may be benign or malignant, primary or secondary. Primary tumors develop from a part of the cord. Secondary tumors start from lung, breast, or other cancer sites, and then spread to the spinal cord. Spinal cord tumors are also classified as *intramedullary* (within the spinal cord) or *extramedullary* (outside the spinal cord). Most tumors occur in the thoracic and cervical areas.

Spinal cord tumors compress the cord, spinal nerve roots, and surrounding blood vessels. Manifestations relate to how fast or slow the tumor grows, the tumor site, and spinal nerve involvement. Slow-growing tumors allow the cord to adapt to the compression. Symptoms do not appear until the tumor is quite involved. Metastatic tumors usually grow quickly, causing symptoms to appear sooner.

Pain is often the first sign and is described as localized or radiating. Localized pain accompanies metastatic tumors involving the vertebrae. Radiating pain follows a path along the spinal nerve root. There are also motor and sensory deficits on one side of the body. Motor deficits include weakness and clumsiness; sensory deficits consist of numbness, tingling, and coldness in an extremity. Bladder involvement causes urinary frequency, urgency, and difficulty voiding.

The diagnosis of a spinal cord tumor begins with a history and neurologic exam. This is followed by a CT scan, MRI, or myelogram to visualize the tumor. A lumbar puncture can identify the presence of tumor cells in the CSF.

Spinal cord tumors are treated by surgical excision and radiation therapy. Surgery is most successful for extramedullary tumors. Intramedullary and metastatic tumors may be only partially removed due to their location or invasiveness of surrounding tissues. Surgery is followed by radiation therapy. Severe pain is managed by inserting an epidural catheter for continuous narcotic analgesic administration. Corticosteroids are given to control edema of the cord.

Assessments and nursing interventions are similar to those described for patients with an SCI or surgery for a herniated intervertebral disk. Care is different depending on whether the patient has a benign or metastatic tumor. Discharge teaching includes how the family can provide physical care and manage pain. (See Chapter 12 for cancer pain control methods.) Refer the patient and family to the Spinal Cord Tumor Association (SCTA) or local support groups for emotional support.

Note: The references and resources for all chapters have been compiled at the back of the book.

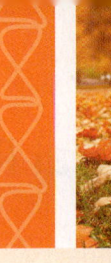
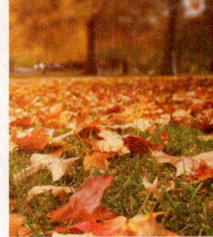

Chapter Review

KEY POINTS

- **Concept:** Multiple sclerosis is the most frequent cause of nontraumatic chronic neurologic disability in young adults. Over time it progressively destroys the brain, optic nerves, and spinal cord.
- Multiple sclerosis (MS) is a chronic demyelinating neurologic disorder that affects young to middle-aged adult women twice as often as men. Patients with MS experience periods of exacerbation and remission, with remissions occurring less often as the disease progresses.
- Disease-modifying therapies such as interferon and glatiramer (Copaxone) and corticosteroids may shorten the exacerbation periods. Symptom management includes baclofen (Lioresal) for muscle spasticity, amantadine (Symmetrel) for fatigue, and gabapentin (Neurontin) for neuropathic pain.
- **Concept:** Parkinson disease (PD) is a slow progressive neurodegenerative movement disorder, resulting from a loss of dopamine. Levodopa is the most common drug used to increase dopamine levels in patients with PD.
- Parkinson disease has three characteristic manifestations: rigidity, tremor, and bradykinesia. As the disease progresses, referrals to physical, occupational, and speech therapists; pain management specialist; and mental health counselors can assist with lifestyle adaptations.
- PD is managed with dopaminergics, dopamine agonists, anticholinergics, and MAOIs. Patients taking levodopa–carbidopa (Sinemet), a dopaminergic, for several years can develop the "on–off" phenomenon. In the "off" period the patient experiences a worsening of the signs and symptoms.
- Myasthenia gravis (MG) is an autoimmune disorder of the peripheral nerves characterized by fatigue and severe skeletal muscle weakness. Life-threatening emergencies include myasthenic or cholinergic crisis, usually caused by undermedication or overdosage.
- Huntington disease and amyotrophic lateral sclerosis (ALS) are progressive neurologic disorders. ALS often advances rapidly and is invariably fatal.
- Cranial nerve disorders include trigeminal neuralgia and Bell palsy. Trigeminal neuralgia causes severe facial pain, and Bell palsy results in unilateral paralysis of the face muscles.
- **Concept:** Spinal cord injuries involve damage to the neurons of the spinal cord. They not only cause loss of independence but also pose numerous long-term physical and psychologic challenges for the patient and family.
- Spinal cord injuries (SCIs) are usually the result of a traumatic event. They occur most often in young adult males from motor vehicle accidents. In a complete SCI, there is total loss of motor and sensory function below the level of injury. In an incomplete SCI, there is variable loss of motor and sensory function below the level of injury.
- Spinal shock is the temporary loss of all reflexes below the level of injury.
- Autonomic dysreflexia is a hypertensive crisis resulting from an exaggerated sympathetic response. It occurs in patients with SCI above T_6 and results from triggers such as blocked urinary catheter or fecal impaction.
- SCI at C_4 or higher threatens the patient's respiratory function, which can result in respiratory distress. The patient may require a tracheostomy and mechanical ventilation. Patients with tetraplegia have an increased risk for urinary tract infections and pneumonia.
- Patients with herniated intervertebral lumbar disk may be treated conservatively or most often by a lumbar laminectomy. Key preventive activities focus on using proper body mechanics.

PEARSON NURSING STUDENT RESOURCES

Find additional materials at **nursing.pearsonhighered.com**.

Clinical Reasoning Care Map

Caring for a Patient With Herniated Intervertebral Disk

NCLEX-PN® Focus Area: Physiologic Integrity

Case Study: A 50-year-old woman is thrown over the handlebars of her bicycle and sustains an intervertebral injury at C_5 and C_6. At the hospital, a CT scan shows damaged ligaments and herniation of the C_7 disk. She is sent home with a cervical collar to stabilize the area. Two weeks later she complains of insomnia, acute pain in her neck and shoulders, and numbness and tingling in her left hand. She is concerned about when she can return to work.

Nursing Diagnosis: Impaired Physical Mobility

COLLECT DATA

Subjective   Objective

_____   _____

_____   _____

_____   _____

_____   _____

Does this present a threat to the patient's safety?

If yes, the priority intervention to address this threat would be:

_____

Nursing Care

_____

_____

_____

_____

_____

_____

_____

Interprofessional team members to include when planning care:

_____

How would you document this?_____

_____

Data Collected
(use only those that apply)

- Insomnia
- Decreased ability to use left hand
- Pain in the neck and shoulders
- Concern about returning to work
- BP 110/78, P 68
- Complains of muscle weakness in left arm
- Unable to ride her bicycle at home
- Decreased reflexes in left arm

Nursing Interventions
(use only those that apply; list in priority order)

- Teach her to not lift objects or twist neck.
- Increase fiber in the diet.
- Instruct her to sleep on a firm mattress.
- Consult with physical therapist for mobility plan.
- Instruct her to keep the cervical collar on at all times.
- Encourage six to eight glasses of water per day.
- Give analgesics around the clock.

Compare your answers and documentation to those provided on the companion website.

NCLEX-PN® Exam Preparation

TEST-TAKING TIP Be familiar with the relationship of functional abilities as they relate to specific levels of spinal cord injuries.

1 A patient is admitted with a spinal cord injury at C_4. Which of the following nursing diagnoses is the highest priority for this patient?

1. Ineffective Breathing Pattern
2. Impaired Urinary Elimination
3. Low Self-Esteem
4. Risk for Injury: Stress Ulcers

2 The nurse is caring for a patient with multiple sclerosis. Which one of these medications should the nurse expect to give if the patient develops urinary frequency?

1. Amantadine (Symmetrel)
2. Dexamethasone (Decadron)
3. Dantrolene (Dantrium)
4. Propantheline (Pro-Banthine)

3 The patient with Parkinson disease is being taught about taking carbidopa–levodopa (Sinemet). What teaching points should the nurse emphasize? **Select all that apply.**

1. Report the "on–off" effect.
2. Change position slowly.
3. Report blurred vision or a rash.
4. Avoid taking medication with meals.
5. Monitor the color of your urine.
6. Increase fluid intake.

4 The nurse is caring for a patient who has sustained a spinal cord injury above the sixth cervical vertebrae. Which of the following stimuli could trigger autonomic dysreflexia?

1. Bladder distention
2. A headache
3. Sneezing
4. Cold feet

5 If a patient is developing Guillain–Barré syndrome, what manifestation should the nurse expect to find first?

1. Weakness in the arms
2. Hypotension
3. Dysphagia
4. Numbness in the lower extremities

6 What functional ability should the nurse expect a patient with a spinal cord injury at the fifth cervical vertebrae to achieve?

1. Use a voice-controlled wheelchair
2. Can self-transfer
3. Operate an electric wheelchair
4. Operate a manual wheelchair

7 When caring for the patient with a herniated lumbar disk, which intervention should the nurse implement?

1. Encourage the patient to sit in a comfortable chair.
2. Elevate the patient's head and place a small pillow under the knees.
3. Place the patient in a low Fowler's position.
4. Turn the patient once a shift.

8 The nurse is caring for a patient with myasthenia gravis. When planning the patient's care, what action is most important for the nurse to implement?

1. Note any complaints by the patient of changes in vision.
2. Administer medications on a strict time schedule.
3. Perform the patient's care quickly because of tiring easily.
4. Monitor for facial muscle weakness.

9 Which one of the following self-care strategies should the nurse teach to the patient with trigeminal neuralgia?

1. Increase fluid intake.
2. Chew on the affected side.
3. Monitor calorie intake.
4. Ways to avoid trigger points.

10 The nurse is caring for a patient who has just had a myelogram (water-soluble dye was used). What teaching point should the nurse emphasize to the patient?

1. Avoid coughing or sneezing.
2. Stay flat in bed for 8 to 12 hours.
3. Drink plenty of fluids.
4. Avoid eating for 6 hours.

Answers and rationales for Review Questions appear in Appendix I.

CHAPTER 40
Caring for Patients With Eye and Ear Disorders

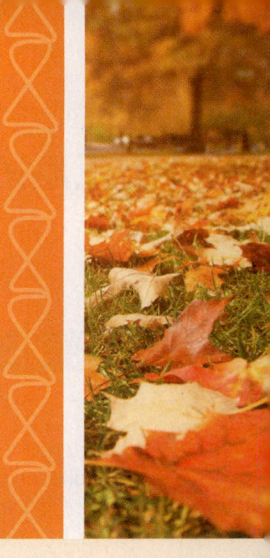

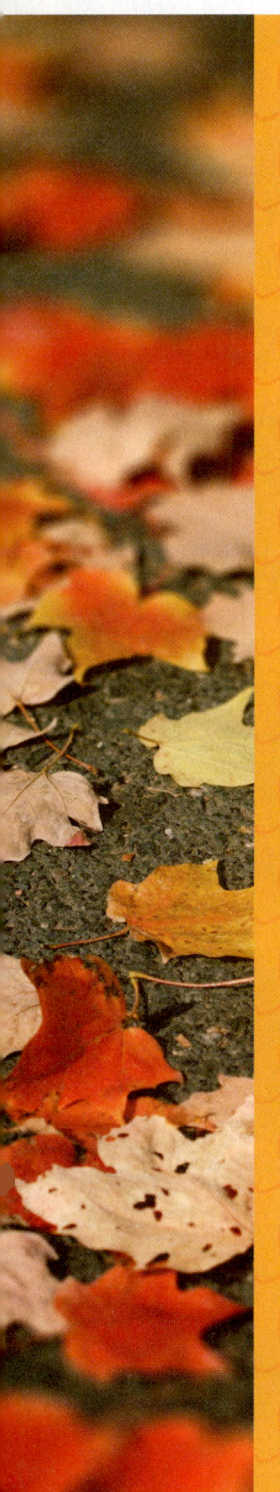

BRIEF OUTLINE

EYE DISORDERS
**Infectious or Inflammatory
Eye Disorders**
Eye Trauma
Refractive Errors
Cataracts
Glaucoma

Detached Retina
Age-Related Macular Degeneration
Diabetic Retinopathy
Enucleation
Blindness
EAR DISORDERS
External Otitis

Impacted Cerumen
and Foreign Bodies
Otitis Media
Otosclerosis
Inner Ear Disorders
Hearing Loss

APPLIED LEARNING OUTCOMES

After completing this chapter, you will be able to:

1. Describe the pathophysiology and manifestations of common eye and ear disorders.
2. Administer prescribed medications safely and effectively for patients with eye and ear disorders.
3. Provide appropriate nursing care for a patient having eye or ear surgery.
4. Use the nursing process to provide individualized care for patients with problems that affect vision or hearing.
5. Reinforce appropriate teaching content for the patient with eye or ear disorders.

KEY TERMS

The key terms are defined on the pages listed below.

SPECIAL FEATURES

Vision and hearing are special senses that allow us to experience the world in which we live. The eyes allow us to see by providing a pathway for light, color, and images to reach the brain. The ears allow us to hear by providing a pathway for sounds to reach the brain. The special senses warn us of danger and protect us from injury. In addition, specialized structures within the ear help maintain position sense and balance. Deficits in the special senses may limit self-care, mobility, independence, communication, and relationships with others.

EYE DISORDERS

Key Concept Structures of the external eye are vulnerable to trauma and infection. While these problems are usually minor, they can cause significant pain, scarring and clouding of the cornea, and impaired or lost vision.

Infectious or Inflammatory Eye Disorders

The normally protective structures of the eye—the eyelids, eyelashes, and conjunctiva—may become inflamed or infected because they are constantly exposed to the environment.

DISORDERS AFFECTING THE EYELID

Blepharitis, inflammation of the eyelid, may be caused by an infection or by dermatitis. The eyelid is irritated and itchy. The eyelid margins are red, crusted, and scaly. A *hordeolum* (*sty*) is an infection of the sebaceous glands of the eyelid, usually caused by *Staphylococcus aureus* (Figure 40-1A■). A sty is red and painful. It may affect either the external or internal lid margin. *Chalazion* is a painless cyst or nodule of the eyelid (Figure 40-1B).

CONJUNCTIVITIS

Conjunctivitis (inflammation of the conjunctiva) is a common eye disease. It is usually caused by bacteria such as *Staphylococcus* or an adenovirus and is spread by direct contact, for example, from hands, tissues, or towels. Acute conjunctivitis, also known as "pink eye," is usually mild, with redness, itching, tearing, and discharge of the eye (Figure 40-2■).

Some conjunctival infections, such as gonorrhea and trachoma, can damage the cornea, threatening vision. *Trachoma* is a major cause of blindness in sub-Saharan Africa, the Middle East, and parts of Asia.

DISORDERS AFFECTING THE CORNEA

The clear cornea transmits and helps focus light and images onto the retina. It also protects the internal eye. The cornea has no blood supply. Scarring or ulceration of the cornea can lead to blindness.

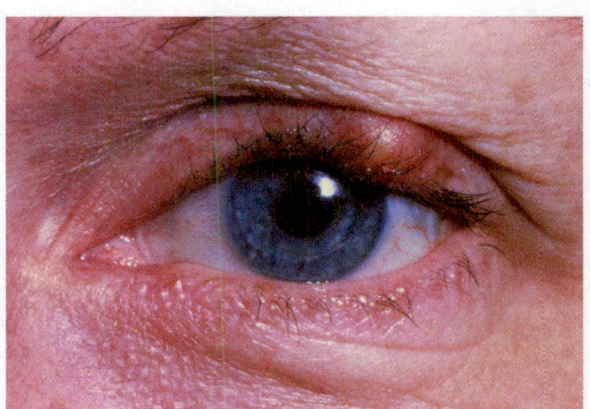

A

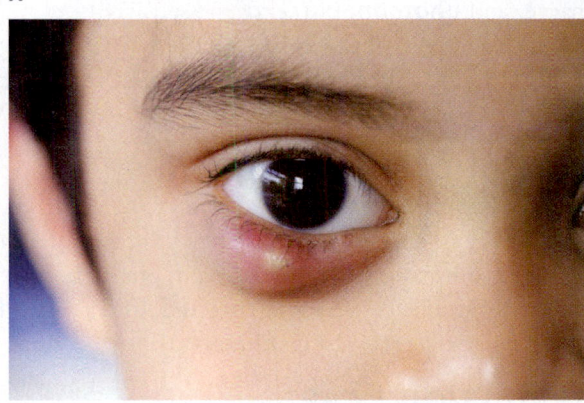

B

Figure 40-1. ■ **(A)** Hordeolum (sty). (Source: Sue Ford/Science Source.) **(B)** Chalazion. (Source: SPL/Science Source.)

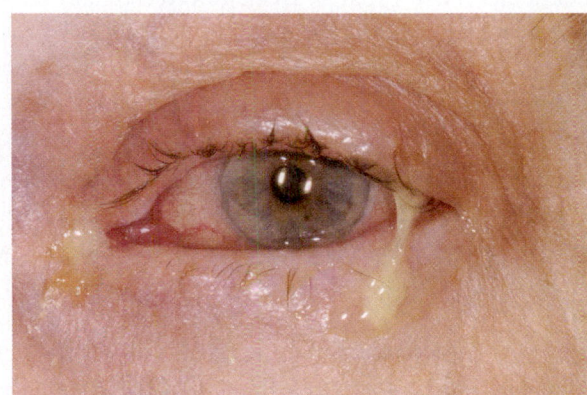

Figure 40-2. ■ An eye with acute conjunctivitis. (Source: Dr. P. Marazzi/Science Source.)

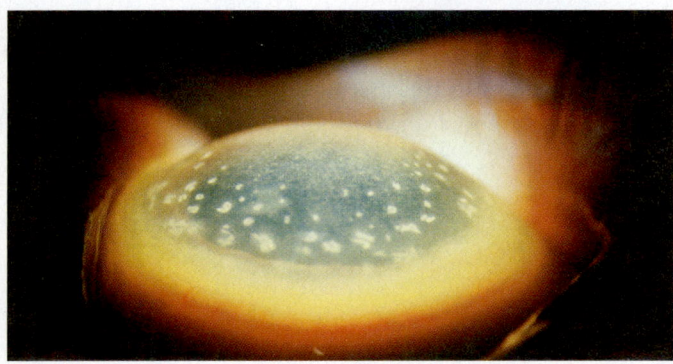

Figure 40-3. ■ Corneal ulcers. (Source: Gilman, CRA / Custom Medical Stock Photos, Inc.)

Keratitis is inflammation of the cornea, usually caused by infection, lack of tears, or trauma. **Corneal ulcers** (Figure 40-3■) may be caused by infection, trauma, or misuse of contact lens. Herpes viruses such as herpes zoster (shingles) can cause corneal ulcers. Corneal ulcers may be superficial or deep. Scarring may occur, clouding the cornea. If the cornea is perforated, infection of the internal eye and vision loss may result.

Inflammation of the cornea causes discomfort, tearing, discharge, and **photophobia** (extreme sensitivity to light). *Blepharospasm* (spasm of the eyelid and inability to open the eye) may develop. Sudden, severe eye pain may indicate corneal perforation.

UVEITIS AND IRITIS

Uveitis is inflammation of the middle vascular layer of the eye. *Iritis* (inflammation of the iris only) is more common. The patient complains of severe eye pain, photophobia, and blurred vision. The pupil is constricted, and the limbus (where the cornea meets the conjunctiva) is red.

COLLABORATIVE CARE

Prompt treatment of infectious or inflammatory eye disorders is important to preserve vision. Corneal ulcers are medical emergencies that must be referred to an ophthalmologist promptly for treatment.

Most of these disorders can be diagnosed by the history and examination of the eye. Usually, no diagnostic tests are required, although the following tests may be ordered:

■ *Fluorescein stain with slit lamp examination* will show corneal ulcers or abrasions, which appear green with staining.
■ *Conjunctival or ulcer scrapings* may be examined or cultured.

Medications

Topical anti-infectives applied as eyedrops or ointments often are ordered to treat eye infections. Antihistamines or corticosteroids may be prescribed when the eye is inflamed but no infection is present. Patients with uveitis may

be given eyedrops to keep the pupil dilated and reduce discomfort.

Corneal Transplant

When the cornea is scarred and opaque (see Figure 40-3), a corneal transplant can restore vision. Corneas may be taken from cadavers under the age of 65 who died as a result of acute trauma or a noninfectious illness. Transplant rejection is low because the cornea has a limited blood supply, which limits the patient's exposure to rejection antibodies. The patient's scarred cornea is removed, and the graft is sutured in place. The sutures remain in place for up to a year. The eye is patched for 24 hours after surgery. The patient must avoid activities that can increase intraocular pressure, such as straining to have a bowel movement, bending over, and lifting or pushing heavy objects. Eyedrops are ordered to reduce inflammation and prevent infection. Nursing care of the patient undergoing eye surgery is discussed later in this chapter.

Complementary Therapies

Careful cleansing of the lid margins using a "no-tears" baby shampoo is often recommended for marginal blepharitis. Soaking the lids with warm saline compresses before cleansing may ease removal of the crusts and exudates seen in blepharitis and conjunctivitis. Eye irrigation may be ordered to remove the purulent discharge associated with conjunctivitis. Local heat applications may be used to treat hordeolum or chalazion.

NURSING CARE

The nursing care for patients with infections and inflammatory eye disorders may involve direct care. More often, care focuses on prevention and patient teaching. Nurses working in outpatient surgical centers provide care to patients undergoing corneal transplant.

PRIORITIZING NURSING CARE

Priority nursing care for patients with infectious and inflammatory eye disorders focuses on preventing complications such as impaired vision and promoting healing. Nursing care also includes reducing pain, preventing further infection, and patient teaching.

HEALTH PROMOTION

Careful and frequent hand washing is essential to prevent the spread of infection from one eye to the other, to patients, and to family members. Teach the patient about correct eye care, including the importance of not sharing makeup, towels, or contact lenses. Emphasize the importance of not using old makeup, which can cause eye infections. Instruct contact lens users proper care and cleaning techniques. If the patient develops keratitis or corneal abrasion, the patient should not wear contact lenses until the cornea has healed.

ASSESSING

Ask the patient to describe the symptoms, their onset, and any relationship between the symptoms and an injury or exposure to an infection or allergen. Inquire about the effect on vision and any associated symptoms, such as chills or fever. Identify the date of the patient's most recent eye examination. Ask about corrective lens use, including the type of lenses. Obtain past medical history, especially any chronic diseases, previous eye problems, and current medication use.

Test vision (with patient wearing corrective lenses if normally worn) using a Snellen chart (see Chapter 5, Figure 5-4) or Rosenbaum chart. The Rosenbaum chart (see Chapter 37, Figure 37-11) is held 12 to 14 in. from the eyes, with vision assessed in the same manner as with the Snellen chart. Inspect the eye, including the conjunctiva, lids, and surrounding tissues. Check pupil size and response to light and accommodation.

DIAGNOSING, PLANNING, AND IMPLEMENTING
Risk for Infection

Expected outcome: Will remain free from infection.

- Instruct to wash hands thoroughly before inserting or removing contact lenses or instilling any eye medications. Teach to avoid touching or rubbing the eyes. *Hand washing is the single most important measure to prevent transmission of infection to the eye.*
- Emphasize the importance of proper contact lens care, including periodic lens removal and cleaning. *Improper cleaning and wearing contact lenses longer than recommended are major risk factors for infection and corneal damage.*
- If the cornea perforates, place the patient in the supine position; close the eye; and cover it with a dry, sterile dressing. Notify the physician immediately. *Corneal perforation can lead to loss of eye contents.*

clinicalALERT

Suspect corneal perforation with complaints of sudden, severe eye pain and photophobia.

Acute Pain

Expected outcome: Will state pain is absent or at tolerable level.

- Administer analgesics routinely in the first 12 to 24 hours after corneal surgery. *The outer portion of the eye, the cornea in particular, is extremely sensitive. Giving analgesics on a schedule prevents pain from becoming severe.*

- Patch both eyes if necessary. *Patching both eyes reduces eye movement and irritation of the affected eye.*
- Teach the patient to apply warm compresses for 15 minutes, three to four times a day. *Warm compresses reduce inflammation and promote comfort.*
- Instruct to use dark sunglasses with ultraviolet (UV) protection when out of doors, even on cloudy days. *Bright light can cause eye pain in patients with an inflammation or infection.*
- Advise to avoid excessive reading or other close tasks. *Eye rest also promotes comfort.*

Risk for Injury

Expected outcome: Will remain free from injury.

- Discuss the effect of an eye patch on depth perception and peripheral vision. Teach the patient to scan from side to side and to be careful when judging distances or speed. *Patching one eye affects depth perception, increasing the risk for falling, traffic accidents, or other trauma.*
- Instruct not to rub or scratch the eye. *Rubbing or scratching may spread infection or damage a corneal graft.*
- Teach how to apply an eye shield at night. *An eye shield helps prevent inadvertent rubbing or trauma of the eye during sleep.*
- Teach patients to use eye protection during activities that can damage the eye. *Trauma increases the risk of infection and scarring of the cornea.*

MANAGING NURSING CARE

As appropriate and allowed by the designated duties and responsibilities of assistive personnel, the nurse may delegate nursing care activities such as assisting with activities of daily living (ADLs) for patients with infectious or inflammatory eye disorders.

EVALUATING

To evaluate the effectiveness of nursing care, collect data about the appearance of the eye and vision (using a chart to measure visual acuity). Determine whether the patient demonstrates proper contact lens care and uses appropriate technique to instill eyedrops.

DOCUMENTING

Documentation includes the appearance of the eye and noted visual deficits. Record patient teaching about eye care, contact lens care, and the ability to instill eyedrops.

CONTINUITY OF CARE

Teach all patients about hand washing and proper eye care. Instruct patients to use a new, clean cotton-tipped swab or cotton ball for each eye when cleansing eyelids. Teach how to instill eyedrops and ointments. If an eye patch is ordered, be sure the patient or a family member knows how to apply it and where to obtain necessary supplies.

Teach contact lens users how to care for and clean the lenses. Stress the importance of periodically removing lenses, even extended-wear lenses. In general, lenses should be removed at night. Advise the patient who has a corneal abrasion or keratitis to avoid wearing contact lenses until the cornea has healed completely.

Stress the importance of follow-up appointments after a corneal transplant. Reinforce teaching about how to prevent increased intraocular pressure (e.g., avoiding straining, vomiting, coughing, and lifting). Instruct the patient and family to promptly report inflammation, graft cloudiness, or increased pain to the physician.

Eye Trauma

Any part of the eye, especially the exposed parts, can be affected by trauma. Foreign bodies, abrasions, and lacerations are the most common types of eye injury.

A *corneal abrasion* is a "scratch" of the cornea. Contact lenses, eyelashes, small foreign bodies, and fingernails often cause corneal abrasions. Corneal abrasions are extremely painful, causing photophobia and tearing. They usually heal rapidly without scarring.

Burns can affect the outer portion of the eye. Chemicals such as ammonia, oven and drain cleaners, and acids from car batteries commonly burn the eye. Thermal burns often occur in an explosion. UV light burns may be called other names depending on the source, such as snow blindness or welder's-arc burn. A burn causes pain and affects vision. Eyelids are swollen, and the conjunctiva is red and edematous; it may slough. The cornea often appears cloudy or hazy.

The eye may be *perforated* by metal flakes produced by high-speed drilling or grinding; glass shards; or weapons such as gunshots (including BBs), arrows, and knives. The layers of the eye can close after being penetrated by a small or sharp object. In these cases, the injury may not be apparent. Eye perforations cause pain, partial or complete loss of vision, and possibly bleeding or loss of eye contents.

Blunt eye trauma is often caused by sports injuries. The injury may be minor, such as lid *ecchymosis* (black eye) or *subconjunctival hemorrhage* (bleeding into the conjunctiva). These minor injuries typically do not need to be treated. *Hyphema*, bleeding into the anterior chamber of the eye, causes a reddish tint to the patient's vision and visible blood in the anterior chamber. The eye orbit may be fractured by blunt trauma. The patient experiences **diplopia** (double vision) and pain with eye movement. The eye appears sunken (*enophthalmos*).

COLLABORATIVE CARE

The extent of injury caused by trauma is determined by eye exam. Unless immediate treatment is required, as with a chemical burn, vision is evaluated with corrective lenses if normally worn. Eye movement is evaluated unless a penetrating object is present (Box 40-1■). The lid and conjunctiva are inspected for foreign objects and lacerations. A topical anesthetic may be used to relieve eye pain and photophobia before inspection. *Fluorescein staining* can help identify the presence of foreign bodies and abrasions. *Ophthalmoscopic examination* is done to detect bleeding or trauma to the interior chamber. Facial x-rays and computed tomography (CT) scans are used to identify orbital fractures or the presence of foreign bodies within the globe.

The eye is irrigated with sterile saline to remove small foreign bodies. Copious amounts of fluid are used to flush the eye when a chemical burn occurs. A special contact lens irrigating unit or a bottle of irrigant with intravenous tubing held to flush all eye surfaces may be used. During irrigation, fluid is directed from the inner canthus of the

---

BOX 40-1	ASSESSMENT

The Cardinal Fields of Vision

Eye movement is assessed using the *six cardinal fields of vision* (see figure).

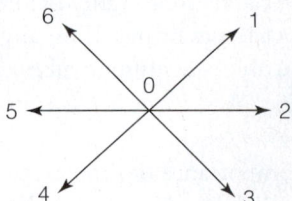

Ask the patient to follow a pen or your finger while keeping the head still. Move the pen or your finger through the six fields one at a time, returning to the central starting point and pausing before proceeding to the next field (see figure). The eyes should move through each field without involuntary movements.

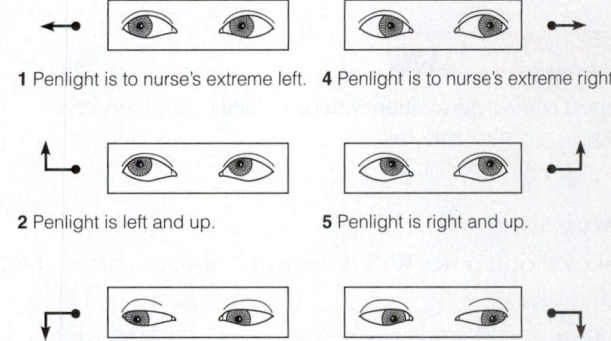

1 Penlight is to nurse's extreme left.   4 Penlight is to nurse's extreme right.

2 Penlight is left and up.   5 Penlight is right and up.

3 Penlight is left and down.   6 Penlight is right and down.

Six Cardinal Fields of Vision

eye to the outer. The patient's head is tipped slightly to the affected side to prevent contamination of the other eye. A sterile, moistened, cotton-tipped applicator or other instrument may be used to remove a foreign body. After the procedure, a topical antibiotic ointment is applied. An eye patch may be applied to keep the eye closed for approximately 24 hours.

Penetrating wounds usually require surgery. Narcotic analgesics, sedatives, and antiemetic drugs are given to relieve pain and anxiety and prevent vomiting, which increases intraocular pressure.

NURSING CARE

Nursing care for patients with eye trauma focuses on protecting the eye and preserving vision. It is important to teach people about ways to prevent eye injuries.

Impaired Tissue Integrity: Ocular

Expected outcome: Ocular injury will heal without complications.

- Assess and record vision in each eye and both eyes, with and without corrective lenses. *The initial assessment provides a baseline and data about the effect of the injury on the patient's vision.*
- Assess eye(s) and surrounding tissues for foreign bodies, burns, penetrating injury, or blunt trauma. *Eye trauma may be hidden by other injuries.*
- Immediately irrigate the eye if a chemical burn is suspected. *Irrigation to remove the chemical is of higher priority than assessment of the eye.*
- Remove loose foreign bodies using a moist, sterile, cotton-tipped applicator. *Prompt removal of foreign bodies may prevent corneal abrasion.*
- For a severe or penetrating injury, place the patient on bed rest and stabilize the injured eye by applying an eye pad or gauze dressing loosely over both eyes. Stabilize any penetrating object if possible. *These measures reduce eye movement and can help preserve vision.*
- After treatment, apply eyedrops or ointment and an eye pad or shield as ordered. *An eye pad is often applied to the affected eye to reduce pain and photophobia and to promote healing.*

CONTINUITY OF CARE

Teaching people how to prevent eye injuries is an important nursing responsibility. Teach employees and people participating in high-risk sports and activities how and when to use eye protectors. Stress the importance of using seat belts and air bags to prevent eye injury in car crashes. Teach patients to immediately flush the eye with copious amounts of water if a chemical splash occurs. Loose, visible foreign bodies can be removed using a clean, moistened, cotton-tipped swab. If an abrasion or penetrating or blunt injury is suspected, loosely cover the eye with sterile gauze and immediately seek medical attention. Instruct patients not to remove objects that penetrate the eye. Both eyes should be patched to prevent movement until medical help is obtained.

After an injury, reinforce teaching about follow-up treatment. Discuss the ordered medications, including how to instill eyedrops and ointments. Stress the need to avoid rubbing or scratching the eye. Teach the patient or family how to apply the eye pad or shield if ordered. If ordered, instruct the patient to avoid activities that increase intraocular pressure, such as lifting, straining, or bending over, to prevent further eye damage.

Refractive Errors

Changes in the shape of the cornea, lens, or the eyeball affect the focus of light on the retina. The result is blurred or indistinct vision. These *refractive errors* or defects are the most common cause of impaired vision. Common refractive errors include *myopia* (nearsightedness), *hyperopia* (farsightedness), and *astigmatism.* The causes and effects of these errors are summarized in Table 40-1 ■. Refractive errors often are detected through routine vision screening. The refractive error can usually be corrected with eyeglasses or contact lenses.

memory**ALERT**

Myopia means that you see near objects clearer and decreases with age. In contrast, *hyperopia* increases with age and means that you see far objects clearer.

Several surgical procedures have been developed to correct refractive errors. *Radial keratotomy* uses a series of shallow radial incisions in the cornea to flatten it. In a *photorefractive keratectomy (PRK)*, a very thin layer of corneal tissue is shaved to reshape the cornea. *Laser in situ keratomileusis (LASIK)* is similar. A thin flap of the cornea is lifted, and then the center of the cornea is shaved to flatten it (Figure 40-4 ■). The flap is then replaced; it is held in place by the eye's natural stickiness. These surgeries require only minutes to complete and are done on an outpatient basis.

Nurses can help identify patients with refractive disorders and encourage them to seek treatment. Check the vision of patients who have difficulty reading printed material, identifying objects, or following visual directions using a standard eye chart. First test each eye, and then test vision using both eyes (see Chapter 5). Refer patients whose vision is poorer than 20/40 in either or

TABLE 40-1	Common Refractive Errors		
PROBLEM	**CAUSE**	**EFFECT**	**CORRECTION**
Myopia (nearsightedness)	Abnormally long eyeball	Light rays focus in front of the retina. Distant objects are unclear. Focus improves as the object is closer to the eye.	Concave corrective lenses Radial keratotomy Photoreceptive keratectomy Laser in situ keratomileusis
Hyperopia (farsightedness)	Abnormally short eyeball	Light rays focus behind the retina.	Convex corrective lenses Laser thermokeratoplasty
Presbyopia	Impaired accommodation of the lens caused by aging	Close objects are unclear. Able to focus on distant objects through accommodation.	Laser thermokeratoplasty
Astigmatism	Irregularities in the curvature of the cornea and lens	Light rays are imperfectly focused on the retina.	Requires correction only when refractive error affects vision

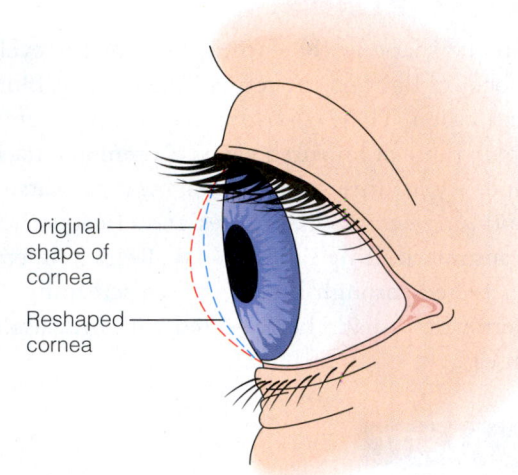

Original shape of cornea

Reshaped cornea

Figure 40-4. ■ LASIK surgery corrects refractive error by flattening the cornea of the eye.

both eyes to an optometrist or ophthalmologist for further evaluation. The primary nursing diagnosis is Disturbed Sensory Perception, but additional nursing diagnoses may be appropriate:

■ Risk for Injury related to inability to clearly see traffic signs and directions
■ Self-Care Deficit related to visual impairment

Discuss the effect of eyeglasses on depth perception, and advise the patient to be careful on stairs until he or she is used to the lenses. If contact lenses have been prescribed, teach and have the patient demonstrate how to insert, remove, and care for them. Emphasize the importance of proper care to prevent eye infections or corneal abrasion. For patients who have had surgical correction of their vision, provide verbal and written instructions about post-operative care and follow-up. Teach the patient and significant others how to instill prescribed eyedrops.

> **Key Concept** Cataracts, glaucoma, age-related macular degeneration, and diabetic retinopathy are leading causes of impaired vision in the United States. Usually these conditions cannot be prevented, but treatment can slow their progression, preserving vision.

Cataracts

A **cataract** is clouding of the lens of the eye that impairs vision. Cataracts are common, and most people over age 65 have some cataracts. The cataract affects vision in only a few of these people, however. Cataracts usually affect both eyes, but tend to develop at different rates. Risk factors for cataracts include exposure to sunlight (UV-B rays), cigarette smoking, heavy alcohol consumption, congenital conditions, eye trauma, diabetes mellitus, and drugs such as corticosteroids and chlorpromazine (Thorazine).

PATHOPHYSIOLOGY AND MANIFESTATIONS

Most cataracts are *senile cataracts*, caused by aging. As the lens ages, its cells become less clear. First, this usually affects the edges of the lens, gradually spreading toward the center. Eventually, the entire lens may be clouded. When only a portion of the lens is affected, the cataract is called *immature*. A *mature cataract* involves the entire lens.

As a cataract matures, both near and distance vision are affected. Details become obscured (Figure 40-5 ■). The clouded lens scatters light rays, causing problems with glare and difficulty adjusting between light and dark environments. With a mature cataract, the pupil appears cloudy gray or white rather than black.

COLLABORATIVE CARE

The diagnosis of a cataract is made based on the history and eye examination. As the cataract matures, the *red reflex* (reddish-orange glow seen in the pupil when a beam of

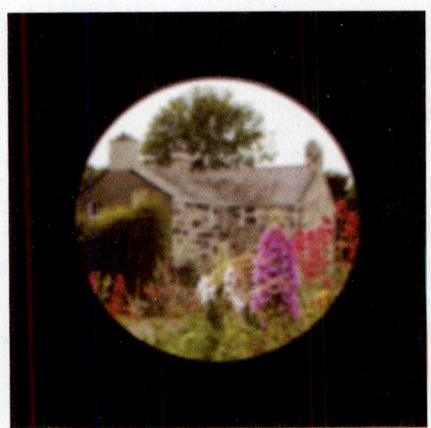

Figure 40-5. ■ Blurring of near and distant vision with a cataract. (Source: Cordelia Molloy / Science Source.)

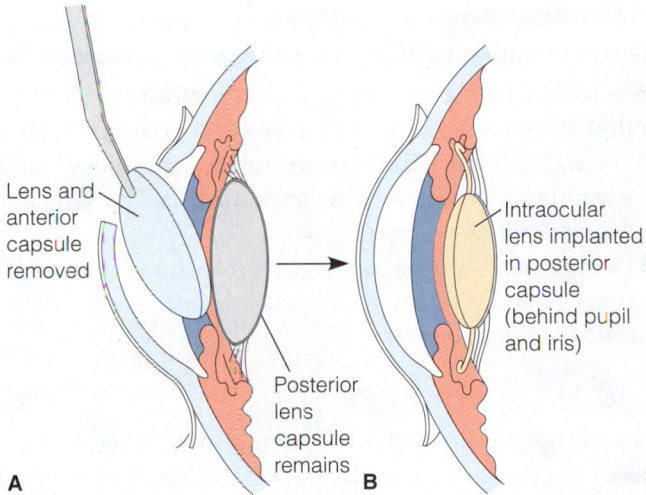

Lens and anterior capsule removed

Posterior lens capsule remains

Intraocular lens implanted in posterior capsule (behind pupil and iris)

A　　　　　　　　　　　B

Figure 40-6. ■ Cataract removal with intraocular lens implant. (**A**) The lens and anterior capsule are removed. (**B**) The intraocular lens is implanted within the posterior capsule behind the pupil.

light is directed into it) is lost. The location and extent of a cataract can be seen with ophthalmoscopic examination. No special diagnostic or laboratory procedures are required.

Cataracts are treated by surgical removal. This is an elective surgery, usually delayed until the cataract interferes with the patient's ADLs and enjoyment of life. Cataract surgery is usually done on an outpatient basis, using local anesthesia. The clouded lens is removed through a small incision in the cornea (Figure 40-6■). An *intraocular lens* is implanted during the surgery to replace the light-focusing function of the diseased lens and restore clear vision and depth perception.

NURSING CARE

Nursing care for patients with cataracts focuses on teaching/learning needs in both the pre- and postoperative periods. Cataract surgery is usually done as an outpatient procedure, using local anesthesia. Box 40-2■ outlines nursing care of the patient having eye surgery.

BOX 40-2　NURSING CARE CHECKLIST

Eye Surgery

Before Surgery

☑ Provide routine preoperative care as indicated (see Chapter 10).

☑ Assess understanding of the procedure. Clarify information as needed.

☑ Orient to the environment.

☑ Assess vision in the unaffected eye before surgery.

☑ Reinforce teaching about postoperative restrictions to prevent increased intraocular pressure: Avoid vomiting, straining at stool, coughing, sneezing, lifting more than 5 lb, and bending over at the waist.

☑ Remove all eye makeup and contact lenses or glasses. Store them in a safe place.

☑ Administer preoperative medications and eyedrops or ointments as ordered.

After Surgery

☑ Assess and document vital signs, level of consciousness, comfort, and eye dressing for bleeding or drainage.

☑ Maintain the eye patch and shield as ordered.

☑ Place in semi-Fowler's or Fowler's position or as ordered.

☑ Intervene as necessary to prevent vomiting, coughing, sneezing, or straining.

☑ Immediately report sudden, sharp eye pain to the physician.

☑ Approach the patient on the unaffected side.

☑ Place all personal articles and call bell within easy reach.

☑ Assist with ambulation when allowed.

☑ Administer eyedrops and other medications as ordered.

☑ Teach the patient and family:

　a. How to instill eyedrops and about ordered medications.

　b. How and when to apply eye patch and eye shield.

　c. To avoid scratching, rubbing, touching, or squeezing the affected eye.

　d. How to prevent constipation and straining and about activity limitations.

　e. Symptoms that should be reported to the physician, including eye pain or pressure, redness or cloudiness, drainage, decreased vision, floaters or flashes of light, or halos around bright objects.

　f. To wear sunglasses with side shields when outdoors.

　g. To make and keep recommended follow-up appointments.

☑ Arrange or refer the patient for assistance with other health care needs (e.g., insulin injections) as needed after discharge.

Deficient Knowledge: Cataracts

Expected outcome: Will state knowledge of postoperative care.

- Provide information about cataracts and their surgical removal. Explain that cataracts usually are removed only when they interfere with vision and ADLs. *This helps the patient decide about surgery.*
- Demonstrate a caring, understanding attitude toward concerns about vision. *Accepting the patient's fears promotes trust and reduces anxiety.*

CONTINUITY OF CARE

Patients usually are discharged home within hours after cataract surgery. Provide verbal and written instructions about postoperative care and directions for follow-up appointments. Include a family member in the teaching. Teach the patient and family how and when to instill the prescribed eyedrops. Instruct the patient to avoid reading, lifting, or strenuous activity; to leave the eye dressing in place; and to take prescribed medications during the initial 24-hour period. During the return visit, reinforce teaching about activity limitations to prevent increased intraocular pressure, protecting the operative eye, and symptoms of complications. Instruct to report eye pain, worsening of vision, headache, nausea, or itching and redness of the affected eye to the physician.

Glaucoma

Glaucoma is a disease characterized by increased intraocular pressure and gradual loss of vision. It is a "silent" thief of vision: Peripheral vision is lost so slowly that it often is not noticed until late in the disease. This vision loss is permanent. Glaucoma is a leading cause of blindness worldwide and affects certain populations (Box 40-3■).

PATHOPHYSIOLOGY AND MANIFESTATIONS

Aqueous humor fills the space between the lens and the cornea. It is produced by the ciliary body and flows through the pupil into the anterior chamber. From there, it drains through the trabecular mesh into the canal of Schlemm. The normal intraocular pressure of 10 to 20 mm Hg is

BOX 40-3	POPULATION FOCUS

Glaucoma

- Open-angle glaucoma occurs more frequently in African Americans over the age of 40 and in Mexican Americans over the age of 60. African Americans, Mexican Americans, Native Americans, and people with a family history of glaucoma should be screened every 2 years over the age of 40.
- Angle-closure glaucoma occurs more frequently in older adults and in people of Asian ancestry.

maintained by a balance between aqueous humor production and drainage. When this balance is disrupted, intraocular pressure increases.

In *open-angle glaucoma*, aqueous humor drainage through the trabecular meshwork into the canal of Schlemm is obstructed (Figure 40-7A■). The amount of fluid in the eye increases. As a result, intraocular pressure increases. The increased pressure damages retinal neurons and the optic nerve. Peripheral vision is gradually lost, and the visual field narrows (Figure 40-8■). Both eyes are usually affected. Untreated glaucoma eventually leads to blindness.

In *angle-closure glaucoma*, the angle between the cornea and the iris closes, completely blocking drainage of aqueous humor from the eye (see Figure 40-7B). Intraocular pressure increases abruptly, damaging the retina and the optic nerve. Clinical manifestations of chronic open-angle and angle-closure glaucoma are similar. However, there are significantly different manifestations with acute angle-closure glaucoma, as listed in Box 40-4■.

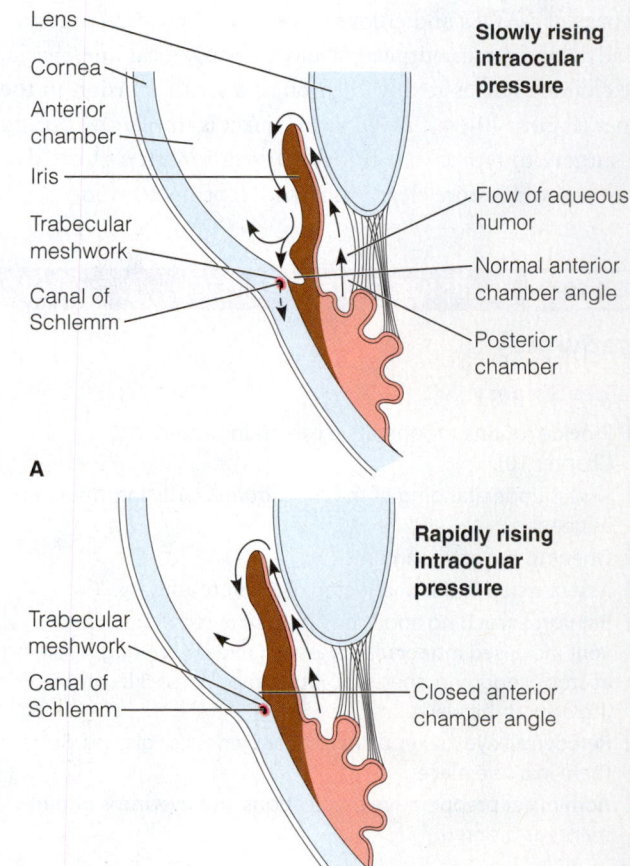

Figure 40-7. ■ Types of glaucoma. (**A**) Chronic open-angle glaucoma. Drainage of aqueous humor through the trabecular meshwork is impaired. (**B**) Angle-closure glaucoma. The angle between the cornea and the iris closes, completely blocking aqueous humor drainage.

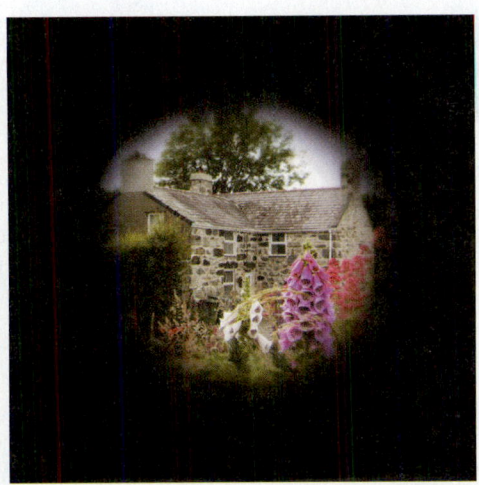

Figure 40-8. ■ Narrowing of the visual field with glaucoma. (Source: Cordelia Molloy / Science Source.)

BOX 40-4	MANIFESTATIONS OF GLAUCOMA

Chronic Open-Angle and Angle-Closure Glaucoma
- Painless
- Gradual loss of peripheral vision
- Difficulty adapting from light to dark
- Blurred vision
- Halos around lights
- Difficulty focusing on near objects

Acute Angle-Closure Glaucoma
- Abrupt onset of eye pain and headache
- Nausea and vomiting
- Blurred vision with halos around lights
- Affected eye red, cornea clouded
- Dilated, fixed (nonreactive) pupil

clinicalALERT

Angle-closure glaucoma is a medical emergency. Without prompt treatment, the affected eye will become blind. Immediately report manifestations of acute angle-closure glaucoma to the physician.

Acute angle-closure glaucoma usually affects one eye and occurs suddenly. Episodes often occur when the pupil dilates (in darkness or with emotional upset), closing the angle. Angle-closure glaucoma can recur; therefore it is *vital* to avoid medications that can dilate the pupil. A patient who has experienced an episode of angle-closure glaucoma in one eye is at risk for developing it in the other eye.

memoryALERT

Mydriatics (drugs that dilate pupils) such as atropine must be avoided in patients with angle-closure glaucoma. Remember "d" is in both mydriatic and dilate.

COLLABORATIVE CARE

Although glaucoma cannot be cured, it can be controlled and vision can be preserved if it is diagnosed and treated early. Routine eye examinations are recommended for early detection.

Diagnostic Tests

- *Tonometry* is done to measure the intraocular pressure. Tonometry screening is recommended for all people over the age of 60. The intraocular pressure is measured with a tonometer (Figure 40-9 ■).
- *Funduscopy* with an ophthalmoscope is done to assess for fundus pallor and optic disk cupping. These changes are important findings in diagnosing glaucoma.
- *Gonioscopy* uses a gonioscope to measure the depth of the anterior chamber and helps differentiate between open-angle and angle-closure glaucoma.
- *Visual field testing* is used to identify loss of peripheral vision. The visual field is the entire area seen by the eye when focused on a central point.

Medications

Drugs often are used to reduce intraocular pressure and preserve vision. Most are administered as eyedrops, but some drugs are available as ointments. Several drug classes are used, including drugs that affect pupil size or the production of aqueous humor. Table 40-2 ■ outlines commonly used drugs and their nursing implications.

Acute angle-closure glaucoma is an ocular emergency that requires immediate intervention. Diuretics are given intravenously to lower intraocular pressure rapidly. Acetazolamide, a carbonic anhydrase inhibitor, and osmotic diuretics, such as mannitol, are used. Fast-acting miotic drops such as pilocarpine are also used to constrict the pupil and help open the angle.

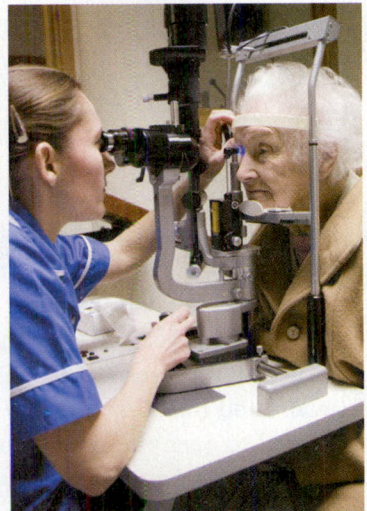

Figure 40-9. ■ An eye professional uses a tonometer to indirectly measure the intraocular pressure of a patient's eye. (Source: Life-in-View / Science Source.)

TABLE 40-2	**Giving Medications Safely: Glaucoma**		
DRUG/CLASS	**PURPOSE**	**NURSING IMPLICATIONS**	**PATIENT TEACHING**
Adrenergic agonists ■ Apraclonidine (Iopidine) ■ Brimonidine (Alphagan)	Adrenergic agonists reduce intraocular pressure by reducing aqueous humor production and increasing its absorption.	Avoid use in patients with acute angle-closure glaucoma, cardiac arrhythmias, or coronary artery disease. Report itching, lid edema, and discharge from the eyes.	Report any change in vision or eye pain that may indicate acute angle-closure glaucoma; contact the doctor immediately.
Beta-blockers ■ Timolol (Timoptic) ■ Betaxolol (Betoptic) ■ Carteolol (Ocupress) ■ Levobunolol (Betagan) ■ Metipranolol (OptiPranolol)	Beta-blockers decrease intraocular pressure by reducing the production of aqueous humor. They do not affect vision like miotics and adrenergic agonists do.	Report contraindications such as asthma, COPD, heart block, and heart failure. After instilling drops hold pressure over lacrimal sac to prevent systemic absorption. Report side effects such as bradycardia, hypotension, and difficulty breathing.	After instilling drops, hold pressure over lacrimal sac to keep the drug from entering your blood. Vision may be blurry at first but will improve. Report worsening vision, difficulty breathing, and sweating to the doctor.
Prostaglandin analogs ■ Latanoprost (Xalatan) ■ Bimatoprost (Lumigan)	Analogs reduce intraocular pressure by increasing the outflow of aqueous humor. Over time they permanently darken the iris and the skin around the eyelids, and increase the growth of the eyelashes.	Administer once daily at bedtime. Report side effects such as burning, stinging, or redness of the eye.	Instill drops at bedtime, as vision blurs after using the drops. These drugs darken the iris and skin around the eyelids permanently, but they are not harmful. Report eye discomfort or redness to the doctor.
Carbonic anhydrase inhibitors ■ Dorzolamide (Trusopt) eyedrops ■ Acetazolamide (Diamox), PO, IV	Carbonic anhydrase inhibitors reduce aqueous humor production, lowering intraocular pressure. Intravenous acetazolamide rapidly reduces intraocular pressure in acute angle-closure glaucoma.	*Dorzolamide* Instill 10 minutes apart from other topical ophthalmic drugs. Report adverse or allergic effects, such as conjunctivitis or redness and itching of the lid. *Acetazolamide* Monitor daily weight, intake and output, vital signs, and serum electrolyte values.	*Dorzolamide* Instill 10 minutes apart from other topical ophthalmic drugs. Notify the physician if prolonged eye irritation continues. *Acetazolamide* Drink 2–3 quarts of fluid daily and change positions slowly to prevent dizziness on standing.

Surgery

Surgery is indicated when chronic open-angle glaucoma cannot be controlled by medication or for treating acute angle-closure glaucoma. The main purpose of surgery is to lower intraocular pressure. The most common surgeries used to manage patients with chronic open-angle glaucoma are *laser trabeculoplasty* and *trabeculectomy*. In laser trabeculoplasty, a laser is used to open drainage into the canal of Schlemm by burning holes into the trabecular meshwork. During trabeculectomy, a permanent fistula is created to drain aqueous humor from the anterior chamber of the eye. For angle-closure glaucoma, a noninvasive procedure called *laser iridotomy* is done. The laser makes multiple small perforations in the iris, allowing aqueous humor to drain from the posterior chamber into the canal of Schlemm.

Complementary Therapies

Kava must be used cautiously in patients with glaucoma because it causes pupil dilation, which can increase intraocular pressure.

NURSING CARE

Glaucoma is a chronic disease that requires lifelong management. The nurse must help the patient and family understand the nature of the disease and its potential to cause blindness.

PRIORITIZING NURSING CARE

Reduced vision caused by the glaucoma can affect the patient's ability to provide self-care as well as manage other conditions, such as diabetes. Glaucoma increases the patient's risk for injury due to altered peripheral vision. The psychologic effects of a chronic disease can increase anxiety.

HEALTH PROMOTION

Early vision screening can reduce the severity and potential damaging permanent effects of glaucoma. It is important to educate the public about risk factors for glaucoma, such as increased age and higher incidence in African Americans, Mexican Americans, and Asians. Eye examinations should be done in people over 40 every 2 to 4 years. Anyone with a family history or over age 60 should be examined every 1 to 2 years.

ASSESSING

Nursing assessment related to glaucoma focuses on identifying patients at risk. Ask about vision, including recent changes, difficulty seeing at night, and halos around lights. Inquire about a family history of glaucoma or any previous episodes of angle-closure glaucoma and the date of the most recent eye examination.

Inspect the eye for possible redness or clouding of the cornea. Assess vision (with corrective lenses if worn) using a standard eye chart. Assess pupil response to light (see Chapter 5). Evaluate peripheral vision (Box 40-5■).

IDENTIFYING POTENTIAL COMPLICATIONS

Untreated glaucoma can lead to irreversible peripheral vision deficits. As the disease progresses, blindness may occur.

DIAGNOSING, PLANNING, AND IMPLEMENTING

Deficient Knowledge: Ocular Care

Expected outcome: Will verbalize understanding of glaucoma and demonstrate appropriate eye care.

- Provide detailed verbal and written instructions about the ordered drugs. *Written instructions reinforce teaching and are a resource for the patient.*
- Teach how to instill eyedrops, and have the patient show you that he or she can do so. *Impaired vision, manual dexterity, or mobility may interfere with the ability to get drops into the eye. In some cases, a family member may need to do this for the patient.*
- If taking other medications, ensure that the patient can identify each and can take the appropriate dose if the drug is in injectable or liquid form. *Impaired vision and coexisting chronic diseases may make it difficult for the patient to read medication labels or to draw up or pour an accurate dose.*

BOX 40-5	ASSESSMENT

Visual Fields by Confrontation

- Face the patient, seated about 2 ft apart.
- Instruct the patient to cover the right eye and focus on your face.
- Cover your left eye, and focus on the patient's face.
- Midway between the patient and you, bring a light-colored object into the field of vision from the side (see figure).

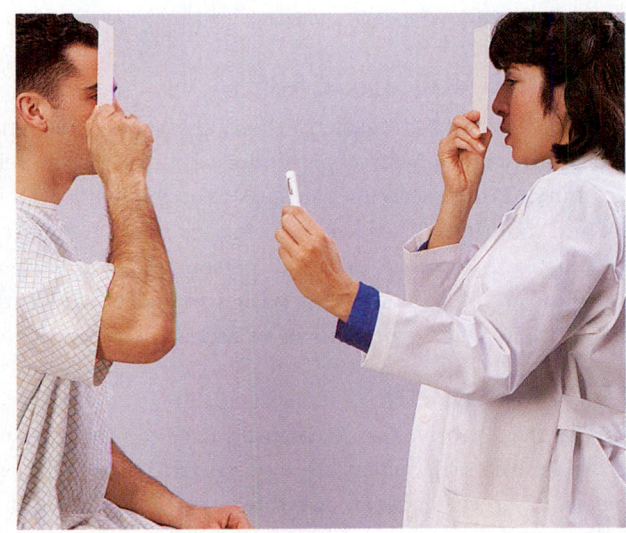

- Ask the patient to indicate when the object is seen.
- Check all visual fields of both eyes in this manner.

- Emphasize the importance of keeping all follow-up appointments to monitor intraocular pressure and vision. *Inadequate treatment can allow vision loss to continue.*

Risk for Injury

Expected outcome: Will remain free from injury.

- Assess the ability to provide self-care. Provide assistance as needed. *Patients may be reluctant to ask for help, believing that they should be able to perform these familiar tasks.*
- Alert caregivers and housekeepers not to move items in the patient's room. *Unexpected changes in the environment increase the risk for falls.*
- With the patient's permission, raise the side rails on the bed. *Raised rails help remind the patient to ask for help until the environment is familiar.*

clinicalALERT

Keep traffic areas free of clutter to reduce the risk of injury in patients with visual impairments.

Anxiety

Expected outcome: Will report less anxiety.

- Assess for evidence of anxiety. Repeated expressions of concern or denial that altered vision will affect the patient's life are indicators of anxiety. *Identifying and acknowledging anxiety helps the patient recognize and deal with it.*
- Discuss the effects of glaucoma and possible vision loss on lifestyle and roles. *This allows the patient to express concerns and fears. It also provides an opportunity to suggest alternative activities and assistive devices.*

MANAGING NURSING CARE

As appropriate and allowed by the designated duties and responsibilities of assistive personnel, the nurse may delegate nursing care activities such as assisting with ADLs, meal and fluid intake, and ambulation for the patient with glaucoma. Ensure that assistive personnel have a clear understanding of ways to assist with ambulation and with meals, such as placing utensils in an accessible position.

EVALUATING

Evaluate the effectiveness of nursing care for the patient with glaucoma by identifying any visual deficits. Determine whether the patient can safely perform ADLs and instill eyedrops as ordered. Identify the patient's knowledge about taking ophthalmic medications, the importance of follow-up care, and the date of the next vision exam.

DOCUMENTING

Documentation includes the level of visual deficits and ability to perform ADLs and instill eyedrops. Record patient teaching about medications, warning signs of acute angle-closure glaucoma, and importance of regular eye examinations.

CONTINUITY OF CARE

Discuss the prescribed drugs, including the name, dose, timing, and possible adverse effects. Teach the patient how to instill eyedrops. Stress the importance of continuing treatment and keeping scheduled eye examinations with intraocular pressure measurements.

Discuss the risks, warning signs, and management of future attacks with the patient who has had an episode of acute angle-closure glaucoma. If a permanent vision loss has resulted, discuss the effect of loss of vision on depth perception and safety.

If a significant amount of vision in both eyes has been lost, help identify changes in the home that can help the patient remain safe and independent. Suggest removing scatter rugs and small items of furniture to allow the patient to navigate safely in this already familiar environment. Refer to local and national resources that can help with assistive devices and modifications of the home.

NURSING CARE PLAN
Patient With Glaucoma and Cataracts

Lila Rainey is an 80-year-old widow who lives alone in the family home. She has worn glasses for myopia since she was a young girl. Four years ago she was diagnosed with chronic open-angle glaucoma, for which she takes timolol (Timoptic) 0.5%. Recently, she has had increasing difficulty reading and watching television. She no longer drives at night because the glare of oncoming headlights makes it very difficult for her to see. Mrs. Rainey is now being admitted to the day surgery unit for a cataract removal and intraocular lens implant in her right eye.

Assessment

Mrs. Rainey is alert and oriented, though apprehensive about surgery. Vital signs are BP 134/72; P 86; R 18. Assessments of other body systems are essentially normal. Mrs. Rainey's pupils are round, equal, and react briskly to light and accommodation. Her conjunctivae are pink; sclera and corneas are clear. The red reflex in the right eye is diminished. Her visual acuity is 20/150 OD (right eye) and 20/50 OS (left eye) with corrective lenses. Her intraocular pressures are 16 mm Hg OD and 12 mm Hg OS. The nurse reviews the operative procedure with Mrs. Rainey, answering her questions and telling her what to expect after surgery.

Nursing Diagnosis

The following priority nursing diagnoses are established for this patient:

- *Risk for Injury* related to myopia and lens extraction
- *Anxiety* related to anticipated surgery
- *Deficient Knowledge* related to a lack of information about postoperative care

Expected Outcomes

The expected outcomes for the plan of care are that Mrs. Rainey will:

- Experience no injury and regain sufficient vision to perform ADLs.
- Demonstrate a reduced level of anxiety.
- Demonstrate eyedrop instillation postoperatively.
- Verbalize postoperative care, including signs of complications to be reported.

Planning and Implementation

The following interventions are implemented for Mrs. Rainey:

- Place call light and personal care items within easy reach.

- Encourage expression of fears about surgery and its potential effect on vision.
- Explain all procedures related to surgery and recovery.
- Instruct her to avoid shutting eyelids tightly, sneezing, coughing, laughing, bending over, lifting, or straining to have a bowel movement.
- Instruct to wear glasses during the day and an eye shield at night to prevent injury to the surgical site.
- Explain and demonstrate the procedure for administering eyedrops.
- Provide verbal and written instructions about postoperative care, including follow-up examinations, potential complications, and actions to take in response.

Evaluation

Mrs. Rainey is discharged 3 hours after surgery. She is visibly relieved the following morning when the eye patch is removed, and her vision is better than before surgery, even without her glasses. Mrs. Rainey instills her own eyedrops before discharge and relates an understanding of the postoperative care and safety precautions. Mrs. Rainey's daughter plans to visit her mother several times a week to help with household chores. Mrs. Rainey understands the chronic nature of her glaucoma and says that her vision is too important for her to neglect her timolol drops and routine eye exams.

Critical Thinking in the Nursing Process

1. Mrs. Rainey was taught to hold pressure over the lacrimal sac, at the corner of the eye near the bridge of the nose, for several minutes after instilling her timolol eyedrops. Why?
2. Timolol drops are not appropriate for all patients. Which common chronic conditions would contraindicate the use of timolol drops and why?
3. What community resources would you suggest to Mrs. Rainey if she did not have a close family member to assist with housework?

Note: Discussion of Critical Thinking questions appears on the companion website.

Detached Retina

The retina contains the photoreceptors of the eye that allow us to see light and images. A **retinal detachment** is separation of the retina from the choroid, the vascular layer of the eye. Retinal detachment can occur spontaneously or result from trauma. The vitreous humor shrinks with aging, increasing the risk for detached retina.

PATHOPHYSIOLOGY AND MANIFESTATIONS

The retina can remain intact but separate from the choroid or tear and fold back on itself (Figure 40-10■). A break or tear in the retina allows fluid to seep between the retina and

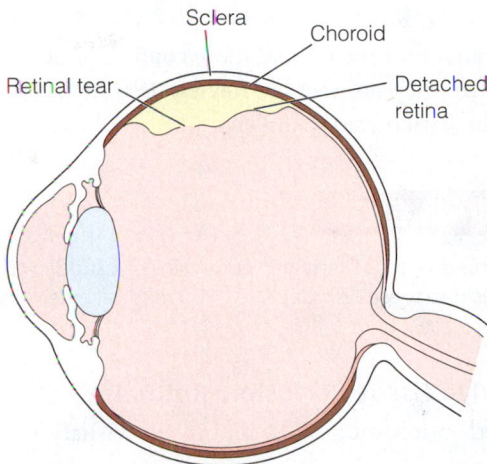

Figure 40-10. ■ Detached retina.

choroid, separating these layers. If the layers remain separated, the neurons of the retina become ischemic and die, causing permanent vision loss. For this reason, retinal detachment is a medical emergency that requires prompt treatment.

A detached retina is painless. The patient may sense that a curtain or veil is being drawn across the vision. The affected area of vision relates to the area of detachment. Because light rays cross as they pass through the lens, a detachment in the upper part of the eye affects vision in the lower part of the visual field. Other common manifestations of a detached retina include floaters (irregular, dark lines or spots in vision) and flashes of light.

COLLABORATIVE CARE

A detached retina is a medical emergency and must be treated immediately to maintain vision. Diagnosis is determined by the patient's symptoms and examination of the eye. Until definitive treatment is available, the patient's head is positioned so that the detached portion of the retina is lower than the rest of the eye.

Retinal detachment is often treated in an ophthalmologist's office. Several procedures are used to reestablish contact between the retina and the choroid. Pneumatic retinopexy involves injecting a gas into the vitreous cavity and positioning the patient so that the gas bubble pushes the detached portion of the retina against the choroid. Either laser therapy or cryotherapy, which uses a supercooled probe, may be used to initiate scarring that will "weld" the layers together. A surgical procedure, *scleral buckling*, creates an indentation or fold in the sclera, bringing the choroid into contact with the retina.

NURSING CARE

Early identification and treatment of a detached retina are vital to preserve sight. Most eye disorders cause a gradual loss of vision. Promptly report rapid changes in vision to the physician. Remember that retinal detachment is painless; patients may seem to be more confused than concerned about what they are seeing. Review Box 40-2 for nursing care of the patient requiring eye surgery.

Ineffective Tissue Perfusion: Retinal

Expected outcome: Will report no visual loss in the affected eye.

■ Position the patient with the area of detachment dependent. For instance, if vision is lost in the upper outer portion of the left eye, indicating an inferior medial retinal detachment of the left eye, place the patient on the right side in a supine position. *Correct positioning allows the vitreous humor to press on the detached area, bringing the retina closer to blood vessels in the choroid and preserving retinal perfusion until treatment is available.*

Anxiety

Expected outcome: Will report less anxiety.

■ Maintain a calm, confident attitude while providing priority care. *Maintaining a calm but urgent manner helps reassure the patient.*

■ Reassure the patient that a detached retina is treatable, usually on an outpatient basis. *Reassurance helps relieve the fear of permanent vision loss.*

■ Explain all procedures fully, including the reason for positioning. *Complete explanations help relieve anxiety and promote understanding.*

■ Allow supportive family members or friends to remain with the patient as much as possible. *Additional support helps reduce anxiety.*

Evaluate the effectiveness of nursing care by collecting data on the extent of any visual deficits before and after treatment. There should be an absence of floaters or flashes of light. Identify the degree to which anxiety has been controlled or decreased.

CONTINUITY OF CARE

After treatment for a detached retina, stress the importance of positioning as ordered. The patient may be instructed to maintain a position with the affected area of the eye inferior to maintain contact between the retina and the choroid.

The patient who has had a spontaneous retinal detachment has an increased risk of future detachments. Discuss early symptoms, and emphasize the importance of seeking immediate treatment if they occur. Emphasize the need to maintain follow-up treatment with the ophthalmologist.

If the retina remains detached, discuss safety measures to accommodate the loss of vision and changes in depth perception.

Age-Related Macular Degeneration

Age-related macular degeneration is a common cause of impaired vision and blindness in adults over age 65. With aging, the neurons of the macula (the area of central vision) may atrophy or separate from the choroid. Other risk factors related to macular degeneration include female gender, smoking, and a family history.

When the macula is damaged, central vision becomes blurred and distorted, but peripheral vision remains intact (Figure 40-11 ■). Distortion of vision in one eye is a common early symptom; straight lines appear wavy or distorted. Macular degeneration particularly affects activities that require close central vision, such as reading and sewing. Vision and retinal examination are done to diagnose macular degeneration, along with the Amsler grid, which identifies distortion of central vision.

Laser treatment or photodynamic therapy may slow macular degeneration, but often no effective treatment is available. Large-print books and magazines, the use of a magnifying glass, and high-intensity lighting can help the patient to cope with reduced vision.

Promptly report new or rapid loss of central vision, because early treatment may help preserve vision and slow

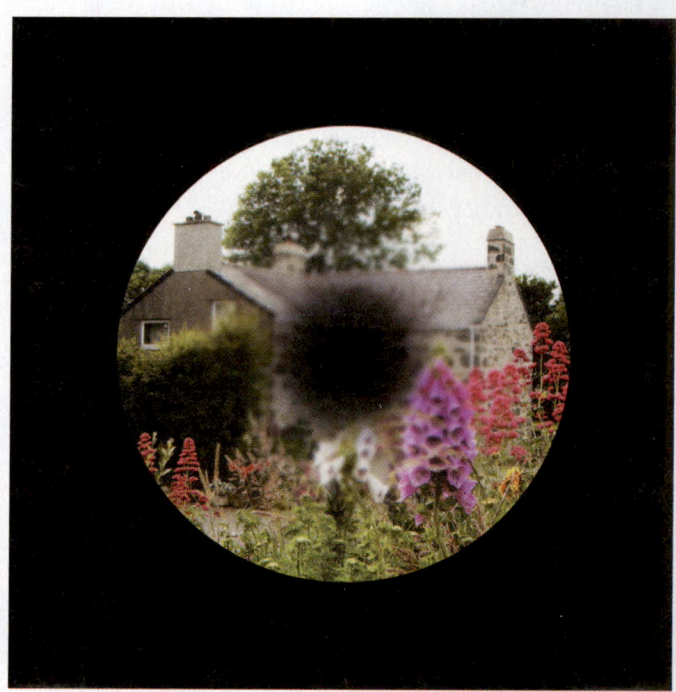

Figure 40-11. ■ Blurred central vision occurs in age-related macular degeneration. (Source: Cordelia Molloy / Science Source.)

the disease. Help patients with slowly progressive vision loss to adapt by recommending visual aids and other coping strategies.

Diabetic Retinopathy

Approximately 85% of diabetics develop *diabetic retinopathy*, a disorder affecting the capillaries of the retina. The capillaries are no longer able to transport blood and oxygen to the retina. Retinopathy develops about 15 years after being diagnosed with either type 1 or type 2 diabetes mellitus. It is the leading cause of new blindness in people ages 20 to 74.

Initially, the venous capillaries dilate and develop microscopic aneurysms that may leak or rupture. These cause edema and small hemorrhages into the retina. As the disease progresses, large areas of the retina become ischemic, and new blood vessels form, spreading over the surface of the retina and into the vitreous body. These vessels are fine and fragile. They may leak or rupture, causing bleeding into the vitreous body. The vessels also increase the risk for a detached retina.

A yearly eye examination is recommended for all adults with diabetes. Laser treatment may be done to seal microaneurysms and destroy new, fragile blood vessels. Treatment slows the disease progress but does not cure it.

The nursing care focus for diabetic retinopathy is on education. Stress the importance of regular eye examinations for all patients with diabetes. Teach the patient to report promptly any change in vision, including blurring; black spots (floaters), cobwebs, or flashing lights in the visual field; or a sudden loss of vision in one or both eyes. Emphasize that controlling blood glucose levels and maintaining blood pressure within normal limits will help limit diabetic retinopathy or slow its progress.

Enucleation

Occasionally, an eye must be removed. This procedure is known as *enucleation*. After the eye is removed, the conjunctiva and eye muscles are sutured to a round implant inserted into the orbit to maintain its shape. A permanent prosthesis is individually designed to closely resemble the patient's other eye. The prosthesis can be fitted 1 to 2 months after surgery. Often, it is difficult to discern which eye is functional and which is the prosthesis.

> **clinicalALERT**
> Don't make the mistake of charting, "Pupils equal, round, and react to light and accommodation (PERRLA)" on a patient with an eye prosthesis!

Postoperative nursing care includes teaching, psychologic support, and observing for potential complications.

The patient may be instructed to apply warm compresses and instill antibiotic ointment or drops postoperatively.

Blindness

Visual impairment ranges from blindness to decreased visual acuity that can be corrected with refractive lenses. *Blindness* is defined as severely limited vision that cannot be corrected. Total blindness usually means the patient cannot see light at all. In practical terms, a person who needs assistive devices or help from others for normal activities of daily living due to impaired vision is considered blind. Most blindness is preventable with early recognition and treatment of common eye disorders such as cataract and glaucoma.

Nurses can foster independence in the hospitalized patient who is blind by doing the following:

- Orient to the environment verbally and physically. Describe the patient's room using a central point such as the bed. Lead the patient around the room, identifying chairs, sink, bathroom, and other landmarks. Be sure that objects such as chairs, personal items, and clothing are not moved within the room unless the patient moves them. Leave doors either fully open or closed as the patient wishes, but, to preserve safety, do not leave doors partially open. Keep the room and hallways free of clutter where the patient will be ambulating.
- Notify staff of a patient with impaired vision with a sign above the bed and in report.
- Use verbal communication freely. Describe activities going on around the patient. Introduce yourself as you enter the room, and let the patient know when you are leaving. Explain what you are going to do before doing it. Use a normal tone of voice when speaking directly to the patient.
- Provide other sensory stimuli such as radio and television as desired by the patient.
- Orient to food trays, describing the position of food items on the plate and tray using the face of a clock as a reference (unless the patient has always been blind and cannot visualize a clock face).
- When assisting with ambulation, offer your arm or elbow for the patient to grasp as you walk slightly ahead. Do not hold the patient's arm. Verbally describe the environment, such as "There will be two steps up five feet ahead."
- Do not be afraid to ask what assistance the patient desires.
- For the patient with a new loss of sight, refer for services as appropriate. Persons who are blind can receive mobility training, assistance with relearning of self-care activities, education about communication tools, and vocational and other forms of rehabilitation. State, local, and national agencies help coordinate services for the blind. Many assistive devices are available, including guide or pilot dogs, computer services, talking books and tape players, and low-vision aids.

EAR DISORDERS

Key Concept For a person to hear, sound waves must enter the external ear and travel through the ear canal to vibrate the tympanic membrane and bony structures of the middle ear, which activate receptors of the cochlea. Trauma or disease to any part of this pathway can affect hearing.

Disorders of the external ear can alter sound wave conduction and hearing. The most common disorders of the external ear include infection or inflammation, trauma, and obstruction of the ear canal with *cerumen* (wax).

Middle ear disorders may be either acute or chronic. They require immediate treatment to prevent damage and scarring of the middle ear structures, which could result in conductive hearing loss. Otitis media and mastoiditis are the common conditions affecting the middle ear.

Common inner ear disorders include labyrinthitis and Ménière disease. They are less common than external and middle ear disorders.

External Otitis

Disorders of the external ear—such as external otitis and impacted cerumen—can affect sound conduction and hearing. **External otitis**, or *swimmer's ear*, is inflammation of the ear canal. Swimmers, divers, and surfers are particularly prone to external otitis. Wearing a hearing aid or earplugs, which hold moisture in the ear canal, also is a risk factor.

PATHOPHYSIOLOGY AND MANIFESTATIONS
External otitis usually is caused by bacteria. Cerumen (earwax) is water repellent and has an antibacterial effect. Moisture, cleaning, or drying of the ear canal can remove earwax, increasing the risk of infection.

External otitis causes ear pain, which may be severe, and a feeling of fullness in the ear. Manipulating the outer ear increases the pain. Drainage may be present. The ear canal appears inflamed and swollen.

COLLABORATIVE CARE
Treatment of otitis externa usually includes:

- Thorough cleaning of the ear canal, particularly if drainage or debris is present.
- Treating the infection with a topical antibiotic.
- Topical corticosteroid drops (often combined with the antibiotic) to relieve the pain, itching, and swelling.
- Teaching to prevent future episodes of swimmer's ear (Box 40-6■).

BOX 40-6	PATIENT TEACHING

Tips to Prevent External Otitis

- Stay out of the water for 7 to 10 days or until completely healed.
- When you resume water activities, use earplugs, a tight-fitting swim cap, or a wetsuit hood to keep water out of the ears or protect the ear from cold water temperatures.
- After swimming, dry the outer ear with a towel, and then use a hair dryer on the lowest setting several inches from the ear to dry ear canals.
- Do not insert cotton swabs or any other object into the ear canals.

NURSING CARE

External otitis can cause severe pain and discomfort, but rarely requires hospitalization. The nurse teaches the patient about the disorder, comfort measures, and strategies to prevent future episodes.

PRIORITIZING NURSING CARE
The priority of care of patients with external otitis focuses on impaired tissue integrity. In addition, the nurse needs to teach the patient about managing external otitis at home.

HEALTH PROMOTION
It is important to educate people who spend a significant amount of time in the water about ways to prevent otitis externa. Review the guidelines listed in Box 40-6.

ASSESSING
When assessing a patient with external otitis, ask about ear cleaning practices and participation in water sports or activities. Have the patient describe ear pain, including its character, timing, aggravating factors (e.g., pulling or moving the auricle of the ear), and relieving factors. Assess hearing in both ears, using the whisper test (see Chapter 5) or an audiometer. Inspect the external ear for drainage, redness, or evidence of trauma. Using an otoscope, insert the speculum just inside (no more than 1 cm) the canal to inspect for redness, swelling, drainage, or trauma.

DIAGNOSING, PLANNING, AND IMPLEMENTING
Impaired Tissue Integrity

Expected outcome: Patient's tissue integrity will return to normal.

BOX 40-7   NURSING CARE CHECKLIST

Instilling Eardrops

- ☑ Wash hands.
- ☑ Warm the drops by holding the bottle or putting it in a pocket for about 5 minutes before instilling.
- ☑ Place the patient on the unaffected side or tilt the head toward the unaffected side.
- ☑ Partially fill the ear dropper with medication.
- ☑ Using the nondominant hand, straighten the ear canal by pulling the pinna of the ear up and back.
- ☑ Instill the prescribed number of drops into the ear canal.
- ☑ Keep the patient on the side for about 5 minutes after putting in the drops.
- ☑ Loosely place a small piece of cotton in the opening to the ear canal for 15 to 20 minutes.

■ Teach patients not to clean the ear canal with a toothpick, cotton-tipped applicator, or other tool. *This damages the skin and disrupts the protective cerumen, allowing infection to develop.*

■ Teach how to instill prescribed eardrops (Box 40-7 ■). *The medication is more effective when it is allowed to reach the inner portion of the ear canal.*

■ Instruct to avoid getting water in the affected ear until it is fully healed. Cotton balls may be used while showering to prevent water from entering the ear canal. Instruct to avoid water sports and activities until allowed by the primary care provider. *Moisture in the ear canal can interfere with healing.*

EVALUATING

To evaluate the effectiveness of teaching related to external otitis, have the patient demonstrate instilling eardrops. Review knowledge and willingness to avoid water sports until healing is complete. Have the patient describe measures to prevent future episodes of external otitis.

DOCUMENTING

Documentation includes any hearing deficits, ability to instill eardrops, and knowledge about preventative strategies.

CONTINUITY OF CARE

The patient is ultimately responsible for following the prescribed treatment and preventing future episodes of external otitis. Provide verbal and written instructions for the prescribed medications. Teach the patient how to prevent recurrent episodes. Inform all patients that ear canals rarely need cleaning beyond washing the external opening with soap and water. Teach patients of all ages not to clean ear canals with any implement.

Instruct the patient to report any increase in pain, swelling, or redness around the ear; fever; malaise; or increased fatigue to the primary care provider.

Impacted Cerumen and Foreign Bodies

The ear canal is narrow and curved. It can become obstructed by earwax or foreign objects such as insects.

As earwax dries, it moves out of the ear canal. In some people, however, it accumulates. Older adults in particular are at risk for *impacted* (tightly wedged) cerumen. With aging, earwax becomes harder and drier. Attempting to remove earwax with cotton-tipped swabs often packs it more deeply into the ear canal.

Ear canal obstruction interferes with sound conduction and hearing. The patient reports a sensation of fullness and **tinnitus** (ringing) in the ear. A foreign body or impacted cerumen can be seen using an otoscope.

Treatment focuses on clearing the canal. The canal may be irrigated to clear the obstruction. Impacted wax, objects, or insects may need to be removed using an ear curette, forceps, or other implement. Mineral oil or topical lidocaine drops are used to immobilize or kill insects before they are removed.

clinicalALERT

If a foreign body such as a bean or an insect occludes the canal, do not irrigate with water. Water may cause the object to swell, making it more difficult to remove.

Teaching is important to prevent obstruction of the ear canal with earwax. Advise the patient with impacted cerumen to use mineral oil or commercial products to soften wax and remove it by irrigating the canal with water. Stress the risk of impacting cerumen against the eardrum if cotton-tipped swabs are used to clean the ear canal. The swab also may break and lodge in the canal. If eardrops have been prescribed, teach the patient and a family member how to instill them.

Otitis Media

Middle ear disorders can lead to permanent hearing loss without effective treatment. **Otitis media**, inflammation or infection of the middle ear, is the most common middle ear disorder. It usually affects infants and young children but can occur in adults. While the eardrum protects the middle ear from the environment, the eustachian tube connects it with the nasopharynx. Organisms can enter the middle ear from the nose and throat through the eustachian tube.

PATHOPHYSIOLOGY AND MANIFESTATIONS

Upper respiratory infection (URI) and eustachian tube dysfunction are risk factors for otitis media. The eustachian tube is narrow and flat, normally opening only during yawning and swallowing. Allergies or URI can cause it to swell, impairing its function.

Serous otitis media occurs when the eustachian tube is obstructed for a long time. Air in the middle ear is gradually absorbed, causing negative pressure in the middle ear. The negative pressure draws serous fluid from the capillaries into the space.

Manifestations of serous otitis media include decreased hearing and a "snapping" or "popping" sensation in the affected ear. The eardrum moves less freely and may appear retracted ("sucked in") or bulging. Fluid or air bubbles may be seen behind the drum. Changes in atmospheric pressure (e.g., flying or underwater diving) can cause acute pain, bleeding into the middle ear, rupture of the eardrum, or rupture of the round window.

Acute otitis media usually follows URI. Swelling of the eustachian tube impairs drainage of the middle ear. Mucus and serous fluid collect in the middle ear. Bacteria enter from the nasopharynx, growing and multiplying in this fluid. The infection causes an immune response, and pus forms in the middle ear. The pus increases pressure in the middle ear and can rupture the eardrum.

Acute otitis media causes pain, often severe, in the affected ear. The patient may have a fever and complain of hearing loss, dizziness, vertigo (discussed later in the chapter), and tinnitus. The eardrum is red and inflamed or dull and bulging (Figure 40-12■). It does not move normally and may rupture, causing purulent drainage.

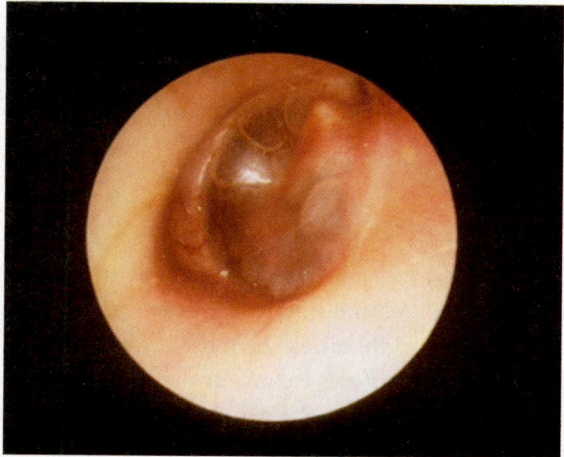

Figure 40-12. ■ A red, bulging tympanic membrane of otitis media. (Source: Southern Illinois University / Science Source.)

COMPLICATIONS

Acute mastoiditis may develop when acute otitis media is not effectively treated. Pus fills the air cells of the mastoid process of the temporal bone, which is next to the middle ear. Acute mastoiditis destroys these air cells, causing recurrent earache and hearing loss on the affected side. The mastoid process (behind the ear) is tender and may be swollen, red, and inflamed. The patient may complain of tinnitus, headache, and fever. Acute mastoiditis may lead to meningitis, although this condition occurs rarely.

Chronic otitis media is a permanent perforation of the eardrum. Middle ear infections are recurrent, and structures of the middle ear are destroyed. Severe conductive hearing loss may result.

COLLABORATIVE CARE

Otitis media is usually diagnosed by the patient's history and the physical examination. A *pneumatic otoscope* is used to examine the eardrum. A puff of air is blown into the ear canal; this normally causes slight movement of the eardrum. In otitis media, the drum moves less freely. A diagnostic test called *impedance audiometry* may also be done to assess movement of the eardrum and middle ear structures.

Medications

Acute otitis media is treated with antibiotic therapy, especially amoxicillin or azithromycin for 5 to 10 days. (See Chapter 9 for more information about antibiotic treatment.) Mild analgesics such as acetaminophen are recommended to relieve pain and reduce fever. Although decongestants may be used to improve eustachian tube function, they show minimal effectiveness in treating serous otitis media. (See Chapter 22 for more information about and the nursing implications of decongestants.) Acute mastoiditis needs aggressive treatment with intravenous antibiotics and possibly myringotomy.

Autoinflation

The patient with eustachian tube dysfunction may learn to open the tube by performing the Valsalva maneuver or by forcefully exhaling through the nose against closed nostrils. Also, the patient is taught to avoid air travel and underwater diving.

Surgery

Surgery may be done to relieve pressure in the middle ear and prevent spontaneous eardrum rupture. In a *tympanocentesis*, a needle is inserted through the eardrum to draw fluid and pus out of the middle ear. *Myringotomy*, surgical drainage of the middle ear, may be done. Patients who do not respond to antibiotics may need *ventilation (tympanostomy) tubes* inserted during myringotomy. This procedure allows ventilation and drainage of the middle ear during healing. The tube eventually comes out of the ear, and the eardrum heals. While the tube is in place, it is important to avoid getting any water in the ear canal. A *mastoidectomy*, removal of infected air cells, bone, and pus, may be done on a patient with mastoiditis.

Complementary Therapies

Complementary therapies may help promote comfort in the patient with otitis media. A drop of lavender oil on cotton in the ear canal helps relieve discomfort. A warm cloth or a chamomile tea bag steeped in warm water can be used to apply heat to the side of the face or ear, reducing pain. A naturopathic practitioner may prescribe remedies such as pulsatilla, belladonna, or aconite.

NURSING CARE

Patients with otitis media are commonly seen and treated in community settings. The nursing role focuses on prevention and teaching.

PRIORITIZING NURSING CARE

Pain and the risk of damage to the middle ear are priority nursing care problems for the patient with otitis media. Untreated middle ear infections can cause serious complications that require surgery for treatment. Box 40-8■ outlines nursing care of the patient having ear surgery.

HEALTH PROMOTION

Health promotion focuses on teaching patients to seek immediate medical attention when severe ear pain with or without drainage exists. This is especially important when these manifestations accompany a URI.

ASSESSING

Collect data about the onset and duration of symptoms, including pain, popping or snapping sensations in the ear, and any drainage from the ear. Ask about any recent URIs. Move the auricle of the ear, asking how movement affects the pain. The pain of otitis media usually does not change with manipulation of the external ear. Inspect the patient's throat for redness, swelling, or drainage. Obtain the patient's temperature. Assess hearing in both ears, using the whisper test or an audiometer. If trained, use an otoscope to inspect the ear canal and eardrum. Inspect and palpate the mastoid process for tenderness.

IDENTIFYING POTENTIAL COMPLICATIONS

Three complications—chronic otitis media, mastoiditis, or eardrum perforation—can develop when otitis media is recurrent or untreated.

DIAGNOSING, PLANNING, AND IMPLEMENTING
Acute Pain

Expected outcome: Will state pain is absent or at tolerable level.

- Assess pain for severity, quality, and location. Encourage the use of mild analgesics every 4 hours as needed to relieve pain and fever. *Pain assessment is essential to*

BOX 40-8	NURSING CARE CHECKLIST

Ear Surgery

Before Surgery

☑ Provide routine preoperative care as ordered (see Chapter 10).
☑ Assess hearing or verify that hearing has been assessed before surgery.
☑ Discuss postoperative communication strategies.
☑ Explain postoperative restrictions such as avoiding blowing the nose, coughing, and sneezing. Instruct to leave the mouth open if coughing or sneezing is necessary.

After Surgery

☑ Provide routine postoperative care as ordered (see Chapter 10).
☑ Assess for bleeding or drainage from the affected ear. Note the color, character, and amount of any drainage.
☑ Assess for nausea; administer antiemetics as ordered to prevent vomiting.
☑ Elevate the head of the bed and position the patient on the unaffected side.

☑ Assess for vertigo or dizziness, especially with movement. Avoid unnecessary movements such as turning. Ensure safety during ambulation.
☑ Assess hearing.
☑ Stand on the patient's unaffected side to communicate. Use alternate strategies, such as writing, when needed.
☑ Remind to avoid coughing, sneezing, or blowing the nose.
☑ Provide instructions for home care.
   a. Avoid showers, shampooing, and immersing the head until approved by the physician.
   b. Keep the outer earplug clean and dry, changing it as needed. Do not remove inner ear dressing until ordered by the physician.
   c. Avoid blowing the nose; if you need to cough or sneeze, keep the mouth open.
   d. Do not swim, dive, or travel by air until allowed by the physician.
   e. You may need to take an antiemetic/antihistamine drug for up to 1 month after surgery.
   f. Notify the physician if you develop a fever, bleeding, increased drainage, increased dizziness, or decreased hearing.

determine the source of the pain. Nonprescription drugs help relieve pain and reduce fever.

- Advise the patient to apply heat to the affected side of the face and head unless contraindicated. *Heat dilates blood vessels, promoting fluid reabsorption and reducing swelling.*
- Instruct the patient to avoid air travel, rapid changes in elevation, or diving. *A rapid change in pressure can increase the patient's pain and damage the inflamed middle ear.*
- Instruct to promptly report abrupt pain relief to the physician. *Abrupt pain relief may mean the eardrum has ruptured, releasing pressure from the middle ear.*

Deficient Knowledge: Otitis Media

Expected outcome: Will verbalize treatment and prevention of otitis media.

- Stress the importance of completing the full course of antibiotic therapy. *Taking the entire ordered antibiotic is important to eliminate the infection and prevent antibiotic-resistant bacteria from developing.*
- Inform the patient that the antibiotic may cause diarrhea, vaginitis, or thrush. Unless contraindicated, instruct the patient to eat 8 oz of yogurt with live bacterial cultures daily during antibiotic therapy. *Antibiotics destroy normal body flora as well as infectious organisms. Live yogurt cultures help restore these beneficial microbes, preventing superinfection.*
- Stress the importance of keeping follow-up appointments. *Follow-up is important to confirm cure of the infection and prevent complications.*
- Instruct the patient with ventilation tubes to avoid swimming, diving, or submerging the head while bathing. *Water can enter the middle ear through the ventilation tubes.*

MANAGING NURSING CARE

As appropriate and allowed by the designated duties and responsibilities of assistive personnel, the nurse may delegate nursing care activities such as assisting with ADLs for the patient with otitis media.

EVALUATING

Evaluate the effectiveness of care by collecting data on the presence of any hearing deficits, ear pain, and drainage. Identify the patient's understanding of the treatment plan and symptoms to report to the primary care provider. Also, determine knowledge about follow-up visits and compliance with prescribed treatment.

DOCUMENTING

Documentation includes improvement of symptoms; hearing ability; and teaching about antibiotics, preventive measures, and postoperative care if surgery was done.

CONTINUITY OF CARE

Teach about otitis media, its causes and prevention, and any specific treatment. Provide verbal and written instructions about the ordered antibiotic, its effects, recommended timing (with or without food, doses evenly spaced throughout the day), and possible side effects. Discuss the symptoms of allergic or adverse reactions that should be reported to the physician.

If surgery has been performed, teach the patient and family members about postoperative care. Discuss postoperative precautions, such as avoiding water in the ear canals and sudden changes in air pressure.

Otosclerosis

Otosclerosis is a hereditary disorder that usually affects White females. Abnormal bone forms, immobilizing the stapes and causing a conductive hearing loss.

Hearing loss usually begins in adolescence or early adulthood. Both ears are affected. Air conduction of sound is lost. However, sound is conducted through bone. As a result, the patient may be able to use a telephone but have difficulty conversing in person. The patient also may experience tinnitus. Otosclerosis may be treated with surgical reconstruction of the middle ear.

Education and referral of the patient to appropriate community agencies are important nursing care priorities for the patient with otosclerosis. For the patient who has surgery, nursing care is similar to that for other patients undergoing ear surgery (see Box 40-8).

Inner Ear Disorders

Inner ear disorders occur less frequently than other ear disorders. Labyrinthitis and Ménière disease are the most common diseases of the inner ear.

PATHOPHYSIOLOGY AND MANIFESTATIONS

The inner ear (or labyrinth) contains the semicircular canals that help maintain balance and the neural receptors for hearing. Inner ear disorders affect balance and may cause permanent hearing loss. **Vertigo**, a sensation of whirling or movement when there is none, is the key symptom of inner ear disorders.

clinicalALERT

Vertigo is a disorder of equilibrium (balance). It can be disabling, causing falls, injury, and difficulty walking. *Dizziness,* on the other hand, is a feeling of unsteadiness, lack of balance, light-headedness, or movement within the head. It is not as severe as vertigo.

Labyrinthitis

Labyrinthitis is inflammation of the inner ear. It may be caused by bacteria or viruses. Labyrinthitis is uncommon. It causes severe vertigo, hearing loss, and *nystagmus* (rapid involuntary eye movements). Nausea and vomiting often accompany the vertigo. Falling is a significant risk if the patient attempts to stand.

Ménière Disease

Ménière disease is a chronic inner ear disorder caused by excess fluid and pressure in the labyrinth of the inner ear. Its onset may be gradual or sudden. Patients with Ménière disease have recurring attacks of vertigo with tinnitus and gradual hearing loss. The hearing loss usually affects one ear, although the other ear also may be affected. Attacks of severe vertigo occur abruptly and are unpredictable, lasting from minutes to hours.

COLLABORATIVE CARE

There is no cure for inner ear disorders. Treatment focuses on managing symptoms and preventing permanent hearing loss.

Several diagnostic tests may be done to identify inner ear disorders.

- *Electronystagmography* is used to assess involuntary eye movements (nystagmus) in response to the stimuli of warm and cool water instilled into the ear canal.
- *X-rays* and *CT scans* of the inner ear structures may be done.
- *Glycerol test* is done by giving the patient oral glycerol to decrease pressure in the inner ear.

Hearing improves temporarily in patients with Ménière disease. Patients with labyrinthitis or an acute attack of Ménière disease may need hospitalization to manage the vertigo and its effects. Hydrochlorothiazide, a diuretic, may be used to reduce inner ear pressure. Drugs such as meclizine (Antivert), prochlorperazine (Compazine), or hydroxyzine (Vistaril) are given to relieve vertigo and nausea. If nausea and vomiting are severe, intravenous fluids may be used to maintain fluid and electrolyte balance. Bed rest in a quiet, darkened room with minimal sensory stimuli and minimal movement provides the most comfort for the patient.

The patient with Ménière disease may be placed on a low-sodium diet to reduce the frequency of attacks. Tobacco, which can precipitate an attack, is avoided, along with alcohol and caffeine.

Surgery may be necessary to relieve excess pressure in the inner ear or to block transmission of stimuli related to balance and vertigo. There is a risk of hearing loss when surgery is required. After surgery, the patient is positioned to minimize ear pressure and vertigo. Movement is restricted, and the patient is assisted during ambulation. Antiemetics and antivertigo drugs are used to manage the nausea and vertigo after surgery. Complications include infection and leakage of cerebrospinal fluid.

NURSING CARE

The patient with inner ear disorders has multiple nursing care needs related to the manifestations of the disease. Persistent episodes of dizziness, tinnitus, balance problems, or hearing loss should be reported to a health care provider. Patients diagnosed and treated early may have a lower risk for injury.

PRIORITIZING NURSING CARE

Nursing care for the patient with inner ear disorders focuses on reducing the risk for injury and promoting normal sleep patterns. Attacks of vertigo may occur without warning. They can be so severe that the patient cannot remain upright. Persistent tinnitus can interrupt sleep and rest.

HEALTH PROMOTION

Health promotion focuses on identifying people with possible inner ear disorders. It is important for people with constant dizziness, balance problems, tinnitus, or hearing loss to report these problems to a health care provider. Identifying and treating inner ear problems early may reduce the potential for injury.

ASSESSING

Assess the effects of the disorder on balance and the ability to safely ambulate. Assess hearing, using the whisper test (see Chapter 5). Ask about tinnitus, including pitch, tone, quality, and duration. Refer for a complete hearing and ear examination if this has not been done. Assess for nystagmus by having the patient follow an object through the six cardinal fields of vision (see Box 40-1). Nausea and vomiting may interfere with nutrition. Ask about usual food and fluid intake, and assess height and weight, skin color and condition, and for other signs of nutritional status. Discuss the effect of the disorder on the patient's life. Unpredictable attacks of vertigo, tinnitus, and hearing loss can affect lifestyle, employment, sleep, rest, and ability to cope.

DIAGNOSING, PLANNING, AND IMPLEMENTING
Risk for Injury

Expected outcome: Will remain free from injury.

- Ask the patient not to get up without assistance during acute attacks of vertigo. *During attacks of vertigo, assistance reduces the risk of falling.*

- Teach the patient to avoid sudden head movements or position changes. *Sudden movement may precipitate an attack of vertigo.*
- Administer drugs as ordered, including antiemetics, diuretics, and sedatives. *These medications may reduce the frequency, severity, and duration of attacks.*
- Teach the patient who senses an oncoming attack to take the prescribed medication and lie down in a quiet, darkened room. *This decreases the risk of injury and may reduce the duration and severity of the attack.*
- Instruct the patient to pull to the side of the road and wait for the symptoms to subside if an attack occurs while driving. *This is vital to protect the safety of the patient and others.*
- Discuss the importance of wearing a MedicAlert bracelet or necklace. *A MedicAlert bracelet or tag helps ensure appropriate treatment if the patient is unable to answer questions or respond in an emergency.*
- Discuss the effect of one-sided hearing loss on the ability to identify sound direction. Encourage the patient to use other senses as well, for example, when crossing the street. *When hearing is lost in one ear, sound perception and the ability to identify its direction change.*

clinicalALERT

During an acute attack of vertigo, keep the patient on bed rest with side rails raised and the call light within easy reach.

Sleep Deprivation

Expected outcome: Will report relief from symptoms of sleep deprivation.

Tinnitus can interfere with concentration, relaxation, and sleep.

- Discuss options for masking tinnitus:
  a. Ambient noise from a radio or sound system
  b. A masking device or white-noise machine
  c. A hearing aid that produces a tone to mask the tinnitus
  d. A hearing aid that amplifies ambient sound

  Masking the perception of tinnitus may allow the patient to focus on something other than the sound.

- Suggest that the patient discuss possible medications to treat tinnitus with the physician. *Drugs, including antidepressants such as nortriptyline (Aventyl, Pamelor), taken at bedtime may relieve tinnitus and promote rest.*

MANAGING NURSING CARE

As appropriate and allowed by the designated duties and responsibilities of assistive personnel, the nurse may delegate nursing care activities such as assisting with ADLs,

meal and fluid intake, and ambulation for the patient with inner ear disorders. Ensure that assistive personnel have a clear understanding of the importance of monitoring for dizziness or balance problems during ambulation.

EVALUATING

To evaluate the effectiveness of nursing care, assess for the presence of symptoms of inner ear problems. Determine the patient's ability to remain safe during periods of vertigo. Discuss the patient's understanding of the disease and measures to reduce the frequency and severity of attacks. Discuss coping strategies the patient can use to manage the effects of the disorder on lifestyle.

DOCUMENTING

Documentation includes noting manifestations of dizziness, tinnitus, balance problems, or hearing loss. Effectiveness of interventions to relieve these symptoms is noted. Record patient and family teaching about strategies to reduce and cope with the attacks, safety, medications, and possible community resources.

CONTINUITY OF CARE

Safety is a primary focus of teaching for home care. Teach the patient to change positions slowly, especially when ambulating. Turning the whole body rather than just the head helps to prevent vertigo. Because attacks can be unpredictable, the patient should not ambulate alone unless in a safe environment. Instruct to sit down immediately when vertigo occurs and lie down if possible. Teach about prescribed medications, providing both verbal and written instructions about their use, desired effects, and possible adverse effects and precautions. Suggest the following resources: Better Hearing Institute and Self-Help for Hard of Hearing People.

If the patient has had surgery, provide information about postoperative care and follow-up. Teach techniques to minimize postoperative vertigo and associated nausea. Surgery may cause permanent hearing loss in the affected ear; discuss safety and communication strategies.

Hearing Loss

Hearing loss impairs the ability to communicate in a world filled with sound and hearing individuals. Approximately 10 million adults in the United States are hearing impaired. Hearing loss is more common in older adults, affecting a quarter to a third of older adults. Up to 70% of long-term care residents have impaired hearing.

PATHOPHYSIOLOGY AND MANIFESTATIONS

Hearing loss is classified as conductive, sensorineural, or mixed, depending on what portion of the auditory system is affected. A hearing deficit can be partial or total, congenital or acquired. It may affect one or both ears. Some types of hearing loss affect the ability to hear specific frequencies of sound.

Conductive Hearing Loss

Anything that affects sound transmission from the external opening of the ear to the inner ear causes a *conductive hearing loss*. Obstruction of the ear canal, for example, by impacted cerumen, is the most common cause. Other causes of conductive loss include perforated eardrum; damage to the ossicles of the middle ear; and fluid, scarring, or tumors of the middle ear. The patient with a conductive hearing loss benefits from sound amplification by a hearing aid.

Sensorineural Hearing Loss

Disorders that affect the inner ear or the auditory pathways of the brain may cause a *sensorineural hearing loss*. Trauma, infection, diseases such as Ménière disease, ototoxic medications, and prenatal exposure to rubella can lead to sensory hearing loss. In the United States, noise exposure is the major cause. Exposure to a high level of noise, for example, standing close to the stage or speakers at a rock concert, damages the hair cells of the organ of Corti. Ototoxic drugs such as aspirin, furosemide (Lasix), vancomycin (Vancocin), streptomycin, aminoglycoside antibiotics, antimalarial drugs, and chemotherapy such as cisplatin (Platinol) also damage the hair cells.

Sensory hearing losses usually affect the ability to hear high-frequency sounds more than low-frequency sounds. This affects speech discrimination and communication, especially in a noisy environment. Hearing aids may not help because they amplify speech and background noise.

Presbycusis

With aging, the hair cells of the cochlea degenerate, causing progressive hearing loss. Hearing begins to decline in early adulthood and progresses with time. **Presbycusis** is a type of sensorineural loss. Initially, loss of high-pitched tones and conversation occurs. Because hearing loss is gradual, the patient and family may not realize the extent of the deficit. Hearing aids and other amplification devices are useful for most patients with presbycusis.

memoryALERT

Presbycusis causes loss of high-frequency tones and understanding of consonants such as *t, p,* or *s.* Talking louder does not help the patient hear or understand speech better.

COLLABORATIVE CARE

Hearing evaluation includes gross tests of hearing (e.g., the whisper test), the Rinne and Weber tests, and audiometry.

- The *Rinne and Weber tests* (Box 40-9■) compare sound conduction by air and through bone. Bone conduction of sound is better than air conduction with a conductive hearing loss. With a sensory hearing loss, both air and bone sound conduction are affected.
- *Audiometry* is used to quantify hearing deficits. Specific sound frequencies are presented to each ear by either air or bone conduction to identify the type and pattern of hearing loss.

Amplification

A hearing aid or other amplification device can help many patients with hearing loss. These devices amplify sound, increasing the sound level so it can be heard by the patient. This improves the perception and interpretation of the sound. Hearing aids must be individually prescribed by an audiologist. To be effective, proper design and fit as well as regular maintenance are necessary. Only 20% of people with a hearing deficit who might benefit from a hearing aid actually use it.

The least noticeable style of hearing aid fits entirely in the ear canal. It allows telephone use and can be worn during exercise. Because it is small, good manual dexterity is needed to insert it, clean it, and change the batteries. Patients with impaired dexterity and older adults may be unable to use this type of hearing aid. An in-ear hearing aid fits into the external ear (Figure 40-13A■). It is larger, is easier to handle, and provides greater amplification than the in-canal style of hearing aid.

The behind-the-ear hearing aid is easier to manipulate (Figure 40-13B). For the patient who wears glasses, it can be integrated into the earpiece of the eyeglasses. With both the in-canal and in-ear style, cleaning is important. Small openings may become plugged with wax, interfering with sound transmission.

Patients with profound hearing loss may require a body hearing aid. The microphone and amplifier of this aid are contained in a pocket-sized case that the patient clips onto clothing, slips into a pocket, or carries in a harness. The receiver is attached by a cord to the case and clips onto the ear mold, which delivers the sound to the ear canal.

For the patient who does not have a hearing aid, an assistive listening device, or "pocket talker," with a microphone and MP3 player–type earpieces, is useful. Pocket talkers are available over the counter and are relatively inexpensive. The earpiece requires no special fitting, and the external microphone allows the patient to focus on the desired sound rather than simply amplifying all sounds.

Surgery

Surgery such as stapedectomy or tympanoplasty may be done to correct damage to the middle ear. The patient with a sensorineural hearing loss may require a cochlear implant

| **BOX 40-9** | **ASSESSMENT** |

The Rinne and Weber Tests

The Rinne and Weber tests are used to help determine whether hearing loss is conductive or sensory.

■ *The Rinne test:* Strike the tines of a tuning fork on the heel of your hand to start it vibrating (see Figure A). Place the base of the tuning fork behind the ear, on the mastoid bone. Ask the patient to tell you when the sound is no longer heard, and then quickly move the tuning fork in front of the ear canal.

Ask if the patient can hear the sound. If the patient says yes, air conduction of sound is better than bone conduction, the normal finding.

■ *The Weber test:* Place the base of the vibrating tuning fork on the middle of the top of the patient's head (see Figure B). Ask where the patient best hears the sound. Sound is normally heard equally in both ears.

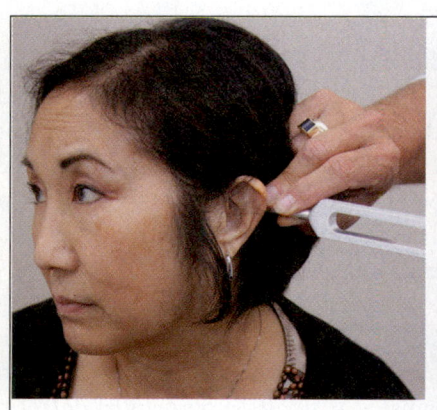
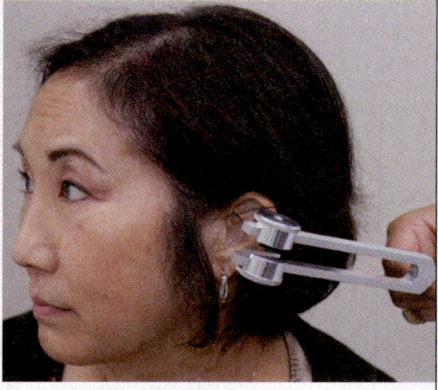

A   Rinne Test (Patrick Watson, Pearson Education.)

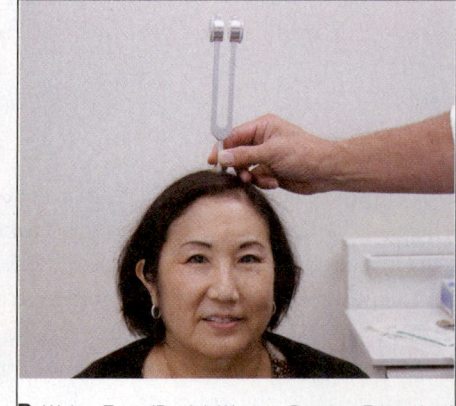

B   Weber Test (Patrick Watson, Pearson Education.)

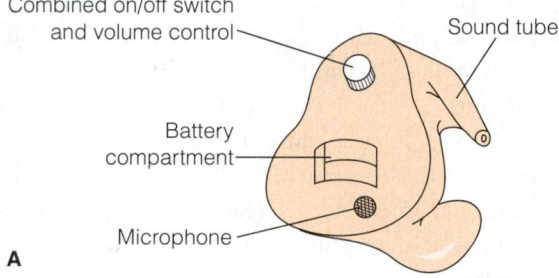

A

Combined on/off switch
and volume control

Sound tube

Battery
compartment

Microphone

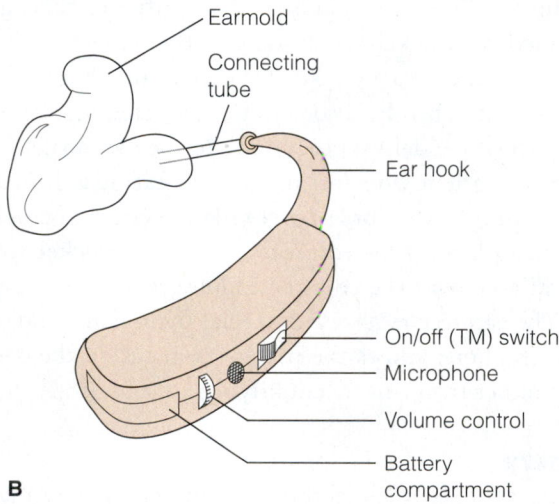

B

Earmold

Connecting
tube

Ear hook

On/off (TM) switch

Microphone

Volume control

Battery
compartment

Figure 40-13. ■ Types of hearing aids. (**A**) An in-ear hearing aid. (**B**) A behind-the-ear hearing aid.

to allow sound perception. Cochlear implants provide sound perception but do not restore normal hearing. The patient can recognize warning sounds such as automobiles, sirens, telephones, and doors opening or closing. They also are alerted to speech so they can focus on the person speaking. Many patients can learn to interpret the perceived sounds as words, especially when the hearing loss occurs in adulthood.

NURSING CARE

Planning and implementing nursing care for the patient with a hearing deficit focuses on the type and extent of hearing loss and on how well the patient has adapted to the loss. It also considers the availability of hearing aids and the patient's ability and willingness to use them.

PRIORITIZING NURSING CARE

Priority nursing care for a patient with a hearing loss focuses on the type and extent of hearing loss, impaired communication, and social isolation. It is important to identify the patient's willingness to use assistive devices and finances to purchase them.

HEALTH PROMOTION

Education is vital to help prevent hearing loss. Promote environmental noise control and ear protection. The Occupational Health and Safety Administration requires ear protection in workplaces that exceed 85 decibels. It is essential to teach about:

- Care of ears and ear canals, including cleaning and treatment of ear infections.
- Use of earplugs when swimming or diving.
- Use of ear protectors when operating loud equipment, shooting firearms, or when exposed to loud noise.
- Never placing hard objects into the ear canal.
- Monitoring for side effects with ototoxic medications.

ASSESSING

Patients with a hearing loss often display signs that caregivers can recognize. Voice volume frequently increases, and the patient positions the head with the better ear toward the speaker. Be alert for signs of impaired hearing such as cupping an ear, difficulty understanding verbal communication when the person cannot see the speaker's face, difficulty following conversation in a large group, and withdrawal from social activities. The patient may appear unsociable or paranoid.

Inspect the external ear canal and eardrum, using an otoscope. Perform the whisper test and Rinne and Weber tests to evaluate hearing. Document findings, and recommend an audiologist for further evaluation if indicated.

DIAGNOSING, PLANNING, AND IMPLEMENTING
Impaired Verbal Communication

Expected outcome: Will use effective communication techniques.

- Encourage the patient to talk about the hearing loss and its effect on ADLs. *Listening to and providing support encourage the patient to develop coping strategies.*
- Provide information about hearing loss and available services to the patient and family. *Information about hearing aids, amplification devices, and other services helps the patient plan ways to compensate for the loss.*
- Replace batteries in hearing aids on a regular and as-needed basis. *Hearing aid batteries last approximately 1 week.*
- If the hearing aid has a toggle switch for microphone/telephone, be sure it is in the appropriate position. *This ensures proper amplification with the hearing aid.*

clinicalALERT

Check hearing aids for patency, cleaning out earwax as needed.

- Use a wave of the hand or tap on the shoulder to get the patient's attention before beginning to speak. *This allows the patient to focus on the person speaking.*
- When speaking, face the patient and keep the hands away from the face. Avoid making the patient look into

glare or standing so that your face is in shadow. Trim mustaches so the lips are visible. *People with a hearing loss often use lip-reading consciously or unconsciously to help understand spoken words.*

- When speaking, use a low voice pitch with normal loudness. The voice tends to become higher in pitch when loudness increases. *The ability to hear higher pitch tones often is lost; lowering the voice pitch allows the patient to hear it more clearly.*
- Speak at a normal rate, and do not overarticulate. Use shorter sentences and pause at the end of each sentence. Rephrase sentences as necessary. *Changing the pace of speech may make conversation more difficult to follow and to lip-read. Using short sentences and pausing gives the patient time to interpret the message. Some words are more difficult to perceive than others; rephrasing often clarifies the message for the patient.*
- Use nonverbal and written communication as needed. *Nonverbal cues and written messages may improve understanding.*
- Ask the patient to repeat important information. *This helps ensure that the patient understood the information.*
- Tell other staff about the patient's hearing loss and effective communication strategies. *Consistent use of effective communication strategies decreases the patient's frustration.*

clinicalALERT

Reduce the noise in the environment before speaking with the patient.

Social Isolation

Expected outcome: Will interact with others and participate in activities.

- Help the patient identify the extent and cause of social isolation. *Identifying the hearing deficit as a contributing factor to a sense of isolation may prompt the patient to seek ways to improve hearing.*
- Encourage interaction with friends and family on a one-to-one basis in quiet settings. *Conversations in small groups and quiet settings are easier for the patient to follow and participate in.*
- Treat the patient with dignity. Remind friends and family that hearing loss does not mean loss of mental faculties. *Inappropriate responses to questions and comments can lead others to think of the patient as "stupid" or demented.*
- Involve the patient in activities that do not require acute hearing, such as checkers and chess. *Activities such as these allow social interactions without the stress of straining to hear.*
- Obtain a pocket talker or encourage the patient and family to do so.
- Refer to an audiologist for evaluation and possible hearing aid fitting.

■ Refer to resources such as support groups and senior citizen centers. *These groups provide new social outlets.*

MANAGING NURSING CARE

As appropriate and allowed by the designated duties and responsibilities of assistive personnel, the nurse may delegate nursing care activities such as assisting with ADLs for the patient with hearing loss. Ensure that assistive personnel have a clear understanding of the ways to communicate with the patient.

EVALUATING

Listen to the patient's responses, and observe behavior, interactions with others, and signs of anxiety or stress to help determine the effectiveness of nursing interventions for the patient with hearing loss.

DOCUMENTING

Documentation includes noting behaviors such as increased voice volume, cupping an ear, or positioning the head with the better ear toward the nurse. Also note the patient's withdrawal from social situations. Record patient and family teaching about caring for a hearing aid, strategies to cope with a hearing loss, and possible community resources.

CONTINUITY OF CARE

Help the patient learn to manage and cope with hearing loss. Discuss evaluation by an audiologist to determine the usefulness of a hearing aid. Teach the patient how to use, care for, and maintain a hearing aid. Encourage the patient to acknowledge the deficit and ask people to speak clearly and repeat statements as needed. Voicing a preference for individual visits and small group interactions rather than large social functions can help the patient to remain connected to friends and family.

Referral to an audiologist may be useful for evaluation of hearing and the possible need for hearing aids. National organizations such as the American Academy of Audiology, American Speech-Language-Hearing Association, and National Deaf Education Center can provide education and assistance.

Note: The references and resources for all chapters have been compiled at the back of the book.

Chapter Review

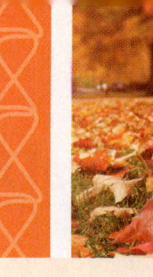

KEY POINTS

- **Concept:** Structures of the external eye are vulnerable to trauma and infection. While these problems are usually minor, they can cause significant pain, scarring and clouding of the cornea, and lost or impaired vision.
- Acute conjunctivitis or "pink eye" is highly contagious and often caused by *Staphylococcus* or *Haemophilus*. Preventing the spread of the infection is a key nursing role.
- **Concept:** Cataracts, glaucoma, age-related macular degeneration, and diabetic retinopathy are leading causes of impaired vision in the United States. Usually these conditions cannot be prevented, but treatment can slow their progression, preserving vision.
- Age, smoking, and diabetes increase the risk for cataracts. Removing the clouded lens and implanting an intraocular lens is the treatment of choice.
- Glaucoma is a gradual increase of intraocular pressure and impaired drainage of aqueous humor, causing a loss of peripheral vision. The most common form is open-angle glaucoma, which is controlled with medications. Acute angle-closure glaucoma is a medical emergency, requiring immediate treatment to lower intraocular pressure and preserve eyesight.
- Age-related macular degeneration causes loss of central vision. Smoking, aging, and being Caucasian are increased risk factors.
- Diabetic retinopathy is the leading cause of new blindness in people ages 20 to 74 that results in the destruction of the retinal blood vessels. Laser surgery is the treatment of choice.
- **Concept:** For a person to hear, sound waves must enter the external ear and travel through the ear canal to vibrate the tympanic membrane and bony structures of the middle ear, which activate receptors of the cochlea. Trauma or disease to any part of this pathway can affect hearing.
- Most outer and middle ear conditions are minor and treatable, but can lead to conductive hearing loss if ignored. Otitis media is the most common middle ear disorder. Acute otitis media can lead to chronic otitis media, mastoiditis, or eardrum perforation.
- Inner ear disorders cause vertigo and possibly hearing loss. Patients with vertigo are at risk for falls and often experience nausea and vomiting that can interfere with nutrition and ADLs.
- The two major types of hearing loss are conductive and sensorineural. Hearing loss associated with age is called presbycusis. Hearing aids are used to treat hearing loss.
- Inspect the ear canal of patients who complain about recent hearing loss, especially if the patient is older or wears a hearing aid or earplugs. Impacted cerumen can interfere with sound conduction and hearing.

PEARSON NURSING STUDENT RESOURCES

Find additional materials at **nursing.pearsonhighered.com**.

Clinical Reasoning Care Map

Caring for a Patient With Age-Related Hearing Loss
NCLEX-PN® Focus Area: Coping and Adaptation

Case Study: Carl Aaron is an 85-year-old retired logger who has been caring for his disabled wife in their home for the past 3 years. Mr. Aaron has osteoarthritis, which now makes it difficult for him to continue providing all the care his wife requires. They move into a care center where his wife can receive nursing care while he resides in the assisted living wing.

Nursing Diagnosis: Impaired Verbal Communication

COLLECT DATA

Subjective	Objective
_____	_____
_____	_____
_____	_____
_____	_____
_____	_____
_____	_____

Does this present a threat to the patient's safety?

If yes, the priority intervention to address this threat would be:

_____

Nursing Care

_____
_____
_____
_____
_____
_____
_____
_____

Interprofessional team members to include when planning care:

_____

How would you document this?_____

_____

Compare your answers and documentation to those provided on the companion website.

Data Collected
(use only those that apply)

- Proximal interphalangeal (PIP) and distal interphalangeal (DIP) joints swollen, cool, and hard bilaterally
- Weber test, no lateralization
- Answers not always appropriate to the question
- *Rinne test* (air conduction greater than bone conduction)
- Appears depressed
- Mental status exam is normal
- Frequently asks nurse to repeat questions
- Ear canals clean, no redness, small amount of dark earwax noted
- C/O hip pain when ambulating
- Audiometric testing reveals significant hearing loss consistent with presbycusis
- BP 144/86, P 78, R 18
- Expresses concerns about wife's care
- Ignores conversation at his table during meals about wife's care

Nursing Interventions
(use only those that apply; list in priority order)

- Teach Mr. Aaron how to use and care for hearing aids.
- Provide a schedule of small group activities for Mr. Aaron.
- Supplement verbal with nonverbal communication strategies.
- Obtain a temperature-controlled heating pad to promote comfort.
- Use a pocket talker as needed until hearing aids are available.
- Ask Mr. Aaron's family to obtain headphones for radio and television use.
- Administer ordered nonsteroidal anti-inflammatory drug (NSAID) every 6 hours.
- Use effective communication techniques.
- Encourage Mr. Aaron to shower on arising to relieve morning stiffness.
- Face Mr. Aaron when speaking with him.
- Facilitate one-on-one interactions between Mr. Aaron and other residents.
- Speak distinctly in a low voice.

NCLEX-PN® Exam Preparation

1   A patient arrives in the outpatient clinic with a possible corneal abrasion. What diagnostic test would confirm this diagnosis?

1. Tonometry
2. Visual field testing
3. Facial x-rays
4. Fluorescein staining

2   A patient arrives in the emergency department with a possible detached retina. What intervention should the nurse implement first?

1. Place the patient in dependent position.
2. Discuss follow-up treatment with an ophthalmologist.
3. Provide care in a calm manner.
4. Notify the physician immediately.

3   The nurse is teaching a patient the correct method for administering eardrops. Place the steps in the correct order that the patient should do them.

1. Tilt the head toward the unaffected side.
2. Instill the ordered number of drops.
3. Pull the pinna (auricle) upward and backward.
4. Place a loose cotton ball in the ear canal for 15 to 20 minutes.
5. Partially fill the ear dropper with medication.
6. Warm the drops by holding the bottle.

4   The nurse is caring for an older patient who has a severe hearing impairment. What would be an appropriate nursing intervention?

1. Encourage the patient to learn sign language.
2. Write out questions and responses.
3. Reduce environment noise before speaking with the patient.
4. Raise the voice to a higher pitch.

5   A patient is being taught about taking timolol (Timoptic). Which of the following side effects should the patient report to a health care provider?

1. Darkening of the iris
2. Stinging in the eyes
3. Bitter taste in the mouth
4. Difficulty breathing

6   A patient in the outpatient clinic has possible acute otitis media. Which of the following manifestations should the nurse report immediately to the health care provider?

1. Hearing loss in the affected ear
2. Tenderness behind the ear
3. Vertigo
4. Tinnitus

7   When educating a patient about acute angle-closure glaucoma, what point should the nurse emphasize to the patient about this condition?

1. Immediately report symptoms to the physician.
2. Do not use medications that cause pupil constriction.
3. Wear sunglasses when outdoors.
4. Lie down for 30 minutes until symptoms disappear.

8   Immediately after cataract surgery, it is important for the nurse to place the patient in what position?

1. Flat in bed
2. Turned on affective side
3. High Fowler's position
4. Semi-Fowler's position

9   During the nurse's initial assessment of an older woman with open-angle glaucoma, what symptoms might the history reveal?

1. Light flashes in both eyes
2. Difficulty focusing on near objects
3. Acute severe eye pain
4. Watery drainage from both eyes

10   When teaching the patient about Ménière disease, which of the following diet changes should the nurse emphasize?

1. Avoid foods high in sodium.
2. Increase the amount of green leafy vegetables.
3. Reduce the intake of milk and milk products.
4. Increase fluid intake before meals.

Answers and rationales for Review Questions appear in Appendix I.

Thinking Strategically About …

You are an LPN/LVN working on a neurologic unit at a major hospital. You will be assisting the RN in caring for the following patients.

Mr. Wong Lee is a 50-year-old tugboat mechanic who is married with three sons. He has been through rehabilitation twice for alcoholism, but continues to drink. Mr. Lee takes an anticoagulant for chronic atrial fibrillation. While attending a family reunion, Mr. Lee joins a game of softball. During the end of the second inning, the batter hits a ball that strikes Mr. Lee in the head. He stumbles and drops to the ground but eventually gets up on his own and insists that he feels fine. Two weeks later, after an evening of socializing and drinking, Mr. Lee develops a headache. He attributes it to a hangover, but the headache becomes steadily worse the next day. He becomes confused and disoriented. His wife takes him to the local emergency department where a CT scan is performed. The diagnosis of subdural hematoma is made, and Mr. Lee is transferred to the neurosurgical unit. Mr. Lee undergoes surgery for burr holes and evacuation of a hematoma. After 3 days in the critical care unit, Mr. Lee is transferred to the neurologic unit.

Physical assessment findings on admission to the neurologic unit include T 98.5°F (37.0°C), BP 160/72, P 62, and R 14. Mr. Lee continues to be disoriented and states he has headache that is relieved with oral pain medication.

Mrs. Josephine Smith, a 62-year-old patient is recovering from a stroke that left her with weakness on the right side and slight slurred speech. She is stable and plans to be transferred to a rehabilitation facility tomorrow.

Mr. Hines, a 28-year-old, was admitted last evening for observation after a sports-induced head injury. Mr. Hines and his wife are active in many outside sports. He routinely wears appropriate helmets and safety equipment. Yesterday while rock climbing he was hit on the head by a small falling rock. He did not lose consciousness. He was brought to the emergency room by his wife. Mr. Hines's vital signs and neurologic exam are stable, and he should be discharged this morning.

Mr. Mullins, a 58-year-old construction worker, underwent surgery 2 days ago for herniated lumbar disk involving L_4 and L_5. Mr. Mullins was in pain for some time preoperatively and is upset that he is still experiencing pain at 5–6 postoperatively. This is Mr. Mullins' first hospitalization.

CRITICAL THINKING

- What are factors in Mr. Lee's history that make intracranial bleeding more likely after a minor head injury?

- Mrs. Smith has been started on a daily dose of Coumadin. Why is long-term anticoagulant therapy recommended after a stroke?

- Compare the risks for complications between Mr. Lee and Mr. Hines.

PRIORITIES IN NURSING CARE

As you leave the report room at 0730, the night nurse tells you that Mr. Mullins is upset with the care that the night CNA provided and wants to speak to the charge nurse. She adds that Mr. Lee has complained of constipation and is sitting on the commode trying to have a bowel movement. The unit secretary tells you that the doctor is asking for a set of vital signs on Mr. Hines and that Mrs. Smith would like something for back pain.

- In what order would you address these needs and why?

MANAGEMENT OF CARE

- Postoperatively, Mr. Lee keeps trying to pull out his IV, remove his dressing, pull out his Foley catheter, and get out of bed without assistance. Knowing he is a risk for infection and increased ICP, what are the nursing implications indicated for Mr. Lee and in general for any patient with an increased ICP?

- Which members of the interprofessional team would have been involved in Mrs. Smith's care when she is transferred to the rehabilitation facility?

- Knowing this is Mr. Mullins's first hospitalization and that he was upset about his care earlier, what approach will you use in providing care today?

DELEGATING

- As Mr. Hines prepares for discharge, what aspects of his preparation can be delegated to the CNA?

PATIENT TEACHING

- Describe what teaching needs to be provided for Mr. Lee's wife and sons to assist in coping with this event?

- What discharge teaching should be provided to Mr. Hines and his wife?

CULTURAL CARE STRATEGIES

- If Mr. Wong Lee had recently emigrated from China, how might his assessment and care be impacted?

DOCUMENTATION

- Write a focused note to document that Mr. Mullins was upset about his care last evening.

Note: Because you were not present to witness any altercation, it is important to document what a patient tells you in a nonaccusing manner.

Note: Discussion of Unit questions appears on the companion website.

UNIT XI
Disrupted Musculoskeletal Function

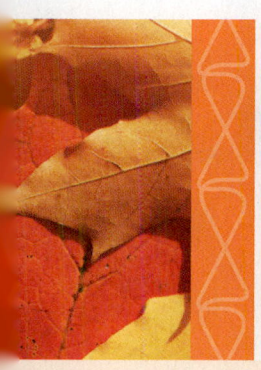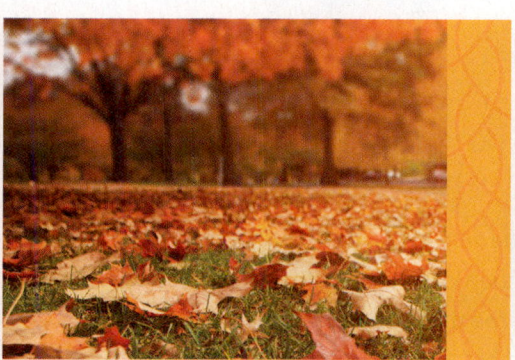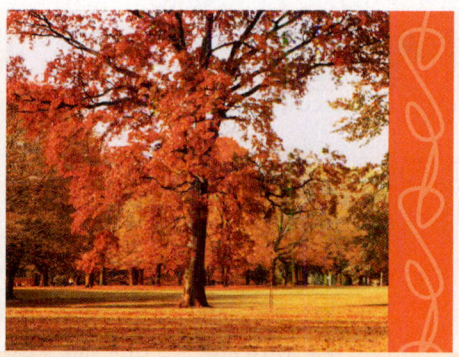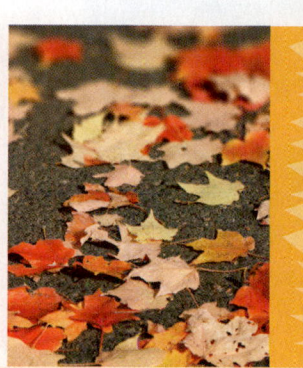

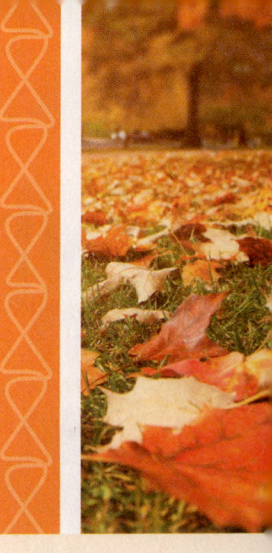

CHAPTER 41

The Musculoskeletal System and Assessment

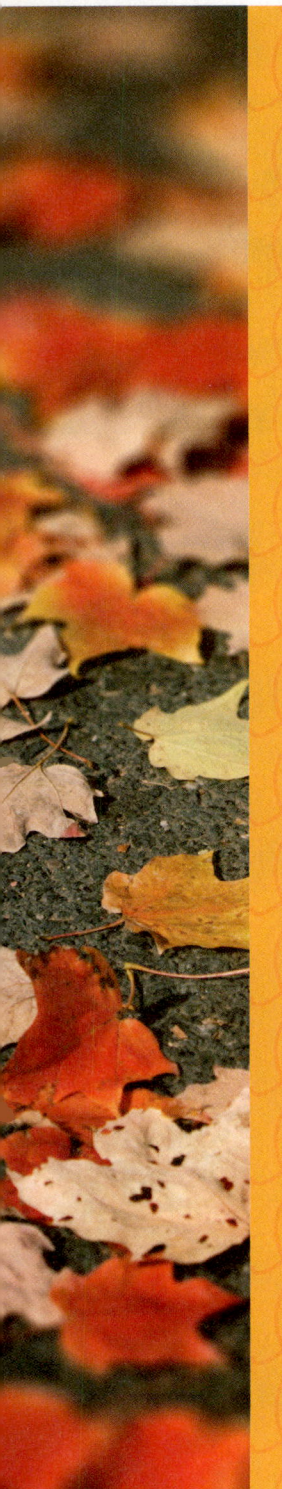

BRIEF OUTLINE

Structure and Function of the   **Assessment**
   Musculoskeletal System

APPLIED LEARNING OUTCOMES

After completing this chapter, you will be able to:

1. Describe the structure and function of the musculoskeletal system.
2. Identify age-related changes in the musculoskeletal system.
3. Perform and document focused health history and physical assessment of the musculoskeletal system, demonstrating sensitivity and respect for the uniqueness of the individual.
4. Recognize and document alterations in musculoskeletal structure and function, reporting findings within the interprofessional team as appropriate.
5. Provide nursing care and evidence-based teaching for patients undergoing diagnostic tests for musculoskeletal system disorders.

KEY TERMS

The key terms are defined on the pages listed below.

Structure and Function of the Musculoskeletal System

Key Concept Intact structure and function of the musculoskeletal system is vital to the ability to perform physical exercise and usual daily living activities independently.

The musculoskeletal system includes bones and joints of the skeleton, connective tissues such as tendons and ligaments, and the skeletal muscles. It allows us to remain upright and to move and protects our vital organs.

BONES

The human skeleton has 206 bones (Figure 41-1■). Bones provide structure and support soft tissues. They protect vital organs from injury. Bones are classified by shape (Figure 41-2■):

- *Long bones,* such as those in the arms and legs, have a shaft, called a *diaphysis,* and two broad ends, called *epiphyses.*
- *Short bones* include those of the wrist and ankle.
- *Flat bones,* including skull bones, the sternum, and ribs, are thin and flat; most are curved.
- *Irregular bones* vary in size and shape. They include the vertebrae, the scapulae, and the bones of the pelvis.

Bone cells include *osteoblasts* (cells that form bone), *osteocytes* (cells that maintain bone), and *osteoclasts* (cells that resorb bone). Bones also contain collagen (a type of connective tissue) and minerals (primarily calcium and phosphate). They are covered with *periosteum,* a double-layered connective tissue that contains blood vessels and nerves.

There are two types of bone: *Compact bone* is smooth and dense, whereas *spongy bone* contains spaces. Both types are found in almost all bones of the body. Compact bone forms the shaft of long bones and the outside layer in other types of bones. The spongy sections of bones contain bone marrow. *Red bone marrow,* found mostly in flat bones such as the sternum, ribs, and ileum, makes blood cells and hemoglobin. *Yellow bone marrow,* found in the shaft of long bones, primarily contains fat and connective tissue.

Bones that are being used and subjected to stress (e.g., weight-bearing activity) are constantly remodeled. In this process, bone is resorbed and new bone is deposited. Bone remodeling is regulated by hormones, the effects of gravity, and mechanical stress from the pull of muscles. Without activity and stress on the bones, more bone is resorbed and less new bone is formed.

JOINTS, LIGAMENTS, AND TENDONS

Joints, also called *articulations,* are where two or more bones meet. They hold the skeleton together while allowing the body to move. The three primary types of joints are:

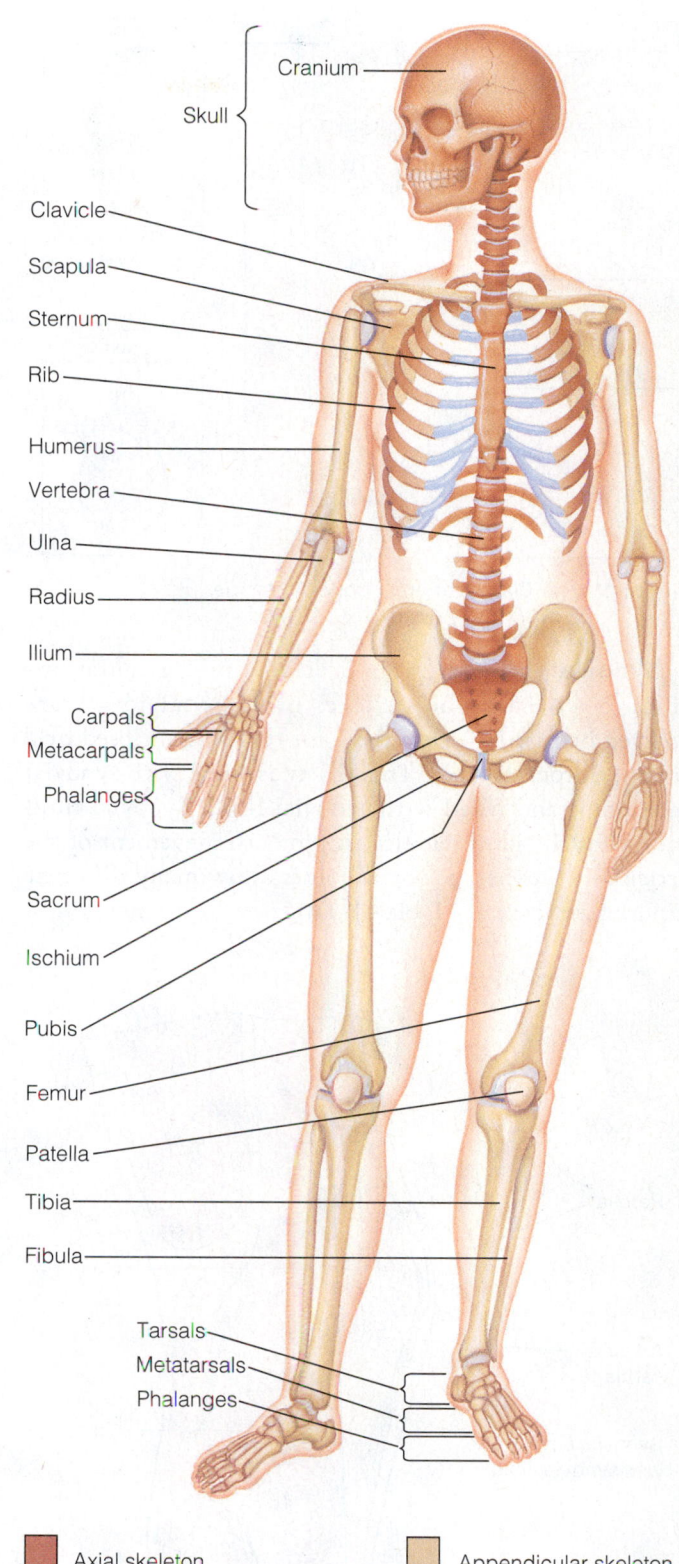

Figure 41-1. ■ Bones of the human skeleton.

1. *Synarthrosis*—immovable joints (e.g., skull sutures)
2. *Amphiarthrosis*—slightly movable joints (e.g., vertebral joints)
3. *Diarthrosis* or *synovial*—freely movable joints (e.g., joints of the limbs, shoulders, hips)

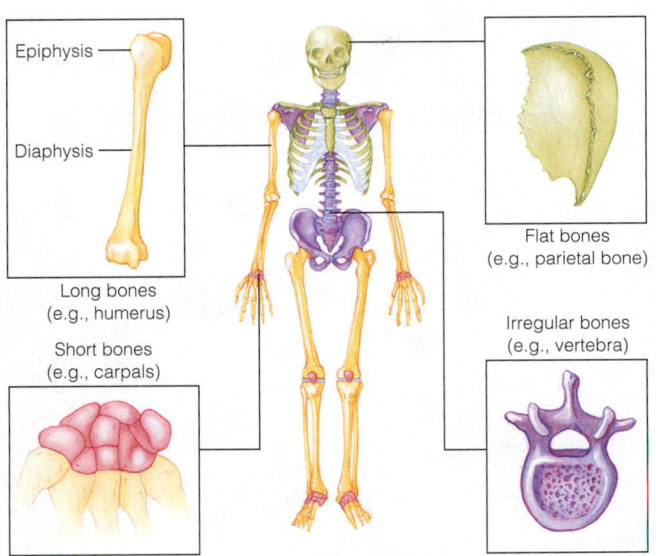

Figure 41-2. ■ Classification of bones by shape.

TABLE 41-1	Movements of Synovial Joints
MOVEMENT	**DESCRIPTION**
Abduction	Movement away from the midline of the body
Adduction	Movement toward the midline of the body
Extension	Straightening of a limb at a joint
Flexion	Bending of a limb at a joint
Dorsiflexion	Bending of the ankle to bring top of foot toward the shin
Plantar flexion	Straightening of the ankle to point toes down
Pronation	Turning of the forearm to place the palm down
Supination	Turning of the forearm to place the palm up
Eversion	Turning out
Inversion	Turning in
Circumduction	Movement in a circle
Internal rotation	Movement inward on a central axis
External rotation	Movement outward on a central axis

Synovial joints are found at all limb articulations (Figure 41-3 ■). The surfaces of synovial joints are covered by cartilage, and the joint cavity is enclosed by a tough, fibrous capsule. This cavity is lined with synovial membrane and filled with synovial fluid. Synovial fluid lubricates the joint, facilitating smooth movement of the articulating bones. Synovial joints allow many different kinds of movements (Table 41-1 ■).

Ligaments are bands of connective tissue that connect bones to bones. They prevent excessive joint movement, provide joint stability, and enhance joint strength. *Tendons* are fibrous connective tissue bands that connect muscles to bones and enable the bones to move when skeletal muscles contract. *Bursae* are small sacs of synovial fluid that cushion and protect bony areas that are at high risk for friction, such as the knee and the shoulder.

MUSCLES

There are three types of muscle tissue: skeletal muscle, smooth muscle, and cardiac muscle. *Skeletal muscle,* also known as *voluntary muscle,* allows voluntary movement. Both *smooth muscle* and *cardiac muscle* are involuntary muscle; their movement is controlled by internal mechanisms. The muscles of the bladder wall, gastrointestinal system, and bronchi are smooth muscle. Cardiac muscle is in the heart.

Skeletal muscles are thick bundles of parallel fibers (Figure 41-4 ■). Each muscle fiber is a bundle of smaller structures called *myofibrils.* Myofibrils are strands of smaller repeating units called *sarcomeres,* which allow the muscle to contract. The cells of skeletal muscle are *excitable;* that is, they can receive and respond to a stimulus.

Skeletal muscle contracts when motor neurons release acetylcholine, a neurotransmitter. This produces an action potential (electrical impulse) that spreads through the muscle fiber, causing it to contract. The more fibers that contract, the stronger the muscle contraction. Muscle fibers

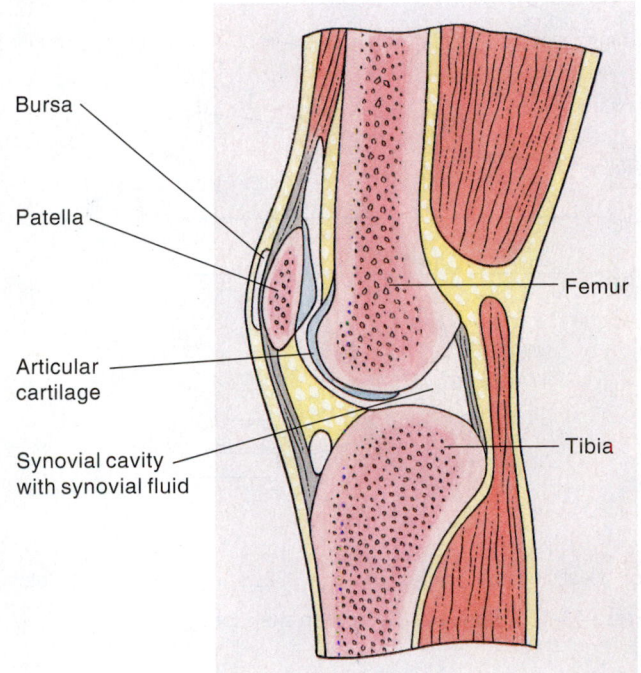

Figure 41-3. ■ Structure of the knee, a synovial joint.
(Source: "Figure 38.06—Structure of a Synovial Joint (knee)" from *Medical Surgical Nursing: Critical Thinking in Patient Care,* 5e by Priscilla LeMone; Karen Burke; and Gerene Bauldoff. Published by Pearson Education, © 2011.)

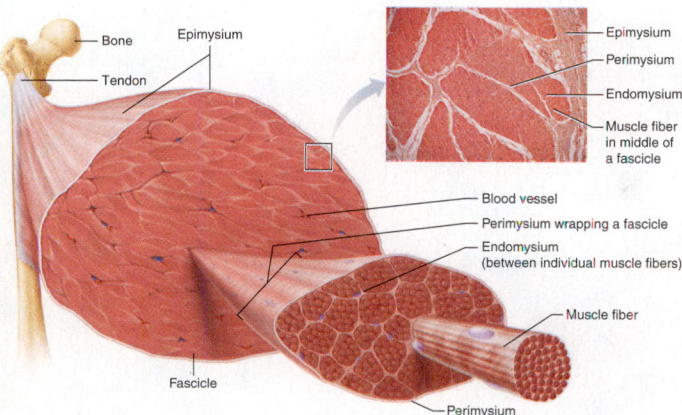

Figure 41-4. ■ Structure of skeletal muscle. (Source: "Figure 9.01—Connective Tissue Sheaths of Skeletal Muscle: Epimysium, Perimysium, and Endomysium" from *Human Anatomy & Physiology*, 9e by Elaine N. Marieb and Katja Hoehn. Published by Pearson Education, © 2013.)

extend when they relax. Extension also occurs in response to a stimulus. Skeletal muscles can be moved through conscious, voluntary control or by reflex activity. Muscle fibers return to their resting length after shortening or lengthening in response to stimuli. There are approximately 600 skeletal muscles in the body (Figures 41-5 ■).

Nerve impulses maintain muscle tone. Lack of use causes muscle atrophy, whereas regular exercise increases the size and strength of muscles. Prolonged strenuous activity can cause a buildup of lactic acid and muscle fatigue.

CHANGES IN THE OLDER ADULT

Aging commonly affects the musculoskeletal system. Although some musculoskeletal system changes appear to relate to the aging process itself, others result from decreased activity, lifestyle factors, or pathophysiologic processes.

Older adults, women in particular, tend to lose bone mass with aging. Joint and disk cartilage dehydrates and loses its flexibility as well. Together, these changes contribute to a loss of height (an average of about 1.5 to 2 in.) and a stooped posture. The hips and knees are somewhat flexed, and the head is tilted slightly backward to maintain eye contact. This posture changes the older adult's center of gravity, increasing the risk for falls. Dehydration of joint cartilage contributes to degenerative joint disease (osteoarthritis) in older adults. Affected joints tend to stiffen and lose range of motion (ROM). Cartilage deteriorates, and pieces of cartilage may be loose in the joint space, contributing to joint pain and stiffness. Ligaments and tendons lose flexibility with aging, increasing the risk of tears and joint instability.

Reduced activity levels, decreased muscle cell innervation, and endocrine changes associated with aging contribute to skeletal muscle atrophy in the older adult.

Muscle tone decreases, as does muscle strength and stamina. Maintaining an active lifestyle and specific exercises such as weight training help counteract these changes, maintain muscle mass, and prevent osteoporosis.

Assessment

Key Concept Manifestations of musculoskeletal injuries and disorders may be detected during a general health assessment as well as during focused and functional musculoskeletal assessments.

This section focuses on assessment of the musculoskeletal system. Assessment data may be collected as part of a comprehensive health assessment of the patient or may be obtained from a patient with a complaint or disorder related to musculoskeletal function.

Pain and limited mobility are the primary manifestations of musculoskeletal trauma and disorders. Because the neurologic and musculoskeletal systems are closely interrelated, a neurologic disorder may have musculoskeletal effects (e.g., a stroke or multiple sclerosis). Assessment of neurologic function is presented in Chapter 37.

HEALTH HISTORY

Explore the patient's chief complaint (e.g., wrist pain), inquiring about the onset of the problem, its duration and specific manifestations, and its effect on function and ability to maintain activities of daily living (ADLs). Ask about any precipitating events such as trauma (e.g., a fall, motor vehicle crash, hyperextension of a joint), repetitive use, or other associated events. Explore complaints of pain, determining the location and any radiation of the pain, its character (sharp, dull, aching, constant, or intermittent), duration and timing, factors that aggravate or relieve the pain, and the effect of the pain on function (e.g., resulting movement limits, ability to complete ADLs, and effect on occupation and other life roles). Inquire about associated complaints, such as fever, fatigue, weight changes, rash, or swelling. Explore past injuries or related or similar problems and treatment measures (prescribed or self-care) and their effectiveness.

PHYSICAL EXAMINATION

Depending on the circumstances, physical assessment of the musculoskeletal system may be very focused or may include overall assessment of musculoskeletal structure and function. In most cases, the practical/vocational nurse focuses on collecting assessment data related to the patient's primary problem/complaint.

Begin by assessing the patient's posture, gait, ability to walk and change directions with or without assistive devices, and ability to sit and rise from a chair.

(Text continues p. 1058.)

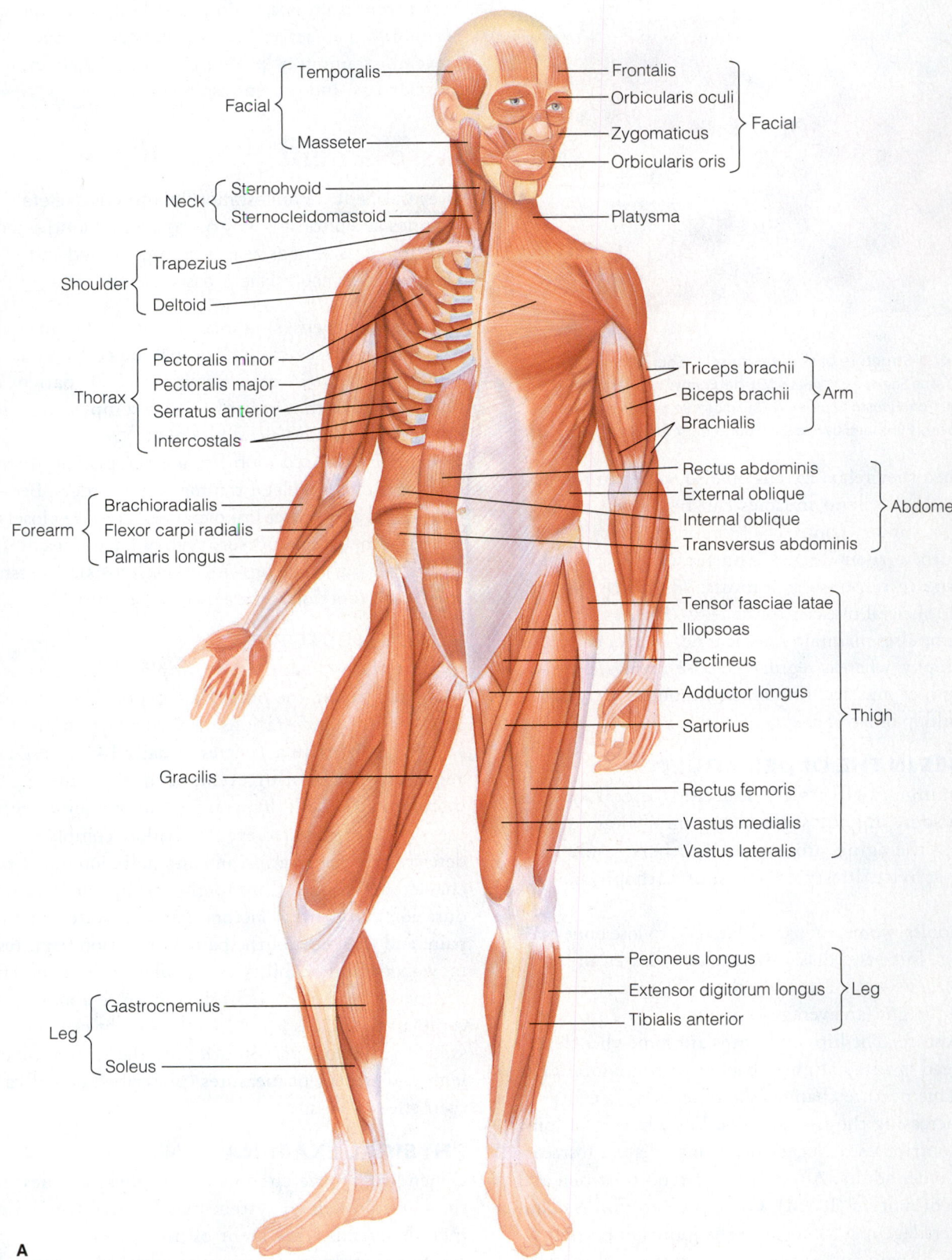

Figure 41-5. ■ (**A**) Muscles of the anterior body.

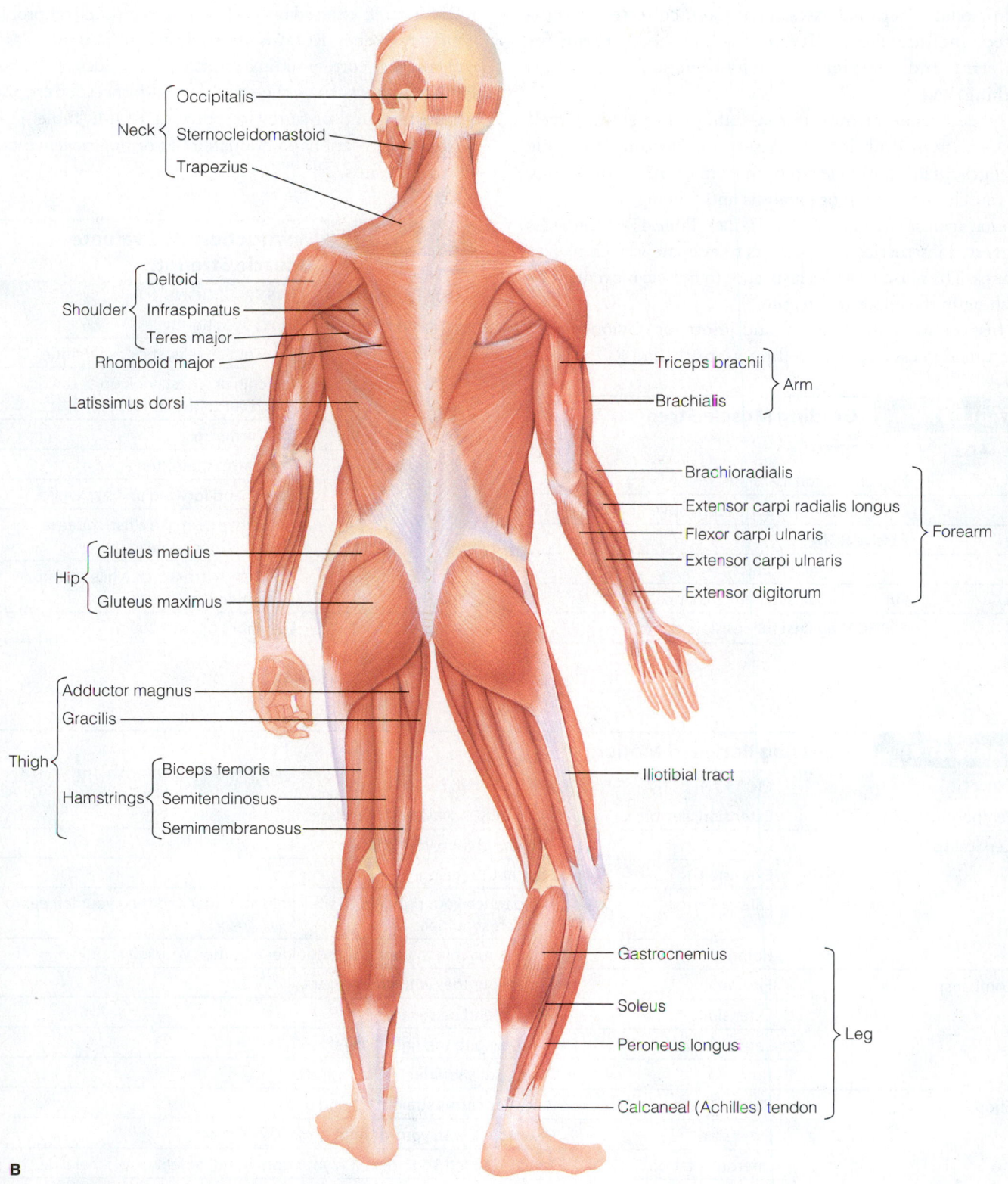

Neck
- Occipitalis
- Sternocleidomastoid
- Trapezius

Shoulder
- Deltoid
- Infraspinatus
- Teres major

Rhomboid major

Latissimus dorsi

Triceps brachii
Brachialis
} Arm

Brachioradialis
Extensor carpi radialis longus
Flexor carpi ulnaris
Extensor carpi ulnaris
Extensor digitorum
} Forearm

Hip
- Gluteus medius
- Gluteus maximus

Thigh
- Adductor magnus
- Gracilis
- Hamstrings
  - Biceps femoris
  - Semitendinosus
  - Semimembranosus

Iliotibial tract

Gastrocnemius
Soleus
Peroneus longus
Calcaneal (Achilles) tendon
} Leg

B

Figure 41-5. ■ **(B)** Muscles of the posterior body.

Additional functional assessment data, collected as indicated, include the ability to manipulate clothing for toileting and complete other hygiene activities (e.g., bathing) and ADLs.

Inspect general muscle mass and symmetry, as well as equality of limb length. Assess and document muscle strength, grading muscle strength from 0 to 5, with 0 being no muscle contraction or paralysis and 5 being full range of motion against resistance (Table 41-2■). Table 41-3■ provides suggested instructions for patients to evaluate various muscle groups. The nurse provides resistance to muscle movement by pushing in the opposite direction.

Inspect and palpate bones and joints for obvious deformity, tenderness or pain, swelling, warmth, and ROM. Joint ROM is often assessed only when a musculoskeletal problem is present. When ROM is assessed, it is important to assess and compare corresponding joints on both sides of the body. Palpate joints such as the shoulders and knees for **crepitus**, a grating sound or sensation, during ROM. Table 41-4■ provides instructions to evaluate the normal movements for the major joints.

TABLE 41-2	Grading Muscle Strength
GRADE	**DESCRIPTION**
0	No contraction; paralysis
1	Contraction felt but no limb movement
2	Passive ROM
3	Full ROM against gravity
4	Full ROM against some resistance
5	Full ROM against full resistance

TABLE 41-3	Instructions to Evaluate Muscle Strength
MUSCLE GROUP	**INSTRUCTIONS**
Eyes and lids	Close eyes tightly.
Facial muscles	Blow out cheeks, stick out tongue.
Neck	Put chin on chest, look up at ceiling, touch ear to the shoulder.
Deltoid	Hold arms up.
Biceps, triceps	Bend arm, straighten arm.
Wrist	Bend hand forward and backward.
Fingers	Shake hands, make a fist, squeeze nurse's fingers, spread fingers.
Gluteal and leg	Alternately cross legs while sitting, straighten leg.
Ankle and foot	Bend foot up and down.

TABLE 41-4	Assessing Range of Motion	
JOINT(S)	**MOTION**	**PATIENT INSTRUCTIONS**
Temporomandibular (TM)	Extension, flexion	Open mouth wide and then close it.
Cervical spine	Flexion	Put your chin to your chest.
	Extension	Look at the ceiling.
	Lateral flexion	Try to touch your right ear to your right shoulder and then your left ear to your left shoulder.
	Rotation	Touch your chin to your right shoulder and then your left shoulder.
Lumbar spine	Flexion	Touch your toes with your fingers.
	Extension	Slowly bend backward.
	Lateral flexion	Bend torso to the right and left.
	Rotation	Twist your shoulders right and left.
Shoulders	Flexion	Raise your arms straight up and out.
	Extension	Reach back with your straight arm.
	Internal rotation	Touch your left shoulder with your right hand; repeat with other side.
	Abduction	Raise your arm straight out to the side.
	Adduction	Move your straight arm across your chest.
Elbows	Flexion	Touch your hands to your shoulders.
	Pronation	With elbows bent, turn your hand palm down.
	Supination	With elbows bent, turn your hand palm up.

(continued)

TABLE 41-4	Assessing Range of Motion *(continued)*	
JOINT(S)	**MOTION**	**PATIENT INSTRUCTIONS**
Fingers	Flexion	Make a fist.
	Extension	Open your hand.
	Abduction	Spread your fingers.
	Adduction	Close your fingers.
Hips	Flexion	Bring your knee to your chest.
	Extension	Reach behind you with your foot.
	Abduction	With your leg straight, move it out to the side.
	Internal rotation	Bend your knee and swing it toward your other leg.
	External rotation	Bend your knee and swing it out to the side.
Knees	Flexion	Bend your knee.
	Extension	Straighten your leg.
Ankles	Dorsiflexion	Pull your toes up toward your head.
	Plantar flexion	Point your toes toward the floor.
	Inversion	Turn the sole of your foot inward.
	Eversion	Turn the sole of your foot outward.
Toes	Flexion	Curl your toes.
	Extension, abduction	Spread your toes.

clinicalALERT

Never attempt to move a joint past its normal range of motion for the patient or past the point at which pain is experienced.

Several special physical assessment maneuvers may be performed with additional training and as indicated. The *bulge sign* may be used to assess for fluid in the knee joint. With the patient supine, milk upward on the medial side of the knee and then tap the lateral side of the patella while observing for a fluid bulge (Figure 41-6■).

The *Thomas test* may be performed when a hip flexion contracture is suspected. The reclining patient is asked to bring one knee up to the chest while keeping the other leg straight. With a hip flexion contracture, the extended leg rises off the examining table.

Box 41-1■ presents an example for documenting a focused musculoskeletal assessment.

DIAGNOSTIC TESTS

Diagnostic tests are often used to assist in diagnosing musculoskeletal disorders. Laboratory testing may include measures of inflammation, selected serum electrolytes and enzymes, and markers of autoimmune disorders. Table 41-5■ identifies laboratory studies that may be used to diagnose musculoskeletal disorders with their nursing implications.

Radiologic studies, x-rays in particular, are commonly used to diagnose musculoskeletal trauma and bone and

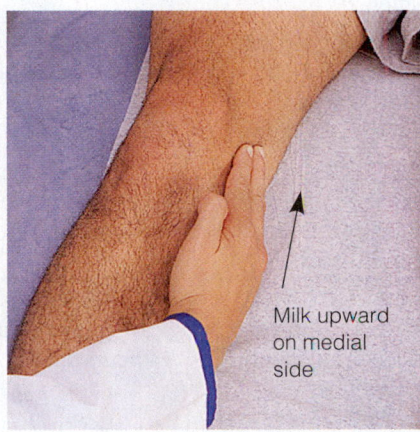
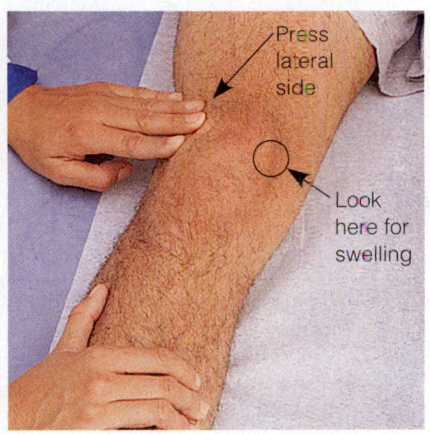

Figure 41-6. ■ Checking for the bulge sign at the knee. (Source: Pearson Education.)

Patient: Mary Simmons presents at her primary care practitioner's office complaining of right elbow pain.

Assessment note: Sharp, intermittent R elbow pain began approximately 6 days ago. No known injury; does relate that she has been taking tennis and golf lessons for the past 3 months and is playing both sports several times a week. Pain aggravated by movement and lifting. No previous known injuries or history of similar problems. Describes self as healthy and physically active. Denies history of joint swelling, pain, or arthritis symptoms. No known chronic diseases or medications. No known allergies. Appears healthy; weight appropriate for height. No joint swelling, warmth, or erythema noted; proximal R elbow tender to palpation. Arm strength 5/5 bilaterally; pain experienced on flexion and extension against resistance. Full ROM all upper extremity joints; no crepitus noted.

joint disorders. Other imaging studies such as CT or MRI may be used to provide more detailed images. Other diagnostic tests may require withdrawal of fluid from a synovial joint for examination (*arthrocentesis*), using a fiberoptic scope to directly examine a joint (*arthroscopy*) or procedures to evaluate impulse conduction along a nerve or muscle. Table 41-6■ outlines imaging studies and other diagnostic procedures commonly used for patients with suspected musculoskeletal trauma or disorders along with related nursing care.

Note: The references and resources for all chapters have been compiled at the back of the book.

TABLE 41-5	Laboratory Tests to Evaluate Musculoskeletal Disorders		
TEST	**NORMAL VALUE**	**EXPLANATION**	**NURSING IMPLICATIONS**
Alkaline phosphatase (ALP)	42–136 unit/L; slightly higher in older adult	ALP is an enzyme found in bone, liver, and other cells of the body. ALP levels rise during bone healing and with bone tumors.	Instruct the patient to fast for 12 hours before the test.
Antinuclear antibodies (ANA), anti-DNA antibodies	Negative at a 1:20 dilution	Antinuclear and anti-DNA antibodies attack antigens in cell nuclei and are found in autoimmune disorders such as systemic lupus erythematosus (SLE).	No special patient preparation is required for these blood tests.
Calcium (Ca^{2+})	4.5–5.5 mEq/L or 9–11 mg/dL	Adequate total body calcium is vital to maintain bone mass. Blood levels increase when calcium is released from the bone.	The patient may be instructed to withhold all calcium preparations for 8–12 hours before the test.
C-reactive protein (CRP)	Negative Positive—more than 1:2 titer	CRP is an abnormal protein that is a sensitive indicator of inflammation.	No special patient preparation is required for this blood test.
Erythrocyte sedimentation rate (ESR)	0–20 mm/hr	The ESR measures the rate at which RBCs settle out of blood. The rate increases in inflammation.	No special patient preparation is required for this blood test.
Phosphorus (P)	1.7–2.6 mEq/L or 2.5–4.5 mg/dL	Phosphorus is primarily combined with calcium in bones and teeth. Calcium and phosphorus have an inverse relationship; when blood levels of one increase, the other decreases.	Fasting for 4 to 8 hours may be recommended prior to this blood test.
Rheumatoid factor (RF)	Negative	RF is a test used to autoantibodies found in patients with rheumatoid arthritis and other connective tissue diseases.	No special patient preparation is required for this blood test.
Uric acid	Women: 2.8–6.8 mg/dL Men: 3.5–8.0 mg/dL	Uric acid is the end product of protein metabolism, excreted by the kidneys and in feces. Elevated levels are found in gout, a metabolic disorder in which urate crystals are deposited in joints and other tissues.	Purine-rich foods such as organ meats, scallops, and sardines are restricted for 24 hours prior to the test.

TABLE 41-6	Diagnostic Tests to Evaluate Musculoskeletal Disorders	
TEST	**DESCRIPTION**	**NURSING RESPONSIBILITIES**
Arthrocentesis	Arthrocentesis, insertion of a needle into the joint capsule to withdraw joint fluid, is used to obtain synovial fluid for examination or to remove excess fluid. Fluid may be sent for synovial fluid analysis, or culture and sensitivity if an infection is suspected.	■ Apply a pressure dressing to the site after the procedure. Instruct the patient to report any bleeding, fluid leakage, or excessive pain to the health care provider.
Arthroscopy	**Arthroscopy** uses a flexible fiberoptic endoscope to view joint structures and tissues. This procedure is used to identify and repair torn tendons or ligaments, an injured meniscus, inflammatory joint changes, and damaged cartilage.	■ Instruct the patient about orders for fasting and medication use prior to the procedure. ■ After the procedure, assess pain and neurovascular status (color, temperature, pulses, movement, and sensation) of the extremity. Assess for bleeding and swelling; apply ice as prescribed. Teach about prescribed activity restrictions and recommendations for resuming use of the joint.
Bone mineral density, bone absorptiometry	Used to diagnose osteoporosis by measuring bone mineral density. Bone density exams help predict fracture risk by comparing the individual's bone mass to that of a healthy 25- to 35-year-old person.	■ These procedures expose the patient to very small amounts of radiation. No special preparation is required.
Bone scan	A nuclear medicine procedure that evaluates the amount of an injected radioactive isotope taken up by bones to reveal "hot spots" where uptake is increased (e.g., a malignant tumor or infected area) or "cold spots" where uptake is reduced (e.g., an area of bone that has decreased blood flow).	■ No special preparation is required, although the patient should be well hydrated. Instruct the patient to drink additional water after the isotope is injected and before the scan is obtained. Advise the patient to remove metal objects, jewelry, and keys prior to the scan.
X-ray	Used to evaluate bone density and structure and joint structure. Contrast medium may be injected to help visualize specific features.	■ Plain x-ray films and CT scans require no special preparation.
CT scans	CT scans produce computer-generated images with significantly more detail than standard x-rays allow. May be done to detect small fractures and bone erosions, to evaluate bone density, to evaluate the spinal column, and to detect tumors.	■ Ask female patients of childbearing age if there is any chance they could be pregnant; alert the physician and radiologic technician if there is. ■ If contrast will be used, assess for allergies to iodine, shellfish, or radiologic contrast media; notify the physician or radiologist if present.
Electromyography (EMG)	This test uses electrodes inserted into skeletal muscle to measure its electrical activity at rest and during contraction. It is useful for diagnosing neuromuscular disorders.	■ Instruct the patient not to drink fluids containing caffeine or to smoke for 3 hours before the test, and not to take any medications before the test unless specifically directed by the physician.
Magnetic resonance imaging (MRI)	Uses a strong magnetic field and radio waves to produce a detailed image of bone and muscle structures. MRI may be used to evaluate soft tissue injuries, degenerative disk changes in the spine, and joint inflammation and injuries.	■ Ask about the presence of any metallic implants (e.g., a pacemaker or joint prosthesis), or other metallic objects (piercings, shrapnel). Notify the physician if present. Ask if patient is pregnant; if so the test is not performed. Patients who are claustrophobic may require an antianxiety agent prior to MRI.
Musculoskeletal ultrasound (US)	Ultrasound procedures use echoes from high-frequency sound waves to evaluate tissues. Musculoskeletal ultrasound is used to help diagnose muscle and tendon tears, bleeding into muscle, soft tissue, or joints, tumors, and joint abnormalities.	■ This noninvasive test requires no special preparation, although the patient may be asked to remove jewelry in the area to be examined.

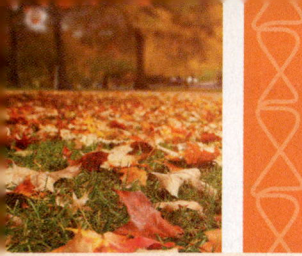

Chapter Review

KEY POINTS

- **Concept:** Intact structure and function of the musculo-skeletal system is vital to the ability to perform physical exercise and usual daily living activities independently.
- Bones and muscles and the structures that connect them (tendons, ligaments, and joints) provide structure to the body, allow people to remain upright, and allow movement.
- **Concept:** Manifestations of musculoskeletal injuries and disorders may be detected during a general health assessment as well as during focused and functional musculo-skeletal assessments.

- The musculoskeletal and neurologic systems are closely related in function. Neurologic disorders may have musculoskeletal manifestations.
- Aging affects both the structure and function of the musculoskeletal system, increasing the risk for traumatic injury due to falls.
- Imaging studies such as x-rays, CT scans, and arthroscopy are widely used to diagnose musculoskeletal trauma and disorders.

PEARSON NURSING STUDENT RESOURCES

Find additional materials at **nursing.pearsonhighered.com**.

NCLEX-PN® Exam Preparation

1. In reviewing an x-ray report that states "distal epiphyseal fracture of the radius," the nurse correctly interprets this as meaning a fracture:
   1. close to the elbow.
   2. of the shaft of the radius.
   3. at the wrist end of the bone.
   4. that has broken the skin.

2. The physician's orders for a patient after hip replacement surgery are to maintain the operative leg in a position of abduction. The nurse positions the patient:
   1. with the legs together and bent at a 60° angle.
   2. on the side, with the knees bent.
   3. supine, with the knees crossed.
   4. with the leg positioned away from the center of the body.

3. Which of the following instructions are appropriate to provide when assessing hand strength? **Select all that apply.**
   1. "Shake hands."
   2. "Move the hand up (extended)."
   3. "Spread the fingers against resistance."
   4. "Make a fist."
   5. "Flex the hand against resistance."

4. When assessing range of motion of the patient's knee, the nurse notes a grating sound. This is appropriately charted as:
   1. crepitus.
   2. synovitis.
   3. erythema.
   4. inflammation.

5. The nurse preparing a patient for a bone scan provides which of the following instructions?
   1. "You should have nothing to eat for 8 to 12 hours before the procedure."
   2. "When the injection is given, you will be instructed to drink four to six glasses of water."
   3. "After the procedure, it is important to avoid close contact with others for 4 hours to avoid exposing them to radiation."
   4. "This test is noninvasive; no special preparation is required."

Answers and rationales for Review Questions appear in Appendix I.

CHAPTER 42

Caring for Patients With Musculoskeletal Trauma

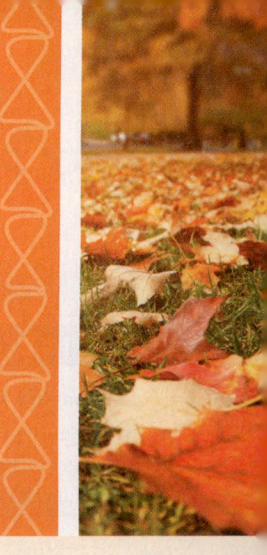

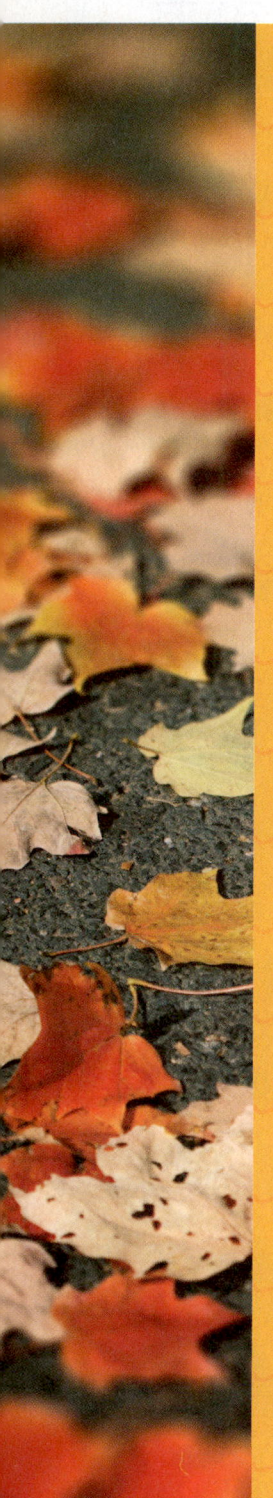

BRIEF OUTLINE

Soft Tissue Trauma

Fractures

Hip Fracture

Joint Trauma and Injury

Amputation

APPLIED LEARNING OUTCOMES

After completing this chapter, you will be able to:

1. Use knowledge of risk factors for and mechanisms of musculoskeletal trauma when teaching and caring for patients in any health care setting.

2. Safely and appropriately assess patients with musculoskeletal trauma, including the patient's perception of the injury, its impact on lifestyle, and expectations for care.

3. Describe how fractures are classified.

4. As a member of the health care team, coordinate and provide individualized and evidence-based care for patients who have experienced musculoskeletal trauma.

5. Safely and effectively care for patients with a fracture or amputation, recognizing and reporting manifestations of common complications and implementing nursing strategies to prevent complications.

6. Document and communicate care for patients experiencing musculoskeletal trauma, using electronic medical records and other communication methods as appropriate.

KEY TERMS

The key terms are defined on the pages listed below.

amputation, 1082
compartment
  syndrome, 1068
contracture, 1082
contusion, 1065

dislocation, 1080
fracture, 1067
gangrene, 1082
hematoma, 1065
phantom limb pain, 1082

reduction, 1071
sprain, 1065
strain, 1065
traction, 1071
trauma, 1065

SPECIAL FEATURES

PATHOPHYSIOLOGY ILLUSTRATED: Fracture Healing, 1069
NURSING CARE PLAN: Patient With Hip Fracture, 1079
CLINICAL REASONING CARE MAP: Caring for a Patient With a Below-Knee Amputation, 1088

Key Concept Musculoskeletal injury, from minor strains to amputation, affects comfort and interferes with mobility and daily living activities. An extended period of recovery and rehabilitation may be required to recover previous function.

Musculoskeletal **trauma** occurs when tissues are subjected to more force than they are able to absorb. The severity of trauma depends on both the amount of force and the location of impact, because different parts of the body can withstand different amounts of force. For example, small bones in the hand cannot absorb as much energy as the femur. Many external sources can cause trauma, and the force can vary in severity. A step off the curb, a fall, being tackled in a football game, and a motor vehicle crash are a few examples.

Musculoskeletal trauma ranges from mild to severe, for example, soft tissue injury, fracture, or complete amputation. It often affects surrounding tissues. A bone fracture can affect the function of muscles, tendons, and ligaments that attach to it.

Nurses can play a major role in trauma prevention. Teach children and young adults the importance of using safety equipment—such as automobile seat belts, bicycle helmets, football pads, proper footwear, protective eyewear, and hard hats—to prevent or decrease the severity of injury from trauma.

Older patients are at higher risk for musculoskeletal trauma due to falls. Assess the home for potential hazards such as poorly lighted stairs or no hand railings. Encourage removing throw rugs and clutter from travel areas. Discuss using bath mats and installing grab bars in bathrooms. Advise wearing shoes with good treads to decrease the risk of slipping.

Soft Tissue Trauma

Key Concept Soft tissue injury is common, often associated with recreational activities or repetitive motions. Nursing care includes assessing the circumstances and impact of the injury as well as circulation and neurologic status distal to the injury, and teaching prescribed treatment and rehabilitation.

Sprains, strains, and other soft tissue damage are common injuries. The lower back and cervical spine are the most common sites for muscle strains. The ankle is the most commonly sprained joint, usually caused by inversion of the foot.

PATHOPHYSIOLOGY AND MANIFESTATIONS

A **contusion**, the simplest musculoskeletal injury, is bleeding into soft tissue resulting from blunt force. With significant bleeding, a **hematoma** forms. A contusion causes swelling and discoloration (a bruise), which initially appears purple or blue ("black-and-blue"). As blood cells break down and are reabsorbed, the mark becomes brown, then turns yellow, and finally disappears.

A **sprain** is a ligament injury. Sprains are caused by a twisting motion that overstretches or tears the ligament. Sprains are graded by the extent of damage:

- *Grade I (mild)*—overstretching with minimal tearing of the ligament and little effect on joint function
- *Grade II (moderate)*—partial tear of the ligament with inflammation and mild to moderate joint instability
- *Grade III (severe)*—complete tearing of the ligament with joint instability and loss of joint function

A **strain** is a microscopic tear in the muscle that causes bleeding into the tissues. A strain (or "pulled muscle") occurs when a muscle is forced to extend past its elasticity. Strains may be caused by inappropriate lifting or by a sudden acceleration–deceleration injury, such as a motor vehicle crash. Nurses and other health care workers are at significant risk for strains associated with patient care activities (Box 42-1■). The characteristics of sprains and strains are compared in Box 42-2■.

BOX 42-1	MUSCULOSKELETAL INJURIES AMONG NURSES

Nurses and other hospital workers experience work-related musculoskeletal injuries twice as often as workers in other U.S. industries; injuries are even more frequent in long-term care settings. Nurses and nursing assistive personnel are at the greatest risk for lost work time due to musculoskeletal pain and back pain (Centers for Disease Control and Prevention [CDC], 2013). Manual patient handling—that is, manually lifting, moving, and repositioning of patients—is identified as the single greatest risk factor for health care worker injuries. It often requires excessive physical effort and places the nurse in an awkward position such as kneeling, squatting, leaning over a bed, or twisting the torso while lifting. It also places the patient at risk for injury when the task exceeds the health care worker's limits to perform safely.

Some interventions, such as back belts and body mechanics training, have not been shown to be effective (Gropelli & Corle, 2010). Using mechanical lifts and transfer devices, in contrast, are identified as effective measures to reduce injuries. In one study, nurses who had ready access to mechanical lifts reported work-related low back pain half as often as those without lifts (Lee et al., 2013). Proper use of these devices also maximizes the safety and comfort of patients during handling.

Nurses share responsibility with their employers for ensuring access to and safely using mechanical lifts and transfer devices. The Occupational Safety and Health Administration (OSHA) publishes guidelines safe patient handling for nursing homes. These guidelines are available at the OSHA website (2009).

BOX 42-2 CHARACTERISTICS OF SPRAINS AND STRAINS

Sprain
- Ligament injury
- Joint instability
- Pain, swelling, discoloration
- Increased pain with joint use

Strain
- Muscle tear
- Swelling, local tenderness
- Sharp or dull pain
- Increased pain with muscle contraction

COLLABORATIVE CARE

Musculoskeletal ultrasound is performed to determine the extent of tissue damage. An x-ray may be done to rule out fracture. If further evaluation is necessary, an MRI may be done.

Soft tissue trauma is treated with measures to decrease swelling, alleviate pain, and encourage rest and healing. Use the acronym RICE to remember initial measures to treat the injury: *Rest, Ice, Compression,* and *Elevation.* The patient is instructed to avoid using the injured area. A splint may be applied. Ice is applied for the first 48 hours, after which heat can be applied. A compression dressing, such as an Ace bandage, may be applied. The injured extremity should be elevated to the level of the heart to increase venous return and decrease swelling. If the lower extremity is injured, crutches are provided. A knee injury also requires a knee immobilizer. If the upper extremity is injured, a sling is provided.

Nonsteroidal anti-inflammatory drugs (NSAIDs) and analgesics, including acetaminophen or narcotics, may be ordered to manage pain and reduce the inflammatory response.

NURSING CARE

PRIORITIZING NURSING CARE

Teaching measures to promote comfort, prevent further injury, and allow healing are the priorities for nursing care for the patient with soft tissue trauma.

HEALTH PROMOTION

Teach and encourage patients to use appropriate equipment and safety devices such as helmets, pads, and braces when engaging in high-risk activities such as contact sports, roller blading, or skateboarding.

ASSESSING

Ask about the mechanism of injury, when it occurred, and protective devices that were being used at the time of injury (e.g., seat belt or air bag). Obtain specific information about pain, including location, character, intensity, and

aggravating and relieving factors. Ask about the effect of the injury or pain on use of the extremity and ability to bear weight. Also ask about movement and sensation distal to the injury, especially numbness, tingling, or inability to move. Inquire about previous injuries and self-care measures that have been used for this injury (e.g., analgesics, ice or heat, wrapping, or rest).

Inspect the injured area for redness, swelling, or deformity. Assess active range of motion (ROM) of affected joints.

clinicalALERT

Do not attempt to move an injured joint beyond the point of comfort. If fracture is suspected, immobilize the joint and do not assess range of motion until the fracture has been ruled out. This is especially important when there is a risk of cervical spine fracture.

Palpate for swelling, warmth, tenderness, deformity, and crepitus (a grating sensation or sound). Check capillary refill, pulses, movement, and sensation distal to the injury.

IDENTIFYING POTENTIAL COMPLICATIONS

Promptly report complaints of numbness, tingling, weakness, or inability to move distal to the injury, as these may be signs of nerve damage. Circulation may be impaired if the extremity is cool or pale. Check capillary refill and peripheral pulses and report these assessment findings immediately.

DIAGNOSING, PLANNING, AND IMPLEMENTING
Acute Pain

Expected outcome: Will use analgesic and nonanalgesic measures appropriately to manage comfort.

The pain of soft tissue injuries is caused by tissue damage and edema.

- Instruct to rest the injured extremity. *Rest allows the injured muscle or ligament to heal.*
- Apply ice to the injury. *Ice causes vasoconstriction and decreases swelling in the injured area. It may also numb the tender area.*
- Maintain compression dressing, such as an Ace bandage. *A compression dressing decreases swelling, edema, and pain.*
- Elevate the extremity 2 in. above the heart. *Elevating the extremity promotes venous return and decreases swelling.*
- Teach the acronym RICE to remember acute injury care: rest, ice, compression, elevation. *Acronyms help memory. Knowing the treatment plan decreases anxiety and pain.*
- If pain continues after several days, instruct to apply heat. *Heat increases blood flow and venous return, decreasing edema and pain. Heat is avoided immediately after the injury, as it can lead to increased bleeding into the tissues.*
- Advise to take aspirin or NSAIDs on a regular basis (around the clock as recommended) with food.

When a therapeutic blood level is maintained, these drugs reduce inflammation, relieving pain. Taking the drug with food reduces gastrointestinal upset.

- Instruct to use analgesics (over the counter or prescribed) to maintain comfort, preventing pain from becoming severe. *Severe pain increases muscle tension and can make it more difficult to relieve pain with medications.*

Impaired Physical Mobility

Expected outcome: Will demonstrate correct use of assistive devices.

- Teach correct use of crutches, canes, or slings if prescribed. *Using correct technique increases the safety and effectiveness of these devices.*
- Remind to rest injured extremity. *Using the extremity can delay healing and increase the risk of further injury.*
- Encourage follow-up with primary care provider. *Severe sprains may require further treatment such as a brace or surgical intervention.*

EVALUATING

To evaluate the effectiveness of nursing care, assess pain, safety when ambulating, and knowledge of home care.

DOCUMENTING

Document assessment data and emergent care provided. Also document teaching, including the patient's apparent understanding of instructions and willingness to comply with self-care measures.

CONTINUITY OF CARE

Teach about ordered medications, splints, dressings, and assistive devices. Always assess use of assistive devices. If the device is inappropriate, the risk of falling can be increased. Older adults often have less muscle mass in the upper extremities; a walker may be safer than crutches. Specify when to schedule a follow-up appointment with the care provider. Explain that activity limitations will be evaluated at the follow-up appointment. Reinforce the RICE acronym. Emphasize the importance of rest to allow complete healing. Instruct to report any complications, such as numbness, coolness of the limb, or severe pain, to the physician immediately.

Fractures

> **Key Concept** Fractures place the patient at risk for complications and may require surgery or other invasive measures for healing. Nurses focus on promoting comfort, preventing and promptly recognizing complications, and teaching for patients with fractures.

A **fracture** is a break in the continuity of a bone. Fractures vary in severity according to the location and the type of fracture.

PATHOPHYSIOLOGY

A fracture occurs when bone is subjected to more force than it can absorb. Fractures may result from a direct blow, a crushing force, a sudden twisting motion, a severe muscle contraction, or a disease that has weakened the bone (*pathologic fracture*).

Types of Fractures

Fractures are classified in a number of different ways (Table 42-1 ■). A *closed* or *simple fracture* is the most common. *Open* or *compound fractures* disrupt the skin over the fracture, allowing bacteria to enter the wound.

TABLE 42-1	Types of Fractures
FRACTURE TYPE	**DESCRIPTION**
Closed (simple)	Skin over fracture remains intact.
Open (compound)	Broken bone protrudes through skin.
Comminuted	Bone fragments into many pieces.
Compression	Bone is crushed.
Impacted	Broken ends of bone are forced together.
Depressed	Broken bone is pressed inward (e.g., the skull).
Spiral	Jagged break occurs due to twisting force.
Greenstick	Incomplete break occurs along the length of the bone.

This increases the risk of complications such as infection or nerve damage. *Complete fractures* involve the entire width of the bone, whereas *incomplete fractures* do not. In a *stable (nondisplaced) fracture,* the pieces of bone remain in alignment. In an *unstable (displaced) fracture,* the bones move out of correct alignment.

The direction of the fracture line is also used to classify fractures. The fracture line may be *oblique,* at a 45-degree angle to the bone, *spiral,* or along the lengthwise plane of the bone (*greenstick fracture*).

clinicalALERT

Spiral fractures are often associated with abuse (e.g., someone deliberately twisting the patient's arm). Be alert for other evidence of abuse, such as bruises of various color and age, a record of frequent emergency care for traumatic injuries, and x-ray reports of multiple healed fractures. Notify the charge nurse and physician if abuse is suspected.

Fracture Healing

Fracture healing is affected by age, physical condition, and the type of fracture. When a bone fractures, blood vessels tear and a hematoma forms between the fractured bone ends and around bone surfaces (Figure 42-1A■). Bone and tissue damage cause a local inflammatory response. Clotting factors within the hematoma form a fibrin meshwork (Figure 42-1B). Within 48 hours, fibroblasts and new capillaries growing into the fracture form *granulation tissue* that gradually replaces the hematoma. Phagocytes remove cell debris. Bone-forming cells called *osteoblasts* migrate to the fracture site, where they build a web of collagen fibers from both sides of the fractured bone. Chondroblasts lay down patches of cartilage as a base for bone growth. This *fibrocartilaginous callus* connects bone fragments, splinting the fracture (Figure 42-1C). Osteoblasts continue to form collagen fibers and bone matrix, which are gradually mineralized with calcium and mineral salts to form *bony callus* (Figure 42-1D). Osteoblasts promote new bone formation. *Osteoclasts* migrate to the repair site to remove damaged and excess bone in the callus (Figure 42-1E). This process usually continues for 2 to 3 months. In the final phase of healing, excess callus is removed and new bone is laid down along the fracture line. As the bone heals and again is subjected to the mechanical stress of everyday use, osteoblasts and osteoclasts remodel the repair site along the lines of force.

Healing time varies with the individual. An uncomplicated fracture of the arm or foot can heal in 6 to 8 weeks. A fractured vertebra takes at least 12 weeks to heal. A fractured hip may require 12 to 16 weeks.

MANIFESTATIONS AND COMPLICATIONS

Common manifestations of fractures are listed in Box 42-3■. Fractures are frequently accompanied by soft tissue injuries that involve muscles, blood vessels, nerves, or skin. The extent of soft tissue injury depends on the amount of energy or force transmitted to the area.

Although most fractures are uncomplicated, serious complications can develop. A fractured pelvis or femur may cause significant bleeding and hypovolemic shock. Up to 4.5 L of blood can be lost with a pelvic fracture, for example. Open fractures may be complicated by infection. Significant tissue trauma may accompany open fractures. The fractured bone may damage peripheral nerves, affecting movement and sensation distal to the fracture. Blood flow to a portion of fractured bone may be disrupted, causing necrosis. Blood vessel damage and immobility increase the risk for developing deep venous thrombosis. Other serious complications such as compartment syndrome, fat embolism, and delayed union are discussed next.

Compartment Syndrome

A *compartment* is a space enclosed by a fibrous membrane or fascia. Compartments within the limbs may enclose and support bones, nerves, and blood vessels. **Compartment syndrome** occurs when excess pressure restricts blood vessels and nerves within a compartment. It may be caused by bleeding or edema within the compartment or by external compression of the limb by a too-tight cast or dressing. Nerve compression causes severe pain and paresthesias (burning, tingling, or loss of sensation). Impaired tissue perfusion may lead to necrosis. Because major arteries are outside muscle compartments, arterial pulses often remain normal, even though circulation to the muscle and nerves is significantly impaired. Unless promptly relieved, compartment syndrome may lead to loss of the limb and sepsis. Compartment syndrome usually develops within the first 48 hours of injury, when edema is at its peak. Manifestations of compartment syndrome are shown in Box 42-4■.

BOX 42-3	MANIFESTATIONS OF FRACTURES

- ■ Deformity
- ■ Swelling, ecchymosis (bruising)
- ■ Pain
- ■ Tenderness, guarding, immobility
- ■ Numbness
- ■ Crepitus
- ■ Muscle spasms

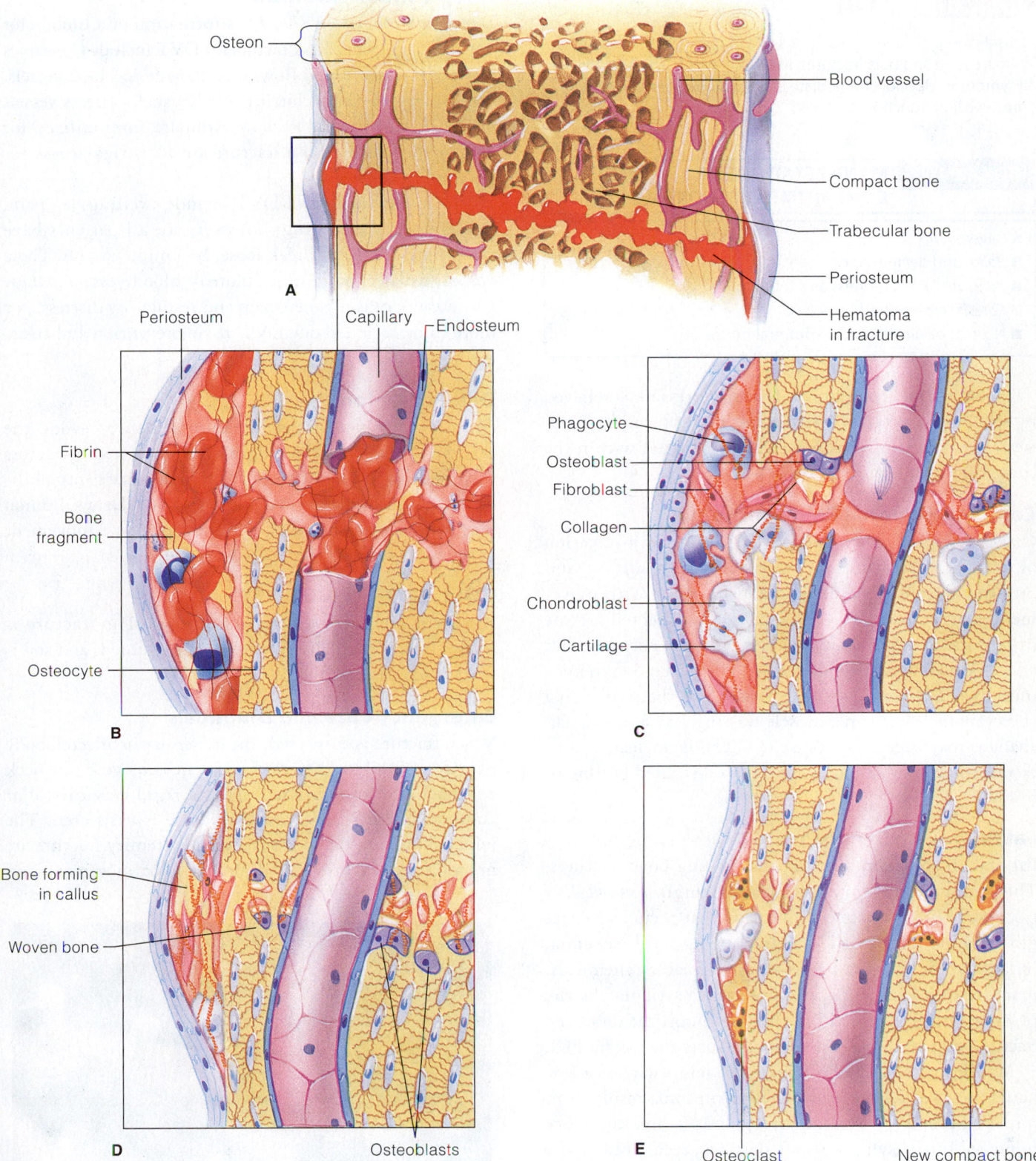

Figure 42-1. ■ Pathophysiology Illustrated: Fracture healing. (**A, B**) When a fracture occurs, bleeding from damaged blood vessels causes a hematoma and local swelling. Clotting factors form a fibrin meshwork. (**C**) Healing begins within 48 hours, as new capillaries form and bone-forming cells (osteoblasts) migrate to the site. A web of collagen fibers forms to connect bone fragments. (**D**) Osteoblasts form collagen and bone matrix; calcium and mineral salts accumulate to form spongy bone. (**E**) As healing continues, the bone is remodeled until the damaged portion appears the same as uninjured parts.

clinicalALERT

Closely monitor for manifestations of compartment syndrome with forearm and tibia fractures. Notify the physician promptly if symptoms develop. Immediate intervention is necessary to preserve limb function.

BOX 42-4	MANIFESTATIONS OF COMPARTMENT SYNDROME

- Severe *pain*
- *Pallor* and decreased capillary refill; later cyanosis
- *Paresthesias* (numbness and tingling)
- *Paresis* (weakness) or paralysis
- Normal or diminished peripheral *pulses*

If compartment syndrome develops, pressure is relieved by removing the tightly fitting cast or performing a *fasciotomy,* a surgical procedure to relieve pressure within the compartment.

Complex Regional Pain Syndrome

Complex regional pain syndrome (CRPS) is a complication of musculoskeletal injury leading to severe, diffuse, and burning extremity pain. The pain increases with movement. It is more severe than would be expected for the injury and is accompanied by vasomotor changes that affect skin color and temperature. The affected extremity initially is red, warm, and edematous, later becoming cool and cyanotic. Over time, muscle wasting and skin and nail changes may occur. The cause of CRPS is unclear; it may be due to nervous system damage or a disrupted healing or immune process.

Fat Embolism Syndrome

Fat emboli are commonly released in long bone fractures. They are usually asymptomatic and benign. *Fat embolism syndrome (FES)* is a rare complication that occurs when fat globules lodge in small vessels, causing local ischemia, inflammation, and the release of inflammatory chemicals. Fracture of a long bone, the femur in particular, is the primary risk factor for FES. Early immobilization of the fracture (e.g., surgical stabilization) reduces the risk for FES.

Manifestations of FES usually develop within a few hours to a week after injury. The symptoms result from impaired blood flow, tissue injury, and the inflammatory response. Initial symptoms are dyspnea, tachypnea, and a drop in oxygen saturation. Manifestations of acute respiratory distress may develop. Altered cerebral perfusion causes confusion and changes in level of consciousness. Normal clotting is disrupted, and petechiae (pin-sized purplish spots that do not blanch with pressure) develop on the skin, soft palate, and conjunctiva.

Deep Venous Thrombosis

Deep venous thrombosis (DVT) is formation of a blood clot within a large vein. Risk factors for DVT include (1) venous stasis (decreased blood flow), (2) damage to blood vessels, and (3) altered blood clotting. DVT usually affects vessels of the legs or pelvis. Patients who are immobilized for an extended time after a fracture are at particular risk for developing DVT.

The manifestations of DVT include swelling, leg pain, tenderness, or cramping; however, not all patients have symptoms. Clots can break loose, becoming emboli. These emboli usually lodge in pulmonary blood vessels (*pulmonary emboli*), causing chest pain and respiratory distress. For more information about DVT, their prevention and treatment, see Chapter 18.

Delayed Union

Delayed union is prolonged healing of bones beyond the expected time. Bone healing may be impaired by factors such as delayed fracture reduction, inadequate immobilization, infection, chronic disease, and age. Delayed union may lead to *nonunion,* with persistent pain and movement at the fracture site.

COLLABORATIVE CARE

A fracture requires prompt treatment. The fracture is *reduced* (the normal alignment of bone restored) and stabilized as soon as possible.

Emergency Care and Diagnosis

When fracture is suspected, the extremity or affected body part is immobilized before the patient is moved. The neck and back are immobilized using a rigid cervical collar and backboard if a vertebral fracture is suspected. The joints above and below a suspected extremity fracture are immobilized (Figure 42-2■). Pulses, color, movement, and

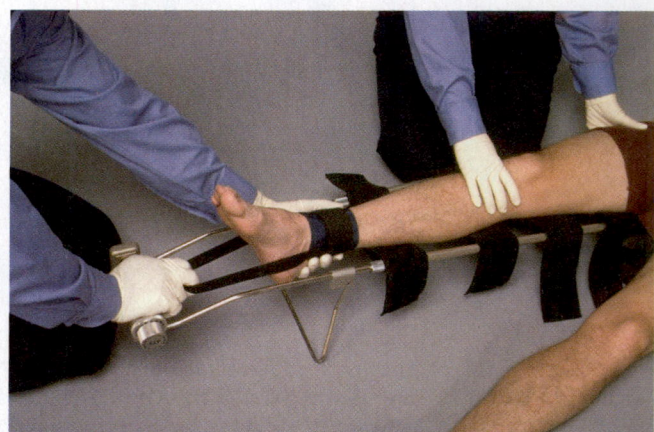

Figure 42-2. ■ Emergency medical technicians apply a traction splint to immobilize the lower leg. (Source: Michal Heron, Pearson Education.)

sensation of the extremity are checked both before and after splinting. Open wounds and fractures are covered with a sterile dressing.

On arrival in the health care setting, x-rays of the affected body part are usually obtained to confirm the diagnosis of a fracture.

Fracture Reduction

Before the fractured bone is stabilized for healing, **reduction** (restoring the bone to its normal alignment) must be done. In *closed reduction*, external manipulation is used to reposition the bone. Local or regional anesthesia or conscious sedation is usually given before closed reduction. The fracture is then immobilized with a splint, cast, or traction. An x-ray may be done to verify proper position, and pulses, movement, and sensation are assessed distal to the fracture. An *open reduction* is done in surgery. The bone is exposed and realigned; nails or screws may be used to maintain its position.

Casts

A *cast* is a rigid device used to immobilize broken bones and promote healing. Casts may be made of plaster or fiberglass. The joints above and below the fracture are immobilized by the cast so the bone will not move during healing. The cast is applied over a thin cushion of padding and molded to the normal contour of the body. Until the cast is completely dry, care is taken to avoid placing pressure on it; simply palpating a wet cast with the fingertips can leave dents that may cause pressure sores. A plaster cast may need up to 48 hours to dry, whereas a fiberglass cast dries in less than 1 hour. The type of cast applied depends on the location of the fracture (Figure 42-3■). Nursing care and teaching for patients with casts is outlined in Box 42-5■.

Significant swelling under a cast can impair blood flow and damage nerves and tissues of the extremity. If this occurs, the cast may be split down both sides to relieve the pressure. The two halves of the cast are then held in place with Velcro straps to keep the fracture immobilized.

Traction

Muscle spasms can pull bones out of alignment after a fracture. **Traction** applies a straightening or pulling force to return or maintain the fractured bones in normal position. Various types of traction may be used:

1. *Manual traction* is applied by physically pulling on the extremity. It is often used to reduce a fracture or dislocation. Other types of traction use ropes, pulleys, and weights to maintain alignment of the bones.
2. *Skin traction* (also called *straight* traction) applies the pulling force through the patient's skin. It is noninvasive and is relatively comfortable for the patient (see Figure 42-2).

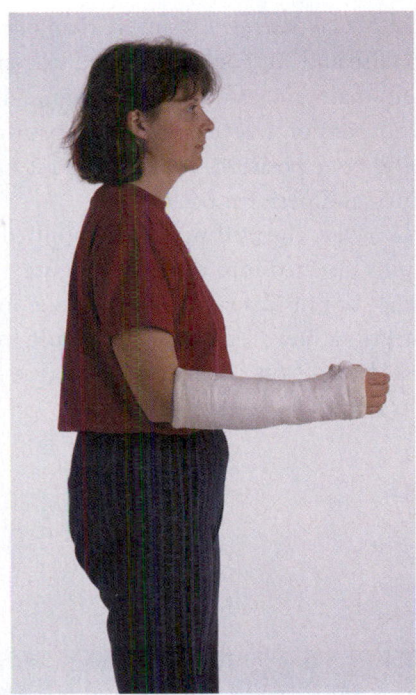

Figure 42-3. ■ A short arm cast that also immobilizes the thumb is used to stabilize a wrist fracture. (Source: Pearson Education.)

BOX 42-5	NURSING CARE CHECKLIST

Cast Care

☑ Frequently assess pulses, color, movement, and sensation of the affected extremity.
☑ Promptly report increased or severe pain; changes in pulses, color, movement, or sensation distal to the cast; or a "hot spot" or drainage on the cast.

Patient and Family Teaching

☑ The cast dries from the inside out; do not use a blow dryer to speed drying; do not cover the cast while it is drying.
☑ A sensation of warmth during drying is normal.
☑ Keep the cast clean and dry; use plastic wrap as needed to protect it.
☑ If a fiberglass cast gets wet, dry it with a blow dryer on cool setting.
☑ Notify your doctor immediately if you develop increased pain, coolness, color changes, increased swelling, or loss of sensation in the injured limb.
☑ Do not put anything into the cast.
☑ Relieve itching by blowing cool air into the cast with a blow dryer on a cool setting.
☑ A sling may help distribute the weight of the cast evenly around the neck; do not roll the sling because this may impair circulation.
☑ Use crutches as taught to prevent weight bearing on the affected leg.
☑ The cast will be removed with a cast saw. You will feel its vibration, but the saw will not cut the skin.

3. *Balanced suspension traction* uses more than one force of pull to raise and support the injured extremity off the bed and maintain its alignment (Figure 42-4A■). Balanced suspension traction increases mobility while maintaining bone position. It also makes it easier to change linen and perform back care.

4. In *skeletal traction,* the pulling force is applied directly through pins inserted into the bone (Figure 42-4B). The presence of pins inserted into the bone increases risk of infection, however, and it may cause more discomfort. Box 42-6■ outlines nursing care for patients in traction.

Surgery

Surgery may be required to align and stabilize a fractured bone. External fixation is the simplest form of surgery used to immobilize a fracture. An *external fixator* uses a frame connected to pins inserted into the bone (Figure 42-5■). The pins require care similar to that of skeletal traction pins. The patient is monitored for infection, and frequent neurovascular assessment is performed.

Internal fixation is usually done in a surgical procedure called an *open reduction and internal fixation (ORIF)*. In this procedure, the fracture is directly reduced, and a nail, screws, plates and screws, or pins are inserted to hold the bones in

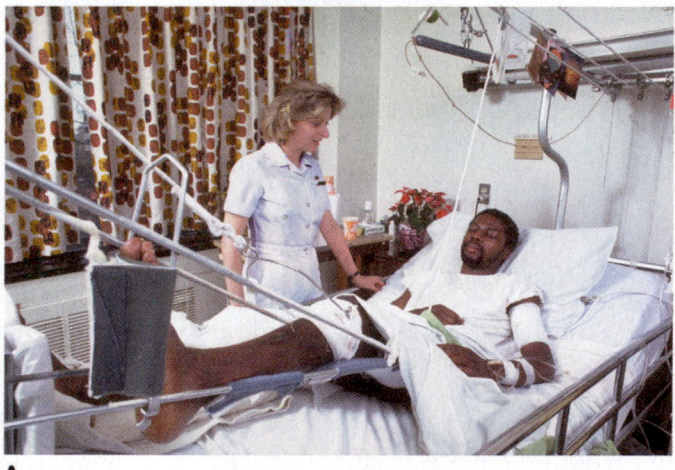

A

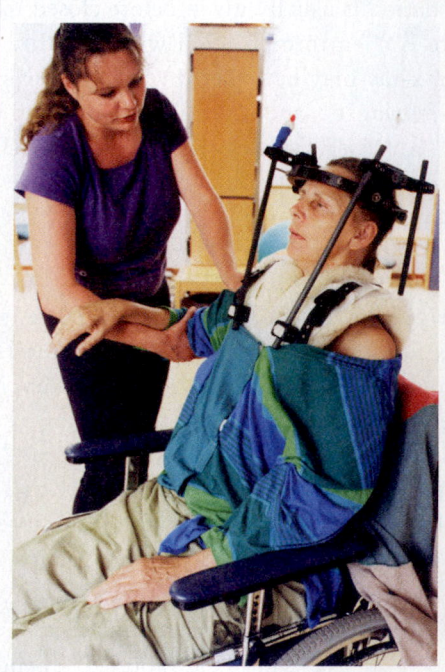

B

Figure 42-4. ■ Traction is applying a pulling force to restore or maintain bone alignment for fracture healing. (**A**) Balanced suspension traction is commonly used for fractures of the femur. (**B**) Skeletal traction, in which the pulling force is applied directly to the bone, may be used to treat fractures of the spine. (Source: A and B, Pearson Education.)

BOX 42-6	NURSING CARE CHECKLIST

Traction

☑ Maintain the pulling force and direction:

　☑ Center patient on the bed; maintain body alignment with the direction of pull.

　☑ Ensure that nothing is lying on or obstructing the ropes.

　☑ Do not allow knots to come in contact with the pulley.

　☑ Ensure that weights hang freely and do not touch the floor.

☑ For skin traction:

　☑ Frequently assess pulses, color, sensation, and movement distal to wrappings; notify the physician or rewrap (if ordered) as necessary.

　☑ Remove weights only if intermittent traction has been ordered and to rewrap bandages.

☑ Frequently assess skin, bony prominences, and pressure points for irritation or breakdown.

☑ Protect pressure sites with padding and protective dressings.

☑ For skeletal traction:

　☑ Never remove weights.

　☑ Frequently assess neurovascular status, skin, and pin insertion sites.

　☑ Provide pin site care as ordered (or per protocol).

　☑ Report signs of infection, such as redness, drainage, and increased tenderness.

　☑ Report manifestations of complications of immobility, including pressure ulcers, DVT, atelectasis or pneumonia, paralytic ileus, and constipation.

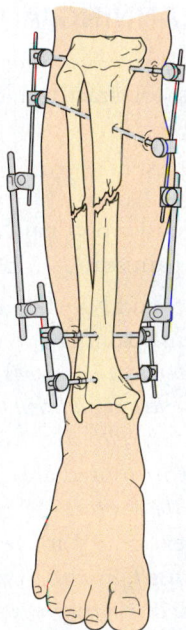

Figure 42-5. ■ In external fixation, pins placed through the bone above and below the fracture site to immobilize the bone. External fixation rods hold the pins in place.

place (Figure 42-6■). Open fractures and hip fractures are frequently repaired with ORIF. Nursing considerations for a patient undergoing ORIF are outlined in Box 42-7■.

Other Interventions

Analgesics and NSAIDs are ordered to relieve pain after a fracture. Parenteral analgesics or patient-controlled analgesia (PCA) may be used for the first 24 to 48 hours. (See discussion of PCA and management of acute pain in Chapter 8.)

Stool softeners may be given and dietary fiber increased to decrease the risk of constipation secondary to narcotics and immobility. An antiulcer drug such as a histamine blocker, proton-pump inhibitor, or antacid may be ordered

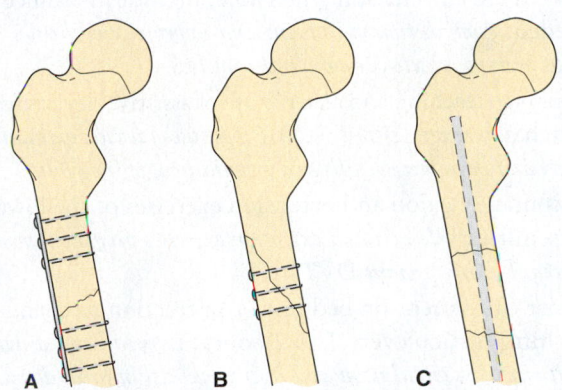

Figure 42-6. ■ Internal fixation. (**A**) A plate and screws used to stabilize an oblique fracture. (**B**) Screws inserted through the fracture site maintain its alignment. (**C**) A medullary nail is inserted into the bone to stabilize a segmental fracture.

BOX 42-7	NURSING CARE CHECKLIST

Open Reduction and Internal Fixation (ORIF)

Before Surgery

☑ Provide routine preoperative care.

☑ Maintain positioning as ordered.

☑ Assess and manage pain. Promptly report pain that is increasing in severity, unexpected, or unrelieved by ordered analgesia.

☑ Frequently assess pulses, temperature, color, movement, and sensation of affected extremity.

☑ Reinforce teaching.

After Surgery

☑ Provide routine postoperative care, assessing vital signs, mental status, lung sounds, and bowel sounds as ordered or indicated (see Chapter 10).

☑ Frequently assess neurovascular status; promptly report changes to the charge nurse or physician.

☑ Assess amount, color, and odor of wound drainage (on dressing and in surgical drain such as Hemovac).

☑ Maintain alignment of affected extremity as ordered.

☑ Collaborate with physical therapists to promote mobility as soon as allowed.

to prevent gastrointestinal bleeding. Antibiotics may be given, particularly with open or complex fractures.

Electrical bone stimulation may be used to treat fractures that are not healing appropriately. An electrical current is used to increase the migration of osteoblasts and osteoclasts to the fracture site. Mineral deposition increases, promoting bone healing.

NURSING CARE

PRIORITIZING NURSING CARE

The priorities for nursing care of the patient with a fracture include teaching, managing pain and impaired mobility, and preventing complications.

HEALTH PROMOTION

Teach and encourage patients of all ages to use safety equipment such as seat belts, protective pads, goggles, and helmets as appropriate. Discuss the importance of adequate daily calcium intake and regular exercise in maintaining strong, healthy bones. Older adults are at particular risk for fractures. See Box 42-8■ for health promotion measures to reduce an older adult's risk of fracture.

ASSESSING

Obtain information about circumstances of the injury. Assess pain in the injured extremity using a standard pain scale. Evaluate the effectiveness of analgesia in relieving pain.

BOX 42-8 **FOCUS ON OLDER ADULTS**

Reducing Fracture Risk

Falls are the most common cause of fractures in older adults. Hip fractures are the leading cause of hospitalization for injuries in older adults. The clavicles and wrists are also commonly fractured. Fractures in older adults can lead to loss of functional ability or death. Fall-related deaths are usually related to complications from prolonged immobility, not the act of falling.

A number of measures can reduce the risk of falling and fracture:

- Encourage children, adolescents, and younger adults to maintain an adequate calcium intake to prevent osteoporosis (see Chapter 43).
- Remove scatter rugs and obstacles in traffic areas of the home.
- Paint a contrast stripe on the edge of stair steps.
- Provide night-lights and transition lighting between bedroom and bath.
- Install grab bars in the bath and railings on stairs.
- Teach to turn using a series of small steps.
- Instruct to wear well-fitting shoes or hard-soled slippers when ambulating.
- Encourage regular aerobic and strength-training exercises.
- Review medication regimen with the physician.
- Teach safe use of assistive devices such as canes and walkers.

Compare the quality of pulses in the affected limb to those of the unaffected limb. Assess sensation proximal and distal to the fracture. Check skin color and temperature in the extremity. Assess motion distal to the fracture site.

IDENTIFYING POTENTIAL COMPLICATIONS

Increasing pain or pain that is not effectively relieved by analgesia may indicate a complication such as compartment syndrome or infection. Numbness, tingling, and changes in sensation or movement distal to the fracture may indicate nerve damage or compartment syndrome. Indicators of impaired circulation include a cool, pale extremity with weak or absent pulses. Edema, warmth, and a bluish or purple tinge may indicate venous pooling.

memoryALERT

Frequent neurovascular checks, often called CMS checks, are an important nursing care responsibility for patients with musculoskeletal injuries. Remember:

- *Color* (or cardiovascular)—compare the color, temperature, and pulses of the affected extremity to the unaffected extremity.
- *Movement*—ask the patient to move the affected extremity distal to the injury (e.g., "wiggle your toes").
- *Sensation*—check sensation distal to the injury (touch, sharp) and compare this to the unaffected extremity.

DIAGNOSING, PLANNING, AND IMPLEMENTING

Nursing implications for fractures of specific bones are listed in Table 42-2■.

Acute Pain

Expected outcome: Will report pain at a level of 2 or lower on a standard 0 to 10 pain scale.

- Administer analgesics and NSAIDs as ordered on a regular basis to prevent intense pain. *Pain is more effectively relieved if analgesics are given before pain becomes severe. NSAIDs have an anti-inflammatory effect in addition to their analgesic effect, so may be used concurrently with other pain medications.*
- Splint and support the injured area. *Splinting helps relieve pain by immobilizing the fracture.*
- Elevate the injured extremity above the heart. *Pain is caused by the fracture itself, as well as muscle spasms and swelling. Elevating the extremity promotes venous return and decreases edema, which decreases pain.*
- Apply ice. *Ice causes vasoconstriction, decreasing swelling. It may also numb the area.*
- Move gently and slowly, supporting the fractured extremity above and below the fracture when moving. *Gentle movement and support of the injured tissue reduces the risk of muscle spasms.*
- Encourage distraction and other adjunctive pain relief measures such as meditation and visualization. *These measures promote relaxation and reduce the intensity of pain.*

Impaired Physical Mobility

Expected outcome: Will demonstrate correct use of exercises and assistive devices before discharge.

- Teach and assist with active ROM exercises of the unaffected limbs and joints. *ROM helps prevent muscle atrophy and maintain strength and joint function.*
- Teach isometric exercises, and encourage them every 4 hours. *Isometric exercises help prevent muscle atrophy.*
- Encourage ambulation when able; provide assistance as needed. *Ambulation maintains and improves circulation and helps prevent muscle atrophy and bone loss.*
- Reinforce teaching and observe use of assistive devices (canes, crutches, walkers, slings, etc.). *Proper use of devices maintains safety and helps prevent falls and complications of immobility.*
- Encourage flexion and extension exercises of the lower extremities. *Flexion and extension exercises promote venous return, helping prevent DVT.*
- Assist the patient on bed rest or in traction to change or shift position every 1 to 2 hours. *Turning and weight shifts increase circulation and help prevent skin breakdown.*
- Encourage frequent use of incentive spirometer, deep breathing, and coughing. *Immobilized patients have an increased risk for developing atelectasis and pneumonia due to retained respiratory secretions.*

TABLE 42-2	Nursing Implications for Specific Fractures		
FRACTURE	**USUAL TREATMENT**	**NURSING IMPLICATIONS**	**PATIENT TEACHING**
Clavicle	Clavicular strap (see Figure 42-7 ■) or surgical repair	■ Frequently assess neurovascular status of injured arm.	■ Applying the clavicular strap; skin care ■ Wrist and elbow ROM exercises
Humerus	Hanging arm cast, traction, or ORIF, depending on location and severity	■ Frequently assess neurovascular status of injured arm.	■ Cast care, sling application ■ Finger and shoulder ROM exercises
Forearm, wrist, and hand	Posterior splint and sling; short arm cast; or finger splint	■ Frequently assess neurovascular status of injured hand. ■ Compartment syndrome is a risk.	■ Manifestations of complications to report ■ Elevate arm ■ Finger exercises
Femur	Skeletal traction followed by internal or external fixation	■ Frequently assess vital signs and neurovascular status of affected leg. ■ Bleeding may lead to shock. ■ Assess respiratory status; fat embolism is a risk.	■ Pain management ■ Reporting signs of complications ■ Gluteal, quadriceps, and ROM exercises of lower legs, feet, and toes ■ Pin site or incision care ■ Use of assistive devices for non–weight-bearing activities as allowed
Tibia or fibula	Long leg cast for 3–4 weeks, followed by short leg cast. External fixation device or ORIF may be used.	■ Frequently assess neurovascular status; blood vessels or nerves may be damaged. ■ Compartment syndrome is a risk. ■ Assess knee; bleeding into joint may occur.	■ Weight-bearing restrictions as ordered ■ Cast, pin, or incision site care ■ Crutch walking
Ankle and foot	Closed reduction and short leg cast or splint; ankle fracture may require ORIF	■ Assess neurovascular status of distal foot and toes.	■ Cast care, crutch walking
Skull	Observation for simple fracture; surgical elevation of depressed skull fracture	■ Frequently assess neurologic status: level of consciousness, mental status, pupil response to light, extremity movement and strength, vital signs. ■ Promptly report neurologic changes.	■ Observations for altered mental or neurologic status ■ Prescribed activity restrictions ■ Preventing future head injuries
Face	Monitoring; ORIF if severely displaced	■ Monitor airway and breathing. ■ Monitor neurologic status as noted earlier. ■ Promptly report changes.	■ Pain management ■ Effect of swelling on appearance and expected changes ■ Indications or options for plastic surgery
Spine	Immediate immobilization. For nondisplaced fractures, cervical collar, halo immobilizer, thoracic brace, or body cast. For displaced fractures, surgical stabilization, and skeletal traction	■ Frequently assess extremity movement and sensation. Promptly report changes to the physician. ■ Maintain spinal immobilization and alignment. ■ Provide good skin care. ■ See Chapter 39 for more information.	■ Skin care under the brace ■ Pin site care ■ Length of immobilization ■ Preventing complications of immobility

(continued)

TABLE 42-2	Nursing Implications for Specific Fractures *(continued)*		
FRACTURE	**USUAL TREATMENT**	**NURSING IMPLICATIONS**	**PATIENT TEACHING**
Rib	Analgesia and respiratory care to prevent atelectasis or pneumonia. Fracture of two or more adjacent ribs in two or more places causes *flail chest*. Flail chest is discussed further in Chapter 23.	■ Frequently assess respiratory status (rate, depth, and equality of chest movement, breath sounds). ■ Provide adequate pain relief to encourage deep breathing. ■ Encourage use of incentive spirometer.	■ Pain management ■ Avoid rib belt or tape unless ordered by the physician. ■ Splint chest with hand or pillow to cough and deep breathe. ■ Use of incentive spirometer ■ Contact the doctor if fever or shortness of breath develops.
Pelvis	Bed rest on firm mattress; if unstable or displaced, pelvic sling followed by surgery	■ Closely monitor for bleeding and shock. ■ Monitor neurovascular status of lower extremities. ■ Report hematuria, rectal bleeding, or blood in feces. ■ Logroll for comfort.	■ Pain management ■ Activity restrictions ■ Contact the doctor for blood in urine or feces, difficulty voiding or defecating. ■ Report numbness, tingling, or weakness of lower extremities to the doctor.

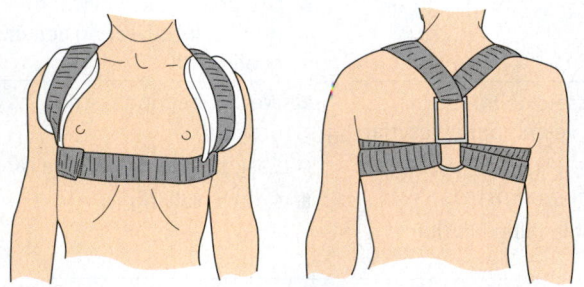

Figure 42-7. ■ A clavicular strap to immobilize a fractured clavicle.

Risk for Ineffective Peripheral Tissue Perfusion

Expected outcome: Circulation will remain effective, as evidenced by normal temperature, color, and sensation of extremities.

Tissue perfusion can be affected by bleeding, edema, compartment syndrome, and immobility.

■ Perform CMS checks every 1 to 2 hours, promptly reporting abnormal or unexpected findings. *Unrelenting pain, pallor, diminished distal pulses, paresthesias, and paresis are indicators of compartment syndrome. Note that pulses may remain strong with compartment syndrome.*

■ Monitor the extremity for edema and swelling. Assess cast for tightness. *Edema can cause the cast to become too tight; a tightly fitting cast affects distal circulation.*

■ If the cast is too tight, prepare to assist with bivalving. *Bivalving (splitting the cast) relieves pressure caused by a too-tight cast.*

■ Unless contraindicated, elevate the injured extremity above the heart. *Elevating the extremity increases venous return and decreases edema.*

■ Administer anticoagulants as ordered. *Anticoagulants may be ordered to reduce the risk for DVT. See Chapter 18 for more information about the nursing implications of anticoagulant therapy.*

■ Apply antiembolism stockings or pneumatic compression boots. *These devices increase venous return, decrease blood pooling, and decrease the risk of DVT.*

MANAGING NURSING CARE

Nursing care activities for the patient with a fracture that may be assigned to nursing assistive or personnel with documented training and competence include vital signs, positioning, hygiene measures, and assisting with allowed activities.

EVALUATING

To evaluate the effectiveness of nursing care, collect data related to pain and the effectiveness of analgesia, safety and mobility, and tissue perfusion. Assess learning and ability to safely use assistive devices as ordered.

DOCUMENTING

Document assessment findings, including neurovascular status, before and after fracture reduction. Also document level of pain before and after interventions, as well as analgesia provided. If traction is used, note type of traction and amount of weight applied. Record any drainage noted on cast, from incision, or from pin sites. Document skin care and measures to prevent complications. Also document all teaching and discharge instructions and the patient's understanding of information. Note the patient's ability to demonstrate techniques such as crutch walking.

CONTINUITY OF CARE

The needs for teaching and home care vary, depending on the type and severity of the fracture and its location. For example, a patient with a simple fracture of the tibia may need only teaching about cast care and crutch walking. An older patient may have more teaching needs, as well as referral to home care nurses and community services.

Teach about ordered activity restrictions. If a cast has been applied, discuss cast care and dealing with irritants such as itching. Instruct about slings, crutches, or a walker as appropriate. Instruct to elevate the extremity to reduce swelling. Ice may be applied initially to reduce both pain and edema. Instruct to perform ROM exercises of affected extremity as allowed. Teach the importance of eating well-balanced meals to promote healing. Stress the importance of follow-up care, and provide information about manifestations of complications to report to the physician.

Suggest resources for patients who need an extended period of immobilization or limited activities:

- Home care agencies for wound care and monitoring healing
- Physical therapy to evaluate home safety and suggest modifications as needed and to teach crutch walking, limited weight bearing, transferring, and other activities
- Local medical suppliers for equipment and supplies such as slings or braces, crutches, walkers, wheelchairs, overhead trapeze units, shower chairs, elevated toilet seats, grab bars, and bedside commodes
- Local pharmacies for dressing supplies
- Fitness equipment suppliers for rehabilitation needs such as hand or ankle weights for strengthening exercises

Hip Fracture

Hip fractures are a significant problem, especially in older adults. Decreased bone mass and muscle strength, slowed reflexes, and medications that can affect cognition or balance all contribute to the increased risk for hip fracture in older adults. Osteoporosis and loss of bone mass can lead to spontaneous hip fracture or one resulting from minor trauma such as stepping off a curb. Hip fracture often leads to loss of independence and restricted activity, even after healing is complete.

PATHOPHYSIOLOGY AND MANIFESTATIONS

A hip fracture is a break of the femur at the head, neck, or trochanteric regions (Figure 42-8■). Fractures of the head or neck of the femur are called *intracapsular fractures; extracapsular fractures* are fractures of the trochanteric region. Most hip fractures occur in the neck or trochanteric regions. When the head or neck of the femur is involved, impaired

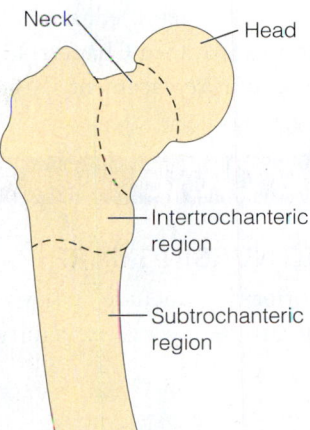

Figure 42-8. ■ Hip fractures usually occur in the neck or trochanteric regions of the femur; the head of the femur (which fits into the hip socket of the pelvis) is less frequently involved.

blood supply to the bone increases the risk of poor healing and *avascular necrosis.*

Manifestations of a hip fracture include pain, which often radiates to the knee, and inability to bear weight on the affected leg. Muscle spasms cause shortening and external rotation of the affected lower extremity.

COLLABORATIVE CARE

A hip fracture is usually diagnosed by the history, physical examination, and an x-ray of the affected hip. Buck's traction (a type of skin traction) may be applied to reduce muscle spasm until surgery can be done.

An ORIF or hip replacement procedure is performed to promote mobility, decrease pain, and prevent complications. Fixation is accomplished by securing the femur with pins, screws, nails, or plates (Figure 42-9A■). ORIF works well for fractures in the trochanteric area. If the femoral head or neck is fractured, a prosthesis is inserted to replace the femoral head (Figure 42-9B). This procedure is called an *arthroplasty.* If both the femoral head and the hip socket

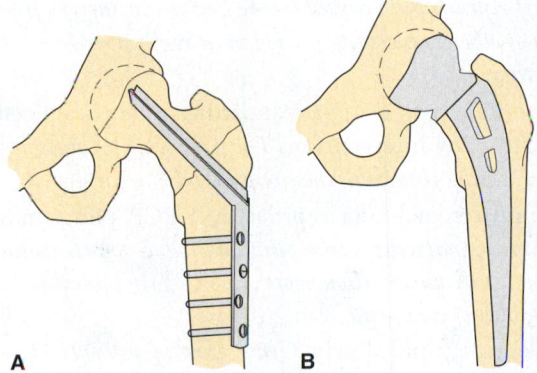

Figure 42-9. ■ Procedures to repair a hip fracture. (**A**) In an ORIF, a surgical nail or screw is used to stabilize an intertrochanteric hip fracture. (**B**) A hip prosthesis is used if the femoral head is damaged or its blood supply is impaired.

(the acetabulum) must be replaced, a *total hip replacement* or *arthroplasty* is performed. (See Chapter 43 for more information about total joint replacement.)

NURSING CARE

PRIORITIZING NURSING CARE

Nursing care priorities include relieving pain, maintaining circulation to the injured extremity, and increasing mobility.

ASSESSING

Careful assessment is vital both before and after surgery. Monitor vital signs frequently, and report changes from baseline. Monitor temperature, reporting any elevation. Increased temperature may indicate wound infection, respiratory infection, or sepsis. Assess color, temperature, capillary refill, pulses, and movement and sensation of affected leg, comparing findings with the unaffected leg. Report changes to the charge nurse or physician. If surgery has been performed, assess the wound for healing, drainage, and signs of infection or inflammation. Promptly report shortening and internal rotation of the affected leg, which could indicate dislocation of the affected hip.

DIAGNOSING, PLANNING, AND IMPLEMENTING

Nursing care of a patient with a hip fracture is challenging. After age 50, the risk of hip fracture increases every year. Many patients with a hip fracture are older and have several underlying health problems.

Acute Pain

Expected outcome: Will report pain at a level of 2 or lower on a standard pain scale.

- Ask about location and nature of pain. *It is important to differentiate pain caused by the fracture or surgery from pain of other causes such as angina, a respiratory infection, or intestinal ileus.*
- Ask to rate pain using a standardized pain scale before and after any intervention. *The pain scale provides a means of evaluating the effectiveness of pain relief measures.*
- Administer analgesia as ordered. A PCA pump may be ordered. *Analgesics relieve pain and reduce muscle tension and spasm. PCA pumps allow more effective pain control with lower total doses of analgesia.*
- Move gently and slowly. *Gentle turning prevents severe muscle spasms.*
- Encourage distraction, deep breathing, relaxation, and other adjunctive pain relief measures. *Adjunctive measures improve the effectiveness of analgesics.*

Impaired Physical Mobility

Expected outcome: Will demonstrate appropriate use of assistive devices with supervision.

Maintaining mobility is important to prevent complications of immobility (e.g., atelectasis, pressure sores, and DVT), especially in older adults.

- Encourage isometric exercises and flexion and extension exercises of the feet, ankles, elbows, shoulders, and knees every 4 hours. *These exercises help maintain muscle tone and promote venous return from the extremities.*
- Work with physical therapy to promote activities as allowed. *The physical therapist can help mobilize the patient when weight bearing is limited and can provide assistive devices and teaching about their appropriate use.*
- Assist and encourage ambulation per the physician's orders. *Ambulation helps prevent muscle atrophy and other complications of immobility.*
- Apply antiembolism (TED) hose or pneumatic compression devices (PCDs) as ordered. Remove hose or the PCD at least every 8 hours to inspect the skin. *TED hose and PCDs promote venous return from the lower extremities, reducing the risk of DVT.*
- Administer anticoagulants as ordered and monitor for adverse effects (bleeding). *Anticoagulants may be ordered to reduce the risk of DVT. Although the risk for bleeding is low, it is important to monitor for abnormal bleeding of the wound, gums, gastrointestinal tract, or other sites.*

Risk for Infection

Expected outcome: Will remain free of signs of infection.

- Use sterile technique for dressing changes. *Sterile technique reduces contamination of the wound by infectious organisms.*
- Assess wound color, healing, and the presence of any drainage. *Redness, swelling, and purulent drainage may indicate infection.*
- Promptly report any temperature elevation, tachycardia, or signs of wound infection to the physician. *Prompt identification and treatment of a wound infection promote healing and may prevent the development of osteomyelitis.*

MANAGING NURSING CARE

Nursing care activities such as measuring vital signs and intake and output, positioning, and assisting with activities of daily living (ADLs) for the patient with hip fracture may be assigned to assistive personnel with appropriate training and documented competence.

EVALUATING

Collect data regarding level of pain and pain relief, ability to resume physical mobility, wound healing, and skin integrity to evaluate the effectiveness of nursing care for the patient with a fractured hip.

DOCUMENTING

Document pre- and postoperative assessment data, including neurovascular assessments of the affected leg and indicators of complications such as lung sounds, incisional drainage, and skin condition. Also document pain level and the effectiveness of measures to relieve pain. Record activity and teaching.

CONTINUITY OF CARE

Hip fracture in the older adult can lead to loss of independence and long-term disability. Box 42-8 outlines teaching to help prevent hip fractures. Helping the patient regain independence in ADLs is a priority in planning for discharge. Box 42-9■ outlines assessment data to help determine an older adult's ability to return to his or her previous living situation after a hip fracture.

Explain activity restrictions. Teach how to limit the amount of weight placed on the affected extremity. Discuss the importance of sitting in a high, firm chair to minimize hip flexion; a raised toilet seat is also helpful. Encourage equipping a shower with a rail to aid stability and prevent falls. If a walker is needed, teach how to use it. Explain that the walker should not be carried. Instruct the patient to lift it, advance it, and then take two steps. If a cane is needed, teach how to use it to reduce weight bearing on the affected side. Stress the importance of well-balanced meals, and explain all ordered medications.

The patient who is cognitively impaired does not learn as effectively and is less able to independently perform ADLs after hip fracture. The stress of the injury and surgery may also worsen manifestations of dementia. Teaching needs to be very focused, presented in brief sessions, and repeatedly reinforced. Temporary or permanent placement in a long-term care facility may be necessary after a hip fracture. This may also be the case if the primary caregiver is cognitively impaired. Discharge planning needs to begin on admission

to the hospital. Provide information and referrals for home care services or long-term care facilities as appropriate. Recommend facilities that provide physical therapy and structured activities to promote independence and recovery.

BOX 42-9	ASSESSMENT

Assessing for Discharge: Hip Fracture

- Ability to independently or with assistance manage ADLs and to use assistive devices such as a walker, elevated toilet seat, grab bars, or shower seat
- Cognitive function of patient and primary caregiver; understanding of activity and weight-bearing limitations; understanding of complications to report to the physician
- Home environment has adequate lighting, grab bars in bathroom, and level floors; note barriers to independence (stairs, small bathrooms, or deep tubs for bathing)
- Resources for and availability of home health and rehabilitation services as needed

NURSING CARE PLAN
Patient With Hip Fracture

Stella Carbolito, 74 years old, lives alone. While walking to the market, Mrs. Carbolito falls and breaks her left hip. She is transported by ambulance to the nearest hospital.

Assessment

On admission, Mrs. Carbolito's left leg appears shorter than her right, and it is externally rotated. Distal pulses are present and strong bilaterally; both legs are warm. Mrs. Carbolito complains of severe pain but denies any numbness or burning. She can wiggle the toes on her left leg and has full movement of her right leg. Her vital signs are T 98.0°F (36.6°C); P 100; R 18; BP 120/58. X-ray shows a fracture of the left femoral neck. Mrs. Carbolito is admitted with an order for 10 lb of straight leg traction. An ORIF is planned for the following day.

Nursing Diagnosis

Mrs. Carbolito's nurse, Maria Davis, identifies the following nursing diagnoses:

- *Acute Pain* related to fracture and muscle spasms
- *Impaired Physical Mobility* related to bed rest and left hip fracture
- *Risk for Peripheral Neurovascular Dysfunction* related to fracture and swelling

Expected Outcomes

The expected outcomes for Mrs. Carbolito's care specify that she will:

- Verbalize adequate pain control.
- Relate an understanding of the purpose of traction and surgery.
- Demonstrate exercises as taught.
- Report increased pain, numbness, tingling, or weakness to the nurse.

Planning and Implementation

The following nursing interventions are planned and implemented:

- Assess pain using a standard scale before and after giving analgesics.
- Give analgesics on a regular basis as ordered to control pain.
- Document color, pulses, temperature, movement, and sensation in left leg every 2 to 4 hours.

- Apply straight leg (Buck) traction as ordered.
- Teach deep breathing and relaxation techniques, as well as isometric and flexion/extension exercises.
- Discuss the purpose of traction and surgery to repair the hip fracture.

Evaluation

Two days after surgery, Mrs. Carbolito is out of bed and in a hip chair. Her pain is effectively managed with the ordered analgesic and relaxation exercises. She does isometric and flexion/extension exercises when reminded. Plans are being made for Mrs. Carbolito's discharge to her daughter's home. A community nurse and physical therapist will visit, and the hospital social worker has ordered a trapeze for her bed, an elevated toilet seat and cushion for her chair, and a walker.

Critical Thinking in the Nursing Process

1. What preoperative teaching does Mrs. Carbolito need before the planned ORIF of her left hip?
2. Explain why Mrs. Carbolito was placed in traction when she was going to the operating room anyway.
3. List all the departments in the hospital that will be involved in Mrs. Carbolito's care. Describe their roles.

Note: Discussion of Critical Thinking questions appears on the companion website.

Joint Trauma and Injury

> **Key Concept** The joints and their associated structures (ligaments, tendons, and muscles) are at risk for injury and damage due to trauma or overuse. Treatment is often conservative, involving rest followed by physical therapy. Nurses are often responsible for teaching about prescribed splints, activity limitations, and measures to prevent future injuries.

Joints, the weakest part of the skeleton, can be damaged when subjected to forcible stretching or twisting. Ligaments, tendons, and muscles that support the joint may be stretched or torn, joint cartilage may be damaged, or the joint itself may be dislocated.

DISLOCATION

A **dislocation** is loss of contact between two bones of a joint. Dislocations usually follow trauma such as a fall or blow during contact sports or activities such as skiing. Joint disease (e.g., arthritis) can cause a spontaneous dislocation. *Subluxation* is partial separation of the bones of a joint. Although any joint may be affected, shoulder dislocations are the most common. Dislocation causes pain, deformity, and limited motion of the affected joint.

REPETITIVE USE INJURIES

Repetitive use injuries result from overuse of or repeated stress on a joint without adequate recovery time. They can result in disability and lost work time.

Carpal tunnel syndrome is a common work-related injury that results from inflammation and swelling of structures in the wrist joint. The carpal tunnel is a canal through which tendons and the median nerve pass from the wrist to the hand. Inflammation and swelling narrow this space, compressing and irritating the nerve. Numbness and tingling of the thumb, index finger, and middle finger of the affected hand develop. The hand is weak, and "falls asleep" at night, with pain that is relieved by shaking or massaging the hand and fingers. The patient may have difficulty holding utensils or performing precise activities with the affected hand.

Bursitis is inflammation of a bursa, a padlike sac that prevents friction between tissues such as ligaments, tendons, and bone. Bursae in the shoulder, hip, leg, and elbow may become inflamed, causing local tenderness and pain with joint movement. The patient guards the joint to decrease pain.

Epicondylitis (also called *tennis elbow* or *golfer's elbow*) is inflammation of a tendon where it inserts into the bone. Repeated trauma that causes tears, bleeding, and inflammation of the tendon can lead to epicondylitis. Its manifestations include point tenderness, pain radiating down the forearm, and a history of repetitive use.

ROTATOR CUFF INJURIES

Rotator cuff injuries are common. The rotator cuff is the group of muscles that control arm movement. Rotator cuff disorders include tendinitis, bursitis, and partial and complete muscle tears. These injuries can be acute or may result from repetitive use injury or degenerative changes of the involved tissues.

Manifestations of rotator cuff damage include shoulder pain, which may be worse at night or when lying on the involved shoulder. Range of motion, abduction and flexion in particular, increases pain and is often limited.

KNEE INJURIES

The knee is vulnerable to ligament tears, meniscal injury, and patellar dislocation. These injuries are frequently associated with sports activities that lead to falls or abnormal twisting of the knee joint. The medial collateral ligament (MCL) and the anterior cruciate ligament (ACL) are commonly injured. The menisci, two C-shaped plates of cartilage within each knee joint, act as shock absorbers. A tear of the medial meniscus is a common knee injury. The patella, or knee cap, can become partially or completely dislocated.

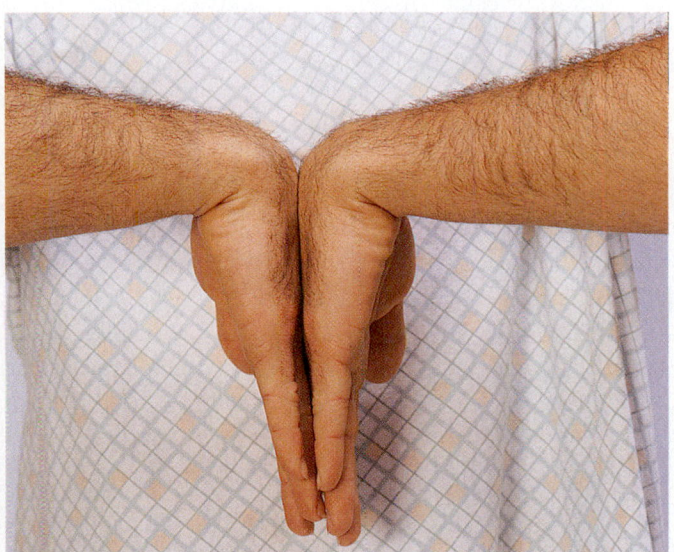

Figure 42-10. ■ Phalen test. The wrist is flexed 90 degrees with the fingers extended. Finger numbness during the test may indicate carpal tunnel syndrome. (Source: Pearson Education.)

The patient with a knee injury often relates a history of an acute injury, with immediate pain, a tearing or popping sensation, or the knee "giving out." Swelling of the affected joint may develop immediately or over several hours after the injury.

COLLABORATIVE CARE

Joint injuries are often diagnosed by history and physical examination. X-rays, MRI, ultrasound, or, in some cases, arthroscopy may be used to confirm the diagnosis. Special maneuvers, such as the Phalen test for carpal tunnel syndrome (Figure 42-10■), may be performed.

Treatment usually includes joint rest; the affected joint may be immobilized or a splint applied. Weight bearing may be restricted for knee injuries. NSAIDs, moist heat, and physical therapy are often prescribed. Surgery may be necessary to treat carpal tunnel syndrome or to repair rotator cuff or knee injuries.

NURSING CARE

Nursing care for joint injuries usually occurs in a community-based care setting.

PRIORITIZING NURSING CARE

A primary focus of nursing care for joint injuries is patient teaching.

ASSESSING

Inquire about circumstances of injury, if known. Ask about pain, including its location, character, timing, and activities or movements that aggravate or relieve the discomfort. Examine the affected joint, including comparing its color and size to the corresponding unaffected joint. Palpate the joint for tenderness, crepitus, temperature, and swelling. Instruct or assist the patient to move the joint through its normal ROM, stopping and noting where pain is experienced. Do not move the affected joint beyond that point. When a joint dislocation is suspected, assess color, temperature, pulses, movement, and sensation of the limb distal to the affected joint.

DIAGNOSING, PLANNING, AND IMPLEMENTING

Acute Pain

Expected outcome: Will use analgesic and nonanalgesic measures appropriately to promote comfort and healing.

■ Encourage use of an appropriate splint or joint immobilizer. *Splinting maintains joint alignment and reduces pain and inflammation.*

■ Teach safe application of ice or heat to the affected joint as indicated. *Ice causes vasoconstriction and numbs the tender area; heat decreases swelling by increasing venous return. Inappropriately applied, both ice and heat can damage tissues.*

■ Instruct about using NSAIDs as ordered. *Taken on a regular basis (not as needed for pain), NSAIDs decrease swelling and inflammation, reducing pain.*

■ Teach use of assistive devices such as a splint, sling, or crutches, to reduce stress on the affected joint or minimize weight bearing. *When used appropriately, assistive devices help minimize use of and stress on the affected joint, promoting joint rest and healing. When used inappropriately, these assistive devices can increase the risk of further injury or damage.*

■ Instruct not to discontinue treatment abruptly. *Stopping treatment abruptly may cause the injured joint to become reinflamed.*

Impaired Physical Mobility

Expected outcome: Will verbalize an understanding of potential benefits of physical and occupational therapy.

■ Refer to physical therapy for appropriate exercises. *The physical therapist can teach exercises to strengthen supportive joint tissues and maintain joint mobility.*

■ Suggest occupational therapy. *Occupational therapy can help the patient learn new ways to perform tasks to prevent recurring symptoms.*

EVALUATING

To evaluate the effectiveness of nursing care, assess the patient's knowledge and understanding of the disorder and its treatment.

DOCUMENTING

Document assessment data and teaching provided for the patient to promote self-care.

CONTINUITY OF CARE

Stress the importance of following recommendations for immobilization of the affected joint. If a brace or sling is prescribed, discuss skin care and ways to prevent skin-to-skin contact, particularly in the axillary area. Refer to physical therapy for exercises to strengthen muscles and supportive structures of the joint to reduce the risk of future injuries.

Teach about the specific joint injury or disorder and its causes and treatments. Rehabilitation may be necessary to restore independence. Help identify ways to avoid activities that increase risk of injury. Suggest that an environmental risk manager or ergonomic specialist evaluate the patient's workstation and recommend measures to reduce the risk of repetitive use injuries. Wrist supports or an ergonomic keyboard may be useful for the patient who uses a computer extensively. Appropriate desk and chair height are also important in maintaining correct anatomic position while working. Provide information about sources for braces or other assistive devices.

Amputation

> **Key Concept** Amputation, the partial or total removal of an extremity, has significant physical and psychosocial effects on the patient and on the family. In addition to providing care and support for the patient and family, the nurse is actively involved with the interprofessional team for optimal patient care and rehabilitation.

Amputation is partial or total removal of a body part. It may be the result of a chronic illness (e.g., peripheral vascular disease or diabetes) or due to trauma. Injuries experienced during military service have resulted in more than 1,200 young adults who have lost a major limb and nearly 400 with loss of a hand, foot, fingers, or toes. Regardless of the cause, amputation is devastating. Adapting to amputation may take a long time and significant effort.

Peripheral vascular disease (PVD) is the major cause of lower extremity amputation. Peripheral neuropathy in patients with diabetes also increases the risk for amputation.

Trauma is the major cause of upper extremity amputation. Men have a significantly higher risk of traumatic amputation than women.

PATHOPHYSIOLOGY AND MANIFESTATIONS

Impaired blood flow and untreated infection that causes **gangrene** (tissue death) can lead to amputation. In PVD, circulation to the extremities is impaired. This leads to edema and tissue damage. Healing is also impaired. Minor injuries and stasis ulcers can become infected because altered immune function can allow bacteria to invade and proliferate. In peripheral neuropathy, loss of sensation frequently leads to unrecognized injury and infection. Untreated infection can lead to gangrene and amputation. The level of amputation is determined by the extent of tissue damage and remaining healthy tissue. When possible, joints are preserved for better function of the extremity. Figure 42-11■ illustrates common sites of amputation.

A limb may be partially or completely severed by acute trauma. In some cases, the severed limb may be reattached. Extensive tissue damage, however, may make reattachment impossible.

COMPLICATIONS

Potential complications of amputation include infection, delayed healing, and contracture.

Infection

Infection is a risk after amputation. The patient who is older, has diabetes, or has PVD is at a particularly high risk for infection. Local manifestations of infection include drainage, odor, redness, positive wound cultures, and increased discomfort at the suture line. Systemic manifestations include chills and fever, tachycardia, and possibly a fall in blood pressure. If any of these manifestations develop, immediately notify the charge nurse or physician. Pneumonia may develop, with a productive cough, pain on deep inspiration, and malaise. Provide good skin care, maintain aseptic technique during dressing changes, and encourage coughing and deep breathing to prevent infection.

Delayed Healing

Delayed healing is healing that occurs at a slower rate than expected. Infection or impaired circulation can lead to delayed healing. It is a particular risk in older patients who are more likely to have chronic diseases, such as diabetes or PVD. Poor nutrition and smoking are also risk factors for delayed healing. Notify the physician if the wound is not healing appropriately or if the stump is cool to the touch.

Contractures

A **contracture** is abnormal flexion and fixation of a joint caused by muscle atrophy and shortening. Contracture of the joint above the amputation is a common complication. Measures to prevent contractures are outlined in Box 42-10■.

Phantom Limb Pain

Most amputees experience phantom limb sensations after surgery. These sensations include tingling, numbness, or itching of the amputated limb. When the sensations are painful, they are called **phantom limb pain**. Phantom limb pain more frequently affects people who had pain in the amputated limb prior to its removal than those who did not. However, the cause of phantom limb pain is unknown.

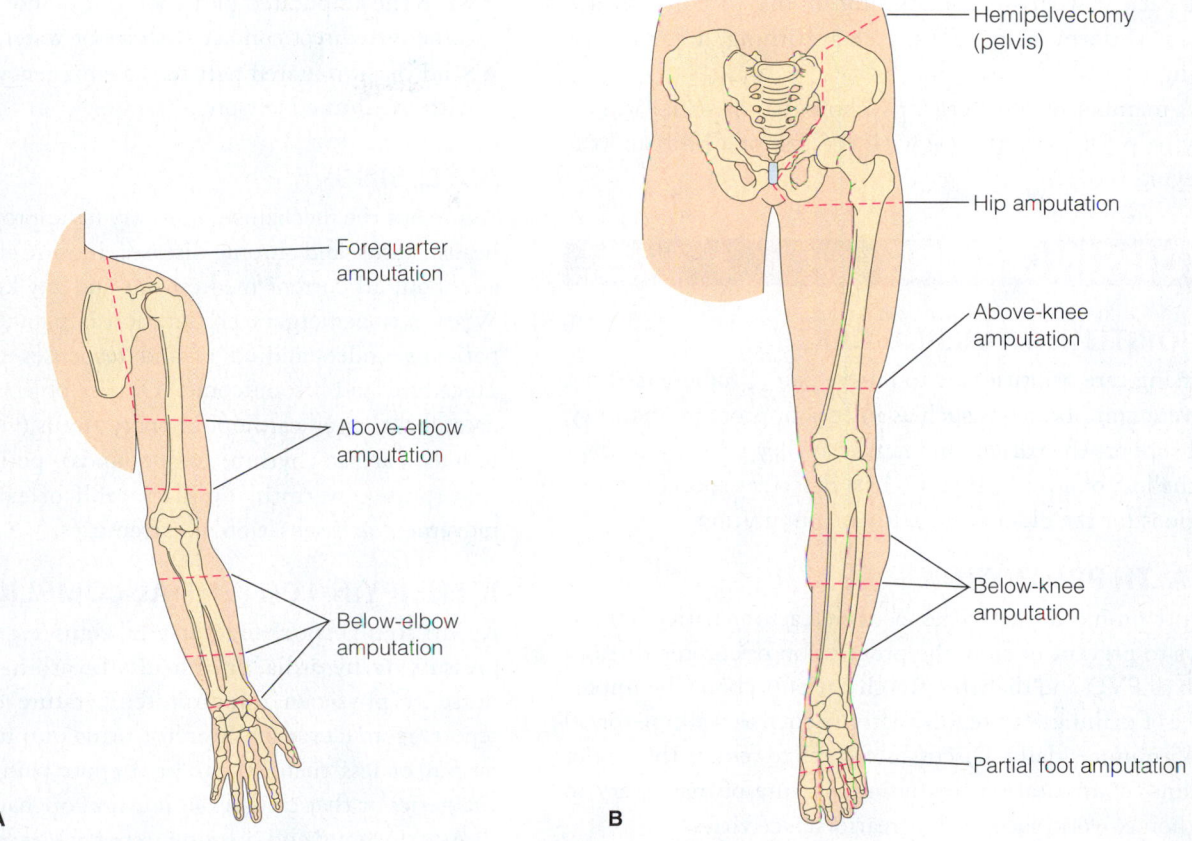

Figure 42-11. ■ Common sites of amputation. (**A**) The upper extremities and (**B**) the lower extremities.

BOX 42-10	NURSING CARE CHECKLIST

Preventing Contractures After Amputation

☑ Encourage joint extension.

☑ With above-knee amputation, place in prone position several times daily; do not elevate stump on pillows after the first 24 hours.

☑ For below-knee amputation, elevate foot of bed, keeping knee extended.

☑ Position upper extremities using the same principles.

☑ Provide active or passive ROM exercises every 2 to 4 hours for all joints.

☑ Use trapeze on bed frame to encourage frequent position changes.

☑ Teach importance of moving and ROM exercises.

☑ For a thigh or above-knee amputation, avoid sitting for prolonged periods.

☑ Teach postural exercises to compensate for loss of weight on affected side.

The missing extremity feels crushed, trapped, twisted, or burning. Management of phantom pain is challenging, often requiring referral to a pain clinic and a comprehensive pain management program.

COLLABORATIVE CARE

After amputation, the wound may be open (*guillotine*) or closed (*flap*). Open amputations are done when an infection is present. The end of the stump (remaining portion of the limb) is left open to drain. Continuous skin traction is applied to the limb. When the infection has cleared, the wound is closed.

In a closed amputation, a flap of skin is formed to cover the end of the wound. A compression dressing is applied to the stump after amputation to reduce edema, prevent infection, and promote healing. The dressing helps mold the stump to fit a prosthesis and helps prevent edema. The patient with a closed amputation may return from surgery with a temporary prosthesis. Limited weight bearing may be allowed within a week or two after surgery. The patient is referred to a *prosthetist* (a professional who makes and fits artificial limbs), who discusses available prosthetic options. The prosthesis is custom made and fitted to the patient. Some patients may have several prostheses made for different functions, depending on their age, occupation, and activity level.

Physical and occupational therapy are provided to help regain optimal function. The patient with a leg amputation is taught how to use crutches or a walker for ambulation.

The patient with an arm amputation may need to relearn how to perform many ADLs, such as bathing, dressing, and eating.

A member of the clergy, psychologist, or social worker may help the patient cope with the loss of a limb and the grieving process.

NURSING CARE

PRIORITIZING NURSING CARE

Nursing care priorities are to relieve pain, promote healing, prevent complications such as infection, promote mobility, and support the patient and family as they grieve and adapt to the loss of a limb. Box 42-11 describes special considerations for the older adult with an amputation.

HEALTH PROMOTION

Health promotion activities focus on teaching patients about ways to prevent or slow the progression of chronic diseases such as PVD and diabetes. Teach patients about the importance of maintaining regular activity such as walking for 30 to 45 minutes daily. Discuss measures to reduce the risk of traumatic amputation, including safe use of machinery in the home, workplace, and recreational activities.

Provide information about emergency care for traumatic amputation:

- Keep the victim in a supine position with the legs elevated.
- Apply firm pressure to the bleeding area.
- Wrap the amputated part in a clean cloth (soaked in saline solution if available), and place in a clean plastic bag.

BOX 42-11 FOCUS ON OLDER ADULTS

Amputation

Holistic nursing care is especially important for the older patient with an amputation.

- Kidney and liver function decline with aging, increasing the risk of adverse drug effects. Closely monitor response to medications.
- Reduced blood flow prolongs wound healing, and immune function often declines with aging, increasing the risk for infection. Monitor for local and systemic signs of infection.
- Slowed reflexes and gait alterations may disrupt balance. Introduce assistive devices in stages.
- A walker may be more appropriate than crutches, because older patients have less upper body strength. Address safety issues, such as the risk for falling.
- Assess the need for in-home assistance and make appropriate referrals to visiting nurses and home health aides.

- Keep the amputated part cool, but do not allow it to come into direct contact with ice or water.
- Send the amputated part to the emergency department with the injured person.

ASSESSING

Ask about the mechanism of injury (as appropriate), current health status, and chronic diseases. Inquire about pain. Also ask about all current medications and any known allergies. When a nonemergent amputation is planned, explore the patient's understanding of and responses to the planned procedure and its outcome. Obtain objective assessment data, focusing on cardiopulmonary status (vital signs, heart sounds, cardiac rhythm, lung sounds), peripheral circulation (pulses, warmth, capillary refill of extremities), and movement and sensation of extremities.

IDENTIFYING POTENTIAL COMPLICATIONS

Report significant changes in vital signs (e.g., a fall in blood pressure, tachycardia, or difficulty breathing) to the charge nurse or physician. Monitor temperature every 4 hours, reporting an elevation. Monitor urine output, reporting an output of less than 30 mL/hr. Report pain unrelieved by analgesics or that changes in location or character.

Assess wound and dressing, reporting excessive or bright red drainage that could indicate hemorrhage. Monitor wound healing, assessing for redness, swelling, purulent drainage, or evidence of a hematoma.

DIAGNOSING, PLANNING, AND IMPLEMENTING
Acute Pain

Expected outcome: Will report pain at a level of 2 or lower on a standard pain scale.

- Administer analgesics as ordered. A PCA pump may be used initially. *Postoperative pain can be compounded by muscle spasms, swelling, and phantom pain. PCA pumps increase patient control over and allow early relief of pain before it intensifies.*
- Splint and support injured area. *Splinting reduces muscle spasm and decreases edema, relieving pressure and pain.*
- Unless contraindicated, elevate the stump for 24 hours. *Elevating the stump promotes venous return and decreases edema, which will decrease pain.*
- Frequently reposition, turning slowly and gently. *Repositioning relieves pressure on tissues. Slow, gentle turning helps prevent severe muscle spasms.*
- Encourage distraction, meditation, deep breathing, and relaxation exercises. *These adjunctive measures help the patient refocus, reducing the intensity of pain, including phantom pain.*

Risk for Infection

Expected outcome: Will remain free of signs of infection.

- Change wound dressing as ordered, using aseptic technique. *Aseptic technique prevents contamination of the wound with bacteria.*
- Protect wound and dressing from contamination by urine or feces. *A high above-knee or hip amputation wound can be contaminated during toileting, increasing the risk for infection.*
- Administer antibiotics as ordered. *Antibiotics inhibit bacterial growth and help prevent or eliminate infection.*
- Teach stump-wrapping techniques. *Correctly wrapping the stump improves circulation, reducing the chance of infection.*
- Report elevated WBC count. *The WBC count rises as the body tries to rid itself of infection.*

Grieving

Expected outcome: Will express thoughts and feelings about loss of the limb and its function.

- Encourage verbalization of feelings, asking open-ended questions. *Open-ended questions allow discussion of feelings and communicate a willingness to listen.*
- Maintain eye contact and actively listen. *Eye contact and active listening communicate respect for the patient and his or her feelings.*
- Reflect on the patient's feelings. *Reflection statements, such as "You seem angry," allow the patient to recognize feelings and validate their presence.*
- Allow unlimited visiting hours, if possible. *Unlimited visiting hours promote increased social supports.*

Disturbed Body Image

Expected outcome: Will acknowledge change in appearance and body function.

- Encourage verbalization of feelings, and validate that feelings are real and appropriate. *This allows communication of fears and lets the patient know the nurse is willing to listen.*
- Allow to wear clothing from home. *Familiar clothing provides emotional comfort and helps the patient retain a sense of identity.*
- Encourage looking at the stump. *Looking at and touching the stump helps the patient face fear of the unknown and move from denial to acceptance.*
- Encourage participation in stump care. *Active participation in care increases self-esteem and independence.*
- Offer visitation by another amputee. *A support person who has experienced the same change provides hope for regaining independence.*
- Encourage active participation in rehabilitation. *Active participation in rehabilitation increases independence and mobility.*

Impaired Physical Mobility

Expected outcome: Will demonstrate correct use of prescribed exercises and assistive devices.

- Perform ROM exercises on all joints. *ROM exercises help prevent contractures that limit mobility.*
- Maintain postoperative dressing (rigid or compression). *Postoperative dressings help mold the stump and promote healing.*
- Frequently turn and reposition. Place the patient with a lower extremity amputation in the prone position every 4 hours. *Repositioning increases blood flow to muscles. The prone position helps prevent hip contracture.*
- Teach crutch walking or the use of assistive devices. *These devices allow more rapid resumption of activity.*
- Encourage active participation in physical therapy. *Physical therapy may initially be fatiguing; continuing participation increases energy level and activity tolerance.*

MANAGING NURSING CARE

Nursing care activities such as measuring vital signs and intake and output, assisting with ADLs and skin care, and promoting mobility for the patient with an amputation may be assigned to assistive personnel with appropriate training and documented competence.

EVALUATING

To evaluate the effectiveness of nursing care for the patient with an amputation, assess pain and the effectiveness of relief measures. Note the presence or absence of wound infection or a complication such as pneumonia. Also note the patient's and family's response to the wound and the loss of a body part. Assess physical mobility and participation in physical therapy.

DOCUMENTING

Document continuing assessment data, including condition of the incision and the stump. Also document nature and amount of pain and the effectiveness of analgesia. Record the patient's and family's responses to the amputation, to teaching, and to the prospect of a prosthesis.

CONTINUITY OF CARE

Assess knowledge of care needs, activity restrictions or special needs, and resources for home care. Discuss home management—who is responsible for household activities such as cleaning and cooking. Inquire about arrangements that have been made for home care activities and ADLs. Evaluate use of prescription and nonprescription medications, paying particular attention to interactions and drugs that may affect balance, mental alertness, or appetite. Ask about social habits, such as cigarette smoking, alcohol use, or other drug use, that may affect healing or the ability to provide self-care.

Assess the home environment for potential safety hazards and access to care needs, such as:

- Scatter rugs
- Stairs between living areas of the house
- Grab bars to facilitate toileting and bathing
- Clean water and other needs for wound care

Teach stump bandaging to prepare for fitting the prosthesis. Discuss positioning to prevent contractures. Teach stump exercises to maintain joint mobility and muscle tone of the affected limb. Encourage resumption of physical activities as soon as possible. Discuss household modifications to promote independence, such as grab bars in the bathroom, faucets with single-handle controls for water flow and temperature, and handheld shower heads and shower chairs for bathing. Encourage to contact local and national agencies and support groups.

Note: The references and resources for all chapters have been compiled at the back of the book.

Chapter Review

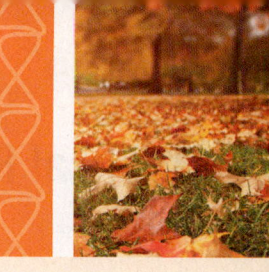

KEY POINTS

- **Concept:** Musculoskeletal injury, from minor strains to amputation, affects comfort and interferes with mobility and daily living activities. An extended period of recovery and rehabilitation may be required to recover previous function.
- Common complications of immobility, such as pneumonia and DVT, are a risk for patients with musculoskeletal injuries.
- With all musculoskeletal injuries, assessment of circulation, movement, and sensation distal to the injury is important both initially and as part of continuing care.
- **Concept:** Soft tissue injury, including sprains and strains, is common, often associated with recreational activities or repetitive motions. Nursing care includes assessing the circumstances and impact of the injury as well as circulation and neurologic status distal to the injury, and teaching prescribed treatment and rehabilitation.
- **Concept:** Fractures are a common musculoskeletal injury. While usually uncomplicated, fractures place the patient at risk for complications and may require surgery or other invasive measures for healing. Nurses focus on promoting comfort, preventing and promptly recognizing complications, and teaching for patients with fractures.
- Fractures may be stabilized for healing with a cast, by surgical insertion of pins or plates, or using traction. Skin and wound care are important to prevent infection and complications of immobility.
- Complications of fracture include infection, compartment syndrome, fat embolism syndrome, and deep venous thrombosis. Prompt identification and treatment of potential complications is critical for the patient's recovery and rehabilitation. Nurses need to recognize and appropriately respond to manifestations of complications.
- Hip fractures are a significant risk in older adults and can lead to loss of independence. Provide meticulous nursing care focusing on rehabilitation from the time of hospital admission to full recovery.
- **Concept:** The joints and their associated structures (ligaments, tendons, and muscles) are at risk for injury and damage due to trauma or overuse. Treatment is often conservative, involving rest followed by physical therapy. Nurses are often responsible for teaching about prescribed splints, activity limitations, and measures to prevent future injuries.
- Carpal tunnel syndrome is a common repetitive use injury that can impair fine motor function of the hands. Prevention is the best treatment.
- **Concept:** Amputation, the partial or total removal of an extremity, has significant physical and psychosocial effects on the patient and on the family. In addition to providing care and support for the patient and family, the nurse is actively involved with the interprofessional team for optimal patient care and rehabilitation.
- Loss of a body part causes grieving and disturbs body image. Many ADLs need to be relearned after amputation.

PEARSON NURSING STUDENT RESOURCES

Find additional materials at **nursing.pearsonhighered.com**.

Clinical Reasoning Care Map

Caring for a Patient With a Below-Knee Amputation
NCLEX-PN® Test Focus Area: Psychosocial Integrity: Coping and Adaptation

Case Study: John Rocke is a 45-year-old divorced man with a history of poorly controlled diabetes mellitus. He lives alone in a second-floor apartment. Two days ago, Mr. Rocke underwent a left below-knee amputation as a result of gangrene of his left foot, a consequence of his diabetes.

Nursing Diagnosis: Ineffective Individual Coping

COLLECT DATA

Subjective	Objective
_____	_____
_____	_____
_____	_____
_____	_____
_____	_____
_____	_____

Does this present a threat to the patient's safety?

If yes, the priority intervention to address this threat would be:

_____

Nursing Care

_____
_____
_____
_____
_____
_____
_____
_____

Interprofessional team members to include when planning care:

_____

How would you document this? _____

_____

Compare your answers and documentation to those provided on the companion website.

Data Collected
(use only those that apply)

- Vital signs stable
- Stump splinted; covered by soft dressing
- Wound healing without signs of infection
- Refuses ROM exercises and turning
- Complaining of severe pain
- Yells "Get out! I don't want anyone to see me like this" when anyone enters room
- Tolerating 1,800-calorie American Diabetes Association (ADA) diet

Nursing Interventions (use only those that apply; list in priority order)

- Request a change from PRN analgesia to a PCA pump.
- Encourage verbalization of feelings.
- Teach the importance of moving and ROM exercises to prevent contractures.
- Contact the physician for a referral to a psychologist or social worker.
- Encourage turning and lying prone.

NCLEX-PN® Exam Preparation

TEST-TAKING TIP   Be familiar with the parameters of pain assessment, because patients experiencing musculoskeletal trauma frequently have severe pain.

1 The nurse is caring for a patient who has a new cast. Which of the following are appropriate nursing care measures? **Select all that apply.**
1. Use a hot blow dryer to apply heat to dry the cast.
2. Cover the extremity and cast with a blanket to prevent chilling.
3. Elevate the extremity on a pillow to reduce swelling.
4. Handle the cast with the palms of the hands only.
5. Pad rough edges of the cast to prevent skin excoriation.

2 When caring for a patient with an above-knee amputation, it is important for the nurse to encourage the patient to spend time in:
1. the prone position.
2. the supine position.
3. a flexed position.
4. a position of comfort.

3 The nurse is admitting a patient who fell at home and is now complaining of right hip pain and an inability to put weight on the right leg. When conducting a focused admission assessment, the LPN/LVN appropriately:
1. assesses passive ROM of the knee on the affected leg.
2. compares movement of the affected leg with the unaffected leg.
3. assesses for a positive Homans sign on the affected side.
4. compares pulses on the affected leg with those on the unaffected leg.

4 The nurse is caring for a patient who has just had surgery to repair a fracture of the tibia. The patient's leg is in a cast and the patient is receiving PCA morphine for pain. The patient continues to complain of severe pain and paresthesias in the foot. The nurse should:
1. elevate the leg above the heart.
2. bivalve the cast.
3. immediately notify the physician.
4. request an increase in the dose of morphine.

5 When educating the patient with a sprained ankle about home care, the nurse should teach the patient the acronym:
1. BRAT.
2. RICE.
3. RACE.
4. ROSE.

6 The nurse is caring for a patient who earlier in the day had surgery to repair a fractured femur. The patient's temperature has been elevated since the previous shift. Current assessment findings include a temperature of 101.5°F, facial petechiae, and confusion. The nurse recognizes these as possible manifestations of:
1. hemorrhage.
2. infection.
3. compartment syndrome.
4. fat embolism syndrome.

7 The nurse is caring for a patient who has recently had a below-knee amputation of the left leg. The nurse knows that the most common cause for amputation of the lower extremities is:
1. motor vehicle crashes.
2. accidents involving machinery at work.
3. bone cancer.
4. peripheral vascular disease.

8 Which of the following nursing care activities are appropriate for the patient in skeletal traction? **Select all that apply.**
1. Position the patient to maintain alignment of the body with the direction of pull.
2. Cleanse pin sites per unit protocol.
3. Assist the patient to the bedside commode for toileting.
4. Release the weights when repositioning the patient in bed.
5. Slide, do not lift, the patient when repositioning.

9 The nurse is caring for a patient with an admitting diagnosis of compound fractures of the radius and ulna. Which of the following nursing measures should the nurse consider as a priority?
1. Obtain temperature every 4 hours; report PO temperature greater than 100°F.
2. Apply ice to the cast for the first 24 hours.
3. Provide information about physical and occupational therapy after discharge.
4. Encourage use of nonpharmacologic measures to promote comfort.

10 Which of the following types of traction increases the patient's mobility while maintaining appropriate bone position?
1. Balanced suspension
2. Straight traction
3. Skin traction
4. Skeletal traction

Answers and rationales for Review Questions appear in Appendix I.

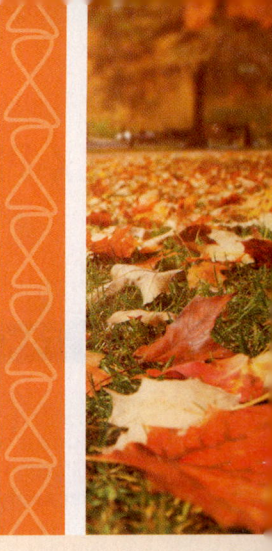

CHAPTER 43

Caring for Patients With Musculoskeletal Disorders

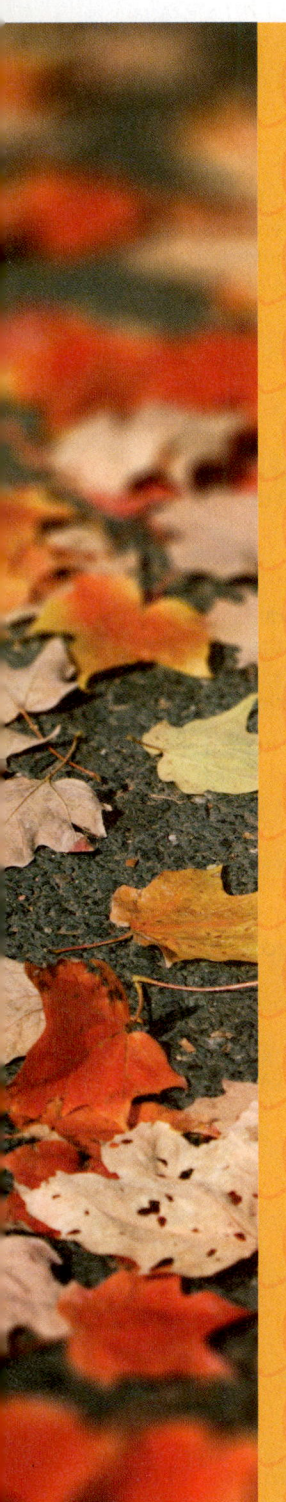

BRIEF OUTLINE

BONE DISORDERS
Osteoporosis
Paget Disease
Osteomalacia
Osteomyelitis
Bone Tumors
JOINT AND CONNECTIVE TISSUE DISORDERS

Osteoarthritis
Rheumatoid Arthritis
Systemic Lupus Erythematosus
Gout
Lyme Disease
Ankylosing Spondylitis

OTHER MUSCULOSKELETAL DISORDERS
Fibromyalgia
Low Back Pain
Common Foot Disorders

APPLIED LEARNING OUTCOMES

After completing this chapter, you will be able to:

1. Relate the effects of common musculoskeletal disorders to the normal structure and function of the musculoskeletal system.
2. Relate the pathophysiology of common musculoskeletal disorders to manifestations and potential complications of the disorder.
3. Perform focused assessments of patients with impaired musculoskeletal function, identifying expected findings and appropriately responding to abnormal or unexpected assessment data.
4. As a member of the health care team, participate in the collaborative care for patients with musculoskeletal disorders.
5. Provide individualized nursing care for patients with musculoskeletal disorders, respecting patients' expressed values, needs, and priorities.
6. Provide evidence-based teaching and home care for patients with musculoskeletal disorders.

KEY TERMS

The key terms are defined on the pages listed below.

SPECIAL FEATURES

Key Concept Musculoskeletal disorders can affect the patient's physical mobility, body image, comfort, and ability to provide self-care. Nurses provide physical care, teaching for self-care, and psychosocial support for the patient and family.

Bone Disorders

Key Concept A variety of disorders can affect the strength and integrity of bone, leaving the patient at risk for fractures. Promoting comfort, maintaining safety, and preventing injuries are priority nursing responsibilities when caring for patients with these disorders.

Osteoporosis

Osteoporosis, literally defined as "porous bones," is a bone disorder in which bone mass is lost. Bones become more fragile, increasing the risk of fractures. Osteoporosis is usually associated with aging. Eighty percent of those affected are women, and most are over the age of 60.

Although the cause of osteoporosis remains unclear, several risk factors have been identified. Some risk factors cannot be changed; others can be changed. Box 43-1 lists risk factors for osteoporosis. Ethnic background affects the risk for developing osteoporosis as well (see Box 43-2).

PATHOPHYSIOLOGY
Bone is constantly being remodeled over a person's lifetime, with old bone being replaced by new bone. Peak bone mass is achieved at about age 35. After that, the balance between bone loss and bone formation is altered. More bone is lost than is gained, and bone mass is lost. In women, bone loss accelerates

---

BOX 43-1   RISK FACTORS FOR OSTEOPOROSIS

Risk Factors That Cannot Be Changed
- Older age, female gender
- Caucasian or Asian heritage
- Small physical stature
- Family history of osteoporosis

Risk Factors That Can Be Changed
- Decreased estrogen/testosterone levels
- Poor nutrition: low lifetime calcium intake, vitamin D deficiency
- Smoking, excess alcohol intake
- Sedentary lifestyle
- Medications (corticosteroids, anticonvulsants)

BOX 43-2   FOCUS ON DIVERSITY

Risk for Osteoporosis
Although patients of all backgrounds are at risk for developing osteoporosis, ethnicity affects the risk. Among women age 50 and older:
- Non-Hispanic White and Asian women have the highest risk, with an estimated one in five affected by osteoporosis and more than half with low bone mass.
- Among Hispanic women, 1 in 10 are affected by osteoporosis and nearly half have low bone mass.
- Black women have a lower incidence, with 1 in 20 affected by osteoporosis and just over one-third with low bone mass.

---

during menopause, slowing after age 60. Men also lose bone mass with aging, although the rate of loss is slower than it is in women. Loss of bone tissue weakens its structure, increasing the risk of fracture. Bone loss affects primarily spongy bone; because of this, patients with osteoporosis are at particular risk for fractures of the spine and the neck of the femur.

MANIFESTATIONS AND COMPLICATIONS
Osteoporosis is often asymptomatic. When present, its usual manifestations are loss of height, progressive curvature of the spine, low back pain, and fractures.

Height is lost as vertebral bodies collapse. Characteristic dorsal **kyphosis** (exaggeration of the normal posterior curve of the thoracic spine) and cervical lordosis develop, causing the "dowager hump" often associated with aging. The abdomen tends to protrude and knees and hips flex as the body attempts to maintain its center of gravity (Figure 43-1).

A fracture may be the first obvious sign of osteoporosis. Some fractures are spontaneous. Others may result from everyday activities (twisting, bending, lifting, rising from bed). These are known as **pathologic fractures**, fractures that occur with minimal or no trauma. Wrist and vertebral fractures are common. Hip fractures associated with osteoporosis often interfere with the ability to maintain normal activity and live independently.

COLLABORATIVE CARE
The care of the patient with osteoporosis focuses on stopping or slowing the process, relieving the symptoms, and preventing complications. Proper nutrition and exercise are important components of treatment.

Bone mineral density (BMD) measurements can help predict the risk for fracture. All women age 65 and older and men age 70 and older should undergo BMD testing. Testing may be done earlier if the patient has risk factors such as a family history of osteoporosis, low body weight, or a prior fracture with minimal trauma. CT scanning of the spine, hip, forearm, or tibia may also be used to evaluate fracture risk.

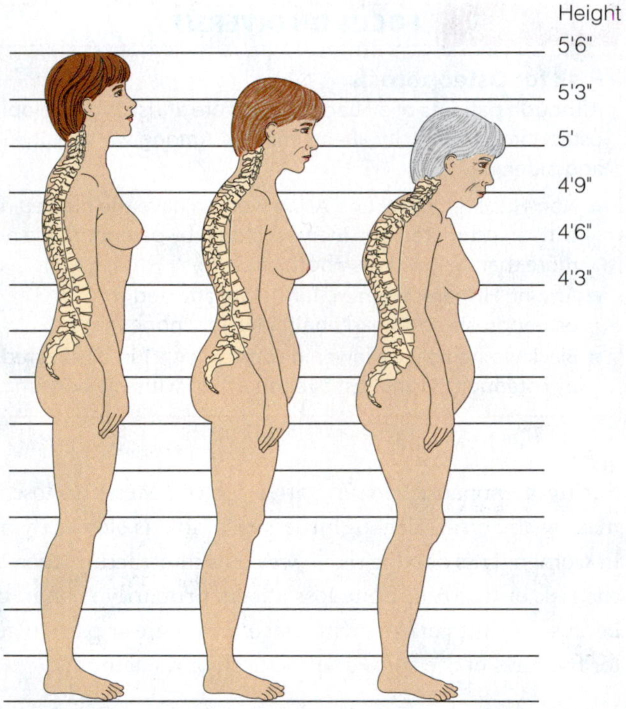

Figure 43-1. ■ Changes in height, posture, and spinal curves caused by osteoporosis.

Calcium and Vitamin D

Calcium and vitamin D are vital to preventing osteoporosis. Adequate calcium and vitamin D intake in the older adult may slow bone loss and reduce fracture risk. Adequate calcium intake before age 30 to 35 increases peak bone mass and reduces the risk of osteoporosis later in life. Calcium needs change over the lifetime. See Table 43-1 ■ for calcium intake recommendations. Box 43-3 ■ lists foods high in calcium. Vitamin D is important for calcium absorption and bone health. It also contributes to muscle function and

TABLE 43-1	Recommended Daily Calcium Intake
AGES	**MILLIGRAMS OF CALCIUM**
0–6 months	200
6 months to 1 year	260
1–3 years	700
4–8 years	1,000
9–18 years	1,300
19–50 years	1,000
Pregnant or lactating	1,000–1,300
51 and older	1,200

BOX 43-3	FOODS HIGH IN CALCIUM

- Dairy products (best source):
  - Milk, yogurt
  - Cheese
- Tofu
- Sardines, with bones
- Clams, oysters
- Canned salmon
- Spinach, greens
- Broccoli, cauliflower, bok choy
- Green beans
- Dark molasses

balance, reducing the risk of falls. A daily intake of 600 IU of vitamin D is recommended until age 70; 800 IU of vitamin D is recommended for those 70 years and older. Exposure to sunlight produces vitamin D; it can also be found in vitamin D–fortified milk and cereals.

Calcium supplements are available in many forms. A combination of calcium with vitamin D is recommended, particularly for older adults who may have limited sun exposure.

Medications

In addition to calcium and vitamin D, a number of drugs are available to prevent and treat osteoporosis. Bisphosphonates are commonly used to treat osteoporosis. These drugs inhibit bone resorption and increase bone density. They significantly reduce the incidence of fractures due to osteoporosis. Estrogen or hormone replacement therapy (HRT) or selective estrogen receptor modulators (SERMs) may be ordered to prevent or treat bone loss in postmenopausal women. These drugs are discussed in Chapter 32. Other drugs that may be used to prevent or treat osteoporosis include:

- Calcitonin, a hormone that promotes the movement of calcium into bone
- Parathyroid hormone, which also increases bone mass
- Sodium fluoride, a mineral, stimulates new bone formation. Its effectiveness in preventing and treating osteoporosis is unknown.

Table 43-2 ■ outlines the nursing implications of bisphosphonates and calcitonin.

Other Therapies

Physical therapy and rehabilitation may be ordered to improve function and reduce the risk of falls in patients with osteoporosis. Training for safe movement and daily living activities, including posture, lifting, and

TABLE 43-2	Giving Medications Safely: Osteoporosis		
CLASS/DRUGS	**PURPOSE**	**NURSING IMPLICATIONS**	**PATIENT TEACHING**
Bisphosphonates ■ *Alendronate* (Fosamax) ■ Etidronate (Didronel) ■ Ibandronate (Boniva) ■ Pamidronate (Aredia) ■ Risedronate (Actonel) ■ Tiludronate (Skelid) ■ Zoledronic acid (Reclast, Zometa)	The bisphosphonates slow bone turnover, increasing the bone density and reducing the risk of fractures. They are used to prevent and treat osteoporosis.	Give oral preparations with water on arising, 30–60 minutes before food or other medications. Hold calcium supplements and foods high in calcium for 2 hours after giving the drug. Instruct to avoid lying down for 30–60 minutes after taking the drug. When administered by intravenous infusion, monitor for manifestations of thrombophlebitis. Report changes in renal function studies (BUN and creatinine) and serum electrolytes to the physician.	Take oral forms with clear water only; avoid eating or drinking for 30–60 minutes as recommended. Do not lie down until after you have eaten breakfast. Report heartburn or difficult or painful swallowing to your health care provider. Report tingling around the mouth or numbness and tingling of fingers or toes. Take calcium and vitamin D supplements as instructed.
Calcitonin ■ Calcitonin (Fortical, Miacalcin)	Calcitonin prevents further bone loss and increases bone mass in osteoporosis if adequate calcium and vitamin D are consumed. Calcitonin may be used in combination with a bisphosphonate or by patients who cannot use bisphosphonates.	Observe for possible anaphylactic reaction for 20 minutes after giving; have resuscitation equipment available. Alternate nostrils daily when giving by nasal spray. Report nausea and vomiting, anorexia, mild flushing of the hands or feet, and urinary frequency. Teach how to handle and inject the drug at home.	Take in the evening to reduce side effects. Warm nasal spray to room temperature before using. Rhinitis (runny nose) is common with calcitonin nasal spray. Nasal sores or itching may occur. Report nosebleed to your health care provider. Nausea and vomiting will improve as treatment continues. Be sure to consume adequate calcium and vitamin D.

Note: Medications identified in *italics* are among the 200 most frequently prescribed drugs in the United States.

ambulation, is provided. When necessary, the patient is taught how to safely use assistive devices such as a walker. An exercise program that includes activities to promote bone and muscle strength is prescribed.

NURSING CARE

PRIORITIZING NURSING CARE

Nursing care focuses on preventing osteoporosis itself and preventing injuries in patients who have osteoporosis.

HEALTH PROMOTION

To prevent osteoporosis, stress the importance of maintaining an adequate calcium intake. Milk and milk products provide the best calcium sources (see Box 43-3 for additional sources). When a calcium supplement is used, recommend one that also contains vitamin D to help the body absorb and use calcium.

Teach the importance of regular physical activity that includes weight bearing to prevent bone loss. Suggest walking for 20 minutes or more five or more days per week. Discuss behaviors such as not smoking, avoiding excess alcohol intake, and limiting caffeine intake to prevent osteoporosis. Recommend that patients with a significant risk for osteoporosis talk to their primary care provider about bone-density testing.

ASSESSING

Ask about known risk factors for osteoporosis, age of menopause, usual activity level, and history of previous fractures or back pain. Measure height, comparing with height in early adulthood. Observe for spinal curvature.

IDENTIFYING POTENTIAL COMPLICATIONS

Promptly report complaints of pain, swelling, bruising, crepitus, or other manifestations of a fracture, even if no known trauma has occurred.

DIAGNOSING, PLANNING, AND IMPLEMENTING
Risk for Injury

Expected outcome: Will remain free of injury.

■ Assess the environment for safety hazards. *The patient with osteoporosis is at risk for fracture, even with minor trauma. Removing scatter rugs and maintaining clear pathways can reduce the risk of fracture related to falls or tripping.*

■ Advise to use the handrail on stairways and take precautions when walking on slippery surfaces. *The patient's center of gravity is affected by kyphosis, increasing the risk for imbalance and falls.*

■ Keep bed in low position. Use side rails as indicated to remind the patient to avoid getting up alone. Provide nighttime lighting to toilet facilities. *Most falls are preventable, particularly in hospitals and long-term care facilities.*

■ Avoid using restraints. *Restraints may increase the risk of falling and the risk of injury due to a fall. Patients may also fracture osteoporotic bones when pulling against restraints.*

■ Encourage weight-bearing exercises for 30 to 40 minutes at least four times a week. *Weight-bearing exercises such as walking or low-impact aerobics promote bone growth. Swimming (including walking on the bottom of the pool) is not a weight-bearing activity.*

■ Encourage older adults to use assistive devices as needed to remain active and independent. *Walking sticks, canes, and other tools help the patient engage in activities that promote bone growth.*

■ Teach older patients about safety and fall precautions. *Helping identify and correct safety hazards in the home can reduce the risk of falls, fractures, and potential disability.*

■ Evaluate medication regimen for drugs that may increase the risk of falling (some antihypertensives, antianxiety agents, antihistamines, or sedatives). *Many drugs may cause orthostatic hypotension or sedation, increasing the risk for falling.*

■ Teach about safe use of prescribed medications such as bisphosphonates and calcitonin. *These drugs, although effective for treating osteoporosis, have significant adverse effects and require careful patient education.*

Imbalanced Nutrition: Less Than Body Requirements

Expected outcome: Will verbalize ways to increase calcium intake to recommended levels.

■ Teach all patients recommended calcium intake for their age (see Table 43-1). *An adequate calcium intake is vital to prevent and treat osteoporosis.*

■ Provide a list of foods high in calcium (see Box 43-3) and help identify ways to include these foods in the diet. *Calcium obtained through the diet is an effective way to maintain adequate calcium levels in the body.*

■ Teach patients using calcium supplements to read and follow directions for timing in regard to meals. All supplements should be taken in divided doses (two to three times daily). *Taking calcium supplements at the appropriate time and in divided doses increases their absorption and effectiveness.*

Pain

Expected outcome: Will report pain at a level of 2 or lower on a standard 0 to 10 pain scale.

■ Assess acute or new complaints of pain. *Acute pain usually results from a fracture, such as compression fracture of the vertebrae.*

■ Give acetaminophen or anti-inflammatory drugs as indicated for pain. *Acetaminophen is often well tolerated by older adults. Regular doses of nonsteroidal anti-inflammatory drugs (NSAIDs) can help manage chronic pain.*

■ Apply heat to the painful area, being careful to avoid burning the patient. *A controlled heating pad (e.g., Aqua-K) may offer temporary pain relief. To avoid the "rebound effect," remove the heating pad every 20 to 30 minutes.*

■ Assist physical therapy to plan an exercise regimen. *Exercise is vital to maintain bone mass, but modifications may be necessary to promote comfort.*

MANAGING NURSING CARE

Teach assisting personnel the importance of providing gentle support when moving and caring for patients with osteoporosis. Many older adults with osteoporosis are in residential and long-term care settings where direct care is provided by assistive personnel.

EVALUATING

Evaluate the patient's knowledge and understanding of fall and injury prevention measures. Have the patient relate calcium-rich foods and ways to incorporate these foods into the diet. Ask the patient to restate drug safety measures and adverse effects to be reported to the physician.

DOCUMENTING

Document continuing focused assessments, including any new complaints of pain or other evidence of injury. Also document all teaching and the patient's understanding of the information. Note measures to promote a safe environment.

CONTINUITY OF CARE

Teaching about osteoporosis is important to prevent the disease and its consequences. Stress the importance of maintaining the recommended daily calcium intake.

Discuss safety and fall prevention with the patient who has osteoporosis and with caregivers. Advise to remove scatter rugs and clutter from walkways in the house. Instruct to use a night-light or graduated lighting from the bedroom to the bathroom to reduce the risk of nighttime falls. Discuss placing grab bars in strategic locations such as the shower and next to the toilet to reduce the risk of falling.

Provide a list of local and national resources, such as medical equipment supply retailers and osteoporosis support groups and foundations. The National Osteoporosis Foundation and the Osteoporosis and Related Bone Diseases National Resource Center have many patient information pamphlets and resources. Refer to a health care provider, social services, or occupational therapy as indicated for bone density testing, home care services, or rehabilitation.

Paget Disease

Paget disease of the bone, also called osteitis deformans, is a progressive disorder characterized by fragile, misshapen bones. The cause of this disease is unknown, but both genetic and environmental factors are thought to contribute.

PATHOPHYSIOLOGY AND MANIFESTATIONS

In Paget disease, the activity of *osteoclasts* (which break down and resorb bone) increases in one or more bones. This stimulates activity in *osteoblasts* (cells that form new bone) to replace lost bone. However, the new bone formed is structurally abnormal, so it is soft, weak, and prone to fractures. Paget disease commonly affects the femur, tibia, pelvis, vertebrae, and skull, although any bone can be affected. Involved bones enlarge and become deformed. Skin over the affected bone is often warm, due to increased blood flow to the area. The manifestations of Paget disease are listed in Box 43-4■. People with Paget disease of the bone have an increased risk of developing a malignant bone tumor, although the risk remains relatively small.

COLLABORATIVE CARE

Treatment goals for patients with Paget disease are to manage and minimize symptoms, improve function, and slow the disease progress to limit disability. Diagnostic testing includes obtaining serum alkaline phosphatase levels, x-rays of involved bones, and a bone scan.

Bisphosphonates are prescribed to suppress bone resorption and prevent fractures. These drugs effectively relieve bone pain and often relieve manifestations of the disease for a year or longer. Calcitonin may be ordered for patients who are unable to tolerate bisphosphonates. (See Table 43-2 for the nursing implications of these drugs.) Acetaminophen or NSAIDs may be used to help relieve pain associated with complications such as bone or joint deformities. Some patients may eventually need surgery to repair fractures or replace affected joints (the hip or knee).

NURSING CARE

The nurse's role in Paget disease is primarily educational. Provide verbal and written information about the disorder, stressing that it does not usually spread to uninvolved bones. Teach about prescribed medications, precautions for their safe use, and adverse effects to report to the physician. Advise the patient that effective treatment of the disorder usually relieves associated bone pain. When analgesics are necessary, teach the patient to take NSAIDs on a regular basis to maintain their anti-inflammatory and analgesic effect. Discuss measures to maintain mobility and safety, including use of assistive devices as recommended.

Osteomalacia

Osteomalacia, also known as *adult rickets,* is a metabolic bone disease that affects the structure and integrity of bone.

PATHOPHYSIOLOGY AND MANIFESTATIONS

Osteomalacia results from inadequate mineralization of bone. Calcium and phosphate are the primary minerals in bone. When insufficient amounts of calcium or phosphate are available, the bone does not harden normally and is unable to bear weight. Weight-bearing bones are deformed and pathologic fractures occur. Osteomalacia is commonly caused by a lack of vitamin D. Vitamin D, obtained from certain foods and ultraviolet (UV) radiation from the sun, is necessary to maintain calcium and phosphate levels in the body. Inadequate intake or impaired absorption (e.g., related to gastrectomy) are risk factors for osteomalacia, as are limited sun exposure, and chronic kidney or liver disease. Manifestations of osteomalacia are listed in Box 43-4.

COLLABORATIVE CARE

Bone x-rays and laboratory tests are used to diagnose osteomalacia. X-rays show the effects of bone demineralization. Serum calcium levels may be low or normal; alkaline phosphatase is usually elevated. Treatment focuses on correcting the underlying cause and ensuring adequate vitamin D,

---

BOX 43-4	MANIFESTATIONS OF PAGET DISEASE AND OSTEOMALACIA

Paget Disease
- Bone pain
- Deformity
- Abnormal gait
- Pathologic fractures (upper femur, pelvis)
- Compression fractures
- Kyphosis, loss of height

Osteomalacia
- Bone pain
- Difficulty changing positions (lying to sitting; sitting to standing)
- Muscle weakness
- Waddling gait
- Dorsal kyphosis
- Pathologic fractures

calcium, and phosphate intake. Patients with osteomalacia are usually placed on calcium and vitamin D supplements. Phosphate supplements may also be ordered.

NURSING CARE

Nursing care for patients with osteomalacia is similar to that provided for patients with osteoporosis. Teaching is critical, particularly for older adults who may be at risk for developing osteomalacia due to lack of sun exposure, dietary deficiencies, and impaired intestinal absorption as a consequence of aging. Encourage older adults to take calcium with vitamin D supplements if they are unable to get adequate amounts in the diet or their daily sun exposure is limited. Teach safety measures to prevent falls. Advise patients with bone pain and muscle weakness to use assistive devices such as a walker or cane when ambulating. Encourage patients to participate in a supervised exercise program or to discuss physical therapy with their primary care provider.

Osteomyelitis

Osteomyelitis is an infection of the bone. It is usually caused by *Staphylococcus aureus* bacteria, although other pathogens can also infect the bone. Osteomyelitis can occur at any age but usually affects children under age 12 and adults over age 50. Prosthetic joint implants and devices used to stabilize fractures are increasingly associated with osteomyelitis. Box 43-5■ lists common risk factors for osteomyelitis. The older adult is at risk for several reasons: reduced immune function, chronic diseases, impaired circulation, and a higher risk of pressure ulcers.

PATHOPHYSIOLOGY AND MANIFESTATIONS

Pathogens usually enter the bone through an open wound, such as an open fracture or a gunshot or puncture wound. Bacteria may also spread to the bone from a local tissue infection. After entry, bacteria lodge and multiply in the bone, causing an inflammatory and immune system response. Phagocytes attempt to contain the infection. In the process, they release enzymes that destroy bone

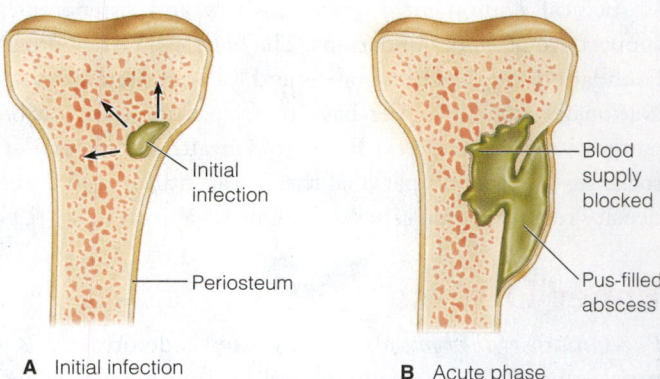

Figure 43-2. ■ Osteomyelitis. **(A)** Bacteria enter and multiply in the bone. **(B)** The infection spreads to other parts of the bone. If the infection reaches the outer part of the bone, the periosteum separates from the surface of the bone.

tissue. Pus forms, followed by edema and vascular congestion. Canals in the marrow cavity of the bone allow the infection to spread to other parts of the bone. If the infection reaches the outer margin of the bone (Figure 43-2■), it raises the periosteum of the bone and spreads along the surface. Pus and edema disrupt the blood supply to the bone, leading to ischemia and, eventually, necrosis of the bone. Blood and antibiotics cannot reach the bone tissue, making it difficult to treat the infection.

The diagnosis of osteomyelitis is often not made until the infection has become chronic. A surgical wound or fracture that does not heal may be the initial sign of infection. Box 43-6■ lists the manifestations of osteomyelitis. The older adult may have less specific symptoms, presenting instead with confusion and vague complaints.

COLLABORATIVE CARE

Early diagnosis and treatment of osteomyelitis with antibiotic therapy is important to prevent bone necrosis.

Diagnostic Tests

■ The *white blood cell (WBC) count* and *erythrocyte sedimentation rate (ESR)* are elevated, nonspecific signs of infection.

BOX 43-5	RISK FACTORS FOR OSTEOMYELITIS

- Open fracture
- Gunshot or deep puncture wound
- Orthopedic surgery
- Soft tissue infection
- Pressure ulcers
- Impaired immune function
- Venous stasis or arterial ulcers of the legs
- Diabetes mellitus

BOX 43-6	MANIFESTATIONS OF OSTEOMYELITIS

- Acute or chronic bone pain of increasing intensity
- Chills and fever
- General malaise, fatigue
- Anorexia, nausea, vomiting
- Swollen, tender regional lymph nodes
- Limited weight bearing in extremity
- Redness, swelling, heat, tenderness over site
- Purulent drainage and ulceration at the site

- *Blood* and *tissue cultures* are obtained to identify the infecting organism.
- *X-rays, MRI, CT scan,* or *ultrasound* are performed to identify the infection site.
- A *bone scan* may be ordered to help identify active infection.

Medications

Antibiotics are initially given intravenously. This may be continued after discharge from the hospital, or an oral antibiotic may be used. Treatment is continued for 4 to 6 weeks.

Surgery

Surgery may be done to obtain a specimen for culture. It may also be done to *debride* the area (remove foreign material and dead or damaged tissue). In surgical debridement, the periosteum is excised and the *cortex* (outer portion of the bone) is drilled to release the pressure from accumulated pus. After irrigation, drainage tubes connected to an irrigation system may be inserted to keep the cavity clean. After surgery, the nurse is responsible for instilling and removing dilute antibiotic solutions through the drainage tubes.

clinicalALERT

Use strict sterile technique when caring for a wound irrigation to prevent additional contamination of the infected bone.

NURSING CARE

PRIORITIZING NURSING CARE

Priority nursing diagnoses for the patient with osteomyelitis focus on preventing further infection, maintaining comfort, and limiting mobility. Because osteomyelitis can be difficult to treat, it is also important to address emotional responses to the disease.

Risk for Infection

Expected outcome: Infection will remain limited to affected bone, with no evidence of extension.

The patient with osteomyelitis is at risk for spread of the infection along the bone as well as superinfection due to compromised immune status.

- Maintain strict hand hygiene practices. *Careful hand hygiene helps prevent spread of infection to vulnerable patients.*
- Use sterile technique when caring for the dressing and irrigation setup. *Using sterile technique during dressing changes and when irrigating the wound significantly reduces the risk for introducing new bacteria to the wound.*

- Assess for manifestations of further infection, including fever, redness, swelling, purulent drainage, and pain. *The patient is at risk for superinfection (infection with organisms that normally do not cause disease) due to compromised immune status.*
- Administer prescribed antibiotics at specified times. *Maintaining optimal blood levels of antibiotic are important to effective treatment of the infection.*
- Maintain optimal calorie and protein intake. *Maintaining the patient's nutritional status is vital to optimal immune function and healing.*

Pain

Expected outcome: Will report pain at a level of 2 or lower on a standard pain scale of 0 to 10.

- Frequently assess pain, using a standard pain scale. Assess effectiveness of prescribed analgesics, reporting pain that is not adequately relieved or that changes in character or location. *Pain unrelieved by previously effective analgesic doses may indicate a complication, such as impaired blood flow and necrosis of bone tissue. Prompt intervention is necessary to preserve the bone and limb.*
- Provide analgesics on a scheduled basis over 24 hours rather than as needed. *Scheduled analgesic doses allow maintenance of constant blood levels.*
- Offer analgesic 20 to 30 minutes before tests, procedures, or exercises. *Premedicating allows time for the medication to take effect before a procedure.*
- Splint or immobilize the affected extremity and handle the affected area gently. *Splinting or immobilizing the involved extremity provides support and reduces pain caused by movement.*
- Use adjunctive strategies (e.g., distraction, relaxation) for pain management. *Muscle or joint pain may be relieved with measures that promote relaxation and vasodilation, such as warm, moist packs or heating pads to the involved extremity.*
- Provide assistive devices (e.g., a splint, walker, or crutches) for ambulation. *Assistive devices help support the involved extremity and reduce weight bearing when ambulating.*

Hyperthermia

Expected outcome: Temperature will remain within the normal range.

- Monitor temperature every 4 hours and during periods of chilling. Report fever to the charge nurse or physician. *A sudden rise in temperature or continued elevation may indicate a lack of response to treatment. Blood cultures may be ordered when an acute temperature elevation occurs.*
- Keep environment cool and provide light clothing and bedding during fever. *A cool environment and light clothing promote comfort when the temperature is elevated.*
- Promote fluid intake of 2,000 to 3,000 mL/day. *The patient with an elevated temperature needs additional fluid to replace losses through perspiration.*

Impaired Physical Mobility

Expected outcome: Will use assistive devices as needed to prevent further injury to affected extremity.

- Keep the affected limb in functional position when immobilized. *Keeping the affected extremity in functional position reduces the risk of contractures.*
- Avoid weight bearing on the affected extremity. *Stress on the weakened bone can lead to pathologic fractures.*
- Assist with active or passive range-of-motion (ROM) exercises every 4 hours. *ROM exercises help maintain normal joint mobility.*

CONTINUITY OF CARE

Reinforce teaching about medications and wound management at home. Emphasize the importance of taking all antibiotics as prescribed. Instruct to use pain medications as needed to prevent pain from becoming severe. Discuss possible drug side effects, and provide information about managing these effects. For example, increase fluid and fiber intake to prevent constipation caused by many analgesics, and consume 8 ounces of live-culture yogurt to help prevent diarrhea and yeast infections (mouth or vagina) often associated with prolonged antibiotic therapy.

Teach wound care as needed. Refer for home health services as appropriate. Provide a list of resources for wound care supplies, such as local medical suppliers. Teach general principles of infection control, including the importance of good hand washing, especially after toileting or contact with wound drainage.

Rest or limited weight bearing is generally ordered for the affected limb. Bed rest is recommended for vertebral osteomyelitis until back pain has eased enough to allow ambulation. Teach how to avoid complications of immobility.

Suggest frequent position changes, keeping skin and linens clean and dry, and active ROM exercises for unaffected joints.

Emphasize the importance of good nutrition. An adequate supply of calories, protein, and other nutrients is necessary for immune function and healing. Suggest frequent small meals and the use of supplements such as Ensure.

Stress the need to keep all follow-up appointments to ensure complete eradication of the infection.

Bone Tumors

Bone tumors (or *neoplasms*) may be either benign or malignant, primary or secondary. Benign bone tumors are more common than malignant and tend to grow slowly. Malignant tumors grow rapidly and metastasize to other tissues. *Primary* bone tumors are rare in adults, occurring more frequently in adolescents. *Metastatic* bone tumors (i.e., seeded from a tumor elsewhere in the body) are more common in adults, often originating from tumors of the prostate, breast, kidney, thyroid, and lung.

PATHOPHYSIOLOGY AND MANIFESTATIONS

Primary bone tumors are classified by the tissue from which they arise: bone (*osteogenic*), cartilage (*chondrogenic*), collagen (*collagenic*), and bone marrow (*myelogenic*) (Table 43-3■).

Primary tumors cause bone breakdown (*osteolysis*), which weakens the bone, resulting in fractures. Malignant bone tumors invade and destroy adjacent bone tissue by producing substances that promote bone resorption or by interfering with a bone's blood supply. Benign bone tumors, unlike malignant ones, have a symmetric, controlled growth pattern. As they grow, they push against neighboring bone tissue. This weakens the bone's structure until it is unable to withstand the stress of ordinary use and frequently causes pathologic fracture.

TABLE 43-3	Primary Bone Tumors		
TUMOR	**TISSUE ORIGIN**	**SITE**	**POPULATION AFFECTED**
Benign bone tumors			
Osteochondroma (most common benign tumor)	Cartilage	On bone surface near growth plate; long bones	Children and adolescents
Enchondroma	Cartilage	Long bones; hands, feet, humerus, femur	Adolescents and young adults
Osteoid osteoma	Bone	Long bones; may also affect hands, fingers, or spine	Children to young adults; 3:1 males to females
Malignant bone tumors			
Osteosarcoma (most common malignant bone tumor, 45% of bone sarcomas)	Bone	Long bones around the knee (distal femur, proximal tibia), other long bones (proximal humerus)	Adolescents and young adults; males more frequently than females
Ewing sarcoma	Bone	Shaft of long bones; flat bones	Adolescents and young adults
Chondrosarcoma (accounts for 20%–25% of sarcomas)	Cartilage	Flat bones (pelvis, scapula), shaft of long bones	Adults and older adults

BOX 43-7	MANIFESTATIONS OF BONE TUMORS

- Deep bone pain; worse at night and at rest
- Redness, warmth, swelling over the affected bone
- Enlarging mass over affected bone
- Muscle weakness or atrophy
- Fever

Bone tumors are usually identified when an injury brings the mass to the patient's attention. Box 43-7■ lists the common manifestations of bone tumors.

COLLABORATIVE CARE

Because symptoms are usually vague, tumor diagnosis may be delayed. Laboratory testing often shows elevated serum alkaline phosphatase and calcium levels, as well as a high red blood cell count. Diagnostic tests to identify the tumor location and extent of bone and surrounding tissue involvement include x-rays, CT scan, and MRI. A biopsy is performed to identify the type of tumor cells.

Malignant bone tumors are treated with a combination of surgery, chemotherapy, and radiation therapy. Whenever possible, surgery is performed to remove the tumor. The tumor itself may be excised, or the affected limb amputated. To avoid amputation, a bone graft or metal prostheses is often used to replace missing bone. Care of the patient undergoing amputation is presented in Chapter 42.

Chemotherapeutic drugs are given to shrink the tumor before surgery, to prevent recurrence after surgery, or to treat tumor metastasis.

Radiation therapy may be used in combination with chemotherapy. After surgery, it is used to eradicate any remaining tumor cells. Radiation therapy is also frequently used to control pain in metastatic bone lesions. Chemotherapy, radiation therapy, and their nursing implications are discussed in Chapter 12.

NURSING CARE

Nursing care needs for the patient with a bone tumor focus on both the physical aspects of care and the psychosocial effects of the diagnosis and its treatment.

PRIORITIZING NURSING CARE

Pain related to the tumor is a priority for nursing interventions.

Acute Pain

Expected outcome: Will report pain at a level of 2 or lower on a standard pain scale of 0 to 10.

- Assess pain, including location, intensity (ask the patient to rate the pain on a standard pain scale), quality or type, aggravating and relieving factors, and duration. *An accurate assessment of pain is necessary to help determine its cause and to evaluate the effectiveness of interventions.*
- Develop strategies for controlling acute pain (from surgery, fracture, or inflammation) and malignant pain (from tumor growth and spread). *Effective pain management is based on the acuity and intensity of the pain.*
- Encourage use of both pharmacologic and nonpharmacologic methods to prevent pain from becoming intense. *Pain relief measures are more effective when used to control pain before it becomes intense.*
- Provide assistive devices (e.g., canes, walkers, crutches) when ambulating. *Assistive devices reduce pain by supporting weight during ambulation.*
- Provide regular rest periods between scheduled treatments. *Rest reduces muscle tension and pain.*

Impaired Physical Mobility

Expected outcome: Will demonstrate correct use of assistive devices and exercises.

- Teach correct use of trapeze. *Using the trapeze helps strengthen the biceps of the arm and allows patients to reposition themselves, get out of bed, and perform other activities.*
- Begin muscle-strengthening and active and passive ROM exercises immediately after surgery. A continuous passive motion (CPM) machine may be used after surgery on an extremity. *Muscle-strengthening and ROM exercises maintain joint function and prevent muscle wasting.*
- Assist the patient who has leg surgery or amputation with exercises to strengthen the triceps muscles of the arms and with quadriceps and gluteal setting exercises and leg raises. *Muscle-strengthening exercises prepare the patient for using assistive devices (e.g., crutches) for ambulation and other activities until a prosthesis is fitted.*
- Refer to physical or occupational therapy for fitting of and teaching about assistive devices such as a cane, crutches, or a walker. *Assistive devices promote mobility and reduce the risk of falling.*

Disturbed Body Image

Expected outcome: Will acknowledge impact of loss on current roles and relationships.

- Listen to and support the patient who is grieving loss of a limb or other changes such as hair loss associated with treatment. *The patient who has lost a body part or experienced a change in body image will go through a grieving process.*
- Allow time for open discussions of feelings about changes in body image and potential changes in social and personal life. *Open and accepting discussion helps the patient work through grieving and begin coping with the changes.*

Grieving

Expected outcome: Will express thoughts, feelings, fears, and spiritual beliefs about loss.

- Listen actively and encourage verbalization of feelings and concerns about the diagnosis and treatment. *Active listening promotes trust and provides an opportunity for the patient and family to work through accepting the diagnosis.*
- Present information in a matter-of-fact manner, taking time to listen to and address concerns. Discuss expected effects and potential side effects of surgery, chemotherapy, and radiation therapy. *Accurate and appropriate information empowers the patient and family to make decisions about treatment.*
- Refer to a counselor, the clergy, or, as appropriate, hospice services. *The patient with a malignant bone tumor faces the very real possibility of dying as a result of the disease, particularly when the tumor is metastatic from another site. Trained professionals can help the patient and family identify and express their feelings and work through the grieving process.*

CONTINUITY OF CARE

Teach about the disease, its potential consequences, and treatment options. Provide information about how to minimize treatment side effects. Depending on the location of the tumor and planned treatment, modifications of the home environment may be necessary. Discuss potential barriers to mobility, such as stairs or lack of access to transportation. Help identify a network of support people who can assist with coping, care, and treatment as needed. If surgery has been performed, teach wound care, demonstrating dressing changes and stump care (if amputation has occurred). Provide a list of local resources for obtaining supplies. Discuss activity and weight-bearing restrictions. Refer to physical therapy for teaching about ambulation and appropriate muscle-strengthening exercises. Ensure that the patient who has experienced an amputation is working with or has a referral to a prosthetic specialist. For the patient with metastatic disease, discuss hospice services and support groups for patients with cancer.

JOINT AND CONNECTIVE TISSUE DISORDERS

> **Key Concept** Arthritis can have many different causes and effects. Nurses focus on educating the patient and family about the disease and its management, promoting mobility, and helping patients adapt to limitations caused by the disorder.

The term **arthritis**, which literally means inflammation of a joint, is often used for any disorder that causes pain and stiffness of the musculoskeletal system. *Rheumatism* is another term used to describe pain in the joints and related tissues. Some arthritic disorders are limited to the joint and surrounding tissues; others are more widespread systemic diseases. Several, such as rheumatoid arthritis and systemic lupus erythematosus, are *connective tissue disorders*.

Connective tissue is the most abundant and widely distributed body tissue. It connects body parts; provides support; forms bones, cartilage, and the walls of blood vessels; and attaches muscles to bones. Connective tissue diseases have diverse manifestations. Arthritic disorders, regardless of their cause, can create problems of mobility, deformity, and disability.

Osteoarthritis

Osteoarthritis (OA) is a degenerative joint disease characterized by progressive loss of joint cartilage in synovial joints. It is the most common type of arthritis and is a leading cause of disability in older adults. It affects men and women equally. Risk factors for OA include age, repetitive joint use or trauma, heredity, obesity, and congenital or acquired defects.

PATHOPHYSIOLOGY

OA affects the entire joint: the cartilage, bone, synovial membrane, and ligaments, muscles, and tendons that surround the joint. The joint cartilage loses its strength and elasticity and is gradually destroyed. As the cartilage erodes and ulcerates, the underlying bone is exposed. The bone thickens in exposed areas, and cysts develop. Cartilage-coated *osteophytes* (bony outgrowths) change the anatomy of the joint. As these spurs or projections enlarge, small pieces may break off, leading to mild inflammation of the joint.

The hips, knees, lumbar and cervical vertebrae, and interphalangeal joints of the fingers, wrist, and big toe joint of the foot are affected most frequently by OA.

MANIFESTATIONS AND COMPLICATIONS

The onset of OA is usually gradual and insidious, and the course is slowly progressive. Localized joint pain (**arthralgia**) is the most common symptom of OA. After periods of immobility (e.g., on awakening in the morning or after an automobile ride), involved joints may stiffen. ROM of the joint decreases as the disease progresses, and grating or crepitus may be noted during movement. Bony overgrowth may cause joint enlargement (Figure 43-3■). Enlarged joints

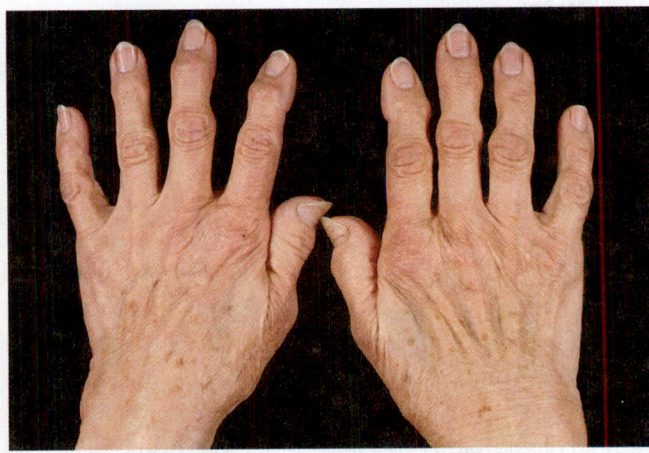

Figure 43-3. ■ Typical changes of osteoarthritis in the interphalangeal joints. (Source: © L. Samsumi/Custom Medical Stock Photo.)

are characteristically bony hard and cool on palpation. The manifestations of OA are listed in Box 43-8■.

OA of the spine may cause disks between the vertebrae to degenerate with narrowing of the joint spaces. Degenerative disk disease may be complicated by a *herniated disk,* protrusion of the *nucleus pulposus* (the internal jellylike mass) of the disk. Herniation can compress nerve roots, causing severe pain and muscle weakness. See Chapter 39 for further discussion of disk disorders. Loss of cartilage between the processes of the vertebrae causes localized pain, stiffness, muscle spasm, and limited ROM. Osteophytes may form on these processes, increasing pain and muscle spasm.

COLLABORATIVE CARE

The diagnosis of OA is based on the history and on physical and x-ray examination of affected joints. Initially, the joint space narrows. As the disease progresses, bone density increases, osteophytes are seen at the joint periphery, and bone cysts may be noted.

Patients with OA are encouraged to lose weight if obese and to remain physically active. Exercise helps maintain muscle tone and joint support and promotes weight loss. Exercise in water (non–weight bearing) may help patients

with OA of the knees or hips. Heat applied locally to affected joints can relieve discomfort. Box 43-9■ provides selected complementary therapies that may be beneficial for patients with OA.

Medications

The pain of OA can often be managed with mild analgesics such as acetaminophen or over-the-counter NSAIDs such as ibuprofen (Motrin) or naprosyn (Aleve). Acetaminophen is preferred for use in older patients because it has fewer toxic side effects. NSAIDs are discussed in more detail in the section of this chapter on rheumatoid arthritis. Nonprescription topical creams, patches, and sprays such as Bengay, Icy Hot, Aspercreme, Sportscreme, and others can provide local pain relief. Capsaicin cream can reduce joint pain and tenderness when applied topically to affected joints such as the knees or hands. Teach patients to avoid getting these products in the eyes, nose, or mouth or applying to any open skin. Instruct the patient to use topical products no more than three or four times a day and to stop using if severe irritation develops.

In some cases, a long-acting corticosteroid mixed with a local anesthetic may be injected directly into the affected joint. Although this procedure relieves pain, it can increase cartilage breakdown if done frequently. For OA of the knee, hyaluronan, a component of synovial fluid, may be injected directly into the knee joint. Although its long-term effects are unknown, this injection may relieve pain and improve function for up to a year.

Surgery

Surgery may be done when pain and limited joint motion interfere with ADLs. *Arthroscopy* may be done for OA of the knee. Using an arthroscope, the joint is inspected, and damaged cartilage and osteophytes can be removed.

BOX 43-8	MANIFESTATIONS OF OSTEOARTHRITIS

- Deep, aching pain in affected joints
- Pain aggravated by use, relieved by rest
- Joint stiffness after periods of immobility
- Limited ROM
- Joint crepitus with movement
- *Heberden nodes* on distal interphalangeal (DIP) joints
- *Bouchard nodes* on proximal interphalangeal (PIP) joints

BOX 43-9	COMPLEMENTARY THERAPIES

Osteoarthritis

Many complementary therapies may help relieve the discomfort of osteoarthritis (OA) and maintain mobility. Refer the patient to a trained practitioner or naturopathic physician. Selected complementary therapies for OA include:

- Acupuncture
- Aromatherapy: massage or compress of cypress or rosemary to affected joints
- Supplements: glucosamine and chondroitin
- Herbs: natural anti-inflammatories such as willow bark
- Magnets over affected joints
- Reflexology
- Therapeutic touch
- Yoga

Nursing care of the patient undergoing arthroscopy is outlined in Table 41-6.

Arthroplasty, reconstruction or replacement of a joint, is often done when the patient has severely restricted mobility and pain at rest. In most cases, both surfaces of the affected joint are replaced with prosthetic parts in a procedure known as a *total joint replacement.* Joints that may be replaced include the hip, knee, shoulder, elbow, ankle, wrist, and joints of the fingers and toes.

In a *total hip replacement,* the joint surfaces of the acetabulum and femoral head are replaced (Figure 43-4A ■). The entire head of the femur and part of the femoral neck are removed and replaced with a prosthesis. In a *total knee replacement* (Figure 43-4B), the femoral side of the joint is replaced with a metallic surface and the tibial side with polyethylene.

Infection is the major complication of total joint replacement surgery. It impairs healing and can lead to failure and removal of the prosthesis. Other potential complications include impaired circulation to the affected limb, thromboembolism, nerve damage, and dislocation of the joint. Box 43-10■ outlines nursing care for the patient undergoing total joint replacement. See Chapter 10 for more information about the patient undergoing surgery.

NURSING CARE

OA frequently complicates pain management and interferes with mobility in both home and institutional settings. It is rarely the primary nursing care problem unless the patient is having joint surgery for the effects of OA.

PRIORITIZING NURSING CARE

Teaching and assisting the patient with OA to manage discomfort and maintain mobility are the priorities for nursing care.

HEALTH PROMOTION

Although OA cannot, at this time, be prevented, discuss the importance of maintaining a normal weight and engaging in regular, daily exercise to reduce the risk of developing it.

ASSESSING

Nursing assessment of the patient with OA focuses on the effects of the disease on daily living activities (functional assessment). Inquire about pain, its timing, location, effect on sleep and rest, and measures used for relief. Ask about limitations in mobility and activities related to stiffness or pain.

Observe the patient's gait, ability to sit and rise from sitting, and performance of activities such as manipulating clothing, performing hygiene and grooming activities, and eating. Assess joints for swelling, tenderness, warmth, and redness. Also assess ROM, noting limitations and the presence of crepitus or complaints of pain with movement.

IDENTIFYING POTENTIAL COMPLICATIONS

The patient with severely limited mobility is at risk for skin breakdown. Carefully assess skin, paying close attention to areas such as the buttocks and sacrum, heels, and bony prominences. Joint contractures are a risk with OA; the patient may often limit joint movement to avoid pain. The hips and knees are often affected, changing the patient's center of balance and gait. Assess for joint contractures by comparing the patient's ROM with the expected ROM of the joint.

The patient who frequently uses aspirin or an NSAID to manage pain is at risk for developing upper GI bleeding. Assess appetite and inquire about nausea. Also assess for abdominal distention, pain, and tenderness, and check feces for evidence of blood. Report manifestations of GI bleeding to the charge nurse or physician.

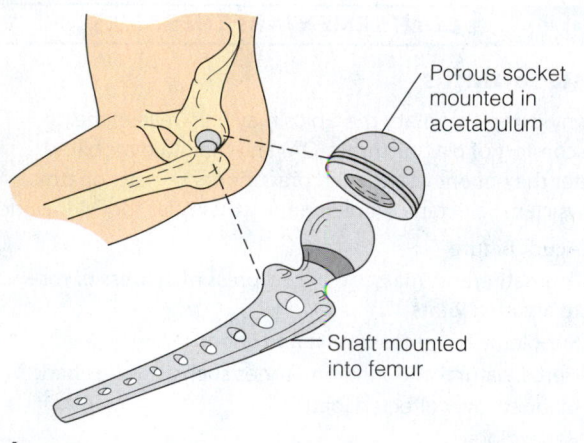

Porous socket mounted in acetabulum

Shaft mounted into femur

A

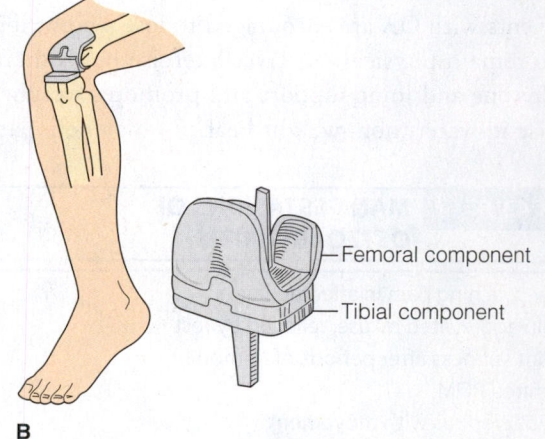

Femoral component

Tibial component

B

Figure 43-4. ■ In a total joint replacement, both surfaces of the affected joint are replaced. (**A**) Total hip replacement. (**B**) Total knee replacement.

BOX 43-10   NURSING CARE CHECKLIST

Total Joint Replacement

Before Surgery

☑ Provide routine preoperative care and teaching.

☑ Reinforce teaching about postoperative activity restrictions and exercises as indicated.

☑ Teach use of overhead trapeze for changing positions.

☑ Teach postoperative pain management, including use of patient-controlled analgesia (PCA) or other anticipated analgesic delivery systems, stressing the importance of reporting unrelieved or increasing pain.

☑ Teach or provide ordered skin preparation such as shower, shampoo, and skin scrub with antibacterial solution.

☑ Administer preoperative medications as ordered.

After Surgery

☑ Provide routine postoperative care.

☑ Monitor vital signs, temperature, pain status, and level of consciousness every 4 hours or more frequently as indicated. Report significant changes to the charge nurse or physician.

☑ Assess neurovascular status (color, temperature, pulses and capillary refill, movement, and sensation) of the affected limb hourly for the first 12 to 24 hours and then every 2 to 4 hours. Report abnormal findings immediately.

☑ Frequently assess for bleeding. Empty and record wound suction drainage every 4 hours. Reinforce the dressing as needed. Report significant bleeding to the charge nurse or physician.

☑ Maintain intravenous infusion as ordered. Monitor intake and output during the initial 24 to 48 hours or more as indicated. Report urine output of less than 30 mL/hr for 2 or more hours.

☑ Maintain extremity position as ordered.

☑ Encourage frequent use of incentive spirometer, deep breathing, and coughing.

☑ Assist out of bed as soon as allowed. Reinforce teaching about weight-bearing restrictions on affected extremity.

☑ Initiate physical therapy and exercises as prescribed.

☑ Use sequential compression devices or antiembolism stockings as ordered.

☑ For total hip replacement, prevent hip flexion greater than 90 degrees and adduction of the affected leg. Provide a seat riser for toilet or commode.

☑ Report signs of hip prosthesis dislocation, including pain or shortening and internal rotation of the affected leg.

☑ For total knee replacement, use a continuous passive range-of-motion (CPM) device or range-of-motion exercises as prescribed.

☑ When CPM is ordered, set prescribed degree of flexion and extension and speed of movement per instructions.

☑ With the machine in extension, pad the CPM with sheepskin before placing the extremity in the CPM. Adjust frame length and foot plate to the extremity; align joints with frame joints.

☑ Disable electric bed controls as indicated to maintain alignment of the extremity with the CPM. Elevate the head of the bed up to 20 degrees if allowed.

☑ Start CPM, observing rate, degree of flexion, and patient responses. Maintain CPM as ordered, frequently assessing comfort, incision, skin condition, and neurovascular status.

☑ Reinforce teaching about postdischarge exercises and activity restrictions. Emphasize the importance of scheduled follow-up physician visits.

☑ For patients requiring additional nursing care and rehabilitation after discharge, assist with transfer to a long-term care or rehabilitation facility. Provide complete and accurate data to nursing staff of the receiving facility.

☑ Make referrals as needed to home health agencies and physical therapy.

DIAGNOSING, PLANNING, AND IMPLEMENTING

Chronic Pain

Expected outcome: Will verbalize and use appropriate ways to manage pain.

■ Administer analgesic or anti-inflammatory medication as needed or on a regular schedule as ordered. *Analgesics reduce the perception of pain; anti-inflammatory drugs reduce local inflammation, swelling, and pain in affected joints.*

■ Teach use of splints or other devices on affected joints as needed. *The pain of OA is often relieved by joint rest.*

■ Apply heat to painful joints using the shower, a tub or sitz bath, warm packs, hot wax dips, heated gloves, or *diathermy,* which uses high-frequency electrical currents to generate heat. *Heat reduces muscle spasm, relieving pain. Moist heat penetrates deeper than dry heat; diathermy delivers heat to deeper body tissues.*

■ Emphasize the importance of proper posture and good body mechanics for walking, sitting, lifting, and moving. *Good body mechanics and posture reduce stress on affected joints.*

■ Encourage the overweight patient to lose weight. *Excess weight places abnormal stress on joints, particularly the knees.*

■ Encourage use of nonpharmacologic measures such as progressive relaxation, meditation, visualization, and distraction. *These adjunctive pain-relief measures can reduce muscle tension and spasm, promoting comfort.*

Impaired Physical Mobility

Expected outcome: Will appropriately use exercise and assistive devices to maintain mobility.

■ Teach active and passive ROM exercises as well as isometric, progressive resistance exercises. *These exercises help maintain muscle tone and strength and mobility of affected joints and prevent contractures.*

- Encourage participation in low-impact aerobic exercises such as water aerobics. *Aerobic exercise improves endurance and cardiovascular fitness.*
- Provide analgesics or other pain-relief measures before exercise or ambulation. *With decreased pain, exercise tolerance improves.*
- Teach good body mechanics and encourage to avoid heavy lifting. *Good body mechanics reduce the stress on joints.*
- Encourage planned rest periods during the day. *Rest reduces fatigue, pain, and joint stress.*
- Teach use of ambulatory aids such as a cane or walker as ordered. *These devices help relieve some weight bearing and stress on affected joints.*

Self-Care Deficit

Expected outcome: Will identify and use techniques and assistive devices to maintain ADLs.

- Assist with ADLs as needed. *OA can significantly interfere with ADLs such as cooking, brushing hair, bathing, and toileting. Minimal assistance can promote self-esteem and as much independence as possible.*
- Refer to an occupational therapist for exercises and assistive devices. *The occupational therapist can identify measures that will help the patient remain independent.*
- Help obtain assistive devices such as long-handled shoehorns, zipper grabbers, long-handled tongs or grippers for retrieving items from the floor (Figure 43-5 ■), jar openers, and special eating utensils. *These devices can promote independence in performing ADLs.*

MANAGING NURSING CARE

In addition to helping the patient with activities of daily living (ADLs; e.g., dressing, toileting, eating), assistive nursing personnel with appropriate education and training may be assigned to provide passive ROM and other exercises as prescribed. Ensure that caregivers understand the importance of gentle handling of affected limbs and never moving joints beyond limits of comfortable movement.

EVALUATING

To evaluate the effectiveness of nursing care, collect data regarding ability to manage pain, maintain mobility, and perform ADLs.

DOCUMENTING

Document assessment data and any changes from baseline assessment. Record level of pain and the effectiveness of analgesic and anti-inflammatory medications to reduce pain. Note mobility and any restrictions or needed accommodations to maintain mobility.

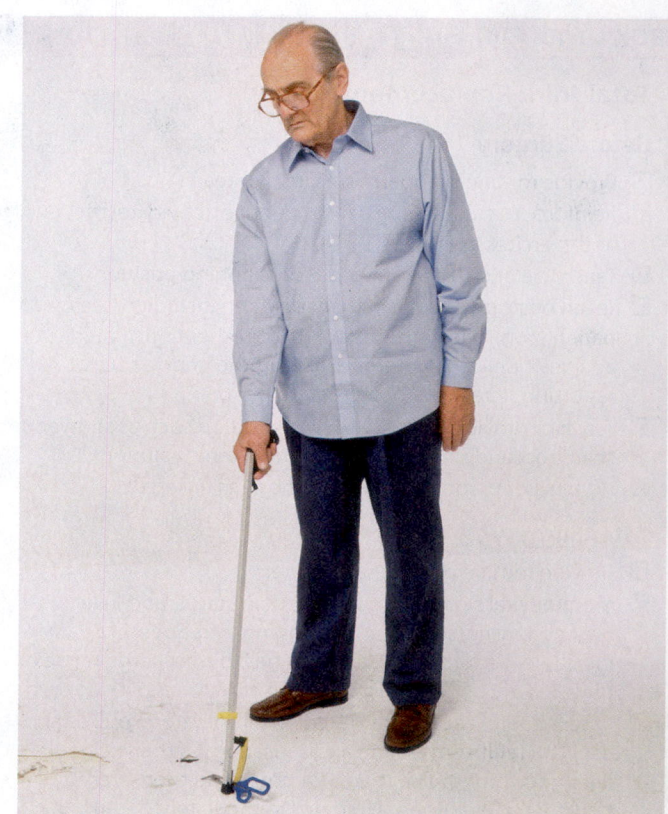

Figure 43-5. ■ An older man with arthritis uses long-handled tongs to pick up an object on the floor. (Source: Dorling Kindersley Media Library.)

CONTINUITY OF CARE

With environmental modifications and assistive devices, the patient with OA can often remain home and independent. Assess the home for hazards to mobility, such as scatter rugs. Identify the need for assistive devices such as handrails, grab bars, walk-in shower stall, or shower chair and handheld shower head. Help obtain and install assistive devices as indicated.

Teach ways to help maintain joint function and mobility:

- Exercise helps maintain joint mobility and develops supportive muscles and tendons. Walking is an effective low-impact, aerobic exercise.
- Do not overuse or stress affected joints.
- Balance exercise with rest of affected joints.
- If obese, lose weight to decrease stress on weight-bearing joints.
- Sit in a straight chair without slumping; avoid soft chairs or recliners.
- Sleep on a firm mattress or use a bed board.

Teach about prescribed or over-the-counter medications for OA. Discuss their use, side effects, and any particular precautions specific to the medication. Also discuss nonpharmacologic pain-relief measures such as heat, rest, massage, relaxation, and meditation.

If arthroplasty has been done, reinforce teaching about activity and weight bearing. Teach use of splints, braces, slings, or other devices to maintain the desired limb position during healing. Discuss assistive devices such as overhead trapeze for getting out of bed, elevated toilet seats, and chairs to use and avoid when sitting. Encourage practice of prescribed exercises. Observe and reinforce teaching as needed for using crutches or a walker.

Discuss possible complications, including signs of infection or dislocation, and instruct to notify the physician promptly if these occur. Refer for home care, physical or occupational therapy, or other community resources as indicated. See the Clinical Reasoning Care Map at the end of this chapter for an opportunity to use the nursing process to plan care for a patient with OA and total hip replacement.

Rheumatoid Arthritis

> **Key Concept** Inflammatory joint disorders such as rheumatoid arthritis are systemic and often chronic, potentially leading to significant disability. Care is multidimensional, involving medications and strategies to promote and maintain optimal function.

Rheumatoid arthritis (RA) is a chronic, systemic inflammatory disorder that primarily affects the joints. It is an autoimmune connective tissue disorder of unknown cause. Genetic factors are known to contribute. RA affects more women than men and usually develops between the ages of 30 and 50 years. Usually, multiple joints are affected. The disease has periods of remission and exacerbation.

PATHOPHYSIOLOGY AND MANIFESTATIONS

In RA, an antigen (e.g., a virus) triggers abnormal immune response. Antibodies produced in this immune response attack antigens in host tissues, including blood, collagen, cartilage, and other proteins and tissues. These autoantibodies, known as *rheumatoid factors (RFs),* bind with tissue antigens to form immune complexes. Complement and other immune factors are activated, prompting an inflammatory response in involved tissues. White blood cells attracted to the area ingest the immune complexes. In the process, they release enzymes that destroy joint tissue.

The resulting inflammation damages the synovial membrane of the joint and affects surrounding tissues. Affected joints are swollen, red, and painful. Joint tissue is destroyed by an extensive network of new blood vessels (vascular tissue known as *pannus*) in the synovial membrane. Pannus erodes the cartilage and bone of affected joints and invades surrounding tissues, including ligaments and tendons (Figure 43-6■).

RA is a systemic disease that affects other tissues as well as joints. Symptoms such as fatigue, anorexia, weight loss, and

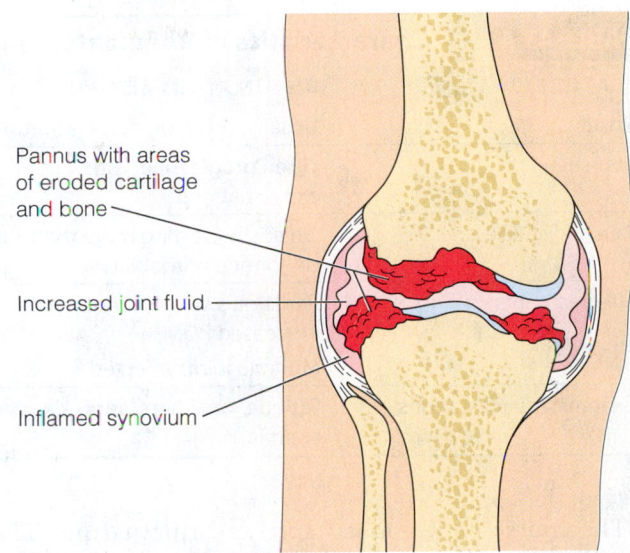

Figure 43-6. ■ Joint inflammation and destruction in rheumatoid arthritis.

Labels: Pannus with areas of eroded cartilage and bone; Increased joint fluid; Inflamed synovium

nonspecific aching and stiffness often occur before typical joint changes are evident. Joint manifestations of RA often develop slowly and insidiously. Joint swelling with stiffness, warmth, tenderness, and pain are typical. The pattern of joint involvement is usually *polyarticular* (involving multiple joints) and *symmetric.* The joint and systemic manifestations of RA are listed in Box 43-11■. Clinical features of RA and OA are compared in Table 43-4■.

BOX 43-11	**MANIFESTATIONS OF RHEUMATOID ARTHRITIS**

Joint
- Swelling, warmth, tenderness, and pain; usually affects PIP and metacarpophalangeal (MCP) joints of fingers, wrists, knees, ankles, and toes
- Limited ROM
- Morning stiffness lasting more than 1 hour
- Joint destruction and deformity (see Figure 43-7):
  - *Swan-neck deformity:* flexion of DIP joint with hyperextension of PIP joint
  - *Boutonniere deformity:* hyperextension of DIP joint with flexion of PIP joint
  - *Ulnar deviation and subluxation* of MCP joints
  - Carpal tunnel syndrome
  - Hallux valgus and hammertoe deformities of the foot

Systemic
- Fatigue, weakness
- Anorexia, weight loss
- Low-grade fever
- Anemia
- *Rheumatoid nodules:* firm subcutaneous tissue nodules over elbow, MCP joints, toes

TABLE 43-4	Characteristics of Rheumatoid Arthritis and Osteoarthritis	
FEATURE	**RHEUMATOID ARTHRITIS**	**OSTEOARTHRITIS**
Onset	Usually insidious, may be abrupt	Insidious
Course	Often progressive, with remissions and exacerbations	Slowly progressive
Pain and stiffness	On arising, lasting more than 1 hour; after prolonged immobility	After activity or periods of immobility; short duration
Affected joints	Red, hot, swollen; tender to palpation; decreased ROM Multiple joints affected	May be swollen; cool and bony hard to palpation; decreased ROM One or several joints affected
Systemic manifestations	Fatigue, weakness, anorexia, weight loss, fever, anemia	Fatigue

The course of RA is variable and fluctuating. The disease progresses more rapidly in its early stages than later. Destruction of affected joints and problems of immobility are the primary complications of RA (Figure 43-7 ■). Patients with severe RA may develop vasculitis (blood vessel inflammation), pleuritis (inflammation of the pleura covering the lungs), or pericarditis (inflammation of the pericardium covering the heart).

COLLABORATIVE CARE

The diagnosis of RA is based on the history, physical exam, and diagnostic tests. There is currently no cure for RA; however, current treatment regimens can often significantly limit joint damage and preserve function. Treatment goals are to relieve symptoms, prevent joint destruction and disability, and improve well-being and function. A multidisciplinary approach is used, with a balance of rest, exercise, physical therapy, and treatments to modify the disease process. For the older adult, less emphasis may be placed on preventing joint deformity and more emphasis on maintaining function.

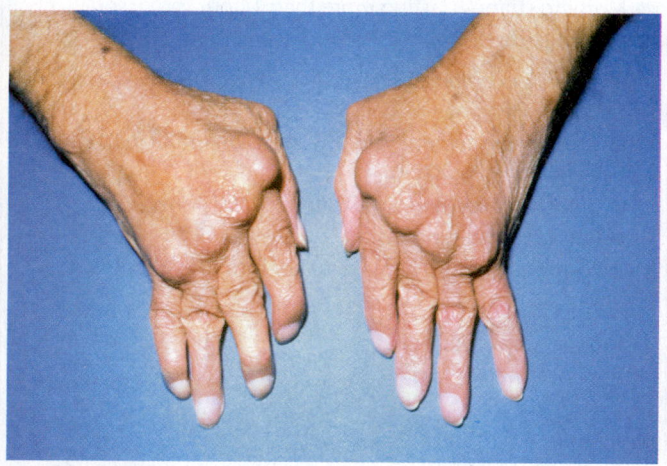

Figure 43-7. ■ Typical hand deformities associated with rheumatoid arthritis. (Source: James Stevenson/Science Source.)

Diagnostic Tests

- *Rheumatoid factors (RFs)* and *anti-CCP antibodies* are present in most people with RA.
- *ESR* is typically elevated, often markedly.
- *Synovial fluid* aspirated from inflamed joints is analyzed.
- *X-ray* of affected joints shows characteristic joint changes as the disease progresses.

Medications

A variety of drugs and drug groups are used to manage RA. Aspirin and other NSAIDs and mild analgesics are used to help manage the signs and symptoms of the disease (see Table 43-5 ■). Because some NSAIDs have been associated with an increased risk for heart attack, they are used with caution.

Low-dose corticosteroids are used to rapidly reduce pain and inflammation. Corticosteroids relieve symptoms and appear to slow the progression of joint destruction. However, when used long-term, corticosteroids have many adverse effects, including an increased risk for infection, poor wound healing, osteoporosis, and gastrointestinal bleeding. See Table 35-3 for nursing responsibilities and patient teaching related to corticosteroid therapy.

A diverse group of drugs called disease-modifying antirheumatic drugs (DMARDs) are used to slow or prevent joint destruction. Although their effects may not be apparent for several weeks or months, these drugs actually reduce disease activity. These drugs include synthetic (or nonbiologic) DMARDs such as methotrexate, sulfasalazine, and antimalarial agents and biologic DMARDs such as anti-tumor necrosis factor-α, abatacept, and rituximab. They may be used individually or in combination. All these drugs are fairly toxic, and close monitoring is necessary during the course of therapy. Treatment with biologic DMARDs suppresses the immune response, increasing the risk for infection and certain cancers. Nursing care and patient teaching related to DMARDs is outlined in Table 43-5; also see Table 11-7 for more information about immunosuppressive drugs.

TABLE 43-5	Giving Medications Safely: Rheumatoid Arthritis		
CLASS/DRUGS	**PURPOSE**	**NURSING IMPLICATIONS**	**PATIENT TEACHING**
Aspirin and nonsteroidal anti-inflammatory drugs (NSAIDs)			
■ Aspirin (Ecotrin, others) ■ *Celecoxib* (Celebrex) ■ *Etodolac* (Lodine) ■ *Ibuprofen* (Motrin, others) ■ *Indomethacin* (Indocin) ■ *Nabumetone* (Relafen) ■ *Naproxen* (Aleve, Anaprox, Naprosyn) ■ *Piroxicam* (Feldene) ■ *Sulindac* (Clinoril) ■ *Tolmetin* (Tolectin) ■ Others	Aspirin and NSAIDs are used to manage arthritis and other causes of inflammation. Although each is different, all inhibit prostaglandin synthesis, reducing inflammation. NSAIDs are more costly than aspirin but may be effective with fewer daily doses than aspirin. For most, adverse effects are similar to aspirin. Although aspirin interferes with blood clotting and may help prevent heart attack or stroke, NSAIDs may increase the risk of heart attack or stroke when used in large doses for a long time.	Obtain baseline weight and vital signs. Assess for contraindications such as allergy or bleeding disorders. Carefully monitor patients who are older or have reduced kidney function for toxicity. Give with food or milk to minimize gastric effects. Report possible adverse effects such as GI bleeding; impaired kidney function; and CNS effects.	Take as ordered to maintain a constant blood level for the best effect. It may take several weeks for the full effect to occur. Take with food or milk. Weigh weekly; report sudden weight gain of more than 3–5 lb to your doctor. Report changes in vision, hearing, mood, or urination; or bloody urine, bloody vomitus, or blood in stool to your doctor. Avoid alcohol while taking NSAIDs. Do not take aspirin while using other NSAIDs. Use acetaminophen as needed for pain relief.
Disease-modifying antirheumatic drugs (DMARDs)			
Nonbiologic DMARDs: ■ *Methotrexate* (Rheumatrex, Trexall) ■ *Hydroxychloroquine* (Plaquenil) ■ Sulfasalazine (Azulfidine) Biologic DMARDs: ■ Abatacept (Orencia) ■ Adalimumab (Humira) ■ Anakinra (Kineret) ■ Etanercept (Enbrel) ■ Infliximab (Remicade) ■ Leflunomide (Arava) ■ Rituximab (Rituxan)	DMARDs reduce joint destruction and slow the progression of RA. These drugs require several weeks or even months of therapy before a response is seen, so are given together with NSAIDs or corticosteroids until their effect is evident. All these drugs suppress the immune response to a certain extent, increasing the risk for infection.	Administer the drug as ordered. Monitor assessment and lab data (CBC, liver function tests, kidney function tests) for evidence of adverse or toxic effects. Promptly report abnormal or unexpected laboratory results or assessment findings. Monitor for signs of infection (e.g., fever, malaise), promptly reporting signs to the care provider. Some of these drugs may cause heart failure; monitor for shortness of breath, dyspnea, dependent edema, neck vein distention, and other signs of heart failure, notifying the physician if noted.	Take the drug exactly as ordered. Several weeks of therapy are necessary before the desired effect is seen; do not stop taking the drug unless directed to do so by your physician. Some of these drugs are given by injection. Report local reactions such as redness or itching to your physician; do not stop taking the drug unless instructed to do so by your doctor. Keep appointments for follow-up, blood tests, and other screening as ordered (e.g., eye examination every 6 months if taking hydroxychloroquine [Plaquenil]). These drugs increase your risk for infection; avoid crowds or people who are ill. Call your doctor if you develop signs of infection, changes in skin color (pallor, jaundice), difficulty breathing, or other unexpected symptoms.

Note: Medications identified in *italics* are among the 200 most frequently prescribed drugs in the United States.

Surgery

Surgery may be done to relieve pain and repair or replace joints damaged by RA. *Arthrodesis* (joint fusion) may be used to stabilize joints such as cervical vertebrae, wrists, and ankles.

Arthroplasty, or total joint replacement, may be necessary in cases of gross deformity and joint destruction. Total joint replacement and nursing care needs of patients undergoing this surgery were discussed in the previous section on osteoarthritis.

Other Therapies

A balanced program of rest and exercise is important to maintain muscle strength and joint mobility for patients with RA. Regular rest periods during the day may be helpful. Dynamic strength training is used to improve muscle strength without increasing joint stress. Low-impact aerobic exercises, such as swimming and walking, are helpful without increasing joint inflammation or prompting acute episodes. A program of 30 minutes of moderately intense activity most days of the week improves both muscle strength and well-being in patients with RA.

Heat and cold are used for their analgesic effects. Moist heat is generally the most effective. Warm tub baths or a shower is often recommended as a way of providing moist heat. Splints and assistive devices such as a cane, walker, or raised toilet seat may be prescribed to provide joint rest.

For most patients with RA, an ordinary, well-balanced diet is recommended. Some patients may benefit from substituting usual dietary fat with omega-3 fatty acids found in certain fish oils.

NURSING CARE

Patients with RA have multiple nursing care needs. In addition to its physical manifestations, the disease has many psychosocial effects. It is a chronic disease that often requires long-term management. Pain and fatigue can interfere with the ability to perform expected roles, such as home maintenance or job responsibilities. Other people may not understand the total body effects of RA or realize that it is different than OA.

PRIORITIZING NURSING CARE

RA is a chronic, systemic disease. Nursing care priorities are on relieving pain and discomfort, managing fatigue, and teaching the patient how to live with the disease.

HEALTH PROMOTION

Although RA cannot be prevented, nurses can promote health by helping the patient prevent disability by becoming an effective self-care manager. Teach patients to respect pain as a warning signal, modifying their activity when it occurs. Refer to physical and occupational therapy for training on use of the strongest muscles and joints for an activity. Use assistive devices to avoid joint stress and activities that require a tight grip (e.g., unscrewing a jar lid, wringing a cloth).

ASSESSING

Assessment of the patient with RA focuses on the progress of the disease and its effect on functional abilities (see Box 43-12). To assess the status of the disease, collect data such as the following:

- Pain level; number of affected joints
- Duration of morning stiffness
- Redness, heat, and swelling of affected joints
- Other symptoms such as fatigue, weakness, anorexia, or fever

IDENTIFYING POTENTIAL COMPLICATIONS

Observe and palpate affected joints for deformity. Many of the drugs used to manage RA have significant adverse effects, requiring observation and monitoring. Ask the patient about sore throat, frequent infection, bleeding gums, easy bruising, black or bloody-appearing stools, and changes in skin color or the color of urine. Monitor appetite, urine, and fecal output. Report abnormal or unexpected laboratory results to the care provider.

DIAGNOSING, PLANNING, AND IMPLEMENTING
Chronic Pain

Expected outcome: Will verbalize an understanding of measures to promote comfort and relieve pain.

The pain of active RA is constant. It affects self-care and daily living activities and contributes to fatigue.

- Encourage to adjust activities according to pain level. *Pain is an indicator of stress on inflamed joints. Increasing pain indicates a need to decrease activity.*
- Teach use of heat or cold for pain relief. A warm shower, tub bath, warm compresses, or paraffin dips can be used to apply heat. If heat increases pain and swelling during periods of acute inflammation, cold packs may be more effective. *Both heat and cold have analgesic effects and can help relieve associated muscle spasms.*
- Discuss the relationship between inflammation and pain and the importance of taking anti-inflammatory medications as ordered. *Anti-inflammatory agents reduce chemical mediators of inflammation and swelling, relieving pain.*
- Encourage use of other nonpharmacologic pain-relief measures such as visualization, distraction, meditation, and progressive relaxation techniques. *These techniques can reduce muscle tension and help the patient focus away from the pain, decreasing the intensity of the pain experience. See Chapter 8 for further discussion of chronic pain management and adjunctive pain-relief measures.*

Fatigue

Expected outcome: Will plan activities to reduce fatigue while maintaining desired roles and responsibilities.

- Encourage a balance of regular physical activity with periods of rest. *Aerobic exercise promotes joint function as well as a sense of well-being and restful sleep. Both joint and whole-body rest are important to reduce the inflammatory response.*

- Assist to prioritize activities, scheduling the most important ones early in the day. *Prioritizing allows the patient to maintain activities that are meaningful and important.*
- Help identify tasks that can be delegated to others. *Enlisting the help of family and friends can help the patient maintain those activities that are important.*

Ineffective Role Performance

Expected outcome: Will verbalize ways to manage life roles and responsibilities within limitations of the disease.

- Discuss effects of the disease on career and other life roles. *Discussion helps the patient accept changes and begin to identify strategies for coping with them.*
- Encourage discussion of feelings about the disease and its effect on patient and family roles. *Open discussion helps family members identify and accept feelings about losses and changes.*
- Listen actively to concerns, acknowledging their validity. *Demonstrating acceptance of these feelings and concerns promotes trust.*
- Help identify strengths to use in coping with role changes. *Past coping strategies and family strengths can be used to deal with necessary role changes.*
- Encourage patient to make decisions and assume personal responsibility for disease management. *Patients who assume an active role in managing their disease maintain a greater sense of self-control and self-esteem.*

Disturbed Body Image

Expected outcome: Will acknowledge actual change in appearance and function.

- Encourage discussion about the effects of RA, both physical and psychosocial. *Verbalization helps the patient identify feelings and provides an opportunity to validate these feelings.*
- Involve patient in decision making and provide choices whenever possible. *Autonomy enhances the sense of control.*
- Discuss clothing and adaptive devices that promote independence. *Independence enhances self-esteem.*
- Provide positive feedback for self-care activities and adaptive strategies. *Positive reinforcement encourages the patient to continue adaptive measures and maintain independence.*
- Refer to self-help groups, counseling and support groups, the Arthritis Foundation, and other agencies for support, assistive devices, and literature. *These groups can help the patient develop strategies to cope with the effects of RA, enhancing self-concept, body image, and independence.*

MANAGING NURSING CARE

When assigning assistive personnel to provide or assist with care for patients with RA, ensure that assigned personnel have an understanding of the systemic nature of the disease and its manifestations, as well as the importance of protecting acutely inflamed joints.

EVALUATING

To evaluate the effectiveness of nursing care for a patient with RA, collect data such as quality and quantity of rest; effective use of NSAIDs and analgesics; ability to maintain ADLs and usual roles; statements about body image and coping with disease effects.

DOCUMENTING

Document continuing assessment data, including the appearance, swelling, and movement of inflamed joints. Record fatigue level and the ability of the patient to perform ADLs. Document all teaching provided and the patient's and family's understanding and acceptance of information. Note specific instructions for medication use, recommended activity, and measures to rest inflamed joints.

CONTINUITY OF CARE

The patient has the primary responsibility for managing RA. Assessment and teaching are vital to prepare for this responsibility. Box 43-12■ outlines assessment data to collect related to home care.

Teach about the disease and its systemic effects. Stress the importance of following all aspects of the treatment plan. Encourage active involvement in planning care.

Help identify strategies to balance rest and exercise. Instruct to reduce exercise and increase rest if pain and stiffness increase. Teach to use heat and cold to promote comfort and activity.

safety**ALERT**

Remember that the patient with RA is vulnerable to quackery and unproven alternative treatment strategies. Maintain open lines of communication to encourage discussion of these options and possible experimental therapies with the treatment team.

BOX 43-12	**ASSESSMENT**

Assessing for Home Care: Patient With Rheumatoid Arthritis

- Ability to perform ADLs; need for help or assistive devices; ability to cope with activity limitations and economic effects; acceptance of assistance from others
- Understanding of RA and its effects; prescribed medications; activity and rest recommendations; long-term management
- Home environment: stairs, environmental barriers that limit independence (e.g., small bathrooms, deep tubs for bathing); energy-saving features (e.g., easily loaded clothes washer and dryer, easy-to-clean floors)

Family and Caregivers
- Ability and willingness to assist with ADLs and household tasks; acceptance of rest needs and altered roles and relationships
- Financial resources for prescribed drugs and treatments

Teach about prescribed medications. Emphasize the need to take NSAIDs as ordered, not on an as-needed basis for pain. Discuss potential adverse effects of DMARDs and their management. Review Table 43-5 for patient and family teaching about medications. Emphasize the importance of keeping regular follow-up appointments to monitor the disease and treatment.

Suggest assistive devices to maintain independence. Include ambulatory aids, such as canes and walkers, and self-care aids, such as handheld showers, long-handled brushes and shoe horns, and eating utensils with oversized or special handles. Discuss clothing options to help maintain independence, such as elastic waist pants without zippers, Velcro closures, zippers with large pull tabs, and slip-on shoes. Refer to local and community agencies as indicated.

NURSING CARE PLAN
Patient With Rheumatoid Arthritis

Janice James, 42 years old, first noticed vague joint pain, fatigue, poor appetite, and general malaise about 6 weeks ago. Her symptoms have continued, and she reports feeling very stiff in the mornings, often lasting until 10:00 or 11:00 a.m. She sees her nurse practitioner (NP) when she notices that her knuckles and finger joints are not just achy but also swollen and hot. The NP tentatively diagnoses RA and refers Mrs. James to a rheumatology clinic.

Assessment
Mrs. James's past medical history reveals only the usual childhood diseases and three uncomplicated pregnancies and deliveries. Mrs. James states that she is allergic to penicillin.

Objective assessment data reveals swelling of PIP and MCP joints of both hands. The second and third PIP and second MCP joints on the right hand appear red and shiny and are hot, spongy, and tender to palpation. Mrs. James can extend her fingers to 180 degrees but cannot make a complete fist with either hand. Her grip strength is weak bilaterally. Wrist ROM is limited in all directions. Mrs. James's knees also appear swollen, and flexion is slightly limited.

Blood work shows ESR 52 mm/hr and hematocrit 30%. She has a positive RF and anti-CCP test.

Nursing Diagnosis
The following nursing diagnoses are identified for Mrs. James:

- *Pain* related to joint inflammation
- *Impaired Home Maintenance* related to fatigue
- *Activity Intolerance* related to the effects of inflammation
- *Readiness for Enhanced Self-Health Management* related to therapeutic regimen

Expected Outcomes
The expected outcomes are that Mrs. James will:

- Verbalize effective pain-management strategies.
- Verbalize a plan to reduce her responsibilities for home maintenance.
- Express a willingness to plan rest breaks during the day.
- Demonstrate understanding of the prescribed treatment and the importance of compliance for both short- and long-term benefit.

Planning and Implementation
The following nursing interventions are implemented over the first 6 weeks of Mrs. James's care at the rheumatology clinic:

- Teach ways to relieve pain and morning stiffness, including:
  a. Take NSAIDs at equal intervals throughout the day.
  b. Take morning NSAID dose with milk and crackers about 30 minutes before arising.
  c. Perform ROM exercises in shower or bathtub.
- Teach ways to minimize joint stress while performing ADLs.
- Discuss delegation of household tasks to other family members.
- Explore ways to incorporate 30-minute rest breaks into work schedule.
- Reinforce teaching about disease process, prescribed drugs and their effects, and the importance of balanced rest and exercise.

Evaluation
After 6 months, Mrs. James's "morning sickness" now lasts about 45 minutes, and her hand and wrist ROM have improved. She has had difficulty scheduling rest periods at work and has had to struggle to delegate household tasks. "I don't look sick to the kids, and they seem to think housecleaning is a terrible imposition on their time. It's often easier to just do it myself than to fight about it. Besides, that way it gets done right." Mrs. James has faithfully followed her treatment plan, keeping her scheduled appointments and maintaining contact with the treatment team.

Critical Thinking in the Nursing Process

1. Explain the normal inflammatory process and relate this to the inflammatory joint changes Mrs. James experienced. Discuss the systemic effects of inflammation on Mrs. James as well.
2. When Mrs. James experiences an acute exacerbation of her disease 1 year later, the rheumatologist orders prednisone, 40 mg daily. The effect is dramatic in

relieving Mrs. James's pain and stiffness. She asks why the physician did not prescribe this drug in the first place. How will you respond?

3. After Mrs. James's acute exacerbation, the rheumatologist prescribes methotrexate. What short- and long-term adverse effects of this drug will you teach Mrs. James about?

Note: Discussion of Critical Thinking questions appears on the companion website.

Systemic Lupus Erythematosus

Systemic lupus erythematosus (SLE) is a chronic inflammatory connective tissue disease. It affects multiple body systems. It is usually a mild and episodic condition; in some patients, however, it is a rapidly fatal disease.

SLE is much more common in women than in men. It is more common and severe in people of African ancestry, and is more common in Asians and Hispanics than it is in Caucasians. Its cause is unknown, but genetic, environmental, and hormonal factors play a role in its development.

PATHOPHYSIOLOGY

In SLE, autoantibodies are produced that target normal body cells and cell components such as DNA, blood cells, and proteins involved in normal coagulation. These autoantibodies react with their antigens to form immune complexes. These complexes are then deposited in the connective tissue of blood vessels, lymphatic vessels, and other tissues. This causes an inflammatory response that damages the tissues. Immune complexes are frequently deposited in and damage the kidneys. Other affected tissues include the musculoskeletal system, brain, heart, spleen, lung, GI tract, skin, and peritoneum.

MANIFESTATIONS AND COMPLICATIONS

Early in the disease, the manifestations of SLE mimic those of RA, including fever, anorexia, malaise, weight loss, and joint pain, inflammation, and stiffness. Skin manifestations are common. SLE was named for its characteristic red *butterfly rash* across the cheeks and bridge of the nose (Figure 43-8■). This rash was thought to resemble the bite of a wolf, hence *lupus* (wolf) *erythematosus* (red). Many patients with SLE are photosensitive. A diffuse rash on skin exposed to the sun is common. Because SLE affects many body systems, its manifestations can be diverse (Figure 43-9■).

The course of SLE is mild and chronic in most patients, with periods of remission and exacerbation. The number and severity of exacerbations tend to decrease with time.

Patients with SLE may have difficulty carrying a pregnancy to term. They also have an increased risk for infections, which may be severe. Infections such as pneumonia and septicemia are the leading cause of death in patients

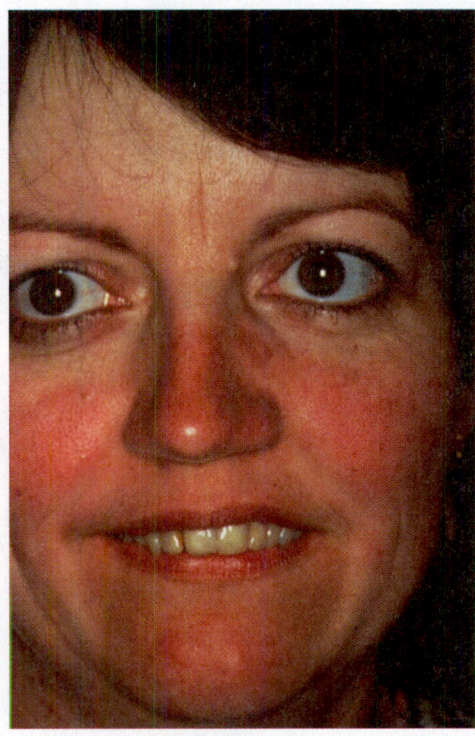

Figure 43-8. ■ The butterfly rash of systemic lupus erythematosus. (Source: Pearson Education.)

with SLE, followed by the effects of kidney or central nervous system involvement.

COLLABORATIVE CARE

The diagnosis of SLE is based on the history and physical exam, along with diagnostic tests. As with RA, effective management requires teamwork, with active participation by the patient and the multidisciplinary health care team.

Diagnostic Tests

- Testing for autoantibodies is done. *Antinuclear* and *anti-DNA antibody testing* are relatively specific indicators but may not be positive in some patients with SLE.
- *C-reactive protein (CRP)* levels are elevated during acute exacerbations.
- The *ESR* is often elevated, and the complete blood count (CBC) shows anemia and low RBC, WBC, and platelet counts.
- *Urinalysis* and renal function studies such as the *serum creatinine* and *blood urea nitrogen (BUN)* may be ordered to assess for kidney damage.

Medications

Acetaminophen, aspirin, and NSAIDs are often used to manage joint pain and inflammation, fever, and fatigue. Table 43-5 outlines nursing responsibilities for aspirin and NSAIDs. The antiplatelet actions of aspirin make it particularly useful for patients with SLE, because it also helps prevent thrombosis. NSAIDs may increase the risk for

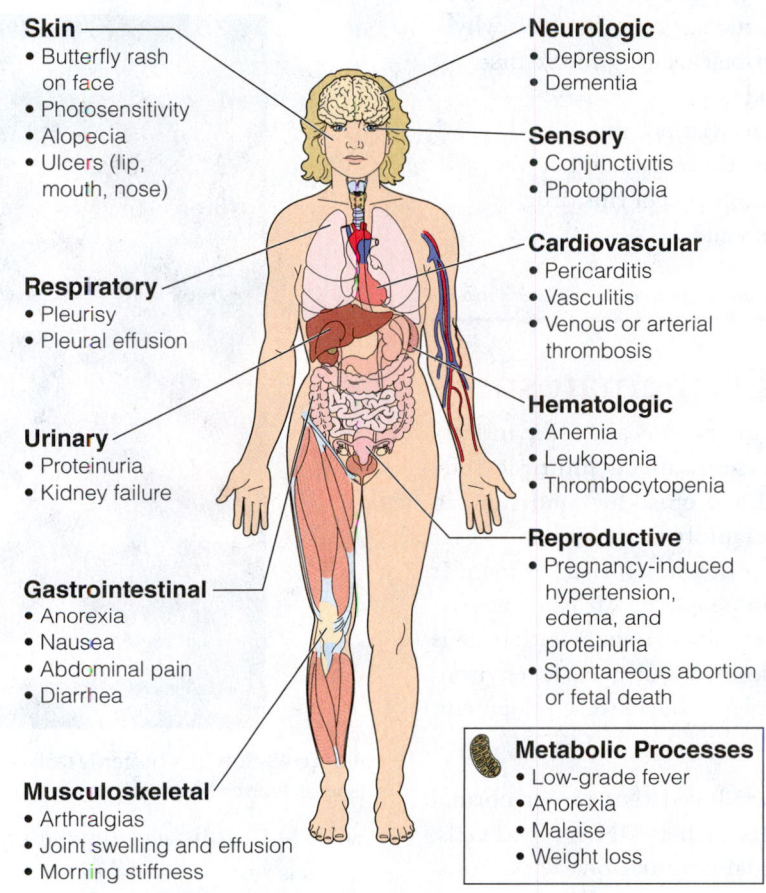

Skin
- Butterfly rash on face
- Photosensitivity
- Alopecia
- Ulcers (lip, mouth, nose)

Respiratory
- Pleurisy
- Pleural effusion

Urinary
- Proteinuria
- Kidney failure

Gastrointestinal
- Anorexia
- Nausea
- Abdominal pain
- Diarrhea

Musculoskeletal
- Arthralgias
- Joint swelling and effusion
- Morning stiffness

Neurologic
- Depression
- Dementia

Sensory
- Conjunctivitis
- Photophobia

Cardiovascular
- Pericarditis
- Vasculitis
- Venous or arterial thrombosis

Hematologic
- Anemia
- Leukopenia
- Thrombocytopenia

Reproductive
- Pregnancy-induced hypertension, edema, and proteinuria
- Spontaneous abortion or fetal death

Metabolic Processes
- Low-grade fever
- Anorexia
- Malaise
- Weight loss

Figure 43-9. ■ The multisystem effects of systemic lupus erythematosus.

kidney injury, so they are used with caution. Antimalarial drugs such as hydroxychloroquine (Plaquenil) may be ordered. Hydroxychloroquine can damage the retina of the eye; for this reason, an ophthalmologic exam is done every 6 months during treatment.

Corticosteroid drugs are used to treat severe and life-threatening manifestations of SLE. Some patients require long-term corticosteroid therapy to manage symptoms and prevent major organ damage. These patients have a high risk for corticosteroid side effects, such as cushingoid effects, weight gain, hypertension, infection, accelerated osteoporosis, and hypokalemia. Immunosuppressive agents may be used alone or in combination with corticosteroids. These drugs increase the risk for infection and malignancy and have other toxic effects.

Other Therapies

Because of photosensitivity associated with SLE, sun exposure should be avoided. Sunscreens with a sun protection factor (SPF) rating of 15 or higher are recommended when out of doors. Some physicians recommend avoiding oral contraceptives, because estrogen can trigger an acute episode of SLE.

Patients with lupus nephritis who develop end-stage kidney disease are treated with dialysis (hemodialysis or peritoneal dialysis) and kidney transplantation. These treatment strategies are discussed in Chapter 29.

NURSING CARE

Many of the nursing care needs and priorities for the patient with SLE are similar to those for patients with RA. This section focuses on the needs related to dermatologic symptoms of lupus, the increased risk for infection, and health maintenance problems.

Impaired Skin Integrity

Expected outcome: Will demonstrate an understanding of optimal skin and wound care.

Skin lesions are a common manifestation of SLE. They disrupt skin integrity and can be disfiguring.

■ Discuss the relationship between sun exposure and disease activity, both dermatologic and systemic. *It is important for the patient to understand that sun exposure can worsen both skin and systemic manifestations of SLE.*

- Help identify strategies to limit sun exposure:
  a. Avoid being outside when sun is most intense (10:00 a.m. to 3:00 p.m.).
  b. Use an adequate amount of sunscreen with an SPF of 15 or higher.
  c. Reapply sunscreen after swimming, exercising, or bathing.
  d. Wear loose clothing with long sleeves and wide-brimmed hats when outside.

  These strategies can help the patient maintain a normal lifestyle while helping to prevent acute episodes.
- Keep skin clean and dry; apply therapeutic creams or ointments to lesions as ordered. *These measures promote healing and reduce the risk of infection.*

Risk for Infection

Expected outcome: Will remain free of infection.

- Wash hands on entering room and before providing direct care. *Hand washing is the best defense against transmitting infection.*
- Use strict sterile technique in caring for intravenous lines and indwelling urinary catheters or performing any wound care. *Aseptic technique reduces the risk of contamination by microorganisms.*
- Monitor temperature and vital signs every 4 hours. Report signs of infection, including tenderness, redness, swelling, and warmth. *Prompt identification of an infection allows early initiation of appropriate treatment.*
- Report abnormal laboratory values. *Increased WBCs may indicate infection; changes in liver or renal function studies, myocardial enzymes, or other laboratory values may indicate organ system involvement.*
- If necessary, use protective isolation. *Treatment with corticosteroids or immunosuppressive agents impairs the ability to fight infection. Protective isolation may be necessary to prevent infection.*
- Instruct family members and visitors to avoid direct contact with the patient when they are ill. *A "minor" upper respiratory infection can be a significant illness for the patient with SLE.*
- Help ensure adequate food intake, offering supplementary feedings as indicated or maintaining parenteral nutrition if necessary. *Adequate nutrition is important for healing and immune system function.*
- Teach the importance of good hand washing after using the bathroom and before eating. *Hand washing reduces the risk of infection with endogenous organisms.*
- Provide good mouth care. *Good oral hygiene reduces the risk of infection from oral bacteria.*

CONTINUITY OF CARE

Teach about SLE and its potential effects. Both physical manifestations of SLE and psychosocial issues can affect the ability to effectively manage the disease. Encourage discussion about the impact of the disease. Refer the patient and family to counseling as needed. Provide information about community and social service agencies and local support groups.

Discuss the importance of skin care. Instruct to avoid irritating soaps, shampoos, or chemicals (e.g., hair dyes and permanent wave solution) to prevent excessive drying of the skin. Encourage use of hypoallergenic products. Stress the importance of limiting sun exposure, use of appropriate sunscreen, and wearing protective clothing. For patients with hair loss, discuss using wigs, turbans, or other head coverings. Remind that the hair will regrow during remission.

Stress the importance of avoiding exposure to infection. Encourage to avoid crowds and infectious people. Teach the importance of adequate rest and nutrition and avoiding stress to increase resistance to infection.

Teach about treatment plan, including rest and exercise, medications, and follow-up appointments. Stress the importance of contacting the physician promptly if symptoms of an exacerbation develop. Encourage to wear a MedicAlert bracelet or tag with their condition and therapy such as corticosteroids or immunosuppressive drugs.

Discuss family planning. Oral contraceptives may be contraindicated; provide information about alternative means of birth control. Pregnancy is not contraindicated; however, the patient should tell her women's health care practitioner about her SLE and notify her primary care physician of her pregnancy.

Gout

> **Key Concept** Gout is an inflammatory arthritis caused by excess uric acid in the body. Treatment focuses on reducing uric acid levels to prevent acute attacks and potential long-term effects.

Gout is a metabolic disorder that causes urate crystals to accumulate in joints and surrounding tissues. It affects more men than women, and its incidence increases with age.

Gout is characterized by episodes of acute inflammatory arthritis triggered by crystallization of urate within the joints. It develops in response to an excess of uric acid in the body, with high uric acid levels in the blood (hyperuricemia) and urate crystals in synovial fluid and other tissues.

PATHOPHYSIOLOGY AND MANIFESTATIONS

Uric acid is the breakdown product of purine metabolism. Normally, uric acid production and excretion are balanced, with most of what is produced each day excreted via the kidneys and the rest in the feces. The serum uric acid level is normally between 3.5 and 8.0 mg/dL in men and 2.8 and

6.8 mg/dL in women. At levels greater than 8.0 mg/dL, urate crystals may form. Crystals tend to form in peripheral tissues of the body, where lower temperatures increase the risk of crystal formation.

Acute gouty arthritis typically occurs abruptly, usually at night, and often involves the first metatarsophalangeal joint (great toe). The affected joint becomes red, hot, swollen, and exquisitely painful and tender. The patient may also have fever, chills, and general malaise.

Acute attacks last from days up to several weeks and typically subside spontaneously. The initial acute attack is usually followed by a period of months or years without manifestations. As the disease progresses, urates are deposited in various other connective tissues. Urate deposits in subcutaneous tissues cause the formation of small white nodules called **tophi**. Deposits of crystals in the kidneys can form urate kidney stones and result in kidney failure.

COLLABORATIVE CARE

The classic presentation of acute gout is so distinctive that the diagnosis is often based on the history and physical exam. *Serum uric acid* is nearly always elevated, usually above 8.5 mg/dL. Fluid aspirated from the inflamed joint shows typical needle-shaped urate crystals.

Treatment focuses on relieving an acute attack and preventing recurrent attacks.

Medications

NSAIDs are used to treat an acute attack of gout. Indomethacin (Indocin) is the most frequently used NSAID for gout. Aspirin is avoided because it may interfere with uric acid excretion. Review Table 43-5 for nursing implications for NSAIDs.

Colchicine, a drug that inhibits the deposition of urate crystals in tissues, may also be ordered to stop an acute attack. The use of colchicine, however, is limited by side effects such as abdominal cramping, diarrhea, nausea, or vomiting. Colchicine may be used in smaller doses (with fewer side effects) to prevent attacks of gout.

Drugs to promote uric acid excretion or block its production may be ordered to prevent attacks. *Uricosuric* drugs block reabsorption of uric acid in the kidney tubules, promoting its excretion and reducing serum levels. Allopurinol affects purine metabolism, decreasing the production of uric acid (see Table 43-6■).

TABLE 43-6	**Giving Medications Safely: Gout**		
CLASS/DRUGS	**PURPOSE**	**NURSING IMPLICATIONS**	**PATIENT TEACHING**
■ Colchicine	Colchicine prevents urate crystals from being deposited in tissues. It does not lower serum uric acid levels. It is available in combination with a uricosuric agent, probenecid. Plain colchicine is used to treat an acute attack of gout; combination therapy is used to prevent further attacks.	Assess for contraindications, such as serious GI, kidney, liver, or heart disease. Administer by mouth on an empty stomach. Report nausea, vomiting, or diarrhea to the physician; these side effects may require stopping the drug.	Drink 3–4 quarts of liquid per day. Report reactions such as GI distress, fatigue, bleeding, easy bruising, or recurrent infections to your doctor. Avoid using alcohol while you are taking this drug.
Xanthine oxidase inhibitors ■ Allopurinol (Zyloprim) ■ Febuxostat (Uloric)	Xanthine oxidase inhibitors reduce uric acid production, lowering serum uric acid levels. They are used for patients with manifestations of gout, including acute attacks, tophi, and kidney stones.	Monitor intake and output. Increase fluids to 3 L/day. Report adverse effects such as nausea, diarrhea, and rash. Give with meals. Report abnormal kidney and liver function tests, CBC, and prothrombin time or international normalized ratio to the physician. Discontinue drug and notify the physician immediately if a rash or fever develops.	Stop the drug and report skin rash, painful urination, bloody urine, eye irritation, or swelling of lips or mouth to your doctor. Take after meals. Drink 3–4 quarts of fluid daily. Report abnormal bleeding, bruising, fatigue, pallor, sore throat, or frequent infections to your doctor. Acute gout may occur when you start this drug; continue drug as ordered. Do not take a double dose if you miss a dose. Use caution when driving, operating machinery, or performing other activities that require alertness; may cause drowsiness.

(continued)

TABLE 43-6	Giving Medications Safely: Gout *(continued)*		
CLASS/DRUGS	**PURPOSE**	**NURSING IMPLICATIONS**	**PATIENT TEACHING**
Uricosuric drugs ■ Probenecid (Benemid)	Probenecid inhibits the tubular reabsorption of urate, increasing the excretion of uric acid and decreasing serum uric acid levels.	Give after meals or with milk. Monitor intake and output. Increase fluid intake to at least 3 L/day. Report adverse effects such as headache, dizziness, nausea and vomiting, flank pain, fever, hives, pruritus, and abnormal lab values.	Do not take aspirin or products containing aspirin while taking probenecid. Use acetaminophen for relief of mild pain. Drink at least 3 quarts of fluids per day.
■ Sulfinpyrazone (Anturane)	Sulfinpyrazone improves uric acid excretion, reducing serum uric acid levels. It is used to prevent recurrent attacks of acute gout and treat chronic gout.	Give with meals or antacid. Monitor diabetic patients for hypoglycemia. Monitor for bleeding in patients receiving warfarin. Encourage fluid intake of at least 3 L/day. Do not give concurrently with aspirin. Report signs of peptic ulcer disease to the physician promptly.	Drink at least 3 quarts of fluid per day. Take with meals to minimize gastric distress. Do not take aspirin; use acetaminophen for relief of mild pain. Report epigastric pain, nausea, or black stools to the physician promptly. Discontinue the drug immediately.

Note: Medications identified in *italics* are among the 200 most frequently prescribed drugs in the United States.

Other Therapies

During an acute attack of gout, rest of the affected joint is ordered. The affected joint may be elevated, and hot or cold compresses may be applied for comfort, although often the patient is unable to tolerate any pressure on the joint.

A liberal fluid intake (3 or more L per day) is ordered.

Patients with gout are advised to limit their intake of purine-rich foods such as organ meats and certain seafoods (e.g., sardines and shellfish), drinks sweetened with high-fructose corn syrup, and alcohol. Intake of low-fat or nonfat dairy products and vegetables, including purine-rich vegetables such as spinach, asparagus, cauliflower, and mushrooms, is encouraged. The obese patient is advised to lose weight, but fasting is contraindicated. Alcohol intake and specific foods that tend to precipitate attacks are avoided.

NURSING CARE

PRIORITIZING NURSING CARE

Pain is a primary focus for nursing assessment and interventions during an acute attack of gout.

Acute Pain

Expected outcome: Will report pain at a level of 2 or lower on a standard scale of 0 to 10.

- Ask the patient to rate pain using a standard pain scale. Note the location and quality of the pain. *Acute gout causes exquisite tenderness of the affected joint. Accurate assessment of pain facilitates evaluation of treatment measures.*
- Position for comfort. Elevate the joint or extremity (usually the great toe) on a pillow, maintaining alignment. *Elevating the joint improves blood return, relieving some of the edema.*
- Protect the affected joint from pressure, using a foot cradle to keep covers off the foot. *Affected joints are so tender that even the weight of a sheet can be unbearable.*
- Administer prescribed anti-inflammatory and antigout medications as ordered. In the initial period, colchicine may be given hourly. *These medications reduce the acute inflammatory response, gradually relieving discomfort.*
- Administer analgesics as prescribed. *Analgesics are often ordered until the acute inflammation is relieved.*
- Monitor for desired and adverse effects of medications. Report adverse effects to the physician. *Anti-inflammatory and antigout medications can have significant side effects that may require a change of therapy.*
- Maintain joint rest. *Rest and immobilizing the affected joint help reduce joint inflammation.*

CONTINUITY OF CARE

Without appropriate treatment between episodes of acute gout, recurrences are likely. Teaching is a vital nursing responsibility for the patient with gout.

Teach about the disease and its manifestations. Advise that initial attacks cause no permanent damage, but recurrent attacks can lead to permanent damage and joint destruction. Discuss other potential effects of continued hyperuricemia, including tophaceous deposits in subcutaneous and other connective tissues. Discuss the risk for kidney damage and stones.

Teach about prescribed medications. Stress the need to continue medications until discontinued by the physician, even if there are no symptoms. Discuss potential side effects of the drugs and their management. Instruct to drink about 3 quarts of fluid per day and to avoid using alcohol. Instruct to avoid over-the-counter medications without talking to the physician. Encourage to keep scheduled follow-up appointments.

Lyme Disease

Lyme disease is an inflammatory disorder caused by a spirochete, *Borrelia burgdorferi,* which is usually spread by ticks. It is the most commonly reported tick-borne illness in the United States. Although Lyme disease is usually seen in children, adults can also be affected. Geographically, Lyme disease is more common in the Northeast, upper Midwest, and along the Pacific Coast. Ticks that act as vectors for Lyme disease are usually carried by mice or deer. The usual time of onset is the summer months.

PATHOPHYSIOLOGY AND MANIFESTATIONS

Borrelia burgdorferi enters the skin at the site of the tick bite. After an incubation period of up to 30 days, it migrates outward in the skin, forming a characteristic lesion called *erythema migrans.* It may spread via lymph or blood to other skin sites, nodes, or organs.

Erythema migrans is the initial manifestation of Lyme disease (Figure 43-10■). This flat or slightly raised red lesion at the site of the tick bite expands over several days (up to a diameter of 50 cm), with the central area clearing as it expands. Systemic symptoms such as fatigue, malaise, fever, chills, and muscle pain often accompany the initial lesion. As the disease spreads, secondary skin lesions develop, as do migratory musculoskeletal symptoms, including muscle and joint pain, and tendonitis. Headache and stiff neck are common. If untreated, the patient may develop chronic arthritis, myocarditis, meningitis, encephalitis, and other neurologic manifestations.

COLLABORATIVE CARE

A number of antibiotics may be used to treat Lyme disease. Treatment may be continued for up to 1 month to ensure that the organism has been eradicated. Aspirin or another NSAID may be prescribed to relieve arthritic symptoms. The affected joint may be splinted to rest the joint. When the knee is involved, weight bearing may be restricted and the patient instructed to use crutches.

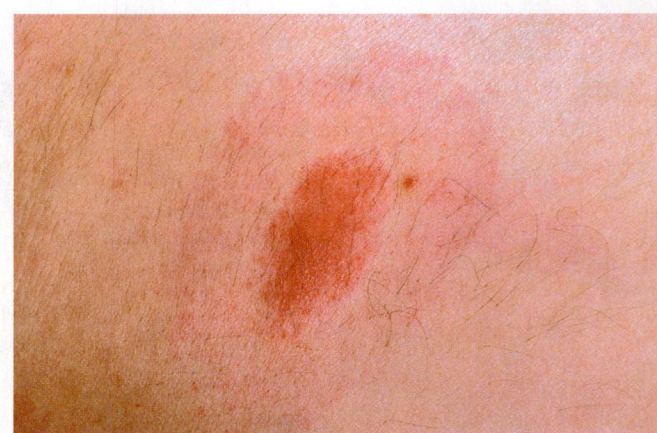

Figure 43-10. ■ Erythema migrans, the lesion characteristic of early Lyme disease. (Source: E.R. Degginger / Science Source.)

NURSING CARE

The nursing role in treating Lyme disease is primarily educational. Teach about the disease and its transmission. Emphasize the importance of completing the full course of antibiotic therapy. Discuss possible adverse effects of treatment and their appropriate management. Teach the patient with arthritic manifestations about using NSAIDs, including the importance of maintaining a consistent schedule of doses rather than taking the medication only as needed for pain.

Nurses can take a major role in educating the public about Lyme disease and its prevention. Box 43-13■ provides important information about preventing Lyme disease.

BOX 43-13 | **PATIENT TEACHING**

Preventing Lyme Disease

- Avoid tick-infested areas, particularly tall grasses and dense brush.
- When walking or working in potentially infested areas, wear clothing that completely covers the extremities (e.g., long pants tucked into boot tops or long socks and long-sleeved shirts tucked into pants).
- Use an insect repellent such as diethyltoluamide (DEET) or permethrin on skin and clothing.
- Inspect skin and clothing for ticks after you have been outside.
- Protect pets with tick collars and inspect them frequently for ticks.
- Remove any ticks found on the body or pets immediately. Grasp the mouth portion of the tick with fine tweezers where it enters the skin, and pull steadily and firmly until the tick releases. Do not twist or jerk.
- Put the tick in alcohol and save it for future examination in case you develop symptoms. Do not crush the tick.
- Wash the affected area thoroughly with soap and water; apply an antiseptic.
- If you develop flulike symptoms or a "bull's-eye" rash around the tick bite, notify a physician immediately.

Ankylosing Spondylitis

Ankylosing spondylitis is a chronic inflammatory arthritis that primarily affects the spine, causing pain and progressive stiffening. The cause of ankylosing spondylitis is unknown. Heredity plays a role in its development. It affects men more often than women.

The onset of ankylosing spondylitis is usually insidious. Patients may complain of persistent or intermittent bouts of low back pain. The pain is worse at night, followed by morning stiffness that is relieved by activity. Pain may radiate to the buttocks, hips, or down the legs. As the disease progresses, back motion is limited, the lumbar curve is lost, and the thoracic curvature is accentuated. In severe cases, the entire spine is fused, preventing any motion. Patients with ankylosing spondylitis may also develop arthritis in other joints, primarily the hip, shoulders, and knees. Systemic manifestations include anorexia, weight loss, fever, and fatigue. Many patients develop uveitis, inflammation of the iris and the middle, vascular layer of the eye.

Physical therapy and daily exercises are important to maintain posture and joint ROM. NSAIDs relieve pain and stiffness and allow the patient to perform necessary exercises.

As with other chronic arthritic disorders, the primary nursing role in ankylosing spondylitis is providing supportive care and education. Encourage to maintain a fluid intake of 2,500 mL or more per day. Suggest performing exercises in the shower because warm, moist heat promotes mobility.

Uveitis may cause photophobia and blurred vision in the affected eye. Provide indirect lighting and a darkened room for photophobia. If vision is significantly impaired, use appropriate measures such as:

- Orient to surroundings; do not move furniture or place objects in usual pathways.
- Introduce yourself verbally when entering the room. Tell patient what you are doing during procedures.
- Assist during ambulation by allowing patient to hold your elbow.

OTHER MUSCULOSKELETAL DISORDERS

Key Concept Musculoskeletal disorders characterized by chronic pain and discomfort have both physical and psychosocial effects. Nurses provide support and education so the patient can be an active partner in managing his or her condition.

Fibromyalgia

Fibromyalgia is a common rheumatic syndrome of musculoskeletal pain, stiffness, and tenderness. It usually affects women over the age of 50. It may be precipitated or aggravated by stress, sleep disorders, trauma, or depression.

The cause of fibromyalgia is unknown, and its pathophysiology is unclear. A gradual onset of chronic, achy muscle pain is typical. The pain may be localized or involve the entire body. The neck, shoulders, lower back, and hips are often affected. Tenderness is present, usually in small, localized trigger points. Local tightness or muscle spasm may also occur. Systemic manifestations of fibromyalgia include fatigue, sleep disruptions, headaches, and an irritable bowel. Pain and fatigue are aggravated by exertion.

This disorder may resolve spontaneously or become chronic and recurrent. The patient with fibromyalgia needs reassurance of that the disorder is real and treatable. Treatment focuses on improving function and quality of life rather than on eliminating pain. A program of structured aerobic exercise, stretching exercises, and heated pool treatments with or without exercise has been shown to be beneficial. Other therapeutic measures include local heat, massage, and sleep improvement. Amitriptyline, a tricyclic antidepressant, has been found to promote better sleep and relieve symptoms of fibromyalgia. Other antidepressant drugs may also be effective in treating the symptoms of fibromyalgia. Pregabalin (Lyrica) is an anticonvulsant drug used to treat neuropathic pain that helps relieve fibromyalgia pain in some patients.

Nursing care for patients with fibromyalgia is supportive and educational, provided in community settings such as clinics and other primary care settings. It is important to validate concerns and reassure patients that their symptoms are not "all in the head." This syndrome is recognizable and manageable; its course is not progressive. Teach about the disorder. Provide verbal and written instructions about management strategies. Instruct to take prescribed medications at bedtime, because they may cause drowsiness. Caution about driving while taking the medication.

Low Back Pain

Back pain is the leading cause of disability among adults under age 45. In most cases, low back pain is nonspecific, without an identifiable anatomic explanation, and involves the lumbar, lumbosacral, or sacroiliac areas of the back. Low back pain caused by degenerative disk disease and herniated vertebral disks is covered in Chapter 39.

PATHOPHYSIOLOGY AND MANIFESTATIONS

Low back pain is often multifactorial in origin, related to one or more of the following:

- *Local pain* is often caused by fractures, strains, or sprains.
- *Referred pain* is caused by disorders of organs in the abdomen or pelvis, such as gastrointestinal or genitourinary disorders or an abdominal aortic aneurysm.
- *Pain of spinal origin* is associated with pathology of the spine such as disk disease or arthritis.
- *Radicular back pain* radiates from the back to the leg along a nerve root. It is sharp pain that may be aggravated by movement, such as coughing, sneezing, or sitting.
- *Muscle spasm pain* is associated with many spine disorders. This type of back pain is dull and may be accompanied by abnormal posture and taut spinal muscles.

Low back pain may range from mild discomfort lasting a few hours to chronic, debilitating pain. Acute pain is usually caused by an activity such as lifting and bending or twisting.

COLLABORATIVE CARE

Low back pain is usually diagnosed by the history and physical exam. X-rays, CT scan, and MRI are ordered only when a potentially serious underlying condition is suspected.

Most patients with acute low back pain need only short-term treatment. Ice packs or ice massage can be applied or rubbed over the painful area for 15 minutes every hour or more. Moist, warm towels or a heating pad can be used as an alternative to ice therapy.

Prolonged rest is not recommended. In fact, increased activity helps to restore function and may increase endorphin levels. Exercise is initiated early and increased gradually. Physical therapy frequently is used in combination with exercise. Diathermy (deep heat therapy), ultrasonography, hydrotherapy, and transcutaneous electrical nerve stimulation (TENS) units may be used to reduce the muscle spasms and relieve pain.

Other treatments include chiropractic manipulation of the spine to reduce spasms and pain. *Back school* is a rehabilitation program that teaches about the anatomy of the spine and ways to decrease the risk of recurring back injury.

Low back pain can often be managed with NSAIDs and analgesics. Muscle relaxants may also be ordered. For intense, intractable pain, a steroid solution may be injected into the epidural space. This helps decrease the swelling and inflammation of the spinal nerves.

NURSING CARE

PRIORITIZING NURSING CARE

Because low back pain is often chronic in nature, teaching the patient measures to reduce the risk of injury and manage the discomfort is a priority for nursing care.

Readiness for Enhanced Self-Health Management

Expected outcome: Will become an active partner in managing low back pain.

- Discuss use of nonprescription analgesics and NSAIDs for low back pain. Instruct the patient to initially take analgesics or NSAIDs on a routine schedule. *Mild analgesics or NSAIDs may help the patient remain active, preventing muscle deconditioning that can occur with prolonged rest.*
- Encourage the patient to stay active and continue daily living activities as allowed by symptoms. *There is little evidence of a benefit to bed rest, but there is evidence that staying in bed for more than one to two days can actually increase pain and cause joint stiffness and muscle weakness.*
- Instruct about appropriate use of heat or cold to relieve back pain. Teach about the "rebound phenomenon" of prolonged heat therapy. *Applying heat for longer than 30 minutes causes a reverse effect known as the rebound phenomenon. Although cold (e.g., an ice pack or massage with ice) may be used, there is little evidence for its effectiveness in relieving back pain.*
- Teach appropriate body mechanics in lifting and reaching. Instruct to plan the lift, keep the object being lifted close to the body, and avoid twisting when lifting. Encourage to obtain help when lifting. *Using good body mechanics can prevent many back injuries.*
- Encourage to avoid prolonged standing or sitting, lying prone, and wearing high heels. *These activities exacerbate back pain.*
- Encourage an exercise program to strengthen abdominal and back muscles. Teach or refer for teaching about exercises such as partial sit-ups with the knees bent and knee–chest exercises to stretch hamstrings and spinal muscles. Instruct to do each exercise five times, gradually increasing to 10 repetitions. Advise to stop any exercise that increases pain, and seek professional advice before continuing. *Prescribed back exercises, such as the pelvic tilt, partial sit-ups, and back rolls, strengthen back and abdominal muscles, reducing the risk of back injury and pain.*
- Discuss the use of complementary and alternative therapies in treating acute low back pain. *Spinal manipulation (chiropractic) has been shown to be equally effective to conventional medicine for treating low back pain.*
- Suggest workplace or environmental modifications to minimize stress on the lower back. *Lumbar supports in chairs, adjustments to chair or table height, and rubber floor mats help prevent back strain or injury.*
- Encourage obese patients to lose weight. *Obesity changes the center of gravity and increases the risk of injury when lifting.*
- Encourage to stop smoking. *Smoking contributes to disk degeneration and the risk of injury.*

CONTINUITY OF CARE

Back pain is a common problem. Nurses can make an impact on this significant problem by teaching health practices to prevent back pain. Teach safe lifting, bending, and turning during physical activity. Stress the importance of using large muscle groups of the legs to lift rather than bending and lifting with the smaller muscles of the back. Teach other aspects of good body mechanics, including posture, sleeping on a firm mattress, and sitting in chairs that provide good support. Discuss the positive effect of maintaining optimal body weight and good physical fitness.

In industrial and work settings, nurses should be alert for situations that increase the risk of back pain and injury. Office workers should have chairs with appropriate seat height and length and back support. Modifications of work space or machinery may be necessary for industrial workers to avoid excess stresses on back muscles. Finally, it is important to remember that back pain is a leading cause of lost work time for nurses themselves. Remind coworkers to use good body mechanics and to seek help when lifting or moving patients.

Common Foot Disorders

Foot disorders often cause pain or difficulty in walking. These disorders may be congenital, related to a systemic disorder, caused by wearing poorly fitting, confining, or high heeled shoes, or due to physical stress on the foot. Women are more frequently affected by foot disorders than men. Common foot disorders are summarized in Table 43-7 ■.

COLLABORATIVE CARE

Corrective shoes are often ordered for patients with foot disorders. Orthotic devices that cushion and stretch the affected joints may be placed within shoes or between the toes. Analgesics may be ordered, or corticosteroid drugs are

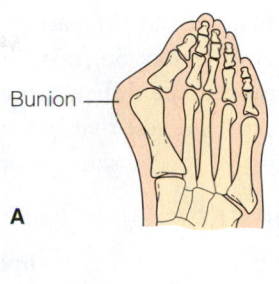
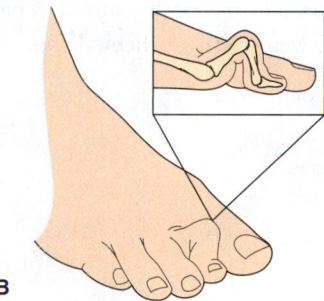

Figure 43-11. ■ (A) Hallux valgus (bunion). **(B)** Hammertoe.

injected into the affected joints to relieve acute inflammation. A bunionectomy may be done to treat hallux valgus. Surgery may also be done to correct hammertoe.

NURSING CARE

The focus and priority for nursing care of the patient with a foot disorder is managing discomfort associated with the disorder and teaching measures to maintain mobility. Instruct the patient to wear appropriate or corrective footwear. Provide information about resources for obtaining a proper shoe fit. Suggest shoes such as running or walking shoes that provide arch support and ample toe room. Also suggest protective pads to wear over bunions, calluses/corns,

TABLE 43-7	Common Foot Disorders	
DISORDER	**DESCRIPTION**	**MANIFESTATIONS**
Hallux valgus (bunion)	Enlargement and lateral displacement of the great toe (Figure 43–11A ■)	■ Lateral deviation of the great toe with MTP joint enlargement ■ Joint pain ■ Calluses ■ Limited joint ROM, possible crepitus
Hammertoe	Flexion of the PIP joint with hyperextension of the MTP and DIP joints (Figure 43-11B); the second toe usually affected	■ Pain ■ Inability to straighten toe ■ Callus on sole of the foot; corn on flexed PIP joint
Plantar fasciitis	Inflammation of the plantar fascia that connects the heel bone to the toes and creates the arch of the foot	■ Severe foot pain with first steps on arising in the morning or after a period of inactivity ■ Aggravated by walking barefoot, climbing stairs

and the ball of the foot. Advise the patient to remove pads and inspect feet every other day. Suggest use of a mirror or a helper to inspect areas that are difficult to see. Teach proper foot care. If appropriate, suggest that the patient seek evaluation by a podiatrist for special shoes or orthotics.

CONTINUITY OF CARE

Teach patients in all age groups the importance of well-fitting footwear. Discuss with women in particular the long-term effects of wearing high-heeled shoes with constricting toes. Suggest alternatives for stylish footwear, and encourage patients to wear supportive and nonrestrictive footwear at all times. Discuss the possible effects of bunions on balance, and talk about safety measures to prevent falls and injury. Teach techniques to relieve pressure on affected joints as discussed in the nursing care section.

Note: The references and resources for all chapters have been compiled at the back of the book.

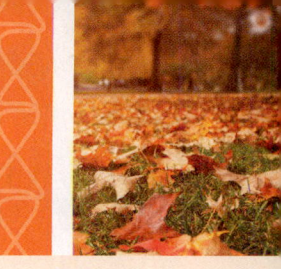

Chapter Review

KEY POINTS

- **Concept:** Musculoskeletal disorders can affect the patient's physical mobility, body image, comfort, and ability to provide self-care. Nurses provide physical care, teaching for self-care, and psychosocial support for the patient and family.
- **Concept:** Bone disorders affect the strength and integrity of affected bones, leaving the patient at risk for fractures. Promoting comfort, maintaining safety, and preventing injuries are priority nursing responsibilities when caring for patients with bone disorders.
- Prevention is a key strategy for osteoporosis. Stress the importance of adequate calcium intake throughout the life span, and encourage menopausal patients to discuss preventive measures with their health care provider.
- Osteomyelitis, infection of the bone, is difficult to treat; prevention and early identification are vital. Promptly report general signs of infection, as well as redness, heat, wound drainage, continued pain, and refusal to use or bear weight on an extremity.
- Benign bone tumors and metastasis of tumors from other locations are more common than primary malignancy of the bone.
- **Concept:** Arthritis can have many different causes and effects. The nursing focus in caring for patients with arthritis is educating the patient and family about the disease and its management, promoting mobility, and helping patients adapt to limitations related to the disorder.

- Most people develop osteoarthritis as they age. The pain and joint effects of OA are localized and are managed symptomatically with balanced rest and activity.
- **Concept:** Inflammatory joint disorders such as rheumatoid arthritis are systemic and often chronic, potentially leading to significant disability. Care is multidimensional, involving medications and other strategies to promote and maintain optimal function.
- RA is a systemic inflammatory disease. Its management is directed toward reducing inflammation and preventing joint destruction.
- Systemic lupus erythematosus is a systemic connective tissue disease with symptoms similar to RA. It is less likely to cause joint crippling but has more widespread effects than RA in many people. Reducing inflammation is a priority in both disorders.
- **Concept:** Gout is an inflammatory arthritis caused by excess uric acid in the body. Treatment focuses on reducing uric acid levels to prevent acute attacks and potential long-term effects.
- **Concept:** Musculoskeletal disorders characterized by chronic pain and discomfort have significant physical and psychosocial effects. The nursing focus is on providing support and education so the patient can be an active partner in managing his or her condition.

PEARSON NURSING STUDENT RESOURCES

Find additional materials at **nursing.pearsonhighered.com**.

Clinical Reasoning Care Map

Caring for a Patient With Osteoarthritis and Total Hip Replacement

NCLEX-PN® Focus Area: Physiologic Integrity: Physiologic Adaptation

Case Study: Robert Cerulli is a 72-year-old retired commercial fisherman who has significant degenerative changes in both hip joints. He is admitted for a right total hip replacement; a left total hip replacement is planned to follow in 6 to 12 months.

Nursing Diagnosis: Impaired Physical Mobility

COLLECT DATA

Subjective	Objective
_____	_____
_____	_____
_____	_____
_____	_____
_____	_____
_____	_____

Does this present a threat to the patient's safety?

If yes, the priority intervention to address this threat would be:

_____

Nursing Care

_____
_____
_____
_____
_____
_____
_____
_____
_____

Interprofessional team members to include when planning care:

_____

How would you document this? _____

_____

Compare your answers and documentation to those provided on the companion website.

Data Collected
(use only those that apply)

- Takes carbidopa/levodopa (Sinemet 25-100) four times a day for Parkinson disease
- No other chronic medical conditions
- No known medication allergies
- Does not smoke; consumes only small amounts of alcohol
- Alert and oriented
- Speech is soft but clear
- Vital signs: BP 116/64; P 68 regular; R 18; T 97.4°F (36.3°C) PO
- Color good, skin warm and moist
- Peripheral pulses strong and equal in upper extremities; slightly weaker but equal in lower extremities
- Feet cool to touch, good capillary refill
- Walks with a limp; shuffling gait noted

Nursing Interventions
(use only those that apply;
list in priority order)

- Perform passive ROM exercises of unaffected extremities every shift.
- Maintain right hip abduction with abduction pillow.
- Help change position every 2 hours; encourage use of overhead trapeze to shift positions.
- Encourage frequent quadriceps-setting exercises and plantar and dorsiflexion of feet.
- Maintain sequential compression device and antiembolic stocking as ordered.
- Remind to use incentive spirometer hourly for first 24 hours and then every 2 hours while awake.
- Collaborate with physical therapy team to teach use of walker for safe ambulation.
- Assess pain hourly first 24 to 48 hours postoperatively, and as needed thereafter.
- Assist out of bed three times a day after the first 24 hours.
- Assess the surgical site frequently; report signs of excess bleeding or inflammation.
- Monitor temperature every 4 hours.
- Teach to use patient-controlled analgesia (PCA) and monitor effectiveness.
- Assess pulses, color, movement, and sensation of right foot hourly for the first 24 hours, then every 2 hours for 24 hours, and then every 4 hours.

NCLEX-PN® Exam Preparation

1 When caring for a patient who sustained a gunshot wound to the femur 4 days ago, which of these assessments requires immediate nursing intervention?

1. Soiled dressing
2. Tenderness, swelling, redness over incision site
3. Increased capillary refill
4. Pain rated 2/10 (2 on a scale of 0 to 10)

2 A patient diagnosed with osteoporosis and a right hip replacement is preparing for discharge. All of the following are important discharge instructions; place them in order of priority.

1. Use of walker and elevated toilet
2. Pain medication
3. List of calcium-enriched foods
4. Smoking cessation programs and tools
5. Schedule for increasing activity

3 A nurse teaches the mother of a 4-year-old child how to prevent Lyme disease. Which of these statements indicates that further teaching is necessary?

1. "We are going camping, but I'll make sure she stays out of the brush."
2. "Even though it's warm, I'll make her wear long pants."
3. "If a tick gets on my child, I'll pull it off immediately and squash it."
4. "I'll buy some insect repellant before we leave on our vacation."

4 When assessing a patient who has osteoarthritis, the nurse should expect to observe which of these findings?

1. Superficial, sharp pain
2. Stiffness after joint use
3. Full ROM
4. Crepitus with movement

5 Which of the following is an appropriate goal for teaching of a patient with SLE?

1. Experiences no joint pain or inflammation.
2. States rationale for maintaining vegetarian diet.
3. Uses SPF 15 or higher sunscreen when outside.
4. Relates importance of splints to prevent joint damage.

6 The nurse is teaching a patient who is recovering from an acute gout attack about his prescription for sulfinpyrazone (Anturane). Which statement by the patient would indicate an understanding of the instructions?

1. "I'm going to drink less water so I won't swell up."
2. "I'll take aspirin every 4 hours until my toe no longer hurts."
3. "I'll let my doctor know if my stomach begins to hurt."
4. "I will take my medicine on an empty stomach."

7 A patient is diagnosed with chronic low back pain. The physician has asked the nurse to provide information related to this condition. Which of the following nursing diagnoses would the nurse be expected to address?

1. Disturbed Body Image
2. Readiness for Enhanced Self Health Management
3. Hopelessness
4. Acute Pain

8 The nurse is teaching a patient with rheumatoid arthritis about the prescribed drug, celecoxib (Celebrex). Which of the following statements does the nurse include? **Select all that apply.**

1. "Always take this drug with food or milk to avoid gastric upset."
2. "Take the drug as needed to manage pain and stiffness."
3. "Contact your doctor if you develop stomach or abdominal pain."
4. "You may use acetaminophen as needed for pain."
5. "Like aspirin, this drug reduces your risk for heart attack."

9 An x-ray done on a patient admitted to the emergency department with an injury to the right tibia shows a mass in the tibia. The patient asks the nurse if this means his leg will need to be amputated. The appropriate response by the nurse is:

1. "The prospect of amputation must be frightening to you."
2. "Do you have other symptoms of bone cancer?"
3. "Most bone tumors are benign. I'm sure you won't need anything that drastic."
4. "Bone masses usually occur secondarily to cancer elsewhere. Treatment will focus on the primary tumor."

10 A patient newly diagnosed with fibromyalgia says "I'm so scared this disease is going to make it impossible to do the things I enjoy if it gets worse." How should the nurse respond?

1. "Fibromyalgia is not a progressive disease. Let's talk about what you can do to manage its symptoms."
2. "I understand your fear. Tell me how you feel about this diagnosis."
3. "In many cases, medications can prevent progression of the disorder. Let's go over your medications and how to use them."
4. "Many people live long and active lives with fibromyalgia."

Answers and rationales for Review Questions appear in Appendix I.

Thinking Strategically About…

You are an LPN/LVN working the day shift at a rehabilitation hospital. You are responsible for providing care, administering medications, and making sure your assigned patients arrive at their therapy classes on time. You are assigned to the following patients.

Nancy is a 53-year-old teacher from a small town 70 miles away. She has smoked a pack of cigarettes a day for 30 years and drinks one or two glasses of wine with dinner each evening. She does not routinely exercise. Nancy has had symptoms of menopause for 8 years, but she has never been on estrogen therapy. Both Nancy's mother and her 60-year-old sister have osteoporosis. Nancy has been having continuous low back pain that is unrelieved by mild analgesics. The pain is worse when bending over and returning to an upright position. She has a noticeable "hump" on her upper back and is 1 in. shorter than her stated height. She has full range of motion in all extremities.

When asked about her diet, Nancy reports that she has never been a "milk drinker," even as a child. She indicates that on a typical day, she takes in only one-half to one dairy serving. Nancy is admitted to the rehabilitation hospital for treatment of her osteoporosis including exercise, medication, and nutrition instruction.

Kevin, a 22-year-old college student, received compound fractures of the left femur, fibula, and tibia during a motorcycle accident. The injury resulted in such widespread tissue loss that the left leg was amputated above the knee. Kevin has been active in basketball and downhill skiing in the winter and water skiing in the summer. He is depressed and feels his life is over. He was admitted to rehabilitation to regain mobility with a prosthetic leg.

Ralph, a 72-year-old retired bank executive, fell when getting out of the shower. He sustained a fractured femoral neck and underwent a total hip replacement two weeks ago. He was admitted to the rehabilitation hospital to gain mobility. He plans to return home with his wife.

CRITICAL THINKING

- Why is Nancy shorter that she was as a younger adult?

- What will you say to Kevin when he tells you his life is over?

- Many older adults die within a short time after a hip fracture. What is the main cause of fracture-related death and what can be done to prevent it?

PRIORITIES IN NURSING CARE

- What physical activities should the nurse encourage for Nancy and why?

- What is the priority intervention when planning care for Kevin?

- Besides encouraging mobility, what are other priority interventions for Ralph?

MANAGEMENT OF CARE

- Discuss the management of dietary needs and exercise therapy for Nancy.

- To organize care for Kevin and Ralph on an hourly basis, what information will you need to obtain from their care plans?

DELEGATING

- What care in a rehabilitation hospital can be delegated to the CNA during the day shift?

PATIENT TEACHING

- What knowledge deficits can the nurse identify for Nancy?

- Before discharge, what teaching must be provided for Ralph and his wife regarding ensuring a safe home environment?

REPORTING

- What observations of Kevin need to be made and reported to the RN daily?

Note: Discussion of Unit questions appears on the companion website.

UNIT XII
Disrupted Integumentary Function

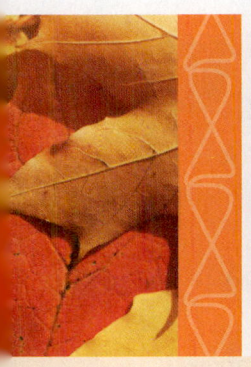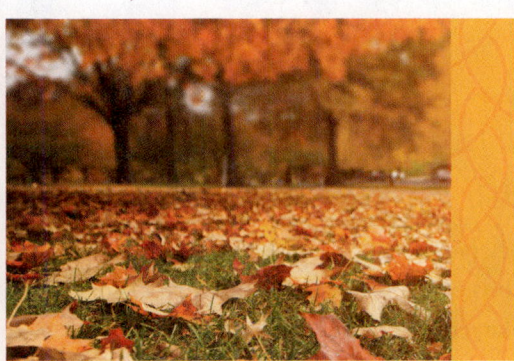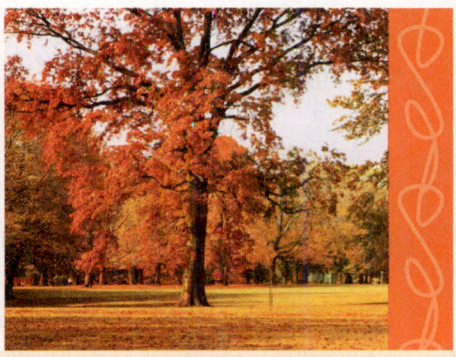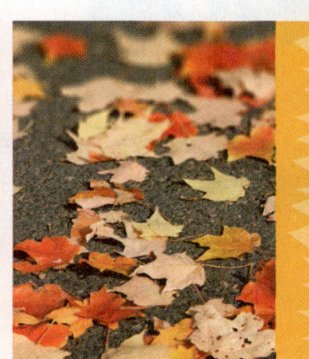

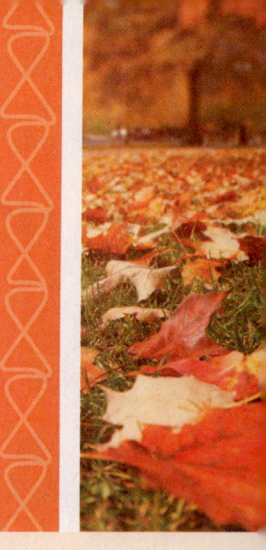

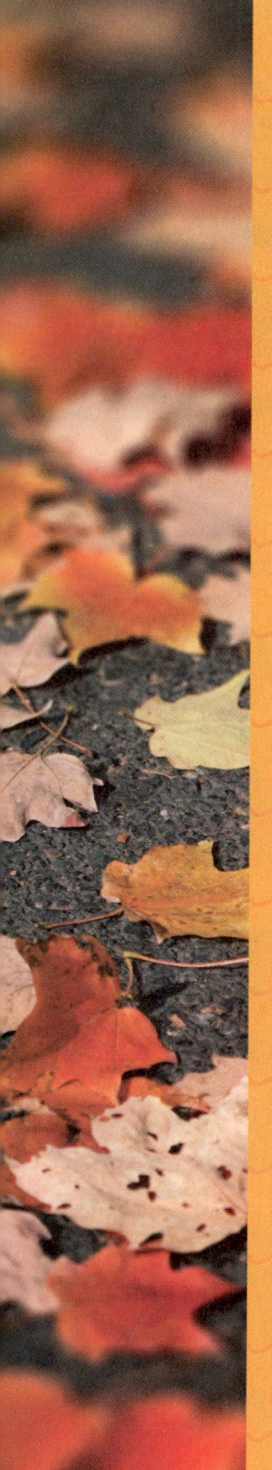

CHAPTER 44

The Integumentary System and Assessment

BRIEF OUTLINE

Structure and Function of the Integumentary System

Assessment

APPLIED LEARNING OUTCOMES

After completing this chapter, you will be able to:

1. Identify the structure and functions of the skin and its appendages.
2. Describe factors that influence skin color.
3. Collect subjective and objective assessment data for patients with integumentary disorders.
4. Describe skin changes in the older adult.
5. Implement nursing responsibilities for common diagnostic tests for patients with integumentary disorders and report results to appropriate health care providers.

KEY TERMS

The key terms are defined on the pages listed below.

Structure and Function of the Integumentary System

Key Concept The integumentary system is the body's first line of defense against environmental hazards. The skin is separated and insulated from the rest of the body by the subcutaneous layer. However, it is connected to the rest of the body by the circulatory network of blood and lymphatic vessels.

The skin, glands, hair, and nails make up the integumentary system. The skin provides an external covering for the body, separating the body's organs and tissues from the external environment. The skin contains receptors for touch and sensation, helps regulate body temperature, and assists in fluid and electrolyte balance. It provides cues to racial and ethnic background, conveys emotional responses, and helps determine self-concept, roles, and relationships. Functions of the skin, glands, hair, and nails are described in Table 44-1 ■. Factors such as allergies, infection, infestation, and cancer can cause disorders of the integumentary system.

THE SKIN

The skin has a surface area of 15 to 20 square feet and weighs about 9 pounds. It has been estimated that each square inch of skin contains 15 feet of blood vessels, 4 yards of nerves, 650 sweat glands, 100 oil glands, 1,500 sensory receptors, and more than 3 million cells that are constantly dying and being replaced.

The skin is composed of two regions: the epidermis and the dermis (Figure 44-1 ■). The **epidermis**, the surface or outermost part of the skin, is made up of several layers of epithelial cells. The deepest layer of the epidermis contains cells that produce melanin and keratin. *Melanin* forms a shield to protect nerve endings in the dermis from the damaging effects of ultraviolet light. *Keratin* is a fibrous, water-repellent protein that makes the epidermis tough and protective. The outermost layer of the epidermis makes up about 75% of the epidermis's total thickness. It consists of about 20 to 30 sheets of dead cells filled with keratin fragments arranged in "shingles" that flake off as dry skin. The **dermis**, the second, deeper layer of skin, is made up of a flexible connective tissue. This layer is richly supplied with blood cells, nerve fibers, and lymphatic vessels. Most of the hair follicles, sebaceous glands, and sweat glands are located in the dermis.

The color of the skin is the result of varying levels of pigmentation. *Melanin,* a yellow-to-brown pigment, is darker and is produced in greater amounts in persons with dark skin color than in those with light skin. Exposure to the sun causes a buildup of melanin and a darkening of the skin in people with light skin. *Carotene* (a yellow-to-orange pigment) is more abundant in the skins of persons of Asian ancestry, and together with melanin accounts for their golden skin tone. The epidermis in Caucasian skin has very little melanin and is almost transparent. The color of their red blood cells shows through, lending Caucasians a pinkish skin tone.

Skin color is influenced by emotions and illnesses. **Erythema** (a reddening of the skin) may occur with embarrassment such as blushing, fever, hypertension, or inflammation. It may also result from a drug reaction, sunburn, or other factors. **Cyanosis** (bluish discoloration of the skin and mucous membranes) results from poor

TABLE 44-1	Functions of the Skin and Its Appendages
STRUCTURE	**FUNCTION**
Epidermis	Protects tissues from physical, chemical, and biologic damage Prevents water loss and serves as a water-repellent layer Stores melanin, which protects tissues from harmful effects of the ultraviolet radiation in sunlight Converts cholesterol molecules to vitamin D when exposed to sunlight Contains phagocytes, which prevent bacteria from penetrating the skin
Dermis	Regulates body temperature by dilating and constricting capillaries Transmits messages via nerve endings to the central nervous system
Sebaceous (oil) glands	Secrete sebum, which lubricates skin and hair and plays a role in killing bacteria
Eccrine sweat glands	Regulate body heat by excretion of perspiration
Apocrine sweat glands	Unknown
Hair	Cushions the scalp. Eyelashes and cilia protect the body from foreign particles. Provides insulation in cold weather
Nails	Protect the fingers and toes, aid in grasping, and allow for various other activities, such as scratching the skin, picking up small items, peeling an orange, and so on

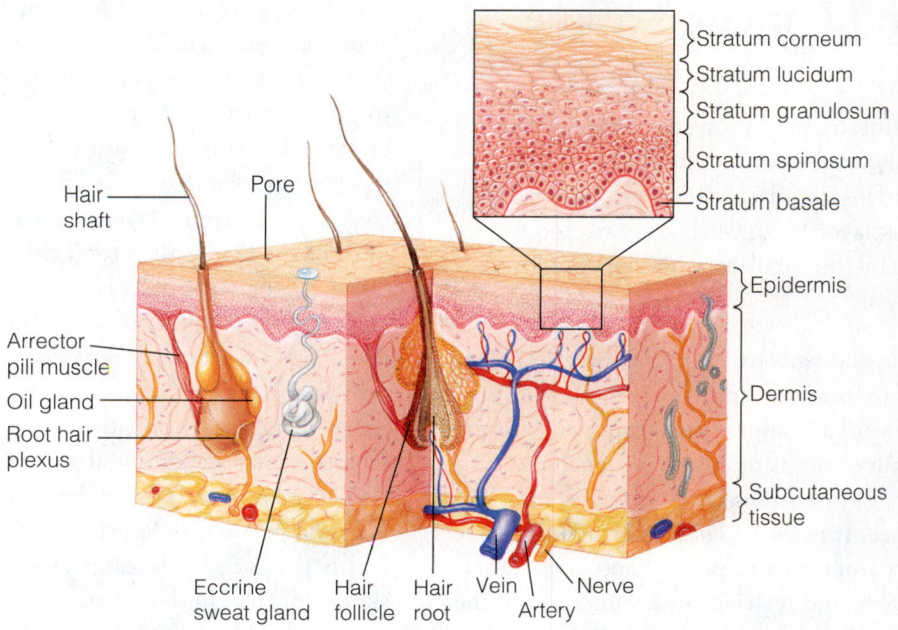

Stratum corneum
Stratum lucidum
Stratum granulosum
Stratum spinosum
Stratum basale

Epidermis

Dermis

Subcutaneous tissue

Hair shaft

Pore

Arrector pili muscle

Oil gland

Root hair plexus

Eccrine sweat gland

Hair follicle

Hair root

Vein

Artery

Nerve

Figure 44-1. ■ Anatomy of the skin.

oxygenation of hemoglobin or lack of adequate hemoglobin or RBCs. **Pallor**, or paleness of skin, may occur with shock, fear, or anger, or in anemia and hypoxia. **Jaundice** is a yellow-to-orange color visible in the skin and mucous membranes; it most often results from a liver disorder.

Glands of the Skin

The skin has three types of glands: sebaceous (oil) glands, sweat glands, and ceruminous glands. Each of these glands has a different function (see Table 44-1).

Sebaceous glands are found all over the body except the palms and soles. These glands secrete an oily substance (*sebum*) that softens and lubricates the skin and hair. Sebum also protects the body from infection by killing bacteria. The secretion of sebum is stimulated by hormones, especially androgens.

There are two types of sweat glands: eccrine and apocrine. Eccrine sweat glands are found mostly on the forehead, palms, and soles. The production of sweat is regulated by the sympathetic nervous system and serves to maintain normal body temperature. Apocrine sweat glands are found in the axillae, breast areolae, and genital areas. They secrete a thick milky substance that causes odor when mixed with bacteria on the skin. Ceruminous glands are modified apocrine sweat glands. They are found in the skin of the external ear and secrete yellow-brown waxy cerumen. This substance provides a sticky trap for foreign materials.

THE HAIR AND NAILS

Hair is distributed and scattered all over the body, except the lips, nipples, parts of the external genitals, the palms of the hands, and the soles of the feet. Hair is produced by a hair

bulb, and its root is enclosed in a hair follicle. The visible hair is composed of dead cells. Many factors, including nutrition and hormones, influence hair growth. Hair in various parts of the body has protective functions. A nail is a modified scale-like epidermal structure. Like hair, nails consist mainly of dead cells. Review Table 44-1 for hair and nail functions.

Assessment

HEALTH HISTORY

The health history may be part of a health screening, total health assessment, or focused on the patient's chief complaint, such as a rash or itching. If the patient has a skin problem, identify its onset, characteristics, course, and severity. Note any precipitating and relieving factors and whether symptoms are associated with specific circumstances. Ask about bathing routine and skin care products.

Ask about any change in health, skin color changes, dryness or oiliness, growth of or changes in warts or moles, the presence of lesions, and delayed wound healing. Determine whether the patient takes hormones, vitamins, steroids, or antibiotics, which may cause skin side effects. For obese patients, inquire about any chafing in areas where moisture accumulates, such as overlapping skin folds.

When the patient complains about itching, ask the patient to describe the type of itching. Inquire about precipitating causes such as medications, soaps, shampoos, cosmetics, skin care products, pets, travel, stress, or diet changes. Ask about skin reactions to insect bites and stings.

In assessing the hair, ask about problems with thinning or baldness, excessive hair loss, change in distribution of hair, use of hair-care products, diet, and dieting. When assessing nail problems, ask about nail splitting or breakage, discoloration, thickness, infection, diet, and exposure to chemicals.

Obtain the patient's past medical history, focusing on previous problems, allergies, surgery, and lesions. Skin, hair, and nail problems may be symptoms of other health disorders, such as cardiovascular, diabetes mellitus, thyroid disease, liver disease, and hematologic disorders. Occupational and social history may provide cues to skin problems; ask the patient about exposure to chemicals at work, travel, use of alcohol, and responses to stress.

Assess the presence of risk factors for skin cancer carefully. These include male gender; age over 50; family history of skin cancer; light-colored hair and eyes; extended exposure to sunlight; tendency to sunburn; history of sunburn or other skin trauma; living in high altitudes or near equator; exposure to radiation, x-rays, coal, tar, or petroleum products; and the use of sun-protection products.

Also explore the risk factors for malignant melanoma. These include a large number of moles, the presence of atypical moles, a family history of melanoma, prior melanoma, repeat severe sunburns, ease of freckling and sunburning, or inability to tan.

PHYSICAL EXAMINATION

The examination should be conducted in a warm, private room. The patient removes all clothing and puts on a gown that allows access to all skin areas. Areas to be examined must be fully exposed but cover the other areas to protect the patient's modesty. Don gloves when palpating open lesions, skin surfaces with possible infection or infestation, or discharge from skin lesions or mucous membranes. Use a ruler to measure the size of lesions. A flashlight may be required to better visualize lesions.

Inspect the skin for pallor, cyanosis, or jaundice. Take special care when assessing the skin color in people with dark skin, such as African Americans, Hispanics, Native Americans, Asians, and Caucasians with deep suntans.

clinicalALERT

In dark-skinned patients, paleness is seen as dull color. The skin may appear dull and darker when cyanosis is present. Jaundice is best assessed on the palms of the hands or sclera of the eyes.

Assess for redness, swelling, and pain related to various rashes, inflammation, infections, and burns. First-degree burns cause painful erythema and swelling. Red, painful blisters occur in second-degree burns and white or blackened areas appear in third-degree burns. Check for *vitiligo,* an abnormal, patchy loss of melanin, over the face, hands, and groin. Assess for *petechiae,* small, reddish-purple pinpoint spots, over the abdomen and buttocks.

Inspect the skin for lesions. Primary and secondary lesions are described and shown in Table 44-2 ■. Look for raised bluish or yellowish bruises. Note bruises that are in varying stages of healing. Assess for lesions that appear in circles, groups, or along the sensory nerves.

TABLE 44-2	Primary and Secondary Skin Lesions		
Macule, Patch 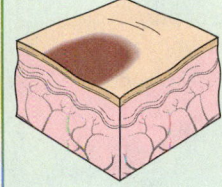	Flat, nonpalpable change in skin color. Macules are smaller than 1 cm, with a circumscribed border, and patches are larger than 1 cm and may have an irregular border. *Examples:* Macules: freckles, measles, and petechiae. Patches: Mongolian spots, port-wine stains, vitiligo, and chloasma.	**Nodule, Tumor** 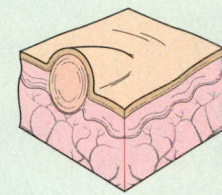	Elevated, solid, hard or soft palpable mass extending deeper into the dermis than a papule. Nodules have circumscribed borders and are 0.5–2 cm; tumors may have irregular borders and are larger than 2 cm. *Examples:* Nodules: small lipoma, squamous cell carcinoma, fibroma, and intradermal nevi. Tumors: large lipoma, carcinoma, and hemangioma.
Papule, Plaque 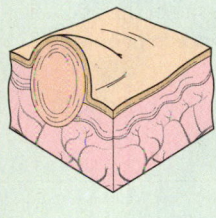	Elevated, solid, palpable mass with circumscribed border. Papules are smaller than 0.5 cm; plaques are groups of papules that form lesions larger than 0.5 cm. *Examples:* Papules: elevated moles, warts, and lichen planus. Plaques: psoriasis, actinic keratosis, and also lichen planus.	**Vesicle, Bulla** 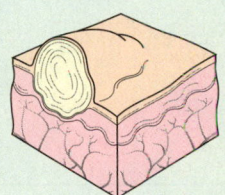	Elevated, fluid-filled, round or oval shaped, palpable mass with thin, translucent walls and circumscribed borders. Vesicles are smaller than 0.5 cm; bullae are larger than 0.5 cm. *Examples:* Vesicles: herpes simplex/ zoster, early chickenpox, poison ivy, and small burn blisters. Bullae: contact dermatitis, friction blisters, and large burn blisters.

(continued)

TABLE 44-2	Primary and Secondary Skin Lesions *(continued)*

Wheal

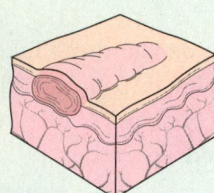

Elevated, often reddish area with irregular border caused by diffuse fluid in tissues rather than free fluid in a cavity, as in vesicles. Size varies.
Examples: Insect bites and hives (extensive wheals).

Scales

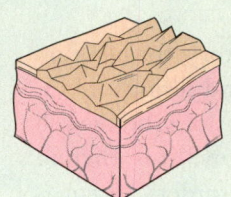

Shedding flakes of greasy, keratinized skin tissue. Color may be white, gray, or silver. Texture may vary from fine to thick.
Examples: Dry skin, dandruff, psoriasis, and eczema.

Pustule

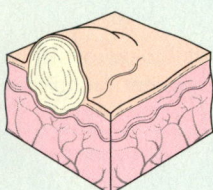

Elevated, pus-filled vesicle or bulla with circumscribed border. Size varies.
Examples: Acne, impetigo, and carbuncles (large boils).

Crust

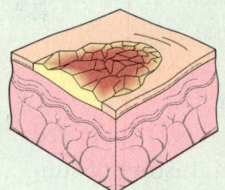

Dry blood, serum, or pus left on the skin surface when vesicles or pustules burst. Can be red-brown, orange, or yellow. Large crusts that adhere to the skin surface are called scabs.
Examples: Eczema, impetigo, herpes, or scabs after abrasion.

Cyst

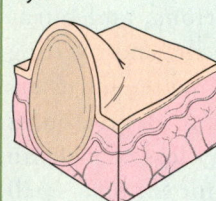

Elevated, encapsulated, fluid-filled, or semisolid mass originating in the subcutaneous tissue or dermis, usually 1 cm or larger.
Examples: Varieties include sebaceous cysts and epidermoid cysts.

Ulcer

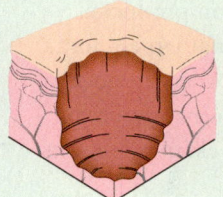

Deep, irregularly shaped area of skin loss extending into the dermis or subcutaneous tissue. May bleed. May leave scar.
Examples: Decubitus ulcers (pressure sores), stasis ulcers, chancres.

Atrophy

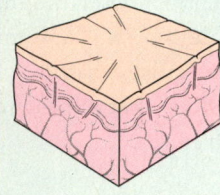

A translucent, dry, paperlike, sometimes wrinkled skin surface resulting from thinning or wasting of the skin due to loss of collagen and elastin.
Examples: Striae, aged skin.

Fissure

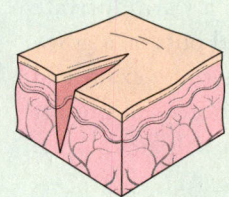

Linear crack with sharp edges, extending into the dermis.
Examples: Cracks at the corners of the mouth or in the hands, athlete's foot.

Erosion

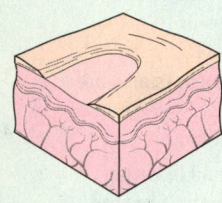

Wearing away of the superficial epidermis causing a moist, shallow depression. Because erosions do not extend into the dermis, they heal without scarring.
Examples: Scratch marks, ruptured vesicles.

Scar

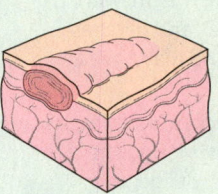

Flat, irregular area of connective tissue left after a lesion or wound has healed. New scars may be red or purple; older scars may be silvery or white.
Examples: Healed surgical wound or injury, healed acne.

Lichenification

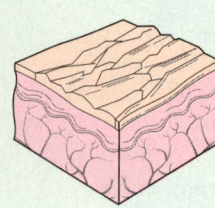

Rough, thickened, hardened area of epidermis resulting from chronic irritation such as scratching or rubbing.
Example: Chronic dermatitis.

Keloid

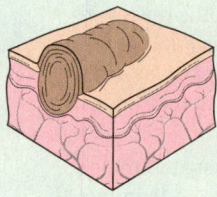

Elevated, irregular, darkened area of excess scar tissue caused by excessive collagen formation during healing. Extends beyond the site of the original injury. Higher incidence in people of African descent.
Examples: Keloid from ear piercing or surgery.

Palpate skin temperature, texture, moisture, and turgor. Note warmth and redness associated with inflammation and coolness related to decreased blood flow. Observe for rough, dry or smooth, oily skin as well as excessive perspiration. Inspect for *tenting* (Figure 44-2■). Tenting is the term used when the skin is pinched gently over the collarbone or back of the hand and remains pinched for a few moments before returning to its normal position. This is a common finding in older adults. Note decreased skin turgor as seen in dehydration. Assess for *edema* (accumulation of fluid in the body's tissues) by depressing the patient's skin over the ankle.

Inspect the distribution and quality of hair. Look for *hirsutism* (excessive hair) or **alopecia** (hair loss). Palpate the hair for coarseness or fineness. Inspect the scalp for lesions such as pustules or scales. Look for *nits* (eggs) seen with head lice adhering to the base of the hair shaft. Note excessive greasy flakes rather than mild dandruff.

Inspect nails for **clubbing** (angle of nail base is greater than 180 degrees; see Figure 23-11). Observe nail surface for inflammation, separation from the nail bed, grooves, pitting, or spoon shape. Inspect for yellowish-colored, bluish-green, or dark nails. Look at the nails for red splinter hemorrhages and pigmented bands, which are normal in 90% of African Americans.

For additional information about assessment techniques, see Chapter 5. See Box 44-1■ for an example of how to document an integumentary assessment.

THE OLDER ADULT

A variety of normal skin changes are seen in the older adult. Loss of subcutaneous tissue, dermal thinning, and decreased elasticity may cause wrinkles and sagging of the skin. The skin is thinner, especially over bony prominences and dorsal surfaces of the hands and feet, and turgor is decreased. Older adults are unable to respond to heat or cold quickly, increasing their risk for heat stroke and hypothermia. (For more information about older adults, see Chapter 4.)

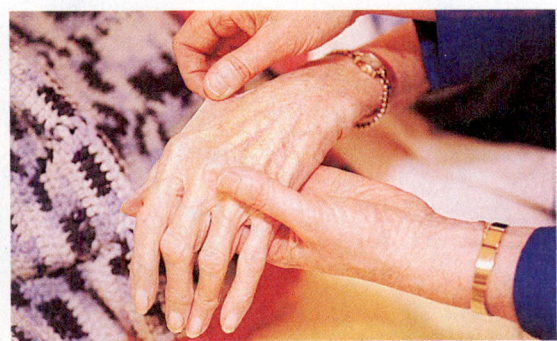

Figure 44-2. ■ Tenting in an older patient.
(Source: Pearson Education.)

BOX 44-1	DOCUMENTATION OF INTEGUMENTARY ASSESSMENT

Patient: A 60-year-old male is seen in an outpatient clinic for psoriasis. States, "This episode is worse than before. I just returned from vacation and this happened." Has a family history of psoriasis.

Assessment note: Raised, red, round plaques noted on anterior part of both arms, back of hands, and scalp. Thick gray scales found between the toes. Toenails yellow with pitting. States, "I just can't seem to stop scratching."

Other age-related changes include the following:

- Dry, itchy skin may result from the reduced number of sweat and oil glands.
- Overall production of melanocytes decreases, whereas abnormal localized proliferations of melanocytes may occur in specific areas. This localized hyperpigmentation may lead to the development of senile lentigines, commonly called "liver spots." These flat, brown macules commonly appear on the arms and hands in areas of sun exposure. Keratoses also result from hyperpigmentation. Seborrheic keratoses are dark, raised lesions. Actinic keratoses are reddish, raised plaques on areas of high sun exposure. They may become malignant.
- Skin tags, small flaps of excess skin, are normal in aging skin.
- Both hair and nail growth decrease with aging. Older men may develop coarse hair in the ears and nose and over the eyebrows. Decreased estrogen levels may cause postmenopausal women to develop dark facial hair over the upper lip and under the chin.
- Hair becomes gray due to a reduction of melanocytes.
- Nails may thicken, yellow, and peel.

DIAGNOSTIC TESTS
Laboratory Tests

Diagnosis of skin problems relies on the patient's history and inspection of the lesion. When diagnosis remains uncertain, other diagnostic procedures are used. The most common test is the skin biopsy. Other tests include stains and cultures to identify bacterial, fungal, and viral infections. Photographs may be taken to document wound healing or to record wounds in suspected abuse cases. Table 44-3■ lists the diagnostic tests, purpose, and nursing implications.

Note: The references and resources for all chapters have been compiled at the back of the book.

TABLE 44-3	Common Diagnostic Tests for Integumentary Disorders	
TEST	**EXPLANATION AND PURPOSE**	**NURSING IMPLICATIONS**
Biopsy	A special biopsy instrument is used to obtain a skin sample of a nodule to rule out malignancy.	Ensure a consent form is signed. Assist with obtaining supplies that the physician will need. Apply dressing and give follow-up instructions. Send specimen to laboratory.
Cutaneous immunofluorescence biopsy	A skin biopsy is obtained and a fluorochrome dye applied. Under a microscope, antibodies become fluorescent. Done to diagnose immune-mediated dermatitis.	Ensure a consent form is signed. Assist with obtaining supplies that the physician will need. Apply dressing and give follow-up instructions. Send specimen to laboratory.
Potassium hydroxide (KOH)	Hair, nail, or scale specimen collected, placed on a glass slide with KOH added, and examined under the microscope. Used to diagnose fungal infections.	Teach patient about purpose of test. Send specimen to laboratory.
Culture and sensitivity	Fluid obtained from intact bullae, pustules, or abscesses to identify bacterial or viral infections and the appropriate medication for treatment.	Explain the purpose and send specimen to laboratory.
Tzanck test	Fluid and cells collected from blisters, placed on slide, stained, and examined microscopically. Used to identify herpes infections.	Explain the purpose and send specimen to laboratory.
Skin scraping	Tissue sample scraped from lesion with a scalpel moistened with oil so skin sticks to blade, transferred to slide, and examined to diagnose fungal infections or scabies.	Explain the purpose and send specimen to laboratory.
Patch test	Suspected allergens applied to normal skin under patches. Reaction ranges from weak with redness or itching to strong with pain and blisters.	Explain purpose and instruct patient to return in 48 hours for removal of patches and evaluation.
Wood's lamp	An ultraviolet light causes organisms such as *Pseudomonas* and fungi to fluoresce.	Explain the purpose of the test and that ultraviolet is not harmful to eyes or skin.

Chapter Review

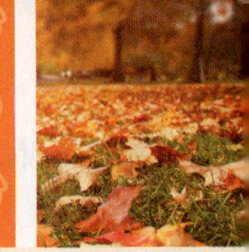

KEY POINTS

- **Concept:** The integumentary system is the body's first line of defense against environmental hazards. The skin is separated and insulated from the rest of the body by the subcutaneous layer. However, it is connected to the rest of the body by the circulatory network of blood and lymphatic vessels.
- The skin and its appendages provide an external covering for the internal tissues and organs, help regulate body temperature, assist in fluid and electrolyte balance, protect tissues, and convey emotions.
- Two layers compose the skin: the epidermis and dermis. Epidermis contains cells that produce melanin and keratin. The dermal layer includes blood cells, nerve fibers, lymph vessels, hair follicles, and sebaceous and sweat glands.
- Primary skin lesions include macule, papule, nodule, vesicle, wheal, pustule, and cyst. Atrophy, scales, ulcer, fissure, scar, and keloid are common secondary lesions.
- In dark-skinned people, paleness and cyanosis may make the skin appear dull and darker. Jaundice is more easily noted in the sclera and palms of the hands.
- Older adults experience loss of subcutaneous tissue, dermal thinning, and decreased elasticity, which increases fragility of skin. These factors increase the risk for pressure ulcers, especially if the older adult has limited mobility or is bedridden.

PEARSON NURSING STUDENT RESOURCES

Find additional materials at **nursing.pearsonhighered.com**.

NCLEX-PN® Exam Preparation

1 Which of the following age-related changes occur in the skin? **Select all that apply**.
1. Increased blood supply
2. Decreased skin elasticity
3. Development of liver spots
4. Appearance of petechiae
5. Increased response to heat
6. Thick yellow nails

2 What technique should the nurse use when inspecting the skin for tenting?
1. Pinch the skin gently over the collarbone.
2. Depress the patient's skin over the ankle.
3. Palpate the patient's skin for moisture.
4. Assess the patient's skin for lesions appearing in a group.

3 Which one of the following risk factors should the nurse ask the patient in regard to a risk factor for skin cancer?
1. Female under 50
2. Dark-colored hair and eyes
3. Living near a lake or river
4. Exposure to radiation

4 An African American patient is admitted with possible hepatitis. Which of the following integumentary manifestations should the nurse expect to find?
1. Yellow color of nailbeds
2. Patches of white spots on face
3. Yellow color of palms of hands
4. Dusky blue color of mucous membranes

5 What diagnostic test should the nurse anticipate to identify a fungal infection?
1. Skin biopsy
2. Skin scraping
3. Patch testing
4. Tzanck test

Answers and rationales for Review Questions appear in Appendix I.

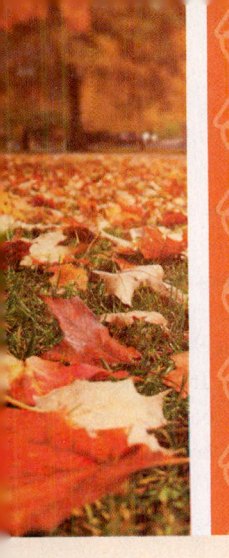

CHAPTER 45
Caring for Patients With Skin Disorders

BRIEF OUTLINE

Common Skin Disorders

Infections and Infestations
 of the Skin

Malignant Skin Disorders

Pressure Ulcers

LEARNING OUTCOMES

After completing this chapter, you will be able to:

1. Use the knowledge about skin changes in the older adult to an increased risk for dry skin, pruritus, skin cancer, and pressure ulcers.

2. Apply the pathophysiology and manifestations to the collaborative care of patients with common skin disorders, infections and infestations of the skin, malignant skin disorders, and pressure ulcers.

3. Use the nursing process to collect data and provide interventions for patients with common skin disorders, infections and infestations of the skin, malignant skin disorders, and pressure ulcers.

4. Provide patient and family teaching appropriate for prevention and self-care of disorders of the skin.

KEY TERMS

The key terms are defined on the pages listed below.

acne, 1137

basal cell carcinoma, 1148

candidiasis, 1142

cellulitis, 1142

dermatitis, 1137

dermatophytes, 1142

folliculitis, 1141

furuncle, 1142

herpes simplex, 1143

herpes zoster, 1143

melanoma, 1148

nevi, 1149

nonmelanoma skin cancers, 1148

pediculosis, 1144

pressure ulcers, 1154

pruritus, 1136

psoriasis, 1136

scabies, 1144

squamous cell carcinoma, 1148

warts, 1143

xerosis, 1136

SPECIAL FEATURES

NURSING CARE PLAN: Patient With Malignant Melanoma, 1153

CLINICAL REASONING CARE MAP: Caring for a Patient With Herpes Zoster, 1159

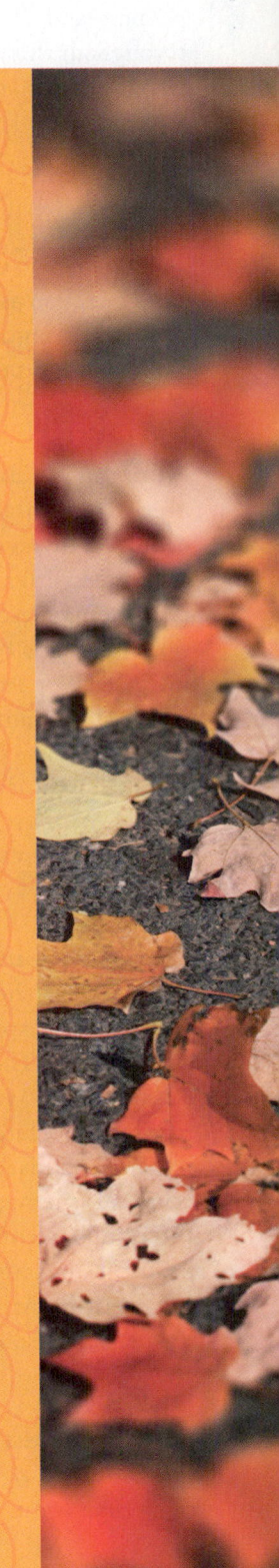

There are many different disorders of the skin. The patient with a minor or benign disorder is often treated in a physician's office or outpatient setting. The patient with a disorder that involves large areas of the body, is chronic, or is malignant may require inpatient care. The nurse collects data about patient needs and implements interventions to meet a wide variety of physical, emotional, and social responses.

Refer to Chapter 44, Table 44-2 for the common primary and secondary skin lesions. These terms are used throughout this and the next chapter. This chapter discusses common disorders of the skin. Chapter 46 discusses burns.

Common Skin Disorders

> **Key Concept**   Pruritus accompanies dry skin (xerosis) and many skin disorders and may result in excoriation and infection as a result of scratching. Patients with psoriasis, a chronic immune skin disorder, often experience pruritus.

PRURITUS

Pruritus is a subjective itching sensation that produces an urge to scratch. It may occur in a small, circumscribed area, or it may involve a widespread area; it may or may not be associated with a rash. Pruritus is not a disorder itself but is rather a manifestation of an underlying irritation or condition. Itching is triggered by heat and prostaglandins and is increased by release of histamine and other chemical mediators. Almost anything in the internal or external environment can cause pruritus. Insects, animals, plants, fabrics, metals, medications, allergies, and emotional distress are among the most common causes. Pruritus may also occur as a secondary manifestation of systemic disorders, such as certain types of cancer, diabetes mellitus, liver disease, and kidney failure.

Pruritus is initiated by a stimulation or irritation of receptors in the junction between the epidermis and dermis. The response by the person is to scratch or rub the affected area. This may irritate the skin and cause further inflammation, setting off a cycle of increasingly intense itching and scratching, called the *itch–scratch–itch* cycle.

The secondary effects of pruritus include skin excoriation, erythema, wheals, changes in pigmentation, and infections. Pruritus that persists may interrupt sleep patterns, because the itching sensation is often more intense at night. Long-term pruritus may be debilitating; broken skin also increases the risk of infection.

DRY SKIN

Dry skin (**xerosis**) is most often a problem in the older adult (see Chapter 44). In older adults, decreased activity of sebaceous and sweat glands reduces the skin's lubrication and moisture retention. However, dry skin may occur at any age as a result of exposure to environmental heat and low humidity, sunlight, excessive bathing, and a decreased intake of liquids.

The primary manifestation of dry skin is pruritus. Other manifestations include visible flaking of surface skin and an observable pattern of fine lines over the area. If the skin has been excessively dry and pruritic for a long period, the patient may have secondary skin lesions and *lichenification* (thickening).

PSORIASIS

Psoriasis is a benign, chronic inflammatory skin disorder. It is characterized by raised, reddened, round circumscribed plaques of varied size, covered by silvery white scales (Figure 45-1 ■). The plaques shed thick gray scales. The lesions may appear anywhere on the body. However, they are most commonly found on the scalp, extensor surfaces of the arms and legs, elbows, knees, sacrum, and around the nails. As with any chronic illness, the skin manifestations may disappear and recur throughout life.

The actual cause of psoriasis is unknown, but evidence suggests it is an autoimmune disorder. Sunlight, stress, seasonal changes, hormone fluctuations, steroid withdrawal, and certain drugs (e.g., beta-blockers, corticosteroids, lithium, and chloroquine) appear to make the disorder worse. About one-third of patients have a family history of psoriasis. Trauma to the skin from surgery, sunburn, or excoriation may also precipitate it. Arthritis is known to develop in about 20% of the patients with psoriasis.

Pruritus is common over the lesions. If the lesions are located in an *intertriginous zone* (between toes, under breasts, or in the perianal region), the psoriatic scales may soften, allowing painful fissures to form. When psoriasis affects the nails, pitting and a yellow or brown discoloration results. The nail may separate from the nail bed, thicken, and crumble, increasing the risk for infection.

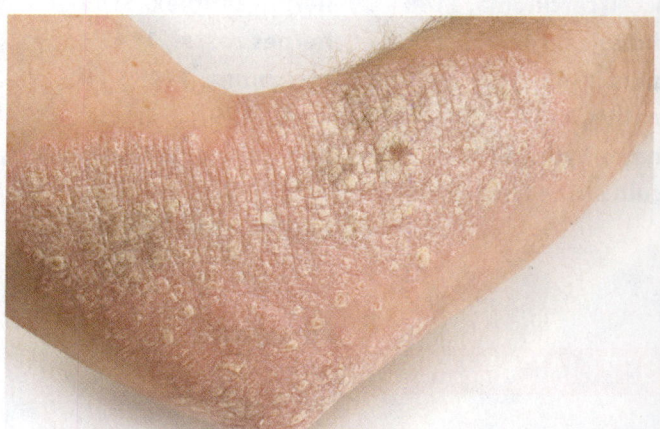

Figure 45-1. ■ The characteristic lesions of psoriasis are raised, red, round plaques covered with thick, silvery scales. (Source: Pearson Education.)

DERMATITIS

Dermatitis is an acute or chronic inflammation of the skin characterized by erythema and pain or pruritus. Various agents or illnesses cause the inflammatory response of the skin. Initial skin responses include erythema, formation of vesicles and scales, and pruritus. Later, irritation from scratching promotes edema, a serous discharge, and crusting. Long-term irritation in chronic dermatitis causes the skin to become thickened, leathery, and darker in color.

Contact (allergic) dermatitis is caused by a hypersensitivity response or chemical irritation. The major sources known to cause contact dermatitis are dyes, perfumes, poison plants (ivy, oak, sumac), chemicals, and metals. Latex dermatitis is a contact dermatitis that is common in the health care field.

Atopic dermatitis is also called *eczema*. The exact cause is unknown, but related factors include depressed cell-mediated immunity, elevated immunoglobulin E (IgE) levels, and increased histamine sensitivity. Patients with atopic dermatitis have a family history of hypersensitivity reactions, such as eczema, asthma, and allergic rhinitis. Characteristic lesions include chronic lichenification, erythema, and scaling, the result of pruritus and scratching. The lesions are usually found on the hands, feet, or flexor surfaces of the arms and legs (Figure 45-2 ■). Scratching and excoriation increase the risk of secondary infections, as well as invasion of the skin by viruses such as herpes simplex.

Seborrheic dermatitis is a chronic inflammatory disorder that involves the scalp, eyebrows, eyelids, ear canals, nasolabial folds, axillae, and trunk. The cause is unknown. This disorder is seen in all ages, from the very young (called "cradle cap") to the very old. Patients taking methyldopa (Aldomet) for hypertension occasionally develop this disorder, and it is a component of Parkinson disease. Seborrheic dermatitis is also frequently seen in patients with AIDS. The lesions are yellow or white plaques with scales and crusts. The scales are often yellow or orange and have a greasy appearance. Mild pruritus is also present.

Exfoliative dermatitis is an inflammatory skin disorder characterized by excessive peeling or shedding of skin. A preexisting skin disorder such as psoriasis, atopic dermatitis, contact dermatitis, or seborrheic dermatitis may be present. Exfoliative dermatitis is also associated with leukemia and lymphoma. Systemic manifestations include weakness, malaise, fever, chills, and weight loss. Scaling, erythema, and pruritus may be localized or involve the entire body. In addition to peeling of skin, the patient may lose the hair and nails.

ACNE

Acne is a disorder of the sebaceous glands. These glands empty into the hair follicles and are open to the skin surface through a pore. They produce sebum in response to direct hormonal stimulation by testicular androgens in men and to adrenal and ovarian androgens in women. Most sebaceous glands are on the face, scalp, and scrotum.

Acne lesions are primarily *comedones* (pimples, whiteheads, and blackheads). Whiteheads are pale, slightly elevated papules. Blackheads are plugs of material that accumulate in the sebaceous glands. Inflammatory acne lesions include comedones, erythematous pustules, and cysts (Figure 45-3 ■). The lesions may itch. The common types of acne are as follows:

- *Acne vulgaris* is common in adolescents and young to middle-aged adults. Many factors once thought to cause acne vulgaris, including high-fat diets, chocolate, infections, and cosmetics, have been disproved (Porth, 2011).
- *Acne rosacea,* chronic facial acne, occurs more often in middle-age and older adults. The lesions begin with erythema over the cheeks and nose. Over years of time, the skin color changes to dark red, and the pores over the area become enlarged.

COLLABORATIVE CARE

Pruritus, dry skin, psoriasis, dermatitis, and acne are most often treated by self-care at home. Treatment focuses on identifying and eliminating or modifying any precipitating

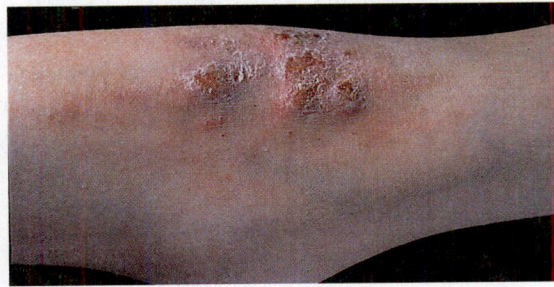

Figure 45-2. ■ Atopic dermatitis or eczema. (Source: © Wellcome Image Library/Custom Medical Stock Photo.)

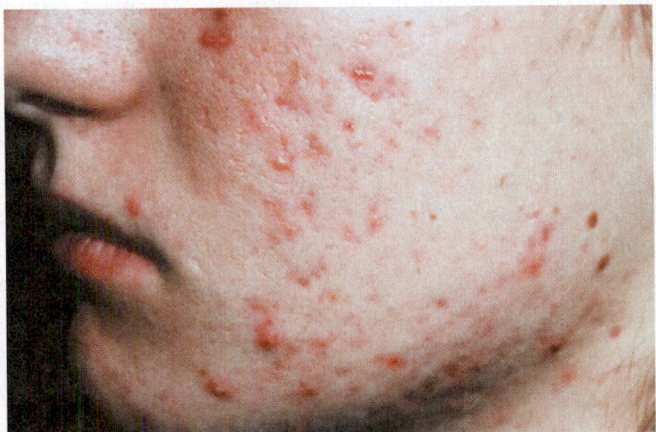

Figure 45-3. ■ Inflammatory acne lesions include comedones, erythematous pustules, and cysts. These lesions often leave scars when they heal. (Source: Pearson Education.)

factors, providing relief from itching and pain, and reducing the risk of further damage to the skin.

Diagnostic Tests

Culture and sensitivity of skin scrapings and studies for fungal infections are conducted by microscopic examination to distinguish pruritus from psoriasis, dermatitis, and other disorders. Cutaneous scratch or patch testing may be performed if allergic reactions are the suspected cause.

If the patient has atypical manifestations, or to differentiate psoriasis from inflammatory or infectious dermatitis, a skin biopsy may be done. Ultrasound tests may be performed to measure skin thickness. Results reveal typical psoriatic changes in the stratum corneum layer (see Figure 44-1) of the epidermis and dermal inflammation.

Medications

PRURITUS   If possible, the patient discontinues all medications to determine whether the pruritus is due to a drug reaction. Oral medications include antihistamines, tranquilizers, and antibiotics. Antihistamines provide relief from pruritus in some patients. Tranquilizers provide sedation, which may relieve the emotional stress associated with pruritus. Systemic antibiotics are used to treat infection resulting from the scratching and excoriation.

Topical medications that contain corticosteroids are often used to relieve pruritus and inflammation. Topical medications may also be administered through therapeutic baths or soaks with agents that relieve pruritus, such as cornstarch, baking soda, or coal tar concentrates (see Box 45-1■). Creams with a topical anesthetic may also be used.

PSORIASIS   Topical corticosteroids, tar preparations, and retinoids decrease inflammation and suppress mitotic activity of psoriatic cells. The most effective topical corticosteroids are potent preparations. They are well absorbed through the skin and are used under an occlusive dressing. Corticosteroids may also be taken systemically or injected directly into the lesions. Tar preparations such as Estar, PsoriGel, and Fototar, applied topically or in a bath, are effective to remove scales and increase remission. They do have the undesirable side effect of staining. A topical retinoid (Tazarotene [Tazorac]) gel results in longer-lasting remissions but may cause skin irritation and pruritus. Calcipotriene (Dovonex), a vitamin D analogue, has been shown to be effective and safe in both short- and long-term treatment of psoriasis. Biologic response modifiers such as etanercept (Enbrel) and infliximab (Remicade) are given by injection to patients with more extensive psoriasis and psoriatic arthritis. Patients with severe cases of psoriasis may receive methotrexate (MTX) or cyclosporine (Neoral).

BOX 45-1	THERAPEUTIC BATHS

Agents Used in Therapeutic Baths

- Saline or tap water
- Antibacterial agents: potassium permanganate, acetic acid, hexachlorophene
- Colloid substances: oatmeal (Aveeno), cornstarch, sodium bicarbonate
- Coal tar derivatives: Balnetar, Zetar, Polytar
- Emollients: Alpha-Keri, Lubath, mineral oil

Therapeutic baths have a variety of uses in treating skin disorders. Depending on the agent used, therapeutic baths soothe the skin, lower the skin bacteria count, clean and hydrate the skin, loosen scales, and relieve itching.

Nursing Responsibilities

- Ensure that the bathwater is at a comfortable temperature that is neither too hot nor too cool (usually 110° to 115°F [43° to 46°C]).
- Fill the tub one-third to one-half full.
- Mix the agent well with the water.
- Assist the patient into and out of the tub to prevent falls.
- Dry the patient by blotting with the towel.

Patient and Family Teaching

- Use a bath mat in the tub: The medications may cause the tub to become slippery.
- Keep the bathroom warm but adequately ventilated.
- Follow directions carefully for the amount of medication to use in the bath.
- Fill the bath one-third to one-half full of water that is at a comfortable temperature.
- Stay in the bath for 20 to 30 minutes, and immerse the areas to be treated.
- Do not get the bathwater in your eyes.
- Dry by blotting (not rubbing) with the towel.
- If the medications cause staining, use old towels or linens.
- If the itching is not relieved or the skin becomes excessively dry, call your health care provider.

Photochemotherapy, using methoxsalen, is a treatment for severe psoriasis. This drug is an antimetabolite that inhibits deoxyribonucleic acid (DNA) synthesis. Exposure to ultraviolet A (UVA) rays activates methoxsalen. It is administered orally, and the patient is exposed to UVA 2 hours later. Treatments are administered two to three times a week for 10 to 20 total treatments. The eyes are covered by dark glasses during the treatment. Treatment causes tanning, and direct sunlight must be avoided for 8 to 12 hours thereafter. If the patient has erythema, the treatments are stopped until the redness and swelling resolve. Photochemotherapy can accelerate aging of exposed skin, induce cataract development, alter immune function, and increase the risk of melanoma.

Ultraviolet B (UVB) light is often used to treat psoriasis. UVB light decreases the growth rate of epidermal cells. Mercury vapor lights or fluorescent UV tubes provide the UVB light. Fluorescent tubes are often arranged in a cabinet so the patient can stand and expose psoriatic lesions more easily. These units may be purchased or constructed to be used in the patient's home. The light therapy is administered in gradually increasing exposure times, until the patient experiences a mild erythema, like a mild sunburn. Treatments are given daily and are measured in seconds of exposure. The eyes are shielded during the treatment. The erythema response occurs in about 8 hours. Careful assessment is necessary to prevent more severe burning, which could exacerbate the psoriasis.

ACNE Treatment for acne is based on the type and severity of the lesions. For acne with comedones, tretinoin (Retin-A) or benzoyl peroxide preparations are prescribed. Azelaic acid (Azelex) may also be used. Benzoyl peroxide preparations are found in over-the-counter medications such as Fostex, Acne-Dome, Desquam-X, Benzagel, Clear By Design, and Xerac BP. These products loosen the comedones. Inflammatory acne is treated with oral or topical antibiotics, such as clindamycin, tetracycline, erythromycin, and minocycline. Severe forms of inflammatory acne are treated with isotretinoin (Accutane), which is effective but has serious side effects. Nursing responsibilities for these medications are discussed in Table 45-1 ■. The treatment for acne lasts months and, in some cases, for the rest of one's life.

Surgery

Dermabrasion of inactive acne lesions can improve the patient's appearance, especially if the scars are flat. The skin is first frozen (and anesthetized) with Freon or ethyl chloride. The lesions are carefully abraded with fine sandpaper or abrasive brushes.

Complementary Therapies

Topical aloe therapy may be used for managing psoriasis, acne, and eczema. Overuse of aloe may result in atopic dermatitis. Goldenseal can be applied topically to treat eczema, acne, and itching. Peppermint oil is applied to the skin to decrease pruritus, but use cautiously because skin irritation and contact dermatitis may develop.

NURSING CARE

Nursing care for the patient with common skin problems focuses on promoting comfort and decreasing the risk of infection. Because patients care for themselves at home, nursing interventions are primarily educational. Teaching focuses on methods of relieving itching and dry skin and preventing infection. Patients with psoriasis require information about medications and light treatments.

PRIORITIZING NURSING CARE

Although pruritus, dry skin, psoriasis, dermatitis, and acne are not life threatening, they may result in physical and emotional distress. Priority nursing care focuses on impaired skin integrity due to the high risk for infection. It is important to include nursing care related to altered body image and possible knowledge deficiency about medication administration.

HEALTH PROMOTION

Activities that promote good health are similar to measures that improve healthy skin. For example, it is important to avoid overexposure to ultraviolet rays, chemical irritants, and radiation. A well-balanced diet and adequate sleep can promote healthy skin, hair, and nails. Exercise increases circulation, causing a healthy glow to the skin. Bathing should be done often enough to remove excess oil and perspiration to prevent odor.

TABLE 45-1	Giving Medications Safely: Acne		
CLASS/DRUGS	**PURPOSE**	**NURSING IMPLICATIONS**	**PATIENT TEACHING**
Antiacne retinoids ■ Tretinoin (Retin-A) ■ Isotretinoin (Accutane)	Tretinoin is a topical agent that decreases comedone formation. Isotretinoin is a vitamin A metabolite that decreases sebum production.	Do not administer to patients with eczema or who are sensitive to the sun. Do not administer to pregnant women. Assess for side effects of redness, scaling, severe erythema with topical use.	Tretinoin: Apply to clean, dry skin. Expect redness and peeling of skin. Isotretinoin: Take pills with food. Avoid taking vitamin A supplements or alcohol with this drug. Use sunscreen and protective clothing when outside. Use a reliable contraceptive for 1 month before, during, and 1 month after the therapy. If visual changes, nausea, vomiting, and headache occur, report manifestations to the physician.

ASSESSING

Assessment data are collected by the nurse to determine the degree of discomfort, the extent to which the skin condition is interfering with the patient's activities of daily living and usual lifestyle, and the risk factors for complications. Box 45-2■ suggests subjective and objective data to collect.

DIAGNOSING, PLANNING, AND IMPLEMENTING
Impaired Skin Integrity

Expected outcome: Will state reduction in pruritus, pain, and reddened skin.

clinical**ALERT**

Use warm—not hot—water because hot water dries the skin and increases itching.

- Recommend that the nails be trimmed short, the environmental temperatures be slightly cool, and loose clothing be worn. *These measures relieve pruritus and decrease the risk of infection.*
- Suggest the following strategies to relieve itching:
  - Rub the pruritic area with the surface of the hand rather than scratching with the nails, briefly apply pressure or cold to help relieve pruritus, and wear cotton gloves at night.

BOX 45-2	ASSESSMENT

Patients With Common Skin Problems

Subjective Data
- Location, duration, and type of itching or skin lesion present
- Ability to sleep at night
- Skin oily or dry, amount of sweating
- Medications used to treat dry skin, itching, or skin lesions
- History of allergies
- History of exposure to environmental substances
- Chronic illness, such as thyroid disorders, diabetes mellitus, or liver disease

Objective Data
- Inspect the entire skin for color and lesions:
  - Redness, swelling, and pain may indicate a secondary infection from itching or may follow phototherapy treatments for psoriasis.
  - Dry, rough skin with visible flaking indicates severe xerosis.
- Palpate the skin for temperature, texture, moisture, and turgor:
  - Increased warmth may indicate infection. Dry skin is rough.
  - Pinch the skin gently over the collarbone or top of the hand; tenting (in which the skin remains in a fold for a few moments) is common in older adults.

- Use distraction or relaxation techniques.
- Wash clothing in a mild detergent and rinse twice. Do not use fabric softeners.
- Avoid using perfumes and lotions containing alcohol, and apply skin lubricants after a bath to help retain moisture.

These strategies relieve itching and prevent excoriation.

- Demonstrate methods of taking therapeutic baths or treatments. Gently rub lesions with a soft washcloth, using a circular motion. *Gentle rubbing reduces the risk of injury to the skin.*
- Dry the skin with a soft towel, using a blotting or patting motion. *Washing or drying the skin with rough linens may excoriate the skin over lesions.*
- Teach the patient and family to watch for and report to the health care provider any complications of treatment, such as excoriation, increased redness, increased skin peeling, or blister formation. *The medications and treatments may cause damage to skin cells through chemical burns or exposure to ultraviolet light. Times and methods of treatment need to be adjusted if these occur.*

Disturbed Body Image

Expected outcome: Will verbalize positive feelings toward self.

- Establish a trusting nurse–patient relationship by verbally and nonverbally expressing acceptance. For example, touching the patient demonstrates that the lesions and the patient's appearance are not offensive. *One's body image is affected not only by self-perception but also by the responses of others. The skin eruptions and lesions, especially chronic ones, often cause patients to isolate themselves from social contacts, withdraw from normal roles and responsibilities, and feel helpless or powerless.*
- Encourage talking about self-perception and questions about the disease and the treatment. *The patient adapts to a changed body image through a process of recognition, acceptance, and resolution. Each person responds individually to changes in body image and loss.*
- Encourage interaction with others through family involvement in care, referral to support groups, and referral to organizations such as the National Psoriasis Foundation. *Acceptance of others is critical to acceptance of self. By becoming involved in care, the family demonstrates love and acceptance. Sharing experiences with others who have the same health problem is a source of strength in adjusting to a visible health problem. Local, state, and national organizations can provide resources and information.*

Deficient Knowledge (Medication Administration)

Expected outcome: Will demonstrate medication administration guidelines.

Teach the patient the following general guidelines for applying topical medications:

- Each time a medication is applied, the skin surface must be clean and dry. Remove creams by washing with tap water. Remove ointments by first washing the skin with mineral oil and then with mild soap and water.
- To apply *gels, creams,* and *pastes:* Squeeze about 1/2 to 1 in. of the medication onto a gloved hand and apply to the affected areas using long strokes until the skin is thinly covered. Exceptions:
  - *Corticosteroids* are usually applied two or three times a day in small amounts and rubbed directly into the skin. If prescribed, cover with a dressing.
  - Medications containing *tar* are applied in the direction of the hair growth. Do not apply these medications to the face, to the genitals, or in skin folds. These medications will stain clothing.
- To apply *lotions:* Shake the bottle well. Pour a small amount into the palm of the hand and pat the medication on the skin. If the lotion is thin, use a gauze pad.
- To apply *sprays:* Hold the container about 6 in. from the skin and apply the medication in a short spray.
- To apply *medicated shampoo:* Rinse the hair. Apply the shampoo, massage into the hair and scalp. Allow it to remain for the prescribed time. Rinse.
- To apply *pastes:* Use enough paste on an applicator (e.g., a wooden tongue depressor) to cover the lesion thinly. *Teaching guidelines ensure accurate administration.*

clinicalALERT

Teach patients using oral corticosteroids to never stop taking the medication abruptly.

MANAGING NURSING CARE

As appropriate and allowed by the designated duties and responsibilities of assistive personnel, the nurse may assign nursing care activities such as assisting with hygiene measures for the patient with pruritus, dry skin, psoriasis, dermatitis, and acne.

EVALUATING

Collect data to determine the patient's knowledge of medications and their use, the patient's degree of comfort, and any changes in the level of skin integrity or involvement.

DOCUMENTING

Document appearance of lesions, effectiveness of pruritic-relief measures, and patient teaching about medications and therapeutic baths.

CONTINUITY OF CARE

In addition to teaching the patient how to administer topical medications, the nurse should provide the following information for self-care:

- Medications and treatments do not cure the disease. They only relieve the symptoms.
- Dry skin increases pruritus, which stimulates scratching. Scratching may in turn cause excoriation, and excoriation increases the risk of infection.
- It may be necessary to change the diet or environment to avoid contact with allergens.

Infections and Infestations of the Skin

Key Concept The skin provides an ideal environment for bacterial and fungal growth. Viral infections of the skin are often difficult to treat. Skin infections and infestations not only involve treating the disorder but also focus on preventing the spread of infection.

The skin's resistance to infections and infestations is provided by normal skin flora, sebum, and the immune response. Disorders may occur from a break in the skin surface, a virulent agent, or decreased resistance due to a compromised immune system.

BACTERIAL INFECTIONS

Bacterial infections of the skin arise from the hair follicle, where bacteria can accumulate and grow and cause a localized infection. If the bacteria invade deeper tissues, they can cause a systemic infection, a potentially life-threatening disorder. Most bacterial infections are treated by a primary care provider, and the patient remains at home for care. Hospital-acquired (nosocomial) infections of wounds or open lesions often result from bacterial infections, especially by methicillin-resistant *Staphylococcus aureus* (MRSA) as discussed in Chapter 9.

Folliculitis

Folliculitis is most often caused by *Staphylococcus aureus.* The infection begins at the skin surface and extends down into the hair follicle. The bacteria release enzymes and chemical agents that cause an inflammation. The lesions appear as pustules surrounded by an area of erythema on the surface of the skin. Folliculitis is found most often on the scalp and extremities, on the face of bearded men, on the legs of women who shave, and on the eyelids (called a *stye*). Although folliculitis may appear without any apparent cause, contributing factors include poor hygiene, poor nutrition, prolonged skin moisture, and trauma to the skin.

Furuncles

A **furuncle** ("boil") is also an infection of the hair follicle. A group of infected hair follicles is called a *carbuncle*. It often begins as folliculitis, but the infection spreads down the hair shaft, through the wall of the follicle, and into the dermis. The causative organism is commonly *Staphylococcus aureus.* Contributing factors include poor hygiene, trauma to the skin, areas of excessive moisture including perspiration, and systemic diseases, such as diabetes mellitus.

A furuncle is initially a deep, firm, red, painful nodule from 1 to 5 cm in diameter. After a few days, the nodule changes into a large, tender cystic nodule. The cysts may contain purulent drainage. Carbuncles are a group of infected hair follicles and have multiple openings onto the skin. They may cause fever, chills, and malaise in addition to the local manifestations.

Cellulitis

Cellulitis is a localized infection of the dermis and subcutaneous tissue. It can occur after a wound or skin ulcer or as an extension of furuncles or carbuncles. The infection spreads as a result of a substance called spreading factor (*hyaluronidase*), which is produced by the causative organism. Hyaluronidase breaks down the fibrin network and other barriers that normally localize the infection in the skin.

The area of cellulitis is red, swollen, and painful (Figure 45-4■). In some cases, vesicles may form over the area of cellulitis. The patient may also experience fever, chills, malaise, headache, and swollen lymph glands.

FUNGAL INFECTIONS

Fungi are plantlike organisms that live in the soil, on animals, and on humans. The fungi that cause superficial skin infections are called **dermatophytes**. In humans, the dermatophytes live on keratin in the stratum corneum, hair, and nails. Superficial fungal infections of the skin are often referred to as *ringworm* or *tinea*. Fungal disorders are also called *mycoses.*

The organism may be transmitted by direct contact with animals or other infected persons or by inanimate objects such as combs, pillowcases, towels, and hats. The onset and spread of the fungal infection is greatest in moist areas, such as in skin folds, between the toes, and in the mouth. Other factors that increase the risk of a fungal infection include the use of broad-spectrum antibiotics that kill off normal flora and allow the fungi to grow, the presence of diabetes mellitus, immunodeficiencies, nutritional deficiencies, pregnancy, increasing age, and iron deficiency.

Dermatophyte (Tinea) Infections

The dermatophyte (*tinea*) infections are named by the body part affected. Those most common in adults are as follows:

- *Tinea pedis (athlete's foot)* affects the soles of the feet, the space between the toes, and the toenail. The lesions vary from mild scaliness to painful fissures with drainage, and they are usually accompanied by pruritus and a foul odor.

- *Tinea cruris* is an infection of the groin that may extend to the inner thighs and buttocks. Also called "jock itch," it is often associated with tinea pedis and is more common in people who are physically active, are obese, and wear tight underclothing.

Candidiasis Infections

Candidiasis infections are caused by *Candida albicans,* a yeastlike fungus. This fungus is normally found on mucous membranes, on the skin, in the vagina, and in the gastrointestinal tract. The fungus becomes a pathogen when certain conditions encourage its growth: an environment of moisture, warmth, or altered skin integrity; systemic antibiotics; pregnancy; birth control pills; poor nutrition; immunosuppression; or diabetes mellitus, Cushing disease, or other chronic debilitating illnesses.

Candidiasis affects only the outer layers of the skin and mucous membranes. It occurs in the mouth, vagina, uncircumcised penis, nails, and deep skin folds. The first sign of infection is a pustule that often burns and itches. As the infection spreads, a white to yellow curdlike substance covers the infected area.

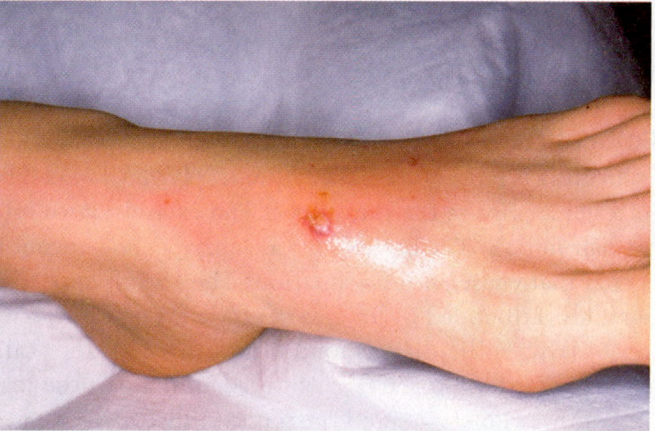

Figure 45-4. ■ Cellulitis is a bacterial infection localized in the dermis and subcutaneous tissue. The involved area is red, swollen, and painful. (Source: Pearson Education.)

VIRAL INFECTIONS

Viruses are pathogens that consist of a ribonucleic acid (RNA) or DNA core surrounded by a protein coat. They depend on live cells for reproduction. The viruses that cause skin lesions either increase cellular growth or cause cellular death. An increase in the incidence of viral skin disorders has been attributed to a variety of causes, including some commonly used drugs such as birth control medications, corticosteroids, and antibiotics.

Warts

Warts (*verrucae*) are lesions caused by the human papillomavirus (HPV). Warts may be found on skin and mucous membranes. Nongenital warts are benign lesions; genital warts may be precancerous. Warts are transmitted through skin contact. Warts may be flat, fusiform (tapered at both ends), or round, but most are round and raised and have a rough, gray surface. Warts resolve spontaneously when immunity to the virus develops. This response may take up to 5 years. There are many different types of HPV. Those most common are described here:

■ A *common wart* may occur anywhere on the skin or mucous membranes. It grows above the skin surface and may be dome-shaped with ragged borders. A flat wart is a small flat lesion, usually seen on the forehead or dorsum of the hand.

■ *Plantar warts* occur at pressure points on the soles of the feet. The pressure of shoes and walking prevents these warts from growing outward. They tend to extend deeper beneath the skin surface than common warts, and they are often painful.

■ *Condylomata acuminata (venereal warts)* occur in moist areas, along the glans of the penis, in the anal region, and on the vulva. They are usually cauliflowerlike in appearance and have a pink or purple color (see Chapter 33, Figure 33-4).

Herpes Simplex

Herpes simplex ("fever blister," "cold sore") infections are caused by two types of herpesvirus: HSV I and HSV II. Most infections above the waist, most commonly on lips, face, and mouth, are caused by HSV I. (Genital herpes infections, which result from either HSV I or HSV II, are classified as sexually transmitted infections and are discussed in Chapter 33.) The virus may be transmitted by physical contact, oral sex, or kissing. The virus lives in nerve ganglia and may cause recurrent lesions in response to sunlight, menstruation, injury, or stress.

The infection begins with a burning or tingling sensation, followed by the development of erythema, vesicle formation, and pain. The vesicles progress through pustules, ulcers, and crusting until healing occurs in 10 to 14 days. The initial infection is often severe and accompanied by systemic manifestations, such as fever and sore throat. Recurrences are more localized and less severe.

Herpes Zoster

Herpes zoster ("shingles") is a viral infection of the skin caused by varicella zoster, the same herpesvirus that causes chickenpox. The varicella virus remains dormant in the sensory dorsal ganglia. Years after the initial chickenpox infection, the virus becomes reactivated. This most often occurs when the patient is immunosuppressed. Once the virus is reactivated, inflammation and painful vesicles develop in the skin area connected to the same sensory dorsal ganglia (Figure 45-5 ■).

Patients with Hodgkin disease, certain types of leukemia, and lymphomas are more susceptible to an outbreak of herpes zoster. Herpes zoster is more prevalent in people who are immunocompromised (e.g., by HIV), those who are receiving radiation therapy or chemotherapy, and those who have had major organ transplants. In people

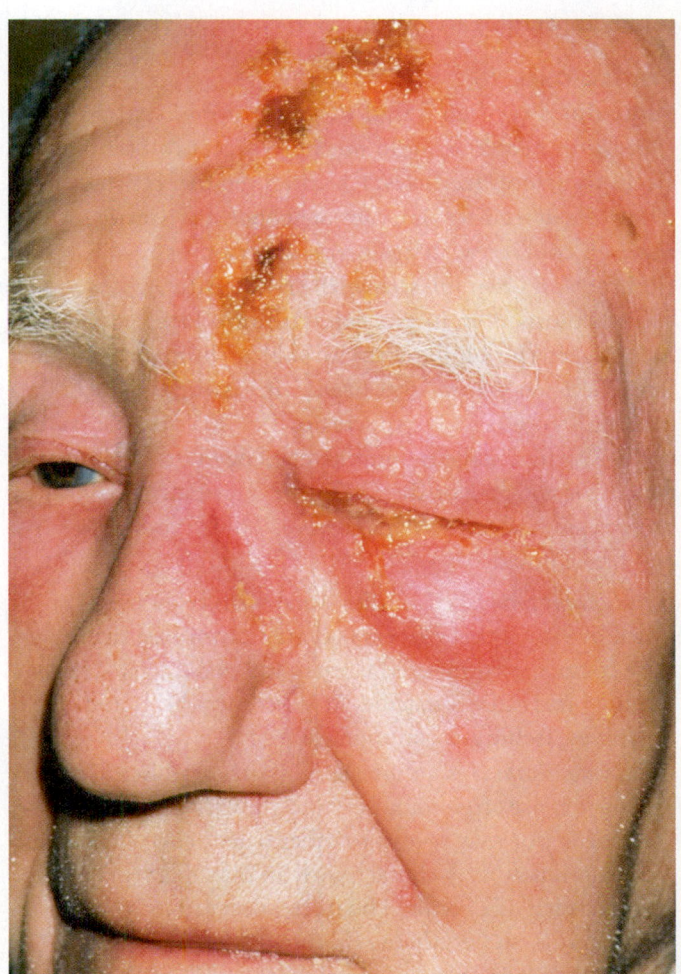

Figure 45-5. ■ The lesions of herpes zoster erupt along the nerve pathway and are extremely painful. (Source: Dr. P. Marazzi/Science Source.)

with HIV infections, the appearance of the lesions may be one of the first manifestations of immune compromise.

The lesions are vesicles with an erythematous base. They usually appear unilaterally on the face, trunk, and thorax; continue to erupt for 3 to 5 days; then crust and dry. Recovery occurs in 2 to 3 weeks. The patient experiences severe pain before and during eruption of the lesions. The older adult is especially sensitive to the pain and often experiences more severe outbreaks of herpes zoster lesions. In most cases, the disease is benign and localized. Complications of herpes zoster include *postherpetic neuralgia* (a sharp, spasmodic pain along the course of one or more nerves) and vision loss. The neuralgia, described as burning or stabbing, results from inflammation of the root ganglia. Permanent loss of vision may follow occurrence of lesions that arise from the ophthalmic division of the trigeminal nerve.

PARASITIC INFESTATIONS

The skin may be invaded by parasites or insects. Infestations affect people of all social classes but are associated with crowded or unsanitary living conditions. Two of the more common parasites are mites and lice.

Pediculosis

Pediculosis is often found in overcrowded living conditions or in people who do not have access to bathing and clothes-washing facilities. Children tend to contract head lice while attending day care or school. Infestation occurs through contact with an infected person or contact with clothing and linen infested with the parasites.

Pediculosis is an infestation with lice. Lice are parasites that ingest the blood of an animal or human host. One louse (a 2- to 4-mm oval organism) is capable of laying hundreds of eggs. All species of lice have a similar life cycle. The first stage is an unhatched egg (a *nit*) laid by the female louse on a hair shaft. The nit is a small pearl-gray or brown egg visible to the naked eye. Three types of lice live on human hosts:

- *Pediculosis corporis* is an infestation with body lice. The lice live in clothing fibers and are transmitted primarily by contact with infested clothes and bed linens. The louse bites cause a macule, followed by wheals and papules. Itching is common.
- *Pediculosis capitis* is an infestation with head lice. The lice are most often found behind the ears and nape of the neck but may spread to other hairy areas of the body. Transmission is by contact with an infected person or object such as a comb. The infestation causes itching, scratching, and erythema (Figure 45-6 ■).
- *Pediculosis pubis* is an infestation with pubic lice ("crabs"). The lice are spread through sexual activity or contact with infested clothing or linens. The infestation causes skin irritation and intense itching.

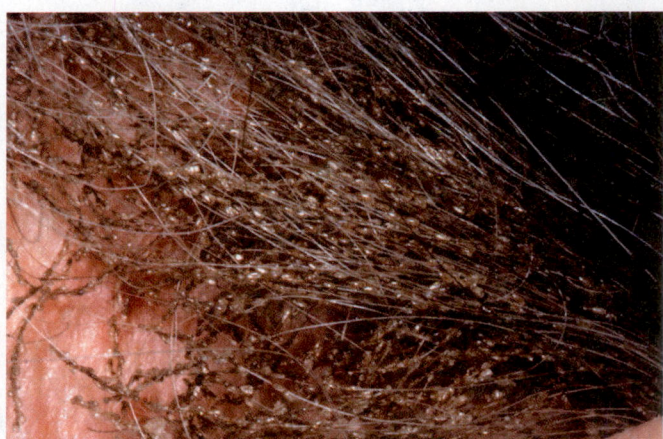

Figure 45-6. ■ Head lice crawling through hair. (Source: © Wellcome Image Library/Custom Medical Stock Photo.)

Scabies

Scabies is an infestation caused by the female mite. It affects people of all races, ages, and socioeconomic classes. Outbreaks of scabies occur frequently in shelters, college dormitories, and long-term care facilities. It is spread from skin-to-skin contact, but the mite can live for 2 days on clothing and bedding.

Scabies is found between the fingers and on the inner surfaces of the wrist and elbow, the axillae, the female nipple, the penis, the belt line, and the gluteal crease. Lesions appear about 2 to 6 weeks after contact with an infected individual. The lesions are small red-brown burrows, about 2 mm in length, sometimes covered with vesicles that appear as a rash. Pruritus is common, especially at night. Excoriations from scratching predispose the person to secondary bacterial infections.

COLLABORATIVE CARE

Patients with infections and infestations of the skin and mucous membranes are usually diagnosed and treated by their primary health care provider and then provide self-care at home. Treatment is focused on identifying the causative agent, administering medications to kill the bacteria or eradicate the organism, and preventing secondary infections. Environments such as day care centers, schools, hospitals, and long-term care facilities that are infested with lice or scabies must be vacuumed and cleaned thoroughly.

Diagnostic Tests

Bacterial infections are diagnosed by a culture and sensitivity of the drainage from a lesion to identify organisms and to target the most effective antibiotic. If the infection is systemic, a blood culture may be conducted to identify the causative organism.

Fungal infections are diagnosed by various methods. Cultures of skin scrapings, nail scrapings, or hairs are done.

Microscopic examination of scrapings may be done to visualize spores and filaments. The affected skin may be inspected under ultraviolet light (called a Wood's lamp); fungal spores fluoresce blue-green.

Laboratory tests may be necessary to differentiate herpes zoster from impetigo, contact dermatitis, or herpes simplex. Cultures of fluids from vesicles and antibody tests are used to identify the herpesvirus types.

When a patient has pediculosis, the hair shaft and clothing are inspected for the lice or the nits, with microscopic examination used for a positive diagnosis. Scabies is diagnosed by skin scrapings and microscopic examination of the mites or their feces.

Medications

BACTERIAL INFECTIONS   The primary treatment for bacterial infections is an antibiotic specific to the organism. The antibiotic is usually administered systemically but may also be applied topically. Multiple furuncles and carbuncles may be treated with cloxacillin, penicillinase-resistant penicillin; the cephalosporins are also often effective. Antibiotic therapy is discussed in Chapter 9.

FUNGAL INFECTIONS   Fungal infections are treated by topical or systemic antifungal medications. Nursing implications for antifungal medications are discussed in Table 45-2■. Dermatophyte infections are usually treated with topical antifungals. Candidiasis infections are treated with nystatin (Mycostatin) in powder, tablet, or vaginal suppository form. Other medications that may be used include ketoconazole and fluconazole, administered orally.

VIRAL INFECTIONS   Most viral skin infections are treated with antiviral medications, and other medications are used to relieve pruritus and pain in patients with herpes zoster. A common method of wart removal is acid therapy, using a colloidal solution of 16% salicylic acid and 16% lactic acid.

The solution is applied to the wart every 12 to 24 hours, and the wart disappears in 2 or 3 weeks. Other methods of eradicating warts are cryosurgery, freezing with liquid nitrogen, and electrodesiccation with an electric cautery. Herpes lesions are treated with acyclovir (Zovirax), an antiviral agent that may be administered topically, orally, or parenterally. Zostavax (a weakened form of varicella-zoster virus) is a vaccine used for adults age 60 years or older to prevent herpes zoster.

PARASITIC INFESTATIONS   Lice are eradicated with topical agents that kill the parasite, such as medications that contain gamma benzene hexachloride, malathion (Prioderm lotion), or permethrin (NIX). Hair infestations are treated with lindane lotion, such as Kwell. A fine-toothed comb is often used to comb the dead nits off the hair shaft. Scabies may be eradicated with a single treatment of Kwell, applied to the entire skin surface.

Complementary Therapies

Tea tree oil, taken from the Australian tea tree (*Melaleuca alternifolia*), has been used to relieve discomfort and speed healing of boils and carbuncles. Most natural food stores carry tea tree oil products. If these products cause allergic reactions, they should be stopped immediately.

NURSING CARE

Nursing care of the patient with a skin infection or infestation focuses on preventing the spread of infection and restoring normal skin integrity. Most patients provide self-care at home. If the hospitalized patient develops a secondary bacterial infection, isolation procedures should be implemented to limit the spread of infection to others.

One of the most effective methods of reducing the spread of infection in any setting is careful hand washing. Health care providers must wash their hands with soap and water

TABLE 45-2	Giving Medications Safely: Fungal Infections		
CLASS/DRUGS	PURPOSE	NURSING IMPLICATIONS	PATIENT TEACHING
■ Nystatin (Mycostatin) ■ Griseofulvin (Fulvicin)	Some drugs interfere with the fungal cell membrane permeability; others interfere with DNA synthesis. They are prepared in many forms: powders, shampoos, suspensions, troches, oral tablets, and vaginal suppositories. Amphotericin B is given intravenously. Assess for known hypersensitivity to these agents.	Assess for side effects: skin rash, gastrointestinal symptoms, and mental status. Administer ketoconazole with food. Shake suspensions well before administering, and ask patients to swish them around in the mouth before swallowing. Tell patients to let oral tablets dissolve in the mouth.	Treatment continues for a long time, but it is important to complete the full prescription. Take griseofulvin with meals high in fat; avoid alcohol and exposure to sunlight. Continue vaginal applications through the menses, and either refrain from sexual intercourse or have partner wear a condom. Your sexual partner must be treated at the same time or the infection will be passed back and forth.

before and after every patient contact, even if gloves are worn. All patients, family members, and visitors should be taught how to wash their hands effectively, and the importance of this procedure should be stressed.

PRIORITIZING NURSING CARE

Nursing interventions for most infections and infestations of the skin focus on providing information so the patient can perform self-care at home (see Continuity of Care). However, the patient with herpes zoster may have increased nursing care needs, including pain, altered sleep, and risk for infection.

HEALTH PROMOTION

The incidence of skin infections and infestations should be reduced with good hygiene practices and avoidance of shared clothing, linens, or towels. It is important to wear clean clothes and avoid walking barefoot in gyms or pools. Careful hand washing and wearing of gloves during treatment is essential to prevent spread of infection or infestation. Pregnant women should avoid contact with any person who has a viral infection.

ASSESSING

The nurse collects subjective and objective assessment data to identify the manifestations of an infection or infestation and to determine the degree to which the patient is at risk for complications. Ask the patient about personal and intimate contact with others who may have been infected or infested, manifestations of increased infection (increased erythema, fever, purulent drainage), and living conditions. Include questions about any chronic illnesses, such as diabetes mellitus, immune disorders, and previous viral infections (including having chickenpox as a child). Inspect the skin, hair, and mucous membranes. Note the location, appearance, and size of lesions; type and color of lesions; and nits. Take and record vital signs. Report abnormal findings.

DIAGNOSING, PLANNING, AND IMPLEMENTING

Acute Pain

Expected outcome: Will state pain is decreased.

- Assess and monitor the location, duration, and intensity of the pain. *Each person experiences and expresses pain differently. Pain tolerance is individualized.*
- Administer prescribed medications regularly and evaluate their effectiveness. *Regular administration prevents the pain from reaching an intensity at which the medication would be less effective.*
- Use measures to relieve pruritus. Administer prescribed antipruritic medications. Apply calamine lotion or cool compresses, if prescribed. Keep the room

temperature cool. *Pruritus is a common problem for these patients, and it may intensify pain. Lotions and cool compresses are often effective in decreasing the itch–scratch–itch cycle.*

clinical**ALERT**

Scratching increases the risk of secondary infection.

- Encourage the use of distraction, such as music or a specific relaxation technique such as progressive muscle relaxation or deep breathing. *Noninvasive methods help the patient manage the pain and also increase the effectiveness of pain medications.*

Sleep Deprivation

Expected outcome: Will awake less frequently during the night.

- Provide appropriate interventions (above) to relieve pain and pruritus. *The pain and pruritus of herpes zoster are often more intense at night, probably as a result of decreased distraction. Analgesics and noninvasive methods of relief may be necessary before bedtime.*
- Maintain a cool environment and avoid heavy bed covers. Use a bed cradle if necessary to keep bed linens off the patient. *Heat and touch intensify pruritus. Pruritus stimulates scratching, which awakens the patient. Pain may then be perceived as being more acute. A cycle is established that interferes with sleep.*

Risk for Infection

Expected outcome: Will remain free of signs of infection.

- Take and record vital signs every 4 hours. Report increased body temperature. Assess skin lesions for increased erythema, formation of pustules, or purulent drainage. Monitor white blood cell (WBC) count. Palpate lymph nodes for enlargement. *Secondary bacterial infections may occur, manifested by fever, changes in lesions or drainage, an increased WBC, or enlarged lymph nodes.*
- Use interventions to decrease the itch–scratch–itch cycle. *Patients with herpes zoster have increased risk for infection because of pruritus, scratching, and skin excoriation. Excoriations from scratching provide a portal for bacterial infection.*
- Institute infection control procedures. Maintain strict isolation for immunocompromised patients. Wear gloves and gown if contact with lesions is likely. Instruct pregnant women (visitors and health care providers) to avoid exposure until lesions have crusted over. *Isolation procedures are instituted for the immunocompromised patient to protect the patient from infection. The patient is also contagious to others who did not have chickenpox or varicella vaccine as a child. The nurse wears gloves and a gown to prevent spreading the infection to self and others. Pregnant women must avoid exposure because the herpesvirus can cross the placental barrier.*

MANAGING NURSING CARE

As appropriate and allowed by the designated duties and responsibilities of assistive personnel, the nurse may assign nursing care activities such as assisting with hygiene measures for the patient with an infectious skin disorder. Ensure that the assistive personnel understand the importance of hand hygiene and preventing the spread of these disorders to other patients and health care workers.

EVALUATING

To evaluate the effectiveness of nursing care for patients with a skin infection or infestation, collect assessment data, evaluating for changes in skin integrity and the need for additional measures to protect skin and underlying tissues from injury. Determine the patient's understanding of medications and their use and of how to prevent transmission of the infection or infestation.

DOCUMENTING

Documentation includes the location, appearance, and size of lesions, as well as the presence of nits. Record measures to protect the skin and patient teaching, including medications and ways to prevent transmission of infection or infestation.

CONTINUITY OF CARE

Planning and teaching for home care are important nursing responsibilities when caring for the patient with a skin infection or infestation. Specific teaching for each type of illness follows.

Bacterial Infections

Teaching focuses on facilitating tissue healing and eliminating the infection. Stress the importance of bathing daily with antibacterial soap, gently washing off crusts during the bath. Warm compresses may be applied to the lesions two or three times a day to increase comfort and decrease swelling. Teach the patient to cover draining lesions with a sterile dressing, to handle soiled dressings or linens according to Standard Precautions, and to wear disposable rubber gloves when changing dressings. Other instructions should be given:

- Maintain good nutrition.
- Carefully wash hands before and after dressing changes.
- Wash all linens and towels in hot water.
- Never squeeze or try to open a lesion. Clean the skin and keep it dry, especially in hot weather. Do not pluck nasal hair or pick the nose.
- Take the full course of prescribed medications until the supply is finished.

Fungal Infections

Many people treat themselves with over-the-counter antifungal medications. It is recommended that the person be diagnosed at the first occurrence. The nurse should provide the following information:

- Fungal infections are contagious. Do not share linens or personal items with others. Use a clean towel and washcloth each day.
- Carefully dry all skin folds, including those under the breasts, under the arms, and between the toes. Do not wear the same pair of shoes every day. Wear cotton socks or hose with cotton feet. Do not wear rubber or plastic-soled shoes. Use talcum powder or an antifungal powder twice a day.
- For vaginal yeast infections: Avoid tight jeans and pantyhose. Wear cotton or cotton-crotch panties. Bathe more frequently, and dry the genital area well. Have your sexual partner treated at the same time you are so you do not pass the infection back and forth.

Viral Infections

The nurse provides the following information:

- The diseases are usually self-limiting and heal completely.
- Do not have contact with children or pregnant women until crusts have formed over the blistered areas in patients with herpes zoster.

Parasitic Infestations

Patient and family teaching is necessary to facilitate treatment at home, to prevent the spread of the infestation, and to dispel the myth that only dirty people have lice. Teach this specific information:

- Wash clothing and linens in soap and hot water, or have them dry-cleaned.
- Iron clothing to kill lice eggs.
- Boil personal care items, such as combs and brushes, to kill parasites.
- Treat all family members and sexual partners.
- Do not use combs, brushes, or hats of others.

  See Clinical Reasoning Care Map on herpes zoster at the end of this chapter.

Malignant Skin Disorders

Key Concept   Nonmelanoma skin cancers do not develop from melanocytes (skin cells that make melanin) as melanoma skin cancers do, but rather they are a neoplasm of the epidermis. Any skin lesion that does not heal should be examined by a health care provider.

The skin is a common site for malignancy. Many of these lesions are found on skin surfaces that have had long-term exposure to the sun or the environment. Skin cancer is the most common of all cancers. This section of the chapter discusses the various types of malignant skin disorders.

NONMELANOMA SKIN CANCER

The skin is a fragile organ and is subject to damage from ultraviolet radiation and chemicals. Over time, this damage results in alterations in cellular structure and function, and malignancies may occur. The two types of **nonmelanoma skin cancers** (named because they do not arise from melanin-producing cells) are basal cell carcinoma and squamous cell carcinoma.

The American Cancer Society estimates that more than 3.5 million new cases of nonmelanoma skin cancer are diagnosed each year. If diagnosed and treated early, 95% to 99% can be cured. Nonmelanoma skin cancer is the most common malignant growth found in fair-skinned people. Of the two types of nonmelanoma skin cancer, basal cell carcinoma is the most common, outnumbering squamous cell carcinoma three to one. Men develop nonmelanoma skin cancer more often than do women, probably because of occupational exposures. Adults between the ages of 30 and 60 have the majority of these cancers. The factors involved in the development of nonmelanoma skin cancer include ultraviolet radiation, chemicals, skin pigmentation, and preexisting pigmented skin lesions.

Ultraviolet radiation from the sun is believed to be the cause of most nonmelanoma skin cancers. Sun rays are thought to either alter DNA or suppress T-cell and B-cell immunity. People who live in higher altitudes receive greater ultraviolet radiation exposure. The amount of clothing worn, the time of day, and the amount of time in the sun also determine the amount of exposure. Exposure to ultraviolet radiation in tanning booths has also been implicated in nonmelanoma skin cancer development.

Certain chemicals have also been associated with nonmelanoma skin cancer. Hydrocarbons, found in mixtures of coal, tar, asphalt, soot, and mineral oils, have been linked with skin cancer. Other factors associated with nonmelanoma skin cancer are the use of ionizing radiation, viruses, and physical trauma. HPV is implicated in the development of squamous cell carcinoma, as is damage to the skin from burns.

Skin pigmentation affects the development of nonmelanoma skin cancer. The more melanin a person has, the more the skin is protected from damaging ultraviolet rays. Thus, African Americans, Asian Americans, and people of Mediterranean descent have a much lower incidence of nonmelanoma skin cancer. People with red hair, fair complexions, and a tendency to freckle or sunburn easily (e.g., those of Scandinavian, Irish, and English ancestry) have a higher incidence.

Most people have many pigmented moles or other lesions on their body, of which most are normal. However, a major risk factor in the development of nonmelanoma skin cancer is a change in an existing lesion or the presence of a premalignant lesion, such as actinic keratosis.

BASAL CELL CARCINOMA

Basal cell carcinoma begins in the basal cell layer of the epidermis, usually on sun-exposed areas of the body, especially the head and neck. Basal cell carcinomas are the most common and the least deadly. They are slow-growing and rarely metastasize, but they can invade nearby areas. They can recur in the same location after treatment.

Nodular basal cell carcinoma is the most common type of basal cell cancer and is usually found on the face, neck, and head. It appears as a smooth, itchy pimple, but as they grow, the skin becomes shiny and either pearly white, pink, or skin-colored. Superficial basal cell carcinoma is a flat papule, often red, which may ulcerate. It is often seen on the trunk or extremities.

SQUAMOUS CELL CARCINOMA

Squamous cell carcinoma is a malignant tumor of the squamous epithelium of the skin or mucous membranes. It occurs most often on areas of skin that are exposed to ultraviolet rays and weather, such as the forehead, helix of the ear, top of the nose, lower lip, and back of the hands. Squamous cell carcinoma may also arise on skin that has been burned or has chronic inflammation. This is a much more aggressive cancer than basal cell cancer, with a faster growth rate and a much greater potential for metastasis if untreated.

Pathophysiology and Manifestations

Squamous cell carcinoma begins as a firm, flesh-colored, or erythematous papule. The tumor may be crusted. As it grows, it may ulcerate, bleed, and become painful. As the tumor extends into the surrounding tissue and becomes a nodule, the area around the nodule becomes *indurated* (hardened) (Figure 45-7■). Recurrent squamous cell carcinoma can be invasive, increasing the person's risk of metastasis.

MELANOMA

Melanoma, also called *cutaneous* or *malignant melanoma,* is a skin cancer that arises from melanocytes, the cells that produce melanin. The incidence of this serious skin cancer

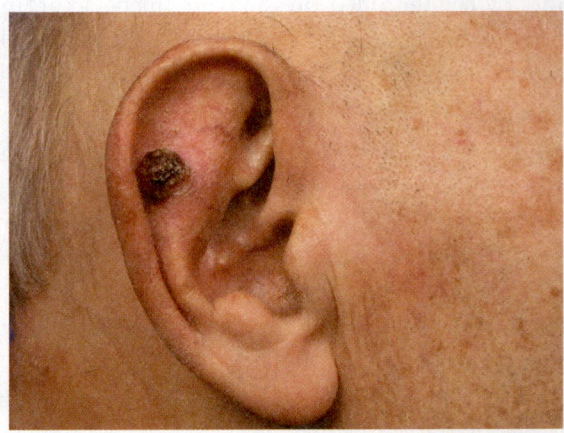

Figure 45-7. ■ As a squamous cell cancer grows, it tends to invade surrounding tissue. It also ulcerates, may bleed, and is painful. (Source: Girand/Science Source.)

is increasing annually; its incidence doubled in the past three decades. Melanoma is the cause of 4% of all skin cancer cases but contributes to a large number of skin cancer deaths. The American Cancer Society estimates that more than 77,000 new melanoma cases will be diagnosed in the United States in 2013.

Pathophysiology and Manifestations

The incidence is highest in Caucasians, people who had severe, blistering sunburns during childhood, and in people who live in sunny climates, burn easily, and visit tanning parlors. However, melanoma may arise from lesions that are already present or from skin that is normally covered with clothing. Although they are still confined to the epidermis, the lesions are flat and relatively benign. However, when they penetrate the dermis, they mingle with blood and lymph vessels and are capable of metastasizing. At this latter stage, the tumors develop a raised or nodular appearance and often have smaller nodules, called satellite lesions, around the periphery.

The prognosis for survival for people diagnosed with malignant melanoma is determined by several variables, including tumor thickness, ulceration, metastasis, site, age, and gender. Younger patients and women have a somewhat better chance of survival. Tumors on the hands, feet, and scalp have a poorer prognosis. Tumors of the feet and scalp may not be noticed and diagnosed until they grow into the dermis.

Precursor lesions for the development of melanoma are congenital nevi, dysplastic **nevi** (moles), and lentigo maligna. *Congenital nevi* are present at birth. They are often slightly raised, with an irregular surface and a fairly regular border. *Dysplastic nevi* (also called atypical moles) appear during childhood and become dysplastic (have abnormal development) after puberty. They most often appear on the face, trunk, and arms but also are seen on the scalp, female breast, groin, and buttocks. They have irregular borders and pigmentation colors. A patient with classic dysplastic nevi has more than 100 nevi, at least one of which is larger than 8 mm in diameter, and at least one has the characteristics of melanoma. *Lentigo maligna* is a tan or black patch on the skin that looks like a freckle. It grows slowly, becoming mottled, dark, thick, and nodular. It is usually seen on one side of the face of an older adult who has had a large amount of sun exposure.

A change in the color or size of a nevus is reported in 70% of people diagnosed with a melanoma. The ABCDE rule is used to assess suspicious lesions:

A = asymmetry; one-half of the nevus does not match the other half

B = border irregularity (edges are ragged, blurred, or notched)

C = color variation or dark black color

D = diameter greater than 5 mm (size of a pencil eraser)

E = evolution (history of skin lesion changing)

During the initial radial phase, which may last from 1 to 25 years (depending on the type), the melanoma grows parallel to the skin surface. During this phase, the tumor rarely metastasizes and is often curable by surgical excision. However, during the next vertical growth phase, atypical melanocytes penetrate into the dermis and subcutaneous tissue, greatly increasing the risk for metastasis and death. When the lesion enters the vertical growth phase, it grows rapidly, and its color changes from a mixture of tan, brown, and black to a characteristic red, white, and blue color. The lesion also develops irregular borders and often has raised nodules and ulcerations (Figure 45-8■).

COLLABORATIVE CARE

Treatment of all skin cancers focuses on removal of malignant tissue using such methods as surgery, curettage and electrodesiccation, cryotherapy, or radiotherapy. These treatments offer a greater than 90% cure rate. The management of melanoma begins with identification, diagnosis, and tumor staging. Besides surgical excision, melanoma is treated with chemotherapy, immunotherapy, radiation therapy, and biological therapies (interleukin-2, interferon, monoclonal antibodies, or therapeutic vaccines containing melanoma antigens).

Diagnostic Tests

Skin cancer is diagnosed by microscopic examination of tissue biopsied from any suspicious lesion. The biopsies are usually done as office procedures under local anesthesia.

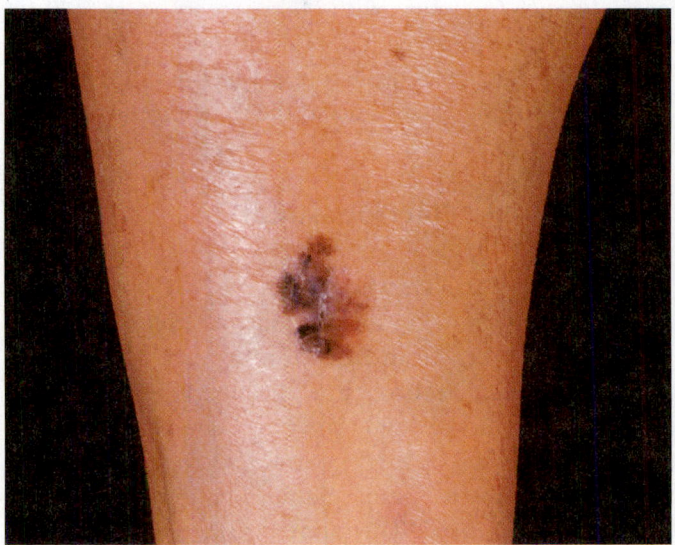

Figure 45-8. ■ Malignant melanoma is a serious skin cancer that arises from melanocytes. (Source: Caliendo, RBP FBPA/Custom Medical Stock Photo.)

Laboratory and diagnostic tests are also conducted to determine whether a melanoma has metastasized.

Liver function tests are done. The combination of an elevated lactic dehydrogenase (LDH), alkaline phosphatase, and aspartate aminotransferase (AST) suggests metastasis to the liver. If liver enzymes are abnormal, a CT scan of the liver is conducted. A complete blood count is done to determine hematologic abnormalities. Serum blood chemistry tests are conducted to identify electrolyte and mineral abnormalities.

Chest x-rays for possible lung metastasis are taken if the patient has respiratory difficulty or hemoptysis. If there is undetermined bone pain, a bone scan is performed. If the patient has headaches, seizures, or neurologic deficits, a CT scan or MRI of the brain is conducted.

The term *microstaging* describes the assessment of the level of melanoma invasion and the maximum tumor thickness. In the Clark system of microstaging, the vertical growth of the lesion is measured from the epidermis to the subcutaneous tissue. In the Breslow system, the vertical thickness is measured from the granular level of the epidermis to the deepest level of tumor invasion. This determination is important, because as the thickness of the melanoma increases, survival rate decreases. Staging of malignant tumors is discussed in Chapter 12.

Surgery

Nonmelanoma skin cancers may be removed through Mohs surgery. In Mohs surgery, thin layers of the tumor are shaved off horizontally. A frozen section of the tissue is stained at each level to determine tumor margins. This is the most accurate method of assessing the extent of nonmelanoma skin cancer, and it conserves the most normal tissue. Cure rates with Mohs surgery are at 99% for primary basal cell cancer and 94% for squamous cell carcinoma. For melanoma, a wide surgical excision that includes the full thickness of the skin and the subcutaneous tissue is the preferred treatment.

Curettage and Electrodesiccation or Cryosurgery

Basal cell cancers less than 2 cm in diameter may be removed with curettage and electrodesiccation. This procedure provides good cosmetic results and preserves normal tissue. However, healing time is longer, and it is difficult to ensure that all tumor margins have been removed. Cryosurgery is noninvasive; liquid nitrogen is used to freeze and destroy the tumor tissue. The area of the tumor is locally anesthetized. Then, liquid nitrogen is applied to the lesion by either a spray or cryoprobes. Cryosurgery is used for some primary basal cell cancers and for low-risk squamous cell cancers.

Radiation Therapy

Radiation is used for lesions that are inoperable because of their location (e.g., on the eyelid, the canthus, or the lip) or their size (between 1 and 8 cm). Radiation is also used for patients who are older and of poor surgical risk. The treatment is given over a 3- to 4-week period in a clinical facility. It does not allow control of tumor margins and may itself cause skin cancer. Small melanoma tumors may be treated with higher dose radiation. Radiation is used for palliation of symptoms for melanoma that has metastasized to brain, bone, and lymph nodes.

Biologic Therapy

Biologic therapy is used to enhance or restore the immune system to fight the cancer. Tumor-specific antigen–antibodies have also recently been identified. Agents such as interferon, interleukin, monoclonal antibodies, bacille Calmette–Guérin (BCG), and tumor vaccines have all shown activity in melanoma, with varying response rates. The effectiveness of these agents alone, in combination with chemotherapy, or in combination with each other is under investigation.

NURSING CARE

Surgical excision is the most common form of treatment for skin cancer. Nursing care and teaching depends on the treatment employed and on the extent of the procedures.

PRIORITIZING NURSING CARE

The diagnosis of skin cancer, especially melanoma, threatens the patient's quality of life. There is fear of metastasis and the possibility of recurrence. Wide excision and the high risk of metastasis from melanoma may require inpatient surgical treatment. Priority nursing care focuses on addressing the patient's anxiety, impaired skin integrity, and feelings of hopelessness and on providing teaching.

HEALTH PROMOTION

Increased incidence of skin cancer requires that nurses be involved in early detection and in teaching preventive behaviors in all settings. The American Cancer Society recommends that people between the ages of 20 and 40 see a dermatologist every three years and those over age 40 have annual skin checkups. Patients with precancerous lesions or with personal risk factors should conduct monthly skin self-examination. Brochures from the American Cancer Society provide photographs of lesions and prevention strategies. Review Box 45-3 ■ for additional suggestions to prevent skin cancer.

ASSESSING

The nurse assesses the skin of patients who seek care for many different health problems and may be the first to

BOX 45-3	PATIENT TEACHING

Preventing Skin Cancer

It is well known that cumulative sun exposure positively correlates with nonmelanoma skin cancers. Many skin cancers can be prevented by limiting exposure to risk factors. Primary prevention behaviors recommended by the American Cancer Society and the Skin Cancer Foundation follow:

- Minimize exposure to the sun between the hours of 10 a.m. and 4 p.m., when ultraviolet rays are the strongest.
- Cover up with a wide-brimmed hat, sunglasses, long-sleeved shirt, and long pants made of tightly woven material when you are in the sun.
- Use a waterproof or water-resistant sunscreen with a sun protective factor (SPF) of 15 or more before every exposure to the sun. Apply sunscreen not only on sunny but also on cloudy days, when ultraviolet rays can penetrate 70% to 80% of the cloud cover.
- Reapply the sunscreen before the protection time is up. If you are at risk for skin cancer, apply sunscreen daily.
- Use sunscreen and protective clothing when you are on or near sand, snow, concrete, or water, which can reflect more than half of the ultraviolet rays onto the skin.
- Avoid tanning booths; UVA radiation emitted by tanning booths damages the deep skin layers.

BOX 45-4	ASSESSMENT

Patients With Skin Cancer

Subjective Data

- Any change in the size, shape, or color of a mole, wart, birthmark, or scar
- Bleeding, crusting, itching, or pain of a mole, wart, birthmark, or scar
- Exposure to hazardous chemicals
- Previous serious sunburn or use of tanning salons
- Knowledge about and frequency of skin examinations
- Previous removal of skin cancer
- Family history of treatment for skin cancer
- Geographic area of residence during lifetime

Objective Data

- Inspect and palpate the entire skin for lesions. Use a good light and stretch the skin as tightly as necessary to better view lesions. Pay special attention to areas covered with hair, skin folds (e.g., under the breasts), the axilla, webs between the fingers and toes, soles of the feet, the area between the buttocks, oral cavity, ear canals, and mucous membranes. Assess for:
  - Skin discoloration or visible swelling
  - Contour, size, and color of moles, warts, birthmarks, and scars
  - Enlarged lymph nodes
  - Areas of ulceration, scaling, crusting, or erosion
- Measure and document all skin lesions on an anatomic chart. If possible, take photographs of any suspicious lesions to use in future comparison.
- Monitor and report results above expected range for liver function tests.

identify suspicious lesions. Assessment data is collected by the nurse to determine factors in the patient's history that may have increased the risk for skin cancer and to identify any skin lesions. Box 45-4■ lists subjective and objective data to collect.

DIAGNOSING, PLANNING, AND IMPLEMENTING
Anxiety

Expected outcome: Will report decreased anxiety level.

- Provide reassurance by sitting quietly with the patient, speaking slowly and calmly, and conveying empathetic understanding by touch. Support the patient's coping mechanisms, such as crying and talking. Use short, simple sentences; focus on the here and now, and provide concise information. *Higher levels of anxiety result in a focus on the present, inability to concentrate, and difficulty understanding verbal communications.*
- Provide accurate information to the patient and family about the illness, treatment, and expected length of recovery. *Accurate information enables a person to make informed decisions.*
- Encourage discussion of expected physical changes and ways to minimize disfigurement through cosmetics and clothing. Provide the patient with strategies for participating in the recovery process. *Coping behaviors differ from person to person and from situation to situation.*

Surgical incisions to remove melanoma may cause disfigurement. Active participation in care provides the patient with some control over the future and is often an effective means of coping with anxiety.

Impaired Skin Integrity

Expected outcome: Skin integrity will improve.

- Monitor for manifestations of infection: fever, tachycardia, and malaise, incisional erythema, swelling, pain, or drainage that increases or becomes purulent. *Intact skin is the first line of defense against infection. Impaired skin integrity increases the risk for infection, causing local and systemic manifestations.*
- Keep the incision line clean and dry by changing dressings as necessary. *Moisture increases the risk of infection.*
- Follow principles of medical and surgical asepsis when caring for a patient's incision. Teach family members and visitors the importance of careful hand washing. Maintain standard precautions if drainage is present.

Aseptic techniques are necessary when caring for any surgical incision to prevent infection. Careful hand washing helps prevent the spread of infection. Nurses must use precautions with blood and body fluids to protect themselves from exposure to HIV.

- Encourage and maintain adequate calories and protein intake in the diet. Suggest a consultation with the dietitian if the patient does not want to eat. *The patient with cancer has increased metabolic needs. If these are not met, healing may be impaired.*

Hopelessness

Expected outcome: Will verbalize concerns about situation.

- Provide an environment that encourages the patient to identify and express feelings, concerns, and goals:
  - Use active listening, ask open-ended questions, and reflect on the patient's statements.
  - Acknowledge and respect the patient's feelings of apathy or anger as expressions of distress.
  - Convey an empathetic understanding of the patient's fears and concerns.
  - Provide opportunities for the patient to express hope, faith, a sense of purpose, and the will to live.
  - Explore the patient's perceptions. Provide information and correct misconceptions if necessary.
  - Encourage the patient to identify support systems and past sources of strength and coping.
  Verbalizing feelings, concerns, and goals allows others to validate or correct them, promotes a therapeutic nurse–patient relationship, and fosters feelings of self-worth. Expressing positive emotions and identifying support systems and effective coping strategies from past crises helps the person resolve the current crisis and develop hope.
- Encourage the patient to participate in self-care, mutual decision making, and goal setting. *Meeting self-care needs and making decisions about one's own care build self-confidence.*
- Encourage focusing not only on the present but also on the future: Review past occasions for hope, discuss personal meaning of hope, establish and evaluate short-term goals with the patient and family, and encourage them to express hope for the future. *Mobilizing the patient's resources strengthens motivation, hope, and the will to live.*

MANAGING NURSING CARE

As appropriate and allowed by the designated duties and responsibilities of assistive personnel, the nurse may assign nursing care activities such as assisting with meals and hygiene measures for the patient with a nonmelanoma or melanoma.

EVALUATING

Evaluating the effectiveness of nursing care for the patient with skin cancer requires ongoing assessment. Collect data about effectiveness of treatment measures, patient's understanding of and compliance with treatments, and effectiveness of medications.

DOCUMENTING

Documentation includes effectiveness of treatment measures, medications, and side effects. Record teaching provided to the patient and family about wound care, regular checkups with a health care provider, and skin self-examination.

CONTINUITY OF CARE

Nurses provide patient and family education for prevention and early detection of skin cancer (see Box 45-3). Numerous brochures are also available from the American Cancer Society, health education and support agencies, and pharmaceutical companies that manufacture sunscreen. Most of this literature is provided free of charge.

Teach the patient or family who is at risk for, or has been diagnosed with, skin cancer how to conduct a self-examination of the skin. Stress that it should be conducted on the same day of each month. Family members can help with areas that are hard to examine (ears, scalp, back, extremities), or the patient can use a mirror. Showing photographs of both normal and cancerous skin lesions may help teach the patient and family what to watch for when doing self-examination. Teach about the following changes:

- Color, especially any lesion that becomes darker or variegated in shades of tan, brown, black, red, white, or blue
- Size, especially any lesion that becomes larger or spreads out
- Shape, especially any lesion that protrudes more from the skin or begins to have an irregular outline
- Appearance, especially bleeding, drainage, oozing, ulceration, crusting, scaliness, or development of a mushrooming outward growth
- Consistency, especially any lesion that becomes softer or is more easily irritated
- Surrounding skin—redness, swelling, or leaking of color from a lesion into the surrounding skin
- Sensation—itching or pain

If any of these changes occurs, the patient should immediately contact the health care provider for further assessment. If treatment is conducted in an outpatient setting, teach the patient and family specific measures for self-care, including how and when to change dressings, the use of aseptic technique and careful hand washing when caring for the wound, symptoms to report (e.g., bleeding, fever, or signs of wound infection), and how to protect the operative site against trauma and irritations. The patient who undergoes extensive surgery will require preoperative and postoperative care as discussed in Chapter 10.

Encourage patients with melanoma to schedule regular medical checkups every 3 months for the first 2 years, every 6 months for the next 5 years, and yearly thereafter. Emphasize that proper self-care combined with regular medical care can help the patient lead a fairly normal life. If assistance for home care is necessary, provide referrals to a community health or home care agency. Refer the patient to a local cancer support group if the patient believes this will be helpful.

NURSING CARE PLAN
Patient With Malignant Melanoma

Pat Malone, age 45, is an insurance broker in Washington. She frequently travels to warm, sunny vacation resorts, where she plays golf and likes to sunbathe. She has a variety of warts and moles but seldom pays attention to them. However, after taking a shower one day, she notices that a mole on her right shoulder looked bigger and darker. She sees her primary care physician, who makes a tentative diagnosis of malignant melanoma and refers her to a dermatologist.

Assessment

Ms. Malone has a family history of skin cancer; her father had several squamous cell cancers removed from his face. She states that the mole has been present for years but that she just noticed yesterday that it is larger and darker. The mole does not bleed or hurt, but sometimes it itches. A complete skin assessment reveals various freckles, warts, and moles. The mole in question is raised, is 3 cm in diameter with irregular borders, and is various shades of brown. Ms. Malone is scheduled for a biopsy of the mole under a local anesthetic the following morning. After the biopsy, histologic examination reveals lentigo maligna melanoma. Staging of the tumor shows a melanoma *in situ,* without metastasis to regional lymph nodes. Ms. Malone undergoes a wide excision of the mole the following afternoon.

Nursing Diagnosis

The following nursing diagnoses are identified for Ms. Malone:

- *Impaired Skin Integrity* related to excision of melanoma from the right shoulder
- *Risk for Infection* related to the surgical wound on the right shoulder
- *Acute Pain* related to wide excision of melanoma on the right shoulder
- *Anxiety* related to diagnosis of skin cancer

Expected Outcomes

The expected outcomes are that Ms. Malone will:

- Demonstrate complete healing of the incision without manifestations of infection.
- Verbalize relief of pain by the time the incision is healed.
- Verbalize fears and concerns about her diagnosis.

Planning and Implementation

The following nursing interventions are implemented following the wide excision of the mole:

- On discharge, provide adequate dressings and tape for the first home dressing change. Include necessary information about where to buy supplies and how many dressing supplies will be needed.
- Reinforce instructions for prescribe antibiotic and pain medication.
- Reinforce teaching about dressing change, manifestations of infection, and phone number of the physician's office. Stress the importance of calling if any abnormal symptoms occur.
- Teach ways to protect the incision from bumps and to protect the site from irritants.
- Stress the importance of lifelong regular health care evaluations to identify any recurrence or metastasis.

Evaluation

Ms. Malone returns to the physician's office 1 week after her surgical incision. Her incision is well approximated without any signs of infection. She is taking her antibiotic four times a day as prescribed and reports that her need for pain medication is decreasing. She says that she is still "scared to death" about having cancer but has joined a local cancer support group. She has gotten a list of skin care guidelines from the American Cancer Society. She plans to quit sunbathing and will use sunscreen and cover up when she plays golf. Ms. Malone makes a follow-up care appointment in 3 months.

Critical Thinking in the Nursing Process

1. Consider reasons why people who notice a change in a skin lesion put off seeking health care. How could this action affect their overall health? What can nurses do to effect change?
2. What would you suggest to Ms. Malone if she called the physician's office and said that the antibiotics are making her sick?
3. Consider nursing interventions that could be implemented for Ms. Malone for a diagnosis of *Powerlessness.*

Note: Discussion of Critical Thinking questions appears on the companion website.

Pressure Ulcers

Pressure ulcers (decubitus ulcers) are ischemic lesions of the skin and underlying tissue caused by external pressure that impairs the flow of blood and lymph (Porth, 2011). The ischemia causes tissue necrosis and eventual ulceration. Pressure ulcers tend to develop over a bony prominence (e.g., heels, greater trochanter, sacrum, and ischia), but they may appear on any part of the body that is subjected to external pressure, friction, or shearing forces. Review Chapter 10, Table 10-5, for a description of surgical positions that might cause pressure ulcers. Pressure causes more damage when it is applied to a small area than when it is distributed over a large surface.

The increased frequency of pressure ulcers in hospitals and long-term care facilities has resulted in infection, loss of function, and pain for patients. These complications increase the length of stay and costs. As a result, the Centers for Medicare and Medicaid will no longer reimburse hospitals for the additional costs associated with pressure ulcers developed during a hospital stay. Pressure ulcers are preventable and nurses play an essential role in their prevention.

PATHOPHYSIOLOGY AND MANIFESTATIONS

Pressure ulcers develop from external pressure that compresses blood vessels or from friction and shearing forces that tear and injure vessels. Both types of pressure cause traumatic injury and start the process for pressure ulcer development.

When a person lies or sits in one position for an extended length of time without moving, pressure on the tissue between a bony prominence and the external surface of the body distorts capillaries and interferes with normal blood flow. If the pressure is relieved, blood flow to the area increases, a brief period of reactive hyperemia occurs, and no permanent damage occurs. However, if the pressure continues, platelets clump in the endothelial cells surrounding the capillaries and form *microthrombi* (very small blood clots). These microthrombi impede blood flow, resulting in ischemia and hypoxia of tissues. Eventually, the cells and tissues of the immediate area and of the surrounding area die and become necrotic.

Alterations in the involved tissue depend on the depth of the injury. Injury to superficial layers of skin results in blister formation. Injury to deeper structures causes the pressure ulcer area to appear dark reddish-blue. As the tissues die, the ulcer becomes an open wound that may be deep enough to expose the bone. The necrotic tissue elicits an inflammatory response. The patient experiences fever and pain and has an increased white blood cell count. Secondary bacterial invasion is common. Enzymes from bacteria as well as macrophages dissolve necrotic tissue, resulting in a foul-smelling drainage.

Shearing forces result when one tissue layer slides over another. The stretching and bending of blood vessels cause injury and thrombosis. Patients in hospital beds are subject to shearing forces when the head of the bed is elevated and the torso slides down toward the foot of the bed. Pulling the patient up in bed also subjects the patient to shearing forces. For this reason, patients are always lifted up in bed. In both cases, friction and moisture cause the skin and superficial fascia to remain fixed to the bed sheet, whereas the deep fascia and bony skeleton slide in the direction of body movement.

Although pressure ulcers may occur in an adult with impaired mobility, those most at risk are older adults with limited mobility, people with quadriplegia, and patients in the critical care setting. Others at risk are patients with fractures of large bones (e.g., hip or femur) and those who have undergone orthopedic surgery or sustained spinal cord injury. Incontinence, nutritional deficit, chronic illnesses (e.g., renal failure and anemia), edema, and infection also create increased risk.

Because of age-related skin changes, the older adult is at increased risk for the development of pressure ulcers. The skin of the older adult has a thicker epidermis, a thinner dermis with decreased vascularity, decreased sebaceous gland activity, and decreased strength and elasticity. The more fragile and less nourished dermal layer is more prone to shear and friction problems. The skin of the older adult responds more slowly to inflammation, and wounds heal more slowly. When pressure ulcers occur, they are more difficult to reverse.

Pressure ulcers are graded or staged to classify the degree of damage. The stages, defined by the National Pressure Ulcer Advisory Panel in Washington, DC, are listed in Box 45-5■.

memoryALERT

Wound edges that are pink usually indicate healing, whereas black wounds indicate necrosis.

COLLABORATIVE CARE

If a patient is at risk for pressure ulcers, the goal is prevention. Ulcers that are already present require collaborative treatment to promote healing and restore skin integrity.

Laboratory tests are conducted to determine the presence of a secondary infection and to differentiate the cause of the ulcer. If the ulcer is deep or appears infected, drainage or biopsied tissue is cultured to determine the causative organism.

| **BOX 45-5** | **PRESSURE ULCER STAGING** |

Stage I

Intact skin with nonblanchable redness of a localized area, usually over a bony prominence. Darkly pigmented skin may not have visible blanching; its color may differ from the surrounding area.

Stage III

Full-thickness tissue loss. Subcutaneous fat may be visible but bone, tendon, or muscle are not exposed. Slough may be present but does not obscure the depth of tissue loss. May include undermining and tunneling.

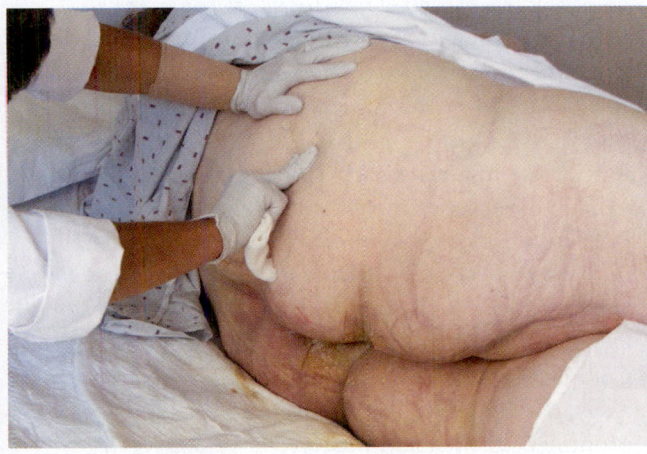

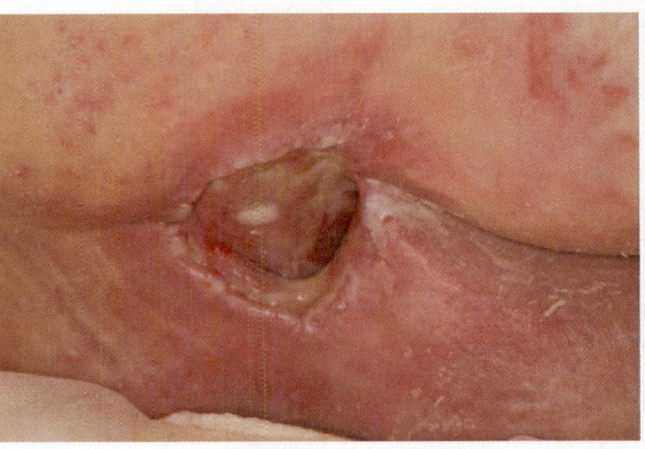

Stage II

Partial-thickness loss of dermis presenting as a shallow open ulcer with a red-pink wound bed, without slough. May also present as an intact or open/ruptured serum-filled blister.

Stage IV

Full-thickness tissue loss with exposed bone, tendon, or muscle. Slough or eschar may be present on some parts of the wound bed. Often includes undermining and tunneling.

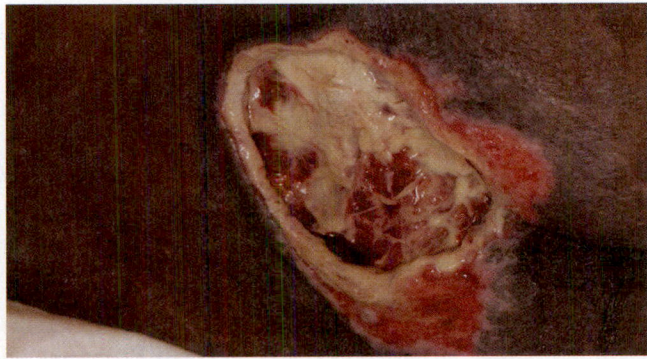

Unstageable

Full-thickness tissue loss in which the base of the ulcer is covered by slough (yellow, tan, gray, green, or brown) and eschar (tan, brown, or black) in the wound bed.

Suspected Deep Tissue Injury

Purple or maroon localized area of discolored intact skin or blood-filled blister due to damage of the underlying soft tissue from pressure and shear. The area may be surrounded by tissue that is painful, firm, mushy, boggy, and warmer or cooler than adjacent tissue.

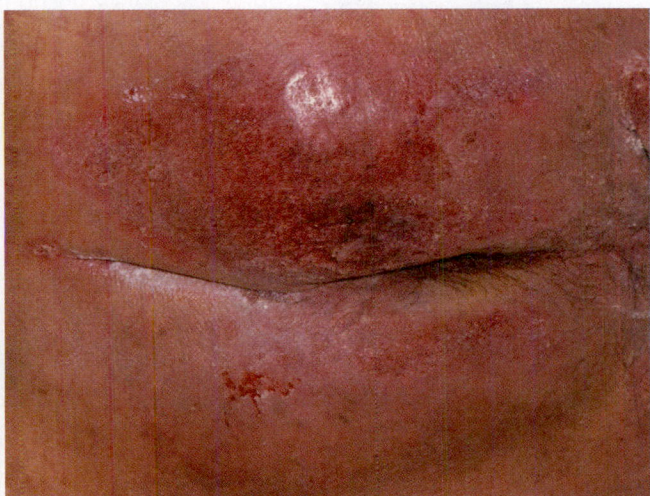

Note: Until enough slough and eschar is removed to expose the base of the wound, the true depth, therefore stage, cannot be determined.

Source: Data from National Pressure Ulcer Advisory Panel. (2007). *Pressure Ulcer Stages.* Washington, DC. Photos: Stage I, B. Slaven / Custom Medical Stock Photo; Stage II, Dr. H.C. Robinson / Science Source; Stages III & IV, Roberto A. Penne-Casanova / Science Source.

Topical and systemic antibiotics specific to the infectious organism are used to eradicate any infection present and to promote healing. Special wound care products and dressings may be used to manage the care of pressure ulcers (Table 45-3 ■). Surgical debridement may be necessary if the pressure ulcer is deep; if subcutaneous tissues are involved; or if an *eschar* (a scab or dry crust) has formed over the ulcer, preventing healing by granulation. Large wounds may require skin grafting for complete closure.

NURSING CARE

The patient with one or more pressure ulcers not only has impaired skin integrity but also is at increased risk for infection, pain, and decreased mobility. Pressure ulcers prolong treatment for other conditions, increase health care costs, and diminish the patient's quality of life.

Risk for Impaired Skin Integrity and Impaired Skin Integrity

Expected outcome: Skin integrity will remain intact or improve.

The following interventions and rationales are adapted from the clinical guidelines of the Agency for Health Care Policy and Research (1992) for identifying adults at risk and treating those with stage I pressure ulcers.

- Identify at-risk individuals and the specific factors that place them at risk.
  - Assess bed- and chair-bound patients, as well as those who cannot reposition themselves, for immobility, incontinence, nutritional status, and altered level of consciousness.

- Assess patients on admission to acute care and rehabilitation hospitals, nursing homes, home care programs, and other health care facilities, using a validated risk assessment tool.
- Document all assessments of risk. *Identifying individuals at risk for pressure ulcers allows reduction of risk factors. Patients who cannot reposition themselves or whose activity is limited to bed or a chair should be assessed. Using a validated assessment tool ensures systematic evaluation and allows reassessment over time. Accurate and complete documentation ensures continuity of care.*
- Participate in a systematic risk assessment that uses a validated risk assessment tool such as the Braden scale. *Patients at risk for pressure ulcers must be identified early so that risk factors can be decreased through intervention. Primary risk factors include immobility, limited activity, and poor nutritional status.*
- Conduct a systematic skin inspection at least once a day, paying particular attention to the bony prominences. *Systematic, comprehensive, and routine skin care decreases incidence. Data from skin inspection are used to design interventions to reduce risk and evaluate outcomes.*
- Clean the skin at the time of soiling and at routine intervals, as frequently as the patient's need or preference dictates. Avoid hot water, use a mild cleansing agent, and clean the skin gently, applying as little force and friction as possible. *Metabolic wastes and environmental contaminants accumulate on the skin and should be removed regularly. Feces and urine cause chemical irritation. Hot water may cause skin injury. Mild cleansing agents are less likely to remove the skin's natural resistance to injury.*

TABLE 45-3	Products Used to Treat Pressure Ulcers
PRODUCT	**PURPOSE**
Skin Prep	Toughens intact skin and preserves skin integrity
Hydrocolloid dressing (e.g., DuoDERM)	May be used for stages I–IV with minimal exudate. Forms a gel when coming in contact with wound exudate. Also forms an occlusive barrier over the ulcer while preventing skin breakdown and promoting healing. Helps prevent friction and shear
Transparent dressing (e.g., OpSite and Tegaderm)	May be used in shallow I–III stage ulcers. Prevents entry of moisture and bacteria but allows oxygen and moisture vapor permeability. Minimizes friction and shear
Alginate dressings such as Sorbsan and SilvaSorb	May be used for stages II–IV ulcers with moderate to heavy drainage and in infected wounds. Forms a gel when comes in contact with wound exudate
Hydrogel dressings such as Intrasite gel	May be used for stages II–IV ulcers. Rehydrates the wound bed and decreases pain. Promotes autolytic debridement
Wet-to-dry gauze dressing with sterile normal saline	Allows necrotic material to soften and adhere to the gauze, so that the wound is debrided
Vacuum-assisted closure (VAC)	Creates a negative pressure to help reduce edema, increase blood supply and oxygenation, and decrease bacterial colonization. Also helps promote moist wound healing and the formation of granulation tissue

- Minimize environmental factors leading to skin drying, such as low humidity and exposure to cold. Treat dry skin with moisturizers. *Well-hydrated skin resists mechanical trauma. Low humidity dries the skin, making it less pliable. Severe dryness is associated with fissures and cracks in the stratum corneum. Moisturizers help reduce dryness of skin.*

clinical**ALERT**

Do not massage over bony prominences. Evidence suggests that massage may lead to deep tissue trauma in at-risk patients.

- Minimize skin exposure to moisture from incontinence, perspiration, or wound drainage. Use materials that absorb moisture and present a quick-drying surface to the skin. Change underpads and briefs frequently. Do not place plastic directly against the skin. *Factors in urine, perspiration, or wound drainage may irritate the skin. Moisture alone can increase the skin's susceptibility to injury.*
- Minimize friction and shearing forces. Use proper positioning, transferring, and turning techniques. Lubricants such as cornstarch or creams, protective films such as transparent dressings and skin sealants, protective dressings such as hydrocolloids, and protective padding may also reduce friction injuries. *Proper positioning can eliminate most shear injury. Friction injuries to the skin occur from moving across a rough surface (e.g., bed linens). Any agent that eliminates contact or decreases friction reduces this risk.*
- For inadequate dietary intake of protein or calories, offer nutritional supplements and support the patient during mealtimes. If dietary intake remains inadequate, enteral or parenteral feedings may be needed. *Poor dietary intake of protein, calories, and iron has been associated with pressure ulcer development.*
- Maintain the patient's current level of activity, mobility, and range of motion. *Frequent turning, repositioning, and movement are essential in reducing risk.*
- Teach patients who can do so to shift their weight every 15 minutes. *Data support that spontaneous movements by older, bedridden patients lower the incidence of pressure ulcers.*

clinical**ALERT**

Reposition all at-risk patients at least every 2 hours, using a written schedule for systematic turning and repositioning. Avoid leaving patients sitting in a chair or wheelchair. Fewer pressure ulcers develop in patients who are turned every 2 to 3 hours.

- For patients on bed rest, use positioning devices, such as pillows, to protect bony prominences. For patients who are completely immobile, use devices that relieve pressure on the heels. The most common method is to raise the heels off the bed. Place any at-risk patient on a pressure-reducing device, such as foam, static air, alternating air, gel, or water mattress. Do not use donut-type devices. *Suspending the heels is the best way to redistribute pressure to those areas. Pressure-reducing devices and beds can reduce the incidence of pressure ulcers. Donut cushions may actually contribute to pressure ulcer development.*

clinical**ALERT**

Avoid placing patients in the side-lying position directly on the trochanter.

- Maintain the head of the bed at the lowest degree of elevation consistent with the patient's medical condition and other restrictions. Limit the amount of time the head of the bed is elevated. *Proper positioning can reduce pressure on body prominences.*
- Use assistive devices, such as a trapeze or bed linen, to move patients in bed who cannot assist during transfers and position changes. *Lifting, rather than dragging, patients up in bed is less likely to cause friction injury.*

CONTINUITY OF CARE

Patient and family teaching focus on prevention of pressure ulcers as discussed. Because many patients at risk for pressure ulcers are older or have other serious illnesses, the nurse may need to teach a caregiver about the following topics:

- Definition, description, and common locations of pressure ulcers
- Risk factors for the development of pressure ulcers
- Skin care
- Ways to avoid injury
- Diet

Depending on the stage of the pressure ulcer, teach the patient or caregiver how to care for ulcers that are already present: how to change wet-to-dry dressings, apply skin barriers, and avoid injury and infection. Referrals to a home health agency or community health department can help the family through the lengthy healing process.

Note: The references and resources for all chapters have been compiled at the back of the book.

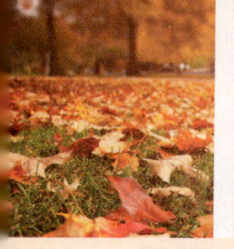
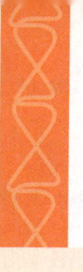

Chapter Review

KEY POINTS

- **Concept:** Pruritus accompanies dry skin (xerosis) and many skin disorders and may result in excoriation and infection as a result of scratching. Patients with psoriasis, a chronic immune skin disorder, often experience pruritus.
- Common skin disorders include pruritus (itching), dry skin, psoriasis, dermatitis, and acne. The goals of patient care are to identify and eliminate precipitating factors, provide relief from itching and pain, and reduce the risk of further damage to the skin.
- **Concept:** The skin provides an ideal environment for bacterial and fungal growth. Viral infections of the skin are often difficult to treat. Skin infections and infestations not only involve treating the disorder but also focus on preventing the spread of infection.
- The skin may be infected or infested with various agents, including bacteria, fungi, viruses, and parasites. Tinea infections, venereal warts, and pediculosis pubis are common sexually transmitted diseases. Treatment is provided to identify the causative agent, administer medications to kill or eradicate the organism, and prevent secondary infections.
- Herpes zoster is believed to follow a childhood infection with chickenpox. It frequently occurs in older adults, causing acute pain.
- **Concept:** Nonmelanoma skin cancers do not develop from melanocytes (skin cells that make melanin) as melanoma skin cancers do, but rather they are a neoplasm of the epidermis. Any skin lesion that does not heal should be examined by a health care provider.
- Nonmelanoma skin cancers (basal cell carcinoma and squamous cell carcinoma) are the most common of all cancers. Skin cancer is the most common malignancy found in fair-skinned Americans. They are believed to be primarily due to damage from ultraviolet radiation from sun exposure. They do not tend to metastasize and are treated by excision.
- Melanoma skin cancers are serious malignancies that do metastasize. Any change in the shape, border, color, size, consistency, or sensation of a nevus (mole) should be immediately evaluated for transformation into a malignant melanoma.
- Staging of malignant tumors such as melanoma is used to determine the type of treatment and prognosis. Patients who need wide excision surgery for a melanoma may require inpatient surgery.
- **Concept:** Skin trauma may be intentional as in the case of plastic surgery or unintentional as from trauma or pressure. Older adults with limited mobility and those who are unable to move have a greater risk for pressure ulcers.
- Pressure ulcers are ischemic lesions of the skin and underlying tissue. They are caused by external pressure or shearing forces that cause ischemia. The most common sites of development are over bony prominences.
- A validated risk assessment tool such as the Braden Scale should be implemented for all hospitalized patients. Nursing interventions are key to reduce risk factors and maintain intact skin.

PEARSON NURSING STUDENT RESOURCES

Find additional materials at **nursing.pearsonhighered.com**.

Clinical Reasoning Care Map

Caring for a Patient With Herpes Zoster
NCLEX-PN® Focus Area: Prevention and Health Maintenance

Case Study: Jesus Rivera is a 34-year-old migrant farm worker living in temporary housing in a rural area of southwestern America. He visits a free clinic and reports that he has not felt well for a week and has had chills and fever. He has painful oozing blisters in a line on his left thorax. His vital signs are T 99°F (37.2°C), P 74, R 22, BP 148/88. He does remember having chickenpox as a child. He is afraid that exposure to pesticides has caused his blisters. The primary health care provider diagnoses Mr. Rivera with herpes zoster and prescribes a topical antiviral medication and an oral pain medication.

Nursing Diagnosis: Risk for Infection

COLLECT DATA

Subjective	Objective
_____	_____
_____	_____
_____	_____
_____	_____
_____	_____
_____	_____

Does this present a threat to the patient's safety?

If yes, the priority intervention to address this threat would be:

_____

Nursing Care

_____
_____
_____
_____
_____
_____
_____

Interprofessional team members to include when planning care:

_____

How would you document this? _____

_____

Data Collected
(use only those that apply)

- Age 34
- Migrant farm worker
- Reports chills and fever
- T 99°F
- BP 148/88
- Open blisters on thorax
- Exposure to pesticides

Nursing Interventions (use only those that apply; list in priority order)

- Provide chickenpox immunization.
- Teach effects of pain medications.
- Report migrant status to local authorities.
- Stress importance of avoiding intimate contact with family members.
- Discuss need for careful hand washing.
- Teach how to apply topical medications.

Compare your answers and documentation to those provided on the companion website.

NCLEX-PN® Exam Preparation

1 A patient diagnosed with psoriasis is preparing for bed. Which nursing intervention should be given the highest priority at this time?

1. Prepare the ordered therapeutic bath.
2. Administer a pain medication.
3. Teach the patient to wear loose clothing.
4. Decrease the temperature in the patient's room.

2 The nurse recognizes that which factors in a patient's history are most likely to be related to a diagnosis of herpes zoster? **Select all that apply.**

1. Cervical cancer
2. Kidney transplant
3. Childhood infection of chickenpox
4. Measles at the age of 20
5. Patient receiving chemotherapy
6. Menstruating female

3 A patient has been receiving antibiotics for 3 days. The nurse should observe for the development of which side effect?

1. Furuncles
2. Candidiasis
3. Tinea pedis
4. Folliculitis

4 Topical acyclovir has been ordered for a patient with genital herpes. What should the nurse teach the patient?

1. Use bare hands when applying the medication.
2. Avoid taking hot baths.
3. Use the medication once a week.
4. Abstain from sexual intercourse.

5 A patient diagnosed with pediculosis corporis returns to the clinic on two separate occasions with complaints of itching. The patient states that all the medicine given to treat the condition was taken as directed. The most important question to ask the patient at this time is:

1. "Are other family members affected by the itching?"
2. "Are you having difficulty sleeping at night?"
3. "Do you have any pets living in your home?"
4. "Did you wash all of your bed linen after taking the medicine?"

6 Which factor increases the risk for the development of nonmelanoma skin cancer?

1. Exposure to ultraviolet radiation
2. Patient is African American
3. Decreased estrogen levels
4. History of blistering sunburn during childhood

7 A patient has developed a small basal cell cancer on the forearm and has been scheduled for cryosurgery. The patient tells you that life is not worth living now that cancer has been found. What is an appropriate nursing diagnosis for this patient?

1. Anxiety
2. Fear
3. Hopelessness
4. Impaired Skin Integrity

8 What is the most important instruction that should be given to patients who are at risk for the development of skin cancer?

1. Self-examination of skin
2. Major risk factors for developing skin cancer
3. Treatments for the various types of skin cancer
4. Prognosis for skin cancer

9 Which of these observations would be most significant when assessing the condition of an older patient who is at risk for a pressure ulcer?

1. Diminished lung sounds
2. Decreased appetite
3. Permanent redness over the sacrum
4. Contracture of the lower extremities

10 What nursing interventions should be included on the care plan for a patient diagnosed with impaired skin integrity? **Select all that apply.**

1. Massage over the bony prominences.
2. Reposition the patient every 2 hours.
3. Use hot water for bathing.
4. Provide a diet high in proteins and calories.
5. Reposition by pulling the patient up in bed.
6. Apply moisture to dry skin.

Answers and rationales for Review Questions appear in Appendix I.

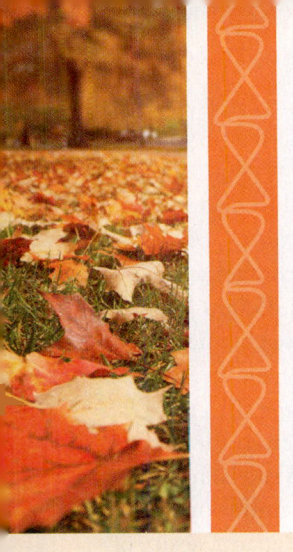

CHAPTER 46
Caring for Patients With Burns

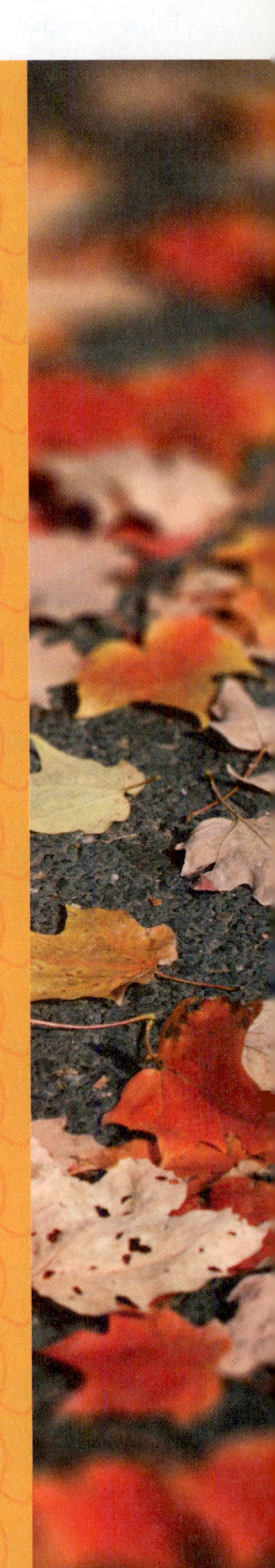

BRIEF OUTLINE

Types of Burn Injury
Classification of Burn Depth
Estimating the Extent of a Burn

Major Burns
Pathophysiology and Manifestations
Collaborative Care

APPLIED LEARNING OUTCOMES

After completing this chapter, you will be able to:

1. Discuss types, classification, extent estimation, and stages of treatment for burns.
2. Describe the pathophysiology of a major burn.
3. Implement collaborative care necessary for the patient with a major burn, including diagnostic tests; medications; fluid resuscitation; respiratory management; nutritional support; wound management; surgery; biologic and biosynthetic dressings; scar, keloid, and contracture prevention; and wound dressings.
4. Use the nursing process to collect data and provide interventions for patients with major burns.
5. Provide patient and family teaching for care of the burn after discharge.

KEY TERMS

The key terms are defined on the pages listed below.

SPECIAL FEATURES

It is estimated that more than 1 million burn injuries occur each year in the United States, resulting in more than 40,000 acute hospitalizations and 3,400 deaths (American Burn Association, 2012). The home is the most common site for fire-related burns. Home fires cause 85% of all fire-related deaths, with about eight people dying in home fires each day. Factors associated with deaths from burns are age (especially children under 4 and adults 65 and older), careless smoking, alcohol or drug intoxication, and physical and mental disabilities.

Burns range from minor loss of the outermost layer of the skin to a complex injury involving all body systems. Treatments vary from simple application of a topical antiseptic agent in an outpatient clinic to an invasive, multisystem, interprofessional health team approach in the sterile environment of a burn center.

Types of Burn Injury

A **burn** is an injury in which a transfer of energy from a heat source to the human body results in tissue loss, damage, or irreversible destruction. Burns may be the result of thermal, chemical, electrical, or radiation damage. Although all four types can lead to generalized tissue damage and multisystem involvement, the causative agents and priority treatment measures are unique to each.

- *Thermal burns* result from exposure to dry heat (flames) or moist heat (steam and hot liquids). They are the most common burns and occur mostly in children and older adults.
- *Chemical burns* are caused by direct skin contact with either acid or alkaline agents. More than 25,000 products found in the home or workplace can cause chemical burns.
- The severity of *electrical burns* depends on the type and duration of current and amount of voltage. Electricity follows the path of least resistance, which in the human body tends to lie along muscles, blood vessels, nerves, and bone. Necrosis of the tissue results from impaired blood flow secondary to blood coagulation at the site of the electrical injury.

memoryALERT

Electrical burns have entry and exit wounds, which are often small. There may actually be widespread tissue damage underneath the wound.

- *Radiation burns* are usually associated with sunburn or radiation treatment for cancer. These kinds of burns tend to be superficial, involving only the outermost layers of the epidermis.

CLASSIFICATION OF BURN DEPTH

After a burn, tissue damage is determined primarily by the extent of the burn (the percentage of body surface area involved) and the depth of the burn (affected layers of underlying tissue). The American Burn Association uses both the extent and depth of burn to classify burns as minor, moderate, or major. Characteristics of burns within each classification are summarized in Table 46-1 ■ and illustrated in Figure 46-1 ■.

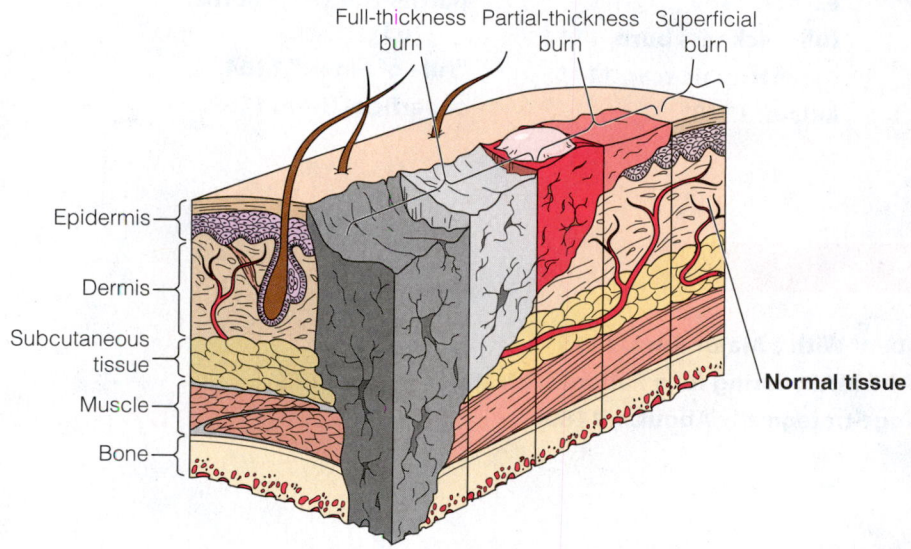

Figure 46-1. ■ Burn injury classification according to the depth of the burn.

TABLE 46-1	Characteristics of Burns by Depth		
CHARACTERISTIC	**SUPERFICIAL**	**PARTIAL THICKNESS**	**FULL THICKNESS**
■ Skin layers lost	Epidermis	Epidermis and dermis	Epidermis, dermis, and underlying tissues
■ Skin appearance over burn	Pink to red and dry; may have local edema	Fluid-filled blisters; bright pink or red with superficial partial thickness. Pale, waxy white with deep partial-thickness burns	Waxy white; dry, leathery, charred
■ Skin function	Present	Absent	Absent
■ Pain sensation	Present	Present	Absent
■ Manifestations at the burn site	Pain; local edema	Severe pain; edema; weeping of fluid	Little pain; edema
■ Treatment	Regular cleaning Topical agent of choice Mild analgesics	Regular cleaning Topical agent of choice May require skin grafting for deep partial-thickness burns	Regular cleaning Topical agent of choice Skin substitutes Excision of eschar Skin grafting
■ Scarring	None; outer layer peels	May occur in deep burns	Of grafted area
■ Time to heal	3–6 days	14 to more than 21 days	Requires skin grafting to heal

A **superficial burn** involves only the epidermal layer. This type of burn most often results from sunburn, ultraviolet light, minor flash injury from a sudden ignition or explosion, or mild radiation burn associated with cancer treatment. Because the skin remains intact, this degree of burn is not calculated into the estimates of burn injury. Patients with superficial burns involving large body surface areas may have chills, headache, nausea, and vomiting. Superficial burns are treated with mild analgesics and the application of water-soluble ointments. Extensive superficial burns, especially in older adults, may require intravenous fluid treatment.

Partial-thickness burns are subdivided into superficial or deep, depending on the depth of the burn.

A *superficial partial-thickness burn* involves the entire dermis. Causes may include a brief exposure to flash flame or dilute chemical agents, or contact with a hot surface. This burn is often bright red and has a moist, glistening appearance with blister formation (Figure 46-2■). The burned area blanches on pressure. Pain in response to temperature and air is usually severe. Pigment changes are common. Analgesics are given, and if large blistered areas are disrupted, skin substitutes may be needed.

A *deep partial-thickness burn* involves the entire dermis plus hair follicles, but sebaceous glands and epidermal sweat glands remain intact. This level of burn may be caused by hot liquids or solids, flash flame, direct flame, intense radiant energy, or chemical agents. The surface of the burned skin appears pale and waxy and may be moist or dry. Large, easily ruptured blisters may

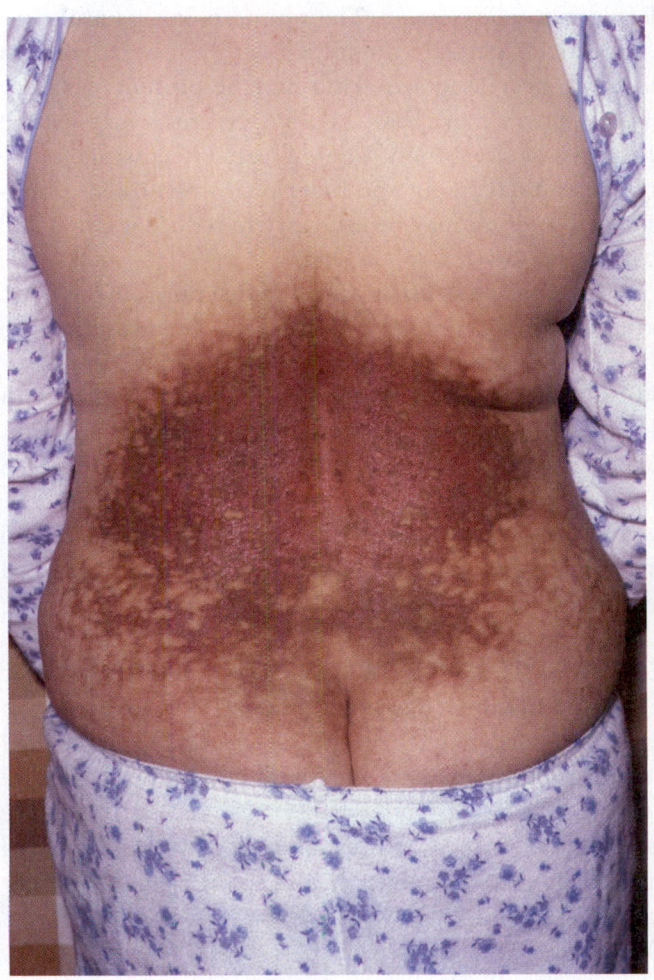

Figure 46-2. ■ Partial-thickness burn injury on the patient's back. (Source: Dr. M.A. Ansary/Science Source.)

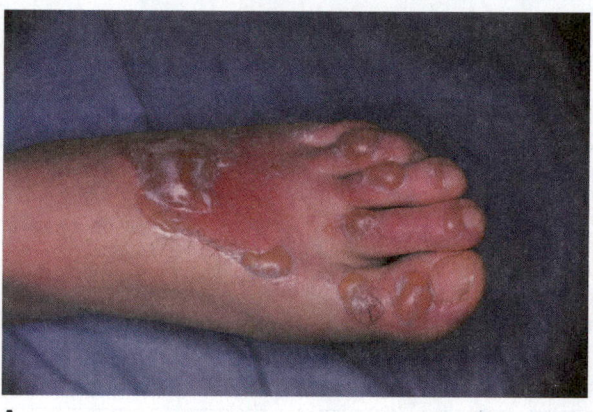

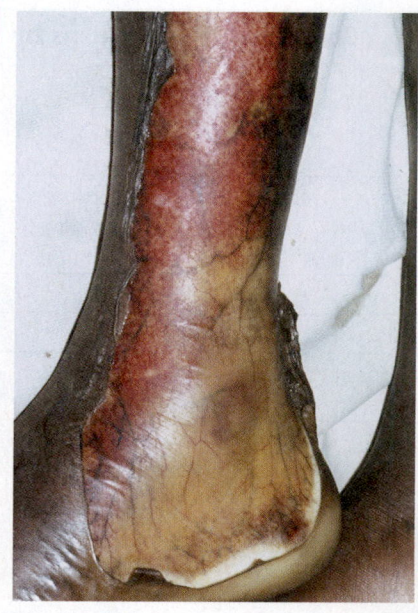

A

B

Figure 46-3. ■ **(A)** Partial-thickness burn injury showing blistering. **(B)** Deep full-thickness burn injury. (Source: A and B, Pearson Education.)

be present. Capillary refill is decreased, but sensation to deep pressure is present. The wound is less painful than a superficial partial-thickness burn, but areas of both pain and decreased sensation may be present. Healing often requires more than 21 days. Necrosis may extend the depth of the wound. Contractures are possible, as are hypertrophic scarring and functional impairment. Excision and grafting may be necessary to reduce scarring and loss of function.

A **full-thickness burn** (third-degree burn) involves all layers of skin (Figure 46-3 ■). The wound may extend into the subcutaneous fat, connective tissue, muscle, and bone. Full-thickness burns are caused by prolonged contact with flames, steam, chemicals, or high-voltage electric current. Depending on its cause, the burn may appear pale, waxy, yellow, brown, mottled, charred, or nonblanching red. The wound surface is dry, leathery, and firm to the touch. Pain and touch receptors are destroyed. Skin grafting is required to heal full-thickness burns.

ESTIMATING THE EXTENT OF A BURN

The **"rule of nines"** is a rapid method of estimating the extent of partial- and full-thickness burns. It is used during prehospital and emergency care phases (Figure 46-4 ■). The head, trunk, arms, legs, and perineum are assigned percentages. For example, a patient with burns of the face, anterior right arm, and anterior trunk has burn injury involving 27% of total body surface area (TBSA). On the patient's admission to a hospital or burn center, more accurate methods for estimating the extent of injury are employed.

Major Burns

Key Concept   The American Burn Association defines a major burn as one that involves more than 25% TBSA in adults less than 40 years of age; more than 10% full-thickness burn; injuries to face, eyes, ears, hands, feet, or perineum; high-voltage electrical injuries; or burn injuries with inhalation injury or major trauma.

PATHOPHYSIOLOGY AND MANIFESTATIONS

The pathophysiologic changes associated with major burns involve all body systems. Extensive loss of skin can result in massive infection, fluid and electrolyte imbalances, and hypothermia. The respiratory system may be compromised by inhaling the products of combustion. Cardiac system dysfunction increases in patients with preexisting cardiovascular disease.

Integumentary System

The burn injury impairs the normal physiologic functions of the skin as discussed in Chapter 44. The prevention of evaporative water loss and bacteria entry as well as maintenance of body warmth is lost. Heat transfer to skin is a complex process. If the microcirculation of the skin remains intact during burning, it cools and protects the deeper portions of the skin and cools the outer surface, once the heat source is removed. With extensive burn injury, however, the microcirculation is lost, and the burning process continues even after the heat source is removed.

The thickness of the dermis and epidermis varies considerably from one area of the body to another. A temperature

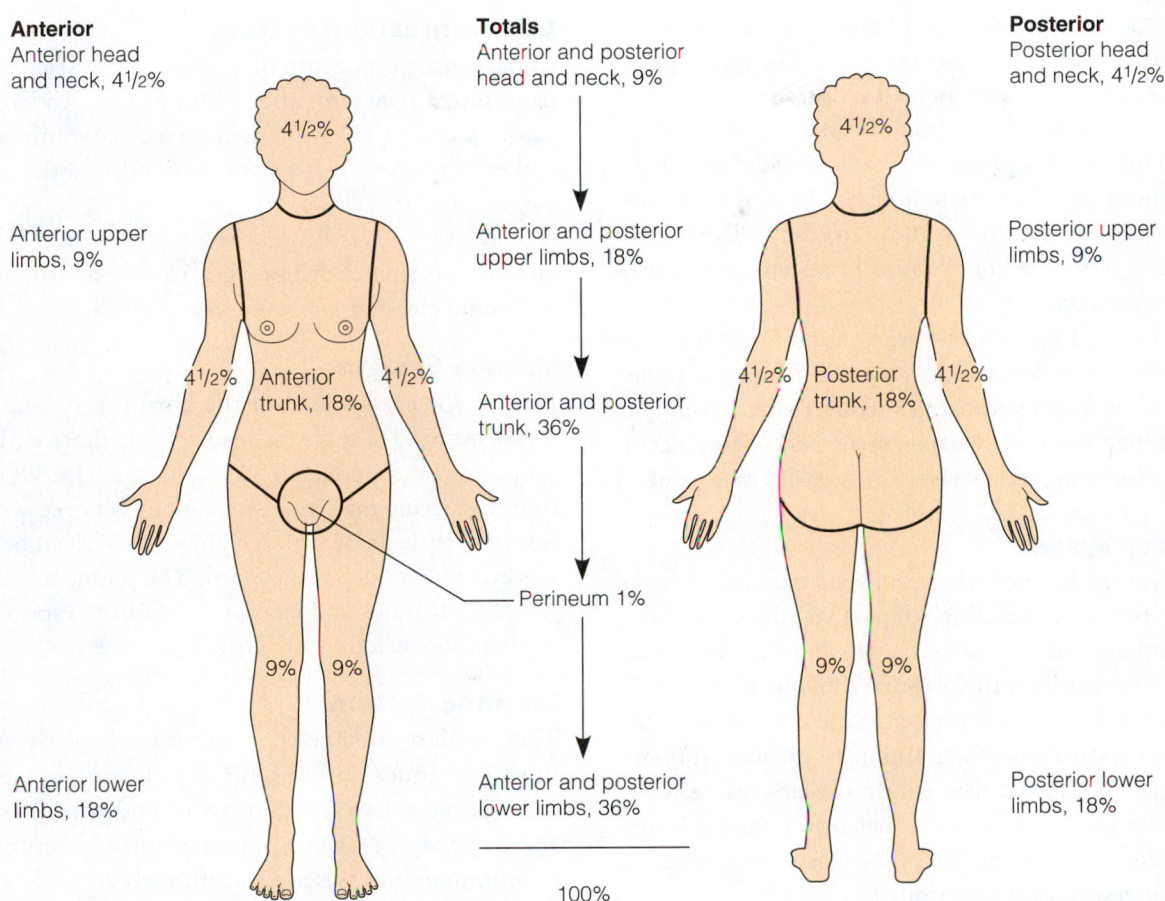

Anterior
Anterior head
and neck, 4¹/2%

Anterior upper
limbs, 9%

4¹/2% | Anterior
trunk, 18%   4¹/2%

Anterior lower
limbs, 18%

Totals
Anterior and posterior
head and neck, 9%

Anterior and posterior
upper limbs, 18%

Anterior and posterior
trunk, 36%

Perineum 1%

Anterior and posterior
lower limbs, 36%

100%

Posterior
Posterior head
and neck, 4¹/2%

Posterior upper
limbs, 9%

4¹/2% | Posterior
trunk, 18%   4¹/2%

Posterior lower
limbs, 18%

9%   9%

9%   9%

4¹/2%

4¹/2%

Figure 46-4. ■ The "rule of nines" is a way to estimate the percentage of TBSA affected by a burn injury. This quick method is useful in emergency situations, but it is not accurate for adults who are short, obese, or very thin.

that damages the medial aspect of the forearm may not cause damage to the skin covering the same person's back.

Cardiovascular System

Major burns affect the cardiovascular system by causing hypovolemic shock (burn shock), cardiac dysrhythmias, cardiac arrest, and vascular compromise. Within minutes of the burn, there is loss of cell wall integrity at the injury site and in the capillary bed. This causes a massive amount of fluid to shift from the intracellular space into the interstitial space. The capillary walls also become more permeable so that fluid leaks from the capillaries at the burn wound site and throughout the body, decreasing intravascular fluid volume. Without adequate fluids in the intracellular and intravascular spaces, the patient becomes hypovolemic. Plasma proteins and sodium escape, further increasing edema formation. Blood pressure falls as cardiac output diminishes. The net result is hypovolemic shock, which is called **burn shock**.

Vasoconstriction occurs as the vascular system attempts to compensate for fluid loss (see Chapter 14). Abnormal platelet aggregation and white blood cell (WBC) accumulation result in ischemia and eventual thrombosis (clotting) in the deeper tissue below the burn. Red blood cells (RBCs) are hemolyzed due to direct damage from the burn. Because plasma fluid is lost rather than RBCs, hemoconcentration develops, which is seen as an elevated hematocrit. Neutrophils accumulate at the burn site, producing an elevated leukocyte count.

The leakage of fluid into the interstitial spaces compromises the lymphatic system, resulting in intravascular hypovolemia and edema at the burn wound site. Edema impairs peripheral circulation and results in necrosis of the underlying tissue. Potassium ions leave the cells due to burn injury and RBC hemolysis. Without adequate potassium to maintain normal cardiac rhythms, the patient is at an increased risk of developing cardiac dysrhythmias.

memory**ALERT**

The loss of intravascular volume causes an increase in blood viscosity that increases the risk for blood clots.

memory**ALERT**

Cells cannot maintain normal electrolytes, resulting in excess sodium within the cell and excess potassium outside of the cell.

Burn shock reverses when fluid is reabsorbed from the interstitium into the intravascular space. The blood pressure rises as cardiac output increases, and urinary output improves. Diuresis continues from several days to 2 weeks postburn. During this phase, the extra cardiac workload may predispose the older patient or the patient with cardiovascular disease to fluid volume overload. Even after capillary integrity is restored, fluid losses continue until the burn wound is closed.

Circumferential burns to the extremities may damage blood vessels, which decreases circulation. Damaged tissue may become edematous, causing further reduction in circulation. When circumferential burns and edema occur together, *compartment syndrome* (see Chapter 42) may result.

Respiratory System

Inhalation injury is a complication that may range from mild respiratory inflammation to massive pulmonary failure. Exposure to toxic chemicals that can cause asphyxia, smoke, and heat initiates the pathophysiologic processes.

Smoke inhalation and poisoning result when toxic gases and soot are deposited on the pulmonary mucosa. Inflammation occurs at localized sites within the airways, cells are destroyed, and the bronchial cilia that help clear the lungs are inactivated. Because of this, the patient may develop bronchial congestion and infection.

Interstitial pulmonary edema develops secondary to the movement of fluid from the pulmonary blood vessels into the interstitial compartment of the lung tissue. Smoke inhalation damages the alveoli, which inactivates surfactant. Without surfactant, the alveoli collapse, leading to atelectasis. Sloughing of the damaged and dead lung tissue occasionally produces debris that may lead to complete airway obstruction.

Upper airway (above the glottis) thermal injury results from the inhalation of heated air. Physical findings include singed facial or nasal hair, black sputum, the presence of soot, charring, edema, blisters, and ulcerations along the mucosal lining of the oropharynx and larynx. The resulting edema in the airway peaks within the first 24 to 48 hours of injury. Ominous signs of hoarseness, labored breathing, or stridor indicate possible airway obstruction due to edema. Because laryngeal reflexes protect the lower airway, thermal injury below the vocal cords is seldom seen. When it does occur, it is typically associated with the inhalation of steam or explosive gases or the aspiration of hot liquids.

Carbon monoxide, produced by incomplete burning of materials, is a colorless, tasteless, odorless gas. It displaces oxygen and binds with hemoglobin, causing carboxyhemoglobinemia. Without oxygen, tissue hypoxia and eventually death occur. The manifestations of carbon monoxide poisoning range from mild visual impairment and headache to coma and death.

Gastrointestinal System

Curling ulcer is an acute ulceration of the stomach or duodenum that may form after a burn injury. Abdominal pain, acidic gastric pH levels, hematemesis (vomiting blood), and occult blood in the stool may indicate the presence of gastric ulcer formation.

Paralytic ileus may occur secondary to burn trauma. The lack of intestinal motility leads to gastric distention, nausea, vomiting, and hematemesis.

Urinary System

During the early stages of the burn injury, massive fluid losses occur. These losses lead to dehydration, hemoconcentration, and decreased urinary output. Dark brown concentrated urine may indicate hemoglobinuria, which is the result of the release of large amounts of dead or damaged erythrocytes after a major burn. The pigments can occlude the renal tubules and cause renal failure, especially when dehydration, acidosis, or shock is also present.

Immune System

The capillary leakage that occurs in the early stages of a burn continues throughout the burn shock phase and impairs the active components of both the cell-mediated and antibody-mediated immune systems. Serum levels of all immunoglobulins are significantly diminished. Serum protein levels remain persistently low until wound closure occurs. These changes in the immune system create a state of acquired immunodeficiency, which places the burn patient at risk for infection for up to 4 weeks after the injury. During this time, infections can develop and cause death despite aggressive antimicrobial therapy.

memoryALERT

Cortisol is released due to the stress of the burn injury, which depresses the immune system and increases the risk of infection.

Metabolism

Two distinct metabolic phases occur as the body responds to the burn injury. The ebb phase, occurring during the first 3 days of the injury, is manifested by decreased oxygen consumption, fluid imbalance, shock, and inadequate circulating volume. These responses protect the body from the initial impact of the injury.

A second phase, the flow phase, occurs when adequate burn resuscitation has been accomplished. This phase is characterized by increased cellular activity and protein catabolism, lipolysis, and gluconeogenesis. The basal metabolic rate (BMR) reaches twice the normal rate. Body weight and heat drop dramatically. Hypermetabolism persists until after wound closure and may reappear if complications occur.

COLLABORATIVE CARE

After stabilization in the emergency department, the patient is transferred to the critical care unit or a specialized burn center. At a burn center, the burn team consists of the nurse, physician, physical and occupational therapists, dietitian, psychologist, and social worker. In both settings, continuous monitoring of laboratory tests, administration of fluids and pharmaceutical agents, pain control, wound management, and nutrition support therapies are the focus of care.

Diagnostic Tests

Laboratory and diagnostic tests are conducted to assess and monitor the patient's response to the burn injury as well as to the treatment prescribed. Cultures of sputum, blood, urine, and wound tissue are done to indicate the presence of infection. Blood is typed and cross-matched upon the patient's arrival to the unit, in case transfusions are required.

- *Urinalysis* is done to evaluate renal perfusion and nutritional status. In catabolic states, nitrogen is excreted in large amounts into the urine. Nitrogen loss is measured through 24-hour urine collections for total nitrogen, urea nitrogen, and amino acid nitrogen. Loss of plasma protein and dehydration lead to proteinuria and elevated urine-specific gravity.
- The *complete blood count* is checked regularly. Hematocrit is elevated secondary to hemoconcentration and fluid shifts from the intravascular compartment during the emergent phase. Hemoglobin is decreased secondary to hemolysis. WBCs are elevated in the presence of infection.
- *Serum electrolytes* are monitored frequently. Sodium levels are decreased secondary to massive fluid shifts into the interstitium. Potassium levels are initially increased but decrease after burn shock resolves, as fluid shifts back to intracellular and intravascular compartments.
- *Total protein* and *albumin* indicate nutritional status during the rehabilitative stage.
- *Renal function* tests are monitored frequently. Blood urea nitrogen increases secondary to dehydration; creatinine levels rise when renal insufficiency is present.
- *Arterial blood gases* (ABGs) are used to monitor oxygen status and acid–base disturbances. The burn-injured patient may have elevated or lowered pH, decreased PCO_2, decreased PO_2, and low-normal bicarbonate levels.
- *Pulse oximetry* allows continuous assessment of oxygen saturation levels. The burn-injured patient may have saturation levels below 95%.

- *Chest x-ray* studies document changes within the first 24 to 48 hours that may reflect the presence of atelectasis, pulmonary edema, or acute respiratory distress syndrome (ARDS). If an upper airway injury is manifested, a *flexible bronchoscopy* permits direct visualization.
- *Electrocardiograms* (ECGs) are necessary to monitor the development of dysrhythmias, especially those associated with hypokalemia and hyperkalemia.

Stages of Burn Injury Care

The treatment for the burn patient is divided into three, sometimes overlapping, stages. At each stage, different groups of nurses, physicians, and other health care specialists collaborate to manage the patient's recovery.

EMERGENT OR RESUSCITATIVE STAGE   This stage lasts from the onset of injury through successful fluid resuscitation. It includes estimating the extent of the burn, instituting initial first-aid measures, and implementing fluid resuscitation therapies. The patient is assessed for shock and respiratory distress. Physicians determine whether the patient is to be transported to a burn center.

ACUTE STAGE   The acute stage begins with the start of diuresis and ends with closure of the burn wound. Hydrotherapy and excision and grafting of full-thickness wounds are performed as soon as possible. Enteral and parenteral nutritional interventions are started early to address caloric needs. Measures to combat infection are implemented, including the administration of topical and systemic antimicrobial agents. Pain management is essential throughout the clinical course of the burn-injured patient. Narcotic agents must be administered before all invasive procedures to maximize patient comfort and to reduce the anxieties associated with wound debridement and intensive physical therapy.

REHABILITATIVE STAGE   This stage begins with wound closure and ends when the patient returns to the highest level of health, which may take years. The primary focus is biopsychosocial adjustment: the prevention of contractures and scars and the patient's successful resumption of work, family, and social roles through physical, vocational, occupational, and psychosocial rehabilitation.

Medications

Burns often cause excruciating pain. In the emergent stages of care, intravenously administered narcotics such as morphine, hydromorphone, or fentanyl are the best means of managing pain. Morphine is the drug of choice. Once the patient has been stabilized, it is appropriate to administer narcotic agents before wound care or intensive exercising routines. Burn treatments can cause high levels of anxiety. Anxiolytics such as midazolam (Versed) and lorazepam (Ativan) are effective when given 1 hour before wound care.

TABLE 46-2	**Giving Medications Safely: Topical Antimicrobial Agents**		
CLASS/DRUGS	**PURPOSE**	**NURSING IMPLICATIONS**	**PATIENT TEACHING**
■ Mafenide acetate (Sulfamylon)	A synthetic antibiotic that appears to interfere with the metabolism of bacterial cells. Effective against many gram-positive and gram-negative organisms. Used to prevent burn wound infections.	Use with caution in patients with renal or pulmonary disease. Assess for itching, swelling, or blisters on unburned areas, which indicate an allergy to the drug. Apply a thin layer with sterile gloves.	When applied, the drug causes pain or burning. Apply one to two times a day until the burn is healed. If symptoms of an allergy develop, stop using the drug and notify your health care provider.
■ Silver nitrate	A bacteriostatic agent that inhibits many different gram-positive and gram-negative organisms. Used as a 0.5% solution in distilled water to prevent burn wound infections.	Apply the solution to gauze dressings every 2 hours and change dressings completely two times a day. Monitor the patient for decreased blood sodium and chloride levels because large amounts of water are absorbed from the dressing site.	Silver nitrate causes the skin and dressings to turn black. Saturate the dressings with the solution every 2 hours, and change all dressings two times a day. Report symptoms of infection, swelling, weight gain, or breathing difficulty to your health care provider.
■ Silver sulfadiazine (Silvadene)	Acts on bacterial cell membranes as a bactericidal. Effective against many gram-negative and gram-positive organisms. Used to prevent burn wound infections.	Monitor WBC because the patient can develop leukopenia.	Apply the drug one to two times a day, completely covering the burn wound.

To eliminate infection on the surface of the burn wound, topical antimicrobial therapy is used, depending on protocol. Many antimicrobial agents are available. The three most widely used are mafenide acetate (Sulfamylon), silver sulfadiazine (Silvadene), and 0.5% silver nitrate soaks. The first two agents are broad-spectrum antibiotics that are supplied in a cream form. The choice of antibiotic is based on the burn depth, wound location, the presence and type of identified bacteria, and whether the wound is treated with an open method (exposing the wound to air) or closed method (covered with bulky dressings) (Table 46-2■).

Other medications that may be used include histamine receptor antagonists or proton-pump inhibitors and antacids to reduce gastric acidity and medications to decrease respiratory mucous production. If unsure about immunization status, tetanus toxoid is given intramuscularly to prevent *Clostridium tetani* infection.

FLUID RESUSCITATION Fluid resuscitation is the administration of intravenous fluids to restore the circulating blood volume during the acute period when capillary permeability is increased. To counteract the effects of burn shock, fluid resuscitation guidelines are used to replace the extensive fluid and electrolyte losses associated with major burn injuries. Fluid replacement is necessary in all burn wounds that involve more than 20% of the TBSA.

Colloids, crystalloids, blood, and blood products are used for fluid resuscitation and maintenance. Crystalloid fluids are administered through two large-bore (14- to 16-gauge) peripheral or central lines. Warmed lactated Ringer's solution is the intravenous fluid of choice during the first 24 hours after burn injury, because it most closely approximates the body's extracellular fluid composition. Infusion rate and amount for the first 24 hours may be determined by using the Parkland formula, in which lactated Ringer's solution is given at 4 mL × kg × % TBSA burn. Hourly urine output is an indicator of effective fluid resuscitation, with 0.5 mL/kg/hr for an adult considered adequate.

Fluid resuscitation rates are adjusted periodically throughout the emergent stage of care. During the fluid resuscitation stage, the patient may require invasive hemodynamic monitoring (see Chapter 17). A pulmonary artery catheter monitors cardiac output, cardiac index, and pulmonary artery wedge pressures. All measurements must be maintained within normal limits to attain adequate fluid resuscitation.

Respiratory Management

Airway management is critical in patients with major burn injuries. The patient's head is elevated to 30 degrees or more to maximize respiratory efforts. To prevent hypostatic pneumonia, turn the patient from side to side every 2 hours. Keep airway passages clear with frequent suctioning, encouraging the patient to use incentive spirometry, and helping the patient cough and deep breathe every 2 hours. The risk of airway obstruction is highest in patients with chest, face, or neck burns. Patients with this type of burn injury will require intubation. Oxygen flow rate is based on ABG results, and humidification of either room air or oxygen is added to prevent the drying of tracheal secretions. The patient may be placed on a face mask, steam collar, T-piece, mechanical ventilation with positive end-expiratory pressure (PEEP), pressure support ventilation, or high-frequency jet ventilation. The goal of all therapies is to maintain adequate tissue oxygenation with the least amount of inspired oxygen flow necessary.

Nutrition

Oral intake can seldom meet the caloric requirements necessary to reverse the excessive protein breakdown and to begin the healing process. Caloric needs may be as great as 4,000 to 6,000 kcal/day. Enteral feedings are started within 24 to 48 hours of the burn injury to offset hypermetabolism, improve nitrogen balance, and decrease length of hospital stay. A gastrointestinal feeding tube is inserted under fluoroscopy, with the tip extending past the pylorus to prevent reflux and aspiration. Enteral feeding is contraindicated in Curling ulcer, bowel obstruction, feeding intolerance, pancreatitis, or septic ileus. When the enteral route cannot be used, a central venous catheter is inserted via the subclavian or jugular vein for the administration of total parenteral nutrition (TPN). (See Chapter 25 for nursing care of the patient receiving enteral feedings or TPN.)

Wound Management

Burn wounds must be cleaned and debrided of necrotic tissue and blisters to promote healing and prevent prolonged inflammation. **Debridement** is the process of removing dead tissue from the wound.

The wound is cleaned with a mild, nonperfumed, antimicrobial soap or wound cleanser solution to remove dead skin and separate eschar. The solution is rinsed off with warm saline or tap water. Body hair is shaved close to the burn wound before debridement to decrease the risk of infection. Intravenous narcotics and anxiolytics are administered during debridement to control pain and anxiety.

Mechanical debridement is performed during hydrotherapy. In this procedure, loose necrotic tissue is gently washed with a washcloth or gauze pad to remove dead skin and **eschar** (a hard crust that forms over the burn wound). Blistered skin is grasped with a dry gauze and gently removed. The edges of blisters or eschar are trimmed with blunt scissors. Wounds should be rubbed hard enough to remove debris yet not cause bleeding. Hydrotherapy measures include showering, using a spray table, or immersion in a tub of water. Prolonged immersion in a tub is used less often because it can lead to chilling after the bath and can increase risk of wound infection.

Enzymatic debridement involves the use of a topical agent to dissolve and remove necrotic tissue. After hydrotherapy, an enzyme of choice is applied in a thin layer directly to the wound and covered with one layer of fine mesh gauze. A topical antimicrobial agent is applied, covered with a bulky wet dressing, and the wound is immobilized with expandable mesh gauze.

SURGERY   Various surgical procedures are performed to treat the burn wound:

- *Surgical debridement* is the process of excising tissue from the burn wound to the level of viable tissue. The most common technique is electrocautery. Debridement may also be performed by using a dermatome to slice off thin layers of damaged skin.

- *Escharotomy* is performed by the physician with a scalpel or by electrocautery. A sterile surgical incision is made longitudinally along the extremity or the trunk to prevent constriction, impaired circulation, and possible gangrene (Figure 46-5 ■).

- *Autografting* is used to effect permanent skin coverage of the wound. Early burn wound excision and skin grafting decrease the hospital stay and enhance rehabilitation. Skin is removed from healthy tissue (donor site) of the burn-injured patient and applied to the burn wound (Figure 46-6 ■). After the autograft is applied, the grafted area is immobilized.

- *Cultured epithelial autografting* is a technique in which skin cells are removed from unburned sites on the patient's body, minced, and placed in a culture medium for growth. With this technique, enough skin can be grown over a period of 3 to 4 weeks to cover an entire human body. The cells are prepared in sheets and attached to petroleum jelly gauze backing, which is applied to the burn wound site.

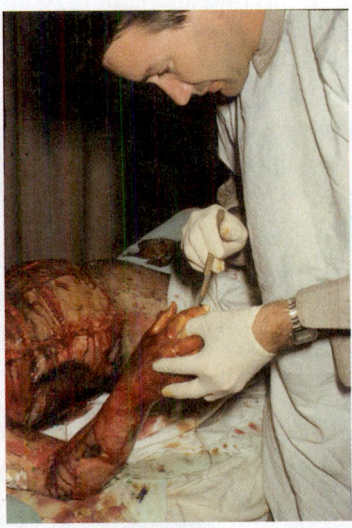

Figure 46-5. ■ Escharotomy. The surgical procedure consists of removing eschar formed on the skin and underlying tissue after severe burns. (Source: © English/Custom Medical Stock Photo.)

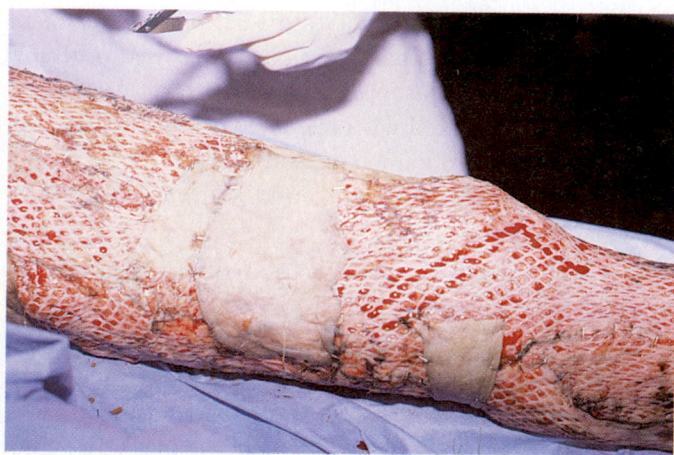

Figure 46-6. ■ Skin graft for burn injury (autograft). (Source: Pearson Education.)

BIOLOGIC AND BIOSYNTHETIC DRESSINGS Biologic dressing and biosynthetic dressing refer to any temporary material that rapidly adheres to the wound bed, promotes healing, or prepares the burn wound for permanent autograft coverage. Ideally, these kinds of dressings should be easy to apply and remove, inexpensive, elastic, able to reduce pain, able to serve as a bacterial barrier, and able to enhance the natural healing process. The dressings are applied to the burn wound as soon as possible. They help eliminate the loss of water through evaporation, reduce infection, and promote wound healing. Biologic and biosynthetic dressings that are currently in use include Biobrane, Dermagraft, Integra, AlloDerm, TransCyte, and Apligraf.

One of the newer treatment methods is the vacuum-assisted closure (VAC) device. VAC consists of a sponge placed over the wound with tubing that connects the sponge to a pump (Figure 46-7 ■). An occlusive, adhesive dressing covers the wound and tubing, sealing the wound to create negative pressure. VAC aids in reducing wound

edema, removing exudate, and improving healing in partial-thickness burns.

SCAR, KELOID, AND CONTRACTURES After a minor burn, the newly formed skin closely resembles its neighboring tissue. The epidermis does not thicken or heighten as a scar. However, when a burn extends into the dermal layer of skin, the skin is repaired through scar formation. Two types of excessive scar may develop. A **hypertrophic scar** is an overgrowth of dermal tissue that remains within the boundaries of the wound. A **keloid** is a scar that extends beyond the boundaries of the original wound. People with dark skin are at greater risk for the formation of hypertrophic scars and keloids. During the healing process, the burn scar shrinks and becomes fixed and inelastic, resulting in **contracture** of the wound (permanent shortening of connective tissue) (Figure 46-8 ■). Once a contracture forms, the tissue resists being stretched, and its inelasticity limits body movement. Positioning, splinting, exercise, and constant pressure application help prevent contractures from forming.

WOUND DRESSINGS After the wound has been cleaned and debrided, it may be dressed by the open or closed method. In the open method, the burn wound remains open to air, covered only by a topical antimicrobial agent. This method allows easy wound assessment. However, it can be used only where strict isolation precautions are followed. Topical agents must be reapplied frequently because they tend to rub off onto the bedding.

In the closed method, a topical antimicrobial agent is applied to the wound site, which is covered with gauze or a nonadherent dressing and then gently wrapped with a gauze roll bandage (Figure 46-9 ■). With the closed method, burn wounds are usually dressed twice daily and as needed. Dressings are applied circumferentially in a distal-to-proximal manner. All fingers and toes are

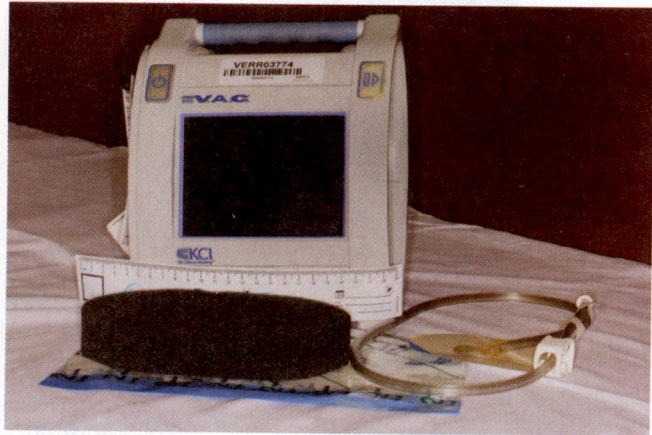

Figure 46-7. ■ Wound vacuum. (Source: Roberto A. Penne-Casanova/ Science Source.)

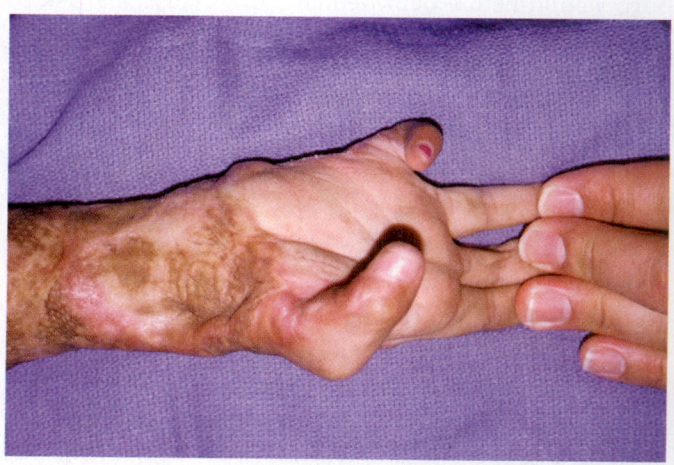

Figure 46-8. ■ Burn contracture. (Source: Pearson Education.)

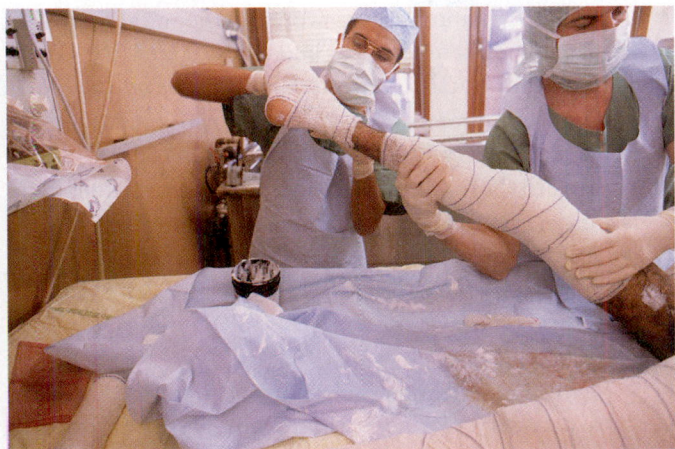

Figure 46-9. ■ Closed method of dressing a burn.
(Source: Boucharlat/Science Source.)

wrapped separately. For wet-to-dry dressings, a thick gauze is applied to maintain moisture and is soaked every 2 hours with the ordered solution.

Splints are used to immobilize body parts and prevent contractures of the joints. They are applied and removed according to schedules established by the physical therapist. Early in the acute phase of care, the physical therapist also prescribes active and passive range-of-motion (ROM) exercises, which are performed during hydrotherapy and every 2 hours at the bedside. Early ambulation is also part of the plan of care once the patient's condition becomes stable.

Applying uniform pressure can prevent or reduce hypertrophic scarring. Tubular support bandages are applied 5 to 7 days postgraft. They maintain a tension ranging from 10 to 20 mm Hg to control scarring. The patient wears custom-made elastic pressure garments such as a Jobst garment for 6 months to 1 year postgraft (Figure 46-10 ■).

Complementary Therapy

Patients with minor burns may apply aloe gel, a clear gel-like substance, three to five times per day. Occasionally, local rashes may develop but will disappear when the gel is discontinued.

NURSING CARE

Key Concept   Primary assessment of the patient with burn injuries focuses on the ABCs, including a patent airway, adequate breathing and oxygenation, and circulation. It is essential to monitor for manifestations of burn shock and to begin fluid resuscitation therapy.

The patient with a burn injury may require care ranging from education for self-care at home to complex care planning involving the multidisciplinary team. The patient and family will experience a wide range of psychologic and

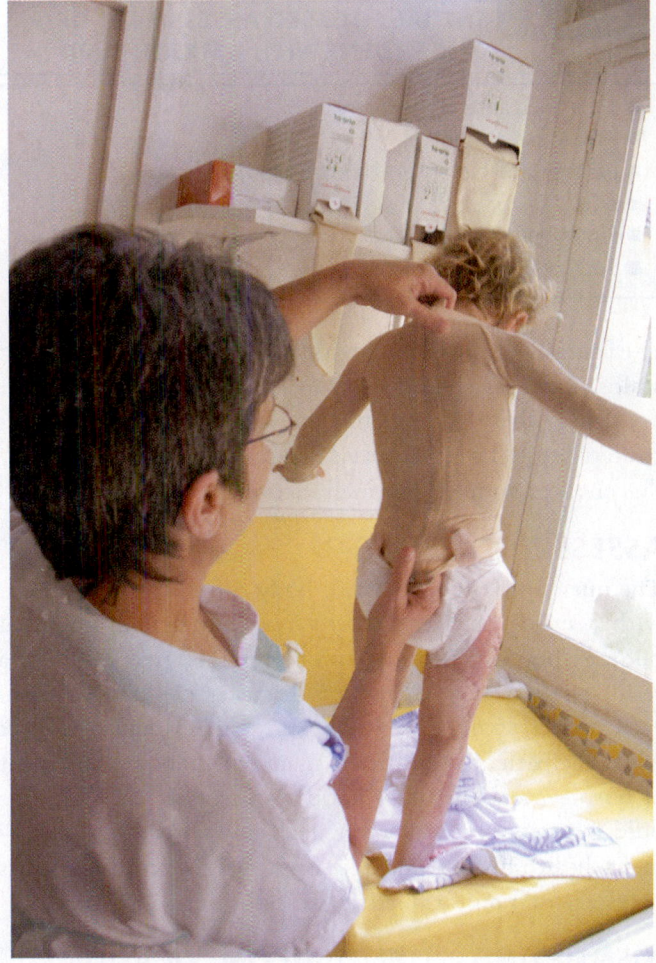

Figure 46-10. ■ The patient may wear a custom-made elastic pressure garment for 6 months to 1 year postgraft.
(Source: AJPhoto/Hôpital de Pédiatrie et de Rééducation de Bullion/Science Source.)

emotional responses. Part of the nurse's role is to support them and to address their concerns.

PRIORITIZING NURSING CARE

During the emergent stage of burn injury care, nursing priorities are fluid resuscitation, maintenance of patent airway, pain, anxiety, and nutrition. In the acute stage, more emphasis is placed on wound care, including skin grafting as needed, pain, prevention of infection, physical and occupational therapy, and nutrition. In the rehabilitative stage, care focuses on assisting the patient to resume a functional role in society. Continuous psychosocial support is essential for the patient and family throughout all stages.

HEALTH PROMOTION

The primary goal is prevention of burn injuries. In the home it is important to (1) install and maintain smoke detectors, (2) have a working fire extinguisher, (3) set water heater temperature no higher than 120°F, and (4) not smoke in bed.

Use caution when cooking with hot water or oils to prevent scalds. Families should develop and practice a home exit fire drill. Advise patients to avoid using flammable liquids to start fires. Have the furnace and wood-burning fireplace flue checked annually for malfunction.

ASSESSING

The nurse initially assesses all body systems of the patient with a major burn to identify not only actual abnormal findings but also potential problems that may occur as a result of the injury. Chapter 5 discusses the assessment of each body system; Box 46-1■ summarizes data to collect when the patient is admitted to an emergency department or burn center. This information is necessary to determine fluid resuscitation, causative agent, any on-the-scene treatment, health history, and age. Body weight on admission is necessary to monitor nutritional status during treatment.

IDENTIFYING POTENTIAL COMPLICATIONS

Complications of the cardiovascular system include burn shock, cardiac dysrhythmias, and compartment syndrome. Common respiratory complications are carbon monoxide poisoning, inhalation injury, pneumonia, and pulmonary edema. Other common problems include acute tubular necrosis, fluid and electrolyte imbalances, Curling ulcer, paralytic ileus, infection, contractures, altered mobility, and malnutrition.

DIAGNOSING, PLANNING, AND IMPLEMENTING

Impaired Skin Integrity

Expected outcome: Will remain free of edema and impaired circulation.

Nursing care for burn injuries focuses on assessing and cleaning the wound and controlling infection.

clinicalALERT

Monitor
Monitor the laboratory data for an increased WBC count.

Report
Report any increase in WBC (of more than 10,000/mm³) to the physician or charge nurse.

- Monitor appearance of burn wound, amount and type of drainage, body temperature, and WBC count. Report changes from usual condition. *Early signs of infection include increased redness and swelling, increased or purulent drainage, fever, and increased WBC.*
- Assist with daily wound care including debridement and hydrotherapy. Explain procedures and administer medications to control pain as prescribed. Keep environment warm. *Wound care is often painful, and the patient is likely to be easily chilled. Hydrotherapy is used to remove topical agents.*
- Apply topical antimicrobial agents as prescribed. Reapply as necessary. *Controlling infection is an essential component in restoring skin integrity for burn wounds.*
- Change dressings as prescribed. When the open method is used, follow strict sterile technique. If the closed method is used, apply in a distal-to-proximal manner. Wrap all fingers and toes separately. *These guidelines are necessary to prevent infection, maintain circulation, and cover all burned areas with dressings.*
- Elevate burned or newly skin-grafted extremities at or above heart level. *This increases venous return and helps to prevent edema.*
- Immobilize skin graft sites for 3 to 5 days. *Immobilization promotes graft adherence and prevents loss of newly grafted skin.*
- Provide special skin care to sensitive body areas:
  - Clean burns involving the eyes with normal saline or sterile water. If contracture of the eyelid develops, apply drops or ointment to the eye *to prevent corneal abrasion.*
  - Gently wipe burns of the lips with saline-soaked pads. Apply an antibiotic ointment as ordered. Assess the mouth frequently, and perform mouth care routinely. If an oral endotracheal tube is in place, reposition it often *to prevent pressure sore formation.*
  - Apply mafenide acetate (Sulfamylon) cream to the nose. Position nasogastric and nasotracheal tubes *to prevent excessive pressure.*
  - Apply mafenide acetate (Sulfamylon) cream to burns of the ears. Do not cover ears with dressings. Do not use pillows. To reduce pressure to the ears, use a foam doughnut. *Burns of the ears are prone to infection. Special positioning devices are used to reduce pressure ulcer formation.*
  - Clean burns of the perineum during hydrotherapy. Assess the area for evidence of infection, and rinse thoroughly after toileting.

Deficient Fluid Volume

Expected outcome: Will maintain adequate circulating volume.

Massive fluid losses occur immediately after the injury and continue throughout the first 2 to 5 days. During this period, nursing care focuses on restoring fluid losses and continuously assessing hemodynamic parameters.

- Assess vital signs frequently. Note increased and weak pulse, decreasing blood pressure, and increased respiratory rate. Document and report changes. *Vital signs change rapidly when fluid resuscitation is inadequate. Those listed indicate decreased fluid volume.*
- Follow prescribed orders for administering intravenous fluids. *Patients with burn shock need fluid replacement to reduce hypovolemia.*
- Monitor intake and output hourly. Report urine outputs of less than 50 mL/hr. *Urine output less than 50 mL/hr indicates decreased circulatory volume and renal perfusion.*
- Weigh daily. *Body weight is used to calculate fluid requirements.*
- Test all stools and emesis for the presence of blood. *Occult blood in stool or emesis indicates gastrointestinal bleeding.*

clinicalALERT

Monitor the patient for fluid volume overload (assess breath sounds, pulse, and blood pressure). Older patients and those with underlying cardiac disease may demonstrate symptoms of heart failure during the fluid resuscitation stage.

Risk for Infection

Expected outcome: Will remain free of signs of infection.

From the onset of the burn injury, the patient is at risk for infection.

- Monitor daily for manifestations of wound infection. *Swelling and redness in intact skin around the burn area; a change in the color, odor, or amount of exudate; and increased pain are early manifestations of infection.*
- Monitor for cough, dyspnea, wheezing, tachypnea, rhonchi, decreased oxygen saturation, and purulent sputum, *which indicate pneumonia.*
- Monitor and record vital signs every 1 to 2 hours. Document and report increased body temperature and pulse. Monitor WBC counts. *Body temperature and pulse increases and increased WBC counts indicate infection.*
- Determine tetanus immunization status. *Patients with burns are at risk for infection caused by* Clostridium tetani.
- Maintain an aseptic environment, using standard precautions. *Strict isolation techniques decrease the risk of secondary infections.*
- Monitor for the presence of urgency, frequency, dysuria, bacteria in urine, and fever. *These are manifestations of urinary tract infections.*

clinicalALERT

If the patient has an indwelling catheter, assess the urine for cloudiness and a foul odor. Obtain a urine culture and sensitivity at least weekly.

Impaired Physical Mobility

Expected outcome: Will maintain mobility to level possible without contractures.

- Perform active or passive ROM exercises to all joints every 2 hours. Ambulate when stable. *Physical therapy begins in the early stages of treatment. As the burn wound heals and new skin tissue forms, the involved area tends to shrink. Contractures significantly limit mobility, especially at joints. Regular exercise prevents further loss of mobility, restores movement, and improves functional status.*
- Apply splints as prescribed. Maintain antideformity positions, and reposition hourly. *Splinting and positioning help prevent contractures.*
- Maintain limbs in functional alignment. *This helps preserve joint mobility.*

clinicalALERT

Assess all patients, especially the older adult, for signs of pressure ulcer formation under a splint.

Imbalanced Nutrition: Less Than Body Requirements

Expected outcome: Will maintain weight within normal limits.

Daily calorie requirements are determined by the dietitian. As soon as possible, enteral feedings are started. Parenteral nutrition is reserved for instances in which enteral feedings are contraindicated.

- Maintain nasogastric/nasointestinal tube placement. *This ensures appropriate absorption of nutrients and prevents aspiration.*
- Maintain enteral/parenteral nutritional support as prescribed. Observe and report any evidence of feeding intolerance. *Diarrhea, vomiting, excessive gastric residue, abdominal distention, absent bowel sounds, and constipation indicate intolerance to the strength or amount of tube feedings.*
- Weigh daily. *The patient's weight is used to measure the adequacy of the nutritional support.*

Acute Pain

Expected outcome: Patient verbalizes a level of acceptable pain.

- Assess level of pain. *With extensive superficial and all partial-thickness burns, the patient experiences excruciating pain.*

Pain tolerance is highly individual. (Pain and pain management are discussed in detail in Chapter 8.)

- Medicate before painful procedures. Determine whether patient-controlled analgesia (PCA) is appropriate. Administer narcotic analgesics as ordered. *Narcotic analgesics are administered regularly to minimize discomfort and also before any painful procedure. An inability to manage pain results in patient feelings of despair and frustration. Invasive procedures and exposed nerve endings increase the patient's pain.*
- Explain all procedures and expected levels of discomfort. *Patients who are prepared for painful procedures experience less stress and are better able to manage pain.*
- Use nonnarcotic pain control along with medications for pain. *Nonnarcotic pain relief methods such as relaxation, distraction, and massage can enhance the therapeutic effects of pain medications.*

Powerlessness

Expected outcome: Will express a sense of control.

- Allow as much control over the surroundings and daily routine as possible, such as choosing times for dressing changes. *The patient with a major burn injury usually endures a lengthy hospital stay. The burn unit is a strange environment, with hospital personnel and even family wearing sterile masks and gowns at patient's bedside; everyone appears different. Feelings of powerlessness during the emergent and acute stages of burn care often pose a challenge to the nurse. Powerlessness results from the belief that one is unable to influence the outcome of a situation.*
- Keep needed items within reach, such as call light, urinal, water pitcher, and tissues. *These items reinforce the patient's feelings of control.*
- Encourage expression of feelings. *Careful listening, a caring presence, and positive reinforcement can help the patient cope.*
- Help set short-term, realistic goals, such as walking from the bedside to the chair twice daily. *Small gains are easier to achieve and allow for ongoing positive reinforcement.*
- Help access support systems, such as spiritual/cultural healing, support group consultation, and psychologic intervention. *Support systems help the patient cope more effectively.*

MANAGING NURSING CARE

As appropriate and allowed by the designated duties and responsibilities of assistive personnel, the nurse may delegate nursing care activities such as assisting with food and fluid intake, measuring intake and output, measuring vital signs, and obtaining daily weights. Before assigning tasks, ensure that the assistive personnel have a clear understanding of the importance of accuracy in measurement and of maintaining strict isolation precautions.

EVALUATING

Evaluate the effectiveness of nursing care by collecting data about wound healing, fluid and electrolyte status, patency of airway, absence of infection, adequate nutrition, pain relief, and absence of complications. Assess the patient's perceptions of ability to control the outcomes of treatment and care. As the burn heals, evaluate effectiveness of exercises and splinting in preventing contractures.

DOCUMENTING

Documentation includes vital signs, appearance of wounds, intake and output, breath and bowel sounds, nutrition intake, CMS of any involved extremity, and effectiveness of pain relief measures. Record patient teaching related to wound care, including skin graft and donor sites, diet, prevention of infection, maintaining hydration status, pain management, and physical activity.

CONTINUITY OF CARE

Patient and family teaching are an important component of all phases of burn care. As treatment progresses, encourage family members to assume more responsibility in providing care. From admission to discharge, teach them to assess all findings, implement therapies, and evaluate progress.

Early in the plan of care, explain to the patient and family the long-term goals of rehabilitation care: to prevent soft tissue deformity, protect skin grafts, maintain physiologic function, manage scars, and return the patient to his or her optimal level of independence. The teaching plan focuses on helping the patient and family prevent dehydration, infection, and pain; maintain adequate nutrition and skin integrity; and restore mobility and psychosocial well-being.

Teach the patient and family how to assess for evidence of fluid volume deficit. Explain the rationale supporting all fluid therapies and emphasize the need to report immediately all signs and symptoms of fluid imbalance: weight loss, scanty urine output, dry mucous membranes.

Explain the rationale about asepsis. Instruct caregivers to protect the patient from exposure to people with colds or infections and to follow aseptic technique meticulously when caring for the wound. Ensure that the patient and family are able to recognize all signs and symptoms of infection: fever, poor wound healing, purulent drainage, malaise.

Consultation with physical therapy begins early in the treatment plan and continues throughout the long-term rehabilitative process. Explain to the patient and family the need for progressive physical activity, and help them establish realistic goals. Also explain the rationale supporting the use of splints, pressure support garments, and other assistive devices, and demonstrate how to apply them. Ensure that the patient and family understand the importance of reporting any evidence of lack of progress.

Identify and answer all questions related to the patient's nutritional therapies and maintaining adequate daily caloric intake. Consult with a dietician early in the treatment plan and throughout rehabilitation.

Encourage the patient and family to express concerns related to pain management. Explain the causes of pain and discomfort and the rationale supporting the use of analgesia. Instruct them to report inadequate pain control. Teach the patient and family alternative pain-control therapies.

Instruct the patient and family in the care of the graft and donor sites. Provide the rationale for use of all pressure support garments. Emphasize the need to report any evidence of inadequate wound healing: altered skin integrity, drainage, swelling, redness.

Encourage the patient and family to express their fears and concerns, and provide referrals to appropriate community resources. The circumstances surrounding the burn injury are often emotionally charged and challenge the nurse to consider all psychosocial implications. Powerlessness, anger, guilt, anxiety, and feelings of loss are common reactions to burn injury. The goal of psychosocial nursing care is to promote functional adaptation, encourage coping mechanisms, and facilitate psychologic adjustment. The burn injury can create dramatic changes in the patient's self-concept, role function, value system, and interpersonal relationships.

Direct the patient and family to occupational therapy, social services, clergy, or psychiatric services as appropriate. Suggest helpful resources such as the American Burn Association, the American Academy of Facial Plastic and Reconstructive Surgery, and the Phoenix Society for Burn Survivors, Inc.

NURSING CARE PLAN
Patient With a Major Burn

Craig Howard, a 39-year-old truck driver, is admitted to the hospital after an accident in which the cab of his truck caught on fire. He was freed from the truck by a passing motorist, who stayed with him until the rescue team arrived and transported him to a local ED. Mr. Howard's wife, Mary, and twin daughters, Jessica and Jane, age 10, have been notified.

Assessment

On his admission to the ED, Mr. Howard is diagnosed with deep partial-thickness and full-thickness burns of the anterior chest, arms, and hands. A quick assessment based on the "rule of nines" estimates the extent of his burn injury at 36% of TBSA. His vital signs are as follows: T, 96.2°F (35.6°C); P, 140; R, 40; BP, 98/60. In the field, the paramedics had inserted a large-bore central line into Mr. Howard's right subclavian vein and started a rapid infusion of lactated Ringer's solution. Mr. Howard is receiving 40% humidified oxygen via face mask. Initial ABGs are as follows: pH, 7.49; PO_2, 60 mm Hg; PCO_2, 32 mm Hg; bicarbonate, 22 mEq/L. Lung sounds indicate inspiratory and expiratory wheezing, and a persistent cough reveals sooty sputum production. A Foley catheter is inserted and initially drains a moderate amount of dark, concentrated urine. A nasogastric tube is inserted and connected to low-intermittent suction. Mr. Howard is alert and oriented and complains of severe pain associated with the burn injuries. The burn unit is notified, and Mr. Howard is prepared for transfer.

Nursing Diagnosis

The following priority nursing diagnoses are established for this patient.

- *Risk for Ineffective Airway Clearance* related to increasing lung congestion secondary to smoke inhalation
- *Deficient Volume Deficit* related to abnormal fluid loss secondary to burn injury
- *Risk for Ineffective Tissue Perfusion (Peripheral)* related to peripheral constriction secondary to circumferential burn wounds of the arms

Expected Outcomes

The expected outcomes established in the nurse's plan of care specify that during the emergent phase of care, Mr. Howard will:

- Demonstrate a patent airway, as evidenced by clear breath sounds; absence of cyanosis; and vital signs, chest x-ray findings, and ABGs within normal limits.
- Demonstrate adequate fluid volume and electrolyte balance, as evidenced by urine output, vital signs, mental status, and laboratory findings within normal limits.
- Demonstrate adequate tissue perfusion, as evidenced by palpable pulses, warm extremities, and normal capillary refill (fingernails).

Planning and Implementation

Ms. Salazar plans and implements the following interventions for Mr. Howard during the emergent phase of care:

- Prepare Mr. Howard for prophylactic nasotracheal intubation to maintain airway patency.
- Initiate fluid resuscitation therapy using the prescribed formula to calculate intravenous fluid rate for the first 24 hours postburn.
- Assist the physician to perform escharotomies of both upper extremities.

Evaluation

The nurse anesthetist has inserted a nasotracheal tube and connected Mr. Howard to a T-piece delivering 40% oxygen. His ABGs have significantly improved. Bronchodilators have been parenterally administered and mucolytic agents added to his respiratory treatments. His tracheal secretions have begun to show evidence of clearing. Hourly urine outputs are 60 to 90 mL, and color and concentration have improved. Blood pressure has increased to 100/64, and the pulse rate has decreased to 100. To improve tissue perfusion of both arms, the physician has performed bilateral escharotomies, and Ms. Salazar has dressed the wounds using sterile procedure. The extremities have demonstrated improved circulation.

Critical Thinking in the Nursing Process

1. Explain the rationale for the immediate insertion of a Foley catheter and nasogastric tube.
2. What is the rationale supporting the intravenous administration of narcotics to control Mr. Howard's pain?
3. What complication is Mr. Howard at risk for developing with burns to his upper arms? Explain why Mr. Howard would need escharotomies of his upper arms.

Note: Discussion of Critical Thinking questions appears on the companion website.

Note: The references and resources for all chapters have been compiled at the back of the book.

Chapter Review

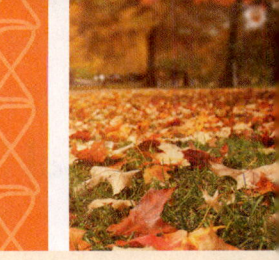

KEY POINTS

- **Concept:** Most burn injuries are minor and treated in emergency departments or clinics. Major burns are often life-threatening injuries that not only interrupt normal physiologic functions of the skin but also may cause multisystem organ damage.
- Burn injuries result from a heat source that causes tissue loss, damage, or irreversible destruction. The heat source may be thermal, chemical, electrical, or radiation.
- The depth of the burn injury determines whether it is classified as superficial, partial thickness, or full thickness. The extent of a burn is determined by using the "rule of nines," which assigns percentages to different parts of the body.
- **Concept:** The American Burn Association defines a major burn as one that involves more than 25% TBSA in adults less than 40 years of age; more than 10% full-thickness burn; injuries to face, eyes, ears, hands, feet, or perineum; high-voltage electrical injuries; or burn injuries with inhalation injury or major trauma.
- Major burn injuries alter the pathophysiology of all body systems. One of the most critical is the shift of fluid into the extravascular space, resulting in a type of hypovolemic shock called burn shock.
- Other pathologic processes affected by major burns include an impaired immune system, altered functions of the skin, inhalation injury, gastrointestinal ulcerations and ileus, renal failure, and hypermetabolism. Each body system must be assessed for alterations and potential complications.
- **Concept:** Primary assessment of the patient with burn injuries focuses on the ABCs, including a patent airway,

adequate breathing and oxygenation, and circulation. It is essential to monitor for manifestations of burn shock and to begin fluid resuscitation therapy.
- Collaborative care focuses on managing the patient through the emergent, acute, and rehabilitative stages. Patients who develop burn shock will require fluid resuscitation using guidelines such as the Parkland formula to replace fluid and electrolyte losses. Hemodynamic monitoring may be used to determine the adequacy of fluid replacement.
- Additional management includes preventing atelectasis, maintaining respiratory function, controlling pain, preventing infection and Curling ulcer, promoting nutrition, and providing wound care.
- Patients with major burn injuries should receive intravenous narcotics such as morphine, hydromorphone, or fentanyl for pain management. Before painful procedures, narcotics and anxiolytics should be given.
- Caloric needs may be as high as 4,000 to 6,000 kcal per day in patients with major burns. When the patient cannot consume an adequate calorie intake, enteral and TPN feedings may be needed.
- Surgical management of burn wounds includes debridement and skin grafting. Biologic and biosynthetic dressings provide temporary coverage until permanent autographs are applied.
- Continual psychologic support of the patient and family is essential throughout convalescence and rehabilitation.

PEARSON NURSING STUDENT RESOURCES

Find additional materials at **nursing.pearsonhighered.com**.

Clinical Reasoning Care Map

Caring for a Patient With Major Burns

NCLEX-PN® Focus Area: Physiologic Integrity: Reduction of Risk Potential

Case Study: Akisha Moore, age 78, was burned over 40% TBSA when her nightgown caught on fire as she was heating coffee in a saucepan. The burns are both partial thickness and full thickness. The partial-thickness burns are covered with large blisters. On admission to the ED, Mrs. Moore is confused. Her blood pressure is 92/62, and her pulse (right wrist is not burned) is 110 and weak. A Foley catheter is inserted, and hourly urine outputs are averaging less than 20 mL per hour. Mrs. Moore is moaning with pain. Her respiratory rate is 36 and shallow, and her temperature is 98°F.

Nursing Diagnosis: Risk for Deficient Fluid Volume

COLLECT DATA

Subjective	Objective
_____	_____
_____	_____
_____	_____
_____	_____
_____	_____
_____	_____

Does this present a threat to the patient's safety?

If yes, the priority intervention to address this threat would be:

_____

Nursing Care

_____
_____
_____
_____
_____
_____
_____
_____

Interprofessional team members to include when planning care:

_____
_____

How would you document this? _____

_____

Compare your answers and documentation to those provided on the companion website.

Data Collected
(use only those that apply)

- Age 78
- 40% TBSA burns
- T 98°F
- BP 92/62
- P 110, weak
- R 36, shallow
- Output averages less than 20 mL/hr
- Moans in pain
- Confused

Nursing Interventions
(use only those that apply; list in priority order)

- Report and continue to monitor vital signs.
- Report and continue to monitor urine output.
- Report and continue to monitor confusion.
- Report and continue to monitor body temperature.
- Administer morphine intravenously as prescribed.
- Determine body weight.
- Monitor IV fluid flow rate.
- Prepare to debride burned areas.
- Cover with a warm blanket.

NCLEX-PN® Exam Preparation

TEST-TAKING TIP Review the disorders that you had difficulty understanding during school. Include the following: etiology, pathophysiology, clinical manifestations, medical treatments, and, most importantly, nursing interventions appropriate for each disorder.

1 During a soccer game, a young student was injured due to a lightning strike. The student began to jerk and speak incoherently. Based on this observation, which body system would be the most affected by the electrical current?

1. Cardiac
2. Pulmonary
3. Urinary
4. Nervous

2 A patient was admitted to the intensive care unit with severe burns to the back and lower legs. The injured skin is dry and leathery, without pain sensations present. What burn depth would the nurse expect the patient to be diagnosed with?

1. Full thickness
2. Superficial partial thickness
3. Superficial
4. Deep partial thickness

3 A patient arrives in the emergency room suffering from burns on the face, arms, and upper torso received in a house fire. Which assessment finding should be reported immediately to the physician?

1. Pain in the arms rated as 6 on a 0 to 10 scale
2. Hoarseness
3. Decreased mobility of the arms
4. Urine output 35 mL per hour

4 An 85-year-old patient, diagnosed with full-thickness burns to the lower extremities, is complaining of severe dyspnea. Crackles are heard in all lung fields with frothy sputum. What would the nurse suspect is occurring with this patient?

1. Acute renal failure
2. Early stages of heart failure
3. Atelectasis
4. Pulmonary edema

5 A patient suffered burns to the anterior trunk and left arm anterior and posterior. Using the "rule of nines," what percent of TBSA was burned?

1. 27%
2. 30%
3. 35%
4. 42%

6 A patient in the intensive care unit with deep partial-thickness burns to the back and left leg is experiencing severe pain. Which of the following medications would the nurse anticipate that the physician would order?

1. Hydromorphone (Dilaudid) by PCA
2. Midazolam (Versed) IV
3. Morphine IV
4. Pantoprazole (Protonix) IV

7 A patient is being discharged after recovering from burns to the upper torso and head. Which teaching point should be emphasized to this patient?

1. Keep dressings on the ears until healed.
2. Encourage a high-fat, low-protein diet.
3. Report any signs of redness or drainage.
4. Apply dressings in a proximal-to-distal manner.

8 Which of these measures should be included in the nursing care plan for a patient with burns to the lower extremities? **Select all that apply.**

1. Meticulous wound care
2. Vital signs every 8 hours
3. Daily weights
4. Range-of-motion exercises
5. Assess peripheral pulses
6. Apply aloe gel to the burn area.

9 A patient with full-thickness burns complains of chills and headache. Which nursing intervention should be the highest priority at this time?

1. Remove the dressings to examine the wound.
2. Obtain a set of vital signs.
3. Notify the physician.
4. Palpate the temperature of the skin.

10 The doctor has ordered silver sulfadiazine (Silvadene) for a patient with a deep partial-thickness burn. What side effect should the nurse anticipate from administering this medication to the patient?

1. Dehydration
2. Pain
3. Bleeding
4. Leukopenia

Answers and rationales for Review Questions appear in Appendix I.

Thinking Strategically About...

You are an LPN/LVN working in a dermatology and plastic surgery clinic. The following patients come for their scheduled appointments.

Geoff, age 69, is retired from the postal service. He has always been an avid participant of outdoor sports, but since his retirement he plays golf four to five times a week. Living in Florida, he enjoys wearing shorts most of the year. In the shower one day, Geoff noticed that a mole on his left lower leg looked bigger and darker. He had just seen a public announcement on television about the dangers of changes in moles. He immediately called the dermatology clinic for an appointment.

With the exception of the nevus that prompted Geoff to come to the clinic, all his moles and freckles are normal. The nevus in question is raised, 3 cm in diameter, has an uneven shape with irregular borders and a nodular surface. It is variegated in color, with various shades from brown to black. The skin surrounding the nevus is slightly erythematous. Geoff states the mole itches sometimes but has never hurt or bled. The surgeon performs a biopsy under local anesthesia.

Marsha, a 21-year-old college student, spent spring break touring with her boyfriend in rural Mexico. Some of the motels they stayed in were not very clean. Four and a half weeks after they returned from Mexico, Marsha developed a red rash in her body creases, especially under her arms. The rash is covered with small blisters and has some small brown wavy lines coming from the center. Marsha states the rash is very itchy. She is to be seen by the dermatologist for confirmation of the diagnosis of scabies and to obtain treatment.

Victor, a 35-year-old farm worker, sustained a third-degree burn on his right lower leg when a motorcycle he was riding fell on him, trapping his leg under the exhaust pipe. He underwent a split-thickness autograft from his right leg. He was discharged from a local hospital 2 weeks ago. Victor comes to the clinic today for an evaluation of wound healing and to determine if further surgery is needed.

CRITICAL THINKING

- Compare the description of Geoff's lesion with the ABCDE skin cancer rule from the American Cancer Society, which outlines warning signs of skin lesions.
- What are some risk factors for Marsha acquiring scabies?
- Why might the surgeon obtain skin from Victor's right leg to graft onto the burn site on his left leg instead of from his abdomen?

PRIORITIES IN NURSING CARE

- If Geoff's biopsy report indicates malignant melanoma, what would you anticipate the treatment to be?
- What precautions need to be discussed with Marsha to prevent the spread of scabies to her friends and roommates?
- If Victor's grafted skin is healing well, what will it look like?

MANAGEMENT OF CARE

- Discuss the staging of Geoff's malignant skin tumor. If Geoff's tumor requires extensive surgery and skin grafting, what interprofessional team members would be involved?
- What measures can be used to help Marsha stop scratching the scabies rash?
- When assessing Victor's wounds, what observations would you anticipate making of the donor site?

DELEGATING

- What part of the care of these three patients can be delegated to the LPN/LVN?

PATIENT TEACHING

- What guidelines should be included when teaching any patient about prevention of skin cancer? Identify credible online resources you can suggest to patients.
- The dermatologist orders lindane lotion to treat Marsha's scabies. What teaching should be provided when giving Marsha a sample of lindane lotion?

CULTURAL CARE STRATEGIES

- Farm workers are especially prone to skin cancer due to sun exposure. What preventive measures must be taken?

DOCUMENTING

- Write a focus note describing Geoff's lesion.

Note: Discussion of Unit questions appears on the companion website.

UNIT XIII
Mental Health Disorders

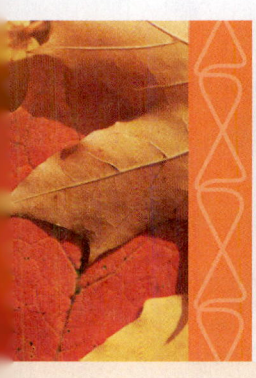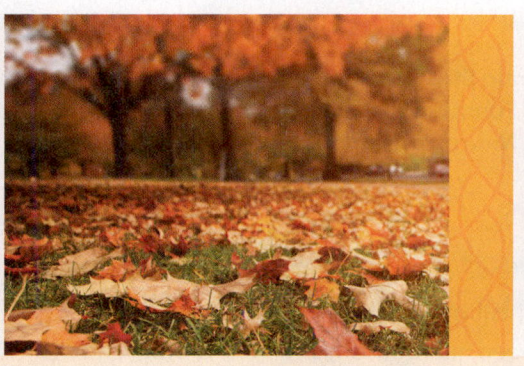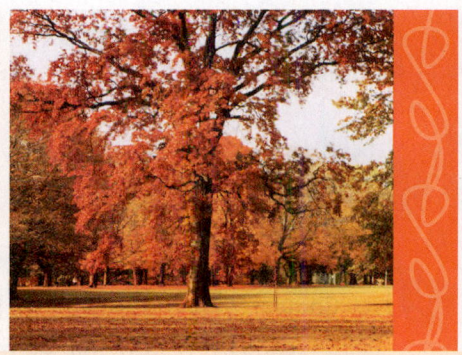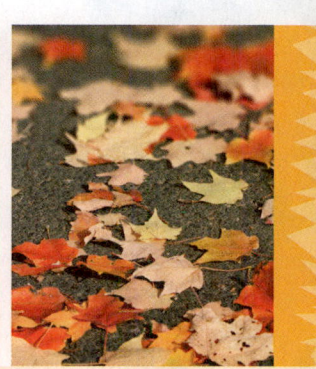

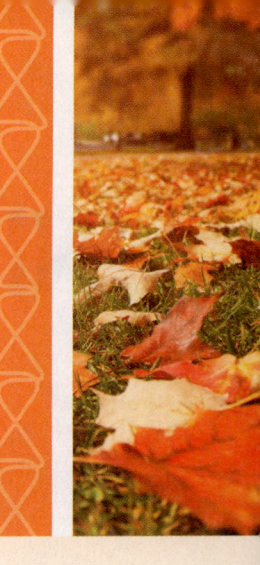

CHAPTER 47
Mental Health and Assessment

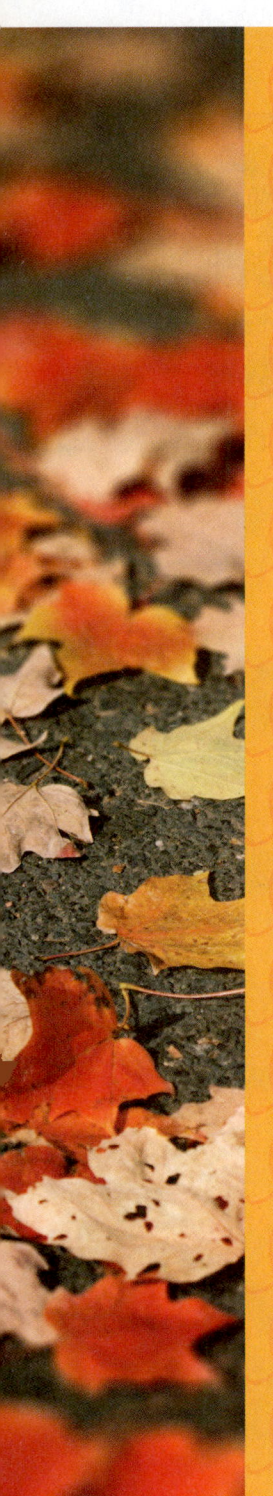

BRIEF OUTLINE

Mental Health

Brain Structure and Function of Brain Neurotransmitters

Mental Disorders Assessment

APPLIED LEARNING OUTCOMES

After completing this chapter, you will be able to:

1. Compare and contrast mental health and mental illness.
2. Describe the relationship between neurotransmission in the brain and mental illness.
3. Discuss the importance of psychosocial assessment.
4. Explain risk factors for mental illness.
5. Explain factors that promote mental health.
6. Perform assessment of subjective and objective psychosocial data.

KEY TERMS

The key terms are defined on the pages listed below.

concrete thinking, 1184	insight, 1183	stigma, 1187
culture, 1188	neuron, 1184	synapse, 1184
family, 1190	neurotransmitters, 1184	
holistic care, 1183	psychosocial, 1188	

Providing **holistic care** (i.e., caring for a person as a whole, including body, mind, and spirit) is one of the foundational values of nursing. Nurses treat patients as whole people. Patients are people who have diseases or disorders, who are people first. Nurses do not define patients by their medical diagnoses or treatments, such as the "asthmatic" or "schizophrenic" or "total hip in room 237." The body, mind, and spirit are integral parts of the whole person. Nurses use the nursing process to treat problems affecting all aspects of the patient: body, mind, and spirit. Refer to a list of nursing diagnoses to find diagnoses in each category.

> **Key Concept** Mental health is an important aspect of the health of each person. Therefore, assessment of patients' mental health status is an essential part of nursing practice.

Nurses encounter patients with psychosocial problems or needs in every area of nursing practice. Patients in the hospital or long-term care settings are likely to have mental health needs as well as physical needs. Nurses who work in the emergency department or trauma care must consider the mental stress of severely injured people and their families. In obstetrics, nurses care for people during the anxiety over the health of their babies and the grief over bad outcomes. Even in the operating room, nurses treat anxiety and knowledge deficits of patients. There is no professional nursing position that involves care only of the patient's body.

Mental Health

In general, there are seven important aspects of a mentally healthy person:

- Accurate assessment of reality
- Healthy self-concept
- Ability to relate to others
- Sense of meaning in life
- Creativity/abstract thinking
- Productivity or contribution to the benefit of others
- Control over one's own behavior
- Adaptability to change and conflict

The ability to determine reality accurately is a basic part of mental health. It includes the abilities to differentiate between what really is and what might be and to reasonably predict the consequences of one's behavior (e.g., knowing that if you hit another person, the person may hit you back).

A healthy self-concept includes a realistic appraisal of the self (abilities, function, appearance) and a positive acceptance of the self as it is. The person in Figure 47-1 ■ demonstrates high self-esteem through pride in her accomplishment.

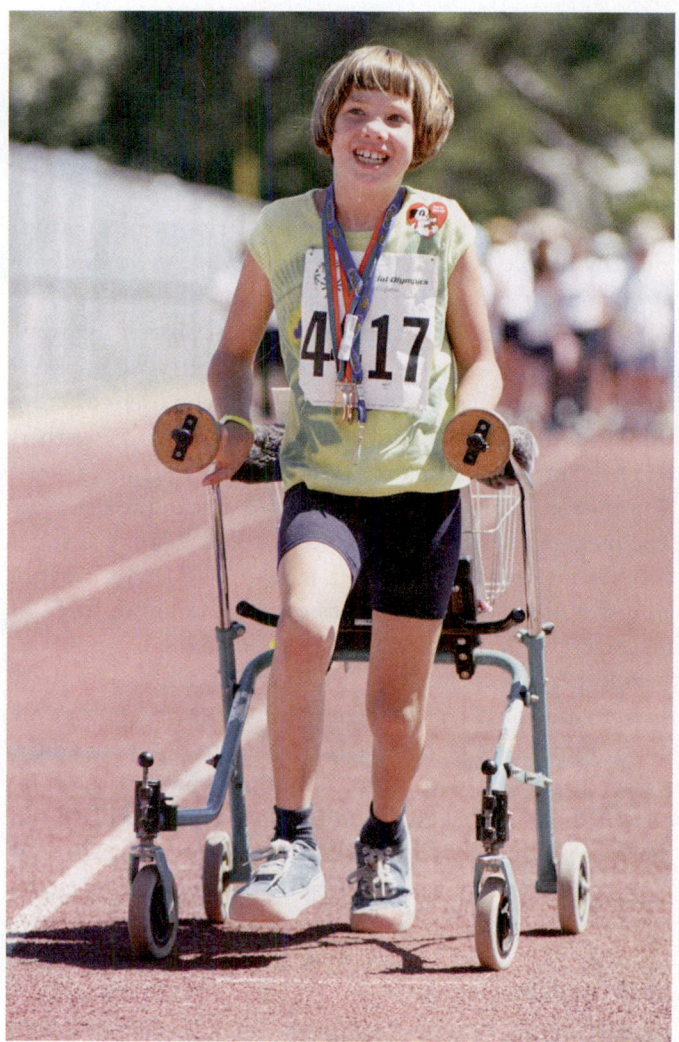

Figure 47-1. ■ This young woman has a healthy concept of herself as an athlete who also has cerebral palsy. She is taking a victory lap at the Special Olympics, wearing her three medals. (Source: © Jonathan Nourok / PhotoEdit.)

Insight, or self-understanding, is important because it allows people to see their own motivations or reasons behind their feelings and behavior. A person lacking insight might refuse to take a medication because it causes his mouth to be dry. With insight, a person could decide that he does not like to take the medication, but because it helps his mental illness, he will take it. Insight is critical for problem solving. Without it people often do not realize that they have a mental illness.

Human beings are creatures who thrive best when they are with others. Love is the most important human emotion. Normal human development is not possible in isolation. People must be able to interact with others in order to flourish. Without the ability to relate to others in a satisfying way, a person cannot be fully healthy.

Humans seek reasons and meaning in life. Many people find a sense of meaning through religion; many others experience meaning through nature. Others may find meaning in philosophy, ethics, or service to others. Spirituality is an important part of what it means to be a person. A fully mentally healthy person will have a sense of what is right and wrong, what is important in life, and what gives life meaning.

A person does not have to be an artist to be creative. Healthy people can solve problems creatively, by thinking of options or possibilities that are not presented in the question. They can interpret experiences abstractly. Some people think *concretely*, meaning literally or without creative options. For example, a person who uses **concrete thinking** may say that the proverb "A rolling stone gathers no moss" means that if a stone rolls it will not collect moss. The answer includes no ideas that were not in the question. The meaning is very literally interpreted. A more abstract thinker might say it means a person who keeps moving around will not accumulate possessions, responsibilities, or maybe even relationships.

Another aspect of mental health is a sense of productivity or contribution. Healthy people want to feel like they are doing something to make a difference to others or to the world. It is healthy to have the feeling that one's actions benefit the family or community. Many people achieve this sense of productivity through their employment. Others may contribute to the well-being of their families by caring for the children or cleaning the house. Some people volunteer for organizations that promote the thriving of their communities, such as exercising dogs at the animal shelter, serving lunches to older people at a meal program, or picking up litter in the neighborhood. Holding a job for money is not a necessary aspect of mental health.

Mentally healthy people can control their behavior, meaning they can balance conflicts with their instincts, conscience, and reality before they act. Healthy people do not act out violently because they are frustrated, nor do they steal something just because they want to have it. Mentally healthy people can delay gratification. They can act in a way that helps someone else, even if it is difficult for themselves. The healthiest people have the integrity to act on their values, even when this is difficult.

Adaptability is critical to success as a person. The one consistent thing around us is that the world is changing. Healthy people can compromise, plan, and be flexible. They can manage conflict successfully. Learning to change is not easy, but if people are healthy they will manage it. Skills are needed for coping with change.

Mental health is a range of behaviors, a relative state instead of an absolute thing. Figure 47-2■ depicts the risks for mental illness and factors that promote mental health. Nobody is at the ultimate level of health in every area all the time. A person can have a range of minimal

to maximal mentally healthy behavior, whether he or she has a mental disorder or not. Just as all people are developing throughout their lives, all people have the potential for increased mental health. Because nurses treat patients holistically, an important aspect of nursing is to promote the mental health and human development of all patients.

Brain Structure and Function of Brain Neurotransmitters

The brain is divided into the cerebrum, the limbic system, the brainstem, and the cerebellum (see Figure 37-2).

The work of the human brain is performed by approximately 100 billion neurons. The neurons are all interconnected, with an average neuron receiving input from 1,000 to 10,000 neighboring neurons. The complex interrelatedness of the human brain is currently incomprehensible. Research is seeking answers to what causes brain disorders such as schizophrenia, depression, and bipolar disorder, and what will treat these disorders specifically and effectively. Although new information is rapidly emerging, some treatments are used because they are effective at relieving patient symptoms, not because their mechanism of action is fully understood.

Human consciousness, behavior, learning, memory, emotion, and creativity are all, to an extent, the result of neurotransmission, the communication between neurons conducted by neurotransmitter chemicals. Neurotransmission must occur for the brain to perform normally.

> **Key Concept**   Neurotransmission is the foundation of mental disorders and their treatment with psychotropic drugs.

Neurotransmitters are chemical messengers that conduct impulses from one neuron to the next. See Figure 47-3■ for a drawing of neurotransmitter function. Neurotransmitters are manufactured in the **neuron** (nerve cell) and are released from the axon (the part of the nerve cell conveying an impulse away from the cell body) into the **synapse** (space between the axon and its target cell's dendrite). The neurotransmitter chemical stimulates the dendrite (the part of the neuron that conveys impulses toward the cell body) of the cell through the synapse.

Each neurotransmitter must fit into a specific receptor site on the surface of the dendrite. The receptor site that is stimulated by the appropriate transmitter opens the ion channel into the dendrite. The ion channel allows for interchange of ions (sodium, potassium, and calcium), which sequentially changes the electrical charge of the cell along the length of the dendrite (depolarization). In this way, an electrical impulse passes from one neuron to the next.

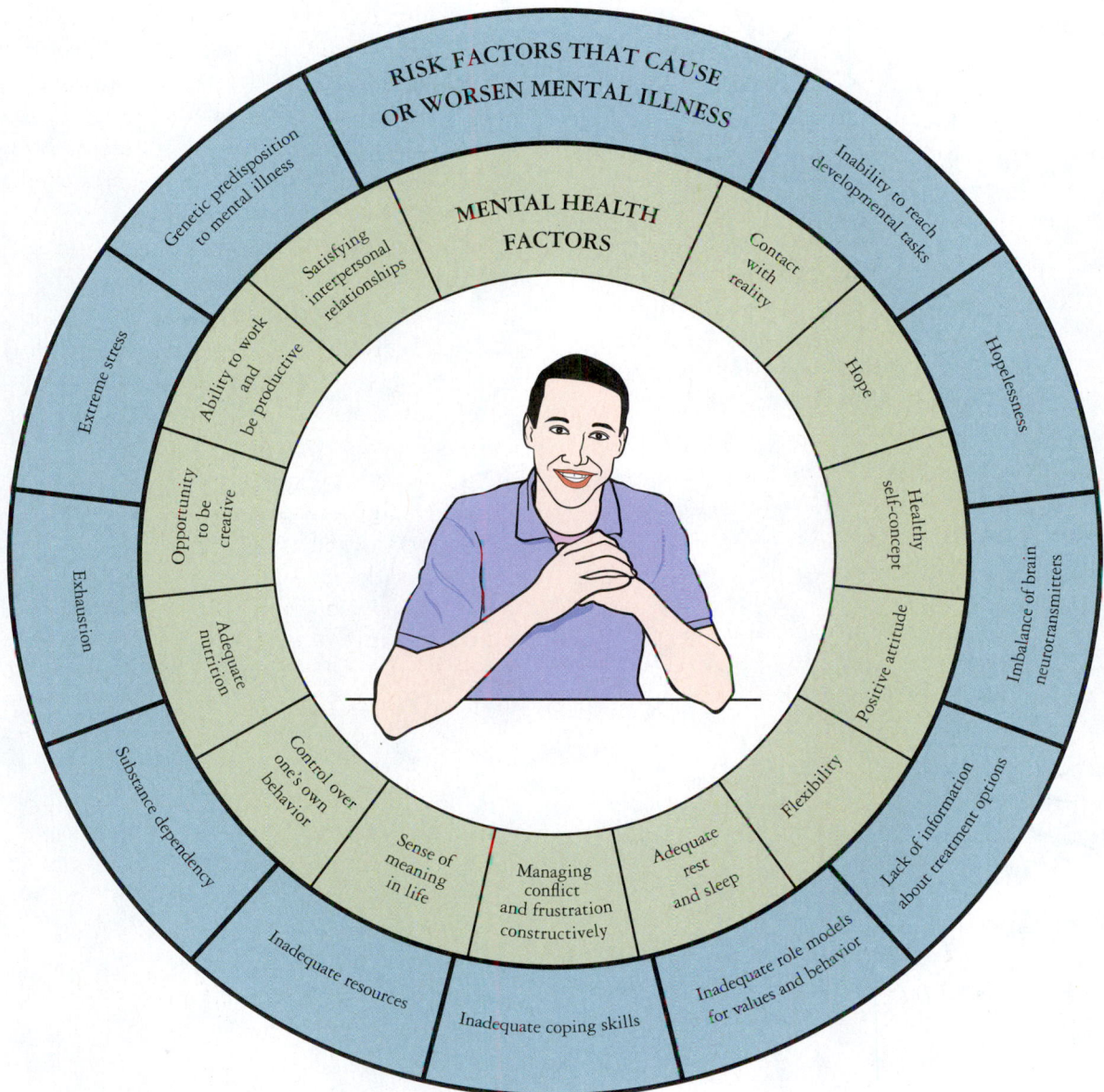

Figure 47-2. ■ Risk factors for mental illness and factors that promote mental health.

After a neurotransmitter is released into the synapse, it either excites or inhibits the next neuron (depending on the neurotransmitter). Then it is either taken back into the axon to be stored for later use (reuptake), or it is broken down and inactivated by enzymes. The most common of these enzymes is monoamine oxidase.

When certain neurotransmitters have abnormally increased or decreased function, mental disorders result. Table 47-1■ lists important neurotransmitters and their relationship to mental disorders.

Mental Disorders

Mental disorders are illnesses with symptoms related to thinking, feeling, or behavior. They are due to genetic, biologic (neurotransmitter or brain structure

abnormalities), environmental, or psychologic influences; most mental disorders are probably the result of an interaction among these factors. These illnesses result in impairment of functioning and other symptoms. Mental disorders are diagnosed according to the diagnostic criteria published in the *Diagnostic and Statistical Manual of Mental Disorders*, 5th edition or *DSM-5* (American Psychiatric Association, 2013). The diagnostic manual is the product of a collaboration of committees of experts working over a decade to integrate current research and expert opinion into a usable diagnostic format. It provides the basis for consistent diagnostic criteria and terminology, and treatment planning for a variety of people with mental disorders. The *DSM-5* allows health care providers from Anchorage to Tallahassee to use the same diagnostic labels for disorders (it is the disorders that are being labeled, not the people).

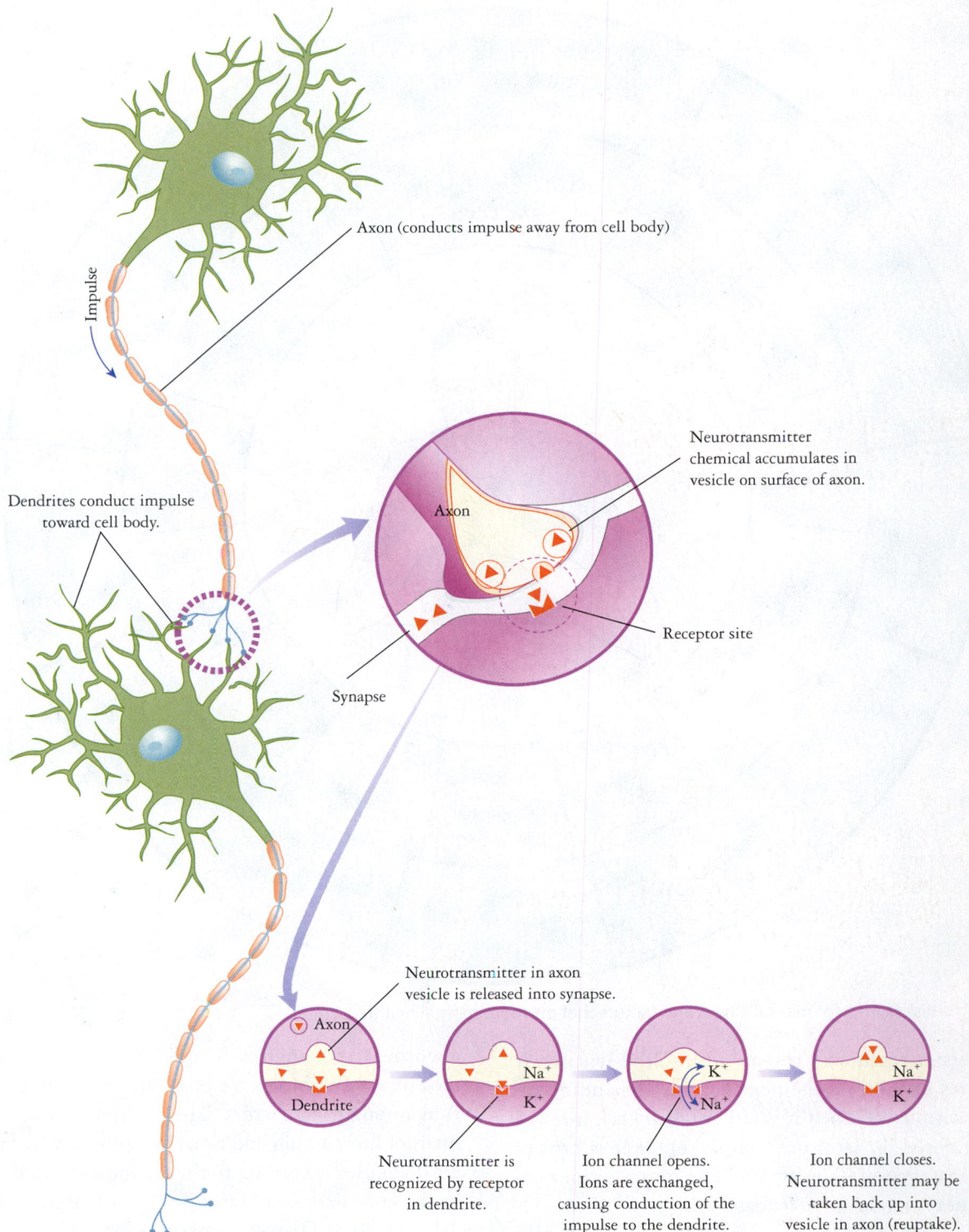

Impulse

Axon (conducts impulse away from cell body)

Neurotransmitter chemical accumulates in vesicle on surface of axon.

Axon

Dendrites conduct impulse toward cell body.

Receptor site

Synapse

Neurotransmitter in axon vesicle is released into synapse.

Axon

Na⁺

K⁺

K⁺

Na⁺

Na⁺

K⁺

Dendrite

Neurotransmitter is recognized by receptor in dendrite.

Ion channel opens. Ions are exchanged, causing conduction of the impulse to the dendrite.

Ion channel closes. Neurotransmitter may be taken back up into vesicle in axon (reuptake).

Figure 47-3. ■ Neurotransmission. *Top inset* shows axon–dendrite interface. *Bottom inset* illustrates step-by-step neurotransmission.

Physicians look at mental disorders in terms of disease processes and medical management. They diagnose and treat schizophrenia, bipolar disorder, and major depressive disorder. While nurses collaborate in interprofessional care, nursing practice is focused on the ways people are affected by these disorders. Nurses treat patients' responses to illness, both physical and mental. Nurses diagnose and treat problems such as ineffective coping, risk for injury, self-care deficit, and nutrition that is less than body requirements.

Mental disorders are a major problem for people all over the world. The incidence of mental disorders is often

TABLE 47-1	Neurotransmitters and Their Relationship to Mental Disorders	
NEUROTRANSMITTER	**PHYSIOLOGIC EFFECTS**	**RELATIONSHIP TO MENTAL DISORDERS**
Acetylcholine	Sleep–wake cycle. Signals muscles to become active.	Decreased in Alzheimer and Parkinson diseases.
Dopamine	Controls complex movements, cognition, motivation, and pleasure. Regulates emotional responses.	Increased in schizophrenia and mania. Decreased in depression and Parkinson disease.
Norepinephrine	Affects attention; learning; memory; and regulation of mood, sleep, and wakefulness.	Decreased in depression. Increased in schizophrenia, mania, and anxiety.
Serotonin	Affects sleep and wakefulness, especially falling asleep. Affects mood and thought processes.	Probably plays a role in thought disorders of schizophrenia. Decreased in depression. Possibly decreased in anxiety and obsessive-compulsive disorder.
Gamma-aminobutyric acid (GABA)	Amino acid that modulates other neurotransmitters.	Decreased in anxiety and schizophrenia.
Glutamate	Amino acid that controls opening of ion channels for calcium, affecting neurotransmission. The major excitatory neurotransmitter in the brain; affects memory, emotions, and cognition.	Implicated in schizophrenia, depression, anxiety, and drug dependency. Increased in Alzheimer disease. Neurotoxicity results from overexposure to glutamate (as in Huntington disease).

underestimated. One reason for this is that the severe impact of mental disorders is not always recognized because people avoid seeking help for mental disorders. They may deny that they are mentally ill, or they may not realize that they are affected. The services they need may actually not be available in their country or area. Some African countries have one psychiatrist for every 9 million people. In Asia some countries have one psychiatrist per 29 million people (WHO, 2012). Mental illness is the leading cause of disability in the United States and Canada, yet many affected people are not treated. Box 47-1■ lists the most common mental disorders in the world. See Box 47-2■ for more details about mental illness.

There is currently no laboratory test to diagnose mental disorders. Technology is available to depict structural and functional brain changes in patients with major mental disorders. See Table 47-2■ for a summary of these methods, which are more often used for research than in individual patient management in psychiatry.

BOX 47-1	FIVE MOST COMMON MENTAL ILLNESSES

- Major depressive disorder
- Alcohol abuse
- Schizophrenia
- Self-inflicted injuries
- Bipolar disorder

THE STIGMA OF MENTAL ILLNESS

Key Concept The stigma of mental illness deters affected people from seeking the treatment they need.

The terms used to refer to people with mental illness (*crazy, nuts, bonkers, one-fry-short-of-a-Happy Meal, wacko, goofy, psycho, mental*, etc.) are different from those used for people with physical illness. What do all these terms have in common? They are all negative and demeaning. When we talk about physical illnesses, we would not use such insulting terms. We would never call a person with diabetes an "insulin junkie" or a "sugar fool." These everyday labels for mentally ill people are inaccurate, inappropriate, and ignorant. They contribute to the stigma and shame associated with mental illness.

Simply talking about mental illness often causes people to laugh nervously. This is because mental illness has a **stigma** (negative attitude marking people as less valuable) in our culture.

It can feel so shameful to have a mental illness that people often refuse to seek treatment, even when that treatment can save their lives. Even physicians sometimes hesitate to give their patients the diagnosis of a mental disorder for fear that the patients will be "labeled" and treated badly as a result.

It is true that people with mental disorders have symptoms and impairment in their functioning (the specifics depend on which disorder they have). However, these

---

BOX 47-2	FACTS ABOUT MENTAL ILLNESS

- Globally, more than 350 million people of all ages have depression, the most common mental disorder.
- One in four people will develop some kind of mental illness at some point in his or her life.
- The largest burden is carried by the 1 in 17 people who has a serious mental illness (schizophrenia, bipolar disorder, or major depressive disorder).
- Mental illness accounts for 15% of the burden of disease in established market economies such as the United States and Canada and 13% in mid- and low-income countries. This is more than the burden of all cancers put together.
- Less than 3% of the world's health care spending is on mental health.
- Although effective treatments are available, fewer than 10% of people with mental illness in the world receive the treatment they need.
- Cultural attitudes and stigma add to the reluctance of mentally ill people to seek help.
- Globally, approximately 1 million people are officially known to have killed themselves each year. The actual number is higher.
- More people in the United States die by suicide than by homicide.
- More than 90% of people who kill themselves have a diagnosable mental disorder (commonly depressive or substance abuse disorders).
- The highest suicide rate is among White males over age 85.
- Approximately 1% of the adult population has schizophrenia.
- Nineteen million Americans ages 18 to 54 have anxiety disorders.
- About 25% of jail inmates in the United States have major mental disorders. In local jails (as compared with state and federal correctional institutions) the percentage is higher.
- At least two-thirds of older adults in nursing homes suffer from a mental disorder, such as major depressive illness.
- Alzheimer disease (AD) affects an estimated 4.5 million Americans. The number of Americans affected by AD has more than doubled since 1980.
- People suffer twice from mental illness: once from the illness itself, and again because they may be shunned by their families, exiled from their communities, and isolated by society (WHO, 2012; National Institute of Mental Health, 2013).

disorders are treatable. Affected people can be and often are successful, productive members of society, such as politicians (including heads of state), artists, teachers, and nurses. The stigma against the mentally ill is certainly not warranted. As patient advocates, nurses should stop using negative labels about people who have mental illnesses and should educate the public that mental illnesses should be treated in the same way as physical illnesses.

There is a human tendency to want to be able to explain the things around us. This may be what makes people who do not truly understand mental illness fill in the blanks in their knowledge with fears and guesses. Nurses must base their practice on evidence, not guesses or stereotypes.

The stigma against mental illness makes nursing assessment of mental symptoms more challenging. Patients may be embarrassed or hesitant to talk about their feelings, ideas, or behavior. Nurses can make it easier for patients to cooperate by taking a confident and competent approach, just as they would when asking patients about bowel movements or urinary output. When a nurse is straightforward and professional, the patient is less likely to be embarrassed.

Assessment

Nurses assess how patients' psychosocial functioning is affected by physical and mental disorders. Both subjective and objective data are important. Nurses, physicians, social workers, therapists, and other members of the interprofessional health care team are involved in promoting the psychosocial health of patients. Psychosocial assessment at a general level is appropriate for all patients. A more specific assessment called a *mental status examination* or *mental status assessment* is appropriate for patients with mental disorders. Both assessments are included in this chapter.

PSYCHOSOCIAL ASSESSMENT

Psychosocial is a broad term that refers to things that affect psychologic and social functioning. Psychologic functions include the following:

- Thinking
- Feelings
- Behavior
- Responses to current stressors

Social functions include the following:

- Relationships with self and others
- Recreation
- Community support
- Cultural attitudes and customs

When a patient is admitted to a health care facility, the nurse may do an initial psychosocial assessment in addition to the physical assessment. Each facility will have its own format. Each aspect of the psychosocial assessment is described in the following paragraphs.

Culture and Family

Information about a patient's family and culture is an important part of the psychosocial assessment, because family and culture affect each person's health attitudes and behaviors related to health and illness. **Culture** is the attitudes, beliefs, customs, and behaviors that are passed from one generation to the next (Figure 47-4 ■). Culture influences how we dress, what we eat, what work we do, our

TABLE 47-2	**Brain Imaging Techniques**		
TEST	**HOW IT WORKS**	**USES AND COMPARISON WITH OTHER METHODS**	**SAMPLE BRAIN IMAGES**
Computerized tomography (CT or CAT) scan of a normal brain	CT scanning relies on the way different tissues deflect x-ray beams that are passed through the subject from numerous points around the circular scanner. CT produces images that represent a "slice" through the body. Done with or without contrast media.	Typically used for visualizing the structure of soft tissues, such as locating tumors or bleeding in the brain. CT technology is more readily available and less expensive than MRI.	(Scott Camazine/Science Source)
Magnetic resonance imaging (MRI) of a normal brain	MRI scanners also produce "slice" images. MRI employs a cylindrical magnet that produces a powerful magnetic field. Radio wave pulses emitted by the scanner interact with atoms in the body affected by the magnetic field, and radio signals rebounding are picked up by the detector.	Used for studying the structure of soft tissues, such as the brain and other organs. MRI produces the most detailed images of soft tissue structures. MRI uses no ionizing radiation. Contraindicated in patients with metal implants (due to strong magnet) and those who fear enclosed spaces. Some hospitals have open MRI machines structured to prevent the claustrophobic feeling of some patients, as opposed to the older style "tube" that encloses the patient.	(BSIP / Getty Images)
Positron emission tomography (PET) scan showing mild Alzheimer disease	PET scanning relies on a radioactive tracer, injected into the bloodstream, to reveal metabolic activity in the brain. As seen here, normal brain metabolic activity produces a roughly symmetric pattern in the yellow areas of left and right cerebral hemispheres.	Used to study metabolic activity in the brain. It can map such functions as glucose uptake in the brain, blood flow, and neurotransmitter activity. The color-coded scan in the example shows brain activity from low (blue) to high (yellow). PET is the most expensive of these scans.	(Copyright © Custom Medical Stock Photo)
Single-photon emission computed tomography (SPECT) scan of a healthy brain	SPECT uses injected isotopes (radionuclides) that emit photons. SPECT creates visual images of brain activity similar to those of PET using a gamma camera that rotates around the head. A computer assembles the image.	Uses similar to PET; SPECT is more widely available and less expensive.	(Charing Cross Hospital/ Science Source)

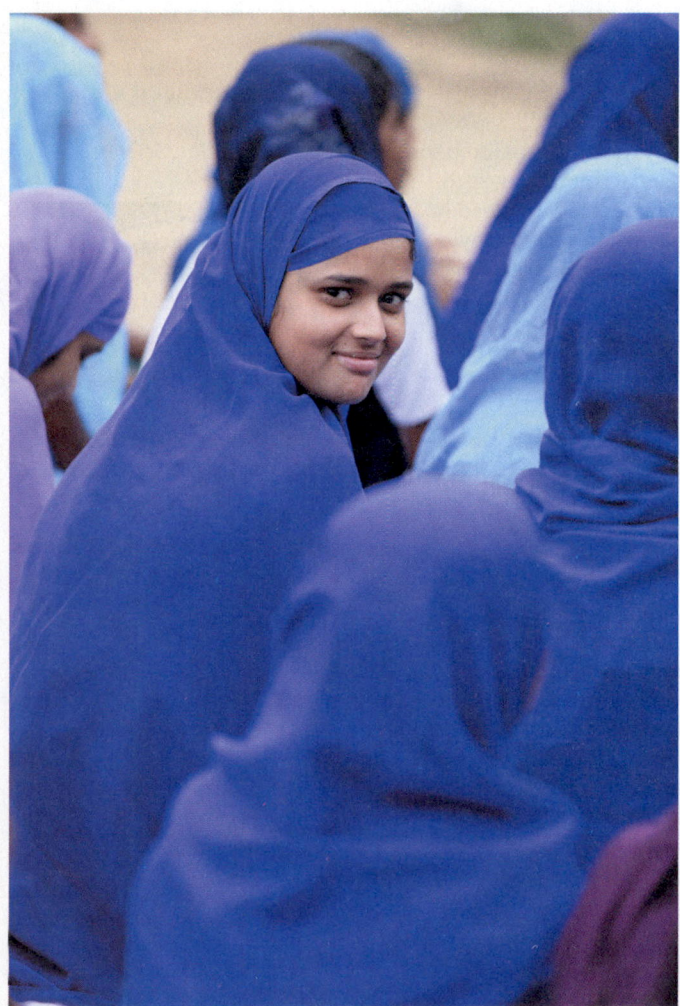

Figure 47-4. ■ Culture affects attitudes, beliefs, customs, and behaviors that are passed from one generation to the next, as with these Muslim girls in India. (Source: © Werli Francois/Alamy.)

religion, the holidays we recognize and celebrate, language, customs, family roles, parenting behavior, the way we relate to other people, how we educate our children, our values, attitudes about right and wrong, and the priorities we set for our lives.

For the purposes of the nurse and the health care system, a patient's **family** can be defined as a group of people who live together or in close contact and who take care of each other and provide assistance for their dependent members (Patterson, 1995). A more recent definition of *family* is an institution where individuals related through biology or enduring commitments participate in roles involving mutual socialization, nurturance, and emotional commitment (Hockenberry & Wilson, 2013). There are many different concepts of family, but the best definition of any patient's family is what the patient says it is. The psychosocial assessment includes the patient's marital status and the members of the patient's household, because this

information helps the health care team understand what family roles and responsibilities the patient has and what kind of support the patient might receive at home.

The patient decides who may visit and who may receive information about the patient's condition. The release of information is noted on a legal document in the patient's medical record.

The languages spoken in the patient's home are an aspect of psychosocial assessment because language affects the patient's ability to relate to and communicate with others. The nurse's ability to communicate with the patient will affect the quality of nursing assessments, some interventions, and teaching. It is important for nurses to know that it requires different skills to understand the technical or medical language than it does to conduct social conversation. Some patients will be independent for everyday communication, but will require a professional interpreter for informed consent or discharge teaching situations. When patients speak English as a nonnative language, even if they speak English well enough to have a social conversation, the nurse should ask whether they need an interpreter for health teaching. When a facility does not have an interpreter on staff, an interpreting agency can be accessed by telephone.

Spirituality and Religion

Religious affiliation is an important psychosocial issue. Patients may have special religious-oriented dietary needs (e.g., Jewish patients who adhere to kosher dietary laws, Muslims who may consume only specific meats prepared according to Halal tradition, Hindus or Seventh-Day Adventists who are vegetarians, Mormons who may not consume caffeine, and many religious traditions that require special foods or restrict foods for certain holy days).

Religion can be especially important to people when they are ill. For example, Catholics and other Christians may want to be visited by their religious priests or ministers when they are sick. The nurse may be able to help patients by asking if they have any religious needs while they are hospitalized. Some people will want to wear items of religious significance (a garment, symbol, amulet, or jewelry). Others may have traditions that require prayer at specified times or certain hygiene practices. Nurses cannot be expected to know about all potential religious or cultural needs, but are expected to know that many people have such needs and that they can discover these issues during the psychosocial assessment.

Reason for Admission

The nurse can find out by reading the chart why the physician has admitted a patient to a health care facility. It is still valuable to ask the patient why he or she was admitted.

The question "What happened that caused you to come to the hospital?" can give the nurse information about the patient's perception of the situation.

Current Medical Problems

Assessing the patient's medical problems might seem misplaced under psychosocial issues. However, medical history is helpful in psychosocial assessment because the patient's health status certainly affects psychosocial functioning. Chronic illnesses provide significant stressors that will challenge the patient's ability to cope when they are discharged. The patient's behavior and relationships with self and others can be affected by health problems. Nurses should consider the patient's whole health status, not only the specific issue for which he or she was admitted, when planning for discharge.

Substance Use

The use of alcohol or drugs as a way to cope with stress is an unhealthy coping mechanism, even if a patient does not have alcohol dependency. (See Chapter 53 to learn more about substance abuse.) The crisis of hospitalization can be an opportunity for a patient to change behavior and to begin new ways of coping. The nurse should ask every patient about alcohol and drug use. Many will underestimate their use. Some will deny use and say that they "never touch a drop." Occasionally, however, a patient will be ready to talk. This is a great opportunity to help patients. If nurses do not ask about alcohol and drug use, the opportunity will be lost.

Another reason to ask about recent alcohol and drug use when patients are admitted is to find out if the patient is currently under the influence of intoxicants. Many prescribed medications interact in potentially dangerous ways with alcohol and other drugs. The physician must be notified immediately if the patient is currently under the influence of alcohol or other intoxicants.

It is also important to determine the history of alcohol use in order to predict the likelihood of alcohol withdrawal syndrome. People who consume large amounts of alcohol regularly are likely to experience elevated vital signs and other symptoms of CNS stimulation if they stop drinking abruptly. Chapter 53 describes alcohol withdrawal in more depth.

Alcohol and street drugs are often used by people with mental illness to treat the bad feelings they have from symptoms of the illness. This behavior is called *self-medication*. Some people who self-medicate with alcohol find it easier to quit drinking when they are given effective treatment for their mental illnesses.

When asking about alcohol or drug use, the nurse must avoid being judgmental. Patients are often embarrassed about these issues and are more likely to speak honestly with a nurse who is accepting of the patient as a person.

Ask how often patients drink rather than if they drink at all. Be careful not to suggest that the "correct" answer is that the patient does not drink. Many people want to give the answer that the nurse wants to hear.

Assess smoking history to determine the risk of respiratory illness and nicotine withdrawal symptoms, such as anxiety, insomnia, and irritability. The surgeon and anesthesiologist should be notified if a surgical patient smokes, due to increased risk of respiratory complications in these patients. A smoking history gives the nurse another opportunity for health teaching.

Patients who drink large amounts of coffee or other caffeinated beverages regularly are at risk for caffeine withdrawal when they are hospitalized. Symptoms of caffeine withdrawal include headache, decreased energy, and constipation.

Support Systems

When people are mentally and psychosocially healthy, they usually have a network of people in their lives. Support systems include people who might be able to help a patient with anything from activities of daily living (ADLs) to shopping, refilling prescriptions, going to see a movie, walking the dog, or checking books out of the library. Information about a patient's social support system is helpful in discharge planning. Social support may come from family, friends, members of religious groups, fellow club members, charitable organizations, neighbors, coworkers, and so forth. When patients do not have an adequate social support system of their own, the nurse should contact a social worker who may need to arrange for help through a public agency.

Self-Concept

Our self-concept affects how we relate to ourselves and to others. Self-concept includes the following:

- Body image
- Role performance
- Identity
- Self-esteem

See Table 47-3 ■ for some questions that can be used to assess a patient's self-concept. A patient with very negative self-concept may need additional assessment for depression.

Coping Skills

Coping skills are the behaviors people use to relieve (cope with) their stress. Some coping skills are healthy and others are not. Knowledge of the patient's usual coping behaviors will help the nurse promote healthy coping behavior or plan for teaching to promote the patient's health. For example, if a patient who has just been diagnosed with cancer usually cries alone in her room when she experiences

TABLE 47-3	Assessing Self-Concept
COMPONENT OF SELF-CONCEPT	**QUESTIONS TO ASK THE PATIENT**
Body image	"How do you feel about your body?"
	"How has the surgery changed the way you feel about yourself?"
	"What do you like or not like about your body?"
Role performance	"Are you able to do all the things that are important to you?"
	"What were you able to do before that you cannot do now?"
	"Can you do [something that is expected during the patient's developmental stage (school, independent adult living, maintaining a relationship, parenting, work, teaching the younger generation)]?"
Identity	"Of all the things you currently do, which ones define who you are the most?"
	"What are the most important things to you?"
	"Tell me five words that describe who you are."
Self-esteem	"How would you describe yourself in 25 words or less?"
	"How do you feel about yourself?"
	"What would you change about yourself if you could?"

stress, the nurse may be able to help this patient talk about her fears and concerns. Learning to talk with others to express feelings and start problem solving might help the patient begin to develop a new healthy way of coping. Table 47-4■ includes some questions to help the nurse assess patients' coping skills.

MENTAL STATUS ASSESSMENT

When asked, "What is the patient's mental status?" the nurse will often reply: "Alert and oriented" or "Oriented times three." Many of the signs and symptoms of mental disorders such as schizophrenia and mood disorders are not covered by the "alert and oriented" assessment. A patient could say, "I am Linda Eby. I am in the hospital. It is Tuesday at 8:00 p.m.," which sounds pretty good, but does this statement show if the patient is experiencing hallucinations, if she feels like killing herself, or if her thinking is disorganized? The major clinical findings of the mental disorders are not covered in a simple assessment of orientation, so a more thorough assessment tool is needed.

Nurses and others on the health care team use mental status assessment to provide a clearer picture of the patient's thinking processes. Because nurses do not read minds, thought processes are best assessed through systematic observation of the patient's speech and behavior. A complete mental status assessment includes the following:

- Appearance (dress, grooming, posture, activity)
- Orientation (to person, place, time, situation)
- Mood and affect (depressed, elated, flat, anxious, changeable, angry)
- Speech characteristics (rate, content logical, pressured, loose associations)
- Thought disorder (delusions, obsessions, phobias)

TABLE 47-4	Assessing Coping Skills
COPING ASSESSMENT	**QUESTIONS TO ASK THE PATIENT**
Past coping behaviors	"What have you done in situations like this in the past?"
	"How do you usually handle problems like this?"
	"How do you manage this at home?"
	"When the stress gets really bad, what do you do?"
	"Do you ever drink when the stress gets too high?"
Plans for coping	"What will you do when this happens again?"
	"What can you do differently the next time that will give you a different result?"
	"Now that we have talked, how will you manage when you go home?"
	"What might work better for you?"

- Hallucinations (auditory, visual, kinesthetic, olfactory)
- Behavior (aggressive, withdrawn, suicidal, homicidal, manipulative, intimidating, confused, intrusive, impulsive)
- Memory (short term and long term)
- Judgment/insight (understands illness, understands need for treatment, able to maintain own safety, able to maintain safety of others)

Note: The references and resources for all chapters have been compiled at the back of the book.

Chapter Review

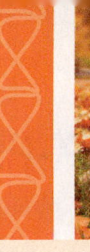
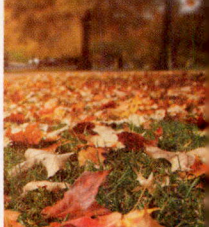

KEY POINTS

- **Concept:** Mental health is an important aspect of the health of each person. Therefore, assessment of patients' mental health status is an essential part of nursing practice.
- Aspects of mental health include accurate assessment of reality, healthy self-concept, ability to relate to others, achieving a sense of meaning in life, creativity, productivity or contribution, control over one's own behavior, and adaptability to change and conflict.
- Holistic care, which is caring for a person as a whole, including body, mind, and spirit, is one of the foundational values of nursing.
- Psychosocial assessment is important because nurses treat the whole patient: body, mind, and spirit. Each aspect of the person affects the others.

- Psychosocial assessment includes patient's thinking, feelings, behavior, coping skills, relationships with self and others, and community support. The nurse should assess some psychosocial issues for every patient.
- **Concept:** Neurotransmission is the foundation of mental disorders and their treatment with psychotropic drugs.
- Mental disorders are brain diseases that affect patients' thoughts, feelings, and behavior.
- **Concept:** The stigma of mental illness deters affected people from seeking the treatment they need.
- Mental status assessment is used to gain information about mental health and the symptoms of mental disorders.

PEARSON NURSING STUDENT RESOURCES

Find additional materials at **nursing.pearsonhighered.com**.

NCLEX-PN® Exam Preparation

1 A patient recently admitted to a long-term care facility is feeling sad and powerless. Which nursing intervention is most likely to promote the patient's mental health?

1. Ask the daughter to stay overnight in the facility with the patient.
2. Give the patient choices about ADLs and introduce the patient to some other residents.
3. Ask the physician to prescribe antianxiety or antidepressant medication.
4. Assign different nurse aides to work with the patient each day.

2 What happens when the brain has too much or too little function of neurotransmitter chemicals?

1. The patient will lose consciousness.
2. The patient will lose control of his or her behavior.
3. The patient may develop a mental disorder.
4. The brain will be completely unable to function.

3 Select the data that are part of a psychosocial assessment. **Select all that apply.**

1. The patient's attitudes about the surgeon and the intensity of surgical pain
2. The patient's coping skills, self-concept, and social support
3. The expected length of stay in the nursing home, patient's daughter's hobbies, and the ages of grandchildren
4. The age at which the patient began sexual activity, and how many steps the patient has to climb to get to his or her apartment
5. The patient's role in the family and the members of the patient's household

4 Which of the following questions by the nurse is most likely to obtain information about the patient's skills for coping with stress?

1. "What would you usually do in a situation like this?"
2. "How many children do you have?"
3. "How do you feel about yourself after the surgery?"
4. "What are your coping strategies?"

5 Which of the following patients has the greatest risk for developing mental illness?

1. A man who is very sad after the death of his dog
2. A 30-year-old woman who lives with her mother while she finishes college
3. A man who is recently unemployed
4. A homeless woman whose mother had a severe mental illness

Answers and rationales for Review Questions appear in Appendix I.

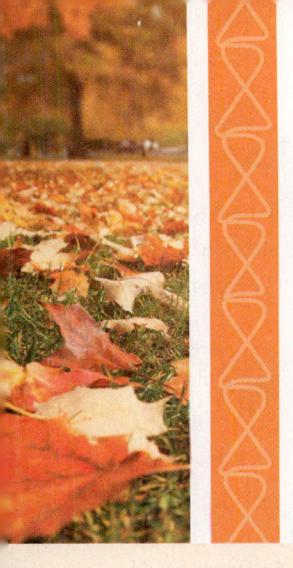

CHAPTER 48
Caring for Patients With Neurocognitive Disorders

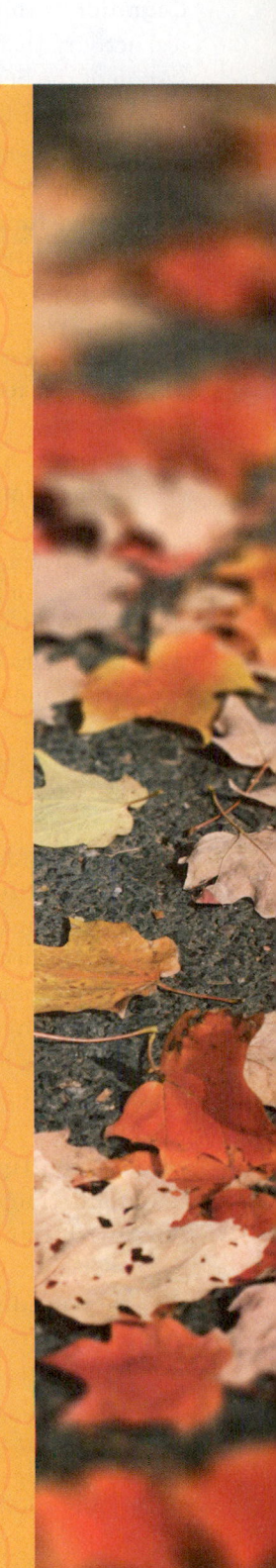

BRIEF OUTLINE

COGNITION	**Memory**	**Types of Dementia**
Changes With Aging	**Delirium**	**Alzheimer Disease**
Neurocognitive Disorders	**DEMENTIA**	

APPLIED LEARNING OUTCOMES

After completing this chapter, you will be able to:

1. Describe cognitive changes that occur with normal aging.
2. Differentiate between delirium and dementia.
3. Identify patients at risk for neurocognitive disorders (NCD).
4. Explain the stages of NCD due to Alzheimer disease and their implications for nursing care.
5. Safely administer medications to patients with Alzheimer disease.
6. Apply the nursing process to the care of patients with NCD.
7. Discuss the impact on the caregivers and families of patients with cognitive disorders.

KEY TERMS

The key terms are defined on the pages listed below.

SPECIAL FEATURES

This chapter is about thinking, some ways it can become disordered, and the ways that nurses can help affected patients. If you can imagine how important it is to you to be able to trust that your perceptions are accurate, to remember people and events, and to understand the world around you, then you will know the impact that cognitive disorders can have.

COGNITION

Cognition is thinking. Cognitive function is a physiological activity that occurs in the cerebral cortex and limbic system of the brain. The American Psychiatric Association (APA, 2013) defines six domains of cognition:

- Complex attention (sustained attentiveness, divided attention, selective attention, and processing speed)
- **Executive function** (planning, decision making, working memory, responding to feedback, correcting errors, overriding habits or inhibitions, and mental flexibility)
- Learning and memory (immediate memory, recent memory [cued or free recall], very long-term memory, and implied learning)
- Language (receptive language and expressive language including naming, word finding, fluency, grammar, and sentence structure)
- Perceptual-motor (includes abilities of visual perception, perceptual-motor, **praxis** [performance of skills], and recognition [as in colors or faces])
- Social cognition (recognition of emotions, social standards and cues, empathy)

Changes With Aging

Aging affects cognition in varying degrees depending upon an individual's genetics, past experiences and living environment, life-long nutrition, and physical health. As the brain ages, a small percentage of neurons are lost, so the brain becomes slightly smaller and loses weight. Slight forgetfulness, especially for recent events, is normal. Problem-solving abilities are slowed. Older adults tend to solve problems based on their past life experiences, which makes them less likely than younger people to try new ways to solve problems. Voluntary movements, reflexes, and reaction time are also slowed due to a decrease in the production of the neurotransmitters that normally assist with impulse conduction. Figure 48-1 ■ depicts normal changes in the aging neurologic system. As people age, they need to consider when to give up activities that require good reflexes and quick reaction time, such as driving cars, climbing ladders, and using dangerous equipment.

Did you ever forget something and wonder whether it is just normal forgetfulness or early signs of a cognitive disorder? Check Table 48-1 ■ to find out.

memoryALERT

Older people move more slowly and are more forgetful because certain specific brain functions naturally become slower. This does *not* mean that brain disorders such as dementia are an expected part of aging.

Neurocognitive Disorders

Cognitive deficits or changes are present in all mental disorders. However, only disorders whose core characteristics are disorders of thinking are included in the category neurocognitive disorders (NCD). The NCDs are conditions in which the impairment in cognition has not been present since birth or early childhood. An NCD (e.g., delirium or dementia) represents a decline from a previously attained functional level (APA, 2013).

The *Diagnostic and Statistical Manual of Mental Disorders,* 5th edition, 2013 (*DSM-5*), includes diagnostic criteria for major and minor neurocognitive disorders such as delirium, dementia, amnestic (memory loss) disorder, NCD with HIV infection, NCD with prion disease, and others. In this chapter, we will focus on the conditions you are most likely to see in nursing practice: delirium and neurocognitive disorder due to Alzheimer disease.

Memory

The two general kinds of memory are procedural memory and declarative memory. **Procedural memory** applies to skills, or physical activities. Some examples of activities in the procedural memory are tooth brushing, eating, tying one's shoes, and other skills that have been repeated frequently over time, such as driving a car. Remember when you first learned to drive? You had to think about every move of your head, hands, and feet. When driving is in your procedural memory, you can referee a fight between the kids in the back seat, order and eat your drive-through dinner, listen to the radio, and still operate the stick shift without a thought about driving.

Declarative memory involves facts. These memories can be discussed (declared) and include standard learning (storing facts), theoretical knowledge (understanding abstract ideas), and memory of personal experiences that occurred at a specific moment in time. Declarative memory is more subject to forgetting. Cognitive disorders affect procedural and declarative memory differently.

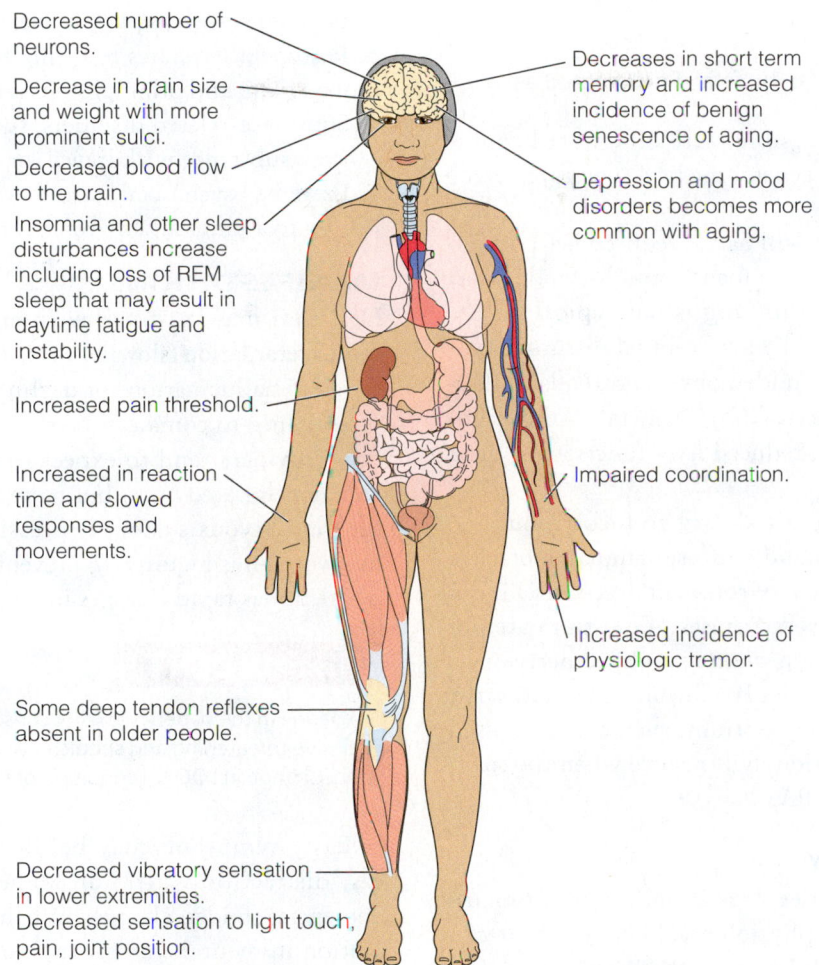

Decreased number of neurons.

Decrease in brain size and weight with more prominent sulci.

Decreased blood flow to the brain.

Insomnia and other sleep disturbances increase including loss of REM sleep that may result in daytime fatigue and instability.

Increased pain threshold.

Increased in reaction time and slowed responses and movements.

Some deep tendon reflexes absent in older people.

Decreased vibratory sensation in lower extremities.
Decreased sensation to light touch, pain, joint position.

Decreases in short term memory and increased incidence of benign senescence of aging.

Depression and mood disorders becomes more common with aging.

Impaired coordination.

Increased incidence of physiologic tremor.

Figure 48-1 ■ Normal changes of aging in the neurologic system.

TABLE 48-1	Am I Just Forgetful, or Is Something Really Wrong?
Use this checklist adapted from the Alzheimer's Association to see the difference between normal brain aging and warning signs of serious mental decline.	
NORMAL MEMORY LAPSE	**SERIOUS WARNING SIGN**
Forgetting where you left your keys or purse	Putting things in odd places, such as keys in the bathtub or laundry in the oven
Searching to find a word that is "on the tip of your tongue"	Forgetting common words or using words that make no sense
Making calculation errors when paying for something	Forgetting how to use numbers
Making an unwise decision	Showing poor judgment in basic daily matters, such as leaving the stove on or wearing mittens and a wool coat on a hot summer day
Momentarily forgetting the date or day of the week or where you were going	Getting lost in your own neighborhood Forgetting where you live or how you traveled to where you are
Forgetting an appointment or someone's name	Asking the same question repeatedly, and repeatedly forgetting the answer
Losing track of why you entered a room or what you planned to say	Struggling to perform a familiar task, such as using the telephone or following a recipe
Choosing not to take a shower today or to skip breakfast	Being unable to perform activities of daily living (bathing, dressing, eating, toileting)

Source: Data from the Alzheimer's Association. (2009). *Know the 10 signs: Early detection matters.* Chicago, IL: Author.

Delirium

Key Concept Delirium can be fatal if not treated early.

Delirium is an acute, reversible state of agitated confusion, which is caused by a general medical (not psychiatric) condition.

A patient with delirium will have a reduced level of consciousness, with less ability to focus thoughts and to pay attention. The change in thinking is not typical for the patient, and it is not caused by a perceptual disturbance or dementia. Delirium has a sudden onset and tends to fluctuate during the day. It is caused by a general medical condition (e.g., kidney injury, reduced liver function, or drug toxicity) (APA, 2013).

It may affect the patient's ability to focus thoughts, recall past events, understand and use language, or have an accurate perception of environmental stimuli. Early recognition is critical. If some causes of delirium are not recognized or treated, the patient may have permanent neurologic damage or may die. If delirium is treated early, it is likely to resolve. Some delirium, such as that caused by severe alcohol intoxication, will resolve when the toxin (alcohol) is metabolized (APA, 2013).

PATHOPHYSIOLOGY

Delirium has multiple causes. It is an indicator of serious, possibly life-threatening physiological changes that can occur at any age. Older adults are at the highest risk, and most affected individuals are over age 65, although children can develop delirium due to a febrile illness. For each individual, the cause is found by determining the risk factors that predispose the person to developing delirium. For example, a patient with delirium who has suddenly stopped drinking alcohol after drinking large daily quantities is probably suffering from alcohol withdrawal delirium. If a patient with advanced liver disease is delirious, he may have an elevated blood ammonia level due to his liver's inability to fully metabolize protein. The ammonia acts as a toxin that causes delirium and damages the brain. Another type of delirium that many have seen is severe alcohol intoxication.

In acute care settings, the onset of delirium often indicates a major underlying biochemical imbalance that might be fatal if untreated. Frequent causes of delirium include:

1. Physical brain disorders, including stroke.
2. Heart disease resulting in low cardiac output or low blood oxygen levels, such as heart failure.
3. Metabolic disorders associated with diabetes, malnutrition (pernicious anemia, folic acid deficiency), renal or hepatic disease, thyroid disease, or other disorders leading to dehydration or electrolyte or acid–base imbalance.
4. Infections, such as pneumonia and urinary tract infection.
5. Postoperative states resulting from anesthesia, blood loss, pain, and other physiologic stressors.
6. Substance-related disorders, such as substance intoxication, substance withdrawal, or drug interactions.
7. Extreme psychosocial stressors, such as grief or relocation to a different environment.

MANIFESTATIONS

Delirium may manifest with either motor agitation or motor retardation (slowing). A sudden onset of severe agitation and hallucinations or declining level of consciousness progressing to coma can be the signs of delirium. Health care providers tend to expect to see delirium in its more common agitated form, but remember that it can also cause central nervous system depression. Immediate medical intervention is required to prevent fatal consequences when a patient has rapid changes in level of consciousness.

clinicalALERT

A change in the patient's level of consciousness (LOC) is potentially life threatening and should always be reported to the physician. Change in LOC is a condition of the highest priority.

Early symptoms may be difficulty paying attention, easy distractibility, and drowsiness. In patients who have dementia, sudden changes in behavior or apparent deterioration in mental status may indicate adverse medication reactions, the onset of infection, or some other physiologic change such as reduced blood flow to the brain. Patients with delirium have an increased mortality rate. All newly admitted older adults should be closely monitored.

COMPLICATIONS

The early symptoms of cognitive disorders are often overlooked, partly because people mistakenly expect older adults to be mentally confused. Another difficulty in recognizing and diagnosing cognitive disorders is that they have symptoms in common with each other, which makes it difficult to tell one disorder from another, or even from the normal changes of aging. It can be especially hard to tell the difference between dementia and delirium, mainly when they occur together in the same person. A person with chronic dementia may develop an infection with no symptoms, and the nurse may only recognize that an abnormality exists when the patient develops delirium secondary to the infection. The recognition of delirium is especially important because this diagnosis carries with it important treatment implications for patient care.

Early diagnosis of delirium is so important because it is an advanced presentation of brain involvement, and treatment must occur as early as possible. Exposure to toxins, including prescription drugs, can cause delirium. An example of this type is postoperative delirium due to drug reaction or slow excretion of drug byproducts (this can happen with anesthetic agents and with drugs used to treat nausea, which act on the central nervous system or with many drugs in kidney failure). Inadequate supply of oxygenated blood to the brain can cause delirium. Examples of this type are heart failure, arterial insufficiency, hemorrhage, and stroke. Infections, such as pneumonia, and even urinary tract infections (which can have severe consequences in older adults) can cause delirium. Obviously, ignoring and postponing treatment of any of these causes can result in dire consequences specific to the individual's pathophysiology, including death.

COLLABORATIVE CARE

Any change in a patient's level of consciousness should be reported to the physician immediately. If delirium is developing, early treatment improves the patient's chance of recovery without permanent cognitive impairment. All surgical patients are at risk and should have their cognitive level assessed frequently. Other patients at high risk for treatable cognitive impairment (delirium) are older adults (over the age of 65); people with diabetes, kidney, liver, or heart disease; and people with alcohol or other substance dependency. Older adults are at risk for having multiple chronic disorders for which they see multiple health care providers. These providers may be prescribing medications without knowledge of what else the patient is taking. Many patients are taking drugs that interact with other drugs or that multiply the effects of those drugs. Patients should be taught to bring a list of all the meds (prescribed and over-the-counter) that they are taking whenever they go to see a doctor. In an emergency, patients may throw all their medication bottles in a bag and bring them to the hospital so the treating physicians will know what they are taking.

Treatment for delirium includes physiologic support (including maintenance of hydration, nutrition, electrolyte balance, oxygenation) as indicated in each patient's situation. Medication regimens should be thoroughly reviewed to detect whether drugs are causing adverse effects. Medications may be discontinued, and dosages may be changed. Environmental support (including a bright, naturally lit room) and reality orientation may be helpful. **Reality orientation** (often called orienting to "person, place, time, and situation") includes nurses introducing themselves each time they enter a patient's room, providing a large clock and calendar that the patient can see easily, and frequent reminders of the name, location, time, and situation of the patient. Constant monitoring of physiologic and mental status is necessary, with an eye toward the onset of further complications. Finally, the patient will need protection from self-injury.

It is better to prevent than to treat delirium. An interprofessional approach to prevention begins with identifying the risk factors. Then, interventions can be planned to prevent each factor that increases risk. The following is a list of risk factors for delirium followed by interventions to prevent them:

- *Cognitive impairment.* Use reality orientation (nurse introduces self at each patient encounter as needed, provide large clock and calendar, remind patient of place and reason for being there).
- *Sleep deprivation.* Initiate a nonpharmacologic sleep protocol, including a 5-minute backrub, a warm drink of herbal tea or milk, and relaxing music. If this is ineffective, then sleeping pills are used.
- *Immobilization.* Use an early mobilization protocol (cooperate with physical therapy), and minimize the use of equipment that requires the patient to be immobilized.
- *Vision impairment.* Use vision aids and other adaptive equipment as indicated, and ensure that patients have their eyeglasses. Explain nursing activities (talking about what you are doing with the patient helps to maintain orientation also).
- *Hearing impairment.* Use amplifying devices, adaptive equipment, and patients' own hearing aids if they have them. If hearing aids are left at home, have family bring them in.
- *Dehydration.* Focus on prevention or early recognition and fluid volume replacement. Older adults may lose their sense of thirst. Offer drinks of various fluids frequently. Have water available at the bedside at all times.

clinical**ALERT**

In addition to the disease processes covered previously, being in the intensive care unit puts patients at high risk of developing delirium. What about intensive care units increases their risk? How can the nurse prevent delirium in these patients?

NURSING CARE

PRIORITIZING NURSING CARE

The priority concern for patients with delirium is the general medical conditions that may cause delirium in the first place. Nurses should identify patients at risk and monitor them carefully (see the program for prevention of delirium mentioned earlier). Notify the physician of any patient's change in level of consciousness or the presence of any of the noted risk factors. The independent nursing priority is providing a safe environment. The environment should have the appropriate amount of sensory stimulation. People with impaired fluctuating cognition are at high risk for injury.

ASSESSING

A classic tool for assessing the mental state of patients is the *Folstein Mini-Mental State Examination.* This brief and easily administered assessment tool has been widely used since the 1970s to document changes in cognitive state (Figure 48-2■). There are 11 items in the whole examination, but a sampling of them is included here.

Each question of the *Folstein Mini-Mental State Examination* (MMSE) provides information about one or more of the domains of cognition. The nurse may use the MMSE to establish a baseline of data about the patient's cognition. It can then be used as a series of assessments to show whether cognition is improving or declining.

The patient's family can be an excellent source of information about the course of the patient's disease. They will know if the onset was slow or quick, whether the patient is oriented at home or not, and whether there are special challenging issues for the patient. Consider the family to be important allies in the care of the patient.

DIAGNOSING, PLANNING, AND IMPLEMENTING
Risk for Injury Related to Impaired Judgment and Disorientation

Expected outcome: Will receive no injuries throughout hospital stay.

- Place the patient in a room with bright natural light. Part of delirium is disturbed sleep patterns. *Patients lose their natural rhythm of day and night. Natural sunlight during the day and darkness (as much as is practical, using*

a small night-light) during the night help to reestablish the day/night wake/sleep cycle. Use nonpharmacologic methods to promote sleep. Also, delusions or hallucinations are often worse in the dark where reality is not easily visible.*

- Approach the patient in a calm, reassuring manner. *The nurse's attitude is "contagious" because if the nurse is anxious, the patient will become anxious. You can lend your calmness to the patient.*
- Observe the delirious patient frequently both day and night. *Delirium causes an inconsistent mental state. In a few minutes, a patient can change and become confused, trying to climb out of bed. Some patients are especially confused at night.*
- Reorient the patient at every opportunity. The room should have a large clock and a calendar. Call the person by name, and introduce yourself each time you enter the room. *People with delirium can be reoriented but may require frequent reorientation. Orientation will decrease the patient's risk for injury.*
- Maintain a safe environment: Keep items that would be dangerous for the patient to ingest out of patient's reach (perfume, soap, water in flower vases, etc.). Keep the space in the room, especially on the patient's way to the bathroom, clear of furniture and clutter. *Inedible things may look edible to a person in delirium. Most falls occur on the way to the bathroom.*

Acute Confusion Related to Chemical, Fluid, or Electrolyte Imbalances

Expected outcome: Will become oriented to person, place, and time and have no more episodes of hallucinations or agitation.

- Orient the patient at every opportunity. Keep a clock and a calendar in the patient's room. Call the person by name and introduce yourself each time you enter the room. *This intervention will help several parts of the process of delirium. The patient will spend more time oriented and less time with disturbed thoughts if the nurse provides orientation interventions frequently. People with delirium have intermittent confusion, which may even include hallucinations, and the disorder can be very frightening for them. Unlike people with long-term disorienting disorders, they can be reoriented, and should be, as often as possible. Do not pretend to believe any hallucination or delusional thoughts a delirious person may have. This only disorients the patient more and is contrary to your goal.*
- Use all your resources, such as the patient, the family, the outpatient medical record, and the hospital pharmacies wherever the patient has been, to determine which medications the patient has been taking at home. Find out all the drugs being taken by the patient, the doses and times, and who prescribed each. Make this information available to the physician. *Polypharmacy (multiple medications especially when prescribed by multiple physicians or other providers)*

Folstein Mini-Mental State Examination, Sample Items

Orientation to Time
"What is the date?"

Registration
"Listen carefully. I am going to say three words. You say them back after I stop.
Ready? Here they are…
APPLE (pause), PENNY (pause), TABLE (pause). Now repeat those words back to me." [Repeat up to 5 times, but score only the first trial.]

Naming
"What is this?" [Point to a pencil or pen.]

Reading
"Please read this and do what it says." [Show examinee the words on the stimulus form.]

CLOSE YOUR EYES

Figure 48-2 ■ Sample from Folstein Mini-Mental State Examination. Data from Folstein, M.F., Folstein, S.E., McHugh, P.R. (1975). Mini-mental state: A practical method for grading the cognitive state of patients for the clinician. *J Psychiatr Res 12*, 189–198; and Cockrell, J.R., and Folstein, M.F. (1988). Mini Mental State Examination (MMSE). *Psychopharm Bull.* 24:689–692.

is a significant cause of delirium. Often older adults have several chronic diseases and are treated by multiple providers. Sometimes the chart at one provider does not include other provider information, so nobody really knows all the meds the patient takes. This is a prescription for drug interactions, overdoses, and delirium.

- When a patient has hallucinations, reassure the patient that they are not real. Keep the patient in reality. Talk about simple things in the here-and-now, such as the weather or what patient had for breakfast. *Patients with delirium may experience frightening hallucinations. The nurse's reassurance that "There are no alligators here. You're safe in the hospital. I'm your nurse. I'm here to help you" may prevent the patient from panicking or becoming agitated. When patients hallucinate, turn on the light so the hospital room can be seen, and simply point out the reality of the situation. Do not pretend to believe hallucinations. This reinforces the hallucination and is not in the patient's best interest. Also, do not argue with them, which makes the patient justify the abnormal perceptions and can reinforce them also. Just tell the simple truth.*

- When you need the patient's cooperation for procedures (e.g., taking vital signs, starting IVs, inserting catheters), approach the patient calmly. Be confident and caring. Explain what you will do in the simplest terms and do it as gently as you can. *If you make yourself trustworthy, the patient can trust you. Your calm demeanor will help calm the patient.*

- Ensure that the patient has full physiologic support. *If patients have a low SaO₂, they may need oxygen; if they are dehydrated, they need fluids; diabetic patients may need fluids, insulin, glucose, or a combination of these. Delirium can be treated by removing its physiological cause (although not all delirium is treatable; sometimes interventions are supportive, to put the patient in the healthiest possible condition).*

MANAGING NURSING CARE

As appropriate and allowed by the designated duties and responsibilities of assistive personnel, the nurse may delegate nursing care activities. For example, the nurse might delegate measuring intake and output, obtaining daily weights, and providing oral and skin care for a patient with fluid volume deficit.

EVALUATING

The patient with delirium should be evaluated for safety issues or injuries. The expected outcome is for patients to suffer no injuries. They should also have mental status (using the MMSE or other consistent tool) evaluated with the goal of improved orientation and recovery from abnormal thoughts (delusions or hallucinations). The nurse must be aware of the general medical condition causing the delirium for each patient and treat that condition as indicated by the physician's orders.

DOCUMENTING

Baseline documentation of the patient's mental status on admission or onset of delirium is important to show where the patient started so changes in condition will be clearly noted. The important points to document regularly on patients with delirium are:

- *Physiological state* pertinent to the condition causing delirium (if the patient has delirium due to decreased hepatic function, the liver function tests should be followed).
- *Mental status,* ideally with a consistent tool.
- The *patient's behavior,* whether he or she is agitated, argumentative, wandering, lethargic, or unarousable is important. If patients seem to be "picking" at the sheets, this may indicate that they see something that is not really there.
- Any *nursing interventions and the patient's response* to them.

DEMENTIA

Dementia is another name for major neurocognitive disorder (NCD). Affected people experience a decline (which can be mild or severe) in any or all of the six domains of cognition: complex attention, executive function, learning and memory, language, perceptual motor function, and social cognition. There are many (over 100) causes of dementia, but 60% to 80% of affected people have NCD due to Alzheimer disease (APA, 2013).

Major neurocognitive disorder is associated with a significant decline in one or more of the six kinds of cognitive functioning. The affected individual, family members, or caregivers notice this decline. Cognitive function is documented to be significantly impaired. The patient's cognitive deficits inhibit independence with activities of daily living (ADLs), such as eating, dressing, and toileting, or instrumental activities of daily living (IADLs), such as using a phone, shopping, driving, and reading. These deficits are not due to another mental disorder, such as depression, or to delirium.

Table 48-2 ■ lists some of the more common causes of dementia. Fifteen percent of people over age 65 in the United States have NCD due to Alzheimer disease, which affects millions of people (patients, families, friends, caregivers). It is progressive, and there is no cure. Because it

TABLE 48-2	Common Causes of Neurocognitive Disorder (NCD)/Dementia
GENERAL CAUSE	**SPECIFIC TYPE OF NCD BY ETIOLOGY/PATHOLOGY**
Neurodegenerative disorders	Alzheimer disease
	Lewy body disease
	Frontal lobe dementia
	Frontal-temporal lobar degeneration (Pick disease)
	Down syndrome
	Amyotrophic lateral sclerosis (ALS or Lou Gehrig disease)
	Parkinson disease
	Huntington disease
Vascular-based dementias	Multi-infarct dementia
	Cardiac disease (cardiovascular disease causing inadequate blood supply to brain)
	Subarachnoid hemorrhage
	Subdural hematoma (chronic)
Toxic or metabolic diseases	Alcoholism or other substance dependency
	Thiamine (vitamin B_1) deficiency
	Cobalamin (vitamin B_{12}) deficiency
	Folate deficiency
	Hyperthyroidism
	Hypothyroidism
	Hypercalcemia
Immunologic diseases	Multiple sclerosis (MS)
	Chronic fatigue syndrome
	Systemic lupus erythematosus
Infections	HIV infection
	Prion infection
	Encephalitis
	Meningitis
	Neurosyphilis
Systemic diseases	Hepatic encephalopathy
	Uremic encephalopathy
	Dialysis dementia
	Wilson disease
Brain trauma	Traumatic brain injury
Tumors	Brain tumors
Ventricular disorders	Hydrocephalus
Seizure disorders	Epilepsy

runs in families, some people watch their parents die slowly from dementia and then spend years dreading or fearing its onset in themselves. No wonder that when they hear the diagnosis, people are often devastated. The ultimate role of nurses in dementia care is to maximize the patient's quality of life. This is a big job.

Types of Dementia

Neurocognitive disorders are named according to their pathophysiological cause (etiology). They are called, "NCD due to … (whatever causes it in this patient)."

Some forms are treatable, such as NCD due to uremia, which can be resolved if kidney function is restored. NCD due to medication use can be treated by stopping or changing the medications a person takes, but most NCDs are not curable or treatable. The three most common types of dementia—NCD due to Alzheimer disease, Lewy body disease, and vascular disease—are not reversible.

Neurocognitive disorder due to **Lewy body disease** is characterized by deposits of alpha-synuclein protein (the Lewy bodies) in the nuclei of brain neurons in the areas that influence memory and motor control. The central feature of NCD due to Lewy body disease is cognitive decline combined with three additional features:

1. Prominent fluctuations in alertness and attention, such as frequent episodes of drowsiness, lethargy, lengthy periods of staring into space, and disorganized speech alternating with being alert and attentive.
2. Recurrent visual hallucinations.
3. Parkinsonian motor symptoms, such as rigidity and the loss of spontaneous movement.

Many people with Lewy body disease also have depression. The similarity between the NCDs due to Parkinson and Alzheimer diseases makes the differential diagnosis of these disorders difficult. It also suggests that there is some relationship among these diseases or that they can occur in the same person, because people with Parkinson and those with Alzheimer diseases can also have Lewy bodies in their brain neurons (National Institute of Neurological Disorders and Stroke, 2013).

Vascular dementia, or NCD due to vascular disease, is also called *multi-infarct dementia* because it is caused by a series of small brain artery occlusions or infarcts (strokes) that cause *ischemia* (low blood and oxygen supply) and tissue death in the brain. The disorder is characterized by a "stair-step" pattern: a sudden decline in function when an infarct occurs, alternating with steady states, unlike the continual decline of Alzheimer disease. The risk factors for vascular dementia are in Box 48-1■.

memory**ALERT**

Compare the risks for vascular dementia with those for other diseases that affect the cardiovascular system, such as stroke and heart attack. Note that they are the same. Once you know this list, you know the risks for cardiovascular diseases in general. Also, the factors that are modifiable (e.g., smoking, obesity, control of blood glucose in diabetes, inactivity) are the basis for teaching patients how to prevent these disorders.

BOX 48-1	RISK FACTORS FOR VASCULAR DEMENTIA

- Advanced age
- History of smoking
- Hypertension
- Hyperlipidemia
- Cardiac dysrhythmias (atrial fibrillation)
- Coronary artery disease
- Sedentary lifestyle
- Diabetes mellitus

Alzheimer Disease

As the number of older adults increases in the world, so does the incidence of dementia. NCD due to Alzheimer disease is becoming an international public health concern. **Alzheimer disease** is a neurologic disorder in which neurofibrillary tangles and beta-amyloid plaques cause deterioration of brain function, characterized by a progressive loss of memory.

The incidence is increased in families with affected members. Genes have been identified that cause Alzheimer disease. Half of all people in long-term care facilities have Alzheimer disease or a related dementia.

Alzheimer disease (a term still in wide use clinically), or Major Neurocognitive Disorder due to Alzheimer disease (the official term in the *DSM-5*), is characterized by two major components and their consequences. People with Alzheimer disease have (1) impaired memory (the inability to learn new things or to remember previously learned information) and (2) one or more additional cognitive disturbances: **aphasia** (disturbance in understanding or expressing language), *apraxia* (impaired ability to carry out motor activities despite functioning nerves and muscles), *agnosia* (failure to recognize or identify objects despite intact sensory function), or disturbance in *executive function* (e.g., planning, organizing, judgment, abstracting). The consequences of the memory and cognitive abnormalities are significant deficits in social or occupational functioning compared with the individual's previous functional level. Unlike delirium, the onset of Alzheimer disease is gradual and accompanied by continuous cognitive decline. These deficits are not due to delirium or other mental or general medical disorders. Some affected people have behavioral disorders. Some do not. The onset is considered "early" if the patient develops Alzheimer disease at or before age 65 and "late" if the onset is after age 65.

The diagnosis of dementia can be confused by the fact that it shares some signs and symptoms with delirium and depression. Table 48-3■ compares and contrasts delirium, dementia, and depression.

PATHOPHYSIOLOGY

Genes on chromosomes 1, 14, 19, and 21 are related to the code for the development of Alzheimer disease. The most characteristic abnormality starts in specific genes on chromosome 19. They control the production of apolipoprotein (APOE). APOE is a protein that transports cholesterol in the blood. The genes responsible for the production of APOE are APOE-e2, APOE-e3, and APOE-e4. People with the gene APOE-e4 have a greater, although not certain, chance of inheriting Alzheimer disease than people with the other APOE types. Inheriting variants

TABLE 48-3	Comparison of Delirium, Dementia, and Depression		
CHARACTERISTICS	DELIRIUM	DEMENTIA	DEPRESSION
Onset	Quick (over hours or days, often at night)	Gradual, over years	May coincide with life events and begin abruptly or slowly
Course	Fluctuates frequently, worse at night	Symptoms slowly progress	Variable but often worse in morning. Usually responds to treatment (causes remission). May be a single episode or multiple episodes over a lifetime
Etiology	Associated with a variety of general medical conditions, surgery, polypharmacy, infections, drugs, alcohol, severe psychosocial stressors	Neurodegenerative disorders, vascular abnormalities, toxic or metabolic disorders, immune abnormalities, infections, systemic diseases, seizure disorders, low pressure hydrocephalus, drugs	Brain neurotransmitter deficit
Orientation, alertness	Fluctuates, disoriented, lethargic or hypervigilant	Progressive impairment in orientation and all cognitive functions	Oriented, short attention span, memory deficit, impaired concentration may look like disorientation
Cognition	Fluctuating, disorganized, fragmented, speech may be slow or fast	Difficulty with abstract thinking, memory impairment, language and perceptual disturbances	May be slowed, may have desire to harm or kill self, may be apathetic, fatigued
Behavior	Psychomotor agitation or psychomotor retardation, or mixed, fluctuating	Apraxia, may have behavior disturbances (refusal to bathe, catastrophic reactions, wandering)	Variable, may have psychomotor retardation, or agitation, risk for suicide
Sleep–wake cycle	Disturbed. Cycle may be reversed	Frequent awakenings, sundowning syndrome (increased confusion at night)	Disturbed. May have frequent awakenings, awaken early, not feeling rested
Progression	Temporary (hours to weeks) if underlying condition is treated; if not, may be fatal	Progressive decline in cognition and abilities. Life expectancy after diagnosis is 8 years	Variable. May be one episode or repeated episodes over a lifetime

of APOE-e4 increases the individual's chance to develop the late-onset type of Alzheimer disease. Geneticists estimate that APOE-e4 is a factor in 20% to 25% of cases of Alzheimer disease (Alzheimer's Association, 2013).

APOE-e4 increases the *risk* of developing Alzheimer disease, whereas a second kind of genetic cause for Alzheimer disease is a deterministic gene. These deterministic genes directly cause anyone who inherits them to develop the disorder in the autosomal dominant pattern. Each offspring of an affected individual has a 50% chance of developing the disorder. Many family members in multiple generations are affected.

The mutations that directly cause Alzheimer disease occur in the genes coding for three proteins: amyloid precursor protein (APP), presenilin-1 (PS-1), and presenilin-2 (PS-2). When Alzheimer disease is caused by these variations, it is called autosomal-dominant Alzheimer disease (ADAD). This dominantly inherited form is the early-onset type. Symptoms nearly always begin before age 60, sometimes during a person's thirties or forties. Deterministic Alzheimer variations have been found in only a few

hundred families worldwide. True ADAD accounts for less than 5% of total cases (Alzheimer's Association, 2013).

Knowing the involved chromosomes is a beginning, but it does not help the clinician determine who will develop Alzheimer disease because in the case of APOE, other factors besides the gene alone determine whether the person at risk will develop the disease. These factors are not known. Genetic testing for the deterministic type is available but is not routinely used.

The diagnosis of Alzheimer disease is based on the clinical signs and symptoms or a postmortem brain biopsy. The biopsy would show beta-amyloid plaques and neurofibrillary tangles. See Figure 48-3 ■ for a look at these characteristic lesions of Alzheimer disease.

The **neurofibrillary tangles** are composed of another protein called *tau*, which is part of the neurons' internal support system. In Alzheimer disease, the tau proteins become entangled. Communication between neurons stops, transportation of nutrients declines, and the neurons die. The tangles appear in the neurons themselves,

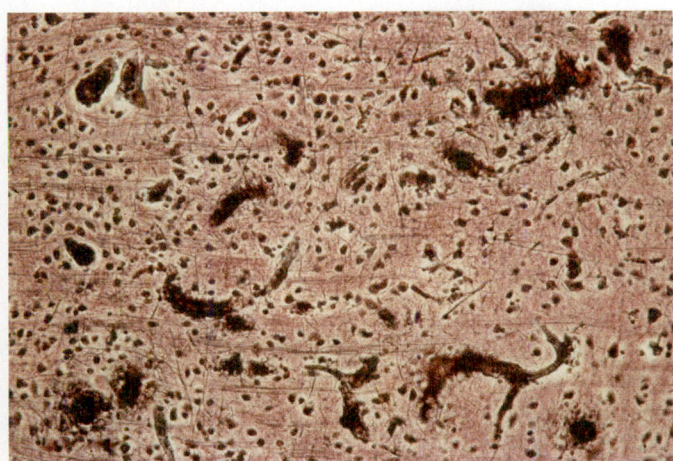

Figure 48-3 ■ Photomicrograph of a section of cerebral cortex of a person with Alzheimer disease. Tau protein neurofibrillary tangles and beta-amyloid plaques are the signature anomalies of the disease. (Source: CNRI/Science Source.)

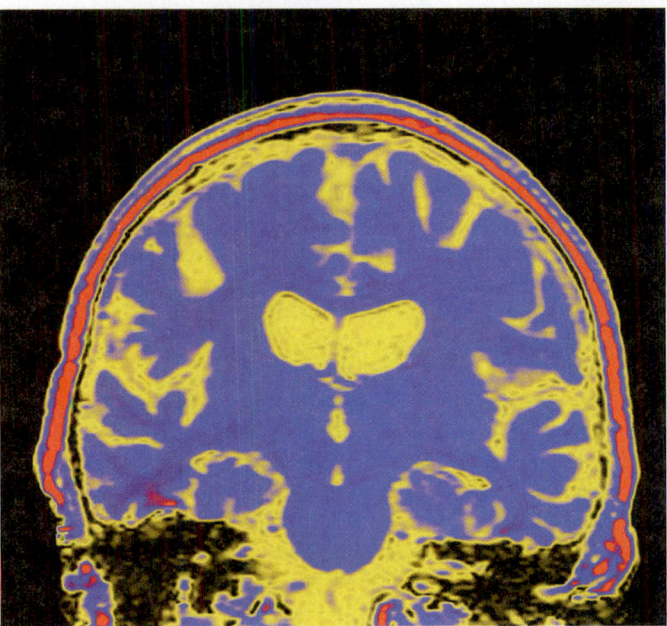

Figure 48-4 ■ MRI of the brain of a person with neurocognitive disorder due to Alzheimer disease. Note the shrunken brain tissue, shown blue here, and the increased fluids, shown here as yellow. The brain also has deep folds on its surface, indicating death and loss of brain tissue. (Source: Dr. W. Crum, Dementia Research Group / Tim Beddow/Science Source.)

and the beta-amyloid plaques occur outside the neurons. They tend to begin to cause symptoms when they accumulate in the parts of the brain most involved with memory. The **beta-amyloid plaques** are the buildup of fragments produced when enzymes act on amyloid protein. Abnormally high levels of beta-amyloid are thought to produce damage to neurons either directly or by eliciting an inflammatory response and ultimately neuron death. It is not known whether these tangles and plaques cause the disease or are a result of the disease process (Eby & Brown, 2009).

Figure 48-4■ depicts an MRI of the brain of a person with NCD due to Alzheimer disease. Note the shrunken brain (blue in this picture), the extra fluid (depicted here as yellow), and the deep folding and shrinking in the Alzheimer brain, all showing loss of brain tissue. Another abnormal finding in Alzheimer disease is the deficiency of the neurotransmitter acetylcholine. When it is lacking, neurotransmission is impaired. Returning acetylcholine to normal levels is the function of some anti-Alzheimer drugs.

Growing evidence links brain health to heart health. Every heartbeat pumps 25% of its volume to the head, where brain cells use at least 20% of the food and oxygen that is carried in the blood. The risk of NCD due to Alzheimer or vascular diseases appears to be increased by conditions that damage the heart or blood vessels. Plaques and tangles are more likely to cause Alzheimer disease if symptoms of stroke or damage to the brain's blood vessels are also present (Alzheimer's Association, 2013).

MANIFESTATIONS

The signs and symptoms of any individual with Alzheimer disease depend on the progression of the disease and how far the individual has advanced. Pathologic changes may precede clinical manifestations by 5 to 20 years. The Alzheimer's Association has developed a list of 10 warning signs that include the most common manifestations of the disease (Box 48-2■). The nursing care of patients with Alzheimer disease depends on the stage and the patient's individual needs. The stages of Alzheimer disease are early, middle, and late. In the course of the disease, specific altered behaviors occur that are typical of the disease; these are discussed later in this chapter.

Patients should be advised that if they recognize any of these signs in themselves or their loved ones, they should see a health care provider. Early diagnosis of Alzheimer disease is an important step toward treatment, care, and support services.

Early Stage

The initial sign of Alzheimer disease is deterioration in memory. It may go unnoticed by family and friends until it becomes too severe for the patient, or sometimes his or her spouse, to cover it up. The early stage usually lasts 2 to 4 years. Antidementia medications are intended to prolong this stage. During this stage, there is a gradually increasing short-term memory impairment, especially for new learning. Patients experience forgetfulness (beyond what is normal or usual for people of their age). They tend to lose initiative and their usual interests. Their judgment is diminished, as is their orientation to geography.

Ten Warning Signs of Alzheimer Disease

1. *Memory loss.* Forgetting recently learned information is one of the most common early signs of dementia. A person begins to forget more often and is unable to recall the information later.

2. *Difficulty performing familiar tasks.* People with dementia often find it hard to plan or complete everyday tasks. Individuals may lose track of the steps involved in preparing a meal, placing a telephone call, or playing a game.

3. *Problems with language.* People with Alzheimer disease often forget simple words or substitute unusual words, making their speech or writing hard to understand. For example, they may forget the word for toothbrush and say, "that thing for my mouth."

4. *Disorientation to time and place.* People with Alzheimer disease can become lost in their own neighborhood, forget where they are and how they got there, and not know how to get back home.

5. *Poor or decreased judgment.* Those with Alzheimer disease may dress inappropriately, wearing several layers on a warm day or little clothing in the cold. They may show poor judgment, like giving away large sums of money to telemarketers.

6. *Problems with abstract thinking.* Someone with Alzheimer disease may have unusual difficulty performing complex mental tasks, such as forgetting what numbers are for and how they should be used.

7. *Misplacing things.* A person with Alzheimer disease may put things in unusual places: an iron in the freezer or a wristwatch in the sugar bowl.

8. *Changes in mood or behavior.* Someone with Alzheimer disease may show rapid mood swings from calm to tears to anger, for no apparent reason.

9. *Changes in personality.* The personalities of people with dementia can change dramatically. They may become extremely confused, suspicious, fearful, or dependent on a family member.

10. *Loss of initiative.* A person with Alzheimer disease may become very passive, sitting in front of the TV for hours, sleeping more than usual, or not wanting to do usual activities.

Source: Data from the Alzheimer's Association. (2009). *10 warning signs of Alzheimer's.* Chicago, IL: Author.

Middle Stage

The second stage of the disease is usually the longest, lasting 2 to 10 years after the diagnosis. Memory loss and mental confusion worsen. As remote memory is lost, the patient has difficulty recognizing close family and friends. Patients may wander, becoming particularly restless in the late afternoon or early evening. They may have difficulty organizing thoughts or thinking logically.

Our case example is Edith, who lived alone in an older apartment building where she had previously been very self-sufficient. She walked to a nearby grocery store, caught the bus to go shopping, did her own laundry in the apartment facilities, wrote letters, cooked for herself, and enjoyed being with and talking to people. She never turned down an invitation to go out. As the disease began to take hold of her, she stayed in more and more. She turned down social opportunities, saying she had to stay in to write to her children. When her children called to find out why she had not written, she said she had been too busy going out. Numerous half-finished letters were found in her apartment. It was evident that she had lost her train of thought and just stopped writing. She stopped going to the apartment complex's laundry facilities and began washing her clothes in the bathtub. Sometimes, she would just put her dirty clothes back into her dresser or hang them back up in the closet. Her apartment was disheveled and she could no longer remember how to cook much except chili and a lemon cake. She had someone else manage her checkbook and pay her bills. She just signed her name.

Source: Nancy Brown in Eby, L., & Brown, N. J. (2009). *Mental health nursing care,* 2nd ed. Upper Saddle River, NJ: Pearson.

In the Ginkgo Evaluation of Memory (GEM) Study, 3,069 community individuals participated in a double-blind placebo-controlled study of whether *ginkgo biloba* would prevent or delay the development of dementia. The study, conducted in five U.S. university medical centers from 2000 to 2008, found no decreased incidence of dementia in *gingko* users and also no postponement of dementia onset as compared with the placebo group.
The study found no evidence for the value of *gingko* for patients with dementia.

Patients in this stage may experience hallucinations, delusional thinking, or illusions. An **illusion** is a misinterpretation of environmental stimuli. Unlike a hallucination where there is not a real object present, an illusion misinterprets something that is there. A patient may look at a bathtub and see a bottomless pit. She might not be able to tell the difference between what is on television and what is in her room. The patient may have expressive or receptive aphasia and apraxia. Behavioral problems at this stage may include agitation and aggressiveness. Patients may *confabulate* or make up stories to explain something that they do not remember or know how to answer.

In this stage, family members often come to the conclusion that they are unable to manage the care of their loved one at home. People who are admitted to long-term care facilities have often experienced severe life stressors.

Consider our patient, Edith, in the middle stage of the disease. When Edith's daughter suspected there was something wrong, she invited her mother to come for a visit. On the first night, Edith got up in the middle of the night and urinated in the bedroom trash basket, thinking it was a toilet. She brought summer clothes and no coat for a visit in November. When her daughter moved her from her old home to a new apartment close by, Edith needed daily supervision. When Edith saw herself in the mirror on her door, she did not recognize herself in the mirror. She told her daughter there was a child living behind the door. Edith sometimes spoke to her daughter as if her daughter were Edith's mother or sister. She called her granddaughter her niece. When asked why she had poured water into a jar of instant coffee, she replied, "I didn't. The coffee just melted." The daughter realized it was time for Edith to receive full-time care when Edith cut the cord of her electric blanket because she could not unplug it. (Fortunately, it was not turned on.)

Source: Nancy Brown in Eby, L., & Brown, N. J. (2009). *Mental health nursing care,* 2nd ed. Upper Saddle River, NJ: Pearson.

Late Stage

The last stage of Alzheimer disease may last 1 to 3 years. In the late stage, the patient has little memory and is thus unable to process new information. Patients may not be able to understand words and forget how to do, and the meaning of, self-care activities. They are likely immobile and incontinent, which is a point at which many families are unable to continue to provide care for their loved one at home. Patients may make repetitious sounds instead of speech and may have difficulty eating and swallowing. Some patients experience **hyperorality**, putting anything within reach into their mouths. Patients at this stage are susceptible to choking, pneumonia, and other infections. Some patients assume the fetal position. The culmination of this stage, of course, is death.

Edith maintained a pleasant demeanor throughout her disease. She laughed inappropriately when she could no longer think of words to say. She had to be dressed, fed, and changed. She died from a stroke less than 10 years from when she was diagnosed.

Source: Nancy Brown in Eby, L., & Brown, N. J. (2009). *Mental health nursing care*, 2nd ed. Upper Saddle River, NJ: Pearson.

ALTERED BEHAVIORS IN ALZHEIMER DISEASE
Wandering

The confusion from dementia often results in a behavior called *wandering*. Patients may walk up and down the halls, may walk around their rooms, or may go outside for a walk and get lost when they forget neighborhood landmarks.

Some patients who live in institutions wander about the nursing home or hospital checking each doorknob for a way to their destination. A wandering patient is in danger of falling, injury, and becoming lost.

Wandering behavior may be motivated by discomfort, the need to use the bathroom, wanting to see family, or searching for something that is meaningful to them. Nurses should be aware of risks but also allow patients to be up and about as much as possible. Sometimes a change of subject is helpful, as in, "The bathroom is this way. Then I'll walk with you to the dining room for lunch." Several patient-tracking mechanisms are on the market to improve the safety of wanderers.

Sundowning Syndrome

Sundowning syndrome is the increased mental confusion in the evening that affects people with Alzheimer disease. The reason may be decreasing light and a resulting confused sensory perception, or it might be that older patients with dementia experience fatigue in the evenings and have reduced resilience. They are less able to tolerate stress.

Refusal to Bathe

Refusal to do any of the activities of daily living, especially bathing, may become a problem behavior. As Alzheimer disease progresses, patients lose certain abilities, including depth perception. They may perceive the bathtub as a bottomless pit or misperceive it in other ways. The process of bathing can also be frightening when an individual the patient does not recognize tries to pull off his or her clothes. Figure 48-5 ■ depicts a woman in the middle stage of Alzheimer disease who does not recognize her daughter.

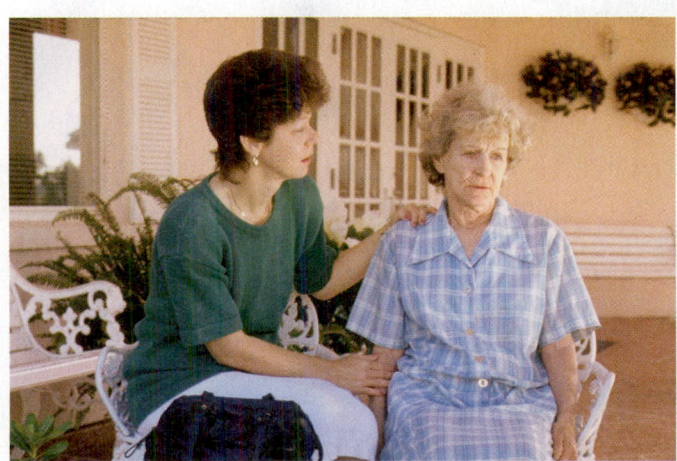

Figure 48-5 ■ This woman in the middle stage of Alzheimer disease has forgotten who her daughter is. Imagine the daughter's feelings. (Source: Michal Heron, Pearson Education.)

Paranoia/Suspicion

Suspicious thinking is to be expected in people with Alzheimer disease. Patients often accuse family members, staff, or roommates of stealing their possessions. One explanation is that they may hide things and, with poor short-term memory, forget where they are. The nurse should not automatically assume that just because a patient has dementia that his or her allegations are false, however. Expensive possessions should, when possible, be locked in a safe place to prevent serious problems.

Catastrophic Reactions

A **catastrophic reaction** is an explosive behavioral or anger response that is totally out of proportion to the situation (Figure 48-6■). These reactions can result in violence, such as hitting, spitting, cursing, screaming, or crying. The overreaction may be due to the difficulty in modulating

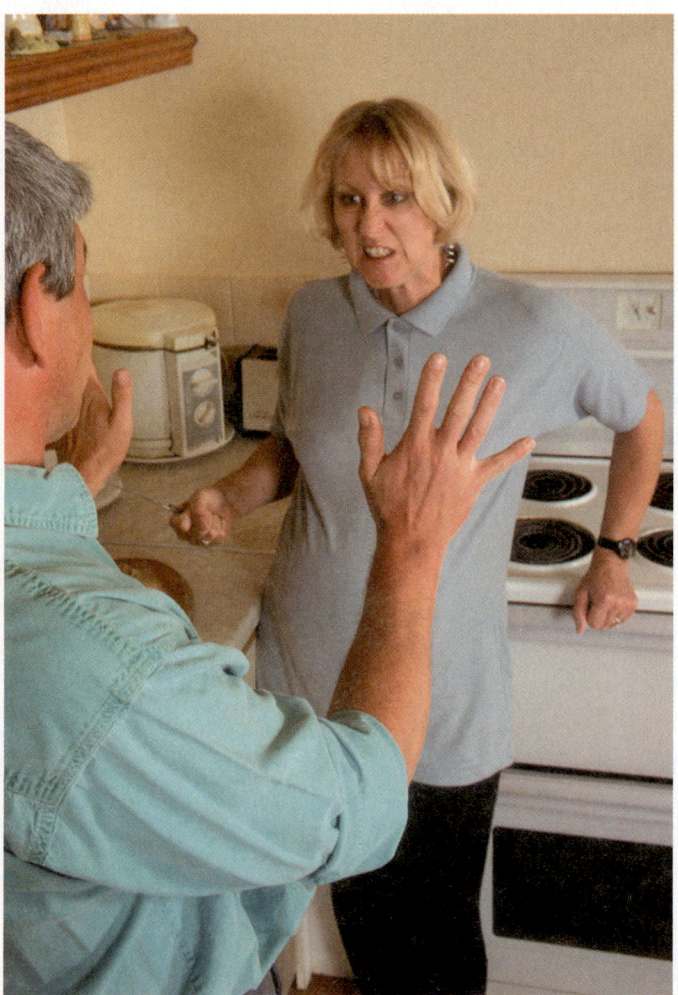

Figure 48-6. ■ A catastrophic reaction is an exaggeration of behavior or anger, beyond what is reasonable in the situation. This woman wielding a whisk may be angry about being unable to find something in the kitchen. (Source: © Angela Hampton Picture Library/ Alamy.)

or controlling behavior and emotions for people with dementia. Their emotions are said to be *labile* or changeable. Dementia makes it impossible for them to respond to multiple stimuli normally. Nurses and caregivers may find that identifying the *precipitating* (beginning or causing) event may be helpful in preventing catastrophic reactions.

Collaborative Care

It truly requires a team to care for a patient with Alzheimer disease. The multidisciplinary team in a long-term care facility may include the patient, nurses, family members, physician, social worker, activity therapist, speech/language pathologist (for swallowing issues), nursing assistant, physical therapist, occupational therapist, and perhaps more. It is crucial to note that a single caregiver cannot "do it all." Each specialty has its expertise to offer. The disorder is complex and challenging for everyone involved, especially for the patient.

The physician usually makes the diagnosis based on the patient's clinical features or the progression of signs and symptoms. A CT scan or MRI would show the typical shrinking of the brain, as seen in Figure 48-4. The definitive diagnosis of Alzheimer disease is by brain tissue pathology (the neurofibrillary tangles and beta-amyloid plaques), and since the tissue is not available until the patient's death, this test is not usually done.

Family members are usually involved in the care of patients at least early in the disorder. It is a challenge for caregivers to remain healthy (Box 48-3■). It is possible, though.

Medications

> **Key Concept** The goal of drug therapy for Alzheimer disease is to prolong the time the patient is in the earlier stages.

Although there is no cure for NCD due to Alzheimer disease, the goal of medication therapy is to prolong the early to middle stages of the disease, postponing the debilitating late stage. Because a decreased amount of the neurotransmitter *acetylcholine* is present in Alzheimer disease, the medications that inhibit the breakdown of acetylcholine are effective in its treatment. These antidementia drugs are in the family called *cholinesterase inhibitors*. Without actually increasing the amount of acetylcholine, they increase the availability of it by inhibiting acetylcholinesterase, the enzyme that breaks it down. Fifty percent of patients using the cholinesterase inhibitors show some temporary improvement with the drugs (Birks, 2009).

Many patients with Alzheimer disease who use cholinesterase inhibitors have improved cognition, behavior, and functioning. They are able to continue to "be themselves"

BOX 48-3   **PATIENT TEACHING**

Ten Ways for Caregivers to Stay Healthy and Reduce Stress

Nurses can be advocates for both patient and caregiver by reminding caregivers that they need to take care of themselves. Caregivers are the most important person in the life of someone with Alzheimer disease, and so maintaining their health and well-being is essential. Teach caregivers the following:

1. *Learn about the disease.* Knowing as much as you can about the disease and care strategies will prepare you for the Alzheimer journey. Understanding how the disease affects the person will help you comprehend and adapt to the changes.
2. *Be realistic about the disease.* It is important, though difficult, to be realistic about the disease and how it will affect the person over time. Once you are realistic, it will be easier for you to adjust your expectations.
3. *Be realistic about yourself.* You need to be realistic about how much you can do. What do you value most? A walk with the person you are caring for, time by yourself, or a tidy house? There is no "right" answer; only you know what matters most to you and how much you can do.
4. *Accept your feelings.* When caring for a person with Alzheimer disease, you will have many mixed feelings. In a single day, you may feel contented, angry, guilty, happy, sad, embarrassed, afraid, and helpless. These feelings may be confusing. But they are normal. Recognize that you are doing the best you can.
5. *Share information and feelings with others.* Sharing information about the disease with family and friends will help them understand what is happening and better prepare them to provide the help and support you need. It is also important to share your feelings. Find someone with whom you feel comfortable talking about your feelings. This may be a close friend or family member, someone you met at an Alzheimer support group, a member of your religious community, or a health care professional.
6. *Be positive.* Your attitude can make a difference in the way you feel. Try to look at the positive side of things.

Focusing on what the person can do, as opposed to the abilities lost, can make things easier. Try to make every day count. There can still be times that are special and rewarding.

7. *Look for humor.* Although Alzheimer disease is serious, you may find that certain situations have a bright side. Maintaining a sense of humor can be a good coping strategy.
8. *Take care of yourself.* Your health is important. Do not ignore it. Eat proper meals and exercise regularly. Find ways to relax and try to get the rest you need. Make regular appointments with your doctor for checkups. You also need to take regular breaks from caregiving. Do not wait until you are too exhausted to plan this. Take time to maintain interests and hobbies. Keep in touch with friends and family so you will not feel lonely and isolated. These things will give you strength to continue providing care.
9. *Get help.* You will need the support that comes from sharing thoughts and feelings with others. This could be individually, with a professional, or as part of an Alzheimer support group. Choose the form of support with which you are most comfortable. It can be hard to ask for and accept practical help. But asking for help is not a sign of inadequate caregiving. You cannot meet all the needs of a person with Alzheimer disease alone. Ask family and friends for help. Most people will be willing to assist you. There may also be programs in your community that offer assistance with household chores, **respite care** (temporary patient care for the purpose of giving the regular caregiver time off), or caregiving tasks. Your local Alzheimer disease association can help you access these.
10. *Plan for the future.* Planning for the future can help relieve stress. Although the person with Alzheimer disease is still capable, review his or her financial situation and plan accordingly. Choices relating to future health and personal care decisions should be considered and recorded. Legal and estate planning should also be discussed. As well, think about an alternate caregiving plan in the event that you are unable to provide care in the future.

---

and to keep up their usual abilities longer (Figure 48-7 ■). However, the brain produces less and less acetylcholine as Alzheimer disease progresses, so the drugs become less effective as decreasing amounts of the neurotransmitter are available. Table 48-4 ■ provides a review of current medications.

Other medications for patients with dementia do not promote cognitive functioning but control the problem behaviors of combativeness and agitation, depression, paranoia, and delusions. These antipsychotic drugs, risperidone (Risperdal), olanzapine (Zyprexa), and haloperidol (Haldol), have been shown to reduce symptoms of hostility, aggression, mistrust, and uncooperativeness in people with dementia. They do not improve memory, depression, or functional ability in these patients. Thus, their value lies in treating the behavioral abnormalities associated

with dementia but not the disorder itself. Antipsychotic drugs should be used with great caution because of their side effects. One important side effect is blocking acetylcholine receptors, reducing the activity of the neurotransmitter already diminished in Alzheimer disease. Cognitive losses may actually accelerate. The antipsychotics may also cause postural hypotension, abnormal body movements, neuroleptic malignant syndrome (acute muscle destruction with high fever and unstable vital signs), abnormal glucose metabolism, dry mucous membranes, constipation, and increased risk of cardiac disease and death in older adults.

Restraints

Key Concept   Patients with dementia in any setting may only be restrained in an emergency involving danger to the patient or others.

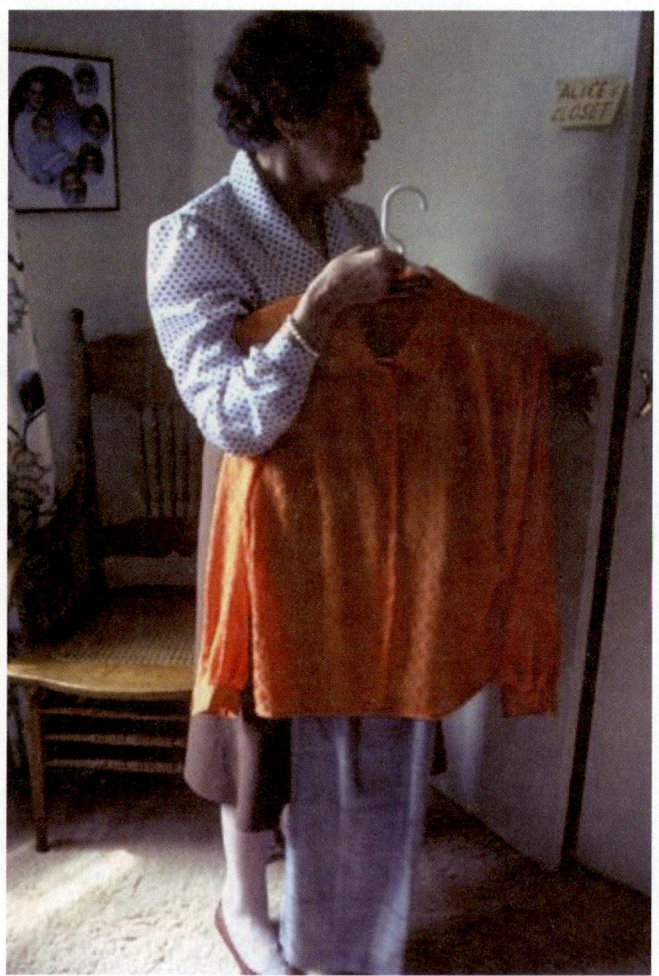

Figure 48-7. ■ Labeling the cabinets, drawers, and closets with their contents can reduce frustration for a patient with Alzheimer disease who forgets where things are at home. (Source: © Rhoda Sidney / PhotoEdit.)

When patients are mentally confused and their behavior is difficult for the staff to manage, restraining the patient is often considered. Restraints should only be used if the patient's behavior is a danger to self or others, or in the case of a medical treatment situation, if the patient is interfering with an important temporary treatment (e.g., removing an endotracheal tube, intravenous line, or dressings from a surgical site). The Centers for Medicare & Medicaid Services (CMS) have a standard for the use of restraint and seclusion of patients. Their standard includes the following (CMS, 2006):

■ In an emergency, a patient may be physically restrained if a physician is not present.
■ The patient must be evaluated face to face within an hour of being restrained for the management of violent or self-destructive behavior. This evaluation must be done by a physician, a registered nurse, or a physician's assistant. The patient's physician or other licensed independent professional must be consulted as soon as possible.
■ The patient or family member must be provided with formal notice of their rights, including freedom from restraints and seclusion when they are used as a means of coercion, discipline, convenience for the staff, or retaliation, at the time of admission.
■ Training about restraint, including behavior management without it, must be provided to staff members.

Nurses can recognize situations that increase patient frustration (and may lead to acting out frustration violently). When patients feel lonely, powerless, or unable to

TABLE 48-4	Giving Medications Safely: Antidementia Agents			
CLASS/DRUG	PURPOSE	USUAL FORM	SIDE EFFECTS	NURSING IMPLICATIONS
■ Donepezil (Aricept)	Cholinesterase inhibitor may slow progress of disease but does not reverse degenerative process.	PO tablets and orally dissolving tablets (ODT) (helpful for patients who choke easily or do not like pills)	Nausea/vomiting, diarrhea, headache, increased gastric acid secretion, bradycardia	Monitor cognitive functions. Monitor heart rate daily. Use NSAIDs with caution. Give at bedtime. Allow ODT to dissolve on tongue and then follow with glass of water. Can be used in late-stage Alzheimer disease (others in early to middle stages only). Has fewer adverse effects than rivastigmine (Birks, 2009).
■ Rivastigmine (Exelon)	Cholinesterase inhibitor	Capsules, oral solution, and now transdermal patch	Nausea/vomiting, weight loss, upset stomach, increased gastric secretion, muscle weakness, sleep disturbances	Nausea/vomiting, weight loss, upset stomach, increased gastric secretion, muscle weakness, sleep disturbances. Remind patient that smoking may decrease blood levels of drug. Use with caution with NSAIDs. Give with food

(continued)

TABLE 48-4	Giving Medications Safely: Antidementia Agents *(continued)*			
CLASS/DRUG	**PURPOSE**	**USUAL FORM**	**SIDE EFFECTS**	**NURSING IMPLICATIONS**
■ Galantamine (Razadyne)	Cholinesterase inhibitor	Tablet, extended-release capsule, oral solution Extended release capsules are given in single daily dose.	Nausea/vomiting, weight loss, diarrhea, sleep disturbances, bradycardia	Monitor cognitive functions. Monitor heart rate daily. Monitor for GI disturbances. Give with morning and evening meals. Give extended-release capsules in AM with food. Single daily dose is easier than multiple daily dosing for most patients. Encourage patient to drink six to eight glasses of water daily.
■ *Memantine* (Namenda)	N-methyl-D-aspartate (NMDA)-receptor antagonist, may reduce brain cell destruction by reducing glutamate-caused extra calcium entering cells.	Tablets and oral solutions, given in twice-daily doses	Dizziness, headache, constipation, confusion, anemia	Monitor cognitive functions. Monitor hemoglobin and hematocrit. Educate the patient and family about the possibility of falls due to dizziness. Give oral solution with syringe provided.
■ Tacrine (Cognex)	Cholinesterase inhibitor	Capsule form, four times per day	Liver damage, nausea, diarrhea, GI bleeding, bradycardia	Second-line drug for Alzheimer disease due to high incidence (one in three) of liver toxicity (Stahl, 2011). Monitor cognitive functions. Monitor heart rate daily. Monitor liver enzymes. Use NSAIDs with caution. Give with food. Four times daily dose is difficult for most patients.

Note: Medications identified in *italics* are among the 200 most frequently prescribed drugs in the United States.

do what they formerly could do, they may feel frustrated. Nurses can try reality orientation, distraction, giving the patient as much decision-making power as possible, or encouraging visitors. Each hospital will have a policy based on CMS standards about restraining patients. Nurses are responsible for acting in accordance with this policy.

NURSING CARE

PRIORITIZING NURSING CARE

It is important for the nurse to recall that Alzheimer disease is an all-encompassing experience for the patient, and it is nearly that for caregivers as well. Family caregivers are so involved and affected by Alzheimer care that they should be also assessed by the nurse.

HEALTH PROMOTION

Health promotion for Alzheimer disease centers on secondary prevention, which is early detection of the disorder. The Alzheimer's Association is an excellent source of information. Their *10 Warning Signs of Alzheimer's* (see Box 48-2) are an excellent way for members of the community to learn whether their own symptoms are just a normal part of aging or possibly significant signs that should be discussed with their health care provider. Community members can be referred to the Alzheimer's Association website; the association's number can also be found in many local telephone books.

ASSESSING

Normal assessments for health must be performed in patients with dementia but should be organized to fit the best time of day, when the patient is most cooperative.

DIAGNOSING, PLANNING, AND IMPLEMENTING

Expected outcomes for patients with cognitive impairment:

■ Freedom from injury to self or others

■ Maintain as much functional (self-care) ability as possible

■ Obtain safe, effective, and comfortable personal care

■ Be able to live life and approach death with dignity

Expected outcomes for family caregivers:

■ Adequate knowledge about Alzheimer disease to know what to expect from the course of the disease and its treatment

- Information about how to manage problem symptoms and behaviors
- Support from peers in their situation (possibly through Alzheimer's Association) and knowledge of available resources in their community
- The ability to maintain physical and mental well-being while being a caregiver

The nurse must be prepared to provide numerous interventions for problem behaviors of Alzheimer disease (Eby & Brown, 2009).

Wandering

Expected outcome: Will cooperate with redirection to positive behavior.

- First, try to understand the patient's agenda. Is he or she hungry, wet, in pain, needing the bathroom, afraid, looking for something, engaging in an old habit (going to work or out to milk the cows)? *If you can find the need, you may be able to meet it (toilet the patient, validate the patient's feelings that this is not his or her house, or validate how it must feel to be ready to go to work). By validating the patient's feelings, you are not agreeing that there are cows here to milk but you are giving the patient the benefit of believing that his or her feelings are real. Why not talk about the cows and how they feel, smell, and sound?*
- After exploring the patient's thought, change the subject to whatever event is about to occur (e.g., dinner). If you are unable to find a reason for the patient's wandering, you can still walk with the patient and talk about old times. *Participating with the patient's thought provides a sense of belonging to the patient. What was it like when she was a nurse or what did he plant in his garden?*
- Put a stop sign on places the patient should not go. If the patient is still at home, put a deadbolt on the outside door, either high or low. Keep pathways free of clutter. Let the patient walk as much as he or she wants. *Stop signs and clear paths provide safety. Walking is good exercise and helps to work out physical tension. Sometimes rocking in a rocking chair can be an alternative to walking, as it gives many people a sense of well-being.*

Sundowning Syndrome

- Keep the house or unit well lit during the day. Provide opportunities for the patient to exercise every day (e.g., going for a walk) so the patient will be tired enough to go to bed. Provide a light evening snack without caffeine. Keep general environmental stimuli low (do not play the television, a radio, and talk loudly on the phone at the same time). Turn the television off if the patient is not watching it. *Turning down the stimuli, especially in the evening, can provide a more pleasant environment for a confused patient and help the patient transition from day to night. The lack of orienting cues during the night can contribute to disorientation.*

Refusal to Bathe

- If possible, determine the reason the patient is reluctant to bathe (could be modesty, previous negative experiences, fear of the bathtub for some perceptual reason, not understanding what you are asking the patient to do, or embarrassment at not being able to bathe independently). *Knowing the reason for refusal allows you to reassure the patient appropriately.*
- Reassure the patient if fear is the reason. Be calm and matter of fact. *Your emotions are contagious, so it helps to model calmness and self-control.*
- Offer assistance. Provide whatever devices the patient needs. Move slowly. Follow the patient's old bath routine as closely as possible. Have everything ready in advance (the water, towels, soap, clothes, etc.). If all else fails, use a sponge bath, or a warm wet-towel bath, and nonrinsing soap. *Many older adults cannot stand again after sitting in a low tub, so devices like a shower chair may be needed. A slow, deliberate pace is calming. In the end, cleanliness and comfort are the goals, so adapting to the patient is important.*

Paranoia/Suspicion

- Remember that being suspicious is not the patient's choice but part of the deterioration of the disease. They have no other explanation for their losses than that someone is stealing things, and they will not respond to reason. Do not argue with the patient's suspicions. Offer to help look for things, or try to divert the patient's attention to something else. Be reassuring instead of argumentative. Consider buying duplicates of frequently lost items. *By responding to the emotion of the patient, rather than their words (which may be confusing), you show caring about the patient's emotional well-being. You can validate the patient's feelings of confusion, "It must be so frustrating not to be able to find things." By recognizing that accusations come from the disease, it will be easier to stay calm and not take the accusations personally.*

Language Difficulties

- Always introduce yourself to the patient by name and role each time you enter the room. Call the patient by name. Approach from the front. *Speaking slowly, calmly, and clearly can help the patient get oriented and process your words.*
- Make simple statements with few words and simple sentences. Allow lots of time for processing what you have said. If the patient does not understand, repeat yourself exactly at least twice before you use new words. *The Alzheimer patient is gradually losing cognition. Repetition of exact words can help the patient process, whereas changing to new words only adds to the confusion and increases processing time.*

- Work on your own listening skills. Show interest in what the patient is saying. Maintain eye contact. Try to supply the word you think the patient is looking for, and encourage the patient to continue trying. Look at the whole of what the patient is saying to find meaning. *These interventions allow you to pick up on nonverbal cues and to convey your caring and interest.*
- Ask the patient to point or describe the idea with different words. Label kitchen cabinets or household drawers indicating what is inside. *Some patients understand written words best. Labeling can prevent the patient from having to look in every drawer in the house to find a comb.*
- Try to use procedural memory. Hand a patient the toothbrush or spoon, or back the patient up to the toilet. *Sometimes starting an action the patient has performed hundreds of times can help the patient make the connection without words.*
- Whatever happens, keep a sense of humor, treat the patient with respect as an adult, and remain calm. *Professionalism is key when a patient has cognitive dysfunction. Your skills at therapeutic communication, especially nonverbal aspects such as positioning, tone of voice, eye contact, and facial expression, will be exercised continually and can contribute greatly to the care these patients need.*

Catastrophic Reactions

- Catastrophic responses are caused by the disease, not the patient's choice. The best approach is to prevent them from happening. The Mayo Clinic recommends using an "ABC" approach to prevent the recurrence of problem behaviors in patients with Alzheimer disease. Look at the *a*ntecedent of the problem behavior (what came directly before the behavior). Then review the *b*ehavior itself. Finally, look at the *c*onsequences of the behavior. *Caregivers too often look at the consequences without considering the antecedent, or what happened before the patient acted like she did. For example, if the patient is on a locked unit and starts screaming whenever she sees your unit keys (perhaps because it reminds her of her loss of freedom), the solution is to keep the keys in your pocket.*
- Do not touch the patient during an outburst. Afterward, gentle touch can be reassuring. Do not hurry patients. Provide opportunities and activities where they can be successful. *Your touch during an outburst may be misinterpreted as part of the catastrophe. The caregivers' role is to provide structure and security, so remain calm.*

MANAGING NURSING CARE

As appropriate and allowed by the designated duties and responsibilities of assistive personnel, the nurse may delegate nursing care activities such as assisting with activities of daily living, for a patient with dementia.

EVALUATING

In evaluating care for patients with Alzheimer disease, it is important to determine whether unmet goals are too high for the patient to reach. A nursing care plan that is realistic and specific to the current needs of the individual patient is the goal. It is far better to plan realistic help to maintain function (or maintain dignity as function declines) than to plan for cognitive improvement or other unrealistic goals.

NURSING CARE PLAN
Patient With Middle-Stage Alzheimer Disease

Rosa White is a 70-year-old female with middle-stage Alzheimer disease. Her 45-year-old daughter Flora has moved in and is caring for her in Rosa's home. Flora had to quit her job due to her mother's increasing safety and care needs. She has finally made the painful decision to place Rosa in a long-term care facility next month. Rosa wanders the house day and night, often asking Flora who she is and what she is doing in her house. She has called the police about Flora more than once. Rosa recently wandered out of the house. When Flora found her several blocks from home and tried to bring her home, Rosa became so hysterical that neighbors came out to see what the problem was. Rosa has trouble thinking of the word she wants and may call objects by names she has made up. She asks Flora the same question over and over. Flora is not getting enough sleep and is tired all of the time. Her mother's repeated questions are irritating to her, but she becomes angry with herself for getting irritated. She has been unable to hire anyone to watch Rosa even while she goes to the store. Long-term care seems the only solution. She wants Rosa to be safe, and Flora wants to rest.

Assessment

On admission, Rosa is well-dressed and clean. She is accompanied by her daughter Flora, who is very attentive to Rosa's needs. Rosa says Flora is her friend and that she (Rosa) is 25 years old and single with no children. Rosa recognizes her own name. She does not know what day it is or where she lives. She is often distracted during the interview. She starts sentences and then stops in mid-thought and giggles. Her speech is hesitant, and she sometimes uses the wrong word or makes up a word.

Flora tells the nurse that she has taken over the household chores. She says her mother cannot cook but does help Flora in the kitchen. Rosa is occasionally incontinent of urine when her daughter misses the signs and does not take her to the bathroom. Flora assists Rosa with bathing, and sometimes Rosa fights being bathed. Flora reports that Rosa wanders around the house at night and has gotten lost in the neighborhood. Flora admits to being very tired.

Nursing Diagnosis

Although there are many nursing diagnoses that can be identified from the case study, the following would have the highest priority:

- Risk for Injury
- Disturbed Sleep Pattern
- Bathing Self-Care Deficit
- Dressing Self-Care Deficit
- Feeding Self-Care Deficit
- Toileting Self-Care Deficit
- Chronic Confusion
- Impaired Verbal Communication

For the caregiver Flora, the priority diagnosis is:

- Caregiver Role Strain related to fatigue and inability to find help with mother's care

Expected Outcomes

Expected outcomes for Rosa include that she:

- Will remain free of injury.
- Will feel rested in the morning.
- Will cooperate with bathing when assisted by caregiver.
- Will answer three yes or no questions appropriately each day.
- Will communicate at least one need a day either verbally or nonverbally.

An expected outcome for Flora is:

- Will establish a schedule for respite from caregiving.

Planning and Implementation

Interventions for these three nursing diagnoses will be integrated, since they are all related to the patient's cognitive impairment.

- The nurse brings Rosa and her daughter Flora to Rosa's new room and introduces her to her roommate. She suggests to Flora that she should bring in some familiar objects for Rosa to place in her room. *Having a scrapbook, photograph album, and some pictures for the wall will help the staff in reminiscence with Rosa. Bringing in her favorite chair and familiar comforter for her bed can ease the transition into a new location.*

- The nurse also suggests that Flora bring in a large calendar and a digital clock that will be easy for Rosa to read. She asks Flora to bring in a photo of Rosa when she was a young woman. *Since Rosa identifies herself as a young woman, this picture—placed outside her door—will help her find her new room more easily. Since Rosa's favorite color is purple, the nurse will place a purple bow next to Rosa's photo to help her to identify her new room.*

- The nurse will communicate to the staff about Rosa's tendency to wander. *The staff will be aware of Rosa's tendency to wander in and out of other residents' rooms. This could be a source of catastrophic reactions with other residents if Rosa is in the room uninvited and rummaging through their belongings. This could result in injury to Rosa if the staff is not watchful. The staff should cooperate for the benefit of all the patients.*

- The nurse asks about favorite activities and learns that Rosa loves to walk outside, likes music, enjoys helping Flora prepare a meal, and can still play Bingo. *All these facts will give the staff examples of diversionary activities that can be used with Rosa when her behavior intrudes upon others. They are also activities that the patient can do successfully to reduce and prevent frustration. Exercise is a very healthful activity, and it is especially good that she already enjoys walking. Exercise/activity should be built into every patient's care plan when possible. It prevents the hazards of immobility while keeping the patient strong (which decreases falls and injuries) and in good spirits.*

- The staff will be aware when floors are wet or when there are articles on the floor that need to be picked up. Clutter will be avoided. The unit will be kept well lit when it starts to get dark outside, so Rosa can still see to walk. Special care will be taken to clear her way to the bathroom. *Most falls occur when the patient is hurrying to the bathroom.*

- The staff will communicate with Rosa in simple sentences. When Rosa does not understand what is said, the directions will be repeated to her, using the same words at least two more times. The staff will avoid using negatives when speaking to Rosa. *It is better to say "Turn around here" than "Do not go there." The second phrase takes more processing because of the negative word "not." Staying positive also reduces patient frustration.*

- The staff will limit Rosa's choices, so she is not overwhelmed. *It will be easier for her to choose between a red dress and a blue dress than to decide on a whole outfit to wear.*

- When Rosa has difficulty remembering a word, the staff will supply it for her and then use the word in a sentence to see if that is what she meant to say. The nurse assured Flora that the staff will always approach Rosa from the front and will not touch her until she sees them. They will speak in a calm manner. *These interventions will help Rosa feel safe and will prevent catastrophic reactions.*

Evaluation

After 2 weeks, Rosa has adjusted to her new surroundings. She is happy to see Flora when she arrives. She still thinks Flora is a friend, but she does recognize her as someone she knows. She is able to show Flora her room. She plays Bingo every Wednesday and sets the table for lunch every day. She has not been injured and follows directions reasonably well if given step-by-step instructions. Staff members take the time to listen to her and help her with her communication. Flora hears Rosa laugh for the first time in months when a staff member has a hard time guessing what object she wants. It is obvious that Rosa feels more at ease in this environment than she did at home where the expectations of her behavior were different. Here she can be herself and not have to struggle with who she used to be.

Critical Thinking in the Nursing Process

1. What factors were involved in Flora's decision to place Rosa in a nursing home? If she had chosen to keep Rosa at home, what adaptations would she have had to make?

2. Discuss the choices of the nursing diagnoses that were considered the most important. Do you agree with those choices? Why or why not?

3. Flora says she feels guilty that Rosa has to be in a nursing home. What community resource might help Flora?

Note: Discussion of Critical Thinking questions appears on the companion website.

Note: The references and resources for all chapters have been compiled at the back of the book.

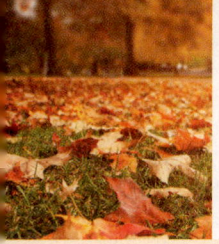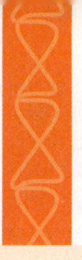

Chapter Review

KEY POINTS

- Cognitive disorders disrupt a person's thinking. The domains of cognition are complex attention, executive function, memory and learning, language, perceptual-motor function, and social cognition.
- Disorders of cognition are not a normal part of aging.
- Delirium has an acute onset, is usually related to some toxicity or pathology outside the brain originally, and is usually treatable if diagnosed and treated early.
- **Concept:** Delirium can be fatal if not treated early.
- Alzheimer disease (the most common dementia) has a slow onset and progression. It is not curable.
- Alzheimer disease is caused by an accumulation of neurofibrillary tangles and beta-amyloid plaques that damage and kill brain cells. There is also a deficiency of the neurotransmitter acetylcholine.
- **Concept:** The goal of drug therapy for Alzheimer disease is to prolong the time the patient is in the earlier stages.

- Alzheimer disease generally has three stages, early, middle, and late. The entire course of the disease may be 5 to 17 years, with the middle stage lasting the longest.
- Nursing care of a patient with Alzheimer disease in the middle to late stages is focused on safety and assisting with activities of daily living.
- **Concept:** Patients with dementia in any setting may only be restrained in an emergency involving danger to the patient or others.
- The families of patients with Alzheimer disease experience a great deal of stress.
- The caregivers of family members with dementia have an especially stressful job and may be diagnosed with Caregiver Role Strain. Nurses can plan and intervene to prevent or treat this.

PEARSON NURSING STUDENT RESOURCES

Find additional materials at **nursing.pearsonhighered.com**.

Clinical Reasoning Care Map

Caring for a Patient With Delirium
NCLEX-PN® Focus Area: Physiologic Integrity

Case Study: Tom Edwards is a 67-year-old European American who is hospitalized for surgery to remove his enlarged prostate gland (a transurethral prostatectomy). Preoperatively he was alert and oriented, and independent with ADLs. He sees a urologist for his prostate problem, a cardiologist for his hypertension, and a family practitioner for his general medical care. In the Post Anesthesia Care Unit, he was oriented to person only, not to place or time. His wife states that he does not know who she is. He has been transferred to the Medical–Surgical Unit where he is expected to stay overnight.

Nursing Diagnosis: Acute Confusion

COLLECT DATA

Subjective	Objective
_____	_____
_____	_____
_____	_____
_____	_____
_____	_____
_____	_____

Does this present a threat to the patient's safety?

If yes, the priority intervention to address this threat would be:

_____

Nursing Care

_____
_____
_____
_____
_____
_____
_____

Interprofessional team members to include when planning care:

_____

How would you document this? _____

Data Collected
(use only those that apply)

- The urologist prescribed several medications.
- The cardiologist prescribed several medications.
- The family practitioner prescribed several medications.
- The patient had sudden onset of change in mental status.
- His symptoms are inconsistent; sometimes he is oriented, sometimes not.
- History of smoking, until 30 years ago.
- The wife states that the patient takes several over-the-counter medications for nasal congestion, GI upset, and occasional headaches.
- The patient states, "I don't know what to do."
- The patient is unable to bathe himself, which he could do before this episode.
- The patient eats a high-salt diet at home.
- His hobby is woodworking.

Nursing Interventions (use only those that apply; list in priority order)

- Teach the patient about unit policies.
- Place frequently used personal items near the bed in easy reach.
- Use simple words and sentences.
- Make a list of all the medications the patient is taking, prescribed and over-the-counter.
- Tell his wife to prepare for nursing-home placement.
- Teach the patient memory-enhancing strategies.
- Tell the patient's wife that because he is sometimes oriented, he is probably not sick, and is doing this for attention.
- Restrain the patient in bed to prevent falls.
- Introduce yourself by name and role each time you enter the room.
- Orient the patient to reality.
- Encourage a family member to stay with the patient when possible.
- Assist the patient with ADLs while he is acutely confused.

Compare your answers and documentation to those provided on the companion website.

NCLEX-PN® Exam Preparation

1 A 60-year-old woman whose mother has Alzheimer disease said to the nurse, "My memory is terrible! I forget where I put my keys, I can't find my cell phone, and the other day I went to the store and forgot half of what I went there for. Am I getting Alzheimer disease?" Select the best response by the nurse.

1. "It does run in families. There are genes for Alzheimer disease on several chromosomes. You should see your physician."
2. "Did you ever remember what you went to the store for?"
3. "How long has this memory abnormality been going on?"
4. "It is not likely that you have Alzheimer disease. Short-term memory gets a little bit worse as we age and when we're under stress."

2 Of the following signs and symptoms, select those that are consistent with delirium. **Select all that apply.**

1. Incurable.
2. Progressive for many years.
3. Sudden onset.
4. Usually treatable if diagnosed early.
5. Affected patients have inconsistent symptoms (confusion may come and go).
6. Caused by neurofibrillary tangles and beta-amyloid plaques in brain.

3 Which of the following patients is at highest risk for a cognitive disorder?

1. A 25-year-old with bladder cancer who sees three different physicians.
2. A 40-year-old who has had chronic inflammatory bowel disease for 25 years.
3. A 65-year-old with alcohol dependency and diabetes.
4. A 70-year-old with iron-deficiency anemia.

4 Which teaching by the nurse would be most appropriate for a patient with Alzheimer disease in the early stage? Teach the patient to:

1. have a place for frequently used items (e.g., keys, wallet or purse, glasses) and to always put them back in the same place to aid memory.
2. use undergarments available in the grocery store or pharmacy to manage incontinence.
3. practice her ADLs carefully so she will not forget them later on.
4. put labels on everyday items such as a toothbrush, comb, and spoons so the patient will remember what they are called.

5 Which nursing intervention is most appropriate for a patient in the middle stage of Alzheimer disease?

1. Provide the patient with written orientation materials about unit policies.
2. Keep the way to the bathroom clear so the patient does not fall.

3. Obtain a physician's order for a sedative in case of a catastrophic reaction.
4. Remind the patient to keep her glasses in their case so they won't get lost.

6 Select the best response by the nurse to a patient's question, "How will that medicine fix my Alzheimer disease?"

1. "It will hopefully put the disease in remission, where you will have no symptoms."
2. "It will help you get your memory back."
3. "The medicines for Alzheimer disease act as sedatives to calm you down."
4. "Alzheimer medicines are made to make the early stages of the disease last longer. They don't really cure the disease."

7 Which available form of medication for Alzheimer disease would be safest for a patient who has difficulty swallowing?

1. Rectal suppository
2. Transdermal patch
3. Oral capsule
4. Oral liquid

8 The nurse has determined that a patient with Alzheimer disease in the middle stage would benefit from validation therapy. When the patient states, "I have to get out of here to feed the cows!" what is the nurse's best response?

1. "Let's talk about your cows."
2. "You are in a nursing home; there are no cows here."
3. "What cows are you talking about? I don't see any cows."
4. "I think it's close to dinner time; let's go to the dining room."

9 When any patient has a sudden change in cognition or level of consciousness, what should the nurse do first?

1. Check the patient's medication list.
2. Withhold the patient's medications until the physician can evaluate them.
3. Notify the physician.
4. Call the patient's family.

10 The nurse is advising a group of caregivers of people with Alzheimer disease. Which is the best advice to help caregivers stay healthy and prevent caregiver role strain?

1. "Be optimistic. The disease might not be as bad for your family member as it is for most people."
2. "Be strong and have confidence in yourself. You don't need anyone else's help. Lots of others have done it."
3. "Learn everything you can about AD so you can have realistic expectations. Accept yourself when you have mixed feelings and accept help from others."
4. "Hire people to be with your family member day and night. You need your sleep."

Answers and rationales for Review Questions appear in Appendix I

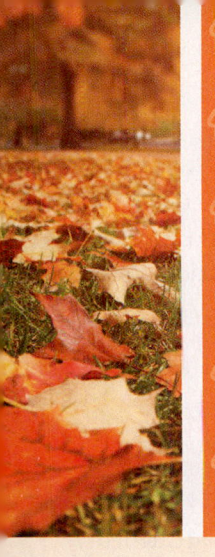

CHAPTER 49

Caring for Patients With Psychotic Disorders

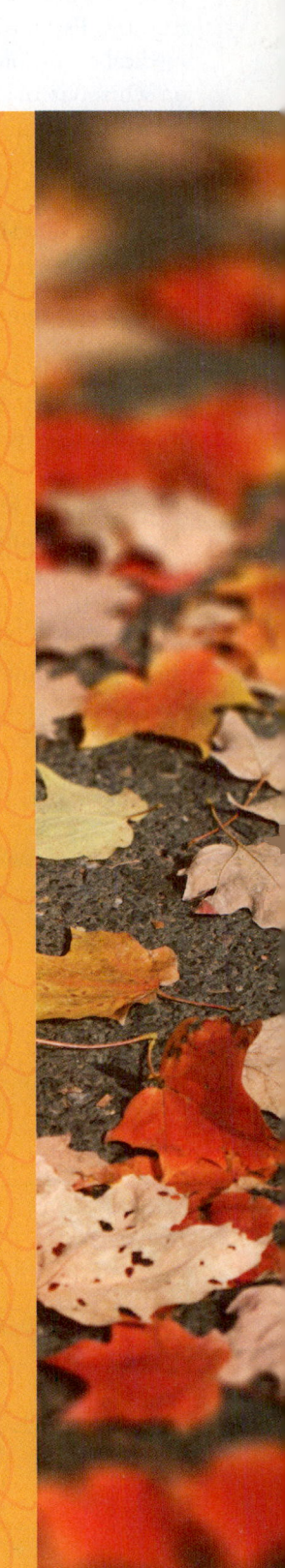

BRIEF OUTLINE

Schizophrenia
Pathophysiology
Manifestations

Collaborative Care

LEARNING OUTCOMES

After completing this chapter, you will be able to:

1. Discuss the major theories about the cause of schizophrenia.
2. Explain the manifestations of schizophrenia.
3. Describe the treatment options for people with schizophrenia.
4. Discuss the impact of schizophrenia on the development and quality of life of affected people.
5. Explain the actions and side effects of antipsychotic drugs.
6. Prioritize the side effects of antipsychotic medications as they relate to patient safety.
7. Explain the recovery model as it applies to recovery from mental illness.
8. Apply the nursing process to the care of patients with schizophrenia or other psychoses.

KEY TERMS

The key terms are defined on the pages listed below.

affect, 1222
akathisia, 1227
anhedonia, 1223
catatonic behavior, 1222
cognitive, 1222
delusions, 1221
dual diagnosis, 1224

dyskinesia, 1226
dystonia, 1226
hallucinations, 1221
insight, 1223
milieu, 1224
negative symptoms, 1220
neologisms, 1222

neuroleptic malignant
  syndrome, 1227
positive symptoms, 1220
prodromal phase, 1223
psychosis, 1220
tardive dyskinesia, 1227

SPECIAL FEATURES

NURSING CARE PLAN: Patient With Schizophrenia, 1235
CLINICAL REASONING CARE MAP: Caring for a Patient With Schizophrenia, 1238

Psychosis refers to a thought disorder that causes the following symptoms: delusions, hallucinations, disorganized speech, and/or disorganized behavior. See Table 49-1■ for definitions of these psychiatric terms. Psychosis is a major feature of schizophrenia, which is the most common thought disorder. There are other disorders that cause psychosis, including schizoaffective disorder, bipolar mania, and depression with psychotic features. Psychosis may also be a symptom of some general medical conditions or drug effects, but this chapter will focus on schizophrenia as the prototype for nursing care of people with psychotic disorders.

Schizophrenia

Key Concept Schizophrenia is a disorder of the brain that affects thinking, mood, and behavior.

Schizophrenia is a complex disorder of the brain's structure and function. While they are experiencing an episode, people have psychosis; personality disorganization; and an impaired ability to interpret reality, to relate to self and others, and to function in daily life. Schizophrenia has a large negative impact on the quality of life of affected people and their families.

More than 2 million people in the United States have schizophrenia. The disorder affects approximately 1% of the adult population in any given year. It affects women, men, people of all ethnicities and nationalities, and people of all socioeconomic classes. The age of onset in males is usually the late teens or early 20s, slightly earlier than in

females. In females, the onset is usually in the 20s or 30s (American Psychiatric Association, 2013). Diagnosis before adolescence is rare. See Box 49-1■ for information about the late onset of schizophrenia in older adults.

PATHOPHYSIOLOGY

Key Concept The pathophysiology behind schizophrenia includes genetic abnormalities, brain structure deviations, and environmental exposures.

A single cause for schizophrenia has not been identified. Schizophrenia has a variety of pathophysiologic processes and associated manifestations. Current theory includes the following components:

BOX 49-1	FOCUS ON OLDER ADULTS

Late-Onset Schizophrenia

The onset of schizophrenia is usually in young people, but it can begin in later life. Those who have a late onset of the disease are more likely to be women. Schizophrenia causes social isolation and all the positive symptoms of usual onset schizophrenia. Affected people tend to have delusions of persecution and hallucinations. This disorder is a chronic long-term illness, and in older people, as in young people, antipsychotic medications can be very effective. Older adult patients tend to respond to lower doses of antipsychotic medications, whether they have the usual or late-onset form. Antipsychotics may increase the risk for cardiovascular disorders and death in older patients with dementia-related psychosis. Psychosis symptoms decrease in the older adult with schizophrenia, probably because brain dopamine decreases with age.

TABLE 49-1	Terms Related to Schizophrenia	
TERM	**DEFINITION**	**EXAMPLE**
Delusion	A false belief that is inconsistent with reality. It is not consistent with what the person's culture or religion accepts as real. It does not respond to reasoning or evidence that it is false.	One patient believes that he is the supreme commander of the entire world's military. Another believes that the CIA is monitoring her conversations through a filling in her tooth.
Disorganized thinking	Thoughts that are not related to each other or to the present situation. The normal flow of thought is disrupted, and thoughts may not form properly. Disorganized thoughts lead to disorganized speech and behavior.	Nurse says, "Would you like some breakfast?" Patient says, "I would like something. I like dogs. I know the rules of fifty-two card games."
Hallucination	A sensory perceptual experience that seems real to the patient but is not related to external stimuli. Most common are auditory, then visual, but they can involve any of the senses.	A patient hears voices commenting on everything he is doing. They tell him that he is bad, stupid, and worthless. Others cannot hear the voices.
Negative symptoms	Manifestations that represent a reduction in normal function, such as reduced movement, thinking, motivation, and expression of emotion.	A patient spends most of his time lying in bed or sitting in a chair. He does not want to go outside. He does not read or listen to music or talk to others. Even when he hears something funny or sad, he shows very little emotion.
Positive symptoms	Manifestations such as delusions, hallucinations, and disorganized thinking that are an excess or distortion of normal function.	A patient believes that the people on TV are talking to him personally. He believes that if he jumped off a roof he would not be hurt because he has super powers.

1. *Neurochemical changes.* Antipsychotic drugs affect the function and availability of neurotransmitters in the brain. These drugs relieve the manifestations of schizophrenia, such as delusional thinking, hallucinations, and disorganized thinking and behavior in most people with the disorder. Therefore, neurotransmitters and their receptors, especially dopamine, norepinephrine, serotonin, GABA (gamma-aminobutyric acid), and glutamate, are altered in schizophrenia. Medical treatment of schizophrenia focuses largely on this area.

2. *Genetic abnormalities.* Schizophrenia is more likely to recur in a family that already has a family member with schizophrenia. Siblings of a person with the disorder are nine times more likely to have schizophrenia than the general population. There is a genetic component, but genetics is not the whole story. It is not purely genetic, because one identical twin can be affected and not the other (even though they have the same genetics). While no single gene causes the disease, people with schizophrenia tend to have higher rates of rare genetic mutations. These gene changes involve any of hundreds of possible different genes and probably disrupt brain development. Schizophrenia can also result when a gene that codes for a brain neurotransmitter mutates. Research implicates several genes that code for susceptibility to schizophrenia. People with one or more of these susceptibility genes may manifest the disease only after they experience some stressor. Interactions between these genes and the environment are necessary for schizophrenia to develop (National Institute of Mental Health, NIMH, 2012).

3. *Changes in brain structure and function.* Imaging studies of the brains of people with schizophrenia have repeatedly shown structural changes. Structural abnormalities include enlargement of the brain ventricles; decrease in the size of the limbic system; and changes in the cell structure in the hippocampus, amygdala, parahippocampal gyrus, entorhinal cortex, and cingulate, which are located in the inferior part of the cerebrum.

4. *Urban living.* People born or raised in an urban area have a greater risk for having schizophrenia than people from rural areas. One reason for the increased number of people with the disorder in cities is that people move to the city for better mental health services. However, the birth rate of affected people in the city is twice that in rural areas (the suburbs have a rate between the two). Are urban dwellers exposed to agents (possibly viruses or pollutants) that increase genetic mutations?

In summary, schizophrenia is caused by abnormalities in brain structure and function. Genetic factors and environmental influences cause these abnormalities. The current disorder that we call schizophrenia is probably more than one distinct disorder. People may have similar symptoms with different causes. More research is required to explain this complicated brain disorder fully.

Treatment of psychosis with antipsychotic medications is based on reducing the function of certain brain neurotransmitters. Table 47-1 shows the various brain neurotransmitters and their relationship to mental disorders.

MANIFESTATIONS

The standard for diagnosis of mental disorders is the *Diagnostic and Statistical Manual of Mental Disorders*, 5th edition (APA, 2013), known as the *DSM-5*. The *DSM-5* diagnostic criteria for schizophrenia include the following:

- Characteristic symptoms: The patient must have two or more of the following:
  Delusions
  Hallucinations
  Disorganized speech
  Grossly disorganized or catatonic behavior
  Negative symptoms
- Seriously impaired self-care, social or occupational function.
- Duration of symptoms must be at least 6 months.
- The symptoms must not be caused by another disorder (depression, bipolar disorder, schizoaffective disorder, or other medical disorder) or drugs.

Key Concept   The disorder is characterized by positive, disorganized, and negative symptoms.

Positive (or *psychotic*) *symptoms* seem to be an excess or distortion of normal functions (APA, 2013). They include hallucinations and delusions.

- **Hallucinations** are sensory perceptions that seem real but occur without external stimuli. The patient may or may not have the insight that these are not real sensory experiences. Auditory hallucinations are the most common in schizophrenia, often experienced by the patient as voices. Approximately 75% of people with schizophrenia hear voices at some time during their illness. Visual hallucinations are the next most common. Hallucinations can also be tactile, gustatory (taste), olfactory (smell), or somatic (involving body sensations, such as electricity).
- **Delusions** are fixed false beliefs. These beliefs persist despite evidence that they are not true. A delusional belief is one not ordinarily accepted by the members of the person's culture or religion. See Table 49-2 ■ for a list of types of delusions, which are categorized by their content.
- *Disorganized symptoms* include disorganized thinking and disorganized behavior.

TABLE 49-2	Types of Delusions	
TYPE OF DELUSION	**CONTENT**	**EXAMPLES**
Grandiose	The affected person has beliefs of inflated powers, knowledge, identity, or relationship to a deity or famous person.	"I am Spiderman."
Delusion of reference	Events, objects, or other people in the immediate environment have a particular and unusual significance.	"The TV newsman is talking to me."
Persecutory	The central belief is that the affected person is being conspired against, harassed, cheated, or persecuted.	"The food here is poisoned."
Somatic	The content of the delusion relates to the structure or function of the patient's body.	"There is a machine inside my body."
Bizarre	The affected person believes clearly improbable ideas that are not derived from real-life experiences.	"My neighbor planted a fish inside my brain that tells me when to drink water."
Thought broadcasting	One's thoughts are being transmitted out loud so other people can hear them.	"I don't want to go to the store. Maybe I'll hurt somebody's feelings if I think they are fat or something."
Thought insertion	One's thoughts are not one's own, but are inserted into one's mind.	"You think I'm bad, but it's not me. The devil puts those ideas there."

■ *Disorganized thinking* is a major feature of schizophrenia. Schizophrenia causes an inability to sort and interpret incoming sensory information and a resulting inability to respond appropriately. Disorganized thinking is demonstrated in disorganized speech. Patients may have incoherent speech (in which subjects change every few words). At its worst, this becomes "word salad" in which words are thrown together without relationship to each other, such as "Dogs, hat, fight, door, happening, machine, quickly." An example of a loose association is "You know I live in the zoo, I like animals, I plan to wear my new shoes when I go on the walk, are you coming?" Sometimes patients make up words called **neologisms** that have no meaning to others. In addition, schizophrenia can affect the thinking process. There are four **cognitive** (thinking) functions affected by schizophrenia:

1. Attention
2. *Executive function* (abstract thinking and problem solving)
3. Awareness of the illness (lack of awareness is called *anosognosia*)
4. Short-term memory

These thinking impairments affect people who have never taken medication, so they are not due to medication side effects. Although the disease affects some aspects of thinking, other aspects remain intact, such as language skills, knowledge of information, and visual–spatial abilities.

■ *Disorganized behavior* lacks goal orientation. The lack of goal orientation makes activities of daily living (ADLs), such as personal hygiene or preparing meals, difficult. Patients may have odd or purposeless behavior, such as walking in circles or pacing. They may dress in unusual ways, perhaps wearing several coats and hats on a hot day. Schizophrenia causes an altered sense of the self and affects movement and behavior. Disorganized behavior may also include unpredictable agitation (pacing, shouting, profanity) or inappropriate personal behavior, such as public masturbation (APA, 2000). It may also include **catatonic behavior** (a marked decrease in response to the environment). Patients with catatonia may have a rigid posture, resisting efforts to be moved. Figure 49-1■ shows a woman with schizophrenia of the catatonic type. People with this type of schizophrenia may have excessive purposeless movement or take on bizarre positions.

Negative symptoms of schizophrenia, in contrast to the positive ones, involve a deficit or decrease of normal functions. Negative symptoms include the following:

■ *Flat affect.* **Affect** is the nonverbal expression of emotion. The person with schizophrenia may have a *blunting* (decrease in) or absence of nonverbal emotional expression, or *flattening* of affect. The person would not show facial expressions or other body language indicating feelings.

■ *Alogia.* Alogia is decreased amount and richness of speech. It is thought that this reflects a reduction in thinking. A person with alogia has brief verbal responses, with

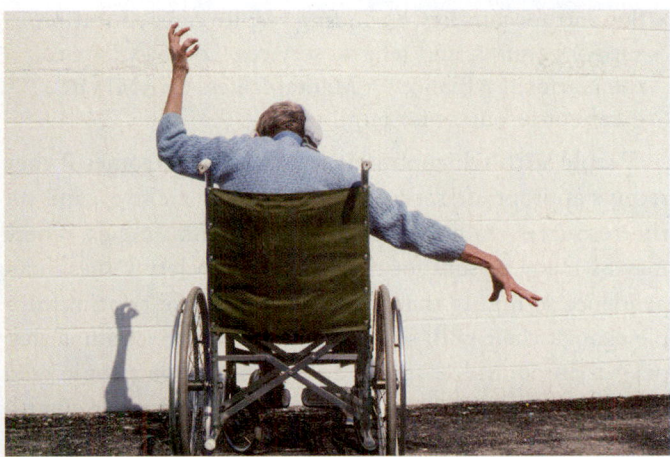

Figure 49-1. ■ This woman has schizophrenia with symptoms of catatonia. Her catatonic symptoms are generalized muscle stiffness, reduced responsiveness, and strange body postures. (Source: Grunnitus Studio/Science Source.)

BOX 49-2	REALITY CHECK ON SCHIZOPHRENIA

"At first it just sounds like wind in the leaves, rustling and soft. Then it becomes voices, whispering then talking louder. If I concentrate I can hear them more clearly."

"I am just here [psychiatric hospital] because I had a fight with my brother. There is nothing wrong with me. You are the one who is crazy!"

"I talk to the animals, you know, through their bellies. I am a vegetarian. I could never hurt them. I know what it is like to be eaten alive."

"The voices are talking to me all the time. They comment on everything, like, 'You want that but it's too good for you, or you are so bad, or that man is going to kill you.'"

"Sometimes I wonder: Did I really see that, or was it in my imagination? Is that a real memory, or not? Is that person trying to kill me? My mother killed herself. I know why."

little emotional expression. The speech may also be very concrete, lacking abstract ideas.

- *Avolition*. Avolition is a lack of motivation. Patients with avolition have difficulty initiating and persisting in goal-directed activities. This symptom can make it difficult for affected people to work or care for themselves.
- **Anhedonia**. Anhedonia is the lack of ability to feel pleasure.

Nursing practice is concerned with the patient's response to illness, so the signs and symptoms, the patient's lived experience of mental illness, are the basis of psychiatric nursing. See Box 49-2■ for a description of the experience of schizophrenia by the real experts (people who are affected by it).

Course of the Disease

In addition to the thought and neurologic symptoms, schizophrenia affects the person's abilities to relate to self and others and to function in society. Most people with schizophrenia do not marry and are more likely than their parents to be unemployed (APA, 2013).

Like many chronic illnesses, schizophrenia is characterized by *exacerbations* when the patient has psychotic and other symptoms and then periods in which the symptoms subside (*remissions*). Many patients experience a **prodromal phase** with early symptoms before a full psychotic episode. If individuals recognize the symptoms of their prodromal phase, treatment with medication may prevent or lessen the psychotic episode to follow. For many individuals, the prodromal phase starts with negative symptoms. Often family members can look back and remember that the patient spent a lot of time in bed or became more distant

or isolated before a psychotic episode. The prodromal symptom for some other people is difficulty sleeping for several nights before the onset of psychosis (APA, 2013).

In the acute phase of the disorder, the affected person may experience hallucinations, delusions, disorganized speech or behavior, and the negative symptoms (alogia, flattened affect, social isolation, loss of motivation, and anhedonia). The affected person is usually unable to maintain employment, participate in school, contribute to household maintenance, or even do ADLs such as personal hygiene and cooking while in an acute episode.

Schizophrenia is associated with a shortened life expectancy. Affected people have a five times greater risk of early death. Suicide is the largest contributor to this excess mortality. Untreated people with schizophrenia who are experiencing depression and psychosis are at risk for suicide. Other risks associated with schizophrenia are accidents, diseases (heart disease, infections, and breast cancer), and homelessness. Homelessness probably contributes to the incidence of accidents and diseases.

The brain disorder in schizophrenia renders many affected people unable to understand that they are mentally ill. This phenomenon is called *anosognosia*. As a result, effective treatments for schizophrenia often are avoided because patients lack the **insight** (self-understanding) to use them. Some health care providers blame the failure of many people with schizophrenia to take their disease seriously or failure to seek treatment on denial. Denial is not the problem. In fact, lack of insight, or anosognosia, is one of the cognitive deficits in schizophrenia. At any given time, 40% of people with schizophrenia are not receiving treatment. These untreated patients are at risk for injury due to poor judgment and disorganized thinking. They may not be able to manage their own basic needs for food or shelter. Because they are so vulnerable, each state has a law making it possible to treat people who are dangerous to themselves or others at state-owned hospitals even if they do not agree to treatment. Some include mental illness and the inability to provide for one's own basic needs as an additional reason for this *civil commitment*.

Early diagnosis and treatment of schizophrenia is important to prevent frequent relapses and rehospitalizations. People with schizophrenia are more likely to respond to treatment if it begins early in their disease process (NAMI, 2013). Early intervention may prevent the worst long-term outcomes (homelessness and death) of this devastating brain disorder.

Patients with schizophrenia often have a **dual diagnosis** (coexisting problems of mental illness and substance abuse). Many people use alcohol or street drugs to medicate themselves for the bad feelings they have with schizophrenia or other serious mental disorders. In combination, mental illness and substance abuse lead to even more homelessness, disease, violence, incarceration, and death. Chapter 53 covers this problem in more depth.

COLLABORATIVE CARE
Continuum of Care
Because schizophrenia is a chronic illness that affects all aspects of life, the best approach to care is on a continuum. A continuum or range of services over time provide assistance for people who have different needs and for individuals as their needs change. A community should provide a continuum of services such as the following:

- Hospitalization for acute episodes.
- Patient education to empower people with mental illness to understand their mental disorders, goals of treatment and medications, so they are able to participate in their own care.
- Case management to ensure that the patient receives appropriate services.
- Resources such as housing, food, medical care, transportation, clothing, employment, and socialization opportunities.
- A range of housing and care options, such as subacute care, day hospitalization, supervised/assisted living, group homes, foster care homes, and individual apartments.
- Outpatient treatment (including mental health clinics and mandatory medication supervision as indicated).

- Support for families, including respite care, education, support groups, and referral services. Local affiliates of the National Alliance on Mental Illness (NAMI) are excellent resources for families.

People with schizophrenia have better outcomes if they receive appropriate services throughout their lives, and yet the resources do not exist in many communities. There may be many reasons for this lack: Our society values independence so highly that we reject the idea of treating people against their will; schizophrenia has such a stigma that people do not value spending tax money on people who suffer from it; and because of their disease, people with schizophrenia are not able to speak for themselves.

Milieu Therapy
For psychiatric inpatients, the environment or **milieu** can be used as part of therapy. Consider the needs of people with psychosis who are having hallucinations, poor judgment about safety, difficulty relating to others, and delusional thinking. The environment should be pleasant, simple, and safe. There should be minimal stimulation: no background music, loud television, loud talking, or flashing lights, because patients already have the stimulation caused by anxiety, fear, or hallucinations.

Consistent nursing staff helps promote development of trust. Nurses also serve as role models for normal behavior. Every interaction in the milieu has the opportunity to be therapeutic. Nurses demonstrate how to interact with other people, how to dress, how to ask someone to change his or her behavior, and how to participate in unit activities. Patients have the opportunity to practice their behavior in the milieu. They also have the opportunity to give and receive feedback on behavior. Peer pressure is a powerful incentive for change.

Patients may need reminders to bathe, comb their hair, or attend group activities. Group activities often include recreation, simple exercise, arts and crafts, music, medication management, substance abuse treatment, relaxation techniques, or watching movies.

Milieu therapy also provides structure for patients' daily living. Meals and group activities are scheduled. Unit policies are followed consistently. Structure offers a predictable environment that is less stressful for a patient with impaired thinking. Ideally, patients are given a role in decision making about activities and unit rules.

Recovery
Some people with mental illnesses are becoming more comfortable being called *consumers* than "mentally ill people" when they are in the community. The consumer movement

(a *consumer* is a person who uses products or services) has started a new way of looking at mental illnesses. The old idea was that people had mental disorders and they alternated between exacerbations and remissions. The goal of treatment was to keep the patient in remission as much as possible. The newer way of looking at mental disorders is that people have a chronic illness, and the goal is recovery from the illness. Even people in recovery have exacerbations (called *relapses*) sometimes. The new part of the idea is that through their behavior and attitudes, people can have an effect on how quickly they recover from an exacerbation or even on whether they have an exacerbation or not. Recovery begins during hospitalization and continues in the community as consumers live each day, trying to keep their behavior as healthy as possible. The recovery model gives more responsibility to consumers, who are providing services (advice, support, education, basic living skills training) for their peers across the nation. Nurses empower consumers with the knowledge and skills they need to explain their feelings and symptoms to their health care providers and to be participants in their care.

Psychopharmacology

Medication is not the only treatment, but it is a cornerstone in the treatment of schizophrenia. Antipsychotic medications help relieve the hallucinations, delusions, and disordered thinking associated with the disorder. The positive symptoms of schizophrenia (hallucinations and delusional thinking) are more responsive to medications than the negative symptoms (alogia, anhedonia, amotivation).

Antipsychotic Agents

Antipsychotic medications (also called *neuroleptics*) are used to treat disorders such as schizophrenia that are characterized by psychosis. They are also used to treat the thought disorders sometimes associated with dementia, mania, or major depression with psychotic features. See Box 49-3■ for a list of antipsychotic medications.

> **Key Concept** Because schizophrenia has different causes in different people, a patient may need to try several different antipsychotics before finding the one that works well.

Ten people with schizophrenia may each have different genetic mutations, or brain structures, or neurotransmitter levels, or may have experienced different stressors or environmental exposures. They are likely to respond to drug therapy differently. An individual may have to try several drugs, each taking many weeks to develop efficacy. This trial process can be demoralizing. The nurse should explain that the health care provider will work with the patient

---

BOX 49-3	ANTIPSYCHOTIC MEDICATIONS

Traditional or Typical Antipsychotics
- Chlorpromazine (Thorazine)
- Fluphenazine (Prolixin)
- Haloperidol (Haldol)
- Loxapine (Loxitane)
- Mesoridazine (Serentil)
- Molindone (Moban)
- Perphenazine (Trilafon)
- Thioridazine (Mellaril)
- Thiothixene (Navane)
- Trifluoperazine (Stelazine)

Atypical Antipsychotics
- Clozapine (Clozaril)
- Olanzapine (Zyprexa)
- Quetiapine (Seroquel)
- Risperidone (Risperdal)
- Paliperidone (Invega)
- Ziprasidone (Geodon)

New-Generation Antipsychotics
- Aripiprazole (Abilify)

until the right treatment is found and that no one will give up hope.

Medication compliance is a major problem for patients with schizophrenia. It can also create problems for nurses, especially when patients do not believe that they are sick. Approximately 80% of those who stop taking their medication after an acute episode have a relapse of psychosis within a year. Even people who continue to take their medications experience relapse at the rate of approximately 30% in a year. Medication clearly improves the quality and quantity of life for people with severe mental illnesses such as schizophrenia. Unfortunately, the people who need medications the most often do not realize this. Also, certain medications cause side effects that combine with lack of insight to further decrease patient compliance.

The antipsychotics are grouped here as either typical (first-generation), atypical (second-generation), or new-generation antipsychotic drugs.

The goals of treatment with antipsychotic agents are to:
- Relieve symptoms of psychosis
- Provide for safety
- Improve patients' function and quality of life

> **Key Concept** Antipsychotic medications have side effects. Some (NMS and TD) are life threatening or longlasting; others (EPS) cause patients discomfort and may discourage compliance with medication therapy.

TYPICAL (FIRST-GENERATION) ANTIPSYCHOTICS The typical antipsychotics tend to be effective in treating psychosis or the positive symptoms of schizophrenia. The typical antipsychotics are especially effective in the treatment of acute psychosis with agitation. The negative symptoms are not very responsive to these medications.

It may take 2 days to 2 weeks for the onset of effects of the typical antipsychotic drugs. Full effect (*efficacy*) may take 4 weeks or longer. Patients and families need to be aware of this, so they do not give up hope and stop taking the medication too soon (Stuart, 2013).

After approximately 12 to 24 months of stable maintenance on antipsychotic medication, patients can be slowly tapered from the drug to assess the need to continue this treatment. Some people with schizophrenia require a lifetime of continuous medication therapy (Stuart, 2013).

Mechanism of Action Psychotic symptoms are thought to be related to excess dopamine activity. Typical antipsychotic medications target the dopamine-2 (D_2) receptors, acting as antagonists to reduce dopamine activity in the brain.

Side Effects Side effects are common and often cause patients to stop taking their medications when they are at home. Management of side effects is a critical part of the care of patients taking these medications.

Extrapyramidal Side Effects Although antagonism of D_2 receptors reduces psychosis, it causes extrapyramidal symptoms (EPS). Box 49-4■ lists extrapyramidal side effects. EPS result from the effects of antipsychotic drugs on the extrapyramidal tracts of the central nervous system, which control involuntary movement. These abnormal movement and muscle tone side effects are listed in Box 49-4.

In the normal nervous system, the neurotransmitters dopamine and acetylcholine must be balanced to maintain normal muscle function. The patient with untreated psychosis has increased dopaminergic activity. The balancing mechanism responds by increasing cholinergic activity. When an antipsychotic medication is given, dopaminergic activity is decreased, but the cholinergic activity is still high, leading to an imbalance. An anticholinergic drug can restore

A. Balance occurs in schizophrenic patient's steady state of high dopamine.

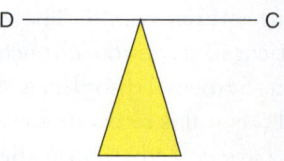

B. Antipsychotic med decreases dopamine activity, putting dopamine, D, and acetylcholine, C, out of balance. Patient has EPS.

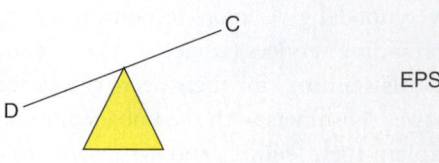

C. Anticholinergic med is given to bring cholinergic activity down, restoring balance and treating EPS.

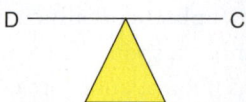

Figure 49-2. ■ Mechanisms of extrapyramidal symptoms (EPS).

this balance and relieve the EPS. See Figure 49-2■ for a diagram of the process of EPS and its treatment. EPS include:

- **Dystonia:** muscular rigidity, abnormal muscle contraction. It can be mild, such as jaw muscle tightening, or as severe as oculogyric crisis (eyes uncontrollably rolled back), torticollis (neck twists head to side and back), and opisthotonos (generalized muscle spasms that result in arching of the back and neck). If the tongue or larynx is involved, choking can result. Dystonia of some kind occurs in approximately 20% of patients taking typical antipsychotics. It usually responds well to anticholinergic medications, which are usually ordered on an as-needed basis for patients new to antipsychotics or after a dose increase. When a choking hazard is present, the anticholinergic medication should be given intramuscularly.
- Pseudoparkinsonism or **dyskinesia** (abnormal movement): stiff, stooped posture (see Figure 39-2); shuffling gait; tremor; slow movements; cogwheel rigidity (jerky, ratchet-like movements of the joints);

BOX 49-4	**EXTRAPYRAMIDAL SIDE EFFECTS FROM ANTIPSYCHOTIC DRUGS**

- *Dystonia:* muscle rigidity
- *Dyskinesia (pseudoparkinsonism):* stiffness, tremors, shuffling gait
- *Akathisia:* restlessness, inability to sit still
- *Tardive dyskinesia:* late-onset permanent movement disorder with involuntary movements of the face and tongue, or less commonly limbs and trunk

masklike facies (loss of facial expression). These symptoms are caused by the imbalance between dopamine and acetylcholine. Dystonia affects 20% of patients taking typical antipsychotics. Antiparkinsonian medications may be used to relieve these symptoms.

- **Akathisia**: restlessness, intense need to move. The patient may report a sense of "jumping out of my skin" or an inability to sit still. Akathisia may cause patients to pace (walk back and forth continuously), fidget with fingers, or move arms and legs while sitting. Akathisia can make rest or sleep impossible for days. It is one of the most common EPS, affecting 25% of patients. It responds poorly to treatment. The antipsychotic medication causing it may have to be changed. The nurse should reassure that patient that this is a medication side effect that will go away and that the nurse understands the patient's need to keep moving (Keltner, Bostrom, & McGuinness, 2011).

- **Tardive dyskinesia** (late onset of abnormal movement) is an extrapyramidal effect that develops after extended antipsychotic drug therapy. The symptoms of tardive dyskinesia (TD) include involuntary movements such as lip smacking, facial grimacing, tongue protrusion, tongue writhing, blinking, or other involuntary movements of the limbs and trunk. The most common TD symptoms involve abnormal involuntary movements of the face and tongue. The symptoms disappear during sleep. Sometimes patients can voluntarily suppress the abnormal movements briefly, but they recur when the patient concentrates on something else.

TD may be due to development of hypersensitivity to dopamine. It is not caused by the same dopamine–acetylcholine imbalance as the other EPS. It does not respond to anticholinergic medications (Keltner, Bostrom, & McGuinness, 2011).

It is important to assess patients on antipsychotic therapy for abnormal involuntary movement with a scale such as the abnormal involuntary movement scale (AIMS) to identify TD early. Table 49-3 ■ shows an example of an AIMS. There is no effective treatment for TD, but it can sometimes be prevented by the use of the lowest effective dose of antipsychotic medication. Changing to another antipsychotic may be able to arrest the progression of TD. TD is irreversible; therefore, early recognition of the signs of TD is a critical nursing function.

EPS are very uncomfortable for patients. When they occur, the antipsychotic dose may be reduced, a different antipsychotic medication may be prescribed, or an anticholinergic or other medication may be used to treat the symptoms. Anticholinergic medications are usually given orally, but may be given intramuscularly in emergent situations. It is the responsibility of the nurse to assess for EPS and to advocate for the patient to obtain relief. See Table 49-4 ■ for a list of drugs used to treat EPS.

Neuroleptic Malignant Syndrome   **Neuroleptic malignant syndrome** (NMS) is a potentially fatal side effect of antipsychotic drugs. The major symptoms are high fever, muscle rigidity, autonomic instability (unstable blood pressure, diaphoresis, pale skin), delirium, inability to speak, tremors, and elevated levels of enzymes that indicate muscle damage (CPK). Temperatures may rise as high as 108°F (42.2°C). It is important for nurses to monitor vital signs of patients receiving antipsychotic medications. Elevated temperature may be the first sign.

Less than 1% of people who take antipsychotic drugs develop NMS, but for these it can be fatal. Early diagnosis and treatment are the keys to patient survival.

Patients are at higher risk for developing NMS if they have dehydration, poor nutrition, or concurrent medical illness. Treatment involves discontinuing antipsychotic drugs and providing supportive treatment for blood pressure changes, muscle breakdown, dehydration, and other symptoms.

NMS is an idiosyncratic reaction to antipsychotic (neuroleptic) drugs. It usually but not always occurs in the first 3 weeks of therapy. It is not a toxic or allergic effect. High-potency typical antipsychotics are most frequently involved.

clinicalALERT

Neuroleptic malignant syndrome is a potentially fatal side effect of antipsychotic drugs. It usually occurs early in therapy. Nurses should assess for high fever, muscle pain, and unstable blood pressure, and report these to the physician immediately. Dehydration increases the risk for NMS, which makes hydration even more important in psychiatric nursing.

Endocrine Side Effects   Dopamine inhibits the hormone prolactin, which promotes breast enlargement and milk production. Typical antipsychotics elevate levels of prolactin because they inhibit dopamine. Chronic prolactin elevation can cause decreased libido (sexual drive), breast enlargement (gynecomastia), and galactorrhea (leakage of milk) in women or men. It can also cause menstrual dysfunction in women.

The incidence of type 2 diabetes is increased in people with schizophrenia, even in those who are not obese. This increase may be in part due to adverse effects on the endocrine system caused by antipsychotic medications. Nurses should be alert for the development of signs and symptoms of hyperglycemia in patients taking antipsychotics.

Monitoring of adverse metabolic effects of atypical (second-generation) antipsychotics should be improved. A recent study showed that 30% of patients on atypical antipsychotics are not tested for metabolic effects. Box 49-5 ■

TABLE 49-3	**Abnormal Involuntary Movement Scale**				
DYSKINESIA SYMPTOMS					
THIS FORM HOLDS FOUR ASSESSMENTS TO SHOW CHANGES OVER TIME.		Date	Date	Date	Date
1. Muscles of facial expression					
2. Lips and area around the mouth					
3. Jaw					
4. Tongue					
5. Upper body (arms, hands, fingers)					
6. Lower body (legs, knees, ankles, toes)					
7. Neck, shoulders, torso, hips					
8. *Overall judgment* Severity of abnormal movements					
EXTRAPYRAMIDAL AND OTHER SYMPTOMS					
1. Rigidity					
2. Tremor					
3. Bradykinesia					
4. Akathisia					
DENTAL PROBLEMS					
1. Current problems with teeth or dentures No = 0, Yes = 1					
2. Does the patient usually wear dentures? No = 0, Yes = 1					

Examination Procedure

Either before or after examination, observe the patient at rest. Abnormal movements can sometimes be suppressed if the patient concentrates on this. The chair used in the examination should be firm and without arms.

1. Ask the patient if there is anything in his or her mouth (gum, candy) and, if so, to remove it.

2. Ask the patient about the current condition of his or her teeth. Ask if he or she wears dentures and, if so, do they bother the patient now? Tongue and mouth movements associated with dental problems may be mistaken for abnormal involuntary movements.

3. Ask the patient whether he or she notices any movements in the mouth, face, hands, or feet. If yes, ask to what extent do they currently bother the patient or interfere with activities.

4. Have the patient sit in a chair with legs slightly apart, hands on knees, and feet flat on the floor. Look at the entire body for movements while the patient is in this position.

5. Ask the patient to sit with hands unsupported (between legs or hanging over knees). Observe hands and other body areas.

6. Ask the patient to open his or her mouth. Observe the tongue at rest in the mouth. Do this twice.

7. Ask the patient to protrude the tongue. Observe for abnormalities of tongue movement. Do this twice.

8. Ask the patient to tap his or her thumb with each finger, one at a time, as rapidly as possible for 10–15 seconds, separately with one hand, and then the other. Observe face and legs. Concentration on finger movements may allow abnormal movements to become evident elsewhere.

9. Flex and extend the patient's arms one at a time. Note any rigidity.

10. Ask the patient to stand up. Observe in profile all body areas again, including hips.

11. Ask the patient to extend both arms outstretched in front with palms down. Observe trunk, legs, and mouth.

12. Have the patient walk a few paces, turn, and walk back to the chair. Observe hands and gait. Do this twice.

Score each item on the following scale. Rate the highest severity observed. None = 0, minimal = 1, mild = 2, moderate = 3, severe = 4.

TABLE 49-4	Anticholinergic Drugs Used to Treat Extrapyramidal Side Effects	
GENERIC (TRADE) NAME	**DRUG CLASSIFICATION**	**AVAILABLE IN INJECTABLE FORM?**
Benztropine (Cogentin)	Anticholinergic	Yes
Biperiden (Akineton)	Anticholinergic	Yes
Diphenhydramine (Benadryl)	Antihistamine (has strong anticholinergic side effects)	Yes
Procyclidine (Kemadrin)	Anticholinergic	No
Trihexyphenidyl (Artane)	Anticholinergic	Yes

includes the potential metabolic effects of antipsychotic medications, which increase patients' risks for cardiovascular disease and diabetes. These risks should be assessed at least annually for every patient on atypical antipsychotics.

Anticholinergic Side Effects   Anticholinergic side effects often result from the use of antipsychotics. See Box 49-6■ for a list of anticholinergic symptoms. Patients taking anticholinergic medications for EPS have an increased risk for these side effects. The patient in Figure 49-3■ has mydriasis (pupil dilation) as an effect of an anticholinergic medication.

Weight Gain   Most of the antipsychotics can cause weight gain. Olanzapine (Zyprexa) causes the highest incidence of weight gain. Weight gain with antipsychotics is associated

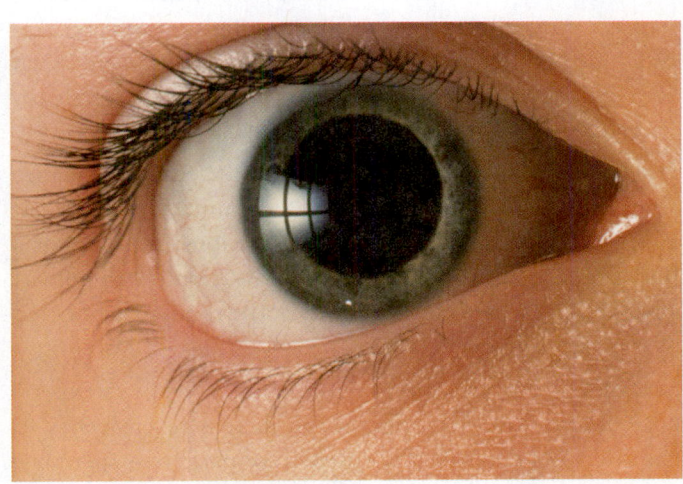

Figure 49-3. ■ This patient has mydriasis (dilated pupils), which is an anticholinergic effect. (Source: Adam Hart-Davis/Science Source.)

with increased appetite, binge eating, carbohydrate craving, decreased satiety, and change in food preferences in some patients. Increased insulin may also contribute to weight gain in people taking antipsychotic drugs.

Obesity is common in people with schizophrenia. They are less likely than the general population to exercise or eat a healthy low-fat diet.

Appetite changes, sedentary lifestyle, and unhealthy food choices all add up to an increased risk for obesity and therefore type 2 diabetes and cardiovascular diseases.

Medical opinion is that the therapeutic effects of these drugs outweigh the importance of weight gain. However, weight gain can be a very important body image, self-esteem, and general health issue for patients.

The best approach to the risk of weight gain is prevention. Nurses can teach patients and their families about this risk and about how to reduce the likelihood of obesity with healthy nutrition and exercise.

Orthostatic Hypotension   The hypotension caused by antipsychotics is an antiadrenergic effect. Normally the blood vessels can respond to changes in body position by constricting, ensuring adequate blood flow to the brain.

BOX 49-5	ASSESSMENT

Metabolic Side Effects of Antipsychotic Drugs

- Blood pressure
- Weight
- Girth
- Glucose
- Total cholesterol
- HDL cholesterol
- LDL cholesterol
- Triglycerides

BOX 49-6	ANTICHOLINERGIC SIDE EFFECTS

- Dry mouth
- Orthostatic hypotension
- Constipation
- Urinary hesitancy or retention
- Pupil dilation (*mydriasis*)
- Blurred near vision
- Dry eyes
- Photosensitivity
- Increased heart rate

When sympathetic alpha-1 receptors are blocked, the vessels are prevented from responding automatically to body position changes.

Orthostatic (position-related) hypotension happens when the individual stands up or changes position quickly. It is also called postural hypotension. Orthostatic hypotension is more likely to occur in older adults. It can create a safety hazard for the patient who becomes dizzy or falls when the blood pressure drops (Keltner, Bostrom, & McGuinness, 2011).

Cardiac Side Effects   Antipsychotics may cause increased heart rate as an anticholinergic side effect. They may also cause prolonged conduction time through the heart's electrical system. On EKG a prolonged QT interval indicates prolonged conduction.

Seizures   The antipsychotics tend to decrease the seizure threshold, so a smaller stimulus is required to cause a seizure in a patient taking these medications. Epilepsy or a history of seizures is not a contraindication for the use of antipsychotic drugs, but the physician should be notified of any such history.

Photosensitivity   Some patients taking antipsychotics experience photosensitivity, which is an increased sensitivity to the effects of the sun. Photosensitive patients experience severe sunburn with minimal sun exposure. Dark-skinned as well as light-skinned patients can experience photosensitivity. They should be counseled to avoid prolonged exposure to sunlight or to wear long sleeves, a hat, or sunscreen on their skin whenever they are outdoors.

ATYPICAL ANTIPSYCHOTICS   The atypical antipsychotics have been used since the 1990s to treat schizophrenia and other psychotic disorders. Their mechanism of action differs from that of the typical agents. The typical agents act largely on dopamine-2 receptors, whereas the atypical agents influence a variety of dopamine receptor sites, serotonin receptors, muscarinic receptors, alpha-receptors, and histamine receptors.

Atypical agents differ from typical antipsychotic agents in several important ways. The atypical agents (Stahl, 2014):

1. Are slightly more effective at treating the negative symptoms.
2. Cause fewer extrapyramidal side effects, including less TD.
3. Are effective against the symptoms of schizophrenia for some people who do not respond to typical agents.

Side Effects   EPS are the side effects most commonly cited by patients as their reason for noncompliance with antipsychotic medications at home. As a group, the atypical agents cause fewer EPS, less prolactin increase, and less TD.

The atypicals treat psychosis effectively in some people who are resistant to the typical antipsychotics. Because of their efficacy and more favorable side effect profile, the atypical antipsychotics are currently prescribed more frequently than typical agents.

While their side effect profile is lower, the atypical antipsychotics as a group are known to cause weight gain, glucose intolerance, EPS, and NMS.

Diabetes   Patients receiving atypical antipsychotics are 9% more likely to have diabetes than people taking typical agents. In one study, the likelihood was significantly increased for patients taking clozapine, olanzapine, or quetiapine. The mechanism may be an increase in insulin resistance in body cells. Patients taking these drugs should be monitored regularly for the development of diabetes. Other risk factors, such as African American, Native American, or Latino ethnicity, obesity, female gender, and family history of type 2 diabetes, increase the patient's risk (Keltner, Bostrom, & McGuinness, 2011). All patients taking atypical antipsychotics should be taught about diabetes risk reduction, including maintaining normal body weight; eating a low-fat, high-fiber, low-salt diet; eating more whole foods and fewer processed foods; and regular aerobic exercise for at least 30 minutes at least 5 days per week.

Agranulocytosis   Even though their side effect profile is favorable, the atypical agents have side effects. The most notable is that clozapine can cause agranulocytosis, a life-threatening decrease in white blood cell (WBC) production. This effect happens to 1% of patients who take clozapine. Therefore, clozapine is used only for patients who are resistant to treatment with other antipsychotics. Treatment resistance is established by failure to respond to at least two different antipsychotic agents. Clozapine is effective in treating 25% to 50% of patients whose symptoms do not respond to typical agents (Stahl, 2014).

clinicalALERT

All patients receiving clozapine should have their WBC measured once per week during the first 6 months of therapy, every other week for months 7 to 12, and every 4 weeks after that, to assess whether their WBC count is stable (Stahl, 2014). If a patient's WBC count drops (indicating bone marrow suppression), clozapine should be permanently discontinued.

NEW-GENERATION ANTIPSYCHOTICS   Unlike the other antipsychotic agents, aripiprazole (Abilify, Abilitat), a dopamine system stabilizer, has a stabilizing and modulating effect on brain dopamine. This drug is intended to reduce dopamine transmission when it is too high and to preserve it when it is too low, thus maintaining the dopaminergic–cholinergic balance. It was hoped that this drug would not cause abnormal involuntary movements (EPS), but it does at a lower rate than other antipsychotics.

DEPOT INJECTION AND OTHER DRUG FORMS   Several antipsychotic agents are currently available in long-acting decanoate (depot injection) form. The depot form of the drug is injected intramuscularly and lasts for several weeks. Haloperidol (Haldol) and fluphenazine (Prolixin) are the typical agents available in depot form. They are supplied in a sesame oil solution. Haloperidol is repeated every 4 weeks, and fluphenazine every 1 to 4 weeks. Risperidone was the first atypical antipsychotic agent available in depot form. It is administered every 2 weeks and is supplied as microspheres suspended in a saline solution. Now olanzapine and ziprasidone are also available in intramuscular form.

The advantages of the long-acting form of antipsychotic drugs relate to compliance with drug therapy. Patients may be able to comply with a clinic visit once every few weeks more consistently than they can take daily oral medications.

Several antipsychotic agents are available in liquid oral concentrate forms. The liquid form can be used to prevent situations in which patients move pills to their cheeks instead of swallowing them, to spit them out later. It is also helpful when the patient has difficulty swallowing pills or prefers the liquid to the pill form. The liquid concentrates must be mixed with a small amount of juice or other liquid to improve the taste.

The newest drug form for antipsychotics is oral disintegrating tablets. Regular oral antipsychotics take 1 to 6 hours to absorb. The disintegrating tablets absorb into the blood within 2 minutes of administration. Such quick absorption is an advantage in patients who have difficulty swallowing or those who have a need for assurance of drug compliance (Keltner, Bostrom, & McGuinness, 2011).

DRUG INTERACTIONS   All antipsychotic agents potentially interact with other CNS agents. There is an additive CNS depressant effect when they are combined with sedatives, narcotics, or alcohol. Antacids can decrease gastrointestinal absorption of the antipsychotics, reducing their effectiveness. Anticholinergic drugs can add to the anticholinergic side effects and decrease the effectiveness of the antipsychotic. Tricyclic antidepressants add to the anticholinergic side effects (Stahl, 2014).

ABUSE POTENTIAL   The antipsychotic medications do not cause euphoria, so there is virtually no abuse potential from these drugs. An overdose of antipsychotic medications is seldom fatal. They also do not cause addiction or dependency. This lack of abuse potential is an important teaching point, because many consumers believe that any drug that affects the mind is addictive.

clinicalALERT

Nurses often hesitate to give PRN medications, perhaps from fear of responsibility for making the decision to give them. If your patient has EPS, do not hesitate to give anticholinergics when they are ordered PRN. EPS are very uncomfortable for patients and are a major reason for noncompliance with antipsychotic medications.

NURSING CARE

PRIORITIZING NURSING CARE

In the acute phase of psychosis, treatment should focus on the patient's basic needs. Safety, nutrition, and rest are the priorities. Acute symptom management is also important.

ASSESSING

In psychiatric nursing, the patient's potential for violence is assessed first because it is a safety issue. Mentally ill people in general are no more violent than the general public, but there are groups of mentally ill people with increased risk for violence toward others. The risk factors for violence are:

- Previous violent acts at home or in treatment
- History of substance abuse, especially if currently under the influence of substances
- Paranoid delusions
- Command hallucinations (commanding the patient to hurt someone)
- History of being a victim of violence (violence can be a learned behavior)

Certain behaviors may suggest that a patient is becoming increasingly agitated and more likely to act out violently. These behaviors include clenched fists, loud talking or yelling, threatening, increasing motor activity (was sitting, then walking, and then pacing back and forth quickly), hitting walls or furniture, and wincing or looking afraid.

Mental Status Assessment

Nurses regularly assess and document the patient's behavior, mood, and thought content (which is reflected in what the patient says). All patients with psychosis should be asked directly if they feel like hurting themselves or others. This important information will remain unknown unless someone asks directly. See Chapter 48 for information about mental status assessment.

Cultural Issues

Interpreting the meaning of patient behaviors can be difficult if the patient is from a different culture from the nurse. Box 49-7 ■ describes cultural sensitivity issues in psychiatric care. The nurse's goal is to see the patient's behavior from the patient's point of view.

Cultural Care in Psychiatric Nursing

It is especially challenging to offer culturally sensitive psychiatric nursing. When the nurse and patient are from different cultures, the nurse may misinterpret behavior that would be considered normal in the patient's culture. For example, in some Latino cultures, people talk to the spirits of their dead relatives. What is intended to be thinking about the loved one's wishes or teachings might appear to be hallucinating to a nurse. Some African and Caribbean cultures recognize witches and sorcerers, which might seem like delusional thinking to an outsider. The nurse should always try to interpret patient behavior relative to the patient's cultural background, rather than through the cultural standards of the nurse. When available, a cultural facilitator who can translate the patient's language and culture-oriented behaviors can be very helpful.

Physical Assessment in the Psychiatric Setting

Although physical assessment plays an important role in nursing in every setting, the psychiatric nurse must be creative when assessing mental and physical health. When patients are hallucinating, they may not be sure what is real and what is not. Physical touching may be perceived as part of a threatening hallucination. Delusional thinking may make even the well-intentioned nurse seem menacing. Physical assessment may be very stressful for the patient. Some patients mistake physical touch for sexual advances. Therefore, only priority physical assessments should be done in the acute psychiatric situation. A physician or nurse practitioner will perform an initial physical assessment as part of the psychiatric patient's admission process. A trusting nurse–patient relationship will make it easier for the nurse to gain patient cooperation for necessary assessments.

Nurses must understand the desired effects and potential side effects of all medications and treatments received by their patients and assess for these. In addition, psychiatric patients may not be able to clearly articulate what is wrong with them. Careful listening is another important nursing skill. When a patient with psychosis says, "The snake is squeezing my chest!" it is possible that this patient is experiencing a heart attack.

The Patient's Family

The patient's family is a critical aspect of psychiatric care. It is important to obtain written permission from patients to communicate with anyone about them, including their family members. Families can make a big difference as allies in treatment for psychiatric patients, yet health care providers often overlook them out of a mistaken sense of

protecting the patient's confidentiality. They are important members of the treatment team.

DIAGNOSING, PLANNING, AND IMPLEMENTING

Data about the patient's mental status, observation of the patient's behavior and interactions with others, physical assessment findings, and information from family all contribute data for establishing nursing diagnoses. Priority nursing diagnoses that often apply to patients with schizophrenia include Risk for Violence: Self-Directed or Other-Directed, Risk for Injury, Ineffective Coping, and Impaired Social Interaction.

Risk for Violence: Self-Directed or Other-Directed

Expected Outcome: Will cause no harm to self or others.

- Avoid touching an actively hallucinating patient. *Touch may be perceived as part of a threatening hallucination, and the patient may hit in self-defense.*
- Intervene early as soon as you have identified increased agitation. Reassure patients that they are safe in the hospital. *Agitation can escalate quickly. Early intervention can prevent the situation from getting worse. Fear may motivate agitation. Patients often benefit from reassurance that they are safe.*
- Avoid confronting patients aggressively about their behavior. When inappropriate behavior arises, tell the patient simply and calmly that the behavior is not acceptable and redirect the patient to another activity. *Patients may not realize that their behavior is inappropriate. Aggressive behavior by the nurse may make patients feel defensive. The nurse's nonverbal behavior should be open and nonthreatening. Hold your hands at your sides. Keep your voice quiet and controlled. Your self-control can be "contagious" to the patient.*
- Start with less restrictive interventions when patients have inappropriate behavior: Try to talk first then redirect, offer meds, isolate/medicate, and restrain last. *Patients have the ethical and legal right to the least restrictive alternative treatment that is effective.*
- Maintain a low-stimulation environment. *Patients with schizophrenia may have difficulty processing multiple stimuli, and extra stimuli may lead to agitation and confusion.*
- Talk with the patient about signs and symptoms of anxiety and agitation and the triggers that start these feelings. Discuss options for appropriate behavior and anxiety management techniques. *If the patient can recognize anxiety and agitation early, the patient can notify staff, who can help identify coping mechanisms to prevent violent acting out. Patients with schizophrenia often have short attention spans and inadequate coping skills and may have impulsive behavior. Cognitive approaches to planning for future episodes help patients try appropriate new behavior.*

- Observe people experiencing paranoia or command hallucinations closely. *Even a person who has a nonviolent personality may act out violently when confronted with an apparently life-threatening hallucination or when terrorized by a paranoid delusion that threatens the person's life. Many people will never be violent unless they are in a life-threatening situation. When people with schizophrenia are violent, usually the violent act is a matter of self-defense from their point of view.*

See Box 49-8■ for help on interacting with patients who are actively hallucinating.

Risk for Injury Related to Psychosis

Expected Outcome: Will have reality-based thinking.

- Provide antipsychotic medications as ordered and monitor effects. *It is the responsibility of nurses to assess the patient's response to medications for the purpose of evaluating their effectiveness.*

- Look for the patient's strengths and abilities when providing nursing care. *When a person has a severe mental illness such as schizophrenia, it is easy to see the pathology. It is important to look for the person's strengths and to acknowledge the normal parts of the person. Even the psychotic patient has coping or survival skills that the nurse can draw on for the patient's benefit.*

- Reinforce reality. Talk about what is really happening. *Even conversations about the simple realities of daily life (the weather, doing laundry, meals, etc.) focus the patient's attention away from disordered thoughts and into the here-and-now. The nurse's role is to help the patient recognize what is real.*

- Do not argue with the patient about delusional thoughts. *Patients do not recognize that they are delusions, and arguments can force the patient to focus on defending the false ideas. Change the subject to reality-based topics.*

- Encourage or assist the patient to express feelings of fear or anxiety. Provide validation for the patient's feelings. *The sense of losing contact with reality can be frightening. Expressing feelings to the nurse who accepts them without judgment and validates how difficult the situation must be can be affirming and helpful to patients.*

Ineffective Coping

Expected Outcome: Will take medications as prescribed, will have behavior choices when frustrated other than acting out frustration physically, and will have stress management strategies.

- Establish a trusting relationship in which the patient is safe to express true feelings, especially negative ones. *The patient may feel that only positive feelings are appropriate and not know an appropriate way to express negative feelings. A nonthreatening relationship provides the opportunity to express unresolved feelings. Verbalizing and discussing feelings can replace aggression as a coping mechanism. A strong reaction to patient's feelings may indicate rejection.*

- Offer medications in a confident way, expecting the patient to take them. *The nurse's confident attitude promotes patient trust.*

- Teach patients stress management techniques such as going to their rooms and doing relaxation exercises. *Practicing new coping behavior teaches adaptive coping skills.*

Impaired Social Interaction

Expected Outcome: Will behave in appropriate ways in social situations (respond verbally, engage in one-to-one conversations with staff and other patients, attend or participate in group meetings). Will maintain contact with family and important friends.

- Approach the patient with an accepting attitude. Be honest and sincere. *Acceptance, honesty, and sincerity promote trust.*

BOX 49-8	NURSING CARE CHECKLIST

Interacting With a Person Who Is Hallucinating

☑ Only one person should interact with the patient at a time. *The patient is having difficulty interpreting stimuli, so it will be easier for the patient to respond to one person.*

☑ Keep environmental noise to a minimum. Do not speak loudly. *The patient is having difficulty filtering sensory stimuli. A low-stimulation environment will make it easier for the patient to differentiate real stimuli from the voices.*

☑ Initially specifically ask the patient about the hallucinations (usually voices) as part of the nursing mental status assessment and what they are saying or telling the patient to do. *It is helpful to know if patients are experiencing voices commanding them to hurt themselves or others.*

☑ Focus on reality. Do not continually ask patients to describe the hallucinations. Do not react to patients' report of hallucinations as if they are real. *Often hallucinations are transitory experiences for patients. Describing the hallucination can form it more clearly in the patient's mind and reinforce it. The nurse's role is to help patients recognize reality, not to further confuse them about their hallucinations or delusions. When the nurse keeps the conversation in reality, reality is reinforced and the hallucinations may be minimized.*

☑ Do not argue with the patient's experience. Share your own perceptions. Reassure the patients that they are safe. *The patient is truly hearing the voices. The goal is to present reality, not to convince the patients that they are wrong. Respectful disagreement can help the patient understand what is real. For example, "I know you hear voices, but I don't hear them." Reassurance may help patients see that they are not in danger and do not need to defend themselves. Focusing on the hallucinations may emphasize them enough to increase their intensity for the patient.*

☑ Avoid touching a person who is actively hallucinating. *During a hallucination, any touch may be perceived by the patient as part of the hallucination. If the hallucination is threatening, the patient may strike out in self-defense.*

- Interact with the patient individually and model appropriate social behavior (body language, topics of conversation). *People with schizophrenia often lack social skills and benefit from role modeling as a way to learn acceptable social behavior.*
- Give positive reinforcement for the patient's voluntary interactions with others. *Positive reinforcement is an effective behavioral approach to behavior change.*
- Encourage the patient to attend group activities in the hospital. Accompany the patient at first if necessary. *The patient may respond positively to encouragement from a trusted nurse.*

MANAGING NURSING CARE

As appropriate and allowed by the designated duties and responsibilities of assistive personnel, the nurse may delegate nursing care activities such as obtaining vital signs, assisting with ADLs as directed, interacting with or supervising behavior of a patient with psychosis.

EVALUATING

When evaluating the effectiveness of nursing care for patients with schizophrenia, the nurse looks to the desired outcomes. The nurse will determine whether the patient:

- Demonstrates reality-based thinking.
- Performs ADLs independently.
- Demonstrates an understanding of medication management.
- States a plan for self-management of stress or frustration.
- Interacts effectively with others.

DOCUMENTING

The nurse should document data that describe patients' mental status and response to medications. Describing patient statements and behaviors is preferable to writing conclusions, because the goal of documentation is to give the reader specific, concise, objective information about patients' responses to their disorders and treatments. For example, documenting, "The patient states that he is Spiderman and plans to jump from roof to roof" illustrates his condition better than "Patient has delusional thinking." Charting "Patient has EPS" is not as clear as "Patient states that his 'jaws feel tight' and he has been pacing the halls for 3 hours."

CONTINUITY OF CARE

As the patient recovers from psychosis and moves into the rehabilitation phase, the intervention focus changes to teaching and psychosocial rehabilitation issues. Medication teaching, group therapies, self-care skills, and social skills become more important. Patients can learn strategies to decrease the likelihood of relapse and increase the likelihood of recovery from schizophrenia. See Box 49-9■ for patient teaching strategies to promote recovery. Learning these strategies can give patients more control over their lives and disease processes. People

---

BOX 49-9	PATIENT TEACHING

Strategies for Recovery or Preventing Relapse of Mental Illness

Discuss the following suggestions for reducing the chance of relapse of mental illness with the patient:

- Learn from your experience. In the past how did you feel in the weeks before you needed to be hospitalized? What feelings or symptoms did you experience? These are the *predictors of relapse* for you. Tell your family about them, and watch for these symptoms. When they happen, get help from your psychiatrist who can change your treatment to help prevent or reduce the severity of the relapse.
- How do you feel about your *medication*? (Look for some positive aspect of patient's attitude and repeat it.) What are your goals for the long term? Whatever you want to accomplish (becoming the president, going to Disneyland) will not happen if you do not take your medication. If medication is part of your treatment, take it. It is what keeps you out of the hospital.
- Know the symptoms of schizophrenia for yourself. Be able to discuss them with your health care provider. Understand what each medication is for, and be able to tell the provider if it is working. You are the expert on how you feel! Tell your prescriber about side effects. Most can be treated.
- Do what you can to decrease the *stress* in your life. Keep your surroundings quiet. Go to a room alone or with one person if you want to. When someone argues with you, go to a quiet place. Know what is most stressful for you. If you know something is really stressful for you, avoid it.
- Know your *resources* and have a plan. Make a list of people who can give help when you need it. For example: Adam can take me to the pharmacy to refill my prescription. Betty can talk when I am lonely or scared. Carlos can take care of my fish if I am too tired. Dad can call the doctor or the hospital if I need to go. Write down all their phone numbers.
- Think of some *things that make you feel better*. Write them on a list. Take it out and do them when you start to feel bad. Maybe you feel better when you take a walk, do relaxation techniques, have a snack, paint, draw, take a nap, look at pictures, listen to music, talk to a trusted person, or pet a dog. The list has to be things you would really do.
- *Avoid risky situations.* Stay away from people who want you to use drugs or alcohol with them. It is too hard to say no. Stay away from negative people who criticize you or make you feel bad about yourself. Avoid situations that increase the voices or your stress.
- *Keep healthy.* Eat right. Sleep regularly. Stay active with hobbies, work or other activities, and exercise.
- *Keep hope alive.* Remember how life is always changing. Do you agree that some days you feel bad and some days you feel better?

---

trying to stay in recovery and prevent relapse should stay out of risky social situations, such as going where people are drinking alcohol or using drugs.

Some people with schizophrenia will continue to have auditory hallucinations after they are discharged. Strategies for stopping these voices include *distraction*, which include listening to music, reading aloud, counting backward from 100, watching television, or describing an object in detail. Some patients report that listening to music through headphones is most effective for overriding voices. *Interacting* is another strategy and includes telling the voices to stop, talking to the voices while pretending to use a mobile phone, and agreeing to listen to the voices at certain times. The *activity* strategy includes walking, doing housework, taking a relaxing bath, playing the guitar, singing, and exercising. The *social* strategy involves talking to a trusted person, phoning a help-line, avoiding large groups of people, going to a drop-in center, and going to a favorite place.

Socialization

Relating to others is a basic human need. It is often difficult for people with schizophrenia to engage in mutually satisfying social relationships. Nurses are role models for normal social behavior. In the community, the nurse can refer the patient to community socialization programs at mental health clinics or encourage the patient to try low-stimulation recreational activities.

People with schizophrenia need a network of social contacts. Nurses cooperate with social workers to provide community resources for patients. Nurses foster relationships and group participation in all settings.

Advocating for Patients

The treatments and knowledge needed to treat schizophrenia already exist. Financial commitment by the government and insurance companies and community priorities must change to bring the resources to the people who need them. The role of nursing in this process is in patient advocacy.

Nurses are experts on the subject of how people are affected by diseases and disorders. Nurses can influence their legislators to prioritize funding for mental illness treatment. Nurses can act collectively through their unions, employers, and professional organizations to influence insurance companies to cover mental illness equally with physical illness (called *mental health parity*). They can advocate in their communities for improved housing and other social services for mentally ill people. They can raise the consciousness of the people in their communities by writing to local newspaper editors about the issue of mental illness treatment. We can work to make the invisible people with mental illness visible so our society can see who truly needs help. Figure 49-4■ shows a depression awareness campaign, organized to raise the consciousness of the community about mental illness.

NURSING CARE PLAN
Patient With Schizophrenia

Anya Daeva is a 30-year-old woman who was diagnosed with schizophrenia 8 years ago. She has been hospitalized several times both for psychiatric admissions and general medical

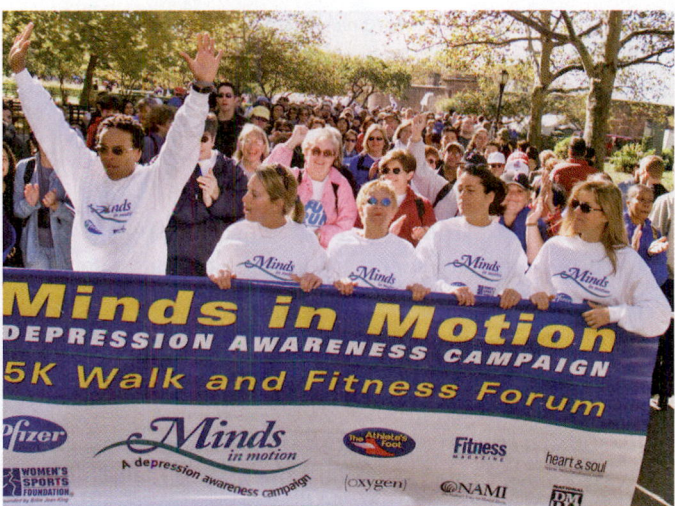

Figure 49-4. ■ Advocacy for the mentally ill includes public awareness activities like this walk sponsored by a depression awareness campaign. (Source: © Robin Weiner / WirePix / The Image Works.)

admissions. When she does not take her Risperdal (risperidone), she has a relapse of psychosis within 2 months. At this time she is experiencing psychosis again and suffered a compound fracture of the humerus and multiple ecchymoses when she ran into traffic. She has been hospitalized on the medical surgical unit since yesterday.

Assessment

The patient's pain is managed by her ordered medications. The circulation, movement, and sensation (CMS) in her fingers distal to the full arm cast are within normal limits. The capillary refill is 2 to 3 seconds. She states, "I was running away from the demons!" She appears to be afraid. She is seen talking when no other people are present, sometimes yelling at unseen others. She has been compliant with taking medications since admission. She told the nurse that when her prescription ran out at home, she felt like she didn't need the medicine any more.

Nursing Diagnosis

The following nursing diagnoses are identified for Ms. Daeva:

- *Risk for Injury Related to Psychosis* secondary to schizophrenia
- *Disturbed Sensory Perception* (auditory) related to hallucinations secondary to schizophrenia
- *Ineffective Coping* related to inadequate coping skills

Expected Outcomes

The patient will:

- Maintain reality orientation (will be oriented to person, place, time, and situation).
- Have brief reality-based conversations with staff every shift.

- State that she has a decrease in frequency and severity of "voices."
- Cooperate by taking all ordered medications during hospitalization.
- Engage in a trusting relationship with the nurse (will keep promises and interact honestly).
- Verbalize her willingness to participate in supervised medication management as an outpatient (after she has been oriented to the program).

Planning and Implementation

The nurse caring for Ms. Daeva will:

- Establish a trusting relationship with the patient.
- Reassure her that she is safe in the hospital, while not arguing with the delusional thinking.
- Reinforce reality.
- Monitor the patient's mental status for improvement in psychotic symptoms (auditory hallucinations and delusional thinking).
- Reinforce the importance of taking antipsychotic medications consistently.
- Ask the hospital social worker to be involved in discharge planning.

Evaluation

After 2 days on the medical surgical unit, Ms. Daeva was still experiencing auditory hallucinations, but they were much less frequent. She complied with all her ordered medications. She was transferred to the inpatient psychiatric unit for 1 week, during which her thinking continued to be intermittently reality based and delusional. The social worker made arrangements for her to be discharged to a supervised apartment living situation, where a staff member would administer her medications.

Critical Thinking in the Nursing Process

1. Why was the social worker asked to participate in this patient's discharge planning?
2. What factors led to this patient's frequent hospitalizations?
3. Why is the nurse planning to have brief conversations with this patient while she is experiencing psychosis?

Note: Discussion of Critical Thinking questions appears on the companion website.

Note: The references and resources for all chapters have been compiled at the back of the book.

Chapter Review

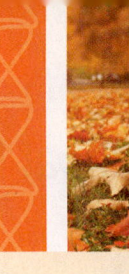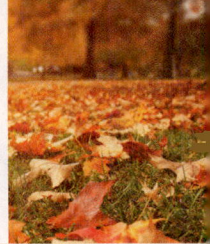

KEY POINTS

- **Concept:** Schizophrenia is a disorder of the brain that affects thinking, mood, and behavior.
- Schizophrenia affects approximately 1% of all people in the United States.
- **Concept:** Schizophrenia is a complex disorder caused by genetic abnormalities, functional and structural abnormalities of the brain, and environmental exposures.
- Schizophrenia affects a person's thinking, mood, and behavior.
- **Concept:** The disorder is characterized by positive, disorganized, and negative symptoms.
- People with schizophrenia have disordered thinking, decreased motivation, difficulty relating to other people and to themselves, and an increased risk of suicide.
- It usually starts in young adulthood and has periods of acute psychosis alternating with periods of reduced or absent symptoms.
- Most people with schizophrenia require a range of services throughout their lives.

- Families are important members of the treatment team.
- Antipsychotic medications work by stabilizing the function of neurotransmitters such as dopamine and glutamate in the brain.
- Antipsychotic medications improve the symptoms of the majority of people with schizophrenia.
- **Concept:** Because schizophrenia has different causes in different people, a patient may need to try several different antipsychotics before finding the one that works well.
- **Concept:** Antipsychotic medications have side effects. Some (NMS and TD) are life threatening or long-lasting; others (EPS) cause patients discomfort and may discourage compliance with medication therapy.
- There is hope for people with schizophrenia. Most people respond well to treatment. Research is promising new medications.

PEARSON NURSING RESOURCES

Find additional review materials at **nursing.pearsonhighered.com**.

Clinical Reasoning Care Map

Caring for a Patient With Schizophrenia
NCLEX-PN® Focus Area: Physiologic Adaptation

Case Study: Craig Koda, age 21, was diagnosed with schizophrenia 6 months ago. He has tried two different antipsychotic medications during this time without full remission of his symptoms. He was admitted to the psychiatric unit through the emergency department today with an exacerbation of psychosis with agitation. His mother states that he resists taking his meds at home, saying that he is "not crazy." He was given an injection of haloperidol 2 mg IM in the emergency department 2 hours ago. Currently he is thrashing in his bed yelling that he is "jumping out of his skin."

Nursing Diagnosis: Risk for Injury Related to Drug Side Effects

COLLECT DATA

Subjective	Objective
_____	_____
_____	_____
_____	_____
_____	_____
_____	_____
_____	_____

Does this present a threat to the patient's safety?

If yes, the priority intervention to address this threat would be:
_____
_____

Nursing Care
_____
_____
_____
_____
_____
_____
_____
_____
_____

Interprofessional team members to include when planning care:
_____
_____

How would you document this? _____
_____

Compare your answers and documentation to those provided on the companion website.

Data Collected
(use only those that apply)

- BP 148/70, P 110, R 24.
- Weight 188 lb.
- Patient states, "I can't hold still!"
- Muscles of legs and arms are stiff.
- Patient's father states, "He is always difficult to get along with."
- Patient is allergic to pollen.
- Refused dinner this evening.
- Patient appears to be in distress.
- Complains of jaw stiffness and discomfort.
- When patient protrudes his tongue, it quivers.

Nursing Interventions
(use only those that apply; list in priority order)

- Tell the patient that he is having a medication side effect called EPS that can be treated.
- Call the physician and ask for an order for a sedative.
- Call the physician immediately to report EPS.
- Encourage the patient to eat some soft foods for dinner.
- Assess VS q1h.
- Expect to give an anticholinergic medication.
- Tell the patient that he is allergic to haloperidol.
- Tell the patient that nothing is wrong and he will be fine.
- Provide a low-stimulation environment.
- Teach the patient about all his medications now.
- Call for the resuscitation team.

NCLEX-PN® Exam Preparation

TEST-TAKING TIP When you prepare for any test, you use your resources. Some people prepare for the NCLEX by using a review book that contains practice questions; some study in groups and discuss difficult concepts; others attend review courses. Do your best to prepare according to your own style. At test time, remember that you have done everything you can to get ready. Your life does not depend on any test score—really.

1. The medical record indicates that a patient is experiencing the negative symptoms of schizophrenia. What would the nurse expect to see?
   1. Hallucinations and delusional thinking
   2. Bizarre behavior
   3. Flat affect and little speech
   4. Difficulty with mental concentration

2. A patient appears to be afraid. He is yelling about aliens and swinging his arms like he is trying to stop something from hitting him in the head. He also yells, "Stop them, stop them!" What is the best way to document this situation? "The patient is:
   1. acting inappropriately and yelling."
   2. a danger to others."
   3. experiencing a frightening hallucination, apparently about aliens attacking him."
   4. yelling, screaming, hitting, and disrupting all the other patients on the unit."

3. When a patient is experiencing a frightening hallucination about aliens, what is the best first response by the nurse?
   1. Reassure the patient that he or she is safe in the hospital and there are no aliens.
   2. Give the patient more medication.
   3. Tell the patient that the aliens are friendly and not to worry.
   4. Move the patient to a private room where he or she will not disturb others.

4. What would the nurse expect to find on a psychiatric unit that uses milieu therapy?
   1. Structured daily activities
   2. A television on a news channel all day for orientation
   3. Plenty of stimulation: loud music and lots of people
   4. Strict rules to control patient behavior

5. Which of the following patients is at greatest risk for violent behavior? A patient who:
   1. is experiencing catatonic symptoms.
   2. has been following the nurse around all day.
   3. refuses to eat or participate in her care.
   4. is pacing the halls, clenching fists, and talking angrily to unseen voices.

6. A patient states that she is the Queen of England and has magical powers. What is this type of thinking called?
   1. Hallucinatory
   2. Manipulative
   3. Delusional
   4. Schizophrenic

7. What is the nurse's best response when a patient newly diagnosed with schizophrenia asks, "What is wrong with me?"
   1. "You are experiencing excessive neurotransmitter amines in your brain synapses."
   2. "You have schizophrenia, which is a brain disorder that affects your thinking."
   3. "You should ask your doctor."
   4. "Nobody really understands schizophrenia."

8. Which of the following symptoms could indicate neuroleptic malignant syndrome in a patient taking an antipsychotic medication?
   1. Dry mouth, orthostatic hypotension
   2. High fever, muscle pain, unstable BP
   3. Urinary retention, dizziness, dry skin
   4. Photosensitivity, abnormal body movements, increased heart rate

9. A patient with schizophrenia probably has excess activity of which brain neurotransmitter?
   1. Epinephrine
   2. Phenylalanine
   3. Dopamine
   4. Meperidine

10. A patient with schizophrenia is experiencing all of the following symptoms. Choose all that are anticholinergic side effects of the psychotropic medications.
    1. Orthostatic hypotension
    2. Dry mouth
    3. Abnormal body movements
    4. Increased heart rate

Answers and rationales for Review Questions appear in Appendix I.

CHAPTER 50

Caring for Patients With Mood Disorders

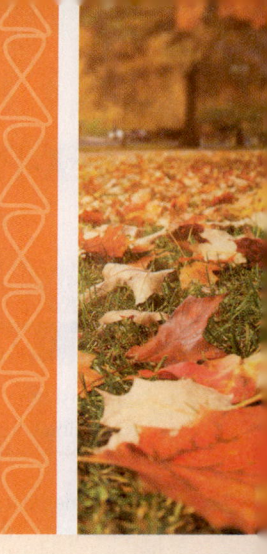

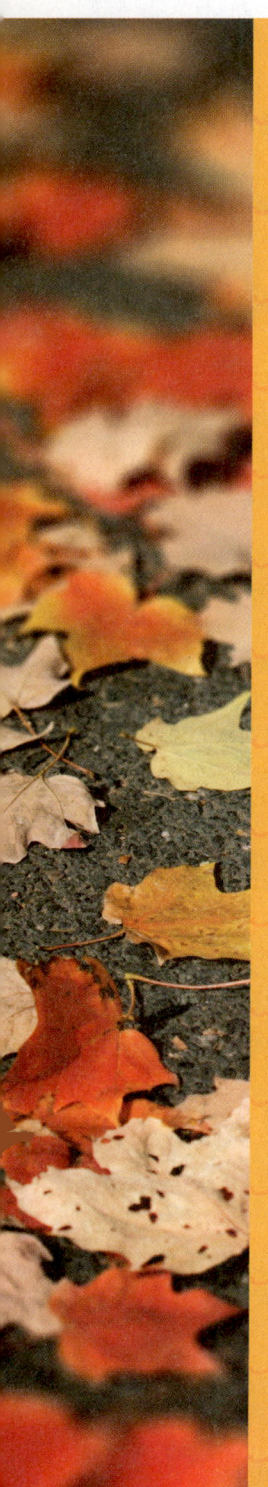

BRIEF OUTLINE

Major Depressive Disorder   **Bipolar Disorder**

APPLIED LEARNING OUTCOMES

After completing this chapter, you will be able to:

1. Explain the pathophysiology of mood disorders in relation to brain neurotransmitters.
2. Prevent safety risks for people with mood disorders.
3. Prioritize nursing care activities for patients with mood disorders.
4. Assess patients for suicidal thinking.
5. Safely and effectively administer antidepressant and mood-stabilizing medications.
6. Discuss the lived experience of people with mood disorders.
7. Apply the nursing process to patients with mood disorders.

KEY TERMS

The key terms are defined on the pages listed below.

affect, 1241
distractibility, 1251
electroconvulsive therapy (ECT), 1249
hypomania, 1250

kindling process, 1254
monoamine oxidase inhibitors (MAOIs), 1248
mood, 1241
pressured speech, 1251

psychomotor agitation, 1243
psychomotor retardation, 1243
suicidal ideation, 1254

SPECIAL FEATURES

NURSING CARE PLAN: Patient With Depression, 1259
CLINICAL REASONING CARE MAP: Caring for a Patient With Bipolar Disorder, 1262

Everyone has had good and bad moods. We can all relate to a range of emotions that people normally experience in the course of their lives. When mood goes beyond the normal range of intensity and when elation and despair are persistent, are not a direct response to life experiences, and interfere with daily functioning and human development, a disorder of mood exists.

Mood is a pervasive and sustained emotion that influences how a person perceives the world. Mood is a relatively constant feeling. There can be *elevated mood*, an exaggerated sense of energy or well-being; *euthymic mood*, which is in the normal range; *dysphoric mood*, which is sad or unpleasant; or *irritable mood*, a mood in which one is easily annoyed, upset, or provoked to anger (American Psychiatric Association [APA], 2013). **Affect** (a'fekt) refers to a person's current expression of emotions. It is more changeable than mood. Affect is evident in nonverbal behaviors, as well as the words a person chooses to use. Even a person with a generally depressed mood can show a temporarily happy affect.

There are several disorders of mood. In this chapter we will use major depressive disorder and bipolar disorder as our prototypes for the nursing management of mood disorders.

Major Depressive Disorder

Because the symptoms of depression are similar to sadness, people often mistake depression (a mental disorder) with sadness (a normal response to a life experience). *Depression* takes sadness and lack of energy and motivation to another level that is not in the usual experience of unaffected people.

The American Psychiatric Association (2013) sets the criteria for the diagnosis of depression and other mental disorders in the *Diagnostic and Statistical Manual of Mental Disorders*, 5th edition, or *DSM-5*. The signs and symptoms of *major depressive disorder* (MDD) occur during a major depressive episode, which for most people with the disorder will recur sporadically over a lifetime. The episode is a change in the person's usual functioning and includes a depressed mood or loss of pleasure in life and a majority of the following symptoms: too much or too little sleep; increased or decreased activity (psychomotor agitation or psychomotor retardation); feeling tired most of the time; feeling useless or guilty; a significant change in weight (gain or loss); having difficulty with mental concentration; or frequent thoughts of death or suicide or an attempt at suicide (APA, 2013).

Depression is not diagnosed if the symptoms are associated with general medical conditions (e.g., hypothyroidism), side effects of substances, or bereavement. Depressive episodes can range from mild to severe, with a range of functional impairment as well.

PATHOPHYSIOLOGY

> **Key Concept**   Depression is caused by genetic abnormalities that interact with the individual's life experiences and environment.

Depression is a multifactorial disorder (i.e., it has a variety of causes). Major depressive disorder has a genetic component, a brain physiology component, and a psychosocial component. Each contributes, but none explains the disorder alone. Because multiple factors cause and affect the disorder, effective treatments often include several treatment interventions for each person. Psychosocial (teaching and counseling) and behavior change as well as physiologic (usually medication) approaches are often used.

Major depressive disorder is 1.5 to 3 times more common among first-degree biologic relatives of affected people than among the general population (APA, 2013). Researchers have found that people who have a variant of the gene that codes for a transporter of serotonin are more likely to develop depression after experiencing a stressful event (Caspi et al., 2003). People inherit the tendency to respond to life stressors with the development of depression. There is no single gene, however, that codes for the patient to have depression (Lohoff, 2010). Complex interactions between a person's genetics and environmental influences impact the development and severity of symptoms of depression (Uder & Mosack, 2011).

Advances in brain imaging have been used to assess brain structure and function of people with depression. Positron emission tomography (PET) shows abnormal function in the prefrontal cortex of the cerebrum and in the limbic system during depressive episodes. Figure 50-1■ shows the PET scan of a brain before and after treatment.

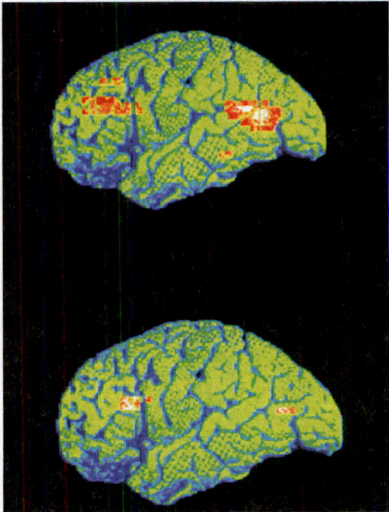

Figure 50-1. ■ Positron emission tomography (PET) scan of a brain before and after treatment for depression. (Source: WDCN/University College London/Science Source.)

There is also evidence that an abnormality in brain neurotransmitter physiology causes depression. Brain neurotransmitters such as serotonin, norepinephrine, dopamine, acetylcholine, and gamma-aminobutyric acid (GABA) are likely involved. In schizophrenia, brain neurotransmitters are overactive. In depression, the opposite is true: The neurotransmitters have reduced function. The fact that antidepressant medications (which increase neurotransmitter availability and function) are often effective is evidence that decreased neurotransmitter function contributes to the cause of depression.

The endocrine system is also involved. The hypothalamus, pituitary, and adrenal glands, together called the *HPA axis*, control the physiologic responses to stress. These glands may be hyperactive in people with depression. The HPA axis also affects the 24-hour day–night cycle of body rhythms (*circadian rhythms*), which include sleep and wakefulness, hormone secretion, mental alertness, and body temperature. In both depression and mania, the normal circadian rhythms are disrupted.

Children show no gender difference in risk, but after puberty, females are 1.5 to 3 times more likely than males to be affected by major depressive disorder. A significant proportion of affected women report a worsening of depressive symptoms in the few days before menstruation. In any given year approximately 7% of people in the United States will have a major depressive episode. Most of these are not diagnosed or treated. The disorder affects people of all ethnicities equally (APA, 2013).

It is common for people with depression to have other disorders simultaneously. The disorders that frequently occur with depression include schizophrenia; substance abuse; eating disorders; anxiety disorders; and general medical conditions such as diabetes, stroke, and heart disease.

Depressive symptoms may be caused by certain medications. Some antibiotics and antifungal, anti-inflammatory, antineoplastic, cardiovascular, and gastrointestinal drugs have been shown to cause depressive symptoms in some people.

Course of the Disease

The disorder may begin at any age. The average age of onset is in the mid-20s, but onset in late life is not uncommon. A major life stressor precedes the first major depressive episode for many people (APA, 2013). However, it is not the stressor alone that causes depression. The person who becomes depressed is probably genetically susceptible to depression after a stressful event. Box 50-1 ■ lists risk factors for the development of depression.

Some people experience only a single episode of depression. Most people continue to have episodes throughout their lives, with a course of exacerbations and remissions

| **BOX 50-1** | **RISK FACTORS FOR DEPRESSION** |

- Previous depressive episode
- Female gender
- Family history of depression
- Stressful life events
- Substance abuse or dependency
- Postpartum period
- History of suicide attempt
- Chronic general medical condition

similar to other chronic disorders. Yet others experience almost a steady state of depressed mood. An untreated episode of depression can last for years.

Some patients experience psychotic symptoms associated with severe depression, such as hallucinations or delusional thinking. This psychotic depression is more disabling and often requires more intensive treatment than a depressive episode without psychotic features.

Peripartum Depression

The *DSM-5* refers to depression that is diagnosed around the time of delivery as *peripartum depression*, as a replacement for the term *postpartum depression*. *Peripartum* is the more accurate term because mood episodes often occur during pregnancy and are usually diagnosed after childbirth. Approximately 3% to 6% of childbearing women experience a major depressive episode during pregnancy or within the 4 weeks following delivery. Women with peripartum major depressive episodes often experience severe anxiety or even panic attacks. These peripartum mood episodes can occur either with or without psychosis and may last for 2 to 3 months. The woman may have a depressed mood, guilt feelings, loss of appetite, and unreasonable fears about the baby or her ability to care for the baby. The episodes with psychotic features are more severe and dangerous. These psychotic episodes may be associated with a loss of interest in the baby or rejection of the baby, agitation, indecision, guilt, an abnormal attitude about body functions, or a morbid fear that the baby will be harmed. A few women have killed their babies or themselves while having hallucinations of voices telling them to do so or delusional thinking that convinces them that the infant would only "be safe with God" or "is possessed by evil." Psychosis can have many other themes, however. Women with previous diagnoses of major depressive disorder or bipolar disorder are more likely to experience peripartum depression or psychosis (APA, 2013). The nurse should advise childbearing women to consult their health providers if they suspect that they are depressed.

The postpartum period is unique in a woman's life in terms of the neurohormonal and psychosocial changes and stressors. Women may experience the "postpartum blues," which is a common and normal situation. It occurs as the result of the abrupt physical and sociologic changes with childbirth and may cause anxiety about baby care and family relationships, tearfulness, and difficulty concentrating. The "postpartum blues" usually begins 3 to 4 days after delivery and resolves within 2 weeks without treatment except for reassurance from the health care team that it is normal and support from significant others. Promoting opportunities for early mother–infant bonding and teaching about the importance of social support for a mother with a newborn are nursing actions that may prevent or facilitate the resolution of an episode of "postpartum blues."

Seasonal Affective Disorder

Seasonal affective disorder (SAD) is depression that is associated with shortened exposure to daylight. It happens in the fall and winter when the days become shorter and resolves in the spring and summer. The symptoms are sleepiness, difficulty awakening in the morning, fatigue, lethargy, irritability, and increased appetite. It is thought to be a result of abnormal melatonin metabolism. The treatment is light therapy (*phototherapy*) (shown in Figure 50-2 ■), which results in a decrease in melatonin in the blood. In light therapy, the patient is exposed to bright light from 2,500 to 10,000 lux each morning for a prescribed amount of time (from 30 minutes to 3 hours). The patient is instructed to orient the head and body toward the light box and then to engage in activities that are illuminated by the light, such as reading, writing, or eating, while not looking directly at the light box itself. Light therapy has been found to be moderately effective for patients with mild to moderate depression, especially that associated with seasonal occurrence (Mayo Clinic, 2013).

MANIFESTATIONS

Major depressive disorder is a disabling disease that affects mood and occupational and personal functioning. An affected person will have a depressed or low mood every day. Other symptoms include *anhedonia* (inability to feel pleasure), weight changes, difficulty sleeping, **psychomotor retardation** (generalized slowing of physical and mental activity associated with mental processes), feelings of worthlessness and guilt, constant fatigue or lack of energy, and recurrent thoughts of death or suicide. Children and adolescents may present with **psychomotor agitation** (increased physical activity associated with mental processes) and irritability. A list of symptoms can never fully describe the human consequences of a disease. See Box 50-2 ■ for statements by people with depression describing their feelings.

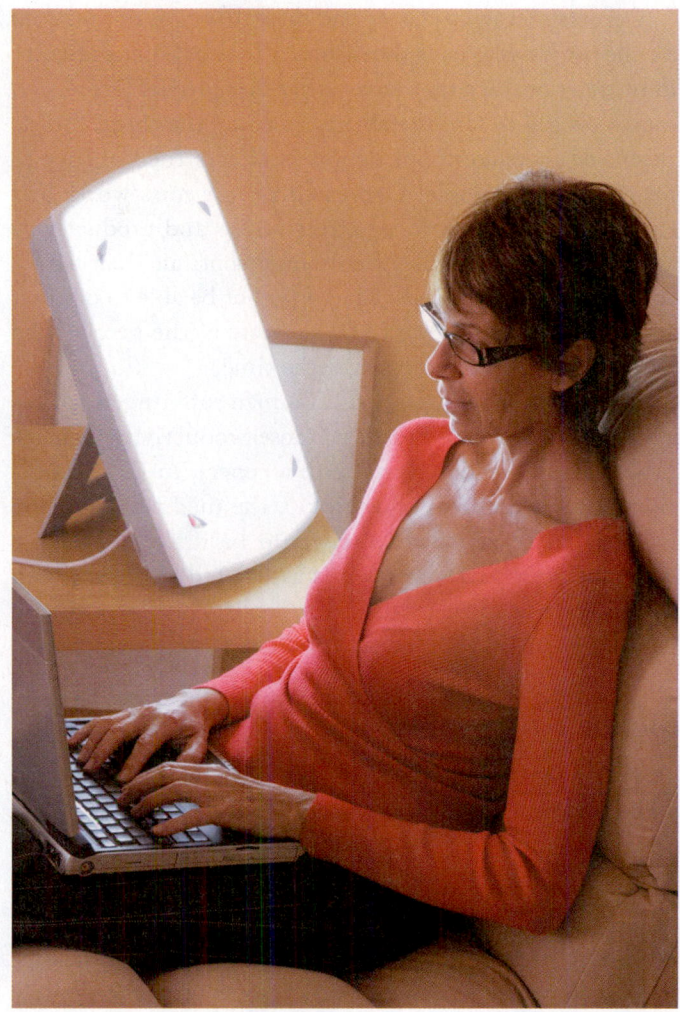

Figure 50-2. ■ Phototherapy is an effective treatment for many people with seasonal affective disorder (SAD). (Source: Bruno Boissonnet/Science Source.)

BOX 50-2	PATIENTS SPEAK THEIR MINDS ON DEPRESSION

"I feel like I'm in a deep dark hole and can't even try to get out."

"Everything worth living for goes out of focus."

"I've been too tired to chew."

"People can be overstimulating, especially when they are cheerful."

"Nothing matters, everything hurts, and you are always alone no matter who is around you."

"People want me to do things that I should really want to do. I just can't get the motivation for it, and it makes me feel guilty."

"My soul left and was replaced with lead."

"When I didn't answer your questions, it was because I didn't have the energy to talk."

"In 1980 I heard a bird call in my front yard. I didn't go outside until later, and saw a cat eating a bird. I could have saved that poor bird. When I am depressed, I think about it and feel so guilty."

Depression causes misery and disability (loss of function) for the people who have the disorder. It also causes difficulty in the relationships they have with other people. Depression causes people to lose the ability to enjoy the things in life that used to make them happy. It affects their ability to relate to other people. Depressed people miss work, lose their jobs, or have reduced effectiveness and productivity at work. Affected people often cannot continue their family and work responsibilities. They may not be able to do their activities of daily living (ADLs). Most of the people who kill themselves are depressed at the time.

Depression has a high cost in human suffering as well as a financial cost to businesses that lose productivity. When a person has depression along with a general medical condition (such as diabetes or a stroke), the medical condition is likely to be worse than it would be if the depression were not present. Depression is associated with increased disability and even increased mortality in hospitalized patients with serious medical conditions.

Stigma

> **Key Concept** Our culture "marks" or stigmatizes people with mental illness as less worthy, intelligent, acceptable, or important than the rest of the population.

Because of the stigma associated with mental illness, people are reluctant to seek help when they have the symptoms of depression. People with depression are less likely to accept treatment, to comply with treatment recommendations, and to continue treatment than are people with general medical conditions without depression. People who belong to ethnic minorities often experience both racism and stigma, which is one reason that Latino immigrants in the United States, statistically at least, are reported to be mentally healthier than their native-born counterparts. Immigrant Latinos may feel too ashamed or afraid to disclose their mental illnesses (NAMI, Multicultural Action Center, n.d.).

The Americans with Disabilities Act has helped some people with mental illnesses receive accommodations that will allow them to continue working with their mental disorders. Unfortunately, many people are afraid to even admit that they are mentally ill. Until mental illness is seen on an equal plane with general medical disorders attitudinally, economically, socially, and politically, it will be under-reported, underdiagnosed, and undertreated.

Because the stigma against mental illness still exists, public education becomes even more important. Nurses and others must educate patients, their families, and communities about the disorder, its outcomes, and treatments.

Knowledge can help people understand treatment, be free from unnecessary guilt, and maintain hope.

Suicide

> **Key Concept** Suicide is a risk for patients with depression. There are factors that increase and decrease the suicide risk for individuals.

In 1996, the World Health Organization urged member nations to create suicide prevention strategies. The U.S. Surgeon General published a call to action in 1999, which included the risks for suicide (Box 50-3■) and the protective factors for suicide (Box 50-4■).

More Americans die each year from suicide than from homicide. An average of 85 Americans die from suicide each day. Suicide rates are highest among older adults. There is no recent change in the rates for this population. Most older suicide victims had been seen by their primary

BOX 50-3	RISK FACTORS FOR SUICIDE

- Depression and other mental disorders or a substance abuse disorder (often in combination with another mental disorder). More than 90% of people who die by suicide have these risk factors.
- Easy access to lethal suicide methods, especially guns. Guns are used in over half of all suicides.
- Previous suicide attempt
- Family history of suicide
- Family violence, including physical or sexual abuse
- Isolation, a feeling of being cut off from other people
- Hopelessness
- History of impulsive and/or aggressive behavior
- Barriers to accessing mental health treatment
- Relationship, social, work, or financial losses
- General medical illness
- Military service; incidence is high among veterans
- Incarceration
- Unwillingness to seek help because of the stigma attached to mental and substance abuse disorders or suicidal thoughts
- Influence of significant people—family members, celebrities, peers who have died by suicide—both through direct personal contact or inappropriate media representations
- Cultural or religious beliefs—for example, the belief that suicide is a noble resolution of a personal dilemma
- Local epidemics of suicide that have a contagious influence
- The feeling of being a burden to others

Source: Data from National Institute of Mental Health. (2010). *Suicide in the U.S.: Statistics and prevention.* Accessed September 30, 2013, from the NIMH website.

| BOX 50-4 | PROTECTIVE FACTORS FOR SUICIDE |

- Effective and appropriate clinical care for mental, physical, and substance abuse disorders
- Easy access to a variety of clinical interventions and support
- Restricted access to guns and other highly lethal methods of suicide
- Family and community support
- Support from ongoing medical and mental health care relationships
- Learned skills in problem solving, conflict resolution, and nonviolent handling of disputes
- Cultural and religious beliefs that discourage suicide and support self-preservation instincts

Source: U.S. Public Health Service. (1999). *The surgeon general's call to action to prevent suicide.* Washington, DC: Author.

| BOX 50-5 | TALKING ABOUT SUICIDE |

A dangerous myth about suicide is that discussing it with someone who is not contemplating suicide may suggest the idea. In fact, most people with depression, whether they are contemplating suicide or not, benefit from talking about their feelings, especially the frightening ones. For people who are contemplating suicide, discussion of their feelings may be the only opportunity for prevention. Depression makes it hard for people to identify and explain their own feelings. Talking about and clarifying these feelings can help a depressed person gain perspective, interrupt negative thinking, or work on problem solving. Active listening is a powerful tool for nurses to use. Patients often express gratitude for the opportunity to express their feelings about suicide.

care provider within a few weeks of their suicide and had been experiencing a first episode of mild to moderate depression. This demonstrates a lost opportunity for identifying suicide risk and preventing suicide (American Foundation for Suicide Prevention, 2013). Patients often benefit from the opportunity to discuss feelings about suicide (Box 50-5■).

The suicide rate in the United States has remained relatively stable since the 1980s. However, the rates for certain groups have increased significantly. The suicide rate among adolescents and young adults has nearly tripled. Among all persons ages 15 to 19, suicides increased 14% from 1980 to 1996. Among African American males in the same age group, the rate increased 105%. Firearms-related suicides account for almost 100% of the increase in adolescent suicide. In the general population, firearms constitute the most common means of suicide in the United States (60% of all suicides). The other two most common means are poisoning (including the overdose of drugs) and suffocation. The National Institute of Mental Health identifies having

a firearm in the home as one of the major risk factors for suicide, since more than half of all suicides are done with firearms (NIMH, 2006). Military personnel are another group at increased risk (twice the risk of the general population), as well as people who are incarcerated, and those who have been exposed to the suicide of others, including their family, peers, or even media personalities (NIMH, 2006). Still, the highest rate of suicide in any group is in older non-Hispanic White males. The suicide rate among older White men with depression is six times higher than the general population (Spires, 2006). The motivations for older men to kill themselves may include feeling alone, the sense of being a burden on other people, and humiliation at loss of independence with ADLs.

One of the most important things to remember about suicide is that most suicide attempts are expressions of extreme distress, not harmless attempts to get attention. A person who appears suicidal needs immediate mental health treatment (NIMH, 2006).

COLLABORATIVE CARE

Effective treatment for depression is available. Once it is accurately identified, depression can usually be treated successfully with medications, psychotherapy, or a combination of somatic and psychosocial therapies. Patients are individuals and respond to treatment differently, but when a patient does not respond to one therapy, there are others to try. The goals of collaborative treatment for depression are for the patient:

- To decrease the depressive symptoms (depressed mood, decreased interest in daily activities, inability to experience pleasure, worthlessness, sleep disturbances, lack of motivation, inability to concentrate, self-harm or suicide).
- To discuss losses with staff and family members.
- To interact willingly with others and to feel positive about these interactions.
- To set realistic personal goals.
- To maintain orientation and mental concentration and to use sound judgments in making decisions.
- To identify areas of self-control over life situations.
- To improve his or her functional level, including self-care abilities and problem-solving skills.
- To prevent recurrence.

There are four commonly used medical treatments for depression:

1. Medication
2. Psychotherapy
3. Electroconvulsive therapy
4. Light therapy (discussed earlier under Seasonal Affective Disorder)

Patients experience the best treatment outcomes when their depression is treated with a combination of medications, cognitive-behavioral or other therapy, patient and family education, and a treatment plan that includes significant others in the patient's life. Electroconvulsive therapy can also be an effective treatment for depression that does not respond to medications.

Medications

Medications have been shown to be effective for all types of depression. However, there is no single medication that works for everyone. There is also no single medication that is better or more effective than the others.

ANTIDEPRESSANT AGENTS   Although antidepressant medications have proven to be effective, they do have limitations. People with depressive symptoms often wait until their symptoms are almost intolerable before they seek help. Antidepressants require 2 to 6 weeks to achieve full effect; often several drugs are tried in an attempt to find effective treatment. Some people experience no improvement with antidepressant medications; others experience intolerable side effects. In other cases, side effects may be useful. For example, a patient with depression who has trouble sleeping may be given an antidepressant with sedating side effects at bedtime.

Depression appears to involve reduced neurotransmitter function in brain synapses and changes in receptors on brain neurons. See Chapter 47 for more information about brain neurotransmitter physiology. Figure 50-3■ diagrams brain neurotransmitters and illustrates the action of antidepressant drugs.

Antidepressants are given orally. Most act on two major brain neurotransmitters, serotonin (5HT) and norepinephrine (NE), which regulate mood. New antidepressants act on dopamine also.

The antidepressants may be organized into four groups:

1. Tricyclic antidepressants (TCAs) and related cyclic agents
2. Selective serotonin reuptake inhibitors (SSRIs)
3. Other, *novel* antidepressants
4. Monoamine oxidase inhibitors

See Table 50-1■ for the nursing implications of antidepressant drugs.

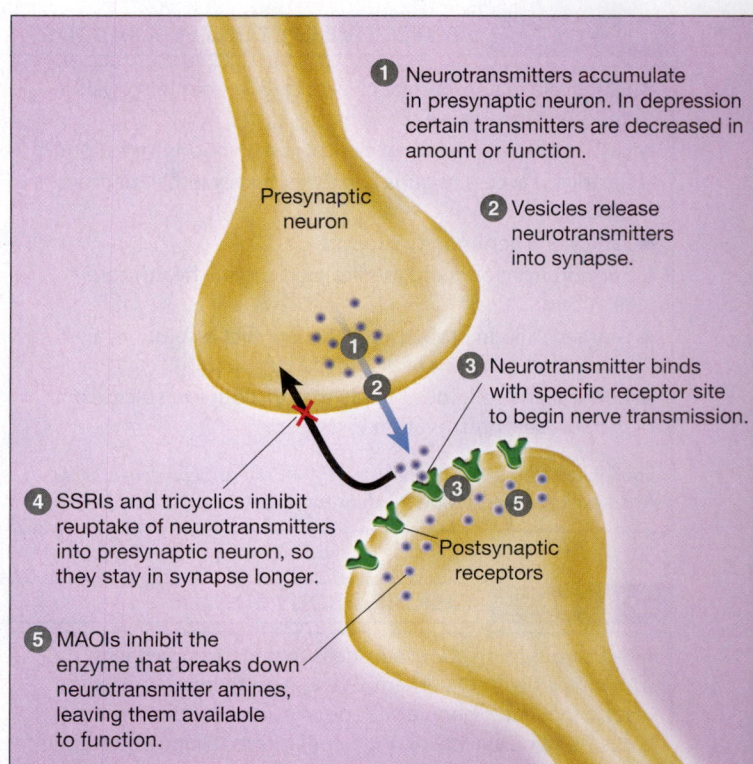

1. Neurotransmitters accumulate in presynaptic neuron. In depression certain transmitters are decreased in amount or function.

Presynaptic neuron

2. Vesicles release neurotransmitters into synapse.

3. Neurotransmitter binds with specific receptor site to begin nerve transmission.

4. SSRIs and tricyclics inhibit reuptake of neurotransmitters into presynaptic neuron, so they stay in synapse longer.

Postsynaptic receptors

5. MAOIs inhibit the enzyme that breaks down neurotransmitter amines, leaving them available to function.

Figure 50-3. ■ Antidepressant agents increase the availability or function of neurotransmitters. (Source: "Figure 10.01—TCAs Inhibit the Reuptake of both Norepinephrine and Serotonin" from *Core Concepts in Pharmacology*, 4e by Leland Norman Holland and Michael Patrick Adams. Published by Pearson Education, © 2014.)

The TCAs were the first choice of treatment for depression from the 1950s until the 1990s. Though useful, they had numerous side effects, including sedation, dry mouth, orthostatic hypotension, increased heart rate, constipation, urinary hesitancy or retention, pupil dilation (mydriasis), blurred near vision, dry eyes, and photophobia.

Since the 1990s, another class of antidepressant, SSRIs, is usually prescribed if a patient has significant suicidal thinking, a history of suicide attempts, or impulse control problems. The SSRIs are usually the first-choice drugs for the treatment of depression because they have fewer side effects than the other types of antidepressants, and they are usually just as effective.

Older adults may experience more severe anticholinergic effects, such as agitation, mental confusion, and paralytic ileus, and are at greater risk for developing orthostatic hypotension when taking TCAs. Older adults respond to lower doses than younger adults, due to slower and less

TABLE 50-1	Giving Medications Safely: Antidepressants		
CLASS/DRUGS	**PURPOSE**	**NURSING IMPLICATIONS**	**PATIENT TEACHING**
Tricyclic and related agents ■ *Amitriptyline* (Elavil) ■ Amoxapine (Asendin) ■ Clomipramine (Anafranil) ■ Desipramine (Norpramin) ■ Doxepin (Sinequan) ■ Imipramine (Tofranil) ■ Maprotiline (Ludiomil) ■ Nortriptyline (Pamelor) ■ Protriptyline (Vivactil) ■ Trimipramine (Surmontil)	Block reuptake of serotonin and norepinephrine. Used to treat depression and as an adjunctive treatment for chronic pain.	Assess for side effects: sedation, orthostatic hypotension, weight gain, anticholinergic effects, tachycardia or cardiac dysrhythmias. Assess vital signs and mental status. Notify the physician if the patient has glaucoma. Assess for suicidal thinking; TCAs can be fatal in overdose. Older adults require lower doses. Use with caution in the older adult, who are more likely to have side effects.	Efficacy takes 2–4 weeks. Take at bedtime to promote sleep and reduce daytime sedation. Make position changes slowly; sit before standing. Do not drink alcohol (causes potentially fatal CNS depression).
Selective serotonin reuptake inhibitors ■ Citalopram (Celexa) ■ Escitalopram (Lexapro) ■ Fluoxetine (Prozac) ■ Fluvoxamine (Luvox) ■ Paroxetine (Paxil) ■ Sertraline (Zoloft)	Inhibit reuptake of serotonin. Used to treat depression; panic disorder (paroxetine); obsessive-compulsive disorder (fluvoxamine, fluoxetine); premenstrual dysphoric disorder; bulimia nervosa (fluoxetine); anxiety (paroxetine); PTSD (sertraline).	Assess for side effects: nausea, loose stools, sexual side effects (decreased libido), headache, anxiety or sedation, insomnia, slight anticholinergic symptoms, orthostatic hypotension. Assess vital signs and mental status. Low potential for harm in overdose. Decrease dose in older adults.	Efficacy takes 2–3 weeks; may take 5 weeks to reach peak effect. Avoid alcohol. Notify the physician if taking herbal medicines (especially St. John's wort or tryptophan).
Novel antidepressants ■ Bupropion (Wellbutrin) ■ Duloxetine (Cymbalta) ■ Mirtazapine (Remeron) ■ Nefazodone (Serzone) ■ Reboxetine (Edronax, Vestra) ■ Trazodone (Desyrel) ■ Venlafaxine (Effexor)	Inhibit reuptake of norepinephrine, dopamine, and/or serotonin. Used to treat depression, insomnia (trazodone), and anxiety disorder (reboxetine) and aid to stop smoking (bupropion).	Assess for S/Es: anxiety, nausea, agitation or sedation, insomnia, weight loss, increased BP (venlafaxine), seizures (bupropion), liver failure (nefazodone), priapism (trazodone). Notify the physician of seizure history. Assess vital signs and mental status.	Same as SSRIs.
Monoamine oxidase inhibitors ■ Isocarboxazid (Marplan) ■ Phenelzine (Nardil) ■ Tranylcypromine (Parnate) ■ Selegiline (Emsam)	Block the enzyme monoamine oxidase that breaks down neurotransmitters. Used to treat depression that is not responsive to other agents.	Can cause hypertensive crisis when the patient eats foods high in tyramine or as a drug interaction occurs with other antidepressants, meperidine, general anesthetics, sympathomimetics, bronchodilators, and methylphenidate. Selegiline is the first MAOI available in a transdermal patch. At its lowest dose (6 mg), the patient does not require the diet restrictions of the other MAOIs. Assess vital signs and mental status. Can be fatal in overdose.	Takes 2–4 weeks for antidepressant effect. The patient must carefully comply with diet restrictions. Call the physician for throbbing headache, pounding heart, or stiff neck. Teach patients using selegiline to remove each patch before applying a new one and to put the new one on a different place to avoid skin irritation.
MAO-A inhibitor ■ Moclobemide (Manerix)	Reversible selective inhibitor of MAO-A. Used to treat depression.	Does not have the hypertensive side effect of MAOIs. Do not give with other MAOIs or narcotics.	No diet restrictions.

Note: Medications identified in *italics* are among the 200 most frequently prescribed drugs in the United States.

efficient metabolism with aging. See Box 50-6■ for more information about older patients taking antidepressants.

Serotonin Syndrome Side effects are not common when SSRIs are taken alone. When SSRIs are combined with antipsychotics, extrapyramidal side effects are increased. Serotonin syndrome, a potentially fatal result of excess serotonin activity, can result from combining SSRIs with each other, MAOIs, St. John's wort, or tryptophan (an amino acid that is a serotonin precursor). The manifestations of serotonin syndrome include changes in mental status, agitation or restlessness, muscle spasms, hyperreflexia, diaphoresis, shivering, tremor, diarrhea, abdominal cramps, nausea, lack of coordination, headache, fever, seizures, and coma (Mayo Clinic, 2013).

clinicalALERT

A 2-week "washout" period should occur between the use of SSRIs or TCAs and MAOIs. If the nurse suspects serotonin syndrome (mental status change, restlessness, muscle spasms, diaphoresis, nausea, diarrhea, lack of coordination, headache, fever, seizures), hold the antidepressant and notify the physician immediately.

As its name implies, the group of novel antidepressants is composed of several unique individual drugs that act in a variety of ways to increase the amount of neurotransmitter available at the synapse.

The **monoamine oxidase inhibitors (MAOIs)** block the enzyme monoamine oxidase that breaks down neurotransmitters in brain synapses, increasing available serotonin and norepinephrine (see Figure 50-3). They take approximately 2 to 4 weeks to have an antidepressant effect. MAOIs are effective antidepressant agents, but they are seldom prescribed because of their serious adverse effects. The MAOIs can cause:

- Hypertensive crisis when combined with foods containing the amino acid tyramine (Box 50-7■).
- Potentially fatal drug interactions with SSRIs, other MAOIs, TCAs, meperidine (Demerol), CNS depressants including general anesthetics, sympathomimetics (such as over-the-counter cold, allergy, and weight loss remedies), methylphenidate (Ritalin), bronchodilators, and some antihypertensives.
- Death in overdose.

clinicalALERT

MAOI drugs can cause hypertensive crisis when combined with other drugs and foods containing tyramine. Symptoms are a throbbing headache, sense of speeding or pounding heart, and stiff neck. If you suspect hypertensive crisis, hold the MAOI, take vital signs, and notify the physician.

BOX 50-6	FOCUS ON OLDER ADULTS

Antidepressants and the Older Adult

Older adults with depression tend to respond well to antidepressant drugs. There are some special considerations for this group, however:

- The older adult requires *lower doses* due to decreased metabolic efficiency.
- Elders are at increased risk for *orthostatic hypotension*, which increases their risks for falls and injury.
- If older adults are *dehydrated*, they are at increased risk for medication side effects.

BOX 50-7	FOODS TO AVOID WHEN TAKING MAOIS

The following foods are high in tyramine and should be avoided by people taking MAOIs:

- Aged cheeses (all cheese is considered aged except cottage, cream, ricotta, and processed cheese slices).
- Foods containing aged cheeses, such as pizza, blue cheese dressing.
- Preserved meats, such as pepperoni, sausage, salami, lunch meats, canned ham, pickled herring, dried fish.
- Liver, other organ meats.
- Broad fava beans, sauerkraut, and banana peel.
- Draft beer (even alcohol-free), red wine.
- Soy sauce, yeast, or protein extract (concentrated) products.
- Although caffeine does not contain tyramine, large amounts of caffeine can cause a sympathomimetic effect. Coffee, cola, and tea should be used in moderation.

Psychotherapy

Psychotherapy is usually used in addition to medication therapy for major depression. Patients tend to have better outcomes when they are treated with a combination of medications and psychotherapy. Some of the psychosocial problems associated with depression (ability to relate to others, motivation, suicidal thinking) can be resolved by medications. Psychotherapy may be used in addition to medications to help the patient learn to live with a chronic depressive disorder, to manage the specific symptoms, to change thinking that makes depression worse, to promote effective coping skills, or for psychosocial rehabilitation. Patients experiencing a mild to moderate depressive episode without psychotic symptoms may benefit from psychotherapy alone.

COGNITIVE THERAPY Cognitive therapy is the most effective psychotherapeutic approach for depression. For depression, the objective of cognitive therapy is to reduce symptoms by identifying and correcting the patient's distorted, negatively biased thinking (Beck & Rush, 1995). According to cognitive theory, depressed people have automatic negative thoughts even in the midst of positive life events. They have negative expectations of their environment, negative perceptions and expectations of self, and negative expectations for the future. Cognitive therapy approaches include identifying the patient's erroneous negative thinking, developing new thinking patterns, and trying new behavior.

BEHAVIORAL THERAPY   Behavioral therapy is often used along with cognitive therapy. The behavioral approach to therapy is based on learning theory. The therapist and patient work together to determine what behaviors to change. The patient practices new ways to behave that are positive, replacing the old dysfunctional behavior. The principle in behavioral therapy is that patients' thinking and feelings will follow positive reinforcement for their new behavior. When people learn to act in a positive, self-confident way, they will feel positive and self-confident. Reinforcement of the patient's successes will promote the persistence of positive effective behavior for coping.

INTERPERSONAL PSYCHOTHERAPY   The interpersonal psychotherapy approach involves identifying and resolving the patient's interpersonal difficulties. Interpersonal problems are viewed as causal or aggravating factors of depression. According to the interpersonal theorists, the difficulties that lead to depression may be social isolation, prolonged grief, or early development of dysfunctional social behavior. The treatment focus is interpersonal relationships and social functioning.

Exercise

Moderate physical exercise has been shown to relieve mild to moderate depressive symptoms. The effects of exercise on depression may be due to the release of endorphins, which cause a sense of well-being. Exercise has proven to be equally as effective as psychotherapy or pharmacotherapy for reducing the signs and symptoms of mild to moderate depression. The ideal amount or form of exercise has not been determined, but even modest exercise has beneficial effects (Cooney et al., 2013). The difficulty with exercise as a treatment for depression is that depressed people do not feel like exercising. Lack of energy and motivation are part of the disease. Regular exercise is also a very good preventive strategy for depression.

Electroconvulsive Therapy

Electroconvulsive therapy (ECT) is the application of electrical current to the brain, which induces a generalized seizure. The procedure is done while the patient is under general anesthesia with muscle relaxation. A series

of treatments are usually prescribed. The exact mechanism of action is not known, but ECT does increase circulating levels of brain neurotransmitters, which may be the way it relieves depression.

ECT is used for patients who have intense, prolonged symptoms with marked disability, especially if the patient has not responded to adequate trials with medications or if psychotic features are present. ECT has been successful in inducing remission in people with severe psychomotor retardation. It may also be used for patients who cannot take medications, or those at imminent risk of suicide or having dangerous delusions. Patients tend to respond more quickly to ECT than they do to medication therapy. Figure 50-4■ shows a man prepared for ECT.

The most common side effects of ECT are transient memory loss and mental confusion. Some patients have had more severe memory loss. Rare mortality associated with the procedure is due to myocardial infarction, stroke, or cardiac rhythm abnormalities. Patients with cardiovascular disease should be treated and carefully assessed for the appropriateness of ECT. Because of the history of misuse of ECT, there is a stigma associated with its use.

Transcranial Magnetic Stimulation

Transcranial magnetic stimulation (TMS) is a relatively new treatment for depression. In the procedure, a series of magnetic impulses are applied to either the left or right

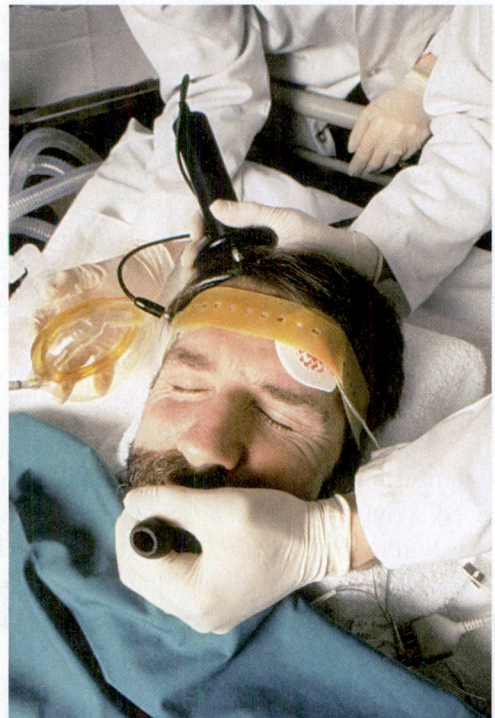

Figure 50-4. ■ A male patient prepared for electroconvulsive therapy. (Source: Will & Deni McIntyre/Science Source.)

dorsolateral prefrontal cortexes of the brain. Some small studies have shown its effectiveness as a new therapy for depression that is resistant to medication treatment. However, in a Cochrane Summary published in 2009, there was no strong evidence for benefit from using TMS to treat depression. Since the published research has all been from studies with small sample sizes, it is possible that benefit may be shown as more people are treated and more data are collected (Rodriguez-Martin et al., 2002).

Bipolar Disorder

Key Concept   People with bipolar disorder in the manic phase have several risks to their safety, including lack of insight, poor judgment, and impulsive behavior.

Bipolar disorder, formerly called *manic-depressive disorder*, is the other major mood disorder. *Bipolar* refers to the experience of both poles of mood: mania and depression. We will present the two major patterns of the disorder, bipolar I and bipolar II. In bipolar I disorder, the individual must experience at least one manic episode that is consistent with the diagnostic criteria discussed in the next subsection, during his or her lifetime. Usually people who have bipolar I have also experienced one or more major depressive episodes, as described in the section on depression. Overall, most people with bipolar I disorder experience more depressive than manic episodes (APA, 2013).

MANIC EPISODE

A manic episode is a distinct period of abnormal and persistently elevated, expansive, or irritable mood, lasting at least a week. This episode of elevated mood includes abnormally increased energy and goal-directed activity. It is severe enough to disturb work or interpersonal function or to require hospitalization to prevent harm to the affected individual or others. The patient may have psychosis as well. The episode represents a significant change in the individual's functioning. During the manic episode, three or more of the following symptoms are present (four if the mood is irritable, not elevated): inflated self-esteem; decreased need for sleep; increased urge to talk; flight of ideas or racing thoughts; easy distractibility; increase in goal-directed activity (at work, at school, socially, or sexually) or psychomotor agitation; and excessive seeking of pleasurable activity that has a high likelihood of painful or negative outcome (buying sprees, gambling, sexual indiscretion) (APA, 2013).

HYPOMANIC EPISODE

People with bipolar I disorder have full manic episodes as described earlier and can also have often have hypomanic episodes, which are less severe than manic episodes (although these episodes are not required for the diagnosis of bipolar I). A hypomanic mood episode has the same diagnostic criteria as the manic episode (as listed earlier), with some differences in severity. While **hypomania** is similar to mania in that it is an episode of abnormally elevated, expansive, or irritable mood, it differs in the following ways: It is shorter (may last 4 days instead of a week); the episode is not as severe as a manic episode; and there are no psychotic symptoms (if psychosis occurs the patient has bipolar I and the episode is mania) (APA, 2013).

BIPOLAR II DISORDER

In bipolar II, the individual has experienced at least one hypomanic episode and one major depressive episode. People with bipolar II disorder do not experience full manic episodes. The recurrent major depressive episodes are more frequent and lengthier than those in bipolar I disorder. The depressive episodes are severe and can be disabling. In bipolar II disorder, people can have episodes with both hypomanic and depressive symptoms, called *mixed episodes* (APA, 2013).

PATHOPHYSIOLOGY

Like major depressive disorder, bipolar disorder has a tendency to recur in families. There is evidence of a genetic etiology, but not of a single gene inheritance. First-degree biologic relatives of a person with bipolar disorder have a 4% to 24% chance of having the disease, the same recurrence rate as depression. Any given manic episode is likely to follow a stressor. Disordered sleep (such as experienced when traveling across time zones or working the night shift) may be a trigger (APA, 2013).

The brain neurotransmitters norepinephrine and dopamine are implicated in the cause of manic episodes. The same monoamine neurotransmitters whose decreased activity is implicated in depression are increased in mania. Hormones also interact with neurotransmitters in mood disorders. Hypothyroidism is correlated with depression and with rapid cycling of mood between depression and mania.

Mania is a biologic condition. Psychosocial factors are more important in the timing of manic episodes than in their cause.

MANIFESTATIONS

The mood a patient feels while in a manic episode may be described as elated, euphoric, high, or unusually good. The mood is characterized by constant and indiscriminate energy and enthusiasm. Frequently the person alternates between elation and irritability. An affected person may play basketball enthusiastically for 24 hours, becoming angry when someone tries to take the ball. Patients may go on an extended shopping spree, buying gifts for everyone on credit, write an entire book, or gamble away an entire paycheck. The flurry of activity seems productive to the patient but can be really disorganized and unproductive. While some people experience the elevated mood of mania as positive, others feel irritable. They may become more argumentative, angry, or aggressive.

Grandiose delusions are common. The patient may believe that he is a famous musician or a successful novelist, without having any skill at music or writing. The patient may feel qualified to give advice on any subject, such as how to conduct brain surgery or send a rocket to Mars. Patients may believe that they are superheroes.

People in mania feel a decreased need for sleep. They may awaken several hours earlier than usual, feeling alert and energetic. When mania is severe, the affected person may go for days with no sleep and not feel tired. They may hold several conversations at the same time or start many projects without finishing any (APA, 2013).

Manic speech is rapid and **pressured speech**, which means that it is so fast and determined that it is difficult to interrupt. The person's expressions may be dramatic or may be related to sounds (usually rhyming) more than words, such as in clang association. The following is an example of *clang association*: "I went to the store, tell me more, open the door, I like to eat cake, may I have a rake?" If irritability is present, the person may make long speeches about angry subjects, such as why anyone would ever want to do nursing care plans. Rapid speech reflects rapid thinking. The person's thinking may be going so fast that the thoughts are disorganized and incoherent. Box 50-8■ describes bipolar disorder in the words of people who experience it.

The affected person is likely to be easily distractible. **Distractibility** is evidenced by an inability to screen out excess or irrelevant sensory stimuli. The person may not be able to distinguish which thoughts are pertinent to the situation and which are not. Manic patients may be distracted from a conversation by someone's clothing, colors, sounds, or even furnishings in the room (APA, 2013).

Unwarranted optimism, grandiosity, and poor judgment characterize the behaviors of affected patients. Patients may spend an entire paycheck on lottery tickets, gamble, drive recklessly, and engage in unsafe sexual behavior, ignoring possible negative consequences. They may act or dress in more exaggerated ways than they normally would. Affected people may spend money they do not have, do illegal things that have serious penalties, or hurt themselves or others in the moment without foreseeing future consequences (APA, 2013).

What may look like an exciting experience at the beginning can be devastating to affected people and their families. Manic episodes impair affected individuals' ability to function and may threaten their lives. Excess energy expenditure without adequate rest, nutrition, and hydration can lead to exhaustion. Often during a manic episode, people will be too busy to eat, thus decreasing their energy supply even more.

People in a manic episode frequently lack insight about their illness and its effects on themselves and others. They often resist treatment. Sometimes involuntary hospitalization is necessary to protect patients from their own behavior. Involuntary hospitalization is indicated when a person is dangerous to self or others.

Course of the Disorder

The average age of onset of a first manic episode in bipolar I is in the early 20s, and mid-20s for bipolar II. Bipolar I affects women and men with equal frequency, while bipolar II affects more women. More than 90% of all individuals who have one manic episode will go on to have more. The exact pattern of recurrence is individual, but without treatment, the average rate of manic episodes is four in 10 years. A few individuals have more rapid cycling (four or more episodes per year). People with bipolar II tend to have more mood episodes over a lifetime than people with either major depressive or bipolar I disorder (APA, 2013).

Some children show a history of behavior problems before their first actual manic episode. Like depressive episodes, manic episodes tend to occur after psychosocial stressors. The episodes usually begin suddenly and last from a few weeks to several months. Manic episodes are briefer and end more abruptly than depressive episodes. A major depressive episode will come immediately before or after a manic episode 50% to 70% of the time. When a manic episode is accompanied by psychosis (hallucinations and delusions), it is more serious and more likely to lead to aggression or suicide (APA, 2013).

Concurrent Disorders

Disorders of substance use occur commonly with bipolar disorder. People who have substance use disorders in addition to bipolar disorder tend to experience more rapid

BOX 50-8	PATIENTS SPEAK THEIR MINDS ON BIPOLAR DISORDER

"Believe me, I have tried every drug I can find. Nothing feels so good as the natural high I get. I am smarter, stronger, quicker, happier, more alive, everything. When I get depressed, I think nothing can feel as bad as that. It is not like being alive. My life is a roller coaster, only more so."

"When Mom first starts to cycle up, she is great. She is so lively and excited, but it scares me. Once she took us to Disneyland, but she fought with some people there and didn't have enough money to get us home. It was so scary."

"Yes, I am feeling better. I am the CEO of Sears. Did you know that I put grocery departments in Sears? You and your family can join all the patients here for free groceries. I will also have free medications for everybody who needs them. Just go to any Sears and mention my name. They'll give you some new clothes for work."

cycling between mania and depression and have more *dysphoric* (unpleasant, unhappy) feelings in the manic phase.

COLLABORATIVE CARE

In the acute phase of a manic episode, the treatment priorities are ensuring patient safety and treating the mood disorder. Medication continues to be the mainstay of treatment for bipolar disorder.

The desired treatment outcomes for patients with bipolar disorder are to:

- Eliminate the symptoms of the mood episode (either depression or mania).
- Stabilize the mood to prevent cycling between depression and mania.
- Improve the patient's self-care ability, function, and quality of life.

Medications

The symptoms of bipolar depression are the same as those in patients who have depression alone (unipolar depression). The depression associated with bipolar disorder does not respond well to antidepressant medications alone.

Antidepressants given with either lithium or divalproex (an anticonvulsant) have been found to be effective in stabilizing mood.

The classes of drugs used to treat manic episodes are mood stabilizers (antimanic agents), anticonvulsants (that act as mood stabilizers), benzodiazepines (to decrease anxiety and agitation while the other drugs are starting to work), and antipsychotics (if the patient has psychotic symptoms). This chapter focuses on the mood-stabilizing, or antimanic, agents. In addition to the mood stabilizer, an antidepressant is often prescribed, often in lower doses than for people who have depression alone. The dose is kept low because antidepressant medications can trigger a manic episode in a person with bipolar disorder.

LITHIUM   Lithium (Li), a naturally occurring element, was the first mood-stabilizing drug. It is a first-line treatment for acute mania due to bipolar disorder and for long-term prevention of recurrent episodes (Table 50-2 ■). Target symptoms of mania include irritability, euphoria, pressured speech, flight of ideas, motor hyperactivity, aggressive behavior, grandiosity, delusions, impulsiveness, and hallucinations.

TABLE 50-2	**Giving Medications Safely: Mood Stabilizers**		
CLASS/DRUGS	**PURPOSE**	**NURSING IMPLICATIONS**	**PATIENT TEACHING**
Lithium - Lithium carbonate - Eskalith - Eskalith CR	To stabilize mood in bipolar disorder, to prevent and treat manic episodes.	Use with caution in older adults, thyroid disease, diabetes. Assess for toxicity. Therapeutic range is 0.5–1.5 mEq/L. Draw levels before morning dose. Check lithium (Li) levels weekly initially and then every 2 months. Monitor weight, stable Na intake, fluid and electrolyte balance, and mental status. Pregnancy category D.	Dehydration and NSAIDs increase risk of toxicity due to increased Li levels. High Na intake increases Li excretion (would decrease Li levels and increase risk for manic episode); maintain stable (not reduced) Na intake, and replace losses due to sweating. Blood tests for Li levels are necessary throughout treatment. Know symptoms of toxicity. Contraceptive teaching.
Anticonvulsant mood stabilizers - Valproic acid (Depakene) - Sodium valproate (Depacon) - Divalproex sodium (Depakote) - Carbamazepine (Tegretol) - Lamotrigine (Lamictal)	To prevent and treat manic episodes. Carbamazepine and lamotrigine are used when valproate is not effective.	Assess for side effects (S/Es): weight gain, tremors, GI upset, transient hair loss, and thrombocytopenia (loss of blood clotting cells). Monitor liver function tests and mental status. Valproate: Mix liquid form with juice to reduce mouth irritation; carbonated beverages increase irritation. Carbamazepine: bone marrow suppression. Lamotrigine: Stevens–Johnson syndrome, discontinue if rash develops, especially in children. Pregnancy category: valproate D, others C.	Avoid alcohol and other CNS depressants. Regular blood tests are necessary to monitor blood cells and liver function. Contraceptive teaching.

Lithium's mechanism of action is not fully understood. It is thought to affect many neurotransmitter functions. It probably corrects an ion exchange abnormality in the neuron and normalizes neurotransmitter functions.

Before a patient starts on lithium therapy, a full history and physical exam should be done, including a pregnancy test. Lithium is excreted by the kidneys and can have toxic effects on renal function, especially when it is at toxic levels. It inhibits several steps in thyroid hormone synthesis and metabolism, so thyroid function should be assessed. Lithium has a narrow therapeutic index, and toxicity is close to therapeutic blood levels.

In acute mania, lithium is effective in 1 to 2 weeks. It may take up to 4 weeks or longer for the symptoms to be fully relieved. A benzodiazepine or other agent may be needed to help the patient during acute mania before the lithium is fully effective.

When the patient is on a maintenance dose of lithium, the frequency and severity of both manic and depressive episodes are decreased. For some people, lithium offers full symptom relief. For many it is only partially effective. The combination of lithium and one of the anticonvulsants may improve mood stability. Some people are not able to tolerate the side effects of lithium, which can be significant. See Box 50-9■ for a list of lithium side effects and toxic effects.

BOX 50-9	LITHIUM SIDE EFFECTS AND TOXICITY

Common Side Effects
- Fine hand tremors
- Polyuria
- Weight gain
- GI discomfort, mild nausea
- Subjective feeling of mental dullness
- Thyroid dysfunction

Early Toxicity (lithium level is greater than 2.0 mEq/L)
- Nausea/vomiting
- Diarrhea
- Coarse hand tremor
- Slurred speech
- Muscle weakness

Severe Toxicity (lithium level is greater than 2.5 mEq/L)
- Mental confusion
- Muscle irritability and decreased coordination
- Fever
- Seizures
- Decreased urine output
- Cardiac dysrhythmias (irregular pulse)
- Severe hypotension
- Coma
- Death

Lithium is a salt. Because of this, the sodium and fluid balances of the body affect lithium levels. The relationship between sodium and lithium is *inverse.* (As the patient's serum sodium decreases, lithium level increases. When the sodium increases, lithium level decreases.) Regular blood tests for serum lithium levels are required to monitor each individual's status.

Patient Teaching   Part of patient education about lithium therapy is how to maintain consistent lithium and sodium levels. For example, if a person taking lithium played basketball for hours, losing sodium through perspiration, he would be at risk for lithium toxicity unless he replaced the lost sodium, maybe with a sports drink or a salty snack. He would also need to replace the water lost during exercise by drinking at intervals during the basketball game. The management of lithium therapy is difficult and can be a challenge for patients.

Treatment Compliance   Compliance with lithium therapy is an important issue. Patients sometimes find the side effects of the drug to be intolerable. There is a relatively high dropout rate for people on lithium therapy. Tolerability of treatment is especially important in bipolar disorder, because people with bipolar disorder expect to live full occupational and social lives.

Trials of several drug combinations may be required before the most effective and agreeable treatment plan for an individual is found. It is no longer necessary for the treatment team to encourage a patient to endure intolerable discomfort in exchange for prevention of mania.

For the patient to have the best possible outcomes, the nurse must ensure that the patient understands the treatment plan. Lifestyle changes are necessary to maintain lithium/fluid and electrolyte balance and to prevent toxicity. People taking lithium require ongoing psychotherapeutic support.

ANTICONVULSANT MOOD STABILIZERS   Some anticonvulsants have proven to be clinically effective both in treating the symptoms of mania and in preventing recurrence of episodes. The anticonvulsant valproate is endorsed as a first-line drug for mood stabilizing in bipolar disorder.

clinicalALERT

Valproate and lithium have been known to cause fetal anomalies and should not be taken by patients during pregnancy or by those who are planning to become pregnant.

Carbamazepine (Tegretol) is another anticonvulsant proven to be effective for the treatment of bipolar disorder. Carbamazepine is used for patients who do not respond to lithium or valproate. It is thought to stabilize mood by inhibiting the **kindling process**. Kindling is the repeated stimulus of brain neurons by stress, which may make the neurons increasingly sensitive to stress and increasingly likely to fire after smaller and smaller stimuli (Kanner, 2011). Like the valproates, carbamazepine increases the amount of stimulus needed to cause seizures or mania. Carbamazepine can cause bone marrow suppression with a decrease in red and white blood cell formation. Patients need to have regular blood cell counts taken while taking this drug.

Psychotherapy

Although bipolar disorder has a largely physiologic etiology, psychosocial therapy is still valuable. Living with bipolar disorder is challenging. At some point in a manic episode, the patient may be feeling so wonderful that taking medications to stop this seems absurd. They may lack the insight to connect untreated mania with its many negative outcomes. Compliance with medication therapy is challenging and often a problem for these patients.

Psychotherapy, in any of the same styles described under depression, can be a valuable tool to help patients with bipolar disorder to discuss and organize their feelings about having a chronic mental illness, consider the dilemmas of treatment, and work on development of insight into the real consequences of untreated bipolar disorder. This therapy is usually used during remissions, when patients can concentrate mentally.

Group Therapy

When the acute phase of mania or depression has passed, patient outcomes shift to coping with the disorder over the long term. Group therapy can be very valuable toward the goal of living with a chronic mental illness (or any chronic illness). The therapy or support group is composed of people who experience the same chronic mental illness. There may or may not be a mental health professional group facilitator. Local affiliates of the National Alliance for Mental Illness have support groups for patients and their families.

NURSING CARE

PRIORITIZING NURSING CARE

Priorities for care for patients with mood disorders include monitoring for safety, treatment-related side effects, patient participation in the treatment plan, and understanding of the disorder and its treatment.

ASSESSING

Mood is reflected in the patient's behavior and speech. When a patient has a mood disorder, a mental status assessment on admission provides baseline information. Over time, briefer

assessments can be made of pertinent parts of mental status and compared with the original assessment to document patient progress and effectiveness of treatment.

Most cases of depression are not diagnosed or treated. Nurses in every area of specialty practice work with depressed people. It makes sense for nurses to routinely do screening assessments for depression. The Geriatric Depression Scale (Box 50-10■) is used for the older adult. The Beck Depression Inventory, short form (Box 50-11■), can be used to identify adults who are likely to be depressed. When the nurse identifies that a patient is at risk for depression, the physician is notified. The patient's cultural background is another important aspect of assessment. See Box 50-12■ for the relationship between culture and symptoms of depression.

Suicide Risk

Only when the nurse is aware of a patient's suicidal thinking, or **suicidal ideation**, can the nurse intervene to help the patient. The nurse can assess the dangerousness of the patient's

BOX 50-10	GERIATRIC DEPRESSION SCALE (SHORT FORM)

1.	Are you basically satisfied with your life?	Yes/**No**
2.	Have you dropped many of your activities and interests?	**Yes**/No
3.	Do you feel that your life is empty?	**Yes**/No
4.	Do you often get bored?	**Yes**/No
5.	Are you in good spirits most of the time?	Yes/**No**
6.	Are you afraid that something bad is going to happen to you?	**Yes**/No
7.	Do you feel happy most of the time?	Yes/**No**
8.	Do you often feel helpless?	**Yes**/No
9.	Do you prefer to stay at home, rather than going out and doing new things?	**Yes**/No
10.	Do you feel you have more problems with memory than most?	**Yes**/No
11.	Do you think it is wonderful to be alive?	Yes/**No**
12.	Do you feel pretty worthless the way you are now?	**Yes**/No
13.	Do you feel full of energy?	Yes/**No**
14.	Do you feel that your situation is hopeless?	**Yes**/No
15.	Do you feel that most people are better off than you are?	**Yes**/No

Scoring: Bold responses indicate depression. A score of 5 or more indicates depression.

Source: Sheikh, J. I., & Yesavage, J. A. (1986). Geriatric depression scale: Recent evidence and development of a shorter form. *Clinical Gerontologist, 5,* 165–172.

BOX 50-11   BECK DEPRESSION INVENTORY (SHORT FORM)

Instructions: This is a questionnaire. On the questionnaire are groups of statements. Please read the entire group of statements in each category. Then pick out one statement in that group that best describes the way you feel today, that is, *right now!* Circle the number beside the statement you have chosen. If several statements in the group seem to apply equally well, circle each one. *Be sure to read all the statements in each group before making your choice.*

A. (Sadness)
3   I am so sad or unhappy that I can't stand it.
2   I am blue or sad all the time and I can't snap out of it.
1   I feel sad or blue.
0   I do not feel sad.

B. (Pessimism)
3   I feel that the future is hopeless and that things cannot improve.
2   I feel I have nothing to look forward to.
1   I feel discouraged about the future.
0   I am not particularly pessimistic or discouraged about the future.

C. (Sense of failure)
3   I feel I am a complete failure as a person (parent, husband, wife).
2   As I look back on my life, all I can see is a lot of failures.
1   I feel I have failed more than the average person.
0   I do not feel like a failure.

D. (Dissatisfaction)
3   I am dissatisfied with everything.
2   I do not get satisfaction out of anything anymore.
1   I do not enjoy things the way I used to.
0   I am not particularly dissatisfied.

E. (Guilt)
3   I feel as though I am very bad or worthless.
2   I feel quite guilty.
1   I feel bad or unworthy a good part of the time.
0   I don't feel disappointed in myself.

F. (Self-dislike)
3   I hate myself.
2   I am disgusted with myself.
1   I am disappointed in myself.
0   I don't feel disappointed in myself.

G. (Self-harm)
3   I would kill myself if I had the chance.
2   I have definite plans about committing suicide.

1   I feel I would be better off dead.
0   I don't have any thought of harming myself.

H. (Social withdrawal)
3   I have lost all of my interest in other people and don't care about them at all.
2   I have lost most of my interest in other people and have little feeling for them.
1   I am less interested in other people than I used to be.
0   I have not lost interest in other people.

I. (Indecisiveness)
3   I can't make any decisions at all anymore.
2   I have great difficulty in making decisions.
1   I try to put off making decisions.
0   I make decisions about as well as ever.

J. (Self-image change)
3   I feel that I am ugly or repulsive-looking.
2   I feel that there are permanent changes in my appearance and they make me look unattractive.
1   I am worried that I am looking old or unattractive.
0   I do not feel that I look any worse than I used to.

K. (Work difficulty)
3   I can't do any work at all.
2   I have to push myself very hard to do anything.
1   It takes extra effort to get started at doing something.
0   I can work about as well as before.

L. (Fatigability)
3   I get too tired to do anything.
2   I get tired from doing anything.
1   I get tired more easily than I used to.
0   I don't get any more tired than usual.

M. (Anorexia)
3   I have no appetite at all anymore.
2   My appetite is much worse now.
1   My appetite is not as good as it used to be.
0   My appetite is no worse than usual.

Scoring: 0–4 = None or mild depression.   5–7 = Mild depression.
8–15 = Moderate depression.   16+ Severe depression.

Source: From Beck, A. T., Ward, C. H., Mendelson, M., et al. (1961). An inventory for measuring depression. *Archives of General Psychiatry, 4,* 561–571. Copyright 1961. American Medical Association.

suicidal thoughts. Fleeting thoughts such as "I feel so bad, I wish I were dead" are not as dangerous as "I have a gun at home, and as soon as I am discharged I plan to shoot myself."

Imagine yourself asking a patient: "Do you ever think about hurting yourself or other people?" This is a hard question. It is socially inappropriate. It is just not polite to talk about suicide or to suggest that a person may be thinking about it. However, the nurse–patient relationship is not social. In this professional relationship, it is the nurse's goal

to assess the patient's safety and to intervene to protect the patient or others as necessary. Nurses must ask "socially inappropriate" questions as part of a mental status assessment in order to provide appropriate care for their patients.

In the general medical setting, every older patient with a chronic illness and every patient who has risk factors for suicide listed in Box 50-3 should be asked: "Do you feel like hurting yourself?" Add "... or other people" if there is a question of delusional or psychotic thinking.

Box 50-12 **FOCUS ON DIVERSITY**

Is Depression the Same Everywhere?

The answer to the question "Is depression the same everywhere?" is yes and no. People from all over the world suffer from depression. According to the World Health Organization, there is a worldwide epidemic of it. However, the signs and symptoms of depression vary from one culture and even subculture to another. Nurses must be aware of this in order to make accurate assessments and interpretations of patient symptoms. African Americans, Asian Americans, and Latinos tend to experience more somatic (physical) symptoms, such as headache, abdominal pain, and body aches than European American patients do. When patients from these cultures have symptoms that are not explained by medical tests, depression should be considered. European Americans are more likely to describe psychologic symptoms, such as sadness and guilt feelings.

The nurse can assess suicidal ideation (thinking) as follows:

1. Start with an assessment of whether the person has suicidal ideation: "Are you thinking about hurting yourself?" or "Do you think about killing yourself?"
2. If patients have suicidal ideation, determine if they have organized their thoughts about it enough to have a plan: "Do you have a plan?"
3. Assess lethality of the plan: "What is your plan?" or "How would you do it?" (more serious if planned means is firearm or hanging).
4. Assess if the patient has access to the planned means of suicide: "Do you have access to a gun? … drugs? (the means in the patient's plan)."
5. *Inform the treatment team.* Failure to report suicidal ideation constitutes breach of the nurse's legal and ethical duty to protect the patient.

Mental Status Assessment

The mental status assessment or mental status exam is the psychiatric equivalent of the physical assessment that is so familiar in the general medical setting. This assessment forms a baseline foundation of information about the patient's specific condition on admission. The assessment is then repeated at appropriate intervals, either in sections of concern or in its entirety. These subsequent data show whether the patient's condition (and mental status is the major determinant of the condition of the patient in the psychiatric setting) is improving or worsening. If the nurse is evaluating the efficacy of antidepressant medications, he or she will assess the patient's mood, psychomotor activity, interaction with others, and appearance. Thus, the mental status assessment constitutes the way the interprofessional team determines the patient's condition on admission, response to treatment, and the progress toward goals.

Mood

One way to monitor a patient's mood over time is to use a mood scale. Ask the patient, "Please rate your mood on a scale of one to ten, where one is the lowest and ten is the best possible mood." Although the numbers themselves do not have real measurement value, the patient's perception of how he or she feels may be quantified in this way. The nurse can compare the numbers over time to see if the patient is feeling better or worse. The mood assessment is done at least once per shift and documented in the nurse's notes.

Appearance and Affect

Other aspects of mental status that are pertinent to a person with a mood disorder are appearance, *affect* (nonverbal expression of mood), behavior, motor activity, and thought processes. The appearance of a person with depression may be disheveled, if the patient does not have the energy to bathe and change clothes. Mania may be expressed with flashy, bright clothing and outrageous makeup and jewelry.

Normal affect is called "broad," meaning that the patient can express a broad range of emotions from happiness to sadness. A person with depression cannot usually express the full range of emotions. Depression limits emotions (and affect) to sadness. This finding is expressed as "blunted affect." Emotions in mania may be restricted to excitement, elation, rage, or irritability.

Psychomotor Activity

Psychomotor activity would be slow (psychomotor retardation) in depression and agitated in mania. The depressed patient may lie in bed all day or sit moving very little. Manic patients may be so active that they are in danger of exhaustion.

Thought Processes

Patients' thought processes also demonstrate how they are affected by mood disorders and how they are responding to treatment. Everyone has occasional thought blocking, in which it is difficult to think of a word that you intended to say. However, thought blocking is very common and more severe in … uh … wait a minute … uh … umm … depression.

Flight of ideas, in which thoughts are moving so fast that the patient's speech jumps from one subject to another frequently, is common in mania. Grandiosity is also common in mania. "I am the world's most famous author, and I will be glad to write my next book about you, if you will give me a candy bar" is a grandiose statement that would much more likely be used by a person in mania than one in depression.

Thought processes might include psychotic features in either severe depression or severe mania. The content in depressive delusions or hallucinations would likely be frightening, persecutory, or very negative ("My boss hates me and wants to kill me"). In mania, delusions or hallucinations would be expansive and fantastic, such as "I will fly on over to my department store to pick up a new TV. No need for a plane."

DIAGNOSING, PLANNING, AND IMPLEMENTING

Common nursing diagnoses for patients with depression include *Impaired Social Interaction, Imbalanced Nutrition, Hopelessness, Powerlessness, Chronic Low Self-Esteem,* and *Self-Care Deficit. Risk for Injury Related to Impaired Judgment* is a common nursing diagnosis for patients with bipolar disorder. Risk for Violence to Self is often seen with major depressive disorder; Risk for Violence to Self or Others is common with bipolar disorder. The interventions listed in Chapter 49 for the patient experiencing Risk for Injury related to psychosis also apply to these patients.

The desired outcomes for patients with psychiatric disorders fall into four categories: thinking (cognition), feeling (mood), physiology, and behavior (acting or coping) (Figure 50-5 ■). Nursing care must be personalized for each individual patient. The suggested interventions in this chapter are based on common concerns for patients with mood disorders. If a patient has different concerns, creativity will be needed. Creativity is one of the cornerstones of nursing.

Risk for Violence: Self-Directed

Expected outcome: Will not harm self.

■ Assess mental status, including suicidal ideation. *Mental status assessment includes information about the patient's mood and whether the patient has psychosis. (Psychosis increases suicide risk due to abnormal reality testing.)*

■ If the patient does have suicidal ideation, assess for plan and whether the patient has the means to complete the plan. *It is more dangerous if the patient has a specific lethal plan and the means to complete it.*

■ Share information about suicidal thinking with the treatment team. *Team must be involved to ensure patient safety.*

■ Remove potentially dangerous items from the patient's area (knives, lighters, razors, belts, glass, etc.).

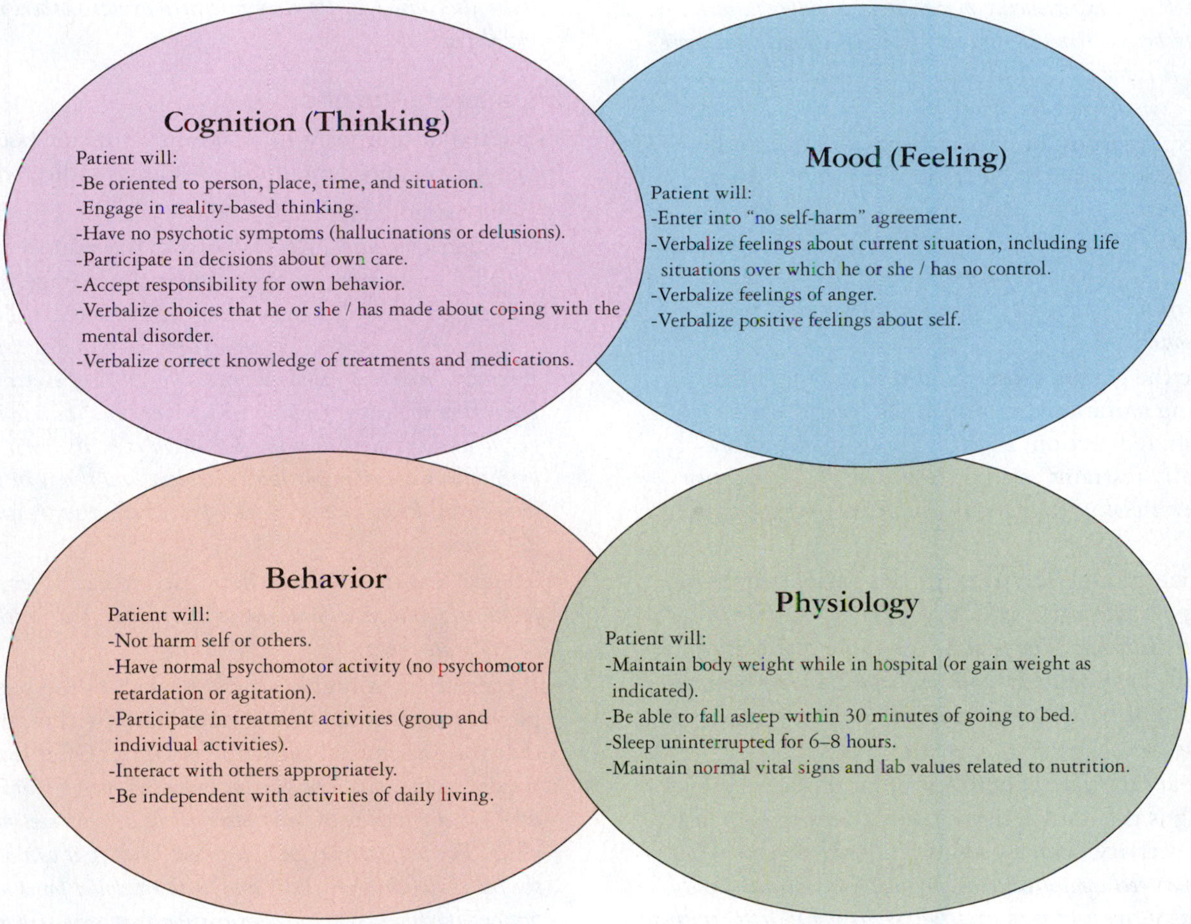

Cognition (Thinking)

Patient will:
-Be oriented to person, place, time, and situation.
-Engage in reality-based thinking.
-Have no psychotic symptoms (hallucinations or delusions).
-Participate in decisions about own care.
-Accept responsibility for own behavior.
-Verbalize choices that he or she / has made about coping with the mental disorder.
-Verbalize correct knowledge of treatments and medications.

Mood (Feeling)

Patient will:
-Enter into "no self-harm" agreement.
-Verbalize feelings about current situation, including life situations over which he or she / has no control.
-Verbalize feelings of anger.
-Verbalize positive feelings about self.

Behavior

Patient will:
-Not harm self or others.
-Have normal psychomotor activity (no psychomotor retardation or agitation).
-Participate in treatment activities (group and individual activities).
-Interact with others appropriately.
-Be independent with activities of daily living.

Physiology

Patient will:
-Maintain body weight while in hospital (or gain weight as indicated).
-Be able to fall asleep within 30 minutes of going to bed.
-Sleep uninterrupted for 6–8 hours.
-Maintain normal vital signs and lab values related to nutrition.

Figure 50-5. ■ Desired outcomes for patients with mood disorders.

Removing dangerous items promotes safety by decreasing the patient's opportunity for impulsive self-harm. People experiencing mania are not likely to harm themselves intentionally, but have impaired judgment, so the nurse must anticipate the risks and must control the environment to promote safety.

■ Assess patient safety frequently during the night. *The patient may feel unsupervised at night.*

■ Remain with the patient who is having feelings about harming self. *The nurse's presence shows regard for the patient's safety and worth. The nurse can prevent harmful behavior. A patient at high risk for suicidal behavior requires constant observation.*

■ Create a "no self-harm" contract with the patient. *Although an agreement by the patient not to harm self is not really binding, it suggests that the patient is in control and responsible for his or her behavior. The contract emphasizes the worth of the patient and the concern by the staff for his or her safety.*

Risk for Violence: Directed at Others

Expected outcome: Will not harm others.

■ Remain calm. *Emotions are contagious. If the nurse is calm, it is easier for patients to remain in control of their behavior.*

■ Provide low-stimulation environment for a manic patient. *People experiencing mania have a reduced ability to filter and process stimuli. The more sensory stimuli, the more difficult it is for the patient to determine what is real and to maintain control over behavior.*

■ Make expectations for patient behavior clear to the patient as soon as possible. Staff must be consistent in expectations of the patient. *Having clear, structured expectations can make it easier for the patient to comply with behavior expectations. Consistency among staff is important to avoid confusion and patient manipulation of staff to change expectations.*

■ Observe the patient closely and respond quickly to increasing agitation. Start with the least restrictive approach: redirection, PRN medication, isolation, and finally restraint as a last resort. *Early intervention may prevent violent behavior and injury to the patient and others.*

■ Minimize group activities for the patient in mania. *Mania puts the patient at risk for sensory overload or overstimulation. The patient may have difficulty responding appropriately with multiple people. One-to-one interactions are less stimulating and easier for the patient to manage.*

■ Provide appropriate opportunities for physical activity. Walking is the ideal activity. The patient may prefer another activity, such as ping-pong or basketball. *The patient may feel compelled to be physically active and would thus find confinement very stressful. Walking is active without being exhausting if prolonged.*

Impaired Social Interaction

Expected outcome: Will interact individually with staff and peers and participate in group activities.

■ Establish a trusting relationship with the patient. *The nurse–patient relationship is the foundation for nursing care and for understanding the patient's needs. When the patient trusts the nurse, he or she has an opportunity to have a sense of emotional security. A patient who feels secure will be more likely to interact positively with others. The nurse provides a role model for how to communicate and behave in an individual relationship.*

■ Spend some time each shift interacting with the patient individually. *The patient may not be able to initiate interactions. The nurse is a role model for appropriate behavior. The nurse's choice to visit with the patient is validating to the patient. Long interactions may be stressful.*

■ Provide structured activities to allow the patient with depression to interact with others. Encourage the patient to participate (arts and crafts groups, listening to music in a group, walking or exercising in a group, discussing medications, reminiscing groups, etc.). *The depressed patient is more likely to be able to interact with others if the situation is structured, because the demands on the individual are less. Positive interactions with others reinforce socializing.*

Imbalanced Nutrition

Expected outcome: Will maintain admission body weight (or gain a specified amount of weight, as indicated).

■ If the patient is lethargic and overweight, offer lighter foods, snacks, and liquids. Discuss the value of regular exercise in improving one's spirits. Encourage the patient to set a plan of regular, light exercise. *The patient may be unable to focus on weight loss until depression is resolved and may be too depressed to think of exercising. It is better to have a regular time for exercise than to try to get up and exercise when the depression is at its worst. Light, brief efforts are more possible to achieve and thus can improve self-esteem. Regular exercise is a proven effective treatment for depression.*

■ The patient may feel too depressed to eat. *Offer fluids frequently and small amounts of nutritious foods as the patient can tolerate them.*

■ If the patient is highly active, pacing, or too busy to eat, provide nutritious "finger foods" (sandwiches, fruit, etc.) that the patient can eat while walking. Offer food and fluids frequently. *The patient has high energy requirements while in a manic phase and may not be able to meet nutritional needs. The patient may be able to eat foods that can be held in the hands when he or she is unable to sit down for a meal. The patient is also at risk for dehydration from excessive activity, especially in hot weather.*

Hopelessness

Expected outcome: Will express feelings and make statements indicating hope that the future can be better.

- Allow the patient to talk about feelings and life events. Use therapeutic communication techniques to help the patient see that he or she has survived difficulties in the past and that he or she has strengths. *The knowledge that one has overcome obstacles before suggests that it is possible to do so again. When the patient recognizes his or her own strengths, it provides a foundation for hope that the current trouble can be overcome.*
- Teach the patient about the disorder and medications and that the treatment team will not give up hope until the patient feels better. *Knowledge that the patient is likely to have a positive response to treatment is hopeful. It may be beneficial to point out that depression has episodes and that this one will eventually resolve. Many patients worry that the staff will abandon them if they do not respond to treatment.*
- See Box 50-13■ for ideas about using therapeutic communication as an intervention for a patient who feels hopeless.

MANAGING NURSING CARE

As appropriate and allowed by the designated duties and responsibilities of assistive personnel, the nurse may delegate nursing care activities such as interacting with patients, assisting or supervising patients with ADLs, or monitoring meals and recording intake.

EVALUATING

In the evaluation phase, the nurse looks back at the desired outcomes to decide whether they were achieved. When patients have mood disorders, the nurse evaluates their cognition, mood, behavior, and physical findings related to these disorders (see Figure 50-5).

DOCUMENTING

Document changes in patients' mental status. These changes will form a record of patients' response to treatment.

CONTINUITY OF CARE

Patients with mood disorders face many challenges related to their disorder and its treatment. Education is an important role for the nurse. The nurse should reinforce patient teaching about medications, side effects, and the interaction between medication and diet or activities. Most patients will need ongoing psychotherapeutic support. Information about support groups, as well as emergency numbers, should be provided. The National Alliance for Mental Illness has support groups in many localities.

BOX 50-13   NURSING CARE CHECKLIST

Talking With a Patient Who Feels Hopeless

☑ Use open-ended questions or broad opening statements when asking the patient to express feelings.

Nurse: "Tell me about how you are feeling."

Patient: "I feel bad."

☑ Clarify the patient's message.

Nurse: "Can you give me some examples of how you feel bad?"

Patient: "I am a failure, I lost my job, I hate myself, and I am so tired of it all."

Nurse: "Do you mean that you are tired of living?"

Patient: "Yes."

☑ Make the implied message explicit. This is very important to do, even if it feels awkward.

Nurse: "Charlie, do you mean that you are thinking about killing yourself?"

Patient: "Well, yes. I think about it a lot."

☑ Clarify and gather data for assessment.

Nurse: "You have a plan?"

Patient: "I have a gun at home."

☑ Validate the importance of the patient's feelings, give information about next steps, and assess the patient's current safety.

Nurse: "Charlie, this is important. I will be talking with Dr. Rodgers and the other team members about your thoughts. We will work on a plan to help you. Are you thinking about hurting yourself here in the hospital?"

Patient: "No."

☑ Obtain a "no self-harm" contract (an agreement with the patient to disclose suicidal feelings before taking action to hurt self).

Nurse: "We want you to be safe. Will you promise me that if you do think you want to hurt yourself while you are here, you will not hurt yourself, but tell me or anyone on the staff first, so we can help you?"

Patient: "OK, I promise. I wish I wanted to live."

☑ Validate the patient's importance, reassure the patient that treatment can help, and offer hope.

Nurse: "You are in the hospital so we can help you through times like this. There are effective treatments for depression, and we will not give up until you feel better. OK?"

Patient: "OK."

NURSING CARE PLAN
Patient With Depression

Ms. G. is a 70-year-old African American widowed woman who is a resident in a long-term care facility. She had a stroke a year ago and has hemiplegia on her right side.

She is right-handed. She has a daughter who lives in another state and a married son with one teenage granddaughter living nearby.

Assessment

The nurse is Craig C., LPN. He assessed that Ms. G. does not feed herself and has little appetite. She is alert and oriented to person and place. She cooperates with having her ADLs done for her, but she does not try to help. When she talks, it is only one or two words at a time. Her face always seems to look sad. Craig has worked with Ms. G. for the 3 months since she has been in this facility. He thinks Ms. G. is depressed. On the Geriatric Depression Scale, she scored 12. In the conversation they had about the depression scale, Ms. G. said that she missed her family.

Nursing Diagnosis

Three priority nursing diagnoses were identified for this patient:

- *Powerlessness* related to disability and impaired communication
- *Self-Care Deficit*, bathing/hygiene, dressing/grooming, feeding, and toileting related to hemiplegia and lack of motivation
- *Impaired Social Interaction* related to lack of motivation and lack of opportunity to socialize with family and peers

Expected Outcomes

The expected outcomes for the plan of care are:

- Patient will identify two areas in which she feels some control.
- Patient will assist with all ADLs and feed herself independently within 2 weeks.
- Patient will interact with the staff, her peers, and her family.

Planning and Implementation

The charge nurse consulted with Ms. G.'s physician about the findings on the Geriatric Depression Scale. The physician agreed that Ms. G. is depressed. She prescribed fluoxetine 20 mg PO each morning. The following interventions were planned and implemented:

- *Offer simple choices first.* Ms. G. is given a choice of clothes to wear each day. She is asked if she wants to take her shower before or after breakfast and where she wants to eat lunch (there are three dining rooms in this facility). She is asked which radio station she wants to listen to.
- *Encourage self-care.* The aides who supervised meals were asked to help her use her left hand to feed herself.
- *Encourage social contact.* The nurse called Ms. G.'s son and encouraged him to visit and to bring his family. He also arranged to visit with Ms. G. for a few minutes himself each day that he worked. (Of course, the nurse would have liked to have more time to talk with her, but this is a real story.) He had Ms. G. put on the list of residents who attend the news group (where the activity aide reads parts of the newspaper each morning).

Evaluation

Two weeks after the plan was started, Craig evaluated its effectiveness. With encouragement, Ms. G. had started to make choices about her clothes, radio stations, social activities, and visitors. She assisted in washing herself during her shower. She tried feebly, but was not much help with dressing. She was able to feed herself about 50% of her meals and was able to call for help to get to the bathroom about 75% of the time.

Within 10 days after starting her new medication, she was smiling, was more interested in her surroundings, had more appetite, and was more active. She is more talkative and enjoys visits from her family.

Critical Thinking in the Nursing Process

1. Why was it important for this patient to make choices?
2. How successful was outcome 2 of Ms. G.'s plan? How might it be adapted after evaluation?
3. How does the range of social interactions that were set up for Ms. G. increase the likelihood that she will meet outcome 3?

Note: Discussion of Critical Thinking questions appears on the companion website.

Note: The references and resources for all chapters have been compiled at the back of the book.

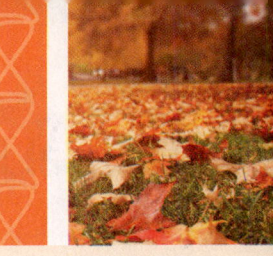

Chapter Review

KEY POINTS

- **Concept:** Depression is caused by genetic abnormalities that interact with the individual's life experiences and environment.
- Mood disorders are caused by an interaction of genetic predisposition, brain function abnormalities, and environmental stressors (biologic and psychosocial factors).
- Depression is the most common mental disorder in the world.
- Nurses in every specialty area work with people who have mood disorders, especially depression.
- **Concept:** Our culture "marks" or stigmatizes people with mental illness as less worthy, intelligent, acceptable, or important than the rest of the population.
- **Concept:** Suicide is a risk for patients with depression. There are factors that increase and decrease the suicide risk for individuals.
- Most people who kill themselves are depressed.
- The suicide rate is highest in the older adult.
- Mood disorders are treatable, and most people respond positively to medications.

- There is a stigma against people with mental disorders.
- Desired outcomes for people with mood disorders are in the areas of cognition, mood, behavior, and physiology.
- People with depression may experience anhedonia, lack of energy, lack of motivation, difficulty relating to other people, and psychomotor retardation, as well as sadness.
- Serious possible side effects are associated with the MAOI antidepressants, including hypertensive crisis when patients combine foods containing tyramine with these drugs.
- Potentially fatal serotonin syndrome can occur when MAOIs are combined with SSRIs or St. John's wort. Symptoms include agitation, unstable BP, muscle spasms, tremor, nausea, abdominal cramps, headache, seizures, and coma.
- **Concept:** People with bipolar disorder in the manic phase have several risks to their safety, including lack of insight, poor judgment, and impulsive behavior.
- Lithium and valproate are both first-line drugs for bipolar disorder.

PEARSON NURSING STUDENT RESOURCES

- Find additional materials at **nursing.pearsonhighered.com**.

Clinical Reasoning Care Map

Caring for a Patient With Bipolar Disorder
NCLEX-PN® Focus Area: Physiologic Integrity

Case Study: David Clay is a 36-year-old European American male patient with a diagnosis of bipolar disorder. He is hospitalized for a surgical repair of an ankle injury he experienced while he was playing basketball. Mr. Clay is a certified public accountant. He is having a manic episode that is less severe than his untreated episodes were, but he has been sleepless for three nights and he stayed home from work yesterday to play basketball all day. He did not eat or drink all day when he was playing basketball. He takes lithium carbonate extended release (Eskalith CR) 450 mg b.i.d. at home, and this is also ordered in the hospital. The morning dose is due now.

Nursing Diagnosis: Risk for Injury related to lithium toxicity

COLLECT DATA

Subjective

_____
_____
_____
_____
_____

Objective

_____
_____
_____
_____
_____

Does this present a threat to the patient's safety?

If yes, the priority intervention to address this threat would be:
_____

Nursing Care

_____
_____
_____
_____
_____
_____
_____

Interprofessional team members to include when planning care:
_____

How would you document this?_____
_____

Compare your answers and documentation to those provided on the companion website.

Data Collected
(use only those that apply)

- Weight 185 lb.
- BP 130/80.
- Pulse 108, irregular.
- Patient states, "My hands won't stop shaking."
- Slept 6 hours last night.
- Skin is warm and dry.
- Patient's mother had bipolar disorder.
- Patient states, "Would you please read the menu to me, I can't see very well."
- When the physical therapist was teaching him to use crutches, the patient was too weak to bear his own body weight on his unaffected leg.
- Patient is allergic to tree pollen.
- Refused dinner last evening and breakfast today.
- Patient's wife states, "He has been under a lot of pressure at work lately."

Nursing Interventions
(use only those that apply; list in priority order)

- Call the physician to request an order for a sleeping pill to help the patient sleep to regain his strength.
- Teach the patient to drink 3 gallons of water daily.
- Look in the patient's chart to find his baseline vital signs.
- Hold the lithium dose that is due now.
- Call the physician to report the presence of symptoms of lithium toxicity.
- Teach the patient and his wife that his strenuous exercise (playing basketball all day) is a good way to improve his cardiovascular fitness.

NCLEX-PN® Exam Preparation

1 What is the best way for the nurse to assess and document how a patient's mood is subjectively responding to treatment over time?
1. Ask the patient to draw a chart of his mood.
2. Measure the mood with the mental status assessment.
3. Ask the patient to rate his mood on a 0–10 scale and document his report regularly.
4. Assess the patient's response to medications, and if the patient responds well to a low dose of medication, his mood is not as depressed as someone who requires a higher dose.

2 A newly married woman confides to the nurse that she tried to commit suicide during high school. She says she is afraid to become pregnant for fear that having a new baby might bring on those feelings again. Select the best information about postpartum depression for this patient.
1. She is no more likely than any other young woman to experience postpartum depression.
2. She was probably just seeking attention in high school and has no risk of future depressive episodes.
3. She is at increased risk for another depressive episode considering her past experience.
4. She is worrying needlessly and should be encouraged to consider pregnancy.

3 A patient complains that every winter she experiences feelings of extreme fatigue and irritability. She has been diagnosed with seasonal affective disorder. The nurse will teach her that the most effective treatment for this type of depression is:
1. light or phototherapy.
2. melatonin supplement.
3. psychoanalysis.
4. electroconvulsive treatment.

4 The nurse reads in the chart that a patient is experiencing anhedonia. What symptom would the nurse expect to find? The patient is:
1. hallucinating.
2. incapable of forming personal relationships.
3. overeating.
4. incapable of feeling pleasure.

5 People suffering from depression are often undiagnosed. The most likely reason for this is that:
1. physicians do not recognize the condition.
2. general practitioners feel under-qualified to treat a mental disorder.
3. patients underreport their feelings, for fear of the stigma of being "mentally ill."
4. physicians do not value the depth of the psychologic feelings a patient reports.

6 A patient has just been started on an antidepressant medication. The patient asked when the medication will work. The best response by the nurse is:
1. "You should feel relief from the depression immediately."
2. "It will take 2 to 6 weeks for the medication to reach its full effect."
3. "The medication usually takes 1 week to reach its potential."
4. "It may be 6 months before you feel the full effects of the medication."

7 What form of behavior would the nurse expect from a patient who is having a manic episode with racing thoughts?
1. Psychomotor agitation
2. Hallucinations
3. Powerlessness
4. Thought blocking

8 A patient with bipolar disorder is pacing constantly today while other patients are having a birthday party. There are music, noise, and food. The patient walks over to the table and starts grabbing handfuls of cake to eat as he paces up and down the halls. The nurse's best response to this behavior would be to:
1. let him continue to pace and eat.
2. medicate him with a PRN antianxiety drug.
3. restrain him in his room.
4. ask him to go outside and take a walk with the nurse.

9 When teaching a patient who takes an MAOI, which foods should the nurse teach the patient to avoid? **Select all that apply.**
1. Aged cheese
2. Bananas
3. Pepperoni pizza
4. Chianti wine
5. All dairy products (milk, cottage cheese)
6. Hot dogs

10 What should the nurse do if a patient scores high on the Geriatric Depression Scale?
1. Tell the patient that he or she is not depressed, and ask if the patient has any questions.
2. Notify the primary care provider, so the patient can be evaluated for depression.
3. Arrange for the patient to be transferred to a psychiatric unit immediately.
4. Teach the patient about what medications he or she will be taking.

Answers and rationales for Review Questions appear in Appendix I.

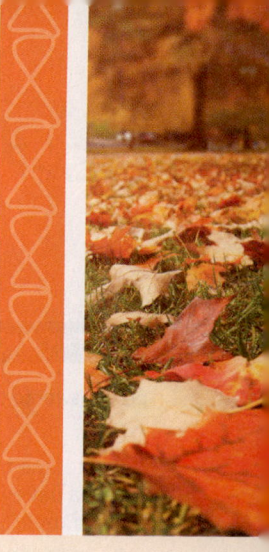

CHAPTER 51

Caring for Patients With Anxiety Disorders

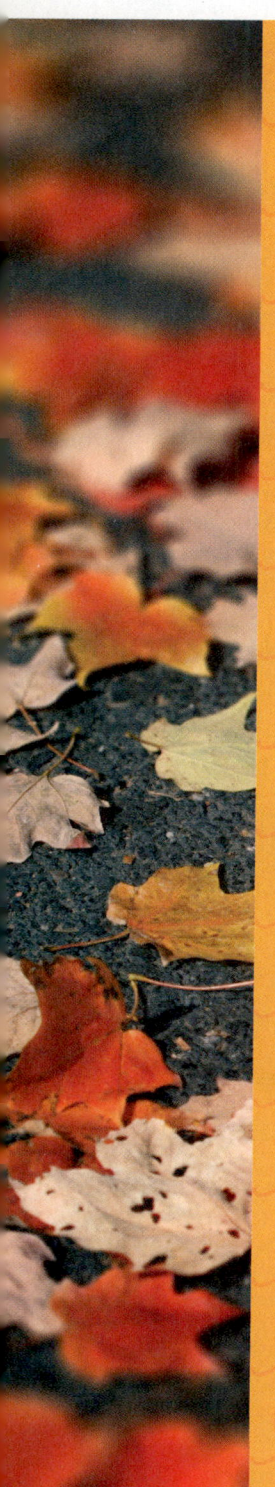

BRIEF OUTLINE

Generalized Anxiety
    Disorder

Panic Disorder

Agoraphobia

Social Anxiety Disorder

Specific Phobias

Obsessive-Compulsive
    Disorder

Posttraumatic Stress
    Disorder

APPLIED LEARNING OUTCOMES

After completing this chapter, you will be able to:

1. Collect subjective and objective data about patients' anxiety.
2. Apply the nursing process to the care of patients with anxiety disorders.
3. Explain the role of coping mechanisms in the management of anxiety.
4. Plan nonpharmacologic nursing interventions to treat or prevent patient anxiety.
5. Safely administer antianxiety (anxiolytic) agents.
6. Explain the nursing role in interprofessional care of patients with anxiety.

KEY TERMS

The key terms are defined on the pages listed below.

SPECIAL FEATURES

Anxiety is a normal response to stress. Everyone has experienced it. **Anxiety** is a feeling of uneasiness or dread and activation of the autonomic nervous system in response to a vague, nonspecific threat. Anxiety is also a feeling of apprehension caused by anticipation of danger (Wilkinson & Ahern, 2009). Anxiety can be an alerting signal that allows the individual to prepare for a threat. However, when anxiety becomes overwhelming; impairs a person's ability to function at home, school, or work; and affects relationships with other people, then it is a disorder. Anxiety disorders are serious medical illnesses that can grow worse if not treated.

PATHOPHYSIOLOGY

Key Concept The experience of anxiety originates in the subcortical or primitive brain, specifically in the limbic system.

During anxiety, there is an increase in blood flow to the limbic system and the cerebral cortex. Figure 51-1■ shows the structures of the limbic system, and Table 51-1■ describes the functions of these structures and what happens when they function abnormally. The limbic system conducts stimuli to the sympathetic part of the autonomic nervous system. Sympathetic stimulation causes the symptoms we recognize as anxiety. From the limbic system, neural messages are also conducted to the cerebral cortex. In the association areas of the cerebral cortex, the individual experiences thoughts about anxiety. Thus, feelings, physiologic responses, and thoughts are all part of the anxiety experience.

Studies of twins and families suggest that there is a genetic influence on the development of anxiety disorders. The Human Genome Project mapped the locations of the 20,000 human genes and in the process did not locate a gene that codes for disorders of anxiety. There are probably multiple genes that code for functions of the sympathetic

nervous system and the thought processes related to it. As with other mental disorders, genetics is not the sole etiology of anxiety disorders. Life experiences also play an important part. Researchers are looking at how genetics and experience interact in anxiety disorders.

From a behavioral point of view, experience can teach people different ways to respond to stressful events. An individual's experiences, in both childhood and adulthood, influence which situations cause anxiety and the severity of the patient's response.

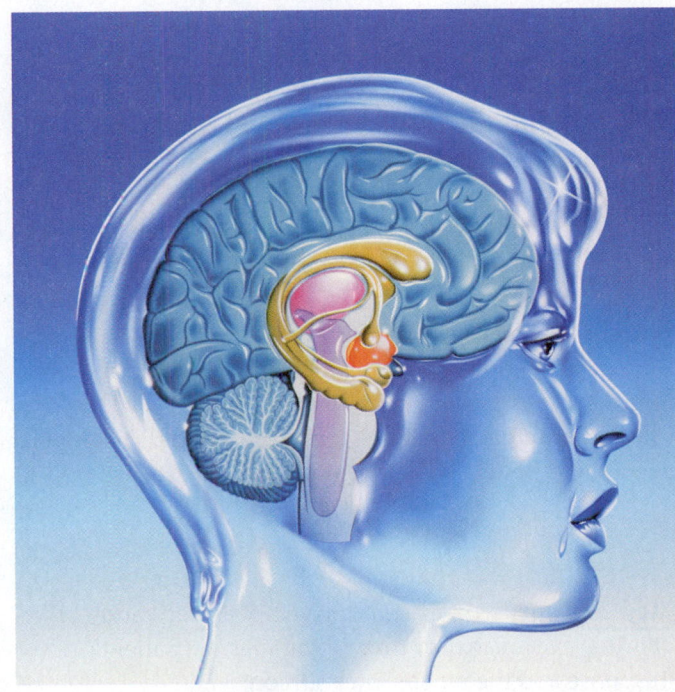

Figure 51-1. ■ The limbic system is surrounded by the cerebral cortex. It plays a role in motivation, emotion, and memory. It is composed of the thalamus, amygdala, hippocampus, and hypothalamus. (Source: John Bavosi/Science Source.)

TABLE 51-1	Functions of the Limbic System	
LIMBIC STRUCTURE	**FUNCTIONS**	**DYSFUNCTIONS**
Thalamus	Relays sensory input from spinal cord. Regulates emotional aspects of sensory experiences.	Obsessive-compulsive disorder (OCD), mood disorders, schizophrenia
Amygdala	Coordinates actions of autonomic nervous system and endocrine system. Involved in control of emotions, nurturing behavior, fear conditioning. Controls memory of fear experiences. Most important site for anxiety response.	Inappropriate fear and rage, anxiety, posttraumatic stress disorder (PTSD)
Hippocampus	Processes information between parts of the brain that receive sensory input and those that translate the input into action. Regulates immune system and memory storage.	Memory and learning impairments
Hypothalamus	Composed of neurons that produce hormones. Integration center. Concentrates dopamine. Converts thinking and feelings into hormones that cause changes throughout the body through the autonomic nervous system.	Excessive thirst and hunger. May be involved in eating disorders and schizophrenia. Implicated in side effects of psychotropic drugs

Cognitive function can affect how a person perceives anxiety-producing stimuli. Therefore, it is the patient's perception of an event that makes the event produce anxiety. Look at the photos in Figure 51-2■. Each represents a situation that causes stress and anxiety for some people. Do some of these situations cause you to feel anxious? If a person focuses her or his thoughts on stressful events, this individual will be more prone to anxiety. Intelligence and the personality trait of introspection may put people at a higher risk for anxiety.

The sympathetic nervous system responds to the stress of fear or anxiety in the same way. Fear has survival value. When a person sees an alligator (Figure 51-3■), fear motivates the person to run away. Anxiety is not as focused and often has no realistic source. Even when the individual experiencing anxiety knows the reason for it, the feeling of **dysphoria** (discomfort and distress) is often out of proportion to the real danger. Low levels of anxiety can arouse the individual's attention and alertness and even make it easier to learn new things, but as anxiety becomes more severe, it causes impairment of function. Anxiety and fear cause the same physiologic responses, which are the result of sympathetic nervous system stimulation (Box 51-1■). Taking a test in nursing school can cause the same physiological responses as being chased by an alligator.

MANIFESTATIONS
Levels of Anxiety

Key Concept   There are four levels of anxiety, and it is the level of anxiety that determines the patient's response and the nurse's intervention.

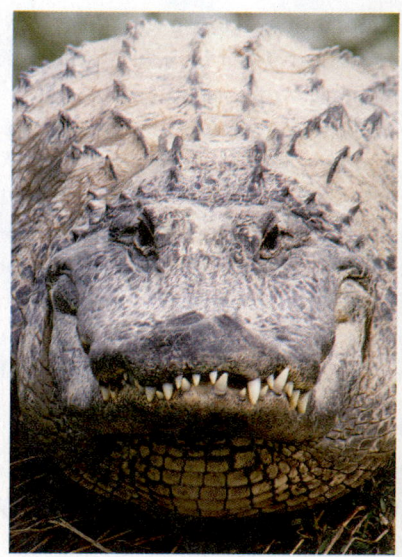

Figure 51-3. ■ The sympathetic nervous system responds in the same way to the fear of an actual alligator that it does to general anxiety. (Source: Art Wolfe / Getty Images, Inc.)

BOX 51-1	MANIFESTATIONS OF SYMPATHETIC STIMULATION

- Increased blood glucose
- Increased heart rate
- Increased blood pressure
- Dilated pupils
- Cool skin
- Diversion of blood flow to the large muscles
- Piloerection (hair "standing on end")
- Decreased GI motility

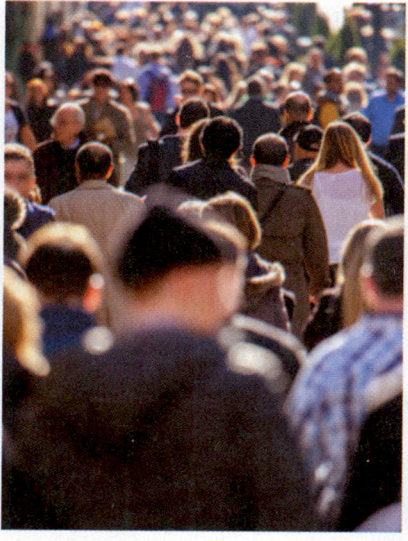
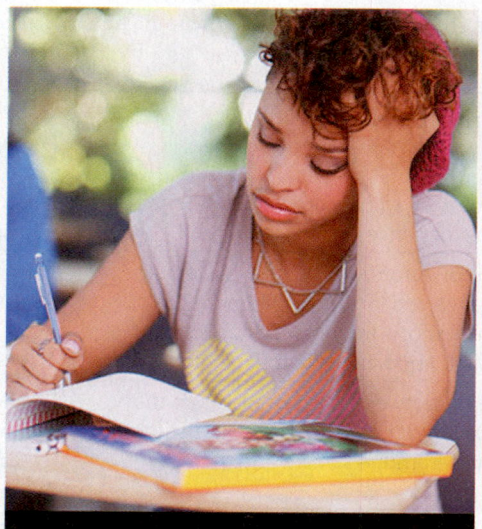
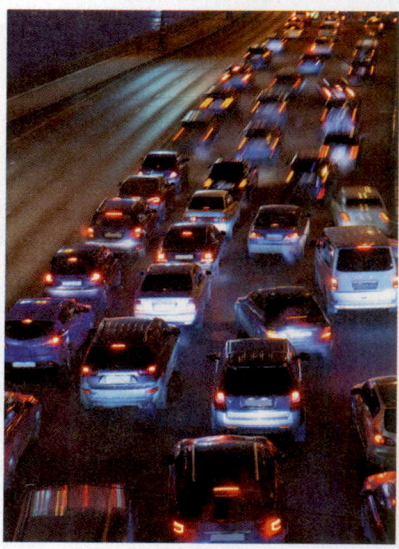

Figure 51-2. ■ Potential anxiety-producing events include being in a crowd, taking a test at school, and driving in heavy traffic. Do some of these events cause you to feel more anxious than others? Individual differences are caused by the cognitive part of anxiety. (Sources: Left: blvdone / Shutterstock. Middle: © OJO Images Ltd / Alamy. Right: Iakov Filimonov/Shutterstock.)

There are four degrees of anxiety (Peplau, 1989). Table 51-2 ■ shows the four levels and the behaviors the nurse might observe in a patient at each level.

The *Diagnostic and Statistical Manual of Mental Disorders* (American Psychiatric Association [APA], 2013) lists three classifications of disorders of anxiety: anxiety disorders, obsessive-compulsive and related disorders, and trauma- and stressor-related disorders (Reichenberg, 2014). There are many different causes of these disorders, but the manifestation they all have in common is anxiety. Anxiety disorders are the most common mental disorders in the United States and Europe.

Generalized Anxiety Disorder

Generalized anxiety disorder (GAD) is classified as an anxiety disorder. It is characterized by excessive anxiety and worry occurring on most days for at least 6 months. There may be any number of different events or activities contributing to the feelings, and the individual finds it difficult to control the anxiety. In addition to the anxiety, the affected person has at least three of the following symptoms: fatigue, irritability, restlessness, difficulty with mental concentration, tension of muscles, or sleep disruption (APA, 2013). Generalized anxiety disorder can occur at any age. It is most common in adults and peaks in middle age, but when children are affected, they only require one of the listed symptoms in addition to anxiety for the diagnosis. It is important for health care workers to know that anxiety disorders can occur in children, because people who

are diagnosed and treated early have a better prognosis for normal development and a good outcome (Reichenberg, 2014). European Americans have a higher incidence than others of generalized anxiety in the United States, and the disorder is more common in developed countries. Although there is no evidence that the tendency for anxiety is culturally related, the subjects of people's worry can be culture specific (APA, 2013).

Affected people will report that they feel significant stress, have difficulty controlling the worry, or have related impairment in social or occupational functioning. In this disorder, the intensity, frequency, and duration of the anxiety are far out of proportion to the realistic likelihood or impact of the feared event. Thoughts of the feared event intrude on the individual's thinking, distracting her or him from other tasks. The focus of worry may shift from one concern to another. A few potential examples of concerns for these individuals are being late, personal performance, illness, family, or job. Generalized anxiety disorder is associated with significant distress and disability, causing 110 million disability days of lost work per year in the United States. Affected adults may be moderately to seriously disabled (APA, 2013).

People with GAD may or may not realize that their anxiety is more intense than makes sense in the situation, but they still cannot control their worries (Reichenberg, 2014). Their anxiety is accompanied by physical symptoms, especially fatigue, headaches, muscle tension, muscle pain, irritability, sweating, nausea, difficulty swallowing, trembling, and hot flashes. Relaxation seems impossible

TABLE 51-2	**Four Degrees of Anxiety**	
DEGREE OF ANXIETY	**SUBJECTIVE EFFECTS**	**OBSERVABLE BEHAVIOR**
Mild	Perceptual field widens slightly. Increased ability to see relationships among data.	Alert, more perceptive, able to recognize anxiety. Promotes motivation and growth.
Moderate	Perceptual field narrows slightly. Concentrates on the immediate focus, ignoring peripheral stimuli. Can change attention if directed.	Able to sustain attention on a focal point. Inattentive to stimuli outside this focus. May talk faster. Vital signs begin to increase (except temperature). Able to recognize and express anxiety.
Severe	Perceptual field is greatly reduced. Does not notice external events. Unable to redirect focus even with outside direction.	Attention is focused on a small part of a specific area. Assumptions made may be erroneous due to incomplete perception. May be unaware of anxiety. Vital signs increasing. Coping/relief measures used.
Panic	Perception is reduced to a detail. Perception is distorted. May jump from one detail to another, as in flight of ideas. Experienced as a threat to survival. Affected person feels dread, terror.	Feelings of unreality, confusion, terror, self-absorption. May be expressed with violence toward self or others. Loss of control. May include pacing or running. Automatic coping/relief behaviors used. Can result in exhaustion if prolonged.

(National Institute of Mental Health [NIMH], n.d.). Box 51-2■ describes patients' feelings about various anxiety disorders in their own words.

Unlike people with other anxiety disorders, people with GAD do not usually avoid situations that are anxiety producing. When the disorder is mild, affected people can function, but at its worst it is very debilitating.

Generalized anxiety disorder affects about twice as many women as men in the general population. In treatment settings, the nurse can expect to see about equal numbers of women and men seeking treatment. In any given year, approximately 3% of the population will have this disorder. Over a lifetime, any individual has about a 9% chance of having it. This disorder is commonly associated with major depressive disorder (APA, 2013).

Panic Disorder

People with panic disorder have recurrent, unexpected panic attacks followed by at least 1 month of persistent concern about having another one. They may worry about the possible complications of the attacks or have a significant behavioral change associated with the attacks (APA, 2013).

A panic attack is characterized by an abrupt episode of intense fear or discomfort. During this episode, four or more of the following are present: sweating; pounding heart, palpitations, or increased heart rate; tremors; chest pain or discomfort; shortness of breath; sensation of choking; nausea or abdominal distress; feeling faint, dizzy, light-headed, or unsteady; chills or hot flashes; abnormal peripheral sensations (numbness, tingling); derealization or feeling detached from oneself; fear of losing control of self or "going crazy"; or fear of dying (APA, 2013).

People with panic disorder may have panic attacks without warning. For some people, the attacks are associated with a predictable stressor. Because there is no way to predict when an attack will occur, people often spend time worrying about when the next one will strike. Unpredictable panic attacks can occur anytime, even during sleep. An attack usually peaks in severity within 10 minutes, but some symptoms last longer. Affected people may feel like they are dying. Untreated, the disorder can be very disabling. Affected people often avoid the site or situation of a previous attack, severely limiting the ability to function. For example, if a person experienced an anxiety attack at a grocery store and another attack on a bus, this individual may not be able to shop for groceries or go to work.

Not everyone who has a panic attack will go on to have panic disorder. Some people have one attack, with no recurrence. In some people, panic attacks are associated with another mental disorder.

BOX 51-2   PATIENTS SPEAK THEIR MINDS ABOUT ANXIETY DISORDERS

Generalized Anxiety Disorder
"I always thought I was just a worrier. I'd feel keyed up and unable to relax. At times it would come and go, and at times it would be constant. I'd worry about what I was going to fix for dinner or what would be a great present for somebody. I just couldn't let something go. I'd have terrible sleeping problems. There were times I'd wake up wired in the middle of the night. I had trouble concentrating, even reading the newspaper or a novel. Sometimes my heart would race or pound, and that would make me worry more. I was always imagining things were worse than they really were; when I got a stomachache, I'd think it was an ulcer" (NIMH, n.d.).

Panic Disorder
"For me, a panic attack is almost a violent experience. I feel disconnected from reality. I feel like I'm losing control in a very extreme way. My heart pounds really hard, I feel like I can't get my breath, and there's an overwhelming feeling that things are crashing in on me. It started 10 years ago, when I had just graduated from college and started a new job. I was sitting in a business seminar in a hotel and this thing came out of the blue. I felt like I was dying. In between attacks there is this dread and anxiety that it's going to happen again. I'm afraid to go back to places where I've had an attack. Unless I get help, there soon won't be anyplace where I can go and feel safe from panic" (NIMH, n.d.).

Agoraphobia
"At first I was uneasy about being in crowds of people, like at the mall or in a really big store. Then I became paralyzed with fear when I got on the bus. I felt trapped, like I would die if I couldn't get off the bus. I lost my job because I couldn't take the bus to get there. I don't feel safe unless I am at home. I never go out alone anymore" (NIMH, n.d.).

Obsessive-Compulsive Disorder
"I couldn't do anything without rituals. They invaded every aspect of my life. Counting really bogged me down. I would wash my hair three times as opposed to once because three was a good luck number and one wasn't. It took me longer to read because I'd count the lines in a paragraph. When I set my alarm at night, I had to set it to a number that wouldn't add up to a 'bad' number. I know the rituals didn't make sense, and I was deeply ashamed of them, but I couldn't seem to overcome them until I had therapy. Getting dressed in the morning was tough, because I had a routine, and if I didn't follow the routine, I'd get anxious and would have to get dressed again. I always worried that if I didn't do something, my parents were going to die. I'd have these terrible thoughts of harming my parents. That was completely irrational, but the thought triggered more anxiety and more senseless behavior. Because of the time I spent on rituals, I was unable to do a lot of things that were important to me" (NIMH, n.d.).

clinicalALERT

People experiencing panic disorder often visit the hospital emergency department several times before they are accurately diagnosed. It may be years before they find out that they have a real, treatable illness (NIMH, n.d.). It is critical for emergency department nurses and physicians to be aware of panic disorder.

Key Concept Many people with treatable anxiety disorder avoid treatment because they do not realize they have a psychiatric problem, do not think they will be believed, or fear the stigma of mental illness.

Imagine a person who comes to the hospital with a terrifying panic episode, believing that she is dying. A physical assessment and EKG show no abnormalities. The episode is resolving by the time the tests are done. The patient is told that there is nothing wrong. The patient may even be told that she has misused the emergency department. This patient is suffering not only the effects of the panic attack but also the humiliation of not being taken seriously. Panic disorder is often associated with other serious disorders such as depression or other mental disorders. Incidence of suicide is increased in people affected by this disorder. The disorder affects three times as many women as men and affects 1% to 2% of the general population. The onset is usually between late adolescence and the mid-thirties, although it can begin at any age (APA, 2013).

Agoraphobia

A **phobia** is a persistent and irrational fear. Agoraphobia is characterized by anxiety about being in places or situations where escape may be difficult (or embarrassing) or when help might not be available in the case of a panic attack. Agoraphobic fears typically include situations that involve being alone away from home in a crowd or standing in line, on a bridge, or traveling in a plane, train, bus, or automobile. The fear-producing situations are avoided, are endured with much anxiety and distress, or require the presence of a companion (APA, 2013).

Agoraphobia is commonly associated with panic disorder. Agoraphobia is more likely to occur in females than in males. It can result in severe impairment in social and occupational functioning when the individual avoids multiple anxiety-producing situations (APA, 2013).

Not everyone who stays home has agoraphobia. Agoraphobia exists when people confine themselves within their homes to avoid overwhelming anxiety. In some cultures, women are expected to remain at home, and their public activities are greatly limited. If a woman from such a culture stays at home, she is acting in accordance with cultural expectations and does not have a mental disorder.

Social Anxiety Disorder

Social anxiety disorder is characterized by a marked and persistent fear of social or performance situations in which embarrassment may occur. Exposure to the social or performance situation (e.g., public speaking or speaking to a supervisor) almost always results in an immediate anxiety reaction. Affected people may fear that they are being watched and judged by everyone in the area. Adults and adolescents with social phobia usually recognize that their fear is excessive; affected children may not. People usually avoid the risky situations but may endure them with dread. Social anxiety disorder only exists if the fear, avoidance, or anxiety about encountering the social situation interferes significantly with the affected individual's daily routine, social, academic, or occupational life or if the person is markedly distressed by the disorder. Anticipatory anxiety may begin weeks before an anticipated social event (APA, 2013).

The symptoms must have lasted for more than 6 months and out of proportion to the danger that is present to make the diagnosis of social anxiety disorder. Temporary social anxiety in childhood or adolescence is quite common and does not constitute social anxiety disorder. Neither does fear of speaking in situations where fear may be justified, such as when the teacher calls on a student who did not do the homework.

Physical symptoms often accompany the anxiety in social anxiety disorder. These include blushing, excessive sweating, nausea, GI distress, tremors, and difficulty talking. Although they realize that their fears are irrational, people with this disorder are unable to control it. Even after they have done the dreaded deed, affected people continue to feel anxious about how they were perceived and judged by others. Making or keeping friends may be difficult. People with social phobia may medicate their symptoms with alcohol or drugs to make it possible for them to endure social situations.

Social Anxiety Disorder

"In any social situation, I felt fear. I would be anxious before I even left the house, and it would escalate as I got closer to a college class, a party, or whatever. I would feel sick at my stomach—it almost felt like I had the flu. My heart would pound, my palms would get sweaty, and I would get this feeling of being removed from everybody else.

"When I would walk into a room full of people, I'd turn red and it would feel like everybody's eyes were on me. I was embarrassed to stand off in a corner by myself, but I couldn't think of anything to say to anybody. It was humiliating. I felt so clumsy; I couldn't wait to get out.

"I couldn't go on dates, and for a while I couldn't even go to class. My sophomore year of college I had to go home for a semester. I felt like such a failure" (NIMH, n.d.).

Specific Phobias

A specific phobia is an excessive fear of a specific object or situation. It might be triggered by the presence, or even the anticipation, of the feared object. Affected people have an immediate anxiety reaction in response to the feared situation, which may take the form of a panic attack. Some examples of specific phobias are animals, flying, heights, or needles. See Table 51-3 ■ for examples of specific phobias and their clinical names. Adults with phobias may or may not recognize that their fears are unreasonable. People usually avoid the phobic stimulus but may endure it with intense anxiety or dread, worrying about it to the extent that their daily routine, occupational or academic functioning, social life, or quality of life are affected. People with phobias experience marked distress (APA, 2013).

Children often have fears that seem irrational to adults. A child with a fear is not diagnosed with a specific phobia unless the fear is specific, is extreme, causes great distress, and has affected school or daily functioning for at least 6 months. Children with phobias may not realize that their fears are irrational. Anxiety in children may be expressed by crying, clinging, the inability to move or "freezing with fear," or tantrums.

People with phobias involving situations or objects that are easy to avoid may not feel the need to seek treatment. A specific phobia is not diagnosed unless the phobia significantly interferes with the individual's functioning or causes severe distress. It often occurs in people who also have other anxiety disorders, mood disorders, and substance-related disorders.

People who have a blood-injection-injury phobia have a history of fainting from a vasovagal response in about 75% of cases (APA, 2013). Nurses should be aware of the possibility of patients fainting during injections or, more frequently, blood draws.

clinicalALERT

The extreme fear in the phobia of blood or needles may result in the *vasovagal response*. The patient's heart and respiratory rates initially increase due to sympathetic stimulation. When the vagus nerve is stimulated, the heart rate and blood pressure fall, potentially resulting in a loss of consciousness. The potential for fainting is one of the reasons that patients should be in a sitting or recumbent position for injections or venipuncture.

The first symptoms of specific phobias usually occur in childhood but can also be in adulthood. Factors that predispose people to develop specific phobias include (APA, 2013):

- Traumatic events such as being trapped in a closet or attacked by an animal.
- Unexpected panic attacks in the feared situation.
- Observing others in the feared situation (seeing someone fall from a height).
- Seeing others demonstrate fear in the situation (mother is afraid of going to the dentist).
- Informational transmission (media coverage of bombing, natural disasters, plane crashes, or repeated parental warnings about dangers of some situation).

The subjects of specific phobias differ from one culture to another. Women are more frequently affected by phobias than men are, at a rate of 2:1. The prevalence of phobias decreases in older adults. Some phobias tend to run in families, especially the fears of blood and injury (APA, 2013).

Social Phobia: Aviophobia

A person with *aviophobia* (fear of flying) stated: "I'm scared to death of flying, and I never do it anymore. I used to start dreading a plane trip a month before I was due to leave. It was an awful feeling when the airplane door closed and I felt trapped. My heart would pound and I would sweat bullets. When the airplane would start to ascend, it just reinforced the feeling that I couldn't get out.... I'm not afraid of crashing. It's just that feeling of being trapped. Whenever I've thought of changing jobs I think 'Would I be under pressure to fly?' These days I only go places where I can drive or take a train. My friends always point out that I couldn't get off a train traveling at high speeds either, so why don't trains bother me? I just tell them it isn't a rational fear" (NIMH, n.d.).

TABLE 51-3	Specific Phobia Names
CLINICAL NAME	**FEARED OBJECT OR SITUATION**
Acrophobia	Heights
Apiphobia	Bees
Astraphobia	Lightning
Aviophobia	Flying
Claustrophobia	Closed spaces
Entomophobia	Insects
Gephyrophobia	Bridge crossing
Hematophobia	Blood
Hydrophobia	Water
Iatrophobia	Doctors
Microphobia	Germs
Monophobia (or autophobia)	Being alone
Mysophobia	Dirt
Nyctophobia	Darkness, night
Pyrophobia	Fire
Xenophobia	Strangers

Obsessive-Compulsive Disorder

The second classification of anxiety disorders is called obsessive-compulsive and related disorders. This group has been changed from the previous classification system due to emerging evidence of the relatedness of disorders such as obsessive-compulsive disorder (OCD), hoarding, and body dysmorphic disorder (Reichenberg, 2014). **Obsessions** are recurrent and intrusive thoughts that caused marked distress. The affected person recognizes that these thoughts are from her or his own mind and tries to ignore or suppress the obsessive thoughts. **Compulsions** are repetitive behaviors or mental acts that the affected person feels driven to perform in response to obsessive thoughts. The objective of these behaviors is to reduce stress or to prevent some dreaded event. The compulsive behaviors are not realistically connected with the situations they are supposed to neutralize, or they are clearly excessive (APA, 2013).

Obsessive-compulsive disorder is characterized by compulsions or obsessions, which the affected person recognizes as excessive or unreasonable. It causes marked distress and takes more than 1 hour each day or significantly interferes with the affected person's daily occupational, academic, or personal functioning (APA, 2013).

Common obsessive thoughts involve dirt and germs, numbers or counting, symmetry and order, ideas that are against the individual's religious beliefs, or sexual thoughts that are disgusting to the affected individual. Some examples of compulsive rituals are cleaning, hand washing, touching or doing things in a certain order, or praying. There is no pleasure for the affected individual in performing the compulsive rituals, only temporary relief from the anxiety caused by not doing these things (NIMH, n.d.). Figure 51-4■ depicts some of these compulsive behaviors.

Many people without OCD have some compulsive behavior, such as checking several times that the stove is really off before leaving home. This behavior does not become OCD until it becomes distressing, consumes over an hour a day, or interferes with the individual's daily life.

OCD usually begins in adolescence or early adulthood. It can begin in childhood. It tends to affect males at an earlier age than females. Affected children often do not realize that the behavior is unreasonable. The majority of affected people experience OCD with a waxing and waning course. The disorder becomes more severe in the presence of stress. OCD occurs more often in first-degree relatives of people with OCD and Tourette disorder than in the general population. OCD occurs in many cultures around the world. It affects approximately 1% to 2% of people at some time in their lives (APA, 2013).

Some people with OCD also have depression or other anxiety disorders. Some have eating disorders. The disorder can involve people so severely that their development or ability to function in their daily lives is affected.

Posttraumatic Stress Disorder

The third classification of anxiety-related disorder is trauma- and stressor-related disorders. Posttraumatic stress disorder (PTSD) is one of these. PTSD was first recognized in war veterans. It is a debilitating condition that follows an extreme traumatic stressor. The traumatic stressor can involve an event that threatens the individual's own life, safety, or personal integrity; witnessing death or serious injury of another; learning about the unexpected, violent death, or serious harm to a significant other; or being repeatedly or traumatically exposed to the repulsive details of a traumatic event (as in police repeatedly exposed to child abuse or first responders to disasters with fatalities). The person's response to the event will involve intense fear, helplessness, or horror. Children respond with agitated or disorganized behavior. The characteristic symptoms of PTSD include the following, which are present for more than 1 month (APA, 2013): persistent reexperiencing of the traumatic event; avoidance of stimuli associated with the trauma; numbing of general responsiveness; increased arousal (difficulty sleeping, nightmares, exaggerated startle response, and hypervigilance or alertness for danger); **depersonalization**, which is the experience of being an outside observer of or detached from oneself; and **derealization**, which is the experience of unreality, distance, or distortion ("This is not real").

Traumatic events that might result in PTSD include, but are not limited to, violent personal assault (sexual assault, physical attack, robbery), military combat, being taken hostage, terrorist attack, torture, imprisonment as a prisoner of war or in a concentration camp, disasters, transportation crashes, or diagnosis of life-threatening illness. Children may develop PTSD as a result of sexual or other

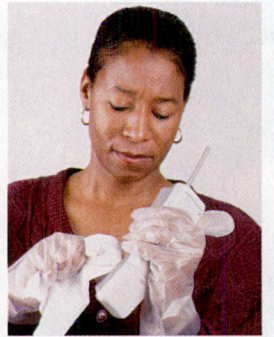
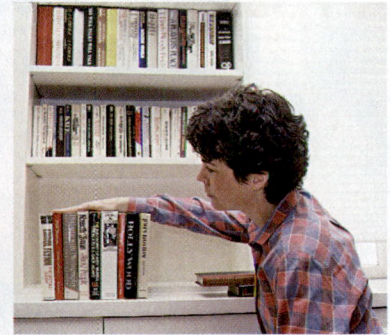

Figure 51-4. ■ These photos show people who suffer from OCD in typical situations: (1) obsessive fear of germs with compulsive cleaning and (2) a woman measuring her books to arrange them "properly." (Sources: Left: © Spencer Grant / PhotoEdit. Right: Pearson Education.)

potentially life-threatening abuse, as well as the stimuli listed earlier. The disorder is more likely to occur and to be more long lasting when the stressor is an intended human action, such as rape or torture (APA, 2013). Some of the people who survived the attack on the World Trade Center on September 11, 2001, have developed PTSD.

People with PTSD can reexperience the traumatic event in various ways. Commonly, the person has repeated intrusive memories or dreams of the event. Some people experience flashbacks in which they relive the event, believing that it is actually happening. A flashback may include sights, sounds, smells, or feelings from the traumatic event.

Affected people feel distressed by situations that remind them of the event and avoid these situations. For example, a person who was raped in an elevator may avoid all elevators. A person who was held in a prison camp with military guards may avoid anyone in uniform. Ordinary events can trigger memories and a flashback in susceptible individuals.

People with PTSD may have difficulty with interpersonal relationships. They may have difficulty trusting or being affectionate. Things they formerly enjoyed may not provide pleasure for them anymore. Irritability, aggression, even violence may be expressed even if they were out of character for the person before the incident. Depression sometimes occurs in people with PTSD, and the rate of suicide is high. As with people affected by other anxiety disorders, people with PTSD may use alcohol and other substances to medicate their anxiety symptoms.

People who experience extreme trauma often have some of the symptoms of PTSD, but the disorder is only diagnosed if symptoms persist for longer than a month. Development of PTSD usually occurs within 3 months of the traumatic experience.

PTSD can occur at any age, and about half of those affected experience complete resolution of symptoms within 3 months. The most important risk factors for development of this disorder are severity of the traumatic event, duration of the trauma, and proximity of the individual's exposure. Approximately 8% of people in the United States will be affected at some time in their lives. The highest rates of occurrence of PTSD are in people who have survived rape, military combat, and captivity, and ethnically or politically motivated imprisonment and genocide (APA, 2013).

MILITARY SEXUAL TRAUMA

The U.S. Veterans Administration has identified a condition called *military sexual trauma* (MST). The experience includes either sexual assault or repeated, threatening sexual harassment that occurred while the veteran was in the military (National Center for PTSD, 2014). Both men and women can be the victims of military sexual trauma, and the perpetrator can be of the same or opposite gender.

The Department of Defense conducted a large study of sexual victimization among active duty populations and found that 78% of women and 38% of men had experienced sexual harassment during a 1-year period. Rates of completed or attempted sexual assault were estimated at 6% for women and 1% for men. The exact rate is difficult to determine due to the strong pressure not to report sexual assault in the military. Research in the Persian Gulf War found that the rates of sexual assault and harassment actually increased during wartime (Suris & Lind, 2012).

Victims of military sexual trauma are at increased risk for PTSD. Men have a 65% risk and women a 45.9% risk of developing PTSD after military sexual trauma (Figure 51-5■). Military sexual trauma causes a greater risk for PTSD than even military combat, which causes PTSD at a general rate of 38.8%. Military veterans with PTSD due to military sexual trauma have higher rates of major depressive disorder, difficulty adjusting after discharge, poorer psychological and physical health, and substance abuse (Burgess, Slattery, & Herlihy, 2013).

The implication for health care providers is that veterans should be assessed carefully for military sexual trauma due to the stigma associated with sexual victimization and the reluctance of victims to report or even acknowledge that it happened. Military camaraderie and the fact that the perpetrators often work closely with the victims make accurate data collection difficult. Rather than asking about "rape" or "sexual harassment," it may be easier for these victims to answer questions such as "While you were in the military, did you ever experience any unwanted sexual attention, like verbal remarks, touching, or pressure for sexual favors?" and "Did anyone ever use force or the threat of force to have sex with you against your will?" The Veterans Administration

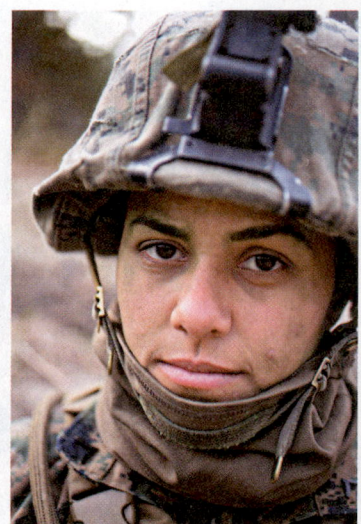

Figure 51-5. ■ Veterans who experience military sexual trauma are at even higher risk to develop PTSD than those who experience combat. (Source: © US Marines Photo/Alamy.)

BOX 51-3	MILITARY SEXUAL TRAUMA

A woman who experienced military sexual trauma said the following: "One of my superior officers was always making sexual jokes or comments to the enlisted women. We just tried to ignore it, or smile so he wouldn't get angry. I had to deliver papers to his tent on a regular basis. I always tried to do it when someone else was there. On the time that he raped me, I couldn't scream, I tried to push him away and tell him not to, but I couldn't even fight too hard because he was my commander. I never felt so helpless. I never felt safe again. Later I thought, 'We are both in the U.S. Army. Who is on my side now?' I never told anyone while I was deployed. I thought they would believe him, or I would get in trouble, or that nobody would believe that it happened at all. When I got out, the nurse at the VA asked me if I had anything like this happen. I was so thankful that someone acknowledged what happened. Now I'm in a women survivors' group. I still have trouble sleeping. I've thought about it every day since it happened. I feel guilty and always afraid. This was the worst thing that happened to me during the war" (Yaeger, Himmelfarb, Cammack, & Mintz, 2006).

mandates universal screening of veterans for a history of military sexual trauma (National Center for PTSD, 2014). Box 51-3■ describes this in a patient's own words.

COLLABORATIVE CARE
Coping With Anxiety
Coping is managing and adapting to stress. People use **coping behaviors** to adapt to or manage stress or change. To control anxiety, people develop patterns of coping behavior. Coping behaviors can be **adaptive** (healthy or likely to lead to positive resolution) or **maladaptive** (unhealthy). Coping behaviors are the conscious ways in which people deal with stress.

A person who uses active problem solving, while considering the rights of others, is using coping behavior adaptively. An example of using adaptive coping behavior is a nurse asking another nurse to help determine why a patient's condition is changing. Maladaptive behavior might be expressed by negative or aggressive behavior toward others. An example of maladaptive active coping behavior is a nurse shouting at a nursing assistant who made a mistake.

UNCONSCIOUS DEFENSE MECHANISMS   Some methods of coping are part of our conscious thoughts, whereas others are unconscious. People use both conscious coping behaviors and unconscious defense mechanisms. These defense mechanisms may also be adaptive or maladaptive. See Table 51-4■ for specific examples of defense mechanisms.

Because the symptom of anxiety is associated with so many different physiologic and psychosocial problems, an accurate diagnosis must be made before treatment begins. It could be dangerous to treat the anxiety caused by hypoxia

with an antianxiety agent. Some general medical disorders that frequently present with anxiety are listed in Box 51-4■.

There are effective treatments for anxiety disorders. Each disorder is treated specifically, but generally the most effective treatments are cognitive-behavior therapy and medications.

Cognitive-Behavior Therapy
Cognitive-behavior therapy (CBT) is based on the idea that how we think (cognition), how we feel (emotion), and how we act (behavior) all affect each other (Figure 51-6■). When CBT is used to reduce anxiety, the patient discovers more adaptive ways to interpret the irrational beliefs and more healthy behavior to replace the unhealthy behavior.

CBT is effective for most anxiety disorders. It has two parts, the cognitive and the behavioral. In the cognitive therapy part, patients are helped to change thinking patterns that contribute to their anxieties. Cognitive therapy includes education about the physiology behind anxiety reactions. It is based on the idea that thinking errors by the patient produce irrational negative beliefs that continue despite evidence to the contrary.

In CBT, patients are taught how to differentiate their thoughts (which may be irrational) from reality. They learn the influence that their thoughts have on their feelings and they are taught how to recognize, observe, and monitor their own thoughts. Patients challenge their own irrational beliefs and prove their own irrational thoughts to be wrong. As a result, their thoughts and beliefs begin to change. For example, in social situations a person may be anxious, may challenge the idea that socializing is awful, and then may go out bowling, to a movie, or for a walk with a friend as a CBT homework assignment. When the patient enjoys the social activity, the person's thoughts begin to change. The homework in CBT involves examining one's own thought processes (especially automatic negative thoughts, or ANTs), thinking about the reality or irrationality of these negative beliefs, and then thinking of a more balanced way to think more rationally.

Albert Ellis (1962) said that we each hold a set of assumptions about ourselves and the world that serve to guide us through life, and determine our reactions to the situations we experience. He said that some people's assumptions are irrational, guiding them to act and react in ways that are self-defeating and decrease their chances of happiness and success.

Some people irrationally assume that they are worthless if everyone they know does not love them. They constantly seek approval and constantly feel rejected. All their interactions are affected by this assumption, so they may leave a great party feeling rejected because they did not receive

TABLE 51-4	Defense Mechanisms	
DEFENSE MECHANISM	**DEFINITION**	**EXAMPLE**
Acting out	Using actions instead of thoughts or feelings to respond to stress or emotional distress	A child who is afraid of being hospitalized kicks the nurse and knocks supplies off the hospital shelf.
Altruism	Dealing with emotional conflict by meeting the needs of others, receiving gratification either vicariously or from the reactions of others	A young man's fiancée leaves him, and he joins the Peace Corps.
Anticipation	Experiencing emotional reactions in advance of a stressful event	When first diagnosed with diabetes, a man begins to experience anticipatory grief for his eventual loss of function and health.
Compensation	Attempt (conscious or unconscious) to overcome perceived inadequacies	A girl who is disappointed to have little athletic skill works hard to excel in academics.
Denial	Refusal to acknowledge a painful reality	A person with alcoholism says, "I don't have a drinking problem, I can quit whenever I want."
Displacement	Transference of a feeling about one person or object to another, usually safer, one	A patient is very angry with his doctor but yells at the nurse.
Dissociation	A breakdown in the usually integrated functions of consciousness, memory, or perception. Detachment from emotional significance	A woman calmly describes her severe sexual abuse in childhood as though she were outside herself watching it happen.
Humor	Emphasis on amusing or ironic aspects of a stressful experience	After making a mistake in front of the class, the teacher makes a joke about it.
Intellectualization	Excessive use of abstract thinking or using generalizations to control disturbing feelings	A man analyzes and explains to a friend the interpersonal dynamics that led to his divorce.
Projection	Attributing one's own unacceptable feelings or thoughts to another	A person who does not like children says, "Children just don't like me."
Rationalization	Concealing the true motivations (even to ourselves) behind our actions with incorrect but acceptable motivations	Instead of admitting that he went to this college to be with his girlfriend, the student says that it is the best college in the state.
Reaction formation	Substituting behavior or feelings that are the opposite of what one actually feels	A woman does not like her supervisor at work, yet she gives the supervisor gifts and compliments.
Regression	Return to an earlier, less stressful level of adjustment	A child returns to bedwetting after being hospitalized.
Repression	Removing unacceptable thoughts or wishes from consciousness	A woman has no memory of being raped but may feel anxious when she goes near the area where it happened.
Sublimation	Diversion of unacceptable feelings into socially acceptable behavior	A person is very angry and runs for hours on the track.
Suppression	Intentionally avoiding thinking about unacceptable or stressful feelings	A woman does not have enough money to pay her bills and keeps herself busy with housework to avoid thinking about money.

enough compliments. According to Ellis, some common irrational beliefs include:

- One should be loved and accepted by everyone he or she knows.
- The idea that one should be thoroughly competent at everything.
- It is catastrophic when things are not the way you want them to be.
- The idea that your past history greatly influences your present life.
- The idea that a perfect solution to human problems exists and it is a disaster if you do not find it.

Cognitive restructuring is a therapeutic technique in which the patient works to change patterns of negative thoughts that occur automatically (automatic negative thoughts, ANTs). Patients are helped to reinterpret their automatic negative anxiety-producing thoughts and negative self-talk. When patients see the basis for the erroneous negative thinking, they can see the situation realistically. Realistic thinking helps patients develop more balanced and reality-based coping strategies; in other words, changing thinking changes behavior and feelings.

For example, a man with panic disorder can learn to replace the thought "I am dying!" with "I'm OK. This is

BOX 51-4   GENERAL MEDICAL CONDITIONS ASSOCIATED WITH ANXIETY

- Hypoglycemia
- Hyperthyroidism
- Asthma
- Pneumonia
- Chronic obstructive pulmonary disease
- Pulmonary embolism
- Encephalitis
- Cardiac dysrhythmias
- Vitamin B_{12} deficiency
- Pheochromocytoma (adrenal tumor)
- Vestibular dysfunction
- Hyperthyroidism
- Neoplasms

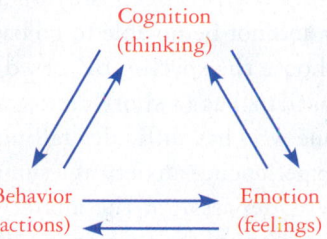

Figure 51-6. ■ Cognitive-behavior therapy is based on the idea that cognition, feelings, and behavior are interrelated.

a panic attack." In CBT, he can discuss his experiences, looking for symptoms and events that come before the panic attacks, to help identify triggers. Finally, he can be helped to find new ways to think about the triggers that start panic attacks, so that he can avoid having them progress into panic.

The goal of the behavioral therapy part of CBT is to change the patient's reaction to anxiety-provoking situations. One behavioral approach is to teach the patient deep-breathing or relaxation techniques to use in situations that they expect will provoke anxiety, thus interrupting the automatic anxiety responses. Homework may include trying dreaded activities to discover whether the dread is irrational or trying new healthy behavior that replaces maladaptive behavior.

Because avoidance of a feared object or situation prevents the person from learning that it is harmless, *exposure* is an important aspect of behavioral therapy for anxiety disorders. In exposure therapy, patients confront the thing they fear. One approach, called *exposure and response prevention*, is often used with people who have OCD. If patients fear dirt and germs, the therapist may encourage them to dirty their hands and then wait a certain amount of time before washing. The therapist helps the patient to cope

with the anxiety that results, and the patient experiences a coping success. With repetition of this technique, the patient will experience a series of successes in surviving being dirty, and the anxiety will decrease over time (NIMH, n.d.).

In another type of exposure exercise, a person with social phobia may be encouraged to spend a certain amount of time in a feared social situation, while fighting the desire to run away. The patient may be asked to try making a small social error to see how others will respond. The therapist then discusses the reaction of others and helps the patient see that the fear of judgment by others is not as brutal as the patient feared. Repeated practice and discussion of feelings and coping techniques with the therapist can help reduce social phobia.

Behavioral therapy alone has long been used effectively to treat specific phobias. The person is gradually exposed to the feared object or situation. Initially, the exposure may only be to pictures of the feared object. Later, when patients feel ready, they confront the actual feared situation in a safe setting. The therapist usually goes with the patient to provide support and guidance (NIMH, n.d.).

Aaron Beck (1967) used CBT to help people with depression and anxiety change illogical thinking processes. He identified the following common illogical thinking processes:

- Selective attention: seeking only the negative features of an event
- Magnification: exaggerating the importance of undesirable events
- Overgeneralization: drawing broad negative conclusions on the basis of a single negative event

CBT or behavioral therapy usually takes about 12 weeks and can be done individually or in groups. As with all psychotherapy, CBT must be directed at the patient's specific concerns; an effective approach for a person who has OCD and intrusive sexual thoughts will not be effective for a person who fears nursing exams.

Promoting Resilience

Resilience is the quality of being hardy or "stress resistant." Resilient people are "survivors" who are able to cope adaptively and seem to flourish despite stress that other people cannot tolerate. Hars, Herrmann, Gold, Rizzoli, & Trombetti (2013) studied older people in the community and discovered several factors that are associated with resilience in the older population. The resilience factors are as follows:

- Self-efficacy (the belief that individuals have control over events in their own lives)
- Regular exercise

- High functional ability
- Independence with activities of daily living
- Good self-rated health
- Positive outlook on life

Health care professionals may be able to promote resilience in patients by supporting their functional abilities and general health. Helping patients make plans to exercise regularly, using activities that are acceptable and available to them, can help improve their resilience. It would also prevent anxiety. This is also evidence of the importance of treating depression in older adults.

Medication

Medications from several classifications treat anxiety effectively. There is some controversy about the use of antianxiety medications, however. As a general rule, people are better off if they can develop the tools to solve their own problems without using drugs to solve problems. This is especially true for people who have transient or low-level anxiety or poor coping skills. The best approach to anxiety treatment for these patients is to promote adaptive coping skills. Medications should not be used when more adaptive approaches could realistically solve the problem.

Despite the potential hazards of antianxiety drugs for a few patients, there are many situations in which they are indicated. Some forms of anxiety, such as specific phobias, respond best to behavioral therapy alone. But most anxiety disorders require a combination of medication and psychotherapy for effective treatment. People with panic disorder may require the long-term prescription of antianxiety drugs if they are not able to function without them.

Nurses should be aware that many people with mental disorders require medications to function. People with depression require antidepressants; those with psychosis require antipsychotics, just as those with anxiety disorders often require antianxiety medications to control their symptoms so they can meet their developmental needs, such as having relationships, working, and going to school. Although the antianxiety medications are contraindicated as a problem-solving approach for the otherwise normal patient, they are required for the well-being of many people with severe anxiety disorders. Nurses must be supportive of these individuals who need medications, because there is a loud message in our culture that says "Just Say No to Drugs" in any situation. There is also a stigma attached to not being able to "handle your problems yourself." The message from mental health care providers is "Take medications if you need them to treat mental disorders."

Nurses should educate patients that if one treatment is not effective, it is worth trying other treatment modalities. A combination of psychotherapy and medications proves to be the most effective for the most people. If one medication is not effective, another one is likely to work. People often must work with their health care providers to find the one that works best for them, which may take time.

ANTIANXIETY AGENTS Benzodiazepines (BZs) are the most widely prescribed drugs in the world today. They are used for anxiety, insomnia, alcohol withdrawal, skeletal muscle relaxation, acute management of seizures, severe agitation, social phobia, generalized anxiety disorder, and panic disorder. They continue to be the mainstay of anxiety management due to their efficacy, rapid onset, and generally favorable side effect profile (Stahl, 2013). See Table 51-5 ■ for information about the BZ drugs.

The target symptoms for the antianxiety (also called *anxiolytic*) drugs are nervousness, sweating, increased heart rate, sense of dread, fearfulness, phobias, compulsiveness, nausea, vomiting, diarrhea, dizziness, irritability, headache, and dry mouth. The target symptoms for sedative-hypnotics are insomnia and sleep disorders. **Insomnia** includes difficulty falling asleep, staying asleep, or awakening too early and not being able to go back to sleep. The provider can choose the specific BZ based on which sleep problem the patient has (a short-acting agent would be best for someone who has difficulty falling asleep). When the patient is experiencing anxiety as a symptom of another disorder, such as depression, the anxiety will probably resolve with treatment of the primary problem.

Mechanism of Action Benzodiazepines are CNS depressants. They enhance the effects of gamma-aminobutyric acid (GABA), which is an inhibitory neurotransmitter. GABA makes the neuron less responsive to excitatory neurotransmitters such as norepinephrine, serotonin, and dopamine. The overall effect is to slow neuronal firing, which results in the CNS depressant properties of the BZs (Stahl, 2013).

Side Effects Benzodiazepines are CNS depressants and have some common side effects. The common side effects include sedation, drowsiness, dizziness, and decreased

TABLE 51-5	Benzodiazepine Antianxiety and Sedative-Hypnotic Agents
DRUG	**DURATION OF ACTION**
Benzodiazepine antianxiety agents	
Alprazolam (Xanax)	Intermediate acting
Chlordiazepoxide (Librium)	Long acting
Clonazepam (Klonopin)	Long acting
Clorazepate (Tranxene)	Long acting
Diazepam (Valium)	Long acting
Halazepam (Paxipam)	Intermediate acting
Lorazepam (Ativan)	Intermediate acting
Oxazepam (Serax)	Intermediate acting
Prazepam (Centrax)	Long acting

coordination. Older adults may have difficulty metabolizing the long-acting BZs and may have increasing blood levels. The shorter-acting agents are a better choice for older adults. They are also more likely to suffer cognitive or memory side effects to long-term BZ therapy than are younger adults.

Occasionally patients will have a **paradoxical response** (contradictory, opposite from expected response) to the BZs. Instead of relaxation, they experience agitation or unstable emotions. Older adults, children, and people with brain damage are at increased risk. When a patient has a paradoxical reaction, the BZ should be discontinued.

Other important concerns with BZs are physical dependence and tolerance:

- Prolonged use of BZs causes a decrease in GABA receptors. Remember that GABA is an inhibiting transmitter. With a reduced capacity for inhibition, CNS stimulation results. When the BZ is discontinued abruptly, the CNS is stimulated and unable to inhibit or regulate itself. The patient experiences all the symptoms of CNS stimulation, including anxiety, agitation, increased blood pressure and pulse, and even possibly seizures. These CNS stimulation symptoms constitute BZ withdrawal. Withdrawal can be prevented by slowly decreasing (tapering) doses, instead of suddenly discontinuing a BZ in a patient who has taken it regularly for an extended period (longer than 2 weeks). The presence of withdrawal does not constitute addiction (addiction is a psychologic process). These are safe drugs that must be prescribed with care and knowledge of their effects. Psychologic dependence occurs when patients believe that they cannot live or function without the drug to treat their anxiety.
- Prolonged regular use also causes tolerance (less response to the same dose, requiring increased doses to give the same effect). Patients become tolerant to the sedative effects relatively quickly. It takes longer to develop tolerance to the antianxiety effect.

Drug Interactions   Overdoses of BZs alone are not commonly fatal. Fatalities involving the combination of BZs and alcohol are relatively common. An additive CNS depressant effect occurs when BZs are taken with CNS depressants such as alcohol, tricyclic antidepressants, MAOIs, anticonvulsants, antihistamines, or antipsychotics.

NON-BENZODIAZEPINE ANTIANXIETY AGENTS   Buspirone (BuSpar) is an effective non-BZ antianxiety agent. It differs from BZs in several ways. It does not bind to the same brain sites. It probably acts as a serotonin agonist. Buspirone is not effective against seizures, muscle spasm, or alcohol withdrawal, nor does it treat panic disorder effectively. Buspirone is not sedating, does not cause euphoria, and has no cross-tolerance with sedatives or alcohol. An example of

cross-tolerance is seen in patients who are tolerant to large amounts of alcohol. They will also be tolerant to BZs, even if they have never taken them before. Buspirone does not cause dependence or withdrawal. It has virtually no abuse potential and is not a controlled substance. It begins to have antianxiety effects within 7 to 10 days but may take up to 6 weeks to achieve full effect.

Propranolol is a blocker of beta-adrenergic receptors (beta-blocker). Rather than acting directly on anxiety, it decreases some anxiety symptoms, such as increased heart rate. It is used in the treatment of social anxiety disorder, for such problems as performance anxiety. See Box 51-5 ■ for a list of the non-BZ antianxiety agents.

NON-BENZODIAZEPINE SEDATIVE-HYPNOTIC AGENTS Zaleplon (Sonata) is a non-BZ sedative-hypnotic for the short-term treatment of insomnia. It binds to the BZ receptor and has a very rapid onset and duration of action. It is most effective for patients who have difficulty falling asleep. Patients who only have 4 hours before they have to get up can take it. It has some effects similar to the BZs: sedation and antianxiety, muscle relaxant, and anticonvulsant properties. It has no morning "hangover" effect.

Zolpidem (Ambien) is also used for short-term insomnia treatment. It is similar to Zaleplon in that it binds to BZ receptors and has fewer side effects than the BZs. This drug has a slightly longer half-life (2.5 vs. 1 hour for Zaleplon). It does not have antianxiety, anticonvulsant, or muscle-relaxant effects. It can cause daytime drowsiness, dizziness, and diarrhea.

Antihistamines, such as diphenhydramine (Benadryl), can be used for their sedating effects. Their advantage is that they do not cause dependence, although they are not as effective as the BZs. With prolonged use, patients become tolerant to the sedating side effect of antihistamines.

BARBITURATES   The barbiturates, such as secobarbital and pentobarbital, are rarely used. The other sedative-hypnotic

---

BOX 51-5   NON-BENZODIAZEPINE ANTIANXIETY AND SEDATIVE-HYPNOTIC AGENTS

Antianxiety Agents
Classification: *Azaspirone*
  Generic name: Buspirone
  Trade name: (BuSpar)
Beta-adrenergic blockers
  Propranolol (Inderal)
Sedative-Hypnotic Agents
Imidazopyridine
  Zolpidem (Ambien)
Pyrazolopyrimidine
  Zaleplon (Sonata)
  Eszopiclone (Lunesta)
Antihistamines
  Diphenhydramine (Benadryl)

agents described earlier are more effective and safer. The barbiturates cause dependence and tolerance, they have a dangerous withdrawal syndrome, they are dangerous in overdose, and they can cause fatalities due to interactions with alcohol and other CNS depressants.

NURSING CARE

PRIORITIZING NURSING CARE

The priority of care with patient with anxiety is to assure patients that their concerns are taken seriously and to help identify triggers of the anxiety. During an acute panic attack, the priority is patient safety.

ASSESSING

During the nursing history, the nurse may identify that the patient has a general medical condition that commonly has anxiety as a symptom. See Box 51-4 for a list of some of these disorders. In these patients, treating the general medical disorder treats anxiety symptoms. For example, if a patient has anxiety symptoms due to hypoxia from an asthma attack, the treatment is her inhaler for bronchodilation, not an antianxiety medication.

The physical symptoms of anxiety usually begin with increased heart rate, blood pressure, and respiratory rate. Hildegard Peplau (1989) described four degrees or levels of anxiety and a syndrome of symptoms that change as anxiety increases. Her idea is adapted in Table 51-2. See this table for a summary of the subjective effects and observable behavior of a person experiencing anxiety. The nurse assesses not only whether the patient has anxiety but also the level of anxiety.

Care plans by nurses include how patients respond to their illnesses and how they respond to their treatments. Nurses must document their objective findings, such as the patients' vital signs and observed behaviors, as well as subjective symptoms such as the patients' statements on how they are feeling. Documentation should also include what factors cause or worsen anxiety if these are observed. In the intervention phase of the nursing process, the nurse will help the patient recognize these factors that increase and decrease anxiety as a way of improving the patient's insight.

Licensed nurses who are responsible for the care of patients who receive medications must know the desired effects and potential side effects of those medications. The nurse assesses the patient's response to medications. See Box 51-6■ for an example of a narrative charting entry on a patient with anxiety by a nurse that included objective and subjective assessment information and how the patient responded to treatment. Note that the nurse tried nonpharmacologic interventions before medicating this patient with her PRN dose of diazepam.

BOX 51-6	NARRATIVE DOCUMENTATION EXAMPLE ON PATIENT WITH ANXIETY

The patient is an 82-year-old woman who has been a resident of a long-term care facility for 1 year, since she had a stroke. She is unable to ambulate due to hemiplegia. She also has a diagnosis of generalized anxiety disorder.

Nurse documentation on narrative notes: Vital signs increased (HR 105, R 24, BP 154/96). Pt. states unable to focus on one activity, moves items around on her bedside table repeatedly. Pt. states: "I am so nervous! I don't know what to do!" Pt. refused a back rub or music to decrease anxiety. PRN dose of Valium 2.5 mg. given 30 min. ago with effective anxiety reduction. Pt. is working on a puzzle and states that she feels better. Ima Nurse, LPN.

If a patient is experiencing an episode of anxiety, the patient's perception of the threat represented by the situation is an important assessment. The nurse should also assess the patient's use of alcohol or drugs as self-medication for anxiety at home. A history of insomnia or the regular use of medications for sleep may indicate chronic anxiety as well. Information about the patient's usual coping methods can be helpful in planning care for the anxious patient. See Box 51-7■ for some questions that might obtain information about the patient's usual coping methods.

The nurse's own anxiety level is another important assessment. When the nurse is anxious, it is much easier for the patient to feel anxious. Anxiety is "contagious" in this way. Nurses need insight and enough self-understanding to know when they are anxious and what situations promote anxiety for them. Then nurses can use their own adaptive coping methods to reduce the anxiety enough to allow for a calm demeanor with the patient. A calm nurse makes it easier for the patient to remain calm.

DIAGNOSING, PLANNING, AND IMPLEMENTING

Anxiety is a nursing diagnosis. Nurses can diagnose and treat the symptom of anxiety independently. When a person has disabling anxiety such as in an anxiety disorder, a physician

BOX 51-7	ASSESSMENT

Questions to Assess Coping Methods

"When you have a lot of stress, what do you do?"
"What do you usually do in situations like this?"
"What usually helps you when this happens?"
"Who can help you at a time like this?"
"Do you ever drink alcohol to help you through stressful times?"
"Where could you go for help?"
"What helps you get through a really bad day?"

makes the diagnosis and care is collaborative. Some common nursing diagnoses for patients experiencing anxiety are *Anxiety, Ineffective Coping,* and *Post-Trauma Syndrome.*

The desired outcomes for people with anxiety are generally on three levels. First, during the *acute phase* of anxiety, the desired outcomes are that the patient will be free from self-inflicted harm and will experience decreased anxiety symptoms. Second, during the *stabilization phase* of therapy, the patient will begin to learn to verbalize own feelings, understand own stress response, and try new methods for anxiety reduction. Finally, *in the community* the patient will develop adaptive methods for coping with stress, use support systems, and demonstrate adequate social and occupational function (Schultz & Videbeck, 2012).

Anxiety

Expected outcome: Will discuss feelings of anxiety and potential desire to harm self.

- Assess for risk of self-harm. *People with some anxiety disorders (especially panic disorder and PTSD) are at risk for suicide.*
- Observe closely and provide safe environment. *People at risk for suicide require close observation, support, and no access to means of self-harm.*
- Have a calm, nonthreatening attitude while caring for patient. *Anxiety is easily transmitted from one person to another. The patient feels more secure when nurse is confident, calm, and nonthreatening.*
- Assure the patient that he or she is safe. Do not leave acutely anxious person alone. *People with high anxiety may fear for their lives. The presence of the nurse can convey a sense of protection and safety.*
- Maintain a low-stimulation environment (avoid loud noise, bright light). *Environmental stimuli can worsen anxiety because high anxiety reduces the patient's ability to filter stimuli.*
- Keep communication simple and direct. *High levels of anxiety make it impossible for the patient to focus on anything more than brief concrete messages.*

Ineffective Coping

Expected outcome: Will verbalize strategies to interrupt anxiety.

- Encourage the patient to express feelings. Provide time for 1:1 interaction and establish a trusting relationship. *Therapeutic use of self by nurse helps establish trust and the foundation for a therapeutic relationship, and 1:1 interaction provides the patient time to express feelings in a nonthreatening place.*
- Use therapeutic communication techniques. *Therapeutic communication techniques help the patient analyze own feelings and actions.*

- Help the patient to explore factors that lead to anxiety. *Understanding what comes before anxiety can begin the process of disarming these precipitating factors and learning to respond to them adaptively without anxiety.*
- Explore options for responding adaptively to stressors, and practice them if possible. *New coping skills can be discussed and planned first but will be best incorporated into the patient's life if an opportunity can be made to practice them.*
- Teach the patient to try five slow deep breaths as a coping mechanism for anxiety or before a possibly anxiety-producing event. *Taking five slow deep breaths can interrupt the sympathetic stimulation the patient is experiencing. Along with slowing the breath, the patient's heart rate will slow and BP may decrease. The patient should practice the five-breath technique so it comes to mind as anxiety is just beginning.*
- Teach the patient to recognize anxiety as it develops and to take control of stopping the anxiety from escalating (relaxation or breathing techniques, exercise, meditation). *If patients can recognize anxiety early while they can still focus on problem solving, they can employ various techniques to reduce anxiety responses. Patient preference indicates which intervention to use. Help patients recognize their own anxiety by describing patient behavior and connecting it to anxious feelings. For example, the nurse could say, "I saw you pacing up and down the hall, or wringing your hands, or shaking, etc. Were you feeling nervous or anxious then?"*
- Teach the patient to use progressive relaxation as a coping strategy. *Progressive relaxation is an effective technique for stress reduction. The directions for assisting the patient through a progressive relaxation exercise are given in Box 51-8 ■. Note that in the directions the nurse tells the patient to first tighten and then relax each muscle group. The tightening shows the contrast between tension and relaxation. The nurse guides the patient through the exercise the first time and then the patient practices it alone. Finally, the patient learns to use the relaxation technique when a stressful situation arises to stop the progression of anxiety.*

Post-Trauma Syndrome

Expected outcome: Will discuss feelings and verbalize situations that increase the sense of threat, fear, or anxiety.

- Assess degree of anxiety or fear and the degree of threat perceived by the patient. *Understanding the patient's perception is necessary for providing appropriate assistance to overcome the fear.*
- Be calm. Stay with the patient. *A calm demeanor on the part of the nurse will help the patient feel calm. The patient's feelings of danger and being threatened may be relieved by the presence of the nurse.*
- Keep communication simple. *A high level of anxiety will make it impossible for the patient to process complicated information.*

BOX 51-8 | PATIENT TEACHING

Progressive Relaxation Exercise

Teach the patient to use progressive relaxation as a way to cope with stress. Explain that progressive relaxation is an exercise involving first tightening and then relaxing the major muscle groups from one end of the body to the other. This exercise can be done with the patient sitting or lying down. Dim the lights. The exercise is best done with the eyes closed to enable the patient to concentrate on relaxation.

The nurse reads the following:

- Take a deep breath in and hold it. Hold it in until it collects all the tension in your body and then slowly let it out. The tension is leaving with the air. Take another slow, deep, relaxing breath. Let out the tension as you let out the air. Now breathe normally.
- Now tighten the muscles in your feet. Your toes are all tightened up. Now let them go. Wiggle the toes and let them relax. Now wiggle your calves and ankles. Point your feet up toward your head and hold them tight. Then point them to the floor and hold tight. Now wiggle your feet and relax them. They are free now. Tighten your thighs. Press them down and feel the tension. OK, shake your legs and loosen them up.
- Contract your abdomen. Hold the muscles down flat. Hold it tight. Now release. Hold your arms close to your body. Closer, tighter. Then release. Shake your arms to loosen them up. Now your hands. Tighten them into fists. Make them tight. Now let them go. Wiggle your fingers. Let them dance as they relax. Last, your mouth. Clench your teeth. Press your tongue to the roof of your mouth. Now let your tongue rest. Open your mouth and take a deep breath.
- Your whole body is relaxed now. Hold your breath in, then let it out, and with it goes that last bit of tension. You are relaxed. You can open your eyes.

- Assist the patient to correct any distortions of thinking. *Reality-based interactions will reinforce the safety of the hospital situation. The nurse can be the patient's source of reality orientation.*
- Help the patient identify coping behaviors that have been useful in the past. *The patient may benefit from using strategies previously found to be successful.*
- Identify supportive people in the patient's life. *Supportive people can help patient cope with current situation and move on to live life fully after the traumatic event.*

EVALUATING

It is not the goal of the nurse to relieve all anxiety. Some anxiety is a necessary protective mechanism that allows people to be alert. Nurses try to help patients understand themselves, so they can learn new coping skills and keep anxiety at a manageable level.

DOCUMENTING

Evaluate effectiveness of nursing interventions by collecting data about and documenting the following: anxiety symptoms, patient safety from self-harm, ability to demonstrate or report the use of new methods for coping with stress, ability to state plans for new adaptive coping methods, ability to state reasons for and side effects of medications for anxiety management, patient report, and behavior observed to indicate that anxiety is reduced.

NURSING CARE PLAN
Patient With Generalized Anxiety Disorder

Mrs. Miedo is a 72-year-old Latina who has lived in a long-term care facility since she had a stroke 10 months ago. She was transferred to the skilled unit when she returned from the hospital to recover from surgery to repair a fractured hip. She was diagnosed with generalized anxiety disorder as a young woman. She had not had severe anxiety symptoms for several years, until after the hip surgery. The nurse in the skilled unit is Eucharia.

Assessment

Mrs. Miedo's heart rate is 110, her respiratory rate is 26, and her BP is 158/98. She is oriented to person and place and is very alert, carefully watching anyone who enters her room. Her skin is pale and cool. She is having surgical pain. She is not sleeping well. When the nurse tried to teach Mrs. Miedo about her medications, she was not able to pay attention. She is restless. Her hands are always busy pulling and twisting the covers on her bed. She stated, "I don't know what to do. I am so nervous. Don't leave me." For Mrs. Miedo's anxiety, the physician ordered diazepam 5 mg PO tid, and an additional 2.5 mg PRN, also tid.

Nursing Diagnosis

The following important nursing diagnosis (among others) is established for this condition:

- *Acute Pain* related to injury and surgery on hip
- *Anxiety* related to unfamiliar situation
- *Ineffective Coping* related to inadequate coping skills in new situation

Expected Outcomes

The expected outcomes for the plan care are that Mrs. Miedo will:

- Experience a manageable level of surgical pain throughout her stay in the skilled unit.
- Have reduced anxiety symptoms (vital signs will be within normal limits, she will state that she feels less nervous or anxious, and she will sleep at least 7 hours per night) within 2 days.
- Be able to express her feelings to the nurse and use strategies to relax herself within 1 week.

Planning and Implementation

The nurse will implement the following interventions:

- Introduce herself and asked if Mrs. Miedo has any questions about her care in the Skilled Unit.
- Give Mrs. Miedo the pain medication that the physician ordered q4h PRN on a regular schedule every 4 hours instead of waiting for her to ask for it.
- Plan Mrs. Miedo's ambulation schedule so she will ambulate when the pain medication is at its peak (about 1 hour after the oral dose).
- Keep environmental stimuli to a minimum. This may include turning off the TV, turning on the radio so Mrs. Miedo can listen to music, and closing the drapes to keep out the bright light.
- Maintain a calm and confident manner with Mrs. Miedo. Keep questions short and communication concrete and simple.
- Check on Mrs. Miedo as often as possible and assign the same nursing assistant to work with her every day.
- Assist the patient with a progressive relaxation exercise.

Evaluation

When Mrs. Miedo took the pain medication on a regular schedule, her pain came under control very quickly. She needed less medication as time went on.

She came to trust the staff in the Skilled Nursing Unit. She was able to call the nurse when she started to feel anxious. Sometimes she needed PRN diazepam, other times she responded to reassurance. She slept 8 hours each night after her pain was under control, and she started taking the antianxiety medication. After 3 days, she no longer needed the additional PRN doses of diazepam. Her behavior indicated that she was feeling more relaxed. She smiled more, and the restlessness resolved. Her vital signs were within normal limits. Her anxiety was under control with the combination of the regular dose of diazepam and the nonpharmacologic nursing interventions. However, she was not able to do the relaxation technique independently.

Critical Thinking in the Nursing Process

1. Explain why the regular dosage of pain medication was better than the PRN dosage for Mrs. Miedo in controlling both her pain and her anxiety.
2. What is the purpose of assigning the same nursing assistant to Mrs. Miedo every day?
3. What factor(s) might prevent Mrs. Miedo from doing self-relaxation exercises independently? Was this outcome realistic for Mrs. Miedo?

Note: Discussion of Critical Thinking questions appears on the companion website.

Note: The reference and resource listings for all chapters have been compiled at the back of the book.

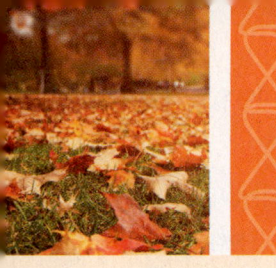
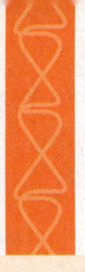

Chapter Review

KEY POINTS

- Anxiety is a universal human experience. It makes people alert to danger and more open to new learning. When it becomes so severe that it affects activities of daily living, occupational functioning, or quality of life, an anxiety disorder is present.
- **Concept:** The experience of anxiety originates in the subcortical or primitive brain, specifically in the limbic system.
- Anxiety disorders are the most common mental disorders in the United States.
- **Concept:** There are four levels of anxiety, and it is the level of anxiety that determines the patient's response and the nurse's intervention.
- **Concept:** Many people with treatable anxiety disorders do not seek help because they do not realize that they have a psychiatric problem, do not think they will be believed, or fear the stigma of mental illness.

- Effective medications and therapies are available to treat anxiety disorders.
- Patient responses to anxiety include physiologic, behavioral, and cognitive changes.
- A calm and confident nurse is most therapeutic with anxious patients.
- It is important for nurses to acknowledge that patients' traumatic experiences have been difficult and that the nurse believes the patient and is there to help.
- Some patient behaviors result in frustration, anger, and anxiety in nurses. Nurses can prevent these reactions by developing insight about how they react to patient behavior.

PEARSON NURSING STUDENT RESOURCES

- Find additional materials at **nursing.pearsonhighered.com**.

Clinical Reasoning Care Map

Caring for a Patient With Severe Anxiety

NCLEX-PN® Focus Area: Psychosocial Integrity

Case Study: Kayla is a 22-year-old European American female patient admitted to the surgical unit of a general hospital with abdominal pain. She had a cholecystectomy yesterday. She told the night nurse that she thinks she might die. She is scheduled for discharge tomorrow.

Nursing Diagnosis: Anxiety

COLLECT DATA

Subjective	Objective
_____	_____
_____	_____
_____	_____
_____	_____
_____	_____
_____	_____

Does this present a threat to the patient's safety?

If yes, the priority intervention to address this threat would be:

_____

Nursing Care

_____
_____
_____
_____
_____
_____
_____
_____
_____

Interprofessional team members to include when planning care:

_____

How would you document this?_____

_____

Compare your answers and documentation to those provided on the companion website.

Data Collected
(use only those that apply)

- Vital signs: T 99°F, P 110, R 20, BP 130/86.
- Patient is married.
- Has 1 child, age 10 months.
- Patient states, "Am I going to die from this?"
- Weight 152 lb.
- Skin is cool, diaphoretic.
- States, "I think my incision is going to tear open."
- Patient's hands are constantly moving, picking at the sheets.
- Nurse stated in report: patient slept approximately 3 hours last night.
- Abdominal incision is well approximated, without exudate.
- Nurse assesses that patient has dry mouth.
- Eyes are glancing around the room, darting from one thing to another.
- Complains of feeling dizzy.

Nursing Interventions (use only those that apply; list in priority order)

- Use progressive relaxation to help the patient relax.
- Keep communication simple and concrete.
- Accept the patient as she is, without judgment.
- Assess coping skills the patient has used successfully in the past.
- Tell the patient that she is fine and that she should quit worrying so much.
- Acknowledge that the patient is anxious.
- Assign a nursing assistant to sit with the patient 24 hours per day.
- Explain the pathophysiology of cholecystitis, the procedure of cholecystectomy, and analgesic therapy in detail.
- Provide comfort measures.
- Encourage the patient to talk about her feelings.
- Be calm and confident with the patient.
- Discuss healthy ways to talk about and relieve anxiety.
- Answer any questions the patient has about her surgical incision.
- Assess the patient's resources for support.
- Give the patient her PRN pain medication to treat the anxiety.
- Give the patient a book to read to distract her from her problems.

NCLEX-PN® Exam Preparation

1 A 30-year-old female patient in the hospital emergency department is experiencing a panic attack. The nurse must provide appropriate nursing actions for this patient. **Select all that apply.**

1. Restrain the patient to keep her safe.
2. Assess for the risk of self-harm.
3. Have a calm approach to the patient.
4. Keep communication simple.

2 A patient started taking lorazepam (Ativan) for anxiety yesterday. The nurse will be assessing for likely side effects. **Select all that apply.**

1. Agitation
2. Sedation
3. Insomnia
4. Decreased muscle coordination

3 A patient expresses nervousness about the MRI he will have in the morning. He is fidgeting with his sheets. The nurse's best first response to the patient is to:

1. bring him his PRN alprazolam (Xanax).
2. validate that the nurse can see that he is anxious and ask him what he thinks is the source of his "nervousness."
3. reassure him that MRIs are safe procedures and nothing to worry about.
4. turn on his television to divert his attention to something else.

4 Which of the following is a true statement about anxiety disorders?

1. People with generalized anxiety disorder often realize that the level of their anxiety is out of proportion to the stimulus, but they cannot control it.
2. Genetics alone is the source of anxiety disorders.
3. Antianxiety medications cause addiction and should not be used.
4. People with a higher level of intelligence are less likely to suffer from anxiety disorders than others.

5 A patient is diagnosed with an anxiety disorder. The physician plans to prescribe a medication and cognitive-behavior therapy. Which medication classification would the nurse expect the physician to prescribe for this patient?

1. Sedative-hypnotic
2. Benzodiazepine
3. Narcotic analgesic
4. Fluoroquinolone

6 When a nursing student starts to enter her patient's room, she bursts into uncontrollable sobbing. She says that her mother died suddenly in that same room 2 months ago. This student is probably experiencing:

1. posttraumatic stress.
2. panic attack.
3. phobic attack.
4. acute stress disorder.

7 A patient is being treated with cognitive-behavior therapy for an anxiety disorder. The cognitive restructuring assists the patient to:

1. avoid the situation or object that produces anxiety.
2. discuss his negative thoughts about certain anxiety-producing situations and objects.
3. replace negative self-talk with more supportive and positive self-talk.
4. accept his negative thoughts about certain situations and objects as being part of his normal life responses.

8 Select the best nursing intervention to assist the anxious patient to adopt effective coping strategies.

1. Teach the patient relaxation and deep-breathing techniques.
2. Leave the patient alone to develop her own plan.
3. Provide reading material on coping strategies.
4. Tell the patient what you would do in similar circumstances.

9 Which question would give the nurse the best information about the patient's usual coping methods?

1. "Why did you let yourself get so sick?"
2. "What are your usual coping behaviors?"
3. "What usually helps you when things like this happen?"
4. "What do you think you should do about this?"

10 A patient is experiencing a moderate level of anxiety about her upcoming surgery. Select the correct nursing actions for this patient. **Select all that apply.**

1. Reassure the patient that there is nothing to worry about.
2. Assess the patient's concerns and knowledge about the surgery.
3. Answer the patient's questions about what to expect after surgery.
4. Help the patient do progressive relaxation.
5. Call the physician to suggest that the surgery should be canceled.

Answers and rationales for Review Questions appear in Appendix I.

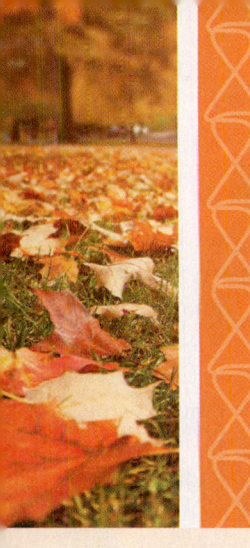

CHAPTER 52

Caring for Patients With Personality Disorders

BRIEF OUTLINE

Personality Disorders

Cluster A Personality Disorders: Odd/Eccentric

Cluster B Personality Disorders: Dramatic/Emotional/Erratic

Cluster C Personality Disorders: Anxious/Fearful

APPLIED LEARNING OUTCOMES

After completing this chapter, you will be able to:

1. Identify the major features of personality disorders.
2. Adapt the nurse–patient relationship to the special concerns of the patient who has a personality disorder.
3. Collect and document information about patient behaviors related to personality disorders.
4. Prioritize the importance of patient behaviors and related nursing actions.
5. Apply the nursing process to patients with personality disorders.

KEY TERMS

The key terms are defined on the pages listed below.

SPECIAL FEATURES

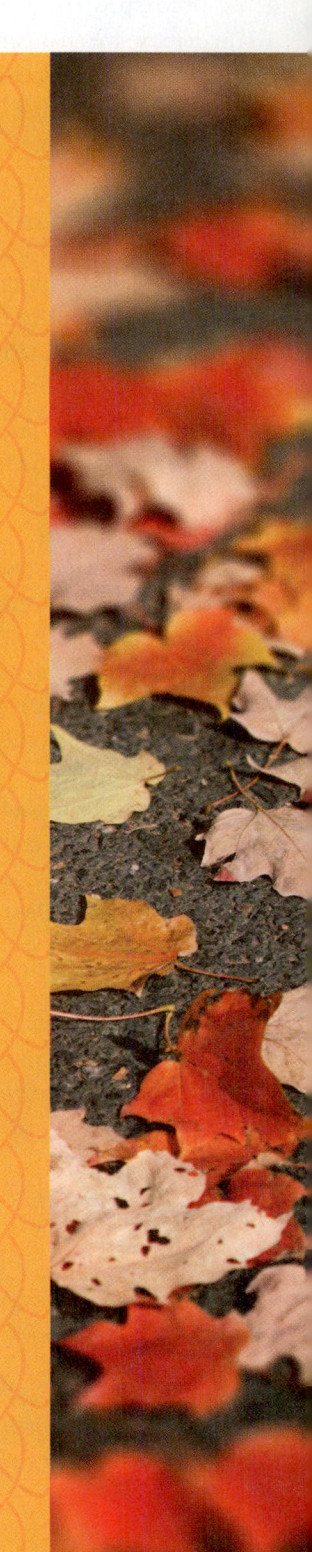

Personality is the relatively stable way in which a person thinks, feels, and behaves. It includes the psychosocial traits and characteristics that make a person an individual.

Personality begins to form in early childhood and continues to develop through young adulthood. The overall pattern of personality is unique to each individual, but there are enough similarities observed in people that generalizations are possible. Personality is affected by genetic predispositions and by life experiences. It affects the defense mechanisms that each individual uses to respond to stress throughout life.

There are five basic personality traits in every person. An individual's personality expresses each trait somewhere along the continuum between its two extremes. Thus, each trait has two extremes or poles. Using the trait of extroversion as an example, a person can be extremely introverted, shy, usually outgoing, dominant, or anywhere on this continuum up to extremely extroverted. Each person tends to have an individual range of behaviors in each of the five personality traits. The five basic personality traits are:

1. *Extroversion: Extroverted* people tend to be energetic, enthusiastic, dominant, sociable, and talkative. *Introverted* people tend to be shy, retiring, submissive, and quiet.
2. *Agreeableness: Agreeable* people tend to be friendly, cooperative, trusting, and warm. On the other end of this continuum, people who are *disagreeable* tend to be argumentative, cold, distrustful, and unkind.
3. *Conscientiousness: Conscientious* people are steady, cautious, dependable, organized, and responsible. *Impulsive* people tend to be disorderly, undependable, and careless.
4. *Emotional stability: Emotionally stable* people are relaxed and contented. *Emotionally unstable* people tend to be nervous, anxious, high-strung, and worrisome.
5. *Openness: Open* people tend to be imaginative, creative, and witty. *Closed* people are simple, concrete, or superficial.

Naturally, each person's personality is unique because of a unique combination of these traits. People think, feel, and behave in various ways also. One of the strengths of the human race is our diversity.

Personality Disorders

> **Key Concept**   Although the normal range of human behavior, feelings, and thought is broad, it is possible for personality to be outside the normal range.

A personality disorder is an enduring pattern of inner experience and behavior that deviates markedly from the individual's culture. A person affected by a personality disorder will have abnormalities in at least two of the following aspects of personality: cognition (ways of thinking about and perceiving the self, others, and things that happen); emotional expression (abnormal range, intensity, stability, and appropriateness of emotional expression); interpersonal functioning (interacting and having relationships with other people at home, at school, at work, or in any setting); and impulse control (inability to control certain emotions or actions that occur suddenly). The problem begins in adolescence or young adulthood and is stable over the long term. The person with a personality disorder will manifest the abnormalities as inflexible and pervasive, affecting interactions in a variety of situations. It leads to impairment in social or work functioning or significant distress for the individual (American Psychiatric Association [APA], 2013).

A person's personality significantly affects how this person responds to life events, including illnesses. A patient's culture also affects the patient's behavior and personality. Box 52-1 ■ describes the importance of considering a patient's cultural background when interpreting behavior.

PATHOPHYSIOLOGY

> **Key Concept**   People with personality disorders can behave irrationally even when their intellect is intact.

Personality disorders are not the same as mental disorders or diseases (Townsend, 2012), although people with mental disorders such as schizophrenia, bipolar disorder, or depression may have personality disorders as well.

Diagnosing personality disorders requires an evaluation of the person's long-term patterns of functioning in a variety of situations. Personality patterns must be persistent to be significant. (APA, 2013).

Box 52-1	**FOCUS ON DIVERSITY**

Personality and Culture

Any judgment about a patient's personality must take into account that person's ethnic, cultural, and social background. People who are immigrants from other cultures are especially at risk of being diagnosed with disorders of mental function and personality when they are acting or thinking in a way that is accepted in their culture of origin but not in their new home. For example, a Cuban immigrant stated to the nurse that her dead father talked to her and told her to be careful when talking to strangers. In the Cuban culture, "talking" with deceased people may mean the same as "This is what my father would have wanted me to do" in the Euro-American culture. The nurse can improve the cultural sensitivity of this patient's care by talking with other Cuban people or learning more about the patient's culture. It can be valuable to have a "culture broker" or person who shares both the nurse's and the patient's culture to interpret cross-cultural issues. This person may be a family member, a language interpreter, clergy, or another employee in the health care setting.

The APA (2013) describes 10 specific types of personality disorders (see Table 52-1 ■). These disorders are grouped into three clusters by their similarities. The clusters are based on similar observed behaviors:

Cluster A. Odd and eccentric
Cluster B. Dramatic and emotional
Cluster C. Anxiety- and fear-based personality disorders

Key Concept   Personality has been attributed to life experience, but brain changes have been found in some people with disorders of personality.

Neuroimaging research found similarities in the limbic system structure among people with conditions characterized by emotional over-reactivity to stress. These disorders include borderline personality disorder, bipolar disorder, and attention-deficit hyperactivity disorder (Stone, 2013). This commonality may explain some of the difficulty health care providers have had in the differential diagnosis of these disorders.

Other experts (APA, 2013; Reichenberg, 2014) developed an alternative model to describe personality disorders. The controversy that moved these psychiatric and psychological experts to view personality disorders differently from the main *DSM-5* model is that the various disorders of personality are in some ways too similar to each other; it can be difficult to choose a diagnosis because the disorders have symptoms that overlap each other; people with one disorder often have symptoms of several disorders; and some of the symptoms are extensions of the normal personality.

It is not important for nurses to have a functional knowledge of this new model because it is not in current use. However, it will probably be the future of diagnosing

personality abnormalities, so it is included here with that in mind. The new model diagnoses personality disorders by how severely the individual's personality is affected in two dimensions:

1. Level of personality functioning
   Self:
   Identity: Experience of oneself should be as unique, with clear boundaries between self and others; self-esteem and accuracy of self-appraisal should be stable; and the person should have the capacity for and the ability to regulate a range of emotional experience.
   Self-direction: Pursuit of coherent and meaningful short-term and life goals; using constructive and socially positive internal standards of behavior; and the person should have the ability to self-reflect productively.
   Interpersonal:
   Empathy: Comprehension and appreciation of others' experiences and motivations; tolerance of differing perspectives; and understanding the effects of one's own behavior on others.
   Intimacy: Depth and duration of connection with others; desire and capacity for closeness; and mutual regard reflected in interpersonal behavior.
2. Pathological personality traits
   The pathological personality traits are organized into five domains: negative affectivity (vs. emotional stability, which is the more normal end of the continuum), detachment (vs. extroversion), antagonism (vs. agreeableness), disinhibition (vs. conscientiousness), and psychoticism (vs. lucidity).

MANIFESTATIONS

Impaired self-identity is a central problem in disorders of personality. Self-identity is a part of normal personality development. It includes an integration of social and occupational roles, chosen values and behaviors, gender roles, beliefs about sexuality and intimacy, personal goals, and political and religious beliefs. An adequately formed identity is necessary for goal-directed behavior and for satisfying interpersonal relationships. With personality disorders, self-identity is often minimal or absent (Boyd, 2011).

Thinking patterns are distorted in personality disorders. The individual's ability to decode stimuli and to interpret environmental events is impaired. Maladaptive thinking patterns cause individuals to misinterpret the actions of others. The misinterpretations result in maladaptive responses by the affected person.

Emotions, in their intensity and quality, appear to be affected by disorders of personality. People with personality disorders have blunted or distorted emotional experiences. They tend to have more negative emotional experiences.

TABLE 52-1	**Personality Disorders by Cluster**
CLUSTER	**PERSONALITY DISORDER**
A: Odd/eccentric	Paranoid personality disorder Schizoid personality disorder Schizotypal personality disorder
B: Dramatic/emotional	Antisocial personality disorder Borderline personality disorder Histrionic personality disorder Narcissistic personality disorder
C: Anxious/fearful	Avoidant personality disorder Dependent personality disorder Obsessive-compulsive personality disorder

Source: Data from American Psychiatric Association. (2013). *Diagnostic and Statistical Manual of Mental Disorders* (5th edition). Washington, DC: Author.

Their ability to function in daily life and even to learn new things is affected.

Behavior is also affected by personality disorders. First, personality disorders cause *impulsive behavior.* These disorders appear to make it more difficult for people to foresee the consequences of their actions or to control their impulses despite probable negative consequences.

Second, these disorders cause *inflexibility of behavior.* Affected people tend to be rigid. They are unable to change their usual behavior when circumstances suggest that a change is indicated. Normally, people learn to change their behavior when they try new behaviors and receive positive reinforcement for the new approach. The inflexibility in personality disorders makes it difficult for people to learn new ways to behave or cope.

This inflexibility traps the patient in vicious cycles of behavior that are self-defeating. Patients become rigid and inflexible in role functions and personal interactions. The inflexibility provokes predicaments, problems, and stress. The problems and stress result in the patient becoming more inflexible. This self-perpetuating circle reduces learning opportunities and alienates other people. See Figure 52-1 ■ for a diagram of this vicious cycle.

COLLABORATIVE CARE

Personality disorders are difficult to treat, because personality is resistant to change. There are no medications that affect personality directly. One thing that the interprofessional team can do to benefit people with personality disorders is to stop stigmatizing them. Personality disorders are among the most stigmatized of mental illnesses. There are jokes about how affected people are difficult to work with and are choosing to have these disorders. We really must extend our respect and care to *all* our patients.

Medications
Pharmacologic treatment of personality disorders is based on treating specific target symptoms rather than the disorder itself. Antidepressants and mood stabilizing drugs can be used to treat symptoms of depression or mood lability (instability). Antipsychotic drugs may be useful if a patient experiences psychosis, which may be a symptom in patients who also have schizophrenia. Antianxiety medications are often used for people with anxiety-based disorders.

Psychotherapy
Cognitive-behavior therapy (CBT) helps many people, but it takes time, commitment, and insight on the part of the patient. Dialectical-behavior therapy is an adaptation of the principles of CBT specifically for people with borderline personality.

Many people with personality disorders lack the insight to realize that they have a problem. People usually do not seek treatment for personality disorders. Patients rarely seek help for personality disorders. These patients are seen in a variety of settings being treated for other things.

NURSING CARE

Often nurses find it frustrating to work with patients who have disorders of personality. Over time these people have developed maladaptive methods of coping with life. These patients can be manipulative, socially inappropriate, and difficult. For these reasons, such patients need all the patience and skill nurses have to offer. Direct communication with clear expectations for patient behavior, and clear and consistent limits, is important for these patients.

To work effectively with patients with personality disorders, nurses must understand themselves first. Nurses must have the insight to know what type of behavior causes them stress, so they can act rather than react to the patient's behaviors. Remember that the goal of the nurse is to provide professional care, not to be the friend of the patient. Objective understanding of personality disorders will help nurses take an objective approach to patient care.

Cluster A Personality Disorders: Odd/Eccentric

PARANOID PERSONALITY DISORDER
Paranoid personality disorder is a pattern of distrust and suspiciousness that other people are acting maliciously toward the affected individual. On the basis of imagined

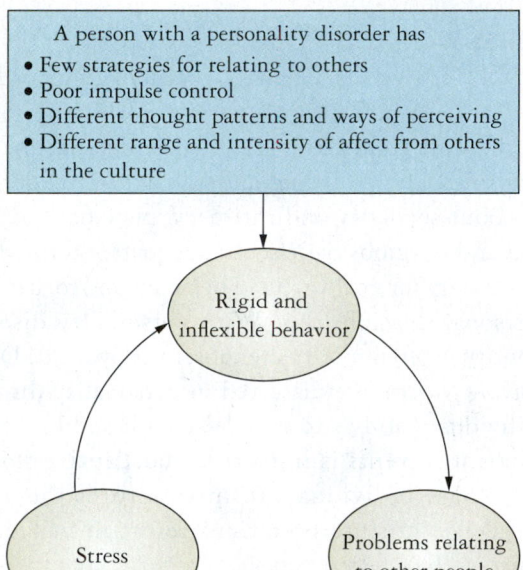

A person with a personality disorder has
- Few strategies for relating to others
- Poor impulse control
- Different thought patterns and ways of perceiving
- Different range and intensity of affect from others in the culture

Rigid and inflexible behavior

Stress

Problems relating to other people

Figure 52-1. ■ Vicious cycle of personality disorders.

evidence, this patient may think that people are plotting against him or her or may attack without reason. The patient may "fight back" when the victim never attacked in the first place. People with paranoid personality disorder often imagine hidden threatening or demeaning messages in innocent remarks or actions. People with this disorder find it difficult to forgive, and they hold grudges (APA, 2013).

Difficulty with interpersonal relationships is a hallmark of this disorder. Affected people tend to be so vigilant to catch the malicious intentions of others, interpreting their actions as deceptive and disloyal, that they cannot form mutually satisfying relationships. They especially distrust the faithfulness or trustworthiness of a partner or friend. The basis of their relationships may be power and control.

This disorder causes a hostile and defensive nature, which is likely to arouse a hostile response in others, confirming the patient's suspicion (APA, 2013). In spite of their aggressive appearance, these patients' inner feelings are often fear and insecurity. These feelings often respond to reassurance about the person's safety. These patients are very aware of power relationships, so they may respond better to information directly from the physician or charge nurse rather than from the staff nurse.

SCHIZOID PERSONALITY DISORDER

The most important features of schizoid personality disorder are a pervasive pattern of detachment from social relationships and a restricted range of emotional expression **(affect)**. People with this disorder of personality appear to receive little satisfaction from being part of a family or group, having little interest in sexual or other intimate relationships. They prefer to be alone and even choose hobbies that can be done in isolation from other people. They lack friends, and they appear indifferent to the opinions of others. People with schizoid personality disorder rarely experience strong emotions such as anger or joy. They may only confide in their parents or sisters and brothers (APA, 2013).

Schizoid personality disorder may cause impairment in occupational as well as social functioning, unless the affected individual can find a suitable job working alone. Affected people find pleasure in few activities.

SCHIZOTYPAL PERSONALITY DISORDER

People with schizotypal personality disorder have a consistent pattern of interpersonal deficits. They have discomfort in and reduced capacity for close relationships. They also have cognitive (thinking) or perceptual distortions and eccentric behavior. The cognitive deficit may be **ideas of reference**, in which patients misinterpret everyday events as having a personal meaning for them. For example, the patient may believe that her thoughts about the plants being dry caused it to rain or that the arrival of the bus

at exactly this moment is because she thought about it coming (APA, 2013).

People with schizotypal personality disorder may be superstitious or preoccupied with paranormal activity that is outside the realm of belief of their culture, such as clairvoyance, telepathy, or mind reading. They may have suspicious or paranoid thoughts. Affect is likely to be restricted or inappropriate. **Inappropriate affect** occurs when the patient has an emotional response that is not culturally appropriate for the situation, such as laughing when someone's pet dies. The thinking, behavior, speech, and appearance of affected people are also likely to be eccentric or peculiar. These patients will probably not have friends. They have excessive social anxiety that does not resolve as people become more familiar. Their social anxiety is more likely to be due to paranoid fears than to negative ideas about themselves (APA, 2013).

COLLABORATIVE CARE

Because personality is such an integral part of the individual's identity, health care providers cannot simply identify a problem, plan an intervention, and make personality changes. Realistic short-term outcomes should be identified. For people affected by the odd/eccentric personality disorders, these outcomes will be related to small changes in thinking patterns and behavior, such as realistic interpretation of events, taking medications, eating meals, and cooperating with treatment. The long-term treatment goals for these patients are improved social skills, reality-based thinking, increased flexibility, and trust.

Social skills training can help these patients behave in more socially appropriate ways, thus making it easier for them to interact in the community. Although these patients do not enjoy being with other people, they require enough interpersonal contact to keep them oriented to reality, but not so much that they cannot cope.

NURSING CARE

PRIORITIZING NURSING CARE

Priorities of care with these patients are to maintain professional boundaries and facility policies and to provide reassurance about the plan of care.

ASSESSING

Collect subjective and objective data about the patient's mental status. Observe and describe the patient's verbal and nonverbal behavior objectively in the chart. Pay particular attention to the patient's anxiety level and ability to cooperate with others. Ask about medications the patient takes at home.

DIAGNOSING, PLANNING, AND IMPLEMENTING
Disturbed Thought Processes

Expected outcome: Will engage in reality-based verbalizations, expressing concerns that are based in reality.

■ Do not ignore the patient's suspicions, but do not overemphasize the fears of the patient either. If the patient is requesting complicated confirmation that the medications are his, the nurse should respectfully and briefly reassure him that they are the correct medications, but not engage in any elaborate unnecessary plans. *Suspiciousness about medications or food being poisoned is common in these types of disorders. It may be enough to tell the patient confidently that the nurse checked these medications personally and they are accurate. The nurse could bring the medications still wrapped in their individual dose wrappers to reassure the patient that they are the correct medications. Because the fears are irrational, excessive and elaborate proof (e.g., bringing in the patient's chart with every medication, calling the pharmacist) does not really help.*

■ Approach patients with a matter-of-fact, professional attitude. *Suspicious/paranoid patients will not respond to a friendly approach by the nurse and may misinterpret friendliness as weakness or deceit.*

■ Reassure patients that they are safe and that the staff is making every effort to provide accurate, quality care for them. *The nurse's confidence may be reassuring to the patient. People with paranoia seem to be aggressive, but their feelings are often based on fear and insecurity.*

■ Adhere strictly to the rules of the organization (e.g., visiting hours, medication times). *Any exceptions may appear to the patient to have a devious intent. Strict adherence may be reassuring that there are limits in which the patient is safe.*

■ Try some corrective statements. Box 52-2■ gives examples of how to adjust unfounded observations toward more realistic thinking.

Impaired Social Interaction

Expected outcome: Will participate in brief interactions with nurse and other health care staff.

■ Make brief and nonthreatening interpersonal interactions with the patient. *Patients who feel suspicious usually feel uncomfortable around other people. They need to interact with others to maintain mental health. Brief interactions may be easier to tolerate.*

■ Assign consistent staff to work with this patient. *Consistent one-to-one relationships promote the patient's ability to form trust.*

■ Provide low-stress opportunities for patients to be with other people, such as eating at a table

BOX 52-2	CORRECTIVE STATEMENTS FOR DISTORTED THOUGHTS

Thought distortion: "This is the worst thing that has ever happened."
Corrective statement: "True, this is a bad thing, but it is not the worst thing that ever happened." (*Giving perspective allows the patient to see the real placement of this stressful event as it relates to life priorities.*)

Thought distortion: "I could *never* do anything so difficult."
Corrective statement: "You have already done challenging things like this before, such as…." (*Giving examples makes the implied generalization specific.*)

Thought distortion: "If only I hadn't made him mad, he wouldn't have beat me up."
Corrective statement: "He is an adult and responsible for his own behavior. You are responsible for your own behavior, not his." (*Stating the mature reality of the situation helps the patient see it from another point of view.*)

Thought distortion: "My boyfriend left me. This will kill me. I can't go on."
Corrective statement: "You have survived disappointments before. You are strong enough to handle this. Let's talk about how you feel." (*Allowing the patient to discuss and examine feelings increases insight and promotes the ability to learn from past experiences and to apply current learning to future situations.*)

Thought distortion: "Nobody understands me."
Corrective statement: "Let's talk about how you feel, so I can understand." (*Suggesting a problem-solving approach promotes adaptive coping.*)

with others at mealtime. *The patient may not really want to socialize with other people, but some contact with other people is important for mental health.*

■ Provide some social skills training, such as redirecting behavior that is socially inappropriate. *If the patient dresses or behaves in ways that the other patients accept, she or he may be more accepted.*

EVALUATING

Collect the following data to determine whether the patient is achieving nursing care outcomes: how the patient interacts with others, verbal and nonverbal behavior, and anxiety level.

DOCUMENTING

Document statements that indicate the patient's thought processes, such as "Leave the light on. I want to see if anyone is coming to get me" or "There is too much going on here. Get me out." Describe the patient's behavior objectively, such as "Patient is in his bathroom with the door closed yelling 'Stay away, don't hurt me!'"

Cluster B Personality Disorders: Dramatic/Emotional/Erratic

ANTISOCIAL PERSONALITY DISORDER

The essential characteristic of *antisocial personality disorder* is a pervasive pattern of disregarding and violating the rights of others. To receive this diagnosis, patients must be at least 18 years old. They must have had conduct disorder by the age of 15. Conduct disorder includes cruelty to people or animals, deceitfulness or theft, destruction of property, and serious violations of rules (APA, 2013). Approximately 1% of females are affected with antisocial personality disorder, whereas 3% of males have the disorder.

People with antisocial personality disorder tend to disregard societal expectations by breaking the law. For example, they may destroy the property of others, harass others, steal, or engage in illegal occupations (drug dealing, dog fighting, selling stolen property). People with this disorder manipulate others for their personal gain or pleasure (for money, sex, and power). They disregard the rights, feelings, and safety of others (APA, 2013).

Impulsiveness is a major feature of antisocial personality disorder. People with this disorder make decisions suddenly, without planning ahead or considering the possible consequences. This leads to frequent change of jobs, residences, and relationships. They may fight repeatedly or assault others frequently, including partners and children. Affected people may be friendly and likable until they are frustrated. This disorder results in disregard for the safety of self or others. Fast, reckless driving, substance use, or irresponsible sexual behavior may illustrate this aspect of the disorder (APA, 2013).

Affected people are irresponsible in all aspects of their lives: family, employment, interpersonal relationships, and finances. People with this disorder tend to be aggressive and irritable. They live in the moment, not concerned with the past or the future. Rules are made for other people, not for them. Figure 52-2■ shows a man with antisocial personality disorder in prison.

People with antisocial personality disorder show little remorse for the negative consequences of their behavior. They may believe that they should do anything necessary to ensure that others will not control them. These patients often blame their victims for weakness or foolishness, without any guilt or sorrow over their suffering or loss (APA, 2013).

Nurses will encounter patients with this disorder much more often in substance abuse treatment or in *forensic* (legal) settings, such as prisons (APA, 2013). The risk of alcoholism is 21 times greater for people with antisocial personality disorder than it is for the general population. Fifteen to twenty-one percent of individuals with

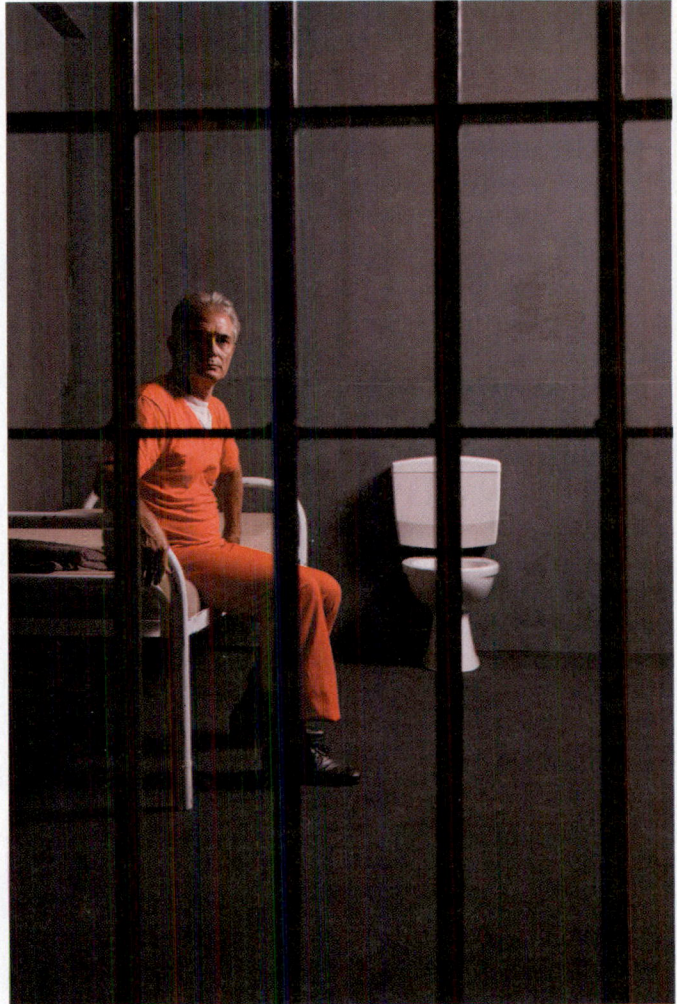

Figure 52-2. ■ People with antisocial personality disorder tend to believe that rules and laws do not apply to them. (Source: © fStop/Alamy.)

alcoholism have antisocial personality (National Institute of Mental Health, n.d.). Health care providers should be aware of the association between these disorders for the purpose of counseling and treating patients who need it. The role of the LPN/LVN with these patients is notifying the physician if the patient makes the nurse aware of either diagnosis.

BORDERLINE PERSONALITY DISORDER

A psychoanalyst named Stern first used the term *borderline personality* in 1938. He was describing patients who seem to be on the border between anxiety and psychosis.

Marsha Linehan is a leading contemporary theorist on borderline personality disorder. She and her colleagues believe that the disorder is caused by an interaction between biologic and social learning influences (nature and nurture). Their research focuses on the behavior patterns in the disorder, which include the following (Koerner & Linehan, 2000; Linehan, 1993):

■ *Emotional vulnerability:* a pattern of difficulty managing negative emotions, high sensitivity to negative emotional stimuli, and slower than normal return to baseline emotional level than the average person

■ *Self-invalidation:* failure to recognize own emotions, thoughts, behaviors; setting unrealistically high expectations for self; makes it impossible for self to be successful; intense shame and self-directed anger; and blames others for unrealistic expectations because the patient has no insight

■ *Unrelenting crises:* experiences frequent, stressful negative events, some caused by self, others not

■ *Inhibited grieving:* tries to overcontrol negative feelings, especially those associated with grieving such as guilt, sadness, shame, and anxiety

■ *Active passivity:* affected person fails to work actively on solving their own life problems and actively seeks help from others for problem solving, resulting in learned helplessness and hopelessness

■ *Apparent competence:* tends to appear to be more competent than he or she really is; may be unable to apply what is learned in one situation to other situations; may fail to display nonverbal cues of early emotional distress

The biosocial theorists propose that borderline personality disorder occurs when a vulnerable individual interacts with an invalidating environment. An invalidating environment is one in which the individual's feelings and emotions are negated, disrespected, or punished; often the environment is abusive. The ultimate invalidation is sexual abuse, which is a common experience of people with the disorder (Linehan, 1993; Stepp, Whalen, Pilkonis, Hipwell, & Levine, 2011).

Borderline personality disorder includes a pattern of impulsiveness and instability in interpersonal relationships, self-image, and emotions. These symptoms begin by early adulthood and are present in a variety of contexts. Affected people have intense fear of abandonment. They make frantic efforts to avoid real or imagined abandonment by others. Being left by others may suggest to people with borderline personality disorder that they are bad. They experience intense fears and inappropriate anger even when separations were to be expected (e.g., when a friend goes on vacation, someone is late for an appointment, or a favorite nurse has a day off work). Patients may even injure themselves in an effort to prevent abandonment (APA, 2013).

Affected people have a pattern of intense and unstable relationships. They may begin by idealizing a potential friend or partner, spending extensive amounts of time with that person, and confiding their innermost thoughts early in the relationship. Then they might unexpectedly change to devaluing the person, saying that the formerly

"perfect" friend or mate does not care enough. People with this disorder are able to cultivate relationships with others. However, they expect that the others will provide nurturance and be there to meet their considerable needs, on demand, at any moment (APA, 2013).

Borderline personality disorder is also characterized by an unstable self-image or sense of self. Life goals, plans, values, sexual identity, and friends may change abruptly and impulsively. The self-image of affected people is based on the feeling that they are bad. They may also have the sense that they do not exist at all or that they have no feelings. This is most likely to occur when they are feeling a lack of support. People with this disorder respond best to a predictable, structured environment (APA, 2013).

Impulsivity is another hallmark of borderline personality disorder. The diagnosis requires impulsivity in at least two areas that are potentially self-damaging (e.g., gambling, spending money irresponsibly, binge eating, unsafe sex, abusing substances, or self-injuring behavior) (APA, 2013).

Self-harm occurs in the majority of people with borderline personality disorder. Completed suicide occurs in 8% to 10% of affected people. Self-injury without suicide intent, such as cutting, scratching, or burning self, occurs much more frequently (Figure 52-3■). Behavior aimed at harming but not killing oneself is called **parasuicidal behavior** (Linehan, 1993) or simply self-harm. Patients with borderline personality disorder tend to see this as a solution: The pain becomes a mechanism for coping.

People with borderline personality disorder also experience unstable emotions. Their baseline low mood is often interrupted with episodes of anger, panic, or despair; rarely do they have periods of well-being or satisfaction. These patients often express intense or inappropriate anger or have difficulty controlling their anger. They may have

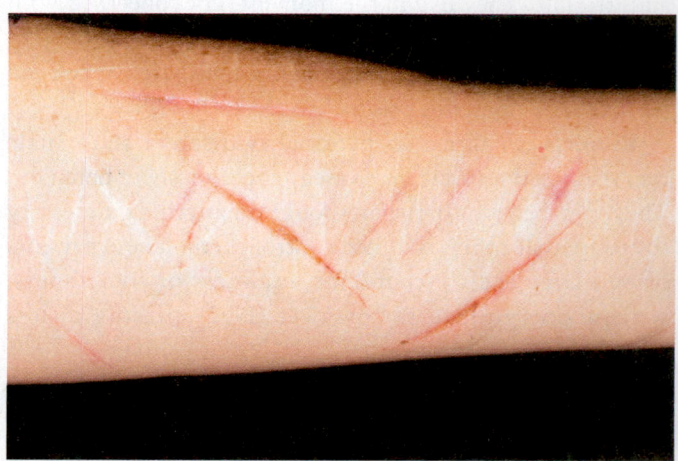

Figure 52-3. ■ Self-injury is used as a coping mechanism by this young man with borderline personality disorder. (Source: © Dr. P. Marazzi / Science Photo Library/Alamy.)

sarcastic or bitter outbursts. Inappropriate angry outbursts are often followed by shame and guilt and contribute to the affected person's feeling of being bad or evil (APA, 2013).

Borderline personality disorder affects men and women in equal numbers. Though it was previously thought that women were more likely to be affected, it seems instead that it affects women more severely. It is associated with substantial mental and physical disability. Borderline personality disorder is five times more common among first-degree relatives of affected people than it is in the general population. Family members are also more likely to have substance-related disorders, antisocial personality disorder, and mood disorders (APA, 2013).

HISTRIONIC PERSONALITY DISORDER

The most important features of histrionic personality disorder are excessive emotionality and attention-seeking behavior. Affected people need to be the center of attention. When they are not, they are uncomfortable or unhappy and will often create a scene to bring attention to themselves (APA, 2013).

Gender role stereotypes can guide the way people express this disorder. Women will dress provocatively or act overly dependent. Men will spend time bodybuilding or exaggerate their sexual exploits. Affected people use physical appearance to draw attention to themselves, as in Figure 52-4■,

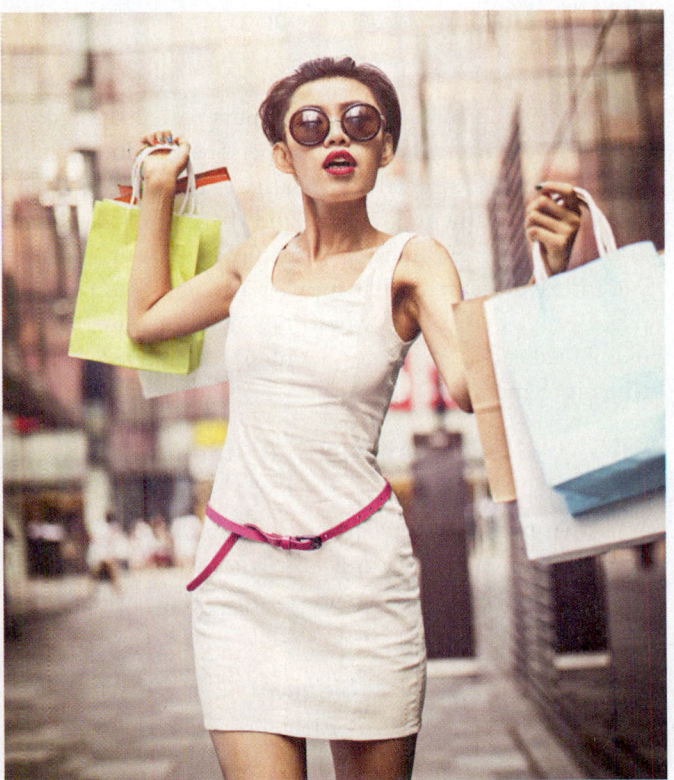

Figure 52-4. ■ Patients with histrionic personality disorder may dress dramatically and express exaggerated emotions. (Source: Ilya Terentyev / Getty Images.)

spending inordinate time, energy, and money on clothes, jewelry, and grooming. Unflattering comments easily upset these people (APA, 2013).

Their emotional expression may be shallow and changeable; their speech is lacking in detail and excessively *impressionistic* (gives a general impression without evidence). An example of impressionistic speech is "He is the greatest man in the world" with no reason given for the greatness. Affected people have strong opinions and express them dramatically, yet there is rarely any foundation for the opinion. Their emotions are exaggerated theatrically, yet they are turned on and off quickly and may seem insincere (APA, 2013). They may embarrass friends and acquaintances by being too intimate, sobbing uncontrollably over minor sentiments, or having temper tantrums.

People with histrionic personality disorder are very suggestible and easily influenced by others. They may be overly trusting, especially of authority figures. They have difficulty achieving close relationships. They may act dependent, while trying to control their partners with emotional manipulation. Affected people often alienate friends with their demands for attention. They may crave novelty and excitement. They have little tolerance for frustration or delayed gratification (APA, 2013).

NARCISSISTIC PERSONALITY DISORDER

Narcissistic personality disorder is characterized by a pervasive pattern of grandiosity, need for admiration, and lack of empathy for others. Affected people have an inflated sense of self-importance. They routinely overestimate their abilities and inflate their accomplishments. They expect that others will have the same high opinion of them. They may be surprised if they do not receive the fame and fortune they think they deserve. Although these patients inflate their own abilities, they tend to underestimate the abilities of others (APA, 2013).

People with narcissistic personality disorder often have fantasies of unlimited success, power, beauty, or ideal love and compare themselves with famous people. Affected people see themselves as superior to others and expect to be so recognized and feel entitled to especially favorable treatment and automatic compliance with their wishes (APA, 2013). They prefer to associate with other "special" people like themselves and may ask to see the head surgeon, head nurse, or head hairdresser. Only the best is good enough.

Affected people tend to exploit others and have little empathy for others' feelings. They present an emotional coldness and lack of reciprocal interest. Narcissistic personality disorder causes people to have arrogant, conceited behavior and attitudes. These people are often envious of others or believe that others are envious of them. They are quick to criticize, yet hate to be criticized. Their interpersonal relationships are usually impaired due to their insensitivity to others' feelings, their need for constant admiration, and their feelings of entitlement. Many people with this disorder also have depression, eating disorders, and substance-related disorders.

COLLABORATIVE CARE

The priority short-term goal for patients with antisocial personality is to prevent harm to self or others. This patient may be manipulative and physically violent, so these issues should be managed first. Other goals include anger management, coping skills, increasing self-awareness (insight), and learning to see an event from another person's point of view. The best personal approach to a patient with this disorder is the most direct one. Nurses should tell the truth, clearly and concisely. The nurse should share perceptions about the emotional consequences of the patient's behavior for others. Group therapy may help patients understand others' feelings. The staff must cooperate to consistently apply the treatment plan and facility policies.

The treatment priority for patients with borderline personality disorder is no self-harm. Other treatment issues are dysfunctional mood and impulsive behavior. Treatment of this disorder is long term. It involves a treatment team of professionals (nurses, psychiatrist, social worker, psychologist, therapists) and the patient working together.

Dialectical-behavior therapy (DBT) (Linehan, 1993) is an approach to treating borderline personality disorder that combines cognitive and behavioral therapies. Treatment may begin with training in *mindfulness,* originally a Zen technique, which is a meditation focusing on the breath. The mindful person observes his or her emotions coming and going without acting on them, focusing on the here and now, not the past or future (Margolies, 2010).

In DBT, a major principle is radical acceptance: accepting life as it is, not how it is supposed to be, and simultaneously accepting the need to change, despite the reality and because of it. DBT strives for a balance between acceptance and change. It is like practicing and learning to live the serenity prayer: accepting the things we cannot change, finding the courage to change the things we can, and using our therapists and supporters to help us distinguish between the two (Linehan, 1993). DBT uses mood monitoring, meditation, and social skills training. Patients actively practice new behaviors for coping and social skills. It is the most effective therapy for borderline personality disorder.

Patients who use self-harming behavior for coping may benefit from alternative choices of behaviors to cope with their stress. The following are some suggestions for "things to try instead of hurting yourself":

- Talk to someone.
- Delay your decision for 5 minutes.

- Hold an ice cube in each hand for 10 minutes.
- Put your hands in a bucket of ice water for 5 minutes.
- Take a hot or cold shower.
- Call a crisis line.
- Mark your arm with red lipstick.
- Yell, scream, or cry.
- Sing very loudly.
- Find a playground and swing as high as you can.
- Count things (ceiling tiles, colors, etc.).
- Masturbate.
- Pound on your bed until you are exhausted.

People with histrionic personality disorder may seek out others to complete their lives and to take care of them. The treatment goal is for patients to begin to focus on themselves for problem solving rather than expecting others to fulfill all their needs.

Patients with narcissistic personality disorder tend to be arrogant and have poor social skills. Treatment goals for them include developing coping skills that involve independent problem solving without exploitation of others.

NURSING CARE

PRIORITIZING NURSING CARE

Priorities include encouraging independent problem-solving and maintaining professional boundaries.

ASSESSING

This group of personality disorders puts patients at risk for violence to themselves (borderline personality) and violence toward others (antisocial personality). Collect data about these patients' mental status and behavior. Document patient behavior specifically and objectively. For example, "Patient is difficult and inappropriate" is subjective and unspecific. A better note would be, "Patient states 'I can't possibly take this medication unless the chief of surgery brings it to me.'"

DIAGNOSING, PLANNING, AND IMPLEMENTING

Sometimes patients with personality disorders in this group can disrupt an entire nursing unit with their behavior. See Box 52-3■ for strategies for preventing these patients from upsetting the unit.

Risk for Self-Directed Violence

Expected outcome: Will not harm self.

- Help the patient identify early internal symptoms of distress (e.g., pounding heart, sense of uneasiness, nervousness). *Identifying the symptoms of distress early can allow the patient time to respond in an adaptive way.*

BOX 52-3   NURSING CARE CHECKLIST

Preventing Personality Disordered Patients From Upsetting the Unit

☑ Make the unit rules clear. *People with some personality disorders (e.g., antisocial, borderline, histrionic, and narcissistic) may not have adaptive social and coping skills. They may be practiced in manipulating people in charge to allow them exceptions to the rules. They may not believe that the rules are for them.*

Example: Unit policy is that televisions are turned off at 10 p.m. A patient wants to watch TV until 3 a.m. "just this once."

☑ Stick to the rules consistently. This means everybody. *When the staff responds to the manipulative patient inconsistently, there is opportunity for the patient to pit the staff against each other.*

Example: One nurse allowed a patient to take pain medication a little bit early, and now the patient refuses to cooperate with any nurse who does not comply with his requests. Some of the nurses sympathize with the patient's apparent pain, others think he is manipulative, and the entire unit is upset.

☑ When a patient is causing the staff to be upset, have a conference. *In the previous situation, some nurses think one thing, others think another, and still others are unaware that there is a controversy. The patient is treated differently every shift. The patient is focusing on manipulating the staff, and the staff is focusing on controlling the patient's behavior. When everyone works together and receives the same information (including the patient), the patient is best served.*

Example: A systematic approach to the situation would include an assessment of the patient's problem (pain) with an appropriate prescription by the physician; an around-the-clock

dosing schedule instead of PRN doses so the patient does not need to ask for the medication; adherence to the schedule by all nurses in the same way; feedback from the patient about how pain is managed.

☑ Include the patient in problem solving. *When a patient's behavior is problematic, the patient has an opportunity to learn how to change to more adaptive behavior only if the patient is included in discussions of problem-solving strategies. Patients with personality disorders can benefit from discussions of how their behavior affects others because they often do not understand others' perspectives.*

Example: A patient asks every staff member to give him coffee. He is drinking 20 cups of coffee a day. His nurse realizes this and tells the rest of the staff to limit the coffee. The patient continues to ask and sometimes he receives coffee, other times he does not. He asks for coffee 50 times a day. When the patient is included in the discussion and is told that he will be given three cups of regular coffee and three cups of decaffeinated coffee each day, and that he can choose when he drinks them, he limits his requests to the designated times.

☑ Maintain professional boundaries. Remember who is the patient and who is the professional. *It is easy to react emotionally when patients act inappropriately or make personal comments. When patients flatter or insult nurses, it is challenging not to respond personally, but it is critical for nurses to respond to patients professionally. The goal is not a friendship with the patient but professional patient care. Maladaptive behavior by the patient is a learning opportunity.*

Example: A patient stated, "I don't want that fat one to be my nurse. I want my favorite nurse." A good response by the nurse is, "Your nurse is Ginger. When you talk like that, it hurts people's feelings."

■ Write the cues of distress listed by the patient on a card and give it to the patient (or the patient can write the list on a card herself). *The patient can refer to the card later in a time of distress. This mechanism for coping is an attempt to replace other maladaptive methods. It takes practice and time for new coping mechanisms to develop.*

■ Teach the patient skills for tolerating distress. The mnemonic "A wise mind ACCEPTS" can help the patient remember new coping behaviors:
  ■ Activities to distract from stress
  ■ Contributing to others such as volunteering or visiting a sick neighbor
  ■ Comparing yourself to people less fortunate than you
  ■ Emotions that are opposite of what you are experiencing
  ■ Pushing away from the situation for a while
  ■ Thoughts other than you are currently thinking
  ■ Sensations that are intense, such as holding ice in your hand

During a stressful situation, the patient is not likely to be able to try new coping behaviors unless there has been advance planning.

■ Use the five senses exercise to help people who have used self-harm for coping to find more enduring and adaptive ways to comfort themselves (Linehan, 1993). The five senses exercise follows:
  1. *Vision* (e.g., go outside and look at the stars or flowers or autumn leaves).
  2. *Hearing* (e.g., listen to beautiful or invigorating music or the sounds of nature or the city).
  3. *Smell* (e.g., light a scented candle, boil a cinnamon stick in water).
  4. *Taste* (e.g., drink a soothing, warm nonalcoholic drink).
  5. *Touch* (e.g., take a hot bubble bath, pet your dog or cat, get a massage).

■ Tell all patients who have thoughts about self-harm or suicide to notify the staff if they feel like hurting themselves. An agreement to notify staff of thoughts of self-harm is called a "no self-harm" contract.

Some nurses write out a statement for the patient to sign that says, "I promise that if I feel like hurting myself I will tell the staff before I do it." *The idea is that patients are stating that they are in control of their own behavior (this is not a legal contract). When the patient tells the nurse of these feelings, the nurse will begin by encouraging the patient to talk about and examine the feelings that led to the self-harm thinking. Alternatives to self-harm are then discussed. The nurse documents the conversation and reports it to the treatment team. The patient has the opportunity to feel the success of problem solving without self-harm.*

Risk for Other-Directed Violence

Expected outcome: Will not harm others and will comply with unit policies.

- Observe the patient for increasing agitation or frustration. *These are the usual precursors to acting out violently (either physically or emotionally). Early redirection can prevent violent acting out behavior.*

- If patients become agitated, direct them away from others into their rooms. *The reduction in sensory stimulation or removal from a frustrating stimulus may help the patient regain control. This action may help the patient learn the coping mechanism of seeking a quiet place.*

- Do not tolerate verbal abuse. Calmly redirect the patient, or state that the behavior is not acceptable. *Verbal abuse may precede violent acting out. Illness is not an excuse for abusing others verbally or otherwise. Patients benefit from the reminder of what appropriate behavior is and from the expectation that they can control themselves. Nurses must role model appropriate behavior. A yelling nurse will not help an agitated patient, even if she or he is yelling something smart. The nurse's calm demeanor is contagious to the patient.*

- Apply the rules consistently. *When patients use manipulation to get staff to change the rules for them, other staff members who uphold the rules are at risk of disapproval or targeting by antisocial patients.*

- When a patient is violent, get help. *When all talk-related and PRN medication interventions have been tried, if a patient is acting out, the nurse should obtain help from the emergency response team, hospital security personnel, or the police.*

Cluster C Personality Disorders: Anxious/Fearful

AVOIDANT PERSONALITY DISORDER

People with avoidant personality disorder have a pervasive pattern of social shyness, feelings of inadequacy, and hypersensitivity to negative evaluation. Affected people would like to have social relationships, but they hesitate to join in social activities because they fear disapproval or rejection. They avoid work or school activities that involve significant contact with other people, because they are preoccupied with thoughts of being criticized or rejected. They view themselves as socially inept, unappealing, or inferior. Their self-esteem is very low. They limit themselves in intimate relationships due to the fear of shame or ridicule. They may have a fearful and tense manner (APA, 2013). In contrast to other personality disorders in which affected people have no desire to socialize with others, people with avoidant personality disorder want to have contact with other people but find themselves unable to take the risk of rejection.

DEPENDENT PERSONALITY DISORDER

A need to be taken care of characterizes dependent personality disorder. These individuals have a pessimistic outlook and tend to minimize their own abilities and strengths. People with this disorder have submissive and clinging behavior and fear separation and abandonment to the degree that they may act incompetent in order to appear to need others. They have difficulty expressing disagreement due to fear of loss of support or approval. Dependent personality disorder is one of the most common disorders seen in mental health clinics (APA, 2013).

People with dependent personality disorder have difficulty making everyday decisions without excessive help and advice from others. They are passive and allow others to take responsibility for major areas of their lives. They submit to the will of others, even if the demands are unreasonable. They make great self-sacrifices and submit to abuse, even though other choices are available. When they are alone, affected individuals feel fearful and helpless because they feel unable to take care of themselves. Their social relationships are limited to the few people on whom they are dependent (APA, 2013).

Like the other personality disorders, dependent personality disorder is difficult to diagnose across cultures. The degree of dependent behavior that is considered normal varies across ages and cultures. So, the cultural expectations of the patient must be considered when interpreting the patient's behavior. An individual must have dependency behavior clearly in excess of what is expected by her or his culture as well as fear of being independent to be diagnosed with this disorder (APA, 2013).

OBSESSIVE-COMPULSIVE PERSONALITY DISORDER

Obsessive-compulsive personality disorder is characterized by a preoccupation with orderliness, perfectionism, and mental and personal control to the extent that they cannot be flexible, open, or efficient. People with this disorder try to maintain a sense of control through painstaking attention to rules, trivial details, lists, and schedules, until the main point of the project is lost. Extraordinary attention is paid to detail and to checking repeatedly for possible mistakes. Affected people are oblivious to the fact that other people find the delays caused by their behavior to be aggravating. They expect themselves to be perfect. When this is not possible, it causes significant stress. They may be so involved in making every detail of a job perfect, that they can never finish it. They insist that everything be done their way, because only they can do things right. They are excessively devoted to work to the exclusion of other activities such as family, friends, and fun (APA, 2013).

They are overly conscientious and inflexible about matters of morality. People with this disorder defer to authority and insist on following rules without exception for any reason. They may criticize themselves without mercy for their own mistakes (APA, 2013).

People with obsessive-compulsive personality disorder may be unable to throw away things that are worn out or worthless, even when they have no sentimental value. Affected people may hoard their resources out of an attitude that spending must be limited to provide for future emergencies.

They are known for being rigid, indecisive, and stubborn. They plan ahead in meticulous detail and will not consider changes to their plans. It is difficult for people with this disorder to consider the perspectives of others. Their expression of emotion is tightly controlled, and they are often uncomfortable around people who are emotionally expressive (APA, 2013).

Obsessive-compulsive personality disorder is not the same as obsessive-compulsive disorder (OCD), which is an anxiety disorder. OCD is characterized by true *obsessions* (uncontrollable desire to continue thinking about an idea or feeling) and *compulsions* (repetitive stereotyped acts done to relieve anxiety that are a response to obsessive thoughts). Obsessive-compulsive personality disorder, because it affects the entire personality, is more pervasive. It affects how the patient perceives and responds to the world on an everyday basis. OCPD defines who the patient is and is less responsive to treatment than OCD.

COLLABORATIVE CARE

Long-term therapy and hard work by the patient are the only effective treatments for personality disorders. Treatment goals for patients with avoidant personality disorder include improving self-esteem, developing a trusting relationship, developing adaptive coping skills, and improving social skills. Symptoms in some people with avoidant personality disorder are reduced when they take antianxiety and antidepressant medications. Dependent personality disorder is seen in various practice settings. These patients expect caregivers to make their decisions for them. The challenge is to support these patients to make their own decisions without giving advice on how to act.

Patients with obsessive-compulsive personality disorder may seek medical help for anxiety or related symptoms. Antianxiety medications may be prescribed. Treatment will focus on how the patient is affected by the disorder in such areas as coping, sleeping, nutrition, and interpersonal relationships.

NURSING CARE

PRIORITIZING NURSING CARE
The focus of care is providing a safe, professional atmosphere in which the patient can express anxieties and identify needs. Personal safety for the patient and staff are the highest priority.

ASSESSING
The physician or psychiatrist will make the medical diagnosis of a personality disorder. The role of the nurse is to help patients deal with the effects of the disorder. Collect information about the patient's functional ability, mental status, and interpersonal relationships. Patients with personality disorders will often not understand how they are affected. Teaching usually does not help, because the problem is lack of insight, not lack of information. Family members may be a source of information about the patient's functional ability at home.

DIAGNOSING, PLANNING, AND IMPLEMENTING
Anxiety
Expected outcome: Will discuss feelings of anxiety and identify situations that precipitate anxiety.

- Help patients identify the situations associated with their anxiety. *Early recognition of anxiety-producing situations will give the patient a chance to take adaptive action.*
- Help anxious or dependent patients practice asking for what they need; give positive reinforcement when they identify their needs. *When patients have a thought distortion about being unworthy of care, they may benefit from a discussion of their perception. Practicing new behavior (asking for help and getting it) can encourage the patient to continue this behavior.*
- Give patients choices about their care whenever possible. *Choices, such as those relating to daily activities (e.g., when to bathe, meal choices, when to ambulate, where to put items at the bedside), can help the patient have a sense of control. A sense of control can decrease anxiety.*
- Encourage patients to express their true feelings. *When patients believe that they are expected to always be compliant and agreeable, regardless of their own feelings, anxiety is worsened. Recognition and expression of feelings is therapeutic.*

■ Reduce environmental stimuli. *Anxiety makes patients more sensitive to noises in the environment. The patient is likely to feel calmer in a calm environment.*

■ Maintain a calm approach to the anxious patient. *The nurse's attitude can be "contagious" in that either calmness or anxiety can be transmitted to the patient.*

■ Promote a trusting relationship with the patient. *A trusting nurse–patient relationship can improve the patient's self-esteem and reduce anxiety.*

EVALUATING

The desired outcomes for patients with personality disorders relate to resolving the effects these disorders have on patients. Nurses will intervene based on the individual patient's needs and evaluate whether the patient achieves the following desired outcomes:

■ Effective, adaptive coping behavior
■ No harm to self or others
■ Adequate sleep to feel rested during the day
■ Appropriate interactions with other people
■ Making positive statements about self
■ Taking initiative to solve problems
■ Following unit rules
■ Asking for help directly and appropriately
■ Reality-based thinking

DOCUMENTING

Documentation focuses on patients' behavior, safety, mental status, and interpersonal interactions. Describe patient behavior and statements that reflect mental status or patients' response to interventions. For example, you might document that a patient sat in bed with her arms around her bent legs and stated, "I can't stay here. I am so scared." Chart your interventions, possibly a brief orientation to the unit and how to call the nurse, and reassurance of the patient's safety. Include the patient's response, "The patient is visibly relaxed and stated, 'Thanks, I feel better now.'"

NURSING CARE PLAN
Patient With Borderline Personality Disorder

Barbara Porter is a 25-year-old European American patient admitted to the urgent care outpatient unit with multiple self-inflicted lacerations on her left forearm.

Assessment

She is oriented to person, place, time, and situation. Barbara is expressing her feelings loudly, crying, "I hurt too much since Bob left me, but nobody cared or understood.

Now they can see my pain. Now he can see how he hurt me." Her short-term and long-term memories are intact. She states that her boyfriend of 2 weeks left her last night, she cried all night, she cut herself multiple times on the left forearm with a leg razor this morning, and she called 911. Her eyes are swollen and red. She states that she does not feel like hurting herself again and agrees to tell the staff if she feels like hurting herself. She stated to the triage nurse: "You and your stupid questions! I know more about all this than you do."

Nursing Diagnosis

■ *Ineffective Coping*

Expected Outcomes

Patient will:

■ Discuss her feelings.
■ List alternatives to self-harm for coping with stress.
■ Not harm herself while she is in the hospital.

Planning and Implementing

A dressing was applied to the patient's left forearm after the physician examined it and determined that no sutures were needed. The dressing is dry and intact. Outpatient psychiatric consultation ordered for this afternoon.

Evaluation

The patient stated that she cut herself to make her "broken heart" from her boyfriend's leaving visible to him and others. She said that she "couldn't hold the pain inside anymore." Alternatives to self-harm for stress management discussed. Barbara said that talking to her mother has helped her in stressful situations in the past. She states emphatically that she will not cut or hurt herself again. She kept her appointment with the psychiatrist in the outpatient clinic adjacent to the hospital.

Critical Thinking in the Nursing Process

1. The charge nurse overheard the patient state, "You and your stupid questions! I know more about all this than you do." How should the nurses interpret this statement? Should the nursing supervisor be notified?

2. What coping mechanism has Barbara used in the past? Is this enough to prevent her from using self-harm in the future?

3. Why did the nurses try to avoid lots of sympathy for Barbara when they provided care for her?

Note: Discussion of Critical Thinking questions appears on the companion website.

Note: The references and resources for all chapters have been compiled at the back of the book.

Chapter Review

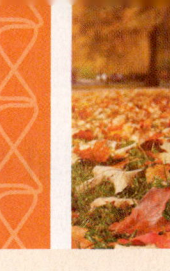

KEY POINTS

- **Concept:** Although the normal range of human behavior, feelings, and thought is broad, it is possible for personality to be outside the normal range.
- Personality disorders cause people to have abnormalities in perception or cognition, emotions, interpersonal functioning, and impulse control.
- **Concept:** People with personality disorders can behave irrationally even when their intellect is intact.
- **Concept:** Personality has been attributed to life experience, but brain changes have been found in some people with disorders of personality.
- Brain imaging technology has found similar abnormalities in the limbic systems of people with disorders of emotional over-reactivity to stress (bipolar disorder, borderline personality disorder, and attention-deficit hyperactivity disorder).
- Nurses often see people with personality disorders when they are hospitalized for reasons other than their personality disorder.
- Personality develops over years starting in childhood and is very resistant to change.
- There is no medication to treat disorders of personality. Medication can be used to treat symptoms, such as anxiety. Some people respond to long-term psychotherapy for changing the pervasive patterns of personality.
- Dialectical-behavior therapy is an effective treatment for many people with borderline personality disorder.
- These disorders appear to make it more difficult for people to foresee the consequences of their actions or to control their impulses despite probable negative consequences.
- Most people with personality disorders do not know that they are affected.
- Nurses can help people with personality disorders achieve personal growth.
- It can be very challenging to care for people with personality disorders. Nurses who work with them must understand themselves and their professional responsibilities to be most effective.
- The most successful nursing interventions will be based on realistic, practical, attainable goals.
- Many people who work very hard on DBT have experienced relief from BPD and other anxiety-based disorders. Keep hope alive!

PEARSON NURSING STUDENT RESOURCES

Find additional materials at **nursing.pearsonhighered.com**.

Clinical Reasoning Care Map

Caring for a Patient With Ineffective Coping
NCLEX-PN® Focus Area: Psychosocial Integrity

Case Study: Ann Lee is a 68-year-old European American female patient. She had acute diverticulitis and was admitted to the general hospital for a partial bowel resection yesterday. Ms. Lee also has dependent personality disorder. She is recovering from her surgery. She is very compliant with requests made by the staff. She has never asked the staff for anything. The physician wrote an order for PRN medication for incisional pain.

Nursing Diagnosis: Ineffective Coping

COLLECT DATA

Subjective	Objective
_____	_____
_____	_____
_____	_____
_____	_____
_____	_____
_____	_____
_____	_____

Does this present a threat to the patient's safety?

If yes, the priority intervention to address this threat would be:

_____

Nursing Care

_____
_____
_____
_____
_____
_____
_____
_____

Interprofessional team members to include when planning care:

_____

How would you document this? _____

_____

Compare your answers and documentation to those provided on the companion website.

Data Collected
(use only those that apply)

- Patient is married.
- BP 158/90, P 110, R 24.
- T 99.0.
- Patient states, "Yes, whatever you say."
- When asked if she needs pain medication, she states, "No, I don't want to bother you."
- When asked if she needs anything she states, "I don't know."
- Weighs 168 lb.
- Awake on all q2h checks during the night.
- Bowel sounds hypoactive.
- Ate 100% of clear liquid breakfast tray.
- Ambulates when asked.
- Abdominal surgical incision is dry and intact, without exudate; incision is well approximated.
- Grimaces and sweats when ambulating or moving in bed.
- States, "What do you think I should do?"

Nursing Interventions
(use only those that apply; list in priority order)

- Tell the patient, "Since you don't seem to want any help, I will leave you alone."
- Call the physician immediately about the vital signs.
- Include offering pain med regularly in the plan of care.
- Ask the patient, "Are you in pain?"
- Say to the patient, "Most people have a lot of pain after surgery. You have signs of pain; does your incision hurt?"
- Visit the patient regularly to determine whether she needs help.
- Say to the patient, "Sometimes people don't like to ask for help. While you are in the hospital, we want to help you, so please tell us what you need."
- Teach the patient now about dressing changes at home.
- Help the patient practice identifying her needs.
- Tell the patient, "It is no trouble to give you some pain medication. I will be glad to get some if you need it."
- Document that the patient is passive, inappropriate, and dishonest.
- Discuss outpatient referral for therapy with treatment team.

NCLEX-PN® Exam Preparation

1. The patient with a paranoid personality disorder responds best to a nurse who uses which of the following approaches?
   1. Friendly, outgoing
   2. Self-confident, matter-of-fact
   3. Shy, hesitant
   4. Quiet, uses brief encounters

2. A patient in a long-term care facility who has cancer also has schizoid personality disorder. The nurse notices that the patient says little to staff members and has no expression in his voice when he speaks. He has no visitors and receives no phone calls. The nurse would conclude that:
   1. this is the patient's usual behavior.
   2. the patient is ashamed of his condition.
   3. the patient is depressed about his diagnosis.
   4. the patient is lonely.

3. As a new resident of an assisted living facility, a patient always refuses to eat in the optional dining room with other residents. She does not attend social functions, preferring to stay in her room. You know that she has a diagnosis of schizotypal personality disorder. The nurse's best approach to this patient would be to:
   1. insist she attend all social functions.
   2. encourage other residents to visit her daily.
   3. invite her to eat at least one meal a day in the dining room.
   4. leave her alone.

4. A patient with antisocial personality disorder yells at the staff frequently. He is very demanding and expects to be exempt from the usual hospital rules. What is the best nursing approach to this patient?
   1. Allow him to break the rules to keep him happy.
   2. Tell him that the rules apply to everyone, including him.
   3. Ask the physician for an order for an anxiolytic medication.
   4. Reassure him that he is safe in the hospital.

5. The treatment priority for a patient with borderline personality disorder is:
   1. teaching appropriate social skills.
   2. preventing self-injury.
   3. teaching problem-solving techniques.
   4. medicating for sleep disturbances.

6. A patient on the psychiatric unit is continually disruptive in any group session by directing all attention to herself. She is constantly asking the other members of the group to help her solve her life problems. She refers to everyone in the group as

her "dearest friends." This patient's behavior is consistent with which personality disorder?
   1. Borderline
   2. Avoidant
   3. Schizotypal
   4. Histrionic

7. A patient is on a medical–surgical unit after gallbladder surgery. He is constantly belittling the nurses taking care of him and wants the surgeon called in the middle of the night to complain about his care. They suspect that he has a narcissistic personality disorder. As night primary nurse, your best approach would be to:
   1. tell him you are sorry he is unhappy with his care. However, you will not call his surgeon, because that is not appropriate. His surgeon will visit in the morning, and he is welcome to voice his complaints at that time.
   2. tell him you will call his surgeon and then do not call. If he asks, tell him no one answered.
   3. tell him he is not the only patient you have to take care of and you do not have time to cater to his every demand.
   4. ask him how you can make him happier with his care. Make an extra effort to meet all his demands.

8. A patient with dependent personality disorder is very anxious. Which of the following nursing interventions are likely to relieve this patient's anxiety? **Select all that apply.**
   1. Establish a trusting nurse–patient relationship.
   2. Teach the patient that he or she does not have to be anxious.
   3. Maintain a calm approach to the patient.
   4. Encourage the patient to express his or her feelings.
   5. Provide a pager so the patient can call the nurse at any time.

9. A hospitalized patient has antisocial personality disorder. Put the following nursing interventions in order of priority for this patient.
   1. Apply hospital rules consistently.
   2. Encourage the patient to participate in outpatient counseling.
   3. Prevent emotional or physical harm to staff.
   4. Encourage the patient to express his needs in socially appropriate ways.

10. Which of the following medications is most likely to be prescribed for someone with obsessive-compulsive personality disorder who is in the hospital?
    1. Anxiolytic
    2. Antidepressant
    3. Antipsychotic
    4. Hypnotic

Answers and rationales for Review Questions appear in Appendix I

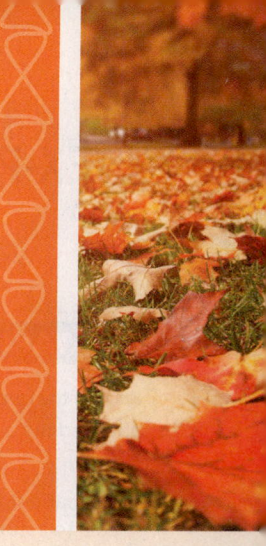

CHAPTER 53
Caring for Patients With Substance Use Disorders

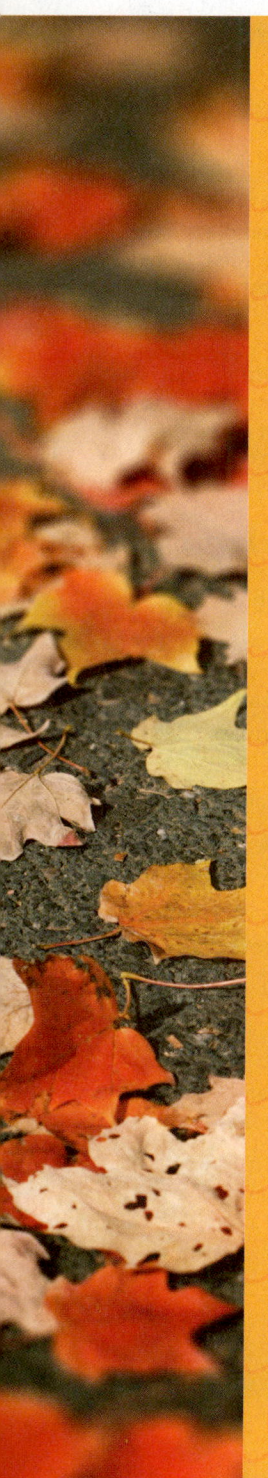

BRIEF OUTLINE

Problem of Substance Abuse
Commonly Abused Substances

Substance Dependency Among Nurses

APPLIED LEARNING OUTCOMES

After completing this chapter, you will be able to:

1. Explain substance use disorders, tolerance, and withdrawal.
2. Collect information from patients who are using commonly abused drugs.
3. Identify adverse effects caused by interactions between commonly abused substances and medications used in medical care.
4. Provide appropriate nursing interventions for a patient in drug or alcohol withdrawal.
5. Apply the nursing process to patients experiencing substance use disorders.

KEY TERMS

The key terms are defined on the pages listed below.

abstinence, 1308
alcoholic, 1306
ataxia, 1305
codependents, 1315
confabulation, 1307
cross-tolerance, 1311
denial, 1303
detoxification, 1312

dual diagnosis, 1315
enabling, 1315
euphoria, 1305
impaired nurse, 1315
intoxication, 1305
Korsakoff syndrome, 1307
labile, 1305
myopathy, 1307

polysubstance abuse, 1309
rehabilitation, 1314
relapse, 1308
tolerance, 1304
Wernicke syndrome, 1307
withdrawal, 1304

SPECIAL FEATURES

NURSING CARE PLAN: Patient With Ineffective Coping, 1317
CLINICAL REASONING CARE MAP: Caring for a Patient With Substance Use Disorder, 1320
UNIT XIII WRAP-UP: Thinking Strategically About..., 1322

Problem of Substance Use

Throughout human history, people have used substances to alter their perceptions; to elevate mood; to relieve pain, fear, anxiety, or boredom; and to aid in religious ceremonies. Alcohol, the most commonly used psychoactive substance, can be used responsibly and enjoyably. However, when substances are abused, they can interfere with people's ability to function normally, cause legal problems, put the drug user or others in danger, and the use will continue despite negative consequences.

> **Key Concept** Substance use is one of the most important health problems of the twenty-first century.

In 2012, 6.4% of the adult population over age 18 of the United States met the diagnostic criteria for a substance use disorder (SAMHSA, 2013). Add to this number the family members, employers, employees, coworkers, people injured or killed by substance abusers, and babies born to women who abuse alcohol and other substances, and it is clear that many people are affected. The annual financial cost to society is in the hundreds of billions of dollars. The toll in human morbidity, mortality, and suffering is staggering. See Figure 53-1 ■ to learn about how often alcohol is a factor in fatal events.

The incidence of substance use peaks in young adults from ages 18 to 25. Substance use does not constitute a substance use disorder unless the diagnostic criteria are present. European Americans are more frequently affected by alcohol and other substance use disorders than African Americans, Asian/Pacific Islanders, or Latinos. Native Americans are affected at the highest rate, however. Substance use disorder is a major public health concern in the United States and the world (SAMHSA, 2013).

The exact number of people with substance use disorders is not known. The reason for this lack of information is that **denial** (refusal to acknowledge the existence of a real situation or feelings) is a common coping mechanism for people with these disorders and for the health professionals who work with them. The stigma of substance abuse is so great that even health care professionals are afraid of it. Substance use disorders can be treated appropriately when we accept that they are physiologic and psychologic diseases and not weaknesses of character.

People with substance use disorders usually do not receive treatment. Health professionals often do not ask the questions that could determine who is affected by substance use. Even when they are aware of patients' substance use, health care providers underreport it. Sometimes health professionals try to avoid stigmatizing patients or are uncomfortable taking about substance use. Sometimes they are not aware of how they can help. This chapter helps the nurse to identify patients with substance-related disorders and provides tools for intervening to help them.

Substance Use Disorders

> **Key Concept** A substance use disorder is a maladaptive pattern of substance use despite adverse outcomes.

A person has a substance use disorder when he or she has a problematic pattern of use (including disordered thinking, behavior, and body function) of any of the substances of abuse, except caffeine. The disorder includes a combination of the following symptoms: The substance is used more often or in higher doses than the person intends; the inability to fulfill major role obligations at work, school, or home; the substance is repeatedly used in physically hazardous situations; a strong desire to use the substance; a recurrent desire to quit or cut down on using the substance; unsuccessful attempts to quit using except for limited periods; continued use even though there are recurrent social or family problems caused by substance use; large amounts of time spent in obtaining, using, and recovering from substance use; or continued use despite knowledge of health problems caused by the substance (APA, 2013).

Compulsive Substance Use

Compulsive behavior is repetitive behavior used for the purpose of reducing distress. It is often undesired by the individual involved. Compulsive substance use is repetitive substance use that represents maladaptive coping behavior. It is part of a substance use disorder.

Commonly Abused Substances

Substances that rapidly alter the mental state, by either stimulating or depressing the central nervous system (CNS), are the most commonly abused. The *DSM-5* (2013) lists 10 substances of abuse:

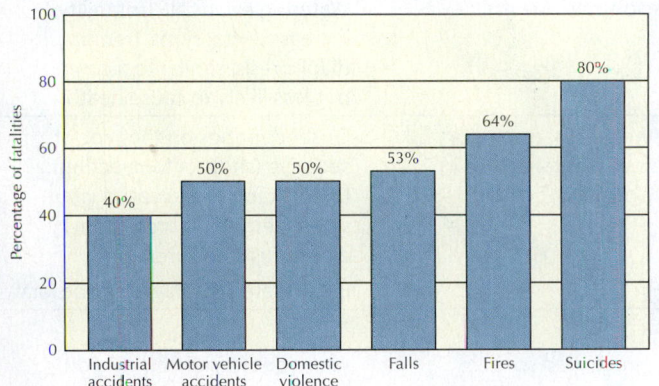

Figure 53-1. ■ Fatal events in which alcohol is a factor.
(Source: From Mental Health Nursing, 6e by Karen Lee Fontaine and J. Sue Fletcher. Published by Pearson Education, © 2009.)

- Alcohol
- Opioids
- Sedatives, hypnotics, and anxiolytics
- Stimulants (amphetamine-type substances, cocaine, and other stimulants)
- Hallucinogens
- Phencyclidine (PCP) and similar drugs
- Inhalants
- Cannabis
- Tobacco
- Caffeine

Tables 53-1 ■ and 53-2 ■ provide summaries of the effects of these substances.

Tolerance and Withdrawal

Key Concept With continued use, the user develops **tolerance** to substances that stimulate or depress the central nervous system. This means that increasing amounts of the substance are needed to achieve the same effect or the same amount causes less effect.

Each of the substances of abuse has its own pattern of tolerance. When an individual uses a CNS depressant regularly, the CNS stimulates itself to maintain homeostasis. Concurrent depression by the substance and stimulation by the CNS create a balance, and the user has fewer CNS symptoms. However, to maintain the desired intoxicant effects, the user must use ever-increasing doses of the substance.

Key Concept When a person uses a CNS depressant or stimulant substance consistently and then stops, the individual will experience **withdrawal** (symptoms related to lack of a substance that has been used heavily for a long time) until the CNS regains homeostasis without the substance.

Withdrawal symptoms vary among the substances of abuse according to their specific actions. For example, when a person is tolerant to a CNS stimulant, the CNS has become depressed to regain homeostasis in the regular presence of a stimulant. A balance is formed. When the stimulant is stopped, the CNS is depressed until homeostasis can be regained. Withdrawal symptoms motivate the user to obtain the substance again. Withdrawal symptoms range from annoying to life threatening, as in alcohol withdrawal. Tolerance and withdrawal are part of the substance use disorder.

ALCOHOL

Ethyl alcohol (ethanol, beverage alcohol) is the most commonly abused substance. It is a CNS depressant that is quickly absorbed into the blood after drinking. Initial symptoms of

TABLE 53-1	Comparison of Commonly Abused CNS Depressants and Stimulants		
DRUG	EFFECTS OF USE	OVERDOSE SYMPTOMS	WITHDRAWAL SYMPTOMS AND THEIR ONSET (AFTER LAST DOSE)
CNS depressants Alcohol (beer, wine, liquor)	Euphoria, loss of inhibition, ataxia, lack of coordination, reduced cognition, impaired judgment, nausea, slurred speech, impairment in attention or memory	Respiratory depression, mental confusion, unconsciousness, death	6–8 hours. CNS irritability, anxiety, increased vital signs, tremors, ataxia, diaphoresis, slurred speech, GI disturbance, disorientation, hallucinations, seizures, death.
Opioids/narcotics (e.g., morphine, meperidine, methadone, oxycodone [OxyContin], heroin)	Analgesia, cough suppression, euphoria, loss of inhibition, lack of coordination, reduced cognition, impaired judgment, apathy, nausea, constipation, constricted pupils	Sedation, respiratory depression, mental confusion, unconsciousness, death	12–72 hours (longer for OxyContin, which is long acting). Watering eyes, CNS irritability, increased vital signs, tremors, diaphoresis, similar to alcohol, but less likely to cause death.
Sedatives, hypnotics, anxiolytics	Sedation, muscle relaxation, apathy, reduced cognition Anxiolytics cause reduced anxiety, muscle relaxation, and less sedation in low doses	Muscle weakness, respiratory depression, mental confusion, unconsciousness, death	Onset depends on the type of sedative (short or long acting). CNS irritability, increased vital signs, tremors, slurred speech, diaphoresis, seizures. Barbiturate withdrawal can be fatal.
CNS stimulants Cocaine, amphetamines, drugs for attention deficit hyperactivity disorder (ADHD)	Local vasoconstriction, sudden rush of euphoria, elation, energy, talkativeness, anorexia, weight loss, elevated vital signs, grandiosity	Chest pain, slurred speech, mental confusion, vomiting, hallucinations, myocardial infarction, severe elevation of BP and P, shock, death	Acute depression, craving drug, fatigue, irritability, suicidal thoughts, loss of pleasure (anhedonia), not life threatening. Withdrawal onset is variable, depending on dose used and degree of tolerance.

TABLE 53-2	Comparison of Hallucinogens, Inhalants, Cannabis, Tobacco, and Caffeine		
SUBSTANCE	**EFFECTS OF USE**	**OVERDOSE SYMPTOMS**	**WITHDRAWAL SYMPTOMS**
Hallucinogens LSD, DMT, mescaline, MDMA (Ecstasy)	Hallucinations and distorted perceptions, distortions of time and space, illusions, emotional lability, tremor, nausea and vomiting, pupil dilation	Panic (may be drug reaction, not OD), seizures (rare)	No withdrawal; may experience flashbacks for several months after last dose
Phencyclidine (PCP)	Bizarre perceptions, disorientation, hallucinations, agitation, grandiosity, withdrawal or agitation or both, paranoia, dilated pupils, nystagmus, hypertension, dry red skin, diminished responsiveness to pain	Seizures, coma, death	No withdrawal
Inhalants and cannabis Inhalants *Hydrocarbons:* glue, gasoline, aerosol spray, solvents *Nitrites:* amyl nitrite, nitrous oxide	*Hydrocarbons:* euphoria, impaired judgment, nystagmus, ataxia, slurred speech, perceptual changes, sense of invulnerability *Nitrites:* prolonged erection or enhanced intercourse	*Hydrocarbons:* stupor, coma, cardiac depression and dysrhythmias, respiratory arrest, renal complications *Nitrites:* panic, hypotension, headache *Both:* brain damage	Similar to alcohol
Cannabis, marijuana, hashish	Euphoria, pleasure, confidence, grandiosity, anxiety, relaxation, sensation of slowed time, impaired judgment and motor coordination, red eyes, dry mouth, increased appetite	None	Irritability, anger, aggression, anxiety, depressed mood, restlessness, insomnia, decreased appetite, weight loss, craving
Tobacco and caffeine Tobacco	Pleasure, alertness, increased BP and P, decreased blood flow to heart muscle	None	Anxiety, depressed mood, anger, craving, increased appetite, sleep disorder
Caffeine	Increased alertness, prolongs ability to work, elevates mood	Anxiety, cardiac dysrhythmias	Headache, fatigue

alcohol **intoxication** (a reversible set of physical, psychologic, and behavioral symptoms caused by the use of the substance) are relaxation, loss of inhibition, **euphoria** (an exaggerated feeling of well-being), and decreased mental concentration. With increased use, symptoms progress to slurred speech, **ataxia** (staggering gait), **labile** (changeable) mood, aggressive behavior, incoherent speech, vomiting, coma, respiratory depression, and death. See Box 53-1■ for manifestations of alcohol intoxication by blood alcohol concentrations.

Pattern of Use

The pattern of use of alcohol varies from one individual to another. Some people start drinking alcohol in childhood or adolescence, some in old age. Some drink daily, starting with "one or two drinks with dinner" and progressing to greater amounts and frequency. Some drink heavily on weekends; others may abstain for long periods and then have a drinking binge.

For most people, drinking alcohol begins for social reasons and continues to be a social event. Some people begin to use alcohol as a coping mechanism, to relieve the everyday stress of life. Using alcohol to cope or to solve problems requires increasing amounts of alcohol over time. In the early stage of alcoholism, the affected individual is likely to deny that alcohol use is a problem, despite the evidence and the tolerance that develops.

BOX 53-1	MANIFESTATIONS OF ALCOHOL INTOXICATION BY BLOOD ALCOHOL CONCENTRATION

BLOOD ALCOHOL CONCENTRATION (G/DL)	MANIFESTATIONS
0.05–0.10 (0.08–0.10 is the legal level of intoxication in most states)	Relaxation, euphoria, decreased inhibitions, impaired judgment, changeable mood, decreased mental concentration, decreased fine motor coordination
0.15–0.25	Slurred speech, decreased motor function, ataxia, mood outbursts, aggressive behavior
0.3	Incoherent speech, mental confusion, stupor, vomiting, labored breathing
0.4	Unconsciousness, coma
0.5	Respiratory depression, death

Alcohol dependency progresses to include memory blackouts during episodes of intoxication. At this stage, the alcohol is no longer a source of pleasure or relief, but a drug that is required by the individual. People in this phase often drink alone or secretly. They experience withdrawal symptoms. They wake up in the morning and need a drink to control tremors (an eye-opener). Denial is still the defense mechanism.

As the disease progresses, the individual completely loses control over the ability to choose whether or not to drink. Side effects include isolation from others, anger, aggression, loss of interest in any activity that previously brought pleasure, and malnutrition. The individual becomes willing to give up everything to maintain the addiction. It is common for people in this phase to lose their jobs, families, friends, and self-respect.

The end stage of alcohol dependency is characterized by emotional and physical disintegration. The individual may experience psychosis. Every body system is affected by life-threatening complications. Abstention from alcohol results in life-threatening withdrawal. Thoughts of suicide are common.

The process of increasing tolerance develops over years of alcohol dependency, until the individual must drink almost constantly to avoid the distressing symptoms of CNS stimulation.

When the alcohol-dependent individual stops drinking, the CNS is still stimulated. The homeostatic mechanism that balanced the depressant effects of the alcohol takes time to return to normal. Meanwhile, the individual suffers withdrawal symptoms. The alcohol withdrawal syndrome includes elevated vital signs; anxiety; tremors; diaphoresis; slurred speech; GI disturbances (vomiting, cramping, diarrhea); ataxia; nystagmus; disorientation; and, at its most severe, hallucinations, seizures, and death.

Note that the symptoms of alcohol withdrawal are generally the opposite of those of alcohol intoxication. The individual takes the CNS depressant substance; the CNS stimulates itself to regain homeostasis. When the substance is withdrawn, the CNS is still stimulated, and the individual has CNS stimulation symptoms until the CNS eventually reestablishes homeostasis without alcohol, and the symptoms subside. Alcohol withdrawal syndrome usually lasts about 4 days. See Table 53-1 for withdrawal symptoms.

Alcohol withdrawal delirium (formerly called delirium tremens or DTs) is diagnosed when withdrawal is associated with severe cognitive symptoms such as confusion, delusions, and terrifying hallucinations. This delirium happens to people with a long (5- to 15-year) history of alcoholism. It is a medical emergency. Alcohol withdrawal delirium is preventable. It occurs when the CNS has stimulated itself to remain conscious under increasing alcohol concentrations. If the risk is identified early and the CNS is allowed to gradually return to its normal state over 2 to 4 days by the administration of a decreasing dose of a CNS depressant drug (usually a benzodiazepine), alcohol withdrawal delirium can be avoided. There are several effective alcohol withdrawal protocols available for physicians to use.

The alcohol-dependent individual (**alcoholic**) may experience many episodes of withdrawal symptoms that he or she treats with alcohol. The statement "I feel bad (nervous, tired, angry, lonely, etc.); I need a drink" may be evidence of withdrawal symptoms. Nurses should be aware that substance withdrawal symptoms are often behind a patient's desire to leave the hospital against medical advice.

Long-Term Physical Effects

Chronic use of alcohol takes a toll on the body. All body systems are affected over a period of years. Figure 53-2■ illustrates the physiologic effects. The gastrointestinal system is one of the first to show the effects of chronic alcoholism. Alcohol causes *gastritis* by inflaming the stomach lining. The protective mucous lining of the stomach is damaged by alcohol, allowing hydrochloric acid to erode the stomach wall. If the vascular structure in the stomach wall is involved, bleeding can occur. Ulcers may form in the stomach. Symptoms include gastric distress, nausea, vomiting, black stools, and abdominal distention. Esophagitis is caused by the irritant effect of alcohol on the esophagus and by frequent vomiting. The primary symptom is esophageal pain.

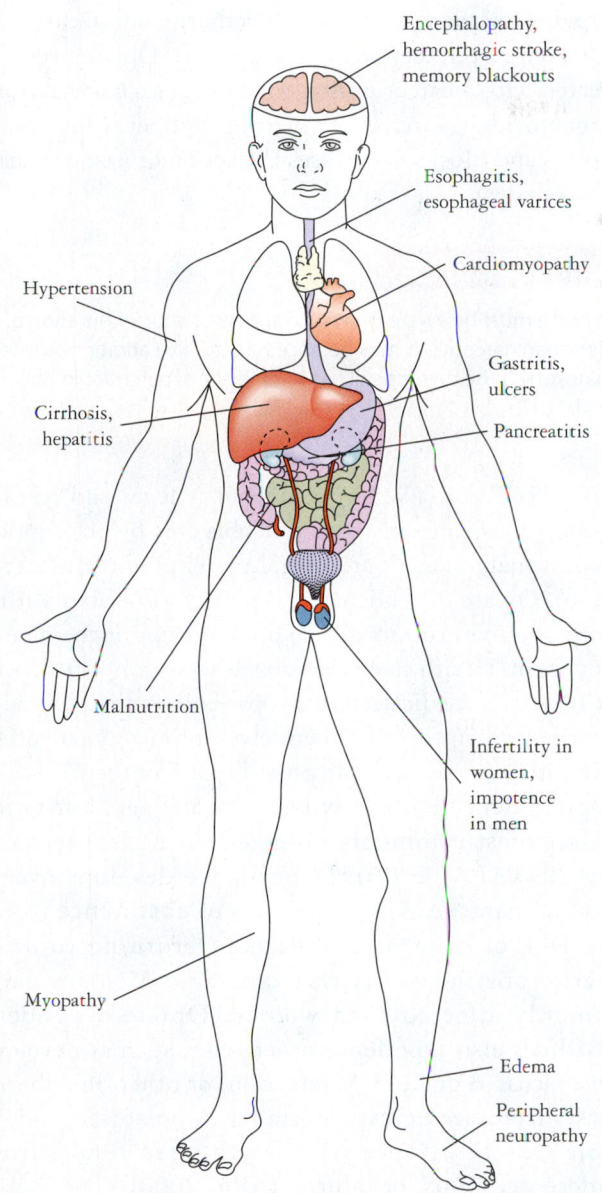

Encephalopathy, hemorrhagic stroke, memory blackouts

Esophagitis, esophageal varices

Cardiomyopathy

Hypertension

Gastritis, ulcers

Cirrhosis, hepatitis

Pancreatitis

Malnutrition

Infertility in women, impotence in men

Myopathy

Edema

Peripheral neuropathy

Figure 53-2. ■ Physiologic effects of alcoholism.

Pancreatitis, either acute or chronic, may also be caused by chronic alcohol use. Chronic pancreatitis leads to pancreatic insufficiency, which causes malnutrition, weight loss, and diabetes mellitus. Acute pancreatitis happens 1 or 2 days after a binge of drinking alcohol. The symptoms include severe, constant epigastric pain, nausea, vomiting, and abdominal distention.

Alcoholic hepatitis affects an already damaged liver, usually after a prolonged binge of excessive alcohol consumption. The patient has right upper quadrant abdominal pain, jaundice, an enlarged liver and spleen, vomiting, weakness, profound fatigue, and possibly ascites.

Cirrhosis of the liver is the worst alcohol-related liver disorder and is the end stage of chronic alcoholic liver disease. In cirrhosis, severely damaged or destroyed liver cells

are replaced by scar tissue, making this disease irreversible. Cirrhosis causes portal hypertension, ascites, *esophageal varices* (varicose veins in the esophagus that can rupture and hemorrhage), and hepatic encephalopathy. *Hepatic encephalopathy*, caused by accumulation of ammonia in the brain, results in impaired mental function and progresses to death.

Cardiomyopathy (muscle abnormality and weakening causing enlargement of the heart), heart failure, and cardiac dysrhythmias may occur. The risk of hemorrhagic stroke is increased. Other cardiovascular manifestations include hypertension (especially diastolic elevation), tachycardia, and edema.

Blackouts are an early sign of alcoholism and reflect neurologic involvement. The affected individual remains conscious and appears to be functioning normally, but is completely unable to remember anything that occurs while intoxicated. After many years of alcohol abuse, a person may develop Korsakoff syndrome and Wernicke syndrome, which affect the entire neurologic system. These syndromes usually occur together and are often called Wernicke–Korsakoff syndrome.

Korsakoff syndrome is a group of symptoms caused by a deficiency in the B vitamins, including thiamine, riboflavin, and folic acid. Amnesia, disorientation to time and place, **confabulation** (falsification of memory to fill in the gaps caused by cognitive deficits), and severe peripheral neuropathy characterize it. Symptoms of the neuropathy include tingling; muscle weakness; sore, burning muscles; abnormal sensation; and pain with movement. The extremities are affected, especially the legs. Because of the extreme pain, care must be taken when moving these patients.

Wernicke syndrome (alcoholic encephalopathy) is characterized by ataxia, paralysis of eye muscles, nystagmus, and mental confusion. It is the result of severe vitamin B_1 deficiency from lack of adequate nutritional intake. Early in the disorder, it may respond well to large doses of parenteral thiamine. If not treated early, it progresses to an irreversible, fatal condition that requires custodial care.

The reproductive system is affected as well. Men may become *impotent*. Women may stop menstruating and become infertile. Further, the unborn child of a pregnant woman may be seriously affected. Box 53-2 ■ describes manifestations of fetal alcohol syndrome.

When the musculoskeletal system is affected, osteoporosis can develop. Also, acute or chronic **myopathy** may occur, characterized by muscle cramps of sudden onset and later development of pain, tenderness, and edema of the skeletal muscles, especially of the legs. In chronic myopathy, there is wasting and weakness of the skeletal muscles.

OTHER CNS DEPRESSANTS

Other depressants of the CNS are similar to alcohol in their effects on the CNS, intoxication symptoms, tolerance

---

BOX 53-2 | **MANIFESTATIONS OF FETAL ALCOHOL SYNDROME**

- Low birth weight
- Microcephaly (small head circumference, small brain)
- Facial anomalies
  - Flat mid-face
  - Flat nasal bridge
  - Small eyes
  - Short palpebral fissures (narrow eye openings)
  - Short nose
  - Flat philtrum (indistinct infranasal depression)
  - Thin upper lip
- Neurodevelopmental disorders
  - Developmental delay
  - Learning disabilities
  - Poor coordination
  - Distractibility/impulsivity

---

effects, and withdrawal symptoms. Table 53-1 provides a profile of the CNS depressants.

The Opiates

Opiates are naturally occurring substances derived from opium (e.g., morphine), semisynthetics (e.g., heroin), and drugs that resemble them (e.g., methadone, meperidine, oxycodone, or codeine). Opiates are narcotic drugs prescribed to relieve pain or diarrhea or to reduce cough. These drugs have alleviated immeasurable human pain, but when abused, they have caused immense suffering as well.

EFFECTS OF OPIATES Opiate drugs can cause physical dependence (tolerance and withdrawal); see Table 53-1. The opiate drugs decrease GI peristalsis, so they can be used therapeutically to treat severe diarrhea. When opiates are abused, constipation can be severe, including fecal impaction. The nausea and vomiting that are commonly caused by opiates are due to stimulation of the medulla of the brain.

In therapeutic doses, opiates have little effect on the heart. Morphine is often used to treat cardiac patients for pain or to divert blood flow to the peripheral circulation, decreasing the work of the heart. In high doses, opiates cause hypotension by affecting the heart or reducing vascular resistance.

Nurses especially need to know about the respiratory effects of opioids. These drugs, which are used therapeutically to suppress cough, depress the respiratory center in the medulla of the brain. Respiratory depression is not likely to happen in therapeutic doses unless the patient is narcotic naive (has not been exposed to opiates recently). With high doses, though, respiratory depression may be life threatening. Chronic respiratory depression predisposes the patient to pneumonia and other respiratory infections.

Opiate overdose is a medical emergency. Death can result from respiratory arrest and hypoxia. Opiate overdose is treated with a narcotic antagonist drug, such as naloxone hydrochloride (Narcan). This drug competes for opiate receptors and blocks or reverses the action of narcotic analgesics (opiates).

clinicalALERT

The nurse must be aware that naloxone has a shorter duration of action than narcotics. It may be necessary to give additional doses of naloxone if the patient still has high levels of narcotics in the blood.

PATTERNS OF USE Whereas alcohol is legal and readily available, the opiates are either available only by prescription (narcotic analgesics) or are illegal under all circumstances (heroin). Opiate dependence is typically associated with a history of crimes committed to obtain drugs or the money to buy them. Health care professionals who are opiate dependent may steal medications from patients or their employers, write prescriptions for themselves, or manipulate other health care providers to write prescriptions for them.

Opioid dependence may begin at any age, but problems are most commonly observed in the late teens or early 20s (APA, 2000). Dependence develops over a period of many years, with periods of **abstinence** (complete lack of drug use). **Relapse** (returning to drug use after abstinence) is very common. Men are more commonly affected than women. Opiate-dependent individuals also experience other risks, such as developing hepatitis B or C, HIV infection, or other bloodborne diseases from needle use. Mortality in opiate-dependent people may be 2% per year. Death often results from overdose, accidents, or injuries (APA, 2000).

Sedative, Hypnotic, or Anxiolytic-Related Drugs

Sedatives, hypnotics, and anxiolytics include the benzodiazepines, the barbiturates, and similar drugs. Prescription sleeping medications and almost all of the anxiolytic (antianxiety) drugs are included. Like alcohol and the opiates, these substances depress the CNS. (For information about anxiety disorders, see Chapter 51.)

OVERDOSE CNS depressant drugs have additive effects when taken together. For example, when people use alcohol and a sedative drug at the same time, the CNS depressant effect is beyond what either substance would cause alone. Although the amount of sedative may be usual and the amount of alcohol may be what the person usually drinks, the two together could cause fatal respiratory depression. It is not uncommon for people to die as a result of this additive effect.

It is common for the substance-dependent individual to have a drug of choice, but to use a variety of other substances, including alcohol. This combination of abused substances is called **polysubstance abuse**. Benzodiazepines alone in overdose are rarely fatal, but barbiturates in overdose are often fatal, due to cardiac or respiratory arrest.

A relatively new, quick-acting sedative drug is flunitrazepam (Rohypnol). It is called the *date rape drug*, because it can rapidly incapacitate a rape victim. One or two tablets dissolved in alcohol can render a person unconscious within minutes. The affected individual then has amnesia for several hours.

CNS STIMULANTS
Cocaine and Amphetamines

The clinical usefulness of this group of drugs is limited to the treatment of attention deficit hyperactivity disorder. Cocaine especially is a popular drug of abuse because of the immediate euphoria it induces. See Table 53-1 for intoxication and withdrawal symptoms.

Hallucinogens

Hallucinogens distort the user's perception of reality. The most common hallucinogens are LSD, mescaline, and PCP (phencyclidine). The CNS effects are unpredictable and may be influenced by the expectations of the user. Some individuals have frightening psychotic experiences. Hallucinations can lead to violent or self-injurious behavior. See Table 53-2 for a comparison of the hallucinogens with other drugs of abuse.

Synthetic or "designer" drugs are popular. MDMA or Ecstasy is derived from amphetamine and methamphetamine, so it acts as both a stimulant and a hallucinogen.

Inhalants

Two kinds of inhalants (hydrocarbons and nitrites) are commonly abused. See Table 53-2 for their effects. The hydrocarbons can induce cardiac depression, renal injury, respiratory depression, and death from cardiac dysrhythmias or accidents while intoxicated (Keltner, 2013).

Cannabis

Delta-9-tetrahydrocannabinol (THC) is thought to be the chemical responsible for the psychoactive effects of marijuana and hashish. See Table 53-2 for its effects.

Cannabis is the most widely used illegal substance in the United States, although its use for medical and even recreational purposes is being legalized in states across the country. It has been therapeutically used to treat the anorexia, nausea, and vomiting associated with AIDS and cancer. While marijuana is being legalized, it still has the potential for abuse and to create a substance use disorder if misused.

Caffeine and Nicotine

It may be surprising to find caffeine and nicotine on the list of substances of abuse. Still, these substances fit the model of dependence defined in the *DSM-5*. Both substances cause tolerance and withdrawal.

Caffeine is the most commonly used stimulant drug. The physiologic effects of caffeine explain why it is so popular as a performance enhancer. It prolongs the time the user can continue to work, improves mental alertness, and elevates mood (Table 53-2). The dose and frequency of use determine the effects and whether the user develops tolerance.

The average coffee drinker consumes 360 to 450 mg of caffeine per day. Intake of more than 600 mg of caffeine per day is considered excessive (Kneisl, Wilson, & Trigoboff, 2013). Caffeine and sugar supply the "energy" in the various energy drinks on the market.

Nicotine dependence is the most common substance dependence in the United States. Smoking is especially common in the population of people who use alcohol and other substances (Figure 53-3 ■) The consequences of smoking are also related to other substances present in tobacco. The incidence of cancer of the lungs, oral cavity, esophagus, pancreas, and prostate is increased significantly in tobacco users. The risk of cardiovascular disease, including stroke, myocardial infarction, and peripheral arterial disease, is increased by tobacco use as well. Accidents related to fire are also a concern (smoking in bed while drinking alcohol can be deadly).

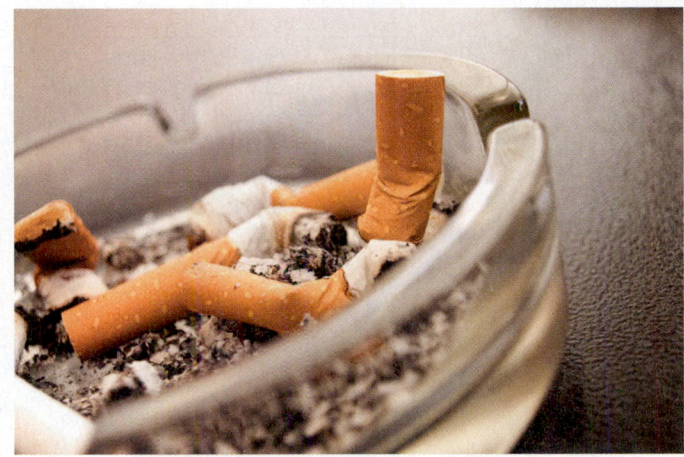

Figure 53-3. ■ Nicotine dependence is the most common substance dependence in the United States. (Source: Sinisa Botas / Shutterstock.)

The risk of cardiovascular disease is significantly reduced when people quit smoking. The physician or nurse should talk to patients who smoke at every office visit about quitting smoking. Even a brief conversation has shown to be motivating to patients to quit smoking. Tobacco withdrawal causes symptoms such as hunger, irritability, and anxiety in many patients. The use of pharmacotherapies is an attempt to minimize these symptoms, to facilitate smoking cessation. Nicotine replacement therapy is the most common strategy. Table 53-3■ shows medications that are used to help patients quit smoking.

Due to the widespread use of caffeine and nicotine, hospitalized patients are likely to experience caffeine or nicotine withdrawal. The headache that patients have after surgery may be better treated with a cup of coffee than medication. Some patients may consider leaving the hospital against medical advice so they can smoke cigarettes. These situations require the nurse's problem-solving skills.

Nurses should acknowledge that physiologic dependence as well as the psychologic habit of smoking make it difficult to quit. Smoking is not a character flaw; it is a significant health issue. Nurses should use the "five As" for every patient who smokes and the "five Rs" to help smokers who are not currently willing to quit:

■ *Ask* the patient about tobacco use.
■ *Advise* the patient to quit.

TABLE 53-3	Giving Medications Safely: Smoking Cessation Agents		
CLASS/DRUG	**PURPOSE**	**NURSING IMPLICATIONS**	**PATIENT TEACHING**
■ Nicotine gum (Nicorette) ■ Lozenges ■ Transdermal patch (NicoDerm, Habitrol, Nicotrol) ■ Nasal spray (Nicotrol NS) ■ Vapor inhaler (Nicotrol inhaler)	Nicotine replacement therapy (NRT) is used to replace nicotine to prevent nicotine withdrawal in patients who smoke.	Monitor for adverse effects: headache, nausea, dizziness. Some adverse effects are route-specific: local irritation. NRT is safely used even in patients with severe cardiac disease. NRT should be offered to all smokers with cardiovascular disease because its risk is so much less than smoking.	Teach the patient to avoid smoking cigarettes or using smokeless tobacco while on NRT. Teach about possible local irritation (mouth with gum and lozenges, skin with patch). Give strategies for reducing irritation (rinse mouth, apply patch on different sites each time).
■ Antidepressant bupropion (Zyban, Wellbutrin)	Increases norepinephrine and dopamine as brain neurotransmitters. Smoking cessation is unrelated to antidepressant effects. Exact mechanism is unknown.	Monitor for side effects: insomnia, dry mouth, blurred vision. Increases seizure potential in patients with epilepsy or head injury, especially at high doses. Monitor for hypertension.	Teach about side effects. The patient may chew sugarless gum to promote saliva secretion. The patient should not stop the drug abruptly. This drug doubles the abstinence rate over placebo and is more effective than the nicotine patch.
■ *Varenicline* (Chantix) ■ e-cigarettes (electronic cigarettes)	Acts on the alpha 4-beta 2-nicotinic acetylcholine receptor where dependency-causing properties of nicotine are mediated. Relieves withdrawal symptoms and cravings while blocking the reinforcing effects of nicotine. Marketed as an aid to quit smoking; research has shown that e-cigarettes are not effective (Grana, Popova, & Ling, 2014).	Monitor for adverse effects: nausea, flatulence, headache, sleep disturbance, lethargy, and joint pain. Monitor for behavior changes, depression, and possibly suicidal thinking if the patient is depressed. FDA has been asked to regulate e-cigs.	Teach about the possibility of agitation or erratic behavior, or depression with suicidal thinking. The odds of quitting smoking are greater with varenicline than with placebo or bupropion. Do not teach patients, especially adolescents (who may be encouraged to continue smoking them) to use them as an aid to quit smoking.

Note: Medications identified in *italics* are among the 200 most frequently prescribed drugs in the United States.

- *Assess* the patient's willingness to make an attempt to quit.
- *Assist* the patient to make an attempt to quit.
- *Arrange* for follow-up contacts to prevent relapse.

The "five Rs" for smokers who are currently unwilling to quit:

- Provide motivational information that is personally *relevant* to the patient.
- Discuss the *risks* associated with smoking and the *rewards* of quitting, such as improvements in functioning and self-efficacy.
- Ask the patient about *roadblocks* or barriers to quitting.
- *Repeat* motivational strategies at every clinic visit because most smokers need to make repeated attempts to quit to be successful.

Steroid Abuse

Among the newer drugs of abuse are the anabolic–androgenic steroids. These are man-made substances related to male sex hormones. *Anabolic* refers to muscle building, and *androgenic* refers to increased masculine characteristics. These drugs are available only by prescription to treat patients with abnormally low testosterone or to treat body wasting in patients with AIDS and other diseases that result in loss of lean muscle mass. Abuse of anabolic steroids can lead to serious health problems, some of which are irreversible.

Anabolic steroids are abused to enhance physical performance and to improve physical appearance. They are taken orally or injected, typically in cycles of weeks or months rather than continuously. Users may combine different types of steroids in an attempt to minimize negative effects.

The major side effects of abusing anabolic steroids include liver tumors, liver cancer, jaundice, edema, hypertension, increased LDL, and decreased HDL. Other side effects include severe acne, tremors, and aggression. Some users have psychiatric symptoms such as mood swings, paranoia, irritability, delusions, and impaired judgment. There are also gender-specific side effects (National Institute on Drug Abuse [NIDA], 2012):

- *For men:* shrinking of the testicles, reduced sperm count, infertility, baldness, breast development, increased risk of prostate cancer
- *For women:* growth of facial hair, male pattern baldness, changes in or cessation of the menstrual cycle, enlargement of the clitoris, deepened voice

Steroid abuse among adolescents has increased since the early 1990s. Although adolescent boys are more likely to abuse steroids, adolescent girls are using steroids in increasing numbers for the purpose of becoming leaner and more muscular. The anabolic steroids cause premature skeletal maturation and accelerated puberty changes. Adolescents who take steroids before their growth spurt is complete may remain short for the rest of their lives. Some people experience depression when they stop taking steroids, which may contribute to dependence on the drugs (NIDA, 2012).

COLLABORATIVE CARE

Medical treatment of the patient in the acute phase of alcohol or sedative withdrawal focuses on physiologic safety issues: symptom management, seizure prevention, stabilizing vital signs, and minimizing the effects of CNS stimulation. Management of the patient in the rehabilitation phase is supportive. Nurses take a cooperative role with physicians, therapists, social workers, and others on the health care team.

Medications

Medical management includes prescription of medications and therefore must include consideration of drug interactions and cross-tolerance. Patients who use drugs or alcohol regularly are at risk for withdrawal, and those who have used drugs or alcohol recently are at risk for additive effects with prescribed drugs.

Nurses and physicians in emergency departments need to know that any patient who is under the influence of drugs or alcohol on arrival is at risk for an overdose of CNS depressants. Patients who are taking narcotics, other CNS depressants (alcohol, barbiturates, sedatives, prescription sleep aids), or illegal drugs that depress the CNS (heroin, "downers") are at high risk for additive CNS depression. Commonly prescribed medications that cause additive CNS depression are the narcotic analgesics, sedatives, benzodiazepines, sleep agents, and anesthetic agents.

A person who is dependent on heroin or alcohol will be tolerant not only to these but to other CNS depressants as well. This phenomenon is called **cross-tolerance**. Cross-tolerance is important to the anesthesiologist, who may find that the patient needs more than the usual anesthetic to put him to sleep. It is also important to physicians and nurses, because patients who are tolerant to CNS depressants may need a higher than usual analgesic dose to relieve pain.

Treatment

There are several theories about chemical dependency and its causes. Current treatment methods are based on the concept that substance dependency is a chronic, progressive medical illness that is characterized by remissions and relapses and that is eventually fatal if untreated. The etiology of substance abuse is a combination of genetic factors and cultural influences (nature and nurture). People who are dependent on substances have learned to use them to cope with their problems. These patients must have new skills to replace the functions substances play in their lives. A promise of abstinence alone is not a long-term solution. The ultimate goals of substance dependency treatment are

(1) abstinence from substance use and (2) development of effective coping mechanisms to replace the need for substances as solutions to problems.

ACUTE PHASE OF TREATMENT   Substance dependency treatment has two major phases: acute and rehabilitation. In the *acute phase*, the person may be in a hospital or another inpatient or outpatient setting. The patient often enters treatment while intoxicated. **Detoxification**, or removal of the substance from the body, begins the acute phase. The withdrawal syndrome also occurs acutely. Medical and nursing support is often needed during withdrawal.

Medications are used in the acute phase of treatment to provide safe withdrawal. For patients whose primary substance of abuse is alcohol, vitamin B_1 is given to prevent Wernicke–Korsakoff syndrome.

The Clinical Institute Withdrawal Assessment for Alcohol Withdrawal (CIWA-Ar Revised) is an assessment tool used for treating alcohol withdrawal symptoms (Sullivan, Sykora, Schneiderman, Naranjo, & Sellers, 1989). The patient is assessed for withdrawal symptoms hourly and treated with a benzodiazepine such as lorazepam to relieve the symptoms. The goal of treatment is to control symptoms without excessive sedation. At first, the patient is likely to have more severe symptoms and require hourly medication, but as the hours pass, the CNS will regain its homeostatic balance, the symptoms will subside, and the medication will no longer be needed. The withdrawal syndrome will be over. The process can take 4 days in a person with a very high tolerance for alcohol. Figure 53-4■ shows the assessment form, which is a good source for the symptoms of alcohol withdrawal. Notice that

(Text continues on p. 1314.)

Clinical Institute Withdrawal Assessment of Alcohol Scale, Revised (CIWA-Ar)

Patient:_____ Date: _____ Time: _____ (24 hour clock, midnight = 00:00)

Pulse or heart rate, taken for one minute:_____ Blood pressure:_____

NAUSEA AND VOMITING—Ask "Do you feel sick to your stomach? Have you vomited?" Observation.

0 no nausea and no vomiting
1 mild nausea with no vomiting
2
3
4 intermittent nausea with dry heaves
5
6
7 constant nausea, frequent dry heaves and vomiting

TREMOR—Arms extended and fingers spread apart. Observation.

0 no tremor
1 not visible, but can be felt fingertip to fingertip
2
3
4 moderate, with patient's arms extended
5
6
7 severe, even with arms not extended

TACTILE DISTURBANCES—Ask "Have you any itching, pins and needles sensations, any burning, any numbness, or do you feel bugs crawling on or under your skin?" Observation.

0 none
1 very mild itching, pins and needles, burning or numbness
2 mild itching, pins and needles, burning or numbness
3 moderate itching, pins and needles, burning or numbness
4 moderately severe hallucinations
5 severe hallucinations
6 extremely severe hallucinations
7 continuous hallucinations

AUDITORY DISTURBANCES—Ask "Are you more aware of sounds around you? Are they harsh? Do they frighten you? Are you hearing anything that is disturbing to you? Are you hearing things you know are not there?" Observation.

0 not present
1 very mild harshness or ability to frighten
2 mild harshness or ability to frighten
3 moderate harshness or ability to frighten
4 moderately severe hallucinations
5 severe hallucinations
6 extremely severe hallucinations
7 continuous hallucinations

Figure 53-4. ■ Clinical Institute Withdrawal Assessment for Alcohol Withdrawal (CIWA-Ar Revised) is used for treating alcohol withdrawal symptoms. (Source: Sullivan, Sykora, Schneiderman, Naranjo, & Sellers, 1989.)

PAROXYSMAL SWEATS—Observation.

0 no sweat visible
1 barely perceptible sweating, palms moist
2
3
4 beads of sweat obvious on forehead
5
6
7 drenching sweats

VISUAL DISTURBANCES—Ask "Does the light appear to be too bright? Is its color different? Does it hurt your eyes? Are you seeing anything that is disturbing to you? Are you seeing things you know are not there?" Observation.

0 not present
1 very mild sensitivity
2 mild sensitivity
3 moderate sensitivity
4 moderately severe hallucinations
5 severe hallucinations
6 extremely severe hallucinations
7 continuous hallucinations

ANXIETY—Ask "Do you feel nervous?" Observation.

0 no anxiety, at ease
1 mild anxious
2
3
4 moderately anxious, or guarded, so anxiety is inferred
5
6
7 equivalent to acute panic states as seen in severe delirium or acute schizophrenic reactions

HEADACHE, FULLNESS IN HEAD—Ask "Does your head feel different? Does it feel like there is a band around your head?" Do not rate for dizziness or lightheadedness. Otherwise, rate severity.

0 not present
1 very mild
2 mild
3 moderate
4 moderately severe
5 severe
6 very severe
7 extremely severe

AGITATION—Observation.

0 normal activity
1 somewhat more than normal activity
2
3
4 moderately fidgety and restless
5
6
7 paces back and forth during most of the interview, or constantly thrashes about

ORIENTATION AND CLOUDING OF SENSORIUM—Ask "What day is this? Where are you? Who am I?"

0 oriented and can do serial additions
1 cannot do serial additions or is uncertain about date
2 disoriented for date by no more than 2 calendar days
3 disoriented for date by more than 2 calendar days
4 disoriented for place/or person

Total **CIWA-Ar** Score _____

Rater's Initials _____

Maximum Possible Score 67

The **CIWA-Ar** *is not* copyrighted and may be reproduced freely. This assessment for monitoring withdrawal symptoms requires approximately 5 minutes to administer. The maximum score is 67 (see instrument). Patients scoring less than 10 do not usually need additional medication for withdrawal.

Figure 53-4. *continued*

severe alcohol withdrawal can cause hallucinations, seizures, and death.

Some health care workers have the attitude that if patients are allowed to suffer agonizing withdrawal, they will "learn a lesson" about why they should stop using drugs. On the contrary, withdrawal causes preoccupation and craving for the substance. There is no ethical justification for allowing patients to suffer needlessly. Alcohol and barbiturate withdrawals can be life threatening.

REHABILITATION PHASE The second phase of substance dependency treatment is **rehabilitation**. This phase continues indefinitely. When patients have detoxified and are abstaining from substance use, rehabilitation begins.

Medications used in the rehabilitation phase of treatment are for the purpose of preventing relapse. Disulfiram (Antabuse) may be prescribed to deter patients from drinking alcohol. It causes a severe, uncomfortable reaction when the patient drinks (flushing, throbbing headache, nausea, and vomiting). Some health care professionals question the ethics of giving a medication that intentionally makes the patient sick. They disagree with the use of negative reinforcement to change behavior.

Methadone, a synthetic opiate, is used as a replacement for heroin for patients with a heroin-use disorder. A regular dose is prescribed, and the patient basically trades one dependency for another. The goal is to prevent the risks of intravenous drug use (methadone is given orally) and the socially inappropriate behaviors associated with obtaining heroin (prostitution, burglary, robbery, etc.). Many people who use methadone lead productive lives.

Naltrexone (ReVia) is an opioid antagonist used to treat opiate overdose. It blocks the effects of any opioids used by the patient. It has been found to reduce the cravings for alcohol in abstinent patients.

Clonidine (Catapres) is an antihypertensive drug. It is given to patients with opiate dependence to prevent some of the symptoms of withdrawal. Nurses should take the patient's blood pressure before each dose and hold the drug if the person is hypotensive.

The tasks of rehabilitation are to:

- Maintain sobriety (abstinence).
- Develop new coping skills.
- Make a plan for relapse prevention.
- Live life with all its responsibilities, joys, and frustrations.

Relapse is common. The best response to relapse is for the person to learn from the experience and to begin again on rehabilitation.

Many people with substance abuse and dependency respond well to treatment. The most popular treatment program is Alcoholics Anonymous (AA). This is a self-help group for alcoholics that is based on 12 steps, thus the

name "Twelve-Step Program." Box 53-3 lists the Twelve Steps of Alcoholics Anonymous. AA itself is for alcoholics only. Other 12-step programs are based on its principles. In all of these anonymous groups, people with similar problems share experience, strength, and hope. The groups offer a sense of community and unconditional support.

There are thousands of AA groups. Refer patients to their local telephone book or directory assistance for the closest meeting. There are also AA meetings for special interest groups, such as nonsmokers, women, lesbians, teachers, and people who want to focus on religious aspects of recovery. Other 12-step programs include Overeaters Anonymous, Narcotics Anonymous, and Cocaine Anonymous.

Substance dependency is certainly a family illness. Al-Anon is a group for family members, especially spouses, of alcoholics. Ala-Teen is a similar group for teenage

---

BOX 53-3 TWELVE STEPS OF ALCOHOLICS ANONYMOUS

We

1. Admitted that we were powerless over alcohol, that our lives had become unmanageable.
2. Came to believe that a Power greater than ourselves could restore us to sanity.
3. Made a decision to turn our wills and our lives over to the care of God as we understood Him.
4. Made a searching and fearless moral inventory of ourselves.
5. Admitted to God, to ourselves, and to another human being the exact nature of our wrongs.
6. Were entirely ready to have God remove all these defects of character.
7. Humbly asked Him to remove our shortcomings.
8. Made a list of all persons we had harmed, and became willing to make amends to them all.
9. Made direct amends to such people whenever possible, except when to do so would injure them or others.
10. Continued to take personal inventory and when we were wrong promptly admitted it.
11. Sought through prayer and meditation to improve our conscious contact with God as we understood Him, praying only for knowledge of His will for us and the power to carry that out.
12. Having had a spiritual awakening as a result of these steps, we tried to carry this message to alcoholics and to practice these principles in all our affairs.

children of alcoholics. ACOA, or Adult Children of Alcoholics, serves people who grew up in alcoholic families. Partners of alcoholics often are **codependents**—they facilitate the alcoholic's problem by allowing for avoidance of the consequences for behavior related to drinking. For example, the codependent may provide excuses for the alcoholic at work or with family. The process of passively helping the substance-dependent patient to continue using the substance is called **enabling**.

DUAL DIAGNOSIS   The term **dual diagnosis** refers to patients who have both a substance use disorder and a serious mental illness. People with severe mental illnesses are at an increased risk for substance use disorders over people without mental illness (SAMHSA, 2013). These individuals have two separate chronic illnesses, and they have a higher level of functional impairment than the general population of people with substance dependency. Many people self-medicate their psychiatric symptoms with alcohol or drugs. Both the mental disorder and the substance use must be treated together.

Substance Dependency Among Nurses

It may seem unlikely for nurses to have problems with substance use, because they should know better. In fact, many nurses do use substances. Some reasons their profession is at especially high risk for substance use disorders are that:

- Nurses see medications as a solution to problems.
- Nurses have access to drugs at work and to physicians who prescribe them.
- Nurses often believe that they should work even when they are tired or sick, so they may use drugs to increase their ability to continue working.
- Nurses experience stress, emotional pain, anger, and frustration, which are symptoms that respond to drugs in the short term.
- Nurses think that if they know about drugs and drug abuse, addiction will not happen to them.

If nurses have adequate understanding of addiction and its early signs, they will be able to identify it earlier in their coworkers and themselves. Signs of an **impaired nurse** (one who is working under the influence of substances) include changes in the nurse's *behavior* (mood changes, irritability, forgetfulness, isolation from coworkers, inappropriate behavior). *Work performance* may be affected (multiple medication errors, missed deadlines, sloppy charting, inattention to detail, absenteeism, poor judgment, volunteering to give other nurses narcotics, excessive wasting of narcotics, patient complaints that pain medications are not effective, tampering with drug packaging, going to the bathroom after administering narcotics). The nurse may also have *signs of drug use or withdrawal* (alcohol on breath, heavy use of breath mints and perfume, red eyes, ataxia, restlessness, anxiety, slurred speech, hyperactivity, family problems that interfere with work, tremors, runny nose).

Substance dependency is a chronic physiologic illness that requires treatment. Affected nurses deserve to be diagnosed and treated before they hurt their patients or themselves. If you suspect that a peer is impaired, notify a manager or hospital supervisor. The nurse is unlikely to be able to manage the problem alone. Check to see if your state board of nursing has a nurse monitoring or treatment program that can help affected nurses recover and return to the profession.

In the acute situation, your duty as a nurse is to protect your patients from an impaired nurse. In the big picture of caring for colleagues in your profession, your duty is to help your peers get treatment. The intervention to reach each of these outcomes is the same: Tell a supervisor (not just the unit charge nurse for the day), so patients will be safe and the nurse will be treated. This is no time to engage in denial.

NURSING CARE

PRIORITIZING NURSING CARE

The priority in caring for patients with acute substance abuse is preventing or treating injury from the substances and the results of their use. Psychosocially, the priority is a nonjudgmental approach when obtaining data and establishing a therapeutic relationship in which the patient can share information and feelings.

ASSESSING

Assess the substance use history of every patient. Notify the physician of recent use or regular use so appropriate measures can be taken to adjust doses of prescribed medications. Nursing assessment questions are listed in Box 53-4■. Note that the substance use assessment does not ask "Do you drink?" Because alcohol and drug use are associated with strong negative attitudes by society and with guilt by users, the patient is most likely to believe that the right answer is "no." People use denial to cope with their substance abuse problems, and they often lie about or underestimate their use. The nurse must present a nonjudgmental attitude and be accepting of patients as people, whether they use drugs or not.

Notice the assessment question that asks the patient what purpose the substance serves. This promotes the nurse's ability to help the patient find other choices for coping or entertainment.

A general screening tool for whether a patient has problems with alcohol is the CAGE questionnaire (Ewing, 1984).

Substance Use

Note: This is a screening assessment. A more thorough assessment would be indicated in a substance abuse treatment setting.

- How many cigarettes a day do you smoke?
- How often do you drink alcohol?
- About how much do you drink?
- What kind of drugs do you use that are not prescribed?
- What is your method of use (oral, smoking, inhaling, injecting)?
- What purpose do these substances serve for you (relaxation, fun, to help you get through the day)?
- Have you had any problems because of drinking or drug use (social, job, or legal)?
- When was the last time you used alcohol or any drug, what was it, and how much?

Further inquiry is indicated if the patient answers "yes" to any one of the following questions:

- Have you ever felt you ought to **C**ut down on your drinking?
- Have people **A**nnoyed you by criticizing your drinking?
- Have you ever felt bad or **G**uilty about your drinking?
- Have you ever had a drink first thing in the morning to steady your nerves or get rid of a hangover (**E**ye-opener)?

DIAGNOSING, PLANNING, AND IMPLEMENTING

Risk for Injury Related to Alcohol Withdrawal

Expected outcome: Will have stable vital signs within the normal range and will not suffer injury due to alcohol withdrawal.

- Take vital signs frequently. If they are elevated (T, P, R, and BP may be involved), medicate with benzodiazepines according to the physician's orders. *Benzodiazepines either treat or prevent symptoms of alcohol withdrawal by balancing the CNS stimulation with a depressant effect until the patient's CNS can return to homeostasis without alcohol. The CIWA assessment tool is the ideal way to treat alcohol withdrawal. The nurse may suggest its use if it is not a policy at the institution.*
- Assess for other withdrawal symptoms (anxiety, mental confusion, agitation, sweating, nausea, vomiting, tremors, and ataxia). *Treat with PRN benzodiazepines as above. If withdrawal is so severe that the patient has hallucinations or seizures, call the physician immediately. These may be symptoms of life-threatening withdrawal.*
- If the patient is nauseated, do not push fluids. Offer small amounts of fluids frequently. Offer high-calorie feedings. *Assess for dehydration. Patients in withdrawal are at risk for fluid and electrolyte disturbances. They are also*

at risk for inadequate nutrition. It is easier for the nauseated patient to take foods and fluids in small amounts than in big meals.

- Maintain a low-stimulation environment for the patient. *Patients in withdrawal are experiencing CNS stimulation. They will be more comfortable and less likely to have a seizure if they are in a quiet room with dim lights.*
- Encourage expression of feelings about drinking or about what the patient is experiencing. *People with alcohol dependency often have difficulty understanding their own feelings. Expressing them can begin the process of behavior change.*

Deficient Knowledge (Substance Abuse and Its Consequences)

Expected outcome: Will list or acknowledge the consequences of substance abuse.

- Assess what patients know and what they need to learn. Teach them about the process of drug abuse and dependency and how people use drugs for coping, recreation, and company. Review the consequences to the patient of substance use. *Because so many people deny the severity of the problem, nurses must be honest about what the consequences are (job loss, divorce, family estrangement, disease of every body system, etc.). When people know what the problem is physiologically and realistically, they can begin to do something about it.*

Ineffective Coping

Expected outcome: Will have a plan for healthy alternatives to substance use for coping.

- Help plan for new healthy coping strategies to replace substance use. *The patient may need to meet new people to make new friends if all of his old friends only get together to drink or use drugs. People need alternatives to substance use when they become too Hungry, Angry, Lonely, or Tired. (HALT is an acronym for feelings that lead to relapse into drug use.)*
- Help make a list of fun, recreational activities. *Patients may not even know what to do for fun. Be sure the list is realistic and includes the patient's preferences (taking a walk, basketball, calling a friend on the phone, listening to music, hiking, bike riding, outdoor work, reading, community service, spiritual activities, dancing, carpentry, painting, and appreciating nature are some ideas).*
- Help patients identify their resources for various needs and stressful situations (e.g., a ride to the grocery store or the doctor's office, help caring for the cat if the patient is in the hospital). His sponsor from AA may be the one to call if he feels like drinking again or if he wants to talk about how hard life is. *A practical list like this may be the thing the patient turns to instead of drinking when he has a problem and cannot think of what to do.*

Other nursing diagnoses that commonly apply to people with substance use disorders are:

- *Compromised or Disabled Family Coping*
- *Chronic Low Self-Esteem*
- *Powerlessness*
- *Fear*
- *Ineffective Denial*
- *Imbalanced Nutrition: Less Than Body Requirements*
- *Disturbed Sleep Pattern*
- *Social Isolation*
- *Spiritual Distress*
- *Disturbed Sensory Perception*
- *Risk for Violence*

EVALUATING

To evaluate whether nursing interventions for patients with substance use disorders are effective, look at the outcomes. Desired outcomes include:

- Patient will have a plan for healthy alternatives to substance use for coping.
- Patient will identify resources for obtaining help when needed (family, friends, AA, social service agencies).
- Patient will identify risk factors for relapse and plan for relapse prevention.
- Patient will identify and verbalize feelings.
- Patient will assume responsibility for own behavior.
- Patient will use peer support to maintain sobriety.

DOCUMENTING

Documentation should include the patient's stated history of substance use, time and description of last drug use, symptoms of intoxication on admission (including smell of alcohol on breath), withdrawal symptoms and their treatment, and the patient's response to medications given. Document any discussions the nurse has with the patient about substance use and its significance to the patient. Most people with substance abuse issues are hospitalized without any mention of substance use at all. Document the topics you have taught the patient and patient's response.

CONTINUITY OF CARE

When people with substance use disorders are discharged from the hospital, there must be follow-up of their substance use issues. Patients may benefit from a written list of telephone numbers for counseling resources, drug abuse treatment, or Alcoholics Anonymous. When a person is not expected to abstain from substance use, the physician must consider this when prescribing medications for use at home. If a patient is going to be discharged with

sedatives or other medications that could interact with drugs of abuse, the physician should discuss risks with the patient.

Nurses should remind patients that they are in control of their own behavior. Patients should be given resources for outpatient support. A promise "never to use again" will not make the person successful. People with substance dependency should always be referred to social services for assistance with discharge planning.

NURSING CARE PLAN
Patient With Ineffective Coping

A 30-year-old woman was hospitalized for hematemesis (vomiting blood) and abdominal pain 3 days ago. The medical diagnosis is acute gastritis due to chronic alcohol use. Her husband is a truck driver and is away from home most of the time.

Assessment

The nurse did a substance use assessment and found that the woman uses alcohol most days. She drinks a bottle of wine at night after her children go to bed. After they go to school, she sometimes has a few drinks in the morning. She drinks because the only time she feels good is when she is drinking. Her parents were both alcoholics. She has no hobbies and states that her only reason for living is her children. The patient states, "I don't even know what I like to do. The only time I feel good is when I'm drunk." Vital signs are T 99.2°F, P 90, R 18, BP 118/80.

Nursing Diagnosis

A priority nursing diagnosis for this patient is:

- *Ineffective Coping*, related to inadequate role modeling and ineffective skills.

Expected Outcomes

The patient will:

- Relate her feelings about alcohol dependency.
- List three resources for help when she needs it.
- Plan for four possible alternatives to drinking alcohol when she is under stress.
- Contact AA while in the hospital and plan to attend a meeting on the day she is discharged.
- List at least three things that she enjoys doing.

Planning and Implementation

The nurse will implement the following interventions:

- Spend time talking with the patient each shift.
- Help the patient make a list of people who can help her in various everyday situations (caring for the children,

driving her to an AA meeting, being available to talk on the phone if she feels lonely).

■ Help the patient make a list of alternatives to drinking. These items will be things that the patient agrees that she would actually do. They may include going for a walk, writing a letter, working outdoors, taking the children to the park or the library, playing a game, listening to music, dancing, exercise, journaling, or volunteering.

■ Show the patient how to find the telephone number of the local AA group in the phone book, and encourage the patient to contact it.

■ Assist the patient to make a list of things she would enjoy doing. The nurse may make suggestions, but the patient should choose the enjoyable things. These also become alternatives to drinking.

Evaluation

The patient was discharged after 6 days in the hospital. She started attending AA, but quit because she did not feel comfortable in the group meetings. Her sponsor convinced her to try an AA group for women only, which she likes and continues to attend. She and her husband are in couple's counseling. He is scheduling his work so he can be at home more often. She has not had any alcohol since she left the hospital 4 weeks ago.

Critical Thinking in the Nursing Process

1. What are the situations that would put this patient at greatest risk for relapse into drinking again?
2. What role did alcohol play in this woman's life?
3. If the patient called the hospital unit and told the nurse that she feels like drinking and doesn't know what to do, what should the nurse say?

Note: Discussion of Critical Thinking questions appears on the companion website.

Note: The references and resources for all chapters have been compiled at the back of the book.

Chapter Review

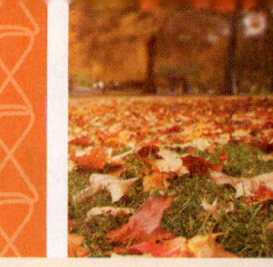

KEY POINTS

- **Concept:** Substance abuse is one of the most important health problems of the twenty-first century.
- **Concept:** Substance use disorder is a maladaptive pattern of substance use despite adverse outcomes.
- The 10 substances of abuse are alcohol; opioids; sedatives, hypnotics, and anxiolytics; stimulants (cocaine, amphetamines, and similar drugs); hallucinogens; phencyclidine (PCP) and similar drugs; inhalants; cannabis; caffeine; and tobacco.
- **Concept:** With continued use, the user develops tolerance to substances that stimulate or depress the central nervous system (CNS). This means that increasing amounts of the substance are needed to achieve the same effect or the same amount causes less effect.
- **Concept:** When a person uses a CNS depressant or stimulant substance consistently and then stops, the individual will experience withdrawal symptoms until the CNS regains homeostasis without the substance.
- The CNS depressant effects of prescribed drugs in the hospital, combined with the effects of drugs or alcohol the patient used before admission, may cause severe respiratory depression.
- People who are tolerant to alcohol or narcotics need more analgesics than normal to obtain pain relief.
- Nurses should assess the substance use history of each patient on admission.
- Understanding the personal consequences of drug and alcohol use is necessary for patient rehabilitation.
- When substance abuse and dependency occur among nurses and other health care professionals, the first responsibility of the nurse is patient safety and the second is to seek help for your colleague.
- The goal of substance use treatment is abstinence from substance use and development of skills to replace drug use for coping, enjoyment, or companionship.
- Patients with substance dependency need referral to social services for assistance and follow-up after discharge.
- Many people respond well to treatment for substance-related disorders: Keep hope alive.

PEARSON NURSING STUDENT RESOURCES

Find additional materials at **nursing.pearsonhighered.com**.

Clinical Reasoning Care Map

Caring for a Patient With Substance Use Disorder
NCLEX-PN® Focus Area: Psychosocial Integrity: Coping and Adaptation

Case Study: A 24-year-old male patient is admitted to the medical–surgical unit with multiple trauma suffered in an automobile accident that happened while he was under the influence of alcohol. He has been on the unit for 4 days. His vital signs are stable now, although he has experienced alcohol withdrawal syndrome during the past several days. The substance use history reveals that he drinks beer every day, usually "about two six-packs or so." The patient states, "I don't have a drinking problem. I can quit whenever I want!"

Nursing Diagnosis: Ineffective Denial

COLLECT DATA

Subjective	Objective
_____	_____
_____	_____
_____	_____
_____	_____
_____	_____
_____	_____

Does this present a threat to the patient's safety?

If yes, the priority intervention to address this threat would be:

_____

Nursing Care

_____
_____
_____
_____
_____
_____
_____

Interprofessional team members to include when planning care:

_____

How would you document this? _____

_____

Compare your answers and documentation to those provided on the companion website.

Data Collected
(use only those that apply)

- Patient states, "I don't have a drinking problem. I can quit whenever I want!"
- Vital signs stable.
- Blood alcohol content on admission 0.24 mg/dL.
- Weight 165 lb.
- Skin warm, dry.
- Requests pain medication (ordered q4h PRN) approximately q1h.
- States "I feel nervous."
- Has insomnia (sleeps less than 4 hours per night).
- Had seizures as a child.
- Poor appetite: eats less than 50% of meals.
- Patient states, "If you don't let me out of here tomorrow, I'm leaving anyway."

Nursing Interventions (use only those that apply; list in priority order)

- Ask the patient why he wants to leave the hospital. If he doesn't say so, ask if he wants to drink alcohol.
- Assess the patient's knowledge about alcoholism.
- Encourage the patient to express his feelings about drinking and alcoholism.
- Teach the patient about the disease of substance dependency.
- Provide effective pain management.
- Minimize the amount of narcotics given to this patient because he is an addict.
- Confront the patient with the reality of the consequences of alcoholism.
- Ask the physician for an order for a sleeping medication for the patient to take now and when he goes home.
- Weigh the patient daily.
- Offer frequent feedings of high-protein foods.

NCLEX-PN® Exam Preparation

1 A patient discovers he needs more than his usual pint of liquor to achieve the same effect. This phenomenon is called:

1. tolerance.
2. intoxication.
3. addiction.
4. abuse.

2 A patient is admitted with a diagnosis of alcohol withdrawal. The nurse expects to find which of the following on assessment?

1. B/P 110/70, P 72, R 20
2. Drowsiness and slow respirations
3. Anxiety, tremors
4. Warm, dry skin

3 A patient is admitted with alcoholic encephalopathy (Wernicke syndrome). The nurse expects to administer which of the following medications?

1. Demerol (meperidine)
2. Valium (diazepam.
3. Thiamine (vitamin B_1)
4. Dilantin (phenytoin)

4 The physical assessment of a patient admitted to the emergency department reveals pinpoint pupils, depressed respirations, and confusion. The physician diagnoses morphine overdose. Treatment includes:

1. Thiamine (vitamin B_1).
2. Narcan (naloxone HCl).
3. Librium (chlordiazepoxide).
4. D5W.

5 A patient is prescribed Xanax (alprazolam) for treatment of anxiety. Which of the following must the LPN/LVN include in the teaching plan? **Select all that apply.**

1. Take the drug every 4 hours.
2. Avoid alcohol while taking the drug.
3. The drug can cause drowsiness.
4. Avoid driving until effects are known.

6 An LPN/LVN suspects her coworker is diverting narcotics from the nursing unit. What action by the nurse would be most effective?

1. Confront the nurse with her suspicions.
2. Notify the physician.
3. Notify the charge nurse.
4. Notify the nursing supervisor.

7 The nurse establishes a nursing diagnosis of *Deficient Knowledge* for a patient with a history of substance abuse. The LPN/LVN reinforces a teaching plan to include:

1. signs and symptoms of withdrawal.
2. consequences to the patient of continued substance abuse.
3. safe levels of drug use.
4. antidotes to opiates.

8 A 28-year-old woman presented to the emergency department for treatment of cocaine intoxication. The nurse expects her to exhibit which of the following behaviors during withdrawal from cocaine?

1. Anxiety
2. Hypertension
3. Depression
4. Seizures

9 The nurse must perform interventions for a patient experiencing alcohol withdrawal. **Select all that apply.**

1. Take vital signs frequently.
2. Provide a low-stimulation environment.
3. Withhold any medications that act on the CNS.
4. Tell the patient that this illness is his punishment for drinking.

10 A 12-year-old male is admitted to the emergency department with mental confusion, ataxia, and silver paint on his hair. What question by the nurse may be most helpful to help the patient describe the cause of his signs and symptoms?

1. "What have you done?"
2. "It looks like you have been 'huffing paint.' Is that what happened?"
3. "Are you using narcotics?"
4. "Why did you do this to yourself?"

Answers and rationales for Review Questions appear in Appendix I.

You are an LPN/LVN working the day shift on an acute psychiatric unit. Your main responsibilities include administering routine medications, assisting patients with ADLs, participating in group activities, and helping to maintain a safe environment. The following are three of the patients on the mental health unit.

Craig, age 21, was admitted to the psychiatric unit Monday morning after an exacerbation of psychosis with agitation. Craig was diagnosed with schizophrenia 6 months ago. He had tried two different medications, but neither relieved all of his symptoms. Craig does not feel he is "crazy" and should not need to take medication all the time. He remains in the psychiatric unit for medication adjustment. At 0830 on Tuesday (the day after admission), Craig was prescribed loxapine 10 mg b.i.d. × 2 doses, 20 mg b.i.d. × 2 doses, and then 30 mg b.i.d.

Mariah, a 22-year-old college student, was admitted to the psychiatric unit 2 days ago after an intentional overdose of Tylenol, sleeping pills, and cold remedies. She is failing all of her college courses and recently discovered her long-term boyfriend was being unfaithful. Mariah stated she really did not want to die, but she is such a failure she did not know what else to do. She expects to be discharged in a few days, but will remain on Zoloft 50 mg daily and plans to attend group therapy on an outpatient basis.

Larry, a 34-year-old, lives alone in a small apartment. He has been working the night shift in the printing area of a local newspaper. Over the past few weeks he has become more rigid in his schedule and work duties. He feels his coworkers are "setting him up" to get him fired. Last night he became physically aggressive toward his supervisor, resulting in the police being called. During the altercation, Larry received a large cut on the right forearm that required stitches. Larry kept insisting that "everyone is out to get him" both at work and in his apartment complex. The police brought Larry to the psychiatric unit for evaluation. Larry has an order for Darvocet N 100 q4 hr PRN for arm pain.

CRITICAL THINKING

- What are two reasons Craig might have developed an acute psychotic episode?

- As you assist Mariah with ADLs, what observations should you make that might indicate a deepening depression?

- Larry is having difficulty shaving because of his injured right arm. When you offer to help, he yells, "Get out of here, you murderer! You can't slit my throat." How will you handle this situation?

COMMUNICATION

- When you are walking Craig to the shower he says to you, "You know I'm not crazy. Why do you think I'm here?" How will you respond?

- At 1:00, Mariah is scheduled to attend a craft class with other patients. After lunch, she states she is too tired and goes to her room. How will you respond to her?

- When you give Larry his medication, he states, "The doctor didn't believe me when I told him my boss was trying to put poison in the sandwich I brought for my dinner. That is why I hit him. You believe me, don't you?" How will you respond to this question?

MANAGEMENT OF CARE

- If today is Thursday morning, how much loxapine would you administer to Craig?

- What time of day should Mariah receive 50 mg of Zoloft?

- Larry requests a pain pill 30 minutes early. He states, "The pain is really bad. The night nurse gave it to me early so you can too." How will you respond to his request?

INTERPROFESSIONAL CARE

- Craig's family feels strongly that they want to care for him at home. A discharge planning conference is being convened. Your RN team leader has asked you to attend, because you have a good relationship with Craig and his mother. Also participating will be the RN, the psychiatric social worker, the home health nurse, and the physician. Craig's mother, father, and older brother will also attend. As the LPN/LVN, what input could you give that would help with the transition from hospital to home?

DOCUMENTING AND REPORTING

- What patient observations should the LPN/LVN working with patients with mental health issues report to the RN?

- Write a focus note documenting Mariah's deepening depression.

Note: Discussion of Unit questions appears on the companion website.

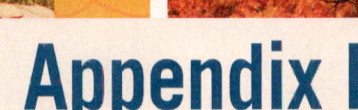

Appendix I

Answers for NCLEX-PN® Review

CHAPTER 1

NCLEX-PN® ANSWERS   (1) 2, 3. Outcome 1. The nurse is providing evidence-based care when using guidelines that have been developed through research and identifying best practices for a patient problem. The nurse is using the Internet as a tool for research. Although guidelines are based on evidence and best practices, they are developed to address a health care situation, not individual patient needs. (2) 2. Outcome 3. The nurse as patient advocate actively promotes the patient's rights to autonomy and free choice. The nurse may speak for the patient, mediate between the patient and other persons, and protect the patient's right to self-determination. In the caregiver role, the nurse plans and implements care. As an educator, the nurse identifies learning needs and teaches to address those needs. When managing care, the nurse prioritizes, assigns, delegates, and supervises care activities. (3) 1. Outcome 2. Quality improvement is a key component when providing safe, effective, and patient-centered care. Delegation is distributing and supervising tasks. A nursing diagnosis is a statement developed by nurses concerning patient needs. Implementation is the step of the nursing process in which nurses perform actions to assist the patient toward wellness. (4) 4. Outcome 7. The LPN/LVN conducts focused initial and ongoing patient assessments, whereas the RN is responsible for conducting the comprehensive assessment. In all instances, assessments must be holistic. Although information from the patient's family may be obtained for both a focused and a comprehensive assessment, this response does not address the full responsibility of the LPN/LVN in assessing patients. (5) 1. Outcome 4, 5. Making a diagnosis is a complex process and always involves uncertainty. Critical thinking and reasoning are used to choose nursing diagnoses that best define the individual patient's health problems. Evaluation is review of actions that have been taken and their effectiveness. Assessment is collection of data about the patient. Planning occurs after the diagnosis has been determined. (6) 2. Outcome 4. Nursing interventions must be specific and individualized. The nurse identifies patient problems and needed interventions and then works with the patient to determine those that are needed and preferred by the individual patient. Interventions can be determined by many members of the interdisciplinary team. Nursing interventions are initiated by nurses. Nursing interventions are based on nursing diagnoses, not medical problems. (7) 1. Outcome 4. Implementation is the action or "doing" phase of the nursing process, when nurses carry out planned activities. Nurses establish outcome criteria in the planning phase. Nurses identify patient problems in the diagnosing phase. Nurses evaluate care after implementation, in the evaluation phase. (8) 3. Outcome 4. Documenting interventions is the final component of implementation, and it is a legal requirement. "If it isn't documented, it isn't done." Setting priorities is an early step. Assessing the patient's condition is done before implementation occurs. Teaching the patient occurs before documentation, and it is documented in the patient record. (9) 4. Outcome 6, 8. Nursing practice is structured by standards and codes of ethics that guide nursing practice and protect the public.

The nursing process is a system that helps nursing practice but is not what protects the public. Physicians' oversight is not what guides nursing practice. Standardized procedures are helpful, but what protects the public and guides nursing practice are standards and codes of ethics. (10) 4. Outcome 7. According to NAPNES Standards for LPNs/LVNs, the LPN/LVN is accountable for care assigned to others. In this instance, the LPN/LVN and the NA are accountable for the care and are responsible for ensuring that appropriate follow-up assessment and care are provided. The LPN/LVN, not the unit charge nurse, did the delegating and so is responsible along with the NA. The LPN/LVN, not the RN team leader, did the delegating and so is responsible along with the NA.

CHAPTER 2

NCLEX-PN® ANSWERS   (1) 2. Outcome 1. High-level wellness is an integrated method of functioning, oriented toward maximizing the individual's potential. Good health, balance, and homeostasis can exist as a relatively passive state of freedom from illness. (2) 1, 2, 4, 5. Outcome 2. A person's health is affected by numerous factors, including culture and ethnicity, education, lifestyle, and socioeconomic background. The patient's choice of health care provider may influence care received, but is not a major determinant of health. (3) 3. Outcome 3. *Healthy People 2020* provides objectives for promoting health of the public and standards by which achievement can be measured. It is not intended as a measurement of individual health or a way to ensure continuity of care, nor does it identify risk factors for disease. (4) 1. Outcome 4. Illness is the highly individualized response a person has to disease. The origin of disease may be biologic; some sources also identify normative and developmental as potential causes of disease. (5) 4. Outcome 5. An acute illness occurs rapidly, lasts for a relatively short period of time, and is self-limiting. It usually responds to self-treatment or to medical–surgical intervention. While acute illnesses may be communicable, this is not true of all acute illness. Acute illnesses are not generally characterized by periods of remission and exacerbation. (6) 1. Outcome 6. Almost all people with a chronic illness need to learn how to manage their disease on a day-to-day basis and live as normally as possible. Most people with chronic illness live independently and do not require pain medication. (7) 3. Outcome 7. Community-based nursing focuses on individual family and health care needs where they live, work, play, worship, and go to school. Community health nursing focuses on the health of a community. Home health nursing provides licensed nursing services in the home. Parish nursing is a type of community-based nursing. (8) 1. Outcome 8. If a conflict arises, the nurse must remain the primary patient's advocate, regardless of any negative response from the family. The goal of advocacy is not to please everyone, but to stand up for the patient. The physician is not responsible for resolving conflicts and may not agree with the patient's desires. (9) 2, 4, 5. Outcome 7. Specific criteria that the patient must meet in order to secure Medicare reimbursement are to have a need for skilled care, be essentially homebound, and have a plan of care. Housekeeping

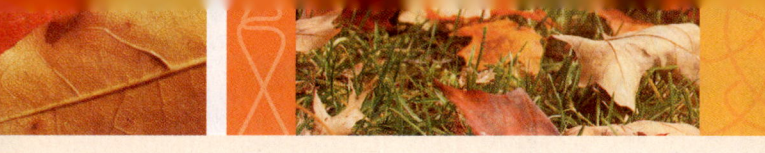
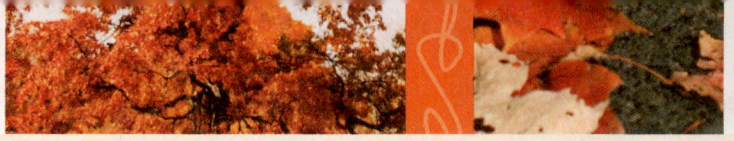

services do not qualify for reimbursement. Income is not a determining factor. **(10) 1.** Outcome 7. Rehabilitation promotes reintegration into the patient's family and community through an interdisciplinary approach that includes in the plan of care physical function, mental health, interpersonal relationship, social interactions, and vocational status. It requires the expertise of a team of health care providers.

CHAPTER 3

NCLEX-PN® ANSWERS   **(1) 1.** Outcome 1, 2. Asking the patient about preferences related to food and other components of caring demonstrates the nurse's consideration of the patient as an individual. The nurse should contact a chaplain only on request of the patient or family. Use of touch varies among cultures; some patients may interpret touch as a threat. Use of children as interpreters is not recommended. **(2) 3.** Outcome 1, 3. Asking the patient to repeat the message allows the nurse to determine whether or not the patient has an accurate understanding of the information being conveyed. This is an appropriate communication strategy for adult patients of all ages and cultures. Speaking loudly and slowly does not increase understanding. While nonverbal communication and gestures may assist to convey the message, they do not help the nurse determine whether the patient has understood the message. **(3) 1.** Outcome 2, 3. Promptly conveying the information regarding the patient's religion demonstrates respect for the patient's wishes, while understanding potential medical care needs. There is no indication in this question that the patient is unable to give permission to treat. Noting the patient's religion in the medical record is appropriate but not the priority. Suggesting legal proceedings is outside the nursing role and fails to convey respect for the patient. **(4) 2.** Outcome 3. Patients with a present orientation to time may have more difficulty making a link between taking a medication now and possible future effects of the disorder. The stem of the question provides no information to support denial or fear on the patient's part. The patient's locus of control is not relevant to the response indicated. **(5) 1.** Outcome 4. Accidents are the leading cause of injury and death in people between ages 15 and 24. Unprotected sex with a variety of people and substance abuse are also major causes of concern for this age group. While increasing numbers of young adults are dealing with obesity, chronic illness and prescription drug use are less frequent concerns in young adults than in middle and older adults. **(6) 1.** Outcome 4. Middle adults often have problems maintaining a healthy weight because they consume the same number of calories as when they were young, while decreasing physical activity. Stressors, chronic illnesses, and normal physiologic changes of aging may contribute, but are much less significant a factor in obesity than an imbalance of calorie intake and use. **(7) 2.** Outcome 5, 7. Women should have a mammogram every 1 to 2 years, beginning at age 50. Men should continue to do testicular self-examination. Vision examinations should be done each year. Regular amounts of exercise are recommended for this age group. **(8) 1, 4, 5.** Outcome 4, 5, 7. The nurse promotes health by teaching and encouraging behaviors to reduce the patient's risk factors for disease. Providing accurate information about recommended health screening promotes health by allowing early identification of health risks. Women should have a mammogram every 1 to 2 years, beginning at age 50. Use of tanning beds is associated with an increased risk for skin cancer. **(9) 3.** Outcome 7. Immunizations are an important measure to prevent illness, even in adults. Cholesterol

screening is recommended every 5 years; pneumococcal pneumonia vaccine is recommended one time for people age 65 and older. While counseling the patient who is overweight about weight loss is appropriate, referral to a commercial weight loss program is outside the nurse's scope of practice. **(10) 4.** Outcome 6. Although not always meeting traditional definitions, people (or even pets) who are significant to the patient are the patient's family. They should be an integral component of care in all health care settings. The decision of family members to step out during nursing care activities or to provide care should be made by the patient and family, not the nurse. Speaking to family about confidential patient matters violates patient confidentiality and, when done without the patient's express permission, violates HIPAA laws.

CHAPTER 4

NCLEX-PN® ANSWERS   **(1) 3.** Outcome 1. The older adult population (age 65 and older) is further divided into three periods: young-old, ages 65–74; middle-old, ages 75–84; and old-old, age 85 and older. Mr. Sanchez falls within the middle-old period, ages 75 to 84. The terms *elderly* and *older adult* are used interchangeably to encompass everyone age 65 and older. **(2) 1.** Outcome 2. Immunity theories are based on the knowledge that the immune system is affected by aging, with decreased defenses against foreign organisms and an increase in chronic illness. Option 2 describes the genetic/biologic clock theories; option 3, the wear and tear theory; and option 4, the programmed aging theory. **(3) 2.** Outcome 3. Ageism is a form of prejudice in which older adults are stereotyped by characteristics of only a small number of their age group; a common myth is that older adults cannot learn new knowledge and skills. The nurse using the nursing process and critical thinking considers each patient as a unique individual. **(4) 4.** Outcome 4. Cognition means the ability to perceive and understand one's world; cognitive function does not normally change with aging. The older adult retains the ability to learn new skills and information. While dementia occurs more frequently in older adults, it is not inevitable. **(5) 2.** Outcomes 4, 5. Older adults like to tell stories about their past during reminiscence, allowing them to relive and restructure life experiences and facilitate achieving ego integrity. This patient's statement provides no information about short-term memory or coping, nor does an isolated statement such as this indicate a tendency to live in the past. **(6) 1.** Outcome 5. When faced with widowhood, the remaining spouse is faced with not only adjusting to the loss of the loved person, but also to living alone. The development of bitterness and sadness versus peace and strength are individually determined. While the individual may gain strength from friends and family, death of a spouse commonly leads to a sense of loss and loneliness. **(7) 4.** Outcome 7. The ability to function safely and independently at home alone depends on a variety of factors, but many older adults can continue living at home with the assistance of home health services, home-delivered meals, and senior transportation. While the patient may choose to participate in activities at a local community center or college, these will not necessarily help the patient remain in his home. **(8) 3.** Outcome 6. The leading causes of death in older adults are cardiovascular disease, cancer, chronic lower respiratory disease, stroke, and Alzheimer disease. **(9) 2.** Outcome 7. Although medications do make life more comfortable for older adults, they carry a risk of drug reactions and interactions that can cause adverse effects, such as dizziness and numbness. These effects

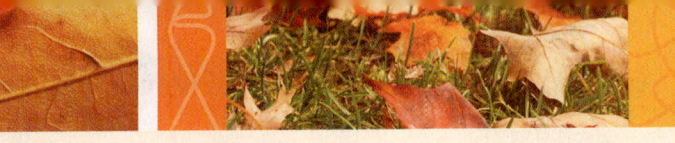

in turn may increase the risk for falling. Temperature, pulse, and respirations provide information about the patient's physical health, not her safety. Unless the nurse is performing home visits, the nurse has few or no opportunities to assess the amount of food and condition of the patient's living quarters. (10) 4. Outcome 7. Nursing care to promote cognition in older adults includes ensuring that eyeglasses and hearing devices are used and that they have clean lenses and good batteries, respectively. Providing a bed bath or stimulation by having the television on and monitoring ambulation do not facilitate cognitive function.

CHAPTER 5

NCLEX-PN® ANSWERS (1) 2. Outcome 1. Objective data are observable or measurable pieces of information (such as the color of urine). Objective data can be seen, heard, touched, or smelled. Subjective data such as the health history are related by the patient. Both objective and subjective data are collected for a comprehensive assessment. *Secondary* is not a term used to describe a type of patient assessment. (2) 3. Outcome 2. A focused assessment addresses a specific patient problem. Assessing a patient with abdominal pain includes assessing bowel movements, temperature, trauma, location, duration, and type of pain. Assessment of the legs, vision, and blood pressure is included in a comprehensive assessment, as well as focused assessments of selected other body systems. (3) 2. Outcome 3. If the patient is very young, very ill, unconscious, or confused, data may be collected from secondary sources, such as family or friends; in all other cases, the patient is the best primary source of information. (4) 4. Outcome 4. Open-ended questions give the patient the chance to provide more information than do closed-ended questions. Questions that can be answered "yes" or "no" are known as closed-ended questions. "Why" questions often make the patient feel threatened or foolish. (5) 3. Outcome 5. Palpation is use of the hands to touch and feel. Light palpation is used for determining pulses, tenderness, skin texture, skin temperature, and skin moisture. Inspection is visual examination; auscultation is listening (e.g., using a stethoscope); and percussion is eliciting a sound by tapping over a body part. (6) 1. Outcome 6. The nurse should wash his or her hands before and after the assessment, even if gloves need to be worn. Setting up the equipment and positioning the patient are components of the assessment, done after washing the hands. A mask is worn only when indicated by a communicable disease; gloves may be worn for selected portions of the physical assessment (e.g., assessing the genitals). (7) Outcome 7. Pulse deficit is 15 (100–85). (8) 2. Outcome 7. Bowel sounds are auscultated by gently placing the stethoscope on the abdomen and listening in all four quadrants. Bowel sounds are clicks or gurgles made as intestinal contents move through the bowel; they should always be present. Inspection, percussion, and palpation are used for complete abdominal assessment, not to assess peristalsis. (9) 3. Outcome 7. Jaundice is a yellow coloration of the skin and mucous membranes. It is caused by liver or gallbladder disease, or by an excessive breakdown of red blood cells. Jaundice is usually first seen in the eyes and then in the skin and mucous membranes. Mottling, erythema (redness), and cyanosis (grayish-blue color) would not be expected findings. (10) 3. Outcome 8. When recording blood pressure, the nurse should write "BP 120/70," not give a detailed description of the assessment method. Data should be organized in a logical way, and inferences or judgments should

be avoided. The word *normal* should not be used; instead, write the specific assessment finding.

CHAPTER 6

NCLEX-PN® ANSWERS (1) 3. Outcome 3. Decreased serum albumin levels in older adults affect drug distribution. There is no effect on absorption, metabolism, or excretion. (2) 1. Outcome 5. This order is missing the number of milligrams so cannot be given as listed. The nurse must call the physician for a complete order because the nurse is unsure when the physician will return to the health care facility. It is inappropriate for the nurse to call the physician for a start time. (3) 2. Outcome 4. Synergism is giving two drugs to cause a greater effect than each drug given separately. Aspirin and an anticoagulant potentiate each other, causing increased risk for bleeding. Nicotine increases the metabolism of anticonvulsants. Alcohol and a sedative drug have an additive effect, increasing sedative effects. (4) 4. Outcome 7. The nurse should question when multiple tablets are prescribed for a single dose. Illegible handwriting should be clarified with the physician who wrote the order. Atypical drug names should always be investigated further. Never use a medication dropper from one medication for another medication. (5) 3. Outcome 2. Because drugs are excreted by the kidneys, anyone with kidney disease is at an increased risk for adverse drug reactions (ADRs). Ages under one or over 65 increase the risk for ADRs. Liver or kidney disease increases the risk of ADR, not croup, pneumonia, or osteoarthritis. (6) 4, 5, 6, 1, 2, 3. Outcome 2. The IV route has the fastest absorption, followed by sublingual, intramuscular (IM), subcutaneous, oral, and transdermal. (7) 3. Outcome 1. Vicodin is a Schedule III controlled substance, not Schedule II, IV, or V. (8) 1. Outcome 4 and 5. Pediatric medication doses are calculated according to the child's body weight. Age, ethnicity, and sex do not affect dose calculation. (9) 4. Outcome 4. A loading dose (giving a larger-than-normal dose) is administered in clinical situations when it is necessary to reach therapeutic drug levels rapidly. This is not called a scheduled, maintenance or therapeutic dose. (10) 2. Outcome 4, 5. Teratogenic drugs are drugs that may cause harm to the fetus and must be avoided in women who are pregnant. It would not affect patients who have renal failure and are under 10 or over 65.

CHAPTER 7

NCLEX-PN® ANSWERS (1) 2. Outcome 1. Females, in general, have more body fat and less body water than males. There is less water available in patients with a higher percentage of body fat. Individuals over the age of 65 also have decreased body water due to higher body fat content. (2) 2. Outcome 2. Antidiuretic hormone (ADH) regulates water excretion in the kidneys. The kidneys are less permeable to water. Copious amounts of dilute urine are produced. Serum osmolality decreases, blood pressure falls slightly, and the thirst mechanism in the brain is activated. (3) 1. Outcome 2, 3. These signs and symptoms indicate a decrease in fluid volume, such as dehydration. Although the patient is at risk for the other problems listed here, the assessment data directly relate to fluid volume status. (4) 4. Outcome 4. Decreased calcium level is manifested by increased muscle excitability. The parathyroid glands, involved in the regulation of calcium in the body, may be inadvertently removed or damaged during a thyroidectomy. Although a positive Chvostek sign may be present in hypomagnesemia, this patient's history does not indicate a risk for this imbalance. Chvostek sign is not a manifestation of sodium or potassium imbalances. (5) 3. Outcome 4. Chronic alcoholism is a principal cause of hypomagnesemia. Excessive antacid use, in contrast, may cause hypermagnesemia. Hypermagnesemia may develop as a result of kidney failure. Lack of sun exposure may lead to hypocalcemia. (6) 1. Outcome 5. The normal pH is 7.35 to 7.45. Respiratory alkalosis (pH greater than 7.45) occurs during hyperventilation. Other values listed are within the normal ranges. (7) 1. Outcome 6. The pancreas secretes bicarbonate into the small intestine. Vomiting, suctioning, and diarrhea contribute to the loss of bicarbonate. Overuse of baking soda increases the bicarbonate levels. Constipation does not affect bicarbonate or electrolyte levels, although its treatment with laxatives or enemas can. Hypomagnesemia is a potential complication of alcohol abuse. (8) 2. Outcome 3, 6. The patient with a potassium imbalance is at risk for cardiac dysrhythmias. Paralytic ileus is a potential result of hypokalemia; fluid retention is associated with sodium imbalances; and kidney stones may be associated with calcium imbalances. (9) 1. Outcome 3. Lasix is a loop diuretic that promotes water loss. Daily weights should be obtained; they are the most accurate measurement for water loss. Intake and output are also measured and compared. The apical pulse and breath sounds may change as excess fluid is eliminated, but they are not measures of the drug's effect. Oral fluid intake is measured for comparison with urinary output, not as an indicator of drug effectiveness. (10) 2. Outcome 3, 6. As the acidosis is corrected, potassium tends to shift from extracellular fluid into the cells. As a result, hypokalemia may develop. The other laboratory values listed are not directly affected by correction of the metabolic acidosis.

CHAPTER 8

NCLEX-PN® ANSWERS (1) 2. Outcome 2. Patients taking codeine, an opioid, for chronic pain have the highest risk for developing pain tolerance because the pain often lasts more than 6 months. Using morphine or patient-controlled analgesia (PCA) after surgery usually does not increase pain tolerance due to the short-term nature of acute pain. Antidepressants do not affect pain tolerance. (2) 1. Outcome 2. Referred pain starts in one site but is perceived in another part of the body. It frequently occurs with visceral pain (pain from body organs lined with viscera), because the pain impulses travel along the same nerve paths. Deep somatic pain occurs from injury to deep body structures, while cutaneous pain is superficial; neither pain types radiate. (3) 1, 3, 5. Outcome 5. Massage, guided imagery, and relaxation are appropriate nonpharmacologic techniques for a patient with cancer pain. A pain diary is used for patients with chronic nonmalignant pain. Hydromorphone is an opioid analgesic and inappropriate for a patient with a pain rating of 4 out of 10. (4) 3. Outcome 7. Phantom limb pain occurs in some individuals after the removal of an extremity. The patient is aware that the part is missing, but the pain can be intense and difficult to treat. Medication should be administered to attempt relief not just report the pain to the charge nurse. Nonpharmacologic approaches are ineffective. (5) 1. Outcome 4. Ibuprofen is an irritant to the gastric mucosa. Patients with gastric ulcer disease should use alternate medications for pain relief. Acetaminophen, meperidine, and codeine do not cause gastric irritation. (6) 4. Outcome 6. Allowing the patient to describe his pain based on a pain scale provides an objective, individualized description of the pain. The nurse can make decisions for intervention based on this assessment. Observing facial expression, taking vital signs, or asking if pain is mild to severe does provide the patient's perception of the pain. (7) 2. Outcome 3. Older adults often have chronic diseases and believe pain is part of growing old; therefore they often do not report pain. All cultures do not respond to pain in the same way. Patients with acute pain are more anxious. Older adults can use a numeric or visual pain scale. (8) 4. Outcome 8. Naloxone blocks the effects of opioid drugs and reverses sedation and respiratory depression that may result from excessive dosages. Ativan, Valium, and Toradol will not reverse respiratory depression but rather add to it. (9) 2. Outcome 7. Alcohol is avoided as it increases the risk for CNS depression. Taking the drug with food helps to reduce GI upset, but it should be taken every 4 hours to reduce pain. The medication is taken until the patient no longer requires it for pain. Taking additional acetaminophen increases the potential for liver toxicity. (10) 3. Outcome 7. Morphine via patient-controlled analgesia (PCA) increases the potential for respiratory depression and must be assessed every 1–2 hours. Decreased peristalsis and constipation are common side effects of morphine, but are not the first priority. Fluids should be increased to at least 3,000 mL/day if not contraindicated. GI bleeding is not a side effect of morphine.

CHAPTER 9

NCLEX-PN® ANSWERS (1) 1. Outcome 5. Urinary tract infections are the leading cause of nosocomial infections, especially in older adults. The patient's Foley catheter was inserted 4 days ago. The 1-week use of the antibiotic is significant, but not as important as the invasive insertion of the Foley catheter. Weight of 150 lb does not increase HIA risk. Peripheral vascular disease increases the susceptibility for a nosocomial infection, but is not a major factor in the hospital stay. (2) 3. Outcome 2. WBC count greater than 15,000 indicates acute infection. Erythrocyte sedimentation rate is increased with infection. The presence of bands means serious infection; the absence means no infection. A positive C-reactive protein indicates inflammation. (3) 4. Outcome 3. Ankle sprains are managed by elevating the limb when sitting to reduce inflammation. Heat or cold therapy is applied for short periods several times a day. Corticosteroids are used for acute hypersensitivity reactions or pain unrelieved by NSAIDs or aspirin. A sprain injury does not need to be cleansed. (4) 2. Outcome 8. The infection is an overgrowth of bacteria due to the side effects of the antibiotic. Nurses cannot diagnose medical conditions. The nurse should address the problem and reassure the patient. Never tell the patient not to worry. "4" is incorrect, because it acknowledges the complaint but doesn't adequately address the patient's concern. (5) 4. Outcome 4, 8. Hand washing is extremely important in preventing infection. Antibiotic treatments should be completed as prescribed. Any fever should be reported because it may indicate an infection. Water intake should be at least 2 1/2 quarts/day to maintain body temperature and metabolism. (6) 1. Outcome 6. Although there is an increase in the growth of vancomycin-resistant organisms, vancomycin is still the drug of choice. Azithromycin, gentamicin, and cephalexin are not used to treat MRSA infection. (7) 1. Outcome 10. Cellulitis is a subcutaneous, connective tissue infection. Antibiotics must be given at appropriate times to decrease the potential damage to the eye. Bed rest is an unlikely order for this patient. IM morphine in frequent doses is contraindicated in older patients because of poor absorption and potential for respiratory depression. Lab values are important, but may be checked at a later time. (8) 2. Outcome 1. Systemic infection produces the enlargement of lymph nodes throughout the body. Localized tenderness, pain when ambulating, and cellulitis are manifestations of local infection. (9) 4. Outcome 7. Herpes zoster is a common infection in older adults. None of the other patients have high-risk factors for herpes zoster. (10) 3, 6. Outcome 9. Chickenpox virus is spread through the air; therefore, the nurse must wear an N95 mask and place a mask on the patient when transporting to another part of the hospital. It is inappropriate to wear a regular mask and gloves only. It is unnecessary to wear sterile gloves. All health care personnel should wash their hands. Family would have to wear gown, N95 mask, and gloves.

CHAPTER 10

NCLEX-PN® ANSWERS (1) 3. Outcome 1. In a thyroidectomy, the diseased thyroid gland is removed (ablation). Because of its location and the nature of the surgery, thyroidectomy is major surgery. Reconstructive surgery rebuilds damaged tissue. This procedure is scheduled, not performed on an emergency basis. (2) 2. Outcome 4. Potassium level of 2.8 is below normal and places the patient at risk for cardiac arrhythmias. All other laboratory values are within normal ranges. (3) 1. Outcome 2. Discussion of risk factors and complications is included in informed consent. Informed consent is the responsibility of the physician. Responses 2 and 3 do not demonstrate respect for the patient's concerns. (4) 2, 1, 5, 3, 4. Outcome 5. Assessment is needed before nursing intervention can be determined. Nursing measures to promote urination are appropriate before notifying the physician or preparing for straight catheterization. (5) 3. Outcome 4, 7. Effective pain management should prevent significant pain and allow the patient to perform deep-breathing, coughing, and leg exercises. Splinting the incision with a pillow when moving, deep breathing, or coughing is appropriate to reduce discomfort. (6) 1. Outcome 5. Primary intention is normal wound healing. The wound edges are approximated and closed by staples or sutures. Wounds healing by primary intention have little or no exudate. Gaping wounds and the presence of granulation tissue describe wounds healing by secondary intention. (7) 2. Outcome 3. The time-out is an important safety measure to prevent surgery on the wrong patient or body part. Equipment required for the surgical procedure should be in place prior to the patient's entry into the operating room. Orientation of the patient to the surroundings is separate from the time-out, which involves all members of the surgical team. The time-out is conducted prior to induction of anesthesia. (8) 3. Outcome 5. Assessment suggests impending shock. The patient should be placed in the shock position to facilitate blood supply to vital organs. Assessing the dressing for bleeding and notifying the physician of the findings are important measures after placing the patient in shock position. Increasing the IV infusion rate of flow requires a physician's order. (9) 4. Outcome 6. The older adult may develop confusion or disorientation related to sensory deprivation if vision and hearing aids are not provided after surgery. The nurse also will document the findings and notify the charge nurse or physician if confusion continues. Bed rest can increase the patient's confusion. (10) 3. Outcome 8. Patients undergoing ambulatory surgery usually are discharged home on the day of surgery.

CHAPTER 11

NCLEX-PN® ANSWERS (1) 3. Outcome 1. Local injections may cause discomfort at the site. A heating pad will soothe the soreness. Redness at the injection site is common and does not indicate a severe reaction. Patients should remain in the clinic for at least 30 minutes after receiving an immunization to monitor for adverse reactions. (2) 4. Outcome 2, 7. HIV viral load is monitored for effectiveness of HAART. Western blot assay is used to confirm HIV diagnosis. Tuberculin skin test would confirm a TB diagnosis. WBC count is within normal limits and is not used to determine HIV treatment effectiveness. (3) 1. Outcome 5. Swelling of the lips may lead to edema in the throat. Breathing difficulties should be assessed immediately. Medication may be administered to counteract the inflammatory process. A medical history is important, as well as patient teaching, after the initial assessment is completed. (4) 2. Outcome 3, 4. Immunosuppressive agents decrease the ability of the immune system to fight infection. Emphasize the need to avoid large crowds and report signs of infection. After surgery, fluids are not restricted to less than 1,000 mL/day. Activity should be increased as tolerated by the patient to prevent post-op complications. Urine output should be normal rather than increased. (5) 2. Outcome 6. Washing the skin is done to hopefully remove any contaminated blood from the body before it infects the nurse. The charge nurse should be notified after washing the skin. Prophylactic medication is given within 2 to 3 hours of the exposure after washing the skin. Follow-up is done at 3 and 6 months after initial exposure. (6) 3. Outcome 7. Primary HIV infection produces few symptoms. Many patients present with sore throat and other flulike symptoms. White patches in the mouth indicate candidiasis. SOB is an early sign of PJP. AIDS dementia complex presents with forgetfulness and difficulty concentrating. (7) 4. Outcome 6. Condoms must be used only one time. Only water-based lubricants should be used to prevent damage to the condom. Oral contraceptives may provide pregnancy protection but have no effect on viral transmission. Anal sex should be avoided because of potential damage to sensitive tissue. Only latex condoms prevent passage of HIV. (8) 2. Outcome 2. The Mantoux is the standard diagnostic test used to identify tuberculosis, a common condition that occurs in patients diagnosed with HIV. MAC is caused by bacteria found in the soil and also affects the respiratory system. Kaposi sarcoma is a cancer. A protozoan, the causative agent for cryptosporidiosis, produces watery diarrhea. (9) 4. Outcome 7. AIDS dementia complex is a progressive disorder, causing mental confusion, motor deficits, and forgetfulness. All of these nursing interventions would be noted on the care plan. With dementia, safety is the priority consideration. (10) 1. Outcome 7. The first priority would be to remove the food from the patient's room. Discuss medications for nausea and appetite enhancement before the next meal. Fluids should be limited with meals to encourage increased solid food consumption.

CHAPTER 12

NCLEX-PN® ANSWERS (1) 2. Outcome 3. The liver is a common site of metastasis from lung tumors; the patient is demonstrating manifestations of liver dysfunction. Although nausea and anorexia may occur as adverse effects of chemotherapy, abdominal pain usually does not. Edema of the face and neck and respiratory symptoms are manifestations of superior vena cava syndrome. Extension of the tumor to involve the diaphragm is unlikely to cause nausea and anorexia. (2) 3. Outcome 2. A diet rich in whole grains, fruits, and vegetables with minimal red and processed meat is associated with a lower risk for colorectal cancer. Although there appears to be a genetic link for many cancers, environmental factors also play a role in development of the disease. Screening is important for early detection of colon cancer, but annual exams are unnecessary due to the slow progression of tumors. (3) 4. Outcome 1, 4. The PSA (or prostate-specific antigen) is a marker for prostate cancer, the most commonly occurring cancer in men. It is not used to screen for other types of cancer or general health. (4) 1. Outcome 6. Family members can provide needed care while the patient adjusts to his diagnosis. The nurse should include the patient in care as much as he will allow. Insisting that the patient care for his colostomy or allowing the patient to avoid watching care are not therapeutic actions. There is no indication that the patient needs counseling to deal with this situational stressor. (5) 4. Outcome 5, 7. Choosing a head cover before losing her hair allows the patient to prepare for the loss and make decisions in a less stressful environment. Drug regimens are chosen based on their effectiveness in eradicating the tumor; adverse effects are common with most regimens. (6) 3, 5. Outcome 6, 8. Small, frequent meals are more palatable when a patient is anorexic. Supplements such as Ensure or powdered drink mixes (e.g., Instant Breakfast) mixed with milk and ice cream provide needed calories for the anorexic patient. Soft, cool foods are usually tolerated better than hot foods. Understanding the importance of maintaining nutritional status does not help the patient deal with anorexia and nausea. Overly large meals or portions often worsen symptoms of nausea and anorexia. (7) 2. Outcome 5. Placing the implant in a lead container prevents radiation exposure. Long-handled forceps reduce the nurse's risk by increasing the distance from the implant. Radioactive materials should not be disposed of in the trash or sewer system because of risk of contamination to individuals and the environment. (8) 3. Outcome 7. Rubbing or scratching increases irritation to the site and increases risk of infection. Skin should be cleansed with clear water; no ointments should be applied unless directed by the physician. Patients receiving external radiation are not radioactive, and therefore are not a risk to others. (9) 1. Outcome 6, 8. Providing antiemetic medication before the treatment reduces the risk of nausea and vomiting. Nutritional needs should be met throughout the course of chemotherapy. (10) 3. Outcome 4, 8. Decreased WBC increases the patient's risk of infection. Temperature elevation is a systemic symptom of infection. Alopecia and nausea and vomiting are not complications of bone marrow depression. The platelet count is usually decreased with bone marrow depression. A platelet count of 200,000 is within normal limits.

CHAPTER 13

NCLEX-PN® ANSWERS (1) 2. Outcome 2. The grief process is highly individual in quality and duration depending on what the loss means to the person experiencing it. The meaning of the loss may be affected by its permanence. Religion and education may affect the individual's coping but do not alter grieving. (2) 2. Outcome 2. In the anger stage, the person resists the loss, often directing his or her anger toward family and health care providers. The stage of denial is characterized by disbelief. In bargaining, the individual seeks to postpone or reverse the loss. In acceptance, the person comes to terms with the

loss and is able to move forward. (3) 1. Outcome 3. The age of the person experiencing the loss influences his or her understanding of and reaction to the loss. An individual's reaction to the loss is also affected by perception of a support system. Responses to loss are less affected by income, self-concept, and employment. (4) 4. Outcome 4. A do-not-resuscitate order is written by the physician for a patient who is near death. The order is usually written based on the wishes of the patient and family. It cannot be initiated by the nurse. (5) 2. Outcome 5. Regardless of the setting, the patient's wishes about death should be respected. Nurses care for the dying patient in intensive care units, emergency rooms, long-term care facilities, and the home. The patient's wishes should be known and followed by the family and caregivers, even if they differ from cultural norms or the wishes of the family. (6) 1. Outcome 5. Hospice is a model of care (rather than a place of care) for patients and their families, emphasizing quality rather than quantity of life for patients as they near the end of life. Hospice care may occur in a variety of settings, including the home and homelike care settings, or in long-term care. Euthanasia is killing prompted by a humanitarian motive. Advance directives are legal documents that specify the patient's wishes for health care. (7) 4. Outcome 7. Providing comfort and care to the dying is an active, desirable, and important component of nursing care. Using data from assessment to plan and provide symptom management is necessary for nurses to provide high-quality end-of-life care. It is neither necessary nor desirable for the nurse to control his or her own emotions or to remain emotionally detached. The nurse also provides comfort and care regardless of whether he or she agrees with the patient's values and beliefs. (8) 2. Outcome 6. Near death, the patient may have periods of apnea and/or Cheyne–Stokes respirations. An accumulation of fluids in the lungs and oropharynx may lead to what is sometimes referred to as the *death rattle*. These respiratory changes are normal at this time. Episodes of tachypnea and coughing are uncommon at this time. Loss of sphincter control and emotional distress are not respiratory changes. (9) 4. Outcome 1. Normal grieving is a combination of intellectual, emotional, physical, spiritual, and social responses and behaviors by which people incorporate an actual, anticipated, or perceived loss. (10) 3. Outcome 7. Spending time listening to patients conveys acceptance of their emotional response to loss. The most appropriate interventions are to listen to how they are feeling and to be present. The other responses do not encourage the patient to share very personal feelings.

CHAPTER 14

NCLEX-PN® ANSWERS (1) 4, 2, 3, 1, and 5. Outcome 3. The nurse should stop the blood immediately and notify the charge nurse. Then start a normal saline infusion with intravenous tubing. Vital signs are then taken. Based on institutional policy, save the blood bag and return it to the lab. (2) 4. Outcome 4. Adult urine output should be no less than 30 mL/hr. The urine output is well below the norm and indicates a problem that should be corrected immediately. First, check the Foley catheter tubing for patency, and palpate the bladder for distention. Notify the charge nurse immediately. The dark color of the urine indicates dehydration due to the patient's blood loss. (3) 2. Outcome 6. Anxiety is the most appropriate nursing diagnosis, because no evidence shows severe blood loss that could account for the restless state. The vital signs are stable, and the dressing is dry. Infection does not develop until 72 hours postoperative. Deficient Knowledge relating to the prognosis of her surgery is important once the anxiety is managed. (4) 3. Outcome 5. The appropriate response is to acknowledge the patient's concern and to make an attempt to ascertain the waiting time. Do not agree or disagree with the long waiting time. The patient may not care that other people need attention or may not understand the levels of triage. Telling the patient that the physician does not have time for him will only increase his anxiety and frustration. (5) 3. Outcome 7. The patient with full-thickness burns of the face is at risk for airway obstruction and must be seen immediately as denoted by a red tag. A patient with an open fracture would be tagged "yellow" and should be treated in less than 2 hours. Contusions are considered minor injuries and are tagged "green." The patient with multisystem trauma is tagged "black" for imminent death. (6) 1. Outcome 1. Cirrhosis of the liver results in the fluid shifting into the interstitial spaces (ascites). This decreases the amount of fluid circulating in the bloodstream, resulting in hypovolemic shock. Anaphylactic shock occurs from a severe allergic reaction. Vital signs indicate that the heart is pumping effectively, so cardiogenic shock is not evident. Septic shock is caused by pathogenic toxins in the blood and results in high fevers. (7) 3. Outcome 2, 4, and 5. Patients should be taught that many reactions are significantly more severe when exposed to the antigen the second time. Precautions should be initiated. MedicAlert bracelets let medical personnel know that the patient is allergic to bee venom. The pharmacist can teach about the antivenom drugs. The patient's immediate family should learn appropriate interventions for handling an anaphylactic reaction. (8) 2, 4, 5. Outcome 5. Heat stroke is characterized by rapid respirations and pulse plus an extremely high temperature (as high as 106°F). Cool skin, profuse sweating, and nausea and vomiting are seen in heat exhaustion. (9) 2. Outcome 2 and 3. Septic shock causes massive vasodilation and reduced blood pressure. When IV fluids are effective, the blood pressure increases. Septic shock is characterized by warm, dry skin and rapid respirations. IV fluids cannot alter these symptoms. Excessive fluid intake would cause rapid respirations and crackles. Heart rhythm is regulated by antidysrhythmic drugs. (10) 4. Outcome 4. Safety tips such as handrails in the bathroom, the removal of all loose rugs from the floors, and night-lights in the rooms in the patient's home should be thoroughly discussed. The patient should be able to maneuver with his walker before discharge. Food preparation and transportation are important once the safety issues are discussed.

CHAPTER 15

NCLEX-PN® ANSWERS   (1) 4. Outcome 3. Sleeping in an upright or semireclining position may indicate impaired pumping of the heart. The other data are irrelevant to cardiac function. (2) 2. Outcome 1. The mitral valve separates the left atrium from the left ventricle. The atrioventricular valve on the right side of the heart is the tricuspid valve; the pulmonic and aortic valves lead from the ventricles to the pulmonary artery and aorta, respectively. (3) 2. Outcome 2. The QRS complex corresponds with ventricular systole (contraction). The P wave corresponds with atrial contraction, and the T wave with repolarization of the ventricles. The ST segment is the period between ventricular polarization as indicated by the QRS complex, and repolarization, as indicated by the T wave. (4) 2, 3, 5.

Outcome 1. Blood vessel length and diameter and the viscosity of the blood affect peripheral vascular resistance, with vessel diameter being the primary factor in determining total peripheral resistance. The number of capillaries, body position, and age of the patient may have minor effects on peripheral vascular resistance but not major effects. (5) 1. Outcome 4. The echocardiogram is an imaging study that helps determine the size and movement of the heart, as well as some structural abnormalities. An echocardiogram is noninvasive, but does not require external electrodes (which are used for an electrocardiogram) or expose the patient to a magnetic field (as does an MRI). It does not required injection of a dye.

CHAPTER 16

NCLEX-PN® ANSWERS   (1) 1. Outcome 3, 6. Many of the statin drugs, including atorvastatin, can impair liver function. Yellowing of the skin and sclera must be promptly reported to the physician to ensure that irreversible liver damage does not occur. Muscle pain can indicate an adverse drug reaction and should be reported. Statins are best taken at bedtime. Limiting fat intake to 30% of total calories is recommended. (2) 3. Outcome 1, 2. Anginal chest pain usually is relieved by rest and sublingual nitroglycerin (or other rapid-acting nitroglycerin preparations), whereas the chest pain associated with an acute myocardial infarction usually continues despite rest or administration of sublingual nitroglycerin. (3) 4. Outcome 4. Disruption of the integrity of the femoral artery by insertion of the catheter and sheath can result in either arterial bleeding or formation of a clot that impairs distal circulation to the affected extremity. The other nursing diagnoses are not supported by the information provided. (4) 2. Outcome 2, 5. Hypotension (low blood pressure) and a urine output of less than 30 mL/hr are indicative of a fall in cardiac output and may indicate inadequate tissue perfusion. The data presented in options 1 and 3 are within normal or expected ranges. A BP of 150/70, while elevated, is not high enough to be of immediate concern. (5) 1. Outcome 2. Creatine kinase (CK) is an enzyme released from necrotic cardiac muscle cells. The blood level of CK rises within hours after an acute myocardial infarction and remains elevated for up to 48 hours. The hematocrit and BUN should remain within normal limits after an MI. Blood glucose levels may increase slightly due to the stress response. (6) 4. Outcome 5, 6. Lifestyle modifications, including dietary changes, can reduce the risk for myocardial infarction in the future. Patients are taught to use no more than 3 nitroglycerine at 5-minute intervals before calling 911 if chest pain is unrelieved. It is neither possible nor desirable to avoid all stress. (7) 3. Outcome 1, 5. The normal adult heart rate is 60 to 100 beats per minute. A rate lower than 60 is bradycardia, a rate greater than 100 is tachycardia. Sinus arrhythmia is an irregular heart rate characterized by increased heart rate on inspiration and decreased heart rate with expiration. (8) 3. Outcome 1, 5. Assessment of the patient is vital to determine whether the apparent heart rhythm is due to a mechanical problem (e.g., a loose monitor lead or wire) and/or is affecting cardiac output. The other actions may be appropriate, based on the patient's status. (9) 2. Outcome 5. Immediate and effective CPR can be lifesaving for the patient who experiences cardiac arrest and sudden cardiac death. Patients who have experienced dysrhythmias and those taking antidysrhythmic medications have an increased risk of future dysrhythmias. It is not within the nurse's scope of practice or responsibility to recommend or provide resources for obtaining an AED. (10) 1, 2, 4. Outcome 5. Correct electrode placement, patient education, and ensuring safe working equipment are important for effective cardiac monitoring. Electrode pads are placed according to the ECG lead selected for monitoring; the midaxillary line generally is avoided to prevent interfering with defibrillation, should it be required.

CHAPTER 17

NCLEX-PN® ANSWERS (1) 1. Outcome 1, 4. Left-sided heart failure affects cardiac output and the availability of blood and oxygen to meet the body's metabolic needs. As a result, fatigue and activity intolerance are common, early manifestations of heart failure. Heart failure is not painful, nor does it usually affect airway clearance. Fluid volume often increases in heart failure due to compensatory mechanisms. (2) 2. Outcome 1. The backward effects of right-sided heart failure affect the venous system and peripheral tissues. Increased pressure in the venous system causes peripheral edema. The heart rate increases, and urinary output may decrease. Pulmonary edema develops with left-sided failure. (3) 3. Outcome 2. A slow pulse may indicate digitalis toxicity. The physician should be notified as diagnostic tests may be necessary to determine the cause of the low pulse rate. Checking the digoxin level and making a decision about digoxin administration is outside the nurse's scope of practice. The drug should not be held for one hour, nor should it be administered without a specific order to do so at this time. (4) 2. Outcome 5. Cheese is high in sodium, as are smoked foods, indicating a need for further instruction about appropriate dietary selections. The other menu selections are appropriate to the diet. (5) 3. Outcome 4. The patient with rheumatic heart disease needs to recognize manifestations of increasing valve dysfunction that may indicate a need for further intervention. Determining the etiology of the disease is not within the nurses' role. While encouraging visitors and assessing for recurring manifestations of strep infection may be appropriate, these are not priority nursing interventions. (6) 4. Outcome 1. Bacterial endocarditis occurs most frequently in patients who have had previous heart or valve damage that affects the flow of blood through the heart. The innermost layer of the heart is affected, and treatment is necessary to reduce the risk of permanent heart valve damage. End-stage heart failure is not a common outcome of bacterial endocarditis. (7) 4. Outcome 1. A pericardial friction rub is a manifestation of pericarditis and therefore an expected assessment finding. Peripheral edema and respiratory wheezes are not expected findings, and should be reported to the physician. Pericarditis typically causes chest pain that increases with movement and breathing. (8) 3. Outcome 4. A collection of fluid or blood in the pericardial sac can obscure or muffle the heart sounds and affect cardiac filling and output. This drop in cardiac output causes the blood pressure to fall. A line of demarcation, loud heart murmur, or irregular pulse of variable intensity are not manifestations of cardiac tamponade, but should be reported to the physician if noted. (9) 1. Outcome 5. The patient needs information about possible complications to be reported to the physician, however, it is not appropriate or expected for the patient to auscultate for heart murmurs. (10) 2. Outcome 3. Mechanical valve replacements necessitate anticoagulant therapy to prevent formation of clots on the valve. Until well regulated, this increases the patient's risk for bleeding. Most patients adjust well to the sound of the mechanical valve if it is noticeable. Cardiac output improves with replacement of the stenosed valve. The coronary arteries, which supply blood to the heart muscle, are not affected by valve surgery.

CHAPTER 18

NCLEX-PN® ANSWERS (1) 4. Outcome 2. When an arterial thrombus develops, blood flow through the artery is occluded. Pain is the primary manifestation of arterial occlusion (tissue ischemia), and the affected extremity is cold and pale due to lack of circulation. Pulses distal to the occlusion are not palpable. Cyanosis and mottling are not seen in an acute arterial occlusion. (2) 1. Outcome 1. Instruct the patient to keep the extremity in a dependent position; gravity helps to maintain blood flow to the distal tissues. Elevating or wrapping the affected extremity can decrease blood flow, not improve it. Exercise is recommended, not simply range-of-motion exercises. (3) 1. Outcome 3. Measuring calf circumference is part of the focused assessment of a patient with DVT. The leg affected by deep venous thrombosis often is larger in diameter than the unaffected extremity. An eye chart, tuning fork, or pulse oximetry unit are not used during focused assessment for DVT. (4) 3. Outcome 7. Stress management is particularly important for patients with Raynaud phenomenon. The patient is encouraged to use relaxation techniques, massage therapy, hobbies, aromatherapy, and counseling to reduce and cope with stress. Elevating the extremity or wearing support hose can interfere with arterial circulation. Repetitive movements are not associated with Raynaud phenomenon. (5) 2, 3. Outcome 6. Protecting the feet and legs from injury is an important part of care for patients with PVD. A heating pad or lamp may burn the patient who has reduced sensation in the feet; elevating the legs further reduces blood flow. (6) 2. Outcome 1. People with stage 1 or stage 2 hypertension commonly have no symptoms other than an increased blood pressure. Hypertension is usually advanced when manifestations are seen. (7) 1. Outcome 7. Based on the lack of symptoms, patients often have difficulty understanding the importance of medication schedules. Hypertension is a chronic disease, requiring long-term management. While lifestyle changes are important in hypertension management, medication is required for effective management of the disease. Range-of-motion exercises are not required in managing hypertension. (8) 4. Outcome 4. Coumadin interferes with liver synthesis of clotting factors, preventing the clot formation. The patient's symptoms and history are consistent with an intracranial bleed and clot formation. The other medications identified are not associated with increased bleeding risk. (9) 3. Outcome 7. Nicotine constricts blood vessels. The smaller the diameter of a vessel, the greater the friction against the walls of vessel and thus the greater impedance to blood flow. Nicotine does not stimulate the blood vessels directly or dilate blood vessels. While it may increase the pulse rate, this is not a major factor in hypertension. (10) 1. Outcome 5. Lower extremities should be warm and dry, with strong, equal pulses. Unequal skin temperature and pulses could indicate occlusion of blood flow to the right leg. The other data are expected findings in the postoperative patient.

CHAPTER 19

NCLEX-PN® ANSWERS (1) 2. Outcome 1, 4. Hemoglobin is the molecule in red blood cells (RBCs) that transports oxygen to the tissues. These levels are significantly lower than normal. Low hemoglobin and hematocrit levels do not increase the patient's risk for clotting or affect the ability to fight infection. (2) 1, 3. Outcome 1, 3, 4. Erythropoietin is a hormone produced by the kidneys that stimulates the production of RBCs in the bone marrow. Patients with renal failure often have low RBC counts and hematocrits. Because hemoglobin is part of the RBC, hemoglobin levels also would be low, not high. The WBC count is unaffected by erythropoietin levels. Erythropoietin is necessary for the production of immature RBCs, so this level would also be decreased. (3) 4. Outcome 2. The spleen is the largest organ of the lymphatic system. It produces lymphocytes, WBCs important for immune function. Drugs are metabolized in the liver; the kidneys are primarily responsible for excretion of wastes. Blood clotting is dependent on platelets and the clotting cascade. (4) 1. Outcome 1, 4. Thrombocytes (platelets) are an important part of the coagulation system, necessary to form stable blood clots. Leukocytes (WBCs) are the primary component of the immune system. RBCs carry oxygen for energy production. Nutrients are carried in the liquid (plasma) portion of the blood. (5) 3. Outcome 5. The patient is at risk for bleeding after bone marrow aspiration, particularly when the iliac crest is used. Bone marrow aspiration does not affect blood volume. The procedure can cause deep bone pain, requiring analgesia for comfort. Bed rest is not necessary after the procedure.

CHAPTER 20

NCLEX-PN® ANSWERS (1) 1. Outcome 2, 4. Patients with sickle cell crisis are in severe pain. Narcotic analgesics should be administered as soon as possible. A physician's order is required for lab analysis. Antibiotics will not relieve the patient's pain. A Foley catheter is not indicated. (2) 3. Outcome 4. Lack of oxygen to the cells results in hypoxia and fatigue. Patients with anemia require frequent rest periods until correction of process can be accomplished. Pernicious anemia does not affect immune function. Increasing iron and fluid intake is not indicated for pernicious anemia. (3) 2. Outcome 1, 4. Thrombocytopenia (low platelet count) places the patient at risk for bleeding. The patient should be protected from injury that could cause bleeding. Risks associated with infection, dehydration, or nutritional deficit are similar for the patient with thrombocytopenia as for other patients; these are not priority nursing care goals. (4) 2. Outcome 1. Contact sports such as hockey, basketball, and baseball place the patient with hemophilia at risk for injury and bleeding. Golf is least likely to result in physical injury. (5) 1, 2, 4, 5. Outcome 3. These interventions promote healing and comfort. Acid pH of citrus juices increases pain and may injure open lesions on mucous membranes. (6) 1. Outcome 1. Coagulation in small blood vessels results in occlusion of small blood vessels and ischemia. Pillows under the knees further occlude vessels and promote ischemia. The other measures are indicated for the patient with DIC. (7) 1. Outcome 2, 3. Radiation therapy (external beam) used to slow the progression of multiple myeloma damages rapidly dividing cells of the skin. Although radiation therapy is not painful, it does have significant side effects. External radiation therapy exposes only the patient to radiation; there is no risk to family members. (8) 2. Outcome 2. Elevation of extremities promotes lymphatic drainage and decreases edema. Antiembolic stockings or pressure devices are not used for upper-extremity edema. The skin should be inspected daily when edema is severe. A low-sodium diet may be recommended, not low potassium. (9) 1. Outcome 1. Enlarged, painless, movable lymph nodes in the cervical area are a symptom of Hodgkin lymphoma. Reed–Sternberg cells and Epstein–Barr virus are associated with Hodgkin lymphoma. Enlarged lymph nodes typically are not painful. (10) 4. Outcome 3, 4. Maintaining isolation precautions as prescribed at all times helps protect a patient with an impaired immune system from infection. Visitors who are ill should not be allowed. Hand hygiene on leaving the patient's room protects other patients, not the patient with leukemia. While evidence of infection should be reported and documented, the goal is to prevent infection.

CHAPTER 21

NCLEX-PN® ANSWERS (1) 1, 2, 5. Outcome 1, 2. Intact airways, an intact thorax able to expand and contract during breathing, and an intact cardiovascular system are vital for the process of respiration, which includes air movement into and out of the lungs, the exchange of gases between the alveoli and blood, and transport of oxygen and carbon dioxide to and from the cells of the body. A concussion, which may involve a momentary loss of memory at the time of the injury, and a torn knee cartilage are unlikely to affect respiratory status. (2) 2. Outcome 1. The cough reflex is ineffective in patients who are comatose or unconscious. Esophageal sphincter tone is not affected in the comatose patient. The gag reflex also may be impaired in the comatose patient. While mouth care is important in a comatose patient, feeding is not appropriate when consciousness is impaired. (3) 4. Outcome 4. The amount of radioactive ion used is small and rapidly excreted; no special precautions to avoid exposure of others to radioactivity are necessary. (4) 3. Outcome 3. An increased anterior–posterior chest diameter is called a barrel chest. It would not be an expected finding in a middle adult. A barrel chest can make auscultation of breath sounds more difficult and may indicate increased residual lung volume. (5) 2. Outcome 4. Bronchodilators, smoking, and caffeine can interfere with PFT results and should be avoided on the morning of the test. Fasting is not necessary, and the test is not painful.

CHAPTER 22

NCLEX-PN® ANSWERS (1) 3. Outcome 2. Antihistamines have many side effects, including drowsiness and a dry mouth. Some patients may have an allergic reaction, with chest tightness or wheezing. Alcohol is contraindicated with most antihistamines, including Chlor-Trimeton. (2) 4. Outcome 4. Moist air helps to loosen secretions and provide comfort for the postoperative tonsillectomy patient. Ice collars are used to decrease the potential for hemorrhage. The head of the bed should be elevated, with the patient's head turned to the side. The airway device must remain in place until the gag reflex returns. (3) 2. Outcome 3. Patients with pertussis are placed in respiratory isolation until about 5 days of antibiotic therapy have been completed. A physician's order is required before administering a narcotic cough suppressant. The disease is diagnosed by nasopharyngeal swab. Contacts of the patient are treated with prophylactic antibiotic therapy. (4) 1. Outcome 2. Although the medical history and physical assessment are important aspects of nursing care, patient allergies to egg products must be ascertained. The influenza vaccine is produced in eggs. (5) 2. Outcome 3. Most viral URIs are self-limiting. Patient teaching that includes self-care should be stressed. Throat cultures are not always required. Antibiotics are not useful in the treatment of viral infections. Monitoring temperature may be done if the patient is febrile. (6) 1. Outcome 1. Impaired verbal communication is a primary nursing diagnosis for a patient with laryngitis. Talking will increase the inflammation of the larynx. There is no need for cough medications or effective coughing techniques with laryngitis. An increase in fluids will not influence the outcome of the condition to a great extent. (7) 3, 2, 1, 4, 5. Outcome 3. All of the answers are important, but controlling the bleeding and maintaining the patient's airway have the highest priority. (8) 2. Outcome 1. Obesity is a major factor for developing sleep apnea. Weight loss should be considered. Alcohol and hypnotics are contraindicated for patients with this condition. During sleep, the tongue relaxes and obstructs the airway. Obstructive sleep apnea is the most common form. (9) 4. Outcome 3. Persistent hoarseness, often without other symptoms such as sore throat, is an early sign of laryngeal cancer. The patient should see his physician promptly, because early tumors often can be removed and the voice preserved. (10) 3. Outcome 5. In a total laryngectomy, the trachea and esophagus are separated and a tracheostomy is formed. There is no risk of choking during eating or drinking.

CHAPTER 23

NCLEX-PN® ANSWERS (1) 2. Outcome 1. Cigarette smoking is strongly associated with chronic bronchitis. The environment such as working in mines, silicone factories, or cotton mills may contribute to this disease. A family history of lung cancer and personal history of having received a pacemaker are not known risk factors for chronic bronchitis. (2) 2. Outcome 7. A positive test indicates presence of antibodies to TB, but does not necessarily indicate active disease and the ability to spread the organism. The husband should be tested because there is a risk of infection with people living in the same household, but there is no evidence that he is positive. Tuberculosis is not a bloodborne disease. (3) 3. Outcome 2. Manifestations of acute asthma attack include chest tightness, wheezing, shortness of breath, and anxiety. Asthma can lead to respiratory distress if not managed properly. The medication effectiveness is also reported. While intake and output may be measured, this is not as important to report as respiratory assessment. LOC is reported only if there is a change in status. (4) 4. Outcome 3, 6. Rinsing the mouth after using the inhaler reduces systemic drug absorption and reduces the risk of thrush associated with some anti-inflammatory drugs used to treat asthma and COPD. Bronchodilators are used to treat acute attacks of asthma and before using anti-inflammatory drugs by MDI. Patients are taught to inhale deeply while compressing the canister to draw the medication into peripheral lung tissues. (5) 4. Outcome 3. COPD patients have increased carbon dioxide in their blood, suppressing it as an effective stimulus for respirations; instead, a drop in blood oxygen levels stimulates the drive to breathe. Low doses of O_2 are useful for the COPD patient, particularly at night. High doses of O_2 suppress the drive to breathe and may result in respiratory failure. Oxygen is flammable and this is one reason the patient should not smoke, however, this is not the best response to this question. (6) 1. Outcome 7. Atelectasis is commonly seen with nonambulatory patients after surgery. Pain medication decreases respirations, which could lead to atelectasis. Increased fluid intake helps liquefy respiratory secretions, reducing the risk of atelectasis. Use of a laxative is unrelated to atelectasis. (7) 2. Outcome 4. A thoracentesis is performed by inserting a needle into the pleural space that surrounds the lungs in order to remove fluid

or air. The mediastinum contains the heart and great vessels. The thoracic cavity refers to the chest. Visceral space is an inappropriate term. (8) 2. Outcome 4, 6. The wound is covered with an occlusive dressing to prevent air from entering the pleural space, and then the physician is notified. Reinsertion of the tube introduces bacteria and other possible contaminants into the pleural space. The chest tube collection device is not emptied while the chest tube is in place. (9) 2, 4, 5. Outcome 1. These measures, along with wearing seatbelts with shoulder harnesses in cars, are important measures to prevent lung and chest trauma. Pneumococcal vaccine is not recommended for young, healthy adults. Exercise, although beneficial, also is not a specific measure to prevent chest and lung trauma. (10) 1. Outcome 5. Restlessness and tachypnea (rapid respiratory rate) are early signs of hypoxia, a component of respiratory failure. Deep coma is a very late sign. Hypotension, tachycardia, and decreased urine output are indicative of decreased cardiac output, a later effect of respiratory failure.

CHAPTER 24

NCLEX-PN® ANSWERS (1) 2. Outcome 2. Saliva contains amylase and lysozyme, enzymes that start the digestion of starch. Dry mouth does not change taste. There is no information in the question to support that the patient needs to drink more fluids or will eat more hard candy. (2) 1. Outcome 1. The cardiac, or lower esophageal sphincter, opens to allow food into the stomach and normally is closed at other times. Stenosis, or tightening of this sphincter, will affect the movement of food from the esophagus into the stomach. As a part of the GI tract, the cardiac sphincter does not affect cardiac output or blood pressure. The pyloric sphincter at the distal portion of the stomach affects emptying of the stomach. (3) 4. Outcome 4. Dullness to percussion generally indicates solid tissue or a mass. The sigmoid colon is found in the left lower quadrant, the liver in the right upper quadrant. A dull percussion tone due to a full bladder is usually noted at midline. Air in the intestine causes a tympanic percussion tone. (4) 3. Outcome 5. In a colonoscopy, a flexible fiberoptic scope is inserted into the large intestine through the anus to visualize the mucous membranes and any abnormalities of the bowel. A colonoscopy does not involve x-rays or use of radiologic contrast, and it is not an ultrasonic examination. (5) 1. Outcome 3. Most food and nutrients are absorbed in the small intestine through the villi and microvilli. Water is absorbed from fecal material in the large intestine to form a solid stool mass. Hydrochloric acid is secreted by specialized cells in the stomach. The liver conjugates bilirubin for elimination as bile.

CHAPTER 25

NCLEX-PN® ANSWERS (1) 3. Outcome 1. Central or upper body obesity is identified by a waist/hip ratio of 1 or higher. Upper body obesity generally is associated with hyperlipidemia. Although the patient may have obese parents (parenteral obesity is a strong risk factor for obesity), that finding does not define upper body obesity. (2) 1. Outcome 3. A weight gain of 1 to 2 lb/week is appropriate. A 1,500-calorie diet does not provide adequate kilocalories to support weight gain; an additional 3,500 calories above metabolic needs is necessary to gain 1 lb. Excessive exercise increases caloric needs and will not promote weight gain. Unsaturated fats and whole-grain

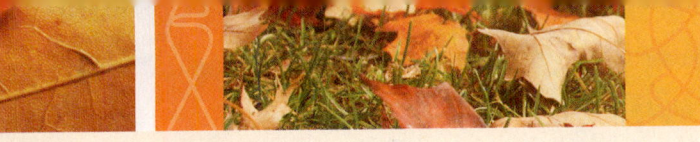

carbohydrates add calories to the diet. (3) 2. Outcome 4. Viscous lidocaine may be used to numb the mucous membranes in the mouth. Never use a strong mouthwash, because many of these contain alcohol that may cause severe burning of the mouth. The gag reflex may be assessed if viscous lidocaine has been swallowed. Raw fruits and vegetables can irritate inflamed mucous membranes and should be limited or avoided. (4) 1. Outcome 1. Early symptoms of oral cancer are painless ulcers. Documenting the lesion and notifying the physician are your next priority. It is not an emergency, nor will you prepare the patient for a biopsy until the diagnosis is made by the physician. It is important for the patient to report any changes in the ulceration. (5) 1, 4. Outcome 4. Remaining upright after eating and raising the head of the bed on blocks reduces regurgitation of gastric contents into the lower esophagus. Continuing prescribed drugs for the full course of treatment is important to heal inflamed tissue of the esophagus. Cigarette smoke, alcohol, peppermint, and chocolate aggravate reflux and symptoms of GERD. (6) 2. Outcome 2. Cancers that erode through the esophageal wall may cause severe hemorrhage. Difficulty swallowing is an early sign of esophageal cancer, which may be followed by choking and weight loss. (7) 2. Outcome 4. During the insertion of the NG tube, the gag reflex may be initiated. Briefly pause, allow the patient a short rest, have him or her sip a small amount of water to help with the insertion, and resume the procedure. Do not initially remove the tube completely; this may increase anxiety and nasal trauma. Placement checks are done after the tube is inserted completely. (8) 4. Outcome 3. Divide 240 mL by 60 mL to calculate the number of hours it will take for the feeding to run. (9) 2. Outcome 4. *Helicobacter pylori* bacteria has been found to increase the incidence of peptic ulcers. It will not affect the acid nor the mucus. Antibiotics are not usually given to prevent the appearance of this organism. (10) 4. Outcome 2. Dumping syndrome is characterized by stomach contents that rapidly flood the small intestine after a meal. Large amounts of water are pulled into the intestines, creating a volume deficit in the blood circulation. Resting after a meal slows down the digestive process. Proteins and fats are absorbed at a slower rate than sugars. Smaller, more frequent meals are generally more tolerated than three large meals.

CHAPTER 26

NCLEX-PN® ANSWERS   (1) 2. Outcome 2. Severe diarrhea can lead to fluid volume deficit and hypovolemia. The first priority for the nurse is to assess fluid volume status (vital signs, orthostatic vitals, skin turgor, moisture of mucous membranes), because maintaining vascular volume is critical to maintain circulation and kidney function. Although the other nursing interventions are important, they are of a lower priority at this time. (2) 4. Outcome 1. Older adults often have a bowel movement every 2 or 3 days. This pattern may be normal for the patient; the nurse assesses for other indications of constipation, such as stool that is very hard or difficult to expel. Laxatives are recommended for treating acute constipation, not promoting a daily bowel movement. Increased fiber consumption promotes bowel function. Although a colonoscopy may be performed to screen for bowel cancer or to diagnose some disorders, it is not indicated for simple constipation. (3) 1. Outcome 1. Rebound tenderness, indicative of appendicitis, is characterized by relief of pain with pressure, followed by increased pain when pressure is relieved. The other descriptors are not characteristic of rebound tenderness. (4)

3. Outcome 4. When using therapeutic communication, the nurse focuses on the patient's concerns. When a colostomy is located in the distal colon, regular, formed bowel movements can usually be established, allowing the patient to simply cap the stoma between evacuations. Responding to this question is within the expected scope of practice and knowledge of the nurse, and referral to an enterostomal therapist for an answer is not necessary. The nurse may provide an educational video to help the patient learn self-care of the colostomy. There is no indication of need for an antidiarrheal medication. (5) 1. Outcome 2. Antidiarrheal medications are not to be used until the cause of diarrhea has been determined because they could worsen or prolong the disease, or lead to complications. They may help prevent fluid and electrolyte imbalances due to severe diarrhea but should be given as ordered. It is not necessary to obtain stool samples or restore fluid and electrolyte balance prior to administering antidiarrheal medications once the cause of diarrhea has been established. (6) 2, 3. Outcome 1, 2. Sulfasalazine increases photosensitivity (the risk for sunburn). It can decrease the effectiveness of oral contraceptives. Sulfasalazine should be taken after, not before, meals. Rash is an adverse effect that should be reported promptly to the physician. The patient should avoid aspirin while on this drug. (7) 3. Outcome 5. Not allowed on this diet are fresh vegetables, rich desserts, raw or fresh fruits, or tough meats. (8) 4. Outcome 2. Increased pain with a rigid, boardlike abdomen may indicate perforation of the bowel and possible peritonitis, a potentially critical complication of bowel obstruction. Hypoactive bowel sounds and fecal-smelling nasogastric tube drainage are expected (although not normal) findings in a patient with a bowel obstruction. A flat, soft abdomen is a normal finding and does not need to be reported. (9) 1. Outcome 3. The passage of flatus and resumption of bowel sounds indicate the return of peristalsis, necessary for safe food introduction. Pain needs to be managed throughout recovery to promote mobility. Promoting mobility, such as in ambulation, will encourage return of normal peristalsis but is not a requirement before introducing food. IV fluids provide fluid and electrolytes but do not provide adequate calories unless total parenteral nutrition is used. (10) 1. Outcome 5. Because colorectal cancer is often a silent disease and treatment at an early stage has a high cure rate, the American Cancer Society recommends routine screening procedures for early detection. This includes annual digital rectal examination for all people over age 50, annual fecal occult blood test for people over age 50, and flexible sigmoidoscopy or colonoscopy at age 50 and every 5 to 10 years thereafter. Screening exams should be early and frequent for patients with IBD, a history of polyps, or a strong family history of colorectal cancer. Bowel cancer usually grows slowly. There may be 5 to 15 years of growth before symptoms occur. Manifestations depend on tumor location, type and extent, and complications. Bleeding is often what prompts patients to seek medical care.

CHAPTER 27

NCLEX-PN® ANSWERS   (1) 2. Outcome 1. Narcotic analgesics are often required for acute pain relief in cholelithiasis. Mild analgesics such as acetaminophen and ibuprofen are less likely to be effective. Codeine is a less effective analgesic than morphine and frequently causes nausea. (2) 2. Outcome 3. Nausea and vomiting after eating may indicate the T-tube is not functioning and/or blockage of the bile ducts. The other options provide expected assessment data. (3) 4. Outcome 2. Low-fat diets decrease stimulation of the gallbladder to release bile, thereby decreasing pain. Sleeping in the prone position and using a heating pad for pain relief are not recommended for patients with cholecystitis. Pain that occurs before meals is unlikely to be related to cholecystitis. (4) 1. Outcome 1. Hepatitis A is transmitted by the oral–fecal route and by consumption of contaminated food or water. Transmission of hepatitis A via blood and body fluids is rare. (5) 3. Outcome 1. Hepatitis B is transmitted through blood and body fluid exposure, including contaminated needles, blood transfusions, and unprotected sexual relations. It is not transmitted via the fecal–oral route. (6) 4. Outcome 4. Alcohol is hepatotoxic and use should be eliminated. The patient is taught to use a soft toothbrush and follow the prescribed diet to reduce the risk of bleeding or other complications of cirrhosis. Difficulty breathing may indicate increasing ascites and should be reported. (7) 1, 2. Outcome 1. Decreased weight and abdominal girth may indicate a decrease in ascites. Urinary output of 30 mL/hr and tea-colored urine are not related to ascites. Increasing shortness of breath may indicate worsening ascites. (8) 2. Outcome 2. Ammonia levels are elevated because of inability of the liver to metabolize protein products. Lactulose decreases the absorption of ammonia from the bowel, reducing blood ammonia levels. Because its action occurs in the bowel, it does not affect urine output or serum potassium levels. Steatorrhea, increased fat content of stool, is unrelated to lactulose. (9) 2, 1, 3, 4, 5. Outcome 4. Narcotic analgesics work quickly to relieve pain. Inserting the nasogastric tube removes gastric secretions that stimulate pancreatic enzyme release. The side-lying position with the head elevated reduces stress on abdominal muscles and tissues. Although these measures are important to promote comfort, they are of lower priority than the first three measures. (10) 2. Outcome 4. Fluid loss associated with vomiting, diaphoresis, third-space shifts, and nasogastric suction is common. Fluid initially is lost from vascular space, potentially impairing cardiac output and tissue perfusion. The other assessments are important, but they do not have as high a priority as maintaining cardiac output and tissue perfusion.

CHAPTER 28

NCLEX-PN® ANSWERS (1) 1. Outcome 2. Flank pain is a possible manifestation of disorders affecting the kidneys or ureters. Questioning about changes in the amount, color, odor, or clarity of urine output is important to help identify if the pain is related to a urologic problem. Questions regarding a history of diabetes, weight changes, and the relationship of pain to sleep may be appropriate follow-up questions, but they are less likely to provide information about the cause of the pain. (2) 3. Outcome 1. The tubule (proximal convoluted, descending, ascending, and distal convoluted) is part of the nephron, the unit of the kidney responsible for urine formation. The kidney receives blood via the renal arteries. Once formed, urine moves from the renal pelvis through the ureters to the bladder, where it collects until voiding occurs. Urinary continence depends on innervation and muscles of the urinary bladder, urethra, and pelvic floor. (3) 4. Outcome 1. Renal function declines with aging as nephron units are lost. This impairs drug excretion, increasing the risk of toxicity. Doses of drugs such as digoxin often need to be lower for older adults. Increased drug levels in the blood are more likely to be found than decreased or inadequate drug levels. Impaired urination is not an adverse effect of this drug. (4) 3, 4, 5. Outcome 3. The

patient voids at the start of the 24-hour period, notes the time of this voiding, and discards this urine, saving all voided urine for the duration of the test. Toilet paper and feces in the saved urine can interfere with test results. (5) 3. Outcome 2. No more than a trace of protein should be present in the urine; this result should be reported to the physician. Protein in the urine does not indicate a need to limit dietary protein intake. The physician may order additional diagnostic tests to determine the cause of proteinuria; this decision, however, is outside the scope of practice for the nurse.

CHAPTER 29

NCLEX-PN® ANSWERS (1) 3. Outcome 5. Assessment to determine whether the bladder is distended is needed before further action is taken or the physician is notified. Additional oral fluids would only be provided if the patient demonstrates signs of dehydration. Catheterization requires a physician's order and is performed only when necessary. (2) 1. Outcome 1. Lack of estrogen after a total hysterectomy results in decreased urethral resistance, placing the patient at risk for stress incontinence. Smoking, exercise, and pregnancy are not identified risk factors for stress incontinence. (3) 2. Outcome 2. Residual urine of 50 mL or less is within normal limits, therefore it is not necessary to notify the physician or institute additional measures to promote urine output or voiding. (4) 3. Outcome 5. Kegel exercises help the patient locate and tighten muscles of the pelvic floor. Orange juice and tea can irritate the bladder muscle, increasing the risk for urge incontinence. Diuretic medications such as furosemide should be taken no later than 4 p.m. to reduce nocturia. Restricting fluids is not recommended for patients with urinary incontinence. (5) 2, 4, 5. Outcome 1. Increasing fluid intake, wearing cotton briefs, and voiding before and after sexual intercourse reduce the risk of colonization of perineal tissues and the lower urethra with bacteria. Although cranberry juice has been shown to reduce the risk of bladder infections, orange juice has not. Wiping from front to back after voiding or defecating is recommended. (6) 1. Outcome 2. Recent infection with group A beta-hemolytic *Streptococcus* is a risk factor for acute glomerulonephritis. The other conditions (pneumonia, gastroenteritis, and influenza) are not associated with a risk of glomerulonephritis. (7) 3. Outcome 5. All urine of patients with urinary calculi should be strained for presence of stones. Stones should be sent to the lab for analysis. Hand hygiene is important when caring for all patients. Increased fluid intake is recommended to prevent further stone formation. A sterile urine specimen is not required to diagnose urinary calculi. (8) 3. Outcome 4. Patient is at risk for urinary tract infection. Signs and symptoms should be reported to the physician promptly. Increased fluid intake is recommended to prevent further stone formation. Adequate calcium intake is important to prevent bone resorption. Dietary measures to maintain acidic or alkaline urine may be recommended based on the composition of the stone. (9) 2. Outcome 3. Protein is decreased to prevent azotemia. A high carbohydrate intake increases calories and spares protein breakdown. Sodium is restricted to reduce fluid retention. High-fat diets are not recommended to reduce cardiovascular risk. (10) 1. Outcome 3. The right arm should be used for blood pressure measurement to avoid injury to the AV fistula on the left arm. The patient is taught to check the fistula for pulsations, remind lab personnel to avoid blood draws on the affected arm, and maintain body and arm positions that promote good blood flow through the fistula.

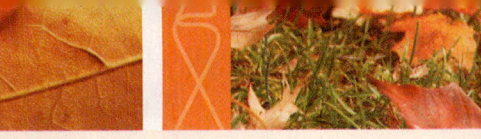
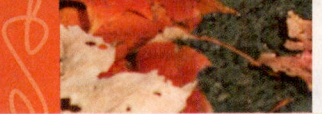

CHAPTER 30

NCLEX-PN® ANSWERS **(1)** 2. Outcome 2. The fallopian tubes contain smooth muscle and are lined with cilia, which facilitate the movement of the ovum to the uterus. Gravity alone would not be effective because the ovum's progress is not direct and would be obstructed; fertilization of an egg is required for implantation in the uterine wall, but not for movement down the tube, and there are no such chemical messengers. **(2)** 2 (**testes**), 4 (**epididymis**), 1 (**vas deferens**), 5 (**seminal vesicle**), 3 (**urethra**). Outcome 1. Sperm are formed in the testes; the epididymis is the secretory duct of the testis, which conducts sperm to the vas deferens, through which they travel to the seminal vesicle where they are stored with the seminal fluid until they are excreted through the urethra. **(3)** 1. Outcome 3. The hormone levels seen are typical of those after menopause, when estrogen levels fall, and FSH levels significantly increase. The levels are not within normal limits but are not a significant abnormality especially for a woman in her mid-40s. **(4)** 3. Outcome 4. The patient will have some abdominal discomfort and may experience shoulder pain after a laparoscopy, but severe pain is unusual and should be reported because it may signal a complication. The other options were all objective data. **(5)** 4. Outcome 5. The PSA results are affected by manipulation of the prostate gland, so it should be drawn either before or at least 2 weeks after a DRE. This question demonstrates how the correct answer must be *fully* correct. True, no written consent is required for a rectal exam, but that answer does not include that the blood test should be done first. True, the doctor will do the exam in the office, but again this answer is incomplete because it lacks the blood test being done first, and the same for option 1, which is true but does not fully answer the question.

CHAPTER 31

NCLEX-PN® ANSWERS **(1)** 4. Outcome 1. Discharge of seminal fluid into the bladder instead of through the urethra (retrograde ejaculation) is common after TURP. Nocturia is voiding more than one time at night. The subjective information presented is not indicative of impotence or decreased libido. **(2)** 2. Outcome 4. Blood clots promote bladder spasms and may obstruct urine flow. Continuous bladder irrigation is titrated to keep the output light pink or clear. When CBI is not used, irrigation may be done as needed to clear blood clots. Irrigation generally does not reduce the urge to void, unless the catheter is obstructed. Large amounts of irrigating fluid can cause hyponatremia, not prevent it. **(3)** 1. Outcome 4. Aspirin would promote excessive bleeding. Tub baths are avoided until the catheter is out, but showers are permitted. Sex should be delayed until healing is complete to avoid excessive bleeding. Extra fluid consumption keeps the bladder clear of blood, clots, and bacteria, thereby preventing painful bladder spasms and infection. **(4)** 4, 3, 1, 2, 5. Outcome 3. Chest pain and difficulty breathing could indicate an embolism or acute cardiac problem and need to be addressed immediately. Blood clots may obstruct the catheter or indicate hemorrhage, requiring attention; restoring urinary flow may relieve the bladder pain and catheter leakage. At this time, the patient's poor appetite is of lowest priority. **(5)** 2. Outcome 2. Frequent ejaculation is thought to relieve congestion in the prostate. Fluids should be increased. This is not an infectious disorder. **(6)** 3. Outcome 3. PSA levels increase in prostate cancer, benign prostatic hypertrophy, and with aging, although the increase is greatest in prostate cancer. When combined with digital rectal examination, the PSA is used to screen for prostate cancer and monitor the response to treatment. **(7)** 1. Outcome 1. Orchiectomy removes the major source of testosterone, which feeds prostate tumor growth. Prostate cancer rarely metastasizes to the testes. **(8)** 3. Outcome 2. Patients should be advised to report an erection that lasts more than 4 hours. This drug is contraindicated with nitroglycerin and other nitrate drugs and is used with caution in men with cardiovascular disease. It should not be taken more than once per day. **(9)** 4. Outcome 3. Acute scrotal pain may indicate testicular torsion, a medical emergency requiring immediate treatment to restore blood flow to the testicle. **(10)** 3. Outcome 1. All young men should be taught to do monthly TSE. This cancer does not usually present with pain, tenderness, blood in the urine, or other symptoms, so TSE is especially important.

CHAPTER 32

NCLEX-PN® ANSWERS **(1)** 1, 3. Outcome 1. HRT is recommended, although the decision to begin HRT is an individual one. HRT reduces the risk of fractures due to osteoporosis. It is associated with a higher, not lower, risk for breast cancer. HRT relieves menopausal symptoms such as hot flashes and night sweats. It does not lower and may actually increase the risk for coronary heart disease. **(2)** 2, 3, 4, 5. Outcome 2. Nonproliferative fibrocystic breast changes do not increase the risk for cancer. 2, 3, and 5 are measures to relieve discomfort. 4 has not been proven but is reported by some to relieve symptoms. **(3)** 1. Outcome 2, 4. Risk factors for cervical cancer include multiple sex partners, early sexual activity, and STIs. Pelvic examinations and Pap smears are important for early detection of cervical cancer but do not reduce the risk. Tamoxifen is used to reduce the risk of breast cancer in women with high-risk factors. **(4)** 2. Outcome 4. Tamoxifen increases the risk for deep venous thrombosis and pulmonary embolism, particularly in women who smoke. **(5)** 1. Outcome 2. The upper outer quadrant, called the tail of Spence, is the most frequent location of breast cancers. When teaching breast self-exam, it is important to teach women to examine the breast tissue all the way to the axillary region. **(6)** 2. Outcome 3. She will need to know how to care for her drainage system. Permanent prostheses are not recommended until the scar is healed, no longer swollen, and not as painful. The arm should not be abducted to the level of the elbow above the shoulder until the drain comes out. She will be encouraged to flex and extend the elbow and do simple ADLs within 24 hours after surgery. **(7)** 4. Outcome 1. The pill is often prescribed to help alleviate symptoms of primary dysmenorrhea. Locally applied heat relieves discomfort. NSAIDs are prostaglandin inhibitors and therefore block one of the main causes of cramping. Orgasm also relieves symptoms in some women. **(8)** 2. Outcome 2. Bleeding in a postmenopausal woman not on hormone replacement is never normal and is the most common symptom of endometrial cancer. **(9)** 4. Outcome 1. Menorrhagia is the appropriate term to describe menstrual bleeding that is excessive in amount or is prolonged. Amenorrhea is the absence of menstruation. Metrorrhagia is bleeding between menstrual periods, whereas Mittelschmerz is midcycle spotting associated with ovulation. **(10)** 3. Outcome 1. PID can cause tubal scarring and blockage, putting her at increased risk for infertility and tubal pregnancy. PID is usually caused by *Neisseria gonorrhoeae* or *Chlamydia trachomatis,* whereas cervical cancer is associated with HPV (genital

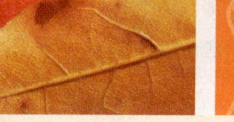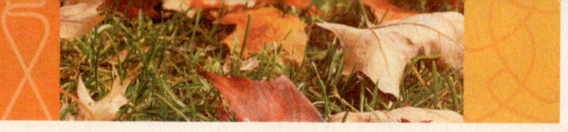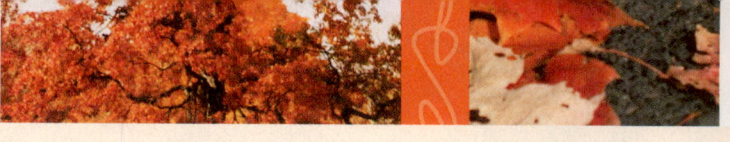

warts). PID is caused by infectious organisms spread during unprotected sex, not by heredity. Toxic shock is caused by *Staphylococcus aureus*; it is related to poor hygiene during menstruation and use of superabsorbent tampons and diaphragms.

CHAPTER 33

NCLEX-PN® ANSWERS (1) 4. Outcome 1. Untreated chlamydia ascends into the upper reproductive tract and is a major cause of PID. Chlamydia is often asymptomatic in women. (2) 2. Outcome 5. Zithromax can be given in a single oral dose. Other antibiotics used for STIs may require multiple daily doses for 7 to 10 days. (3) 1. Outcome 6. Addresses the feelings in the patient statement. 2 and 3 give unsolicited advice, which would block communication. She will receive prescriptions, but to follow her comments with 4 before recognizing her feelings changes the topic, also blocking communication. (4) 4. Outcome 4. Pap smears are important for this patient because certain subtypes of HPV increase the risk for cervical cancer. HPV infection is painless. Warts are removed with topical treatments, not acyclovir. (5) 3. Outcome 2. Patients with gonorrhea often have another STI such as HIV, syphilis, or chlamydia. (6) 1. Outcome 5. Preventing spread of the infection to others is the most important reason for treatment of STIs. Although effective treatment will prevent tertiary syphilis, this is a less important goal than protection of the public health. (7) 1. Outcome 4. Penicillin G IM is the usual treatment for syphilis. If the patient is allergic to penicillin, oral doxycycline (a tetracycline) can be used. (8) 2. Outcome 3. Condoms should be used during all sexual relations to prevent spread of the disease to the partner. Mutual monogamy does not prevent spreading the disease to the sexual partner nor does oral sexual relations. (9) 2. Outcome 6. STIs can be spread by anal, oral, and vaginal intercourse. Some young patients do not consider oral contact to be intercourse, and since it avoids pregnancy, it is seen as a risk-free activity. (10) 1, 3, 4, 5. Outcome 6. These STIs are reportable by law in all 50 states. The other measures, with the exception of cesarean delivery, are important to prevent spread of the disease to sexual partners and reinfection of the patient after effective treatment. Cesarean delivery is not necessary after effective treatment and cure of the infection.

CHAPTER 34

NCLEX-PN® ANSWERS (1) 1. Outcome 1. ADH promotes water retention by the kidneys. ACTH controls cortisol secretion from adrenal cortex; epinephrine is released during stress; and aldosterone regulates blood volume. (2) 3. Outcome 4. Radioactive I-125 is harmless. The patient is not required to fast before the test. Contrast dye is not injected nor is blood drawn. (3) 4. Outcome 3. Increased calcium results from excess secretion of PTH. Increased T_3 and T_4 is found with hyperthyroidism. Liver disease cause decreased serum albumin. Hypofunction of the adrenal cortex would cause decreased aldosterone. (4) 2. Outcome 3, 4. Glycosylated hemoglobin (HbA1c) identifies glucose control during the past 3 months and is useful in diagnosing new-onset diabetes mellitus. The water deprivation test diagnoses posterior pituitary function and the secretion of ADH. 17-Ketosteroids and serum cortisol tests evaluate adrenal cortex function. (5) 4. Outcome 2. Chvostek sign is a facial muscle spasm

when the facial nerve is tapped and indicates tetany. Trousseau sign occurs when blood flow is restricted to lower arm from a blood pressure cuff being inflated. It also indicates tetany. Kernig sign is the inability to extend the leg when the hip is flexed at a 90-degree angle and indicates meningitis.

CHAPTER 35

NCLEX-PN® ANSWERS (1) 4. Outcome 3. Excess cortisol in Cushing syndrome causes increased glucose levels. Serum sodium levels are increased, not decreased. Serum potassium levels are decreased. GH levels are increased in acromegaly. (2) 1. Outcome 5. Hemorrhage is life threatening. Be sure to assess the dressing behind the neck. Observe for edema and increased swallowing. Tetany due to decreased serum calcium levels usually occurs 1 to 7 days postop if the parathyroid glands were damaged. Dehydration does not occur during the immediate postop period and usually is not life threatening. The laryngeal nerve may be damaged during surgery, but this is not life threatening. (3) 1. Outcome 1. Iodine is needed for the production of TH. A decrease in this hormone causes the thyroid to enlarge, goiter, in order to increase the hormone production. Excess TSG causes hyperthyroidism but not a goiter. Deficient calcium and PTH causes hypoparathyroidism. Cushing syndrome results from excess cortisol. (4) 2. Outcome 7. Patients taking steroids like prednisone must never abruptly stop taking their medications. Steroids cause weight gain and sodium retention. Checking pulse rate is important for patients taking thyroid drugs. Nervousness and chest pain are side effects of levothyroxine (Synthroid). (5) 3. Outcome 6. Increased cortisol production by the adrenal cortex causes numerous physical and psychologic changes. The buffalo hump, moon face, edema, and purple striae on the abdomen add to the depression that is typically seen in patients with Cushing syndrome. These patients have fluid volume excess, not deficiency. Although they are at risk for falls, they do not experience activity intolerance. Also, they do not develop constipation. (6) 4. Outcome 6. Hypoparathyroidism can cause bronchospasm and laryngeal spasms, leading to respiratory distress. It is most important to ensure a patent airway first. All other interventions are important but not the highest priority for this patient. (7) 2, 5, 6. Outcome 4. Patients allergic to shellfish, which contain iodine, cannot take potassium iodide (SSKI). SSKI should be mixed in milk or orange juice, and patients should be monitored for bradycardia. Antacids do not interfere with its absorption. SSKI does not cause rash or itching, nor worsen asthma. (8) 1. Outcome 6. Patients with SIADH have a decreased urine output. Urine production must be monitored along with fluid restriction. A high-protein diet is not needed for this patient. SIADH does not alter heart rate, so checking the pulse is not required. The SIADH patient has no increased risk of infection from crowds. (9) 3. Outcome 4. Synthroid is given for hypothyroidism, which causes bradycardia. By taking a thyroid drug, heart rate should return to normal. Decreased appetite and constipation are signs of hypothyroidism. Excessive weight loss could indicate side effects of hyperthyroidism. (10) 2. Outcome 2. With a lack of the mineralocorticoid aldosterone, blood volume and blood pressure are lower, which causes postural hypotension. Multiple bruises are noted with Cushing syndrome. Peripheral edema and SOB are found in many disorders but not in Addison disease.

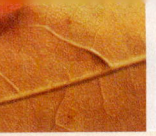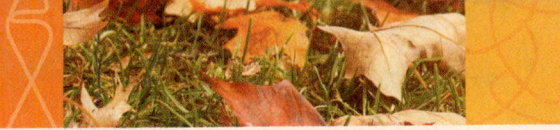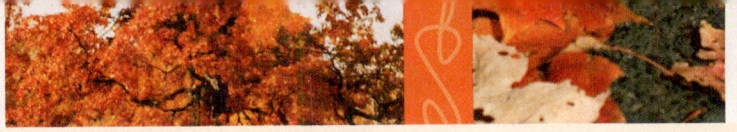

CHAPTER 36

NCLEX-PN® ANSWERS **(1)** 2. Outcome 2, 3, 6. The sliding scale permits periodic monitoring of blood glucose levels to provide better control. Fast-acting insulin (regular insulin) is used with the sliding scale to best mimic the natural action of the pancreas. **(2)** 1. Outcome 5. Patients experiencing Somogyi effect should be taught the symptoms of nighttime hypoglycemia, including tremors, night sweats, and restlessness. A bedtime snack or decreasing the evening dose of intermediate insulin may reduce the risk of developing the effect. **(3)** 3. Outcome 7. During periods of illness, blood glucose levels increase in response to physiologic stress and the body's need for glucose. It is important to continue taking insulin in order to prevent DKA or HHS. **(4)** 4. Outcome 1. Risks for type 2 DM include adults over 65, obesity, sedentary lifestyle, and Hispanic or African American women and Native Americans. The 16-year-old has lower risk due to physical activity. Heredity plays a more important role in the development of type 1 DM. Thyroid disease does not increase risk for DM. **(5)** 1. Outcome 6. Type 1 diabetes is caused by lack of insulin production. These individuals are insulin dependent and cannot be managed with oral antidiabetic medications. **(6)** 2. Outcome 7. The most likely time for a patient to experience hypoglycemia as a result of receiving lispro insulin is 3 to 6 ½ hours after administration. **(7)** 2. Outcome 4. Diabetic ketoacidosis is characterized by hyperglycemia and spillage of ketones in the urine, which causes the classic acetone breath. The skin is very warm and dry as a result of dehydration. Slurred speech occurs with hypoglycemia. The pulse is usually rapid and weak. **(8)** Correct sequence is 5, 2, 4, 1, 3. Outcome 3. Inspect regular insulin for clarity first. Next, NPH insulin is rolled between the palms to mix. Then clean the tops of both vials with alcohol. Inject air into NPH insulin and then the regular insulin. The regular insulin is withdrawn first to avoid mixing of the NPH in the regular insulin vial. **(9)** 4. Outcome 4. Regular soda, a rapid-acting glucose source, is given immediately to a conscious patient with hypoglycemia. Giving insulin would decrease glucose levels further. Glucagon is used only with an unconscious patient. Crackers and cheese are given after glucose levels have returned to normal because they take longer to act. **(10)** Correct teaching points are 1, 4, and 6. Outcome 5, 6, 7. Toenails should be cut straight across to avoid development of ingrown toenails that can lead to infection. Diabetic patients should avoid open-toed shoes and heating pads to prevent injury. Applying lotion between the toes results in a warm, moist environment, which promotes bacterial and fungal growth. Shoes are best bought in the afternoon when feet are the largest. Patients must be taught to use a mirror daily to inspect all sides of the feet.

CHAPTER 37

NCLEX-PN® ANSWERS **(1)** 2. Outcome 3. Older adults report reduced ability to discriminate between blue and green colors. They experience less tear secretion, reduced vision at night, and difficulty focusing on near objects. **(2)** 4. Outcome 4. Paste is used to attach electrodes to the scalp and should be washed out to increase patient comfort. An EEG is noninvasive, so there is no insertion site, nor does it cause nausea and vomiting. Increasing fluid intake is unnecessary. **(3)** 1, 4, and 5. Outcome 1. These are actions of the sympathetic nervous system. Slowing of the heart rate, dilation of skin blood vessels,

and bronchoconstriction are actions of the parasympathetic nervous system. **(4)** 3. Outcome 1, 2. Cranial nerve VIII (vestibulocochlear) is responsible for hearing and equilibrium. Cranial nerve III (oculomotor) controls pupil constriction and eye movement; V (trigeminal) controls chewing and scalp sensations; and XI (accessory) controls neck and shoulder movement. **(5)** 1. Outcome 2. The nurse should ask if the patient was wearing a helmet in order to assess the extent of injury. Difficulty sleeping does not relate to this case. It is important to know if the patient has diabetes, but not the most important for this patient. Taking herbal preparations is not relevant for this patient's situation.

CHAPTER 38

NCLEX-PN® ANSWERS **(1)** 1. Outcome 1. Blunt trauma may cause a contusion of the brain. If the skull is fractured, there may be leakage of cerebrospinal fluid into the ears or nose. Infection is a serious complication of brain injury. Hematomas commonly develop from blood leaking underneath the skin. Headaches and dizziness are commonly seen after a blow to the head. **(2)** 2, 3, 5. Outcome 1. Use of birth control pills, atherosclerosis, and obesity increase the risk for stroke. Persons older than 65, those with excessive alcohol intake, and African Americans also have a higher risk for CVA. **(3)** 2. Outcome 2. It is most important to monitor for CSF leak and hematoma formation. The patient is kept flat afterward for 4 to 8 hours but can move legs. Fluids are increased, not limited. The patient should empty the bladder before the procedure, not necessarily afterward. **(4)** 4. Outcome 4. Phenytoin (Dilantin) causes gingival hyperplasia, which can be prevented by daily oral hygiene. It should be taken with meals. Dilantin does not cause fatigue, weakness, or brownish urine. **(5)** 3. Outcome 3. The earliest sign of increased intracranial pressure is level of consciousness. Irritability, personality changes, restlessness, and disorientation are early manifestations of ICP. Decreased heart rate, slow pupil responses, and projectile vomiting are seen during later stages. **(6)** 1. Outcome 5, 6. Removing a tumor from the occipital lobe requires the patient to be placed in a side-lying position. Assessing for cranial nerve impairment is important after carotid artery surgery. Morphine is never given after a craniotomy, as it could mask signs of neurologic deterioration. Only Tylenol or codeine is given for headache. Vital signs must be monitored every 1 to 2 hours. **(7)** 3. Outcome 6. Status epilepticus is a life-threatening emergency, leading to physical exhaustion and respiratory distress. The first priority is to maintain the airway. Anxiety and risk for injury also need to be addressed in the nursing care plan. There is no risk for cerebral perfusion alterations. **(8)** 4. Outcome 7. Patient education is a priority because most headaches are treatable at home. Helping a patient understand what causes the migraines may help reduce the number of attacks. Diaries, comfort measures during an attack, and stress reduction classes are also important. **(9)** 3. Outcome 1. Meningitis is an inflammation of the spinal cord and meninges. It is usually secondary to an upper respiratory infection. Encephalitis is caused by a virus, in most cases. Brain abscesses occur from middle ear infection. A subdural hematoma is a collection of blood underneath the dura mater. **(10)** 2, 3, 6, 1, 5, 4. Outcome 6. Loosen the gown and turn the patient on his side. If on floor, place pillow under head and clear the area of objects that could cause injury. Provide supplemental oxygen. Pad the side rails as soon as possible.

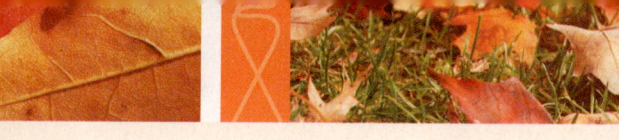

CHAPTER 39

NCLEX-PN® ANSWERS   (1) 1. Outcome 6. SCI at C_4 has a high risk for breathing problems that must be addressed first. The other nursing diagnoses are important, but not the highest priority on admission. (2) 4. Outcome 2. Propantheline (Pro-Banthine) is used to control urinary frequency. Amantadine (Symmetrel) controls fatigue; dexamethasone (Decadron) reduces inflammation; and dantrolene (Dantrium) decreases muscle spasm. (3) 1, 2, 5. Outcome 5. These are important points to teach the patient taking Sinemet. This drug should be taken with food. Sinemet does not change urine color or cause a rash or blurred vision. (4) 1. Outcome 4. Autonomic dysreflexia is an exaggerated sympathetic response in patients with a spinal cord injury above the T_6 level. Stimuli such as bladder or fecal impaction trigger a hypertensive crisis. (5) 4. Outcome 1. Guillain–Barré syndrome causes ascending paralysis that starts in the lower extremities. All other manifestations occur later. (6) 3. Outcome 3. Patients with C_5 spinal cord injuries can expect to operate an electric wheelchair. Patients with C_1–C_3 injuries can operate a voice or sip-n-puff wheelchair only. Patients with C_6 and lower injuries can learn self-transfer, whereas those with C_7 and lower injuries can operate a manual wheelchair. (7) 2. Outcome 5. Elevate the patient's head and place a small pillow under the knees for a herniated lumbar disk to decrease intervertebral pressure. (8) 2. Outcome 6. Patients with dysphagia may not be able to swallow the medication unless it is taken exactly on time. Doses taken too late may cause myasthenic crisis. The nurse must monitor and report vision changes or facial muscle weakness and prevent patient tiring, but these are not the most important actions of those listed. (9) 4. Outcome 5. Patients must understand that stimulating trigger points can initiate an attack. They are taught to chew on the unaffected side unless they cannot eat; then, a high-calorie, high-protein diet is needed. Fluids do not need to be increased. (10) 3. Outcome 6. The patient should have a fluid intake of 2,400 to 3,000 mL in 24 hours to reduce the possibility of headache.

CHAPTER 40

NCLEX-PN® ANSWERS   (1) 4. Outcome 1. Fluorescein stain is placed in the eye, and a slit lamp is used to diagnose a corneal abrasion. (2) 1. Outcome 4. First place the patient in a dependent position to bring the retina closer to the blood vessels, preserving retinal perfusion. While the patient is being positioned, notify the physician. Always approach patients in a calm manner. Teaching occurs after emergency care is implemented. (3) 6, 1, 5, 3, 2, 4. Outcome 2. First warm the drops, tilt the head toward the unaffected side, and then partially fill the ear dropper with the medication. With the nondominant hand, pull the auricle up and backward, instill the drops, and place a loose cotton ball in the ear for 15 to 20 minutes. (4) 3. Outcome 4. It is most important to reduce environmental noise before speaking with the hearing-impaired patient. Speaking in a higher pitch does not help the patient hear. Use written messages when the patient cannot hear. Most older patients are unwilling to learn sign language. (5) 4. Outcome 2. Breathing difficulty, worsening vision, or increased sweating should be reported immediately to a health care provider. Stinging and bitter taste in the mouth are common with dorzolamide (Trusopt). Darkening of the iris develops with latanoprost (Xalatan). (6) 2. Outcome 1. Tenderness behind the ear could indicate acute mastoiditis, a complication of acute otitis media that must be reported immediately. Hearing loss in the affected ear, vertigo, and tinnitus are symptoms of acute otitis media. (7) 1. Outcome 5. Acute angle-closure glaucoma is an emergency condition that must be treated immediately. Darkness and emotional stress cause pupil dilation, which can trigger the condition. Medications and sunlight that cause pupil constriction do not affect this condition. Lying down will not help; it could only make the condition worse. (8) 4. Outcome 3. After surgery, place in semi-Fowler's position to decrease intraocular pressure in the affected eye. (9) 2. Outcome 1. Symptoms of open-angle glaucoma may include blurred vision, difficulty focusing on near objects, and halos around lights. (10) 1. Outcome 5. Because Ménière disease causes a sensation of fullness or pressure in the ears that may be related to edema of the membranous labyrinth, a diet low in sodium is recommended.

CHAPTER 41

NCLEX-PN® ANSWERS   (1) 3. Outcome 1. The epiphysis is the broad end of the bone; distal indicates the end further away from the trunk of the body. A fracture close to the elbow is described as proximal. The shaft of a long bone is known as the diaphysis. A fracture that breaks the skin is described as an open or compound fracture. (2) 4. Outcome 2, 3. Abduction is to move the extremity away from the midline of the body. The legs are in adduction when the knees are together or crossed. Flexion describes bent knees. (3) 1, 3, 4. Outcome 3. Grip and flexion and extension of the fingers against resistance are used to assess hand strength. Extension of the wrist and the ability to make a fist are used to assess wrist and hand range of motion. (4) 1. Outcome 4. Crepitus is a grating sensation or sound. Synovitis and inflammation are conditions that may affect a joint, not manifestations. Erythema is an observed finding. (5) 2. Outcome 5. Drinking a large quantity of water after injection of the radioisotope promotes its distribution; the patient can eat and drink before and during the procedure. No special radiation precautions are necessary because the amount of radioactivity is small. This is an invasive procedure that requires informed consent.

CHAPTER 42

NCLEX-PN® ANSWERS   (1) 3, 4, 5. Outcome 7. Elevating the extremity facilitates venous return and helps prevent edema. Until the cast is completely dry, use only the palms of the hands. Handling with the fingers can leave dents that may cause pressure sores. Rough areas on the edges of the cast should be padded and taped to reduce skin irritation. The cast dries from the inside out; using a blow dryer or covering the cast during drying are not recommended. (2) 1. Outcome 2, 5. The prone position helps to prevent hip contracture. Place the patient in a prone position every 4 hours. The other positions identified may actually promote contracture development. (3) 4. Outcome 2. When assessing a possible fracture, the nurse avoids moving the affected extremity. Peripheral pulses on the affected extremity are compared with corresponding pulses on the unaffected extremity to evaluate circulation to the affected extremity. (4) 3. Outcome 5. The patient has manifestations of compartment syndrome, including pain unrelieved by narcotics and paresthesias. Prompt intervention is required to preserve function of the extremity. Elevating the extremity can further impair circulation to the region. The decision to bivalve the cast is outside

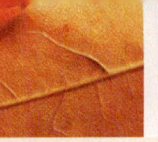
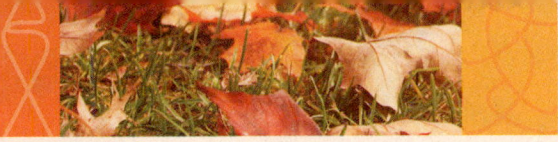
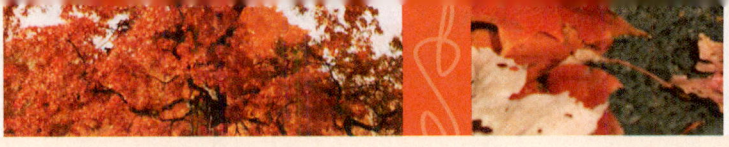

the scope of practice for the nurse. Increasing the morphine dose may alleviate the pain while masking symptoms and delaying treatment of the underlying problem. (5) 2. Outcome 4. Teaching the patient the RICE acronym will help him or her to remember how to care for the injury. (6) 4. Outcome 5. Fracture of a long bone is the principal risk for fat embolism syndrome (FES). The manifestations may include confusion, petechiae, pulmonary edema, and acute respiratory distress syndrome. Hemorrhage may be obvious or manifested by swelling of the thigh or evidence of hypovolemia (tachycardia, restlessness, possible hypotension, decreased urine output). Although fever may be a sign of infection, petechiae on the face or mucous membranes generally are not. Manifestations of compartment syndrome include increasing pain, paresthesias, pallor, and possible decreased pulses distal to the fracture. (7) 4. Outcome 1. Peripheral vascular disease (PVD) is the major cause of amputation of the lower extremities. Upper extremity amputations are more commonly associated with trauma. Bone cancer may lead to amputation of the affected extremity but is a less frequent cause of lower extremity amputation. (8) 1, 2. Outcome 4. When caring for a patient in traction, maintain the pulling force and traction by maintaining the body alignment with the direction of the pull. Pin sites have a risk for infection and are cleansed regularly. Weights are not released on the patient with skeletal traction nor is the patient allowed up to the bedside. Sliding when repositioning increases the risk of skin trauma and excoriation. (9) 1. Outcome 3. Disruption of skin integrity by the fractured bones leads to a significant risk for infection in a compound fracture, making close monitoring of the temperature critical. The other measures identified may be appropriate but are not priority interventions. (10) 1. Outcome 4. Balanced suspension traction increases the patient's mobility while maintaining appropriate bone position. Straight and skin traction use the patient's weight as a counterbalance, and therefore inhibit mobility. Skeletal traction may promote mobility or require that the patient remain immobilized, depending on the fracture site.

CHAPTER 43

NCLEX-PN® ANSWERS   (1) 2. Outcome 3. Osteomyelitis may develop in the patient with open fractures or open wounds near a bone. The nurse should assess for other signs and symptoms of infection including chills, fever, and elevated WBC. Dressings should be changed as ordered. Evaluation of the drainage on the bandage is critical. The dressing should be dry and intact. Capillary refill should be within normal limits. A decreased capillary refill may indicate occlusion. Pain medications should be administered as necessary. (2) 1, 2, 4, 5, 3. Outcome 6. Safety, comfort, and promoting healing are the most important issues for discharge instruction. The walker and elevated toilet seat reduce the risk of falling and dislocation or damage of the hip. Effective pain management promotes activity and healing. Smoking constricts blood vessels and reduces oxygen delivery to tissues, slowing healing. Gradually increasing activities promotes the patient's level of wellness. Calcium supplements may be ordered for the patient, because increased calcium may help prevent further bone loss and promote healing. (3) 3. Outcome 6. The tick should be removed with tweezers without jerking or twisting. It should not be crushed and should be saved in alcohol. (4) 4. Outcome 2, 3. Osteoarthritis affects the entire joint, causing deep, aching pain, stiffness after immobility, limited ROM, and crepitus with movement. (5) 3. Outcome 2, 4. The SLE patient is sensitive to UV light and should

avoid skin exposure, especially when rays are intense. No special diet is prescribed, and joint inflammation is treated as necessary. SLE is a chronic inflammatory disease that affects all body systems. (6) 3. Outcome 4, 6. Sulfinpyrazone may cause peptic ulcers in some patients. Patients should report any symptoms of GI distress to their physician. Water should be increased to at least 3 L per day. Use of aspirin is contraindicated while taking sulfinpyrazone. Probenecid, sulfinpyrazone, and allopurinol are taken with food to prevent gastric upset. (7) 2. Outcome 5. Patients with chronic low back pain need to focus on rehabilitation and learning to manage this chronic condition. Appropriate body mechanics, back exercises, and environmental modifications need to be discussed. The question provides no information to support the other nursing diagnoses. (8) 3, 4. Outcome 4, 6. Celecoxib is an NSAID that is taken on a regular basis to reduce inflammation and pain. It can be taken without regard to meals but may increase the risk for GI bleeding. Abdominal pain, tarry stools, and other manifestations of GI bleed should be promptly reported to the physician. Acetaminophen, an analgesic that works by a different mechanism, can be taken as directed to manage pain while using celecoxib. This and other NSAIDs may increase the risk for heart attack and stroke when taken in prescription strength for long periods. (9) 1. Outcome 5. This statement indicates the nurse's understanding and willingness to discuss the patient's fears about the meaning of the mass. The other statements indicate inappropriate assumptions about the mass by the nurse. (10) 1. Outcome 1, 5. Although patients with fibromyalgia may experience remissions and exacerbations of their symptoms, it is not a progressive disorder. Medications are used as needed to improve sleep and manage symptoms of the disorder.

CHAPTER 44

NCLEX-PN® ANSWERS   (1) 2, 3, 6. Outcome 4. Decreased elasticity, liver spots, and thick yellow nails are common findings in the older adult. Blood supply and temperature regulation decrease rather than increase. Petechiae are an abnormal finding in all adults. (2) 1. Outcome 1, 3. Tenting is seen in older adults and in people with dehydration. The nurse assesses for it by pinching the skin over the collarbone. Edema is assessed by depressing the skin over the ankle. Palpating for moisture and looking for lesions in a group do not relate to tenting. (3) 4. Outcome 3. Exposure to radiation increases the risk for skin cancer. Other factors include men over age 50, light-colored hair and eyes, and living in high altitudes. (4) 3. Outcome 2, 3. Hepatitis often causes jaundice. In dark-skinned patients, jaundice is usually seen in the sclera and palms of the hands. White patches known as vitiligo, cyanosis, or dusky gray color does not occur in hepatitis. (5) 2. Outcome 5. Skin scraping is done to identify a fungal infection. Biopsy is used to rule out malignancy. Allergy testing is done with patch testing. Tzanck test is done to identify herpes infection.

CHAPTER 45

NCLEX-PN® ANSWERS   (1) 1. Outcome 3. The temperature should be decreased to provide comfort for skin lesions but only after the bath is given. Cornstarch or baking soda baths help to relieve itching. Loose-fitting pajamas should be worn to bed after bathing. Medication for itching such as Benadryl may be given, but pain med-

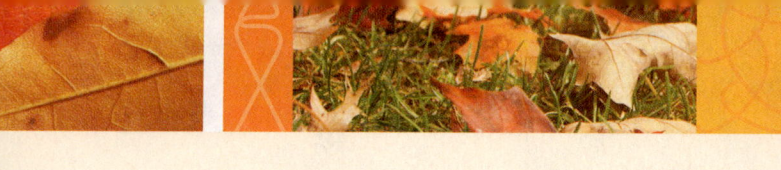
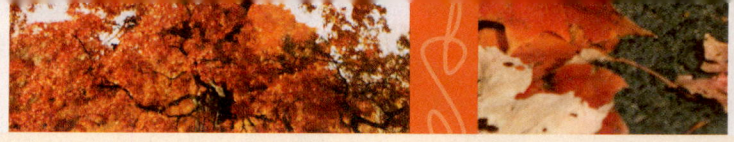

ication is generally not needed for psoriasis. (2) **2, 3, 5.** Outcome 2. Kidney transplant, childhood occurrence of chickenpox, and chemotherapy are all risk factors for herpes zoster. Cervical cancer and measles are important to note in the history but do not cause herpes zoster. Menstruation may trigger an outbreak of herpes simplex. (3) **2.** Outcome 3. Antibiotics may result in superinfections such as mouth fungi, candidiasis. Furuncles are boils, tinea pedis is athlete's foot, and folliculitis is an infection of hair follicles. (4) **4.** Outcome 4. Herpes is a sexually transmitted disease. Abstinence is recommended during an outbreak of the virus. Gloves should be worn to prevent the spread of the infection. The medication should be used daily. The type of bathing does not affect treatment of genital herpes. (5) **4.** Outcome 3. Body lice are transmitted from contact with infested clothing or bed linens. Washing the items decreases the chance of reinfestation. Body lice may affect other family members or pets and can cause itching, especially at night. The best answer reflects the transmission of the lice. The lice must be eradicated from the household objects. (6) **1.** Outcome 2. Most nonmelanoma skin cancers are directly related to exposure to sunlight. Fair-skinned people are at higher risk for skin cancer. Estrogen levels are not directly related. Blistering sunburn during childhood increases the risk of melanoma. (7) **3.** Outcome 3. This patient does not believe life will get better after the surgery, so Hopelessness is the best answer. Anxiety, Fear, and Impaired Skin Integrity are all appropriate diagnoses for some cancer patients. Based on this statement, the patient should be given more information regarding the success rate for cryosurgery and the treatment of basal cell carcinomas. (8) **1.** Outcome 4. Patients should be able to identify changes in their own skin. Treatment and the prognosis for skin cancers need to be discussed after a positive diagnosis. Risk factors should be taught after the skin examination. (9) **3.** Outcome 1. Redness over bony prominences suggests the beginning of skin breakdown. A decreased appetite could lead to a lack of protein and vitamins, which are needed for intact skin. Contractures may also lead to loss of skin integrity due to immobility. Lack of mobility increases the mucous buildup in the lungs, causing a decrease in lung expansion. (10) **2, 4, 6.** Outcome 3. Repositioning patients every 2 hours and providing high-protein and high-calorie diets decreases the likelihood that decubiti will develop. Dry skin needs moisture to prevent cracks and fissures. Massaging the compromised skin may cause damage to the tissues. Hot water may burn the skin. Patients should be lifted up in bed rather than pulled.

CHAPTER 46

NCLEX-PN® ANSWERS (1) **4.** Outcome 2. Electricity follows the path of least resistance. Lightning travels along bones, blood vessels, and nerve fibers. Although lightning may cause abnormal cardiac rhythms, the symptoms exhibited are directly related to the brain and central nervous system. There is a potential for loss of both urinary and pulmonary function, depending on the severity of the electrical discharge. (2) **1.** Outcome 1. With full-thickness burns, the skin appears dry, leathery, and firm to the touch, and pain receptors are destroyed. Partial thickness includes both deep and superficial partial-thickness injuries. Pain is present in various degrees, and the wound has blister formations. Superficial burns only involve the epidermis, causing pink to red coloration with local edema and pain. (3) **2.** Outcome 4. The emergent stage consists of estimating the extent of burn damage, initiating first aid, and assessing for shock and respiratory distress. An inhalation injury is suspected in facial burns when singed facial hair, hoarseness, and black-colored sputum exists. It must be reported immediately to prevent pulmonary complications. Pain and decreased mobility are expected with this type of burn. The urine output is normal. (4) **4.** Outcome 3. During reversal of burn shock, fluids shift from the extracellular spaces to the circulatory system. Older patients may develop excess fluid volume, which is manifested by pulmonary edema. Renal failure can develop, but the manifestations indicate a respiratory problem. Heart failure manifestations depend on which side of the heart is affected. Atelectasis can occur with inhalation injury and reduced mobility, but acute symptoms indicate pulmonary edema. (5) **1.** Outcome 1. The anterior trunk equals 18%, and the anterior and posterior aspect of the left arm equals 9%. (6) **3.** Outcome 3. Morphine by the intravenous route is the drug of choice for managing pain. Hydromorphone by PCA is inappropriate for severe burn injuries because the patient requires continuous analgesia. Midazolam is only used as a preprocedure medication. Pantoprazole is used to reduce gastric acidity. (7) **3.** Outcome 5. Because burn patients have a higher risk for infection, any redness or drainage must be reported. Dressings are not applied to the ears. The patient should eat a diet high in calories and protein. All extremity dressings are applied from in a distal to proximal manner. (8) **1, 3, 4, 5.** Outcome 4. All burn patients should have aseptic wound care and daily weights. Burns to the extremities are at risk for compartment syndrome due to eschar, which can drastically reduce blood flow. It is essential to monitor peripheral pulses for signs of reduced blood flow. Injuries to extremities may also cause contractures so it is important to perform ROM exercises. Vital signs should be checked at least every 4 hours. Aloe gel is only applied to minor burns. (9) **2.** Outcome 4. Infection is a constant threat due to the decreased immune system in patients with major burns. Frequent vital signs are imperative. A set of vital signs should always be obtained before calling the physician. Dressings should be removed during wound care or on specific orders from the doctor. Palpating skin temperature will not add any useful information at this point. (10) **4.** Outcome 3. Leukopenia may develop during the first 2 to 3 days of treatment. The nurse must monitor the patient's WBC. Pain occurs more often with mafenide acetate (Sulfamylon). Dehydration and bleeding do not develop with this drug.

CHAPTER 47

NCLEX-PN® ANSWERS (1) **2.** Outcome 4. Helping the patient in a new environment to identify ways in which she can have control over ADLs and to meet new people to form possible friendships should be helpful to her mental health. It is a mistake to solve social problems with medications when they could be solved with coping mechanisms. The nurse is trying to help this patient cope with her new residence. (2) **3.** Outcome 1. Mental disorders are caused by too little or too much neurotransmitter activity. The brain continues to function and will not lose consciousness, but the symptoms of mental illness occur (which symptoms is dependent on which neurotransmitter is involved). (3) **2, 5.** Outcome 6. The patient's coping skills, self-concept, social support, and family roles are components of a psychosocial assessment. Attitudes about surgery might be helpful in the preoperative assessment of some patients, and the sexual history of patients under other cir-

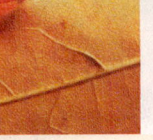
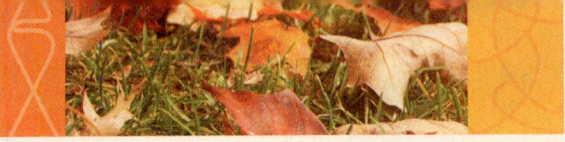
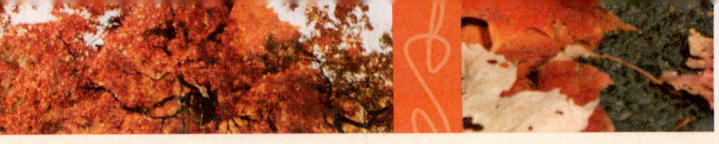

cumstances might be important, but not in the psychosocial assessment. The number of stairs is relevant when a patient will have impaired mobility when returning home from the hospital. (4) 1. Outcome 5. The patient's answer will be what he or she does to cope. Using medical terminology is often confusing for patients. (5) 4. Outcome 3. The homeless woman is under a great deal of stress; she has inadequate resources and inadequate support for coping. She also has a genetic predisposition for mental illness. None of the other options represents the degree of stress of homelessness. They are stressful, but you are asked for the best answer.

CHAPTER 48

NCLEX-PN® ANSWERS (1) 4. Outcome 1. The woman's short-term memory is probably a little worse because she is older or under stress. Just having a mother with Alzheimer disease is stressful. These examples do not constitute a memory abnormality. There is no reason to increase her anxiety about Alzheimer disease without evidence of abnormal memory loss. (2) 3, 4, 5. Outcome 2. 3, Sudden onset; 4, Usually treatable if treated early; and 5, inconsistent symptoms are all true of delirium. Delirium can be curable, and it is not caused by plaques (i.e., Alzheimer disease). (3) 3. Outcome 3. The 65-year-old with alcohol dependency and diabetes. This patient has three risk factors (age, alcoholism, diabetes). The 70-year-old is older, but there is more to dementia than age. Bladder cancer and inflammatory bowel disease do not cause dementia. (4) 1. Outcome 4. In the early stage, patients are still functioning but becoming more forgetful. The patient will not remember things later, no matter how hard she tries now. The patient may not be incontinent, and labels may be helpful for knowing what is in cupboards but will not help the person remember names. (5) 2. Outcome 6. Safety is the most likely issue to arise in the middle stage. The patient may not be able to read. Catastrophic reactions are better prevented than treated with sedatives. (6) 4. Outcome 5. Although the medications may temporarily improve memory, option 2 is not the best choice. The meds do not cause remission or cure. They are intended to prolong the early stage. (7) 2. Outcome 5. There are currently no Alzheimer meds in rectal form, so transdermal is the only choice that leaves out putting the drug in the patient's mouth, which increases the chance of choking. (8) 1. Outcome 6. Validating the patient's feelings is the correct nursing action. He is disoriented, but he feels strongly about something that is left undone. By "validating" or recognizing that the patient's feelings are real, the nurse is helping the patient fulfill a need and is respecting the patient's feelings. This patient is too far in the disease to respond well to reorientation. At this point, reorientation is frustrating. (9) 3. Outcome 6, 5. The physician should be notified first. The physician will diagnose the patient's medical disorder. Delirium, which has a sudden onset, can be fatal if not recognized early. Change in LOC is of the first priority. (10) 3. Outcome 7. Everyone with Alzheimer disease has a declining course, caregivers need help or they cannot be healthy, and few families can afford to hire help day and night. Unrealistic optimism is not helpful.

CHAPTER 49

NCLEX-PN® ANSWERS (1) 3. Outcome 2. Flat affect and little speech are negative symptoms, which represent findings that are "less than" normal behavior. Difficulty with mental concentration

is also a possibility, but this symptom may also be true for various disorders or be a result of a poor night's sleep. (2) 3. Outcome 4. "The patient is experiencing a frightening hallucination, apparently about aliens attacking him" is the most objective, descriptive documentation. (3) 1. Outcome 4. Reassure the patient that he is safe in the hospital and there are no aliens. The nurse should reinforce reality. (4) 1. Outcome 2. Structured daily activities are a part of milieu therapy, in which the environment is therapeutic. (5) 4. Outcome 2. A patient who is pacing the halls, clenching his fists, and talking angrily to unseen voices is probably hallucinating and most likely to be violent. (6) 3. Outcome 2. Delusional thinking (false belief). (7) 2. Outcome 4. "You have schizophrenia, which is a brain disorder that affects your thinking." This correctly answers the patient's question in layperson's terms. Answer 1 is too technical. (8) 2. Outcome 3. High fever, muscle pain, and unstable BP are symptoms of NMS. (9) 3. Outcome 1. Dopamine is the most important brain neurotransmitter in excess in schizophrenia. (10) 1, 2, 4. Outcome 3. These are all anticholinergic side effects. Abnormal body movements are an extrapyramidal side effect.

CHAPTER 50

NCLEX-PN® ANSWERS (1) 3. Outcome 2. The best way to document whether the patient is feeling better is to use the 0–10 mood scale regularly because it shows how the patient rates his or her feelings over time. Drawing a chart is probably an unrealistic expectation. The mental status assessment is objective, not subjective. The dose of medication required for an individual is related to metabolic rate and other physiologic factors, not to the severity of the patient's symptoms. (2) 3. Outcome 3. The patient has a combination of factors that put her at risk for another episode of depression. She has had a previous depressive episode, is female, and has a history of a suicide attempt. With a new baby, she would be experiencing another stressful episode in her life and would be susceptible to postpartum depression. However, she is not more likely than *any* other woman to have depression. Whether she was "seeking attention" in high school is not relevant. This is often used to invalidate psychologic concerns such as depression and suicidal thinking. Avoid the accusation of "seeking attention." Finally, she is at increased risk, and it is not the nurse's responsibility to decide or encourage some people to get pregnant and others not to do so. (3) 1. Outcome 1. Light therapy is the treatment of choice for SAD. It is the loss of light in the day–night cycle that seems to precipitate the symptoms. Melatonin is used to induce sleep, not to treat depression; psychoanalysis is not indicated; and ECT is used for treatment-resistant major depression. (4) 4. Outcome 1. Anhedonia is the medical term for the inability to experience pleasure and is a common symptom of depression. It is the only correct definition. (5) 3. Outcome 2. Patients tend to be quiet about their feelings of depression, so that the physician is not aware of their psychologic state. The most common reason for this is the stigma society has placed on mental illness. It is often seen as a weakness on the part of the depressed person. Physicians can diagnose depression, but for the same reason as patients, they hesitate to document the diagnosis because they want to spare the patient the stigma of mental illness. (6) 2. Outcome 3, 4. It will take 2 to 6 weeks for the maximum effect of the medication to be reached. The other time frames are not correct. It is important for

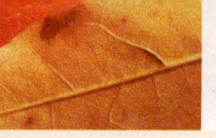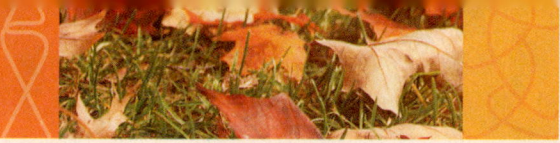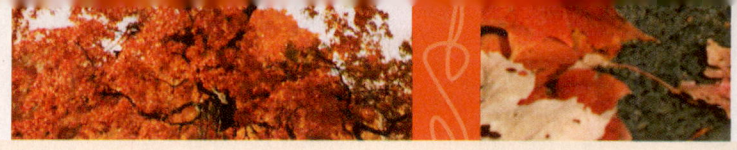

the nurse to know that medication effect is not immediate. (7) 1. Outcome 1. Racing thoughts are moving very fast and are likely to result in fast-moving behavior (psychomotor agitation). There is no reason to expect powerlessness or thought blocking (the opposite of these occur). A person may have hallucinations, but they are not common or necessarily associated with racing thoughts. (8) 4. Outcome 4. People in the manic state do not respond well to excessive environmental stimuli. Removing the patient from the stimulation by taking him outside is the first line of intervention you should try. Walking with him allows him to continue his movement. Talk calmly and softly to help him de-escalate the agitation. Restraint is used only in emergencies. Appropriate behavior is encouraged for patients in the therapeutic milieu as part of therapy. (9) 1, 3, 4, 5. Outcome 4. Foods with tyramine must be avoided when using MAOIs, because they can cause hypertensive crisis in this combination. The fruit of bananas is low in tyramine; the peel is high (and not usually consumed). Milk and cottage cheese are allowed dairy products (low in tyramine). (10) 2. Outcome 3, 4. Notify the physician or nurse practitioner. Option 1 is wrong because a high score indicates that the patient should be further evaluated for depression. Every depressed person does not require treatment in a psychiatric unit. The nurse does not know whether the patient will be taking medication.

CHAPTER 51

NCLEX-PN® ANSWERS (1) 2, 3, 4. Outcome 4. Option 1, restraint is not indicated, it is only used in emergencies. A calm, reassuring approach by the nurse, keeping stimulation to a minimum, is correct. (2) 2, 4. Outcome 5. The benzodiazepines cause sedation, drowsiness, dizziness, and decreased coordination. Options 1 and 3 represent the opposite of expected BZ actions. (3) 2. Outcome 1. This is a response to a specific situation and may not be an anxiety disorder. Validate his feelings and then assess for the source of his anxiety. Does he need more information about the process? Does he fear the results? Is he concerned about being in a small, closed space? Medication is not indicated unless you have tried other options. Telling any patient that, "everything will be all right" is wrong, because you do not know if that is true. Turning on the TV is usually the wrong answer because it is diverting the nurse's responsibility to the TV. (4) 1. Outcome 1. People with generalized anxiety disorder are often aware that they are not responding to situations appropriately, but they are unable to control those feelings without assistance. Genetics is not the only cause of anxiety disorders; anxiety medications are not addictive unless they are misused; they can be very effective; intelligence is positively associated with anxiety. (5) 2. Outcome 5. Benzodiazepine antianxiety agents are the most commonly prescribed drugs for anxiety. A sedative hypnotic is a sleeping pill. Fluoroquinolones are antibiotics. (6) 1. Outcome 2. The nursing student is reliving the trauma of seeing her mother die suddenly in this room. Entering the room triggered the memory of this event. It is common for such episodes to occur within 3 months of the traumatic event. She is experiencing posttraumatic stress. The other options are not real disorders. (7) 3. Outcome 4. The goal of CBT is for the patient to view the situation realistically and replace inappropriate negative self-talk with positive thoughts that are supportive and calming. The other options do not describe reframing or looking in a different way at the stressful thought. (8) 1. Outcome 4.

Relaxation and deep-breathing responses are effective for many different anxiety-producing events. Leaving the patient alone, telling what you would do, or a reading assignment will not give the patient the opportunity to practice the new behavior, which is the most effective way to learn a new coping behavior. (9) 3. Outcome 3. See Box 51-7 for more help with assessing coping skills. Only option 3 asks the patient in layperson's terms how she copes with stress. The other options either blame the patient, talk to her in medical terminology, or assess her future planning, which are not correct. (10) 2, 3, 4. Outcome 2. Option 1 is wrong because false reassurance is not helpful. There is no need to cancel the surgery. It is normal for patients to be anxious about surgery. Nurses can help by assessing for the basis of the anxiety and providing information to ensure that the patient understands what to expect. Progressive relaxation can be an excellent nonpharmacological anxiety relief measure.

CHAPTER 52

NCLEX-PN® ANSWERS (1) 2. Outcome 2. Patients with paranoid personality disorder are suspicious of others. They have more confidence in a nurse who shows self-confidence and treats the patient in a direct, matter-of-fact way. A nurse who is quiet, shy, or even friendly does not inspire as much confidence in a patient with suspiciousness as one who is confident. (2) 1. Outcome 1. The patient with a schizoid personality disorder typically avoids relationships even with caregivers. Not having visitors or receiving phone calls would validate the lack of social relationships. A flat affect is common. This patient is not likely to be ashamed (he lacks insight about having a problem) nor will he be depressed or lonely—this is usual for him. (3) 3. Outcome 3. As a patient with schizotypal personality disorder, this patient would prefer to be alone because of severe social anxiety. The stress of being forced to interact with other residents could precipitate delusional thinking or perceptual alterations. Inviting her to one meal a day should be less threatening. Allow her to move at her own pace, and praise her when she is able to comply. Forcing her into more social contact than she is comfortable with or willing to do will not help her. Ignoring her will not help her either, because it is most healthy for her to have some social contact. (4) 2. Outcome 2. The patient with an antisocial personality disorder is often a very manipulative person to care for. Staff members all need to be consistent in care and in following all unit rules. He is not concerned about safety. Breaking the rules for him will make him worse, not better, and treating his personality with medications is a dangerous lesson for this patient. (5) 2. Outcome 1. Although some of the other choices might be appropriate, your first priority would be to prevent self-injury. Patients with borderline personality disorder commonly respond to stress by cutting or burning themselves. (6) 4. Outcome 2. These behaviors are consistent with the self-centeredness of histrionic personality disorder. People with borderline, avoidant, or schizotypal personalities are not likely to behave in this way. (7) 1. Outcome 3. This patient is demonstrating the symptoms of the narcissistic personality disorder. You may briefly empathize with his stress, but you must consistently lay down the limits with what is appropriate and what is not. You

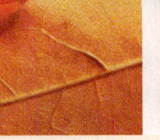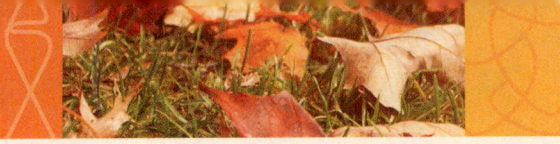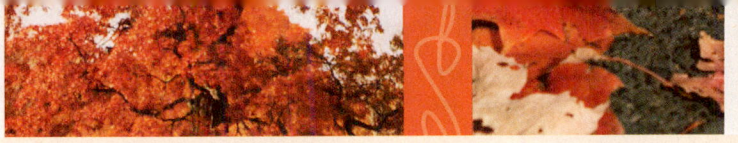

must maintain a professional, no-nonsense approach. Do not lie to the patient, treat him gruffly, or cater to his unreasonable demands. The nurse is a role model for normal behavior. (8) 1, 3, 4. Outcome 4. Patients with anxiety respond well in a trusting relationship, when the nurse is calm, and when they understand their own feelings. Option 2, teaching her that she does not have to be anxious is wrong, because she already knows that, but she cannot help it. And 5, giving her a pager, will not allow her to solve any problem or concern by herself, which is what she needs to learn. (9) 3, 1, 4, 2. Outcome 4. Safety is always a high priority. Consistency is critical for this patient. Learning to express his feelings will be an ongoing effort, and finally, his outpatient care is important but lowest of these priorities at this time. (10) 1. Outcome 4. The obsessive-compulsive behavior in persons with this personality disorder is worsened by anxiety. Hospitalization is likely to be stressful. The question gives us no information that the patient is depressed, is psychotic, or has difficulty sleeping.

CHAPTER 53

NCLEX-PN® ANSWERS   (1) 1. Outcome 1. The body adjusts to constant use of a drug. As consumption continues, larger amounts are needed to give the desired effect. Once tolerance develops, many patients begin use of different, more potent substances. This is the definition of tolerance; it is not intoxication, addiction, or abuse. (2) 3. Outcome 1. When alcohol is withdrawn, the central nervous system is still stimulated. The patient exhibits signs of stimulation, including elevated vital signs, anxiety, tremors, and seizures. Options 1 and 4 represent normal findings. Option 2 is the opposite of the stimulant effects expected. (3) 3. Outcome 1. Alcoholic encephalopathy is caused by vitamin B_1 deficiency related to inadequate nutritional intake. There is no information in the question to indicate that the nurse should expect Demerol (analgesic), valium (BZ), or Dilantin (anticonvulsant). (4) 2. Outcome 5. Opiate overdose results in depressed central nervous system, including marked respiratory depression. Narcan (naloxone HCl) reverses the sedative effects. Thiamine would be given to a person with chronic alcohol use, Librium is for anxiety, and D5W is an unmedicated IV fluid. (5) 2, 3, 4. Outcome 3. The most important point is that patients must be cautioned to avoid combining alcohol and antianxiety drugs. These combinations can result in respiratory depression or cardiac arrhythmias, including cardiac arrest. Options 3 and 4 are also correct because the drug can cause drowsiness, and if so, the patient should not drive until some tolerance to that effect has occurred. There is no reason for option 1, taking the drug every 4 hours, included in the question. (6) 4. Outcome 3. The nursing supervisor usually holds accountability and administrative authority for the unit and is aware of policy related to follow-up of situations in which narcotics are diverted. It is not appropriate to confront the suspect nurse because he or she will be defensive and this will not resolve the problem, the physician is not involved, and the charge nurse does not have the authority to intervene. (7) 2. Outcome 5. Teaching the consequences of continued substance abuse gives the patient information to make choices related to his or her behavior. Avoidance of adverse consequences is the usual reason people quit. The patient would already know about withdrawal, and there are not safe levels of drug use for people with substance use disorders; the antidote for narcotics is not helpful. (8) 3. Outcome 1. Opiates are central nervous system stimulants. When the drugs are withdrawn, the CNS is depressed. All the other options suggest CNS stimulation. (9) 1, 2. Outcome 4. Patients in alcohol withdrawal are experiencing CNS stimulation. Vital signs help assess the extent of this. Holding any CNS medication is not a good idea (the patient may need a BZ), and blaming the patient for his disease is an even worse idea! (10) 2. Outcome 2. The nurse verbalizes the observation that the patient has silver paint on his hair, which is the most commonly used paint type (it has more propellant) used for inhalation. The accusatory answers are wrong, because the nurse should be establishing a trusting relationship with this confused patient. The patient may not know the technical term for his form of drug use.

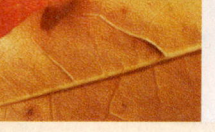
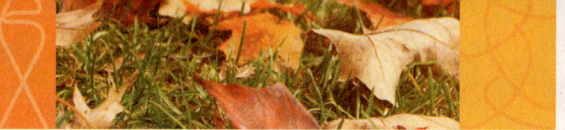
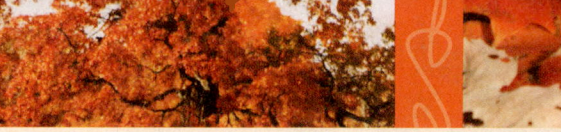

Glossary

(Note: The number(s) in parentheses in boldface after the glossary definition show the chapter(s) in which the term is defined. Words other than key terms that require definitions are italicized in the text and are defined there.)

A

Abscesses: pockets of accumulated pus **(9)**

Abstinence: voluntarily refraining from use of a drug or substance that has been abused or from an activity such as sexual intercourse **(33, 53)**

Acidosis: increased hydrogen ion concentration; a pH of less than 7.36 **(7)**

Acne: disorder of the sebaceous glands **(45)**

Acquired immunodeficiency syndrome (AIDS): last stage of HIV infection **(11)**

Active transport: process by which molecules are moved against a concentration gradient across cell membranes **(7)**

Acuity: the severity of the patient's illness and the level of care required **(2)**

Acute coronary syndrome (ACS): a condition of severe cardiac ischemia **(16)**

Acute illness: illness that occurs rapidly, lasts for a relatively short period of time, and is self-limiting **(2)**

Acute kidney injury: an abrupt and rapid decline in renal function; it is often reversible with prompt treatment **(29)**

Acute myocardial infarction: myocardial cell necrosis (death) due to lack of blood and oxygen **(16)**

Acute pain: temporary pain that has a sudden onset and is localized **(8)**

Acute pulmonary edema: Accumulation of fluid in the interstitial spaces and alveoli of the lungs; may be classified as either cardiogenic (due to acute heart failure) or noncardiogenic **(17)**

Acute respiratory distress syndrome (ARDS): a severe form of respiratory failure due to acute damage to the alveoli **(14, 23)**

Adaptive: related to coping behavior that is healthy **(51)**

Addiction: condition of seeking drugs habitually (other than for a medical purpose) and of not being able to give them up without adverse psychologic and physiologic effects **(8)**

Addison disease: autoimmune destruction of adrenal glands that causes deficient production of corticosteroids and mineral corticoid hormones **(35)**

Addisonian crisis: acute deficiency of cortisol that causes a life-threatening condition **(35)**

Additive: the sum of the effects when two drugs with similar actions are taken **(6)**

Advance directives: legal documents that allow a person to plan for health care and financial affairs in the event of incapacity **(13)**

Adventitious: abnormal (e.g., abnormal breath sounds) **(21)**

Advocate: one who speaks for another **(1)**

Affect: the outward expression of emotion; nonverbal signs of emotion including facial expression, tone of voice, body movements; more transient than mood **(49, 50, 52)**

Ageism: a form of prejudice that stereotypes older adults **(4)**

Agonist: a drug that initiates an action **(6)**

Akathisia: restlessness; intense need to move **(49)**

Alcoholic: alcohol-dependent individual **(53)**

Alkalosis: decreased hydrogen ion concentration; a pH greater than 7.45 **(7)**

Allograft: tissue transplanted between members of the same species **(11)**

Alopecia: hair loss **(44)**

Alterations in health: change in normal health state **(3)**

Alzheimer disease: a neurologic disorder in which neurofibrillary tangles and beta-amyloid plaques cause deterioration of brain function, characterized by a progressive loss of memory **(48)**

Ambulatory surgery: a surgical procedure performed on a nonhospitalized patient under local or general anesthesia **(10)**

Amenorrhea: absence of menstruation **(32)**

Amputation: partial or total removal of a body part **(42)**

Amyotrophic lateral sclerosis (ALS): fatal neurologic disease causing loss of motor neuron function in the spinal cord and brainstem **(39)**

Anabolism: process by which tissues are built up **(9)**

Analgesics: pharmacologic agents used to relieve or reduce pain **(8)**

Anaphylactic shock: shock caused by a severe allergic reaction **(14)**

Anaphylaxis: an acute, immediate allergic reaction **(11, 14)**

Anastomosis: surgical connection of two tubular structures **(25)**

Androgens: male sex hormones **(30)**

Anemia: condition in which the hemoglobin concentration or the number of circulating RBCs is decreased **(20)**

Anergy: lack of response to common antigens given to test for immunocompetence **(11)**

Anesthesia: use of chemical substances to produce loss of sensation, reflex loss, or muscle relaxation during a surgical procedure, with or without the loss of consciousness **(10)**

Aneurysm: localized dilation of a blood vessel **(18, 38)**

Angina pectoris: chest pain that occurs when there is a temporary imbalance between myocardial blood supply and demand **(16)**

Anhedonia: inability to feel pleasure **(49)**

Anorexia: loss of appetite **(25)**

Anorexia nervosa: an eating disorder marked by a disturbed body image, fear of gaining weight, and weight less than 85% of that expected for age and height **(25)**

Anorexia–cachexia syndrome: effect of cancer cells on metabolism; cancer cells divert nutrition to own use and inhibit food intake; they also break down the body's tissue and muscle proteins to support their growth **(12)**

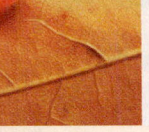
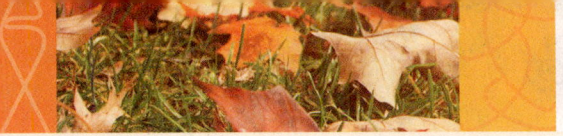
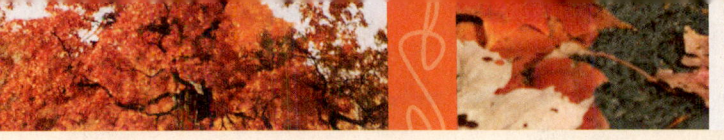

Antagonist: prevents drug action (6)

Antibiotics: medications used to treat bacterial infections (9)

Antibody: an immunoglobulin that binds to and inactivates a specific antigen (11)

Antigen: substance that stimulates an immune response (11)

Anxiety: feeling of uneasiness and activation of the autonomic nervous system in response to a nonspecific threat (51)

Aphasia: the partial or total inability to express or receive and understand speech, as a result of brain damage (38, 48)

Appendicitis: inflammation of the appendix (26)

Arteriosclerosis: disorder characterized by thickening, loss of elasticity, and calcification of arterial walls (18)

Arthralgia: joint pain (43)

Arthritis: inflammation of a joint (43)

Arthroplasty: reconstruction or replacement of a joint (43)

Arthroscopy: use of a flexible fiberoptic endoscope to view and/or repair joint structures and tissues (41)

Ascites: accumulation of serous fluid in the peritoneal cavity (27)

Assessment: collection of data about the patient's individualized health and health care needs; first step of the nursing process (1, 5)

Asthma: a chronic inflammatory airway disorder with recurrent episodes of wheezing, breathlessness, chest tightness, and coughing (23)

Ataxia: staggering or unsteady gait (37, 53)

Atelectasis: an area or areas of alveolar collapse and airlessness (10, 23)

Atherosclerosis: disease in which the lining of medium and large arteries is affected by lesions called atheromas or plaque (16)

Aura: warning sign of a seizure or migraine headache; it may be a bright light, an unusual sound, or an abnormal taste or odor (38)

Auscultation: method of assessment that uses a stethoscope to listen for body sounds (5)

Autoantibodies: antibodies made against self-antigens (11)

Autograft: tissue transplanted from one part of the body to another (11)

Autologous: self (11)

Automatism: repetitive, nonpurposeful actions such as lip smacking or aimless walking (38)

Autonomic dysreflexia: an exaggerated sympathetic response associated with high spinal cord injuries (39)

Autotransfusion: process in which a patient's own blood is collected and reinfused (14)

Azotemia: increased blood levels of nitrogenous wastes, including urea and creatinine (29)

B

Bactericidal: ability to kill microorganisms (9)

Bacteriostatic: ability to inhibit growth of microorganisms (9)

Bariatrics: the medical specialty that focuses on preventing and treating obesity (25)

Barrel chest: a greater anterior–posterior (AP) chest diameter than lateral chest diameter (21, 23)

Basal cell carcinoma: cancer that begins in the basal cell layer of the epidermis, usually on sun-exposed areas of the body (45)

B-cell lymphocytes (B cells): white blood cells responsible for humoral immunity that produce antibodies (11)

Bell palsy: neurologic disorder resulting from inflammation of the facial nerve (39)

Benign: nonmalignant (for tumors): localized growths with well-defined borders; they are frequently encapsulated (12)

Benign prostatic hyperplasia (BPH): enlargement of the prostate gland (31)

Beta-amyloid plaques: the buildup of fragments produced when enzymes act on amyloid protein in the brains of people with Alzheimer disease (48)

Biliary colic: right upper quadrant pain associated with bile duct obstruction (27)

Biotherapy: use of medications that stimulate the patient's immune system to target and destroy cancer cells (12)

Biotransformation: process by which the body changes a drug from its original chemical structure into a form that can be eliminated by the body (6)

Blood pressure: force exerted by blood against the walls of the arteries (15)

Bone marrow transplant (BMT): transplantation of bone marrow from one person to another, or the harvest, preservation, and reinfusion of the patient's own bone marrow (autologous BMT) (20)

Borborygmi: loud, hyperactive bowel sounds (25)

Bradykinesia: slowed voluntary movements and speech (39)

Brain abscess: collection of purulent material within the brain (38)

Brain death criteria: clinical criteria for determining when a patient is dead (14)

Broad-spectrum antibiotics: antibiotics that act against a wide variety of pathogens (9)

Bronchitis: inflammation of the bronchi (23)

Bruit: harsh or musical sound (murmur) heard on auscultation of a blood vessel (18)

Buffers: substances that prevent major changes in pH by either removing or releasing hydrogen ions from a solution (7)

Bulimia nervosa: episodic binge eating and self-induced vomiting, laxative or diuretic use, or excessive exercise (25)

Burn: injury of tissue loss, damage, or irreversible destruction from exposure to a thermal, chemical, electrical, or radiation heat source (46)

Burn shock: type of hypovolemic shock resulting from the shift of a massive amount of fluid into the extravascular space (46)

C

Cancer: disease that results when normal cells mutate into abnormal ones and continue to reproduce within the body (12)

Candidiasis: infections caused by *Candida albicans*, a yeastlike fungus (45)

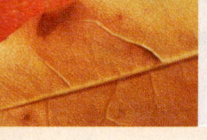
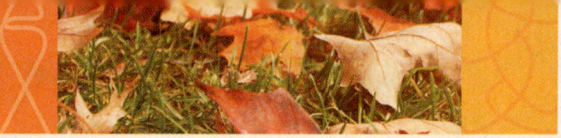
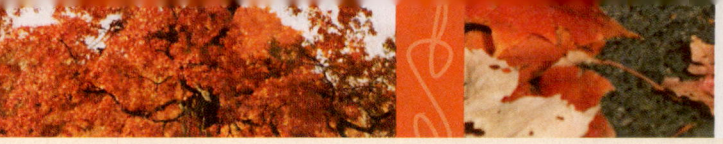

Carcinogenesis: the process in which normal cells are transformed into cancer cells; cancer begins with transformation of a single normally functioning cell into a cancer cell (12)

Carcinogens: cancer-causing agents (12)

Cardiac arrest: cessation of effective heart contractions and blood circulation; usually caused by ventricular fibrillation (16)

Cardiac dysrhythmia: disturbance or irregularity in the electrical system of the heart (16)

Cardiac output: amount of blood pumped from the ventricles in 1 minute (15, 17)

Cardiac reserve: ability of the heart to increase the cardiac output in response to metabolic demand (17)

Cardiac tamponade: compression of the heart by blood or fluid in the pericardial sac (17)

Cardiogenic shock: impaired tissue perfusion caused by pumping failure of the heart (14, 16)

Cardiomyopathy: disorder that affects the structure and function of the heart (17)

Cardioversion: restoration of a normal heart rhythm (normal sinus rhythm) using either electric shock or medications (16)

Carditis: inflammation of the heart (17)

Caregivers: people who provide personal, individual assistance (1)

Carotid endarterectomy: surgical procedure to remove plaque from the carotid artery (38)

Carrier: person who transmits an infectious disease but does not show any clinical manifestations (9)

Catabolism: process by which body tissues are broken down (9, 25)

Cataract: clouding of the lens of the eye (40)

Catastrophic reaction: an explosive behavioral or anger response that is totally out of proportion to the situation (48)

Catatonic behavior: a marked decrease in response to the environment (49)

Ceiling effect: the limit of some drugs to produce a specific effect (6)

Cellulitis: localized infection of the dermis and subcutaneous tissue (9, 45)

Cerebrovascular accident (CVA): sudden loss of neurologic function due to a blood clot or rupture of a cerebral artery; brain attack or stroke (38)

Cerumen: earwax (37)

Chain of infection: set of factors that must exist in order for an infection to develop (9)

Chancre: painless ulcer characteristic of primary syphilis (33)

Cholecystitis: inflammation of the gallbladder (27)

Cholelithiasis: formation of gallstones (27)

Chronic illness: any impairment or deviation from normal functioning that affects more than one body system and that is permanent, leaves permanent disability, is irreversible, requires special teaching for rehabilitation, or requires a long period of care (2)

Chronic obstructive pulmonary disease (COPD): chronic and progressive airflow obstruction caused by chronic bronchitis and emphysema (23)

Chronic pain: pain that lasts longer than 6 months, may not be totally eliminated, or may end only with death; may be malignant (related to cancer) or nonmalignant (8)

Chyme: mixture of partly digested food and digestive juices (24)

Cirrhosis: chronic liver disease that destroys the structure and function of liver lobules (27)

Clinical judgment: process used by nurses and other health care professionals to determine a patient's needs, to identify appropriate interventions to address those needs, and to use patient responses to determine whether new approaches are appropriate (1)

Clonic contractions: alternate contraction and relaxation of muscles, causing jerky movements (38)

Clubbing: enlargement of fingertips characterized by nail base angle of greater than 180 degrees (44)

Codependents: people who enable a person with substance dependency to avoid the consequences of substance use (often by making excuses or taking on their responsibilities) (53)

Cognition: the ability to perceive and understand one's world (4, 48)

Cognitive: thinking and memory (49)

Colectomy: surgical removal of the colon (26)

Collaborator: a person working with others to achieve a goal; the nurse collaborates with the patient and the interprofessional team to provide optimal patient care; effective collaboration requires mutual respect and shared decision making (1)

Collateral circulation: circulation developed to maintain blood flow to a tissue when the primary vessel is obstructed (18)

Colonization: the growth of bacteria on or in a body part (9)

Colostomy: opening of the colon through the abdominal wall to the skin surface (26)

Colposcopy: examination of tissues of the vagina and cervix using a brightly lighted microscope (30)

Comfort measures only order: order indicating that no further life-sustaining interventions are necessary and that the goal of care is a comfortable, dignified death (13)

Community-based nursing: nursing that focuses on culturally competent care and individual and family health care needs in the places where people live, work, play, worship, and go to school (2)

Compartment syndrome: constriction of blood vessels and nerves within a compartment by excess pressure in the compartment (42)

Compliance: distensibility (stretch) of the lungs (21)

Compulsions: repetitive behaviors or mental acts that the affected person feels driven to perform in response to obsessive thoughts (51)

Concrete thinking: literal thinking, without creativity (47)

Concussion: brain injury resulting from violent shaking or impact with an object (38)

Confabulation: falsification of memory to fill in the gaps caused by cognitive deficits (53)

Conjunctivitis: inflammation of the conjunctiva of the eye (40)

Constipation: infrequent or difficult passage of stools (26)

Contraception: the avoidance of pregnancy while having the ability to have heterosexual sexual intercourse (30)

Contractility: the natural ability of cardiac muscle fibers to shorten during systole (15)

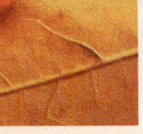
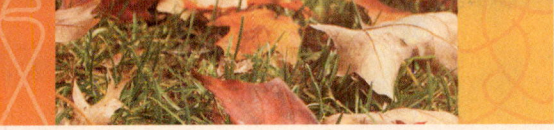
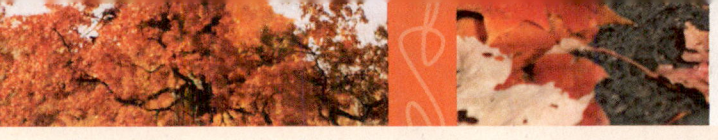

Contracture: abnormal flexion and fixation of a joint caused by muscle atrophy and shortening (42, 46)

Contusion: bleeding into soft tissue resulting from a blunt force (38, 42)

Convulsion: involuntary muscle contraction and relaxation (38)

Coping behaviors: behaviors that help a person manage stress (51)

Corneal ulcers: superficial or deep ulceration of the cornea caused by infection, trauma, or contact lens overuse (40)

Coryza: profuse nasal discharge (22)

Crepitus: a grating sound or sensation (41)

Creutzfeldt–Jakob disease (CJD): a rare, progressive neurologic disease causing brain degeneration (39)

Critical thinking: self-directed thinking that is focused on what to believe or do in a specific situation (1)

Crohn's disease: regional enteritis; a chronic, relapsing inflammatory disorder of the gastrointestinal tract (26)

Cross-tolerance: resistance to the effects of similar types of substances (e.g., alcohol and heroin); for example, a patient who is dependent on any CNS depressant will also be tolerant to other CNS depressants (53)

Cryptorchidism: failure of one or both testes to descend through the inguinal ring into the scrotum (31)

Culture: attitudes, beliefs, customs, and behaviors that are passed from one generation to the next (3, 47)

Cushing syndrome: results from excessive production of corticosteroids from the adrenal glands (35)

Cyanosis: bluish, grayish, or dark purple skin tone caused by reduced oxygen content of the blood (23, 44)

Cystectomy: surgical removal of the urinary bladder (29)

Cystitis: inflammation of the urinary bladder (29)

Cystocele: herniation of the bladder into the vagina (32)

Cytomegalovirus (CMV): a viral infection with the cytomegalovirus that can affect the retina, gastrointestinal tract, or lungs (11)

Cytotoxic T cells: subset of T cells that attack viruses, fungi, and cancer cells (11)

D

Dawn phenomenon: rise in blood glucose levels between 5 and 8 a.m. (36)

Death: irreversible cessation of circulatory and respiratory functions or irreversible cessation of all functions of the entire brain, including the brainstem (13)

Debridement: process of removing dead tissue from a wound (46)

Debulking: surgery to remove a large part of a tumor when complete removal is impossible (38)

Declarative memory: memory involving facts (48)

Deep venous thrombosis (DVT): a blood clot in one or more of the deep veins of the legs, pelvis, arms, or other areas of the body (18)

Dehiscence: separation in the layers of an incisional wound (10)

Dehydration: fluid volume deficit (FVD) due to excessive fluid losses, insufficient fluid intake, or both (7)

Delirium: a temporary condition that alters the level of consciousness (48)

Delusions: false beliefs that are not accepted by one's culture and persist despite evidence that they are false (49)

Dementia: organic disorders that progressively reduce mental function (4)

Demyelination: destruction and degeneration of the myelin sheath covering nerve axons (39)

Denial: refusal to acknowledge the existence of a real situation or feelings as a mechanism for coping with stress (53)

Depersonalization: experience of being an outside observer of, or detached from, oneself (51)

Derealization: experience of unreality, distance, or distortion (51)

Dermatitis: inflammation of the skin characterized by erythema and pain or pruritus (45)

Dermatome: area of the skin supplied by a single sensory nerve (37)

Dermatophytes: tinea (fungal) infections of the skin (45)

Dermis: second, deeper layer of the skin (44)

Desensitization: treatment of an allergy by giving several dilute injections that contain the allergen (11)

Detoxification: removal of a toxic substance from the body (53)

Diabetes insipidus: excessive urination caused by a lack of antidiuretic hormone (ADH) (35)

Diabetes mellitus: chronic disorder of carbohydrate metabolism (36)

Diabetic ketoacidosis (DKA): life-threatening illness occurring in type 1 diabetics, characterized by hyperglycemia, metabolic acidosis, and coma (36)

Dialysate: dialysis solution (29)

Dialysis: diffusion of solutes from higher to lower concentration across a semipermeable membrane (29)

Diaphoresis: profuse sweating (16)

Diarrhea: increase in the frequency, volume, and water content of stool (26)

Diastole: period of ventricular relaxation and filling (15)

Diffusion: process in which molecules move from an area of high concentration to an area of low concentration to become evenly distributed (7)

Dilemma: choice between two unpleasant alternatives (1)

Diplopia: double vision (40)

Disease: disruption in the structure and function of the body or mind (2)

Dislocation: separation of contact between two bones of a joint (42)

Disseminated intravascular coagulation (DIC): condition characterized by abnormal clotting and bleeding (14)

Distractibility: an inability to screen out excess or irrelevant sensory stimuli, causing difficulty with focusing attention (50)

Diverticulitis: inflammation and perforation of a diverticulum, usually in the sigmoid colon (26)

Do-not-resuscitate (DNR) order: order written by the physician for a patient near death, usually based on the wishes of the patient and family that no cardiopulmonary resuscitation be performed for respiratory or cardiac arrest (13)

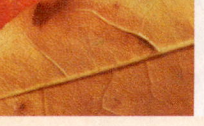
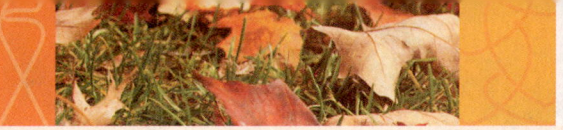
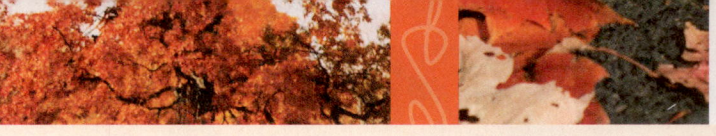

Dopamine: neurotransmitter that controls complex movements, cognition, motivation, and pleasure; it regulates emotional responses (39)

Drain: device that promotes drainage of wound debris and healing from the inside to the outside and decreases the risk of abscess formation (10)

Dual diagnosis: concurrent diagnoses of both a substance use disorder and a mental illness (49, 53)

Durable power of attorney for health care: a legal document written by a competent (mentally healthy) adult that gives another competent adult the right to make health care decisions on the patient's behalf if he or she cannot (13)

Dysfunctional uterine bleeding (DUB): vaginal bleeding that is unusual in amount, duration, or time of occurrence (32)

Dyskinesia: abnormal movement such as shuffling gait, tremor, slow movement, lack of facial expression (49)

Dysmenorrhea: pain associated with menstruation (32)

Dyspareunia: pain during sexual intercourse (32)

Dysphagia: difficult or painful swallowing (22, 25, 37)

Dysphoria: low, uncomfortable mood, but not as low as depression (51)

Dyspnea: difficult or labored breathing (5, 7, 23)

Dystonia: muscle rigidity (49)

Dysuria: difficult or painful urination (28, 29)

E

Ectopic: occurring in an abnormal location (32)

Edema: excess fluid in body tissues (7)

Ejaculation: expulsion of seminal fluid from the male urethra (30)

Electrocardiogram (ECG): graphic record of the heart's electrical activity (15)

Electroconvulsive therapy (ECT): the application of electrical current to the brain, which induces a generalized seizure (50)

Electrolytes: substances that dissociate in solution to form charged particles, or ions (7)

Emancipated minors: individuals under age 18 who are responsible for their own welfare and live independently of their parents (10)

Embolus: blood clot or foreign matter that moves within the vascular system (18)

Emphysema: destruction of alveolar walls leading to large, abnormal air spaces in the lungs (23)

Empyema: a collection of pus in the pleural cavity (23)

Enabling: the process of passively helping the substance-dependent patient to continue using the substance (53)

Encephalitis: an acute inflammation of the white and gray matter of the brain and spinal cord (38)

Endocarditis: inflammation of the endocardium (17)

Endogenous pyrogens: chemicals, bacterial toxins, prostaglandins, and interleukin-1 that act on the hypothalamus to raise body temperature (9)

Endorphins: body's naturally produced morphines (painkillers) (8)

Enteral: within or into the GI tract (25)

Epidermis: outermost part of the skin (44)

Epiglottitis: inflammation of the epiglottis (22)

Epilepsy: chronic pattern of seizure activity; seizure disorder (38)

Epileptogenic focus: group of neurons that fire abnormally, causing a seizure (38)

Epistaxis: nosebleed (22)

Equianalgesic doses: doses of different drugs that have the same analgesic effect when administered to the same individual; drug dosages are equianalgesic if they have the same effect as morphine sulfate 10 mg IM (8)

Erectile dysfunction: impotence; inability to achieve and maintain an erection (31)

Erythema: reddening of the skin (44)

Erythrocytes: red blood cells (19)

Eschar: hard crust that forms over a burn wound (46)

Esophageal varices: enlarged, overdistended veins in the distal esophagus (27)

Estrogens: steroid hormones essential to developing and maintaining female secondary sex characteristics (30)

Ethics: principles of conduct concerned with moral duty, values, obligations, and the distinction between right and wrong (1)

Ethnic group: a group of people who share and are unified by experiences and backgrounds based on such factors as socioeconomic status, religion, education, and residence (3)

Euphoria: an exaggerated feeling of well-being (53)

Euthanasia: (from the Greek for painless, easy, gentle, or good death) a term commonly used to signify killing prompted by a humanitarian motive (13)

Evaluation: the final step of the nursing process, which allows the nurse to determine whether the plan was effective and to continue, revise, or terminate the plan (1)

Evidence-based practices: use of the best current evidence together with clinical knowledge and patient values and preferences to provide optimal care (1)

Evisceration: protrusion of body organs from a wound dehiscence (10)

Exacerbation: time period in some chronic illnesses when symptoms reappear after a remission (2)

Executive function: complex cognitive skills including planning, organizing, judgment, abstracting (48)

Exophthalmos: forward protrusion of the eyeballs (34)

External otitis: inflammation of the ear canal; swimmer's ear (40)

Extracellular fluid (ECF): body fluid located outside of cells (7)

F

Family: a group of people who live together or in close contact and who take care of each other and provide assistance for their dependent members (3, 47)

Fasciculations: involuntary contractions of the voluntary muscles (39)

Female condom: a lubricated polyurethane sheath inserted into the vagina and held in place by a flexible ring around the cervix (33)

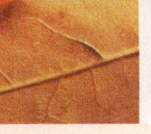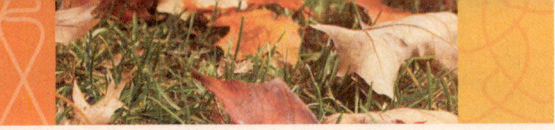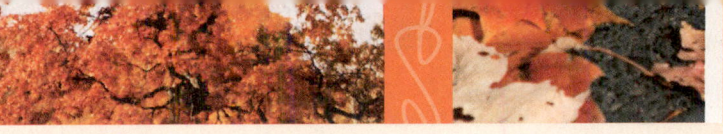

Filtration: process by which water and solutes move across capillary membranes, driven by fluid pressure (7)

Fistula: abnormal tubelike passage from one body cavity to another (9)

Flaccidity: decreased muscle tone (37)

Fluid volume deficit: dehydration, may be due to excessive fluid losses, insufficient fluid intake, or both (7)

Fluid volume excess: greater than normal amount of fluid in the body (7)

Folliculitis: infection that begins at the hair follicle opening and extends down into the follicle (45)

Fracture: break in the continuity of a bone (42)

Full-thickness burn: burn (third-degree) that involves all layers of the skin and may extend into subcutaneous fat, connective tissue, muscle, and bone (46)

Furuncle: boil, infection of the hair follicle (45)

G

Gangrene: tissue death from reduced or absent blood supply (36, 42)

Gastrectomy: partial or total removal or resection of the stomach (25)

Gastritis: inflammation of the stomach lining (25)

Gastroenteritis: inflammation of the stomach and intestines (25)

Gastroesophageal reflux: backward movement of gastric contents into the esophagus (25)

Geriatrics: the area of health care that focuses on the holistic care of older adults, including physiologic, psychologic, and socioeconomic aspects of aging (4)

Gerontologic nursing: care of the older adult (4)

Glaucoma: disorder of increased intraocular pressure and gradual loss of peripheral vision (40)

Glomerular filtration rate: amount of fluid filtered from the blood into the glomerular capsule per minute (28)

Glomeruli: small clusters of capillaries in the kidney (28)

Glomerulonephritis: inflammation of the glomeruli (29)

Gluconeogenesis: process to make glucose in the liver (34)

Glycogenolysis: conversion of glycogen into glucose in the liver and muscles (34)

Glycosuria: presence of glucose in the urine (36)

Goiter: enlargement of the thyroid gland (35)

Gout: a disorder of purine metabolism characterized by the accumulation of urate crystals in joints and surrounding tissues (43)

Grief: emotional response to loss and its changes (13)

Guillain–Barré syndrome: acute progressive inflammation of the peripheral nervous system (39)

Gynecomastia: breast enlargement (31)

H

Half-life: the amount of time needed for elimination processes to decrease the original blood concentration by 50% (6)

Hallucinations: sensory perceptions that seem real but occur without external stimuli; most common is hearing voices (49)

Handoff: transfer of responsibility for care from one individual or care unit to another (10)

Health: state of complete physical, mental, and social well-being, not merely the absence of disease or infirmity (2)

Health care informatics: the management and use of data, information, and knowledge through computer information systems (1)

Health care–associated infections: infections associated with health care delivery in any setting (9)

Health disparities: differences in the incidence and outcomes of diseases and disorders that occur among specific population groups (3)

Health–illness continuum: representation of health as a dynamic process, with high-level wellness at one extreme of the continuum and death at the opposite extreme (2)

Heart failure: inability of the heart to function as a pump to meet the needs of the body (17)

Heat stroke: life-threatening condition in which the body cannot cool itself (14)

Helper T cells: cells that turn on the immune system (11)

Hematemesis: vomiting blood (25)

Hematochezia: bright red blood in the stool (25)

Hematoma: collection of blood within a tissue, organ, or space caused by a break in a blood vessel (38, 42)

Hematuria: blood in the urine (may be microscopic or visible) (28, 29)

Hemiplegia: paralysis on one side of the body (38)

Hemodynamics: the study of the pressures involved in blood circulation (17)

Hemoglobin: oxygen-carrying protein in red blood cells (19)

Hemolysis: destruction of red blood cells (19)

Hemophilia: hereditary clotting factor deficiencies (20)

Hemoptysis: bloody sputum (23)

Hemorrhage: excessive loss of blood (10)

Hemorrhoids: weakening and dilation of veins of the anus or anal canal (26)

Hemostasis: blood clotting (19)

Hemothorax: blood in the pleural space (23)

Hepatic encephalopathy: brain dysfunction related to accumulation of substances normally detoxified by the liver (27)

Hepatitis: inflammation of the liver (27)

Hepatocytes: liver cells (24)

Hepatorenal syndrome: kidney failure associated with end-stage liver disease (27)

Herniated intervertebral disk: injury to the disk between two vertebrae that compresses the nearby spinal nerve root, resulting in motor and sensory changes and pain (39)

Herpes simplex: (fever blisters; cold sores) infections caused by herpes virus I or II (45)

Herpes zoster: (shingles) viral infection of a dermatome section of the skin caused by varicella zoster, the herpes virus that causes chickenpox (45)

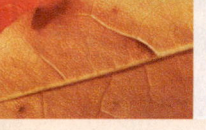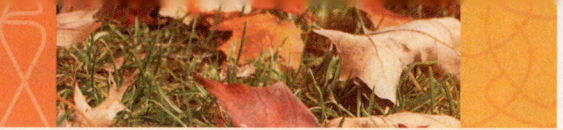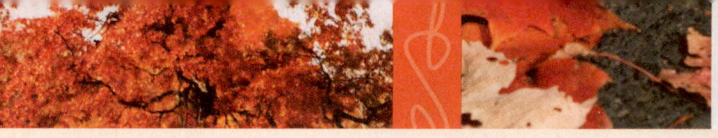

High-level wellness: way of functioning to reach one's maximum potential at a particular point in time (2)

HIPAA (Health Insurance Portability and Accountability Act): laws designed to protect individuals' health information while allowing such information to be shared as needed for effective care (1)

Hirsutism: excessive hair growth or hair growth in unusual places, such as facial hair on women (35)

Histocompatibility: immunologic similarity or compatibility; determines the ability of cells and tissues to survive transplant without rejection (11)

Holistic care: caring for a person as a whole, including body, mind, and spirit (47)

Holistic: health care concerned with the whole person—physical, emotional, and spiritual (1)

Home health care: health and social services provided in the home to people who are chronically ill, disabled, or recovering from an illness (2)

Homeostasis: body's tendency to maintain a state of physiologic balance in the presence of constantly changing conditions (2, 7)

Homonymous hemianopia: loss of vision in half of the visual field (38)

Hormones: chemical messengers of the body (34)

Hospice: model (not a place) of care for patients and families when the patient is faced with a limited life expectancy; it emphasizes quality rather than quantity of life (13)

Human immunodeficiency virus (HIV): retrovirus that causes HIV disease and AIDS (11)

Human papillomavirus: virus causing genital warts, a sexually transmitted disease (11)

Huntington disease: progressive disease of the CNS affecting personality, intellectual function, and movement (39)

Hydronephrosis: abnormal dilation of the renal pelvis and calyces (29)

Hyperglycemia: high blood glucose level (34, 36)

Hyperkalemia: serum potassium level greater than 5.0 mEq/L (7)

Hypernatremia: serum sodium concentration greater than 145 mEq/L (7)

Hyperorality: putting anything within reach into one's mouth (48)

Hyperosmolar hyperglycemic state (HHS): life-threatening illness occurring in type 2 diabetics, characterized by hyperglycemia, severe dehydration, and coma (36)

Hypersensitivity: altered immune response to an antigen that causes harm to the body (11)

Hypertension: blood pressure higher than 140 mm Hg systolic or 90 mm Hg diastolic on three separate readings several weeks apart (18)

Hypertrophic scar: overgrowth of dermal tissue that remains within the boundaries of the wound (46)

Hypervolemia: excess intravascular fluid (7)

Hypoglycemia: low blood glucose level (34, 36)

Hypokalemia: serum potassium level less than 3.5 mEq/L (7)

Hypomania: a short episode of abnormally elevated, expansive, or irritable mood (50)

Hyponatremia: serum sodium less than 132 mEq/L (7)

Hypovolemic shock: shock caused by a decrease in intravascular volume (14)

Hypoxemia: low oxygen levels in the blood (7)

Hysterectomy: removal of the uterus (32)

I

Icteric: related to jaundice (27)

ICU psychosis: acute confusion after 2 to 3 days in the intensive care unit (14)

Ideas of reference: a cognitive deficit in which a person misinterprets everyday events as having a personal meaning; for example, a person may believe that her thoughts about the plants being dry caused it to rain (52)

Ileostomy: opening of the ileum through the abdominal wall to the skin surface (26)

Illness: response a person has to a disease (2)

Illusion: a misinterpretation of environmental stimuli (48)

Immunocompetent: ability of the body's immune system to ward off pathogenic organisms (11)

Immunoglobulins: antibodies produced by B cells (11)

Immunosuppression: inability of the immune system to provide adequate immunity (9)

Impaired nurse: nurse with substance abuse problems, who may exhibit mood changes, irritability, forgetfulness, self-isolation, and inappropriate behavior (53)

Implementation: the fourth step in the nursing process (the "doing" phase) during which the nurse carries out planned interventions (1)

Impotence: erectile dysfunction; inability to achieve and maintain an erection (31)

Inappropriate affect: an emotional response that is not culturally appropriate for the situation, such as laughing when someone's pet dies (52)

Incision and drainage: procedure for draining pus from a wound (9)

Infection: condition in which pathogenic organisms trigger the inflammatory process (9)

Infectious disease: illness that is caused by a microorganism and can be transmitted to another person (9)

Infertility: inability to conceive during a year or more of unprotected intercourse (31, 32, 33)

Inflammation: nonspecific response that occurs when the body experiences any type of injury (9)

Inflammatory bowel disease: chronic bowel disease; includes two closely related disorders, ulcerative colitis and Crohn's disease (26)

Influenza: flu; highly contagious viral upper respiratory disease (22)

Informed consent: a legal document required for certain diagnostic procedures or therapeutic measures, including surgery (10)

Inotropic: strengthening the contraction of the heart (17)

Inpatient surgery: surgical procedure requiring admission to a hospital before and after the procedure (10)

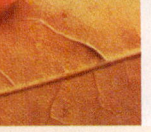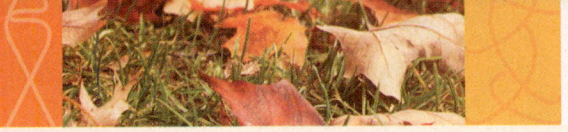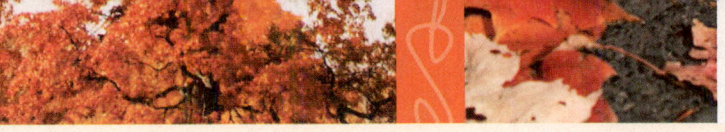

Insight: self-understanding (47, 49)

Insomnia: difficulty falling asleep or staying asleep, or awakening too early (51)

Inspection: method of assessing by observing the patient through the senses of seeing, smelling, and hearing (5)

Intermittent claudication: cramping or aching sensation in the calves, thighs, and buttocks that occurs with activity and is relieved by rest (18)

Interventions: purposeful actions performed by the nurse in implementing patient care (1)

Intoxication: reversible set of physical, psychologic, and behavioral symptoms caused by use of a substance (53)

Intracellular fluid (ICF): body fluid contained within the cells (7)

Intracranial pressure (ICP): pressure exerted within the cranium by the brain, blood, and cerebrospinal fluid (38)

Intraoperative phase: beginning with entry into the operating room and ending with admittance to the postanesthesia care unit (PACU) or recovery room (10)

Invasiveness: an organism's ability to invade the body and cause disease (9)

Ischemia: decreased blood flow to body tissue or organ (14)

Ischemic: inadequate blood and oxygen to meet a tissue's metabolic needs (16)

J

Jaundice: yellowness of the skin, sclera of the eyes, mucous membranes, and body fluids due to deposited bile pigment resulting from excess bilirubin in the blood (27, 44)

K

Keloid: scar that extends beyond the boundaries of the original wound (46)

Keratitis: inflammation of the cornea (40)

Ketonuria: presence of ketones in the urine (36)

Ketosis: buildup of ketones in the body (36)

Kidney failure: condition in which the kidneys are unable to remove accumulated waste products from the blood (29)

Kindling process: the process of small seizure activity that builds up into a major seizure or manic episode (50)

Korsakoff syndrome: group of symptoms caused by a deficiency in B vitamins, including thiamine, riboflavin, and folic acid (53)

Kyphosis: exaggeration of the normal posterior curve of the thoracic spine (43)

L

Labile: changeable (53)

Laparoscopy: exploration of the abdomen using an endoscope (26)

Laparotomy: surgical opening of the abdomen (26)

Laryngectomy: removal of the larynx (voice box) (22)

Laryngitis: inflammation of the larynx (22)

Laryngospasm: spasm of the muscles of the larynx (22)

Leukemia: malignant proliferation of white blood cells (20)

Leukocytes: white blood cells (11, 19)

Leukocytosis: white blood cell count greater than normal (9)

Leukopenia: white blood cell count below normal (9)

Lewy body disease: dementia characterized by deposits of alpha-synuclein protein (the Lewy bodies) in the nuclei of brain neurons in the areas that influence memory and motor control (48)

Libido: sexual desire (30)

Lithotomy position: supine position with the knees flexed and separated (30)

Living will: legal document that formally expresses a person's wishes regarding life-sustaining treatment in the event of terminal illness or permanent unconsciousness (13)

Loading dose: an initial higher-than-normal dose of a drug (6)

Lobules: basic functional units of the liver (24)

Local anesthesia: administration of an anesthetic to a specific area of the body (10)

Loss: occurs when a valued object, person, body part, or situation is lost, removed, or irreversibly changed (13)

Lower body obesity: peripheral obesity, characterized by a waist–hip ratio of less than 0.8 (25)

Lymphadenopathy: swelling and enlargement of the lymph nodes (9, 20)

Lymphatic system: the lymphoid organs, including lymph vessels, lymph nodes, spleen, and thymus (19)

M

Macrophages: mature, large white blood cells that develop from monocytes (9)

Macular degeneration: loss of neurons in the area of central vision of the eye (40)

Maladaptive: having to do with coping behaviors that are unhealthy (51)

Malignant: describes tumors that grow aggressively and do not respond to the body's controls (12)

Malignant lymphomas: cancerous tumors of lymphoid tissue (20)

Malnutrition: long-term nutrient and calorie deficiencies resulting in health problems (25)

Malpractice: harm that results from the actions, or failure to act, of a licensed person (1)

Mammography: x-ray imaging of breast tissue to detect breast cancer (30)

Manifestations: objective and subjective data (signs and symptoms) associated with a specific illness (2, 5)

Marfan syndrome: hereditary disorder affecting connective tissue, bones, muscles, and ligaments (18)

Mastectomy: removal of the breast (32)

Medical–surgical nursing: the health care and illness care of adults (1)

Melanoma: skin cancer that arises from melanocytes, the cells that produce skin pigment (45)

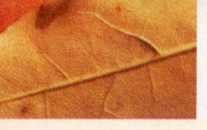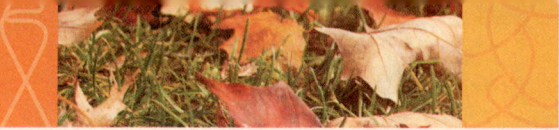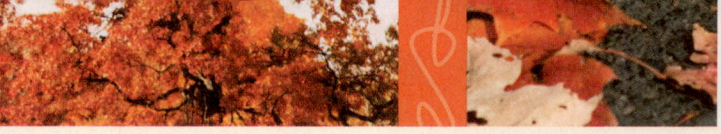

Melena: black, tarry stool that contains blood (25)

Memory cells: cells that provide immunity when reexposed to a past antigen (11)

Meningitis: inflammation of the meninges of the brain and spinal cord (38)

Menopause: period during which menstrual activity permanently ceases (32)

Metabolic acidosis: increased hydrogen ion concentration and a pH of less than 7.35 due to inadequate bicarbonate in relation to the amount of acid in the body (7)

Metabolic alkalosis: decreased hydrogen ion concentration and a pH of greater than 7.45 due to an excess of bicarbonate (7)

Metabolism: biochemical reactions that occur in the body's cells (24)

Metastasis: process by which malignant neoplasms spread to distant sites; a secondary tumor formed by this process (12)

Metrorrhagia: bleeding between menstrual periods (32)

Microalbuminuria: presence of small amounts of albumin in the urine (36)

Milieu: therapeutic environment, or using the environment as part of therapy (49)

Miosis: constriction of one or both pupils (5)

Moderate (or conscious) sedation/analgesia: provides analgesia, amnesia, and depressed consciousness but allows the patient to maintain airway and respirations independently and to respond to verbal commands and physical stimulation (10)

Monoamine oxidase inhibitors (MAOIs): antidepressants that work by blocking the enzyme monoamine oxidase that breaks down neurotransmitters in brain synapses, increasing available serotonin and norepinephrine (50)

Mood: pervasive and sustained emotion that influences how a person perceives the world (50)

Multiple myeloma: malignancy in which plasma cells multiply uncontrollably and infiltrate bone marrow, lymph nodes, and other tissues (20)

Multiple organ dysfunction syndrome: irreversible complication of shock in which the body's systems fail (14)

Multiple sclerosis (MS): chronic, degenerative disease that damages the myelin sheath surrounding the axons of the CNS (39)

Mutation: change in an organism from its original form to a different form (9)

Mutual monogamy: a sexual relationship in which the partners have sex only with each other (33)

Myasthenia gravis: chronic autoimmune disorder that is characterized by muscle fatigue (39)

Mydriasis: dilation of one or both pupils (5)

Myelin sheath: white, fatty substance that insulates and protects some axons (37)

Myocarditis: inflammation of the heart muscle (17)

Myopathy: a condition characterized by muscle cramps of sudden onset, plus pain, tenderness, and edema of skeletal muscles (53)

Myxedema coma: life-threatening form of hypothyroidism (35)

N

Narrow-spectrum antibiotics: antibiotics that act against a few pathogens (9)

Natural killer (NK) cells: white blood cells that can attack viruses and cancer cells (11)

Nausea: a vague but unpleasant sensation of sickness or queasiness (25)

Negative symptoms: a deficit or decrease of normal functions (49)

Neologisms: use of made-up words; symptom of disorganized thinking (49)

Neoplasm: tumor; mass of abnormal cells that grows independently of its surrounding structures and has no physiologic purpose (12)

Nephrons: functional units of the kidney (28)

Nephrotoxins: agents that damage kidney tissue (29)

Neurofibrillary tangles: knotting of a protein called tau, part of the neurons' internal support system; characteristic of Alzheimer disease (48)

Neurogenic shock: shock caused by an interruption to the sympathetic nervous system (14)

Neuroleptic malignant syndrome: a potentially fatal side effect of antipsychotic drugs (49)

Neuron: basic cell of the nervous system (37, 47)

Neuropathic pain: pain caused by damage to the CNS or peripheral nerves (8)

Neurotransmitter: a chemical released during the transmission of an electrical impulse that assists or inhibits the impulse in crossing the synapse (37, 47)

Neutropenia: a decrease in the number of circulating neutrophils (the prevalent white blood cells and an integral component of the immune system) (20)

Nevi: moles (45)

Nociceptors: nerve endings in the body that respond to noxious stimuli (8)

Nocturia: urinating more than one time at night (28, 29)

Nonmelanoma skin cancers: malignant lesions that do not arise from melanin-producing cells; basal cell carcinoma and squamous cell carcinoma (45)

Nonopioids: drugs such as acetaminophen and nonsteroidal anti-inflammatory drugs (NSAIDs) that are used to treat mild to moderate pain (8)

Nursing diagnosis: the second step in the nursing process; a clinical judgment about individual, family, or community responses to actual or potential health problems/life processes (1)

Nursing process: systematic and creative approach to thinking and acting that nurses use as they care for patients (1)

Nutrients: substances in food used for growth, maintenance, and repair of the body (24)

Nutrition: process of ingesting, absorbing, using, and eliminating food (24)

Nystagmus: involuntary eye movements (37)

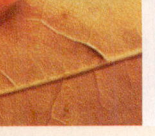
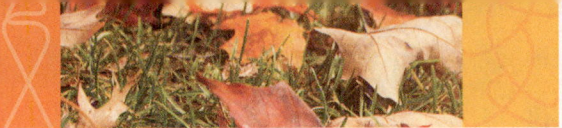
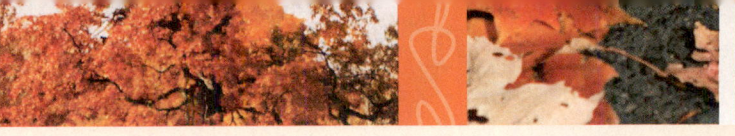

O

Obesity: excess adipose tissue or fat, with body weight above ideal for gender, height, and age (25)

Objective data: observable or measurable pieces of data that can be seen, heard, touched, or smelled (also called *signs*) (5)

Obsessions: recurrent and intrusive thoughts that cause marked distress (51)

Occult: hidden (25)

Oncogenes: genes capable of triggering cancer (12)

Oncology: the study of cancer; oncologists are physicians who specialize in cancer care (12)

Oophorectomy: removal of the ovary (32)

Opioid tolerance: process by which the body requires a progressively greater amount of an opioid drug to achieve the same results (8)

Opioids: drugs derived from opium (e.g., morphine) used to treat moderate to severe pain (8)

Orchiectomy: surgical removal of the testes (31)

Orthopnea: difficulty breathing while lying down (5, 7, 17)

Osmosis: transport process by which water moves across a semipermeable membrane from an area of lower solute concentration to an area of higher solute concentration (7)

Osteoarthritis: degenerative joint disease with progressive loss of joint cartilage in synovial joints (43)

Osteomyelitis: infection of the bone (43)

Osteoporosis: bone disorder characterized by loss of bone mass (43)

Ostomy: a surgically created opening from an organ to the surface of the body (26)

Otitis media: inflammation or infection of the middle ear (40)

Otorrhea: leakage of fluid from the external ear (38)

Outcomes: time-specific, achievable goals (1)

P

Pain: unpleasant sensory and emotional experience associated with actual or potential tissue damage (8)

Pain threshold: point at which each person recognizes pain (8)

Pain tolerance: amount and duration of pain a person can stand before seeking relief (8)

Palliative care: service provided to individuals who have an incurable illness; focused on promoting comfort by alleviating symptoms such as pain, nausea, dyspnea, and anxiety (13)

Pallor: paleness of skin (44)

Palpation: method of assessing by using the hands to touch and feel (5)

Pancreatitis: inflammation of the pancreas (27)

Paracentesis: removal of fluid from the peritoneal cavity (27)

Paradoxical response: contradictory result, opposite from expected effect (51)

Paralytic ileus: slowing or stopping of peristalsis (26)

Paraplegia: paralysis of the lower half of the body (39)

Parasuicidal behavior: behavior aimed at harming but not killing oneself (52)

Parenteral nutrition: intravenous administration of a solution that meets all the patient's nutritional needs (except fiber); hyperalimentation (25)

Parkinson disease: chronic, progressive, degenerative neurologic disease that alters motor coordination (39)

Paroxysmal nocturnal dyspnea: attacks of acute shortness of breath that occur at night, awakening the patient (17)

Partial-thickness burn: burn (second-degree) that involves the entire dermis and may also involve the hair follicles (46)

Pathogens: microorganisms that are capable of producing disease (9)

Pathologic fracture: break in a diseased or weakened bone that occurs with minimal force or trauma (43)

Patient-centered care: care in which the nurse attends to the uniqueness of the individual, planning and adapting care to the needs of that person (1, 3)

Patient-controlled analgesia (PCA): self-administration of opioid medications by a programmed infusion pump (8)

Pediculosis: infestation with lice (45)

Pelvic inflammatory disease (PID): infection of the pelvic organs; often associated with sexually transmitted infections (32)

Peptic ulcer: break in the mucous lining of the gastrointestinal tract where it comes in contact with gastric juice (25)

Percussion: method of assessing by tapping the body to produce sound waves that provide information about underlying body structures or organs (5)

Pericardial effusion: an abnormal collection of fluid between the pericardial layers (17)

Pericardial friction rub: leathery, grating sound produced by the inflamed pericardial layers rubbing against the chest wall or pleura (17)

Pericarditis: inflammation of the pericardium (17)

Perimenopause: the period of several years around menopause during which estrogen levels decline (32)

Perioperative: relating to the period immediately before, during, and after surgery (10)

Peripheral vascular disease (PVD): disorder caused by decreased blood supply to tissues due to arteriosclerosis or atherosclerosis (18)

Peripheral vascular resistance: force that opposes blood flow (15)

Peripheral vascular system: network of blood vessels that carry blood to peripheral tissues and then return it to the heart (15)

Peristalsis: alternating waves of contraction and relaxation of involuntary muscle (24)

Peritonitis: inflammation of the peritoneum, the double-layered membrane that lines the walls and organs of the abdominal cavity (26)

Personality: relatively stable way in which a person thinks, feels, and behaves (52)

Pertussis: an upper respiratory infection also known as whooping cough (22)

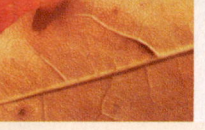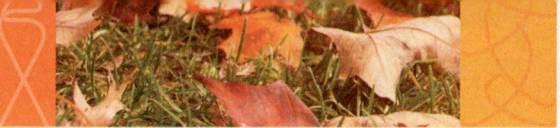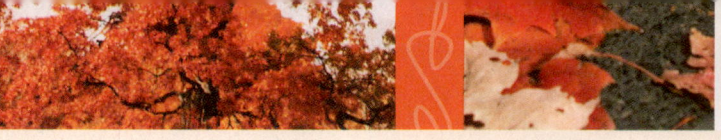

Petechiae: small, flat, purple or red spots on the skin or mucous membranes that do not blanch with pressure (20)

pH: measure of hydrogen ion concentration in a solution; as H^+ concentration increases, the solution becomes more acid and the pH falls; as H^+ concentration decreases, the solution becomes more alkaline and the pH rises (7)

Phagocytosis: process by which phagocytes ingest harmful bacteria and dead tissue cells (9)

Phantom limb pain: pain in a missing extremity resulting from nerve trauma during surgery (42)

Pharmacodynamics: the study of how drugs produce their effects in the body to result in a pharmacologic response (6)

Pharmacokinetics: the study of how drugs are processed by the body (6)

Pharmacology: the study of drugs and their uses in the body (6)

Pharyngitis: acute inflammation of the pharynx; sore throat (22)

Pheochromocytoma: tumor of the adrenal medulla that causes an increased release of catecholamines (35)

Phobia: persistent and irrational fear (51)

Photophobia: extreme sensitivity to light (40)

Planning: the third step in the nursing process, in which the nurse develops a list of nursing interventions (1)

Plasma: the liquid part of the blood (19)

Platelets: small fragments of cytoplasm without nuclei; an essential component of the body's clotting mechanism (19)

Pleural effusion: collection of fluid in the pleural space (23)

Pleuritis: inflammation of the pleura that covers the lung surface and lines the inner chest wall (23)

Pneumatic antishock garment (PASG): inflatable garment applied to trauma victims in the prehospital setting to raise blood pressure (14)

Pneumocystis jiroveci pneumonia: pneumonia caused by a fungus-like organism that rarely causes disease in patients with an intact immune system (11)

Pneumonia: inflammation of the respiratory bronchioles and alveoli (23)

Pneumothorax: accumulation of air in the pleural space (23)

Polycythemia: erythrocytosis; abnormally high red blood cell count and high hematocrit (20)

Polydipsia: excessive thirst (36)

Polyphagia: excessive hunger (36)

Polysubstance abuse: use of a variety of substances to induce an altered physical, mental, or emotional state (53)

Polyuria: excessive urine output (36)

Portal hypertension: elevated blood pressure in the portal venous system (27)

Positive inotropic drugs: group of drugs used to increase cardiac output (14)

Positive symptoms: symptoms of a disorder that are an excess or distortion of normal functions (49)

Postoperative phase: beginning with admission to the postanesthesia recovery area and ending with complete recovery from the surgical intervention (10)

Potentiation: when the action of one drug increases the effect of the second drug (6)

Praxis: performance of skills (48)

Premenstrual syndrome (PMS): complex of symptoms including irritability, depression, edema, and breast tenderness preceding the monthly menses (32)

Preoperative phase: beginning when the decision for surgery is made and ending when the patient is transferred to the operating room (10)

Presbycusis: progressive hearing loss associated with aging (40)

Presbyopia: condition in which the lens of the eye becomes less elastic in older adults, causing decreased near vision (37)

Pressure ulcers: bedsores; decubitus ulcers; ischemic lesions of the skin and underlying tissue caused by external pressure that impairs the flow of blood and lymph (45)

Pressured speech: rapid, persistent speech associated with mania, difficult to interrupt (50)

Primary care: comprehensive, first-contact health and illness care across the life span (2)

Primary hypertension: hypertension with no identified cause (18)

Primary intention: healing that takes place when a wound is uncomplicated and clean and has little tissue loss (10)

Procedural memory: applies to skills or physical activities (48)

Prodromal phase: in schizophrenia, a period of time in which patients have symptoms before they have a full psychotic episode (49)

Prodromal symptoms: warning symptoms that occur before the onset of disease manifestations; for example, prodromal symptoms of herpes outbreaks include burning, itching, tingling, or throbbing at the sites where lesions commonly appear (33)

Professional boundaries: the limits maintained between a person who is vulnerable (the patient) and the person with power (the nurse) (1)

Prophylactic: preventing an infection (9)

Prostatectomy: surgical removal of the prostate gland (31)

Proteinuria: protein in the urine (29)

Pruritus: subjective itching sensation producing an urge to scratch (45)

Psoriasis: chronic, noninfectious skin disorder characterized by raised, reddened, round circumscribed plaques of varied size, covered by silvery white scales (45)

Psychomotor agitation: increased physical activity (50)

Psychomotor retardation: decreased purposeful activity (50)

Psychosis: a disorder of thought that causes delusions, hallucinations, disorganized speech, or disorganized behavior (49)

Psychosocial: psychologic or social factors (47)

Ptosis: drooping eyelid (37)

Pulmonary embolism: sudden blockage of a pulmonary artery that disrupts blood flow to the lungs (23)

Pulmonary hypertension: abnormal elevation of the pulmonary arterial pressure (23)

Purpura: purple rashes caused by blood leaking into the skin; hemorrhage into the tissues (19, 20)

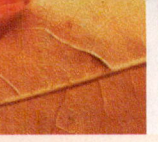
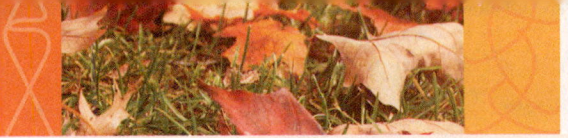
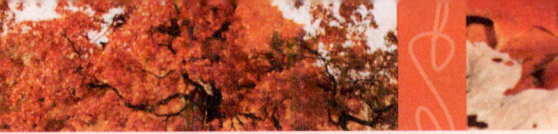
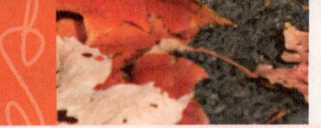

Pyelonephritis: inflammatory disorder affecting the renal pelvis and parenchyma (29)

Pyuria: cloudy, foul-smelling urine that contains pus (28, 29)

Q

Quality improvement: the use of data to evaluate the outcomes of care and to design and test changes to improve the quality and safety of health care systems (1)

R

Rabies: viral infection of the CNS caused by an animal bite (39)

Race: a term used to identify differences in physical characteristics such as skin color, eye shape, and bone structure (3)

Reality orientation: includes frequent reminders of the name, location, time, and situation of the patient (often called orienting to "person, place, and time") (48)

Rectocele: herniation of the rectum into the vagina (32)

Reduction: restoration of normal alignment of a bone or joint (42)

Referred pain: pain that begins in one area of the body but is felt in another part (8)

Reflex: involuntary motor response to a stimulus (37)

Refraction: bending of light rays to focus on the retina (37)

Regurgitation: failure of a valve to close properly, allowing substances (e.g., blood) to flow back through it (17)

Rehabilitation: process of learning to live to one's maximum potential with a chronic impairment, disability, or substance dependency (2, 53)

Relapse: return to drug use after abstinence or of an illness after a period of freedom from symptoms (53)

Relative hypovolemia: hypovolemia resulting from shift of fluids from the intravascular space to the interstitial space (14)

Reminiscence: recalling and telling stories of past; "life review" (4)

Remission: time period in a chronic illness when the disease is present, but there are no symptoms (2)

Renal colic: acute, severe, intermittent flank pain usually associated with renal calculi (29)

Renin–angiotensin–aldosterone system: blood pressure regulation system activated when there is reduced blood flow to the kidneys (14)

Resilience: flexibility in a stressful situation and the ability to return to normal afterward (51)

Respiration: exchange of gases between the person and the environment (21)

Respiratory acidosis: increased hydrogen ion concentration and a pH of less than 7.35 due to carbon dioxide retention (7)

Respiratory alkalosis: decreased hydrogen ion concentration and a pH of greater than 7.45 due to loss of carbon dioxide from the body (hyperventilation) (7)

Respiratory failure: inability of the lungs to oxygenate the blood and remove carbon dioxide well enough to meet the body's needs, even at rest (23)

Respite care: temporary patient care for the purpose of giving the regular caregiver time off (48)

Retinal detachment: separation of the retina from the vascular choroid layer of the eye (40)

Retroperitoneal: behind the peritoneum and outside the peritoneal cavity (24)

Rheumatic fever: a systemic inflammatory disease caused by an abnormal immune response to infection with group A beta-hemolytic streptococci (17)

Rheumatoid arthritis (RA): chronic, systemic inflammatory disorder resulting in persistent inflammation of the synovial tissue that lines joints (43)

Rhinitis: inflammation of the nasal cavities (22)

Rhinoplasty: surgical reconstruction of the nose (22)

Rhinorrhea: discharge of fluid from the nose (38)

Rhizotomy: surgical procedure that severs a nerve root to control pain (39)

"Rule of nines": rapid method of estimating the extent of a burn by assigning percentages to parts of the body (46)

S

Safety: (in health care): the effort to minimize the risk of harm to patients and to providers by examining both individual performance and system effectiveness (1)

Salpingo-oophorectomy: removal of the fallopian tubes and ovaries (32)

Scabies: infestation caused by a mite (45)

Sciatica: pain that occurs along the sciatic nerve (39)

Secondary hypertension: hypertension that results from a known cause (18)

Secondary intention: healing that occurs when a wound is large, gaping, and irregular (10)

Seizure: brief episode of abnormal electrical activity in nerve cells of the brain (38)

Senescence: the process of aging (4)

Sentinel event: any unexpected event in a health care facility that causes death or serious injury to a patient (6)

Septic shock: shock caused by overwhelming infection (14)

Septicemia: presence of bacteria in the blood (14)

Seroconversion: the presence of a disease's antibody in the blood (11)

Sexually transmitted infection (STI): any infection acquired as a result of sexual intercourse or intimate contact with an infected individual (33)

Shock: life-threatening condition characterized by inadequate blood flow to organs, tissues, and cells (10, 14)

Sinusitis: inflammation of the mucous membranes of the sinuses (22)

Sleep apnea: temporary absence of breathing during sleep (22)

Somogyi effect: early morning hyperglycemia after an episode of hypoglycemia at night (36)

Spasticity: increased muscle tone (37)

Spinal shock: temporary loss of reflex activity below the level of the spinal cord injury (39)

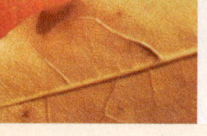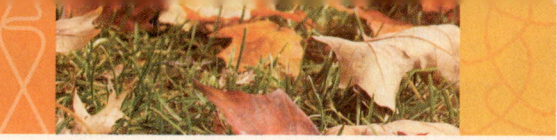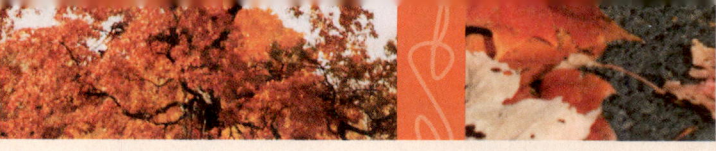

Sprain: injury to a ligament caused by a twisting motion (42)

Squamous cell carcinoma: malignant tumor of the squamous epithelium of the skin or mucous membranes (45)

Staging: system of classifying cancer by tumor size, lymph node involvement, and metastasis to distant sites (32)

Standard: statement or criterion that can be used by a profession and by the general public to measure quality of practice (1)

Standard Precautions: guidelines to protect the health care worker and prevent transmission of infectious organisms to other patients (9)

Status epilepticus: period of continuous tonic–clonic seizures (38)

Statutory law: the law created by federal and state legislatures (1)

Stem cells: immature cells that mature to become red blood cells, white blood cells, and platelets (19)

Stem cell transplant (SCT): transplantation of stem cells from one person to another (20)

Stenosis: narrowing of a valve opening, which obstructs forward blood flow (17)

Stigma: negative attitude marking people as less valuable (47)

Stomatitis: inflammation of the oral mucosa (25)

Strain: microscopic muscle tear that causes bleeding into the tissues (42)

Stridor: high-pitched, harsh sound heard during inspiration, usually caused by partial airway obstruction (22)

Stroke: an emergency condition that causes neurologic deficits from a decreased blood supply to a local area of the brain; also called cerebrovascular accident (CVA) or brain attack (38)

Stroke volume: amount of blood ejected from the heart with each contraction (15)

Subarachnoid hemorrhage: bleeding into the subarachnoid space in the brain (38)

Subjective data: experiences (data) that only the patient can describe, such as pain; also called symptoms (5)

Subtotal thyroidectomy: partial removal of the thyroid gland (35)

Suction: device to promote drainage of fluid from the wound, decreasing pressure on healing tissues and reducing hematoma or abscess formation (10)

Suicidal ideation: thinking about suicide (50)

Sundowning syndrome: behavior characterized by time disorientation and wandering in the evening (4, 48)

Superficial burn: first-degree burn that involves only the epidermal layer of the skin (46)

Superinfection: overgrowth of bacteria that occurs when antibiotics eliminate the body's normal flora (9)

Suppressor T cells: cells that turn off the immune system, limiting the immune response (11)

Synapse: space between two neurons across which an electrical impulse passes (37, 47)

Synergism: when two drugs given together cause a greater response than each drug given separately (6)

Synovial joints: joints in which synovial fluid separates the surfaces of the adjoining bones (41)

Systemic lupus erythematosus (SLE): chronic inflammatory connective tissue disease that affects multiple body systems (43)

Systole: period of ventricular contraction (15)

T

Tardive dyskinesia: late onset of movement disorder; irreversible side effect of antipsychotic medications (49)

T-cell lymphocytes (T cells): white blood cells responsible for cell-mediated immunity (11)

Tetanus: life-threatening disorder of the nervous system caused by an aerobic bacillus, *Clostridium tetani* (39)

Tetany: continuous spasm of the muscles; symptom complex of increased neuromuscular excitability associated with decreased ionized calcium levels (7, 35)

Tetraplegia: paralysis of the arms, legs, and trunk (39)

Thrombocytopenia: platelet count of less than 100,000 platelets/mL of blood (20)

Thrombus: blood clot (18)

Thymectomy: surgical removal of the thymus gland (39)

Thyroid crisis (thyroid storm): extreme state of hyperthyroidism (35)

Tinnitus: ringing in the ears (40)

Tolerance: need for more of a substance to achieve the same effect; diminished effect from continued use of the same amount of a substance (53)

Tonic contractions: contractions in which the body becomes rigid, with the arms and legs extended (38)

Tonsillectomy: surgical removal of the tonsils (22)

Tonsillitis: acute inflammation of the tonsils (22)

Tophi: urate deposits in subcutaneous tissues noted as small white nodules associated with gout (43)

Tort law: the set of laws that deal with injuries that occur to one person through the actions (or failure to take action) of another person (1)

Toxic shock syndrome (TSS): form of septic shock caused by *Staphylococcus aureus* (14)

Toxoid: injection containing a weakened toxin, for example, tetanus toxoid (11)

Tracheostomy: surgical opening into the trachea (22)

Traction: use of a pulling force to reduce a fracture or maintain alignment (42)

Transient ischemic attack (TIA): brief episode of reversible neurologic deficits (38)

Transitional care: facilitation of the transition of chronically ill patients from one health care setting to another or to home (2)

Transmission-Based Precautions: guidelines to prevent spread of infection through the air, by droplet, and through contact (9)

Trauma: injury caused by applying more force to tissue than it is able to absorb (42)

Triage: system to identify who will receive medical attention first (14)

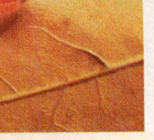
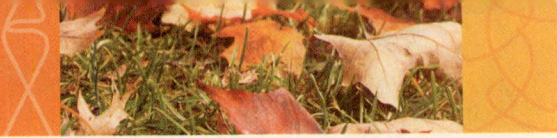
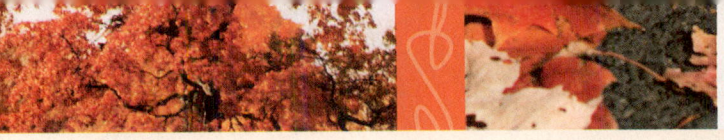

Trigeminal neuralgia: disease of the trigeminal nerve resulting in periodic, severe, one-sided facial pain (39)

Tuberculosis: a chronic infectious disease caused by *Mycobacterium tuberculosis* (23)

Tumor: a mass of abnormal cells that grows independently of its surrounding structures and has no physiologic purpose (12)

Type and cross-match: test to determine donor and recipient ABO types and Rh groups and their compatibility with one another (14)

U

Ulcerative colitis: chronic inflammatory bowel disorder of the mucosa and submucosa of the colon and rectum (26)

Universal protocol: an important safety initiative established by the Joint Commission in 2003 to reduce the "wrong site, wrong procedure, wrong person surgery" risk (10)

Unstable angina (UA): angina occurring with increasing frequency, at rest, or unpredictably, and acute myocardial ischemia with or without muscle tissue damage (16)

Upper body obesity: central obesity, characterized by a waist–hip ratio of greater than 1 in men and greater than 0.8 in women (25)

Uremia: a symptom complex caused by excess metabolic waste products in the blood (29)

Urgency: a sudden, compelling need to urinate (29)

Urinary incontinence: involuntary urination (29)

Urolithiasis: development of stones within the urinary tract (29)

Uterine prolapse: descent of the uterus into the vagina (32)

V

Vaginitis: inflammation or infection of the vagina (32)

Valvular heart disease: deformity of one or more of the heart valves affecting blood flow through the chambers of the heart and/ or to the pulmonary or systemic circulation (17)

Varicose veins: irregular, tortuous veins with incompetent valves (18)

Vascular dementia: condition caused by a series of small brain artery occlusions or infarcts (strokes) that cause *ischemia* (low blood and oxygen supply) and tissue death in the brain (48)

Vasectomy: sterilization procedure in which a portion of the spermatic cord is removed (31)

Vasopressor drugs: drugs used to increase the blood pressure (14)

Venous insufficiency: stasis of venous blood flow in the lower extremities (18)

Venous thrombosis: formation of a blood clot (thrombus) on the wall of a vein, which obstructs the flow of blood back to the heart (18)

Ventilation: air movement into and out of the lungs (21)

Vertigo: sensation of whirling or rotation (40)

Vesicles: blisters (33)

Virulence: power of a microorganism to cause an infection (9)

Vomiting: the forceful expulsion of stomach contents (25)

Vulva: perineal area outside the vagina (33)

W

Warts: verrucae; lesions caused by the human papillomavirus (45)

Wernicke syndrome: alcoholic encephalopathy; characterized by ataxia, paralysis of eye muscles, nystagmus, and mental confusion (53)

Widowhood: loss of a spouse from death (4)

Withdrawal: set of symptoms resulting from discontinuation or reduction of a substance after heavy or prolonged use (53)

X

Xerosis: dry skin (45)

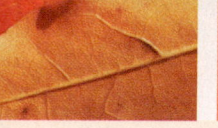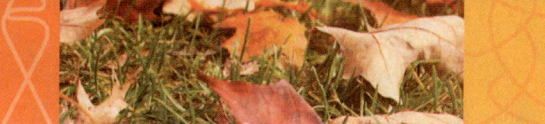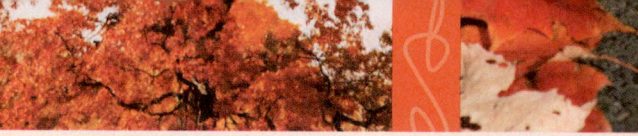

References and Resources

FREQUENTLY USED REFERENCES AND RESOURCES

Abrams, A. C., Pennington, S. S., & Lammon, C. B. (2009). *Clinical drug therapy* (9th ed.). Philadelphia: Lippincott Williams & Wilkins.

Adams, M. P., Holland, L. N., Jr., & Bostwick, P. M. (2011). *Pharmacology for nurses: A pathophysiologic approach* (3rd ed.). Upper Saddle River, NJ: Pearson Prentice Hall.

Adams, M. P., & Urban, C. Q. (2013). *Pharmacology connections to nursing practice* (2nd ed.). Upper Saddle River, NJ: Pearson.

Amer, K. S. (2013). *Quality and safety for transformational nursing core competencies.* Upper Saddle River, NJ: Pearson.

American Cancer Society. (2012). *Cancer facts & figures 2012.* Atlanta, GA: Author.

American Psychiatric Association. (2013). *Diagnostic and statistical manual of mental disorders* (5th ed.). Washington, DC: Author.

Aschenbrenner, A., & Venable, S. (2009). *Drug therapy in nursing* (3rd ed.). Philadelphia: Lippincott Williams & Wilkins.

Berman, A., & Snyder, S. (2012). *Skills in clinical nursing* (7th ed.). Upper Saddle River, NJ: Pearson.

Copstead, L. C., & Banasik, J. L. (2010). *Pathophysiology* (4th ed.). St. Louis, MO: Elsevier/Saunders.

D'Amico, D., & Barbarito, C. (2012). *Health & physical assessment in nursing* (2nd ed.). Upper Saddle River, NJ: Pearson.

Fontaine, K. L. (2011). *Complementary & alternative therapies for nursing practice* (3rd ed.). Upper Saddle River, NJ: Pearson.

Giger, J. N. (2013). *Transcultural nursing: Assessment & intervention* (6th ed.). St. Louis, MO: Elsevier.

Grossman, S., & Porth, C. (2014). Porth's pathophysiology: Concepts of altered health states (9th ed.). Philadelphia, PA: Wolters Kluwer/Lippincott Williams & Wilkins.

Herdman, T. H. (Ed.). (2012). *NANDA International Nursing diagnoses: Definitions & classification, 2012–2014.* Oxford, UK: Wiley-Blackwell.

Huether, S. E., & McCance, K. L. (2012). *Understanding pathophysiology* (5th ed.). St. Louis, MO: Elsevier.

Jarvis, C. (2009). *Physical examination & health assessment* (5th ed.). St. Louis, MO: Mosby.

Kee, J. L. (2014). *Laboratory and diagnostic tests with nursing implications* (9th ed.). Upper Saddle River, NJ: Pearson.

Keltner, N. L., Schwecke, L. H., Bostrom, C. E., & McGuinness, T. (2011). *Psychiatric nursing* (6th ed.). St. Louis, MO: Mosby.

Lehne, R. (2010). *Pharmacology for nursing care* (7th ed.). St. Louis, MO: Saunders.

Longo, D. L., Fauci, A. S., Kasper, D. L., Hauser, S. L., Jameson, J. L., & Loscalzo, J. (Eds.). (2012). *Harrison's principles of internal medicine* (18th ed.). New York: McGraw-Hill.

Marieb, E., & Hoehn, K. (2013). *Human anatomy & physiology* (9th ed.). San Francisco, CA: Pearson Benjamin Cummings.

Martini, F., Nath, J., & Bartholomew, E. (2012). *Fundamentals of anatomy & physiology* (9th ed.). San Francisco, CA: Pearson Benjamin Cummings.

McCance, K. L., & Huether, S. E. (2010). *Pathophysiology: The biologic basis for disease in adults and children* (6th ed.). St. Louis, MO: Elsevier Mosby.

McPhee, S. J., Papadakis, M. A., & Rabow, M. (Eds.). (2012). *Current medical diagnosis & treatment* (51st ed.). New York: McGraw Hill.

Murray, R., Zentner, J., & Yakimo, R. (2009). *Health promotion strategies through the life span* (8th ed.). Upper Saddle River, NJ: Pearson Prentice Hall.

National Center for Health Statistics. (2012). *Health, United States, 11 with special feature on socioeconomic status and health.* Hyattsville, MD: Author.

National Heart, Lung, and Blood Institute, National Institutes of Health. (2012). *Morbidity & mortality: 2012 chart book of cardiovascular, lung, and blood diseases.* Bethesda, MD: Author.

Pender, N. J., Murdaugh, C. L., & Parsons, M. A. (2011). *Health promotion in nursing practice* (6th ed.). Upper Saddle River, NJ: Pearson Prentice Hall.

Porth, C. M. (2011). *Essentials of pathophysiology: Concepts of altered health states* (3rd ed.). Philadelphia: Lippincott Williams & Wilkins.

Rothrock, J. C. (2011). *Alexander's care of the patient in surgery* (14th ed.). St. Louis, MO: Mosby Elsevier.

Spector, R. E. (2013). *Cultural diversity in health and illness* (8th ed.). Upper Saddle River, NJ: Pearson.

Smith, S., Duell, D., & Martin, B. (2012). *Clinical nursing skills: Basic to advanced skills* (8th ed.). Upper Saddle River, NJ: Pearson.

Tabloski, P. A. (2014). *Gerontological nursing* (3rd ed.). Upper Saddle River, NJ: Pearson Prentice Hall.

Tucker, S., & Dauffenbach, V. (2011). *Nutrition & diet therapy for nurses.* Upper Saddle River, NJ: Pearson.

Wells, B., DiPiro, J., Schwinghammer, T., & DiPiro, C. (2012). *Pharmacotherapy handbook* (8th ed.). New York: McGraw Hill.

Wilkinson, J. M. (2013). *Pearson nursing diagnosis handbook* (10th ed.). Hoboken: Pearson.

Wilson, B., Shannon, M., & Shields, K. (2013). *Pearson nurse's drug guide 2013.* Upper Saddle River, NJ: Pearson.

Chapter-Specific References and Resources

CHAPTER 1

Amer, K. (2013). *Quality and safety for transformational nursing: Core competencies.* Upper Saddle River, NJ: Pearson.

American Nurses Association (ANA). (1980). *Nursing: A social policy statement.* Kansas City, MO: Author.

American Nurses Association (ANA). (2001). *Code of ethics for nurses.* Silver Spring, MD: Author.

American Nurses Association (ANA). (2010). *Nursing: Scope and standards of practice.* Silver Spring, MD: Author. Retrieved from Nursebooks.org

American Nurses Association (ANA). (2013). *What is nursing?* Retrieved from http://nursingworld.org/especiallyforyou/whatisnursing

Anderson, F. (2007). Finding HIPAA in your soup: Decoding the privacy rule. *American Journal of Nursing, 107*(2), 66–71.

Benner, P., Hughes, R., & Sutphen, M. (2008). Clinical reasoning, decision making, and action: Thinking critically and clinically. In R. G. Hughes (Ed.), *Patient safety and quality: An evidence-based handbook for nurses* (Chapter 6). Rockville, MD: Agency for Healthcare Research and Quality (US). Retrieved from http://www.ncbi.nlm.nih.gov/books/NBK2643/

Benner, P., Sutphen, M., Leonard, V., & Day, L. (2010). *Educating nurses: A call for radical transformation.* San Francisco, CA: Jossey-Bass.

Blais, K., & Hayes, J. (2011). *Professional nursing practice: Concepts and perspectives* (6th ed.). Upper Saddle River, NJ: Pearson.

Burggraf, V. (2012). Overview and summary: The new millennium: Evolving and emerging nursing roles. *OJIN: The Online Journal of Issues in Nursing, 17*(2), Overview and Summary.

Centers for Medicare and Medicaid Services (CMS). (2013). *Proposed clinical quality.* Retrieved from http://www.cms.gov/Medicare/Quality-Initiatives-Patient-Assessment-Instruments/QualityMeasures/ProposedClinicalQualityMeasuresfor2014.html

Cronenwett, L., Sherwood, G., Barnsteiner, J., Disch, J., & Johnson, J. (2007). Quality and safety education for nurses. *Nursing Outlook, 55*(3), 122–131.

Guido, G. (2010). *Legal & ethical issues in nursing* (5th ed.). Upper Saddle River, NJ: Pearson.

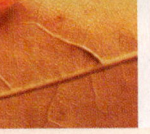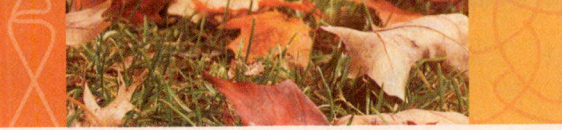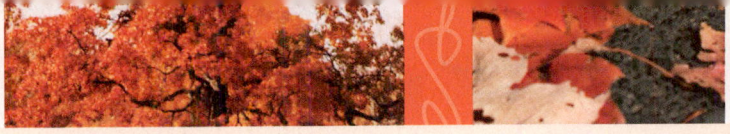

Herdman, T. H. (2012). *NANDA international nursing diagnoses: Definitions & classification, 2012–2014.* Oxford, UK: Wiley-Blackwell.

Howell, W. (2013). *The changing role of nurses.* Health forum: Hospitals and health networks. Retrieved from http://www.hhnmag.com/ hhnmag/jsp/articledisplay.jsp?crpath=HHNMAG/Article/data /03MAR2012/0312HHN_FEA_movingforward&domain=HHNMAG

International Council of Nurses. (2002). *The definition of nursing.* Geneva: Imprimeries Populaires.

(The) Joint Commission. (2013). *National Patient Safety Goals Effective January 1, 2014.* Hospital Accreditation Program. Retrieved from http://www.jointcommission.org/assets/1/6/HAP_NPSG_ Chapter_2014.pdf

Mitchell, P. H. (2008). Defining patient safety and quality care. In R. G. Hughes (Ed.), *Patient safety and quality: An evidence-based handbook for nurses* (Chapter 1). Rockville, MD: Agency for Healthcare Research and Quality (US). Retrieved from http://www.ncbi.nlm.nih.gov/books/ NBK2681/

National Academy of Sciences. (2004). The core competencies needed for health care professionals. In *Health professions education: A bridge to quality* (pp. 45–73). Washington, DC: Author.

National Association for Practical Nurse Education and Service (NAPNES). (2007a). *NAPNES standards of practice for licensed practical/vocational nurses.* Silver Spring, MD: Author.

National Association for Practical Nurse Education and Service (NAPNES). (2007b). *Standards of practice and educational competencies of graduates of practical/vocational nursing programs.* Silver Spring, MD: Author.

National Council of State Boards of Nursing, Inc. (NCSBN). (1996). *Professional boundaries: A nurse's guide to the importance of appropriate professional boundaries.* Chicago, IL: Author.

National Council of State Boards of Nursing, Inc. (NCSBN). (2012). *NCSBN model rules (2012).* Chicago, IL: Author.

Seago, J. A., Spetz, J., Chapman, S., Dyer, W., & Grumbach, K. (2004). *Supply, demand, and use of licensed practical nurses.* San Francisco: Center for Health Workforce, Distribution Studies, University of California.

Sherwood, G., & Barnsteiner, J. (2012). *Quality and safety in nursing: A competency approach to improving outcomes.*

Spector, N. (2005). *Practical nurse scope of practice white paper.* Chicago, IL: NCSBN. Retrieved January 19, 2008, from www.ncsbn.org/ Final_11_05_Practical_Nurse_Scope_Practice_White_Paper.pdf

Tanner, C. A. (2006). Thinking like a nurse: A research-based model of clinical judgment in nursing. *Journal of Nursing Education, 45*(6), 204–211.

CHAPTER 2

Berenson, R., Hammons, T., Gans, D., Zuckerman, S., Merrell, K., Underwood, W., et al. (2008). A house is not a home: Keeping patients at the center of practice redesign. *Health Affairs, 27*(5), 1219–1230.

Berryman, S., Palmer, S., Kohl, J., & Parham, J. (2013). Medical home model of patient-centered health care. *MEDSURG Nursing, (223),* 166–171, 196.

Boult, C., Green, A., Boult, L., Pacala, J., Snyder, C., & Leff, B. (2009). Successful models of comprehensive care for older adults with chronic conditions: Evidence for the institute of medicine's "Retooling for an aging America" report. *Journal of the American Geriatrics Society, 57*(12), 2328–2337.

Centers for Disease Control and Prevention (CDC). (2012a). *Chronic diseases and health promotion.* Retrieved from http://www.cdc.gov/chronicdisease/ overview/

Centers for Disease Control and Prevention (CDC). (2012b). *Ten leading causes of death and injury.* Retrieved from http://www.cdc.gov/injury/ wisqars/pdf/10LCID_All_Deaths_By_Age_Group_2010-a.pdf

Centers for Medicare & Medicaid Services (CMS). (2012). *New home health claims reporting requirements for G codes related to therapy and skilled nursing services* (MLN Matters®, MM7182). Baltimore, MD: Author.

Dunn, H. (1959). High level wellness for man and society. *American Journal of Public Health, 49,* 786–972.

Fielding, J., Teutsch, S., & Koh, H. (2012). Health reform and healthy people initiative. *American Journal of Public Health, 102*(1), 30–33.

Grant, R., & Greene, D. (2012). The health care home model: Primary health care meeting public health goals. *American Journal of Public Health, 102*(6), 1096–1103.

Henderson, S., Princell, C., & Martin, S. (2012). The patient-centered medical home. *American Journal of Nursing, 112*(12), 54–59.

Homes, A. (2011, August). The CNO and the ACO: An alphabet soup of healthcare reform. *Nursing Management,* 46–48.

National Center for Health Statistics. (2012). *Health, United States, 2011: With special feature on socioeconomic status and health.* Hyattsville, MD: U.S. Department of Health and Human Services.

The National Long-Term Care Ombudsman Resource Center. (2011). *Residents' rights.* Retrieved from www.ltcombudsman.org/issues/residents-rights

Naylor, M., Bowles, K., McCauley, K., Maccoy, M., Maislin, G., Pauly, M., et al. (2011). High-value transitional care: Translation of research into practice. *Journal of Evaluation in Clinical Practice, ISSN1365-2753,* 1–7.

Pender, N., Murdaugh, C., & Parsons, M. (2011). *Health promotion in nursing practice* (6th ed.). Upper Saddle River, NJ: Pearson.

Schulman-Green, D., Jaser, S., Martin, F., Alonzo, A., Grey, M., McCorkle, R., et al. (2012). Processes of self-management in chronic illness. *Journal of Nursing Scholarship, 44*(2), 136–144.

Seago, J. A., Spetz, J., Chapman, S., Dyer, W., & Grumbach, K. (2004). *Supply, demand, and use of licensed practical nurses.* San Francisco: Center for Health Workforce, Distribution Studies, University of California.

Strauss, A. (1984). *Chronic illness and the quality of life.* St. Louis, MO: Mosby.

Suchman, E. (1972). Stages of illness and medical care. In E. Jaco (Ed.), *Clients, physicians and illness.* New York: Free Press.

U.S. Department of Agriculture and U.S. Department of Health and Human Services. (2010). *Dietary Guidelines for Americans, 2010* (7th ed.). Washington, DC: U.S. Government Printing Office.

U.S. Department of Health and Human Services. (2010). *Healthy people 2020: Understanding and improving health* (3rd ed.). Washington, DC: U.S. Government Printing Office.

Wier, L., Pfuntner, A., Maeda, J., Stranges, E., Ryan, K., Jagadish, P., et al. (2011). *HCUP facts and figures: Statistics on hospital-based care in the United States, 2009.* Rockville, MD: Agency for Healthcare Research and Quality. Retrieved from http://www.hcup-us.ahrq.gov/reports.jsp

World Health Organization (WHO). (1974). *Constitution of the world health organization.* Geneva: Author.

CHAPTER 3

Adherents.com. (n.d.). *Major religions of the world ranked by number of adherents.* Retrieved from http://www.adherents.com/Religions_By_ Adherents.html

Amer, K. (2013). *Quality and safety for transformational nursing: Core competencies.* Upper Saddle River, NJ: Pearson.

American Cancer Society. (2013a). *Cancer facts & figures 2013.* Atlanta, GA: American Cancer Society.

American Cancer Society. (2013b). *Guidelines for the early detection of cancer.* Retrieved from www.cancer.org/Healthy/FindCancerEarly/ CancerScreeningGuidelines/American-cancer-society-guidelines-for-the-early-detection-of-cancer

Appel, L., Frohlich, E., Hall, J., Pearson, T., Sacco, R., Seals, D., et al. (2011). The importance of population-wide sodium reduction as a means to prevent cardiovascular disease and stroke: A call to action from the American Heart Association. *Circulation, 123,* 1138–1143. Retrieved February 9, 2012, from http://circ.ahajournals.org

Centers for Disease Control and Prevention (CDC). (2010). *Chronic diseases and health promotion.* Retrieved from http://www.cdc.gov/chronicdisease/ overview/

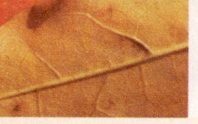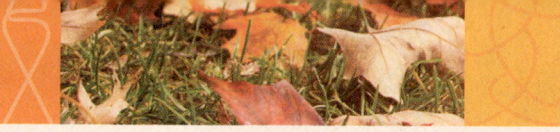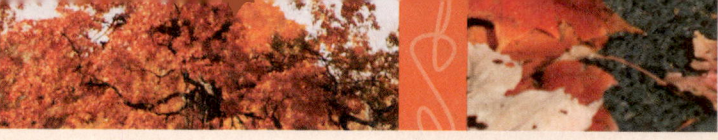

Centers for Disease Control and Prevention (CDC). (2011). CDC health disparities and inequalities report—United States, 2011. *Morbidity and Mortality Weekly Report, 60*(Suppl.), 1–116.

Centers for Disease Control and Prevention (CDC). (2012a). *Fact sheets. Binge drinking.* Retrieved from www.cdc.gov/alcohol/fact-sheets/binge-drinking.htm

Centers for Disease Control and Prevention (CDC). (2012b). *High blood pressure facts.* Retrieved from www.cdc.gov/bloodpressure/facts.htm

Centers for Disease Control and Prevention (CDC). (2012c). Recommended adult immunization schedule—United States, 2012. *Morbidity and Mortality Weekly Report, 61*(4), 1–7.

Duvall, E. (1977). *Marriage and family development* (5th ed.). Philadelphia, PA: Lippincott.

Giger, J., Davidhizar, R. E., Purnell, L., Harden, J. T., Phillips, J., & Strickland, O. (2007). American Academy of Nursing Expert Panel Report: Developing cultural competence to eliminate health disparities in ethnic minorities and other vulnerable populations. *Journal of Transcultural Nursing, 18*(2), 95–102.

Humes, K., Jones, N., & Ramirez, R. (2011). Overview of race and Hispanic origin: 2010. *2010 Census Briefs.* Retrieved from http://www.census.gov/prod/cen2010/briefs/c2010br-02.pdf

Institute for Clinical Systems Improvement (ICSI). (2011). *Health care guideline: Preventive services for adults* (17th ed.). Retrieved from http://www.icsi.org/preventive_services_for_adults/preventive_services_for_adults_4.html

Institute of Medicine of the National Academies (IOM). (2010). Dietary reference intakes for calcium and vitamin D. *Report brief.* Retrieved from http://www.iom.edu/Reports/2010/Dietary-Reference-Intakes-for-Calcium-and-Vitamin-D.aspx

Murray, R., Zentner, J., & Yakimo, R. (2009). *Health promotion strategies through the life span* (8th ed.). Upper Saddle River, NJ: Pearson.

National Center for Health Statistics. (2012). *Health, United States, 2011: With special feature on socioeconomic status and health.* Hyattsville, MD: Author.

The National Long-Term Care Ombudsman Resource Center. (2011). *Residents' rights.* Retrieved from www.ltcombudsman.org/issues/resident-rights

Pender, N., Murdaugh, C., & Parsons, M. (2011). *Health promotion in nursing practice* (6th ed.). Upper Saddle River, NJ: Pearson.

Savett, L. A. (2007). Every clinical encounter is a cultural encounter: Understanding the patient's story. *Creative Nursing, 13*(1), 13–14.

Sherwood, G., & Barnsteiner, J. (2012). *Quality and safety in nursing: A competency approach to improving outcomes.* Oxford, UK: Wiley-Blackwell.

Siantz, M. L. D., & Meleis, A. I. (2007). Integrating cultural competence into nursing education and practice: 21st century action steps. *Journal of Transcultural Nursing 18*(1, Suppl.), 86S–90S

Spector, R. (2013). *Cultural diversity in health and illness* (8th ed.). Upper Saddle River, NJ: Pearson.

Suchman, E. (1972). Stages of illness and medical care. In E. Jaco (Ed.), *Patients, physicians and illness (155–171).* New York: Free Press.

U.S. Department of Agriculture and U.S. Department of Health and Human Services. (2010). *Dietary guidelines for Americans, 2010* (7th ed.). Washington, DC: U.S. Government Printing Office.

U. S. Department of Health and Human Services. (2010). *Healthy people 2020.* Retrieved from www.health.gov

Van Horn, E. R., & Kautz, D. (2007). Promotion of family integrity in the acute care setting. *Dimensions of Critical Care Nursing, 26*(3), 101–107.

Wier, L., Pfuntner, A., Maeda, J., Stranges, E., Ryan, K., Jagadish, P., et al. (2011). *HCUP facts and figures: Statistics on hospital-based care in the United States, 2009.* Rockville, MD: Agency for Healthcare Research and Quality. Retrieved from http://www.hcup-us.ahrq.gov/reports.jsp

World Health Organization (WHO). (1974). *Constitution of the World Health Organization.* Geneva: Author.

CHAPTER 4

ACIP Adult Immunization Workgroup. (2013). Advisory committee on immunization practices (ACIP) recommended immunization schedule for adults aged 19 years and older—United States, 2013. *Morbidity and Mortality Weekly Report, 62,* 9–18.

Administration on Aging, U. S. Department of Health & Human Services. (2007b). *Strategic action plan 2007–2012.* Retrieved from www.aoa.gov

American Cancer Society. (2012). *Cancer facts & figures 2012.* Atlanta: American Cancer Society. Retrieved from www.cancer.org

American Cancer Society. (2013). *Guidelines for the early detection of cancer.* Retrieved from http://www.cancer.org/healthy/findcancerearly/cancerscreeningguidelines/American-cancer-society-guidelines-for-the-early-detection-of-cancer

American Geriatrics Society (AGS). (2012). *AGS beers criteria for potentially inappropriate medication use in older adults.* Retrieved from http://www.americangeriatrics.org/files/documents/beers/PrintableBeersPocketCard.pdf

Appel, L., Frohlich, E., Hall, J., Pearson, T., Sacco, R., Seals, D., et al. (2011, January 13). The importance of population-wide sodium reduction as a means to prevent cardiovascular disease and stroke: A call to action from the American Heart Association. *Circulation, 123,* 1138–1143. Retrieved February 9, 2012, from http://circ.ahajournals.org

Centers for Disease Control and Prevention (CDC). (2010, July 7). *Chronic diseases and health promotion.* Retrieved February 7, 2012, from http://www.cdc.gov/chronicdisease/overview/

Erikson, E. (1963). *Childhood and society* (2nd ed.). New York: Norton.

Federal Interagency Forum on Aging-Related Statistics. (2012). *Older Americans 2012: Key indicators of well-being.* Retrieved from http://www.agingstats.gov/agingstatsdotnet/Main_Site/Data/2012_Documents/Docs/EntireChartbook.pdf

Grossman, S., & Lange, J. (2006). Theories of aging as a basis for assessment. *MEDSURG Nursing, 15*(2), 77–83.

Havighurst, R. J. (1972). *Developmental tasks and education.* New York: David McKay.

Institute of Medicine of the National Academies (IOM). (2010, November). Dietary reference intakes for calcium and vitamin D. *Report brief.* Retrieved from http://www.iom.edu/Reports/2010/Dietary-Reference-Intakes-for-Calcium-and-Vitamin-D.aspx

Kohlberg, L. (1969). Stage and sequence: The cognitive-developmental approach to socialization. In D. Gaslin (Ed.), *Handbook of socialization: Theory and research* (pp. 347–380). Chicago: Rand-McNally.

National Center for Health Statistics (NCHS). (2012). *Health, United States, 2011: With Special Feature on Socioeconomic Status and Health.* Hyattsville, MD: Author.

National Center for Health Statistics (NCHS). (2013). *Life expectancy.* Retrieved from www.cdc.gov/nchs/fastats/lifeexpec.htm

National Institute on Aging, National Institutes of Health. (2012). *2011–2012 Alzheimer's disease progress report: Intensifying the research effort.* Retrieved from http://www.nia.nih.gov/alzheimers/publication/2011-2012-alzheimers-disease-progress-report

Reed, P. (1996). Transcendence: Formulating nursing perspectives. *Nursing Science Quarterly, 9*(1), 2–4.

U.S. Census Bureau, Population Division. (2012). *Table 2. Projections of the population by selected age groups and sex for the United States: 2015 to 2060.* Retrieved from http://www.census.gov/population/projections/

U.S. Department of Agriculture and U.S. Department of Health and Human Services. (2010). *Dietary guidelines for Americans, 2010* (7th ed.). Washington, DC: U.S. Government Printing Office.

CHAPTER 5

Burland, P. (2012). Vascular disease and foot assessment in diabetes. *Practice Nursing, 23*(4), 187–192.

Chester, J. G., & Rudolph, J. (2011). Vital signs in older adults: Age-related changes. *Journal of the American Medical Directors Association, 12*(5), 337–343.

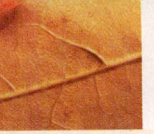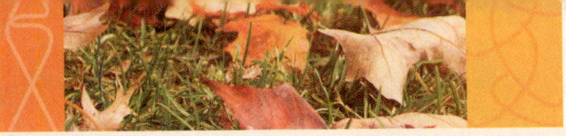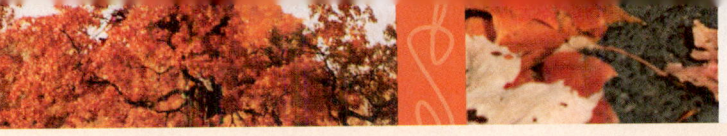

Crampton, J. (2013). Why nurses should use clinical reasoning to diagnose a cough. *Primary Health Care, 23*(7), 18–24.

DiMaria-Ghalili, R., & Amella, E. J. (2012). *Assessing nutrition in older adults. Try this: Best practices in nursing care to older adults, 9.* New York: Hartford Institute for Geriatric Nursing, College of Nursing, New York University. Retrieved from www.ConsultGeriRN.org

Hogan-Quigley, B., Palm, M. L., & Bickely, L. S. (2012). *Bates' nursing guide to physical examination and history taking.* Philadelphia: Lippincott Williams & Wilkins.

Jarvis, C. (2012). *Physical examination & health assessment* (6th ed.). St. Louis, MO: Saunders Elsevier.

Jensen, S. (2011). *Nursing health assessment: A best practice approach.* Philadelphia: Lippincott Williams & Wilkins.

Kresevic, D. (2012). *Nursing standard of practice protocol: Assessment of physical function.* New York: Hartford Institute for Geriatric Nursing. Retrieved from http://consultgerirn.org/topics/function/want_to_know_more

Langdon, R., Johnson, M., Carroll, V., & Antonio, G. (2013). Assessment of the elderly: It's worth covering the risks. *Journal of Nursing Management, 21*(1), 94–105.

Mager, D., & Grossman, S. (2013). Promoting nursing students' understanding and reflection on cultural awareness. *Home Healthcare Nurse, 31*(10), 582–590.

McCullagh, M., & Frank, K. (2013). Addressing adult hearing loss in primary care. *Journal of Advanced Nursing, 69*(4), 896–904.

O'Shea, L. (2010). Differential diagnosis of chest pain. *Practice Nurse, 40*(6), 13–18.

Pessagno, R. (2013). Don't be embarrassed: Taking a sexual health history. *Nursing, 43*(9), 60–64.

Pritchard, M. (2012). Pre-operative assessment of elective surgical patients. *Nursing Standard, 26*(30), 51–56.

Smith, C., & Cotter, V. (2008). *Normal aging changes. Nursing standard of practice protocol: Age-related changes in health.* New York: Hartford Institute for Geriatric Nursing. Retrieved from http://consultgerirn.org/topics/normal_aging_changes/want_to_know_more.

Spector, R. (2013). *Cultural diversity in health and illness* (8th ed.). Upper Saddle River, NJ: Pearson.

Sue, D., & Sue, D. (2012). *Counseling the culturally different: Theory and practice* (6th ed.). New York: John Wiley & Sons.

Swann, J. (2013). Dementia and reminiscence: Not just a focus on the past. *Nursing & Residential Care, 15*(12), 790–795.

Weber, J., & Kelley, J. (2013). *Health assessment in nursing* (5th ed.). Philadelphia: Lippincott Williams & Wilkins.

CHAPTER 6

Abrams, A. C., Pennington, S. S., & Lammon, C. B. (2009). *Clinical drug therapy* (9th ed.). Philadelphia: Lippincott Williams & Wilkins.

Anderson, J. K., & Fox, J. R. (2012). Potential food-drug interactions in long-term care. *Journal of Gerontological Nursing, 38*(4), 38–46.

Berryman, S. N., Jennings, J., Ragsdale, S., Lofton, T., Huff, D. C., & Rooker, J. S. (2012). Beers criteria for potentially inappropriate medication use in older adults. *MedSurg Nursing, 21*(3), 129–132.

Gill, D., Spain, M., & Edlund, B. J. (2012). Crushing or splitting medications unrecognized hazards. *Journal of Gerontological Nursing, 38*(1), 8–12.

Guthrie, P. S. (2010). Combining herbal remedies and prescription drugs. *American Journal of Nursing, 110*(7), 18–19.

Institute of Safe Medicine Practices. (2011). *FDA and ISMP lists of look-alike drug names with recommended tall man letters.* Retrieved October 14, 2013, from http://www.ismp.org/FDA and ISMP lists of look-alike drug names with recommended tall man letters.asp

Institute of Safe Medicine Practices. (2012a). *ISMP's list of error-prone abbreviations, symbols, and dose designations.* Retrieved October 13, 2013, from http://www.ismp.org/ISMP's list of error-prone prone abbreviations, symbols, and dose designations.asp

Institute of Safe Medicine Practices. (2012b). *ISMP's list of high-alert medications.* Retrieved October 14, 2013, from http://www.ismp.org/ISMP's list of high alert medications.asp

The Joint Commission. (2013). *Hospital: 2013 National Patient Safety Goals.* Retrieved October 14, 2013, from http://www.jointcommission.org/hap_2013_npsg/

McCormick, M. J. (2012, May–June). Drug alert: New guidelines for acetaminophen products. *Nursing Made Incredibly Easy,* 49–51.

Messina, B. A., & Escallier, L. A. (2011). Take the "hyper" out of pharmacotherapy. *Nursing 2011, 41*(7), 51–53.

Mitchell, J. F. (2012). *Oral dosage forms that should not be crushed.* Horsham, PA: ISMP.

Phillips, R. M. (2011, January–February). The challenge of medication management in older adults. *Nursing Made Incredibly Easy,* 24–31.

Smith, S. F., Duell, D. J., & Martin, B. C. (2012). *Clinical nursing skills* (8th ed.). Upper Saddle River, NJ: Prentice Hall.

CHAPTER 7

Adams, M., Holland, N., & Urban, C. (2014). *Pharmacology for nurses: A pathophysiologic approach* (4th ed.). Upper Saddle River, NJ: Pearson.

Appel, L., Frohlich, E., Hall, J., Pearson, T., Sacco, R., Seals, D., et al. (2011, January 13). The importance of population-wide sodium reduction as a means to prevent cardiovascular disease and stroke: A call to action from the American Heart Association. *Circulation 2011, 123,* 1138–1143. Retrieved February 9, 2012, from http://circ.ahajournals.org

Centers for Disease Control and Prevention (CDC). (2012, February). Where's the sodium? *Vital Signs.* Retrieved February 23, 2012, from http://www.cdc.gov/vitalsigns/Sodium/index.html

Dewey, M., & Heuberger, R. (2011, September–October). Vitamin D and calcium status and appropriate recommendations in bariatric surgery patients. *Gastroenterology Nursing, 34*(5), 367–374.

Grossman, S., & Porth, C. M. (2014). *Pathophysiology: Concepts of altered health states* (9th ed.). Philadelphia, PA: Lippincott Williams & Wilkins.

Harvey, S., & Jordan, S. (2010, June 30–July 6). Diuretic therapy: Implications for nursing practice. *Nursing Standard, 24*(43), 40–50.

Hogan, M., Gingrich, M., & Nichols, E. (Eds.). (2013). *Fluids, electrolytes, & acid-base balance* (3rd ed.). Upper Saddle River, NJ: Pearson.

Jacobson, R., Peery, J., Thompson, W., Kanapka, J., & Caswell, M. (2010, May–June). Serum electrolyte shifts following administration of sodium phosphates enema. *Gastroenterology Nursing, 33*(3), 191–201.

Lawes, R. (2009). Body out of balance: Understanding metabolic acidosis and alkalosis. *Nursing, 39*(11), 50–54.

McPhee, S., & Papadakis, M. (2012). *Current medical diagnosis & treatment* (51st ed.). New York: Lange /McGraw-Hill.

Mentes, J. (2008). *Hydration management: Nursing standard of practice protocol: Oral hydration management.* Hartford Institute for Geriatric Nursing. Retrieved from http://www.consultgerirn.org/topics

Metheny, N. M. (2012). *Fluid and electrolyte balance: Nursing considerations* (5th ed.). Sudbury, MA: Jones & Bartlett Learning.

Perrin, K. O. (2009). *Understanding the essentials of critical care nursing.* Upper Saddle River, NJ: Pearson.

Pruitt, B. (2010, July). Interpreting ABGs: An inside look at your patient's status. *Nursing, 40*(7), 31–36.

Rosenthal, K. (2009). Tonicity and IV fluids. *Resource Nurse.* Retrieved from http://www.resourcenurse.com/feature_tonicity_fluids.html

Wagner, K., Johnson, K., & Hardin-Pierce, M. (2010). *High-acuity nursing* (5th ed.). Upper Saddle River, NJ: Pearson.

Wells, B., DiPiro, J., Schwinghammer, T., & DiPiro, C. (2012). *Pharmacotherapy handbook* (8th ed.). New York, NY: McGraw-Hill.

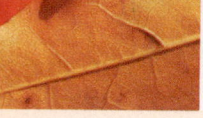
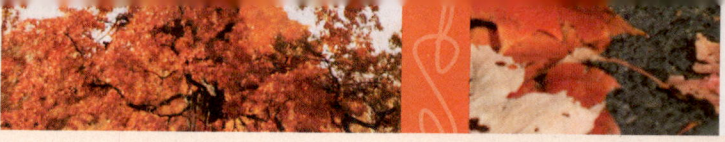

CHAPTER 8

Adams, M. P., & Koch, R. W. (2010). *Pharmacology: Connections to nursing practice*. Upper Saddle River, NJ: Pearson.

American Academy of Pain Medicine. (2012). *AAPM facts and figures on pain*. Retrieved from www.painmed.org

Chapman, S. (2011). Assessment and management of patients with cancer pain. *Clinical Nursing Practice, 10*(10), 28–36.

Cranwell-Bruce, L. A. (2011). Drug treatment for peripheral neuropathy. *MedSurg Nursing, 20*(5), 269–271.

D'Arcy, Y. (2009). Are opioids safe for your patient? *Nursing, 39*(4), 40–44.

D'Arcy, Y. (2010a). Managing chronic pain in acute care. *Nursing, 40*(4), 49–51.

D'Arcy, Y. (2010b). How to manage pain in addicted patients. *Nursing, 40*(8), 60–64.

Gatlin, C. G., & Schulmeister, L. (2007). When medication is not enough: Nonpharmacologic management of pain. *Clinical Journal of Oncology, 11*(5), 699–704.

Jablonski, A. M., DuPen, A. R., & Ersek, M. (2011). The use of algorithms in assessing and managing persistent pain in older adults. *American Journal of Nursing, 111*(3), 34–45.

LeMone, P., & Burke, K. M. (2011). *Medical–surgical nursing* (5th ed.). Upper Saddle River, NJ: Prentice Hall Health.

Lu, D. F., & Herr, K. (2012). Pain in dementia. *Journal of Gerontological Nursing, 38*(2), 8–13.

McCaffery, M., & Pasero, C. (1999). *Pain: Clinical manual*. (2nd ed). St. Louis, MO: Mosby.

McCormick, M. J. (2012, May–June). Drug alert: New guidelines for acetaminophen products. *Nursing Made Incredibly Easy*, 49–51.

Melzack, R., & Wall, P. (1965). Pain mechanisms: A new theory. *Science, 150*, 971–979.

Narayan, M. C. (2010). Culture's effects on pain assessment and management. *American Journal of Nursing, 110*(4), 38–49.

Pasero, C., & McCaffery, M. (2011). *Pain assessment and pharmacologic management*. St. Louis, MO: Elsevier.

Sawhney, M. (2012). Epidural analgesia: What nurses need to know. *Nursing 2012, 42* (8), 36–42.

CHAPTER 9

Aldabagh, B., & Tomecki, K. J. (2010). What's new in MRSA infections. *Dermatology Nursing, 22*(2), 2–9.

Benson, S., & Powers, J. (2011, May–June). Your role in infection protection. *Nursing Made Incredibly Easy*, 36–41.

Centers for Disease Control and Prevention. (2007). *Guideline for isolation precautions: Preventing transmission of infectious agents in healthcare settings*. Retrieved from www.cdc.gov/ncidod/dhqp/gl_isolation.html

Centers for Disease Control and Prevention. (2010a). *Diagnosis and testing of MRSA infections*. Retrieved from www.cdc.gov/mrsa/diagnosis/index.html

Centers for Disease Control and Prevention. (2010b). Use of anthrax vaccine in the United States: Recommendations of the advisory committee on immunization practices. *Morbidity and Mortality Weekly Report, 59*(6), 1–30.

Centers for Disease Control and Prevention. (2011). *Diseases and organisms in healthcare settings*. Retrieved from www.cdc.gov/HAI/Organisms/organisms.html

Centers for Disease Control and Prevention. (2012a). *Avian A influenza virus infections in humans*. Retrieved from www.cdc.gov/flu/avianflu/avian-in-humans.htm

Centers for Disease Control and Prevention. (2012b). *Types of healthcare-associated infections*. Retrieved from www.cdc.gov/HAI/Infection

Delahanty, K., & Myers, F. (2010). 3 bad bugs. *Nursing, 40*(3), 24–31.

Grossman, S., & Mager, D. (2010). Clostridium difficile: Implications for nurses. *MedSurg Nursing, 19*(3), 155–158.

Herron, C. (2012, January–February). Know your WBCs. *Nursing Made Incredibly Easy*, 11–15.

The Joint Commission. (2014). *2014 National patient safety goals*. Retrieved from www.jointcommission.org

Keske, L. A., & Letizia, M. (2010). *Clostridium difficile* infection: Essential information for nurses. *MedSurg Nursing, 19*(6), 329–332.

Schwoen, S. J. (2012). Recognizing and preventing norovirus. *Nursing, 42*(6), 68–70.

Upshaw-Owens, M., & Bailey, C. A. (2012). Preventing hospital-associated infection: MRSA. *MedSurg Nursing, 21*(2), 77–81.

World Health Organization. (2009). *Smallpox*. Retrieved from www.who.int/mediacentre/factsheets/smallpox/en/index.html

CHAPTER 10

Amato-Vealey, E., Barba, M., & Vealey, R. (2008). Hand-off communication: A requisite for perioperative patient safety. *AORN Journal, 88*(5), 763–770.

American Society of Anesthesiologists. (2009). *Continuum of depth of sedation: Definition of general anesthesia and levels of sedation/analgesia*. Retrieved from http://www.asahq.org/For-Members/Standards-Guidelines-and-Statements.aspx

Association of perioperative Registered Nurses (AORN). (2013). *Registered nurse first assistant*. Retrieved from http://www.aorn.org/Advocacy/Issues_and_Initiatives/Legislative_Priorities/Registered_Nurse_First_Assistant.aspx

Ball, K. (2009). Do-not-resuscitate orders in surgery: Decreasing the confusion. *AORN Journal, 89*(1), 140–146.

Benson, E. E., McMillan, D. E., & Ong, B. (2012). Original research: The effects of active warming on patient temperature and pain after total knee arthroplasty. *American Journal of Nursing, 112*(5), 26.

Blais, K., & Hayes, J. (2011). *Professional nursing practice: Concepts and perspectives* (6th ed.). Upper Saddle River, NJ: Pearson.

Brooks, P. B. (2012). Postoperative delirium in elderly patients. *American Journal of Nursing, 112*(9), 38–49.

Collins, A. (2011). Postoperative nausea and vomiting in adults: Implications for critical care. *Critical Care Nurse, 31*(6), 36–45.

Crenshaw, J. T. (2011). Preoperative fasting: Will the evidence ever be put into practice? *American Journal of Nursing, 111*(10), 38.

Gonzales, E., Ledesma, R., McAllister, D., Perry, S., & Dyer, C. (2010). Effects of guided imagery on postoperative outcomes in patients undergoing same-day surgical procedures: A randomized, single-blind study. *AANA Journal, 78*(3), 181–188.

Guido, G. (2010). *Legal & ethical issues in nursing* (5th ed.). Upper Saddle River, NJ: Pearson.

Helms, J. E., & Barone, C. P. (2008, December). Physiology and treatment of pain. *Critical Care Nurse, 28*(6), 38–49.

The Joint Commission. (2010). *The universal protocol*. Retrieved from http://www.jointcommission.org/standards_information/up.aspx

The Joint Commission. (2012). *2013 Hospital National Patient Safety Goals*. Retrieved from http://www.jointcommission.org/standards_information/npsgs.aspx

Kibler, V. A., Hayes, R. M., Johnson, D. E., Anderson, L. W., Just, S. L., & Wells, N. L. (2012). Cultivating quality: Early postoperative ambulation: Back to basics. *American Journal of Nursing, 112*(4), 63.

Potera, C. (2012). Some surgeons disregard advance directives. *American Journal of Nursing, 112*(3), 17.

Rothrock, J. (2011). *Alexander's care of the patient in surgery* (14th ed.). St. Louis, MO: Elsevier.

Tanner, J., Swarbrook, S., & Stuart, J. (2009). Surgical hand antisepsis to reduce surgical site infection. *Cochrane Database of Systematic Reviews*, CD004288.

Winslow, E. H., & Kelly, P. A. (2012). Active warming study. *American Journal of Nursing, 112*(9), 12.

World Health Organization. (2009). *Safe surgery saves lives: The second global patient safety challenge*. Retrieved from http://www.who.int/patientsafety/safesurgery/en/

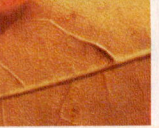
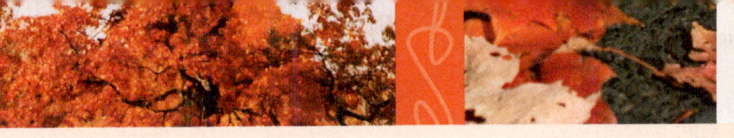

CHAPTER 11

American Academy of Allergy, Asthma & Immunology (AAAAI). (2012). *Allergy statistics*. Retrieved from http://www.aaaai.org/about-the-aaaai/newsroom/allergy-statistics.aspx

Belavic, J. M. (2010, July/August). An update on HIV/AIDS medications. *Nursing Made Incredibly Easy*, 6–10.

Centers for Disease Control and Prevention. (2008). *HIV/AIDS among persons aged 50 and older*. Retrieved from http://www.cdc.gov/hiv/topics/over50/resources/factsheets/over50/htm

Centers for Disease Control and Prevention. (2012a). *HIV/AIDS surveillance reports*. Retrieved from http://www.cdc.gov/hiv/topics/surveillance/htm

Centers for Disease Control and Prevention. (2012b). *HIV in the United States: At a glance*. Retrieved from http://www.cdc.gov/hiv/resources/factsheet/us.htm

Centers for Disease Control and Prevention. (2012c). Recommended adult immunization schedule-United States, 2012. *Morbidity and Mortality Weekly Report, 61*(4), 1–7.

Jang, H., Anderson, P. G., & Mentes, J. C. (2011). Aging and living with HIV/AIDS. *Journal of Gerontological Nursing, 37*(12), 4–7.

Kaufman, C. (2011). The secret life of lymphocytes. *Nursing, 41*(6), 50–54.

Kirton, C. (2011). HIV the changing epidemic. *Nursing, 41*(1), 36–43.

National Institute for Occupational Safety and Health (NIOSH). (2012). *NIOSH fast facts: How to prevent latex allergies*. Retrieved from http://www.cdc.gov/niosh/docs/2012-119/pdfs/2012-119.pdf

Planton, J., Meyer, J. O., & Edlund, B. J. (2012). Recommended routine vaccinations for older adults. *Journal of Gerontological Nursing, 38*(7), 16–20.

UNAIDS (2012). *UNAIDS fact sheet 2012*. Retrieved from http://www.unaids.org.

CHAPTER 12

American Cancer Society. (2012a). *Cancer Facts & Figures for Hispanics/Latinos 2012–2014*. Atlanta, GA: Author.

American Cancer Society. (2012b). *Cancer Prevention & Early Detection: Facts & Figures 2012*. Atlanta, GA: Author.

American Cancer Society. (2012c). *Cancer Treatment & Survivorship: Facts & Figures 2012–2013*. Atlanta, GA: Author.

American Cancer Society. (2013a). *Cancer Facts & Figures 2013*. Atlanta, GA: Author.

American Cancer Society. (2013b). *Cancer Facts & Figures for African Americans—2013–2014*. Atlanta, GA: Author.

Appelbaum, F. (2012). Hematopoietic cell transplantation. In D. Longo, A. Fauci, D. Kasper, S. Hauser, J. Jameson, & J. Loscalzo (Eds.), *Harrison's Principles of Internal Medicine* (18th ed., pp. 958–964). New York: McGraw-Hill.

Brant, J. (2010). Palliative care for adults across the cancer trajectory from diagnosis to end of life. *Seminars in Oncology Nursing, 26*(4), 222–230.

Brittain, K., Loveland-Cherry, C., Northouse, L., Caldwell, C., & Taylor, J. (2012). Sociocultural differences and colorectal cancer screening among African American men and women. *Oncology Nursing Forum, 39*(1), 100–107.

Fulop, T., Larbi, A., Koth, R., de Angelis, F., & Pawelec, G. (2011). Aging, immunity, and cancer. *Discovery Medicine, 11*(61), 537–550.

Gucalp, R., & Dutcher, J. (2012). Oncologic emergencies. In D. Longo, A. Fauci, D. Kasper, S. Hauser, J. Jameson, & J. Loscalzo (Eds.), *Harrison's Principles of Internal Medicine* (18th ed., pp. 2266–2279). New York: McGraw-Hill.

Hoffe, S., & Balducci, L. (2012). Cancer and age: General considerations. *Clinics in Geriatric Medicine, 28*(1), 1–18.

Holt, K. (2011). Common side effects and interactions of colorectal cancer therapeutic agents. *Journal of Practical Nursing, 61*(1), 7–20.

Kluckhohn, F. R., & Strodtbeck, F. L. (1961). *Variations in Value Orientations*. Evanston, IL: Row, Peterson and Company.

Kvåle, K., & Bondevik, M. (2010). Patients' perceptions of the importance of nurses' knowledge about cancer and its treatment for quality nursing care. *Oncology Nursing Forum, 37*(4), 436–442.

Longo, D. (2012). Approach to the patient with cancer. In D. Longo, A. Fauci, D. Kasper, S. Hauser, J. Jameson, & J. Loscalzo (Eds.), *Harrison's Principles of Internal Medicine* (18th ed., pp. 646–654). New York: McGraw-Hill.

McBride, A., & Westervelt, P. (2012). Recognizing and managing the expanded risk of tumor lysis syndrome in hematologic and solid malignancies. *Journal of Hematology & Oncology, 13*(5), 75.

Ness, S., Kokal, J., Fee-Schroeder, K., Novotney, P., Satele, D., & Barton, D. (2013). Concerns across the survivorship trajectory: Results from a survey of cancer survivors. *Oncology Nursing Forum, 40*(1), 35–42.

Ogboli-Nwasor, E., Makama, J., & Yusufu, L. (2013). Evaluation of knowledge of cancer pain management among medical practitioners in a low-resource setting. *Journal of Pain Research, 6,* 71–77.

Palos, G., & Zandstra, F. (2013). Call for action: Caring for the United States' aging cancer survivors. *Clinical Journal of Oncology Nursing, 17*(1), 88–90.

Perry, H. (1993). Mourning and funeral customs of African Americans. In D. P. Irish, K. F. Lundquist, & V. J. Nelsen (Eds.), *Ethnic Variations in Dying, Death, and Grief* (pp. 51–67). Washington, DC: Taylor & Francis.

Riley, B., Culver, J., Skrzynia, C., Senter, L., Peters, J., Costalas, J., et al. (2012). Essential elements of genetic cancer risk assessment, counseling, and testing: Updated recommendations of the national society of genetic counselors. *Journal of Genetic Counseling, 12*(2), 151–161.

Rojas-Cooley, M. T., & Grant, M. (2006). Complementary and alternative medicine: Oncology nurses' experiences, educational interests, and resources. *Oncology Nursing Forum, 33*(3), 581–588.

Rosenblatt, P., Walsh, R., & Jackson, D. (1976). *Grief and Mourning in Cultural Perspective*. New Haven, CT: HRAF Press.

Ross, L., Fletcher, A., Anderson, M., Meade, S., Powe, B., & Howard, D. (2012). Complementary and alternative medicine (CAM) use among men with a history of prostate cancer. *Journal of Cultural Diversity, 19*(4), 143–150.

Rotter, J. (1966). Generalized expectancies for internal versus external control of reinforcements. *Psychological Monographs, 80,* Whole No. 609.

Sausville, E., & Longo, D. (2012). Principles of cancer treatment. In D. Longo, A. Fauci, D. Kasper, S. Hauser, J. Jameson, & J. Loscalzo (Eds.), *Harrison's Principles of Internal Medicine* (18th ed., pp. 689–711). New York: McGraw-Hill.

Tse, M., Wong, A., Ng, H., Lee, H., Chong, M., & Leung, W. (2012). The effect of a pain management program on patients with cancer pain. *Cancer Nursing, 35*(6), 438–446.

Ussher, J., Perz, J., & Gilbert, E. (2012). Changes to sexual well-being and intimacy after breast cancer. *Cancer Nursing, 35*(6), 456–465.

Williams, P., Williams, K., LaFaver-Roling, S., Johnson, R., & Williams, A. (2011). An intervention to manage patient-reported symptoms during cancer treatment. *Clinical Journal of Oncology Nursing, 15*(3), 253–258.

World Health Organization (WHO). (2013). *WHO's pain ladder*. Retrieved from http://www.who.int/cancer/palliative/painladder/en/

CHAPTER 13

American Association of Colleges of Nursing. (2013). *About ELNEC*. Retrieved from http://www.aacn.nche.edu/elnec/FactSheet.pdf

American Association of Retired Persons (AARP). (2010). *End of life: Beginning the conversation*. Retrieved from http://www.aarp.org

American Geriatrics Society. (2007). *The care of dying patients*. Retrieved from http://americangeriatrics.org/products/positionpapers/careofdPF.shtml

American Nursing Association. (2008). *Code of ethics for Nurses with Interpretive Statements*. Silver Spring, MD: Author.

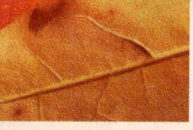
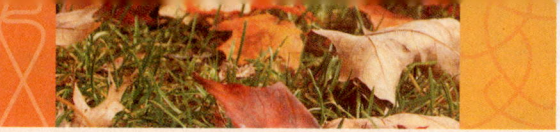
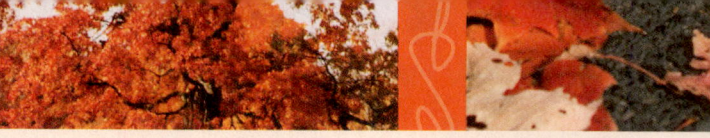

American Nurses Association. (2010). *Nursing's social policy statement: The essence of the profession.* Silver Spring, MD: Author.

American Nurses Association. (2012). *Position statements: Nursing care and do not resuscitate (DNR) and allow natural death (AND) decisions.* Retrieved from http://www.nursingworld.org/MainMenuCategories/Policy-Advocacy/Positions-and-Resolutions/ANAPositionStatements

American Nurses Association. (2013). *Position statements: Euthanasia, assisted suicide and aid in dying.* Retrieved from http://www.nursingworld.org/MainMenuCategories/Policy-Advocacy/Positions-and-Resolutions/ANAPositionStatements

Bowlby, J. (1980). *Attachment and loss. Volume 3: Loss: Sadness and depression.* New York: Basic Books.

Clabots, S. (2012). Strategies to help initiate and maintain the end-of-life discussion with patients and family members. *MEDSURG Nursing, 21*(4), 197–204.

Drumright, K., Julkenbeck, S., & Judd, C. (2012, November–December). Easing pain with palliative care. *Nursing Made Incredibly Easy!, 48–50.* Retrieved from www.NursingMadeIncrediblyEasy.com

Ellershaw, J. (2011). *Care of the dying: A pathway to excellence* (2nd ed.). New York: Oxford University Press.

Erikson, J. (2013). Bedside nurse involvement in end-of-life decision making. *Dimensions of Critical Care Nursing, 32*(2), 65–68.

Field, N., Gao, B., & Padema, L. (2005). Continuing bonds in bereavement: An attachment theory based perspective. *Death Studies, 29*(4), 277–299.

Freeman, B. (2013). CARES: An acronym organized tool for the care of the dying. *Journal of Hospice and Palliative Nursing, 15*(3), 147–153.

Giovanni, L. A. (2012). End-of-life care in the United States: Current reality and future promise—a policy review. *Nursing Economics, 30*(3), 127–134.

Hodo, A., & Buller, L. (2012, August). Managing care at the end of life. *Nursing Management, 28–33.* Retrieved from http://nursingmanagement.com

Hospice Association of America. (2010). *Hospice facts & statistics, November 2010.* Retrieved from http://www.nahc.org/assets/1/7/HospiceStats10.pdf

Hospice Foundation of America. (2005). *The dying process: A guide for caregivers.* Washington, DC: Hospice Foundation of America.

Hospice Foundation of America. (2008). *HFA grief resource page: What is grief?* Retrieved from http://www.hospicefoundation.org/griefAndLoss/

Huggins, M. (2007). Discussing end-of-life care with older patients: What are you waiting for? *Geriatrics Aging, 10*(7), 461–464.

International Council of Nurses. (2006a). *The ICN definition of nursing; the ICN code of ethics for nurses.* Geneva, Switzerland: Author.

International Council of Nurses. (2006b). *Position statement: Nurse's role in providing care to dying patients and their families.* Geneva, Switzerland: Author.

International Council of Nurses. (2012). *Position statement: Nurses' role in providing care to dying patients and their families.* Retrieved from http://www.icn.ch/images/stories/documents/publications/position_statements/A12_Nurses_Role_Care_Dying_Patients.pdf

Johnson, J., & Johnson, M. (2003). *Grief. What it is and what you can do.* Omaha, NE: Centering Corporation.

Kübler-Ross, E. (1969). *On death and dying.* New York: Macmillan.

Kübler-Ross, E. (1978). *To live until we say goodbye.* Englewood Cliffs, NJ: Prentice Hall.

Kübler-Ross, E. (1997). *On death and dying: What the dying have to teach doctors, nurses, clergy, and their own families.* New York: Simon & Schuster.

Lysaght, S., & Ersek, M. (2013). Settings of care within hospice. *Journal of Hospice and Palliative Nursing, 15*(3), 171–176.

Mazanec, P., & Tyler, M. (2003). Cultural considerations in end-of-life: How ethnicity, age, and spirituality affect decisions when death is imminent. *American Journal of Nursing, 103*(3), 50–58.

McHugh, M. E., Arnold, J., & Buschman, P. R. (2012). Nurses leading the response to the crisis of palliative care for vulnerable populations. *Nursing Economics, 30*(3), 140–147.

Perry, H. (1993). Mourning and funeral customs of African Americans. In D. P. Irish, K. F. Lundquist, & V. J. Nelsen (Eds.), *Ethnic Variations in Dying, Death, and Grief* (pp. 51–67). Washington, DC: Taylor & Francis.

Purnell, L. D. (2012). *Transcultural health care: A culturally competent approach* (4th ed.). Philadelphia: F. A. Davis.

Rabbetts, L. (2013). The challenges patients experience in speaking about death: A guide for home healthcare and hospice clinicians. *Home Healthcare Nurse, 31*(2), 58–64.

Sherman, D. W., & Cheon, J. (2012). Palliative care: A paradigm of care responsive to the demands for health care reform in America. *Nursing Economics, 30*(3), 153–162.

Spruill, A. D., Mayer, D., & Hamilton, J. (2013). Barriers in hospice use among African Americans with cancer. *Journal of Hospice and Palliative Care, 15*(3), 136–144.

Steed, M. (2012). Palliative care: Are you asking the right questions? *Nursing 2012, 42*(10), 59–61.

Talamantes, M. A., Lawler, W. R., & Espino, D. V. (1995). Hispanic American elders: Caregiving norms surrounding dying and the use of hospice services. *Hospice Journal, 10*(4): 35–49.

Townsend, M. C. (2011). *Essentials of psychiatric mental health nursing: Concepts of care in evidence-based practice* (5th ed.). Philadelphia: F. A. Davis.

U.S. Department of Health & Human Services. (2013). *Medicare hospice benefits.* Baltimore: Centers for Medicare & Medicaid Services.

Varcarolis, E. M. (2013). *Essentials of psychiatric mental health nursing: A communication approach to evidence-based care* (2nd ed.). St. Louis, MO: Elsevier Saunders.

Wholihan, D., & Anderson, R. (2013). Empowering nursing assistants to improve end-of-life care. *Journal of Hospice and Palliative Nursing, 15*(1), 24–32.

Williams, B. R., Lewis, D. R., Burgio, K. L., & Goode, P. (2012). Wrapped in their arms: Next-of-kin's perceptions of how hospital nursing staff support family presence before, during, and after the death of a loved one. *Journal of Hospice and Palliative Nursing, 14*(8), 541–550.

CHAPTER 14

American Trauma Society. (2012). *Trauma facts.* Retrieved from http://www.amtrauma.org/injury-prevention-programs/trauma-facts/index.aspx

Bartley, M. K., & Shiflett, L. A. (2010). Handle older trauma patients with care. *Nursing, 40*(8), 24–30.

Beach, P. R., Hallett, A. M., & Zarcos, K. (2011). Organ donation after circulatory death: Vital partnerships. *American Journal of Nursing, 111*(5), 32–40.

Bechtel, G., & Davidhizar, R. (1998). Culture, personal space, and health. *Competence Matters, 1*(2), 20. Birmingham, AL: University of Alabama at Birmingham.

Cutugno, C. L. (2011). The 'graying' of trauma care: Addressing traumatic injury in older adults. *American Journal of Nursing, 111*(11), 40–50.

Davis, R. A. (2012). The big chill: Accidental hypothermia. *American Journal of Nursing, 112*(1), 38–48.

Hall, E. (1966). *Hidden dimension.* New York: Doubleday.

Kiwan, M. M. (2011, May–June). Disaster planning: Are you ready? *Nursing Made Incredibly Easy, 18–24.*

Laskowski-Jones, L. (2010). Summer emergencies: Can you take the heat? *Nursing, 40*(6), 24–31.

Morton, P. G., & Fontaine, D. K. (2013). *Essentials of critical care nursing a holistic approach.* Philadelphia: Lippincott Williams & Wilkins.

National Center for Injury Prevention and Control. (2012). *10 leading causes of death by age, United States-2010.* Retrieved from http://www.cdc.gov/ncipc

Tazbir, J. (2012). Early recognition and treatment of sepsis in the medical-surgical setting. *MedSurg Nursing, 21*(4), 205–209.

Wilmot, L. (2010). Shock: Early recognition and management. *Journal of Emergency Nursing, 36*(2), 134–139.

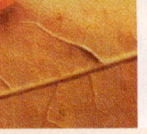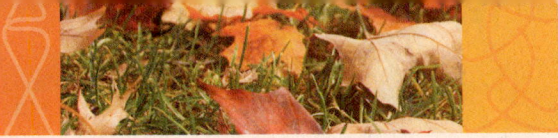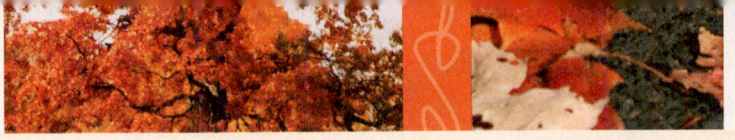

CHAPTER 15

Aponte, J. (2011). The prevalence of asymptomatic and symptomatic peripheral arterial disease and peripheral arterial disease risk factors in the US population. *Holistic Nursing Practice, 25*(3), 147–161.

Burland, P. (2012). Vascular disease and foot assessment in diabetes. *Practice Nursing, 23*(4), 187–192.

Chester, J. G., & Rudolph, J. (2011). Vital signs in older adults: Age-related changes. *Journal of the American Medical Directors Association, 12*(5), 337–343.

Eastwook, J., Doering, L., Dracup, K., Evangelista, L., & Hays, R. (2011). Health-related quality of life: The impact of diagnostic angiography. *Heart & Lung, 40*(2), 147–155.

Ferket, B. S., Spronk, S., Colkesen, E. B., & Hunink, M. G. (2012). Systematic review of guidelines on peripheral artery disease screening. *American Journal of Medicine, 125*(2), 198–208.

Fihn, S., Gardin, J., Abrams, J., Berra, K., Blankenship, J., Dallas, A. P., et al. (2012). Practice guidelines: 2012 ACCF/AHA/ACP/AATS/PCNA/SCAI/STS guideline for the diagnosis and management of patients with stable ischemic heart disease: A report of the American College of Cardiology Foundation/American Heart Association Task Force on Practice Guidelines, and the American College of Physicians, American Association for Thoracic Surgery, Preventive Cardiovascular Nurses Association, Society for Cardiovascular Angiography and Interventions, and Society of Thoracic Surgeons. *Circulation, 126,* e354–e471. Retrieved November 19, 2012, from my.americanheart.org/professional/StatementsGuidelines

Goodridge, E., Furst, C., Herrick, J., Song, J., & Tipton, P. (2013). Accuracy of cardiac rhythm interpretation by medical-surgical nurses: A pilot study. *Journal for Nurses in Professional Development, 29*(1), 35–40.

Höglund, J., Stenestrand, U., Tödt, T., & Johansson, I. (2011). The effect of early mobilization for patient undergoing coronary angiography: A pilot study with focus on vascular complications and back pain. *European Journal of Cardiovascular Nursing, 10*(2), 130–136.

Kreiger, G. (2007). A basic guide to understanding plasma B-type natriuretic peptide in the diagnosis of congestive heart failure. *MedSurg Nursing, 16*(2), 75–79.

Macabasco-O'Connell, A., Meymandi, S., & Bryg, R. (2010). B-type natriuretic peptide (BNP) is useful in detecting asymptomatic left ventricular dysfunction in low-income, uninsured patients. *Biological Research for Nursing, 11*(3), 280–287.

National Cholesterol Education Program. (2002). *Third report of the National Cholesterol Education Program (NCEP) Expert Panel on detection, evaluation, and treatment of high blood cholesterol in adults (Adult Treatment Panel III).* Bethesda, MD: National Heart, Lung and Blood Institute, National Institutes of Health.

Pearson, T. (2010). Ankle brachial index as a prognostic tool for women with coronary artery disease. *Journal of Cardiovascular Nursing, 25*(1), 20–24.

Skalski, J., Allison, T., & Miller, T. (2012). Exercise physiology: The safety of cardiopulmonary exercise testing in a population with high-risk cardiovascular diseases. *Circulation, 126,* 2465–2472. Published online before print October 22, 2012.

Wilcoxson, V. (2012). Early ambulation after diagnostic cardiac catheterization via femoral artery access. *Journal for Nurse Practitioners, 8*(10), 810–815.

CHAPTER 16

Alspach, J. (2012). Editorial: Acute myocardial infarction without chest pain: A life-threatening variant? *Critical Care Nurse, 32*(4), 10–13.

Berg, R., Hemphill, R., Abella, B., Aufderheide, T., Cave, D., Hazinski, M. F., et al. (2010). Part 5: Adult basic life support: 2010 American Heart Association Guidelines for cardiopulmonary resuscitation and emergency cardiovascular care. *Circulation, 122,* S685–S705.

Bermudez, N. (2012). Heart matters. ACS: A triad of troubles sets the stage for MI. *Nursing Made Incredibly Easy, 10*(6), 14–17.

Coventry, L., Finn, J., & Brenner, A. (2011). Sex differences in symptom presentation in acute myocardial infarction: A systematic review and meta-analysis. *Heart & Lung, 40*(6), 477–491.

Cox, B. (2010). Taking the heartache out of angina. *British Journal of Primary Care Nursing: Cardiovascular Disease, Diabetes & Kidney Care, 7*(1), 32–34.

Dechant, L. (2012). UA/NSTEM: Are you following the latest guidelines? *Nursing, 42*(9), 26–34.

DeVon, H., Hogan, N., Ochs, A., & Shapiro, M. (2010). Time to treatment for acute coronary syndromes: The cost of indecision. *Journal of Cardiovascular Nursing, 25*(2), 106–114.

Ellison, D., Williams, M., Moodt, G., & Farrar, F. (2010). Electrodiagnostic studies. *Critical Care Nursing Clinics of North America, 22*(1), 7–18.

Field, J., Hazinski, M., Sayre, M., Chameides, L., Schexnayder, S., Hemphill, R., et al. (2010). Part 1: 2010 American Heart Association Guidelines for cardiopulmonary resuscitation and emergency cardiovascular care. *Circulation, 122,* S640–S656.

Fihn, S., Gardin, J., Abrams, J., Berra, K., Blankenship, J., Dallas, A., et.al. (2012). 2012 ACCF/AHA/ACP/AATS/PCNA/SCAI/STS Guideline for the diagnosis and management of patients with stable ischemic heart disease: A report of the American College of Cardiology Foundation/American Heart Association Task Force on Practice Guidelines, and the American College of Physicians, American Association for Thoracic Surgery, Preventive Cardiovascular Nurses Association, Society for Cardiovascular Angiography and Interventions, and Society of Thoracic Surgeons. *Circulation, 126,* e354-e471.

Flanagan, J., Carroll, D., & Hamilton, G. (2010). The long-term lived experience of patients with implantable cardioverter defibrillators. *MedSurg Nursing, 19*(2), 113–119.

Gallagher, R., Totter, R., & Donoghue, J. (2010). Preprocedural concerns and anxiety assessment in patients undergoing coronary angiography and percutaneous coronary interventions. *European Journal of Cardiovascular Nursing, 9*(1), 38–44.

Go, A., Mozaffarian, D., Roger, V., Benjamin, E., & Berry, J., Borden, W., et al. (2013). AHA statistical update. Heart disease and stroke statistics—2013 update: A report from the American Heart Association. *Circulation, 127,* e6–e245. Retrieved from http://circ.ahajournals.org/content/127/1/e6.full#sec-194

Harold, J., Bass, T., Bashore, T., Brindis, R., Brush, J., Burke, J. A., et al. (2013). ACCF/AHA/SCAI 2013 update of the clinical competence statement on coronary artery interventional procedures: A report of the American College of Cardiology Foundation/American Heart Association/American College of Physicians Task Force on Clinical Competence and Training. *Circulation.* Dallas, TX: American Heart Association. Retrieved from http://circ.ahajournals.org/content/early/2013/05/07/CIR.0b013e318299cd8a.full.pdf

Hawley, C. (2010). Managing patients with recent onset chest pain: Key steps. *British Journal of Primary Care Nursing: Cardiovascular Disease, Diabetes & Kidney Care, 7*(4), 182–186.

Heart disease trends: Women are looking more like men. (2010). Action for Outcomes Series: Cardiovascular Disease in Women. *Healthcare Traveler,* 35–37.

Lee, G., Stub, D., & Ling, H. (2012). Atrial fibrillation in the elderly—not a benign condition. *International Emergency Nursing, 20*(4), 221–227.

Lesneski, L. (2010). Factors influencing treatment delay for patients with acute myocardial infarction. *Applied Nursing Research, 23*(4), 185–190.

Lopes, J., Nogueira-Martins, L., & Barros, A. (2013). Bed and shower baths: Comparing the perceptions of patients with acute myocardial infarction. *Journal of Clinical Nursing, 22*(5–6), 733–740.

McSweeney, J., O-Sullivan, P., Cleves, M., Lefler, L., Cody, M., Moser, D., et al. (2010). Racial differences in women's prodromal and acute symptoms of myocardial infarction. *American Journal of Critical Care, 19*(1), 63–73.

Miller, N. (2012). Heart matters. Warning! Cardiac cath complications. *Nursing Made Incredibly Easy, 10*(4), 8–10.

Milligan, F. (2012). Cardiac rehabilitation: An effective secondary prevention intervention. *British Journal of Nursing, 21*(13), 782–785.

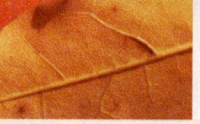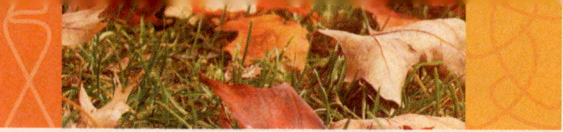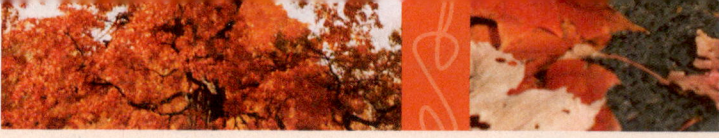

National Center for Health Statistics. (2013). *Health, United States, 2012: With special feature on emergency care.* Hyattsville, MD: Author. Retrieved from http://www.cdc.gov/nchs/data/hus/hus12.pdf

National Cholesterol Education Program. (2002). *Third report of the National Cholesterol Education Program (NCEP) Expert Panel on detection, evaluation, and treatment of high blood cholesterol in adults (Adult Treatment Panel III). Final report.* Bethesda, MD: National Heart, Lung, and Blood Institute, National Institutes of Health.

National Heart, Lung, and Blood Institute (NHLBI). (2013). *Fact book. Fiscal year 2012.* Bethesda, MD: National Institutes of Health.

O'Donnell, S., & Moser, D. (2012). Slow-onset myocardial infarction and its influence on help-seeking behaviors. *Journal of Cardiovascular Nursing, 27*(4), 334–344.

O'Shea, L. (2010). Differential diagnosis of chest pain. *Practice Nurse, 40*(6), 13–18.

Son, H., Thomas, S., & Friedmann, E. (2012). The association between psychological distress and coping patterns in post-MI patients and their partners. *Journal of Clinical Nursing, 21*(15–16), 2392–2394.

Stamps, D., & Carr, M. (2012). Holiday season for a healthy heart. *Critical Care Nursing Clinics of North America, 24*(4), 519–525.

Thanavaro, J., Thanavaro, S., & Delicath, T. (2010). Heath promotion behaviors in women with chest pain. *Heart & Lung, 39*(5), 394–403.

Thygesen, K., Alpert, J., Jaffe, A., Simoons, M., Chaitman, B., & White, H. (2012). Third universal definition of myocardial infarction. *Circulation, 126,* 2020–2035.

Trotter, R., Gallagher, R., & Donoghue, J. (2011). Anxiety in patients undergoing percutaneous coronary interventions. *Heart & Lung, 40*(3), 185–192.

Wier, L., Pfuntner, A., Maeda, J., Stranges, E., Ryan, K., Jagadish, P., et al. (2011). *HCUP facts and figures: Statistics on hospital-based care in the United States, 2009.* Rockville, MD: Agency for Healthcare Research and Quality. Retrieved from http://www.hcup-us.ahrq.gov/reports.jsp

Wu, J., Moser, D., Riegel, B., McKinley, S., & Doering, L. (2011). Impact of prehospital delay in treatment seeking on in-hospital complications after acute myocardial infarction. *Journal of Cardiovascular Nursing, 26*(3), 184–193.

CHAPTER 17

Barnford, M., & Paulus, M. (2011). Dyspnea with comorbid heart failure and COPD. *Clinical Advisory for Nurse Practitioners, 14*(10), 59–65.

Boyoung, H., Fleischmann, K., Howie-Esquivel, J., Stotts, N., & Dracup, K. (2011). Caregiving for patients with heart failure: Impact on patients' families. *American Journal of Critical Care, 20*(6), 431–442.

Cooper, K. (2011). Care of the lower extremities in patients with acute decompensated heart failure. *Critical Care Nurse, 31*(4), 21–29.

Fouse, J., Naylor, M., Bixby, M., & Ratcliffe, S. (2012). Medication problems occurring at hospital discharge among older adults with heart failure. *Research in Gerontological Nursing, 5*(1), 25–33.

Go, A., Mozaffarian, D., Roger, V., Benjamin, E., Berry, J., Borden, W., et al. (2013). AHA statistical update. Heart disease and stroke statistics— 2013 update: A report from the American Heart Association. *Circulation, 127,* e6–e245. Retrieved from http://circ.ahajournals.org/content/127/1/e6.full#sec-194

Hunt, S. A., Abraham, W. T., Chin, M. H., Feldman, A. M., Francis, G. S., Ganiats, T. G., et al. (2005). *ACC/AHA 2005 guideline update for the diagnosis and management of chronic heart failure in the adult: A report of the American College of Cardiology/American Heart Association Task Force on Practice Guidelines (Writing Committee to Update the 2001 Guidelines for the Evaluation and Management of Heart Failure).* Retrieved from American College of Cardiology website:www.acc.org/clinical/guidelines/failure/index/pdf

Is aldosterone antagonist therapy safe? (2013). *Nursing, 43*(2), 12–13.

Jelinek, H., & Warner, P. (2011). Digoxin therapy in the elderly: Pharmacokinetic considerations in nursing. *Geriatric Nursing, 32*(4), 263–269.

Jessup, M., Abraham, W., Casey, D., Feldman, A., Francis, G., Ganiats, T. G., et al. (2009). 2009 focused update: ACCF/AHA guidelines for the diagnosis and management of heart failure in adults: A report of the American College of Cardiology Foundation/American Heart Association Task Force on Practice Guidelines: Developed in Collaboration with the International Society for Heart and Lung Transplantation. *Circulation, 119,* 1977–2016.

Joffe, S., DeWolf, M., Shih, J., McManus, D., Spencer, F., Lessard, D., et al. (2013). Trends in the medical management of patients with heart failure. *Journal of Clinical Medicine Research, 5*(3), 194–204.

Kesscnich, C. (2011). Lab logic. BNP and heart failure: What is the connection? *Nurse Practitioner, 36*(1), 13–14.

Lowey, S. E., Powers, B. A., & Xue, Y. 2013. Short of breath and dying. *Journal of Gerontological Nursing, 39*(2), 43–52.

Luttenberger, K., & DiNapoli, M. (2011). Subacute bacterial endocarditis: Making the diagnosis. *Nurse Practitioner, 36*(3), 31–38.

Makaity, M. (2012). Congestive heart failure: An "F" isn't an option. *Nursing Made Incredibly Easy, 10*(2), 12–24.

Moser, D. K., & Riegel, B. (2008). *Cardiac nursing: A companion to Braunwald's Heart Disease.* St. Louis, MO: Saunders Elsevier.

National Center for Health Statistics. (2013). *Health, United States, 2012: With special feature on emergency care.* Hyattsville, MD: Author. Retrieved from http://www.cdc.gov/nchs/data/hus/hus12.pdf

National Heart, Lung, and Blood Institute (NHLBI). (2013). *Fact book. Fiscal year 2012.* Bethesda, MD: National Institutes of Health.

Nieuwenhuis, M., van der Wal, M., & Jaarsma, T. (2011). The body of knowledge on compliance in heart failure patients: We are not there yet. *Journal of Cardiovascular Nursing, 26*(1), 21–28.

Niklasch, D. (2011). Differential diagnosis of acute heart failure: Brain versus heart. *Advanced Emergency Nursing Journal, 33*(4), 279–287.

Parks, C., Turner, M., Perry, M., Lyons, R., Chaney, C., Hooper, E., et al. (2011). Educational needs: What female patients want from their cardiovascular health care providers. *MedSurg Nursing, 20*(1), 21–28.

Pastor, D., & Moore, J. (2013). Uncertainties of the heart: Palliative care and adult heart failure. *Home Healthcare Nurse, 31*(1), 29–38.

Pfuntner, A., Wier, L., & Stocks, C. (2013). *Most frequent conditions in U.S. Hospitals, 2011* (HCUP statistical brief #162). Rockville, MD: Agency for Healthcare Research and Quality. Retrieved from http://www.hcup-us.ahrq.gov/reports/statbriefs/sb162.pdf

Piamjariyakul, U., Smith, C., Werkowitch, M., & Elyachar, A. (2012a). Part 1: Heart failure home management: Patients, multidisciplinary health care professionals and family caregiver's perspectives. *Applied Nursing Research, 25*(4), 239–245.

Piamjariyakul, U., Smith, C., Werkowitch, M., & Elyachar, A. (2012b). Part 2: Enhancing heart failure home management: Integrated evidence for a new family caregiver educational plan. *Applied Nursing Research, 25*(4), 246–250.

Scherb, C., Head, B., Maas, M., Swanson, E., Moorhead, S., Reed, D., et al. (2011). Most frequent nursing diagnoses, nursing interventions, and nursing sensitive patient outcomes of hospitalized older adults with heart failure: Part 1. *International Journal of Nursing Terminologies 7 Classifications, 22*(1), 13–22.

Seright, T. (2013). Heart matters. Detecting decompensated heart failure. *Nursing Made Incredibly Easy, 11*(3), 12–16.

Wynne, J., Narveson, S., & Littmann, L. (2012). Cardiorenal syndrome. *Heart & Lung, 41*(2), 157–160.

CHAPTER 18

Aponte, J. (2012). The prevalence of peripheral arterial disease (PAD) and PAD risk factors among different ethnic groups in the US population. *Journal of Vascular Nursing, 30*(2), 37–43.

Aronow, W., Fleg, J., Pepine, C., Artinian, N., Bakris, G., Brown, A. S., et al. (2011). ACCF/AHA 2011 expert consensus document on hypertension in the elderly: A report of the American College of Cardiology

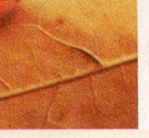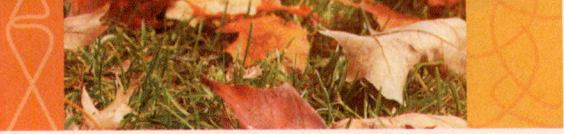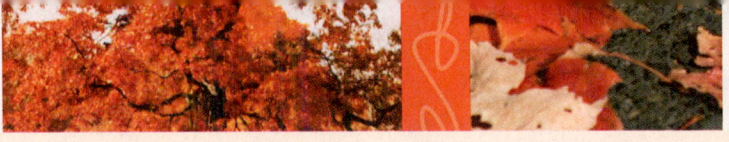

Foundation Task Force on Clinical Expert Consensus Documents. *Circulation, 123,* 2434–2506. Retrieved from http://circ.ahajournals.org

Barrows, K. (2013). Chapter e5: Complementary & alternative medicine. In M. Papadakis & S. McPhee (Eds.), *Current medical diagnosis & treatment 2013.* New York, NY: McGraw-Hill. Retrieved from http://www.access-medicine.com/resourceTOC.aspx?esourceID=1

Centers for Disease Control and Prevention. (2014). High blood pressure facts. Retrieved from http://www.cdc.gov/bloodpressure/facts.htm

Fitzgerald, M. (2011). Hypertension treatment update: Focus on direct renin inhibition. *Journal of the American Academy of Nurse Practitioners, 23*(5), 239–248.

Fournier, M. (2012). Preventing organ damage from hypertensive crisis. *American Nurse Today, 7*(3), 17.

Hartley, M., & Repede, E. (2011). Nurse practitioner communication and treatment adherence in hypertensive patients. *Journal for Nurse Practitioners, 7*(8), 654–659.

Headley, C., & Melander, S. (2011). When it may be a pulmonary embolism. *Nephrology Nursing Journal, 38*(2), 127–152.

Holland, L. N., Adams, M., & Brice, J. L. (2015). *Core concepts in pharmacology,* 4th ed. Upper Saddle River, NJ: Pearson. p. 272. Fig. 18.6.

Lucky, D., Turner, B., Hall, M., Lefaver, S., & deWerk, A. (2011). Blood pressure screenings through community nursing health fairs: Motivating individuals to seek health care follow-up. *Journal of Community Health Nursing, 28*(3), 119–129.

Luehr, D., Woolley, T., Burke, R., Dohmen, F., Hayes, R., Johnson, M., et al. (2012). *Hypertension diagnosis and treatment.* Bloomington, MN: Institute for Clinical Systems Improvement (ICSI).

Meguid, C. (2011). Best practice for deep vein thrombosis prophylaxis. *Journal for Nurse Practitioners, 7*(7), 582–587.

Muirhead, L., Roberson, A., & Secrest, J. (2011). Utilization of foot care services among homeless adults: Implications for advanced practice nurses. *Journal of the American Academy of Nurse Practitioners, 23*(4), 209–215.

National Center for Health Statistics (NCHS). (2013). *Health, United States, 2012: With special feature on emergency care.* Hyattsville, MD: Author. Retrieved from http://www.cdc.gov/nchs/data/hus/hus12.pdf

National Heart, Lung, and Blood Institute (NHLBI). (2006). *Your guide to lowering your blood pressure with DASH* (NIH Publication No. 06-4082). Retrieved from http://nhlbi.hih.gov

National Heart, Lung, and Blood Institute (NHLBI). (2013). *Fact book. Fiscal year 2012.* Bethesda, MD: National Institutes of Health.

National Heart, Lung, and Blood Institute: National High Blood Pressure Education Program. (2004). *The seventh report of the Joint National Committee on prevention, detection, evaluation, and treatment of high blood pressure.* Bethesda, MD: National Institutes of Health.

Okonta, N. (2012). Does yoga therapy reduce blood pressure in patients with hypertension? An integrative review. *Holistic Nursing Practice, 26*(3), 137–141.

Pashikanti, L., & Von Ah, D. (2012). Impact of early mobilization protocol on the medical-surgical inpatient population: An integrated review of literature. *Clinical Nurse Specialist: The Journal for Advanced Nursing Practice, 26*(2), 87–94.

Rigsby, B. (2011). Hypertension improvement through healthy lifestyle modifications. *ABNG Journal, 22*(2), 41–43.

Rooke, T., Hirsch, A., Misra, S., Sidawy, A., Beckman, J., Findeiss, L. K., et al. (2011). 2011 ACCF/AHA focused update of the guideline for the management of patients with peripheral artery disease (updating the 2005 guideline): A report of the American College of Cardiology Foundation/American Heart Association Task Force. *Journal of the American College of Cardiology, 58*(19), 2020–2045.

Ruppar, T., Dobbeis, F., & De Geest, S. (2012). Medication beliefs and antihypertensive adherence among older adults: A pilot study. *Geriatric Nursing, 33*(2), 89–95.

Spencer, A., Jablonski, R., & Loeb, S. (2012). Hypertensive African American women and the DASH diet. *Nurse Practitioner, 37*(2), 41–46.

Stephens, J., Hagler, D., & Clark, E. (2011). Got PAD? Hidden dangers revealed with ABI. *Journal of Vascular Nursing, 29*(4), 153–157.

U. S. Preventive Services Task Force. (2005). Screening for abdominal aortic aneurysm: Recommendation statement. *The American Journal for Nurse Practitioners, 9*(5), 55–60.

U. S. Preventive Services Task Force. (2007). Screening for high blood pressure: U. S. Preventive Services Task Force reaffirmation recommendation statement. *Annals of Internal Medicine, 147*(11), 783–786.

CHAPTER 19

Bostock-Cox, B. (2012). Caring for patients with anaemia of chronic disease. *British Journal of Primary Care Nursing: Cardiovascular Disease, Diabetes & Kidney Care, 9*(2), 62–63.

Byrd, L. (2011). Anemia in elders: Diagnosing & treatment strategies. *Geriatric Nursing, 32*(4), 297–304.

Kaufman, C. (2011). The secret life of lymphocytes. *Nursing, 41*(6), 50–54.

Miller, J., & Starks, B. (2010). Deciphering clues in the CBC count. *Nursing, 40*(7), 52–55.

Rauen, C. (2012). Beyond the bloody mess: Hematologic assessment. *Critical Care Nurse, 32*(5), 42–47.

CHAPTER 20

Adams, K., & Tolich, D. (2011). Blood transfusion: The patient's experience. *American Journal of Nursing, 111*(9), 24–32.

Adegbola, M., Barnes, D., Opollo, J., Herr, K., Gray, J., & McCarthy, A. (2012). Voices of adults living with sickle cell disease pain. *Journal of National Black Nurses Association, 23*(2), 16–23.

American Cancer Society (ACS). (2013). *Cancer facts & figures 2013.* Atlanta, GA: Author.

Bossaer, J., & Cluck, D. (2013). Home health care of patients with febrile neutropenia. *Home Health Care Management & Practice, 25*(3), 115–119.

Brown, M. (2012). Managing the acutely ill adult with sickle cell disease. *British Journal of Nursing, 21*(2), 90–96.

Byrd, L. (2011). Anemia in elders: Diagnosing & treatment strategies. *Geriatric Nursing, 32*(4), 297–304.

Cairo, M. (2011). Mild fatigue follows progressively heavy monthly periods. *Clinical Advisor for Nurse Practitioners, 14*(4), 131–133.

Centers for Disease Control and Prevention (CDC). (2012). *Folic acid recommendations.* Retrieved from http://www.cdc.gov/ncbddd/folicacid/recommendations.html

Coleman, E., Goodwin, J., Coon, S., Richards, K., Enderlin, C., Kennedy, R., et al. (2011). Fatigue, sleep, pain, mood, and performance status in patients with multiple myeloma. *Cancer Nursing, 34*(3), 219–227.

Derbyshire, E. (2012). Strategies to improve iron status in women at risk of developing anemia. *Nursing Standard, 26*(20), 51–57.

Dowling, M., & Kelly, M. (2011). Patients' lived experience of myeloma. *Nursing Standard, 25*(28), 38–44.

Dressler, D. (2012). Coagulopathy in the intensive care unit. *Critical Care Nurse, 32*(5), 48–60.

Farsi, Z., Nayeri, N., & Negarandeh, R. (2012). The coping process in adults with acute leukemia undergoing hematopoietic stem cell transplantation. *Journal of Nursing Research, 20*(2), 99–109.

Filler, K., Kelly, D., & Lyon, D. (2011). Fall risk in adult in patients with leukemia undergoing induction chemotherapy. *Clinical Journal of Oncology Nursing, 15*(4), 369–370.

Foster, C. (2011). Neutropenia. *MedSurg Nursing, 20*(5), 262, 264.

Hardy, D. (2012). Management of a patient with secondary lymphoedema. *Cancer Nursing Practice, 11*(2), 21–26.

Jenerette, C., & Brewer, C. (2011). Situation, background, assessment, and recommendation (SBAR) may benefit individuals who frequent emergency departments: Adults with sickle cells disease. *JEN: Journal of Emergency Nursing, 37*(6), 559–561.

Jenkins, G. (2012). Using dietary education to avoid iron deficiency in at risk patients. *Primary Health Care, 22*(3), 20–21.

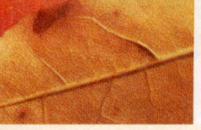
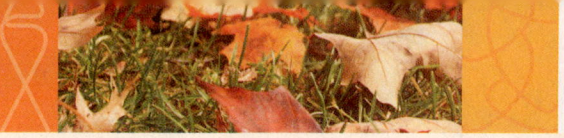
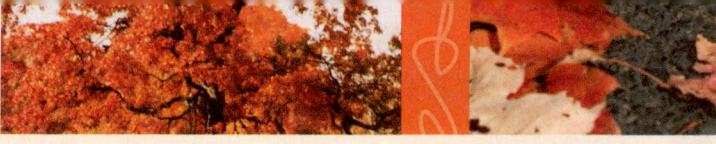

Kaufman, C. (2011). The secret life of lymphocytes. *Nursing, 41*(6), 50–54.

Kelly, M. (2011). Management of multiple myeloma. *World of Irish Nursing & Midwifery, 19*(3), 27–29.

Kelly, M., Dowling, M., & Meenaghan, T. (2011). Young patients with chronic lymphocytic leukaemia. *British Journal of Nursing, 20*(17), S30.

Kessenich, C., & Cronin, K. (2013). Lab logic: Fecal occult blood testing in older adult patients with anemia. *Nurse Practitioner, 38*(1), 6–8.

Konkle, B. (2012). Disorders of platelets and vessel wall. In D. Longo, A. Fauci, D. Kasper, S. Hauser, J. Jameson, J. Loscalzo (Eds.), *Harrison's principles of internal medicine* (18th ed.) (pp. 965–973). New York: McGraw-Hill Medical.

Lambing, A. (2012). Advances in the treatment of patients with hemophilia: Understanding the importance of comprehensive care and of the NP role. *American Journal for Nurse Practitioners, 16*(3–4), 6–14.

Linker, C., & Damon, L. (2012). Blood disorders. In S. McPhee & M. Papadakis (Eds.), *2012 Current medical diagnosis & treatment*. (pp. 475–519) New York: McGraw-Hill.

Maloney, K., & Denno, M. (2011). Tumor lysis syndrome: Prevention and detection to enhance patient safety. *Clinical Journal of Oncology Nursing, 15*(6), 601–603.

Phillips, R. (2012). The mystery of leukemia in older adults. *Nursing Made Incredibly Easy, 10*(1), 39–54.

Radovich, P. (2011). The multiple causes and myriad presentations of thrombocytopenia. *American Nurse Today, 6*(1), 9–12.

Ridner, S., Bonner, C., Deng, J., & Sinclair, V. (2012). Voices from the shadows: Living with lymphedema. *Cancer Nursing, 35*(1), E18–26.

Roper, K., Cooley, M., McDermott, K., & Fawcett, J. (2013). Health-related quality of life after treatment of Hodgkin lymphoma in young adults. *Oncology Nursing Forum, 40*(4), 349–360.

Sheehan, D. (2012). Wound care management of a patient with stage III lymphedema. *Rehabilitation Nursing, 37*(4), 176–179.

Smith, S. (2013). Safe administration of intravenous iron therapy. *Nursing Standard, 27*(31), 45–48.

Stephen, J., & Robertson-Artwork, A. (2012). Adults with sickle cell disease: An interdisciplinary approach to home care and self-care management with a case study. *Home Healthcare Nurse, 30*(3), 172–185.

Todd, M. (2013). Chronic oedema: Impact and management. *British Journal of Nursing, 22*(11), 623–627.

CHAPTER 21

Buccalo, S. (1997). Window on another world: An "English" nurse looks at the Amish culture and their health care beliefs. *Journal of Multicultural Nursing and Health, 3*(2), 53–58.

Davidhizar, R., Bechtel, G., & Giger, J. (1999, April). The influence of time and culture on health patterns. *Competency Matters, 2*(1), 13–15.

Ehrlich, A. (2010). Evidence-based medicine. Radiation from CT scans might increase lifetime risk of cancer. *Clinical Advisor for Nurse Practitioners, 13*(3), 107.

Johnson, C., Anderson, M., & Hill, P. (2012). Comparison of pulse oximetry measures in a healthy population. *MedSurg Nursing, 21*(2), 70–76.

Jonsson, T., Johsdottir, H., Möller, A., & Baldursdottir, L. (2011). Nursing documentation prior to emergency admissions to the intensive care unit. *Nursing in Critical Care, 16*(4), 164–169.

Kayyali, A. (2011). Journal watch. Low-dose CT screening for lung cancer in high-risk patients. *American Journal of Nursing, 111*(11), 60.

Langdon, R., Johnson, M., Carroll, V., & Antonio, G. (2013). Assessment of the elderly: It's worth covering the risks. *Journal of Nursing Management, 21*(1), 94–105.

LeMone, P., Burke, K., & Bauldoff, G. (2015). *Medical–surgical nursing: Critical thinking in patient care* (6th ed.). Hoboken, NJ: Pearson.

Lian, J. (2013). Using ABGs to optimize mechanical ventilation. *Nursing, 43*(6), 46–53.

Munroe, B., & Curtis, K. (2011). Assessment, monitoring and emergency nursing care in blunt chest injury: A case study. *Australasian Emergency Nursing Journal, 14*(4), 257–263.

Nawafleh, H., Al-Sayed Abo Zead, S., & Fayez Al-Maghaireh, D. (2012). Pulmonary function test: The value among smokers and nonsmokers. *Health Science Journal, 6*(4), 703–713.

O'Shea, L. (2010). Differential diagnosis of chest pain. *Practice Nurse, 40*(6), 13–18.

Pruitt, B. (2010). Interpreting ABGs: An inside look at your patient's status. *Nursing, 40*(7), 31–36.

Ranu, H., & Madden, B. (2010). "More is missed by not looking than by not knowing": Endobronchial foreign bodies. *Care of the Critically Ill, 25*(3–4), 79–84.

Saxon, C. (2012). Relevant lung diseases in bronchoscopy. *J.GENCA, 22*(2), 6–12.

Wallace, E. (2012). Is there a role for lung cancer screening? *World of Irish Nursing & Midwifery, 20*(2), 43–44.

CHAPTER 22

American Cancer Society. (2013a). *Cancer facts & figures 2013*. Atlanta, GA: Author.

American Cancer Society. (2013b). *Cancer facts & figures for African Americans 2013–2014*. Atlanta, GA: Author.

Ardilio, S. (2011). Calculating nutrition needs for a patient with head and neck cancer. *Clinical Journal of Oncology Nursing, 15*(5), 457–459.

Barrows, K. (2013). Chapter e5. Complementary & alternative medicine. In M. A. Papadakis, S. J. McPhee, & M. W. Rabow (Eds.), *CURRENT medical diagnosis & treatment 2013*. Retrieved from http://www.access-medicine.com/content.aspx?aID=22146

Brownfield, E., Marsden, J., Iverson, P., Zhao, Y., Mauldin, P., & Moran, W. (2012). Point of care experience with pneumococcal and influenza vaccine documentation among person aged >65 years: High refusal rates and missing information. *American Journal of Infection Control, 40*(7), 672–674.

Centers for Disease Control and Prevention. (2010). *2009 H1N1 Flu*. Retrieved from http://www.cdc.gov/h1n1flu/

Centers for Disease Control and Prevention. (2011). Updated recommendations for use of tetanus toxoid, reduced diphtheria toxoid and acellular pertussis vaccine (Tdap) in pregnant women and persons who have or anticipate having close contact with an infant aged *Morbidity & Mortality Weekly Report, 60*, 1424–1426.

Centers for Disease Control and Prevention. (2012a). Updated recommendations for use of tetanus toxoid, reduced diphtheria toxoid and acellular pertussis vaccine (Tdap) in adults aged 65 years and older—Advisory Committee on Immunization Practices (ACIP), 2012. *Morbidity & Mortality Weekly Report, 61*, 468–470.

Centers for Disease Control and Prevention. (2012b). Pertussis epidemic—Washington, 2012. *Morbidity & Mortality Weekly Report, 61*, 517–522.

Centers for Disease Control and Prevention. (2013a). *Guidance for clinicians on the use of rapid influenza diagnostic tests*. Retrieved from http://www.cdc.gov/flu/professionals/diagnosis/clinician_guidance_ridt.htm

Centers for Disease Control and Prevention. (2013b). *Prevention strategies for seasonal influenza in healthcare settings*. Retrieved from http://www.cdc.gov/flu/professionals/infectioncontrol/healthcaresettings.htm

Cerantola, C., & Happ, M. (2012). Transitional care for communication impaired older adults: ICU to home. *Geriatric Nursing, 33*(6), 489–492.

Cunha, B., Hage, J., & Thekkel, V. (2011). Infection control implications of influenza A and influenza B: Coinfection or cocirculating strains? *American Journal of Infection Control, 39*(8), 701–702.

Dambaugh, L. (2012). A review of influenza: Implications for the geriatric population. *Critical Care Nursing Clinics of North America, 24*(4), 573–580.

Douglas, N. (2012). Sleep apnea. In D. Longo, A. Fauci, D. Kasper, S. Hauser, J. Jameson, & J. Loscalzo (Eds.), *Harrison's principles of internal medicine* (18th ed.). New York: McGraw-Hill.

DTap, Tdap: What's in a name? (2011). *AACN Bold Voices, 3*(1), 15.

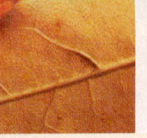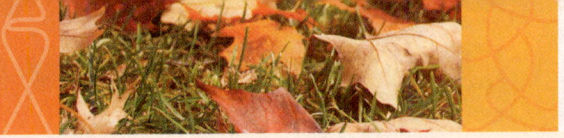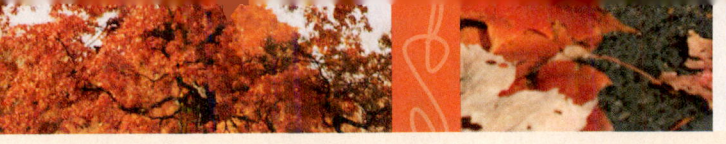

Elfström, M., Karlsson, S., Nilsen, P., Fridlund, B., & Svanborg, E. (2012). Decisive situations affecting partners' support to continuous positive airway pressure-treated patients with obstructive sleep apnea syndrome: A critical incident technique analysis of the initial treatment phase. *Journal of Cardiovascular Nursing, 27*(3), 228–239.

Freeman, S. (2011). Care of adult patients with a temporary tracheostomy. *Nursing Standard, 26*(2), 49–56.

Keenan, C., & Deasy, J. (2011). Communicating Tdap vaccination status to adults. *Clinical Advisor for Nurse Practitioners, 14*(7), 70.

McGrory, A. (2011). Communicating with head and neck cancer patients. *ORL-Head & Neck Nursing, 29*(3), 7–11.

McLaughlin, L. (2013). Taste dysfunction in head and neck cancer survivors. *Oncology Nursing Forum, 40*(1), E4–E13.

National Center for Health Statistics. (2013). *Health, United States, 2012: With special feature on emergency care.* Hyattsville, MD: Author.

Nursing interventions to help protect older adults. (2013). *Nursing, 43*(4), 26–27.

Olyarchuk, L., Willoughby, D., Davis, S., & Newsom, S. (2012). Examining the benefit of vaccinating adults against pertussis. *Journal of the American Academy of Nurse Practitioners, 24*(10), 587–594.

Planton, J., Meyer, J., & Edlund, B. (2012). Recommended routine vaccinations for older adults. *Journal of Gerontological Nursing, 38*(7), 16–20.

Schween, S. (2011). Combating infection. Pertussis: Not just for kids anymore. *Nursing, 41*(10), 61–62.

Seasonal flu taking heavy toll on elderly. (2013). *Hospital Infection Control & Prevention, 40*(2), 22.

Sharma, S., Agrawal, S., Damodaran, D., Sreenivas, V., Kadhiravan, T., et al. (2011). CPAP for the metabolic syndrome in patients with obstructive sleep apnea. *New England Journal of Medicine, 365*(24), 2277–2286.

Shoup, J. (2011). Management of adult rhinosinusitis. *Nurse Practitioner, 36*(11), 22–27.

Smith, H., Peek-Asa, C., Nesheim, D., Nish, A., Normandin, P., & Sahr, S. (2012). Etiology, diagnosis, and characteristics of facial fracture at a midwestern level 1 trauma center. *Journal of Trauma Nursing, 19*(1), 57–65.

Thornton, K., Alston, M., Dye, H., & Williamson, S. (2011). Are saline irrigations effective in relieving chronic rhinosinusitis symptoms? A review of the evidence. *Journal for Nurse Practitioners, 7*(8), 680–686.

Vaccines and immunizations. (2011). *Journal of Practical Nursing, 61*(3), 14–20.

Vokes, E. (2012). Head and neck cancer. In D. Longo, A. Fauci, D. Kasper, S. Hauser, J. Jameson, & J. Loscalzo (Eds.), *Harrison's principles of internal medicine* (18th ed.). New York: McGraw-Hill.

Zastrow, R. (2011). Pertussis on the rise: A troubling picture of waning immunity, with unvaccinated children especially vulnerable. *American Journal of Nursing, 111*(6), 51–56.

CHAPTER 23

Al-Yateem, N. (2012). Child to adult: Transitional care for young adults with cystic fibrosis. *British Journal of Nursing, 21*(14), 850–854.

American Cancer Society (ACS). (2013a). *American cancer society guidelines for the early detection of cancer.* Atlanta, GA: Author.

American Cancer Society (ACS). (2013b). *Cancer facts & figures 2013.* Atlanta, GA: Author.

Ames, N. (2011). Evidence to support tooth brushing in critically ill patients. *American Journal of Critical Care, 20*(3), 242–250.

Aziz, A. (2011). Minimizing respiratory infections through hygiene. *Nursing & Residential Care, 13*(7), 330–333.

Barrows, K. (2013). Ch e5. Complementary & alternative medicine. In M. A. Papadakis, S. J. McPhee, & M. W. Rabow (Eds.), *CURRENT medical diagnosis & treatment 2013.* Retrieved from http://www.accessmedicine.com/content.aspx?aID=22146

Bonk, A. (2012). Management of dyspnea in a patient with lung cancer. *Oncology Nursing Forum, 39*(3), 257–260.

Bostock-Cox, B. (2012). Prescribing established and new therapies in COPD. *Nurse Prescribing, 10*(11), 539–540, 542–544.

Bostock-Cox, B. (2013a, January 21). Distinguishing asthma from COPD in primary care settings. *Independent Nurse,* 28–31.

Bostock-Cox, B. (2013b, April 15). Assessment and management of an exacerbation of COPD. *Independent Nurse,* 14–18.

Carter, D. (2011). Long-term effects of ARDS after ICU stay: Five years later, subtle symptoms persist despite normal lung tests. *American Journal of Nursing, 111*(7), 17.

Centers for Disease Control and Prevention (CDC). (2011). Recommendations for use of an isoniazid-rifapentine regimen with direct observation to treat latent *Mycobacterium tuberculosis* infection. *Morbidity and Mortality Weekly Report, 60*(48), 1650–1653.

Centers for Disease Control and Prevention (CDC). (2012). *Reported tuberculosis in the United States, 2011.* Atlanta, GA: U.S. Department of Health and Human Services, CDC.

Centers for Disease Control and Prevention (CDC). (2013). *TB incidence in the United States, 1953–2011.* Retrieved from http://www.cdc.gov/tb/statistics/tbcases.htm

Clerk, N., Sisson, K., & Antunes, G. (2011). Latent tuberculosis: Concordance and duration of treatment regimens. *British Journal of Nursing, 20*(13), 824–827.

Corbridge, S., Wilken, L., Kapella, M., & Gronkiewicz, C. (2012). An evidence-based approach to COPD: Part 1. *American Journal of Nursing, 112*(3), 46–59.

Day, M. (2011). Action stat. Tension pneumothorax. *Nursing, 41*(1), 72.

Disability higher among geriatric mechanical ventilation survivors. (2011). *AACN Bold Voices, 3*(4), 10.

Dobbin, K., & Howard, V. (2011). Listen closely to detect healthcare-associated pneumonia. *Nursing, 41*(7), 59–62.

Geary, K., & Beckett, G. (2012). Management of seasonal and pandemic flu. *Nurse Prescribing, 10*(10), 488–493.

Global Initiative for Chronic Obstructive Lung Disease (GOLD). (2011). *Global strategy for the diagnosis, management, and prevention of chronic obstructive pulmonary disease.* Vancouver, WA: Author.

Hall, M. (2012). Chronic obstructive pulmonary disease and asthma. *Home Healthcare Nurse, 30*(10), 603–614.

Institute for Clinical Systems Improvement (ICSI). (2011). *Prevention of ventilator-associated pneumonia. Health care protocol.* Bloomington, MN: Author.

Kent, V. (2011). Put a cap on community-acquired pneumonia. *Nursing Made Incredibly Easy, 9*(2), 34–45.

Khalaila, R., Zbidat, W., Anwar, K., Bayya, A., Linton, D., & Sviri, S. (2011). Communication difficulties and psychoemotional distress in patients receiving mechanical ventilation. *American Journal of Critical Care, 20*(6), 470–479.

Laird, P., & Ruppert, S. (2011). Acute respiratory distress syndrome—a case study. *Critical Care Nursing Quarterly, 34*(2), 165–174.

Lareau, S., & Hodder, R. (2012). Teaching inhaler use in chronic obstructive pulmonary disease patients. *Journal of the American Academy of Nurse Practitioners, 24*(2), 113–120.

Lian, J. X. (2013). Using ABGs to optimize mechanical ventilation. *Nursing, 43*(6), 46–53.

McLenon, M. (2012). Acute pulmonary embolism. *Critical Care Nursing Quarterly, 35*(2), 173–182.

Molle, E. (2013). Mucolytic agents for COPD and chronic bronchitis. *American Journal of Nursing, 113*(7), 23.

Moore, D. (2013). Preventing acute hypercapnic respiratory failure in COPD patients. *Nursing Standard, 27*(47), 35–41.

Morgan, J., & Sego, S. (2011). BCG vaccine and latent TB. *Clinical Advisory for Nurse Practitioners, 14*(7), 80–81.

Munroe, B., & Curtis, K. (2011). Assessment, monitoring and emergency nursing care in blunt chest injury: A case study. *Australasian Emergency Nursing Journal, 14*(4), 257–263.

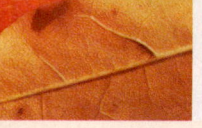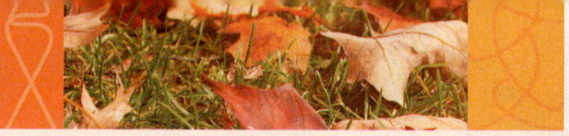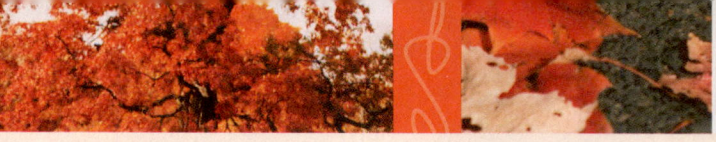

National Heart, Lung, and Blood Institute. (2007). *Expert panel report 3: Guidelines for the diagnosis and management of asthma*. Bethesda, MD: Author.

Parsons, S., Lee, C., Strickert, D., & Trumpp, M. (2013). Oral care and ventilator-associated pneumonia. *Dimensions of Critical Care Nursing, 32*(3), 138–145.

Perry, M. (2012). How the signs and symptoms of common infections vary with age. *Practice Nursing, 23*(4), 176–181.

Pezzotti, W., & Freuler, M. (2012). Using anticoagulants to steer clear of clots. *Nursing, 42*(2), 26–35.

Raviglione, M., & O'Brien, R. (2012). Tuberculosis. In D. Longo, A. Fauci, D. Kasper, S. Hauser, J.L. Jameson, & J. Loscalzo, Eds. *Harrison's principles of internal medicine* (18th ed.), pp. 1340–1359. New York: McGraw Hill Medical.

Ruiz, C. (2011). Thwarting a pneumothorax: The nurse's assessment skills help avoid a worst-case scenario. *American Nurse Today, 6*(5), 32.

Rutt, A. (2012). Hypersensitivity pneumonitis: An occupational hazard. *Journal for Nurse Practitioners, 8*(5), 399–405.

Sanford, D. (2012). Management of a pulmonary artery embolectomy and recurrent embolus. *AANA Journal, 80*(1), 11–15.

Shapiro, A., & Swenson, K. (2011). Nutritional challenges during treatment for lung cancer. *Oncology Nursing Forum, 38*(5), 515–518.

Smith, B., & Tasota, F. (2011). Smoking out the dangers of COPD. *Nursing, 41*(4), 32–40.

Stacy, K. (2012). Withdrawal of life-sustaining treatment: A case study. *Critical Care Nurse, 32*(3), 14–24.

Sveum, R., Bergstrom, J., Brottman, G., Hanson, M., Heiman, M., Johns, K., et al. (2012). *Diagnosis and management of asthma*. Bloomington, MN: Institute for Clinical Systems Improvement.

Vacca, V., Jr., & Jehle, J. (2013). Acute pulmonary embolism. *Nursing, 43*(3), 25–26.

Wallace, E. (2012). Is there a role for lung cancer screening? *World of Irish Nursing & Midwifery, 43*–44.

Wier, L., Pfuntner, A., Maeda, J., Stranges, E., Ryan, K., Jagadish, P., et al. (2011). *HCUP facts and figures: Statistics on hospital-based care in the United States, 2009*. Rockville, MD: Agency for Healthcare Research and Quality.

Willgoss, T., Yohannes, A., Goldbart, J., & Fatoye, F. (2011). COPD and anxiety: Its impact on patient's lives. *Nursing Times, 107*(15–16), 16–19.

CHAPTER 24

Derbyshire, E. (2012). Trans fats; Implications for health. *Nursing Standard, 27*(3), 51–56.

DiMaria-Ghalili, R. A. (2012). *Nutrition in the elderly. Nursing standard of practice protocol: Nutrition in aging*. Hartford Institute for Geriatric Nursing. Retrieved from www.consultgerirn.org/topics/nutrition_in_the_elderly

DiMaria-Ghalili, R. A., & Amella, E. J. (2012). Assessing nutrition in older adults. *Try This: Best Practices in Nursing Care to Older Adults, 9*. The Hartford Institute for Geriatric Nursing, College of Nursing, New York University. Retrieved from www.ConsultGeriRN.org

Heath, H., Sturdy, D., Edwards, T., Griffiths, J., Hylton, B., Jones, V., et al. (2011, January). Promoting older people's oral health. *Nursing Standard, Supplement,* 1–19.

Tucker, S., & Dauffenbach, V. (2011). *Nutrition and diet therapy for nurses*. Upper Saddle River, NJ: Pearson.

U.S. Department of Agriculture and U.S. Department of Health and Human Services. (2010). *Dietary guidelines for Americans 2010* (7th ed.). Washington, DC: U.S. Government Printing Office.

Van der Kramer, V. (2011). Nutrition for older people: Building immunity over the winter season. *Nutrition, 16*(11), S22–24.

Woodward, S. (2012). Assessment and management of constipation in older people. *Nursing Older People, 24*(5), 21–26.

CHAPTER 25

Ahmed, A., & Stanley, A. (2012). Acute upper gastrointestinal bleeding in the elderly. *Drugs & Aging, 29*(12), 933–940.

American Cancer Society (ACS). (2013). *Cancer facts & figures 2013*. Atlanta, GA: Author.

American Cancer Society (ACS). (2014). *Stomach cancer*. Retrieved from http://www.cancer.org/cancer/stomachcancer/detailedguide/stomach-cancer-risk-factors

Avery, A. (2012). Managing obesity in young adults. *Practice Nursing, 23*(6), 291–294.

Best, C., & Evans, L. (2013). Identification and management of patients' nutritional needs. *Nursing Older People, 25*(3), 30–37.

Bissett, S., & Preshaw, P. (2011). Guide to providing mouth care for older people. *Nursing Older People, 23*(10), 14–21.

Burns, B. (2012). Oral care for older people in residential. *Nursing & Residential Care, 14*(1), 26–31.

Centers for Disease Control and Prevention (CDC). (2011). *Guideline for the prevention and control of norovirus gastroenteritis outbreaks in healthcare settings, 2011*. Atlanta, GA: Author. Retrieved from http://www.cdc.gov/hicpac/norovirus/002_norovirus-toc.html

DiMaria-Ghalili, R. A. (2012). *Nutrition in the elderly. Nursing standard of practice protocol: Nutrition in aging*. Hartford Institute for Geriatric Nursing, New York University College of Nursing. Retrieved from http://consultgerirn.org/topics/nutrition_in_the_elderly/want_to_know_more

DiMaria-Ghalili, R. A., & Amella, E. (2012). Assessing nutrition in older adults. *Try This: Best Practices in Nursing Care to Older Adults, 9*. Retrieved from www.ConsultGeriRN.org

Fontaine, K. L. (2011). *Complementary & alternative therapies for nursing practice* (3rd ed.). Upper Saddle River, NJ: Pearson.

Gunther, S., Gue, F., Sinfield, P., Rogers, S., & Baker, R. (2012). Barriers and enablers to managing obesity in general practice: A practical approach for use in implementation activities. *Quality in Primary Care, 20*, 93–103.

Hambridge, K. (2013). Assessing the risk of post-operative nausea and vomiting. *Nursing Standard, 27*(18), 35–43.

Institute for Clinical Systems Improvement (ICSI). (2011). *Prevention and management of obesity (mature adolescents and adults)*. Bloomington, MN: Author.

Karthick, P., Sowmya, T., Raja, K., & Natarajan, R. (2011). Prevalence of disease with epigastric pain with reference to gastric pathology. *Internet Journal of Health, 12*(2), 1.

Metheny, N. (2012). *Fluid and electrolyte balance: Nursing considerations* (5th ed.). Sudbury, MA: Jones & Bartlett Learning.

Moxon, R. (2011). Oesophageal cancer: Symptoms, treatment and nursing role. *Nursing Standard, 25*(32), 50–56.

National Cancer Institute. (2014). *Oral cancer prevention (PDQ$^®$)*. Retrieved from http://www.cancer.gov/cancertopics/pdq/prevention/oral/HealthProfessional#Section_121

National Center for Health Statistics (NCHS). (2013). NCHS Data Brief: Prevalence of obesity among adults: United States, 2011–2012. Retrieved from www.cdc.gov/nchs/data/databriefs/db131.pdf

National Institutes of Health. (2000). *The practical guide: Identification, evaluation, and treatment of overweight and obesity in adults* (NIH Publication No. 00–4084). Bethesda, MD: Author.

Smith, D., Griffin, Q., & Fitzpatrick, J. (2011). Exercise and exercise intentions among obese and overweight individuals. *Journal of the American Academy of Nurse Practitioners, 23*, 92–100.

Sobieraj, D., Coleman, S., & Colman, C. (2011). US prevalence of upper gastrointestinal symptoms: A systematic literature review. *American Journal of Managed Care, 17*(11), e449–e458.

Söderhamn, U. (2012, November). Tools to identify nutritional risk for older people in the home. *Nutrition,* S26–S29.

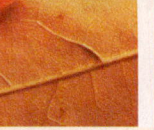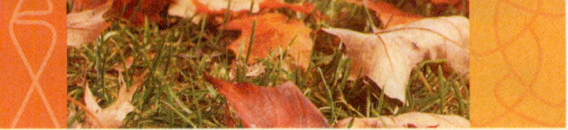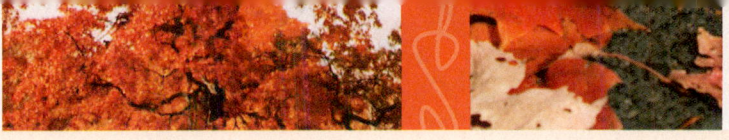

Stake-Nilsson, K., Hultcrantz, R., Unge, P., & Wengström, Y. (2011). Complementary and alternative medicine used by persons with functional gastrointestinal disorders to alleviate symptom distress. *Journal of Clinical Nursing, 21,* 800–808.

Thomas, C., & Taub, L. (2011). Monitoring for and preventing the long-term sequelae of bariatric surgery. *Journal of the American Academy of Nurse Practitioners, 23,* 449–458.

Timms, L. (2011). Effect of nutrition on wound healing in older people: A case study. *British Journal of Nursing, 20*(11), S4–S10.

U.S. Department of Agriculture (USDA), & U.S. Department of Health and Human Services (HHS). (2010). *Dietary guidelines for Americans, 2010* (7th ed.). Washington, DC: U.S. Government Printing Office.

Wright, K., & Hacking, S. (2011). An angel on my shoulder: A study of relationships between women with anorexia and healthcare professionals. *Journal of Psychiatric and Mental Health Nursing, 19,* 107–115.

CHAPTER 26

American Cancer Society (ACS). (2012). *Cancer facts & figures for Hispanics/Latinos 2012–2014.* Atlanta, GA: Author.

American Cancer Society (ACS). (2013a). *American cancer society guidelines for the early detection of cancer.* Retrieved from www.cancer.org

American Cancer Society (ACS). (2013b). *Cancer facts & figures 2013.* Atlanta, GA: Author.

American Cancer Society (ACS). (2013c). *Cancer facts & figures for African Americans 2013–2014.* Atlanta, GA: Author.

Bettany, J., & Gardiner, A. (2013). Inflammatory bowel disease: An overview on assessment. *Nursing and Residential Care, 15*(9), 607–610.

Black, P. (2011a). Coping with common stoma problems in care homes. *Nursing & Residential Care, 13*(3), 126, 128.

Black, P. (2011b). The role of the carer and patient in stoma care. *Nursing & Residential Care, 13*(9), 432–434, 436.

Brittain, K., Taylor, J., Loveland-Cherry, C., Northhouse, L., & Caldwell, C. (2012). Family support and colorectal cancer screening among urban African Americans. *Journal for Nurse Practitioners, 8*(7), 522–533.

Causey, C., & Greenwald, B. (2011). Promoting community awareness of the need for colorectal cancer prevention and screening: A replication study. *Gastroenterology Nursing, 34*(1), 34–40.

Crohn's & Colitis Foundation of America. (2013). *What are Crohns and Colitis?* Retrieved from http://www.ccfa.org/what-are-crohns-and-colitis/

Dalrymple, J., & Bullock, I. (2008, March). Diagnosis and management of irritable bowel syndrome in adults in primary care: Summary of NICE guidance. *BMJ: British Medical Journal, 336*(7643), 556–558.

De Melo, S., Jr., & DiPalma, J. (2012). The role of capsule endoscopy in evaluating inflammatory bowel disease. *Gastroenterology Clinics of North America, 41*(2), 315–323.

Di Sabatino, A., & Corazza, G. (2012). Nonceliac gluten sensitivity: Sense or sensibility? *Annals of Internal Medicine, 156*(4), 309–311.

The diversity of inflammatory bowel disease: Beyond the gut. (2012). *Gastrointestinal Nursing, 10*(4), 22–28.

Duncan, J. (2011). Nursing assessment in inflammatory bowel disease. *Gastrointestinal Nursing, 9*(1), 14–20.

Holt, K. (2011). Common side effects and interactions of colorectal cancer therapeutic agents. *Journal of Practical Nursing, 61*(1), 7–20.

Lichtenstein, G., Hanauer, S., & Sandborn, W. (2009). Practice parameters committee of American College of Gastroenterology. Management of Crohn's disease in adults. *American Journal of Gastroenterology, 104*(2), 465–483.

Martins, L., Tavernelli, K., Sansom, W., Dahl, K., Claessens, I., Porrett, T., et al. (2013). Strategies to reduce treatment costs of peristomal skin complications. *Gastrointestinal Nursing, 10*(10), 24–32.

Richbourg, L. (2012). Food fight: Dietary choices made by people after stoma formation. *Gastrointestinal Nursing, 10*(4), 44–50.

Taylor, R. (2011). What are functional foods and what they can do? *Nursing & Residential Care, 13*(2), 72, 74, 78–81.

Thompson, H., North, J., Davenport, R., & Williams, J. (2011, September 8). Matching the skin barrier to the skin type. *British Journal of Nursing,* S27–S30.

Tucker, S., & Dauffenback, V. (2011). *Nutrition and diet therapy for nurses.* Upper Saddle River, NJ: Pearson.

Walker, H. (2012). Managing abdominal complications due to severe diverticular disease: A team approach. *Gastrointestinal Nursing, 10*(Suppl.), 7–10.

Woodward, S. (2012). Assessment and management of constipation in older people. *Nursing Older People, 24*(5), 21–26.

CHAPTER 27

American Cancer Society (ACS). (2013). *Cancer facts & figures 2013.* Atlanta, GA: Author.

Blann, A. (2012). Making sense of liver function tests. *British Journal of Primary Care Nursing: Cardiovascular Disease, Diabetes & Kidney Care* (Special issue: Chronic Liver Disease), 30–33.

Brooks, K., Scarborough, J., Vaslef, S., & Shapiro, M. (2013). No need to wait: An analysis of the timing of cholecystectomy during admission for acute cholecystitis using the American College of Surgeons National Surgical Quality Improvement Program database. *Journal of Trauma & Acute Care Surgery, 74*(1), 167–174.

Centers for Disease Control and Prevention. (2012). *Epidemiology and prevention of vaccine-preventable diseases* (12th ed., W. Atkinson, S. Wolfe, & J. Hamborsky, Eds.). Washington, DC: Public Health Foundation.

Centers for Disease Control and Prevention. (2013). *Statistics and surveillance. Disease burden from viral hepatitis A, B, and C in the United States.* Retrieved from www.cdc.gov/

Frazer, K., Glacken, M., Coughlan, B., Staines, A., & Daly, L. (2011). Hepatitis C virus infection in primary care: Survey of registered nurses' knowledge and access to information. *Journal of Advanced Nursing, 67*(2), 327–339.

Fullwood, D. (2012). Portal hypertension and varices in patients with liver cirrhosis. *Nursing Standard, 26*(48), 52.

Gee, C. (2011). Pancreatic cancer: A whistle-stop tour. *Gastrointestinal Nursing, 9*(7), 41–45.

Harris, H., & Crawford, A. (2013). Hepatitis goes viral. *Nursing,* 38–43.

Hayes, C. (2011). The here and now of pancreatic cancer. *Gastrointestinal Nursing, 9*(10), 28–33.

Horne, P. (2011). Managing complications in patients with cirrhosis and hepatocellular carcinoma. *American Journal for Nurse Practitioners, 15*(1-2), 28-30–32-34.

Institute of Medicine (IOM). (2010). *Hepatitis and liver cancer: A National Strategy for Prevention and Control of Hepatitis B and C.* Washington, DC: The National Academies Press.

Lacovara, J. E. (2011). Whipple pancreaticoduodenectomy surgery for the treatment of pancreatic cancer. *Medsurg Nursing: Official Journal of the Academy of Medical-Surgical Nurses, 20*(6), 337–339.

Maghlaoui, A. (2012). Challenges and issues in managing hepatitis C. *Nursing Times, 108*(32–33), 18.

Milk thistle. (2012). *Herbs at a glance.* National Center for Complementary and Alternative Medicine. Retrieved from www.nih.gov/nccam

Olson, M., & Jacobson, I. (2011). Role of the nurse practitioner in the management of patients with chronic hepatitis C. *Journal of the American Academy of Nurse Practitioners, 23,* 410–420.

Page, J. (2012a). Nonalcoholic fatty liver disease: The hepatic metabolic syndrome. *Journal of the American Academy of Nurse Practitioners, 24*(6), 345–351.

Page, J. (2012b). Recent developments in the treatment of chronic hepatitis C. *Journal for Nurse Practitioners, 8*(3), 225–230.

Poll, R. (2012). Hepatitis C part 2: Treatment and prevention. *Practice Nursing, 23*(11), 540–546.

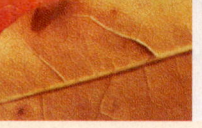
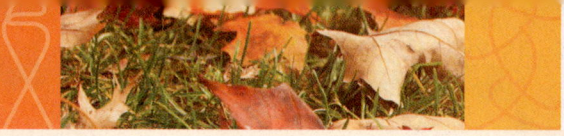

Ross, S. (2008, September). Milk thistle (Silybum marianum): An ancient botanical medicine for modern times. *Holistic Nursing Practice, 22*(5), 299–300.

Runyon, B. (2013). *Management of adult patients with ascites due to cirrhosis: Update 2012.* Alexandria, VA: American Association for the Study of Liver Diseases.

Smith, S. B. (2013). Discharge planning for the patient with chronic pancreatitis. *Gastroenterology Nursing: The Official Journal of the Society of Gastroenterology Nurses and Associates, 36*(6), 415–419.

Windsor, J. (2012). New guidance: Awareness and testing for hepatitis B and C. *Nursing Standard, 27*(15), 35–35.

CHAPTER 28

Bradway, C., & Cacchione, P. (2010). Teaching strategies for assessing and managing urinary incontinence in older adults. *Journal of Gerontological Nursing, 36*(7), 18–26.

Cowdell, F. (2011). Older people, personal hygiene, and skin care. *MedSurg Nursing, 20*(5), 235–240.

Cystatin, C. (2010). *Lab tests online.* Retrieved from www.labtestsonline.org/understanding/analytes/cystatin-c

Dowling-Castronovo, A. (2007). Urinary incontinence assessment in older adults: Part I—transient urinary incontinence. *Try This: Best Practices in Nursing Care to Older Adults from the Hartford Institute for Geriatric Nursing, 11.1*, 1–2.

Dowling-Castronovo, A. (2008). Urinary incontinence assessment in older adults: Part II—established urinary incontinence. *Try This: Best Practices in Nursing Care to Older Adults from the Hartford Institute for Geriatric Nursing, 11.2*, 1–2.

Ruxton, C. (2012). Promoting and maintaining healthy hydration in patients. *Nursing Standard, 26*(31), 50–56.

Smith, C., & Cotter, V. (2008). *Normal aging changes. Nursing standard of practice protocol: Age-related changes in health.* Hartford Institute for Geriatric Nursing. Retrieved from http://consultgerirn.org/topics/normal_aging_changes/want_to_know_more

CHAPTER 29

Ali, B., & Gray-Vickrey, P. (2011). Limiting the damage from acute kidney injury. *Nursing, 41*(3), 22–32.

American Medical Directors Association (AMDA). (2010). *Urinary incontinence.* Columbia, MD: Author.

AUA Foundation. (2011). *Urinary tract infections in adults.* Retrieved from http://www.urologyhealth.org/urology/index.cfm?article=47

Brown, T. (2012). Protection against urinary tract infections seen with cranberry products. *Medscape.* Retrieved from www.medscape.org/viewarticle/767190

Castner, D. (2010). Understanding the stages of chronic kidney disease. *Nursing, 40*(5), 24–32.

Centers for Disease Control and Prevention (CDC). (2012). *National Chronic Kidney Disease fact sheet 2010.* Retrieved from www.cdc.gov/diabetes/pubs/factsheets/kidney/htm

Dailly, S. (2011). Prevention of indwelling catheter-associated urinary tract infections. *Nursing Older People, 23*(2), 14–19.

Dirkes, S. (2011). Acute kidney injury: Not just acute renal failure anymore? *Critical Care Nurse, 31*(1), 37–49.

Dowling-Castronovo, A., & Bradway, C. (2008). *Urinary incontinence. Nursing standard of practice protocol: Urinary incontinence (UI) in older adults admitted to acute care.* Hartford Institute for Geriatric Nursing, New York University. Retrieved from consultgerirn.org/topics/urinary_incontinence

Ehrlich, A. (2011). Stat consult. Urinary tract infection in adults. *Clinical Advisor for Nurse Practitioners, 14*(3), 109.

Evans, M., & Tulaney, T. (2012). Urinary tract infection in older adults. *Nursing, 42*(4), 72.

Fink, H., Ishani, A., Taylor, B., Greer, N., MacDonald, R., Rossini, D., et al. (2012). Screening for, monitoring, and treatment of chronic kidney disease stages 1 to 3: A systematic review for the U.S. Preventive Services Task Force and for an American College of Physicians clinical practice guideline. *Annals of Internal Medicine, 156*(8), 570–581.

Gill, P. (2012). Stressors and coping mechanisms in live-related renal transplantation. *Journal of Clinical Nursing, 21*(11–12), 1622–1631.

Grasso, M. (2012). Extracorporeal shockwave lithotripsy. *Medscape Reference.* Retrieved from http://emedicine.medscape.com/article/444554-overview

Kidney Disease: Improving Global Outcomes (KDIGO) Acute Kidney Injury Work Group. (2012). KDIGO clinical practice guideline for acute kidney injury. *Kidney International, 2*(Suppl.), 1–138.

Leaver, R. (2011). Essential guide to urinary incontinence. *Practice Nurse, 41*(8), 33–36.

Lerma, E. (2011). Acute tubular necrosis. *Medscape Reference: Drugs, diseases, & procedures.* Retrieved from http://emedicine.medscape.com/article/238064-overview

Leung, S., Hunter, K., Parke, B., Sales, A., Molzahn, A., & Davison, S. (2012). Nursing strategies to support self-management in people with chronic kidney disease. *CANNT Journal, 22*(2), 14.

Lewington, A., & Kanagasundaram, S. (2011). *Clinical practice guidelines: Acute kidney injury* (5th ed.). UK Renal Association. Retrieved from www.renal.org/guidelines

Muaai-Bjornson, L., & Macera, L. (2011). Preventing infection in elders with long-term indwelling urinary catheters. *Journal of the American Academy of Nurse Practitioners, 23*(3), 127–134.

National Kidney and Urologic Diseases Information Clearinghouse. (2012). *Kidney disease statistics for the United States* (NIH Publication No. 12–3895). Retrieved from www.niddk.nih.gov

O'Shay, L. (2010). Diagnosing urinary tract infections. *Practice Nurse, 40*(9), 20–25.

Pellatt, G. (2012). Non-containment management options of urinary continence. *Nursing & Residential Care, 14*(2), 68, 70–73.

Perry, M. (2011). Treating symptomatic UTIs in older people. *Practice Nursing, 22*(1), 21–23.

Perry, M. (2012). How the signs and symptoms of common infections vary with age. *Practice Nursing, 23*(4), 176–181.

Peters, R., & Olsen, K. (2010). Kidney disease awareness among high-risk African Americans. *American Journal for Nurse Practitioners, 14*(3), 40–47.

Pratt, R., & Pellowe, C. (2010). Good practice in management of patients with urethral catheters. *Nursing Older People, 22*(8), 25–29.

Racial differences in trends of end-stage renal disease, by primary diagnosis—United States, 1994–2004. (2007). *Morbidity & Mortality Weekly Report.* Bethesda, MD: Centers for Disease Control and Prevention.

Robins, V. (2010). Managing diabetic nephropathy. *Practice Nursing, 21*(2), 84.

Ruxton, C. (2012). Promoting and maintaining healthy hydration in patients. *Nursing Standard, 26*(31), 50–56.

Shaxted, E. (2011). The management of stress urinary incontinence in women. *The AvMA Medical & Legal Journal, 17*(1), 26–28.

Stewart, E. (2010). Treating urinary incontinence in older women. *British Journal of Community Nursing, 15*(11), 526, 528, 530–532.

Tingström, P., Milberg, A., & Sund-Levander, M. (2010). Early nonspecific signs and symptoms of infection in institutionalized elderly persons: Perceptions of nursing assistants. *Scandinavian Journal of Caring Sciences, 24*, 24–31.

Tranter, S. (2011). Cochrane nursing care corner: Nutritional support for acute kidney injury. *Renal Society of Australasia Journal, 7*(1), 36–37.

Urinary diversions. (2011). *MedSurg Nursing, 20*(2), 94–95.

U. S. Renal Data System (USRDS). (2011). *2011 Annual data report: Atlas of chronic kidney disease and end-stage renal disease in the United States.* Bethesda, MD: National Institutes of Health, National Institute of Diabetes and Digestive and Kidney Diseases.

Yaklin, K. (2011). Acute kidney injury: An overview of pathophysiology and treatments. *Nephrology Nursing Journal, 38*(1), 13–19.

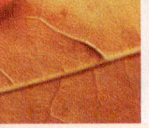
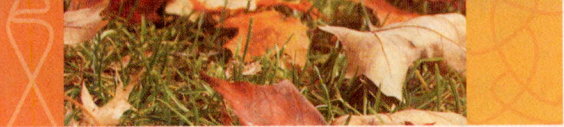
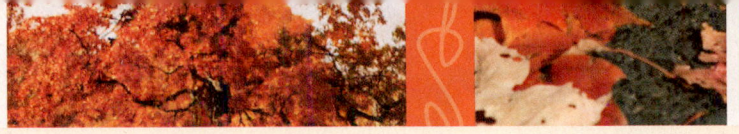

CHAPTER 30

Department of Health and Human Services Office on Women's Health (DHHSOWH). (2012). *Menopause and sexuality, in menopause.* U.S. Department of Health and Human Services Office on Women's Health. Retrieved September 3, 2012, from http://womenshealth.gov/menopause/menopause-sexuality/

Martini, F., Nath, J. L., & Bartholomew, E. F. (2012). *Fundamentals of anatomy and physiology.* San Francisco: Benjamin Cummings.

MedlinePlus. (2012). *Menopause.* U. S. National Library of Medicine, National Institutes of Health. Retrieved September 4, 2012, from www.nlm.nih.gov/medlineplus/menopause.html

National Cancer Institute. (2010). *Prostate cancer: Screening and testing.* Retrieved June 3, 2014, from http://www.cancer.gov/cancertopics/types/prostate

Planned Parenthood. (2014). *Birth control.* Retrieved June 3, 2014, from www.plannedparenthood.org/health-info/birth-control/

Siegfried, N., Muller, M., Deeks, J. J., & Volmink, J. (2011). Male circumcision for prevention of heterosexual acquisition of HIV in men. *Cochrane database of systematic reviews.* Retrieved September 4, 2012, from http://summaries.cochrane.org/search/site/circumcision

CHAPTER 31

American Cancer Society. (2012). *Man to man news.* Retrieved from http://www.cancer.org/acs/groups/content/@editorial/documents/document/acspc-033744.pdf

American Diabetes Association. (2012). *Living with diabetes.* Retrieved from http://www.diabetes.org/living-with-diabetes/complications/mens-health/sexual-health/erectile-dysfunction.html

Cleveland Clinic Disease & Conditions. (2012). *Male incontinence.* Retrieved from http://my.clevelandclinic.org/disorders/male_urinary_incontinence/urology_treatment.aspx

ED Guide. (2008). *Ejaculation. (Ejaculation problems).* Retrieved from http://www.edguidance.com/causes/ejaculation.html

Mayo Clinic Staff. (2011). Prostate laser surgery. *Mayoclinic.com.* Retrieved from http://www.mayoclinic.com/health/prostate-laser-surgery/my00611

National Health Service (NHS). (2012). Causes of testicular cancer. *NHS choices.* Retrieved from http://www.nhs.uk/Conditions/Cancer-of-the-testicle/Pages/Causes.aspx

National Institutes of Health (NIH). (2012). *Prostate enlargement: Benign prostatic hyperplasia.* Bethesda, MD: National Kidney and Urologic Diseases Information Clearinghouse. Retrieved from http://kidney.niddk.nih.gov/kudiseases/pubs/prostateenlargement

National Kidney and Urologic Diseases Information Clearinghouse (NKUDIC). (2012). *Prostatitis: Disorders of the prostate.* Retrieved from http://kidney.niddk.nih.gov/kudiseases/pubs/prostatitis/

Patel, V. R., & Sivaraman, A. (2012). Current status of robot-assisted radical prostatectomy: Progress is inevitable. *Oncology.* Retrieved June 6, 2014, from www.cancernetwork.com/

Testicular Cancer Society. (2012). *Testicular cancer 101.* Retrieved from http://www.testicularcancersociety.org/tc_101.html

Urology Care Foundation. (2011). *Urology A-Z.* Retrieved from http://www.urologyhealth.org/urology/index.cfm?article=34

Yarbro, C. H., Wujcik, D., & Gobel, B. H. (2011). *Cancer nursing: Principles and practice* (7th ed.). Sudbury, MA: Jones & Bartlett.

CHAPTER 32

American Cancer Society. (2012). *Detailed guide: Breast cancer.* Retrieved September 13, 2012, from http://www.cancer.org/Cancer/BreastCancer/DetailedGuide/index

American College of Obstetricians and Gynecologists. (2011). *Dietary changes help relieve PMS symptoms.* Retrieved December 12, 2012, from www.acog.org/~/media/For%20Patients/faq057.pdf

American Society of Plastic Surgeons. (2011). *Report of 2010 reconstructive demographics, breast surgery statistics.* Retrieved December 27, 2012, from http://www.plasticsurgery.org/Documents/news-resources/statistics/2010-statisticss/Patient-Ages/2010-reconstructive-demographics-breast-surgery-statistics.pdf

Breastcancer.org. (2014). *Exercise after surgery.* Retrieved August 14, 2014, from http://www.breastcancer.org/tips/exercise/treatment/surgery

Centers for Disease Control and Prevention. (2012). *National breast and cervical cancer early detection program.* Retrieved September 4, 2012, from www.cdc.gov/cancer/ubccedp/about.htm

Centers for Disease Control and Prevention. (2014a). *Pelvic inflammatory disease (PID)—CDC fact sheet.* Retrieved August 14, 2014, from http://www.cdc.gov/std/pid/stdfact-pid.htm

Centers for Disease Control and Prevention. (2014b). *What should I know about screening?* Retrieved August 14, 2014, from http://www.cdc.gov/cancer/ovarian/basic_info/screening.htm

Chism, L. A. (2014). Guiding your patients through menopause. *American Nurse Today, 9*(1). Retrieved August 14, 2014, from http://www.americannursetoday.com/guiding-your-patients-through-menopause/

Darsareh, F., Taavoni, S., Joolae, S., & Haghani, H. (2012). Massage and aromatherapy for menopausal symptoms. *Menopause, 19*(9), 995–999.

Greenblum, C. A., Rowe, M. A., Neff, D. F., & Greenblum, J. S. (2013). Midlife women's symptoms associated with menopausal transition and early postmenopause quality of life. *Menopause, 20*(1), 22–27.

Komen, S. G. (2014). *Healthy lifestyle for breast cancer survivors.* Retrieved August 14, 2014, from http://www.komen.org/BreastCancer/HealthyWeightampDiet.html

Kosters, J. P., & Gotzsche, P. C. (2008). Regular self-examination or clinical examination for early detection of breast cancer (review). *Cochrane Database Systematic Review* Issue 3, C0003373.

Marrone, J. A., Maddalozzo, G. F., Branscum, A. J., Hardin, K., Cialdella-Kam, L., Philbrick, K. A., et al. (2012). Moderate alcohol intake lowers biochemical markers of bone turnover in postmenopausal women. *Menopause, 19*(9), 974–979.

Mayo Clinic Staff. (2011). *Infertility.* Retrieved December 27, 2012, from http://www.mayoclinic.com/health/infertility

National Cancer Institute. (2012). *HPV and cancer.* Retrieved August 14, 2014, from http://www.cancer.gov/cancertopics/factsheet/Risk/HPV

National Cervical Cancer Coalition. (2013). *HPV/cervical cancer overview.* Retrieved August 14, 2014, from http://www.nccc-online.org/index.php/overview

Osborn, K. S., Watson, A., & Wraa, C. F. (2010). *Medical surgical nursing: Preparation for practice* (Vol. 1). Upper Saddle River, NJ: Prentice Hall.

The Practice Committee of the American Society for Reproductive Medicine. (2012). Endometriosis and infertility: A committee opinion. *Fertility and Sterility, 98*(3), 591–598.

Youngkin, E. Q., Davis, M. S., Schadewald, D. M., & Juve, C. (2013). *Women's health: A primary care clinical guide* (4th ed.). Upper Saddle River, NJ: Pearson.

CHAPTER 33

Brown, T. (2013, February 15). Multidrug-resistant gonorrhea: New treatment guidelines. *Morbidity and Mortality Weekly Report, 62*(6), 93–98.

Centers for Disease Control and Prevention [CDC]. (2009). *Sexually transmitted disease surveillance 2007 supplement: Syphilis surveillance report.* Atlanta, GA: U.S. Department of Health and Human Services.

Centers for Disease Control and Prevention [CDC]. (2013). *CDCs STD guidelines, antibiotic-resistant gonorrhea basic guidelines 2-11-13.* Retrieved from http://www.cdc.gov.std/gonorrhea/arg/references.htm

Dunne, E. F. (2012). *HPV vaccine now recommended for boys and young men.* Retrieved from http://www.medscape.com/viewarticle/59820

Fontaine, K. L. (2011). *Healing practices: Alternative therapies for nursing* (3rd ed.). Upper Saddle River, NJ: Prentice Hall Health.

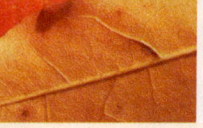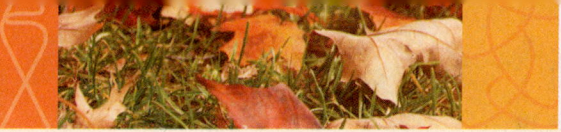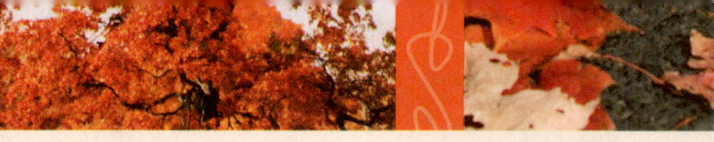

Planned Parenthood Federation of America. (2013). *Sexually transmitted diseases (STDs)*. Retrieved February 28, 2013, from http://www.plannedparenthood.org/healthtopics/stds

Porth, C. M. (2013). *Pathophysiology: Concepts of altered health states* (9th ed.). Philadelphia: Lippincott Williams & Wilkins.

Thomas, L. C. (2009). *Can safer sex be latex safe? Rubber room Listserv*. Retrieved June 16, 2009, from http://www.immune.com/rubber/safesexr.html

CHAPTER 34

Gray-Vickery, P. (2010). Gathering pearls of knowledge for assessing older adults. *Nursing, 40*(3), 34–43.

CHAPTER 35

Crawford, A., & Harris, H. (2012a). SIADH: Fluid out of balance. *Nursing, 42*(9), 50–58.

Crawford, A., & Harris, H. (2012b). Adrenal cortex hormones: Hormones out of kilter. *Nursing, 42*(10), 32–39.

Hurley, S., & Piras, S. E. (2012, November–December). Cushing disease: A disease, a syndrome, or both? *Nursing Made Incredibly Easy*, 38–47.

National Cancer Institute. (2012). *Thyroid cancer: Treatment*. Retrieved from www.cancer.gov/cancertopics/types/thyroid

National Institute of Diabetes and Digestive and Kidney Diseases. (2012). *Acromegaly*. Retrieved from www.endocrine.nddk.nih.gov/pubs/acro/acro.aspx

Simmons, S. (2010). A delicate balance: Detecting thyroid disease. *Nursing, 40*(7), 22–29.

CHAPTER 36

American Diabetes Association. (2004). Insulin administration. *Diabetes Care, 27*(Suppl. 1), S106–S107.

American Diabetes Association. (2008). Nutrition recommendations and interventions for diabetes. *Diabetes Care, 31*(Suppl. 1), S61–S74.

American Diabetes Association. (2012a). Diagnosis and classification of diabetes mellitus. *Diabetes Care, 35*(Suppl. 1), S64–S71.

American Diabetes Association. (2012b). Standards of medical care in diabetes—2012. *Diabetes Care, 35*(Suppl. 1), S11–S63.

Appel, S. J. (2011). Tapping incretin-based therapy for type-2 diabetes. *Nursing, 41*(3), 49–51.

Centers for Disease Control. (2011). *National diabetes fact sheet*. Retrieved from http://www.cdc.gov/diabetes/pubs/pdf/ndfs_2011.pdf

Hughes, L. (2012). Think "SAFE": Four crucial elements for diabetes education. *Nursing, 42*(1), 58–61.

Lange, V. Z. (2010). Successful management of in-hospital hyperglycemia: The pivotal role of nurses in facilitating effective insulin use. *MedSurg Nursing, 19*(6), 323–328.

Longo, R. (2010). Understanding oral antidiabetic agents. *American Journal of Nursing, 110*(2), 49–52.

McEuen, J. A., Gardner, K. P., Barnachea, D. F., Locke, C. L., Backhaus, B. R., & Hughes, S. K. (2010). An evidence-based protocol for managing hypoglycemia. *American Journal of Nursing, 110*(7), 40–45.

National Diabetes Information Clearinghouse. (2012). *Complementary and alternative medical therapies for diabetes*. Retrieved from http://diabetes.niddk.nih.gov/dm/pubs/alternativetherapies/index/aspx

National Institute of Diabetes and Digestive and Kidney Diseases. (2012). *Hypoglycemia*. Retrieved from http://diabetes.niddk.nih.gov/dm/pubs/hypoglycemia/index/aspx

United States Department of Agriculture. (2013). *Choose my plate: Weight management, Decrease portion size*. Retrieved from http://www.choosemyplate.gov/weight-management-calories/weight-management/better-choices/decrease-portions.html

Woo, K. Y., Santos, V., & Gamba, M. (2013). Understanding the diabetic foot. *Nursing, 43*(10), 36–43.

CHAPTER 37

Gray-Vickery, P. (2010). Gathering "pearls" of knowledge for assessing older adults. *Nursing, 40*(3), 34–43.

Rank, W. (2013). Performing a focused neurologic assessment. *Nursing, 43*(12), 37–40.

Vacca, V. M. (2010). How to perform a 60-second neurologic exam. *Nursing, 40*(6), 58–59.

CHAPTER 38

Cahill, J. E., & Armstrong, T. S. (2011). Caring for an adult with a malignant primary brain tumor. *Nursing, 41*(6), 28–34.

Centers for Disease Control and Prevention. (2010). *Traumatic brain injury in the United States: Emergency department visits, hospitalizations, and deaths 2002–2006*. Retrieved from http://www.cdc.gov/traumaticbraininjury/tbi_ed.html

Centers for Disease Control and Prevention. (2011). Surveillance for traumatic brain injury—related deaths—United States, 1997–2007. *Morbidity and Mortality Weekly Report, 60*(SS05), 1–32.

Centers for Disease Control and Prevention. (2012). *Bacterial meningitis*. Retrieved from http://www.cdc.gov/meningitis/bacterial.html

Cook, L. K., & Clements, S. L. (2011). Stroke recognition and management. *American Journal of Nursing, 111*(5), 64–69.

Heavey, E. (2010). An update on meningococcal meningitis. *Nursing, 40*(10), 61–62.

Mink, J., & Miller, J. (2011a). Opening the window of opportunity for treating acute ischemic stroke. *Nursing, 41*(1), 24–33.

Mink, J., & Miller, J. (2011b). Respond aggressively to hemorrhagic stroke. *Nursing, 43*(3), 36–43.

Morton, P. G., & Fontaine, D. K. (2013). *Critical care nursing: A holistic approach* (10th ed.). Philadelphia: Lippincott Williams & Wilkins.

National Cancer Institute. (2012). *SEER stat fact sheets. Brain and other nervous system*. Retrieved from: http://www.cancer.gov

National Institute of Neurological Disorders and Stroke. (2013a). *Headache*. Retrieved from www.ninds.nih.gov/disorders/headache/detail_headache.htm

National Institute of Neurological Disorders and Stroke. (2013b). *Seizures and epilepsy. Hope through research*. Retrieved from www.ninds.nih.gov/disorders/epilepsy/detail_epilepsy.htm

National Institute of Neurological Disorders and Stroke. (2013c). *Stroke. Hope through research*. Retrieved from www.ninds.nih.gov/disorders/stroke/detail_stroke.htm

National Institute of Neurological Disorders and Stroke. (2013d). *Traumatic brain injury: Hope through research*. Retrieved from www.ninds.nih.gov/disorders/tbi/detail_tbi.htm

National Stroke Association. (2013a). *Warning signs of stroke*. Retrieved from http://www.stroke.org/site/PageServer?pagename=SYMP

National Stroke Association. (2013b). *Women and Stroke*. Retrieved from http://www.stroke.org/site/PageServer?pagename=WOMSYMP

Norton, C., Feltz, S. J., Brocker, A., & Granitto, M. (2013). Tackling the long-term consequences of concussion. *Nursing, 43*(1), 50–55.

Simmons, S. (2012). Recognizing and preventing acute stroke in women. *Nursing, 42*(3), 30–36.

CHAPTER 39

Brodkey, M. B., Ben-Zacharia, A. B., & Reardon, J. D. (2011). Living well with multiple sclerosis. *American Journal of Nursing, 111*(7), 40–50.

Cranwell-Bruce, L. A. (2010). Drugs for Parkinson's disease. *MedSurg Nursing, 19*(6), 347–349.

Johnson, C. M. (2012). Managing fatigue in patients with multiple sclerosis. *Nursing, 42*(6), 26–29.

Morton, P. G., & Fontaine, D. K. (2013). *Critical care nursing: A holistic approach*. (10th ed.). Philadelphia: Lippincott Williams & Wilkins.

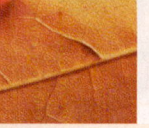
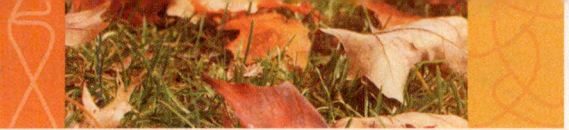
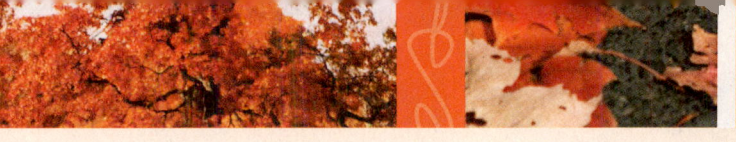

National Institute of Neurological Disorders and Stroke. (2010). *Huntington's disease: Hope through research.* Retrieved from www.ninds.nih.gov/disorders/huntington/detail_huntington.htm

National Institute of Neurological Disorders and Stroke. (2012a). *Multiple sclerosis: Hope through research.* Retrieved from www.ninds.nih.gov/disorders/multiple_sclerosis/detail_multiple_sclerosis.htm

National Institute of Neurological Disorders and Stroke. (2012b). *Myasthenia gravis fact sheet.* Retrieved from www.ninds.nih.gov/disorders/myasthenia_gravis/detail_myasthenia_gravis.htm

National Institute of Neurological Disorders and Stroke. (2012c). *Parkinson's disease: Hope through research.* Retrieved from www.ninds.nih.gov/disorders/parkinsons_disease/detail_parkinsons_disease.htm

National Institute of Neurological Disorders and Stroke. (2012d). *Spinal cord injury: Hope through research.* Retrieved from: www.ninds.nih.gov/disorders/sci/detail_sci.htm

National Spinal Cord Injury Statistical Center. (2012). *Spinal cord injury facts and figures at a glance.* Retrieved from www.nscisc.uab.edu

Nayduch, D. A. (2010). Back to basics: Identifying and managing spinal cord injury. *Nursing, 40*(9), 24–32.

Roberts, B. R. (2010). Caring for patients with Parkinson disease. *Nursing, 40*(7), 58–64.

Simmons, S. (2010). Guillain-Barre syndrome. *Nursing, 40*(1), 24–30.

Snow, M. (2011). Human rabies: Treatment and prevention. *Nursing, 41*(4), 65–66.

CHAPTER 40

Ayers, D. M. (2010). Take a close look at LASIK surgery. *Nursing, 40*(7), 48–51.

Laubach, G. (2010). Speaking up for older adults with hearing loss. *Nursing, 40*(1), 60–62.

National Eye Institutes. (2009a). *Facts about age-related macular degeneration.* Retrieved from www.nei.nih.gov/health/macualrdegen/armd_facts.asp

National Eye Institutes. (2009b). *Facts about cataract.* Retrieved from www.nei.nih.gov/health/cataract/cataract_facts.asp

National Eye Institutes. (2009c). *Facts about glaucoma.* Retrieved from www.nei.nih.gov/health/glaucoma/glaucoma_facts.asp

National Institute on Deafness and Other Communication Disorders. (2010). *Ménière's disease.* Retrieved from www.nidcd.nih.gov/health/balance/pages/meniere.aspx

National Institute on Deafness and Other Communication Disorders. (2011). *Cochlear implants.* Retrieved from www.nidcd.nih.gov/health/hearing/pages/coch.aspx

Turkoski, B. B. (2012). Glaucoma and glaucoma medications. *Orthopaedic Nursing, 31*(1), 37–40.

Yumori, J. W., & Cadogan, M. P. (2011). Primary open-angle glaucoma. *Journal of Gerontological Nursing, 37*(3), 10–15.

CHAPTER 41

Groarke, A. (2012). Falls prevention: Risk assessment and intervention. *World of Irish Nursing & Midwifery, 20*(5), 37–38.

Jarvis, C. (2012). *Physical examination & health assessment* (6th ed.). St. Louis, MO: Saunders Elsevier.

Kresevic, D. (2012). *Nursing standard of practice protocol: Assessment of physical function.* New York: Hartford Institute for Geriatric Nursing. Retrieved from http://consultgerirn.org/topics/function/want_to_know_more

LeMone, P., Burke, K., Bauldoff, G., & Gubrud-Howe, P. (2015). Medical surgical nursing: Clinical reasoning in patient care (6th ed.). Hoboken, NJ: Pearson

Miedany, Y., & Palmer, D. (2012). Musculoskeletal US: Examining the joints. *British Journal of Nursing, 21*(6), 340–344.

Smith, C., & Cotter, V. (2012). *Geriatric nursing protocol: Age-related changes in health.* Retrieved from http://consultgerirn.org/topics/normal_aging_changes/want_to_know_more#item_8

Ultrasound–Musculoskeletal. (2012). *Radiologyinfo.org.* Retrieved from http://www.radiologyinfo.org/en/pdf/musculous.pdf

U.S. Preventive Services Task Force. (2011). Clinical guideline. Screening for osteoporosis: U.S. Preventing Services Task Force recommendation statement. *Annals of Internal Medicine, 154*(1), 356–364.

CHAPTER 42

Bowie, D. (2011). Choosing the right pain relief for patients with soft-tissue injuries. *Emergency Nurse, 19*(2), 28–30.

Centers for Disease Control and Prevention (CDC). (2010). *Hip fractures among older adults.* Retrieved from www.cdc.gov/HomeandRecreationalSafety/Falls/adulthipfx.html

Centers for Disease Control and Prevention (CDC). (2012). *Falls among older adults: An overview.* Retrieved from www.cdc.gov/HomeandRecreationalSafety/Falls/adultfalls.html

Centers for Disease Control and Prevention (CDC). (2013). *Safe patient handling.* Retrieved from www.cdc.gov

Fischer, H. (2010). U.S. Military casualty statistics: Operation New Dawn, Operation Iraqi Freedom, and Operation Enduring Freedom (Congressional Research Service, No. 7-5700). CRS Report for Congress. Retrieved from http://www.fas.org/sgp/crs/natsec/RS22452.pdf

Goebel, A. (2011). Complex regional pain syndrome in adults. *Rheumatology, 50*(10), 1739–1750. Retrieved from http://www.medscape.com/viewarticle/750778

Graham, P., & Dougherty, J. (2012). Oh, their aching backs! Occupational injuries in nursing assistants. *Orthopaedic Nursing, 31*(4), 218–223.

Gray-Micelli, D., & Quigley, P. (2012). *Falls. Nursing Standard of Practice Protocol: Fall Prevention.* Hartford Institute for Geriatric Nursing. Retrieved from http://consultgerirn.org/topics/falls

Groarke, A. (2012). Falls prevention: Risk assessment and intervention. *World of Irish Nursing & Midwifery, 20*(5), 37–38.

Gropelli, T., & Corle, K. (2010). Nurses' and therapists' experiences with occupational musculoskeletal injuries. *AAOHN Journal, 58*(4), 159–166.

Institute for Clinical Systems Improvement. (2006). *Health care guideline: Ankle sprain.* Retrieved from http://www.icsi.org/ankle_sprain_4.html

Jones, C. (2011). Preventing broken hips in care homes. *Journal of Community Nursing, 25*(4), 11–13.

Kemle, K. (2011). Falls in older adults: Averting a disaster. *Clinical Advisor for Nurse Practitioners, 14*(2), 50–56.

Kirkland, L. (2011). Fat embolism. *Medscape Reference.* Retrieved from http://emedicine.medscape.com/article/460524

Lee, S.-J., Faucett, J., Gillen, M., & Crause, N. (2013). Musculoskeletal pain among critical-care nurses by availability and use of patient lifting equipment: An analysis of cross-sectional survey data. *International Journal of Nursing Studies, 50*(12), 1648–1657.

Luke, A., & Ma, C. B. (2012). Sports medicine & outpatient orthopedics. In S. McPhee & M. Papadakis (Eds.), *Current medical diagnosis & treatment* (51st ed.). New York: McGraw Hill.

Miedany, Y., & Palmer, D. (2012). Musculoskeletal US: Examining the joints. *British Journal of Nursing, 21*(6), 340–344.

Montana, C., & Kautz, D. (2011). Turning the nightmare of complex regional pain syndrome into a time of healing, renewal, and hope. *MedSurg Nursing, 20*(3), 139–142.

National Limb Loss Information Center. (2009). *Amputation statistics by cause: Limb loss in the United States.* Retrieved from www.amputee-coalition.org/fact_sheets/amp_stats_cause.html

Occupational Safety and Health Administration (OSHA), U.S. Department of Labor. (2009). *Guidelines for nursing homes ergonomics for the prevention of musculoskeletal disorders.* Retrieved from https://www.osha.gov/ergonomics/guidelines/nursinghome/final_nh_guidelines.pdf

Spratt, D., Cowles, C., Jr., Berguer, R., Dennis, V., Waters, T., Rodriguex, M., et al. (2012). Workplace safety equals patient safety. *AORN Journal, 96*(3), 235–244.

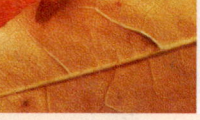

CHAPTER 43

Aletaha, D., Neogi, T., Silman, A., Funovits, J., Felson, D., Bingham, C. O., III, et al. (2010). 2010 Rheumatoid arthritis classification criteria. *Arthritis & Rheumatism, 62*(9), 2569–2581.

American Cancer Society. (2011). *Bone cancer.* Retrieved from http://www.cancer.org/acs/groups/cid/documents/webcontent/003086-pdf.pdf

Centers for Disease Control and Prevention (CDC). (2011a). *Data and statistics. Arthritis related statistics.* Retrieved from www.cdc.gov/arthritis/data_statistics

Centers for Disease Control and Prevention (CDC). (2011b). *Lyme disease.* Retrieved from www.cdc.gov/lyme

Crofford, L. (2012). *Fibromyalgia.* Atlanta, GA: American College of Rheumatology. Retrieved from www.rheumatology.org/practice/clinical

Elliott, M. (2011). Taking control of osteoporosis to cut down on risk of fracture. *Nursing Older People, 23*(3), 30–35.

Firth, J. (2011). Rheumatoid arthritis: Diagnosis and multidisciplinary management. *British Journal of Nursing, 20*(18), 1179–1185.

Firth, J., & Critchley, S. (2011). Treating to target in rheumatoid arthritis: Biologic therapies. *British Journal of Nursing, 20*(20), 1284, 1287–1291.

Goldenberg, D. (2010, May 28). Comprehensive assessment of fibromyalgia and overlapping conditions. *MedscapeCMA Rheumatology.* Retrieved from http://cme.medscape.com/viewarticle/722159/

Hochberg, M., Altman, R., April, K., Benkhalti, M., Guyatt, G., McGowan, J., et al. (2012). American College of Rheumatology 2012 recommendations for the use of nonpharmcologic and pharmacologic therapies in osteoarthritis of the hand, hip, and knee. *Arthritis Care & Research, 64*(4), 465–474.

Huynh, C., Yanni, L., & Morgan, L. (2008). Fibromyalgia: Diagnosis and management for the primary healthcare provider. *Journal of Women's Health, 17*(8), 1379–1387.

Institute for Clinical Systems Improvement. (2012). *Health care guideline: Adult acute and subacute low back pain* (15th ed.). Bloomington, MN: Institute for Clinical Systems Improvement.

Joyce, M. (2012). *Tumors of bones and joints.* Retrieved from http://www.merckmanuals.com/professional/musculoskeletal_and_connective_tissue_disorders/tumors_of_bones_and_joints

Kalish, R. (2012). *Lyme disease.* Atlanta, GA: American College of Rheumatology.

Khanna, D., Fitzgerald, J., Khanna, P., Bae, S., Singh, M., Neogi, T., et al. (2012). 2012 American College of Rheumatology guidelines for management of gout. Part 1: Systematic nonpharmacologic and pharmacologic therapeutic approaches to hyperuricemia. *Arthritis Care & Research, 64*(10), 1431–1446.

Khanna, D., Khanna, P., Fitzgerald, J., Singh, M., Bae, S., Neogi, T., et al. (2012). 2012 American College of Rheumatology guidelines for management of gout. Part 2: Therapy and anti-inflammatory prophylaxis of acute gouty arthritis. *Arthritis Care & Research, 64*(10), 1447–1461.

Manheimer, E., Cheng, K., Linde, K., Lao, L., Yoo, J., Wieland, S., et al. (2010). *Acupuncture for osteoarthritis.* Retrieved from http://summaries.cochrane.org/CD001977/acupuncture-for-osteoarthrits

MossRehab Resource Net. (2010). *Arthritis fact sheet.* Retrieved from http://www.mossresourcenet.org/arthritis/htm

National Osteoporosis Foundation. (2010). *Clinician's guide to prevention and treatment of osteoporosis.* Washington, DC: Author.

National Osteoporosis Foundation. (2011). *Fast facts.* Retrieved from http://www.nof.org

NIH Osteoporosis and Related Bone Diseases National Resource Center. (2012). *Calcium and Vitamin D: Important at every age.* Retrieved from http://www.niams.nih.gov/Health_Info/Bone/Bone_Health/Nutrition/#d

Office of Dietary Supplements (ODS). (2013). *Dietary supplement fact sheet: Calcium.* Bethesda, MD: National Institutes of Health. Retrieved from http://ods.od.nih.gov/factsheets/Calcium-HealthProfessional/#h2

Olson, A. (2007, June). Osteoporosis detection: Is BMD testing the future? *Nurse Practitioner, 32*(6), 20–28.

Paget Foundation. (2012a). *A nurse's guide to the management of Paget's disease of bone.* Retrieved from www.paget.org

Paget Foundation. (2012b). *A physician's guide to the management of Paget's disease of bone.* Retrieved from www.paget.org

Saag, K., Teng, G., Patkar, N., Anuntiyo, J., Finney, C., Curtis, J., et al. (2008, June 15). American College of Rheumatology 2008 recommendations for the use of nonbiologic and biologic disease modifying antirheumatic drugs in rheumatoid arthritis. *Arthritis & Rheumatism, 59*(6), 762–784.

Singh, J., Furst, D., Bharat, A., Curtis, J., Kavanaugh, A., Kremer, J., et al. (2012). 2012 update of the 2008 American College of Rheumatology recommendations for the use of disease-modifying antirheumatic drugs and biologic agents in the treatment of rheumatoid arthritis. *Arthritis Care & Research, 64*(5), 625–639.

Spondylitis Association of America. (2012). *Ankylosing spondylitis.* Retrieved from www.spondylitis.org/about/as.aspx

University of Texas, School of Nursing, Family Nurse Practitioner Program. (2009). *Management of fibromyalgia syndrome in adults.* Retrieved from www.guideline.com

U.S. Preventive Services Task Force. (2011). Screening for osteoporosis: U.S. Preventive Services Task Force recommendation statement. *Annals of Internal Medicine, 154*(5), 356–364.

Vernon, S., & King, R. (2011). Using FRAX to assess the risk that an older person will suffer a fragility fracture. *British Journal of Community Nursing, 16*(11), 534, 536, 538–539.

Walker, J. (2011). Management of osteoarthritis. *Nursing Older People, 23*(9), 14–19.

Walker, J. (2012). Rheumatoid arthritis: Role of the nurse and multidisciplinary team. *British Journal of Nursing, 21*(6), 334–339.

Wolfe, F., Clauw, D., Fitzcharles, M. A., Goldenberg, D., Katz, R., Mease, P., et al. (2010). The American College of Rheumatology preliminary diagnostic criteria for fibromyalgia and measurement of symptom severity. *Arthritis Care & Research, 62*(5), 600–610.

CHAPTER 44

Gray-Vickrey, P. (2010). Gathering 'pearls' of knowledge for assessing older adults. *Nursing, 40*(3), 34–43.

Hess, C. T. (2010). Performing a skin assessment. *Nursing, 40*(7), 66.

CHAPTER 45

Agency for Health Care Policy and Research. (1992). *Pressure ulcers in adults: Prediction and prevention.* Rockville, MD: U.S. Department of Health and Human Services.

American Academy of Dermatology. (2013). *Psoriasis: Tips for managing.* Retrieved from http://www.aad.org/skin-conditions/dermatology-a-to-z/tips/psoriasis-tips-for-managing

American Cancer Society. (2013a). *Melanoma skin cancer.* Retrieved from http://www.cancer.org

American Cancer Society. (2013b). *Skin cancer: Basal and squamous cell.* Retrieved from http://www.cancer.org

Centers for Disease Control. (2010). *Head lice: Treatment.* Retrieved from http://www.cdc.gov/parasites/lice/head/treatment.html

Lawton, S. (2011). Atopic eczema and evidence-based care. *Journal of the Dermatology Nurses' Association, 3*(3), 131–136.

National Eczema Association. (2012). *All about atopic dermatitis.* Retrieved from http://www.nationaleczema.org/living/all_about_atopic_dermatitis.htm

National Pressure Ulcer Advisory Panel. (2007). *NPAUP pressure ulcer stages/categories.* Retrieved from http://www.npuap.org

Nolan, M. E., Beebe, V. R., King, J. M., Bryn, N., & Limaye, K. M. (2011). Nonmelanoma skin cancer: Part 1. *Journal of the Dermatology Nurses' Association, 3*(5), 260–281.

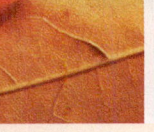
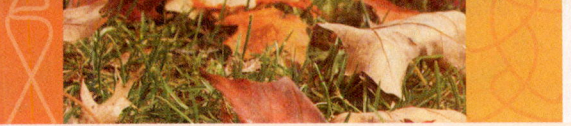
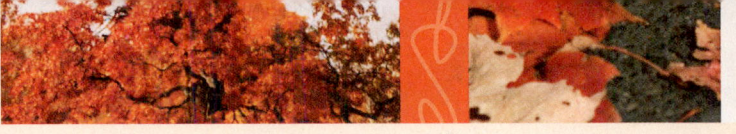

Siegel, V. (2012). Adding patient education of skin cancer and sun-protective behaviors to the skin assessment screening on admission to hospitals. *MedSurg Nursing, 21*(3), 183–184.

CHAPTER 46

American Burn Association. (2012). *Burn incidence and treatment in the United States: 2012 fact sheet.* Retrieved from http://www.ameriburn.org/resources_factsheet.php

Arnstein, P. (2010). What is the best way to cool my patient's burn pain? *Nursing, 40*(3), 61–62.

Centers for Disease Control. (2011). *Fire deaths and injuries: Fact sheet.* Retrieved from http://www.cdc.gov/ncipc/factsheets/fire.htm

Davidge, K. (2008). Older adults and burns. *Geriatrics Aging, 11*(5), 270–275.

Kornhaber, R., & Wilson, A. (2011). Psychosocial needs of burn nurses: A descriptive phenomenological inquiry. *Journal of Burn Care & Research, 32*(2), 286–293.

Laskowski-Jones, L. (2010). Summer emergencies: Can you take the heat? *Nursing, 40*(6), 24–31.

National Fire Protection Association. (2012). *Home safety information.* Retrieved from http://www.nfpa.org

CHAPTER 47

Hockenberry, M. J., & Wilson, D. (2013). *Wong's essentials of pediatric nursing* (9th ed.). St. Louis, MO: Mosby/Elsevier.

Lives restored: Living with major mental illness. (2013, June–December). *New York Times series.* Retrieved August 28, 2013, from http://www.nytimes.com/interactive/science/lives-restored-series.html

Murray, C., & Lopez, A. (1996). *The global burden of disease: A comprehensive assessment of mortality and disability from disease, injuries, and risk factors in 1990 and projected to 2020.* Cambridge, MA: Harvard University Press. [classic]

National Institute of Mental Health. (2013). *Health education: Statistics.* Retrieved October 8, 2013 from www.nimh.gov/statistics/index.shtml

Oulette-plamondon, C., & George, T. P. (2012). Glutamate and psychiatry in 2012-Up, up, and away! *Psychiatric Times.* Retrieved September 8, 2012, from www.psychiatrictimes.com

Patterson, J. (1995). Promoting resilience in families experiencing stress. *Pediatric Clinics of North America, 42*(1), 47–63. [classic]

Raza Bermudo-Soriano, C., Perez-Rodriguez, M. M., Vaquero-Lorenzo, C., & Baca-Garcia, E. (2012). New perspectives in glutamate and anxiety. *Pharmacology and Biochemistry of Behavior, 100,* 752–774.

Sanacora, G., Treccani, G., & Popoli, M. (2012). Towards a glutamate hypothesis of depression: An emerging frontier of neuropsychopharmacology for mood disorders. *Neuropharmacology, 62,* 63–77.

Sorrell, J. M. (2013). Diagnostic and statistical manual of mental disorders, fifth edition: Implications for older adults and their families. *Journal of psychosocial nursing and mental health services, 51*(3), 19–22.

World Health Organization. (2012). *WHO marks 20th anniversary of mental health day.* Retrieved October 8, 2013, from www.who.int/mediacentre/news/notes/2012

CHAPTER 48

Alzheimer's Association. (2009). *10 warning signs of Alzheimer's.* Chicago: Author. Retrieved August 23, 2013, from http://www.alz.org

Alzheimer's Association. (2013). *Alzheimer's disease risk factors.* Retrieved August 30, 2013, from www.alz.org_alzheimers_disease_causes_risk_factors.asp

American Psychiatric Association. (2013). *The diagnostic and statistical manual of mental disorders (DSM-5).* Washington, DC: Author.

Birks, J. (2009). Cholinesterase inhibitors for Alzheimer's disease. *Cochrane Database of Systematic Reviews,* Issue 1, CD005593. doi:10.1002/14651858

Centers for Medicare & Medicaid Services. (2006). *CMS Publishes final patients' rights rule on use of restraint and seclusion.* Washington, DC: Author. Retrieved August 29, 2013, from https://www.cms.hhs.gov/Regulations-and-Guidance/Legislation/CFCsANDCoPs/

Crotty, M., Unroe, K., Cameron, I. D., Miller, M., Ramirez, G., & Couzner, L. (2010). Rehabilitation interventions improving physical and psychosocial functioning after hip fracture in older people. *Cochrane Database of Systematic Reviews,* Issue 1, CD007624.pub3. doi:10-1002/14651858

Eby, L., & Brown, N. J. (2009). *Mental health nursing care.* Upper Saddle River, NJ: Prentice Hall.

Folstein, M. F., Folstein, S. E., & McHugh, P. R. (1975). Mini-Mental State: A practical method for grading the cognitive state of patients for the clinician. *Journal of Psychiatric Research, 2,* 189–198.

Mayo Clinic Staff. (2013). *Mayo Clinic on Alzheimer's disease.* Rochester, MN: Mayo Clinic Health Information. Retrieved August 23, 2013, from www.mayoclinic.com/health/alzheimers-disease

National Institute of Neurological Disorders and Stroke, National Institutes of Health. (2013). *NINDS dementia with Lewy bodies information.* Bethesda: Author. Retrieved August 23, 2013, from http://www.nids.nih.gov/disorders/dementiawithlewybodies/dementiawithlewybodies.htm

Oltmanns, T. F., & Emery, R. E. (2012). *Abnormal Psychology* (7th ed.). Upper Saddle River, NJ: Pearson/Prentice Hall.

Solomons, L., Solomons, J., & Gosney, M. (2013). Dementia and cancer. *Aging Health, 9*(3), 307–319.

Stahl, S. M. (2011). *Essential pharmacology: The prescriber's guide* (4th ed.). Cambridge, MA: Cambridge University Press.

Zheng, L., Mack, W. J., Dagerman, K. S., Hsiao, J. K., Lebowitz, B. D., Lyketsos, C. G., et al. (2009). Metabolic changes associated with second-generation antipsychotic use in Alzheimer's disease patients: The CATIE-AD study. *American Journal of Psychiatry, 166*(5), 583–590.

CHAPTER 49

Eisenberg, D. P., & Berman, K. F. (2010). Executive function, neural circuitry, and genetic mechanisms in schizophrenia. *Neuropsychopharmacology, 35,* 258–277.

Faschinagbauer, K. M., Peden-McAlpine, C., & Tempel, W. (2013). Use of seclusion: Finding the voice of the patient to influence practice. *Journal of Psychosocial Nursing and Mental Health Services, 51*(7), 32–38. doi:10:3928/02793695-20130503-01

Keltner, N. L., Bostrom, C. E., & McGuiness, T. (2011). *Psychiatric nursing.* St. Louis: Mosby/Elsevier.

Klobassa Davidson, N., & Moreland, P. (2012). *Self talk: What are you telling yourself?* Retrieved July 24, 2013, from www.mayoclinic.com

Mayo Clinic Staff. (2012). *Cognitive behavioral therapy in schizophrenia.* Retrieved July 23, 2013 from Mayo Clinic website: www.mayoclinic.com

National Alliance on Mental Illness. (2013). *Schizophrenia/Latest research.* Retrieved July 24, 2013, from www.nami.org

National Association of Cognitive-Behavioral Therapists. (2013). *Cognitive behavioral therapy.* Retrieved July 24, 2013, from http://www.nacbt/whatiscbt.aspx

National Institute of Mental Health. (2012). *Schizophrenia.* Retrieved July 24, 2013, from www.nimh.nih.gov

Pies, R. W. (2013). Psychiatry and the myth of "medicalization." *Psychiatric Times, 30,* 7.

Stahl, S. M. (2014). *Essential psychopharmacology: The prescriber's guide.* 5th ed. New York: Cambridge University Press.

Stuart, G. W. (2013). *Principles and practice of psychiatric nursing* (10th ed.). St. Louis, MO: Mosby.

Substance Abuse and Mental Health Services Administration. (2013). *Schizophrenia.* Retrieved July 24, 2013, from www.SAMHSA.com

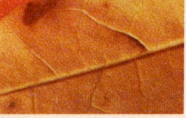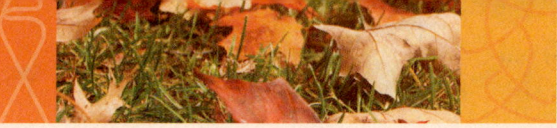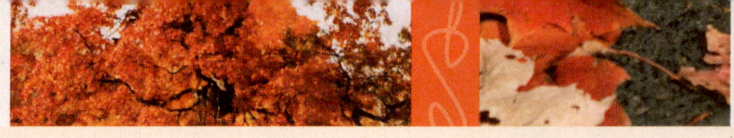

CHAPTER 50

American Foundation for Suicide Prevention. (2013). *Suicide deaths, facts and figures.* Retrieved October 2, 2013, from www.afsp.org

Beck, A. T., & Rush, A. J. (1995). Cognitive therapy. In H. I. Kaplan & B. J. Sadock (Eds.), *Comprehensive Textbook of Psychiatry IV* (Vol. 2). Baltimore: Williams & Wilkins.

Beck, A. T., Ward, C. H., Mendelson, M., et al. (1961). An inventory for measuring depression. *Archives of General Psychiatry, 4,* 561–571. Copyright 1961. American Medical Association.

Caspi, A., Sugden, K., Moffitt, T., Taylor, A., Craig, I., Harrington, H., et al. (2003). Influence of life stress on depression: Moderation by a polymorphism in the 5-HTT gene. *Science, 301,* 386.

Centers for Disease Control and Prevention. (2011). *Web-based Injury Statistics Query and Reporting System (WISQARS). Fatal Injury Reports.* Atlanta, GA: National Center for Injury Prevention and Control. Retrieved September 30, 2013, from http://www.cdc.gov/injury /wisqars/index.html

Columbia University. (2013). *Light therapy.* Retrieved October 24, 2013, from www.columbia.edu/cu/csr/CSRIssues/2009_Fall_issue_pdf

Cooney, G. M., Greig, C. A., Lawtor, D. A., Rimer, J., Waugh, F. R., McMurdo, M., et al. (2013). Exercise for depression. *Cochrane Database for Systematic Reviews,* Issue 9. doi:10. 1002/14651858.CD00436

Holland, L. N., Adams, M., & Brice, J. L. (2015). *Core concepts in pharmacology,* 4th ed. Upper Saddle River, NJ: Pearson.

Kanner, AM. (2011). Depression and epilepsy. *Epilepsia, 52,* s1, 21–27.

Keltner, N. L., Bostrom, C. E., & McGuinness, T. (2011). *Psychiatric nursing* (6th ed.). St. Louis, MO: Mosby/Elsevier.

Khan, A., Faucett, J., Morrison, S., & Brown, W.A. (2013). Comparative mortality risk in adult patients with schizophrenia, depression, bipolar disorder, anxiety disorders, and attention deficit/hyperactivity disorder participating in psychopharmacological clinical trials. *JAMA Psychiatry, 149.* doi:10. 1001/jamapsychiatry

Levinson, D. F., & Nichols, W. E. (2013). *Major depression and genetics.* Stanford School of Medicine. Genetics and Brain Function. Retrieved October 2, 2013, from depressiongenetics.stanford.edu/mddandgenes. html

Lohoff, F.W. (2010). Overview of the genetics of major depressive disorder. *Current Psychiatric Reports,12*(6), 539–546. doi:10. 1007/s11920-010-0150-6

Mayo Clinic Staff. (2013). Monoamine oxidase inhibitors (MAOIs). Retrieved October24, 2013, from mayoclin ic.com/health/maois /MH00072

National Alliance on Mental Illness (NAMI) (n.d.). Multicultural action center. Retrieved August 31, 2014, from www.nami.org

National Institute of Mental Health. (2010). *Suicide in the U.S.: Statistics and prevention.* Accessed September 30, 2013, from the NIMH website

National Institute of Mental Health (2006). *Suicide in the U.S. statistics and prevention.* Washington, DC: Author

Rodriguez-Martin, J. L., Barbanoj, J. M., Schlaepfer, T., Clos, S. S. C., Pérez, V., Kulisevsky, J., et al. (2002). Transcranial magnetic stimulation for treating depression. *Cochrane Database of Systematic Reviews,* Issue 2. Art. No.: CD003493. doi:10.1002/14651858.CD003493- http:// summaries.cochrane.org/CD003493/transcranial-magnetic-stimulation-tms-for-depression#sthash.x0vcLq4b.dpuf

Sheikh, J. I., & Yesavage, J. A. (1986). Geriatric depression scale: Recent evidence and development of a shorter form. *Clinical Gerontologist, 5,* 165–172.

Spires, RA (2006). Depression in the elderly. RNWeb. Retrieved January 15, 2007, from http://www.rnweb/article/articleDetail. jsp?id=329133&searchString=depression

Uder, B. L., & Mosack, V. (2011). Genetics of depression: An overview of the current science. *Issues in Mental Health Nursing, 32*(4), 192–202. doi:10. 3109/01612840

U.S. Public Health Service. (1999). *The surgeon general's call to action to prevent suicide.* Washington, DC: Author.

CHAPTER 51

Beck, A. T. (1967). *Depression: Causes and treatment.* Philadelphia: University of Pennsylvania Press.

Beck, A. T. (n.d.). *Interview.* Retrieved March 7, 2014, from The Beck Institute for Cognitive Behavior Therapy Web site: http://www .beckinstitute.org/history-of-cbt/

Burgess, A. W., Slattery, D. M., & Herlihy, P. A. (2013). Military sexual trauma a silent syndrome. *Journal of Psychosocial Nursing and Mental Health Services, 51*(2), 20–26. doi:10.3928/02793695-20130109-03

Ellis, A. (1962). *Reason and emotion in psychotherapy.* New York: Stuart.

Ellis, A. (n.d.). Retrieved February 23, 2014, from http://www .brainyquote.com/quotes/authors/authors/a/albert_ellis.html

Goodwin, D. W. (1986). *Anxiety.* New York: Oxford University Press.

Hars, M., Herrmann, F. R., Gold, G., Rizzoli, R., & Trombetti, A. (2013). Effect of music-based multitask training on cognition and mood in older adults. *Oxford Journals British Geriatrics Society, Oxford University Press.* doi:10,1093/ageing/aft163

Higgins, E. S., & George, M. S. (2013). *The neuroscience of clinical psychiatry: The pathophysiology of behavior and mental illness* (2nd ed.). Philadelphia: Lippincott, Williams, & Wilkins.

Keltner, N. L., Bostrom, C. E., & McGuiness, T. (2011). *Psychiatric nursing* (6th ed.). St. Louis, MO: Mosby.

National Center for PTSD. (2014). *PTSD overview.* Washington, DC: U.S. Department of Veterans Affairs. Retrieved March 7, 2014, from www. ptsd.va.gov

National Institute of Mental Health. (n.d.). *Anxiety disorders.* Retrieved February 23, 2013, from http://www.nimh.nih.gov/publicat/anxiety .cfm

Peplau, H. (1989). Theoretical constructs: Anxiety, self, and hallucinations. In A. O'Toole & S. Welt (Eds.), *Interpersonal theory in nursing practice. Selected works of Hildegard E. Peplau* (pp. 270–326). New York: Springer.

Reichenberg, L. W. (2014). *DSM-5 essentials: The Savvy Clinician's guide to the changes in criteria.* Hoboken, NJ: Wiley.

Schultz, J. M., & Videbeck, S. L. (2012). *Lippincott's manual of psychiatric nursing care plans* (9th ed.). Philadelphia: Lippincott Williams & Wilkins.

Stahl, S. M. (2013). *Stahl's essential pharmacology: Neuroscientific basis and practical applications.* Cambridge, MA: Cambridge University Press.

Stuart, G. W. (2013). Anxiety responses and anxiety disorders. In G. W. Stuart (Ed.), *Principles and practice of psychiatric nursing* (10th ed.). St. Louis, MO: Mosby.

Suris, A., & Lind, L. (2012). Military sexual trauma: A review of prevalence and associated health consequences in veterans. *Trauma, Violence, & Abuse, 9*(4), 250. Retrieved March 7, 2014, from tva. sagepub.com

Yaeger, D., Himmelfarb, N., Cammack, A., & Mintz, J. (2006). DSM-IV diagnosed posttraumatic stress disorder in female veterans with and without military sexual trauma. *Journal of General Internal Medicine, 21,* S65–S69.

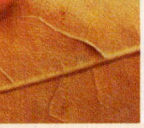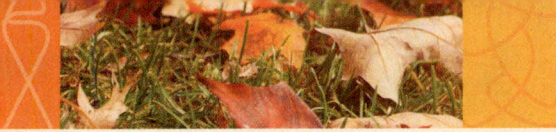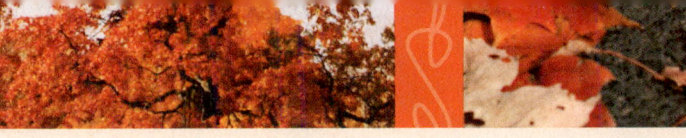

CHAPTER 52

Boyd, M. A. (2011). *Psychiatric nursing: Contemporary practice* (5th ed.). Philadelphia: Lippincott Williams & Wilkins.

Friedman, H. S., & Schustack, M. W. (2010). *Personality: Classical theories and modern research* (5th ed.). Upper Saddle River, NJ: Pearson.

Koerner, K., & Linehan, M. (2000). Research on dialectical behavior therapy for patients with borderline personality disorder. *Psychiatric Clinics of North America, 23*(1), 151–167.

Linehan, M. (1993). *Cognitive-behavioral treatment of borderline personality disorder*. New York: The Guilford Press.

Margolies, L. (2010). Understanding the different approaches to psychotherapy. *Psych Central.* Retrieved March 31, 2014, from http://psychcentral.com/lib/understanding-different-approaches-to-psychotherapy/0003077

Mayo Clinic Staff. (2012). *Personality disorders.* Retrieved March 28, 2014, from http://www.mayoclinic.org/diseases-conditions/borderline-personality-disorder/basics/symptoms/con-20023204

National Institute of Mental Health. (n.d.). *Borderline personality disorder.* Retrieved March 28, 2014, from http://www.nimh.nih.gov/health/topics/borderline-personality-disorder/index.shtml

Reichenberg, L. W. (2014). *DSM-5 essentials: The Savvy Clinician's guide to the changes in criteria.* Hoboken, NJ: Wiley.

Stepp, S. D., Whalen, D. J., Pilkonis, P. A., Hipwell, A. E., & Levine, M. D. (2011, March 28). Children of mothers with borderline personality disorder, identifying parenting behaviors as potential targets for intervention. *Personality Disorders: Theory, Research, and Treatment.* doi:10.1037/A0023081

Stern, A. (1938). Psychoanalytic investigation of and therapy in the borderline group of neuroses. *Psychoanalytic Quarterly, 7,* 467–489.

Stone, M.H. (2013). The brain in overdrive: A new look at borderline personality disorder and related personality disorders. *Current Psychiatry Rep, 15*(10), 399. doi: 10.1007/s11920-013-0399-7

Townsend, M.C. (2012). *Essentials of psychiatric mental health nursing: Concepts of care in evidence-based practice* (7th ed.). Philadelphia: F.A.Davis.

CHAPTER 53

Cassels, C. (2013). 'Bath salts' linked to large number of drug-related ED visits. *Medscape Nurses.* Retrieved April 26, 2014, from http://www.medscape.com/viewarticle/811201?nlid=33883_328&src=wnl_edit_medn_psyc&uac=71504CG&spon=12

Centers for Disease Control. (2014). *Smoking and tobacco use.* Retrieved May 1, 2014, from http://www.cdc.gov/tobacco/

Ewing, J. A. (1984). Detecting alcoholism: The CAGE questionnaire. *Journal of the American Medical Association, 252,* 1902–1907.

Fontaine, K. L., & Fletcher, J. S. (2009). *Mental-health nursing,* 6th ed. Upper Saddle River, NJ: Prentice Hall.

Grana, R. A., Popova, L., & Ling, P. M. (2014). A longitudinal analysis of electronic cigarette use and smoking cessation. *JAMA Internal Medicine, 174*(5), 812–813. doi:10.1001/jamainternmed2014.187

Keltner, N. L. (2013). *Psychiatric nursing* (6th ed.). St. Louis, MO: Mosby.

Kneisl, C. R., Wilson, H. S., & Trigoboff, E. (2013). *Contemporary psychiatric-mental health nursing* (3rd ed.). Upper Saddle River, NJ: Pearson Education.

Mayo-Smith, M. F. (July, 1997). Pharmacological management of alcohol withdrawal. A meta-analysis and evidence-based practice guideline. American Society of Addiction Medicine Working Group on Pharmacological Management of Alcohol Withdrawal. *Journal of the American Medical Association, 278*(2):144–151.

National Institute on Drug Abuse, National Institutes of Health. (2012). *NIDA infofacts: Anabolic steroids.* Retrieved May 1, 2014, http://www.drugabuse.gov/publications/drugfacts/anabolic-steroids

Substance Abuse and Mental Health Services Administration (SAMHSA). (2013). *National survey on drug use and health (NSDUH).* Washington DC: U.S. Department of Health and Human Services.

Sullivan, J. T., Sykora, K., Schneiderman, J., Naranjo, C. A., & Sellers, E. M. (1989). Assessment of alcohol withdrawal: The revised Clinical Institute Withdrawal Assessment for Alcohol withdrawal scale (CIWA-Ar). *British Journal of Addiction, 84,* 1353–1357.

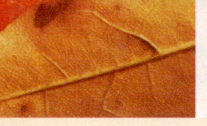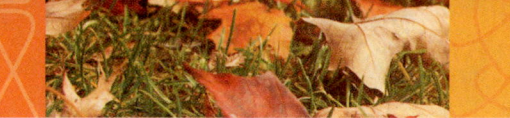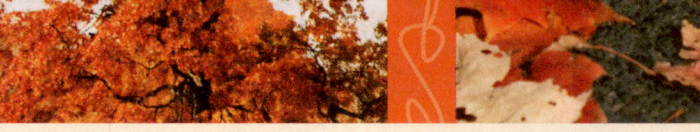

Index

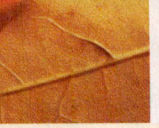
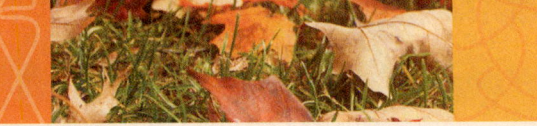
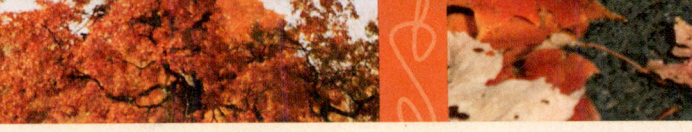

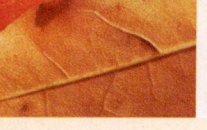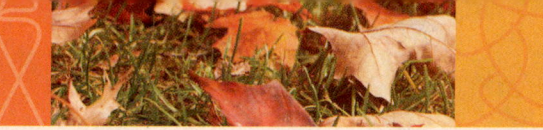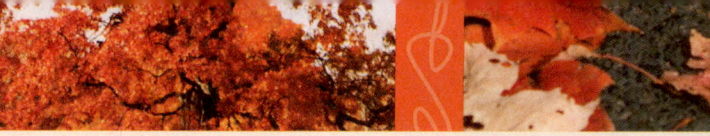

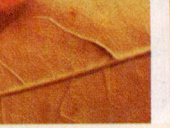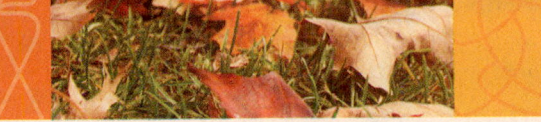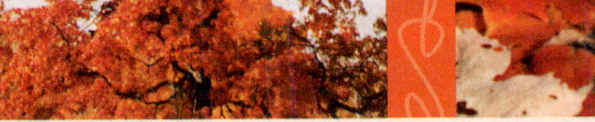

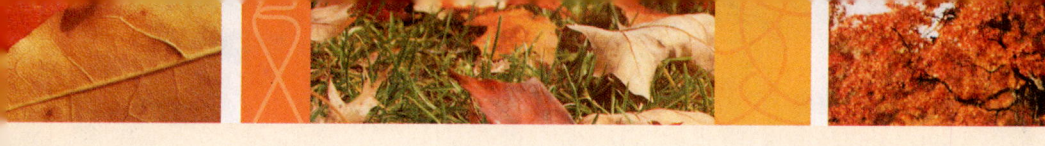
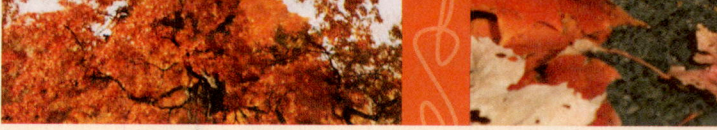

Bone tumors, 1098–1100
    classifications, 1098, 1098*t*
    collaborative care, 1099
    nursing care, 1099–1100
    pathophysiology and manifestations, 1098–1099,
        1098*t*, 1099
Borborygmi, 655
Borderline personality disorder
    collaborative care, 1294
    nursing care, 1294–1296
    nursing care plan, 1298
    pathophysiology and manifestations, 1291–1293,
        1292*f*
Borrelia burgdorferi, 1116
Botanical agents, for cancer, 286*b*
Botulism, 645*t*
Bovine spongiform encephalopathy (BSE), 1007
Bowel
    preoperative preparation, 211
    sounds, 78
Bowel obstruction, 687–689
    collaborative care, 688
    manifestations and complications, 688
    nursing care, 688–689
    pathophysiology, 687, 688*f*
BPH. *See* Benign prostatic hypertrophy (BPH)
Brachytherapy, 278
    caregiver safety in, 279*b*
    nursing care checklist, 280*b*
Bradycardia, 76
Bradykinesia, 998
Bradypnea, 75
Brain, 943–945
    blood supply to, 944
    structure and function, 1184–1185, 1186*f*
        blood-brain barrier, 945
        cerebrospinal fluid, 9
        neurotransmitters in, 1184, 1186*f*, 1187*t*
        regions, 943, 944*f*
        in schizophrenia, 1221
Brain abscess, 985
    collaborative care, 985–986
    nursing care, 986–987
    pathophysiology and manifestations, 984*t*, 985
Brain death, 961
Brain death criteria, 334
Brain herniation, 961
Brain natriuretic peptide (BNP), 4, 355*t*
Brainstem, 944, 944*f*
Brain tumor, 967–971
    classifications, 967, 968*t*
    collaborative care, 968
    nursing care, 969–971
    pathophysiology and manifestations,
        967–968
Brawny edema, 505
Breast(s), 786, 787*f*
    cancer screening, 849–850
    disorders of
        cancer. *See* Breast cancer
        fibrocystic changes, 846–847, 847*f*
        mastitis, 847
        reconstruction, 847
    physical examination, 71*t*, 76–77, 77*f*
        self-examination, 849, 849*f*
Breast biopsy
    nursing care checklist, 851*b*
    techniques, 850, 850*f*
Breast cancer, 847–856

collaborative care, 848–853
    incidence and mortality rates, 847*b*
    metastasis, treatment, 852
    nursing care, 853–856
    in older women, 850*b*
    pathophysiology and manifestations, 848
    risk factors, 847, 848*t*
    risk profile, 850
    screening, 849–850
Breast feeding, in mastitis, 847
Breast reconstruction, 847
Breathing
    diaphragmatic, for pain management, 161
    nursing care
        in head injury with IICP, 965
        in pericarditis, 421
        in postoperative care, 230
        in spinal cord injury, 1111–1112
Breathing exercises, preoperative, nursing care, 212*b*
Brimonidine, for glaucoma, 1030*t*
Broad-spectrum antibiotics, 190
Bromocriptine, for Parkinson disease, 1000*t*
Bronchiectasis, 578
Bronchitis, acute
    collaborative care, 553–554
    nursing care, 554
    pathophysiology and manifestations, 553
Bronchitis, chronic, 572
Bruit, 446
BSE. *See* Bovine spongiform encephalopathy (BSE)
Buccal drug administration, 87, 88*t*
Buddhism, 38*t*
Buffers, 135–136, 136*f*
Bulimia nervosa, 631, 635
Bumetanide, for heart failure, 408*t*
Bundle branches, 350, 350*f*
Bundle of His, 350, 350*f*
Bunion. *See* Hallux valgus
Bupropion, for depression, 1247*t*
Burn, 1162
Burn injury, 1162–1176
    clinical reasoning care map, 1178
    collaborative care, 1167–1171
    depth classifications, 1162–1164
    extent, "rules of nines" estimate, 1164
    eye-related, 1024
    incidence and etiology, 1162
    nursing care, 1171–1175
    nursing care plan, 1175–1176
    pathophysiology and manifestations, 1164–1166
    types of, 1162
    wound management, 1169–1171
        biologic and biosynthetic dressings, 1170
        debridement, 1169
        scar, keloid, and contractures, 1170
        surgery, 1169
        wound dressings, 1170–1171
Burr hole, 963, 963*f*, 968
Bursitis
    collaborative care, 1081
    nursing care, 1081–1082
    pathophysiology and manifestations, 1080
Busulfan, for chemotherapy, 281*t*

C

Caffeine
    common sources and doses, 1309*f*
    effects, 1305*t*, 1309–1311

intake levels, 1309
    overdose and withdrawal symptoms, 1305*t*
Calcipotriene, for psoriasis, 1138
Calcitonin, 128, 881*t*, 882, 1093*t*
Calcitonin-salmon injection, for osteoporosis, 1093*t*
Calcitriol, in calcium imbalance, 128
Calcium
    food sources, 132*b*, 1092*b*
    imbalances. *See* Calcium imbalance
    osteoporosis and, 1092
    recommended daily intake, 1092*t*
    replacement therapy, 130, 130*t*
    serum values, 104*t*
        in calcium imbalances, 128, 129*t*, 129
        in endocrine disorders, 885*t*
Calcium carbonate, 646*t*
Calcium imbalance, 128–132
    causes and manifestations, 129*t*, 129*f*
    collaborative care, 129–131, 130*t*
    laboratory values, 129*t*
    nursing care, 131–132
Calcium replacement therapy, 130, 130*t*
Calymmatobacterium granulomatis, 863*t*
CAM. *See* Complementary and alternative medicine
    (CAM)
Campylobacter jejuni, 1004
Cancer, 268–294. *See also specific cancer*
    carcinogenesis, 270–271
    collaborative care, 275–285
    culturally appropriate care, 300
    early detection and, 273, 273*b*
    emergencies. *See* Oncologic emergencies
    health team, 268
    incidence and trends, 268–269
    manifestations, 273, 274*b*, 274*f*
        possible warning signs, 273*b*
    in middle adult, 42–43
    nursing care, 285–292
    nursing care plan, 293–294
    in older adult, 271, 272*b*
    pain, 153
        nursing care, 166–167, 167*f*
    pathophysiology, 269–270, 270*t*
    patient education, 291–292
        when to call for help, 288*b*
    physiologic effects, 273–280, 283–294
    risk factors, 271–273
    screening guidelines, 273*b*
Candida albicans. See Candidiasis infection
Candidiasis infection
    collaborative care, 1144–1145
    nursing care, 1145–1147
    pathophysiology and manifestations, 1142
Cannabis, 1305*t*, 1309
Capsaicin cream, 157
Captopril, for heart failure, 408*t*
Carbamazepine
    for bipolar disorder, 1252*t*
    for seizure disorder, 982*t*
Carbidopa-levodopa, for Parkinson disease, 1000*t*
Carbohydrates, consistent-carbohydrate diabetes
    meal plan, 920
Carbon dioxide, in acid-base balance, 135
Carbonic acid, 135–136, 136*f*
Carcinogenesis, 270–271, 280
Carcinogens, 271
    drugs, 93
    drugs as, 271, 272
Cardiac catheterization, 358*t*, 425

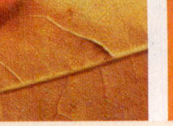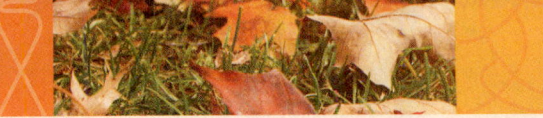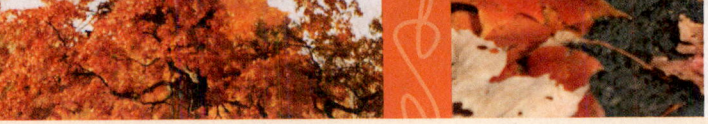

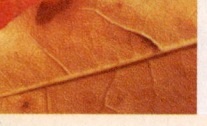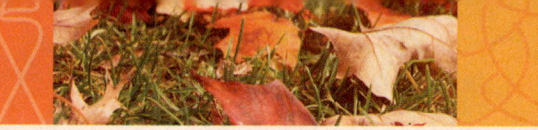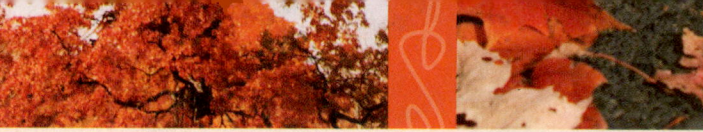

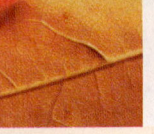
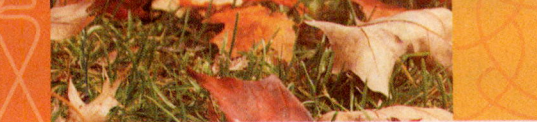
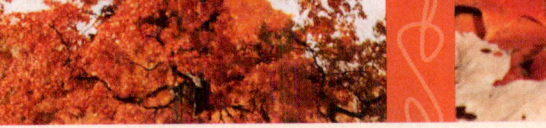

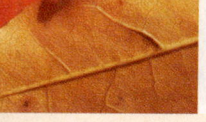
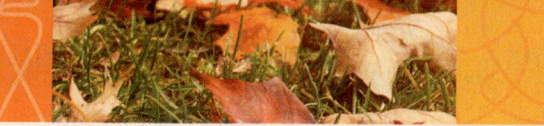
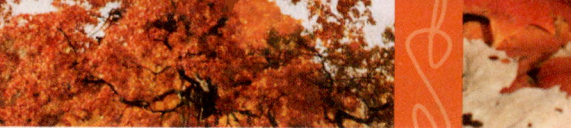

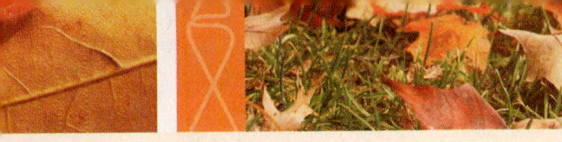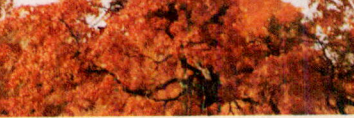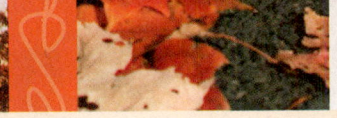

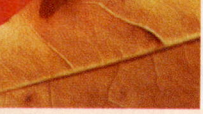
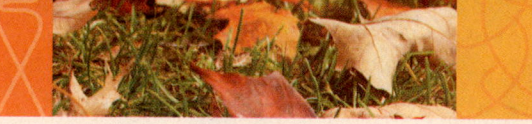
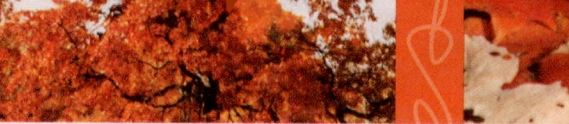

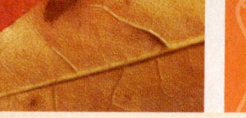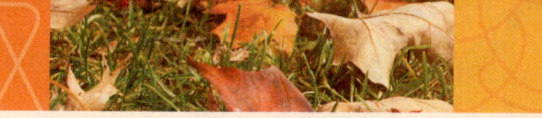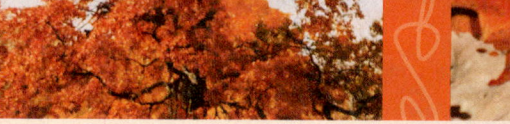

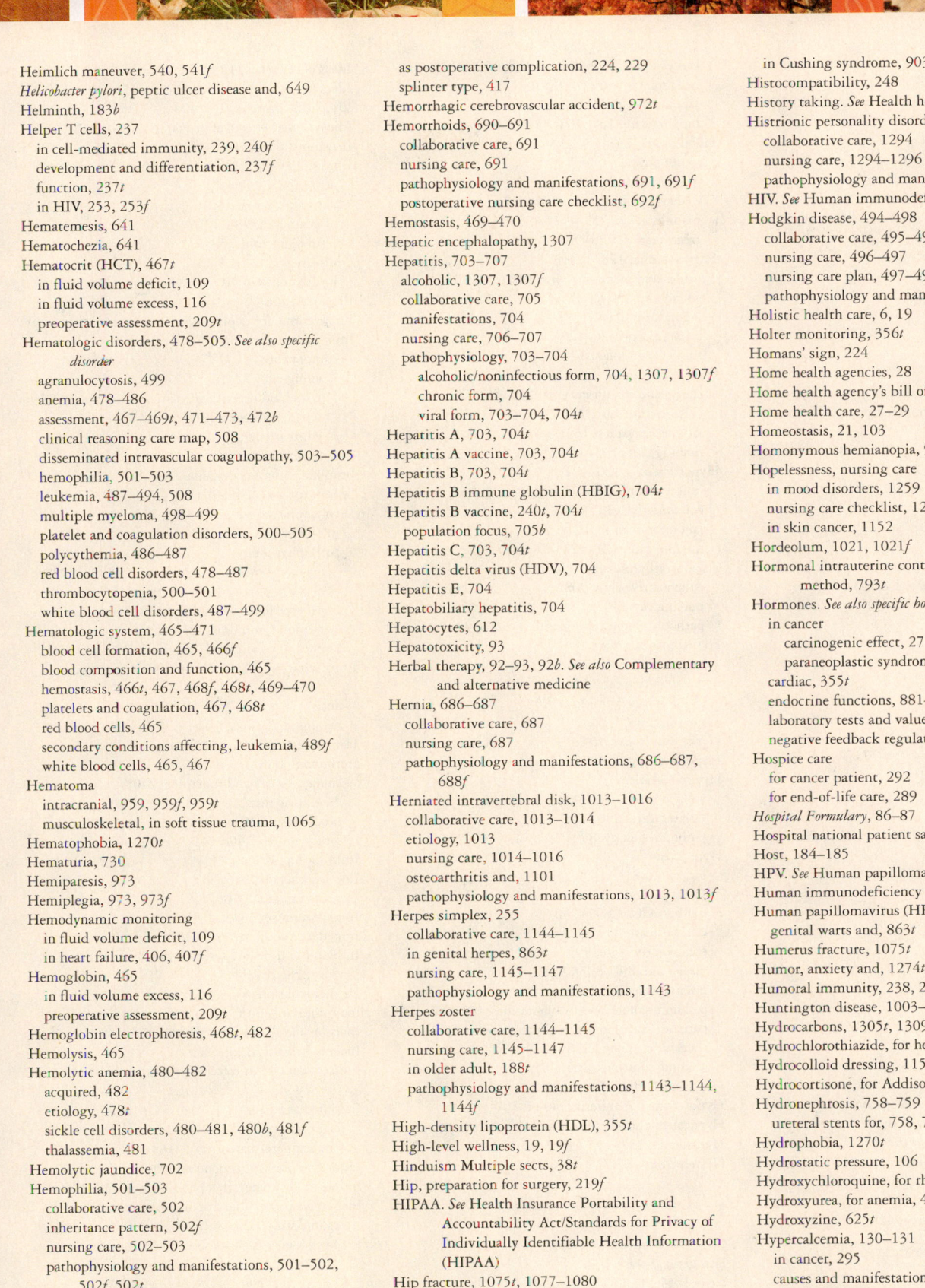

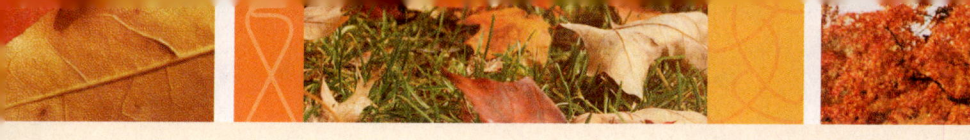

IV therapy (continued)
IV set, 111f
over-the-needle catheter, 111, 112f
procedure checklist, 112b
changing bag, tubing, and dressing site, 112b
initiating infusion, 114b
sites, 112b

J

Jackknife surgical position, 220t
Jacksonian march, 980
Jaundice, 72, 1128
in hepatitis, 704
Jehovah's Witnesses, 39t
Joints, 1053–1054
dislocation and subluxation, 1080
repetitive use injury, 1080
Judaism, 38t

K

Kaposi sarcoma (KS), 255
Kegel exercises, in urinary incontinence, 741b
Keloids, 1130t, 1170
Keratitis, 1022
Keratotomy, 1025
Ketoacidosis, 922–923
Ketoconazole, 193t
Ketone bodies, 914
Ketonuria, 923
Ketosis, in diabetes mellitus, 914
Kidney(s)
in acid-base regulation, 136
function tests, 116
structure and function, body fluid regulation, 107
Kidney failure, 766–776
acute kidney injury, 766–768, 766t, 767f
collaborative care, 768–774
nursing care, 774–776
pathophysiology and manifestations
acute form, 766–768, 766t, 767f
chronic form, 768
multisystem effects if uremia, 769f
Kidney function tests, in hyperkalemia, 125
Kidney and urinary tract disorders
cancer, bladder, 760–766
as surgical risk factor, 207t
Kindling process, 1253–1254
Knee, injury, 1080–1081
Korsakoff syndrome, 1307
Kussmaul respirations, 140
Kyphosis, 75
in osteoporosis, 1091, 1092f

L

Labile mood, in intoxication, 1305
Labyrinthitis
collaborative care, 1041
nursing care, 1041–1042
pathophysiology and manifestations, 1040
Lacrimal apparatus, gland, and ducts, 948
Lactated Ringer's solution, 111t
Laminectomy nursing care checklist, 1015b
Lamotrigine
for bipolar disorder, 1252t
for seizure disorder, 982t
Lansoprazole, 644, 646t

Laryngeal cancer, 542–548
collaborative care, 543
nursing care, 545–548
pathophysiology and manifestations, 542, 543f
population focus, 542b
Laryngeal obstruction
collaborative care, 540, 541f
nursing care, 541
pathophysiology and manifestations, 540
Laryngectomy, 543
nursing care checklist, 544b
tracheostomy following, 544, 544f
Laryngitis
nursing care, 532–534
pathophysiology and manifestations, 529
Laryngospasm, 540
Laser in situ keratomileusis (LASIK), 1025, 1026f
Laser iridotomy, 1030
Laser trabeculoplasty, 1030
LASIK. See Laser in situ keratomileusis
Latanoprost, for glaucoma, 1030t
Latent-stage syphilis, 873
Lateral surgical position, 220t
Latex allergy, 244–245, 245b
LDL. See Low-density lipoprotein
LDS. See Church of Jesus Christ of Latter-Day Saints
Leflunomide, for rheumatoid arthritis, 1107t
Leg. See also Extremities
exercises, preoperative, 212b–213b
preparation for surgery, 219f
Legal considerations, in home health care, 29–30
Legal protections, 13–14
Legal requirement, documenting interventions, 8
Lens, function and structure, 948–949, 948f
Lesions, 73
Lethargic patient, 79
Leukemia, 487–494
classifications, 487, 488t
clinical reasoning care map, 508
collaborative care, 488–491, 490t
etiology and risk factors, 487–488
multisystem effects, 489f
nursing care, 491–494
pathophysiology and manifestations, 487–488, 489f
Leukocytes, 236, 465
Leukocytosis, inflammation and, 176
Leukopenia, 177
Level of consciousness (LOC), 79
altered, in head injury
cerebral edema and, 961
increased intracranial pressure and, 960, 960t
nursing care plan, 967
Glasgow Coma Scale assessing, 961t
Levodopa, Parkinson disease and, 999, 1000t
Levofloxacin, 191t
Levothyroxine sodium, for hypothyroidism, 899t
Lewy body dementia, 1202
LH. See Luteinizing hormone
Libido, 783
Licensing standards, 11
Lichenification, 1130t
Life review, 54
Lifestyle
disease and, 21–22
health effects, 20, 60, 61f, 62
Ligaments, 1053–1054
Light therapy, in seasonal affective disorder, 1243
Limb leads, 355b
Limbus, 948, 948f

Liothyronine sodium, for hypothyroidism, 899t
Lipid profile, 355t
Lipoatrophy, 918
Lipodystrophy, 918
Lisinopril, for heart failure, 408t
Lithium
for bipolar disorder, 1252t, 1253–1254
side effects and toxicity, 1253b
Lithotomy position, 788
for surgery, 220t
Liver cancer, 715
Liver disorders. See also specific disorder
as surgical risk factor, 208t
Liver function tests, in fluid volume excess, 116
Living arrangements for older adult, 57
Living will, 305
Loading dose, 90
Lobules, 612
LOC. See Level of consciousness
Local drug effect, 89–90
Local nerve infiltration, 218
Lockjaw, 1006
Long-term care facilities, 25–26, 26f
nursing care in, 26
Loop diuretics, in fluid volume excess, 117t
Lou Gehrig's disease, 1004
Low back pain
in ankylosing spondylitis, 1117
collaborative care, 1118
nursing care, 1118–1119
pathophysiology and manifestations, 1118
Low-density lipoprotein (LDL), levels and classification, 355t
Lower body obesity, 627
LSD (lysergic acid diethylamide), 1305t, 1309
Lumbar puncture
in head injury, 962b
in infection, 190
Lung abscess, 565–566
Lung auscultation, 75
Lung cancer, 580–584
cell types, 580t
collaborative care, 581
incidence, mortality rate, and risk factors, 582
manifestations and complications, 581
nursing care, 582–584
pathophysiology, 580–581, 582t
pleural effusion in, 581–582
Lung surgery, 582t
in lung cancer, 582
nursing care checklist, 582b
Lungs
in older adult, 70b
physical examination, 71t
Luteinizing hormone (LH), 789t
Lutheran, 39t
Lyme disease
collaborative care, 1116
nursing care, 1116
pathophysiology and manifestations, 1116
prevention, patient education, 1116, 1116b
Lymphadenitis, 505
Lymphadenopathy, 176, 505
Lymphangitis
collaborative care, 506
nursing care, 506
pathophysiology and manifestations, 505
Lymphatic disorders, 505–506. See also specific disorder

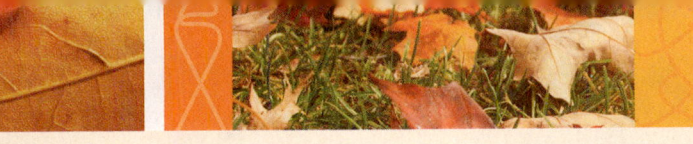
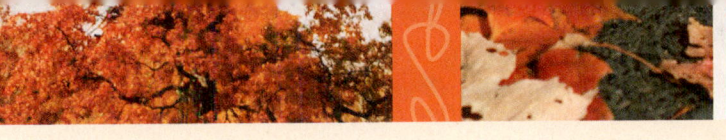

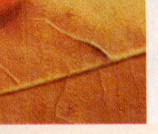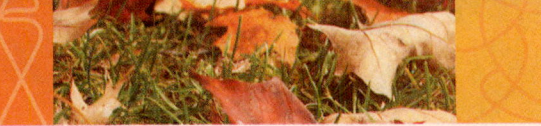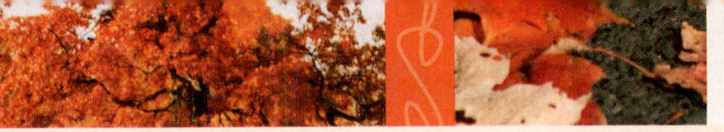

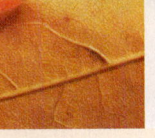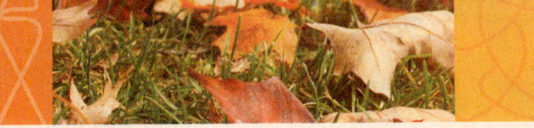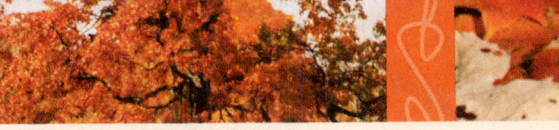

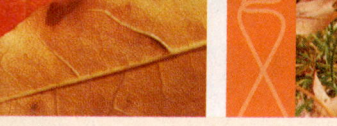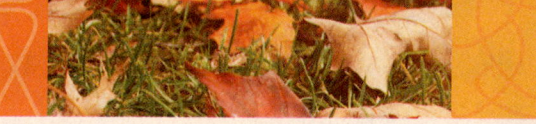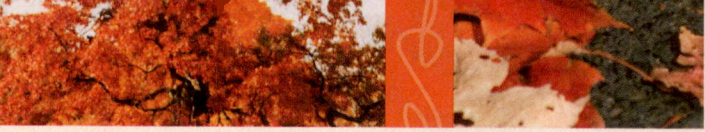

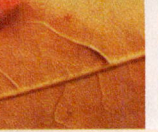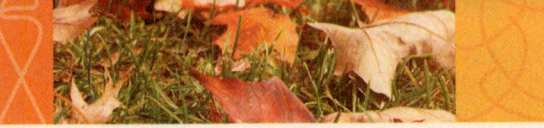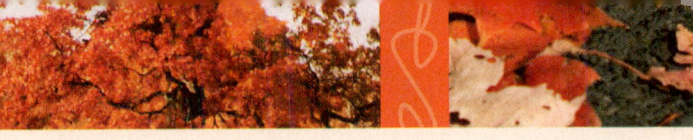

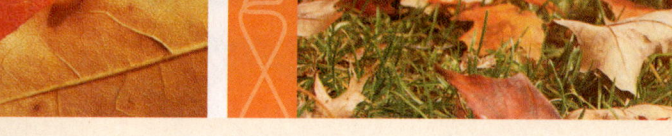
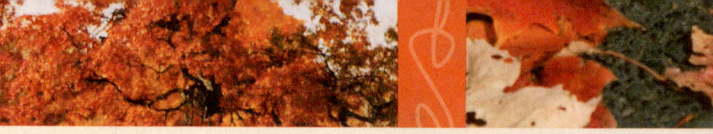

Preoperative care, 206–216
  collaborative care
    diagnostic tests, 208–209, 209*t*
    medications, 209, 210*t*
    physical preparations, 209–211
  nursing care, 211–215, 211*b*
  nursing care plan, 215–216
  patient education, 212–213*b*
  physiology review in, 206
  risk assessment and factors, 206, 207*t*
  withholding of food/fluids in, 211
Presbycusis, 1043
Presbyopia, 952, 1026*t*
Pressure speech, 1251
Pressure ulcers, 1154–1157
  collaborative care, 1154–1156
  nursing care, skin integrity, 1156–1157
  in older adult, 188*t*, 1154
  pathophysiology and manifestations, 1154
  staging, 1155*b*, 1156
Priapism
  nursing care, 812
  pathophysiology, manifestations, and treatment, 812
Primary (simple) acid-base disorders, 138
Primary intention, 223, 223*f*
Primary syphilis, 373*f*, 864*t*, 872
Primidone, for seizure disorder, 982*t*
Prion, 1007
Prioritizing, 5
Privacy invasion, 13
PRK. *See* Photorefractive keratectomy (PRK)
PRN orders, 94
Probenecid, for gout, 1115*t*
Problem solving, 9
Procedural memory, 1196
Prochlorperazine, 625*t*
Procyclidine
  for extrapyramidal side effects of antipsychotics, 1229*t*
  for Parkinson disease, 998
Prodromal phase
  of infection, 184
  of schizophrenia, 1222
Professional boundaries, 15
Progesterone, 789*t*
Programmed aging theory, 53
Projection, anxiety and, 1274*t*
Proliferative phase, of wound healing, 223–224
Promethazine, 625*t*
  for headaches, 989
Prophylactic anti-infective therapy, 190
Propranolol
  for headaches, 988
  for hyperthyroidism, 894*t*
Proprioception, pernicious anemia and, 479
Propylthiouracil, for hyperthyroidism, 894*t*
Prostate cancer, 802–806
  collaborative care, 802–803
  diversity focus, 802*b*
  manifestations and complications, 802
  nursing care, 803–806
  pathophysiology, 802
Prostatectomy
  for prostate cancer, 803
  for urinary incontinence, 740
Prostate gland, 783
Prostatitis, 806
Prosthetist, 1083
Proteolytic enzymes, for pressure ulcer, 1156*t*

Protestant denominations, 38*t*
Prothrombin time (PT), preoperative assessment, 208, 209*t*
Protozoa, 183
Protriptyline, for depression, 1247*t*
Pruritus
  collaborative care, 1137–1139
  nursing care, 1139–1141
  pathophysiology and manifestations, 1136
Psoriasis
  collaborative care, 1137–1139
  nursing care, 1139–1141
  pathophysiology and manifestations, 1136, 1136*f*
Psychiatric hospitals, care settings in, 25
Psychologic influences, pain response, 155
Psychologic status
  in acute pain, 154*t*
  in cancer diagnosis, 275, 277
Psychomotor activity
  in depression, 1241
  in mental status assessment, 1256
Psychomotor agitation, 1243
Psychomotor retardation, 1243
Psychosis, 1220
Psychosocial, 1188
Psychosocial factors, in young adult, 42
Psychosocial function
  assessment, 1188–1192, 1192*t*
  in older adult, 53–54
    changes in, 55, 57, 57*f*
    nursing care to promote, 60*t*
Psychotherapy
  in bipolar disorder, 1254
  in depression, 1249
PT. *See* Prothrombin time (PT)
PTH. *See* Parathyroid hormone (PTH)
Ptosis, 951, 952, 952*f*
PTSD. *See* Posttraumatic stress disorder (PTSD)
PTT. *See* Partial thromboplastin time (PTT)
PUD. *See* Peptic ulcer disease (PUD)
Pulmonary contusion, 594–595
  nursing care, 594–595
Pulmonary edema, in heart failure, 405
Pulmonary embolism, 585–587
  collaborative care, 585
  nursing care, 585–587
  pathophysiology and manifestations, 585–586
  as postoperative complication, 224
Pulmonary hypertension, 587
Pulmonary valve, 349*f*, 350
Pulmonary veins, 349, 349*f*
Pulse
  apical, 76, 76*f*
  peripheral, 72*t*, 78, 78*f*
Pulse deficit, 78
Pupils, 947*t*, 948, 948*f*
  physical examination, 74*b*
Pure Food and Drug Act, 86
Purkinje fibers, 350, 350*f*
Purpura, 500
Purulent drainage, 224
Pustule, 1130*f*
PVD. *See* Peripheral vascular disease (PVD)
Pyelonephritis, 745–749
  collaborative care, 746
  nursing care, 746–749
  in older adult, 745
  pathophysiology and manifestations, 746
  risk factors, 745–746

Pyridostigmine, for myasthenia gravis, 1002, 1003*t*
Pyrophobia, 1270*t*
Pyuria, 730

Q

QRS complex, 356*b*
QT interval, 356*b*
Quality improvement, 4
Quality and Safety Education for Nurses (QSEN), 3
Quinapril, for heart failure, 408*t*

R

RA. *See* Rheumatoid arthritis (RA)
Rabeprazole, 646*t*
Rabies, 1006
Race, 35
Racial factors. *See* Ethnicity
Radial keratotomy, 1025
Radiation, as carcinogen, 271, 272
Radiation pneumonia, 278
Radiation therapy
  adverse effects, 278
  brachytherapy, 278, 279*b*, 279*f*
  in brain tumor, 969
  in Cushing syndrome, 904
  external, 278
  in leukemia, 488
  in malignant lymphoma, 495
  nursing care checklist, 280*b*
  patient/family education, 280*b*
  for prostate cancer, 803
  in skin cancers, 1150
Radioactive iodine (I-131), 894
Radioactive iodine (RAI) uptake test, 886*t*
Radioactive therapy, in hyperthyroidism, 894
Radiography
  in cardiovascular assessment, 357*t*
  in neurologic assessment, 953*t*
RAI. *See* Radioactive iodine (RAI) uptake test
Ramipril, for heart failure, 408*t*
Range of motion, assessment of, 1058*t*
Ranitidine bismuth citrate, 646*t*
Ranitidine, for gastritis, 646*t*
Rationalization, anxiety and, 1274*t*
Raynaud phenomenon
  collaborative care, 450
    nursing care, ineffective protection, 450–451
    pathophysiology and manifestations, 450
Reaction formation, anxiety and, 1274*t*
Reality orientation, 1199
Reboxetine, for depression, 1247
Receptor site action, 89, 89*f*
Recreational drug use, as cancer risk factor, 272–273
Rectal drug administration, 88*t*, 157
Rectocele, 844
Red blood cell disorders
  anemia. *See* Anemia
  polycythemia, 486
Reduction of fracture, 1071
Reed-Sternberg cells, 494
Referred pain, 152–153, 153*f*
Reflex(es), 945
  common, 945–946
  red reflex, 1026–1027
Reflex arc, 945, 946*f*
Reflux incontinence, 739*t*
Refraction disorders, 1026*t*, 1026*f*

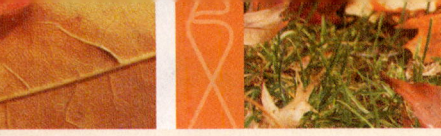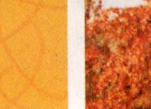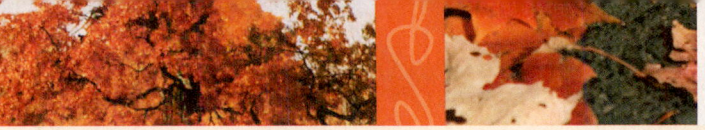

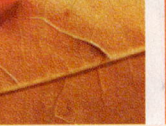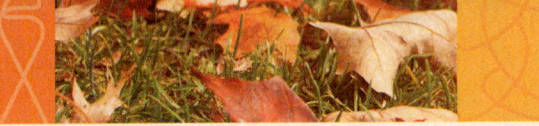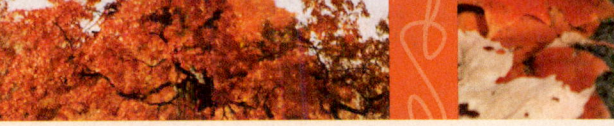

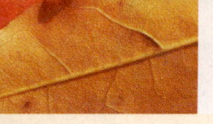
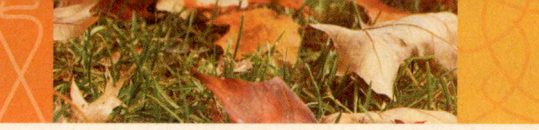
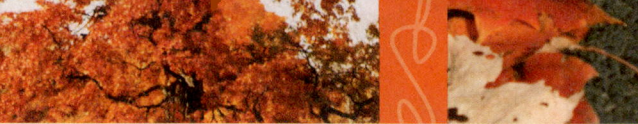

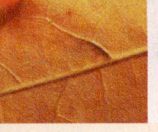
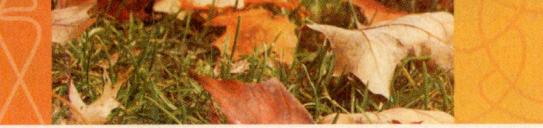
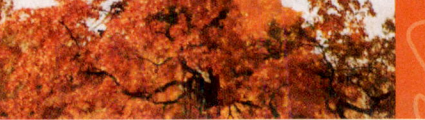
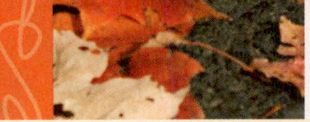

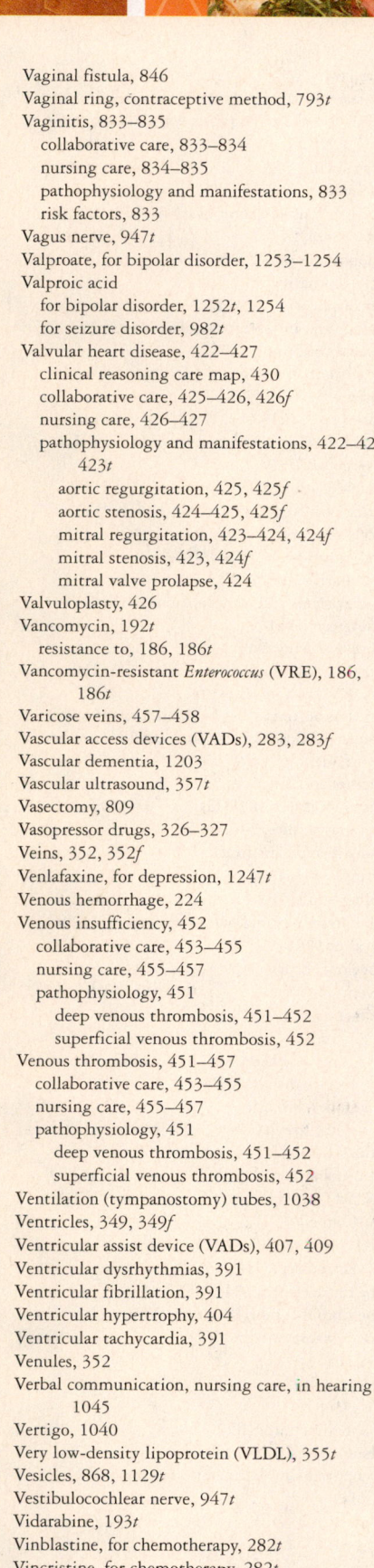

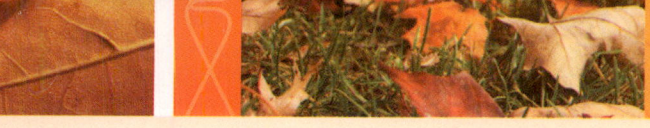

Guide to Special Features

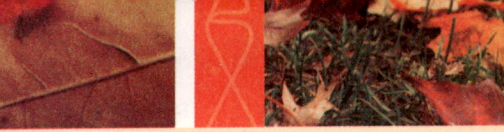
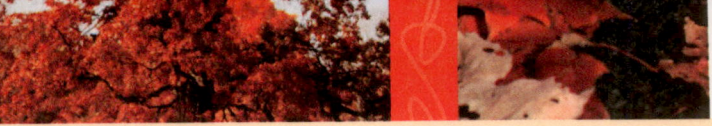

Guide to Special Features

NURSING CARE CHECKLISTS